Solved Papers
Surgery
for PG Students
(Topic Wise)

Solved Papers
Surgery
for PG Students
(Topic Wise)

A must for MS & DNB Surgery Students

Last 10 Years Exams Across Various State Health Universities, AIIMS & DNB

Second Edition

Editor

Arkaprovo Roy
MS (General Surgery)
Professor
Department of Surgery
North Bengal Medical College
Darjeeling, West Bengal, India

Forewords

Shibajyoti Ghosh
Indranil Biswas

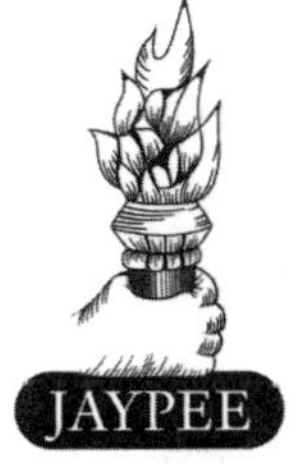

JAYPEE BROTHERS MEDICAL PUBLISHERS
The Health Sciences Publisher
New Delhi | London

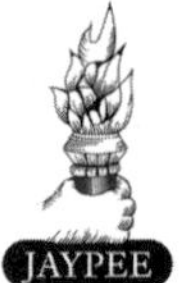

Jaypee Brothers Medical Publishers (P) Ltd

Headquarters
EMCA House, 23/23-B
Ansari Road, Daryaganj
New Delhi 110 002, India
Landline: +91-11-23272143, +91-11-23272703
+91-11-23282021, +91-11-23245672
e-mail: jaypee@jaypeebrothers.com

Corporate Office
4838/24, Ansari Road, Daryaganj
New Delhi 110 002, India
Phone: +91-11-43574357
Fax: +91-11-43574314
e-mail: jaypee@jaypeebrothers.com

Overseas Office
JP Medical Ltd.
83, Victoria Street, London
SW1H 0HW (UK)
Phone: +44-20 3170 8910
e-mail: info@jpmedpub.com

EU GPSR Authorised Representative
Logos Europe, 9 rue Nicolas Poussin
17000, La Rochelle, France
Phone: +33 (0) 6 67 93 73 78
e-mail: contact@logoseurope.eu

Website: www.jaypeebrothers.com
Website: www.jaypeedigital.com

Solved Papers Surgery for PG Students—(Topic Wise)

First Edition: 2024

Second Edition: **2026**

ISBN: 978-93-7202-962-8

Printed at: Sterling Graphics Pvt. Ltd.

Dedicated to

My parents, Shibani Roy and Rajib Roy

Foreword

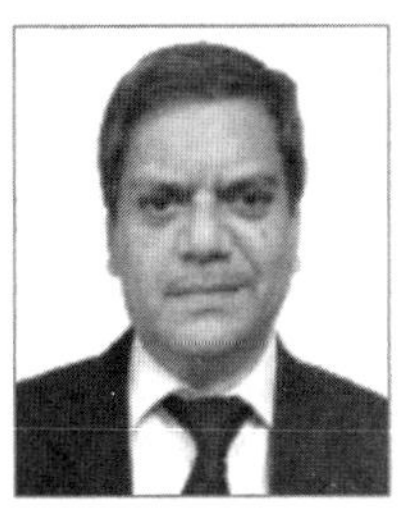

Arkaprovo Roy is known to me since he was a postgraduate trainee in General Surgery. He had always shown a keen interest in academics since his training days. In his teaching career of over 10 years, he has been an examiner several times and always endeavors to give his feedback to the examinees.

Writing a theory examination answer is an essential art both for the student who is well-informed and also for one not so well-informed. In the answer script, the examiner evaluates the knowledge, approach, and the capacity to solve a problem and the personality of the student as a whole.

I hope students will find this book helpful for approaching questions in postgraduate theory examinations, and I wish Arkaprovo Roy all the best in his academic journey.

Shibajyoti Ghosh
MS (General Surgery)
Professor and Head
Department of Surgery
Government Medical College
Kolkata, West Bengal, India

Foreword

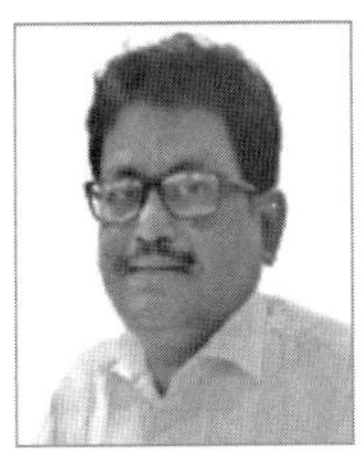

Answering questions in theory papers in a precise and perfect way is an important part in summative assessment. Arkaprovo Roy, a hardworking Academician and Surgeon, has beautifully compiled the answers to questions of theory papers of different universities. Students can utilize this book also in self-directed learning.

Wishing all the best to Arkaprovo Roy for his effort for the students and expecting all the students will be benefitted through this book.

Indranil Biswas
MBBS DVD (Diploma in Venereology and Dermatology) MD (Pharmacology)
Principal
Government Medical College
Kolkata, West Bengal, India

Preface

This endeavor is an overview of the magnificent subject of General Surgery with important questions and concepts that have been accumulated with references based on current editions of standard textbooks like *Bailey & Love Short Practice of Surgery, Sabiston's Textbook of Surgery, Maingot's Abdominal Operations, Schwartz Principle of Surgery, Cameron's Current Surgical Therapy, Oxford Textbook of Surgery, and Washington Manual of Surgery.*

This book has been conceptualized keeping in mind that the postgraduate trainees not only need a good guide for their examinations, but also they will step out into the real world of medical practice as Consultant Surgeons. The purpose of the book is not to spoon-feed the readers with answers to all questions but to provide clues and information, so that the students can perceive the concepts and produce their own answers.

The questions have been arranged chapterwise, and I hope that it will not only guide the MS (Surgery) students, but the DNB Surgery examinees shall also benefit from it.

With all humility and optimism, I hope this book serves its purpose and helps the readers to attain success, both in examination and in life.

All the best!

Arkaprovo Roy

Arkaprovo Roy

Acknowledgments

I must thank my wife Dr Svaresmi Unnithan, my parents, and my in-laws for their constant help and support during the preparation of this book. I must also grateful to my little daughter whose presence gives me the enthusiasm to write the book.

My sincere thanks and gratitude to the following persons for their encouragement in writing the book: Professor Indranil Biswas, Principal, Government Medical College, Kolkata; Professor Anjan Adhikari, Medical Superintendent cum Vice Principal, Government Medical College, Kolkata; Professor Shibajyoti Ghosh, Head, Department of Surgery, Government Medical College, Kolkata; Professors Pratip Kundu, Saibal Mukherjee, Makhanlal Saha, Sukumar Maity, Diptendra Kumar Sarkar, Madhumita Mukhopadhyay, Ramanuj Mukhopadhyay, Drs Somdatta Lahiri, Prasenjit Mukherjee, Parathasarathi Ghosh, Ananya Mondal, Rajarshi Bhattacharyya, Sudeshna Saha Bhattacharyya, Amit Kumar Roy, Parthapratim Guha, Anirban Banerjee, Uttam Mondal, Abhishek Mondal, Arijit Sinha Mahapatra, Yash Sharma, and Rudradeep Banerjee.

I am also grateful to all the members of my unit—Drs Suhas Das, Md Hasanuzzaman, Saptarshi Saha Chowdhury, Subhendu Barman, Rashel Haque, Manik Mondal, Pradipta Mondal, and Praveen Kumar.

My special thanks to Dr Dhritiman Maitra, Associate Professor of Surgery, Medical College, Kolkata; Drs Indrajit Mondal, Siddhartha Bhattacharya, and Anwesh Biswas for helping me in editing this book.

I must convey my gratitude to all my friends from Hindu School who are instrumental encouraging me writing the book.

I would like to express my special gratitude to Shri Jitendar P Vij (Group Chairman), Mr Ankit Vij (Managing Director), Mr MS Mani (Group President), Mr Sabyasachi Hazra (Associate Director-Publishing and Digital Sales), Ms Pooja Bhandari [Director—Production (Books and Journals)], Ms Nikita Chauhan (Publishing Manager), Mr Priyansh Saxena (Development Editor), and the staff of M/s Jaypee Brothers Medical Publishers (P) Ltd, New Delhi, India.

Contents

Basic Surgical Principle

LEARNING OBJECTIVES

- Surgical Safety Checklist
- Various Surgical Incisions of the Abdomen
- Surgical Technique of Closure of Midline
- Anastomosis in Surgery
- Stoma Creation versus Primary Anastomosis after Gut Resection
- Drains in Gastrointestinal Surgery
- Surgical Never Events

SURGICAL SAFETY CHECKLIST

1. Write a note on surgical safety checklist.

SAIMS, Indore 2025; RGUHS, Karnataka 2025; WBUHS 2024, DNB 2024 October

A *Surgical Safety Checklist* is a tool developed to improve the safety of surgical procedures by ensuring that key safety steps are completed before, during, and after surgery. The most widely adopted version is the *WHO Surgical Safety Checklist*, which is divided into three main phases:

1. **Before Induction of Anesthesia (Sign In)**

   Confirm with the patient (if possible) and the surgical team:
   - Patient identity
   - Surgical site and procedure
   - Consent obtained
   - Anesthesia safety check completed
   - Pulse oximeter on patient and functioning
   - Allergies
   - Airway/aspiration risk
   - Risk of blood loss (>500 mL)

2. **Before Skin Incision (Time Out)**

   Entire team introduces themselves and confirms:
   - Patient identity, procedure, and site
   - Anticipated critical events
     - *Surgeon:* What is expected, unusual steps, duration, blood loss
     - *Anesthesia:* Any concerns
     - *Nursing:* Sterility confirmed, equipment issues
   - Has antibiotic prophylaxis been given within 60 minutes?
   - Essential imaging displayed and available

3. **Before Patient Leaves Operating Room (Sign Out)**

   Nurse verbally confirms with the team:
   - Name of the procedure performed
   - Completion of instrument, sponge, and needle counts
   - Specimen labeling (if any)
   - Equipment problems to be addressed
   - Key concerns for recovery and patient management.

BASIC SURGICAL PRINCIPLE

2. Discuss the anatomical basis, advantages and disadvantages of various surgical incisions of the abdomen.
Tripura University 2025; WBUHS 2021 Supplementary

Vertical Incisions

- *Midline incisions or median incisions:*
  - It is mostly favored in exploratory laparotomy as it provides quick access to all areas of abdomen and organs.
  - It allows almost bloodless surgery with a minimum risk of injury to the blood vessels and nerves.
  - Closure is quick and easy.
  - Poor healing.
- *Paramedian incisions:*
  - These incisions are made 2–5 cm lateral to the midline of the abdomen.
  - It provides access to abdominal organs such as the stomach, liver, and spleen.
  - It avoids any neurovascular trauma, limits trauma to rectus abdominis muscle and permits good healing and function restoration.

Transverse Incisions

- Cosmetically better.
- Stronger and less painful.
- Good exposure of upper abdominal organs.
- Mostly used in pediatric patients as their transverse abdominal diameter is more than longitudinal hence providing better exposure.
- Preferred in overweight and have short statured individuals.
- Reduced risk of wound dehiscence.
- Risk of hernia is more.
  - *Pfannenstiel's incisions:*
    - Most common muscle-separating incisions.
    - Frequently used for pelvic genitourinary surgeries.
    - They are commonly used for lower uterine cesarean section (LUCS) as they provide a cosmetically better appearance.
    - Drawback—limited exposure beyond the pelvis.
    - Chance of injury to inferior and superficial epigastric vessels.
  - *Cherney's incisions:*
    - 2–3 cm above the groin area, lower than Pfannenstiel's incisions.
    - Excellent access to the pelvic organs during surgeries of urinary bladder or vaginal repair.
    - As they are a tendon-detaching operation, reattachment of the tendons (fibrous collagen tissue band) is tedious.

- *Maynard's incisions:*
  - These are true muscle-cutting incisions.
  - Excellent exposure to the genital organs.
  - These incisions are made parallel to the traditional Pfannenstiel's incisions.
  - Can be used for cesarean delivery and also for pelvic cancer surgeries.
- *Modified Gibson incisions:*
  - These incisions are specifically made during surgeries related to women's genitourinary system.
  - Most placed on the left paramedian side.

Oblique Incisions

Several oblique incisions are used for specific organ exposures:

- *McBurney's incisions:*
  - Specifically used for appendectomy.
  - They are made at the junction of the middle third and outer third of the spinoumbilical line.
  - The superficial epigastric, as well as perforating branches of the inferior epigastric, may be injured.
- *Lanz incision:*
  - A variation of the traditional Mc Burney's incision, which was made at McBurney's point on the abdomen but transverse.
  - Used to perform an open appendectomy.
  - Some surgeons advocate that the incision is made approximately 2 cm below the umbilicus centered on mid-clavicular-midinguinal line.
- *Subcostal incisions:*
  - These start at the midline 2–5 cm incisions below the lower part of the sternum (breastbone) that extends down outward parallel to the lower edge of the chest-rib.
  - Easy access to the gallbladder and spleen.
  - They are often used in cholecystectomy.
    - *Kocher incision:*
      - It is a subcostal incision which is used to access the gallbladder and the biliary tree.
      - Associated with increase in pain during the postoperative phase due to the cutting of the rectus muscle.
      - The incision closure is in two layers approximating the fascial layers.
    - *Chevron/rooftop incision or modification:*
      - The extension of the subcostal incision to the other side of the abdomen.
      - This may be used for esophagectomy, gastrectomy, bilateral adrenalectomy, hepatic resections, or liver transplantation.
      - Access to the intra-abdominal cavity as well as the retroperitoneal space.
      - Though the bilateral superficial epigastric are damaged, the abdominal wall will have collaterals from the perforating branches through the oblique muscles as well as the inferior epigastric meaning there will be no devascularized tissues.
      - However, if there is another surgery after a Chevron takes place, and the incision is through the lower abdominal wall, there may be an interruption of the inferior epigastric and middle of the abdominal wall with the least amount of collateral blood supply may ultimately be devascularized.
- *Mercedes Benz incision or modification:*
  - The Chevron incision with a vertical incision and break through the xiphisternum.
  - This may be used for the same indications as the Chevron incision, however classically seen in liver transplantation.

A Selection of Common Abdominal Incisions

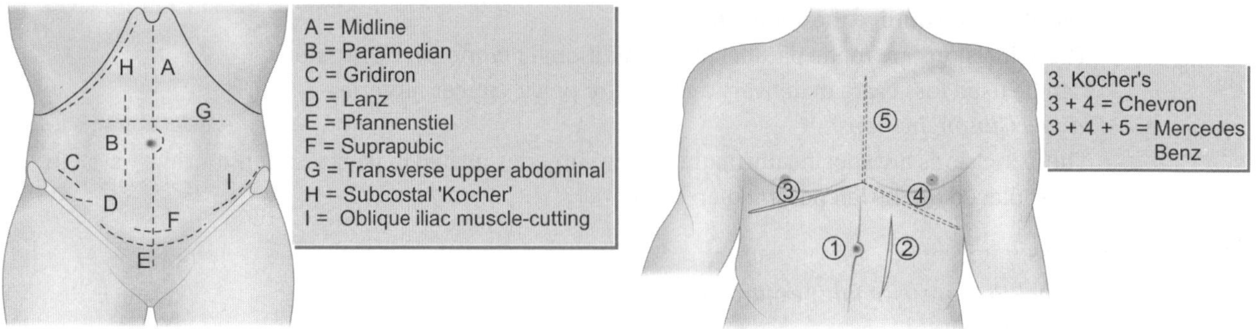

3. Discuss the surgical technique in closure of a midline incision. ***WBUHS 2022***

A midline incision is the most commonly used route of access to the abdominal cavity and hence the ensuing discussion of abdominal closure focuses on this incision. The general technique can be applied to other abdominal incisions (some of which are discussed more briefly below); however, it must be kept in mind that the actual layers composing the abdominal wall vary, depending on the location of the incision.

Midline Incision

- *Peritoneal closure:* A number of randomized, controlled trials have showed that peritoneal closure has no added benefit and thus refrained from though some surgeons believe that closure of the peritoneum reduces adhesions between the abdominal contents and the suture line.
- *Fascial closure:* The technique of fascial closure is highly variable among surgeons; however, the various approaches may be grouped into two primary methods as follows:
  1. *Layered closure:* Sequential closure of each fascial layer individually. The primary advantage of this method is that dehiscence of one layer may not lead to complete wound dehiscence.
  2. *Mass closure:* Continuous fascial closure with a single suture allowing even distribution of tension across the entire suture length, resulting in minimization of tissue strangulation. The goal is approximation of tissue edges to allow scar formation. Excessive tension leads to tissue necrosis and eventual failure of the closure.

The theoretical disadvantage of mass closure is that a single suture is responsible for maintaining the integrity of the closure.

The benefits of mass closure include decreased cost and decreased operating time.

There is no evidence that mass closure is associated with an increased incidence of hernia formation or wound dehiscence.

The small-bite technique (in which the distance between the suture and the wound edge is reduced to 5–8 mm and the distance from stitch to stitch is reduced to 5 mm from the fascial edge) has been shown to be beneficial. This reduces the tissue trauma and infection, as well as reduce the rates of hernia.

At 4 days after closure of a midline laparotomy incision (with a suture length-to-wound length ratio of 4), the incisional wound burst strength was higher with sutures placed 3–6 mm from the wound edge than with those at 1 cm. Incisional burst strength also increased with the number of stitches used.

It is noted that in elective midline closure, the use of a slowly absorbable suture material, continuous closure, small-bite technique resulted in significantly less incisional hernias than a large-bite technique did.

The use of prophylactic mesh in high-risk patients, yielded a significant reduction in the incisional hernia rate.

Often, having the assistant cross the Kocher's allows for better visualization for the surgeon.

Suture material is chosen. For most closures, the authors prefer to use looped polydioxanone (PDS) suture.

Starting at the superior or inferior aspect of the incision, the looped PDS is passed through the vertex of the fascia.

The needle is then passed through the loop locking the stitch in order to anchor the knot or tied if it is not a looped suture.

The suture is subsequently run in a continuous fashion, with each bite including tissue from the linea alba, the rectus sheath, and muscle itself if necessary (preferably avoided) to get an adequate bite.

4. Anastomosis in surgery. *WBUHS 2011*

In surgical jargon, to create an anastomosis is to join together two hollow organs (viscus), usually to restore continuity after resection, or to bypass an unresectable disease process.

While an anastomosis may be end-to-end, equally it could be performed side-to-side or end-to-side depending on the circumstances of the required reconstruction or bypass.

The term reanastomosis is also used to describe a surgical reconnection usually reversing a prior surgery to disconnect an anatomical anastomosis, e.g., tubal reversal after tubal ligation.

Anastomosis are typically performed on:

- *Blood vessels:*
    - Arteries and veins.
    - Most vascular procedures, including all arterial bypass operations (e.g., coronary artery bypass), aneurysmectomy of any type, and all solid-organ transplants require vascular anastomoses.
    - An anastomosis connecting an artery to a vein is also used to create an arteriovenous fistula as an access for hemodialysis.
- *Gastrointestinal (GI) tract:*
    - Esophagus, stomach, small bowel, large bowel, bile ducts, and pancreas.
    - Virtually all elective resections of gastrointestinal organs are followed by anastomoses to restore continuity; pancreaticoduodenectomy is considered a massive operation, in part, because it requires three separate anastomoses (stomach, biliary tract and pancreas to small bowel).
    - Bypass operations on the GI tract, once rarely performed, are the cornerstone of bariatric surgery.
    - The widespread use of mechanical suturing devices (linear and circular staplers) changed the face of gastrointestinal surgery.
- *Urinary tract:*
    - Ureters, urinary bladder, urethra.
    - Radical prostatectomy and radical cystectomy both require anastomosis of the bladder to the urethra in order to restore continuity.
- *Microsurgery:* The advent of microsurgical technique allowed anastomoses previously thought impossible, such as so-called "nerve anastomoses" (not strictly an anastomosis according to the above definition), and operations to restore fertility after tubal ligation or vasectomy.

Fashioning an anastomosis is typically a complex and time-consuming step in a surgical operation, but almost always crucial to the outcome of the procedure.

5. Discuss the role of stoma creation versus primary anastomosis after gut resection. *WBUHS 2018*

Introduction

- Following intestinal resection the surgeon faces a decision of stoma formation or primary anastomosis.
- The conventional view is that it is safer to exteriorize the bowel ends because the presence of peritonitis, inflammation of the bowel wall, and reduced intestinal blood supply unfavorable factors for the healing of the anastomosis which are present mainly in the emergent settings.
- The stoma also allows for adequate healing and rests the distal bowel before subsequent reanastomosis.
- However, stoma formation does not always provide a straightforward solution.

- Stomas may be complicated by poor weight gain, electrolyte imbalance due to high intestinal output, stenosis, prolapse, and excoriation of the surrounding skin.
- Restoration of intestinal continuity involves a second anesthetic and is usually performed once the patient has fully recovered from the acute stage of the illness.
- The alternative to stoma formation is resection followed by primary anastomosis.
- This was once considered a hazardous option because of the risk of anastomotic leakage due to poor healing of intraperitoneal anastomoses, but in recent years, several centers have published encouraging reports in support of this technique.
- Rates of anastomotic leakage and stricture do not seem to be as high as anticipated, and primary anastomosis has been reported as a valid treatment option after bowel resection.
- Stomas can also be created in a patient undergoing primary anastomosis in order to create a fecal diversion, so as to allow rest to the distal bowel.

Advantages of Primary Anastomosis Over Stoma Creation

- Avoids second operation (stoma reversal)
- Less morbid for the patient who otherwise would have had to deal with a stoma
- Avoidance of complications of stoma formation like electrolyte and fluid imbalance, skin excoriation.

Advantages of Stoma Creation Over Primary Anastomosis

- It's a safe option in case of grossly contaminated cases where there is high incidence of anastomotic leak.
- It's a safer option in case of nutritionally debilitated patients.
- A loop stoma can also be used as a diversion to protect distal anastomosis.

6. Drains in gastrointestinal surgery. *WBUHS 2010, 2011, Supplementary 2025, RIMS, Imphal 2012*

Types of drains-based on:

- *Rationale:* Prophylactic and therapeutic drains.
- *Mechanism:*
  - Open and closed drains.
  - Suction drains.
  - Sump suction drains.
- *Drain materials:* Polyurethane, silicone, PTFE etc.

Reasons for the Insertion of a Drain

- To remove unwanted fluid/exudates/pus/gas.
- To allow monitoring of fluid volume and quality.
- To promote tissue apposition.
- To allow diversion of body fluids.
- To facilitate subsequent access to a body space or cavity.
- To allow the injection of dye or contrast to provide diagnostic information about an underlying cavity or fistula.

Things to Watch for in a Patient with Drain

- Is the patient well?
- Has the drain been secured and is still secure?
- Are the signs of infection, excoriation or peritubal leakage at the skin exit site?
- Is the tube kinked or damaged?
- Is the drain connected properly?
- What is draining?—volume, color, nature and smell.
- Has there been any change in the nature or volume of the effluent?
  - Little or no output indicates that the drain is either blocked or that it has served its function.
  - Excessive drainage may indicate formation of a fistula or tissue irritation.
- Is the vacuum for suction drains working?

Common Complications of Drains

- Tissue damage during insertion and removal.
- Erosion into adjacent structures—blood vessels, bowel, anastomoses.
- Skin flap necrosis.
- Visceral herniation through the drain tract.
- Bacterial colonization and infection.
- Loss of fluid and electrolytes (e.g. through a T-tube).
- Pain
- Migration or displacement of the drain (into the body cavity or extrusion)
- Accidental removal
- Blockage
- Fracture of the drain
- Failure of vacuum in suction drains
- Restricted patient mobility.

Key Points

- Use of drain after routine colorectal surgery cannot be recommended.
- The placement of a prophylactic drain following appendicectomy is not indicated, regardless of the severity of appendicitis.
- Prophylactic drain placement cannot be advocated following simple cholecystectomy, either laparoscopic or open.
- Prophylactic drain placement following liver resection is not beneficial and may even be detrimental.
- In upper gastrointestinal and pancreatic surgery there is little evidence to support the use of drains.
- Currently, the placement of drains following incisional hernia repair has to be the discretion of the operating surgeon.
- Percutaneous drainage is the recommended treatment for symptomatic postoperative collections and when there are signs of infection.

---

7. Write a short note on "Surgical Never Events". ***WBUHS 2020***

Introduction

Never Events are patient safety incidents that are considered preventable when national guidance or safety recommendations that provide strong systemic protective barriers are implemented by healthcare providers.

Things to be included:

- *How to create a receptive team culture during interventional procedures:* One where questioning related to safety is welcomed, advice listened to and acted on, and all staff are encouraged to speak up when they have concerns.
- Reducing the risks and enhancing awareness of safety in situations where team members are unfamiliar with each other or with the environment, equipment or procedure
- Developing the use of safety checks, so that they are done because all those participating realize their importance, not because they have been mandated.

Other areas with potential for improvement include:

- *Interruptions and distractions:* These were described as leading to a loss of situational awareness in several cases—reducing these and recognizing how they impact on concentration remain a challenge, despite what has been learned from research and from other industries.
- *Site marking:* More work is needed to identify the best way to mark surgical sites for—hand and foot surgery; angiograms that are side specific; dermatology; and pain injections.
- *Reducing transcription errors:* Removing the need to copy information from one piece of paper to another or from paper to computer remains a challenge. Several cases highlighted that a transcription error may be copied onto all other records including the theatre list.

- *Counting:* Following a Never Event many trusts have added items to their count policies
- *Equipment with covers or caps that come apart:* Several of the cases raised the question of how to handle covers and caps that are passed across the surgical field.
- *Design:* Manufacturers of medical implants, components and devices need to add visual cues to clearly display side and size on their packaging and, if possible, the device itself. The medical device/implant industry should consider using a common size indicator and color code for left and right labelling and packaging. Similarly, manufacturers need to consider designing visual cues for equipment and supplies that are wholly inserted into the surgical field, to help prevent retention of foreign objects.
- *Reducing choice of implants and components:* Lack of familiarity with implants, equipment and consumables was the cause of some of the Never Events reviewed. Reducing the number of different types available would increase staff familiarity with what is being used, as well as reducing the training load.
- *Size and side compatible components:* Where multiple components are used that need to be both size and side compatible, systems and procedures are needed to check compatibility before each component is used.

Example Never Event: Retained guide wire

Definitions and Examples

- *Wrong site surgery:*

  This includes:
  - Wrong level spinal surgery and interventions that are considered surgical but may be done outside of a surgical environment, example-wrong site block (unless being undertaken as a pain control procedure), biopsy, interventional radiology procedures, cardiology procedures, drain insertion and line insertion, example[peripherally inserted central catheter] PICC/Hickman lines.

  But excludes:

  Interventions where the wrong site is selected because of unknown/unexpected abnormalities in the patient's anatomy. This should be documented in the patient's notes.
  - Incidents where the wrong site surgery is due to incorrect laboratory reports/results or incorrect referral letters.
- Wrong implant/prosthesis

  Retained foreign objects after a surgical/invasive procedure:

The London protocol for classifying the contributory factors in healthcare adverse events [Taylor-Adams et al. (2004)].

Factor type	*Influencing/contributory factors*
Institutional context	• Economic and regulatory context • National guidelines and policies
Organizational and management factors	• Trust financial resources and constraints • Organizational structure • Trust policy standards and goals • Safety culture and priorities
Work environment factors	• Staffing levels and skills mix • Workload and shift patterns • Design availability and maintenance of equipment • Design of the work space including noise levels
Team factors	• Verbal communication • Written communication • Supervision and seeking • Team structure (congruence, consistency, leadership, etc.)

Contd...

Contd...

Factor type	***Influencing/contributory factors***
Individual (staff) factors	• Knowledge and skills • Competence • Physical and mental health
Task factors	• Task design and clarity of structure • Availability and use of protocols • Availability and accuracy of test results
Patient factors	• Condition (complexity and seriousness) • Language and communication • Personality and social factors

- Definition of 'Never Events' declares it as an identifiable and preventable medical 'Error' resulting in serious consequences for patients.
- Literal meaning of an 'Error' according to advance English dictionary is a wrong action attributable to bad judgement or ignorance or attention.
- But when we look at the frequency, magnitude, and impact of this Never Event's 'Error' on the patient safety, it is difficult to digest it as a once in a while incidence pertaining to human error.
- It casts doubt on our system which just formally disposes off the case on the basis of anecdotal media coverage and then forgets it.
- Probably, this is the only reason that in spite of lot of action being taken against this problem in past decade, situation is not as good as it should be.
- We cannot deny the fact that on a given day, even the best person can make the worst error, and we cannot make any action hundred percent free of error or free of accident.
- Also, the complex system of surgical management requiring multidisciplinary approach with multiple level of intervention makes it more error prone.
- In such scenario, no magic pill can be expected to improve the patient safety but a comprehensive approach would only help to minimize this grave problem.
- Keeping in view of its magnitude and widespread universal root, strategic approach is required which can be applied right from institution to national and International level.

Surgical Site Infection and Postoperative Complications

LEARNING OBJECTIVES

- Surgical Risk Scores
- Prophylactic Antibiotics and Antibiotic Resistance
- Risk Factors for Surgical Infection
- Surgical Site Infection
- Intra-abdominal Sepsis
- Postoperative Fever
- Antibacterials
- Clavien-Dindo classification

SURGICAL RISK SCORES

1. Discuss various surgical risk scores used for identifying high-risk surgical patients. ***WBUHS 2022, DNB 2021 June***

- The definition of surgical risk is complex and differs depending on the point of view of the assessor and patient.
- Discussion of surgical risk should include the side effects, complications, failure of the procedure to achieve the desired outcome, and the consequences of taking no action.
- There are a number of risk scoring systems that are available, including the American Society of Anesthesiologists (ASA) risk score, Acute Physiology and Chronic Health Evaluation (APACHE) system and Physiological and Operative Severity Score for the enumeration of Mortality and morbidity (POSSUM).
- In Australia, the majority of patients in the public health system are evaluated in a hospital-specific preadmission clinic where surgical risk can be assessed and medical conditions optimized prior to surgery.
- The most common comorbidities increasing the risk of surgery are cardiac, respiratory, and renal but age is also a significant risk factor, with the elderly having a two to five times greater risk of death in comparison to younger patients.

Category	*Physical status*
ASA 1	Normal healthy patient
ASA 2	Patient with mild systemic disease
ASA 3	Patient with severe systemic disease that is not a constant threat to life
ASA 4	Patient with severe systemic disease that is a constant threat to life
ASA 5	Moribund patient not expected to survive with or without surgery

- APACHE II score is a general measure of disease severity based on current physiologic measurements, age, and previous health conditions. The score can help in the assessment of patients to determine the level and degree of diagnostic and therapeutic intervention.
- Interpretation of APACHE II: minimum 0 and maximum 71; increasing score is associated with an increasing risk of hospital death. The advantage of the APACHE is that it can be used throughout the patient's hospital course in monitoring the patient's response to therapy.

Acute Physiology Score (Measured within 24 hours of Admission)

- Alveolar-arterial oxygen difference ($AaDO_2$) or partial pressure of arterial oxygen (PaO_2) [for fraction of inspired oxygen (FiO_2) ≥0.5 or <0.5, respectively]
- Body temperature (rectal)
- Mean arterial pressure
- Blood pH
- Heart rate
- Respiratory rate
- Serum sodium
- Serum potassium
- Creatinine (double point score for acute renal failure)
- Hematocrit
- White blood cell count
- Glasgow Coma Scale (GCS) (15 minus actual GCS)

Parameters used in POSSUM scoring system.

Physiological parameters	*Operative parameters*
• Age • Cardiac signs • Respiratory history • Systolic blood pressure • Pulse • Glasgow Coma Scale • Hemoglobin • White cell count • Urea • Sodium • Potassium • Electrocardiogram	• Operative severity • Operative urgency • Multiple procedures • Total blood loss • Peritoneal soiling • Presence of malignancy • Mode of surgery

The POSSUM system is a two-part scoring system that includes a physiological assessment and a measure of operative severity. The physiological part of the score includes 12 variables, each divided into 4 grades with an exponentially increasing score (1, 2, 4, and 8).

Risk prediction tool	*Description*	*Advantages*	*Disadvantages*
APACHE II	12 variables measured over first 24 hours: • Physiological indices • Comorbidities • Type of admission	• Well known • Individual risk of morbidity and mortality	• Designed for critical care, not for perioperative use • Requires multiple variables and data entries entered over first 24 hours of admission
POSSUM	12 physiological and six operative variables	• Best known • Well validated	Problems with over and underestimation of mortality
Surgical Outcome Risk Tool (SORT)	6 preoperative variables: • Type of surgery • Urgency of surgery • ASA of the patient • UK developed system	Easy and quick to use	• New tool therefore no external validation • Not patient specific, only provides general risk of procedure
The American College of Surgeons (ACS) National Surgical Quality Improvement Program (NSQIP) Surgical Risk Calculator	21 preoperative risk factors	Patient-specific risks	• Does not account for urgency of procedure • Not widely publicized • Not validated for emergency surgery

PROPHYLACTIC ANTIBIOTICS AND ANTIBIOTIC RESISTANCE

2. Prophylactic antibiotics. *WBUHS 2008, MAMC 2022*

Regardless of the antibiotics administered, the goal of treatment is to achieve antibiotic levels at the site of infection that exceed the minimum inhibitory concentration of the pathogens present. Every patient with a serious infection is evaluated daily or more frequently to assess response.

If you do not see a clear improvement within 2–3 days, you should consider the following:
- The first surgical procedure was not enough.
- The first procedure was enough, but complications occurred.
- Superinfection has developed in a new location.
- The choice of medicine is correct, but it is not given enough. Another or different medication is needed. Antibiotic choice is not the most common cause of failure, unless the initial choice was clearly inappropriate, such as failure to provide anaerobes with an intra-abdominal infection.

When choosing an antibiotic for empiric treatment, the following guidelines must be followed:
- Choose an antibiotic that reaches the site of infection.
- Choose antibiotics with high renal and biliary concentrations, especially for urinary tract infection and cholangitis.
- Consider skin, lung, and central nervous system tissue concentrations at these sites for infection.
- Consider toxicity, especially in critically ill patients, where bioavailability and the range of therapeutic and toxic levels are difficult to predict. When starting an antimicrobial with significant toxic side effects, closely monitor blood levels and organ function. If an infection requiring antibiotics is detected, administer antibiotics aggressively. The rate of redistribution in these patients is unpredictable because they usually received aggressive fluid replacement as part of their support or resuscitation.
- Each time you start antibiotic treatment, set a limit for the antibiotic dosing period.

3. Give a brief account of rational use of antibiotics in surgical practice. Comment about prevention of abuse of antibiotics. *WBUHS 2006*

Rational Use of Antibiotics

Antibiotics are the most important weapons in our hands. Each one of them have been invented after spending considerable amount of time, energy, and money.

Indications for Antibacterial Therapy
- *Definitive therapy:* This is for proven bacterial infections. Antibacterials are drugs to tackle bacteria and hence should be restricted for the treatment of bacterial infections only. Based on the reports, a narrow spectrum, least toxic, easy-to-administer, and cheap drug should be prescribed.
- *Empirical therapy:* Empirical antibacterial therapy should be restricted to critical cases, when time is inadequate for identification and isolation of the bacteria and reasonably strong doubt of bacterial infection exists: septicemic shock/sepsis syndrome, immunocompromised patients with severe systemic infection, hectic temperature, neutrophilic leukocytosis, raised erythrocyte sedimentation rate (ESR), etc. In such situations, drugs that cover the most probable infective agent/s should be used.
- *Prophylactic therapy:* Antimicrobial prophylaxis is administered to susceptible patients to prevent specific infections that can cause definite detrimental effect. These include antitubercular prophylaxis, antirheumatic prophylaxis, antiendocarditis prophylaxis, and prophylactic use of antimicrobials in invasive medical procedures, etc. In all these situations, only narrow spectrum and specific drugs are used.

When Choosing an Antibiotic for Empirical Treatment, follow these Guidelines

- Ensure suspected microorganisms are covered. This usually means starting with broad-spectrum antibiotics that can then be tailored and narrowed down to the specific microorganism isolated. If possible, avoid antibiotics with an anaerobic spectrum, because this group of bacteria plays an important role in maintaining the microenvironment of the gastrointestinal tract.
- An antibiotic that reaches the site of infection must be chosen. For urinary tract infection and cholangitis in particular, choose antibiotics with high renal and bile concentrations. For infection at these sites, consider skin, lung, and central nervous system tissue concentrations.
- Consider toxicity, especially in critically ill patients, where bioavailability and the range of therapeutic and toxic levels are difficult to predict. When starting an antimicrobial with significant toxic side effects, closely monitor blood levels and organ function.
- If an infection requiring antibiotics is detected, antibiotics should be used aggressively. The rate of redistribution in these patients is unpredictable because they usually receive aggressive fluid replacement as part of support or resuscitation.
- Each time you start antibiotic therapy, set a time limit for the antibiotic dosing period.

The Molecular Mechanisms by which Bacteria Acquire Resistance to Antibiotics can be Broadly Classified into four Categories

1. Decreased intracellular concentration of antibiotic due to either decreased influx or increased efflux. Most antibiotics are sensitive to this mechanism (*Pseudomonas*/Enterobacteriaceae β-lactams).
2. Neutralization by inactivating enzymes. This is the most common mechanism of antibiotic resistance and affects all β-lactam antibiotics (e.g., β-lactamases from gram-positive and gram-negative bacteria).
3. Change the target affected by the antibiotic. This class affects all antibiotics and is the main resistance mechanism of some specific bacteria [*Pneumococcus*—penicillin or methicillin-resistant *Staphylococcus aureus* (MRSA) to all β-actam antibiotics].
4. Complete removal of the target affected by the antibiotic. Some specific bacteria develop the ability to create new metabolic pathways and completely eliminate a specific target [e.g., vancomycin-resistant enterococci (VRE)].

Prevention of Abuse of Antibiotics

Interventions to improve rational use of antibiotics:

- A mandated multidisciplinary national body to coordinate antibiotic use policies
- Clinical guidelines
- Essential antibiotics list based on treatment choice
- Drug and therapeutics committees in districts and hospitals
- Problem-based learning in pharmacotherapy in undergraduate circulation continuing in-service medical education as a licensure requirement
- Supervision, audit, and feedback
- Independent information on public education about antibiotics
- Avoidance of perverse financial incentives
- Appropriate and enforced regulation
- Sufficient government expenditure to ensure availability of antibiotics and staff

  A patient may fail to respond to an antibiotic for a number of reasons which include:
  - The etiological agent is resistant to the antibiotic
  - The diagnosis is incorrect
  - The choice of antibiotic is correct but the dose and/or route of administration is wrong
  - The antibiotic cannot reach the site of infection
  - There is a collection of pus that should be drained surgically or a foreign body/devitalized tissue that should be removed

  - There is secondary infection
  - Antibiotic fever
  - Noncompliance of the host
- The World Health Organization (WHO) has urged for intensified global commitment to safeguard antibiotics for future generations.
- Antibiotics and other antimicrobial medicines help to treat conditions that would otherwise be fatal; however, antimicrobial resistance which is drug resistance renders these medicines ineffective.
- The WHO has urged the governments and stakeholders to implement policies and practices to prevent and counter the emergence of highly resistant microorganisms. Antimicrobial resistance is not a new problem; however, it is fast becoming more dangerous.
- Antimicrobial resistance also carries enormous social and personal costs. When infections become resistant to first-line antibiotics, treatment must be switched to second and third-line drugs, which are almost always much more expensive and sometimes more toxic.
- The drugs needed to treat multidrug-resistant tuberculosis (MDR-TB) are >100 times more expensive than first-line drugs. In some countries, the high costs are prohibitive and therefore some of these cases can no longer be processed. Similarly, the emergence of human immunodeficiency virus (HIV) resistance to currently effective drugs could destroy the survival hopes of millions of people living with HIV.
- The discovery, development, and distribution of new antibiotics is a long, drawn out and expensive process. When a new antibiotic is available after millions of dollars and years of research, its misuse renders it ineffective in a very short time.
- Misuse of antibiotics by doctors and users has behavioral, educational, ethical, and economic dimensions that require joint and continuous action by all sectors of society. Weak pharmaceutical regulatory mechanisms in most developing countries also allow the availability of antibiotics of questionable quality and the unauthorized sale of these antibiotics.

4. Antibiotic resistance. ***WBUHS 2010, RIMS, Imphal 2012***

- Antibiotic resistance is a type of drug resistance where a microorganism is able to survive exposure to an antibiotic.
- While a spontaneous or induced genetic mutation in bacteria may confer resistance to antimicrobial drugs, genes that confer resistance can be transferred between bacteria in a horizontal fashion by conjugation, transduction, or transformation.
- Thus, a gene for antibiotic resistance that evolves via natural selection may be shared. Evolutionary stress such as exposure to antibiotics then selects for the antibiotic resistant trait.
- Many antibiotic resistance genes reside on plasmids, facilitating their transfer. If a bacterium carries several resistance genes, it is called multidrug resistant (MDR) or, informally, a superbug or super bacterium.
- The increasing prevalence of antibiotic-resistant bacterial infections seen in clinical practice stems from antibiotic use both within human medicine and veterinary medicine.
- Any use of antibiotics can increase selective pressure in a population of bacteria to allow the resistant bacteria to thrive and the susceptible bacteria to die off.
- As resistance toward antibiotics becomes more common, a greater need for alternative treatments arises.

Causes

- Evolutionary pressure from their use has played a role in the development of multidrug resistance varieties and the spread of resistance between bacterial species.
- Antibiotics are sold over the counter without a prescription, which also leads to the creation of resistant strains.
- Misuse and overuse of antibiotics.
- Addition of antibiotics to livestock feed.

- Household use of antibacterials in soaps and other products, although not clearly contributing to resistance, is also discouraged (as not being effective at infection control).
- Also unsound practices in the pharmaceutical manufacturing industry can contribute toward the likelihood of creating antibiotic-resistant strains.
- The procedures and clinical practice during the period of drug treatment are frequently flawed; usually no steps are taken to isolate the patient to prevent reinfection or infection by a new pathogen, negating the goal of complete destruction by the end of the course.
- Certain antibiotic classes are highly associated with colonization with "superbugs" (highly antibiotic resistant bacteria) compared to other antibiotic classes. The risk for colonization increases if there is a lack of sensitivity (resistance) of the superbugs to the antibiotic used and high tissue penetration, as well as broad-spectrum activity against "good bacteria".
- In the case of MRSA, increased rates of MRSA infections are seen with glycopeptides, cephalosporins, and especially quinolones.
- In the case of colonization with *Clostridium difficile,* the high-risk antibiotics include cephalosporins and in particular quinolones and clindamycin.

Natural Occurrence

- There is evidence that naturally occurring antibiotic resistance is common.
- The genes that confer this resistance are known as the environmental resistome. These genes may be transferred from nondisease-causing bacteria to those that do cause disease, leading to clinically significant antibiotic resistance.
- Inappropriate prescribing of antibiotics has been attributed to a number of causes, including people who insist on antibiotics, physicians who simply prescribe them as they feel they do not have time to explain why they are not necessary, and physicians who do not know when to prescribe antibiotics or else are overly cautious for medical legal reasons.
- Antibiotic resistance has been shown to increase with duration of treatment; therefore, as long as a clinically effective lower limit is observed (that depends upon the organism and antibiotic in question), the use by the medical community of shorter courses of antibiotics is likely to decrease rates of resistance.
- Compliance with once-daily antibiotics is better than with twice-daily antibiotics. Patients taking less than the required dosage or failing to take their doses within the prescribed timing results in decreased concentration of antibiotics in the bloodstream and tissues, and in turn, exposure of bacteria to suboptimal antibiotic concentrations increases the frequency of antibiotic resistant organisms.
- Poor hand hygiene by hospital staff has been associated with the spread of resistant organisms, and an increase in handwashing compliance results in decreased rates of these organisms.

Role of Other Animals

- Drugs are used in animals that are used as human food, such as cattle, pigs, chickens, and fish. There has been extensive use of antibiotics in animal husbandry.
- Historically this use has been little regulated, because very little restrictive legislation or regulatory limitations exist.
- These drugs can affect the meat, milk, and eggs produced from those animals and can be the source of super bugs. For example, farm animals, particularly pigs, are believed (though not proven) to be able to infect people with MRSA.
- The resistant bacteria in animals due to antibiotic exposure can be transmitted to humans via three path ways, those being through the consumption of meat, from close or direct contact with animals, or through the environment.
- However, complete cooking of meat inactivates bacteria, whether or not they are antibiotic-resistant.
- The WHO concluded that antibiotics as growth promoters in animal feeds should be prohibited, in the absence of risk assessments.

Mechanisms

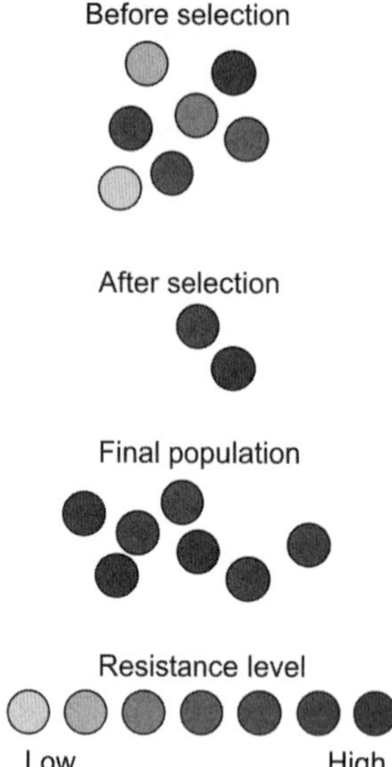

The four main mechanisms by which microorganisms exhibit resistance to antimicrobials are:

1. *Drug inactivation or modification:* For example, enzymatic deactivation of penicillin G in some penicillin resistant bacteria through the production of β-lactamases
2. *Alteration of target site:* For example, alteration of penicillin-binding protein (PBP)—the binding target site of penicillins—in MRSA and other penicillin-resistant bacteria
3. *Alteration of metabolic pathway:* For example, some sulfonamide-resistant bacteria do not require para aminobenzoic acid (PABA), an important precursor for the synthesis of folic acid and nucleic acids in bacteria inhibited by sulfonamides, instead, like mammalian cells, they turn to using preformed folic acid.
4. *Reduced drug accumulation:* By decreasing drug permeability and/or increasing active efflux (pumping out) of the drugs across the cell surface.

There are three known mechanisms of fluoroquinolone resistance.

1. Some types of efflux pumps can act to decrease intracellular quinolone concentration.
2. In gram-negative bacteria, plasmid-mediated resistance genes produce proteins that can bind to deoxyribonucleic acid (DNA) gyrase, protecting it from the action of quinolones.
3. Finally, mutations at key sites in DNA gyrase or topoisomerase IV can decrease their binding affinity to quinolones, decreasing the drug's effectiveness.

Prevention

- Rational use of antibiotics may reduce the chances of development of opportunistic infection by antibiotic resistant bacteria due to dysbacteriosis.
- Vaccines do not have the problem of resistance because a vaccine enhances the body's natural defenses, while an antibiotic operates separately from the body's normal defenses. Nevertheless, new strains may evolve that escape immunity induced by vaccines; e.g., an updated influenza vaccine is needed each year.
- While theoretically promising, antistaphylococcal vaccines have shown limited efficacy, because of immunological variation between *Staphylococcus* species, and the limited duration of effectiveness of the antibodies produced. Development and testing of more effective vaccines is under way.

Phage Therapy

- Phage therapy, an approach that has been extensively researched and used as a therapeutic agent. Bacteriophages or "phages" are viruses that invade bacterial cells and, in the case of lytic phages, disrupt bacterial metabolism and cause the bacterium to lyse. Phage therapy is the therapeutic use of lytic bacteriophages to treat pathogenic bacterial infections.

- Bacteriophage therapy is an important alternative to antibiotics in the current era of MDR pathogens.
- Discovery of the structure of the viral protein PlyC is allowing researchers to understand the way it kills a significant range of pathogenic bacteria.

Applications

Antibiotic resistance is an important tool for genetic engineering. By constructing a plasmid that contains an antibiotic resistance gene as well as the gene being engineered or expressed, a researcher can ensure that when bacteria replicate, only the copies that carry the plasmid survive. This ensures that the gene being manipulated passes along when the bacteria replicates.

- The most commonly used antibiotics in genetic engineering are generally "older" antibiotics that have largely fallen out of use in clinical practice. These include ampicillin, kanamycin, tetracycline, and chloramphenicol.

SURGICAL SITE INFECTIONS

5. Risk factors for surgical site infection. *WBUHS 2007*

Risk Factors for Surgical Site Infection According to the Three Main Determinants of Such Infection

Microorganism	*Local wound*	*Patient*
• Remote site infection • Long-term care facility • Recent hospitalization • Duration of the procedure • Wound class • Intensive care unit patient • Previous antibiotic therapy • Preoperative shaving • Bacterial number, virulence, and antimicrobial resistance	*Surgical technique:* • Hematoma/seroma • Necrosis • Sutures • Drains • Foreign bodies	• Age • Immunosuppression • Steroids • Malignancy • Obesity • Diabetes • Malnutrition • Multiple comorbid conditions • Transfusions • Cigarette smoking • Oxygen • Temperature • Glucose control

6. Surgical site infection. *Tripura University 2025; RGUHS Karnataka, 2025; WBUHS 2008, 2009, 2021*

Introduction

- Surgical site infections (SSIs) are infections present in any location along the surgical tract after a surgical procedure.
- SSIs are the most common nosocomial infection in our population and constitute 38% of all infections in surgical patients. By definition, they can occur anytime from 0 to 30 days after the operation or up to 1 year after a procedure that has involved the implantation of a foreign material (mesh, vascular graft, prosthetic joint, and so on). Incisional infections are the most common; they account for 60–80% of all SSIs and have a better prognosis than organ/space-related SSIs do.
- *Staphylococcus aureus* remains the most common SSI pathogen, followed by coagulase-negative staphylococci, enterococci, and *Escherichia coli*. However, in clean-contaminated and contaminated procedures, *E. coli* and other Enterobacteriaceae are the most common cause of SSIs. In addition, some emerging organisms have become more common in recent years. Vancomycin-resistant enterococci (VRE) and gram-negative bacilli with

unusual resistance were isolated more frequently. Of particular interest is the increase in *Candida* species as a cause of SSIs and surgical infections in general.

Types

Surgical site infection usually occurs within 30 days of surgery. The Centers for Disease Control and Prevention (CDC) describes three types of SSIs:

1. Shallow incision SSI. This infection occurs in the area of the skin where the incision was made.
2. Deep incision SSI. This infection occurs under the incision area of the muscle and surrounding tissues.
3. SSI of the organ or chamber. This type of infection can occur in any area of the body except the skin, muscles, and surrounding tissues that were involved in the surgery. It includes a body organ or the space between organs.

Signs and Symptoms

Any SSI may cause redness, delayed healing, fever, pain, tenderness, warmth, or swelling.

These are other signs and symptoms of some types of SSIs:

- Superficial incisional SSI can produce pus from the wound area. Pus samples can be cultured to determine the bacteria causing the infection.
- Deep incisional SSI can also produce pus.
- The wound may reopen on its own, or the surgeon may reopen the wound and find pus inside the wound.
- SSI of an organ or space may indicate purulent discharge coming through the skin from a drain placed into the body space or organ. A collection of pus, called an abscess, is an enclosed area of pus and decaying tissue surrounded by inflammation. An abscess can be seen when the surgeon reopens the wound or with special X-rays.

Causes and Risk Factors

Postoperative infections are caused by bacteria. The most common of them are *Staphylococcus, Streptococcus*, and *Pseudomonas* bacteria.

The degree of risk of SSI is related to the type of surgical wound you have. Surgical wounds can be classified as follows:

- *Clean wounds:* These are not inflamed or contaminated and do not involve incision of an internal organ.
- *Clean contaminated wounds:* They show no signs of infection during surgery, but involve cutting into an internal organ.
- *Contaminated wounds:* These include cutting an internal organ, where the contents spill from the organ into the wound.
- *Dirty wounds:* These are wounds with a known infection at the time of surgery.

Other Risk Factors

- Having surgery that lasts >2 hours
- Having other medical problems or diseases
- Being an elderly adult
- Being overweight
- Smoking
- Having cancer
- Having a weak immune system
- Having diabetes
- Having emergency surgery
- Having abdominal surgery

Risk factors for surgical site infection according to the three main determinants of such infection:

Microorganism	*Local wound*	*Patient*
• Remote site infection • Long-term care facility • Recent hospitalization • Duration of the procedure • Wound class • Intensive care unit patient • Previous antibiotic therapy • Preoperative shaving • Bacterial number, virulence, and antimicrobial resistance	*Surgical technique:* • Hematoma/seroma • Necrosis • Sutures • Drains • Foreign bodies	• Age • Immunosuppression • Steroids • Malignancy • Obesity • Diabetes • Malnutrition • Multiple comorbid conditions • Transfusions • Cigarette smoking • Oxygen • Temperature • Glucose control

Prevention

- Stop smoking before surgery
- Control blood sugar
- Also, avoid shaving in the skin area that the surgeon is planning to operate through

Preventive Measures

Timing of action	*Microorganism*	*Local*	*Patient*
Preoperative	• Shorten preoperative stay • Antiseptic shower preoperatively • Appropriate preoperative hair removal or no hair removal • Avoid or treat remote site infections • Antimicrobial prophylaxis	Appropriate preoperative hair removal or no hair removal	• Optimize nutrition • Preoperative warming • Tight glucose control (insulin drip) • Stop smoking
Intraoperative	• Asepsis and antisepsis • Avoid spillage in gastrointestinal cases	*Surgical technique:* • Hematoma/seroma • Good perfusion • Complete debridement • Dead spaces • Monofilament sutures • Justified drain use (closed) • Limit use of sutures/foreign bodies • Delayed primary closure when indicated	• Supplemental oxygen • Intraoperative warming • Adequate fluid resuscitation • Tight glucose control (insulin drip)
Postoperative	• Protect incision for 48–72 hours • Remove drains as soon as possible • Avoid postoperative bacteremia	Postoperative dressing for 48–72 hours	• Early enteral nutrition • Supplemental oxygen • Tight glucose control (insulin drip) • Surveillance programs

Microorganism Related

- Microorganisms causing SSI can be either exogenous or endogenous.
- Exogenous microorganisms come from the operating team or from the environment around the surgical site (operating room, equipment, air, water, and so on).
- Endogenous microorganisms come either from the bacteria present in the patient at the surgical site or from bacteria present at a different location (e.g., remote site infection and nasal colonization).

- Two primary measures exist to control the bacterial load in the surgical site: aseptic and antiseptic methods and antimicrobial prophylaxis.

Treatment
- Most SSIs can be treated with antibiotics.
- Sometimes additional surgery or procedures may be required to treat the SSI.

7. Surgical site infection—classification. ***AIIMS, Bhopal 2023***

Surgical Site Infection (SSI)—Classification

Surgical site infection is an infection that occurs after surgery in the part of the body where the surgery took place. The Centers for Disease Control and Prevention (CDC) classifies SSIs into *three main categories* based on the depth and extent of infection.

1. **Superficial Incisional SSI**
    - *Involves:* Only the *skin and subcutaneous tissue* of the incision.
    - *Timing:* Occurs within *30 days* of the operation.
    - *Clinical signs:*
        - Redness (erythema)
        - Warmth
        - Swelling
        - Pain or tenderness
        - Pus or other drainage
        - Positive wound culture

    Must not involve deeper tissues (fascia or muscle).
2. **Deep Incisional SSI**
    - *Involves: Deep soft tissues* such as *fascia and muscle layers.*
    - *Timing:*
        - Within *30 days* of surgery *without an implant.*
        - Within *90 days* if *implant is placed.*
    - *Clinical signs:*
        - Fever or localized pain/tenderness
        - Deep purulent drainage
        - Dehiscence (wound opens up)
        - Abscess formation (confirmed clinically or radiologically)
3. **Organ/Space SSI**
    - *Involves:* Any part of the *anatomy (organs or spaces)* that was opened or manipulated during surgery, *excluding the incision itself.*
    - *Timing:* Same as deep SSI (30 or 90 days depending on implant).
    - *Clinical signs:*
        - Purulent drainage from drain or wound leading to organ/space
        - Positive culture from fluid or tissue from organ/space
        - Evidence of infection on imaging or reoperation

Examples: Peritonitis after abdominal surgery, empyema after thoracic surgery, brain abscess after craniotomy.

Type	*Involves*	*Timing*	*Examples*
Superficial incisional	Skin and subcutaneous tissue	Within 30 days	Red, warm, pus at incision
Deep incisional	Fascia and muscle layers	30 or 90 days	Dehiscence, deep abscess
Organ/space	Internal organs/spaces	30 or 90 days	Intra-abdominal abscess, empyema

INTRA-ABDOMINAL SEPSIS

8. Intra-abdominal sepsis. ***WBUHS 2010***

9. Discuss the current definition, evaluation and management of intra-abdominal sepsis.
AIIMS, Bhubaneswar 2024

Introduction

An intra-abdominal sepsis may lead to septicemia, septic shock, and multiple organ dysfunction syndrome.
Intra-abdominal sepsis may occur in:

- The peritoneal cavity
- The retroperitoneum
- An organ

Definition

Intra-abdominal sepsis is defined as a life-threatening organ dysfunction caused by a dysregulated host response to infection originating from within the abdominal cavity. It typically results from peritonitis or intra-abdominal abscesses, often due to conditions like gastrointestinal perforation, appendicitis, diverticulitis, or postoperative complications.

Causes

Surgical Causes

- Acute infections such as acute appendicitis, acute cholecystitis, acute tubo-ovarian infection, and acute diverticulitis
- Acute infections supervening on acute inflammation, e.g., acute necrotizing pancreatitis followed by infection and acute necrotizing enterocolitis
- Perforations, e.g., appendicular, peptic, tuberculous and enteric perforations and diverticulitis with perforation. Patients on steroid therapy and nonsteroidal anti-inflammatory drugs (NSAIDs) are vulnerable.
- Hollow visceral injury by accidental trauma, or during an operation, endoscopy or an interventional radiologic procedure.
- Strangulation, infarction, or ischemic gangrene of bowel with or without perforation.
- Anastomotic dehiscence
- Postoperative sepsis due to breakdown of intraoperative asepsis, especially in a patient who is diabetic, malnourished, immunocompromised or neutropenic, or in a patient who is on steroids or chemotherapy.

Medical Causes

- Spontaneous bacterial peritonitis in preexisting liver disease
- Nephrotic syndrome
- Systemic lupus erythematosus (SLE)
- Malignancy
  - *Bacteriology:*
    - May be monobacterial—due to pneumococci or β-hemolytic streptococci or *Staphylococcus aureus*
    - May be polybacterial—gram-negative bacilli—*E. coli* being the most common
    - Anaerobes such as Bacteroides fragilis, anaerobic cocci, and clostridia are frequently encountered
  - Fungus is isolated with immunocompromised patients

Clinical Features

- Pain
- Tenderness, guarding, abdominal distension, and absent bowel sounds
- Restricted abdominal movement with respiration

- Tachycardia, pyrexia, and tachypnea
- May be features of shock

Laboratory Studies
- Leukocytosis, hemoconcentration, and electrolyte disturbances
- Liver functions, renal profile, or coagulation parameters may be deranged
- Blood culture may be helpful
- Procalcitonin level has some help

Imaging Studies
- X-ray chest—pneumonic patch, collapse, pleural effusion, and pneumoperitoneum
- X-ay abdomen—air fluid level
- Ultrasonography (USG)—can detect intra-abdominal abscess, distended bowel loops, and interloop collections
- CT and contrast-enhanced CT (CECT)—best diagnostic tool to diagnose pancreatic and peripancreatic abscess. Extraluminal air is diagnostic of infection in acute necrotizing pancreatitis.
- MRI—for detecting complications of gallstone disease, pancreatitis, etc.
- Doppler USG, CECT with angiography, and MRA—help in evaluation of vascular pathology related to intra-abdominal sepsis.
- USG/CT-guided paracentesis or laparoscopy—useful in diagnostic dilemma.

Local Treatment
- In de novo intra-abdominal sepsis, after initial resuscitation, an aggressive prompt surgical intervention should be instituted.
- Patients who have been operated earlier for intra-abdominal sepsis are treated by percutaneous CT-guided drainage with wide multiple pigtail drains or sump drains.

Contraindications to Conservative Approach
- Multiple pockets of pus
- Very thick pus
- Considerable necrosis
- Absence of a "safe-window"
- Overwhelming septicemia

Surgery is Essential in
- Intra-abdominal sepsis where percutaneous drainage is not possible or has failed.
- In patients with infected pancreatic necrosis after delaying surgery as much as possible.
- All other patients with intra-abdominal sepsis.

Guidelines for Surgery
- Once the decision of surgery is made, it should be carried out without any delay.
- The perforation should be closed, if possible. The septic focus is eradicated totally or eradicated as much as possible.
- If the infective focus is localized and cannot be eradicated, a diversion stoma is fashioned.
- Thorough copious irrigation of peritoneal cavity is essential.
- In selected cases with severe sepsis and considerable local necrosis with large number of pockets of pus laparostoma may have to be resorted to.

General Treatment
- Fluid and electrolyte administration
- Inotropic support if needed
- Appropriate antibiotic therapy with broad-spectrum coverage
- Chest physiotherapy

- Nutritional support
- Organ support

Newer Aspects

- To prevent multiple organ failure
- To prevent thrombosis in microcirculation one can use antithrombin IV, tissue factor pathway inhibitor, and activated protein C

10. Intra-abdominal infection.

11. Investigations for intra-abdominal infection. ***WBUHS 2008***

Definition

Infections that spread beyond the cavity of origin into the peritoneum and are associated with abscess formation or peritonitis.

Primary	*Secondary*	*Tertiary*
Spontaneous bacterial peritonitis without abdominal or gastrointestinal lesions	• Occurs as a result of spillage of intestinal organisms through a physical hole in the digestive tract or through a necrotic intestinal wall • May be community acquired or treatment related	Peritonitis in a critically ill patient that persists or recurs at least 48 hours after apparently adequate treatment of primary or secondary peritonitis

Microbiology

Abscesses or secondary peritonitis. Healthcare-associated intra-abdominal infection, usually caused by nosocomial organisms, especially at the surgical site and within a specific hospital and ward.

- *Community-acquired infections:*
  - Infections derived from stomach, duodenum, biliary system, and proximal small bowel:
    - Gram-positive and gram-negative aerobic and facultative bacteria
- *Distal small bowel:*
  - Gram-negative facultative and aerobic bacteria
  - Anaerobes
- *Large bowel:*
  - Facultative and obligate anaerobic bacteria
  - Streptococci and enterococci commonly present
- Tertiary peritonitis:
  - Coagulase-negative staphylococci
  - *Pseudomonas*
  - *Candida*
  - Enterococci

Clinical Features

- Difficult to diagnose in a critically ill patient because the history is usually not taken and physical signs are masked by loss of consciousness.
- Consider making the diagnosis in the appropriate clinical setting in patients with otherwise unexplained signs of sepsis or organ dysfunction:
  - Recent abdominal surgery
  - Source of arterial embolism
  - Peripheral vascular disease
  - Thrombotic disorder
  - Recent arteriography
  - Anterior splanchnic circulatory disorder (e.g., use of vasopressors or prolonged shock)

- Unexpected dyspnea or supraventricular tachycardia occurring 3–4 days after abdominal surgery, new renal dysfunction, or elevated bilirubin or transaminases should all raise suspicion of intra-abdominal infection.

Investigations

- Microbiological
- *Blood cultures:*
  - Often negative
  - Polymicrobial or anaerobic bacteremia should increase the possibility of anaerobic infection
    - *Community-acquired infections:* Gram stain is of no value
    - *Healthcare-associated infections:* Gram stain can be valuable for *S. aureus* or *Enterococcus* spp. to determine the need for specific treatment.
- *Radiological:* Definitive diagnostic approach to intra-abdominal infection
  - *X-ray of the abdominal cavity:*
    - Look for free gas, intestinal obstruction, or subtle signs of intestinal ischemia
    - Water-soluble contrast studies can show leaks
    - Contrast injection into drains, fistulas, or sinuses can help demonstrate the anatomy of complex infections and check the adequacy of abscess drainage.
  - *Ultrasound:*
    - Portable and virtually risk-free advantage
    - *Useful:*
      - Detection of abscesses and fluid accumulation
      - Instruction in percutaneous drainage procedures
      - Detection of free fluid
      - Evaluation of the gall tree
    - *Disadvantages:*
      - Depends on the user
      - Difficult to perform in patients with abdominal ligaments or paralytic ileus
  - *CT abdomen:*
    - With intravenous (IV) and oral or rectal contrast, most causes of secondary peritonitis are easily diagnosed
    - Requires removal of a potentially unstable patient from the intensive care unit
    - Relative contraindications:
      - *Renal dysfunction:* Contrast media can worsen renal dysfunction
      - Paralytic ileus
    - A negative CT usually indicates a very low probability of a process that can be reversed by surgical intervention, but intestinal ischemia cannot be ruled out, especially in the early stages.
  - *Invasive examinations in the intensive care unit:*
    - Careful examination of surgical wounds with a sterile culture stick or gloved hand can often identify collections of infected material immediately adjacent to the incision.
    - *Diagnostic peritoneal lavage:*
      - May reveal bacteria, white blood cells, bile, or intestinal contents
      - A blood smear indicates acute intestinal ischemia
    - *Diagnostic laparoscopy:*
      - Difficult
      - Experience with critically ill patients is largely anecdotal

Management

- Physiological resuscitation
- Systemic antibiotics
- Source control

POSTOPERATIVE FEVER

12. Postoperative fever. ***WBUHS 2008***

13. Enumerate the causes of postoperative fever. Discuss its management.
Tripura University 2024; DNB 2021 June

Introduction

- Postoperative fever is a common condition challenging to find the right diagnosis, because it can be a hall mark of serious underlying conditions.
- Between 40 and 50% of surgical patients develop postoperative fever depending on type of surgery but only a small percentage turn out to be due to infection.

Causes

Category	*Day*	*Description*
Wind	POD 1–2	The lungs, i.e., pneumonia, aspiration, and pulmonary embolism Once attributed to atelectasis, but this has been shown to be inaccurate
Water	POD 3–5	Urinary tract infection, related to indwelling catheter (during surgery or currently, i.e., Foley catheter)
Wound	POD 5–7	Surgical site infection, which in obstetrics or gynecology, may refer to the uterus
Walking	POD 4–6	Deep vein thrombosis or pulmonary embolism
Wonder drugs or "What did we do?"	POD 7+	Drug fever and infections related to intravenous lines

Causes of Fever

Workup: Complete blood count (CBC) with differential, chest X-ray (CXR), two blood cultures, urinalysis, and urine culture

- Atelectasis (POD 1–2)
  - The most common cause of postoperative fever
  - *Risk factors:* Longterm immobilization, smoking, and lung diseases
  - *Symptoms:* Low fever, noise when listening, tachycardia, and tachypnea
  - *Treatment:* Bronchoscopy
- Pneumonia (POD 1–2)
  - *Risk factors:*
    - Use of respiratory protective equipment (*Pseudomonas* and *Klebsiella*)
      - *Treatment:* Aminoglycosides + penicillin
    - Aspiration
      - *Treatment:* Nasogastric tube (NGT) for decompression and oxygenation
  - *Symptoms:* Cough, discharge of sputum; vitals: fever, ↑ respiratory rate (RR)
  - *Findings:* CXR infiltrate and leukocytes on CBC
- Urinary tract infection (UTI) (POD 3+)
  - 5% chance for each day the Foley catheter is in place
  - *Symptoms:* Burning sensation during urination; no pain if the Foley is still inside
  - *Risk factors:* Prostatic hyperplasia, diabetes, catheters, and urinary retention
  - *Microorganisms: Pseudomonas, Serratia, Enterococcus, E. coli, Proteus*, and *Klebsiella*
  - *Findings:* Leukocyte esterase and nitrite changes in UA; growth of urine culture, and leukocytes in CBC
  - *Treatment:* Remove Foley, add fluids, and antibiotics

- Wound (POD 5+)
  - *Symptoms:* >2 cm redness, swelling, heat, and pain around the incision site
  - *Microorganisms: Staphylococcus* most common
  - *GI infections: E. coli, Bacteroides,* and *Enterococcus*
  - *Genitourinary (GU) infections: Pseudomonas* and *Proteus*
  - *Care:* Drain and moisten the bandage twice a day
  - *Other complications:* Hematoma, seroma, and detachment (facial opening)
- Deep vein thrombosis (DVT) (POD 7+)
  - *Symptoms:* Leg swelling, tender superficial veins, chest pain, tachycardia, tachypnea, shortness of breath (SOB)
  - *Investigations:* Doppler, venogram, and CT (looking for pulmonary artery occlusion)
  - *Treatment:* Ambulatory, SCDs, systemic heparin, and consult cardiologist
- *Medications:* A medication reaction can happen at any time
- *Linear infections:*
  - IV lines come out after 72 hours
  - *Symptoms:* Fever, leukocytosis in CBC, bacteremia in blood, and (+) culture of at the top of the line
  - *Microorganisms: S. aureus* and *S. epidermidis*
  - *Treatment:* Line removal and ± IV antibiotics
- *Peritonitis:*
  - Perforation of the digestive tract, abdominal pain, fever, and sepsis
  - *Studies:* KUB (Check Free Air)
  - *Treatment:* NPO with NGT, IV antibiotics, and surgery for abdominal irrigation
  - *Complications:* Formation of abscesses
  - *Treatment:* Localize by CT scan or gallium study (X-rays during injection radioactive gallium into the bloodstream), sewage, and antibiotics

Fever Occurring Few Hours Postoperative

- Thyroid storm
- Addisonian crisis
  - *Treatment:* Restart steroid therapy for Addison's disease
- Alcohol withdrawal
  - Low grade fever, tremors, and seizures
  - *Wernicke's encephalopathy:* Confusion, nystagmus, and ataxia
  - *Korsakoff's psychosis:* Confabulation and amnesia caused by damage to mammillary bodies
  - *Treatment:* Thiamine
- Anastomotic leak
- *Clostridium perfringens* wound infection

ANTIBACTERIALS

14. Antibacterials.

Should be administered as soon as infection is suspected and preferably before surgery (to minimize the risk of surgical wound infection).

Selection of antibacterial agents for community-acquired infections:

- Should be active against enteric gram-negative aerobic and facultative bacilli and β-lactam-susceptible gram positive cocci.
- For infections of the distal small intestine and colon, antibacterial drugs should cover anaerobes. The same recommendation applies to proximal gastrointestinal perforations when there is obstruction.

- Avoid agents used to treat nosocomial infection in the intensive care setting, except in high-risk patients.
- Addition of antibacterial agents covering enterococcal infections does not benefit patients with community acquired infections.
- *Appropriate treatments include:*
    - Cefazolin or cefuroxime plus metronidazole
    - Metronidazole and a quinolone (e.g., moxifloxacin or gatifloxacin)
- Broader-spectrum antibacterial drugs should be given to high-risk patients
    - *Risk factors:*
        - Advanced APACHE II
        - Poor nutritional value
        - Major cardiovascular disease
        - Failure to achieve adequate source control
        - Immunosuppression
        - Suitable systems are:
            - Piperacillin/tazobactam
            - Imipenem/cilastatin, meropenem
            - Third or fourth-generation cephalosporins plus metronidazole
            - Ciprofloxacin plus metronidazole
            - Aztreonam plus metronidazole

Selection of Antibacterial Agents for Healthcare-associated Infections

- More resilient vegetation routinely encountered
- The organisms found are similar to those seen in other nosocomial infections
- Treatment should be based on the local hospital flora and its resistance
- Enterococcal masking agents should be used when enterococci are isolated from patients with healthcare-associated infections
- The role of antibiotics in tertiary peritonitis is poorly defined
- Little evidence that they significantly change the outcome
- Some recommend the use of narrow-spectrum agents based on culture results and sensitivity and avoidance of agents with antianaerobic activity
- Some data suggest that the use of anaerobic antibiotics increases intestinal colonization with *Candida* and vancomycin-resistant enterococci.

Duration of Therapy

- *Not >24 hours for:*
    - Bowel injuries due to penetrating, blunt, or iatrogenic trauma that are repaired within 12 hours
    - Intraoperative contamination of operative field by enteric contents
    - Acute perforations of stomach, duodenum, and proximal jejunum in absence of antacid therapy or malignancy
- *For patients with established infections:*
    - Until resolution of signs of infection occurs. This assessment should be based on signs of sepsis and return of GI function
    - If source control is adequate the role of antibiotics is largely adjuvant and the course can usually be restricted to 5–7 days.
    - Further investigation is indicated or patients with persistent or recurrent clinical evidence of intra-abdominal infection after 5–7 days of therapy.

Source Control

Physical measures to eradicated focus of infection, prevent ongoing contamination, and ultimately to restore optimal anatomy and function:

- Drainage

- Debridement
- Definitive management

Successful source control and antibiotic management is associated with resolution of clinical features of systemic inflammation and reversal of organ dysfunction. Progression or failure of resolution of organ dysfunction suggests persistence of the disease and the need for further intervention.

Drainage

- Abscess formation isolates the infection from the surrounding sterile tissues, but has the disadvantage of preventing the influx of host immune cells and antibiotics.
- Drainage becomes a controlled sinus or fistula
- Percutaneous ultrasound or CT-guided drainage is the primary procedure to control localized, and radio logically defined sites of infection.
- Can also be used as a temporary procedure to decompress infected retroperitoneal masses in patients with necrotizing pancreatitis, allowing surgical treatment to be delayed until it becomes safer.
- *Indications for surgery:*
  - Failure of percutaneous drainage
  - Collections that have a significant solid tissue component and require cleaning
  - Simultaneous control of a continuous source of pollution
  - If the local protection of the peritoneum did not contain the site of infection causing generalized peritonitis

Debridement

- Unlike drainage, which removes the fluid component of the infection, debridement is the physical removal of infected or necrotic solid matter.
- Cleansing is required less frequently in patients with intra-abdominal infection
- Key indicators of this provision:
  - Intestinal infarction
  - Infected peripancreatic necrosis

Deciding when to act has relative risks and benefits. Thus, the benefits of early resection of necrotic bowel far outweigh the risks. In contrast, in infected retroperitoneal necrosis, the bacterial load is lower and organisms associated with the necrotic tissue have less access to the circulation. In addition, early detection is difficult because the boundary between viable and nonviable tissue is poor. As a result, there is a tendency to intervene immediately rather than immediately.

15. Antibiotics in abdominal surgery current guideline and practices. ***WBUHS 2022***

Surgical antimicrobial prophylaxis is an accepted part of surgical practice in some procedures to prevent infections at the surgical site and optimize postoperative recovery. The use of antimicrobials for the prevention of infection must be weighed against any harm associated with their use (such as allergic and adverse drug reactions) and potential contribution to the development of antimicrobial resistance.

Classification of Surgical Wounds

Classification of surgical wound	*Criteria*
Clean	Uninfected operative wounds in which no inflammation is encountered and the respiratory, gastrointestinal, and genital or urinary tracts are not entered (and no break in aseptic technique). Clean wounds are primarily closed and, if necessary, drained with closed drainage. Operative incisional wounds that follow nonpenetrating (blunt) trauma should be included in this category if they meet the criteria

Contd....

Contd.…

Classification of surgical wound	*Criteria*
Clean-contaminated	Operative wounds in which the respiratory, gastrointestinal, genital (including female and male reproductive tracts), or urinary tracts are entered under controlled conditions and without unusual contamination. Specifically, operations involving the biliary tract, appendix, vagina, and oropharynx are included in this category, provided no evidence of infection or major break in technique is encountered
Contaminated	Major breaks in sterile technique (e.g., open cardiac massage), gross spillage from the gastrointestinal tract, or the incision encounters acute and nonpurulent inflammation (including necrotic tissue without evidence of purulent discharge). Open, fresh, or accidental wounds are also included in this category
Dirty (or infected)	Existing clinical infection or perforated viscera as well as old traumatic wounds with retained devitalized tissue. This definition suggests that the organisms causing postoperative infection were present before the operation. In these cases, antibiotic treatment in addition to prophylaxis is required

Preoperative Considerations

- Consider each patient's individual risk factors, including the need for prophylaxis. Antibiotic selection/dosing may need to be modified depending on patient factors (e.g., immunosuppression, presence of prostheses, allergies, renal function, obesity, malnutrition, diabetes, malignancy, infection at another site, colonization with multidrug-resistant bacteria, and preexisting pathologies).
- Consider surgical wound classification (clean, contaminated, and dirty) when determining the need or choice of antibiotic prophylaxis.
- Refer to surgical antimicrobial prophylaxis
- Prescribing guideline for further information.
- Preexisting infections (known or suspected)—if present, use a regimen appropriate for the procedure rather than a prophylactic regimen, but ensure the regimen has activity against the organisms most likely to cause postoperative infection.
- Adjust the timing of the therapeutic dose to achieve appropriate plasma and tissue concentrations at the surgical incision and during the procedure, if in doubt, consult the infectious disease (ID) or antimicrobial stewardship (AMS) team.
- Prevention of enterococcal endocarditis is indicated in patients with high-risk heart disease undergoing abdominal, gastrointestinal, and biliary surgical procedures.

Practice Points

- *Timing and administration of antibiotics:* Surgical prophylaxis of antibiotics must be administered preoperatively to achieve effective plasma and tissue concentrations at the time of incision.
- Administration of any antibiotic after a skin incision reduces effectiveness. IV cefazolin can be administered within 5 minutes and should be administered no later than 60 minutes before the skin incision. IV gentamicin can be given over 3–5 minutes and should be given within 120 minutes before surgery. An IV infusion of metronidazole can be administered over 20 minutes and must be completely administered within 120 minutes of the surgical incision.
- The maximum concentration in plasma and tissues is reached at the end of the infusion. IV infusion of vancomycin should be administered at 1 g over at least 60 minutes and 1.5 g over at least 90 minutes.
- Vancomycin should be administered 15–120 minutes before the skin incision. This ensures adequate concentration during the incision and allows detection of potential infusion-related toxicity prior to induction.
- The infusion can be stopped after a skin incision.
- *Obese patients—use cefazolin:* Consider increasing the dose of cefazolin (3 g) in adult patients weighing
    - >120 kg. *Gentamicin*—For adult patients with a body mass index of 30 kg/m^2 or more, calculate the dose of gentamicin based on adjusted body weight (up to 100 kg). *Vancomycin*—Consider increasing the dose of vancomycin (1.5 g) in adult patients weighing >80 kg.

- High MRSA risk (defined as MRSA colonization or infection or repeated stay or current long-term hospitalization with high MRSA prevalence or living in an area or elderly care facility with high MRSA prevalence or current residence or residence in the last 12 months in detention facility): Add vancomycin.
- Repeat dosing a single preoperative dose is sufficient for most procedures; however, repeat intraoperative doses are advisable: for prolonged surgery (>4 hours from the time of first preoperative dose) when a short acting agent is used (e.g., cefazolin dose should be repeated after 4 hours), or if major blood loss occurs (e.g., >1,500 mL in adults), following fluid resuscitation.
- When measuring the time to the second intraoperative dose, measure the time from the first preoperative dose instead of the surgical incision.
- *Special considerations for colorectal surgery:* There is evidence that oral nonabsorbable antibiotics such as neomycin can improve outcomes in elective colorectal resections. Neomycin 500 mg tablets are available through a special access scheme. The recommended dose is 1 g (2 × 500 mg tablets) on the day before surgery at 13:00, 15:00, and 22:00.

16. Describe the Clavien-Dindo classification of postoperative complications. Write in brief about the prevention and diagnosis of postoperative deep venous thrombosis of lower limbs. ***WBUHS 2025***

The Clavien-Dindo (CD) classification is a standardized system for grading the severity of postoperative surgical complications, first proposed in 1992 and refined in 2004. It focuses on the therapeutic intervention required to treat the complication rather than the specific type or organ involved, making it simple, reproducible, and applicable across surgical fields. The system ranges from Grade I (mild, often requiring no therapy) to Grade V (death), with subgrades for situations involving organ-space infections or long-term disabilities. It has been validated in large cohorts and is widely used in clinical trials and outcome reporting to enable comparisons between procedures, centers, and therapies.

The classification is summarized in the table below:

Grade	*Definition*	*Examples*	*Therapy required*
I	Any deviation from the normal postoperative course without the need for pharmacologic treatment or surgical, endoscopic, or radiological interventions. Acceptable limits include wound infections treated in the outpatient setting, hematomas requiring no intervention, and transient elevations in laboratory values	Superficial wound infection resolved with local care; minor atelectasis managed with physiotherapy	None or symptomatic (e.g., antiemetics, antipyretics, analgesics, diuretics, electrolytes, physiotherapy). Blood transfusions and nutritional support are also allowed
II	Complication requiring pharmacologic treatment with drugs other than those allowed for Grade I (e.g., antibiotics, blood products beyond transfusion, or total parenteral nutrition)	Infectious complications requiring antibiotics; deep vein thrombosis treated with anticoagulants	Drug therapy (e.g., antibiotics for pneumonia or wound infection)
III	Complication requiring surgical, endoscopic, or radiological intervention	Anastomotic leak requiring reoperation; hematoma needing drainage	• *IIIa:* Intervention under local anesthesia (nonoperative, e.g., percutaneous drainage) • *IIIb:* Intervention under general anesthesia (e.g., surgical revision)
IV	Life-threatening complication requiring intermediate care or intensive care unit (ICU) management	Organ failure such as acute respiratory distress syndrome or acute kidney injury	• *IVa:* Single-organ dysfunction (e.g., dialysis for kidney failure) • *IVb:* Multiorgan dysfunction (e.g., sepsis leading to respiratory and cardiac failure)
V	Death of the patient	Any complication resulting in mortality	None (patient dies)

Prevention of Postoperative Deep Vein Thrombosis (DVT) in Lower Limbs

Postoperative DVT risk is elevated due to immobility, surgical trauma, and patient factors like age >60, obesity, cancer, or prior VTE. Guidelines (e.g., ASH 2019) emphasize risk stratification and multimodal prophylaxis for hospitalized surgical patients.

- *Pharmacological:* Low-molecular-weight heparin (LMWH, e.g., enoxaparin) or fondaparinux is recommended for most moderate- to high-risk patients (e.g., orthopedic, abdominal surgery). Start pre- or postoperatively; duration 7–14 days or until mobile. Direct oral anticoagulants (e.g., rivaroxaban) are alternatives in select cases. Avoid in high bleeding risk.
- *Mechanical:* Intermittent pneumatic compression (IPC) devices or graduated compression stockings (GCS) for all patients; preferred when anticoagulation is contraindicated. Combine with pharmacological for high-risk (e.g., hip/knee arthroplasty).
- *Nonpharmacological:* Early mobilization (within 24 hours), hydration, and leg elevation. Aspirin may suffice for low-risk orthopedic procedures.

Prophylaxis reduces VTE incidence by 50–70%; tailor to individual bleeding/thrombosis risk.

Diagnosis of Postoperative Deep Vein Thrombosis (DVT) in Lower Limbs

Postoperative DVT is often asymptomatic (up to 50% of cases), with symptoms like unilateral leg swelling, pain, warmth, or erythema appearing in 50%. Suspect in high-risk patients; fatal PE may be the first sign.

- *Clinical Assessment:* Use Wells score (e.g., +3 for calf swelling >3 cm, +1.5 for tenderness) to stratify probability (low <2, moderate 2–6, high >6).
- *D-dimer:* High-sensitivity test to rule out in low/moderate probability (negative excludes DVT); elevated in 90% of postoperative cases but nonspecific.
- *Imaging:*
  - *Duplex ultrasound:* First-line, noninvasive; sensitivity/specificity >95% for proximal DVT. Perform on postoperative days 3–7 or if symptoms arise.
  - *Venography:* Gold standard for equivocal cases (e.g., pelvic veins) but invasive/rarely used.
  - *MRI:* For iliofemoral or abdominal veins if ultrasound inconclusive.

CHAPTER 3

Nutrition

LEARNING OBJECTIVES

- Assessment of Nutrition, Artificial Nutritional Support
- Nutritional Augmentation in Surgical Patients
- TPN, Enteral Feeding
- Immunonutrition
- PEG

Recommendations

Level 1:
- Patients with chronic malnutrition benefit from nutritional support
- *Enteral nutrition:*
  - It is preferred over parenteral nutrition in patients with a functional GI tract
  - It should be initiated within 18 hours of injury in burn patients
  - It should be initiated within 24 hours of admission in the critically ill
- *Immunonutrition should be utilized in:*
  - Severely injured abdominal/thoracic trauma patients (ISS >18, ATI >20) when given in conjunction with early feeding and adequate protein/calorie support
  - Malnourished elective GI surgical patients (albumin <3.5 g/dL for upper GI tract and <2.8 g/dL for lower GI tract)
  - Immunonutrition should involve an initial 5–7-day course with subsequent reevaluation

Level 2:
- Patients with severe closed head injury who do not tolerate gastric feedings within 48 hours of injury should receive postpyloric feedings
- Nutritional assessments (such as 24-hour UUN and indirect calorimetry studies) should be performed weekly and support titrated to meet the patient's needs
- Of the visceral protein markers, serial determination of serum prealbumin is the most sensitive indicator of appropriate nutritional support

Level 3:
- Incompletely resuscitated patients should not receive direct small bowel feedings due to the risk for GI intolerance and possible intestinal necrosis
- In blunt or penetrating trauma patients undergoing laparotomy, direct small bowel feeding access should be obtained and enteral feeding begun within 12–24 hours of injury
- Intragastric feeding of severe closed head injury patients should be attempted within 12 hours of admission
- Elective surgery patients with an anticipated NPO status of 7 days or greater should receive supplemental nutritional support
- In severely injured patients, parenteral nutrition should be started by day 7 if the patient is not tolerating at least 50% of their estimated caloric requirement enterally

(ATI: Abdominal Trauma Index; GI: gastrointestinal; ISS: Injury Severity Score; NPO: nothing by mouth; UUN: urinary urea nitrogen)

1. How will you assess the nutritional status of a surgical patient? Define and classify artificial nutritional support (ANS). Give an account of enteral nutrition and its advantages and drawbacks.

WBUHS 2015, DNB 2021 June

Introduction

- The first task when considering perioperative nutritional recommendations is to assess whether or not the patient has malnutrition.
- The basic principle of dietary and nutritional assessment in the general population is discussed elsewhere.
- Important aspects of nutritional assessment that pertain to surgical patients are reviewed in the following text.

Based upon expert consensus, a diagnosis of malnutrition requires that the patient exhibits two or more of the following:

- Insufficient energy intake
- Weight loss
- Loss of muscle mass
- Loss of subcutaneous fat
- Localized or generalized fluid accumulation that may sometimes mask weight loss
- Diminished functional status as measured by handgrip strength

History and Physical Examination

- Several aspects of the past medical history are of particular importance, including chronic disease (particularly diabetes), infection, recent hospitalization, and prior surgery (particularly gastrointestinal surgery).
- A history of weight loss or gain is important.
- Any recent losses or gains (and whether they were purposeful or not) prior to the hospital stay should be assessed.
- The details of the current hospitalization also play a central role.
- Newly admitted trauma patients who are otherwise well have drastically different needs from patients who have had surgery several weeks in the past but have remained hospitalized due to complications.
- In addition to collecting information on current medications, nonprescription medicines and other supplements should be noted.
- The use of dietary supplements, such as protein shakes, should also be determined.
- Any allergies or food intolerances should also be noted. A diet history should be collected from the patient, family, or care facility.
- Although there are several methods of dietary assessment, the most useful and straightforward may be to assess the usual intake on an average day before hospitalization or before the onset of the current illness.

In addition to vital signs and a general physical examination, the following should be noted:

- Height and weight [calculate body mass index (BMI) using weight in kg divided by height in meters squared, or using a nomogram]
- *General:* Loss of subcutaneous fat, any generalized fluid accumulation
- *Head and neck exam:* Hair loss, bitemporal wasting, conjunctival pallor, xerosis, glossitis, bleeding or sores on the gums and oral mucosa, angular cheilosis or stomatitis, dentition
- *Cardiovascular:* Evidence of heart failure or high-output state
- *Neck:* Thyromegaly
- *Extremities:* Edema, loss of muscle mass
- *Neurologic:* Evidence of peripheral neuropathy, reflexes, tetany, mental status, handgrip strength

- *Skin:* Ecchymoses, petechiae, pallor, pressure ulcers, assessment of surgical wound healing and signs of surgical site infection (if postoperative).
- Signs of specific nutritional deficiencies should also be sought. Appropriate micronutrient levels should be investigated depending on clinical exam findings.

Several clinical tools are available to quickly assess and score nutrition status:

- The Subjective Global Assessment of Nutritional Status is a brief tool that includes history and physical examination findings, and allows standardized assessment.
- The Nutritional Risk Screening tool (NRS 2002) can be applied rapidly and used to screen for poor baseline nutritional status.
- *Assessing protein status:*
  - Assessing protein status is particularly important in the surgical patient because of the close relationship between protein status and wound healing, and because protein–calorie malnutrition can be treated with supplementation as discussed below.
  - Protein status is affected by previous intake, muscle mass, duration of current illness, blood loss, wound healing, infections, and gastrointestinal absorption.
  - Three serum measures of protein status have differing half-lives.
  - These serum components do not directly indicate nutritional status, but rather reflect the severity of illness and must be used in conjunction with other clinical data such as the duration of the current surgical illness to be useful in determining therapy.
    - *Serum albumin* has the longest half-life at 18–20 days and is the most extensively used parameter. Low serum albumin (<2.2 g/dL) is a marker of a negative catabolic state, and a predictor of poor outcome. Surgical stress, other acute stresses, hepatic disease, and renal disease decrease serum albumin levels.
    - *Serum transferrin* has an intermediate half-life of 8–9 days, reflecting protein status over the past 2–4 weeks. Transferrin also reflects iron status, and low transferrin should be considered an indicator of protein status only in the setting of normal serum iron.
    - *Serum prealbumin (transthyretin)* has the shortest half-life at 2–3 days. Although prealbumin responds quickly to the onset of malnutrition and rises rapidly with adequate protein intake, the level can be altered in the acute phase response due to acute or chronic inflammation. In general, inflammatory cytokines reduce the level of prealbumin synthesis by the liver, and it can also be reduced with renal and hepatic disease. Therefore, serum prealbumin is the least helpful of the three for assessing overall nutritional status.
  - *Other laboratory studies:*
    - In addition to assessing protein status, a few other laboratory studies may be helpful.
    - Electrolytes, glucose, and blood urea nitrogen (BUN)/creatinine help assess overall clinical and fluid volume status and need to be obtained if parenteral (intravenous) nutrition will be instituted.
    - Iron levels should be measured in the setting of unexplained anemia, as should specific vitamin levels if clinically indicated (e.g., B_{12}/folate in macrocytic anemias, others based upon specific physical signs).
    - Serum calcium, magnesium, and phosphorous should also be assessed periodically, particularly in the setting of poor oral intake or diarrhea.

Artificial Nutrition Support

It refers to the administration of nutrient solutions by the enteral or intravenous (parenteral) routes.

- *Enteral feeding includes the use of oral supplements and tube feeding:*
  - The method of tube feeding may be by nasogastric, nasojejunal, percutaneous endoscopic gastrostomy (PEG), percutaneous endoscopic jejunostomy (PEJ), or fine-needle jejunostomy.

Feeding method	Advantages	Disadvantages	Indications
Continuous	• May improve tolerance • May reduce risk of aspiration • Increased time for nutrient absorption	• Feeding pump required • May restrict ambulation • More expensive	• Initiation of feeding in critically ill patients • Promote tolerance • Compromised gastric function • Feeding into small bowel • Intolerance to other feeding methods
Cyclic	• Facilitates transition of support to oral diet • Allows daytime ambulation • Encourages patient to eat normal meals and snacks	• Feeding pump required • May require high infusion rates • May promote intolerance	• Transitioning from enteral nutrition (EN) to oral nutrition (enhance appetite during the day) • Supplement inadequate oral intake • Free patient from enteral feedings during the day
Intermittent	• Feeding pump may not be required • May enhance quality of life • Allows greater mobility between feedings • More physiological • May be better tolerated than bolus feeding	• Increased risk for aspiration • Gastric distention • Delayed gastric emptying	• Intolerance to bolus administration • Initiation of EN without feeding pump
Bolus	• More physiological • Feeding pump not required • Inexpensive and easy administration • Limits feeding time • Patient is free to move about, participate in rehabilitation therapies, and live a relatively normal life • More likely patient will receive all of formula	• Increased risk of aspiration • Hypertonic, high-fat, or high-fiber formulas may delay gastric emptying or result in osmotic diarrhea	• Recommended for gastric feeding • Normal gastric function

- *Parenteral nutrition may be administered by peripheral or central veins.*

2. Write in short on preoperative assessment and optimization of nutrition in surgical patient.

WBUHS 2025 Supplementary

Preoperative Assessment and Optimization of Nutrition in Surgical Patients

Pre-operative nutritional assessment and optimization are critical for improving surgical outcomes, reducing complications, and promoting faster recovery. Proper nutrition helps ensure that the patient's body is in the best possible condition to handle surgery and heal afterward.

Nutritional Assessment

A comprehensive nutritional assessment should be performed prior to surgery, including:

- *Screening for malnutrition:* Tools like the *Malnutrition Universal Screening Tool (MUST)* or *Nutritional Risk Screening (NRS)* help identify patients at risk of malnutrition.
- *Clinical evaluation:* Assessing weight loss, muscle mass, appetite, and any signs of nutritional deficiencies (e.g., anemia, low albumin levels).
- *Dietary history:* Understanding the patient's usual intake, including any specific dietary restrictions, comorbidities (e.g., diabetes, gastrointestinal disorders), or alcohol use.

Optimization of Nutrition

Once malnutrition or nutritional risk is identified, steps should be taken to optimize the patient's nutritional status:

- *Oral nutritional supplements (ONS):* If the patient can tolerate oral intake, high-protein, calorie-dense supplements are often used to improve nutritional intake.
- *Enteral nutrition:* In patients who cannot eat orally but have a functional gastrointestinal tract, enteral feeding (e.g., via a nasogastric or PEG tube) can provide adequate calories and nutrients.
- *Parenteral nutrition (PN):* In patients who cannot tolerate enteral feeding (e.g., severe bowel obstruction), intravenous nutrition is considered, though it carries higher risks and costs.

Specific Nutritional Interventions

- *Protein and calorie intake:* Ensuring adequate protein (to support tissue healing and immune function) and calorie intake is critical, especially in patients with high nutritional needs (e.g., cancer, burns).
- *Micronutrients:* Correcting any deficiencies in vitamins and minerals (e.g., vitamin D, folate, zinc) is essential, as these are key for wound healing and immune function.
- *Managing blood glucose:* For diabetic patients, controlling blood glucose levels through appropriate nutrition and insulin management reduces surgical risks and improves recovery.

Timing of Nutritional Optimization

- *Preoperative period:* Ideally, nutritional optimization should start 7–10 days before surgery. In urgent situations, even a few days of nutritional support can be beneficial.
- *Postoperative nutrition:* Postsurgery, nutrition should be gradually introduced, starting with clear liquids and advancing to solids, while closely monitoring for complications.

Other Considerations

- *Hydration:* Ensuring adequate hydration, especially in patients with dehydration due to illness or surgery-related factors.
- *Managing comorbidities:* Optimizing conditions like anemia or electrolyte imbalances to reduce surgical risks.

3. What are the methods of assessment of nutritional status? What are the modes of artificial nutritional support? Enumerate the advantages and disadvantages of enteral nutrition. ***RGUHS, Karnataka 2025; WBUHS 2023***

Introduction

- The first task when considering perioperative nutritional recommendations is to assess whether or not the patient has malnutrition.
- The basic principle of dietary and nutritional assessment in the general population is discussed elsewhere.
- Important aspects of nutritional assessment that pertain to surgical patients are reviewed below.
  Based upon expert consensus, a diagnosis of malnutrition requires that the patient exhibit two or more of the following:
  - Insufficient energy intake
  - Weight loss
  - Loss of muscle mass
  - Loss of subcutaneous fat
  - Localized or generalized fluid accumulation that may sometimes mask weight loss
  - Diminished functional status as measured by handgrip strength

History and Physical Examination

- Several aspects of the past medical history are of particular importance, including chronic disease (particularly diabetes), infection, recent hospitalization, and prior surgery (particularly gastrointestinal surgery).
- A history of weight loss or gain is important.
- Any recent losses or gains (and whether they were purposeful or not) prior to the hospital stay should be assessed.

- The details of the current hospitalization also play a central role.
- Newly admitted trauma patients who are otherwise well have drastically different needs from patients who have had surgery several weeks in the past but have remained hospitalized due to complications.
- In addition to collecting information on current medications, nonprescription medicines and other supplements should be noted.
- The use of dietary supplements, such as protein shakes, should also be determined.
- Any allergies or food intolerances should also be noted. A diet history should be collected from the patient, family, or care facility.
- Although there are several methods of dietary assessment, the most useful and straightforward may be to assess the usual intake on an average day before hospitalization or before the onset of the current illness.

In addition to vital signs and a general physical examination, the following should be noted:

- Height and weight (calculate body mass index [BMI] using weight in kg divided by height in meters squared, or using a nomogram)
- *General:* Loss of subcutaneous fat, any generalized fluid accumulation
- *Head and neck exam:* Hair loss, bitemporal wasting, conjunctival pallor, xerosis, glossitis, bleeding or sores on the gums and oral mucosa, angular cheilosis or stomatitis, dentition
- *Cardiovascular:* Evidence of heart failure or high-output state
- *Neck:* Thyromegaly
- *Extremities:* Edema, loss of muscle mass
- *Neurologic:* Evidence of peripheral neuropathy, reflexes, tetany, mental status, handgrip strength
- *Skin:* Ecchymoses, petechiae, pallor, pressure ulcers, assessment of surgical wound healing and signs of surgical site infection (if postoperative).
- Signs of specific nutritional deficiencies should also be sought. Appropriate micronutrient levels should be investigated depending on clinical exam findings.

Several clinical tools are available to quickly assess and score nutrition status:

- The Subjective Global Assessment of Nutritional Status is a brief tool that includes history and physical examination findings, and allows standardized assessment.
- The Nutritional Risk Screening tool (NRS 2002) can be applied rapidly and used to screen for poor baseline nutritional status.
- *Assessing protein status:*
  - Assessing protein status is particularly important in the surgical patient because of the close relationship between protein status and wound healing, and because protein-calorie malnutrition can be treated with supplementation as discussed below.
  - Protein status is affected by previous intake, muscle mass, duration of current illness, blood loss, wound healing, infections, and gastrointestinal absorption.
  - Three serum measures of protein status have differing half-lives.
  - These serum components do not directly indicate nutritional status, but rather reflect the severity of illness and must be used in conjunction with other clinical data such as the duration of the current surgical illness to be useful in determining therapy.
- *Serum albumin* has the longest half-life at 18–20 days and is the most extensively used parameter. Low serum albumin (<2.2 g/dL) is a marker of a negative catabolic state, and a predictor of poor outcome. Surgical stress, other acute stresses, hepatic disease, and renal disease decrease serum albumin levels.
- *Serum transferrin* has an intermediate half-life of 8–9 days, reflecting protein status over the past 2–4 weeks. Transferrin also reflects iron status, and low transferrin should be considered an indicator of protein status only in the setting of normal serum iron.
- *Serum prealbumin (transthyretin)* has the shortest half-life at 2–3 days. Although prealbumin responds quickly to the onset of malnutrition and rises rapidly with adequate protein intake, the level can be altered in the acute

phase response due to acute or chronic inflammation. In general, inflammatory cytokines reduce the level of prealbumin synthesis by the liver, and it can also be reduced with renal and hepatic disease. Therefore, serum prealbumin is the least helpful of the three for assessing overall nutritional status.

- *Other laboratory studies:*
  - In addition to assessing protein status, a few other laboratory studies may be helpful.
  - Electrolytes, glucose, and blood urea nitrogen (BUN)/creatinine help assess overall clinical and fluid volume status and need to be obtained if parenteral (intravenous) nutrition will be instituted.
  - Iron levels should be measured in the setting of unexplained anemia, as should specific vitamin levels if clinically indicated (e.g., B_{12}/folate in macrocytic anemias, others based upon specific physical signs).
  - Serum calcium, magnesium, and phosphorous should also be assessed periodically, particularly in the setting of poor oral intake or diarrhea.

Enteral Nutrition

- In general, the enteral route is preferred over the parenteral route. Enteral feeding is simple, physiologic, relatively inexpensive, and well tolerated by most patients.
- Enteral feeding maintains the GI tract cytoarchitecture and mucosal integrity (via trophic effects), absorptive function, and normal microbial flora.
- This results in less bacterial translocation and endotoxin release from the intestinal lumen into the bloodstream.
- Enteral feedings are indicated for patients who have a functional GI tract but are unable to sustain an adequate oral diet.
- Enteral feedings may be contraindicated in patients with an intestinal obstruction, ileus, GI bleeding, severe diarrhea, vomiting, enterocolitis, or a high-output enterocutaneous fistula.
- Choice of appropriate feeding site, administration technique, formula, and equipment may circumvent these problems.

Routes for Administration of Enteral Feeding

- Nasoenteric and postpyloric feeding
- Gastrostomy
- Jejunostomy

Feeding tubes: Nasogastric, nasojejunal, gastrostomy, and jejunal tubes are available for the administration of enteral feeds. Percutaneous gastrostomy tubes can be placed endoscopically or under fluoroscopy.

Enteral feeding products:

- A variety of commercially available enteral formulas are available. Standard solutions provide 1 kcal/mL; calorically concentrated solutions (>1 kcal/mL) are available for patients who require volume restriction. The available dietary formulations for enteral feedings can be divided into polymeric (blenderized and nutritionally complete commercial formulas), chemically defined formulas (elemental diets), and modular formulas.
  - Blenderized tube feedings can contain any food that can be blenderized. Caloric distribution of these formulas should parallel that of a normal diet.
  - Nutritionally complete formulas (standard enteral diets) vary in protein, carbohydrate, and fat composition. Several formulas use sucrose or glucose as carbohydrates and are suitable for lactose-deficient patients. Commercial formulas are convenient, sterile, and inexpensive. They are recommended for patients with minimal metabolic stress and normal gut function.
  - Chemically defined formulas (elemental diets). The nutrients are provided in predigested and readily absorbed form. They contain protein in the form of free amino acids or polypeptides. They are hyperosmolar, which may cause cramping and diarrhea. Elemental diets are efficiently absorbed in the presence of compromised gut function. However, they are costlier.
  - Modular formulations are designed for use in specific clinical situations (e.g., pulmonary, renal, or hepatic failure or immune dysfunction).

- Bolus feedings are reserved for patients with nasogastric or gastrostomy feeding tubes. Feedings are administered by gravity, begin at 50–100 mL every 4 hours, and are increased in 50-mL increments until goal intake is reached (usually 240 to 360 mL every 4 hours). Tracheobronchial aspiration is a potentially serious complication because feedings are prepyloric. To reduce the risk of aspiration, the patient's head and body should be elevated to 30–45 degrees during feeding and for 1–2 hours after each feeding. The gastric residual volume should be measured before administration of the feeding bolus. If this volume is greater than 50% of the previous bolus, the next feeding should be held. The feeding tube should be flushed with approximately 30 mL of water after each use. Free water volume can be adjusted as needed to treat hypo- or hypernatremia.
- Continuous infusion administered by a pump is generally required for nasojejunal, gastrojejunal, or jejunal tubes. Feedings are initiated at 20 mL/hour and increased in 10- to 20-mL/hour increments every 4 to 6 hours until the desired goal is reached. The feeding tube should be flushed with approximately 30 mL of water every 4 hours. Feedings should be held or advancement should be slowed if abdominal distension or pain develops.
- Conversion to oral feeding. When indicated, an oral diet is resumed gradually. In an effort to stimulate appetite, enteral feeding can be modified by the following measures:
  - Providing fewer feedings.
  - Holding daytime feedings.
  - Decreasing the volume of feedings. When oral intake provides approximately 75% of the required calories, tube feedings can be stopped.
- Administration of medications. Many oral medications can be administered through feeding tubes. The elixir form is preferred but is not always available. Medications that are not suitable for administration through a feeding tube include the following:
  - Enteric-coated medications.
  - Drugs in gelatinous capsules.
  - Medications that are designed for sublingual use.
  - Most sustained-release medications.
- For some patients, the entire day's feeding can be infused over 8–12 hours at night to allow the patient mobility free from the infusion pump during the day.

Enteral Feeding

Feeding method	*Advantages*	*Disadvantages*	*Indications*
Continuous	• May improve tolerance • May reduce risk of aspiration • Increased time for nutrient absorption	• Feeding pump required • May restrict ambulation • More expensive	• Initiation of feeding in critically ill patients • Promote tolerance • Compromised gastric function • Feeding into small bowel • Intolerance to other feeding methods
Cyclic	• Facilitates transition of support to oral diet • Allows daytime ambulation • Encourages patient to eat normal meals and snacks	• Feeding pump required • May require high infusion rates • May promote intolerance	• Transitioning from enteral nutrition (EN) to oral nutrition (enhance appetite during the day) • Supplement inadequate oral intake • Free patient from enteral feedings during the day
Intermittent	• Feeding pump may not be required • May enhance quality of life • Allows greater mobility between feedings • More physiological • May be better tolerated than bolus feeding	• Increased risk for aspiration • Gastric distention • Delayed gastric emptying	• Intolerance to bolus administration • Initiation of EN without feeding pump

Contd...

Contd...

Feeding method	*Advantages*	*Disadvantages*	*Indications*
Bolus	• More physiological • Feeding pump not required • Inexpensive and easy administration • Limits feeding time • Patient is free to move about, participate in rehabilitation therapies, and live a relatively normal life • More likely patient will receive all of formula	• Increased risk of aspiration • Hypertonic, high-fat, or high-fiber formulas may delay gastric emptying or result in osmotic diarrhea	• Recommended for gastric feeding • Normal gastric function

4. Calculate the composition of 3:1 total parenteral nutrition (TPN) formula required for a 70-kg man with an enterocutaneous fistula. How do you monitor a patient receiving TPN? ***WBUHS 2023***

- *Determine fluid energy requirements:*
  Fluid = 35 mL/kg/day = 35 × 70 = 2,450 mL/day
  Calories = 30 kcal/kg/day = 2,100 kcal/day
- *Calculate amount of protein and carbohydrate needed (g):*
  Protein = 1.5 g/kg/day = 1.5 × 70 = 105 g/day
  Carbohydrate = 3 mg/kg/min = 3 × 70 × 1,440 min/day = 302,400 mg or 302.4 g/day
  Always keep <5 mg/kg/min to avoid hyperglycemia and liver dysfunction
- *Energy provided by protein and carbohydrate:*
  Protein = 4 kcal/g = 4 × 105 = 420 kcal/day
  Carbohydrate = 3.4 × 302.4 = 1,028.2 kcal/day
- *Calculate amount of fat needed:*
  Total calories = Calories from protein + carbohydrate + fat
  2,100 = 420 + 1,028.2 + calories from fat

  Calories from fat = 2,100 – (420 + 1,028.2)
  = 651.8 kcal

  Fat given as intravenous (IV) fat emulsion:
  Fat = 9 kcal/g
  Thus, total fat = 652/9 = 72.4 g

Protein	Carbohydrate	Fat
420/2,100 × 100 = 20%	1,028.2/2,100 × 100 = 48.95%	651.8/2,100 × 100 = 31.03%
- *Volume of each macronutrient*
  Standard concentrations are 10% amino acids, 70% dextrose, 20% fat emulsion
  Amino acid = 10% → 105 × 100/10 = 1,050 mL

  Dextrose = 70% → 302.4 × 100/70 = 432 mL

  Intravenous fat emulsion = 20% → 72.4 × 100/20 = 362 mL

  Total volume = 1,050 + 432 + 362 = 1,844 mL
  Additives: Electrolytes, vitamins, trace minerals

  Add 606 mL of water to reach total fluid requirement of 2,450 mL/day

Some Ways to Monitor a Patient Receiving TPN

- *Vital signs:* Monitor the patient's vital signs, including temperature, heart rate, blood pressure, respiratory rate, and oxygen saturation, to detect any signs of infection, dehydration, or other complications.

- *Fluid balance:* Monitor the patient's fluid balance, including input and output, to ensure that the patient is receiving the correct amount of fluids and electrolytes.
- *Blood glucose:* Monitor the patient's blood glucose levels regularly to ensure that the TPN is not causing hyperglycemia or hypoglycemia. Adjustments to the TPN may be necessary to maintain blood glucose levels within a normal range.
- *Electrolytes:* Monitor the patient's electrolyte levels, including sodium, potassium, and magnesium, to ensure that they are within normal ranges. Adjustments to the TPN may be necessary to maintain normal electrolyte levels.
- *Liver and kidney function:* Monitor the patient's liver and kidney function regularly to detect any potential damage or dysfunction caused by the TPN.
- *Weight:* Monitor the patient's weight regularly to ensure that the TPN is providing adequate nutrition and that the patient is not experiencing significant weight loss or gain.
- *Infection control:* Follow proper infection control procedures, including hand hygiene and aseptic technique, to prevent infections associated with TPN.
- In addition to these measures, close collaboration between the healthcare team, including pharmacists, dietitians, and nurses, is essential to monitor the patient receiving TPN and ensure their safety and well-being.

5. Discuss nutritional augmentation in surgical patients. ***WBUHS 2020***

The surgical patient with established malnutrition should begin aggressive nutrition at least 7–10 days before surgery. Those patients in whom eating is not anticipated beyond the first 5 days following surgery should receive the benefits of early enteral or parenteral feeding depending on whether the gut can be used.

Nutritional Assessment

- Nutritional Risk Screening 2002

Impaired nutritional status		***Severity of disease***	
Absent 0	Normal nutritional status	Absent 0	Normal nutritional requirements
Mild 1	Weight loss >5% in 3 months 50–75% of usual food intake over last week	Mild 1	Hip fracture cirrhosis, DM, benign Cx hemodialysis, COPD
Moderate 2	Weight loss >5% in 2 months BMI 18.5–20.5 with impaired general condition 25–50% of usual food intake over last week	Moderate 2	Major abdominal surgery stroke, PNA, malignancy
Severe 3	Weight loss of >5% in 1 month weight loss >15% in 3 months BMI <18.5 with impaired general condition 0–25% of usual food intake over last week	Severe 3	Head injury bone marrow transplant ICU admission

(BMI: body mass index; COPD: chronic obstructive pulmonary disease; DM: diabetes mellitus; ICU: intensive care unit; PNA: pneumonia)

- Preoperative serum albumin <3.0 mg/dL
    - *Preoperative fasting:* An 8–12-hours fast depletes almost all glycogen stores.
    - *Carbohydrate loading:*
        - Surgical stress causes postoperative insulin resistance, immunosuppression, and increased patient discomfort.
        - Patient outcomes may be improved by a shorter fasting period preceded by prescribed carbohydrate intake.
        - Studies have reported that postoperative insulin sensitivity is preserved by carbohydrate drinks (100 g the night before surgery and 50 g 2 hours before surgery) or intravenous glucose (5 mg/kg/min), possibly through suppression of fat and glucose oxidation and attenuation of pyruvate dehydrogenase kinase.
    - *Preoperative nutritional support and immunonutrition:*
        - International guidelines recommend nutritional support for severely malnourished patients 7–14 days before elective major surgery.

- Severely malnourished patients have at least one of the following: weight loss >10–15% within 6 months; BMI < 18.5 kg/m^2; or serum albumin below 30 g/L without hepatic or renal dysfunction.

Preoperative	***Intraoperative***	***Postoperative***
Ensure adequate hydration	Maintain fluid balance	Encourage early oral intake
• Avoid excessive tasting • Allow fluid intake up until 2 hours before surgery • Replace further losses in those with enterocutaneous fistulas and high-output stomas	• Avoid excessive fluid therapy during surgery • Use balanced fluid (e.g., Hartmann's) • Use monitoring to guide fluid administration • Blood transfusion as indicated for blood loss	• Early resumption of oral intake • Stop IV fluids once oral intake established • Aim for a state of zero fluid balance • If oral intake inadequate supplement with IV fluid • If oral intake delayed, consider EN/PN

(EN: enteral nutrition; IV: intravenous; PN: parenteral nutrition)

- Identification of malnourished patients and prehabilitation prior to surgery
- If the gut works, use it after 24 hours postoperation
- Enteral > parenteral

6. Discuss the role of nutrition and its methods in surgical patients. ***RIMS, Imphal 2022***

7. Discuss indications and technique of supplementing nutrition in surgical patients. ***WBUHS 2017, 2019***

Nutrition plays a crucial role in the management and recovery of surgical patients. Adequate nutritional support before, during, and after surgery significantly influences patient outcomes, wound healing, immune function, and the risk of complications.

Preoperative Nutrition

Goal: Optimize the patient's nutritional status to improve surgical outcomes and reduce the risk of complications.

- *Malnutrition risk assessment:* Patients undergoing major surgery are screened for malnutrition, which is associated with increased morbidity and mortality.
- *Immunonutrition:* Supplementation with nutrients like arginine, omega-3 fatty acids, and nucleotides before surgery can modulate the immune response and improve recovery.
- *Carbohydrate loading:* Preoperative intake of carbohydrate-rich fluids can reduce insulin resistance and improve postoperative recovery.

Intraoperative Considerations

- *Nutritional status monitoring:* In prolonged or complex surgeries, especially in critically ill patients, maintaining metabolic balance is important.
- *Glucose control:* Maintaining euglycemia helps reduce infection risks and improve healing.

Postoperative Nutrition

Goal: Promote healing, prevent complications, and support recovery.

- *Early enteral nutrition (EEN):* Initiating feeding within 24–48 hours postsurgery improves gut integrity, reduces infections, and shortens hospital stay.
- *Parenteral nutrition (PN):* Used when enteral feeding is not possible, but associated with higher risks of infection and metabolic complications.
- *Protein requirements:* Increased protein intake (1.2–2.0 g/kg/day) is needed to support tissue repair and immune function.
- *Micronutrient support:* Zinc, vitamin C, vitamin A, and other nutrients are essential for collagen formation and wound healing.

Special Considerations

- *Surgical stress response:* Surgery induces a catabolic state, increasing energy and protein needs.
- *Chronic illness and comorbidities:* Diabetic, cancer, or elderly patients may require tailored nutritional interventions.
- *Enhanced recovery after surgery (ERAS) protocols:* Emphasize early nutrition, reduced fasting, and use of nutritional supplements.

Consequences of Poor Nutrition

- Increased risk of:
  - Wound dehiscence and infections
  - Prolonged hospital stay
  - Reoperation or readmission
  - Mortality

Indications

- The patient's premorbid state (healthy or otherwise)
- Poor nutritional status (current oral intake meeting <50% of total energy needs)
- Significant weight loss (initial body weight less than usual body weight by 10% or more or a decrease in inpatient weight by >10% of the admission weight
- The duration of starvation (>7 days' inanition)
- An anticipated duration of artificial nutrition (particularly TPN) of longer than 7 days
- The degree of the anticipated insult, surgical or otherwise
- A serum albumin value <3.0 g/dL measured in the absence of an inflammatory state
- A transferrin level of <200 mg/dL
- Anergy to injected antigens

Clinical Sequelae of Impaired Nutrition

- Numerous studies have clearly shown an increased incidence of nosocomial infection, longer hospital stay, and increased mortality in patients with significant unintentional weight loss (>10%) before their acute illness.
- Even in an individual with initially normal nutritional status, after 7–10 days of inanition, the body's ability to heal wounds and to support normal immune function begins to be impaired.
- Such deficits include diminished complement and immunoglobulin production, poor cellular immunity, and impairment of various aspects of leukocyte action, including chemotaxis, phagocytosis, and oxidative burst.
- Other consequences of inadequate nutrition in the postoperative period include poor tissue repair and wound healing and loss of muscle function and strength as a result of progressive muscle wasting, which may contribute to reduced ventilatory performance and prolonged ventilator dependence.
- Overall, malnutrition will be limiting to all aggressive surgical and medical therapies.

Techniques of Supplementation of Nutrition

- *Enteral nutrition:*
  - In general, the enteral route is preferred over the parenteral route. Enteral feeding is simple, physiologic, relatively inexpensive, and well tolerated by most patients.
  - Enteral feeding maintains the GI tract cytoarchitecture and mucosal integrity (via trophic effects), absorptive function, and normal microbial flora.
  - This results in less bacterial translocation and endotoxin release from the intestinal lumen into the bloodstream.
  - Enteral feedings are indicated for patients who have a functional GI tract but are unable to sustain an adequate oral diet.
  - Enteral feedings may be contraindicated in patients with an intestinal obstruction, ileus, GI bleeding, severe diarrhea, vomiting, enterocolitis, or a high-output enterocutaneous fistula.

- Choice of appropriate feeding site, administration technique, formula, and equipment may circumvent these problems.

- *Routes for administration of enteral feeding:*
    - Nasoenteric and postpyloric feeding
    - Gastrostomy
    - Jejunostomy
- *Feeding tubes:* Nasogastric, nasojejunal, gastrostomy, and jejunal tubes are available for the administration of enteral feeds. Percutaneous gastrostomy tubes can be placed endoscopically or under fluoroscopy.
- *Enteral feeding products:* A variety of commercially available enteral formulas are available. Standard solutions provide 1 kcal/mL; calorically concentrated solutions (>1 kcal/mL) are available for patients who require volume restriction. The available dietary formulations for enteral feedings can be divided into polymeric (blenderized and nutritionally complete commercial formulas), chemically defined formulas (elemental diets), and modular formulas.
    - Blenderized tube feedings can contain any food that can be blenderized. Caloric distribution of these formulas should parallel that of a normal diet.
    - Nutritionally complete formulas (standard enteral diets) vary in protein, carbohydrate, and fat composition. Several formulas use sucrose or glucose as carbohydrates and are suitable for lactose-deficient patients. Commercial formulas are convenient, sterile, and inexpensive. They are recommended for patients with minimal metabolic stress and normal gut function.
    - Chemically defined formulas (elemental diets). The nutrients are provided in predigested and readily absorbed form. They contain protein in the form of free amino acids or polypeptides. They are hyperosmolar, which may cause cramping and diarrhea. Elemental diets are efficiently absorbed in the presence of compromised gut function. However, they are costlier.
    - Modular formulations are designed for use in specific clinical situations (e.g., pulmonary, renal, or hepatic failure or immune dysfunction).
    - Bolus feedings are reserved for patients with nasogastric or gastrostomy feeding tubes. Feedings are administered by gravity, begin at 50–100 mL every 4 hours, and are increased in 50-mL increments until goal intake is reached (usually 240–360 mL every 4 hours). Tracheobronchial aspiration is a potentially serious complication because feedings are prepyloric. To reduce the risk of aspiration, the patient's head and body should be elevated to 30°–45° during feeding and for 1–2 hours after each feeding. The gastric residual volume should be measured before administration of the feeding bolus. If this volume is greater than 50% of the previous bolus, the next feeding should be held. The feeding tube should be flushed with approximately 30 mL of water after each use. Free water volume can be adjusted as needed to treat hypo- or hypernatremia.
    - Continuous infusion administered by a pump is generally required for nasojejunal, gastrojejunal, or jejunal tubes. Feedings are initiated at 20 mL/hour and increased in 10–20 mL/hour increments every 4–6 hours until the desired goal is reached. The feeding tube should be flushed with approximately 30 mL of water every 4 hours. Feedings should be held or advancement should be slowed if abdominal distension or pain develops.
    - *Conversion to oral feeding:* When indicated, an oral diet is resumed gradually. In an effort to stimulate appetite, enteral feeding can be modified by the following measures:
        - Providing fewer feedings
        - Holding daytime feedings
        - *Decreasing the volume of feedings:* When oral intake provides approximately 75% of the required calories, tube feedings can be stopped.
    - *Administration of medications:* Many oral medications can be administered through feeding tubes. The elixir form is preferred but is not always available. Medications that are not suitable for administration through a feeding tube include the following:
        - Enteric-coated medications

- Drugs in gelatinous capsules
- Medications that are designed for sublingual use
- Most sustained-release medications
- For some patients, the entire day's feeding can be infused over 8–12 hours at night to allow the patient mobility free from the infusion pump during the day.

Indications for Parenteral Nutrition

Therapy	*Efficacy shown*	*Efficacy not shown*
Primary therapy	• Gastrointestinal cutaneous fistulas • Renal failure (acute tubular necrosis) • Short bowel syndrome • Acute burns • Hepatic failure (acute decompensation superimposed on cirrhosis)	• Crohn's disease • Anorexia nervosa
Supportive therapy	• Acute radiation enteritis • Acute chemotherapy toxicity • Prolonged ileus • Weight loss preliminary to major surgery	• Before cardiac surgery • Prolonged respiratory support • Large wound losses
Area under intensive study		• Patients with cancer • Patients in sepsis

Parenteral Nutrition

TPN solutions must be administered through a central venous catheter. A dedicated single-lumen catheter or a multilumen catheter can be used. Catheters should be replaced for unexplained fever or bacteremia.

Routes of Administration for TPN

- Peripheral (PPN) given via a medium-caliber cannula in a peripheral vein; maximum calorie input limited by the maximum osmolarity of the solution given into a peripheral vein; avoids the risks of central venous cannulation; usually used for short-term supplementation
- Central (TPN) given into a central vein [superior vena cava (SVC) or brachiocephalic]; may be via a dedicated tunneled line (e.g., Hickman line), a conventional central venous cannula, or a peripherally inserted central venous catheter (PICC line); maximum calorie input only limited by volume of fluid that can be infused; carries risks of central venous catheterization

Administration of TPN

- Introduction of TPN should be gradual. For example, approximately 1,000 kcal is provided the first day. If there is metabolic stability (i.e., normoglycemia), this is increased to the caloric goal over 1–2 days.
- TPN solutions are delivered most commonly as a continuous infusion. A new three-in-one admixture bag of TPN is administered daily at a constant infusion rate over 24 hours. Additional maintenance IV fluids are unnecessary, and total infused volume should be kept constant while nutritional content is increased.

Cyclic administration of TPN solutions may be useful for selected patients, including:

- Those who will be discharged from the hospital and subsequently receive home TPN
- Those with limited IV access who require administration of other medications
- Those who are metabolically stable and desire a period during the day when they can be free of an infusion pump
- Cyclic TPN is administered for 8–16 hours, most commonly at night. This should not be done until metabolic stability has been demonstrated for patients on standard, continuous TPN infusions.

8. What are the indications and contraindications of parenteral nutrition? How will you monitor a patient who is on parenteral nutrition support? ***WBUHS 2025***

Indications for Parenteral Nutrition

Therapy	*Efficacy shown*	*Efficacy not shown*
Primary therapy	• Gastrointestinal cutaneous fistulas • Renal failure (acute tubular necrosis) • Short-bowel syndrome • Acute burns • Hepatic failure (acute decompensation superimposed on cirrhosis)	• Crohn's disease • Anorexia nervosa
Supportive therapy	• Acute radiation enteritis • Acute chemotherapy toxicity • Prolonged ileus • Weight loss preliminary to major surgery	• Before cardiac surgery • Prolonged respiratory support • Large wound losses
Area under intensive study		• Patients with cancer • Patients in sepsis

Contraindications of Parenteral Nutrition

Absolute Contraindications

These are rare but important:

- *Functioning gastrointestinal tract:*
  - If the GI tract can be used (even partially), enteral nutrition (EN) is preferred.
  - Using PN unnecessarily increases risks and costs.
- *Hemodynamic instability:* In critically ill patients with unstable blood pressure (e.g., septic shock), initiating PN can worsen outcomes.
- *Severe fluid overload:* In cases like pulmonary edema or heart failure, the extra fluid from PN may worsen the condition.

Relative Contraindications/Conditions Requiring Caution

These do not absolutely prohibit PN, but require careful assessment:

- *Uncontrolled hyperglycemia:* PN solutions are high in glucose; giving PN without controlling blood sugar can cause complications.
- *Severe electrolyte imbalance:* PN can exacerbate conditions like hypokalemia, hypophosphatemia, or hypomagnesemia unless corrected beforehand.
- *Severe liver disease:* Risk of hepatic complications (fatty liver, cholestasis); need close monitoring.
- *Sepsis or bacteremia:* Risk of catheter-related bloodstream infections; PN may worsen infection if not managed properly.
- *Renal failure (without dialysis):* Accumulation of fluid and nitrogenous waste; need a modified PN formula.
- *Metabolic instability:* Conditions like refeeding syndrome require correction and gradual initiation of PN.

Other Considerations

- *Short-term nutritional needs:* If a patient will resume oral/enteral feeding within 5–7 days, PN may not be necessary.
- *Lack of venous access:* Safe administration of PN requires central venous access in most cases.
- *Patient refusal or end-of-life care:* In palliative settings, PN may be inappropriate or not aligned with care goals.

Monitoring a patient on parenteral nutrition (PN) support involves a systematic approach to ensure nutritional needs are met, prevent complications, and optimize outcomes. Below is a concise guide to monitoring such patients, based on clinical best practices:

Baseline Assessment (Before Starting PN)

- *Nutritional status:* Assess weight, BMI, muscle mass, and nutritional deficiencies (e.g., vitamins, minerals).
- *Laboratory tests:* Obtain baseline blood work, including:
  - Complete blood count (CBC)
  - *Comprehensive metabolic panel (CMP):* electrolytes (sodium, potassium, chloride, magnesium, calcium, phosphate), glucose, liver function tests (LFTs), kidney function (BUN, creatinine).
  - Lipid panel (triglycerides, cholesterol).
  - Micronutrient levels (e.g., vitamin D, B_{12}, iron, zinc, selenium) if deficiency is suspected.
- *Medical history:* Review underlying conditions (e.g., short bowel syndrome, intestinal failure), allergies, and contraindications.
- *Catheter assessment:* Ensure proper placement of the central venous catheter (CVC) via imaging (e.g., chest X-ray) and check for infection risks.

Ongoing Monitoring

- *Clinical monitoring*
  - *Vital signs:* Monitor daily for fever, tachycardia, or signs of infection (e.g., redness, swelling at catheter site).
  - *Fluid balance:* Track intake and output (urine, stool, drains) to assess hydration and prevent fluid overload or dehydration.
  - *Weight:* Measure daily or every 2–3 days to evaluate nutritional adequacy and fluid status.
  - *Catheter care:* Inspect the CVC site for signs of infection, thrombosis, or dislodgement. Ensure sterile dressing changes per protocol.
- *Laboratory monitoring*
  - *Daily (initially, then taper based on stability):*
    - Electrolytes (sodium, potassium, chloride, bicarbonate).
    - Glucose (to detect hyperglycemia or hypoglycemia).
    - BUN and creatinine (kidney function).
  - *Weekly (or as indicated):*
    - LFTs (ALT, AST, alkaline phosphatase, bilirubin) to monitor for PN-associated liver disease (PNALD).
    - Triglycerides (for lipid emulsion tolerance).
    - CBC to assess for anemia or infection.
  - Periodic (every 1–3 months or as needed):
    - Micronutrient levels (e.g., zinc, copper, selenium, vitamins A, D, E, K).
    - Markers of nutritional status (e.g., prealbumin, albumin, though these may be less reliable in inflammation).
- *Nutritional adequacy*
  - Assess if PN meets caloric and protein needs (e.g., 25–35 kcal/kg/day and 1.2–2.0 g/kg/day protein, adjusted for condition).
  - Monitor for signs of overfeeding (e.g., hyperglycemia, hypertriglyceridemia) or underfeeding (e.g., weight loss, muscle wasting).
  - Evaluate tolerance to PN (e.g., gastrointestinal symptoms if partial enteral feeding is used).

Complication Monitoring

- *Infections:* Watch for catheter-related bloodstream infections (CRBSI). Symptoms include fever, chills, or leukocytosis. Culture blood from the catheter and peripheral site if infection is suspected.
- *Metabolic complications:*
  - Electrolyte imbalances (e.g., hypokalemia, hypophosphatemia in refeeding syndrome).
  - Hyperglycemia (adjust dextrose or add insulin if needed).
  - Hypertriglyceridemia (reduce lipid dose if triglycerides >400 mg/dL).

- *Hepatobiliary complications:* Monitor for PNALD (e.g., steatosis, cholestasis) via LFTs and bilirubin. Consider cycling PN or adjusting lipid formulations (e.g., fish oil-based emulsions).
- *Bone health:* Long-term PN patients may need bone density scans due to risk of metabolic bone disease.

Adjusting PN

- Tailor PN formula based on lab results, clinical status, and nutritional goals.
- Transition to enteral/oral feeding when feasible, gradually reducing PN to minimize complications.
- Involve a multidisciplinary team (dietitian, pharmacist, physician) to optimize PN composition and delivery.

Patient Education and Follow-up

- Educate patients/caregivers on catheter care, signs of complications, and adherence to PN schedule (especially for home PN).
- Schedule regular follow-ups with a nutrition support team to reassess PN needs and monitor long-term outcomes.

Frequency of Monitoring

- *Inpatient:* Daily clinical and lab monitoring initially, then adjust based on stability.
- *Outpatient/home PN:* Weekly to biweekly labs initially, then monthly once stable, with regular clinic visits.

9. Complications of parenteral nutrition. ***Tripura University 2024; WBUHS 2011, 2013***

Catheter Issues in Parenteral Nutrition

Many different types of venous catheters are available for central infusion, and which is most appropriate for a given patient depends on many factors.

- *Catheter sepsis:*
  - Catheter sepsis is potentially the most lethal complication in patients receiving TPN.
  - This problem is directly related to catheter care.
  - Organisms causing line infections are generally 80% *Staphylococcus* (50:50 *aureus* versus *epidermidis*), 15% yeast, and 5% gram-negative bacteria.
  - Staphylococcal infections are generally related to catheter care, whereas yeast probably reaches the catheter through the gut.
  - Additional factors influencing the incidence of line sepsis include the presence of a percutaneous stoma (e.g., a colostomy or tracheostomy), preexistent malnutrition with an increased susceptibility to infection, corticosteroid administration, recent broad-spectrum antibiotic therapy, concurrent chemotherapy, or severe neutropenia (e.g., in acute leukemia).
  - Fungemia is the most serious type of line infection, with the entry site of *Candida*, the most common fungal pathogen, most probably being the GI tract. It is important to treat colonization with yeast (defined as two positive site cultures, e.g., urine and skin) in a critically ill patient aggressively with either fluconazole or amphotericin to avoid further complications such as line sepsis.
  - For patients receiving long-term TPN who may have limited access options remaining because of multiple previous lines, line salvage becomes even more attractive.
  - For *Staphylococcus epidermidis* or gram-negatives, antibiotic therapy is effective in 60–70% of patients.
  - At times a fibrin sheath at the catheter tip may be a nidus, and dissolution with tissue plasminogen activator or urokinase may be useful.
  - Line tract infections can be more difficult to eradicate. In general, if *Staphylococcus aureus* or yeast is documented on blood culture, the line should simply be removed and IV antimicrobial therapy subsequently administered because these organisms are too virulent and dangerous to treat in lesser fashion.
- *Catheter thrombosis and other complications:*
  - *Catheter failure* as a result of clogging and lack of function because of an intraluminal thrombus or a fibrin tip sheath is quite common. This problem can often be corrected by instillation of tissue plasminogen activator

or urokinase and can be avoided by administering long-term prophylactic low-dose heparin (usually 6,000 U/bag) or by the use of low-dose warfarin (1–2 mg/day).

- Thrombosis of the great veins (subclavian, SVC) occurs much less frequently, although some series report an incidence as high as 5–10%.
- Other catheter complications include pneumothorax, vascular injuries (arterial or venous lacerations, delayed arteriovenous fistulas), brachial plexus injury, chronic pain, thoracic duct injury after left-sided cannulation, air embolism, and catheter embolism. Erosion of the catheter into the bronchus, right atrium, or other structures may occur.
- Septic venous thrombosis is a life-threatening complication, and if antibiotics and anticoagulation are not successful, excision of the involved vein or Fogarty catheter embolectomy may occasionally be successful.
- Hydrothorax results from catheter malposition and administration of fluid into the thoracic cavity.

Home Parenteral Nutrition

A major contribution of parenteral nutrition has been the ability to maintain patients in a functional state for decades with minimal oral intake. Unlike the continuous-infusion approach appropriate for a hospitalized patient, home parenteral alimentation is generally cycled and performed overnight over an 8–14-hour period.

- *Metabolic complications of long-term administration of TPN:*
  - *Liver disease:*
    - Hepatic dysfunction is commonly observed in patients receiving TPN, and these disorders occupy a spectrum ranging from simple elevations in liver function test results to cirrhosis.
    - Most often, if hyperbilirubinemia occurs acutely in a patient receiving TPN, the cause is generally sepsis.
    - Factors responsible for liver disease attributable primarily to TPN administration, as opposed to other causes, remain unclear and are a source of controversy.
    - Hepatic steatosis, cholestasis (presumably from lack of enteral stimulation and reduced release of cholecystokinin), and the presence of chronic inflammation have all been implicated as relevant mechanisms.
    - Predisposing factors include short gut syndrome (ileal disease or resection), a history of bacterial overgrowth, and recurrent sepsis or a chronic inflammatory state.
    - Short-bowel syndrome alone seemed an insufficient risk factor unless combined with a chronic inflammatory state such as Crohn's disease.
    - TPN-specific factors include excessive glucose or insulin administration (with increased hepatic lipogenesis), excessive lipid administration (sequestration in hepatocytes), and alterations in fatty acid metabolism leading to the release of arachidonate-derived inflammatory leukotrienes.
    - Deficiencies in particular nutrients, such as carnitine, choline, taurine, cysteine, and S-adenosyl methionine, have also been implicated in TPN-related liver disease.
    - In infants dependent on TPN, hepatic dysfunction is a more serious and potentially lethal disease, and it may have a pathophysiology different from that seen in adults. It is frequently associated with cholestasis. Even when enteral feeding is begun and TPN is discontinued, hepatic dysfunction may persist and progress to cirrhosis and death.
  - *Metabolic bone disease:*
    - In various studies, 40% to nearly 100% of patients administered TPN over prolonged periods have decreased bone mineral density (BMD) or histologic evidence of bone disease.
    - Some individuals can be shown to have increased urinary calcium or phosphate excretion, decreased parathyroid hormone (PTH) levels, or vitamin D deficiency as possible mechanisms, but even in these patients there is poor correlation with BMD.
    - Patients at greatest risk are postmenopausal women, patients with longstanding malnutrition or malabsorption (e.g., Crohn's disease), those with preexisting liver disease, or patients receiving steroids.
    - Some TPN-specific mechanisms postulated to contribute to bone loss are TPN-induced hypercalciuria, in which fixed acids generated by metabolism are buffered by bone calcium carbonate, and calcium

diuresis induced by hyperglycemia or excessive sodium. TPN-associated deficiency states, such as calcium or magnesium (magnesium deficiency may decrease PTH release and vitamin D formation), copper (a cofactor for lysyl oxidase and collagen synthesis), boron, or silicon, have also been suggested to play a role.

- Pamidronate, a second-generation agent shown to be effective in randomized trials in inhibiting postmenopausal osteoporosis, can be administered IV to TPN patients in the outpatient setting (30 mg/200 mL 5% dextrose in water over a 2-hour period) every 3 months, with minimal toxicity.

10. Immunonutrition in surgical patients. *WBUHS 2014*

Introduction

Oral or enteral dietary supplementation with arginine, omega3 fatty acids, and nucleotides (known as immunonutrition) significantly improve outcomes in patients undergoing elective surgery. The objective of the study was to determine the impact on hospital costs of immunonutrition formulas used in patients undergoing elective surgery for gastrointestinal cancer.

Carbohydrate overfeeding	
• Hyperglycemia • Hypercarbia • Hypertriglyceridemia • Hyper- or hypokalemia • Hypomagnesemia	• Respiratory in sufficiency • Immunosuppression • Hepatic steatosis or "fatty liver" • Failure to wean from mechanical ventilation • Increased susceptibility to infection
Lipid overfeeding	
• Hyperlipemia • Hypoxia	• Increased susceptibility to infection • Increased postoperative mortality
Protein overfeeding	
• Azotemia • Elevated creatinine	Acute renal failure

Type	*Modification*	*Rationale*
Diabetic	• High fiber • Low simple sugar • High fat	Decreased risk of hyperglycemia
Hepatic	• Low protein • High branch-chain amino acid	Decreased encephalopathy
Pulmonary	• High fat • High calorie	Decreased CO_2 production
Renal	• High calorie • Low electrolyte	Decreased fluid and electrolyte overload
Immune-enhancing	• L-arginine • Glutamine • Omega-3 fatty acids • Ribonucleic acid	• Improved wound healing • Decreased infectious complications • Decreased hospital length of stay • Decreased mortality

Major Ingredients

These are glutamine, L-arginine, nucleotides, and omega-3 fatty acids. Few human studies have investigated individual enteral components and outcome.

Glutamine

- Glutamine is a conditionally essential amino acid and the preferred fuel for rapidly replicating cells such as gastrointestinal mucosal cells (enterocytes and colonocytes) and immune cells (lymphocytes and macrophages).
- It is a precursor for nucleotide synthesis, a substrate for hepatic gluconeogenesis, a precursor of the antioxidant glutathione, and essential to the renal handling of ammonia.
- Patients under catabolic stress are at risk for glutamine deficiency as a result of their increased metabolic demand for this amino acid, inadequate nutritional intake, and the relative instability of this amino acid in standard protein solutions.
- An association between high-dose glutamine and decreased mortality has been identified. Further prospective, randomized trials are necessary to recommend widespread utilization of glutamine in nutritional support.

Arginine

- L-arginine, a dibasic amino acid, has numerous important roles in the transport, storage, and excretion of nitrogen, formation of nitric oxide; mediation of macrophage function after injury; and regulation of wound healing.
- Meta-analyses of arginine-containing enteral nutrition formulas have demonstrated a decreased incidence of infectious complications, a shorter hospital length of stay, and fewer ventilator days.
- Such differences were most marked in the surgical patient subpopulation and less so in the critically ill. Further prospective, randomized trials are necessary to recommend widespread utilization of arginine in nutritional support.

Nucleotides

- Nucleotides serve as the building blocks of deoxyribonucleic acid (DNA) and ribonucleic acid (RNA). Nucleotides are required for catalysis, energy transfer, and coordination of hormonal signals.
- In the absence of an adequate nucleotide supply, replication of rapidly growing cells (such as gastrointestinal mucosa and lymphocytes or macrophages) is downregulated.

Omega-3 Fatty Acids

- Of the long-chain fatty acids, the omega-3 polyunsaturated fatty acids appear to have the greatest potential for clinical benefit in modulating immune response and improving patient outcome.
- These fatty acids are precursors of the prostacyclins, thromboxanes, prostaglandins, lipoxins, and leukotrienes.
- Unlike glutamine, L-arginine, and nucleotides, the omega-3 fatty acids do not directly stimulate the immune system, but compete with arachidonic acid (an omega-6 fatty acid) for cyclooxygenase metabolism. The ratio of omega-3 to omega-6 fatty acids appears to be important to optimizing immune function.
- The omega-3 family of fatty acids has been shown to reduce the development of atherosclerosis and incidence of myocardial infarction, reduce hypertension, and improve outcome from various proinflammatory states.

11. Enteral nutrition. ***WBUHS 2010***

The need for nutritional support should be assessed continually in patients preoperatively and postoperatively:

- In general, the enteral route is preferred over the parenteral route. Enteral feeding is simple, physiologic, relatively inexpensive, and well tolerated by most patients. Enteral feeding maintains the GI tract cytoarchitecture and mucosal integrity (via trophic effects), absorptive function, and normal microbial flora. This results in less bacterial translocation and endotoxin release from the intestinal lumen into the bloodstream.
- Enteral feedings are indicated for patients who have a functional GI tract but are unable to sustain an adequate oral diet.
- Enteral feedings may be contraindicated in patients with an intestinal obstruction, ileus, GI bleeding, severe diarrhea, vomiting, enterocolitis, or a high-output enterocutaneous fistula.
- Choice of appropriate feeding site, administration technique, formula, and equipment may circumvent these problems.

Feeding tubes: Nasogastric, nasojejunal (e.g., Dobhoff), gastrostomy, and jejunal tubes are available for the administration of enteral feeds. Percutaneous gastrostomy tubes can be placed endoscopically or under fluoroscopy.

Enteral feeding products:

- A variety of commercially available enteral formulas are available. Standard solutions provide 1 kcal/mL; calorically concentrated solutions (>1 kcal/mL) are available for patients who require volume restriction. The available dietary formulations for enteral feedings can be divided into polymeric (blenderized and nutritionally complete commercial formulas), chemically defined formulas (elemental diets), and modular formulas.
- Blenderized tube feedings can contain any food that can be blenderized. Caloric distribution of these formulas should parallel that of a normal diet.
- Nutritionally complete formulas (standard enteral diets) vary in protein, carbohydrate, and fat composition. Several formulas use sucrose or glucose as carbohydrates and are suitable for lactose-deficient patients. Commercial formulas are convenient, sterile, and inexpensive. They are recommended for patients with minimal metabolic stress and normal gut function.
- Chemically defined formulas (elemental diets). The nutrients are provided in predigested and readily absorbed form. They contain protein in the form of free amino acids or polypeptides. They are hyperosmolar, which may cause cramping and diarrhea. Elemental diets are efficiently absorbed in the presence of compromised gut function. However, they are costlier.
- Modular formulations are designed for use in specific clinical situations (e.g., pulmonary, renal, or hepatic failure, or immune dysfunction).

Enteral Feeding Protocols

- Bolus feedings are reserved for patients with nasogastric or gastrostomy feeding tubes. Feedings are administered by gravity, begin at 50–100 mL every 4 hours, and are increased in 50-mL increments until goal intake is reached (usually 240–360 mL every 4 hours). Tracheobronchial aspiration is a potentially serious complication because feedings are prepyloric. To reduce the risk of aspiration, the patient's head and body should be elevated to 30°–45° during feeding and for 1–2 hours after each feeding. The gastric residual volume should be measured before administration of the feeding bolus. If this volume is greater than 50% of the previous bolus, the next feeding should be held. The feeding tube should be flushed with approximately 30 mL of water after each use. Free water volume can be adjusted as needed to treat hypo- or hypernatremia.
- Continuous infusion administered by a pump is generally required for nasojejunal, gastrojejunal, or jejunal tubes. Feedings are initiated at 20 mL/hour and increased in 10–20 mL/hour increments every 4–6 hours until the desired goal is reached. The feeding tube should be flushed with approximately 30 mL of water every 4 hours. Feedings should be held or advancement should be slowed if abdominal distension or pain develops. For some patients, the entire day's feeding can be infused over 8–12 hours at night to allow the patient mobility free from the infusion pump during the day.
- *Conversion to oral feeding:* When indicated, an oral diet is resumed gradually. In an effort to stimulate appetite, enteral feeding can be modified by the following measures:
  - Providing fewer feedings
  - Holding daytime feedings
  - *Decreasing the volume of feedings:* When oral intake provides approximately 75% of the required calories, tube feedings can be stopped.
- *Administration of medications:* Many oral medications can be administered through feeding tubes. The elixir form is preferred but is not always available. Medications that are not suitable for administration through a feeding tube include the following:
  - Enteric-coated medications
  - Drugs in gelatinous capsules

- Medications that are designed for sublingual use
- Most sustained-release medications

Complications

- *Metabolic complications:* Abnormalities in serum electrolytes, calcium, magnesium, and phosphorus can be minimized through vigilant monitoring.
  Hyperosmolarity (hypernatremia) may lead to the development of mental lethargy or obtundation. Hyperglycemia may occur in any patient but is particularly common in individuals with preexisting diabetes or sepsis. Insulin should be used to control serum glucose level.
- Clogging can usually be prevented by careful routine flushing of the feeding tube. Wire stylets should not be used to unclog a feeding tube because of the risk of tube perforation and injury to the GI tract.
- Tracheobronchial aspiration of tube feeds may occur with patients who are fed into the stomach or proximal small intestine and may lead to the development of pneumonia. Patients at particular risk are those with central nervous system abnormalities and those who are sedated.
  Testing tracheal aspirates with glucose strips or adding methylene blue (1 mL/L) to the tube feeds aids in assessing for aspiration. Historically, jejunal feeding has been the preferred route for patients who are at risk for aspiration. High gastric residuals as a result of outlet obstruction, dysmotility, intestinal ileus, or bowel obstruction may limit the usefulness of nasogastric or gastrostomy feeding tubes.
- Diarrhea occurs in 10–20% of patients; however, other causes of diarrhea (e.g., *Clostridium difficile* colitis) should be considered. Diarrhea may result from an overly rapid increase in the volume of hyperosmolar tube feedings, medications (e.g., metoclopramide), a high-fat diet, or the presence of components not tolerated by the patient (e.g., lactose).
  If other causes of diarrhea can be excluded, the volume or concentration of tube feedings should be decreased. In surgical patients, *C. difficile* is a frequent cause of diarrhea due to the common use of perioperative antibiotics. Diagnosis can be confirmed with a *C. difficile* toxin assay or colonoscopy.
  Treatment includes stopping unnecessary antibiotics, followed by either oral or IV metronidazole or vancomycin orally or as a retention enema.

12. Percutaneous endoscopic gastrostomy. *WBUHS 2010*

Introduction

- Percutaneous endoscopic gastrostomy (PEG) is now the preferred method for long-term feeding in patients who are unable to swallow or who require supplemental nutrition or chronic gastric decompression.
- PEG may be preferable to surgical gastrostomy since it is safe, less expensive, and less invasive.
- PEG and PEJ are contraindicated only in patients with total esophageal obstruction, massive ascites, or intra-abdominal sepsis.

Steps

- Prior to the procedure, a single dose of prophylactic cephalosporin (or equivalent) should be given intravenously.
- The patient is placed in the supine or semi-Fowler position, after which the abdomen is prepared and draped using sterile technique. The endoscope is then passed into the stomach, which is distended with air insufflation.
- The assistant then presses on the abdomen with a finger and the impact against the anterior gastric wall should be noted. Ideally, this point should be 2–3 cm below the left costal margin.
- It is critical that the assistant's finger be clearly observed to indent the stomach.
- In patients with thin abdominal walls, light transillumination from within the stomach to the skin surface may aid in identifying a safe landmark.
- A polypectomy snare is passed through the endoscope channel.
- The selected site on the abdominal wall is then infiltrated with local anesthesia.
- If desired, the fine needle used to anesthetize the skin can be inserted into the abdomen at the intended gastrostomy site; observation of the needle's clean entry into the stomach suggests the position is adequate.

- After making a small incision (approximately 5 mm) in the skin, the assistant then inserts a 14 gauge IV cannula through the incision; the IV cannula must be seen to enter the stomach.
- The snare is then tightened around the cannula and the inner stylet is removed. In the "pull technique", a long looped suture is placed through the cannula, after which the snare is released.
- The suture is then firmly grasped with the polypectomy snare.
- The endoscope and the tightened snare are removed together, bringing the suture out of the patient's mouth.
- The suture is secured to a well-lubricated 20F or 24F gastrostomy tube at its tapered external end.
- The assistant then pulls on the suture until the attached tube exits the abdominal wall.
- The endoscope is then reinserted and used to view the tube's inner bolster as the stomach is loosely seated against the abdominal wall and the tube is properly positioned.
- The endoscope is then removed and the tube is secured in place on the abdominal wall, usually with an external Silastic crossbar or disc.

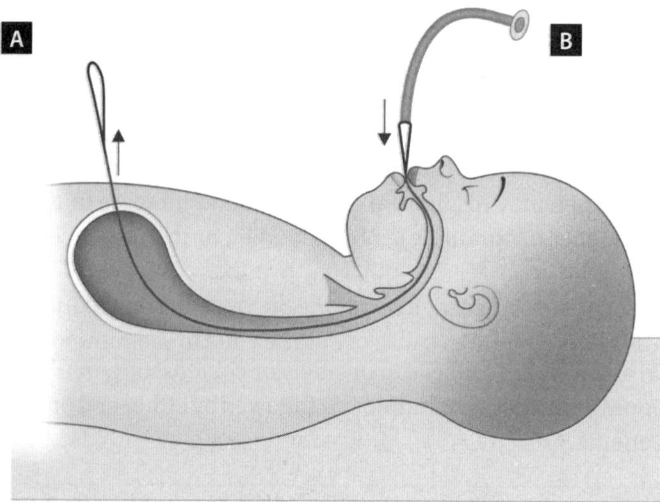

(A) After the looped wire is retrieved out of the esophagus and mouth, it is secured to the Silastic (Ponsky) gastrostomy down the esophagus and out of the abdominal wall by the loop wire; (B) The tube's bumper is pulled flush against avoid a buttonhole necrosis.

Two Other Techniques can be used for PEG Placement

- In the "push technique", in lieu of a suture a guidewire is inserted through the cannula and pulled out of the patient's mouth.
- The gastrostomy tube is then pushed over the wire until it exits the abdominal wall.
- Finally, in the "introducer technique", the stomach is inflated, the site of insertion selected, and the IV cannula introduced into the stomach as described above.
- A J-tipped guidewire is then passed through the cannula into the stomach after which the cannula is removed.
- An introducer with a peel-away sheath is then passed over this wire, allowing removal of the wire and introducer.
- A Foley catheter or other similar gastrostomy tube is then placed through the sheath, its balloon is inflated, and the sheath is removed.
- The catheter is then secured to the abdominal wall.
- The PEG procedure can be extended to include jejunostomy (PEG-J) in patients who fail to tolerate gastric feedings due to severe gastroesophageal reflux or gastroparesis.
- While enteral feeding by PEG-J is intuitively believed to decrease the incidence of aspiration when compared with PEG feedings, most series report aspiration pneumonia to occur in only 0–5% of patients with PEG feedings—even for the neurologically impaired patient.

CHAPTER 4

Fluid, Electrolyte, and Acid–Base Balance

LEARNING OBJECTIVES

- Metabolic Alkalosis
- Blood Gas Components
- Metabolic Acidosis
- Hypokalemia and Hyponatremia
- Flow Directed Fluid Therapy
- Perioperative Fluid Management
- Postoperative Fluid Management in GI Surgery

1. A previously healthy 55-year-old man undergoes laparoscopic cholecystectomy for cholelithiasis and has prolonged paralytic ileus with frequent vomiting (skin turgor was diminished) with dry mucus membrane and orthostatic hypotension, laboratory values were: arterial blood gas (ABG): pH—7.56, partial pressure of oxygen (pO_2) 85, partial pressure of carbon dioxide (pCO_2) 50, Na 132, K 3.1, Cl 80, HCO_3 42, urine: Na 2, K 5, Cl 16. Give the diagnosis and therapy. Discuss the best regimen for routine maintenance of fluid for surgical patients. ***WBUHS 2017***

Arterial Blood Gas

pH—7.56, pO_2 85, pCO_2 50, Na 132, K 3.1, Cl 80, HCO_3 42

- *Urine:* Na 2, K 5, Cl 16.
- ABG shows uncompensated metabolic alkalosis.
- Urine shows dehydration
- Diagnosis is contraction alkalosis

Treatment

Treatment consists of NaCl infusion to correct extracellular fluid (ECF) volume contraction and administration of K^+ to replace urinary losses.

Metabolic alkalosis can be corrected partially with the following:

- Potassium supplementation
- Potassium-sparing diuretics
- Nonsteroidal anti-inflammatory drugs
- *Angiotensin-converting enzyme (ACE) inhibitors:*
    - Intravenous (IV) fluid therapy for routine maintenance refers to the provision of IV fluids and electrolytes for patients who cannot meet their needs by oral or enteral routes, yet are otherwise well in terms of fluid and electrolyte balance and handling (i.e., they are essentially euvolemic with no significant electrolyte deficits, ongoing abnormal losses, or complex internal redistribution issues).
    - However, even when prescribing IV fluids for more complex cases, there is still a need to account for patients' routine maintenance requirements, providing IV fluid maintenance prescriptions that are then adjusted to account for their more complex fluid or electrolyte problems.

- Estimates of routine maintenance requirements are therefore essential for any patient on continuing IV fluid therapy.
- The goal of fluid therapy is to preserve the normal body water volume and its electrolyte composition:
  - Maintenance therapy replaces the ongoing daily losses of water and electrolytes occurring via physiologic processes (urine, sweat, respiration, and stool), which normally preserve homeostasis.
  - For calculating the minimum amount of fluid per day, a formula based on body weight is recommended: 1,500 mL is the minimum water intake with 15 mL fluid per kg to be added for the actual weight minus 20 kg. This formula can be used for older adults who are normal weight, underweight, or overweight.

Routine Maintenance Fluids for Surgical Patients

- One group that frequently receives IV fluids which are essentially for "routine maintenance" is postoperative patients, although early after surgery many such patients have fluid redistribution issues and either deficits or more frequently excesses consequent to imbalances in fluid and electrolyte loss versus provision during the operation itself.
- Advances in surgery, anesthesia and perioperative care, however, have reduced the length of time that patients need to be nil by mouth (NBM) both prior to and following surgery and so even after major abdominal operations, gastrointestinal function returns rapidly.
- Early postoperative oral intake is often therefore possible and the absence of bowel sounds per se does not mean that food and drink will not be tolerated. Generally, nasogastric (NG) tubes are only indicated for drainage in the presence of true ileus or gastric dysfunction (e.g., delayed gastric emptying after pancreatic surgery) and indeed, in many cases, morbidity from NG tubes may exceed benefit.
- The aim when giving routine maintenance fluids is to provide enough fluid and electrolytes to meet insensible losses (500–1,000 mL), maintain normal status of body fluid compartments and enable renal excretion of waste products (500–1,500 mL).
- Routine maintenance provision should nearly always be a short-term measure since inappropriate therapy risks volume overload and electrolyte and acid–base disturbance particularly hyponatremia.

Choice of IV Fluids for Maintenance

A variety of fluids can be used to meet routine maintenance needs although there is considerable debate about the optimal ones to use.

Isotonic Saline

- *Sodium chloride 0.9%,* with or without additional potassium, is one of the most commonly used IV fluids in UK practice. It is distributed throughout the ECF compartment with perhaps only 25% of the infused volume remaining in the intravascular compartment. In recent years, questions have been raised as to whether it is suitable for routine maintenance purposes since the high sodium content could promote a degree of unnecessary sodium and water retention and the high chloride content will promote some degree of hyperchloremia. This may then lead to hyperchloremic acidosis and/or significant reductions in renal blood flow and glomerular filtration rate as well as gastrointestinal mucosal acidosis and ileus.
- *Glucose 5% solution:* Glucose 5% solution provides a useful means of giving free water for, once the glucose is metabolized, the fluid is distributed throughout total body water. It is therefore a potentially useful means of correcting or preventing simple dehydration and the glucose content will also help to prevent starvation ketosis, although it is important to recognize that it will not make much of a contribution to covering a patient's overall nutritional needs. The use of 5% glucose will increase risks of significant hyponatremia, particularly in children, the elderly, patients on diuretics, and those with excess antidiuretic hormone (ADH) due to osmotic and nonosmotic stimuli (a problem seen quite frequently in hospitalized patients).
- *Glucose salines:* There are many different IV fluids containing glucose and saline in different concentrations but the two most commonly used in general areas of UK hospital practice are glucose 4% with sodium chloride (either 0.18% or 0.45%). Both are available with or without potassium at various concentrations). The use of glucose 4%

with sodium chloride 0.18% or even glucose 4% with sodium chloride 0.45% will promote hyponatremia if given rapidly or in excess, although both are less likely to cause this than glucose 5% alone.

- *Balanced crystalloid solutions:* Balanced crystalloids are distributed throughout the ECF and therefore have similar properties to sodium chloride 0.9% in terms of plasma volume expansion and overall fluid distribution. However, they have theoretical advantages over sodium chloride 0.9% in that they contain somewhat less sodium and significantly less chloride.

A number of newer balanced crystalloid solutions are likely to appear on the market, better tailored to meet the theoretical requirements for maintenance. When prescribing these fluids it is essential to specify the "maintenance" version where appropriate since there may be other versions of the fluids designed for resuscitation of replacement. The fact that some balanced solutions contain lactate or other buffers is not likely to alter their usefulness for routine maintenance.

Recommendations

If patients need IV fluids for routine maintenance alone, restrict the initial prescription to:

- 25–30 mL/kg/day of water
- Approximately 1 mmol/kg/day of potassium, sodium, and chloride
- Approximately 50–100 g/day of glucose to limit starvation ketosis (this quantity will not address patient's nutritional status)

For patients who are obese, adjust the IV fluid prescription to their ideal body weight. Use lower range volumes per kg (patients rarely need more than a total of 3 L of fluid per day) and seek expert help if their body mass index (BMI) >40 kg/m^2

- Consider prescribing less fluid (for example, 20–25 mL/kg/day fluid) for patients who:
  - Are older or frail
  - Have renal impairment or cardiac failure
  - Are malnourished and at risk of refeeding syndrome

Assessment and Monitoring of Fluid Balance

Parameter	*Significance*
History	Alerts to likelihood of fluid deficit (e.g., vomiting/diarrhea/hemorrhage) or excess (e.g., from intraoperative fluids)
Weighing	24-hour change in weight (performed under similar conditions)—best measure of change in water balance; simple to carry out by bedside
Fluid balance charts	Inherent inaccuracies in measurement and recording; does not measure insensible loss; large cumulative error over several days; good measure of changes in urine output, fistula loss, gastric aspirate, etc.
Urine output	<30 mUh is commonly used as indication for fluid infusion, but in the absence of other features of intravascular hypovolemia, it is usually due to the normal oliguric response to surgery. Urine quality (e.g., urine: plasma urea or osmolality ratio) is just as important, particularly in the complicated patient
Blood pressure	Cuff measurements may not always correlate with intra-arterial monitoring; does not necessarily correlate with flow; affected by drugs, etc.; nonetheless, a fall is compatible with intravascular hypovolemia, particularly when it correlates with other parameters such as pulse rate, urine output, etc.
Capillary refill	Slow refill compatible with, but not diagnostic of volume deficit; can be influenced by temperature and peripheral vascular disease
Autonomic responses	Pallor and sweating, particularly when combined with tachycardia, hypotension and oliguria are suggestive of intravascular volume deficit, but can also be caused by other complications, e.g., pulmonary embolus or myocardial infarction
Skin turgor	Diminished in salt and water depletion, but also caused by aging, cold, and wasting
Dry mouth	Usually due to mouth breathing, but compatible with salt and water depletion
Sunken facies	May be due to starvation or wasting from disease, but compatible with salt and water depletion

Contd...

Contd...

Parameter	***Significance***
Serum biochemistry	Indicates ratio of electrolytes to water in the extracellular fluid and is a poor indicator of whole body sodium status; hyponatremia most commonly caused by water excess; if change in water balance over 24 hours is known, then change in serum sodium concentration can guide sodium balance. Hypokalemia nearly always indicates the need for potassium supplementation, and blood bicarbonate and chloride concentrations measured on point-of-care blood gas machines are useful in patients with acid-base problems including iatrogenic hyperchloremia
Urine biochemistry	Urine sodium concentration reflects renal perfusion and a low value (<20 mmol/L) indicates renal hypoperfusion. Measurement of urine sodium allows assessment of postoperative sodium mobilization (see text). Urine potassium measurement is helpful in assessing the cause of refractory hypokalemia. Urine urea excretion increases several fold in catabolic states (e.g., sepsis) and is an indication for provision of additional free water to avoid hypernatremia and uremia.

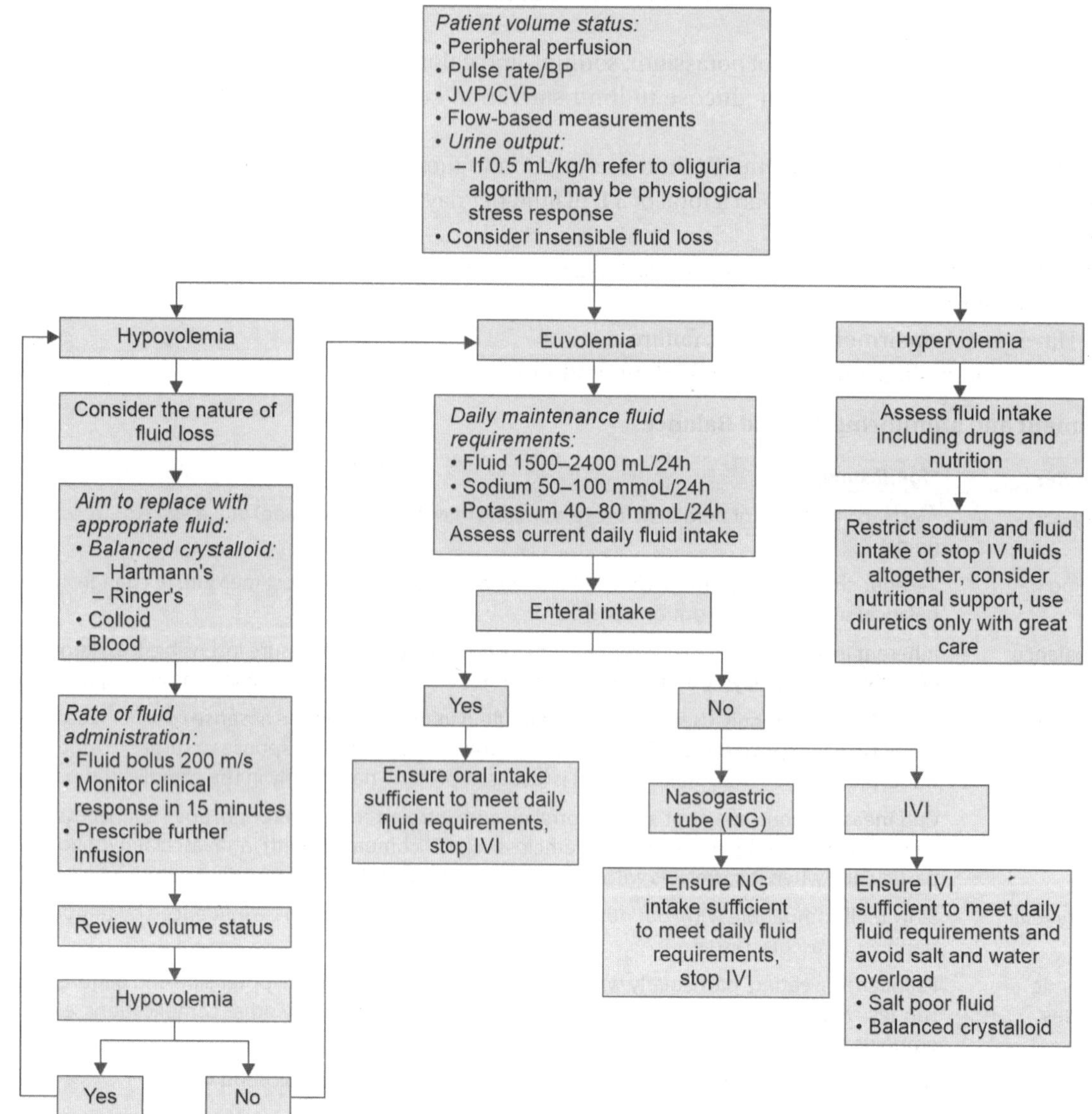

(BP: blood pressure; CVP: central venous pressure; IVI: intravenous infusion; JVP: jugular venous pressure)

BLOOD GAS ANALYSIS AND GUIDELINE FOR FLUID THERAPY

2. Enumerate components of blood gas analysis and their significance in patients' management. ***WBUHS 2020***

3. Treatment of metabolic acidosis. ***SAIMS, Indore 2025; WBUHS 2020***

4. Clinical features and management of hypokalemia. ***AIIMS, Patna 2025; WBUHS 2020***

The components of an ABG analysis are partial pressure of arterial oxygen (PaO_2), arterial oxygen saturation (SaO_2), hydrogen ion concentration (pH), partial pressure of arterial carbon dioxide ($PaCO_2$), HCO_3^-, base excess, and serum levels of hemoglobin (Hb), lactate, glucose, and electrolytes (sodium, potassium, calcium, and chloride).

The following are normal ranges for results of a blood gas test: pH: 7.35–7.45, PaO_2: 80–100 mL of mercury (mm Hg), $PaCO_2$: 35–45 mm Hg

The utilization of an ABG analysis becomes necessary in view of the following advantages:

- Aids in establishing diagnosis
- Guides treatment plan
- Aids in ventilator management
- Improvement in acid/base management; allows for optimal function of medications
- Acid/base status may alter electrolyte levels critical to a patient's status

Rules for rapid clinical interpretation of ABG:

- *Look at pH:* <7.40—acidosis; >7.40—alkalosis
- If pH indicates acidosis, then look at $PaCO_2$ and HCO_3^-
- If $PaCO_2$ is ↑, then it is primary respiratory acidosis.
- If $PaCO_2$ is ↓ and HCO_3^- is also ↓→ primary metabolic acidosis
- If HCO_3^- is ↓, then anion gap (AG) should be examined.

Metabolic acidosis results from the accumulation of nonvolatile acids, reduction of renal acid excretion, or loss of alkali.

CAUSES OF METABOLIC ACIDOSIS

Increased anion gap	*Normal anion gap (hyperchloremic)*
• *Increased acid production:* – *Ketoacidosis:* - Diabetic - Alcoholic - Starvation – Lactic acidosis – Toxic ingestion (salicylates, ethylene glycol, methanol) • Renal failure	• *Renal tubular dysfunction:* – Renal tubular acidosis – Hypoaldosteronism – Potassium-sparing diuretics • *Loss of alkali:* – Diarrhea – Ureterosigmoidostomy – Carbonic anhydrase inhibitors • Administration of HCl (ammonium chloride, cationic amino acids)

Metabolic acidosis has few specific signs. The appropriate diagnosis depends on the clinical setting and laboratory tests.

- The AG (normal = 12 ± 2 mmol/L) represents the anions, other than Cl^- and HCO_3^-, that are necessary to counterbalance Na^+ electrically:

$$AG\ (mmol/L) = Na^+\ (mmol/L) + [Cl\ (mmol/L) + HCO_3^-\ (mmol/L)]$$

  It is useful diagnostically to classify metabolic acidosis into increased or normal AG metabolic acidosis.
- Treatment of metabolic acidosis must be directed primarily at the underlying cause of the acid–base disturbance. Bicarbonate therapy should be considered in patients with moderate-to-severe metabolic acidosis only after the primary cause has been addressed. The HCO_3^- deficit (mmol/L) can be estimated using the following equation:
  - HCO_3^- deficit (mmol/L) = body weight (kg) × 0.4 × {[desired HCO_3^- (mmol/L)] – [measured HCO_3^- (mmol/L)]}
  - This equation serves to provide only a rough estimate of the deficit because the volume of HCO_3^- distribution and the rate of ongoing H^+ production are variable.

Hypokalemia

Clinical Manifestations

- Mild hypokalemia [K^+ >3 mmol/L] is generally asymptomatic.
- The symptoms present with severe K^+ deficiency [K^+ < 3 mmol/L (11.7 mg/dL)] and are primarily cardiovascular.
- Early electroencephalogram manifestations include ectopy, T-wave depression, and prominent U waves.
- Severe depletion increases susceptibility to reentrant arrhythmias.

Treatment

- In mild hypokalemia, oral replacement is suitable. Typical daily therapy for the treatment of mild hypokalemia in the patient with intact renal function is 40–100 mmol KCl orally in single or divided doses.
- Parenteral therapy is indicated in the presence of severe depletion, significant symptoms, or oral intolerance. K^+ concentrations (administered as chloride, acetate, or phosphate) in peripherally administered IV fluids should not exceed 40 mmol/L), and the rate of administration should not exceed 20 mmol (78 mg)/h.
- However, higher K^+ concentrations [60–80 mmol/L (234–312 mg/dL)] administered more rapidly (with cardiac monitoring) are indicated in cases of severe hypokalemia, for cardiac arrhythmias, and in the management of diabetic ketoacidosis.
- Administration of high K^+ concentrations via subclavian, jugular, or right atrial catheters should be avoided because local K^+ concentrations may be cardiotoxic.
- Hypomagnesemia frequently accompanies hypokalemia and generally must be corrected to successfully replenish K^+.

5. Clinical approach to hyponatremia. ***WBUHS 2019***

6. Write short note on postoperative hyponatremia. ***RIMS, Imphal 2012***

7. Etiology and management of hyponatremia. ***KIIT University, Odisha. 2025***

Causes

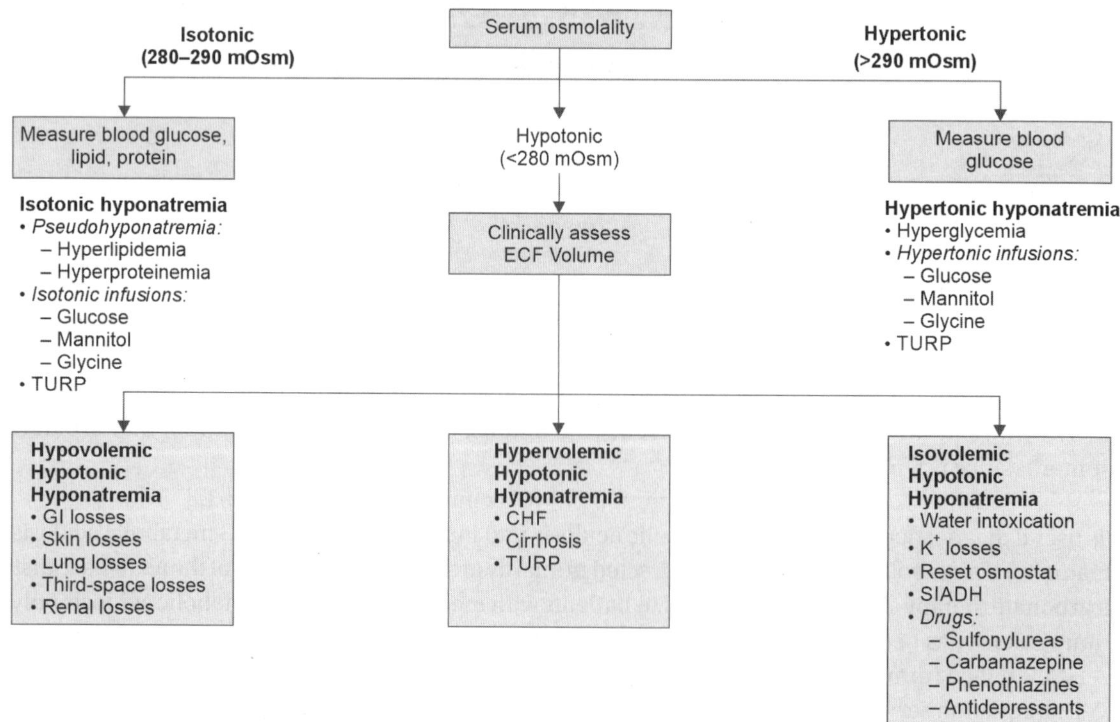

(CHF: congestive heart failure; ECF: extracellular fluid; GI: gastrointestinal; SIADH: syndrome of inappropriate antidiuretic hormone secretion; TURP: transurethral resection of the prostate)

Treatment

- Isotonic and hypertonic hyponatremia correct with resolution of the underlying disorder.
- Hypovolemic hyponatremia can be managed with administration of 0.9% NaCl to correct volume deficits and replace ongoing losses.
- Water intoxication responds to fluid restriction (1,000 mL/day).
- For SIADH (syndrome of inappropriate antidiuretic hormone secretion), water restriction (1,000 mL/day) should be attempted initially. The addition of a loop diuretic (Furosemide) or an osmotic diuretic (Mannitol) may be necessary in refractory cases.
- Hypervolemic hyponatremia may respond to water restriction (1,000 mL/day) to return Na^+ to greater than 130 mmol/L.
  In cases of severe congestive heart failure, optimizing cardiac performance may assist in Na^+ correction. If the edematous hyponatremic patient becomes symptomatic, plasma Na^+ can be increased to a safe level by the use of a loop diuretic while replacing urinary Na^+ losses with 3% NaCl. A reasonable approach is to replace approximately 25% of the hourly urine output with 3% NaCl.
  Hypertonic saline should not be administered to these patients without concomitant diuretic therapy.
  Administration of synthetic brain natriuretic peptide (BNP) is also useful therapeutically in the setting of acute heart failure (because it inhibits Na^+ reabsorption at the cortical collecting duct and inhibits the action of vasopressin on water permeability at the inner medullary collecting duct).
- In the presence of symptoms or extreme hyponatremia (Na^+ <110 mmol/L) hypertonic saline (3% NaCl) is indicated. Serum Na^+ should be corrected to approximately 120 mmol/L. The quantity of 3% NaCl that is required to increase serum Na^+ to 120 mmol/L can be estimated by calculating the Na^+ deficit:

  $$Na^+ \text{ deficit (mmol)} = 0.60 \times \text{lean body weight (kg)} \times [120 - \text{measured serum } Na^+ \text{ (mmol/L)}]$$

- Central pontine demyelination occurs in the setting of correction of hyponatremia. The risk factors for demyelination are controversial but appear to be related to the chronicity of hyponatremia (>48 hours) and the rate of correction. The serum Na^+ should be increased by no >12 mmol/L in 24 hours of treatment.
- For acute hyponatremia (<48 hours), the serum Na^+ may be corrected more rapidly (i.e., Na^+ = 1–2 mmol/h). The patient's volume status should be carefully monitored over this time, and the serum Na^+ should be determined frequently (every 1–2 hours). Once the serum Na^+ concentration reaches 120 mmol/L and symptoms have resolved, administration of hypertonic saline can be discontinued.

8. "Flow-guided intraoperative fluid therapy has been shown to reduce complications and hospital stay in patients undergoing major abdominal surgery"—Discuss. Criticize the basis of recent advances the role of colloids as resuscitation fluid. ***WBUHS 2017***

Flow-guided Intraoperative Fluid Therapy

Commonly used colloids include:

- Gelatins
- Hetastarch
- Albumin
- Plasma protein fraction
- Dextran

There has been criticism of research, however, because tests involved a single colloid type only, but the conclusions drawn were applied to the whole classification of colloids. Those who support the use of colloids argue that because in hypovolemia the intravascular space is the site of injury, fluid resuscitation should be aimed at the optimal restoration of the intravascular space.

Advantages and Disadvantages

- Colloids are better than crystalloids at expanding the circulatory volume because their larger molecules are retained more easily in the intravascular space and increase osmotic pressure.

- However, excessive use of colloids can precipitate cardiac failure, and pulmonary and peripheral edema. Although the pulmonary edema caused by excessive use of colloids is delayed in comparison with that caused by crystalloids, it is more sustained.
- Schierhout and Roberts (1998) also found that fluid resuscitation using colloids can cause pulmonary edema as well as anaphylactic shock and they can lead to a small increase in the rate of death.
- Gelatins can cause anaphylactic reactions and there is concern regarding the possible transmission of bovine spongiform encephalopathy.
- In addition, colloids are required for fluid challenges, as 200 mL of colloid solution will reexpand intravascular volume by 200 mL.

Comparisons

- The selection of the type of fluid to use depends on the primary origin of the exact kind of fluid loss, the condition of the patient, and the preference of the prescribing clinician.
- It is generally agreed that colloid solutions act more promptly to secure homeostasis, but some studies did indicate that crystalloid solutions are adequate for volume replacement.
- Rapid colloid infusion increased blood volume and therefore cardiac output more effectively than crystalloid infusion.
- Patients who received colloids experienced reduced fluid requirements, superior hemodynamics performance, and shortened intensive care requirements in comparison with those who received crystalloids.
- However, the Cochrane Report (Alderson et al., 2001) states that there is no evidence to indicate that use of colloids, although effective at expanding the circulation, improves mortality in the critically ill patient. The same report goes so far as to suggest that there is little justification for the use of colloids outside the context of randomized controlled trials.
- A systematic review highlights the need for further trials and indicates that insufficient data is available to suggest abandoning the use of colloids in practice.
- It is important to remember that the choice of fluid for resuscitation is only one small part of measures taken in the quest for reduced mortality.
- There is little conclusive evidence that mortality or morbidity outcomes are affected by the choice of either colloid or crystalloid fluid and mortality has not been found to be related to the specific fluid used for resuscitation.

In summarizing these most recent recommendations and with addition of the literature that emerged over the past couple of years, the following conclusions can be drawn.

- *Colloids at large:* There has not been a clear benefit associated with the use of expensive colloids compared to inexpensive crystalloids. Colloids as a whole have, however, shown to have increased mortality in patients with traumatic brain injury (TBI). No indications currently exist for the routine use of colloids over crystalloids.
- *Albumin:* There is no evidence to support the unique benefit of use of albumin as a resuscitation fluid. With the inclusion of the latest ALBIOS trial, mortality benefit in sepsis has not thus far been proven. In light of the cost and limited shelf life, the use of albumin as a resuscitation fluid is not supported.
- *Hydroxyethyl starch (HES):* The benefit of using HES has been refuted. To the contrary, HES is associated with increased harm. Though it is not clearly associated with increase in mortality, evidence clearly shows increased acute kidney injury (AKI) and use of renal replacement therapy (RRT) associated with the use of HES. It is further associated with coagulopathy and increased use of blood transfusion. The effects seem to be dose-dependent, but no consensus has been reached as to a safe dose of HES. As such, the use of HES in resuscitation should be avoided.
- *Dextran and gelatins:* Other synthetic colloids (dextran and gelatins) are not well studied in the literature. Although there is no evidence showing harm beyond what is seen with other colloids, there is also no evidence showing benefit. In light of the lack of evidence, and the theoretical potential for adverse effect, the suggestion is not to use gelatins or dextran.

9. Recent strategy in assessment of monitoring of IV fluids and electrolytes' need in perioperative period. ***WBUHS 2021***

Flow-guided intraoperative fluid therapy has been shown to reduce complications and hospital stay in patients undergoing major abdominal surgery.

Flow-guided Intraoperative Fluid Therapy

Commonly used colloids include:
- Gelatins
- Hetastarch
- Albumin
- Plasma protein fraction
- Dextran

There has been criticism of research, however, because tests involved a single colloid type only but the conclusions drawn were applied to the whole classification of colloids. Those who support the use of colloids argue that because in hypovolemia the intravascular space is the site of injury, fluid resuscitation should be aimed at the optimal restoration of the intravascular space.

Advantages and Disadvantages
- Colloids are better than crystalloids at expanding the circulatory volume because their larger molecules are retained more easily in the intravascular space and increase osmotic pressure.
- However, excessive use of colloids can precipitate cardiac failure, and pulmonary and peripheral edema. Although the pulmonary edema caused by excessive use of colloids is delayed in comparison with that caused by crystalloids, it is more sustained. Schierhout and Roberts (1998) also found that fluid resuscitation using colloids can cause pulmonary oedema as well as anaphylactic shock and they can lead to a small increase in the rate of death.
- Gelatins can cause anaphylactic reactions and there is concern regarding the possible transmission of bovine spongiform encephalopathy.
- In addition, colloids are required for fluid challenges, as 200 mL of colloid solution will re-expand intravascular volume by 200 mL.

In summarizing these most recent recommendations and with addition of the literature that emerged over the past couple of years, the following conclusions can be drawn.
- *Colloids at large:* There has not been a clear benefit associated with the use of expensive colloids compared to inexpensive crystalloids. Colloids as a whole have, however, shown to have increased mortality in patients with TBI. No indications currently exist for the routine use of colloids over crystalloids.
- *Albumin:* There is no evidence to support the unique benefit of use of albumin as a resuscitation fluid. With the inclusion of the latest ALBIOS trial, mortality benefit in sepsis has not thus far been proven. In light of the cost and limited shelf life, the use of albumin as a resuscitation fluid is not supported.
- *HES:* The benefit of using HES has been refuted. To the contrary, HES is associated with increased harm. Though it is not clearly associated with increase in mortality, evidence clearly shows increased AKI and use of RRT associated with the use of HES. It is further associated with coagulopathy and increased use of blood transfusion. The effects seem to be dose-dependent, but no consensus has been reached as to a safe dose of HES. As such, the use of HES in resuscitation should be avoided.
- *Dextran and gelatins:* Other synthetic colloids (dextran and gelatins) are not well studied in the literature. Although there is no evidence showing harm beyond what is seen with other colloids, there is also no evidence showing benefit. In light of the lack of evidence, and the theoretical potential for adverse effect, the suggestion is not to use gelatins or dextran.

10. Perioperative fluid management. ***WBUHS 2013***

Goals of Fluid Administration

- O_2 delivery/blood flow—perfusion
- Maintain electrolyte composition
- Glycemia
- Body temperature

Requirement of Fluid Depends on

- Type of patient
- Type of surgery
- Amount of trauma
- Acute injury versus elective operation
- Anesthetic, positioning

Classic Fluid Management

- Deficits
- Maintenance
- Third space
- Blood loss
- *Deficits:*
  - Preoperative NPO (hourly maintenance × duration)
  - Preoperative bowel preparation (1–1.5 L)
  - Preoperative blood loss (trauma) or fluid loss (burns) Typically replaced over first 2–4 hours
- *Maintenance:*
  - 4 mL/kg/h for first 10 kg of body weight
  - 2 mL/kg/h for second 10 kg of body weight
  - 1 mL/kg/h for each kg of body weight above 20 kg
- *Replace fluid losses:*
  - Third space 2–10 mL/kg/h
  - *Blood losses:*
    - 3-to-1 ratio of crystalloid to estimated blood loss (EBL)
    - 1-to-1 for colloid or blood (or hypertonic saline)

11. Describe the concept of zero fluid balance in perioperative fluid management. ***WBUHS 2016***

- Use fluid management technologies to deliver individualized goal-directed fluid therapy.
- Avoid crystalloid excess (salt and water overload). "Maintenance" fluid, if utilized, should be limited to <2 mL/kg/h including any drug infusions. The use of isotonic-balanced electrolyte solution (e.g., Hartmann's) will minimize hyperchloremic acidosis.

Aims by the End of Surgery

- Patient's core temperature is normal (circa 37°C).
- No evidence of hypovolemia, tissue hypoperfusion, or hypoxia
- No evidence of hypervolemia or excess fluid ("zero balance")
- Hb >7 g/dL.
- No clinically significant coagulopathy
- *Minimal use of vasopressors:*
  - *Predictors of poor outcome include:* Greater age, higher ASA (American Society of Anesthesiologists) status, high blood loss, longer than expected surgery, evidence of hypovolemia or hypoperfusion (e.g., metabolic

acidosis, blood lactate >2 mmol/L, central venous O_2 <70%), greater use of vasopressors, high volumes of IV fluids (>3.5 L total), positive fluid balance (>2 L positive on day of surgery).

- *The enhanced recovery partnership recommends that all anesthetists caring for patients undergoing intermediate or major surgery should have cardiac output measuring technologies immediately available and be trained to use them.*
- The use of intraoperative fluid management technologies are recommended from the outset in the following types of cases:
  - Major surgery with a 30-day mortality rate of >1%.
  - Major surgery with and anticipated blood loss of greater than 500 mL.
  - Major intra-abdominal surgery.
  - Intermediate surgery (30-day mortality >0.5%) in high-risk patients (age >80 years, history of left ventricular failure (LVF), myocardial infarction (MI), cerebrovascular accident (CVA), or peripheral arterial disease)
  - Unexpected blood loss and/or fluid loss requiring >2 L of fluid replacement.
  - Patients with ongoing evidence of hypovolemia and/or tissue hypoperfusion (e.g., persistent lactic acidosis)

12. Write the postoperative IV fluid protocol after major GI surgery and the composition of Ringer's lactate.
WBUHS 2021

Enhanced recovery programs (ERPs) aim to implement multimodal pathways in the perioperative period to reduce the risk of perioperative organ dysfunction and morbidity through such aims as encouraging early mobilization. Overall goals of fluid management should be to maintain euvolemia while avoiding excess water, salt, and electrolyte imbalance.

- Because of the risk of inducing hyperchloremic acidosis in routine practice, when crystalloid resuscitation or replacement is indicated, balanced salt solutions, e.g., Ringer's lactate/acetate or Hartmann's solution should replace 0.9% saline, except in cases of hypochloremia, e.g., from vomiting or gastric drainage.
- Solutions such as 4%/0.18% dextrose/saline and 5% dextrose are important sources of free water for maintenance, but should be used with caution as excessive amounts may cause dangerous hyponatremia, especially in children and the elderly. These solutions are not appropriate for resuscitation or replacement therapy except in conditions of significant free water deficit, e.g., diabetes insipidus.
- To meet maintenance requirements, adult patients should receive sodium 50–100 mmol/day and potassium 40–80 mmol/day in 1.5–2.5 L of water by the oral, enteral, or parenteral route (or a combination of routes). Additional amounts should only be given to correct deficit or continuing losses. Careful monitoring should be undertaken using clinical examination, fluid balance charts, and regular weighing when possible.
- Details of fluids administered must be clearly recorded and easily accessible.
- When patients leave theater for the ward, high-dependency unit (HDU), or intensive care unit (ICU), their volume status should be assessed. The volume and type of fluids given perioperatively should be reviewed and compared with fluid losses in theater including urine and insensible losses.
- In patients who are euvolemic and hemodynamically stable, a return to oral fluid administration should be achieved as soon as possible.
- In patients requiring continuing IV maintenance fluids, these should be sodium poor and of low enough volume until the patient has returned their sodium and fluid balance over the perioperative period to zero. When this has been achieved the IV fluid volume and content should be those required for daily maintenance.
- The hemodynamic and fluid status of those patients who fail to excrete their perioperative sodium load, and especially whose urine sodium concentration is <20 mmol/L, should be reviewed.

- In high-risk patients undergoing major abdominal surgery, postoperative treatment with IV fluid and low-dose dopexamine should be considered, in order to achieve a predetermined value for systemic oxygen delivery, as this may reduce postoperative complication rates and duration of hospital stay.
- In patients who are edematous, hypovolemia if present must be treated followed by a gradual persistent negative sodium and water balance based on urine sodium concentration or excretion. Plasma potassium concentration should be monitored and where necessary potassium intake adjusted.
- Nutritionally depleted patients need cautious refeeding orally, enterally, or parenterally, with feeds supplemented in potassium, phosphate, and thiamine. Generally, and particularly if edema is present, these feeds should be reduced in water and sodium. Though refeeding syndrome is a risk, improved nutrition will help to restore normal partitioning of sodium, potassium, and water between intra- and extracellular spaces.
- Surgical patients should be nutritionally screened, and NICE (National Institute for Health and Care Excellence) guidelines for perioperative nutritional support adhered to. Care should be taken to mitigate risks of the refeeding syndrome.

Lactated Ringer's is composed of sodium chloride 6 g/L, sodium lactate 3.1 g/L, potassium chloride 0.3 g/L, and calcium chloride 0.2 g/L. Lactated Ringer's contains ions of sodium 130 mEq/L, potassium 4 mEq/L, calcium 2.7 mEq/L, chloride 109 mEq/L, and lactate 28 mEq/L.

1 L of Ringer's Lactate Solution Contains

- 130–131 mEq of sodium ion = 130 mmol L^{-1}
- 109–111 mEq of chloride ion = 109 mmol L^{-1}
- 28–29 mEq of lactate ion = 28 mmol L^{-1}
- 4–5 mEq of potassium ion = 4 mmol L^{-1}
- 2–3 mEq of calcium ion = 1.5 mmol L^{-1}

Shock and Hemorrhage

LEARNING OBJECTIVES

- Classification of Shock
- Endotoxic Shock
- Distributive Shock
- Biomarkers of Sepsis
- Hemorrhagic Shock

CLASSIFICATION OF SHOCK

1. Classify shock and discuss the pathophysiology of septic shock. How do you manage it?
SAIMS Indore, 2025; RIMS, Imphal 2022

2. Discuss the pathophysiology of endotoxic shock and discuss the role of vasoactive drugs in shock.
WBUHS 2023

Classification of Shock—According to Bailey and Love

Classification of Shock

- Hypovolemic shock
- Cardiogenic shock
- Obstructive shock
- Distributive shock
- Endocrine shock

Other Classification

- *Cardiogenic:* Shock caused as a result of cardiac pump failure
  Causes:
  - Myocardial infarction
  - Arrhythmias (atrial fibrillation, ventricular tachycardias, bradycardias, etc.)
  - Mechanical abnormalities (valvular defects)
  - Extracardiac abnormalities [pulmonary embolism (PE), pulmonary hypertension (HTN), and tension pneumothorax]
- *Hypovolemic:* Shock caused by decreased preload due to intravascular volume loss
  Causes:
  - Hemorrhagic trauma, gastrointestinal (GI) bleeding, hemorrhagic pancreatitis, and fractures
  - Fluid loss induced—diarrhea, vomiting, and burns
- *Distributive:* Shock as a result of severely diminished systemic vascular resistance (SVR)
  The three subtypes are:
  1. *Septic:* Secondary to an overwhelming infection
  2. *Anaphylactic:* Secondary to an overwhelming infection
  3. *Neurogenic:* Secondary to a sudden loss of the autonomic nervous system function

- *Combined:*

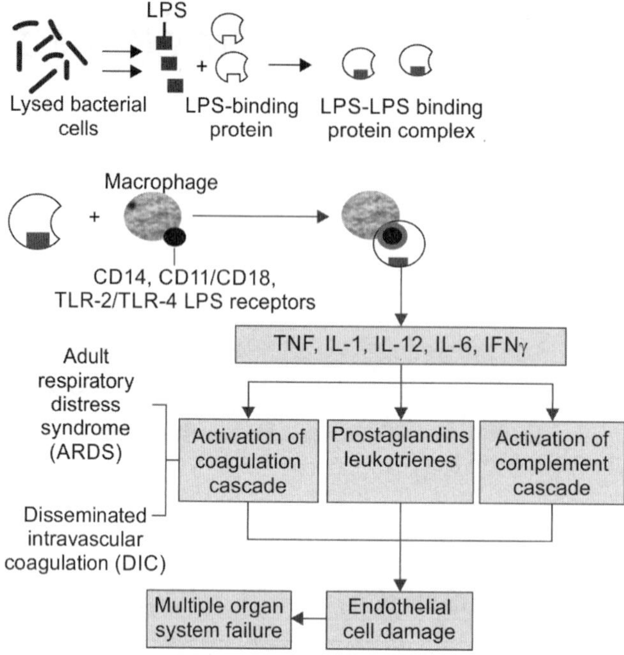

(IFN: interferon; IL-1: interleukin-1; LPS: lipopolysaccharide; TLR: toll-like receptor; TNF: tumor necrosis factor)

Septic Shock-mediated Inflammatory Cascade

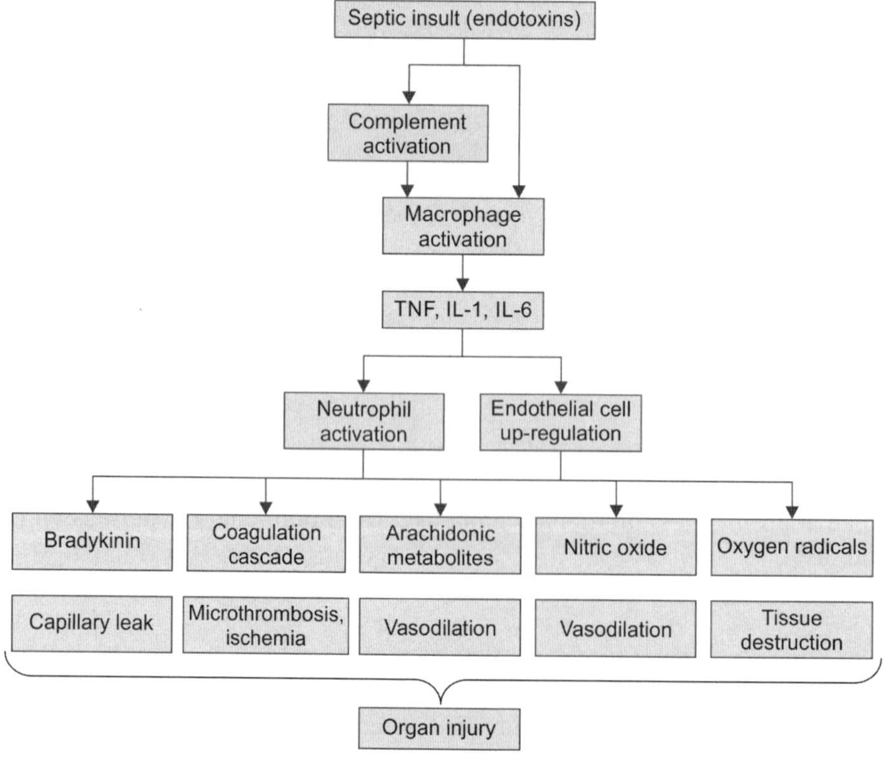

(IL-1: interleukin-1; TNF: tumor necrosis factor)

PATHOPHYSIOLOGY OF ENDOTOXIC SHOCK

General Clinical Signs

- Flu-like symptoms—fever, chills, general malaise, irritability, and lethargy
- Tachycardia and hypotension
- Hyperventilation
- Site of infection may or may not be evident

Cardiovascular

- Systemic vasodilation and hypotension [systolic (sys) <90 mm Hg]
- Tachycardia (>100 beats/min)
- Increased cardiac output (hyperdynamic), although contractility is depressed; hypodynamic in late shock
- Ventricular dilation; decreased ejection fraction
- Loss of sympathetic responsiveness
- Hypovolemia due to vascular leakage; central venous pressure (CVP) may be decreased or increased depending upon fluid resuscitation.
- Compromised nutrient blood flow to organs; decreased organ oxygen extraction

Pulmonary and Renal

- Hyperventilation with respiratory alkalosis
- Pulmonary HTN and edema
- Hypoxemia [arterial partial pressure of oxygen (pO_2) <50 mm Hg]
- Reduced pulmonary compliance; increased work
- Respiratory muscle failure
- Renal hypoperfusion; oliguria
- Acute tubular necrosis and renal failure

Other

- Disseminated intravascular coagulation (DIC)
- Blood dyscrasias:
  - Leukopenia
  - Thrombocytopenia
  - Polycythemia
- Central and peripheral nervous dysfunction
- Increased lactate occurs early.

Protocol for Resuscitation of Adult Hypotensive Patients with Suspected Sepsis

- Culture-relevant body fluids, including blood
- Infuse a balanced electrolyte solution of 500 mL/15 min. Monitor the systolic blood pressure response.
- Insert a central venous or pulmonary artery catheter.
- If after a 500-mL bolus of saline, the patient remains hypotensive and CVP is <8–12 mm Hg or pulmonary artery wedge pressure (PAWP) is <8–12 mm Hg, infuse another 500-mL bolus of fluid; repeat as needed.
- If CVP is >15 or PAWP is 15–20 and the patient remains hypotensive (<65 mm Hg), start an infusion of the inotrope dobutamine or dopamine. The goal is a mean systemic pressure >65 mm Hg and a pulse rate <120 beats/min.
- Determine the cardiac index and SVR.

- If after infusion of fluid and inotropes, SVR is <600, infuse a vasopressor—either norepinephrine or vasopressin—to increase SVR.
- Monitor mixed venous oxygen saturation and urine output as an indication that therapeutic interventions have improved perfusion.

Diagnostic Studies

Blood	Complete blood count, amylase, lipase, renal function, liver function, serum lactate, and arterial blood gases
Roentgenograms	Chest, abdomen, and plain films of areas with suspected soft-tissue infection
Advanced imaging	Ultrasound, computerized tomography, magnetic resonance injury, and nuclear imaging

A Simple Algorithm to Match the Therapeutic Response to the Patient's Clinical Condition

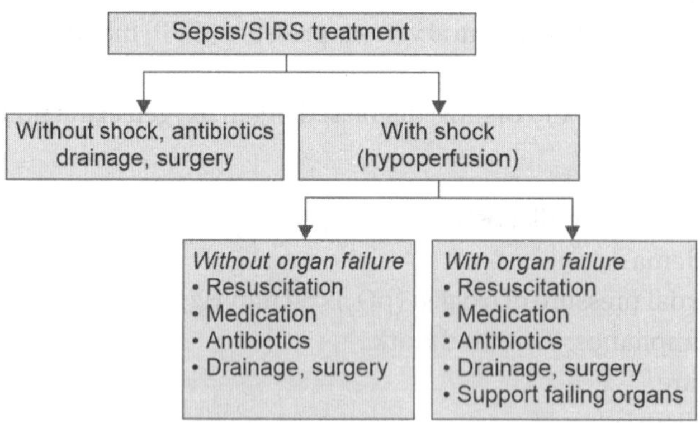

(SIRS: systemic inflammatory response syndrome)

Tools to Evaluate Cardiovascular Profile in Shock

Myocardial function	*Vasomotor tone/fluid responsiveness*	*End-organ perfusion*
• TTE/TOE • Transpulmonary thermodilution—PAC, PiCCO, and LiDCO	• Dynamic fluid responsiveness • SVR • Transpulmonary thermodilution	• Mentation • Urine output • Mottling of skin • Lactate/metabolic status • $SvO_2/ScvO_2$ • CO_2gap

(LiDCO: lithium dilution cardiac output measurement; PAC: pulmonary artery catheter; PiCCO: pulse contour cardiac output; $ScvO_2$: central venous oxygen saturation; SvO_2: venous oxygen saturation; SVR: systemic vascular resistance; TOE: transesophageal echocardiogram; TTE: transthoracic echocardiogram)

Algorithm for the Use of Vasoactive Therapy in Shock

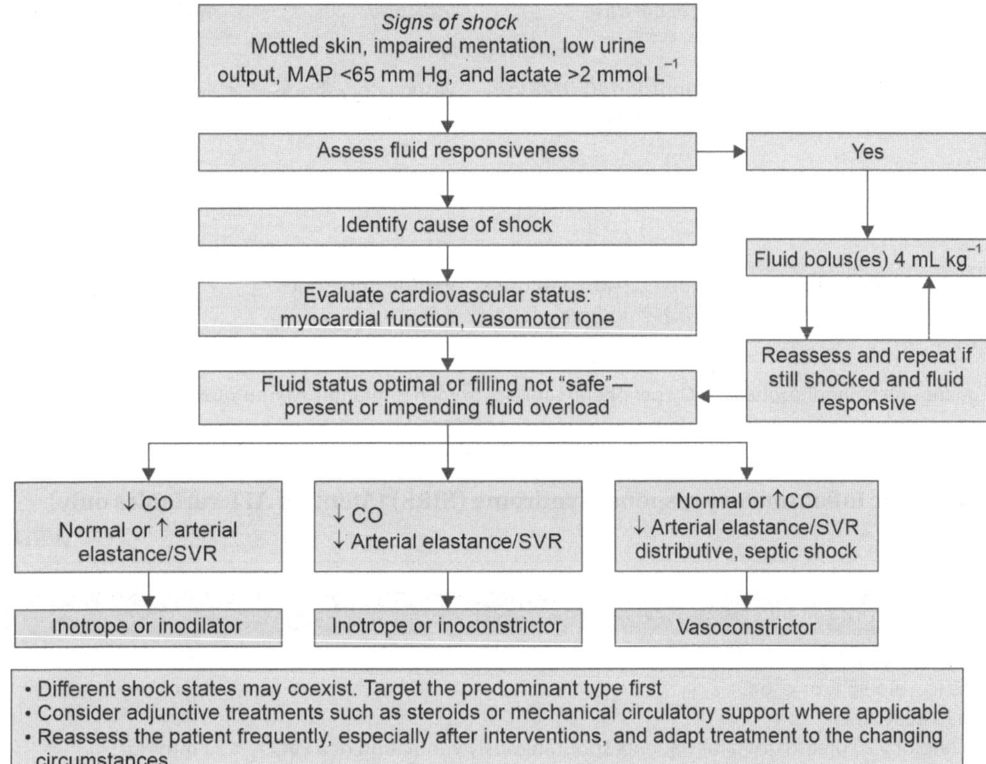

(MAP: mean arterial pressure; SVR: systemic vascular resistance)

Vasopressors in Clinical Use

Drug	*Site of action*	*Usual dose*	*Indication*	*Major adverse effects*
		Catecholamines		
Noradrenaline	Strong α_1 and modest B	0.01–0.5 μg/kg/min	First line in septic shock	• Tachyarrhythmias • Severe peripheral/visceral ischemia
Adrenaline	B: 0.01–0.1 μg/kg/min α_1: >0.1 μg/kg/min	0.01–0.3 μg/kg/min	Cardiogenic shock, vasodilatory shock, cardiac arrest, and severe bradycardia	• Tachyarrhythmias • High glucose/lactate • Severe peripheral/visceral ischemia
Phenylephrine	Strong α	0.4–4 μg/kg/min	Hypotension	• Reflex bradycardia • Severe peripheral/visceral ischemia
Metaraminol	Strong α_1: Stimulates noradrenaline release	Boluses of 0.5–1 μg	Hypotension secondary to vasodilation	• Reflex bradycardia • Severe peripheral/visceral ischemia
Dopamine	$D_{1,2}$: 1–5 μg/kg/min B: 5–10 μg/kg/min α_1: 10–15 μg/kg/min	1–15 μg/kg/min	Vasodilatory shock Severe bradycardia	• Tachyarrhythmias • Severe peripheral/visceral ischemia • Immunosuppression
Vasopressin	V_{1a}, V_{1b}, and V_2	0.01–0.04 U/min	Second line in septic shock	Severe peripheral/visceral Ischemia

Contd...

Contd...

Drug	*Site of action*	*Usual dose*	*Indication*	*Major adverse effects*
		Noncatecholamines		
Terlipressin	V_{1a} (V_{1b}) > V_2	Infusion 20–160 µg/h or boluses 1–2 µg q.d.s	Vasodilatory shock—acute liver failure	Severe peripheral/visceral ischemia
Angiotensin II	AT_X, AT_2	5–200 ng/kg/ min	Vasodilatory shock	• Tachyarrhythmias • Severe peripheral/visceral ischemia
Methylene blue	cGMP blocker	Bolus 2 µg/kg, infusion 0.2–2 µg/kg/h	Vasodilatory shock	• Falsely low SpO_2 readings • Methemoglobinemia • Pulmonary vasoconstriction

(cGMP: cyclic guanosine monophosphate; SpO_2: peripheral capillary oxygen saturation; ATx: autotoxin; AT_2: angiotensin)

3. Criteria for systemic inflammatory response syndrome (SIRS) (Mention ALL variables only).

WBUHS 2013, 2021

Criteria for four categories of SIRS.

Two or more of the following:
- Temperature (core) >38°C or <36°C
- Heart rate >90 beats/min
- Respiratory rate of >20 breaths/min for patients spontaneously ventilating or a $PaCO_2$ < 32 mm Hg
- White blood cell count >12,000 cells/mm^3 or <4,000 cells/mm^3 or >10% immature (band) cells in the peripheral blood smear

Sepsis:
- Same criteria as for SIRS but with a clearly established focus on infection in severe sepsis
- Sepsis associated with organ dysfunction and hypoperfusion
- Indicators of hypoperfusion:
  - Systolic blood pressure <90 mm Hg
  - >40 mm Hg fall from normal systolic blood pressure
  - Lactic acidemia
  - Oliguria
  - Acute mental status changes

Septic shock: Patients with severe sepsis who:
- Are not responsive to intravenous fluid infusion for resuscitation
- Require inotropic or vasopressor agents to maintain systolic blood pressure

4. Pathogenesis of sepsis-induced hypotension.

WBUHS 2014

- Hypotension is a serious sign of sepsis. In general, hypotension can be caused by a decrease in blood volume, a decrease in vascular tone, or a decrease in cardiac output; the hypotension of sepsis can be caused by reductions in all three parameters. Initially, sepsis usually reduces blood volume by increasing capillary leakage, so the administration of fluids is an early priority during treatment.
- In sepsis, the blood volume is not only reduced. It is redistributed ineffectively. Fluid resuscitation will usually refill the underperfused arteries. In septic shock, poor vascular tone has been added to the patient's other systemic problems. In shock, the administration of large amounts of fluids will not succeed in restoring normal blood pressure.

5. Distributive shock. ***WBUHS 2014***

- Distributive shock as a result of severely diminished SVR.
- Distributive shock is a medical condition in which abnormal distribution of blood flow in the smallest blood vessels results in inadequate supply of blood to the body's tissues and organs.
- *Septic:* Secondary to an overwhelming infection
- *Anaphylactic*
- *Neurogenic:* Secondary to a sudden loss of the autonomic nervous system function
- *Pathophysiology:*
  - The cause of inadequate tissue perfusion (blood delivery to tissues) in distributive shock is a lack of normal responsiveness of blood vessels to vasoconstrictive agents and direct vasodilation.
  - *There are four types of distributive shock.*
    1. The most common—septic shock:
       - It is caused by an infection, most frequently by bacteria, but viruses, fungi, and parasites have been implicated.
       - Infection sites most likely to lead to septic shock are the chest, abdomen, and genitourinary tract.
       - In septic shock, the blood flow in the microvasculature is abnormal with some capillaries underperfused and others with normal to high blood flow.
       - The endothelial cells lining the blood vessels become less responsive to vasoconstrictive agents, lose their glycocalyx (normal coating) and negative ionic charge, become leaky, and cause extensive overexpression of nitric oxide.
       - The coagulation cascade is also disrupted. The tissue factor that initiates the clotting cascade is produced by activated monocytes and the endothelial cells lining the blood vessels, while antithrombin and fibrinolysis are impaired.
       - DIC can result from the thrombin produced in the inflammatory response.
       - The ability of red blood cells to change shape decreases and their tendency to clump together increases, inhibiting their flow through the microvasculature.
    2. In anaphylactic shock, low blood pressure is related to decreased SVR triggered primarily by a massive release of histamine by mast cells activated by antigen-bound immunoglobulin E and also by increased production and release of prostaglandins.
    3. Neurogenic shock is caused by the loss of vascular tone normally supported by the sympathetic nervous system due to injury to the central nervous system, especially spinal cord injury.
       Rupture of a hollow organ, with subsequent evacuation of contents in the peritoneal cavity, could also determine neurogenic shock, a subtype of distributive shock. This happens due to the widespread peritoneal irritation by the ruptured viscus contents, as in peptic ulcer perforation, with consequent strong vagal activation, and generalized extensive peripheral vasodilatation and bradycardia.
    4. Distributive shock associated with adrenal crisis results from inadequate steroid hormones.

Elbers and Ince have identified five classes of abnormal microcirculatory flow in distributive shock using side-stream dark field microscopy.
Class I: All capillaries are stagnant when there is normal or sluggish venular flow.
Class II: There are empty capillaries next to capillaries that have flowing red blood cells.
Class III: There are stagnant capillaries next to capillaries with normal blood flow.
Class IV: Hyperdynamic flow in capillaries adjacent to capillaries that are stagnant.
Class V: There is widespread hyperdynamic flow in the microcirculatory system.

Treatment

- The main goals of treatment in distributive shock are to reverse the underlying cause and achieve hemodynamic stabilization.

- Immediate treatment involves fluid resuscitation and the use of vasoactive drugs, both vasopressors and inotropes.
- Hydrocortisone is used for patients whose hypotension does not respond to fluid resuscitation and vasopressors.
- Opening and keeping open the microcirculation is a consideration in the treatment of distributive shock; as a result, limiting the use of vasopressors has been suggested.
- Control of inflammation, vascular function, and coagulation to correct pathological differences in blood flow and microvascular shunting has been pointed to as a potentially important adjunct goal in the treatment of distributive shock.
- Patients with septic shock are treated with antimicrobial drugs to treat the causative infection. Some sources of infection require surgical intervention including necrotizing fasciitis, cholangitis, abscess, intestinal ischemia, or infected medical devices.
- Anaphylactic shock is treated with epinephrine.

BIOMARKERS OF SEPSIS

6. Write a short note on biomarkers of sepsis. ***WBUHS 2023***

Introduction

- Sepsis remains a leading cause of death in critically ill patients, despite efforts to improve patient outcome.
- Early diagnosis and prompt initial management such as early goal-directed therapy are key to improve sepsis outcome.
- For early detection of sepsis, biological markers (biomarkers) can help clinicians to distinguish infection from host response to inflammation. Ideally, biomarkers can be used for risk stratification, diagnosis, monitoring of treatment responses, and outcome prediction.
- More than 170 biomarkers have been identified as useful for evaluating sepsis, including C-reactive protein, procalcitonin, various cytokines, and cell surface markers.
- Recently, studies have reported on the usefulness of biomarker-guided antibiotic stewardships.
- However, the other side of these numerous biomarkers is that no novel single laboratory marker can diagnose, predict, and track the treatment of sepsis. The purpose of this review is to summarize several key biomarkers from recent sepsis studies.
    - *Characteristics of ideal sepsis biomarkers:*
        - *Role of biomarkers:*
            - Screening patients at risk of sepsis
            - Establish early diagnosis that helps the initial management of sepsis.
            - Risk stratification to identify patients at risk of poor outcome.
            - Monitoring the response of intervention
            - Predict outcomes
        - *Requisites for useful biomarkers:*
            - Objectively measured
            - Have reference standard
            - Reproducibility of test
            - Have well-known kinetics
            - Cost-effectiveness
            - Reflect normal biologic process, pathologic process, or pharmacologic response to therapy

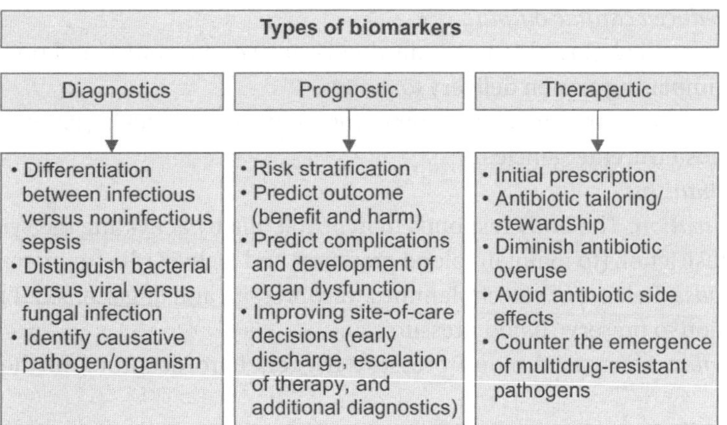

List of Biomarkers of Sepsis

- *Acute-phase proteins:*
  - CRP
  - Procalcitonin
  - Pentraxin 3 (PTX3)
  - Lipopolysaccharide-binding protein (LBP)
- *Cytokines and chemokines:*
  - IL-1RA, IL-1β, IL-2, IL-6, MCP-1
  - TNF-α, TNFR1/2
  - HMGBP1
- *Cell surface markers:*
  - Soluble CD14 (presepsin)
  - Neutrophil CD64 index (CD64in)
  - mHLA-DR (monocyte HLA-DR levels)
  - CD-163
- *Receptor markers:*
  - *VEGF:*
    - Soluble VEGF-receptor 1 (sFLT)
    - Soluble urokinase plasminogen activator (suPAR)
    - sTREM-1
    - Soluble receptor for advanced glycation end products (RAGE)
- *Coagulation:*
  - Activated partial thromboplastin time (aPTT) waveform analysis
  - Protein C receptor
  - Thrombomodulin
- *Endothelial damage:*
  - Heparin-binding protein
  - E-selectin
  - Neopterin
  - ICAM-1, VCAM-1
  - Angiopoietin-1 and 2
  - *Syndecan-1 and 2*
- *Vasodilation:* Copeptin (AVP precursor)
- *Cell damage:*
  - MicroRNA
  - Microparticles
- *Cell repair:* Procollagen III amino propeptide

(AVP: arginine vasopressin; CRP: C-reactive protein; HMGBP1: high mobility group box 1; ICAM-1: intercellular adhesion molecule 1; IL-1β: interleukin-1β; IL-1RA: interleukin-1 receptor antagonist; MCP-1: monocyte chemoattractant protein-1; mHLA-DR: monocyte human leukocyte antigen; sTREM-1: soluble triggering receptor expressed on myeloid cell-1; TNF: tumor necrosis factor; TNFR: tumor necrosis factor receptor; VCAM-1: vascular cell adhesion molecule 1; VEGF: vascular endothelial growth factor)

- Biomarkers promise to transform sepsis from a physiologic syndrome to a group of distinct biochemical disorders.
- This transformation could aid therapeutic decision-making, and hence improve the prognosis for patients with sepsis, but will require an unprecedented degree of systematic investigation and collaboration.

7. Discuss the pathophysiology and management of hemorrhagic shock. ***KIIT University, Odisha 2025***

Pathophysiology of Hemorrhagic Shock

Hemorrhagic shock is a life-threatening condition caused by significant blood loss, leading to inadequate tissue perfusion and oxygenation. The pathophysiology can be broken down into several key stages and mechanisms:

- *Hypovolemia and reduced cardiac output:*
  - Blood loss reduces circulating blood volume, decreasing venous return and preload. This leads to reduced cardiac output, impairing oxygen delivery to tissues.
  - Common causes include trauma (e.g., penetrating injuries, fractures), gastrointestinal bleeding, ruptured aneurysms, or obstetric emergencies.
- *Compensatory mechanisms:*
  - *Sympathetic activation:* The body responds to hypovolemia by activating the sympathetic nervous system, causing vasoconstriction (to maintain blood pressure) and tachycardia (to increase cardiac output).
  - *Hormonal response:* Release of catecholamines, vasopressin, and angiotensin II promotes vasoconstriction and fluid retention to preserve blood pressure.
  - *Baroreceptor reflex:* Decreased blood pressure triggers baroreceptors, further enhancing sympathetic outflow.
- *Cellular and organ effects:*
  - *Tissue hypoxia:* Reduced oxygen delivery leads to anaerobic metabolism, causing lactic acidosis and accumulation of metabolic byproducts.
  - *Microvascular dysfunction:* Prolonged hypoperfusion damages endothelial cells, leading to capillary leak, edema, and worsening tissue ischemia.
  - *Systemic inflammatory response:* Hypoxia and tissue injury trigger cytokine release, contributing to systemic inflammatory response syndrome (SIRS) and potential multiorgan dysfunction.
- *Stages of hemorrhagic shock:*
  - *Class I (≤15% blood volume loss):* Minimal symptoms; heart rate may be normal or slightly elevated.
  - *Class II (15–30%):* Tachycardia, tachypnea, and mild hypotension; patient may be anxious or restless.
  - *Class III (30–40%):* Marked tachycardia, hypotension, oliguria, and altered mental status.
  - *Class IV (>40%):* Life-threatening; profound hypotension, minimal urine output, and coma or death if untreated.
- *Coagulopathy:* Blood loss dilutes clotting factors, while tissue injury activates the coagulation cascade. Hypothermia, acidosis, and dilution from fluid resuscitation can exacerbate trauma-induced coagulopathy, forming the "lethal triad" (coagulopathy, hypothermia, acidosis).
- *Multi-organ failure:* Prolonged hypoperfusion leads to organ ischemia, particularly affecting the brain, heart, kidneys, and liver. If uncorrected, this progresses to irreversible shock and death.

Management of Hemorrhagic Shock

The management of hemorrhagic shock focuses on controlling bleeding, restoring blood volume, and optimizing tissue perfusion while addressing complications. Key steps include:

- *Initial assessment and stabilization:*
  - *Airway and breathing:* Ensure a patent airway and adequate oxygenation. Administer supplemental oxygen or intubate if necessary (e.g., in unconscious patients or severe respiratory distress).
  - *Control bleeding:* Apply direct pressure to external bleeding sites, use tourniquets for extremity hemorrhage, or stabilize fractures (e.g., pelvic binders). For internal bleeding, urgent surgical or interventional radiology consultation is needed.
  - *Vascular access:* Establish large-bore intravenous (IV) lines or intraosseous access for rapid fluid administration.
- *Fluid resuscitation:*
  - *Permissive hypotension:* In trauma patients with uncontrolled bleeding, maintain a lower blood pressure (e.g., systolic BP ~80-90 mm Hg) to avoid disrupting clots until hemorrhage is controlled. This does not apply to patients with traumatic brain injury, where higher BP is needed to maintain cerebral perfusion.
  - *Crystalloids:* Use balanced crystalloids (e.g., lactated Ringer's or normal saline) for initial resuscitation. Avoid over-resuscitation to prevent hemodilution and clot disruption.

- *Blood products:* Transfuse packed red blood cells (PRBCs) early for significant blood loss. Use a balanced transfusion strategy (1:1:1 ratio of PRBCs, fresh frozen plasma, and platelets) to address coagulopathy, especially in trauma-induced massive hemorrhage.

- *Definitive hemorrhage control:*
  - *Surgical intervention:* Urgent surgery (e.g., laparotomy, thoracotomy) or interventional radiology (e.g., embolization) is required for internal bleeding sources like splenic rupture or pelvic fractures.
  - *Damage control surgery:* In unstable patients, perform rapid, limited surgery to control bleeding and contamination, followed by stabilization in the ICU before definitive repair.
- *Correcting the Lethal Triad:*
  - *Coagulopathy:* Administer fresh frozen plasma, platelets, and cryoprecipitate as needed. Consider tranexamic acid (TXA) within 3 hours of injury to reduce bleeding in trauma patients.
  - *Hypothermia:* Actively warm the patient using warmed fluids, blankets, or forced-air warming devices to maintain normothermia.
  - *Acidosis:* Correct acidosis by improving perfusion and oxygenation. Sodium bicarbonate is rarely needed unless pH is critically low.
- *Monitoring and support:*
  - *Hemodynamic monitoring:* Use vital signs, urine output, lactate levels, and base deficit to guide resuscitation. Invasive monitoring (e.g., arterial line, central venous pressure) may be needed in critical cases.
  - *Organ support:* Address complications like acute kidney injury or respiratory failure with appropriate interventions (e.g., dialysis, mechanical ventilation).
  - *Labs:* Monitor hemoglobin, hematocrit, coagulation parameters (INR, PTT), and arterial blood gases to guide therapy.
- *Special considerations:*
  - *Trauma:* Follow Advanced Trauma Life Support (ATLS) guidelines, prioritizing rapid assessment and hemorrhage control.
  - *Nontraumatic hemorrhage:* For conditions like gastrointestinal bleeding, use endoscopy or embolization. For obstetric hemorrhage, consider uterine artery embolization or hysterectomy.
  - *Medications:* Avoid vasopressors in early hemorrhagic shock, as they may worsen tissue perfusion. Use them only in specific cases (e.g., neurogenic shock) after volume resuscitation.
- *Postresuscitation care:*
  - Monitor for complications like transfusion-related acute lung injury (TRALI), infections, or abdominal compartment syndrome.
  - Transition to ICU care for ongoing monitoring and optimization of organ function.

CHAPTER 6

Blood Coagulation

LEARNING OBJECTIVES

- ➤ Physiology of blood coagulation
- ➤ Coagulopathy in trauma patients

1. Physiology of blood coagulation and its importance in surgery. *WBUHS 2024, RIMS, Imphal 2022*

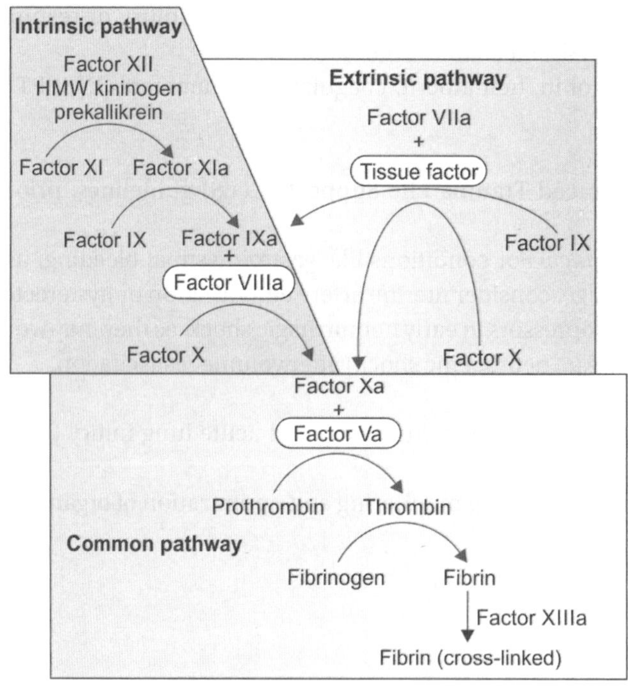

(HMW: high molecular weight)

Blood Coagulation Cascade

- Plasma zymogens are sequentially converted to active proteases (arrows).
- Nonenzymatic protein cofactors (ovals) are required at several stages of the cascade.
- Factors IX and X and prothrombin are activated on phospholipid surfaces.
- Thrombin cleaves fibrinogen, yielding fibrin monomers that polymerize to form a clot.
- Coagulation is a complex equilibrium among thrombotic, anticoagulant, and fibrinolytic processes.
- Disruption of these processes can lead to severe hemorrhagic or thrombotic complications.

Disorders of Coagulation

- *Acquired factor deficiencies* in surgical patients commonly result from a nutritional deficiency (e.g., vitamin K) or from medical conditions such as liver failure and disseminated intravascular coagulation (DIC).
  - *Vitamin K deficiency:*
    - It leads to the production of inactive, noncarboxylated forms of prothrombin, factors VII, IX, and X, and proteins C and S.
    - The diagnosis should be considered in a patient with a prolonged partial thromboplastin time (PTT) that corrects with a 50:50 mixture of normal plasma.
    - Vitamin K deficiency can occur in patients without oral intake within 1 week, with biliary obstruction, with malabsorption, and in those receiving antibiotics or warfarin.
- *Sepsis:*
  - Sepsis stimulates the coagulation cascade, whereas levels of anticoagulant factors such as protein C, protein S, and antithrombin (AT) III are decreased.
  - This represents an imbalance in hemostasis, causing microvascular thrombi to form.
  - These thrombi further amplify injury and cause distal tissue ischemia and hypoxia.
  - Therapy with activated protein C (APC) has been reported to decrease mortality in patients with severe sepsis as defined by an Acute Physiology and Chronic Health Evaluation (APACHE) II score ≥25.
- *Liver dysfunction:*
  - It leads to complex alterations in coagulation through decreased synthesis of all clotting factors and inhibitors except von Willebrand factor (vWF).
  - Coagulopathy can be worsened by thrombocytopenia from associated hypersplenism.
  - Spontaneous bleeding is infrequent, but coagulation defects should be corrected prior to invasive procedures.
  - Fresh frozen plasma (FFP) administration often improves the coagulopathy transiently.
- *Disseminated intravascular coagulation:*
  - Disseminated intravascular coagulation has many inciting causes, including sepsis, extensive trauma or burns, necrotic tissue, intravascular antibody-antigen immune reactions, malignancies, liver failure, obstetric complications, and intravascular prosthetic devices.
  - The pathogenesis of DIC is due to the inappropriate generation of thrombin within the vasculature, leading to the formation of fibrin thrombi, platelet activation, and fibrinolytic activity.
  - DIC often presents with complications from microvascular thrombi that involve the vascular beds of the kidney, brain, lung, and skin.
  - Laboratory findings in DIC include thrombocytopenia, hypofibrinogenemia, increased fibrinogen degradation products (FDPs), and prolonged thrombin time (TT) and PTT.
  - Therapy begins with treatment of the underlying cause.
  - Management of hemodynamics and oxygenation is critical.
  - Correction of coagulopathy with platelet transfusions, FFP, and cryoprecipitate should be undertaken for bleeding complications but should not be given empirically.
- *Inherited factor deficiency disorders:*
  - *Hemophilia:*
    - It is an inherited factor deficiency of either factor VIII (hemophilia A) or factor IX (hemophilia B—Christmas disease).
    - The severity of the disease depends on the factor activity level.
    - The diagnosis is suggested by patient history and an elevated PTT, normal prothrombin time (PT), and normal bleeding time. Factor activity assays confirm the diagnosis.
    - Minor bleeding can often be controlled locally without the need for factor replacement therapy. DDAVP (1-deamino-8-D-arginine vasopressin) stimulates the release of vWF into the circulation, which increases factor VIII levels two- to six-fold.

- This may control minor bleeding in patients with mild disease. Major bleeding (e.g., during a surgical procedure) requires factor VIII replacement.
- Cryoprecipitate contains factor VIII, vWF, and fibrinogen and can be used to treat patients with hemophilia A for control of bleeding.
- Purified factor IX is the treatment of choice for *hemophilia B.*

- Other inherited factor deficiencies account for fewer than 10% of severe factor deficiencies. Deficiencies of factor XII, high-molecular-weight kininogen (HMWK), or prekallikrein do not cause bleeding and require no treatment.

- *Inherited hypercoagulable disorders* place patients at risk for thrombosis and include deficiencies in the body's anticoagulants (AT, protein C, and protein S deficiencies), hyperhomocysteinemia, and prothrombin gene mutations. Indications for anticoagulation depend on the type, severity, and clinical situation of the disorder.
  - *Antithrombin deficiency:*
    - Antithrombin deficiency is an autosomal dominant disorder that presents with recurrent venous thromboembolism, usually in the second decade of life.
    - Assays for AT levels are typically decreased in the setting of acute thrombosis and also if the patient is receiving heparin.
    - Patients with acute thromboembolism or previous history of thrombosis are typically anticoagulated. AT-deficient patients should have the AT level restored to >80% of normal activity with AT concentration prior to operation or childbirth.
  - *Protein C deficiency and protein S deficiency:*
    - They are risk factors for venous thrombosis.
    - In a state of protein C or S deficiency, factors Va and VIIIa are not adequately inactivated, thereby allowing unchecked coagulation.
    - Besides the inherited type, protein C deficiency is encountered in patients with liver failure and in those who are receiving warfarin therapy.
    - Symptomatic patients are treated with heparin (or LMWH) anticoagulation followed by warfarin therapy.
    - In individuals with diminished protein C activity, effective heparin anticoagulation must be confirmed before warfarin initiation because warfarin transiently lowers protein C levels further and potentially worsens the hypercoagulable state.
    - Patients with protein C or S deficiency but with no history of thrombosis typically do not require prophylactic anticoagulation.
  - *Activated protein C resistance (factor V Leiden):*
    - It is a genetic mutation in factor V that renders it resistant to breakdown by APC, placing patients at an increased risk for thromboembolism.
    - Routine preoperative screening in asymptomatic patients is unnecessary.
    - Therapy for venous thrombosis consists of anticoagulation with heparin followed by warfarin therapy.
    - The role of long-term warfarin anticoagulation for patients with a single thrombotic event is undefined.
- *Acquired hypercoagulable disorders:*
  - *Antiphospholipid antibodies* are immunoglobulins that are targeted against antigens composed in part of platelet and endothelial cell phospholipids.
  - *Antiphospholipid antibody disorders* may be detected by lupus anticoagulant, anticardiolipin, or other antiphospholipid antibodies. Patients with these antibodies are at risk for arterial and venous thrombosis, recurrent miscarriages, and thrombocytopenia.
  - Other acquired hypercoagulable states include malignancies, pregnancy or the use of estrogen therapy, intravascular hemolysis (e.g., hemolytic anemia or after cardiopulmonary bypass), and the localized propensity for thrombosis in arteries that have recently undergone endarterectomy, angioplasty, or placement of prosthetic vascular grafts. Along with effective anticoagulation therapy, treatment should be directed at any identified underlying risk factor.

2. Coagulopathy in trauma patients. ***WBUHS 2021***

Introduction

- Trauma remains a leading cause of death and disability in adults in spite of advances in resuscitation, surgical management, and critical care.
- Between 25 and 35% of injured civilian trauma patients develop a biochemically evident coagulopathy upon arrival in the emergency department, in spite of improved efficiency of trauma systems, military and civilian, in reducing the time interval between acute injury and treatment.
- Coagulopathy may be the result of physiologic derangements such as acidosis, hypothermia, or hemodilution related to fluid or blood administration; however, an acute coagulopathy can also occur in severely injured patients independent of, or in addition to, these factors.
- Several terms are used in the literature to refer to this condition, including acute traumatic coagulopathy (ATC), early coagulopathy of trauma (ECT), trauma-induced coagulopathy (TIC), and acute coagulopathy of trauma shock.

Mechanism

- Acute intrinsic coagulopathy arising in severely injured trauma patients is now termed trauma-induced coagulopathy and is an emergent property of tissue injury combined with hypoperfusion. Mechanisms contributing to TIC include anticoagulation, consumption, platelet dysfunction, and hyperfibrinolysis.
- Hemorrhagic shock from blood loss is a critical cause of mortality in severely injured patients. Contributing to blood loss is an intrinsic dysregulation of the blood coagulation system now named trauma-induced coagulopathy.
- TIC arises in the presence of both tissue hypoperfusion from blood loss and severe anatomical tissue injury and, when present, is strongly and positively associated with mortality. The physiological environment in which TIC arises is a complex mixture of inflammation, anticoagulation, and cellular dysfunction of mixed etiology.
- Several key processes, including dysfunction of natural anticoagulant mechanisms, platelet dysfunction, fibrinogen consumption, and hyperfibrinolysis, have been identified as primary components of TIC. In addition, specific effects of blood dilution from resuscitation fluids, environmental hypothermia, and acidosis can modulate clot formation, adding more layers of complexity to TIC.

Anticoagulation

- Anticoagulation is a primary component of TIC. It was initially described as an increased international normalized ratio (INR) by Brohi et al. in severely injured trauma patients measured on arrival at the emergency department.
- Activated partial thromboplastin time (aPTT) was also elevated in patients with severe injury and there was tissue hypoperfusion as measured by the base deficit, although changes in this assay lagged behind changes in INR.
- The investigators presumed that elevations in INR and aPTT were independent of dilution by fluid resuscitation or environmental influences due to the limited resuscitation fluids received by these patients before sampling.
- The thrombin–thrombomodulin–protein C anticoagulant system was implicated as a potential primary mechanism of anticoagulation.
- The anticoagulant properties of APC are derived by its degradation of activated factors V and VIII, producing reduced concentrations and activities.
- Other anticoagulant mechanisms may contribute to the pathomechanism of TIC. Endogenous auto-heparinization, possibly related to the shedding of the endothelial glycocalyx, has been suggested by the ability to reverse anticoagulation in the presence of heparinase in whole blood from TIC patients.
- Measurement of fibrinopeptides, liberated either by thrombin or from degradation by plasmin, has shown a relatively greater increase of plasmin relative to thrombin activation during the initial encounter with trauma patients.

- It is clear that anticoagulation, either directly from the thrombin–thrombomodulin–APC system or through thrombin activation and factor consumption, is an important component of TIC.

Platelet Dysfunction

There is a rapidly growing body of support for a prominent role of platelet dysfunction in the pathophysiology of TIC.

Fibrinogen Consumption and Fibrinolysis

- After its activation by thrombin, fibrinogen spontaneously polymerizes from its individual monomers to form an insoluble polymeric fibrin mesh to stop blood loss at sites of vascular injury. This process, along with platelet-induced clot contraction, is the primary component of secondary hemostasis.
- There is strong evidence that the consumption of fibrinogen and fibrinolysis by the action of plasmin is a key mechanistic component of TIC.

Combining Injury and Shock to Produce TIC

- Observational clinical data have demonstrated that TIC is most common in severely injured trauma patients who are subjected to a high degree of both anatomical tissue injury and hypoperfusion from hemorrhagic shock.
- A synergistic effect of materials released from tissue injury with inflammation and anticoagulant factors induced by endothelial injury and tissue hypoxia likely mediates this relationship to produce TIC.
- There is evidence that circulating intracellular contents such as histones, known to be released from injured tissue, are associated with TIC.
- In a small study of 37 multiple trauma patients, patterns of elevated histones and extracellular DNA derived from activated neutrophils followed leukocyte counts, interleukin-6 (IL-6) levels, and myeloperoxidase levels and were associated with subsequent sepsis, multiple organ failure, and death.
- Neurohormonal and endothelial activation in response to acute blood loss may also be involved in the development of TIC.
- Although specific mechanisms of shock-induced endothelial activation and dysfunction have not yet been elucidated, there is emerging evidence that disruption of the endothelial glycocalyx barrier (indicated by syndecan-1 release) plays an important role in the endothelial response to traumatic shock.
- Three proinflammatory cytokines, interferon-γ (IFN-γ), IL-1β, and fractalkine, were negatively associated with plasma syndecan-1 levels, presumably by their binding and activation of the endothelium.
- Glycocalyx shedding and associated loss of endothelial barrier function also presumably promotes leukocyte recruitment and activation, liberation of injurious reactive oxygen species, and endothelial cell damage, as demonstrated by the damaging effect of incubating leukocytes captured from trauma patients on endothelial progenitor cells in vitro.

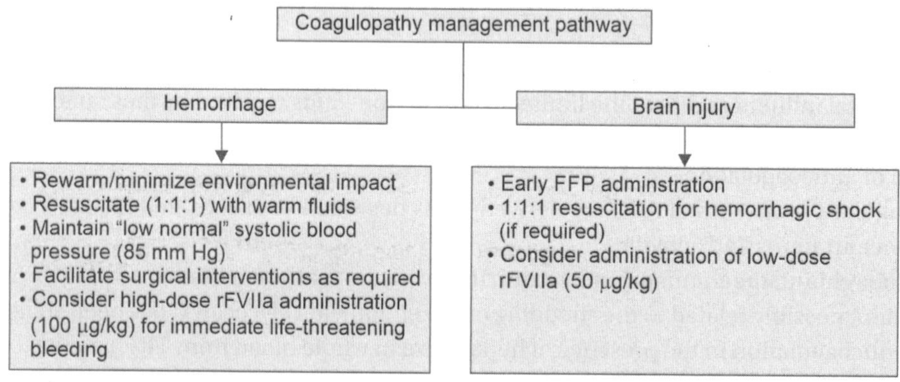

(rFVIIa: recombinant activated factor VII; FFP: fresh frozen plasma)

Blood Transfusion

LEARNING OBJECTIVES

- Blood component separation and their role in surgery
- Blood substitutes
- How will assess the amount of blood loss in surgical practice?
- Changes in stored blood
- Autologous blood transfusion
- Allogenic blood transfusion
- Massive blood transfusion
- Platelet-rich plasma
- Complications of blood transfusion
- TRALI

BLOOD COMPONENTS

1. Blood component separation and their role in surgery. ***WBUHS 2015, 2022, Rajiv Gandhi Institute of Health Sciences 2019***

2. Role of blood components in surgery. ***WBUHS 2016***

Anticoagulants Preservative Solutions

- Anticoagulants prevent blood clotting
- Preservatives provide nutrients for cells
- *Heparin:*
  - Rarely if ever used anymore
  - Anticoagulant ONLY
  - Transfuse within 48 hours, preferably 8

Anticoagulants

	CPD or CP2-D	CPD-A1
Storage time	21 days	35 days
Temperature	1–6°C	1–6°C
	Slows glycolytic activity	
Adenine	None	Substrate for ATP synthesis
Volume	450 ± 10%	
Dextrose	Supports ATP generation by glycolytic pathway	
Citrate	Prevents coagulation by binding calcium	

(ATP: adenosine triphosphate; CPD: citrate–phosphate–dextrose; CPDA-1: CPD-adenine; CP2D: citrate–phosphate–double dextrose)

Additive Solution (AS)

- Primary bag with satellite bags attached
- One bag has AS
- Unit drawn into citrate-phosphate-dextrose (CPD) anticoagulant
- Remove platelet-rich plasma (PRP) within 72 hours
- *Add AS to red blood cells (RBCs), ADSOL, which consists of:*
    - Saline
    - Adenine
    - Glucose
    - Mannitol
- Extends storage to 42 days
- Final hematocrit approximately 66%

Changes Occur during Storage

Shelf life = expiration date

- At end of expiration must have 75% recovery
- At least 75% of transfused cells remain in circulation 24 hours after transfusion

Storage Lesion

- Biochemical changes which occur at 1–6°C
- Affects oxygen dissociation curve, increased affinity of hemoglobin for oxygen
    - Low 2,3-diphosphoglycerate (2,3-DPG), increased O_2 affinity, less O_2 released
    - pH drops causes 2,3-DPG levels to fall
    - Once transfused RBCs regenerate adenosine triphosphate (ATP) and 2,3-DPG
- Few functional platelets present
- Viable (living) RBCs decrease
- Significant for infants and massive transfusion
- Summary of biochemical changes
    - pH decreases
    - 2,3-DPG decreases
    - ATP decreases
    - Potassium increases
    - Sodium decreases
    - Plasma hemoglobin increases

Preparation of Components

- Collect unit within 15 minutes to prevent activation of coagulation system
- Draw into closed system—primary bag with satellite bags with hermetic seal between
- If hermetic seal broken transfuse within 24 hours if stored at 1–4°C, 4 hours if stored at 20–24°C
- Centrifuge—light spin, platelets suspended
- Remove PRP
- Centrifuge PRP heavy spin
- Remove platelet poor plasma
- Freeze plasma solid within 8 hours
- Thaw plasma at 1–4°C—precipitate forms
- Centrifuge, express plasma leaving cryoprecipitate (CRYO); store both at –18°C
- RBCs-CPD—21 days, ADSOL—42 days—1–6°C

One unit of whole blood can produce:
- Packed red blood cells (PRBCs)
- Fresh frozen plasma (FFP)
- CRYO
- Single donor plasma (SDP)—CYRO removed
- Platelets

- *Sterile docking device joins tubing:*
  - Used to add satellite bags to maintain original expiration of component
  - May be used to pool components

Quality control:
- Requires certain number of blood products to be tested at regular intervals
- Usually 4 per month
- Must ensure product preparation results in a component that meets the regulatory agencies guidelines for number or quantity
- Blood separated into components to specifically treat patients with product needed
- *Advantages of component separation:*
  - Allow optimum survival of each component
  - Transfuse only component needed

Transfusion practice:
- Transfusion requires doctor's prescription
- All components MUST be administered through a filter
- Infuse quickly, within 4 hours
- D (Rh)-negative require D-negative cellular products
- ABO identical preferred, ABO compatible can be used
- "Universal donor"—RBCs group O, plasma AB

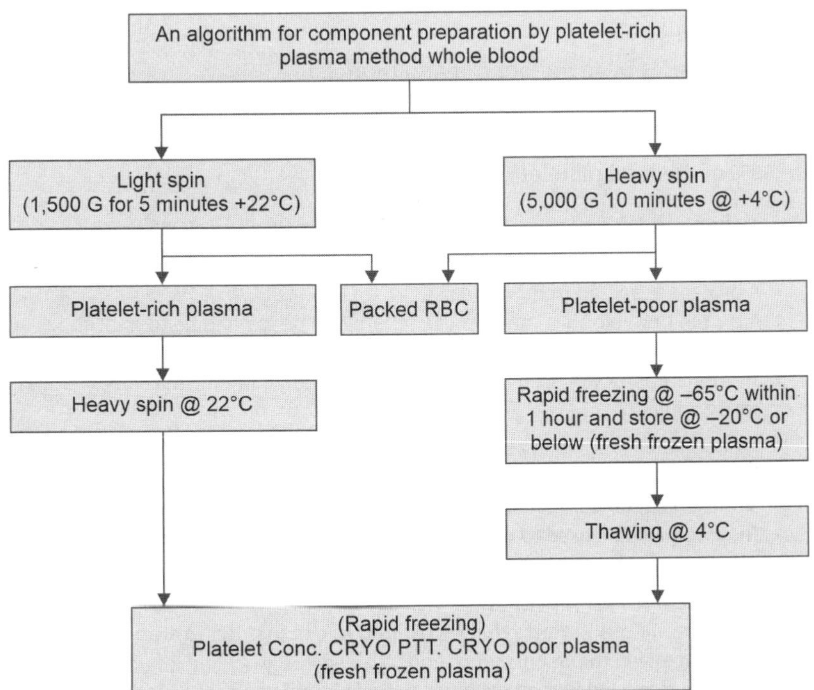

(CRYO: cryoprecipitate; PTT: partial thromboplastin time; RBC: red blood cell)

Buffy Coat Method

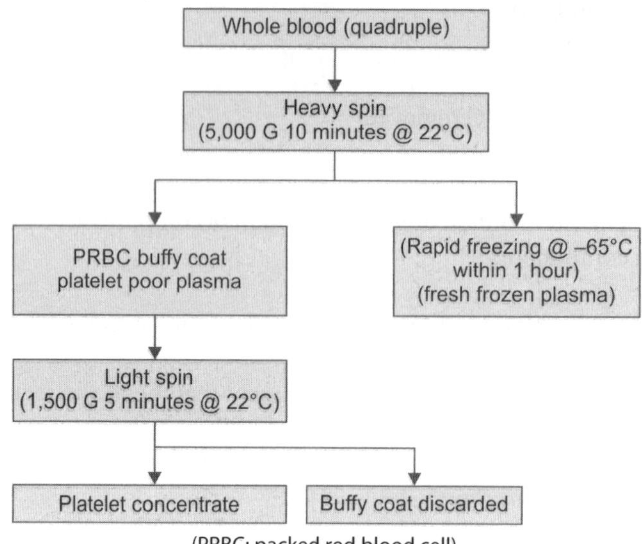

(PRBC: packed red blood cell)

- Whole blood is collected into 350 mL or 450 mL double/triple/quadruple or penta bags containing CPD-adenine (CPDA-1) or supplement solution.
- After blood collection, the components must be separated within 5–8 hours.
- The composition room must be a separate disinfected room.
- All precautions must be taken to avoid contamination of erythrocytes, such as tapping the ends of the segment, proper balancing of opposite bags, following the standard programs, and protocols described in the cold centrifuge manufacturer's manual.
- The program is basically run in two rounds with a heavy spin (e.g., 5,000 G for 10–15 minutes) and a light spin (e.g., 1,500 G for 5–7 minutes).
- Heavy and light rotation varies by manufacturer and model.
- Here "G" is the relative centrifugal force calculated from revolutions per minute (RPM) and rotor length.
- The use of a fully automatic component separator enables the production of small volumes of buffy coat (BC) with a recovery of 90% of the total platelets.

Whole blood	**Fractions**
Plasma	*Albumin:* Up to 4% of plasma • A protein extracted from plasma • Albumin from blood is sometimes used in volume expanders to treat shock and severe burns • These preparations may contain up to 25% albumin • Minute amounts are used in the formation of many other medicines, including some formulations of erythropoietin *Immunoglobulins:* Up to 3% of plasma • Protein fractions that may be used in some medicines that fight viruses and diseases, such as diphtheria, tetanus, viral hepatitis and rabies • They may also be used to guard against some medical conditions that threaten the life of a developing baby and to counteract the effects of snake or spider venom *Clotting factors:* <1% of plasma • There are various proteins that help blood to clot in order to stop bleeding • Some are given to patients who tend to bleed easily • They are also used in medical glues to seal wounds and stop bleeding after surgery • One combination of clotting factors is known as cryoprecipitate • Some clotting factors are now made from nonblood sources

Contd....

Contd....

Whole blood	***Fractions***
Red blood cells	*Hemoglobin:* 33% of red blood cells • It is a protein that transports oxygen throughout the body and carbon dioxide to the lungs • Products being developed from human or animal hemoglobin could be used to treat patients with acute anemia or massive blood loss *Hemin:* <2% of red blood cells • An enzyme inhibitor derived from hemoglobin that is used to treat a group of rare genetic blood disorders (known as porphyria) that affect the digestive, nervous, and circulatory systems
White blood cells	*Interferons:* These are a tiny fraction of white blood cells • Protein that fights certain viral infections and cancers • Most interferons are not derived from blood • Some are made from fractions of human white blood cells
Platelets	At present, no fractions from platelets are being isolated for direct use in medical treatment

Role of Components

Suggested Transfusion Guidelines for Plasma

- Treatment of multiple or specific coagulation factor deficiency with an abnormal prothrombin time and/or activated partial thromboplastin time (PTT)
- *Abnormal specific factor deficiency in the presence of one of the following:*
  - Congenital deficiency of antithrombin III; prothrombin; factors V, VII, IX, X, and XI; protein C or S; plasminogen or antiplasmin
  - Acquired deficiency related to warfarin therapy, vitamin K deficiency, liver disease, massive transfusion, or disseminated intravascular coagulation
  - Also indicated as prophylaxis for the above if a surgical/invasive procedure is planned
- *Unwarranted indications:*
  - Empirical use during massive transfusion if the patient does not exhibit clinical coagulopathy
  - Volume replacement
  - Nutritional supplement
  - Hypoalbuminemia

CRYO

It is useful in treating factor deficiency (hemophilia A), von Willebrand's disease, and hypofibrinogenemia and may help treat uremic bleeding. Each 5- to 15-mL unit contains >80 units of factor VIII and about 200 mg of fibrinogen. CRYO is usually administered as a transfusion of 10 single units.

Suggested Transfusion Guidelines for RBCs

- Hemoglobin <8 g/dL or acute blood loss in an otherwise healthy patient with signs and symptoms of decreased oxygen delivery and two or more of the following:
  - Estimated or anticipated acute blood loss of >15% of total blood volume (750 mL in a 70-kg male)
  - Diastolic blood pressure <60 mm Hg
  - Systolic blood pressure drop >30 mm Hg from baseline
  - Tachycardia (>100 beats/min)
  - Oliguria/anuria
  - Mental status changes
- Hemoglobin <10 g/dL in patients with a known increased risk for coronary artery disease or pulmonary insufficiency who have sustained or are expected to sustain significant blood loss
- *Symptomatic anemia with any of the following:*
  - Tachycardia (>100 beats/min)
  - Mental status changes

  - Evidence of myocardial ischemia, including angina
  - Shortness of breath or dizziness with mild exertion
  - Orthostatic hypotension
- *Unfounded/questionable indications:*
  - To increase wound healing
  - To improve the patient's sense of well-being
  - Hemoglobin between 7 and 10 g/dL (or hematocrit from 21 to 30%) in an otherwise stable, asymptomatic patient
  - Mere availability of predonated autologous blood without medical indication.

Granulocyte transfusions have been used for profound granulocytopenia (<500/mm^3) with evidence of infection (e.g., positive blood culture, persistent temperature higher than 38.5°C) unresponsive to antibiotic therapy. Daily transfusions are given until the infection is under control or the granulocyte count is greater than 1,000/mm^3.

Indications for Leukocyte-reduced Blood Components

- To decrease the incidence of subsequent refractoriness to platelet transfusion caused by human leukocyte antigens (HLA) alloimmunization in patients requiring long-term platelet support
- To provide blood components with reduced risk for transmission of cytomegalovirus (CMV)
- To prevent subsequent febrile nonhemolytic transfusion reactions in patients who have had one documented episode
- To decrease the incidence of HLA alloimmunization in nonhepatic solid-organ transplant candidates

Platelet Transfusions

Indications: Platelet transfusions are used to control bleeding that is caused by thrombocytopenia or platelet dysfunction and to prevent spontaneous bleeding in situations of severe thrombocytopenia.

Suggested Transfusion Guidelines for Platelets

- Recent (within 24 hours) platelet count <10,000/mm^3 (for prophylaxis)
- Recent (within 24 hours) platelet count <50,000/mm^3 with demonstrated microvascular bleeding ("oozing") or a planned surgical/invasive procedure
- Demonstrated microvascular bleeding and a precipitous fall in the platelet count
- Adult patients in the operating room who have had complicated procedures or have required >10 units of blood *and* have microvascular bleeding; giving platelets assumes that adequate surgical hemostasis has been achieved
- Documented platelet dysfunction (e.g., prolonged bleeding time >15 minutes; abnormal platelet function tests) with petechiae, purpura, microvascular bleeding ("oozing"), or a surgical/invasive procedure
- *Unwarranted indications:*
  - Empirical use with massive transfusion when the patient is not exhibiting clinically evident microvascular bleeding
  - Prophylaxis in patients with thrombotic thrombocytopenic purpura/hemolytic-uremic syndrome or idiopathic thrombocytopenic purpura
  - Extrinsic platelet dysfunction (e.g., renal failure, von Willebrand's disease).

Use of Anticoagulants

Principles and indications: Anticoagulation is used to prevent and treat thrombosis and thromboembolic events. The risk of thromboembolic and bleeding complications caused by anticoagulants should be carefully considered before starting therapy.

- *Special indications for anticoagulant therapy:*
  - Atrial fibrillation
  - Mechanical heart valve prostheses

- Venous thromboembolism
- Prevention of stroke
- Acute occlusion of an artery or graft

- *Heparin:*
  - Unfractionated heparin [molecular weight (MW) 10,000–20,000] increases the effect of AT, resulting in more rapid inhibition of thrombin, factor Xa, and other coagulation proteases.
  - Low-molecular-weight heparin (LMWH) formulations (enoxaparin, dalteparin and tinzaparin) are depolymerized to give 3,000–7,000 Daltons.
  - The anticoagulant effect of LMWH is largely due to inhibition of factor Xa, and LMWH inhibits thrombin less than unfractionated heparin.
- *Direct thrombin inhibitors* are a class of compounds that bind to free and fibrin-bound thrombin. These substances prevent the activation of thrombin coagulation factors, fibrin formation, and platelet aggregation.
  - *Hirudin:* An anticoagulant originally derived from leeches and formulated as lepirudin and bivalirudin.
  - *Lepirudin:* Recombinant hirudin, which binds irreversibly to thrombin and provides effective anticoagulation
  - *Bivalirudin:* It is a truncated form of recombinant hirudin that targets only the thrombin active site.
  - *Argatroban:* It is a synthetic thrombin inhibitor that is also approved for the treatment of heparin- induced thrombocytopenia (HIT). The treatment is done under the supervision of PTT. Elimination is primarily hepatic and should be used with caution in patients with hepatic impairment.

Fibrinolytic Therapy

- *Indications and contraindications:*
  - Thrombolytic therapy is most often used for iliofemoral deep venous thrombosis (DVT), superior vena caval thrombosis, pulmonary embolism (PE) resulting in a hemodynamically unstable patient, acute thrombosis of peripheral, mesenteric and coronary arteries, acute vascular graft occlusion, thrombosis of hemodialysis access grafts, and occlusion of venous catheters. Dosage depends on the agent and the indication.
  - Tissue plasminogen activator (alteplase) or recombinant analog (reteplase) and urokinase (abbokinase) are used to break up catheter, and venous and peripheral arterial thrombi.

Transfusion Products for Coagulopathy

- FFP contains all clotting factors. However, factors V and VIII are not necessarily stable during the thawing process and cannot be reliably recovered from FFP.
- Therefore, it can be used to correct coagulopathies due to any other coagulation factor deficiency and is particularly useful when multiple factor deficiencies are present (e.g., liver disease or massive transfusion).
- The effect of FFP is immediate and usually lasts about 6 hours. Factor VIII and IX deficiencies are best treated with special factor concentrates.

Contraindications to Fibrinolytic Therapy

- *Absolute contraindications:*
  - Intolerable ischemia (for arterial thrombosis)
  - Active bleeding (not including menses)
  - Recent (<2 months) stroke or neurosurgical procedure
  - Intracranial pathology such as neoplasm
- *Relative contraindications:*
  - Recent (<10 days) major surgery, major trauma, parturition, or organ biopsy
  - Active peptic ulcer or recent gastrointestinal bleeding (within 2 weeks)
  - Uncontrolled hypertension (blood pressure >180/110 mm Hg)
  - Recent cardiopulmonary resuscitation
  - Presence or high likelihood of left heart thrombus
  - Bacterial endocarditis

- Coagulopathy or current use of warfarin
- Pregnancy
- Hemorrhagic diabetic retinopathy
- *Recombinant human factor VIIa (rhFVIIa):*
  - Mainly used in patients with hemophilia or factor VIII inhibitors
  - The use of RhFVIIa in blunt trauma patients requiring massive transfusions has been shown to reduce total transfusion requirements.
  - Its use also tended to reduce the incidence of multiple organ failure and acute respiratory distress syndrome (ARDS).

BLOOD SUBSTITUTES

3. Blood substitutes. ***WBUHS 2011, RIMS, Imphal 2012***

4. Changes in stored blood. ***WBUHS 2021***

5. What are the changes that occur in store blood? Write in short on blood substitute. ***WBUHS 2023***

Changes that Occur in Stored Blood

- Increased K^+ ions in plasma (Na-K pump inhibited by cold)
- Decrease dextrose and changed to lactic acid
- Decrease platelet count
- RBCs are swollen and become spherical
- Decrease clotting factors VII, VIII, IX
- Decrease 2,3-DPG leads to decrease oxygen supply to the cell which results in hypoxia.

A blood substitute (also called artificial blood or blood surrogates) is a substance used to mimic and fulfill some functions of biological blood, usually in the oxygen-carrying sense. It aims to provide an alternative to blood transfusion, which is transferring blood or blood-based products from one person into another.

First-generation Blood Substitute

- The main categories of such oxygen-carrying blood substitutes are hemoglobin-based oxygen carriers (HBOC) and perfluorocarbon-based oxygen carriers (PFBOC).
- An oxygen-carrying blood substitute, sometimes called artificial hemoglobin, is an artificially made RBC substitute whose main function is to carry oxygen, as natural hemoglobin.
  - The use of oxygen-carrying blood substitutes is often called oxygen therapeutics to differentiate from true blood substitutes.
  - The initial goal of oxygen-carrying blood substitutes is merely to mimic blood's oxygen transport capacity.
  - There is additional longer range research on true artificial RBCs and white blood cells (WBCs) which could theoretically compose a blood substitute with higher fidelity to human blood.
- There are two basic approaches to constructing an oxygen therapeutic.
  1. The first is perfluorocarbons (PFC), chemical compounds which can carry and release oxygen. The specific PFC usually used is perfluorodecalin.
  2. The second is hemoglobin derived from humans, animals, or artificially via recombinant technology.

Stroma-free Hemoglobin

- Stroma-free hemoglobin has been investigated as an oxygen carrier since the 1940s, when researchers realized that native hemoglobin is not antigenic. A solution containing stroma-free hemoglobin has many advantages over RBCs, including the ability to withstand sterilization and a shelf life of approximately 2 years at room temperature for some products.

- Solutions of acellular hemoglobin are not as effective at oxygenation as PRBCs because of their high affinity for oxygen. RBCs have adapted to release oxygen at an oxygen half saturation pressure of hemoglobin (p50) of approximately 26.5 mm Hg. This is due to the allosteric effect of 2,3-bisphosphoglycerate (2,3-BPG), which shifts the oxyhemoglobin dissociation curve to the right. In the absence of 2,3-BPG, stroma-free hemoglobin has a p50 of 12–14 mm Hg.
- Unmodified free hemoglobin, when infused rapidly, splits into dimers and is cleared by glomerular filtration and uptake by the reticuloendothelial system.
  - When free hemoglobin was used initially, it caused a substantial increase in oncotic pressure because of its hyperosmolarity.
  - Unfortunately, the initial attempts at transfusing stroma-free hemoglobin produced renal dysfunction, coagulopathy, and hypertension.
  - Several approaches have been tried to decrease the avidity with which hemoglobin binds to oxygen.
  - These adaptations include the addition of organic phosphate to serve the function of 2,3-BPG and ATP, cross-linking dimers of hemoglobin tetramers and polymerizing the tetramers to decrease oncotic pressure and prevent glomerular filtration.
  - Hypertension has remained a significant adverse effect of stroma-free hemoglobin.
- Diaspirin cross-linked hemoglobin (DCLHb) is the prototype molecule of this category of blood substitutes. It consists of cross-linking between the two alpha chains that lend stability to the molecule. The cross-linking agent is bis(dibromosalicyl) fumarate (DBBF). DCLHb made from outdated human blood has a shelf life of approximately 9 months when frozen and 24 hours when refrigerated. The intravascular half-life is 2–12 hours and is dose-dependent.

Next-generation Blood Substitutes

- Polyethylene glycol (PEG) hemoglobin was a conjugated bovine hemoglobin that was evaluated for use in cancer therapy to increase tumor oxygenation and enhance the efficacy of radiation and chemotherapy. However, at present, production of this product has been discontinued.
- Hemospan also known as MP4OX, is a PEG-conjugated human hemoglobin currently undergoing clinical trials in the US and Europe. At relatively low concentrations, Hemospan (MP4OX) is capable of transporting large amounts of oxygen.
- Pyridoxylated hemoglobin-polyoxyethylene conjugate (PHP) is a conjugated hemoglobin developed by Apex Biosciences that completed a phase III trial in August 2009 in patients with shock associated with systemic inflammatory response syndrome.

For HBOC cross-linked with enzymes, there has been an effort to synthesize compounds that not only perform the function of carrying oxygen, as do the molecules mentioned previously, but also harbor some of the enzyme activity that normal RBCs possess. Polymerized hemoglobin has been cross-linked with catalase and superoxide dismutase to form a compound that in animal models can not only carry oxygen but also remove oxygen radicals that are responsible for ischemia reperfusion injuries.

- Polyhemoglobin has also been cross-linked with tyrosinase to form a soluble complex that can carry oxygen and decrease the systemic levels of tyrosine. This agent can help to increase the efficacy of chemotherapy and radiation therapy in tumor tissue and in a melanoma model has been shown to delay tumor growth without having significant adverse effects.
  - The ultimate RBC substitute would contain not only hemoglobin but also other contents of the RBC also encapsulated in an artificial membrane.
  - However, production of such a product would be extremely challenging.
  - Efforts have been made to use polylactide, a biodegradable polymer that is converted to lactic acid in the body, to create artificial RBCs.
  - These cells contain hemoglobin along with the RBC enzyme complement including superoxide dismutase, methemoglobin reductase, and catalase.

Potential uses:

- If such a blood substitute were indeed developed, it would presumably play a major role in the setting of trauma care and for elective surgeries.
- It would also benefit patients with medical conditions who are in need of long-term blood transfusions, such as patients with myelodysplastic syndrome and aplastic anemia.
- These products could also be used as organ preservatives to prevent or decrease reperfusion injury to donor organs.
- Religious and ethnic groups with concerns regarding the use of human-derived blood products may accept these substances, which would provide a significant patient care advance.

Adverse effects:

- Adverse effects associated with HBOC include hypertension, abdominal pain, skin rash, diarrhea, jaundice, hemoglobinuria, oliguria, fever, and stroke.
- Laboratory anomalies such as an elevation in lipase levels.
- Although most of these side effects were transient and clinically asymptomatic, many clinical trials involving these agents have been discontinued or held due to the associated adverse effects.

ASSESSMENT AND MEASUREMENT OF BLOOD LOSS

6. How will assess the amount of blood loss in surgical practice? ***WBUHS 2021***

Methods of Determining Acute Blood Loss

Assessment of blood loss must be related to the preexisting circulating blood volume, which can be derived from the patient's weight:

- Infant 80–85 mL/kg
- Adult 65–75 mL/kg

Measuring Blood Loss

- *Blood clots:* The size of a fist is approximately 500 mL.
- *Swelling in case of closed fracture:* Moderate swelling in case of closed tibial fracture corresponds to 500–1,500 mL of blood loss. Moderate swelling in a fractured femoral shaft corresponds to 500–2,000 mL of blood loss.
- *Weighing swabs:* In the operating room, blood loss can be measured by weighing tampons after use and subtracting their dry weight. The total amount obtained (1 g = 1 mL) is added to the amount of blood collected in the suction or drainage bottles. In extensive wounds and surgeries, blood loss is greatly under-estimated because water evaporates from the swab samples before each batch is weighed. Rapid transfer of discarded tampons into polythene bags reduces this source of error.
    - For operations such as radical mastectomy or partial gastrectomy, it may be necessary to multiply the total weight of the tampon by a factor of 1.5.
    - For prolonged surgery on larger wounds, such as abdominal-thoracic or abdominal surgery, it may be necessary to multiply the measurement total by two.
- *Hemoglobin level:* This is estimated g/100 mL (g/dL), normal values are 12–16 g/100 mL (12–16 g/dL). Bleeding does not change immediately, but after a few hours the level decreases as interstitial fluid flows into the vascular compartment to restore blood volume.
- *Measurement of central venous pressure:* Continuous measurement of tissue oxygen tension.

STORED BLOOD

7. Changes in stored blood.

General

- Whole blood contains RBC, plasma, proteins, coagulation factors, WBC, platelets, electrolytes, dissolved gases.
- Additives to donated whole blood are aimed at prolonging the shelf life before transfusion, and minimized degradation of blood product during storage.

Additives

- *Anticoagulant:* CDP; CPDA-1
- SAG-M (saline-adenine-glucose-mannitol)
- *ADSOL:*
  - Adenine prolongs shelf life to 35 days (energy substrate)
  - Citrate →↓Ca^{2+} (anticoagulate blood)
  - Phosphate buffers pH
  - Glucose/dextrose for Embden-Meyerhof glycolysis pathway

Storage temperature: 4°C to ↓metabolic activity of RBC, ↓bacterial colonization

Time for storage: 28 days—measured as the maximum storage time which allowed the survival of >70% of RBC 24 hours after infusion.

Changes with Storage

- RBCs undergo a series of biochemical fluctuations during 35–42-day storage period at 1°–6°C. The sodium/potassium pump is immobilized causing a decrease in intracellular potassium with an increase in cytoplasmic sodium levels, glucose levels decline, and acidosis occurs as a result of low pH levels.
- Blood bank storage resulted in: ↓ Na^+, Cl^-, 2,3-DPG and ATP—↑ lactate, pyruvate, ammonia, plasma HB, intracellular Na, phosphate
- *2,3-DPG and ATP:*
  - During the first 3 weeks of storage the content of 2,3-DPG and ATP decreases.
  - In the presence of adenosine the concentration of 2,3-DPG is maintained for periods up to 6 weeks at 4°C. On reincubation at 37°C after storage for 3 weeks at 4°C, red cells lose their ability to utilize glucose.
  - This can be restored by adenosine; the ability to utilize glucose appears to be related to levels of ATP within the cell.
  - Restoration can occur after 6 weeks of storage in the presence of adenosine.
- *Effect of storage on RBC function:* One of the RBC's principal functions is O_2 delivery; increases in O_2 affinity in stored RBCs, reflecting progressive decreases in 2,3-DPG over the weeks of storage; O_2 delivery by stored RBCs is deficient even early after processing and before significant decline in 2,3-DPG.

White Blood Cell

- Granulocytes lose phagocytic and bactericidal properties within 4–6 hours of collection
- Antigenic properties maintained

Platelets

- Nonfunctional within 48 hours of blood stored at 4°C
- Change shape from discoid → spherical

Factor V and VIII

Decrease with storage:

- Factor V → ↓by 50% at 21 days
- Factor VIII → exponential decrease to 75% at 24 hours → 30% after 21 days

Biochemical Changes

- ↓ATP: Energy substrate derived from adenine; glucose/dextrose
- Levels fall with time in storage, slower than ↓2,3-DPG, ↑K^+: Progressive impairment of Na^+/K^+ ATPase results in ↓RBC K^+ →↑extracellular K^+ → ~30 mmol/L at 28 days
- ↑Lactate
- ↓Na^+
- ↓Ca^{2+}
- ↓Glucose
- ↓pH → 6.8 at 28 days
- Free Hb: RBC lysis in storage →↑free Hb →haptoglobin/hemopexin (mop-ups) saturable
- 1.7% at collection → 30% at 28 days

Bacteria

- 3/1,000 contaminated by bacteria
- *Pseudomonas* species/*Yersinia enterocolitica* can proliferate at 4°C

Immunity

- Microaggregates cause binding of fibronectin and ↓macrophage activity and altered antigen presenting capability.
- Much of the stored blood may lack a component vital for it to deliver oxygen to the tissues. Nitric oxide, which helps keep blood vessels open, begins breaking down as soon as blood goes into storage.
- Total Hb-bound NO and SNO-Hb decreased markedly from 0 hour (fresh RBCs) to 3 hours.

"Banked blood is truly a national treasure that needs to be protected. It can be life-saving, and in some cases, it may be making things worse. In principle, a solution to the nitric oxide problem, to put it back, needs to be proven in a clinical trial."

ALLOGENIC BLOOD TRANSFUSION

8. Discuss the classification, indications and complications of allogeneic blood transfusion. ***WBUHS 2025***

Classification of Allogeneic Blood Transfusion

Allogeneic blood transfusion refers to the transfusion of blood or blood components *donated by another individual.*

Based on Blood Component Transfused:

Component	*Description*
Whole blood	Contains red cells, plasma, platelets, and clotting factors. Rarely used today
Packed red blood cells (PRBCs)	Used to increase oxygen-carrying capacity
Platelets	For prevention/treatment of bleeding due to thrombocytopenia
Fresh frozen plasma (FFP)	Contains all clotting factors; used in coagulopathies
Cryoprecipitate	Rich in fibrinogen, factor VIII, vWF; used in DIC, hemophilia A, etc.
Leukocyte-reduced Blood	Filters out most white blood cells; reduces febrile reactions and alloimmunization
Irradiated blood products	Prevents transfusion-associated graft-vs-host disease (TA-GVHD)
Washed red cells	Removes plasma proteins; used in IgA deficiency or allergic reactions

Indications of Allogeneic Blood Transfusion

Packed RBCs

- Symptomatic anemia (Hb <7–8 g/dL or as clinically indicated)
- Acute blood loss (e.g., trauma, surgery)
- Chronic anemia unresponsive to other treatments (e.g., renal failure)

Platelets

- Platelet count <10,000/μL (prophylaxis)
- <50,000/μL before invasive procedures or active bleeding
- Platelet dysfunction (e.g., due to antiplatelet drugs)

Fresh Frozen Plasma (FFP)

- Coagulation factor deficiencies (e.g., liver disease, DIC)
- Reversal of warfarin (when prothrombin complex not available)
- Massive transfusion protocols

Cryoprecipitate

- Hypofibrinogenemia (<100 mg/dL)
- von Willebrand disease (when specific concentrates unavailable)
- Hemophilia A (in emergencies)

Complications of Allogeneic Blood Transfusion

A. Acute Complications (Within 24 Hours)

Complication	Cause	Features
Hemolytic transfusion reaction (Acute)	ABO incompatibility	Fever, chills, back pain, hemoglobinuria, renal failure
Febrile non-hemolytic reaction	Cytokines from donor WBCs	Fever, chills (most common reaction)
Allergic reaction (mild to anaphylaxis)	Reaction to plasma proteins	Urticaria to severe hypotension, bronchospasm
Transfusion-related acute lung injury (TRALI)	Donor anti-leukocyte antibodies	Non-cardiogenic pulmonary edema, dyspnea, hypoxia
Septic reaction	Bacterial contamination (esp. platelets)	Fever, chills, hypotension, shock
Transfusion-associated circulatory overload (TACO)	Rapid transfusion volume	Hypertension, dyspnea, pulmonary edema

B. Delayed Complications (Days to Weeks Later)

Complication	Cause	Features
Delayed hemolytic reaction	Minor antigen incompatibility	Mild anemia, jaundice
Alloimmunization	Development of antibodies to donor antigens	Future transfusion complications
Iron overload (hemosiderosis)	Multiple transfusions	Organ dysfunction (liver, heart, pancreas)
Graft-vs-host disease (TA-GVHD)	Donor lymphocytes attack host	Fever, rash, pancytopenia (often fatal)
Infectious disease transmission	HIV, HBV, HCV, syphilis, malaria, etc.	Variable, depends on pathogen

AUTOLOGOUS BLOOD TRANSFUSION

9. Autologous blood transfusion. *WBUHS 2021*

10. Discuss different types of Autologous Blood Transfusion. *WBUHS 2022*

Autotransfusion

It is a process of collecting a patient's own shed blood, cleaning it, and giving back the washed RBCs.

Autologous Blood

Blood donated and received by the same person.

Types of Autologous Blood Transfusion

- *Autologous (acute) normovolemic hemodilution:*
  - This technique involves collecting a patient's blood (2–4 units) into anticoagulant-containing storage bags at the outset of surgery, accompanied by intravenous replacement with crystalloids or colloids to maintain normovolemia.
  - The patient's whole blood can then be transfused later in the case as needed. The evidence on the overall efficacy of autologous normovolemic hemodilution is conflicting with respect to blood savings and transfusion avoidance, but it appears to be safe and efficacious in centers that make routine use of this technique.
- *Preoperative autologous donation:*
  - In general, preoperative autologous donation limits (but does not eliminate) the infectious, immunologic, and hemolytic complications of allogeneic blood transfusion. Although accepted by patients and many surgeons, preoperative autologous donation is encumbered by unexpected disadvantages.
  - These disadvantages include patient inconvenience and the cost of processing the blood. Because many patients require no blood, up to one third of collected units are discarded.
  - Patients are frequently rendered anemic at the time of their operation, increasing the likelihood that transfusion will be necessary. Even though these patients would be transfused with their own blood, risk is still present.
  - The most common cause of hemolytic transfusion reactions is clerical error, and predonated blood is not exempt. Changes in blood during storage may render patients susceptible to complications, such as TRALI (transfusion-related acute lung injury), even if the transfused blood is their own.
- *Intraoperative autotransfusion/cell salvage:*
  - Cell salvage is an effective method of transfusion avoidance. Shed blood is collected from the operative field and mixed with an anticoagulant. It is concentrated and washed or filtered, then returned to the patient.
  - Harmful contaminants, such as potassium, fat, and free hemoglobin, are removed from the salvaged blood; the washed blood is returned via a 40-μm blood filter. Blood obtained from the thoracic cavity via chest tubes in a closed system can be processed and autotransfused in a similar manner. However, this is much less frequently done.
  - Relative contraindications to cell salvage include the following: malignancy, bacterial contamination of the surgical site, cesarean delivery, and sickle cell disease.
  - However, improvements in processing, particularly the use of leukocyte-depletion filters, have made cell salvage possible in anecdotal cases complicated by the contraindications described above and are supported by in vitro data.
  - Nonetheless, most practitioners still hew to the existing guidelines for the use of scavenged blood.

Benefits of Autotransfusion

- Lower risk of clerical error
- Significant reduction in blood-borne infection

- Fresh RBCs
- Better oxygen transfer
- More cost-effective medicine

Mechanism of Autotransfusion

- As bleeding starts to occur, blood is collected through a suction line and collected in a sterile reservoir. The collected blood is then washed with a specialized instrument to remove contaminants and debris. This washed blood can now be safely returned to the patient, thus decreasing the risk and need for banked blood.
- By collecting all of the patients' blood that was lost, the patient is able to avoid complications associated with blood bank transfusions and can get on the right track to a healthy recovery

Autotransfusion can be utilized in many other surgical procedures including:

- Cardiothoracic surgery
- Vascular surgery
- Orthopedic surgery
- General surgery
- Gynecological surgery
- Urological procedures
- Trauma
- Organ transplantation procedures
- Selected neurosurgical procedures.

MASSIVE BLOOD TRANSFUSION

11. Write down the definition, complications and management of massive blood transfusion. ***WBUHS 2022***

12. How do you prevent and manage complications of massive blood transfusion?
WBUHS 2018, RIMS, Imphal 2022

Massive transfusion is defined as the transfusion of blood products that are greater in volume than a patient's normal circulating blood volume in a period of <24 hours.

This creates several risks not encountered with a lesser volume or rate of transfusion.

- *Coagulopathy* might arise as a result of platelet or coagulation factor depletion. This has led to the use of transfusion ratios in the trauma setting that involve the transfusion of platelets and FFP in concert with PRBCs.
- *Hypothermia* can result from massive volume resuscitation with chilled blood products but can be prevented by using blood warmers. Hypothermia can lead to cardiac dysrhythmias and coagulopathy.
- *Citrate toxicity* can develop after massive transfusion in patients with hepatic dysfunction. Hypocalcemia can be treated with intravenous administration of 10% calcium gluconate.
- Electrolyte abnormalities, including acidosis and hyperkalemia, can rarely occur after massive transfusions, especially in patients with preexisting hyperkalemia.

Many centers have established *massive transfusion protocols (MTPs)* which make use of these ratios. Although no definitive ratios are standardized, ratios of 1:1 or 1:2 FFP: PRBC are common.

The algorithm for MTP at Barnes-Jewish Hospital is shown below: In it, prepacked boxes serve to maintain the proper ratio of clotting factor and platelets to RBCs during situations requiring rapid volume expansion. Additionally, they remove confusion and human error that may result when actively calculating proper ratios during an emergency.

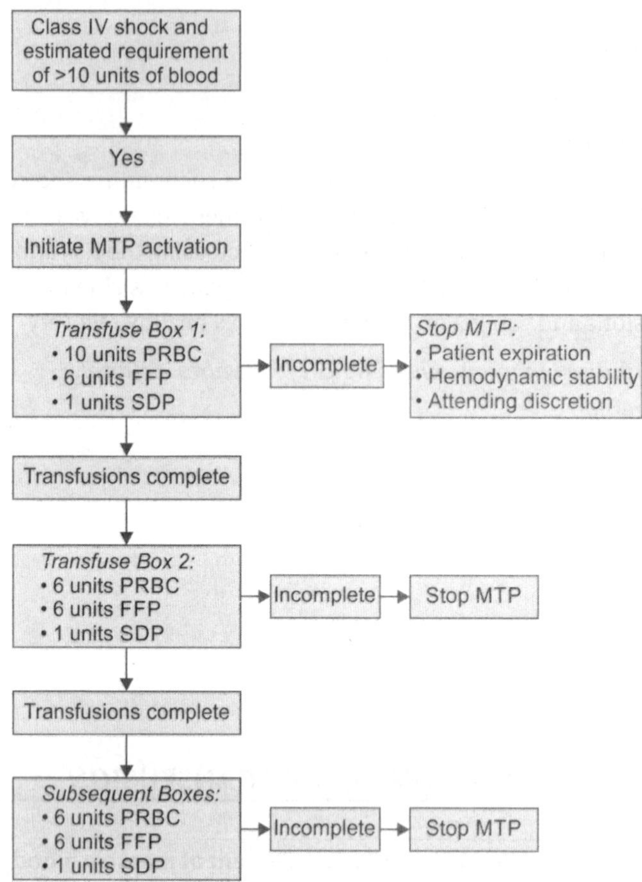

(FFP: fresh frozen plasma; MTP: massive transfusion protocol; PRBC: packed red blood cell; SDP: single donor plasma)

Complications

- Complications of massive transfusion include metabolic and hemostatic abnormalities, immune hemolysis and air embolism which can result in a patient presenting with cardiac arrhythmia or cardiac arrest.
- Massive transfusion is an independent risk factor for developing multi-organ failure.
- *The complications associated with massive transfusion are dependent on the following factors:*
  - Number of units transfused
  - Rate of transfusion
  - Patient factors
- *Some of the complications of massive transfusion include:*
  - Hypothermia
  - Dilutional coagulopathy
  - Hypocalcemia, hypomagnesemia, citrate toxicity
  - Metabolic acidosis
  - Hyperkalemia
  - Air embolism

Prevention of Complications

- All efforts should be initiated to avoid RBC transfusion in patients at risk for acute lung injury (ALI) and ARDS after completion of resuscitation (level 2)
- All efforts should be made to diagnose and report (TRALI) to the blood bank because it has emerged as a leading cause of transfusion associated morbidity and mortality, despite underdiagnosis and underreporting (level 2)

- Blood warmers should be used as the rapid transfusion of multiple units may reduce the core temperature and can lead to cardiac arrhythmias.
- Clinically significant hypocalcemia usually does not occur unless the rate of transfusion exceeds 1 unit every 5 minutes.
- *To minimize the risk of hyperkalemia:*
  - Use of <5 days stored blood
  - Wash unit before transfusion
  - *To prevent volume overload:* Careful monitoring of volume status and diuretic therapy

Management of Complications

- Use of warmer
- Calcium injection
- Use of diuretics
- Treatment of arrhythmias

PLATELET-RICH PLASMA

13. Application of platelet-rich plasma (PRP) in surgical practice. ***WBUHS 2021 Supplementary***

Introduction

- Platelet-rich plasma consists of two elements: Plasma, or the liquid portion of blood, and platelets, a type of blood cell that plays an important role in healing throughout the body.
- Platelets are well-known for their clotting abilities, but they also contain growth factors that can trigger cell reproduction and stimulate tissue regeneration or healing in the treated area.
- PRP is simply blood that contains more platelets than normal.

Application

- After creating PRP from a patient's blood sample, that solution is injected into the target area, such as an injured knee or a tendon.
- In some cases, the clinician may use ultrasound to guide the injection.
- The idea is to increase the concentration of specific bioproteins or hormones, called growth factors, in a specific area to accelerate the healing process.

The mechanism behind PRP injections is not completely understood. Studies show that the increased concentration of growth factors in PRP may stimulate or speed up the healing process, shortening healing time for injuries, decreasing pain, and even encouraging hair growth.

Uses

PRP injections are used for a range of conditions, from musculoskeletal pain and injuries to cosmetic procedures.

- *Tendon, ligament, muscle, and joint injuries:*
  - PRP injections may be able to treat a range of musculoskeletal injuries and conditions. For example, chronic tendon injuries such as tennis elbow or jumper's knee can often take a long time to heal, so adding PRP shots to a treatment regimen can help to stimulate the healing process, decrease pain and enable a return to activities sooner.
  - It can also be used in chronic plantar fasciitis.
  - It can be used in osteoarthritis.
- *Post-surgical healing:*
  - It can be used to accelerate healing after jaw or plastic surgeries.
  - Now, postsurgical PRP injections have expanded to help heal muscles, tendons, and ligaments, as procedures on these tissues have notoriously long recovery times.

COMPLICATIONS OF BLOOD TRANSFUSION

14. Complications of blood transfusion. ***DNB 2021 June***

Complications of Blood Transfusion

Complications from a single transfusion include:

- Incompatibility hemolytic transfusion reaction
- Febrile transfusion reaction
- Allergic reaction
- Infection
    - Bacterial infection (usually due to faulty storage)
    - Hepatitis
    - HIV
    - Malaria
- Air embolism
- Thrombophlebitis
- Transfusion-related acute lung injury (usually from FFP)

Complications from massive transfusion include:

- Coagulopathy
- Hypocalcemia
- Hyperkalemia
- Hypokalemia
- Hypothermia.

15. Describe various blood products and plasma expanders used for treatment in a patient with shock following polytrauma. What are the complications associated with blood transfusion?

DY Patil Education Society, Deemed to be university, 2020.

Blood Products

Blood products are derived from donated human blood and are critical in managing hemorrhagic shock in polytrauma patients, where significant blood loss leads to hypovolemia, impaired oxygen delivery, and coagulopathy. They are often used in a balanced resuscitation approach, such as massive-transfusion protocols with ratios like 1:1:1 (plasma:platelets:packed red blood cells) to mimic whole blood and prevent dilutional effects from excessive fluids. Below are key blood products and their descriptions:

- *Whole blood (e.g., low titer O+ Whole blood - LTOWB):* This is unseparated blood containing red blood cells (RBCs), plasma, and platelets in their natural ratios. It is administered in 1–2 units (approximately 550–1100 mL) via rapid infusion, often prehospital or in emergency settings. Benefits include simultaneous restoration of oxygen-carrying capacity (hemoglobin 13–15 g/dL), volume expansion, and hemostasis through coagulation factors and functional platelets. It supports clot formation, reduces mortality in hemorrhagic shock, and is logistically simpler than component therapy. However, it requires refrigeration (1–6°C) with a 35-day shelf life, and platelet activity declines after 14 days. Evidence shows no clear superiority over component therapy for mortality, but it may lead to faster shock resolution and lower transfusion volumes.
- *Packed red blood cells (PRBCs):* Concentrated RBCs separated from whole blood, used to replace lost oxygen-carrying capacity in anemic or bleeding patients. Typically transfused in units of 250-300 mL, often in combination with plasma or platelets. In trauma, they are a core component of resuscitation for patients with hemoglobin <7-10 g/dL or ongoing hemorrhage. Benefits include improving tissue oxygenation and perfusion without adding excess volume.

- *Fresh frozen plasma (FFP):* Plasma frozen within 8 hours of collection, rich in coagulation factors (e.g., fibrinogen, factors II, V, VII, VIII, IX, X, XI), proteins, and anticoagulants. It is thawed before use (shelf life 4–5 days post-thaw) and dosed at 1–2 units (~500 mL) for coagulopathy correction. In polytrauma, it addresses trauma-induced coagulopathy, restores endothelial integrity, and prevents hyperfibrinolysis. Prehospital administration reduces 24-hour mortality (risk ratio 0.69) and 30-day mortality by 9.8% in high-risk patients, especially with transport >20 minutes. Higher ratios (e.g., 1:1 FFP:PRBC) improve survival compared to lower ratios.
- *Liquid plasma (LP):* Never-frozen plasma stored at 1–6°C with a 26-day shelf life, containing higher fibrinogen levels than dried forms. Used similarly to FFP for volume expansion and hemostasis in hemorrhagic shock, particularly in urban prehospital settings. It corrects coagulopathy without RBC replacement, is cost-effective ($50–100/unit), and is scalable for EMS. Short-dated units can be returned to blood banks to minimize waste.
- *Dried plasma (DP, freeze-dried or lyophilized):* Dehydrated plasma reconstituted with sterile water in 2–7 minutes, with coagulation factors comparable to FFP (10–20% lower concentration but similar clot strength). Stored at room temperature for 2+ years, making it ideal for austere or rural prehospital use (e.g., type AB or low-titer A). It expands volume, restores clotting factors, and reduces capillary leak. Benefits include logistical superiority (no cold chain), reduced waste, and effectiveness in coagulopathy management. Cost is higher ($500–1500/unit), but offset by stability; pending broader FDA approval in the US.
- *Platelets:* Concentrated platelets from whole blood or apheresis, used to enhance clotting in patients with thrombocytopenia or platelet dysfunction (e.g., <50,000/µL). Transfused in units equivalent to 4–6 donor pools. In trauma, they are part of high-ratio protocols (e.g., higher PLT:PRBC ratios) to improve 24-hour and 30-day survival. They prevent ongoing bleeding but have a short shelf life (5–7 days).

Plasma Expanders

Plasma expanders are non-blood fluids used to increase intravascular volume rapidly, stabilizing hemodynamics in hypovolemic shock from polytrauma. They are initial choices for resuscitation, especially when blood products are unavailable, but excessive use can cause dilutional coagulopathy, acidemia, and edema. Crystalloids are preferred first-line due to cost and availability, while colloids provide more sustained expansion. In trauma, goals include restoring volume to maintain organ perfusion without overloading.

Crystalloids

These are salt-based solutions that distribute across body compartments, requiring larger volumes (e.g., 3:1 ratio to blood loss) for effective expansion.

- *Normal saline (0.9% sodium chloride):* Isotonic solution for initial fluid resuscitation in shock. Used in boluses (e.g., 1–2 L) to replace volume in bleeding patients. *Benefits:* Readily available, inexpensive, and effective for short-term stabilization. Risks include hyperchloremic acidosis with large volumes.
- *Lactated Ringer's (Ringer's lactate):* Balanced isotonic solution with sodium, chloride, lactate, potassium, and calcium. Preferred in trauma and burns for its physiologic pH and electrolytes, reducing acidosis risk. Administered similarly to saline; evidence shows no mortality difference vs. colloids in critically ill patients.
- *Dextrose solutions (e.g., 5% Dextrose in water—D5W):* Hypotonic solution providing free water and glucose. Used for dehydration or as a medication carrier, but less common in acute shock due to risk of hyponatremia.
- *Hypertonic saline (with or without Dextran):* Concentrated saline (3–7.5%) sometimes combined with dextran for osmotic pull. Improves 24-hour survival but no long-term mortality benefit over isotonic fluids; not routinely recommended.

Colloids

These contain larger molecules that stay intravascular longer, drawing fluid in via oncotic pressure, requiring smaller volumes (1:1 ratio to blood loss).

- *Albumin:* Human-derived protein (5% or 25% solutions) from plasma, used when crystalloids fail, in hypoalbuminemia, burns, or sepsis. Provides sustained expansion, maintains oncotic pressure, and reduces capillary leak. Avoid in traumatic brain injury, heart failure, or renal issues due to risks of overload or coagulopathy.

- *Hydroxyethyl starch (HES):* Synthetic starch polymer for volume expansion in hypovolemia. Efficient but associated with kidney injury and coagulopathy; use limited in modern guidelines.
- *Gelatins (e.g., Polygeline):* Collagen-derived solutions like succinylated gelatin. Used in emergencies for rapid expansion in shock or surgery. Short half-life (2–4 hours), cost-effective, but risks allergic reactions and limited efficacy data.
- *Dextrans:* Glucose polymers that expand volume and improve microcirculation. Used sparingly due to risks of anaphylaxis, renal failure, and interference with blood typing.

In practice, start with crystalloids (e.g., 1–2 L boluses), transition to blood products for unstable patients or massive hemorrhage (>40% blood volume loss).

Complications of Blood Transfusion

Complications from a single transfusion include:

- Incompatibility haemolytic transfusion reaction
- Febrile transfusion reaction
- Allergic reaction
- Infection
  - Bacterial infection (usually due to faulty storage)
  - Hepatitis
  - HIV
  - Malaria
- Air embolism
- Thrombophlebitis
- Transfusion-related acute lung injury (usually from FFP).

Complications from massive transfusion include:

- Coagulopathy
- Hypocalcaemia
- Hyperkalaemia
- Hypokalaemia
- Hypothermia.

TRANSFUSION-RELATED ACUTE LUNG INJURY

16. TRALI: Definition, mechanism, and management. ***WBUHS 2021***

Definition

TRALI is defined as new ALI that occurs during or within 6 hours of transfusion, not explained by another ALI risk factor. Transfusion of part of one unit of any blood product can cause TRALI.

Mechanism

The cause of TRALI is currently not fully understood. About 80–85% of cases are thought to be immune-mediated. Antibodies directed toward HLA or human neutrophil antigens (HNA) have been implicated. Women who are multiparous develop these antibodies through exposure to fetal blood; transfusion of blood components obtained from these donors is thought to carry a higher risk of inducing immune-mediated TRALI. Previous transfusion or transplantation can also lead to donor sensitization. To be at risk of TRALI via this mechanism, the blood recipient must express the specific HLA or neutrophil receptors to which the implicated donor has formed antibodies. A two-hit hypothesis has been suggested wherein preexisting pulmonary pathology (i.e., the first hit) leads to localization of neutrophils to the pulmonary microvasculature. The second hit occurs when the aforementioned antibodies are transfused and attach to and activate neutrophils, leading to release of cytokines and vasoactive substances that induce noncardiac pulmonary edema.

A nonimmune mechanism has been studied and proposed by Silliman, involving the accumulation of bioactive lipids in stored blood components (red cells, platelets, plasma) that possess neutrophil priming capabilities.

TRALI is typically associated with plasma products such as FFP. It can also occur in recipients of PRBCs both in adult and pediatric patients.

Treatment

TRALI should be suspected and investigation considered for patients fulfilling the following criteria:

- Hypoxia
- Bilateral pulmonary infiltrates on chest X-ray (CXR)
- Lacking clinical evidence of fluid overload or other cause of pulmonary shadowing
- Occurrence during or within 6 hours of blood component transfusion
- Supportive care is the mainstay of therapy in TRALI
- Oxygen supplementation is employed in all reported cases of TRALI and aggressive respiratory support is needed in 72% of patients
- Intravenous administration of fluids as well as vasopressors, are essential for blood pressure support
- Use of diuretics, which are indicated in the management of transfusion-associated circulatory overload (TACO), should be avoided in TRALI
- Corticosteroids can be beneficial.

CHAPTER 8

Anesthesia and Critical Care

LEARNING OBJECTIVES

- Local Anesthesia
- Regional Anesthesia
- Incentive Spirometry
- Management of Cardiac Arrest During Surgery
- Pain Relief in Surgery
- Invasive and Noninvasive Techniques of Postoperative Analgesia
- Postoperative Ventilatory Support

1. Pharmacological advances in local anesthetics (LAs) in surgical practice. *WBUHS 2015*

- Local anesthetics can be defined as drugs that reversibly block transmission of a nerve impulse, without affecting consciousness.
- All of the amide LAs harbor varying levels of cardiovascular system (CVS) and central nervous system (CNS) toxicity that is still a major complication seen today.
- *Ropivacaine* is indicated for local anesthesia including infiltration, nerve block, and epidural and intrathecal anesthesia in adults and children over 12 years. It is also indicated for peripheral nerve block and caudal epidural in children 1–12 years for surgical pain. It is also sometimes used for infiltration anesthesia for surgical pain in children.
- Ropivacaine is often coadministered with fentanyl for epidural analgesia, e.g., in pregnant women during labor.
- Compared to bupivacaine, *levobupivacaine* is associated with less vasodilation and has a longer duration of action. It is approximately 13% less potent (by molarity) than racemic bupivacaine and has a longer motor block onset time.
- Levobupivacaine is indicated for local anesthesia including infiltration, nerve block, ophthalmic, epidural, and intrathecal anesthesia in adults, and infiltration analgesia in children.

Short-acting Local Anesthetics for Spinal Anesthesia

- *Heavy prilocaine:* Prilocaine 2% hyperbaric solution for injection was associated with faster discharge times than a hyperbaric formulation of another LA in one small single-center, double-blind, randomized study. Use of this preparation may allow service improvement through benefits to individual patients or service delivery.
- *2-chloroprocaine:* Chloroprocaine (2-chloroprocaine, CP) has been one candidate to replace lidocaine for short procedures, despite the fact that neurologic sequelae have been described following the intrathecal injection of large doses of preservative-containing CP intended for epidural use.

It is also used in transurethral resection of prostate (TURP).

The Association of Anesthetists of Great Britain and Ireland (AAGBI) Safety Guideline

Management of severe local anesthetic toxicity		
Recognition	*Signs of severe toxicity:* • Sudden alteration in mental status, severe agitation or loss of consciousness, with or without tonic-clonic convulsions • *Cardiovascular collapse:* Sinus bradycardia, conduction blocks, asystole and ventricular tachyarrhythmias may all occur • Local anesthetic (LA) toxicity may occur sometime after an initial Injection	
Immediate management	• Stop Injecting the LA • Call for help • Maintain the airway and if necessary, secure it with a tracheal tube • Give 100% oxygen and ensure adequate lung ventilation (hyperventilation may help by increasing plasma pH in the presence of metabolic acidosis) • Confirm or establish intravenous access • *Control seizures:* Give a benzodiazepine, thiopental or propofol in small incremental doses • Assess cardiovascular status throughout • Consider drawing blood for analysis, but do not delay definitive treatment to do this	
Treatment	*In circulatory arrest* • Start cardiopulmonary resuscitation (CPR) using standard protocols • Manage arrhythmias using the same protocols, recognizing that arrhythmias may be very refractory to treatment • Consider the use of cardiopulmonary bypass if available	*Without circulatory arrest* Use conventional therapies to treat: • Hypotension • Bradycardia • Tachyarrhythmia
	Give intravenous lipid emulsion (following the regimen overleaf) • Continue CPR throughout treatment with lipid emulsion • Recovery from LA-induced cardiac arrest may take >1 hour • Propofol is not a suitable substitute for lipid emulsion • Lidocaine should not be used as an anti- arrhythmic therapy	*Consider intravenous lipid emulsion (following the regimen overleaf)* • Propofol is not a suitable substitute for lipid emulsion • Lidocaine should not be used as an anti-arrhythmic therapy
Follow-up	• Arrange safe transfer to a clinical area with appropriate equipment and suitable staff until sustained recovery is achieved • Exclude pancreatitis by regular clinical review. Including daily amylase or lipase assays for two days • Report cases as follows: – In the United Kingdom to the National Patient Safety Agency (via www.npsa.nhs.uk) – In the Republic of Ireland to the Irish Medicines Board (via www.imb.ie) – If Lipid has been given, please also report its use to the international registry • Details may also be posted at www lipidrescue.org	

2. Regional anesthesia. ***WBUHS 2006***

Introduction

- Regional anesthesia is anesthesia that affects only a large part of the body, such as a limb. Regional anesthetic techniques can be divided into central and peripheral methods.
- The key techniques are the so-called neuraxial blocks (epidural anesthesia and spinal anesthesia).
- Peripheral techniques can be further divided into plexus blocks, such as the brachial plexus block, and single nerve blocks.
- Regional anesthesia can be done with a single injection or with a continuous catheter, through which the drug is administered over a longer period of time, e.g., a continuous peripheral nerve block. Finally, regional anesthesia can be performed by injecting LAs directly into a vein in the arm (provided the tourniquet prevents venous flow).

- This is called an intravascular regional technique (Bier block). Another example of regional anesthesia is tumescent anesthesia.
- In tumescent anesthesia, a diluted LA solution is pumped into the subcutaneous tissues of the area requiring surgery.
- Regional anesthesia usually uses LAs to block nerve supply to a part of the body, such as a limb, so that patients do not feel pain.

Indications and Applications

- Regional anesthetic can be used to provide an anesthetic without feeling (including pain) so that a surgical operation can be performed, or to provide pain relief after the operation.
- It can also be used to treat chronic pain.
- In some cases, regional anesthesia can be used in place of general anesthesia. For example, it can be used to treat pain during a cesarean section procedure.
- Nerve blocks can be used for various purposes in veterinary medicine, including the diagnosis of lameness in horses and the diagnosis of navicular disease.
- Routine regional anesthetic can also be used in some cases, such as in labor and childbirth. An epidural or a combined spinal epidural can be used to relieve pain during childbirth.

Complications

- Unlike a small LA infiltration, which allows suturing of a wound or excision of a skin lesion, regional anesthesia can involve large doses of local anesthesia or administration of local anesthesia very close to or directly in the CNS.
- Therefore, there is a risk of complications of LA toxicity (such as seizures and cardiac arrest) and spinal shock-like syndrome.
- Most regional anesthetic techniques fail 1–10% even in skilled hands. Therefore, general anesthesia may be necessary even if the procedure was originally planned to be performed with a regional technique.
- For these reasons, regional anesthesia should always be performed only in an environment that is fully equipped and staffed to ensure safe general anesthesia when necessary.

3. Write short note on epidural anesthesia. ***Rajiv Gandhi Institute of Health Sciences 2019; RIMS, Imphal 2012.***

Introduction

Epidural anesthesia is regional anesthesia that blocks pain in a particular region of the body. The goal of an epidural is to provide analgesia, or pain relief, rather than anesthesia which leads to total lack of feeling. Epidurals block the nerve impulses from the lower spinal segments.

Indications

Injecting medication into the epidural space is primarily performed for analgesia.

For analgesia alone, where Surgery is not contemplated. An epidural injection or infusion for pain relief (e.g. in child birth) is less likely to cause loss of muscle power, but has to be augmented to be sufficient for surgery.

- As an adjunct to general anesthesia. This may reduce the patient's requirement for opioid analgesics. This is suitable for a wide variety of surgery, for example gynecological surgery (e.g. hysterectomy), orthopedic surgery (e.g. hip replacement), general surgery (e.g. laparotomy) and vascular surgery (e.g. open aortic aneurysm repair).
- As a sole technique for surgical anesthesia. Some operations, most frequently Caesarean section, may be performed using an epidural anesthetic as the sole technique. This can allow the patient to remain awake during the operation.
- For post-operative analgesia, after an operation where the epidural technique was used as either the sole anesthetic or was used in combination with general anesthesia. Analgesics are given into the epidural space typically for a few days after surgery, provided a catheter has been inserted. Through the use of a patient-controlled

epidural analgesia (PCEA) infusion pump, a person has the ability to give themselves an occasional dose of pain medication through an epidural catheter.

- Treatment of back pain. Injection of analgesics and steroids into the epidural space may improve some forms of back pain.
- Treatment of chronic pain or palliation of symptoms in terminal care, usually in the short- or medium-term.

Epidural Analgesia during Childbirth

Advantages	*Disadvantages*
• Better pain relief than other pain medication • Fewer babies needing naloxone to counter opiate use by the mother • Decreased maternal hyperventilation and increased oxygen supply to baby • Decreased circulating adrenocorticotropic hormone and decreased fetal distress	• More use of instruments to assist with the birth • Increased risk of Caesarean section for fetal distress • Longer delivery (second stage of labor) • Increased need for oxytocin to stimulate uterine contractions • Increased risk of very low blood pressure • Increased risk of muscular weakness for a period of time after the birth • Increased risk of fluid retention • Increased risk of fever

Epidural analgesia has been demonstrated to have several benefits after surgery, including:

- Effective analgesia without the need for systemic opioids.
- The incidence of postoperative respiratory problems and chest infections is reduced.
- The incidence of postoperative myocardial infarction ("heart attack") is reduced.
- The stress response to surgery is reduced.
- Motility of the intestines is improved by blockade of the sympathetic nervous system.
- Use of epidural analgesia during surgery reduces blood transfusion requirements.

Complications

- Failure to achieve analgesia or anesthesia occurs in about 5% of cases, while another 15% experience only partial analgesia or anesthesia
- The following factors are associated with failure to achieve epidural analgesia/anesthesia
  - Obesity
  - Multiparity
  - History of a previous failure of epidural anesthesia
  - History of regular opiate use
  - Cervical dilation of more than 7 cm at insertion
  - The use of air to find the epidural space while inserting the epidural instead of alternatives such as saline or lidocaine
- Accidental dural puncture with headache. This may cause cerebrospinal fluid (CSF) to leak out into the epidural space, which may in turn cause a post dural puncture headache (PDPH). Most cases resolve spontaneously with time.
- Delayed onset of breastfeeding and shorter duration of breastfeeding.
- Bloody tap.
- Catheter misplaced into a vein.
- High block, as described above.
- Catheter misplaced into the subarachnoid space. This may result in a high block, or, more rarely, a *total spinal*, where anesthetic is delivered directly to the brainstem, causing unconsciousness and sometimes seizures.
- Neurological injury lasting less than 1 year.
- Epidural abscess formation.
- Epidural hematoma formation.
- Neurological injury lasting longer than 1 year.
- Paraplegia.

- Arachnoiditis.
- Death (extremely rare, less than 1 in 100,000).

4. Incentive spirometry. ***WBUHS 2008***

Introduction

- An incentive spirometer is a medical device used to improve lung function in patients.
- It is given to patients who have undergone any surgery that impairs breathing, especially lung surgery itself, but also generally to patients recovering from cardiac or other surgery that involves a prolonged period of anesthesia and prolonged recovery in bed.
- A stimulus spirometer is also given to patients recovering from rib injuries to minimize fluid accumulation in the lungs.
- The patient inhales from the device as slowly and deeply as possible.
- The indicator shows how well the patient and the lungs are working by showing a constant inspiratory vacuum. The patient is usually asked to do several repetitions a day while measuring his progress with a meter.

Incentive Spirometry

- It is a technique that encourages voluntary deep breathing by providing visual feedback on the volume of inhalation.
- Using a special spirometer, the patient inhales until a predetermined volume is reached and then maintains the inspiratory volume by holding the breath for 3–5 seconds. Incentive spirometry reduces the risk of atelectasis and lung consolidation.

How to Use?

1. Sit or lie comfortably in a comfortable position.
2. Hold the incentive spirometer in an upright position with both hands.
3. Slide the cursor (located in the left column when looking at the spirometer) to the desired level. For example, start with 1,250 mL and slowly increase as treatment progresses.
4. Place the mouthpiece in your mouth and close your lips around it.
5. Keep your lips tightly closed around the mouthpiece and inhale slowly and as deeply as possible. The piston under the indicator should now rise to the top of the post.
6. Hold your breath for at least 3 seconds and let the piston falls back to the bottom of the column.
7. Cough after each deep breath to clear the airways of mucus.
8. Rest for a few seconds and repeat steps 2–8, 10 times for each waking hour.

According to a randomized controlled trial, it is not clear whether incentive spirometry is better than controlled deep breathing.

5. Management of cardiac arrest during surgery. ***WBUHS 2007, WBUHS 2025 Supplementary***

Perioperative Cardiac Arrest—Causes and Management

A sudden unsuspected cessation of effective cardiac pump function is termed cardiac arrest (CA). In the perioperative period it occurs more frequently during general anesthesia (GA) (5.5/10,000) than regional anesthesia (1.5/10,000).

Perioperative cardiac arrest may be due to:

- Medication related (β-blocker, antiarrhythmic drugs, and anticholinesterase)
- Airway or ventilation (esophageal intubation, hypoxia, and N_2O without O_2)
- Electrolyte and metabolic disturbance (potassium, calcium, etc.)
- Hypovolemia and blood loss

In general, there are four basic mechanisms of cardiac arrest:

1. Ventricular fibrillation (VF)
2. Ventricular tachycardia leading to pulseless (VT)
3. Asystole
4. Pulseless electrical activity (PEA)

Majority of in hospital CA are VF/VT but perioperative cardiac arrest are mainly asystole, usually asystole have poor prognosis in CA but in the perioperative period prognosis is better as majority are due to temporary increased parasympathetic activity (peritoneal pull and anticholinesterase without atropine).

Perioperative Cardiac Arrest Management

- Basic life support (BLS)
- Advanced life support (ALS)

An ultra-quick rapid assessment to conform collapse, unconscious state is due to CA is made. It includes carotid, femoral pulses pallor, cyanosis, unconsciousness (if not in GA), and presence of any secretion in upper airway.

Once confirmed, call for help.

Begin BLS Immediately

Basic life support includes three components:

1. Airway patency (jaw thrust-chin lift, oropharyngeal airway, and tracheal intubation)
2. Ventilation by self-inflating bag or intubation. Lung should be inflated 8–10 times/min with tidal volume of 7 mL/kg with adequate spacing
3. Chest compression with heel of dominant hand in center of sternum rate of 100/min.

Continue cardiopulmonary resuscitation (CPR) till defibrillator available and personnel trained in ALS are present.

Advance Life Support

- Starts with intubation and ventilation and use of defibrillator.
- Peripheral venous access is made and various vasopressors and antiarrhythmics are administered.
- In case of asystole and PEA transvenous pacing may be required.
- If hypovolemic administer fluid [Ringer's lactate/normal saline (RL/NS).
- CPR is continued throughout the process.

Drugs Used

- *Vasopressor:* Epinephrine and vasopressin
- *Antiarrhythmics:* Atropine, lidocaine, amiodarone, and magnesium
- *Others:* Calcium gluconate, sodium bicarbonate, potassium chloride, and calcium chloride

Monitoring

- Arterial pulse and pressure
- Coronary perfusion pressure
- End tidal CO_2
- Venous blood gas
- Electrocardiogram (ECG)

How long to resuscitate: 15–30 minutes.

6. Pain relief in surgery. ***WBUHS 2009***

7. Postoperative pain management. ***WBUHS 2011***

Introduction

- Most people have some pain after surgery.
- Pain can be harmful if it is not relieved after surgery.

- Pain can make it hard for the patient to take deep breaths, move, and walk.
- This can cause problems such as blood clots and pneumonia.

Pain Control after Surgery

- Keep patient's pain under control.
- Patient should be comfortable so that he or she can sleep, deep breath, walk, and visit with others.
- Manage pain to help the patient heal after surgery.

Different Medicines used to Control Pain

- After surgery, different medicines can be used to control pain. They work together so that less medicine is needed while getting better pain control.
- *Pain medicines:* Patient may be given one or more different pain medicines, such as opiate and nonsteroidal anti-inflammatory drugs (NSAIDs).
- *Antianxiety medicines*
- *Antinausea medicines*
- *Patient-controlled analgesia (PCA):*
  - PCA is a special pump that has pain medicine in it that connects to patient's intravenous (IV) tube.
  - When patient feels pain, he or she pushes a button, and the pump gives a measured dose of medicine into your bloodstream.
  - Only patient should push the button, not the family members or friends.
- *Epidural analgesia:*
  - Epidural analgesia is another way by which a pain medicine is given.
  - A small plastic tube called an epidural catheter is placed in patient's back just before surgery.
  - A small pump is attached to the epidural catheter.
  - The pump puts a small amount of analgesic medicine through the catheter in back of the patient at a set rate.
  - One can use epidural medicine until the pain has eased enough to take pain pills by mouth.
- *Local anesthetic block* can also be used.

Acute Postoperative Pain Relief

- Requires an expert team approach
- Pain levels must be measured regularly
- Analgesia is best given before pain breaks through
- A combination of analgesics gives best result
- Opioids should not be withheld
- The dose of analgesia used must be adequate to control the pain

Techniques for Postoperative Pain Relief

- Regular intramuscular injections—may get pain breakthrough
- Local anesthetic block—ideal if it works
- Indwelling epidural—good pain control; opioids may depress respiration
- Continuous infusions—reduce oscillations in pain relief but risk overdose
- PCA—pain relief titrated to patient's need.

8. Describe the invasive and noninvasive techniques of postoperative analgesia. ***WBUHS 2021 Supplementary***

Postoperative Pain Management

- Surgical procedures cause tissue damage which along with the presence of drains, tubes, and postoperative complications results in pain.
- Pain management in a perioperative setting refers to actions before during and after a procedure that is intended to reduce or eliminate pain before discharge.

Hyperalgesia in Incisional Pain is Mediated by

- Sensitization of A and C fiber nociceptors
- Conversion of silent A delta nociceptors to mechanically sensitive fibers after incision

Noninvasive Techniques

- *Opioid therapy:*
  - Highly effective in relieving moderate to severe postop pain
  - Do not have a ceiling effect
  - Available as a wide variety of formulation
  - But there are many dose limiting side effects such as nausea vomiting sedation, somnolence, and respiratory depression
  - *Transdermal:* Fentanyl buprenorphine
  - *Intranasal:* Fentanyl, sufentanil, diamorphine, and ketamine
  - *Oral submucosal:* Fentanyl
  - *Sublingual:* Buprenorphine and sufentanil
- *Needle-free PCA:* Transdermal system using iontophoresis to allow rapid transfer of fentanyl to the circulation
- *Multimodal analgesia:*
  - The concurrent use of more than one class of anesthetic agent or technique to target different mechanisms of analgesia.
  - Paracetamol, NSAIDs, LAs, gabapentinoids, ketamine, and glucocorticoids are used mostly

Invasive Methods

- *Epidural techniques:*
  - Safe and effective method for management of acute postoperative pain and even considered as the gold standard for postoperative pain management.
  - *The main indications for epidural analgesia are:*
    - High-risk patient scheduled for open major surgeries
    - Extensive surgeries involving large areas of the body
    - Labor analgesia
- *Perineural techniques:*
  - Highly effective and superior to IV opioid techniques
    - Single injection peripheral nerve block
    - Catheter techniques

    As effective as epidural but less invasive with better adverse effects profile

Infiltrative Techniques

- Epidural and perineural catheter techniques are very effective in controlling postoperative pain but these techniques require the expertise of an anesthesiologist.
- Thus local application of an LA to the surgical site is a rational approach to block pain transmission from afferent nociceptive barrage.
- Local anesthetics inhibit inflammatory response to injury and may therefore reduce the risk of hyperalgesia.
  - Simple and inexpensive
  - Good safety profile
  - Can be used alone or as a part of multimodal regimens depending on the severity of postoperative pain

Wound Catheter Infusions

Also called surgical site catheter infusions and it involves catheters placed in a number of sites including subcutaneous, subfascial, preperitoneal, intraperitoneal, subacromial, intraosseous, intra-articular, and others

Local Infiltration Techniques

- It is not just infiltration of LAs but a multimodal optimization package
- Was mainly introduced for pain control after total hip arthroplasty

Intraperitoneal Local Anesthetics for Abdominal Surgery

- *In colorectal surgery:* Ropivacaine infusion through a preperitoneally placed catheter
- *In cesarean section:* Subfascial catheter

Transversus Abdominis Plane Block

- Useful in bowel surgeries, hernia repair, umbilical surgeries, etc.
- It is safe and efficacious

9. Postoperative ventilatory support. ***WBUHS 2010***

Mechanical ventilation is often utilized and required in patients with postoperative respiratory failure.

The indications for tracheal intubation include:

- Inadequate oxygenation or ventilation
- Inadequate airway patency or protection
- Excessive secretions
- Increased work of breathing, and
- Impaired physiologic reserve.

Early intubation should be the goal to avoid airway and hemodynamic compromise, preferably in the presence of someone specifically trained in routine and difficult airway management. Equipment for managing difficult airways must be readily available, and placement should always be confirmed with an end-tidal carbon dioxide detector.

Modes of Mechanical Ventilation

Volume-limited Modes

- *Assist-control (A/C) ventilation:*
  - It creates a predetermined tidal volume at a specified rate.
  - As the machine detects the inspiratory effort of each patient, it outputs the set tidal volume.
  - If the patient's breathing rate is below the machine and the set rate, the ventilator will start a breathing rate that replaces the difference between the set rate and the patient's breathing rate.
  - Air-conditioned ventilation minimizes the work of breathing, because the ventilator helps all breaths (hence the term full support); therefore, this mode is however inconvenient when the patient's breathing and the ventilator are synchronized.
  - Respiratory alkalosis may occur in nervous patients due to hyperventilation.
- *Intermittent mandatory ventilation (IMV):*
  - It is like A/C ventilation, delivers a preset tidal volume at a set rate.
  - IMV does not assist spontaneous respiratory efforts; it is commonly used with pressure support.

Pressure-limited Modes

- *Pressure-support ventilation:*
  - It produces a preset inspiratory pressure but not a preset pressure.
  - Constant inspiratory pressure continues until the inspiratory gas flow falls below a predetermined level and the expiratory valve opens.
  - Thus, tidal volumes occur only when the patient is breathing spontaneously.
  - It allows the patient to maintain control over the time of inhalation and exhalation and thus the volume of the breath; As a result, this mode is most comfortable for spontaneously breathing patients.
  - Disadvantages of pressure support ventilation are:
    - All ventilation depends on the efforts of the patient, and
    - A sudden increase in airway resistance reduces the volume of breathing.
  - A small amount (5–8 cmH_2O) of pressure support ventilation is routinely used to eliminate airflow resistance caused by the endotracheal (ET) tube and ventilator inspiratory valves.
- *Pressure-control ventilation:*

- It produces a predetermined inspiratory pressure (as opposed to tidal volume) at a predetermined rate.
- This mode is used in patients with poor (low) pulmonary compliance who develop high inspiratory pressures when ventilated using the more traditional methods described previously.
- Thus, the advantage of this mode is that it allows the physician to regulate airway pressure and thus minimize barotrauma.
- Disadvantage is that tidal volume varies with compliance.
- For example, a sudden increase in airway resistance (cough, thick secretions, ET tube kink, and Valsalva maneuver) increases airway pressure and lowers tidal volumes to dangerously low levels.

- *Bilevel ventilation:*
  - Spontaneous breathing ventilator support is a type of ventilator that allows the patient to breathe at two levels [positive end-expiratory pressure (PEEP)] at the same time.
  - The time at the lower level of the PEEP may be limited, allowing the patient to take all their breaths at the upper level of PEEP, and then the pressure will be released just long enough for the lung volume to drop (airway pressure release ventilation).
  - In some cases, spontaneous breathing may take place at both levels of the PEEP.
  - There is evidence to support that spontaneous breathing improves patient comfort and respiratory synchronization.

High-frequency Oscillatory Ventilation (HFOV)

- Uses significantly higher speeds (180–300/min) and smaller tidal volumes than conventional installations.
- The result is a relative decrease in diaphragm motion, lung motion, and airway pressure.
- The physical mechanisms responsible for gas movement are complex and incompletely understood.

Ventilator Management

- *Choice of ventilator mode:* Patient needs should be matched with the appropriate ventilator mode by considering each mode's advantages and disadvantages.
- *Fraction of inspired oxygen (FiO_2)* should be adjusted to ensure adequate arterial oxygenation, which is a blood hemoglobin saturation of 92% in lighter-skinned individuals and 95% in darker-skinned patients. The lowest possible FiO_2 (ideally ≤0.40) should be used to achieve these levels of arterial saturation to prevent pulmonary oxygen toxicity.
- *Tidal volume:* There is no consensus on the optimal tidal volume for the postoperative patient who requires short-term mechanical ventilatory support. However, in acute respiratory distress syndrome (ARDS), low tidal volumes are associated with improved survival.
- *Ventilatory rate:* Once the tidal volume has been determined, the rate is chosen (typically 8–16 breaths per minute) to provide adequate minute ventilation (the product of rate and tidal volume). The rate is adjusted to optimize arterial pH and partial pressure of arterial carbon dioxide ($PaCO_2$); an end-tidal CO_2 monitor is useful in this regard.
- *Inspiratory-expiratory (I:E) ratio:*
  - The normal I:E ratio is 1:2–1:3.
  - Longer expiratory times allow patients with obstructive pulmonary disease (high compliance) to fully exhale and avoid gasping.
  - In contrast, longer inspiratory times that reduce peak airway pressure are beneficial for patients with low lung compliance.
  - Reverse ventilation uses respiratory stacking using I:E ratio of 1:1–4:1.
  - Only used in patients with severe established lung disease. Inverse proportional ventilation is thought to improve gas exchange due to progressive recruitment of alveoli (average airway pressure is higher, keeping a greater number of alveoli open for a greater percentage of the respiratory cycle). Inverse proportional ventilation is most often used in conjunction with pressure controlled ventilation.
- *Positive end-expiratory pressure:*

- It increases functional residual capacity, increases lung compliance, and improves ventilation-perfusion compatibility by opening airways and recruiting partially collapsed alveoli.
- PEEP of 5 cmH_2O is considered physiological; larger amounts are used for moderate or severe hypoxemia.
- PEEP significantly increases intrathoracic pressure and thus decreases CO, decreases venous return to the heart, increases airway pressure and changes pulmonary vascular resistance.
- PEEP levels above 15 cmH_2O significantly increase the risk of barotrauma and spontaneous pneumothorax.
- PEEP administered to a spontaneously ventilated patient without an inspiratory pause is called continuous positive airway pressure (CPAP).

- *Sedation and neuromuscular paralysis:*
  - In mechanically ventilated patients, sedation is often needed to manage anxiety, allow for rest, and to synchronize breathing.
  - The need for paralysis is rarely necessary, except for those with severe respiratory failure who benefit from improved pulmonary compliance due to reduced elastic recoil in the chest wall.
  - If paralytics are needed, they should be stopped as soon as possible, as prolonged use can lead to paresis that can last for weeks or months
  - *Prone positioning* is one of several techniques that may have benefit as "rescue" strategies in patients with severe acute lung injury or ARDS.

Mechanical ventilation is associated with significant morbidity, mortality, and costs of care. Therapies available to reduce this burden are listed here.

Concurrent Evidence-based Therapies

- Semirecumbency
- Peptic ulcer disease prophylaxis
- Deep venous thrombosis prophylaxis
- Holding sedation such that patients can follow commands once a day
- Daily assessment of respiratory function
- Tight glucose control <110 mg/dL

Criteria for Extubation

Parameter	***Value***
PaO_2 on FiO_2	>80 mm Hg on <0.6
$PaCO_2$	<45 mm Hg
Respiratory rate	<35
Tidal volume	>5 mL/kg
Vital capacity	>10 mUkg
Minute ventilation	<10 L/min
Negative inspiratory force	–20 cmH_2O or more negative
Rapid shallow breathing index	<80

(FiO_2: fraction of inspired oxygen; PaO_2: partial pressure of arterial oxygen)

CHAPTER 9

Trauma

LEARNING OBJECTIVES

- Triage, Coagulopathy of Trauma
- Head Trauma
- Chest Trauma
- Abdominal Trauma—Blunt Abdominal Trauma, Splenic Trauma, Liver trauma, Duodenal Injury, Pancreatic Injury, Colorectal Injury
- Renal and Urethral Injury
- Level I Trauma Center

TRIAGE

1. Triage in disaster and principles of a polytrauma patient. *WBUHS 2019*

Triage levels and color coding: A color-coded tagging method to categorize disaster victims in the field has been almost universally adopted and incorporated into existing triage systems.

1. *Red triage tag ("immediate" or T1 or priority 1):* Patients whose lives are in immediate danger and who require immediate treatment.
2. *Yellow triage tag ("delayed" or T2 or priority 2):* Patients whose lives are not in immediate danger and who will require urgent, not immediate, medical care.
3. *Green triage tag ("minimal" or T3 or priority 3):* Patients with minor injuries who will eventually require treatment.
4. *Black triage tag ("expectant" or no priority):* Patients who are either dead or who have such extensive injuries that they cannot be saved with the limited resources available.

The "expectant" category can be the most challenging for caregivers from an ethical and emotional standpoint. While it is logical to help the greatest number of victims in a disaster, it is difficult to walk away from a person who is on the verge of succumbing to severe injuries.

Patients need to be reassessed repeatedly, and initial color-coded triage designations can change over time.

START (Simple Triage and Rapid Transport)

START is a civilian triage system that was first developed in California in the early 1980s. It has since become the de facto standard of disaster triage for the US Department of Defense.

SALT (Sort–Assess–Lifesaving Interventions–Treatment/Transport)

It was developed in response to a lack of scientific evidence about the effectiveness of mass casualty systems. In response to this lack of evidence, the CDC (Centers for Disease Control and Prevention) created an advisory committee that analyzed existing systems and recommended a national standard. SALT has the backing of several national organizations such as the American College of Emergency Physicians, the American College of Surgeons (ACS) Committee on Trauma, the American Trauma Society, and the National Association of EMS Physicians.

2. Describe briefly the acute coagulopathy of trauma (ACoT); rationale of damage control resuscitation (DCR) in civilian trauma. ***WBUHS 2021***

Acute coagulopathy of trauma shock (ACoTS) is caused by a combination of tissue injury and shock. It may occur without significant fluid administration, clotting factor depletion, or hypothermia.

- ACoTs occur in patients with shock and is characterized by systemic anticoagulation and hyperfibrinolysis, dilution, acidemia and consumption of coagulation proteases do not appear to be significant factors at this stage.
- There is evidence to implicate activation of the protein C pathway in this process.
- Diagnosis of acute coagulopathy currently relies on laboratory assessment of clotting times.
- These tests do not fully characterize coagulopathy and have significant limitations, which reduce their clinical utility.

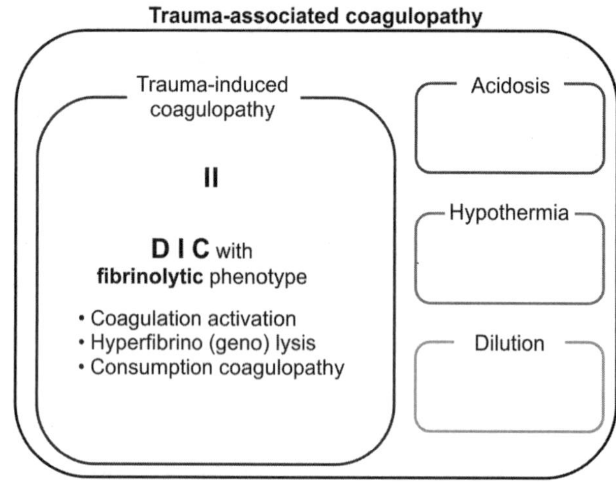

(DIC: disseminated intravascular coagulation)

PATHOPHYSIOLOGY OF TRAUMA-INDUCED COAGULOPATHY

Trauma-induced coagulopathy is generated by the following pathophysiological mechanisms:

- *Coagulation activation:*
  - Procoagulants in the systemic circulation
  - Impairment of endogenous anticoagulant activity
  - Thrombin generation in the systemic circulation
- *Hyperfibrino(geno) lysis:*
  - Acute release of tissue-plasminogen activator (t-PA)-induced hyperfibrinolysis
  - Coagulation activation-induced fibrinolysis
- *Consumption coagulopathy:*
  - Transfusion requirements, incidence of organ dysfunction, critical care stay, and mortality, all are increased in acute coagulopathy.
  - Recognition of an early coagulopathic state has implications for the care of shocked patients and the management of massive transfusion.
  - Identification of novel mechanisms for traumatic coagulopathy may lead to new avenues for drug discovery and therapeutic intervention.

Damage Control Resuscitation

Damage control resuscitation (DCR) is a systematic approach to the management of the trauma patient with severe injuries. It starts in the emergency room and continues through the operating room and the intensive care unit (ICU).

Components of DCR

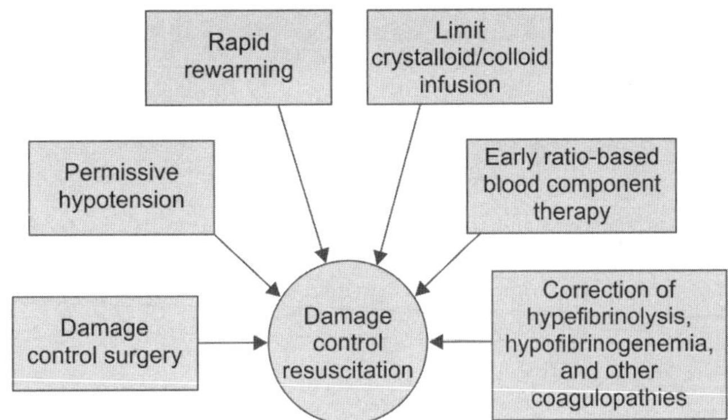

- Coagulopathy observed in trauma patients was thought to be a resuscitation-related phenomenon.
- Replacement of lost and depleted coagulation factors has been the mainstay of resuscitation in hemorrhagic shock for decades.
- Damage control surgery (DCS) was introduced 20 years ago to combat traumatic coagulopathy. It consists of three stages: abbreviated surgery to control bleeding and contamination, ICU resuscitation, and elective reoperation with definitive surgery.
- DCS resuscitation strategy focused on rapid reversal of acidosis and prevention of hypothermia through the first two phases. However, direct therapy of coagulopathy has not been emphasized in DCS.
- A better understanding of the pathophysiology of recent trauma-induced coagulopathy guides the patient to manage this coagulopathy immediately during major trauma resuscitation.
- DCR is a strategic approach to the extreme trauma patient. It consists of balanced resuscitation, hemostatic resuscitation and prevention of acidosis, hypothermia, and hypocalcemia.
- In balanced resuscitation, fluid administration is limited and hypotension is allowed until definitive hemostatic measures are initiated:
  - In the initial stages of resuscitation, it is recommended to give blood products consisting of fresh frozen plasma, packed red blood cells, and platelets in a proportion similar to whole blood.
  - The DCR strategy is currently the most cost-effective procedure for trauma-induced coagulopathy and may change the treatment strategy for trauma patients.
  - DCS is now integrated as part of DCR. DCR as a structured intervention begins immediately in the emergency room after a rapid initial assessment and continues with DCS through the operating room to the ICU.
  - Starting from scratch with performing DCS, DCR allows the trauma surgeon to correct traumatic coagulopathy.
  - The effect of coagulopathy reversal in massively bleeding patients may change the surgical strategy for DCS.

HEAD TRAUMA

3. Glasgow Coma Scale (GCS). ***WBUHS 2009***

Initial management of head injury focuses on hemodynamic stabilization through establishment of an adequate airway, ventilation, and support of circulation, followed by the rapid diagnosis and treatment of intracranial injuries.

A rapid but systematic neurologic examination is performed on the scene and is repeated frequently during transport and on initial presentation to the emergency room. Examination focuses on the three components of the GCS—eye opening, verbal response, and motor response. This score indicates injury severity and measures changes in the impairment of consciousness.

Glasgow Coma Scale.	
Component	*Points*
Eye opening:	
Spontaneous	4
To voice	3
To stimulation	2
None	1
Motor response:	
To command	6
Localizes	5
Withdraws	4
Abnormal flexion	3
Extension	2
None	1
Verbal response:	
Oriented	5
Confused but comprehensible	4
Inappropriate or incoherent	3
Incomprehensible (no words)	2
None	1

Note: Glasgow Coma Score (GCS) = best eye opening + best motor response + best verbal response. If patient is intubated, the verbal score is omitted, and an addendum of "T" is given to the best eye opening + best motor response score.

- *Mild injury:* GCS 14–15
- *Moderate injury:* GCS 9–13
- *Severe injury:* GCS 3–8

4. What is GCS in adults and children? State its significance and fallacies. ***WBUHS 2021***

The GCS is used to describe the general level of consciousness in patients with traumatic brain injury (TBI) and to define broad categories of head injury:

- The GCS is divided into three categories—eye opening (E), motor response (M), and verbal response (V).
- The score is determined by the sum of the score in each of the three categories, with a maximum score of 15 and a minimum score of 3, as follows:

$$GCS\ score = E + M + V$$

- The GCS has limited applicability to children, especially below the age of 36 months. Consequently, the pediatric GCS, a separate yet closely related scale, was developed for assessing younger children.

GCS in Adults

Eye Opening Scores

- 4—Spontaneously
- 3—To verbal command
- 2—To pain
- 1—No response

Best Motor Response Scores

- 6—Obeys command
- 5—Localizes pain
- 4—Flexion withdrawal
- 3—Flexion abnormal (decorticate)
- 2—Extension (decerebrate)
- 1—No response

Best Verbal Response Scores

- 5—Oriented and converses
- 4—Disoriented and converses
- 3—Inappropriate words; cries
- 2—Incomprehensible sounds
- 1—No response

Generally, brain injury is classified as:

- Severe, GCS < 8–9
- Moderate, GCS 8 or 9–12 (controversial)
- Minor, GCS ≥13

Tracheal intubation and severe facial/eye swelling or damage make it impossible to test the verbal and eye responses. In these circumstances, the score is given as 1 with a modifier attached (e.g., "E1c", where "c" = closed, or "V1t" where *t* = tube). Often the 1 is left out, so the scale reads Ec or Vt.

A composite might be "GCS 5tc". This would mean, for example, eyes closed because of swelling = 1, intubated = 1, and leaving a motor score of 3 for "abnormal flexion".

The GCS has limited applicability to children, especially below the age of 36 months (where the verbal performance of even a healthy child would be expected to be poor).

Consequently, the Pediatric Glasgow Coma Scale was developed for assessing younger children.

Glasgow Coma Score in Children

Eye Opening

Score	Age 1 year or older	Age 0–1 year
4	Spontaneously	Spontaneously
3	To verbal command	To shout
2	To pain	To pain
1	No response	No response

Best Motor Response

Score	Age 1 year or older	Age 0–1 year
6	Obeys command	
5	Localizes pain	Localizes pain
4	Flexion withdrawal	Flexion withdrawal
3	Flexion abnormal (decorticate)	Flexion abnormal (decorticate)
2	Extension (decerebrate)	Extension (decerebrate)
1	No response	No response

Best Verbal Response

Score	Age >5 years	Age 2–5 years	Age 0–2 years
5	Oriented and converses	Appropriate words	Cries appropriately
4	Disoriented and converses	Inappropriate words	Cries
3	Inappropriate words; cries	Screams	Inappropriate crying/screaming
2	Incomprehensible sounds	Grunts	Grunts
1	No response	No response	No response

Significance	Fallacies
• Most widely recognized of all conscious level scoring systems in the world • Has face validity (looks like it should work) • Quick • Reproducible (this is controversial, in one study 38% of the cases the GCS scores were the same and in 33% of cases the scores varied with >2 points) • Skewed toward motor score, which is good since this is the most reliable measure of short-term prognosis in TBI • The distinction between a motor score of 2, 3, and 4 is a very useful clinical indicator of the severity of TBI, and the area of brain function that has been affected. • Correlates with adverse neurological outcomes such as brain injury, neurosurgical intervention, and mortality	• Controversies in literature • There is poor interobserver reliability • Reproducibility is poor (only 50% in neurosurgeons) • There is little evidence demonstrating validity and reliability of the GCS • Not proven to be better than unstructured clinical judgment • There are numerous other neurological scoring systems that have demonstrated similar or greater validity and reliability, e.g., the FOUR score, AVPU in children • GCS 8 does not reliably correlate with the presence or absence of airway reflexes

(AVPU: Alert, Verbal response, response to Pain, Unresponsive; FOUR: Full Outline of UnResponsiveness; GCS: Glasgow Coma Scale; TBI: traumatic brain injury)

5. Transient Loss of Consciousness Following RTA – Approach. ***WBUHS 2021 Supplementary***

6. Describe your approach in case of transient loss of consciousness following RTA. ***WBUHS 2024***

Introduction

- Head injury accounts for 3–4% of emergency department attendances.
- Annual mortality is estimated at 9 per 100,000.
- RTAs are the leading cause of head injury, being responsible for up to 50% of cases.
  - *Assess airway:*
    - Elicit verbal response
    - Protect cervical spine
  - *Establish stable airway:*
    - Endotracheal intubation
      - *Consider:*
        - Airway adjuncts
        - Gum elastic bougie
        - Laryngeal/surgical airway
  - *Supplemental oxygen:*
    - Assisted ventilation
    - Consider tube thoracostomy
  - *Assess breathing:*
    - Physical examination (PE)
    - Pulse oximetry

Glasgow Coma Scale.

Event	Response	Score
Eye opening	• Spontaneously • To verbal command • To painful stimulus • Do not open	4 3 2 1
Verbal command	• Normal-oriented conversation • Confused • Inappropriate words only • Uncomprehensive sounds • No sounds • Intubated patients	5 4 3 2 1 T
Motor response	• Obeys command • Localizes pain • Withdrawl flexion • Abnormal flexion • Extension • No motor response	6 5 4 3 2 1

- *Assess circulation shock?*
    - PE
    - Vital signs [blood pressure (BP), heart rate (HR), respiratory rate (RR)]
        - Two large-caliber IVs
        - 1–2 L warm crystalloid infusion
- *Consider tension pneumothorax*
- *Immediate evaluation for bleeding*
    - PE
        - External loss
        - Multiple long bones
    - *Chest X-ray:* Intrathoracic loss
    - *Pelvic X-ray:* Retroperitoneal loss
    - *Focused abdominal sonography for trauma (FAST):* Intra-abdominal loss
- *Assess disability/neurologic condition*
    - GCS
    - Moving all extremities
- *Specific hemorrhage control:*
    - Control external loss
    - Tube thoracostomy
    - Splint/stabilize fractures
    - Decrease pelvic volume—wrap
    - Operating room
    - Angiography

- Secondary survey
- Radiographic evaluation
- Laboratory studies
- Urinary/gastric catheters

Indications for CT imaging within 1 hour	*Indications for CT imaging within 8 hours*
• GCS < 13 at any point • GCS < 15 at 2 hours • Focal neurological deficit • Suspected open, depressed, or basal skull fractures • More than one episode of vomiting • Post-traumatic seizure	• Age >65 years • Coagulopathy (e.g., aspirin, warfarin, riboflavin use) • Dangerous mechanism of injury (e.g., fall from a height, road traffic accident) • Retrograde amnesia >30 minutes

Primary Brain Injury

Concussion: Mildest

Colorado Classification

I. Confusion

II. Amnesia

III. *Loss of consciousness:*

- Noncontrast computed tomography (NCCT)—normal
- Self-resolving

Diffuse Axonal Injury

- Most severe
- Shearing force between grey and white matter
- Patient comatose
- NCCT—normal

- Magnetic resonance imaging (MRI)—punctate hemorrhage at gray and white matter junction
- Worst prognosis

Intracranial hemorrhage	*Extradural hemorrhage*
• Intraparenchymal hemorrhage • Most common • Most common site—Temporal region • Hematoma—Resolves • Coalesce and increase in site—Surgical drainage	• Middle meningeal artery is the source • Young patients • High-velocity impact • Transient loss of consciousness with lucid interval • *Contralateral hemiparesis, reduced conscious level, and ipsilateral pupillary dilatation: The* cardinal signs of brain compression and herniation

Management

- *Indications of craniotomy:*
  - >5-mm midline shift
  - >1-cm thickness
  - Fall in GCS >2 points
  - Fixed/dilated pupil
  - Intracranial pressure (ICP) >20 mm Hg

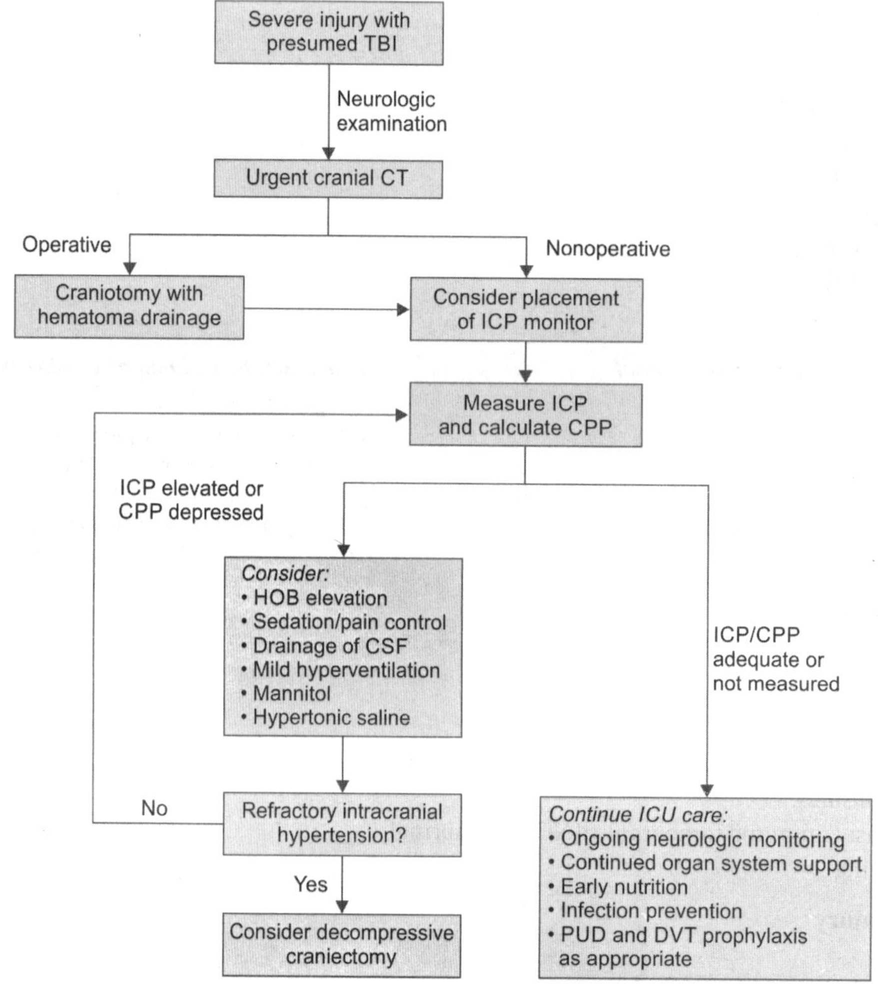

(CPP: cerebral perfusion pressure; CSF: cerebrospinal fluid; CT: computed tomography; DVT: deep venous thrombosis; HOB: head of bed; ICP: intracranial pressure; ICU: intensive care unit; PUD: peptic ulcer disease; TBI: traumatic brain injury)

CHEST TRAUMA

7. Complications of chest trauma. ***WBUHS 2010, 2020***

- *Chest wall injury:*
  - Sucking wound and open pneumothorax
  - Rib fracture, hemothorax, flail chest, deformed chest, respiratory distress
- *Lung injury:*
  - Lung contusion, hemothorax, pneumothorax (usually hemopneumothorax)
  - Empyema thoracis
- *Major airway injury:* Surgical emphysema, massive pneumothorax
- *Esophageal injury:* Mediastinal sepsis, septicemia, pneumothorax
- *Cardiac injury:* Cardiac tamponade, myocardial contusion/laceration
- *Great vessel injury:* Hypovolemia, shock
- *Terminal complication:* Acute respiratory distress (ARD)

8. Enumerate the "dangerous dozen" of thoracic trauma. Describe the management of immediate life-threatening conditions. ***Rajasthan University of Health Sciences 2025; WBUHS 2021***

Major Thoracic Injuries are known as the Deadly Dozen

- The Lethal Six (airway obstruction, tension pneumothorax, cardiac tamponade, open pneumothorax, massive hemothorax, and flail chest) are immediate, life-threatening injuries that require evaluation and treatment during primary survey.
- The Hidden Six (thoracic aortic disruption, tracheobronchial disruption, myocardial contusion, traumatic diaphragmatic tear, esophageal disruption, and pulmonary contusion) are potentially life-threatening injuries that should be detected during secondary survey.

Immediate Life-threatening Conditions

- *Airway obstruction:*
  - Early preventable trauma deaths are often due to lack of or delay in airway control.
  - The most common cause in the unconscious patient is obstruction caused by the tongue.
  - Dentures, teeth, secretions, and blood can contribute to airway obstruction in trauma.
  - Bilateral mandibular fracture, expanding neck hematoma producing deviation of the pharynx and mechanical compression of the trachea, laryngeal trauma such as thyroid or cricoid fractures, and tracheal injury include other causes of airway obstruction.
  - These patients need intubation (with simultaneous protection of the cervical spine).
  - Early intubation is very important, particularly in cases of neck hematomas or possible airway edema.
  - Airway edema can be insidious and progressive and can make delayed intubation more difficult if not impossible.
- *Tension pneumothorax:*
  - A tension pneumothorax develops when a "one-way-valve" air leak occurs, either from the lung or through the chest wall.
  - The most common causes are:
    - Penetrating chest trauma
    - Blunt chest trauma with parenchymal lung injury that did not spontaneously close
    - Iatrogenic lung punctures and mechanical positive pressure ventilation
  - The patient is panicky, with:
    - Tachypnea
    - Dyspnea
    - Distended neck veins (similar to pericardial tamponade)

- Clinical examination can reveal tracheal deviation (a late finding—not necessary to clinically confirm diagnosis), hyperresonance and absent breath sounds over the affected hemithorax.
- Tension pneumothorax is a clinical diagnosis and treatment should not be delayed by waiting for radiological confirmation.
- Treatment consists of immediate decompression and is managed initially by rapidly inserting a large-bore needle into the second intercostal space in the midclavicular line of the affected hemithorax.
- This is immediately followed with a chest tube insertion.

▪ *Pericardial tamponade:*
  - In a shock patient with enlarged jugular veins, pericardial tamponade must be differentiated from tension pneumothorax.
  - Most often it is a result of penetrating trauma.
  - Clinical diagnosis can be simple or very difficult.
  - All patients with near-cardiac penetrating injury and shock should be considered cardiac unless proven otherwise.
  - The classic diagnostic Beck triad consists of increased venous pressure, decreased arterial pressure, and dull heart sounds.
  - Pulsus paradoxus and Kussmaul's sign may still indicate pericardial tamponade.
  - In a subclinical case, a high index of suspicion and further diagnostic studies are necessary (chest X-ray showing an enlarged heart chamber or echocardiography showing fluid in the pericardial sac).
  - In cases where there has been heavy bleeding from other sites, jugular veins may be flat.
  - Pericardiocentesis has a high potential for iatrogenic cardiac injury and should be used as a temporary measure in a transport situation [under electrocardiogram (ECG) monitoring].
  - The correct immediate treatment for tamponade is surgery (sternotomy or left thoracotomy) if time permits in the operating room, otherwise in the emergency room.

▪ *Open pneumothorax (sucking chest wound):*
  - This is because the chest is wide open (over 3 cm) and the blood flow between the chest and atmospheric pressure is equalized.
  - As the blood flow is equalized, air builds up in the hemithorax, leading to deep hypovolemic and hypoxic conditions.
  - The signs and symptoms are typically proportional to the defect size.
  - The initial management is to immediately close the defect with sterile occlusion dressing tape on three sides to act like a flutter-type valve.
  - If the patient is not intubated, a chest tube should be placed in a location remote to the site of injury.
  - If definitive treatment is needed, the patient should be admitted to the operating room and referred early.

▪ *Massive hemothorax:*
  - Accumulation of blood in a hemithorax can significantly compromise respiratory efforts by compressing the lung and preventing adequate ventilation.
  - Such massive accumulation of blood presents as hemorrhagic shock, unilateral absence of breath sounds, dullness to percussion, and flat neck veins.
  - The treatment consists of correcting the hypovolemic shock, insertion of an intercostal drain, and in some cases intubation.
  - Blood in the pleural space should be removed as completely and rapidly as possible in order to prevent ongoing bleeding, empyema or late fibrothorax.
  - Initial drainage of >1,500 mL of blood or ongoing hemorrhage of >200 mL/h over 3–4 hours are generally considered indications for urgent thoracotomy.

▪ *Flail chest:*
  - It occurs when part of the chest wall lacks bony continuity with the rest of the chest.
  - This condition is usually caused by blunt trauma associated with multiple rib fractures (two or more ribs breaking in two or more places).

- The diagnosis is clinical.
- The chest wall should be observed for paradoxical movement of the chest segment during multiple breaths and coughing.
- The patient is also at high risk of immediate or delayed pneumothorax or hemothorax. Standard treatment consisted of mechanical ventilation in an "internal splint" of the chest until fibrous union of the fractured ribs occurred.
- Currently, treatment consists of oxygen administration, adequate analgesia, and physical therapy. Breathing is reserved for patients with respiratory failure.
- Surgery is another treatment option for thoraco-thoracic joint pain after it was previously dismissed because the underlying pathology was emphysema.
- It has now been shown that a select group of people with isolated, severe chest injuries and operations benefit from internal surgery.

9. Discuss the management of chest injury. ***KIIT University, Odisha 2025***

Management of Chest Injury in Blunt Trauma

Chest injuries from blunt trauma, such as those from motor vehicle accidents or falls, can range from minor rib fractures to life-threatening conditions like tension pneumothorax or massive hemothorax. Effective management involves rapid assessment, stabilization, and targeted interventions based on the injury's severity and the patient's clinical status. Below is a structured approach to managing chest injuries, focusing on blunt trauma, as derived from standard trauma protocols.

- *Initial assessment and stabilization*

  Chest injuries are evaluated as part of the primary survey in trauma care, following the *ABCDE* approach (Airway, Breathing, Circulation, Disability, Exposure). Immediate life-threatening conditions are addressed promptly.

  - *Airway:*
    - Ensure a patent airway. If compromised (e.g., due to facial trauma or unconsciousness), secure with intubation or advanced airway techniques.
    - Suspect airway obstruction in patients with stridor or severe respiratory distress.
  - *Breathing:*
    - Assess respiratory rate, oxygen saturation, and chest symmetry. Look for signs of hypoxia or respiratory failure.
    - Administer high-flow oxygen (10–15 L/min via non-rebreather mask) to maintain $SpO_2 \geq 94\%$.
    - *Identify and treat immediate threats:*
      - *Tension pneumothorax:* Signs include hypotension, distended neck veins, tracheal deviation, and absent breath sounds on the affected side. Treat with immediate needle decompression (2nd intercostal space, midclavicular line) followed by chest tube insertion (thoracostomy, 4th–5th intercostal space, anterior axillary line).
      - *Open pneumothorax:* Cover with a three-sided occlusive dressing to create a flutter-valve effect, followed by chest tube placement.
      - *Flail chest:* Multiple rib fractures causing paradoxical chest wall movement. Provide analgesia (e.g., intercostal nerve blocks, epidural) and consider mechanical ventilation if respiratory failure occurs.
      - *Massive hemothorax:* Significant blood in the pleural cavity (e.g., >1500 mL initially or >200 mL/h). Insert a large-bore chest tube (36–40 Fr) and prepare for possible surgical exploration (thoracotomy) if ongoing bleeding persists.
  - *Circulation:*
    - Control external bleeding and assess for hemorrhagic shock (e.g., from hemothorax or cardiac injury).
    - Obtain IV access and initiate fluid resuscitation cautiously (avoid over-resuscitation in permissive hypotension until bleeding is controlled).

    - Transfuse blood products early in massive hemorrhage (balanced 1:1:1 ratio of PRBCs, plasma, and platelets).
  - *Disability and exposure:*
    - Assess for associated neurological injuries (e.g., traumatic brain injury) and expose the patient to identify all injuries while preventing hypothermia.
- *Diagnostic evaluation*
  Once life-threatening conditions are addressed, perform a secondary survey and diagnostic workup to identify specific injuries.
  - *Physical examination:*
    - Inspect for chest wall deformity, bruising, or open wounds.
    - Palpate for crepitus, subcutaneous emphysema, or rib tenderness.
    - Auscultate for diminished or absent breath sounds.
  - *Imaging:*
    - *Chest X-ray (CXR):* First-line imaging to detect pneumothorax, hemothorax, rib fractures, or widened mediastinum (suggesting aortic injury).
    - *Focused Assessment with Sonography for Trauma (FAST):* Extended FAST (eFAST) assesses for pneumothorax (absent lung sliding) or hemothorax.
    - *CT chest with contrast:* Gold standard for stable patients to evaluate for pulmonary contusion, rib fractures, vascular injuries (e.g., aortic disruption), or diaphragmatic rupture. Use if suspicion of occult injuries persists despite normal CXR.
    - *Echocardiography:* If cardiac tamponade or myocardial injury is suspected (e.g., muffled heart sounds, hypotension, or ECG changes).
  - *Other tests:*
    - *Arterial blood gas (ABG):* To assess oxygenation and ventilation status.
    - *ECG:* To evaluate for cardiac contusion (arrhythmias, ST changes).
    - *Bronchoscopy:* For suspected tracheobronchial injury (persistent air leak or large pneumothorax).
- *Specific management of common chest injuries:*
  Management depends on the specific injury identified. Below are key chest injuries and their treatments:
  - *Rib fractures:*
    - *Analgesia:* Critical to prevent hypoventilation. Use multimodal pain control (NSAIDs, opioids, intercostal nerve blocks, or thoracic epidural).
    - *Pulmonary toilet:* Encourage deep breathing, coughing, and incentive spirometry to prevent atelectasis or pneumonia.
    - *Surgical fixation:* Considered in severe flail chest with respiratory compromise or displaced fractures causing ongoing pain or lung injury.
  - *Pneumothorax:*
    - *Simple pneumothorax:* Small (<20% lung volume) and asymptomatic cases may be observed with supplemental oxygen. Larger or symptomatic cases require chest tube insertion.
    - *Tension pneumothorax:* Immediate needle decompression followed by chest tube placement.
    - *Persistent air leak:* May indicate tracheobronchial injury; consider bronchoscopy or surgical repair.
  - *Hemothorax:*
    - *Chest tube drainage:* For significant hemothorax (>500 mL). Monitor output; persistent bleeding (>200 mL/h for 2–4 hours or >1500 mL initially) indicates need for thoracotomy.
    - *Video-assisted thoracoscopic surgery (VATS):* For retained hemothorax or evacuation of clots in stable patients.
    - *Exploratory thoracotomy:* Indicated for massive hemothorax, ongoing bleeding, or suspected vascular/cardiac injury.

- *Pulmonary contusion:*
  - *Supportive care:* Optimize oxygenation, restrict fluids to avoid pulmonary edema, and monitor for acute respiratory distress syndrome (ARDS).
  - *Ventilation:* Noninvasive positive pressure ventilation (NIPPV) or mechanical ventilation if severe hypoxia develops.
- *Flail chest:*
  - *Analgesia and respiratory support:* As above. Intubation and positive pressure ventilation may be needed for severe cases.
  - *Surgical stabilization:* Rib fixation improves outcomes in patients with respiratory failure or persistent pain.
- *Cardiac tamponade:*
  - *Pericardiocentesis:* Emergent drainage for hemodynamic instability (guided by ultrasound if possible).
  - *Subxiphoid pericardial window or sternotomy:* For definitive management, especially if ongoing bleeding is suspected.
- *Aortic Injury:*
  - *Suspect in high-velocity trauma:* Widened mediastinum on CXR or CT findings (e.g., pseudoaneurysm).
  - *Management:* Urgent endovascular repair (thoracic endovascular aortic repair, TEVAR) or open surgery in specialized centers. Control blood pressure (beta-blockers, e.g., esmolol) to reduce aortic wall stress.
- *Diaphragmatic injury:*
  - *Diagnosis:* Often missed on initial CXR; CT or laparoscopy confirms rupture.
  - *Surgical repair:* Via laparotomy or thoracotomy, depending on associated injuries.

- *Damage control approach:*
  In unstable patients with multiple injuries, adopt a damage control strategy:
  - Address life-threatening chest injuries (e.g., chest tube for hemothorax, packing for bleeding).
  - Defer definitive repairs (e.g., rib fixation) until the patient is stabilized.
  - Use temporary closure techniques and transfer to ICU for resuscitation.
- *Adjuncts and supportive care:*
  - *Antibiotics:* Not routine for chest tubes unless contamination is suspected (e.g., open chest wounds). Use broad-spectrum antibiotics (e.g., cefazolin) in penetrating trauma or surgical cases.
  - *Tetanus prophylaxis:* Administer if open wounds are present.
  - *Thromboprophylaxis:* Start low-molecular-weight heparin (e.g., enoxaparin) in hospitalized patients once bleeding risk is low to prevent venous thromboembolism.
  - *Rehabilitation:* Early mobilization and physiotherapy to restore lung function and prevent complications like pneumonia.
- **Indications for Surgical Intervention**
  - *Thoracotomy:*
    - *Emergency thoracotomy:* For cardiac arrest due to penetrating trauma, massive hemothorax, or suspected cardiac injury. Performed in the trauma bay or operating room.
    - *Urgent thoracotomy:* For ongoing bleeding (>200 mL/hr via chest tube), large retained hemothorax, or great vessel injury.
  - *VATS:* For stable patients with retained hemothorax, empyema, or diagnostic evaluation of diaphragmatic injuries.
  - *Sternal/rib fixation:* For severe flail chest or nonhealing fractures causing chronic pain.
- *Non-operative management:*
  Many blunt chest injuries (e.g., small pneumothorax, rib fractures, pulmonary contusion) can be managed non-operatively in stable patients:
  - Monitor in a high-dependency unit or ICU for high-risk injuries (e.g., multiple rib fractures in elderly patients).
  - Serial imaging (CXR, CT) to assess resolution or progression.
  - Optimize pain control and respiratory support to avoid complications.

- *Special considerations:*
  - *Elderly patients:* Higher risk of morbidity due to reduced respiratory reserve. Aggressive pain management and early mobilization are critical.
  - *Pediatric patients:* More flexible chest wall; significant internal injury may occur without rib fractures. Use pediatric-specific protocols for imaging and intervention thresholds.
  - *Associated injuries:* Blunt chest trauma often occurs with head, abdominal, or orthopedic injuries. Prioritize based on hemodynamic and clinical status.

10. What is flail chest? Mention physiological changes that develop after flail chest. Outline its management.
WBUHS 2021 Supplementary

11. Flail chest. ***WBUHS 2009, 2015***

12. What is flail chest? What are the types of flail chest? How will you manage a patient with an anterior flail chest?
DY Patil Education Society, Deemed to be University. 2024.

Definition

Flail chest is a life-threatening medical condition that occurs when a segment of the rib cage breaks under extreme stress and becomes detached from the rest of the chest wall. It occurs when multiple adjacent ribs are broken in multiple places, separating a segment, so a part of the chest wall moves independently.

Types of Flail Chest

Flail chest can be classified based on:

1. *Based on the location of rib fractures:*
   - *Anterior flail chest*
     - Fractures occur in the *front (anterior)* part of the ribs.
     - Often involves *costochondral junctions* or sternum.
     - May be associated with *sternal fractures.*
   - *Lateral flail chest*
     - Fractures along the *side (lateral)* of the rib cage.
     - Most common type due to direct trauma (e.g., car accidents, falls).
     - Leads to a clearly visible paradoxical movement.
   - *Posterior flail chest*
     - Fractures occur in the back (posterior) ribs.
     - Less obvious clinically due to muscle coverage.
     - May be missed unless imaging is done.
2. *Based on the number and pattern of rib fractures:*
   - *Classic (Segmental) flail chest*
     - At least *three or more consecutive ribs* are fractured in *two or more places.*
     - This forms a free-floating segment of the chest wall.
   - *Nonclassic or incomplete flail chest*
     - Less than three ribs involved or not fractured in two places.
     - Still may cause paradoxical movement if instability is significant.
3. *Based on the cause or mechanism*
   - *Blunt trauma-induced flail chest*
     - Most common.
     - Caused by direct impact (e.g., MVCs, falls).

- Penetrating trauma-related flail chest
  - Less common.
  - Caused by stab wounds or gunshots that create instability in the chest wall.

4. *Based on association with other injuries:*
   - *Isolated flail chest:* Only the chest wall is involved, without underlying organ injury.
   - Complicated flail chest
     - Associated with:
       - Pulmonary contusion (very common)
       - Pneumothorax or hemothorax
       - Cardiac injury or great vessel injury

Physiological Changes

- During normal inspiration, the diaphragm contracts and intercostal muscles pull the rib cage out. Pressure in the thorax decreases below atmospheric pressure, and air rushes in through the trachea. The flail segment will be pulled in with the decrease in pressure while the rest of the rib cage expands.
- During normal expiration, the diaphragm and intercostal muscles relax increasing internal pressure, allowing the abdominal organs to push air upward and out of the thorax. However, a flail segment will also be pushed out while the rest of the rib cage contracts.
- A flail segment of the chest wall will negatively affect respiration in three ways: ineffective ventilation, pulmonary contusion, and hypoventilation with atelectasis. There is ineffective ventilation because of increased dead space, decreased intrathoracic pressure, and increased oxygen demand from injured tissue.

Treatment

Treatment of the flail chest initially follows the principles of advanced trauma life support.

Further treatment includes:

- Good analgesia, including intercostal blocks; narcotic pain relievers should be avoided as much as possible.
- It helps improve ventilation, increase breathing capacity, and increase blood oxygenation.
- If the segment is small and breathing is not compromised, treat the high-dependency unit (HDU) patient with appropriate analgesia.
- Encourage early movement and vigorous physical therapy. Blood gas analysis should be done regularly.
- Positive pressure breathing, careful adjustment of ventilator settings to avoid pulmonary barotrauma.
- Chest tubes as needed.
- Adjusting the position to make the patient as comfortable as possible and relieve pain
- Aggressive pulmonary toilet
- Positive pressure endotracheal intubation is necessary in more severe cases.
- Surgical fixation can help significantly shorten the duration of ventilatory support and preserve lung function.

---

13. Hemopneumothorax. ***WBUHS 2007***

Hemopneumothorax is a combination of two conditions: pneumothorax, or air in the chest cavity, and hemothorax (also called hemothorax), or blood in the chest cavity.

Pathogenesis

- A puncture of the chest wall can result in hemothorax, pneumothorax, or both.
- The pleural space is anatomically located between the visceral membrane, which is firmly attached to the lungs, and the parietal membrane, which is firmly attached to the chest (thoracic and intercostal muscles, intercostal muscles).
- The pleural space contains pleural fluid. This liquid holds the two membranes together by surface tension, just as a drop of water between two sheets of glass prevents them from separating.

- Therefore, when the intercostal muscles move the chest outward, the lungs are also pulled in, causing the pressure in the lungs to decrease and the air to be drawn into the bronchi when we inhale.
- The state of the pleura remains constant in the negative pressure state (compared to atmospheric pressure).
- If the rib cage, and thus the pleural space, is punctured, blood, air, or both can enter the pleural space. Air/blood rushes into the chamber to equalize the pressure with atmospheric pressure.
- As a result, the fluid breaks down and the two membranes no longer stick to each other. As the chest moves outward, it no longer pulls on the lungs.
- Thus, the lungs cannot expand, the pressure in the lungs never decreases, and air is drawn into the bronchi. Breathing is not possible.
- A diseased lung with a lot of elastic tissue shrinks into a so-called collapsed lung.

Treatment
- Tube thoracostomy
- Commonly, surgery is needed to close off whatever injuries caused the blood and air to enter the cavity (e.g., stabbing, broken ribs).

---

14. Underwater seal drainage. ***WBUHS 2021 Supplementary***

Introduction

Chest drains also known as underwater sealed drains (UWSD) are inserted to allow draining of the pleural spaces of air, blood, or fluid, allowing expansion of the lungs and restoration of negative pressure in the thoracic cavity. The underwater seal also prevents backflow of air or fluid into the pleural cavity.

Technique

Tube Thoracostomy
- The tube is inserted in an area described as the "safe zone", a region bordered by the lateral border of pectoralis major, a horizontal line inferior to the axilla, the anterior border of latissimus dorsi, and a horizontal line superior to the nipple.
- More specifically, the tube is inserted into the fifth intercostal space slightly anterior to the midaxillary line.
- The free end of the tube is usually attached to an underwater seal, below the level of the chest. This allows the air or fluid to escape from the pleural space and prevents anything returning to the chest.
- Chest tubes are usually inserted under local anesthesia.

Indications
- *Pneumothorax:* Accumulation of air or gas in the pleural space
- *Chylothorax:* A collection of lymphatic fluid in the pleural space
- *Empyema:* A pyogenic infection of the pleural space
- *Hemothorax:* Accumulation of blood in the pleural space
- *Hydrothorax:* Accumulation of serous fluid in the pleural space
- *Postoperative:* For example, thoracotomy, esophagectomy, cardiac surgery

Contraindications
- Refractory coagulopathy
- Diaphragmatic hernia
- Hepatic hydrothorax
- Scarring in the pleural space (adhesions)

Complications
- Major insertion complications include hemorrhage, infection, and reexpansion pulmonary edema.
- Injury to the liver, spleen, or diaphragm is possible if the tube is placed inferior to the pleural cavity. Injuries to the thoracic aorta and heart can also occur.

- Minor complications include a subcutaneous hematoma or seroma, anxiety, shortness of breath (dyspnea), and cough (after removing large volume of fluid).
- Subcutaneous emphysema indicates backpressure created by a clogged drain or insufficient negative pressure.

ABDOMINAL TRAUMA

15. NOMAT (Nonoperative management of solid organ injuries due to blunt abdominal trauma)

Definition

It is nonoperative management of solid organ injury due to blunt abdominal trauma.

Introduction

Abdominal trauma is regularly encountered in the emergency department. It is one of the leading causes of death and disability. Identification of serious intra-abdominal injury is often challenging. Most affected age group of blunt trauma abdomen is 15–30 years and prevalence is 13%.

Types of Abdominal Trauma

- Blunt trauma
- Penetrating trauma—Stab and gunshot injury

Common Solid Organ Injury

- Spleen
- Liver
- Kidney

Prehospital Care

- The goal of prehospital care is to deliver the patient to hospital for definitive care.
- Maintain airway and start intravenous (IV) line.
- Care of spinal cord
- Rapid transport the patient to trauma center

Initial Assessment and Resuscitation

Primary Survey

- A—Airway
- B—Breathing
- C—Circulation
- D—Disability
- E—Exposure

Emergency Care

- IV fluid
- Control external bleeding
- Dressing of wound
- Give high-flow oxygen
- Immobilize the patient with a fractured pelvis
- Keep the patient warm
- Analgesic
- Catheterization
- Nasogastric tube

Secondary Survey

- General and systemic examination
- Special attention to back, axilla, perineum

- Per rectal examination—sphincteric tone, bleeding, perforation
- Foley's catheter—monitor urine output
- Nasogastric tube

AMPLE History

- A—Allergy
- M—Medication
- P—Past medical history
- L—Last meal
- E—Event (what happened)

Examination

- *Palpation:* Mass, tenderness, peritonitis, rib fracture
- *Auscultation:* Bowel sound

Investigations

- FAST
- X-ray chest and abdomen
- USG
- CT scan
- Paracentesis
- Diagnostic peritoneal lavage (DPL)
- Diagnostic laparoscopy

Splenic Injury

- Most common intra-abdominal organ injury
- Commonly arterial hemorrhage
- *Conservative management:*
  - Hemodynamic stability
  - Negative abdominal examination
  - Absence of contrast extravasation in CT
  - Absence of other indication of laparotomy
  - Grade I–III injury (subcapsular hematoma, laceration <3 cm)

Splenic Injury Scale

Grade	Injury	Description
I	Laceration	Capsular tear, <1 cm parenchymal depth
II	Hematoma	• Subcapsular, 10–50%, surface area • Intraparenchymal, <5 cm in diameter
	Laceration	1–3 cm parenchymal depth, which does not involve a trabecular vessel
III	Hematoma	• Subcapsular, >50% surface area or expanding; ruptured subcapsular or parenchymal hematoma • Intraparenchymal hematoma >5 cm or expanding
	Laceration	>3 cm parenchymal depth or involving trabecular vessels
IV	Laceration	Laceration involving segmental or hilar vessels producing major devascularization (>25% of spleen)
V	Laceration	Completely shattered spleen
	Vascular	Hilar vascular injury which devascularizes spleen

- *Monitoring:* Serial abdominal examination and hematocrit are essential. Success rate of conservative management >80%.

Liver Injury

- Second-most common solid organ to be injured.
- Usually venous bleeding; 85% of all hepatic injury due to trauma are stable.
- CT scan is the mainstay of diagnosis in a stable patient.

Nonoperative management:

- Hemodynamically stable
- No other intra-abdominal injury require surgery
- Less than 2 units' PRBC transfusion
- Hemoperitoneum <500 mL on CT
- Grade I–III

Renal Injury

Diagnosis:

- History, clinical examination
- *Presentation:* Shock, hematuria, pain

Imaging: X-ray KUB, ultrasonography (USG) abdomen, CT scan abdomen

Management:

- About 85% of blunt renal injury can be managed conservatively.
- *Renal contusion:* Manage conservatively.

16. How do you manage a patient with blunt trauma abdomen who is in shock? ***WBUHS 2024***

Management of a Patient with Blunt Trauma Abdomen in Shock

Blunt trauma to the abdomen can cause serious internal injuries, leading to hemorrhagic shock due to organ rupture (e.g., spleen, liver), vascular injury, or bowel perforation. Managing such a patient requires a systematic approach following *Advanced Trauma Life Support (ATLS)* guidelines to ensure rapid stabilization, diagnosis, and definitive treatment.

Primary Survey (ABCDE Approach)

A—Airway and Cervical Spine Control

- Ensure a patent airway by suctioning secretions and assessing for obstruction.
- If the patient has altered consciousness (GCS ≤8), intubation is necessary.
- Protect the cervical spine with a rigid collar until cervical injury is ruled out.

B—Breathing and Oxygenation

- Assess for pneumothorax, hemothorax, or flail chest, which may worsen shock.
- Provide high-flow oxygen (15 L/min) via a non-rebreather mask or initiate mechanical ventilation if needed.

C—Circulation and Hemorrhage Control

- Insert two large-bore (16G or 14G) IV cannulas or a central line if peripheral access is difficult.
- Start aggressive fluid resuscitation with crystalloids (Ringer's lactate or normal saline, 1–2 L bolus).
- Initiate blood transfusion (O-negative or cross-matched blood) if there are signs of ongoing hemorrhage.
- Consider using massive transfusion protocols (1:1:1 ratio of PRBCs, plasma, and platelets) if hemorrhagic shock is suspected.
- Monitor blood pressure, heart rate, and urine output (goal: ≥0.5 mL/kg/h).

D—Disability (Neurological Status)

- Check Glasgow Coma Scale (GCS) to assess neurological function.
- Look for signs of head injury or spinal cord involvement.

E—Exposure and Environmental Control

- Fully expose the patient to identify other injuries, while preventing hypothermia with warm IV fluids and blankets.

Secondary Survey (Focused Trauma Assessment)

History and mechanism of injury: Obtain information on the type and force of impact (e.g., motor vehicle accident, fall, assault).

Physical examination:

- *Signs of peritoneal irritation:* Guarding, rigidity, rebound tenderness.
- *Signs of internal bleeding:* Abdominal distension, bruising (e.g., Cullen's sign, Grey-Turner's sign).
- *Pelvic instability:* Suggests associated fractures, which can cause massive blood loss.

Bedside imaging and laboratory tests:

- *FAST (Focused Assessment with Sonography for Trauma):* Rapid bedside ultrasound to detect free intraperitoneal fluid (blood).
- *CT abdomen with IV contrast (if stable enough for transport):* Identifies organ injuries, retroperitoneal bleeding.
- *X-rays:* Chest and pelvis to assess for associated injuries.
- *Arterial Blood Gas (ABG):* To assess for metabolic acidosis (suggesting ongoing shock).
- *Hemoglobin and hematocrit:* To estimate blood loss.
- *Coagulation profile and cross-matching:* Prepare for transfusion if needed.

Definitive Management Based on Diagnosis

Unstable patient with positive fast → emergency laparotomy

- If the patient remains in shock despite resuscitation and has a positive FAST scan (free fluid), immediate damage control surgery is indicated.
- *Common injuries requiring surgery:*
  - *Splenic rupture:* Splenectomy or splenorrhaphy
  - *Liver laceration:* Packing, hemostasis, or partial resection
  - *Bowel perforation:* Resection with primary anastomosis or diversion
  - *Major vascular injury:* Ligation or repair

Stable patient with positive FAST → Further Imaging (CT Abdomen)

- If the patient stabilizes after resuscitation, a CT scan helps define the injury and plan non-operative management.

Unstable patient with negative FAST → Consider other causes of shock

- Retroperitoneal hematoma (e.g., Pelvic Fracture) → May require angiographic embolization.
  - Spinal or Neurogenic Shock → Needs careful fluid management and vasopressors.

Postoperative or ICU Care

- ICU monitoring for ongoing bleeding, multi-organ dysfunction, and sepsis
- Continue resuscitation with fluids and blood products as needed
- *Monitor for complications:*
  - Acute kidney injury (AKI)
  - Abdominal compartment syndrome
  - Sepsis and multi-organ failure

17. Write notes on diagnostic modalities of blunt abdominal trauma. ***WBUHS 2016***

- FAST should be the initial diagnostic modality to evaluate for hemoperitoneum.
- CT is accurate in determining the presence of injury and delineating the need for operation in blunt abdominal trauma. It should be reserved for hemodynamically stable patients.

- DPL is accurate in diagnosing intraperitoneal injury but has a limited role nowadays.
- Bowel, diaphragm, and pancreas injuries are difficult to exclude with any of the three diagnostic modalities.
- CT, FAST, and DPL play complementary roles in blunt abdominal trauma diagnostic algorithms.

Recommendations

1. *Level I:*
   - *DPL:* Positive—exploratory laparotomy.
   - *CT scan:* Hemodynamically stable patients with equivocal findings on PE, associated neurologic injury, or multiple extra-abdominal injuries. Patients with a negative CT should be admitted for observation.
   - CT is the diagnostic modality of choice for nonoperative management of solid visceral injuries.
   - In hemodynamically stable patients, DPL and CT are complementary diagnostic modalities.
2. *Level II:*
   - FAST may be considered as the initial diagnostic modality to exclude hemoperitoneum. If FAST is negative, DPL and CT have complementary roles.
   - When DPL is done, clinical decisions should be based on the presence of gross blood on initial aspiration (i.e., 10 mL) or microscopic analysis of lavage effluent.
   - Hemodynamically stable patients with a positive DPL—follow-up CT scan should be considered, if there is pelvic fracture or suspected injuries to the genitourinary tract, diaphragm, or pancreas.
   - Hemodynamically unstable patients with a positive FAST—exploratory laparotomy

     Hemodynamically stable patients with a positive FAST—follow-up CT to decide nonoperative management of select injuries

     Surveillance studies (i.e., DPL, CT, repeat FAST) are required in hemodynamically stable patients with indeterminate FAST results.
3. *Level III:*
   - Objective diagnostic testing (i.e., FAST, DPL, CT) is indicated for patients with abnormal mentation, equivocal findings on PE, multiple injuries, concomitant chest injury, or hematuria.
   - Patients with seatbelt sign (SBS) should be admitted for observation and serial PE to be done. Detection of intraperitoneal fluid by FAST or CT in a patient with SBS mandates either DPL to determine the nature of the fluid or exploratory laparotomy.
   - CT is indicated for the evaluation of suspected renal injuries.
   - A negative FAST should prompt follow-up CT for patients at high risk for intra-abdominal injuries (e.g., multiple orthopedic injuries, severe chest wall trauma, neurologic impairment).
   - Splanchnic angiography may be considered in patients who require angiography for the evaluation of other injuries (e.g., thoracic aortic injury, pelvic fracture).

18. What are the approaches and indication for laparotomy in patient with blunt trauma abdomen?

KIIT University, Odisha, 2024

Indications for Laparotomy in Blunt Abdominal Trauma

Laparotomy is a critical intervention in blunt abdominal trauma, reserved for cases where non-operative management is not feasible or has failed. The decision is based on clinical presentation, hemodynamic status, and diagnostic findings from tools like FAST (Focused Assessment with Sonography for Trauma), DPL (Diagnostic Peritoneal Lavage), or CT imaging. Key indications include:

- *Hemodynamic instability or uncontrolled hemorrhage:* This is a primary indication, particularly when associated with positive FAST or DPL showing hemoperitoneum. For instance, in hemodynamically unstable patients with evidence of intra-abdominal bleeding, immediate laparotomy is mandated.
- *Signs of peritonitis:* Diffuse abdominal tenderness, rigidity, or rebound tenderness on physical examination signals potential hollow viscus injury or contamination, necessitating exploration.

- *Clinical deterioration during observation:* In patients initially managed non-operatively, worsening vital signs, development of peritonitis, or failure to improve (e.g., requiring >2 units of blood transfusion due to solid organ injury) warrants laparotomy.
- *Specific diagnostic findings:*
  - Active extravasation or contained hematoma adjacent to major vessels on CT.
  - Hollow viscus injury (e.g., bowel perforation suggested by free air, unexplained free fluid, bowel wall thickening, or mesenteric hematoma on CT).
  - Major pancreatic ductal injury (confirmed by imaging like MR pancreatography).
  - Intraperitoneal bladder rupture (confirmed by cystography).
  - Diaphragmatic tear (e.g., evident on chest radiograph or high suspicion with negative non-invasive tests).
  - Persistent urinary leakage or hematuria from renal fragmentation.
- *Special considerations:* In cases of multiple-system injuries, pelvic fractures with expanding hematomas, or closed head injuries complicating assessment, laparotomy may be indicated if non-operative approaches fail. For retroperitoneal hematomas, exploration depends on zone: all Zone I (central) must be explored; Zone II (perinephric) only if expanding or pulsatile; Zone III (pelvic) often managed with packing or embolization rather than routine exploration.

Not all positive findings (e.g., free fluid on FAST in stable patients) require immediate laparotomy; these may be followed with CT or observation if the patient is hemodynamically stable.

Surgical Approaches for Laparotomy in Blunt Abdominal Trauma

The standard approach is an exploratory laparotomy via a midline incision, allowing comprehensive access to the peritoneal cavity for hemorrhage control, injury assessment, and repair. The procedure emphasizes rapid control of life-threatening issues, with a potential shift to damage control surgery in unstable patients.

- *Incision and entry:* A generous midline laparotomy incision is made from the xiphoid process to the pubic symphysis (or midway to the umbilicus if pelvic packing is anticipated). The peritoneum is entered carefully to avoid iatrogenic injury. Broad-spectrum antibiotics are administered preoperatively.
- *Initial hemorrhage control:* Upon entry, evacuate blood/clots and pack all four quadrants and the pelvis. Clamp vascular structures if needed. If the patient is in hemorrhagic shock, prioritize packing to allow resuscitation before full exploration.
- *Systematic exploration:* Eviscerate the small bowel for inspection. Perform a thorough evaluation of intra-abdominal contents, including solid organs (liver, spleen, kidneys), hollow viscera, mesentery, and diaphragm. Suture obvious hollow viscus injuries. Explore retroperitoneum based on hematoma zones (as noted above). Use specific maneuvers for exposure:
  - *Mattox maneuver (left medial visceral rotation):* For left-sided injuries, mobilize the left colon, spleen, and pancreas medially to access the aorta, celiac axis, superior mesenteric vessels, left kidney, iliac vessels, and ureter.
  - *Cattell-Braasch maneuver (right medial visceral rotation):* For right-sided injuries, mobilize the right colon and small bowel to access the inferior vena cava, right kidney, ureter, and iliac vessels. Include Kocher maneuver for duodenal and pancreatic head exposure.
  - Enter the lesser sac for posterior stomach and pancreas visualization.
- *Damage control surgery:* In coagulopathic, hypothermic, or acidotic patients, abbreviate the procedure: control bleeding (e.g., packing, ligation) and contamination (e.g., staple bowel ends), then temporarily close the abdomen (e.g., with negative pressure dressing) for later definitive repair. Avoid complex reconstructions initially.
- *Closure and adjuncts:* After repair, close the fascia with absorbable suture; use drains if needed. In contaminated cases, continue antibiotics for 5–7 days. For pelvic bleeding, consider preperitoneal packing via a separate incision or postoperative angiography/embolization.

Laparoscopy is rarely used in blunt trauma due to limitations in visualization and risk of complications like air embolism, though it may have a role in diagnosing diaphragmatic injuries in select stable cases. Non-operative alternatives like angiography with embolization are preferred for stable patients with solid organ bleeding to avoid laparotomy when possible.

19. Discuss grades of splenic injury and their various modalities of management. ***KIIT University, Odisha 2025***

Splenic injury is one of the most common abdominal injuries, especially in blunt trauma (e.g., road traffic accidents). The spleen is a highly vascular organ, so injuries can lead to life-threatening hemorrhage.

To guide diagnosis and treatment, the *American Association for the Surgery of Trauma (AAST)* has classified splenic injuries into *Grades I to V.*

Grades of Splenic Injury (AAST—Revised 2018)

Grade	*Injury description*
Grade I	• Subcapsular hematoma <10% of surface area • Capsular laceration <1 cm depth
Grade II	• Subcapsular hematoma 10–50% of surface area • Intraparenchymal hematoma <5 cm • Laceration 1–3 cm depth without trabecular vessel injury
Grade III	• Subcapsular hematoma >50% or expanding • Intraparenchymal hematoma >5 cm or expanding • Laceration >3 cm depth or involving trabecular vessels
Grade IV	• Laceration involving segmental or hilar vessels with major devascularization (>25% of spleen)
Grade V	• Completely shattered spleen • Hilar vascular injury with devascularization of entire spleen

Modalities of Management

- Nonoperative Management (NOM)
  - Preferred in *hemodynamically stable patients*, especially with *low-grade (I–III) injuries*
  - Close monitoring in ICU/trauma ward
  - Serial hemoglobin monitoring
  - Bed rest, observation, and repeat imaging if needed
  - *Advantages:* Preserves splenic function, avoids surgery
  - *Indications:*
    - Hemodynamic stability
    - No other indications for laparotomy
    - Patient can be observed in a monitored setting
- Angioembolization
  - Used for active bleeding, contrast blush on CT, or pseudoaneurysm
  - Minimally invasive
  - Often used with NOM to control bleeding
  - Can help avoid surgery even in Grade III–IV injuries

Operative Management

- Indicated in:
  - Hemodynamic instability despite resuscitation
  - Peritonitis
  - Massive hemoperitoneum
  - Failure of NOM or angioembolization

Types of Surgery:

- Splenorrhaphy (splenic repair)—for low-grade injuries
- Partial splenectomy—rarely done
- Total splenectomy—for shattered spleen or hilar injury (Grade V)

Postsplenectomy Care

- Risk of *overwhelming postsplenectomy infection (OPSI)*, especially in children
- Vaccinations required:
  - Pneumococcal
  - Meningococcal
  - *Haemophilus influenzae* type b (Hib)
- Ideally given before surgery or within 14 days postoperative

LIVER TRAUMA

20. What are the grades of liver injury? Discuss the management algorithm of liver injury with active bleed. DY Patil Educational Society 2020

21. Management of liver trauma . KGMU Lucknow 2025

Introduction

- Liver is the *most commonly injured solid organ* in abdominal trauma (both blunt and penetrating).
- Due to its *large size, friable parenchyma, and dual blood supply* (hepatic artery and portal vein).
- *Mortality* mainly due to *massive hemorrhage* and *associated injuries.*

Grading of Liver Injury (AAST - American Association for the Surgery of Trauma Classification, 2018)

Grade	Description	Extent / Criteria
Grade I	Minor injury	• Subcapsular hematoma <10% surface area • Laceration <1 cm deep
Grade II	Mild injury	• Subcapsular hematoma 10–50% surface area, intraparenchymal <10 cm • Laceration 1–3 cm deep, <10 cm long
Grade III	Moderate injury	• Subcapsular hematoma >50% or ruptured hematoma • Intraparenchymal hematoma >10 cm or expanding • Laceration >3 cm deep
Grade IV	Severe injury	Parenchymal disruption involving 25–75% of a hepatic lobe or 1–3 Couinaud segments within a single lobe
Grade V	Critical injury	• Parenchymal disruption of >75% of hepatic lobe or >3 Couinaud segments • Juxtahepatic venous injury (retrohepatic IVC or major hepatic veins)
Grade VI	Hepatic avulsion	Total hepatic avulsion (fatal)

Pathophysiology of Bleeding in Liver Trauma

- *Source:* hepatic artery, portal vein, hepatic veins, or parenchymal oozing.
- *Patterns:*
  - *Capsular tears → minor bleeding*
  - *Deep parenchymal tears → major bleeding*
  - *Hepatic venous or IVC injury → torrential bleed*

Clinical Presentation

Findings	Features
History	Blunt trauma (RTA, fall) or penetrating injury
Symptoms	Right upper quadrant pain, abdominal distension, shock
Signs	Hypotension, tachycardia, tenderness, guarding, signs of peritonitis
Others	Associated rib fractures (esp. right lower ribs), shoulder tip pain (diaphragmatic irritation)

Diagnosis/Investigations

Investigation	Findings/Role
FAST (Focused Assessment with Sonography in Trauma)	Free intraperitoneal fluid (first-line in unstable patients)
CT Abdomen with IV contrast	Gold standard in hemodynamically stable patients – defines grade, active bleeding, pseudoaneurysm, bile leak
Diagnostic peritoneal lavage (DPL)	Used rarely now; positive for gross blood
Laboratory	Hb drop, LFT derangements (AST/ALT markedly raised)

Management Algorithm of Liver Injury

- *Initial Assessment (ATLS Principles)*
  - *Airway* with cervical spine control
  - *Breathing* – oxygenation, ventilation
  - *Circulation* – control hemorrhage, IV fluids, blood transfusion
  - *Disability* – neurological assessment
  - *Exposure* – full examination, keep patient warm
- *Determine Hemodynamic Stability*

Stable	Unstable
Normal BP and HR after resuscitation	Persistent hypotension despite fluids/blood
Can undergo imaging (CT)	Needs urgent surgical or angiographic intervention

F. Management Algorithm in Liver Injury with Active Bleed

Step 1: Resuscitation

- Two large-bore IV lines / central access
- *Massive transfusion protocol* if required (PRBC:FFP:Platelet = 1:1:1)
- Correct acidosis, hypothermia, coagulopathy ("lethal triad")

Step 2: Evaluate Stability

- *Hemodynamically stable → CT with contrast*
  - *Active contrast extravasation* = active arterial bleed
  - *Contained hematoma* = non-expanding injury

Step 3: Definitive Management

Non-Operative Management (NOM)

(Preferred for hemodynamically stable patients — even for high-grade injuries)

Components:

- Intensive monitoring (vitals, Hb, LFTs)
- Serial clinical exams and imaging
- Bed rest and gradual mobilization
- *Transfusion support as needed*
- *Adjunct:* Angioembolization for active bleed or pseudoaneurysm

Success rate: >85–90% for Grades I–III, and many Grade IV–V injuries if stable

Angiographic (Interventional Radiology) Management

Indications:

- Active contrast extravasation (arterial bleed) on CT
- Persistent bleeding despite hemodynamic stability
- Pseudoaneurysm or arteriovenous fistula

Procedure:

- *Selective hepatic artery embolization* using coils, gelfoam, or glue
- Controls bleeding while preserving liver parenchyma

Operative Management

Indications:

- Hemodynamic instability despite resuscitation
- Peritonitis or hollow viscus injury suspected
- Massive hemoperitoneum or expanding hematoma with active bleeding
- Failed non-operative/embolization management

Surgical Techniques (Stepwise Approach)

Technique	*Purpose / Indication*
Manual compression	Initial control of hemorrhage
Perihepatic packing	Temporizing measure in damage-control surgery
Pringle's maneuver	Occlude hepatoduodenal ligament (portal triad) to stop inflow bleeding (portal vein + hepatic artery)
Direct suture repair (hepatorrhaphy)	Control of laceration with absorbable sutures ± hemostatic agents
Topical hemostatics	Fibrin glue, Surgicel, gel foam
Resectional debridement / Segmentectomy	For devitalized tissue or uncontrolled segmental bleeding
Total vascular isolation	For uncontrolled hepatic venous or retrohepatic IVC bleeding
Damage control surgery	For unstable patient – packing, temporary closure, ICU resuscitation, relook after 24–48 hr

Postoperative and Conservative Care

- ICU monitoring
- Serial Hb, LFT, coagulation profile
- Broad-spectrum antibiotics
- Watch for complications (bile leak, abscess, rebleed)
- Early enteral nutrition

Complications of Liver Injury

Early	*Late*
Hemorrhage, shock, coagulopathy	Bile leak, biloma, biliary peritonitis
Infection, abscess	Post-traumatic cyst or pseudoaneurysm
ARDS, sepsis	Secondary hemorrhage
Liver failure (rare)	Portal hypertension (very rare)

22. Classify duodenal injuries. *WBUHS 2025*

23. Give an outline of the management of duodenal injuries. *WBUHS 2021*

24. Traumatic duodenal injury. *WBUHS 2014*

Introduction

Duodenal injuries are uncommon after blunt and penetrating trauma but can be challenging to diagnose and manage. Most are caused by penetrating mechanisms occurring in 6.7% of penetrating abdominal cases, most of which are the result of gunshot wounds. The associated mortality is significant.

In those that present with a blunt hollow visceral injury, 12% are located in the duodenum. The mortality after blunt duodenal injury ranges from 11.4 to 14.8%.

Mechanism of Injury

Blunt injuries are presumably caused by a blow to the epigastrium by a narrow object, resulting in contusion of the wall or a blowout secondary to acute elevation of intraluminal pressure.

The classic description is the abdomen being struck by a steering wheel, or in children, a bicycle handlebar.

Clinical Features and Diagnosis

- Although duodenal injuries after penetrating trauma are found at laparotomy, their identification after a blunt mechanism can be challenging and therefore require a high index of suspicion to avoid missed injuries.
- Because of the retroperitoneal location of a significant portion of the duodenum, PE findings may be limited.
- Even full-thickness perforations of the duodenum may not demonstrate peritoneal signs unless the perforation involves an intraperitoneal segment.
  - The mainstay of evaluation for duodenal injury has become abdominal CT, with a low threshold for operative exploration.
  - Findings on CT that reflect possible duodenal injury include thickened duodenal wall, air or fluid outside the bowel lumen, and contrast extravasation if oral contrast was administered.
  - Low-grade injuries resulting in a duodenal hematoma can be identified by CT, although it is important also to evaluate the pancreas because of a high rate of concomitant injury.

Duodenum Injury Scale

Grade	*Type of injury*	*Description of injury*
1	• Hematoma • Laceration	• Involving single portion of duodenum • Partial thickness, no perforation
II	• Hematoma • Laceration	• Involving more than one portion • Disruption <50% of circumference
III	Laceration	• Disruption 50–75% of circumference of D2 • Disruption 50–100% of circumference of D1, D3, D4
IV	Laceration	• Disruption >75% of circumference of D2 • Involving ampulla or distal common bile duct
V	• Laceration • Vascular	• Massive disruption of duodenopancreatic complex • Devascularization of duodenum

Management

Duodenal Perforation

- It can be difficult to diagnose.
- Patients often complain only of vague back or flank pain, and symptoms can evolve slowly.
- Plain radiographic signs suggestive of perforation include evidence of retroperitoneal gas, blurring of the right psoas muscle, and leftward scoliosis.
- Upper gastrointestinal (GI) fluoroscopy using water-soluble contrast may also show evidence of a leak.
- The diagnostic modality of choice, however, is CT using oral and IV contrast, with the oral contrast administered in the trauma bay. Operative therapy depends on the degree of injury, but complete mobilization of the duodenum (Kocher maneuver) is essential for proper visualization and repair.
- Most defects (approximately 80%) can be repaired primarily in two layers, with a transverse closure to avoid luminal narrowing. Closed suction drainage placed around the repair is strongly recommended to control any anastomotic leak.
- Nasoduodenal decompression should be initiated.

- Alternatively, antegrade or retrograde (preferred) tube duodenostomy can be performed in conjunction with tube gastrostomy and feeding jejunostomy, the so-called triple tube drainage.

Complex Duodenal Injuries

- They are an operative challenge, and management remains controversial, especially in the presence of tissue devitalization.
- Whenever possible, debridement with primary repair should be performed. The repair should be protected via triple tube drainage or pyloric exclusion with diverting gastrojejunostomy.
- For large defects not amenable to primary closure, a retrocolic Roux-en-Y duodenojejunostomy is an option.
- Finally, pancreaticoduodenectomy (Whipple procedure) should be reserved only for the most complex injuries, including duodenal devascularization or severe combined injuries involving the pancreatic head and bile duct. This procedure has a very high morbidity and mortality in the trauma setting.
- In the damage control setting, the use of a duodenostomy tube or resection leaving the GI tract in discontinuity is highly effective for controlling contamination temporarily.

25. Outline the management algorithm for traumatic pancreatic injury. ***WBUHS 2021 Supplementary***

Classification of Pancreatic Trauma

Grade or type	***Condition***
AAST-OIS : American Association for the Surgery of Trauma Organ Injury Scale	
Grade I: • Hematoma • Laceration	• Minor contusion without ductal injury • Superficial laceration without ductal injury
Grade II: • Hematoma • Laceration	• Major contusion without ductal injury or tissue loss • Major laceration without ductal injury or tissue loss
Grade III: Laceration	• Distal transection or pancreatic parenchymal injury with ductal injury
Grade IV: Laceration	• Proximal transection or pancreatic parenchymal injury involving the ampulla
Grade V: Laceration	• Massive disruption of the pancreatic head
JAST: Japanese Association for the Surgery of Trauma	
Type I: Subcapsular injury	• Maintained continuity of capsule • No leak of pancreatic juice
Type II: Superficial injury	• Parenchymal injury <1/2 • No main pancreatic duct injury
Grade or type	***Condition***
Type IIIa: Simple deep injury	• Parenchymal injury >1/2 • No main pancreatic duct injury
Type IIIb: Complex deep injury	• Parenchymal injury >1/2 • With main pancreatic duct injury

Algorithm for Management of Pancreatic Trauma

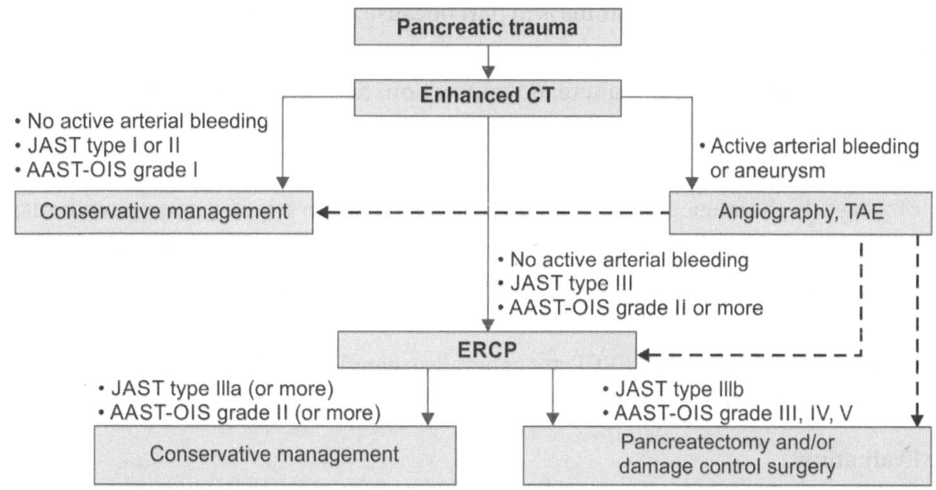

(AAST–OIS: American Association for the Surgery of Trauma Organ Injury Scale; CT: computed tomography; ERCP: Endoscopic retrograde Cholangiopancreatography; JAST: Japanese Association for the Surgery of Trauma; TAE: transcatheter arterial embolization)

26. Outline the management of pancreaticoduodenal injury. ***WBUHS 2007***

27. Discuss the management of combined pancreaticoduodenal injuries. ***WBUHS 2025***

Introduction

Detection and surgical management of duodenal and pancreatic injuries is a difficult one to manage. Delay in diagnosis is common due to nonspecific clinical findings and high incidence of associated injuries. Moreover, the low incidence of injuries to the duodenum and pancreas prevents from acquiring a large clinical experience which results in a low index of suspicion.

Diagnosis

- The approach to pancreatic and duodenal injuries begins with the evaluation of the injured patient.
- Management of hemodynamic instability and penetrating abdominal injuries requires little preoperative evaluation. Diagnosis of blunt injuries in hemodynamically stable patients can be more difficult.
- Common mechanisms include deceleration injuries with blunt force to the epigastrium and crush injuries.
- Initial PE findings may be subtle and include persistent abdominal pain and tenderness with or without peritonitis. They may be overshadowed by findings associated with major chest, abdominal, and pelvic injuries.
- Duodenal injuries missed on initial evaluation often develop into peritonitis and shock within a few days of injury. Plasma amylase or lipase levels should be measured in all patients with suspected pancreatic and duodenal injuries. Although a single elevated value is not diagnostic for pancreatic injury, serial evaluation showing elevated amylase or lipase activity with peritonitis demands further evaluation or exploration.

Imaging Investigations

- Initial plain radiographs are of little use in the diagnosis of pancreatic or duodenal injuries. Signs such as retroperitoneal air, obliteration of the right psoas shadow, and mild spine scoliosis are subtle or absent.
- FAST examination is helpful in identifying hemoperitoneum in hemodynamically unstable patients, it is not helpful in locating the source of bleeding or in diagnosing retroperitoneal injuries.
- Contrast-enhanced CT (CECT) is helpful in case of an early suspicion of retroperitoneal duodenal injury. An extraluminal gas or is contrast extravasation diagnostic for duodenal perforation. False-negative studies occur.

- Preoperative identification of blunt pancreatic injuries in the absence of clear indications for laparotomy is difficult. Delayed presentation of symptoms is in part because of the requirement of pancreatic secretions to be activated by infection or small bowel contents.
- CT findings may be normal or show pancreatic transection, hemorrhage, phlegmon and peripancreatic fluid. Initial CT scans may not define pancreatic injuries and should be repeated for patients with persistent abdominal pain, fever, or chemical evidence of pancreatitis.
- Endoscopic retrograde cholangiopancreatography (ERCP) is used in selected patients with suspected pancreatic injuries for which other diagnostic maneuvers are equivocal. The value of ERCP is to exclude main pancreatic duct injury in the patient with CT and chemical evidence of pancreatitis but with minimal clinical signs and symptoms.
- Pancreatic duct injuries identified by ERCP are generally treated surgically. Treatment of pancreatic duct injury by ERCP-placed stents in select patients with a prohibitive operative risk has been reported.

Preoperative Evaluation

- Pancreatic and duodenal injuries are often discovered at the time of laparotomy. In such cases, the principles of trauma surgery priority pertain, with control of life-threatening hemorrhage and control of enteric spillage. Damage control maneuvers should be considered early and abbreviated laparotomy performed to avoid acidosis, hypothermia, and coagulopathy.
    - A systematic examination of the abdomen is performed.
    - Complete evaluation of the duodenum and pancreas is indicated for the presence of upper or central retroperitoneal hematoma, air, or bile staining.
    - Intraoperative indications of pancreatic injury include peripancreatic fluid, subcapsular hematoma, hemorrhage, parenchymal disruption, pancreatic fluid leak, and fat necrosis.

Intraoperative evaluation of the duodenum requires examination of anterior and retroperitoneal surfaces from the pylorus to the mesenteric vessels and inspection of the fourth portion of the duodenum to the left of the mesenteric vessels.

Complete evaluation of the pancreas requires visualization of the head, body, and tail. Because the duodenum and pancreas are intimately associated, examination of both structures proceeds simultaneously.

The presence of penetrating injury to the anterior surface of the pancreas requires assessment of the main pancreatic duct.

Upfront exploration identifies injury in most cases of penetrating trauma. Although technically possible, intraoperative ERCP is often prohibited by time constraints and inability to cannulate the major papilla endoscopically.

Modified Lucas Classification of Pancreatic Injury

Class I: Simple superficial contusion or peripheral laceration with minimal parenchymal damage; any portion of the pancreas can be affected, but the main pancreatic duct is intact.

Class II: This includes deep laceration, perforation, or transaction of the neck, body, or tail of the pancreas, with or without pancreatic duct injury.

Class III: This includes severe crush, perforation, or transaction of the head of the pancreas, with or without pancreatic duct injury.

Class IV: Combined pancreaticoduodenal injuries, subdivided into:

- Minor pancreatic injury
- Severe pancreatic injury and duct disruption

Type of injury	Treatment
Class I	Control of bleeding and simple external drainage without repair of capsular lacerations + put a closed suction drain
Class II	Distal pancreatectomy + splenectomy, some surgeons prefer additional Roux-en-Y pancreaticojejunostomy to prevent pancreatic fistula, but a visible pancreatic duct is best managed by ligation with a transfixing suture; oversewing or stapling at the end of the pancreas and using simple buttress or seal-the-cut margin are sufficient
Class III	Simple external drainage, even if there is a suspected isolated pancreatic duct injury, provided there is no devitalization and ampulla is intact.
Class IV	• Define the integrity of the CBD, pancreatic duct, and the ampulla and the viability of the duodenum • If the CBD and ampulla are shown to be intact, the duodenal laceration is repaired, and the pancreatic injury is treated according to the site of the injury. Localized ischemia at the site of the duodenal injury should be debrided before primary duodenal closure • With a severe injury to the duodenum—diversion of gastric and biliary contents from the duodenal repair is advised by some—like duodenal "diverticulization" procedure with primary closure of the duodenal wound, a vagotomy, an antrectomy with an end to side gastrojejunostomy, a T-tube CBD drainage, and a tube duodenostomy • Another procedure is pyloric exclusion • Pancreaticoduodenectomy is needed when: – Extensive devitalization of the head of the pancreas and duodenum so that reconstruction is not possible – Ductal disruption of the pancreatic head in association with injuries to the duodenum and distal CBD – Injury to the ampulla of Vater, with disruption of the MPD from the duodenum – Uncontrollable bleeding from vessels in the head of the pancreas – Inaccessible exsanguinating retropancreatic portal or SMV injury

(CBD: common bile duct; SMV: superior mesenteric vein)

Complications

- Exsanguination is the most common cause of death associated with pancreatic and duodenal injuries.
- Other causes of death include multiple organ failure and sepsis. Mortality from combined pancreatic and duodenal injury approaches 30%.
- Both pancreatic and duodenal fistula are often encountered following injury. Lateral duodenal fistulas are difficult to manage and rarely close spontaneously.
- Intra-abdominal abscess

28. Principles of management of colorectal injuries. *WBUHS 2019, RIMS, Imphal 2022*

Etiology

- *Penetrating trauma:* This is the most common type of trauma seen, and is usually due to:
  - High velocity missiles
  - Rectal impalement injuries result when a patient falls on a penetrating object or using foreign bodies for sexual satisfaction.
  - Iatrogenic injuries due to uterine perforation during curettage of the uterus, use of endoscopies whether diagnostic or during polypectomies or other rectal instrumentations
  - During surgical operations for urologic or gynecologic operations
- *Blunt trauma:* This is rare due to the protected situation of the anus and rectum, and it is usually associated with fracture pelvis. The most common cause is motor vehicle accidents followed by falls and crush injuries.

Diagnosis

Intra-abdominal injuries are diagnosed as any abdominal trauma by the presence of manifestations of peritoneal irritation, free intraperitoneal fluid or air, and/or by assuring the presence of penetration into the peritoneal cavity.

Rectal, anal canal, and perineal trauma are diagnosed by proper inspection and per rectal examination of the patient.

- The presence of bleeding per rectum is a very important sign.
- The presence of different types of urethral injuries as well as different types of fracture pelvis should stimulate the surgeon to properly examine and even sigmoidoscope for the rectum and the pelvic colon.

Investigations

- Recently CT abdomen and to a lesser extent the ultrasound examination are the initial investigations of choice.
- Sigmoidoscope (the preferred method of investigation) for the rectum and the pelvic colon
- If an enema is to be used, water-soluble contrast (gastrografin) is a must.
- A CT abdomen and pelvis with double or at least IV contrast is indispensable for proper diagnosis.

Treatment

Direct laceration closure: This necessitates the presence of the following conditions:

- Small tear <2 cm after debridement of the large bowel wound
- Minor spillage reaching to a distance <5 cm all around the lacerating wound
- Interference in a time <8 hours from wound inflection
- Unloaded colon
- No other large bowel injuries
- No other organ injuries
- No hemodynamic shock or a status of imperfect tissue perfusion (e.g., septic shock)

Contraindications of primary closure:

- Patient is or has been in shock (systolic <80 mm Hg).
- The interval between injuries and closure is >8 hours.
- More than one organ injured
- Injuries at two different locations of the large bowel
- Massive colonic destruction
- Massive contamination
- Presence of prosthetic material or the necessity of its insertion

Resection Anastomosis/Stoma

- Resection of the injured area with direct anastomosis of the small bowel to the transverse colon
- In cecal injuries, end ileostomy with long Hartmann closure.
- Double-barrel colostomy at the site of injury (instead of exteriorization of the repaired injured colon) is done in transverse colon or the sigmoid colon if the injury is in a mobile area with long mesentery.
- *Resection with endcolostomy and mucosal fistula or Hartmann pouch:* This is done if the injury is at a site where mobility of the distal limb is limited while mobility of the proximal limb is free.
- Suture closure with proximal diversion

Principles of Management of Rectal Injuries

- The injury in the rectum is detected by a rigid sigmoidoscope.
  - Whether in the intraperitoneal segment or in the extraperitoneal one
  - The extraperitoneal space for the rectum is divided into retroperitoneal high up in the abdomen and subperitoneal low in the presacral space. Direct per rectal repair is done in low injuries (subperitoneal spaces) with possible drainage of the presacral space through an incision situated midway between the coccyx and the anus. This is especially indicated in posterior injuries.

- Direct repair through abdominal exploration is done in injuries of the intraperitoneal segment or in the retroperitoneal segment, with possible use of suction drainage of the presacral space if the injury is posteriorly located, and drainage of the Douglas pouch if it is anteriorly located as is usually the case. A proximal complete fecal diversion is a must in all situations.
- Removal of all retained feces by irrigation should be done.

29. Recent concept of management of penetrating injuries of abdomen. *WBUHS 2016*

Penetrating Abdominal Injury

The management of abdominal trauma varies according to the following factors:

- Mechanism and location of injury
- Hemodynamic and neurologic status of the patient
- Associated injuries
- Institutional resources

Priorities

Patients with significant penetrating abdominal injury tend to fall into three major categories:

Presentation	*Injury type*	*Management priority*
1. Pulseless	Major vascular injury	• Emergency laparotomy • Consider emergency department (ED) thoracotomy
2. Hemodynamically unstable	• Vascular and/or solid organ injury and/or • Hemorrhage from other sites	Identify and control hemorrhage
3. Hemodynamically normal	• Hollow viscus injury • Pancreas or renal	Identify presence of gastrointestinal, diaphragmatic, or retroperitoneal injury

The appropriate investigations and management pathway vary with each of these clinical presentations.

The management of abdominal trauma varies according to the following factors:

- Mechanism and location of injury
- Hemodynamic and neurologic status of the patient
- Associated injuries
- Institutional resources

Adjuncts the initial evaluation of the trauma patient can provide clues to significant intraperitoneal injury:

- *Chest X-ray:* An erect chest radiograph may identify subdiaphragmatic air. This must be interpreted with some caution in the absence of peritonitis, as air may be entrained into the peritoneal cavity with a stab or gunshot wound. However, it certainly signals peritoneal penetration and warrants further investigation.
- *Nasogastric tube:* Blood drained from the stomach will identify gastric injury.
- *Urinary catheter:* Macroscopic hematuria indicates a renal or bladder injury; microscopic injury suggests but is not pathognomonic of ureteric injury.
- *Rectal examination:*
  - Rectal blood indicates a rectal or sigmoid penetration.
  - Proctoscopy and sigmoidoscopy should be performed (see below)

Options for Evaluation

Further evaluation requires the use of one or more of the following diagnostic modalities:

- Serial PE
- Local wound exploration (LWE)
- DPL
- Ultrasound (FAST)

- CT scan
- Laparoscopy
- Laparotomy

FAST

- A positive FAST indicates peritoneal penetration, but it is poor at discriminating for injuries requiring intervention.
- A negative FAST does not exclude significant abdominal injury.

CT Scan

- CT scanning is finding more and more of a role in the evaluation of penetrating abdominal injury.
- CT gives the best assessment of retroperitoneal structures.
  - The CT features of penetrating bowel injury are:

Signs of peritoneal violation	*Signs of bowel injury*	*Other signs of intraperitoneal injury*
• Free intraperitoneal air • Free intraperitoneal fluid • Wound track extending through peritoneum	• Wound track extending to bowel wall • Bowel wall defect • Bowel wall thickening • Intraluminal contrast leak (not free intraperitoneal air—may have been entrained through peritoneal wall)	• Intravenous contrast extravasation • Diaphragmatic tear

Laparoscopy

- A full trauma laparoscopy for the evaluation of penetrating injury requires general anesthesia and complete examination of intraperitoneal contents, including visualization of the whole small bowel and intraperitoneal colon.
- In most studies, laparoscopy has a significant false-negative values, primarily from missed bowel injuries.
- Laparoscopy is also limited in the evaluation of retroperitoneal injury.
- Laparoscopy is the diagnostic method of choice for the diagnosis of suspected diaphragmatic injury. Many diaphragmatic lacerations can also be repaired via the laparoscope.
- Laparoscopy may also have a role in patients who have localized tenderness or develop a white cell count or fever without generalized peritonitis after a period of clinical observation.
- Laparoscopy may be useful to confirm that a wound is tangential and does not enter the peritoneal cavity—although many of the methods above have advantages over laparoscopy for this indication.

Laparotomy

Exploratory laparotomy for all penetrating abdominal wounds still has a role in resource-limited environments, or occasionally in cases of multicavitary injuries.

RENAL AND URETHRAL INJURY

30. Classify renal injury. Discuss clinical features and management of a patient having injury to left kidney following blunt trauma in left loin.

31. Grade renal trauma. Discuss principles of management in renal trauma. ***RGUHS 2019***

Types of Closed Renal Trauma

These include (A) subscapular hematoma; (B) laceration; (C) avulsion of one pole; and (D) avulsion of the renal pedicle.

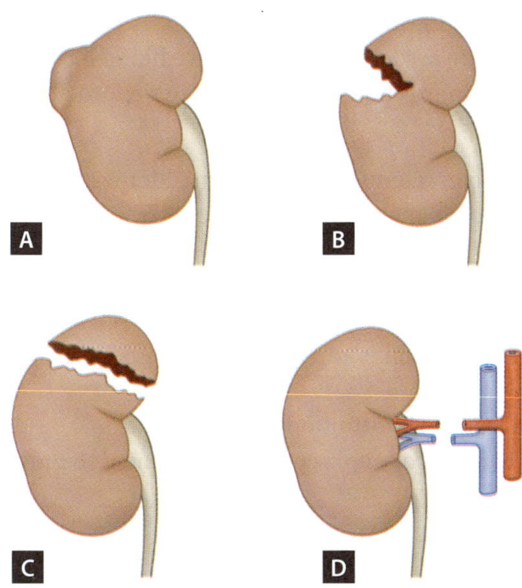

Classified According to the Organ Injury Scaling (OIS) Committee Scale

Minor	I	• Contusion • Hematoma	• Microscopic or gross hematuria, urological studies normal • Subcapsular, nonexpanding without parenchymal laceration
	II	• Hematoma • Laceration	• Nonexpanding perirenal hematoma confined to renal retroperitoneum • <1 cm parenchymal depth of renal cortex without urinary extravasation
Major	III	Laceration	>1 cm depth of renal cortex, without collecting system rupture or urinary extravasation
	IV	• Laceration • Vascular	• Parenchymal laceration extending through the renal cortex, medulla, and collecting system • Main renal artery or vein injury with contained hemorrhage
	V	• Laceration • Vascular	• Completely shattered kidney • Avulsion of renal hilum which devascularizes kidney

Clinical Features of Closed Renal Trauma

- There are local pain and tenderness, sometimes with superficial soft-tissue bruising.
- *Hematuria:* Hematuria may not appear until days after the injury. Profuse bleeding may cause clot colic.
- *Severe delayed hematuria:* Sudden hematuria between the third day and third week after trauma in a recovering patient is caused by a clot becoming dislodged.
- *Meteorism:* Abdominal distension 24–48 hours after renal injury is probably a result of retroperitoneal hematoma implicating splanchnic nerves.

Management and Treatment

- Watchful treatment of closed renal trauma is often successful. Consider the possibility of injury to other organs at an early stage.
- Crossmatch blood and secure IV access if there, is any evidence of hypovolemic shock or continuing hemorrhage.
- Advise bed rest while there is macroscopic hematuria and restrict activity for a week after the urine clears.
- Administer appropriate analgesia.
- Keep hourly observations.
- Antibiotics should be given to prevent infection of hematoma.
- Check the urine passed for hematuria and chart the result.
- Urgent intravenous urography (IVU) or contrast-enhanced
- CT will clarify the extent of renal damage and show that the other kidney is normal.
- Blood should be sent for grouping and serum saved for crossmatching in all cases.

Surgical Treatment in Closed Renal Trauma

- Exploration of the kidney may be associated with massive blood loss as the hematoma is opened.
- Check that the contralateral kidney is functioning because nephrectomy is a possibility.

Complications

- Heavy hematuria may lead to clot retention requiring bladder washout.
- Pararenal pseudohydronephrosis may occur weeks later from a combination of complete cortical tear and ureteric obstruction caused by scarring.
- Hypertension, resistant to drugs, resulting from renal fibrosis, may occur long after injury. Nephrectomy may be necessary.
- Post-traumatic aneurysm of the renal is rare. There is loin pain and a nontender swelling may be felt if the aneurysm is large.
- Congestion of parenchyma leads to intermittent hematuria.
- Aortography is diagnostic. Excision or nephrectomy is indicated to prevent fatal rupture of the aneurysm.

---

33. Urethral injury. ***WBUHS 2009, 2015***

---

33. Management of urethral injury. ***WBUHS 2008***

Introduction

- Urethral injuries are associated with 4–14% of all pelvic fractures and are more common in cases of bilateral pelvic injuries.
- Diagnosis of urethral injury is made by a high index of suspicion in the presence of blood at the urethral meatus, inability to urinate, or a palpable full bladder on abdominal examination. When blood is present at the meatus, retrograde urethrography aids in the diagnosis of urethral injury. In the presence of minor urethral injury, a catheter can be placed by an experienced urologist with or without the aid of a cystoscope.

Classification

- Urethral injuries are classified as those confined to the posterior urethra (above the urogenital diaphragm) or the anterior urethra (below the urogenital diaphragm).
- Posterior urethral injuries are further subclassified as type I (urethral stretch), type II (urethral disruption proximal to the urogenital diaphragm), or type III (proximal and distal disruption of the urogenital diaphragm).

Management

Posterior Urethral Injury

- For treatment of posterior urethral injuries, early endoscopic realignment has become more accepted as an excellent initial option.
- Realignment of the damaged urethra with a stented Foley catheter can lead to either complete healing of the urethral injury or need for future endoscopic treatment of developed urethral strictures.
- If realignment of the damaged urethra cannot be achieved, then suprapubic catheterization, followed by delayed combined antegrade and retrograde endoscopic repair or open surgical repair, is undertaken.

Anterior Urethral Injury

- Anterior urethral injuries are often isolated and associated with straddle injuries.
- The bulbar urethra is typically the site of injury.
- Primary realignment with a Foley catheter is the best initial treatment.
- In cases of severe anterior urethral injury, a suprapubic catheter may be required, followed by delayed open surgical repair.

Principles of End-to-end Urethroplasty

- Adequate perineal exposure
- Freeing of corpus spongiosum proximal and distal to injury for tension-free anastomosis.

- Excision back to normal urethra
- Spatulation of urethral ends
- Anastomosis with interrupted sutures
- Transanastomotic silastic catheter plus suprapubic cystostomy
- Perineal drain

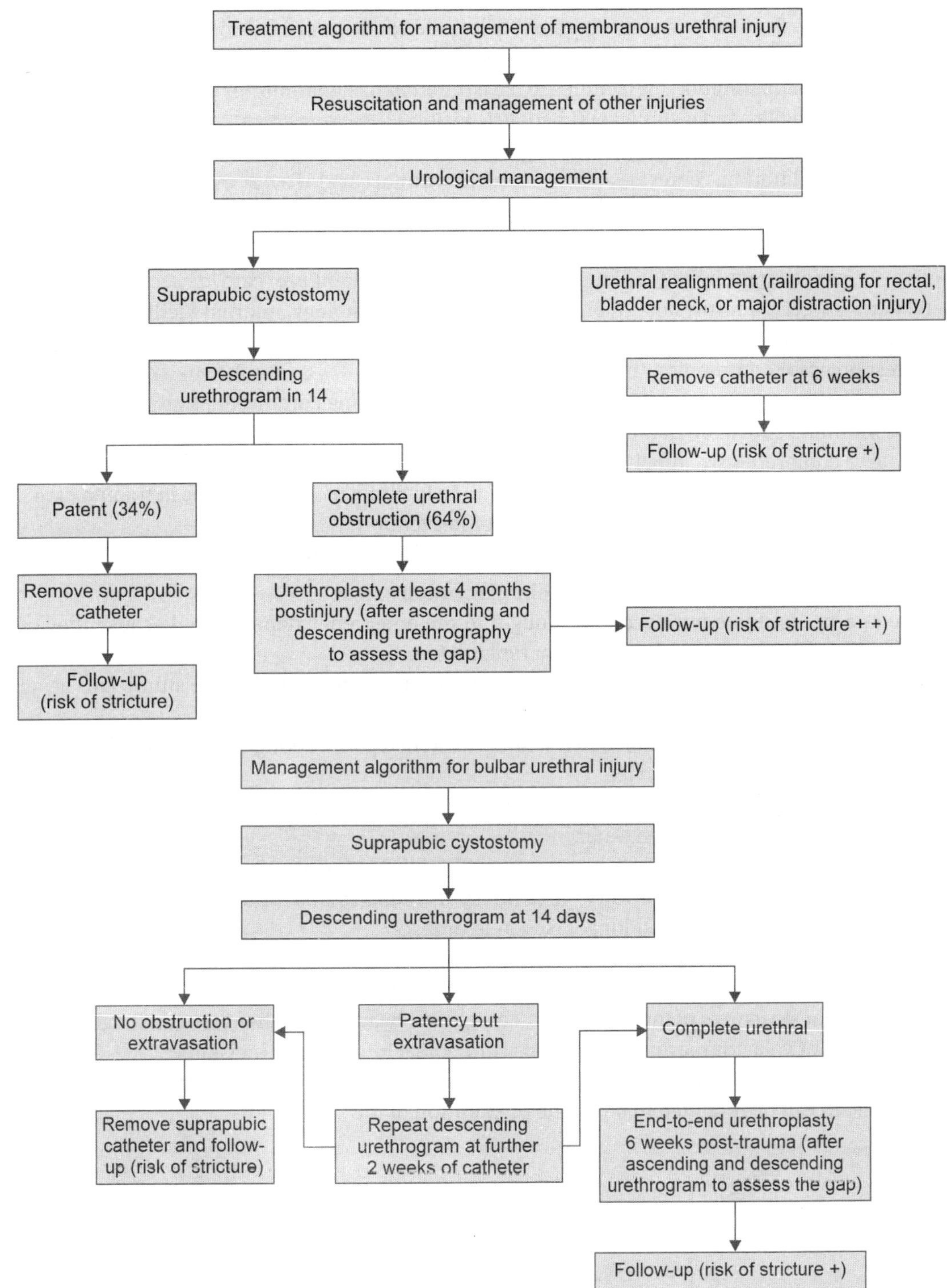

LEVEL I TRAUMA CENTER

34. Elements of level I trauma center. How to preserve and transport an amputated part for possible reimplantation? ***WBUHS 2022, 2025***

Trauma Center Levels

Trauma categories vary from state to state. Outlined below are common criteria for Trauma Centers verified by the ACS and also designated by states and municipalities. Facilities are designated or verified as adult and/or pediatric trauma centers. It is not uncommon for facilities to have different designations for each group (i.e., a trauma center may be a level I adult facility and also a level II pediatric facility).

Level I: Level I trauma center is a comprehensive regional resource that is a tertiary care facility central to the trauma system. A level I trauma center is capable of providing total care for every aspect of injury—from prevention through rehabilitation.

Elements of Level I Trauma Centers

- 24-hour in-house coverage by general surgeons, and prompt availability of care in specialties such as orthopedic surgery, neurosurgery, anesthesiology, emergency medicine, radiology, internal medicine, plastic surgery, oral and maxillofacial, and pediatric and critical care.
- Referral resources for communities in nearby regions
- Provides leadership in prevention, public education to surrounding communities
- Provides continuing education of the trauma team members
- Incorporates a comprehensive quality assessment program
- Operates an organized teaching and research effort to help direct new innovations in trauma care
- Program for substance abuse screening and patient intervention
- Meets minimum requirement for annual volume of severely injured patients

Transport of an Amputated Part for Possible Reimplantation

- Amputated parts should be retrieved and brought to the emergency department because they can provide a valuable source of tissue, even if the part is not replantable.
- Bleeding vessels in the stump should not be clamped. Hemostatic control of the stump can be achieved with compressive dressing and elevation.
- The amputated part should be wrapped in a saline-moistened gauze sponge placed in a plastic bag. The plastic bag should be sealed and placed on ice.
- The amputated part should not be placed directly on ice because this could result in a frostbite injury to the vessels.
- The part should not be immersed in water.
- Recommended ischemia times for reliable success with replantation are 12 hours of warm and 24 hours of cold ischemia for digits and 6 hours of warm and 12 hours of cold ischemia for major replants, although successful replantation has been reported after longer ischemia times.
- In order to minimize ischemia time, the amputated part can be prepared on a back table before the patient is brought to the operating room. If the amputated part is grossly contaminated, it can be prepared with gentle irrigation.
- The neurovascular structures of the fingers can be exposed by making either bilateral longitudinal incisions in the midaxial line or volar zigzag and dorsal veins with dorsal longitudinal incisions.
- Usually, preparation of the amputated part can be performed before the patient arrives in the operating room, or a second team can be recruited to begin the preparation of the stump.

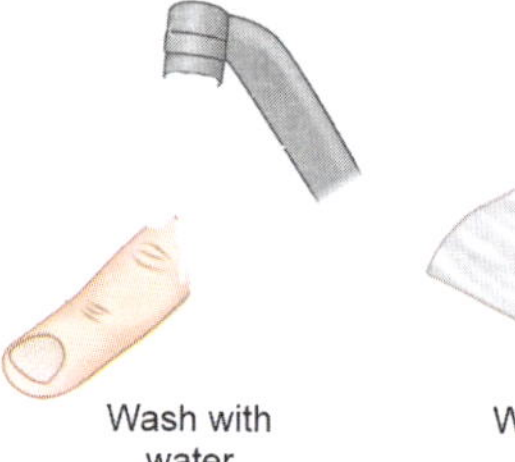

Wash with water

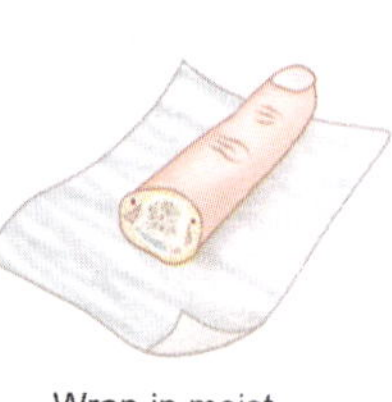

Wrap in moist qauze

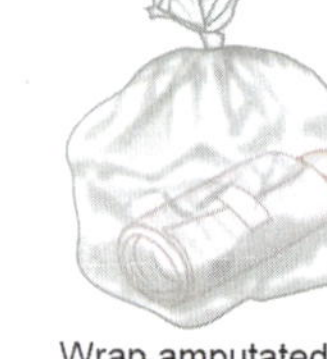

Wrap amputated part in dry plastic bag

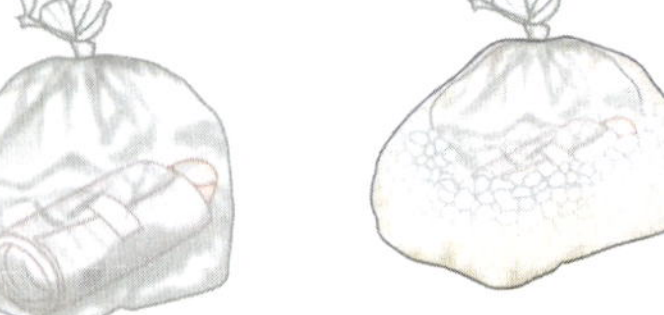

Bag with amputated part place in another bag with ice

CHAPTER 10

Metabolic Response to Trauma

LEARNING OBJECTIVES

- Metabolic Response to Trauma
- ERAS

METABOLIC RESPONSE TO TRAUMA

1. Describe the neuroendocrine response to trauma. Write the local and systemic changes following 50% burn.

Endocrine response to trauma: Changes occur to circulating concentrations of many hormones following injury. These changes take place as a result of direct stimulation of the various glands that produce the hormones and also because normal negative feedback mechanisms are altered as part of the response to injury.

Factors Mediating the Metabolic Response to Injury

Acute inflammatory response	*Endothelial cell activation*	*Nervous system*	*Endocrine response*	*Bacterial infection*
Inflammatory cells (macrophages, monocytes, and neutrophils)	Adhesion of inflammatory cells	Afferent nerve stimulation	Increased secretion of stress hormones	
Proinflammatory cytokines and other inflammatory mediators	Vasodilatation		Decreased secretion of anabolic hormones	
	Increased permeability			

Hormonal Changes in Response to Trauma

Hormonal change	*Pituitary*	*Adrenal*	*Pancreas*	*Others*
Increased secretion	• GH • ACTH • Prolactin • ADH/AVP	• Adrenaline • Cortisol • Aldosterone	Glucagon	• Rennin • Angiotensin
Unchanged secretion	• TSH • LH • FSH			
Decreased secretion			Insulin	• Testosterone • Estrogen • Thyroid hormones

(ACTH: adrenocorticotropic hormone; ADH: antidiuretic hormone; AVP: arginine vasopressin; FSH: follicle-stimulating hormone; GH: growth hormone; LH: luteinizing hormone; TSH: thyroid-stimulating hormone)

Causes of Fluid Loss Following Trauma

Nature of fluid	*Mechanism*	*Contributing factors*
Blood	Hemorrhage	• Site and magnitude of tissue injury • Poor surgical hemostasis • Abnormal coagulation
Electrolyte-containing fluids	Vomiting	• Anesthesia/analgesia (e.g., opiates) • Ileus
	Nasogastric drainage	• Ileus • Gastric surgery
	Diarrhea	• Antibiotic-related infection • Enteral feeding
	Sweating	Pyrexia
Wafer	Evaporation	Prolonged exposure of viscera during surgery
Plasma-like fluid (third-space fluid losses)	Capillary leak/sequestration in tissues	• Acute inflammatory response • Infection • Ischemia-reperfusion syndrome

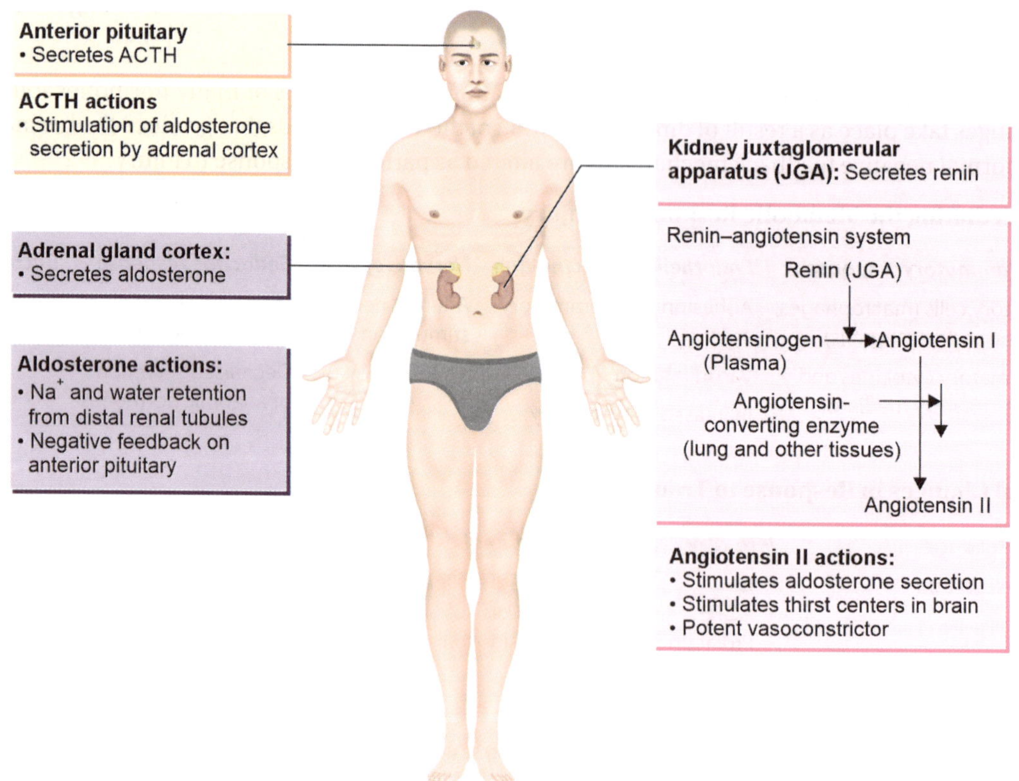

(ACTH: adrenocorticotropic hormone)

Urinary Changes during the Metabolic Response to Injury

- Reduced urine volume in response to hypovolemia and antidiuretic hormone (ADH) release
- Low urinary sodium and increased urinary potassium excretion due to aldosterone release
- Increased urinary nitrogen excretion due to the catabolic response to injury

Neuroendocrine Response Altogether

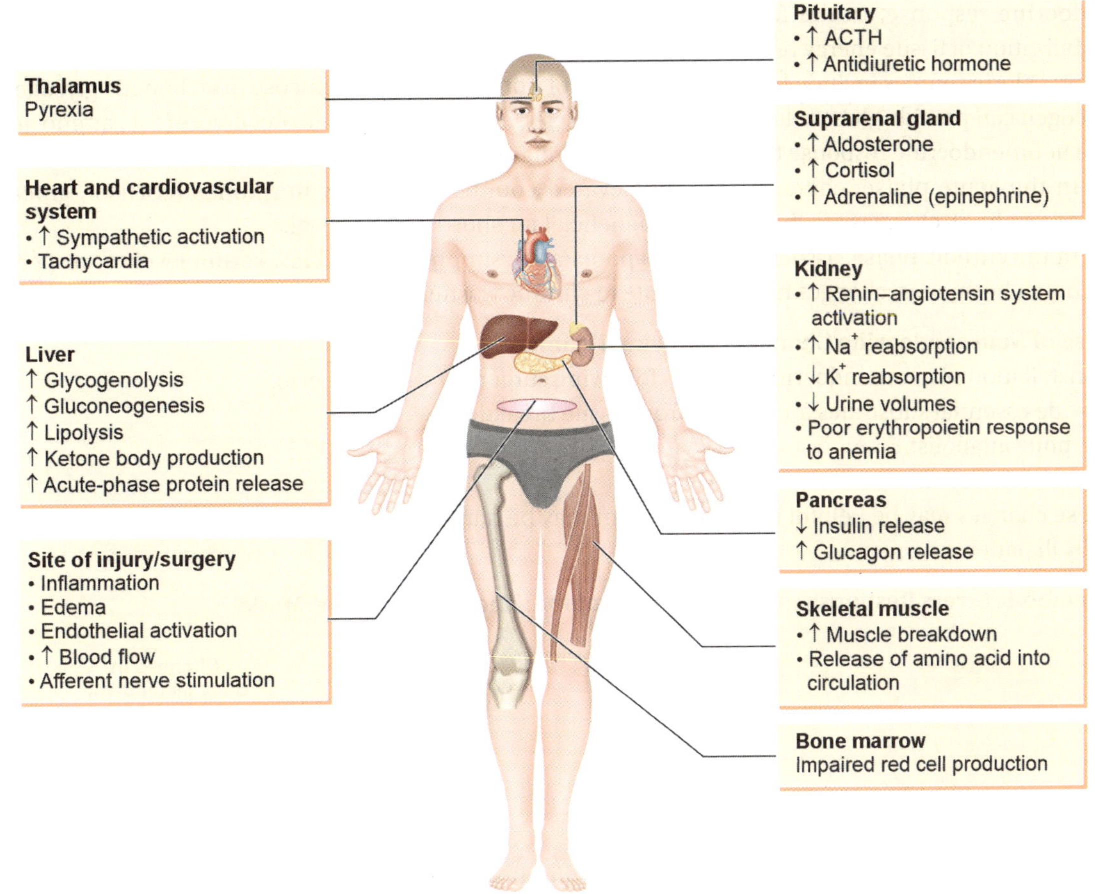

(ACTH: adrenocorticotropic hormone)

2. Describe the neuroendocrine response to trauma and its clinical implications in surgical patients. ***WBUHS 2025***

3. Metabolic response to trauma. ***RGUHS Karnataka 2025; WBUHS 2015***

4. Write in detail about the post-traumatic stress response.
DY Patil Education Society, Deemed to be University, 2024

Introduction

- Following accidental or deliberate trauma, a characteristic series of changes occur both locally at the site of injury and within the body generally.
- These changes are intended to restore the homeostasis of the body.
- The magnitude of the metabolic response is generally proportional to the severity of tissue injury and the presence of ongoing stimulation.
- The response of injury has probably evolved to aid recovery by mobilizing substrate and mechanism of preventing infection and by activating the recovery process.
- Although the metabolic response aims to return an individual to health, a major response can damage organs distant to the injured site itself.

Mediators of Metabolic Response to Injury

- Neuroendocrine mediators
- Immunological mediators

Neuroendocrine Mediators

- Endocrine response, in the form of increased catecholamines, glucocorticoids, and glycogen, leads to mobilization of tissue energy reserve.
- These caloric sources include fatty acid and glycerol from lipid reserve, glucose from hepatic glycogen (muscle glycogen can provide glucose for the involved muscle), and gluconeogenic precursors (e.g., amino acids).
- The neuroendocrine response to severe injury is biphasic.
  - In the acute phase, characterized by elevated counter-regulatory hormones (cortisol, glucagon, and adrenaline), changes are thought to be beneficial for short-term survival.
  - In the chronic phase, associated with hypothalamic suppression and low serum levels of respective target organ hormones, changes may contribute to chronic wasting.

Purpose of Neuroendocrine Changes Following Trauma

The constellation of neuroendocrine changes following surgery or trauma acts to:

- Provide essential substrates for survival from tissue breakdown.
- Postpone anabolism
- Optimize host defense

These changes may be helpful in short term but may be harmful in long term, especially to severely injured or critically ill patients.

The Metabolic Stress Response to Surgery and Trauma: The 'ebb and flow' Model

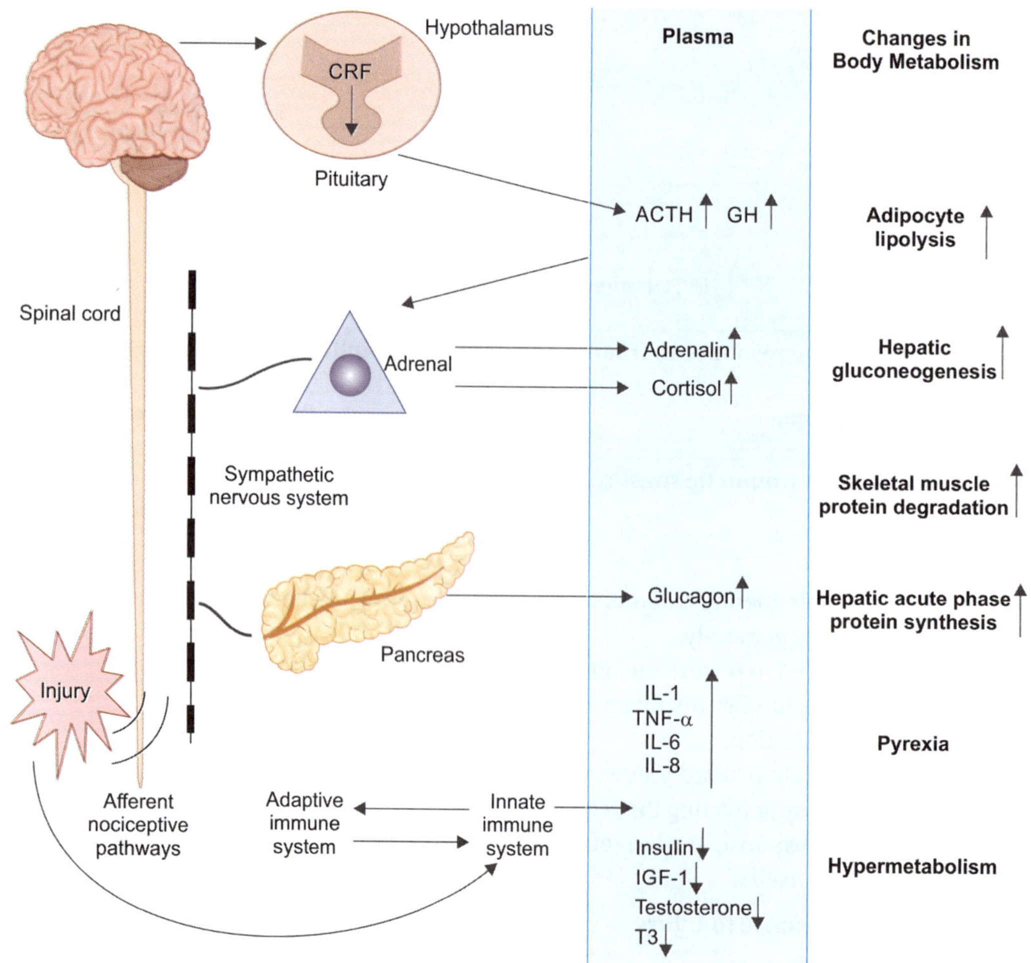

(ACTH: adrenocorticotropic hormone; CRF: chronic renal failure; GH: growth hormone; IGF: insulin-like growth factor; IL: interleukin; T3: tri-iodothyronine; TNF: tumor necrosis factor)

Immunological Mediators

Immunological mediators are grouped into two categories:

1. Pro-inflammatory mediators
2. Anti-inflammatory mediators

Pro-inflammatory Mediators

- Rapid onset of response in trauma driven by pro-inflammatory cytokines, e.g., IL-1, IL-6, and tumor necrosis factor (TNF)-α.
- Broadly related to injury severity, most severe in sepsis, burns, and major trauma
- Varies in severity between individuals (genetic)
- Causes catabolism, muscle breakdown, immunosuppression, and organ dysfunction/failure
- Counterbalanced by antagonist response but the balance may be imperfect
- Prolonged by sepsis and other secondary insults (hemorrhage, massive transfusion, acidosis, surgery, crush syndrome, and ischemia reperfusion)
- Can become chronic
- Associated with most late deaths from injury or surgery in developed health systems

Anti-inflammatory Mediators

- Within hours of upregulation of pro-inflammatory cytokines, endogenous cytokine antagonists (IL-54, 5, 9, and 13 and TGF-β) act to control the initial pro-inflammatory response and limit any systemic organ damage caused by it.
- The degree of secondary anti-inflammatory response varies between individuals, probably on a genetic basis.
- If the anti-inflammatory response dominates or is accentuated and prolonged in critical illness, it is characterized as a compensatory anti-inflammatory response syndrome (CARS), resulting in immunosuppression and increased susceptibility to opportunistic (nosocomial) infection. Further sepsis with its associated catabolism results.
- CARS can be prolonged by ongoing critical illness as a part of an ongoing vicious cycle of chronic critical illness.

Agonist and Antagonist: An Uncertain Balance

- Thus, both the initial inflammatory response to tissue injury and the secondary modulating response can be seen to different degrees in different individuals or at different stages of the critical illness.
- Either circumstances can cause harm and rapid restoration of homeostasis and preventing secondary inflammation or sepsis are key therapeutic principles that influence late outcomes as well as immediate ones.

Responses to Trauma

The responses to trauma can be divided into two phases:

1. Ebb phase
2. Flow phase

The ebb phase occurs immediately after trauma and lasts for 24–48 hours followed by the flow phase. After this comes the anabolism phase.

- *Ebb phase (up to 24–48 hours) is characterized by:*
    - Hypovolemia
    - Decreased basal metabolic rate (BMR)
    - Reduced cardiac output
    - Hypothermia
    - Lactic acidosis
- *Flow phase (may last for weeks) is characterized by:*
    - *Hypermetabolism:* The majority of trauma patients demonstrate energy expenditure approximately 15–25% above predicted healthy response values.
    - *Alternation in skeletal muscle and protein metabolism:*
        - Provides amino acids for the metabolic support of central organs/tissues.
        - Is mediated at a molecular level mainly by activation of the ubiquitin-proteasome pathway

    - Is inevitable to some degree but is prolonged by sepsis in particular
    - Can result in immobility and contribute to prolonged recovery, poor healing, hypostatic pneumonia, and death if prolonged and excessive
  - *Alternation in hepatic protein metabolism:* The acute phase protein response
  - Insulin resistance

Alternation in Hepatic Protein Metabolism

The acute phase protein response:

- The hepatic acute phase response represents a reprioritization of body protein metabolism toward the liver and is characterized by:
  - *Positive reactants [e.g., C-reactive protein (CRP)]:* Plasma concentration increased
  - *Negative reactants (e.g., albumin):* Plasma concentration decreased

Anabolic Phase

- Recovery phase
- Restoration of lean body mass, weight, and well-being

Changes in Body following Major Surgery Critical Illness

- Catabolism leads to a decrease in fat mass and skeletal muscle mass.
- Body weight may paradoxically increase because of the expansion of fluid within the extracellular fluid space.
- It is now possible to maintain body weight and nitrogen equilibrium following major elective surgery. This can be achieved by enhanced recovery after surgery (ERAS) protocol.

Avoidable factors that compound the metabolic response to injury during elective surgery are:

- Continuing hemorrhage/volume loss
- Hypothermia
- Tissue edema
- Tissue underperfusion
- Starvation
- Immobility

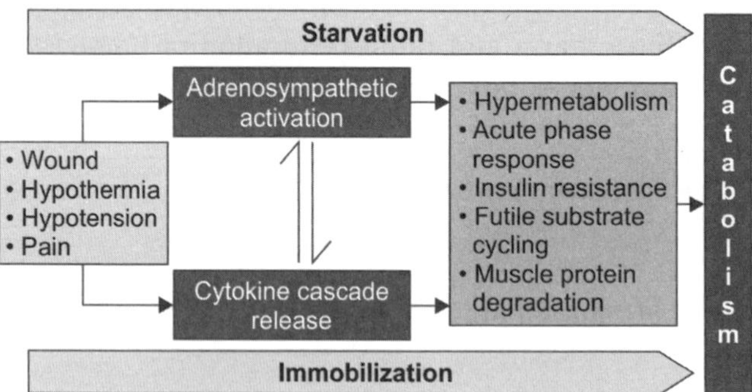

5. Write in short on different avoidable factors that compound the metabolic response to trauma. ***WBUHS 2025 Supplementary***

Factors mediating the metabolic response to injury:

The acute inflammatory response	*Endothelial cell activation*	*Nervous system*	*Endocrine response*	*Bacterial infection*
Inflammatory cells (macrophages, monocytes, neutrophils)	Adhesion of inflammatory cells	Afferent nerve stimulation	Increased secretion of stress hormones	
Pro-inflammatory cytokines and other inflammatory mediators	Vasodilatation		Decreased secretion of anabolic hormones	

Avoidable Factors that Compound the Metabolic Response to Trauma (Short Note)

- *Delayed resuscitation:* Inadequate fluid or blood replacement worsens shock and tissue hypoxia.
- *Hypoxia:* Poor oxygenation increases anaerobic metabolism and lactic acidosis.
- *Hypothermia:* Low body temperature impairs coagulation and increases metabolic demands.
- *Pain and anxiety:* Elevate stress hormones (e.g., cortisol, catecholamines), intensifying the catabolic response.
- *Infection and sepsis:* Trigger excessive inflammatory responses, worsening tissue damage and metabolic imbalance.
- *Poor nutritional support:* Increases protein catabolism and delays wound healing.
- *Repeated surgical interventions:* Each procedure can prolong the stress response and metabolic burden

ENHANCED RECOVERY AFTER SURGERY

6. Discuss the concepts behind enhanced recovery after surgery. ***WBUHS 2022, AIIMS, Raipur 2024***

7. What is enhanced recovery after surgery (ERAS) protocol? What are the preoperative and postoperative strategies of ERAS? What are the inclusion and exclusion criteria? ***WBUHS 2023***

8. Write in short about enhanced recovery after surgery (ERAS) protocol. ***KIIT University, Odisha 2025; AIIMS, Raipur 2025***

9. Describe ERAS protocols and their impact on patient outcomes after major Colorectal/HPB/urological surgery. ***Maharashtra University of Health Sciences 2025.***

ERAS

- Modern understanding of the metabolic response to surgical injury and the mediators involved has led to a complete reappraisal of traditional perioperative care, and the process is known as ERAS.
- Compared with traditional perioperative care, the ERAS program represents a fundamental shift in the process of care by including multiple interventions that attenuate surgical stress, maintain physiological function, and expedite return to baseline. While each intervention has a small effect, all together they have a stronger synergetic impact.
- In modern surgery, a major goal is to actively reduce the need for a homeostatic response by minimizing the primary insult via minimal access and by "Stress Free" preoperative care.
- ERAS protocols are multimodal perioperative care pathways designed to achieve early recovery after surgical procedures by maintaining preoperative organ function and reducing the profound stress response following surgery.

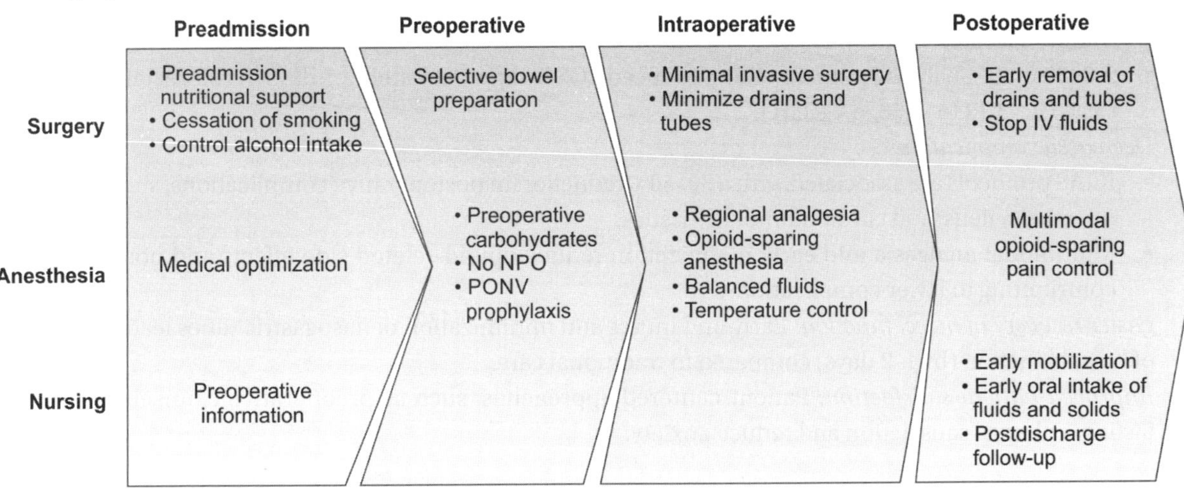

(IV: intravenous; NPO: nil per os; PONV: postoperative nausea and vomiting)

- The first ERAS protocol was established in 2001 by a group of surgeons from northern Europe.
- Their primary goal was to optimize surgical outcomes through the implementation of evidence-based medicine and best practices in patients undergoing colonic resections.
- The major positive consequence of implementing ERAS pathways is the improvement of patient outcomes at decreased costs.
- It has been demonstrated that ERAS positively influences patient subjective well-being with better health-related quality of life, less pain or fatigue, and better patient satisfaction.
- ERAS is also well accepted and supported by medical and nursing staff.

Inclusion criteria	• Age >18 years • Patients diagnosed with primary colorectal carcinoma • Patients who underwent elective laparoscopic colorectal resection following a protocol of enhanced recovery after surgery • Normo-nourished patients (MNA-SF score ≥12) • ASA I, II, and III
Exclusion criteria	• Age <18 years • Malnutrition (MNA-SF score <12) • Inflammatory bowel disease • Rectal cancer patients who had neoadjuvant radiotherapy or chemotherapy • Acquired or congenital immunodeficiency • Preoperative infection • Pregnancy • Emergency setting • Conversion to open surgery • Multivisceral resections • ASA IV

(ASA: American Society of Anesthesiologists MNA-SF: Mini Nutritional Assessment Short-Form)

Impact on Patient Outcomes

The impact of ERAS protocols on outcomes after colorectal, HPB, and urological surgeries has been extensively studied. Below is a summary of key findings:

Colorectal Surgery

- *Reduced length of hospital stay (LOS):*
  - ERAS protocols significantly shorten LOS, typically by 1–3 days, compared to conventional care. For example, studies report an average LOS of 4–6 days for colorectal surgery under ERAS versus 6–10 days with traditional care.
  - A 2020 meta-analysis found that ERAS reduced LOS by approximately 2.5 days in colorectal surgery patients (95% CI: -3.12 to -1.88, $p < 0.001$).
- *Decreased complications:*
  - ERAS protocols are associated with a 30–50% reduction in postoperative complications, such as surgical site infections, ileus, and cardiopulmonary issues.
  - Multimodal analgesia and early mobilization reduce opioid-related side effects and postoperative ileus, contributing to fewer complications.
- *Faster recovery of bowel function:* Early oral intake and minimization of nasogastric tubes lead to earlier return of bowel function (by 1–2 days) compared to traditional care.
- *Improved patient satisfaction:* Patient-centered approaches, such as preoperative counseling and reduced fasting, enhance satisfaction and reduce anxiety.

- *No increase in readmissions:* Despite shorter LOS, ERAS protocols do not significantly increase readmission rates, with studies showing comparable or lower readmission rates (e.g., 5–10% in ERAS vs. 8–15% in conventional care).
- *Mortality:* ERAS protocols are associated with no increase in mortality and, in some studies, a slight reduction in perioperative mortality due to fewer complications.

Hepatobiliary (HPB) Surgery

- *Reduced LOS:*
  - In HPB surgeries (e.g., liver resection, pancreaticoduodenectomy), ERAS protocols reduce LOS by 1–4 days. For example, LOS after pancreatic surgery may decrease from 10–14 days to 6–10 days.
  - A 2019 systematic review reported a mean reduction of 2.7 days in LOS for liver surgery under ERAS ($p < 0.05$).
- *Lower complication rates:*
  - ERAS protocols reduce complications such as delayed gastric emptying and postoperative infections by 20–40%. For pancreatic surgery, ERAS reduces pancreatic fistula rates in some studies.
  - Goal-directed fluid therapy and early drain removal are particularly impactful in reducing complications.
- *Faster functional recovery:* Early mobilization and nutrition improve functional recovery, with patients resuming normal activities 1–2 weeks earlier compared to conventional care.
- *Challenges in HPB:* HPB surgeries are complex, and adherence to ERAS protocols can be lower due to patient frailty or surgical complexity. However, even partial adherence improves outcomes.
- *Mortality and readmissions:* No significant increase in mortality or readmissions is reported, with some studies showing a slight decrease in 30-day mortality.

Urological Surgery

- *Reduced LOS:*
  - In major urological procedures (e.g., radical cystectomy, prostatectomy, nephrectomy), ERAS protocols reduce LOS by 1–3 days. For example, LOS after radical cystectomy may decrease from 8–12 days to 5–9 days.
  - A 2021 study on radical cystectomy reported a mean LOS reduction of 2.1 days with ERAS ($p < 0.01$).
- *Decreased complications:*
  - ERAS protocols reduce complications such as urinary tract infections, ileus, and wound infections by approximately 20–30%.
  - Multimodal analgesia and early catheter removal are key contributors to reduced morbidity.
- *Improved pain management:* Nonopioid analgesia (e.g., epidural or regional blocks) reduces postoperative pain scores and opioid consumption, improving patient comfort.
- *Enhanced recovery:* Early mobilization and oral intake accelerate return to baseline function, particularly in prostatectomy and nephrectomy patients.
- *Readmissions and mortality:* Readmission rates remain comparable to conventional care (5–15%), with no significant increase in mortality.

Specific Considerations Across Specialties

- *Cost-effectiveness:* ERAS protocols reduce healthcare costs by decreasing LOS and complications. Studies estimate cost savings of $1,000–$5,000 per patient in colorectal and HPB surgeries.
- *Compliance and implementation:* Higher compliance with ERAS protocols correlates with better outcomes. However, adherence varies (50–80% in most studies) due to institutional barriers or patient factors.
- *Patient populations:* ERAS benefits are consistent across diverse populations, including elderly patients, though outcomes may be less pronounced in frail or high-risk patients.
- *Oncological outcomes:* In colorectal and urological cancers, ERAS does not compromise oncological outcomes (e.g., margin status, recurrence rates) and may improve recovery for adjuvant therapies.

10. What are the components of the ERAS protocol? What are the barriers in its implementation? *WBUHS 2016*

Components are:

Preoperative	*Intraoperative*	*Postoperative*
• Preadmission counseling • Fluid and carbohydrate loading • No prolonged fasting • No or selective bowel preparation • Antibiotic prophylaxis • Thromboprophylaxis • No premedication	• Short-acting anesthetic agents • Midthoracic epidural anesthesia • No drains • Avoidance of salt and water • Overload	• No nasogastric tube • Prevention of nausea and vomiting • Avoidance of salt and water overload • Early removal of catheter • Early oral nutrition • Nonopioid analgesia • Early mobilization • Stimulation of gut motility • Audit of compliance and outcomes

Preoperative Recommendations

- Preoperative counseling and training
- A curtailed fast (6 hours to solids and 2 hours to clear liquids) and preoperative carbohydrate loading
- Avoidance of mechanical bowel preparation
- Deep vein thrombosis prophylaxis using low-molecular-weight heparin
- A single dose of prophylactic antibiotics covering both aerobic and anaerobic pathogens

Perioperative Recommendations

- High (80%) inspired oxygen concentration in the perioperative period
- Prevention of hypothermia
- Goal-directed intraoperative fluid therapy

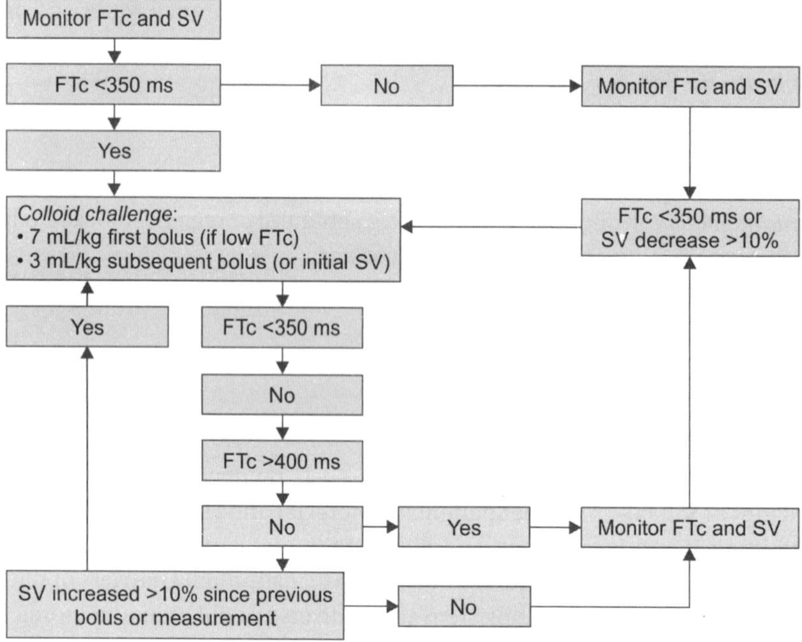

(FTc: flow time corrected; SV: stroke volume)

- Preferable use of short and transverse incisions for open surgery
- Avoidance of postoperative drains and nasogastric tubes
- Short duration of epidural analgesia and local blocks

Postoperative Recommendations

- Avoidance of opiates and the use of paracetamol and nonsteroidal anti-inflammatory drugs (NSAIDs)
- Early commencement of postoperative diet
- Early and structured postoperative mobilization
- Administration of restricted amounts of intravenous fluid
- Regular audit

Barriers to Implementation and Functioning of ERAS Programs

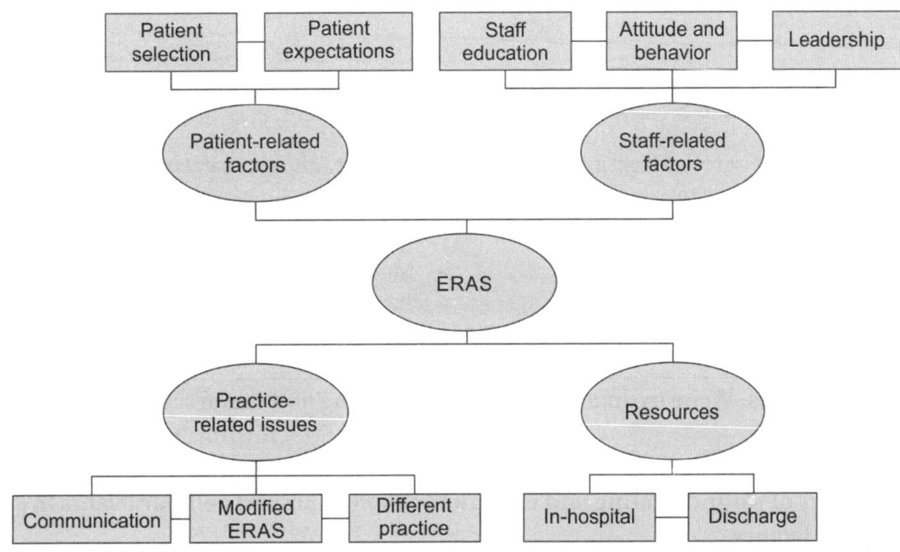

(ERAS: enhanced recovery after surgery)

CHAPTER 11

Wound

LEARNING OBJECTIVES

- Definition; Classification; Factors Affecting Wound Healing; and Biological Process of Wound Healing
- Biofilm in Wound Management
- Recent Advances in the Management of Open Wound; Vacuum-assisted Closure (VAC) and Negative-pressure Wound Therapy (NPWT)
- Methods of Promoting Soft Tissue Healing

1. Define and classify wounds. Write in detail about wound healing and factors affecting wound healing.
AIIMS, Raipur 2024; NTRUHS, Vijayawada 2024

2. Discuss the physiology of wound healing and explain the molecular and cellular events in each phase and the influence of systemic factors.
WBUHS 2025

3. Describe the biological process of wound healing. What are the factors affecting wound healing?
Ayush University, Chhattisgarh, 2025; MUHS, Maharashtra 2025; Srimanta Sankaradeva University, Assam 2025

4. Write briefly about phases of wound healing. How do you manage untidy wounds?
Rajiv Gandhi University of Health Sciences, Karnataka, January 2025

5. What are the facilitating and interfering factors in wound healing? How can adverse scars be prevented and managed?
WBUHS 2023

Definition

Wound can be defined as an injury, usually involving division of tissue or rupture of the integument or mucus membrane, due to external violence or some mechanical agency rather than disease.

Classifications

General wounds are classified as being:

- Superficial (loss of epidermis only)
- Partial thickness (involve the epidermis and dermis)
- Full thickness (involve the dermis, subcutaneous fat, and sometimes bone)

According to level of contamination a wound can be classified as:

- *Clean wound*—a wound made under sterile conditions where there are no organisms present in the wound and the wound is likely to heal without complications.
- *Contaminated wound*—where the wound is as a result of accidental injury where there are pathogenic organisms and foreign bodies in the wound.

- *Infected wound*—where the wound has pathogenic organisms present and multiplying showing clinical signs of infection, where it looks yellow, oozing pus, having pain, and redness.
- *Colonized wound*—where the wound is a chronic one and there are a number of organisms present and very difficult to heal as in a bedsore.

Open wounds can be classified according to the object that caused the wound. The types of open wound are:

- Incisions or incised wounds, caused by a clean, sharp-edged object such as a knife, razor, or glass splinter.
- Lacerations, irregular tear-like wounds caused by some blunt trauma. Lacerations and incisions may appear linear (regular) or stellate (irregular). The term *laceration* is commonly misused in reference to incisions.
- Abrasions (grazes), superficial wounds in which the topmost layer of the skin (the epidermis) is scraped off. Abrasions are often caused by a sliding fall onto a rough surface.
- Avulsions, injuries in which a body structure is forcibly detached from its normal point of insertion. A type of amputation where the extremity is pulled off rather than cut off.
- Puncture wounds, caused by an object puncturing the skin, such as a splinter, nail, or needle.
- Penetration wounds, caused by an object such as a knife entering and coming out from the skin.
- Gunshot wounds, caused by a bullet or similar projectile driving into or through the body. There may be two wounds, one at the site of entry and one at the site of exit, generally referred to as a "through-and-through".

Closed wounds have fewer categories, but are just as dangerous as open wounds. The types of closed wounds are:

- Hematomas, also called a blood tumor, caused by damage to a blood vessel that in turn causes blood to collect under the skin.
- Hematomas that originate from internal blood vessel pathology are petechiae, purpura, and ecchymosis. The different classifications are based on size.
- Hematomas that originate from an external source of trauma are contusions, also commonly called bruises.
- Crush injury, caused by a great or extreme amount of force applied over a long period of time.

Surgical Wounds

- *Class I—Clean:* Uninfected operative wound where no inflammation is encountered and respiratory, gastrointestinal (GI), genital, and urinary tracts are not entered. Wounds are primarily closed, and a drain (if needed) is connected to a closed system.
- *Class II—Clean contaminated:* Have no signs of infection at the time of surgery but do involve repairing or removing an organ. Example of this type of wound include surgery on lungs, appendix, and vaginal procedure.
- *Class III—Contaminated:* Open, fresh, and accidental wound from surgery with a major break in sterile technique or gross spillage from GI tract; incision in which acute, nonpurulent inflammation is encountered (including necrotic tissue without evidence of purulent drainage, such as dry gangrene).
- *Class IV—Dirty/infected:* Old traumatic wounds with retained devitalized tissue; procedures with existing clinical infection (purulence already present in wound) or perforated viscera.

Local and systemic impediments to wound healing.

Systemic	*Local*
Malnutrition	Wound infection
Diabetes mellitus	Wound necrosis
Drugs (steroids and cytotoxins)	Foreign bodies
Obesity	Wound hypoperfusion and hypoxia
Shock	Repeat trauma
Immunodeficiency	Irradiated tissue
Renal failure	Neoplasm

Intrinsic or Local Factors

- *Ischemia and hypoxia are common contributing causes of nonhealing wounds:*
  - Atherosclerosis or local vascular damage in the form of trauma or vasculitis leads to ischemia and subsequent hypoxia in the wound. Hypoxia leads to a decrease in collagen synthesis, inhibits fibroblast migration, and increases the susceptibility of the wound to infection.
  - Wound infection slows healing. Diabetes, malnutrition, malignancy, steroids, or other immunosuppressive treatments can weaken the host's immune system. If the wound is allowed to persist, wound infections lead to increased tissue destruction and alter the effect of cytokines on wound healing.
  - The presence of foreign bodies and necrotic tissue can delay wound healing.
  - Chronic venous insufficiency causes persistent venous hypertension and chronic edema of the lower extremities. These factors in turn lead to pericapillary fibrosis, tissue ischemia, and the release of superoxide radicals, which presumably lead to wound healing in chronic venous insufficiency limbs.
  - Ionizing radiation directed at the wound causes abnormal wound healing.
  - Edema and acute swelling, especially around joints, can lead to skin breakdown and complete skin loss.

Extrinsic or Systemic Factors

- Malnutrition alters everyday recovery via the oblique and the direct consequences of nutrition and mineral deficiency.
- An instance is the affected person with medical or subclinical scurvy (nutrition C deficiency); such a person produces inadequately hydroxylated collagen, and the healed wound turns into substantially weakened as a result.
- Diabetes mellitus is thought to have an effect on recovery adversely at each degree and in each segment of the recovery process.
- Steroids and antineoplastic capsules can markedly lessen the rate and great of the recovery process. Vitamin A appears to reason a partial reversal of the destructive consequences of steroids on recovery.
- Smoking contributes to not on time wound recovery with the aid of using inflicting cutaneous vasoconstriction, lowering the oxygen-wearing ability of hemoglobin, and contributing to atherosclerosis.
- Collagen vascular sicknesses are frequently observed with the aid of using a vasculitic component, which ought to be managed earlier than recovery can begin.
- Cleansing sellers inclusive of chlorhexidine gluconate or povidone-iodine or chemical substances can also additionally impair wound recovery with the aid of using affecting mobileular migration.
- Repetitive trauma, intentional or otherwise, from shearing or strain forces frequently results in a failure in recovery. Wound regions over strain factors frequently require stabilization of the overlying pores and skin envelope with outside taping or splinting.
- Wounds in sufferers with renal disorder and liver disorder frequently heal extra slowly because of persistent protein deficiencies and decreased capacities for protein synthesis.
- Hematopoietic disorders, sickle mobileular disorder, with its excessive prevalence of ankle wounds and leukocytoclastic and granulomatous processes, and mycosis fungoides are related to poorly recovery wounds. Maximal clinical remedy for the underlying ailment is wanted to impact significant recovery.

[Enumerate phases of wound healing. *DNB 2017, December*]

Biological Process of Wound Healing

This process is divided into predictable phases: Blood clotting (hemostasis), inflammation, the growth of new tissue (proliferation), and the remodeling of tissue (maturation). Sometimes blood clotting is considered to be part of the inflammation stage instead of its own stage.

- *Hemostasis (blood clotting):* Within the first few minutes of injury, platelets in the blood begin to stick to the injured site. This activates the platelets, causing a few things to happen. They change into an amorphous shape, more suitable for clotting, and they release chemical signals to promote clotting. This results in the activation of fibrin, which forms a mesh and acts as "glue" to bind platelets to each other. This makes a clot that serves to plug the break in the blood vessel, slowing/preventing further bleeding.

- *Inflammation:* During this phase, damaged and dead cells are cleared out, along with bacteria and other pathogens or debris. This happens through the process of phagocytosis, where white blood cells "eat" debris by engulfing it. Platelet-derived growth factors are released into the wound that cause the migration and division of cells during the proliferative phase.
- *Proliferation (growth of new tissue):* In this phase, angiogenesis, collagen deposition, granulation tissue formation, epithelialization, and wound contraction occur.
  - In angiogenesis, vascular endothelial cells form new blood vessels.
  - In fibroplasia and granulation tissue formation, fibroblasts grow and form a new temporary extracellular matrix (ECM) through the secretion of collagen and fibronectin.
  - At the same time there is a re-epithelialization of the epidermis, where epithelial cells proliferate and crawl over the wound bed, which protects the new tissue.
  - When a wound contracts, myofibroblasts reduce the size of the wound by attaching to the edges of the wound and contracting by a mechanism similar to that of smooth muscle cells. When the cells' roles are close to complete, unneeded cells undergo apoptosis.
  - In this phase, angiogenesis, collagen deposition, granulation tissue formation, epithelialization, and wound contraction occur.
    - In angiogenesis, vascular endothelial cells form new blood vessels.
    - In fibroplasia and granulation tissue formation, fibroblasts grow and form a new, provisional ECM by excreting collagen and fibronectin.
    - Concurrently, re-epithelialization of the epidermis occurs, in which epithelial cells proliferate and "crawl" stop the wound bed, providing cover for the new tissue.
  - In wound contraction, myofibroblasts decrease the size of the wound by gripping the wound edges and contracting using a mechanism that resembles that in smooth muscle cells.

Maturation (Remodeling)

During maturation and remodeling, collagen is realigned along tension lines, and cells that are no longer needed are removed by programmed cell death, or apoptosis.

Managing Untidy Wounds

- *Control bleeding:* Apply direct pressure with a clean cloth or sterile dressing to stop bleeding. Elevate the limb if possible, unless it causes significant pain or worsens the injury.
- *Clean the wound:* Rinse the wound thoroughly with clean water or a saline solution to remove dirt, debris, or foreign objects. Avoid harsh antiseptics like hydrogen peroxide unless needed, as they can damage tissue. If debris remains, do not force it out.
- *Assess severity:* Untidy wounds often require professional care, especially if they're deep, gaping, heavily contaminated, or involve structures like tendons or bones. Signs of infection (redness, swelling, warmth, pus, or fever) or impaired function (e.g., inability to move a finger) warrant immediate medical attention.
- *Dress the wound:* If medical care is not immediately needed, apply a sterile, non-stick dressing or bandage. For large or oozing wounds, use an absorbent dressing and secure it without applying excessive pressure. Dressings should be changed daily or if they become wet or soiled.
- *Prevent infection:* Keep the wound clean and dry. Avoid picking at it. If prescribed antibiotics or antiseptic ointments by a doctor, use them as directed.
- *Medical care:* Most untidy wounds need thorough evaluation due to the risk of infection or complications. Debridement may be needed. Tetanus vaccination may be updated if needed (typically if it's been over 5–10 years).
- *Monitor healing:* Watch for signs of infection or poor healing (e.g., increasing pain, swelling, or foul odor). Follow-up with a healthcare provider as advised.

6. Describe the role of Biofilms in wound management. ***WBUHS 2014 [Define biofilm. DNB -2017, December]***

Introduction

- The term *biofilm* is used to describe a community of microorganisms encased within an extracellular polymeric matrix, which accumulates at a surface. Biofilms play a significant role in a large number of infections in humans, and due to the intrinsic resistance of these structures to an array of antimicrobial agents and host defense mechanisms, such diseases can be difficult to treat effectively.
- In the absence of specific antibodies, the polysaccharide component of the biofilm matrix also blocks complement activation. If antibodies are present, the polymeric matrix generally renders them ineffective.
- It has been shown that the biofilm matrix is also able to inhibit chemotaxis and degranulation by polymorphonucleocytes (PMNs) and macrophages and also depress the lymphoproliferative response of monocytes to polyclonal activators.
- Not only are host defenses unable to deal effectively with biofilms, but also their persistence can cause tissue damage (e.g., lung tissue in cystic fibrosis). Contact with a surface triggers the expression of a panel of bacterial enzymes that catalyze the formation of sticky polymers that promote colonization and protection.
- The structure of biofilms is such that immune responses may be directed only at those antigens found on the outer surface of the biofilm, and antibodies and other serum proteins often fail to penetrate into the biofilm.
- In addition, PMNs are unable to effectively engulf bacteria growing within a complex polymer matrix attached to a solid surface. This causes the PMNs to release large amounts of proinflammatory enzymes and cytokines, leading to chronic inflammation and destruction of nearby tissues (i.e., chronic inflammation). Bacteria that may be embedded within the wound biofilm matrix are likely to be resistant to both immunological and nonspecific defense mechanisms of the body.
  - It has been estimated that biofilms are associated with 65% of nosocomial infections. So why are biofilm-related infections such a problem to treat? The challenge arises as a consequence of the following several factors:
    - *Biofilms display innate resistance to antimicrobial agents, thus protecting associated bacteria.*
    - *Biofilms increase the opportunity for gene transfer between and among bacteria.*
  - Antibiotics are used to treat bacterial infections. However, biofilm-related infections do not succumb so easily to this form of treatment, because they provide a protective mechanism that renders bacterial cells less susceptible to both antibiotics and biocides. However, on removal of these cells from the matrix of the biofilm, they are equally susceptible to biocides. There have been a number of models used to determine resistance in biofilms, and the results of these studies have highlighted a number of the factors thought to contribute to the ability of a biofilm to tolerate high concentrations of antibiotics. These include:
    - Impaired penetration of an antibiotic into the biofilm matrix
    - Reduced growth rate of bacteria in biofilms, which renders them less susceptible to antibiotics (they change from being physiologically active in the planktonic state to sessile in the biofilm state).
    - Altered microenvironment within the biofilm (e.g., pH and oxygen content), which reduces the activity of an antimicrobial agent. There is evidence of gradients of physiological activity within a biofilm in response to antibiotic treatment. This would suggest that the response to antibiotics will vary according to the location of specific cells within a biofilm ecosystem.
    - Altered gene expression.
    - *Quorum sensing (QS):*
      - It has been documented as being involved in antibiotic resistance, but its role is currently unclear, which justifies the need for additional research in this area.
      - QS involves the production of signaling molecules within a bacterial population that enables bacteria to communicate with each other and initiate a response to their surrounding environment once a critical population density (quorum) has been reached.

- In a wound environment, many different bacteria live together in often dense populations, and this provides an ideal situation for QS to occur.
- Communication in this way allows bacteria to coordinate their behavior and, if necessary, change physiologically to enable them to adapt to a new environment (e.g., a wound).
- Adaptive responses of bacteria within a wound environment may be associated with nutrient availability, competition with other microorganisms, and the avoidance of host defense mechanisms.
- Adaptation to a wound environment via QS may involve bacteria secreting protective extracellular polymeric substance (EPS) and increasing the production of enzymes that facilitate their tissue invasion.

- *Reduced biofilm-specific phenotype:*
  - Wounds are susceptible to microbial contamination from both exogenous and endogenous sources including the nose, skin, mouth, and the gut, and it is likely that such organisms are involved in the evolution of microbial communities in wounds.
  - Early contaminants on a wound surface are most likely to be skin flora (e.g., *Staphylococcus epidermidis*) that adhere to the wound, proliferate, synthesize EPSs, and form a "healthy" biofilm. It is at this point that the host initiates a normal immune response and maintains a "homeostasis" at the site of contamination.
  - It is conceivable, based on documented evidence, that gram-negative bacilli may then colonize the biofilm—these organisms utilize available oxygen and provide growth factors that enable anaerobes to establish within the biofilm thus forming a complex but stable polymicrobial "climax" community often termed *microbial homeostasis.*
  - A climax community is a collection of microorganisms within a "quasi" steady state, implying stable associations and integrations of function between microbial populations. In this situation, the progression to wound healing may become compromised by the biofilm community.
  - At this stage, the microorganisms, while interfering with the wound healing process, may not necessarily induce any clinical signs of infection, although there may be subtle signs that indicate bacterial imbalance (e.g., change in wound color or odor together with the presence of devitalized tissue and ischemia).
  - The combined effects of the antimicrobial agent and the host immune response are likely to improve conditions for healing where bacterial imbalance is evident. Without control of microbial progression, a transition from an early "healthy" biofilm to a "pathogenic" wound biofilm may develop and ultimately lead to clinical infection.
  - While the net pathogenic effect of the biofilm community exceeds the host's immune response, wound healing is likely to be compromised.

Scientific and clinical research in the area of wound biofilms and the associated bacterial interactions is now warranted to better understand the impact on wound healing.

7. Vacuum-assisted wound management. ***WBUHS 2019, DNB 2021 June, DNB 2017 December***

8. Discuss the indications, contraindications and complications of negative pressure wound therapy. ***WBUHS 2024***

Vacuum-assisted closure of a wound is a type of therapy to help wounds heal. It is also known as wound VAC. During the treatment, a device decreases air pressure on the wound. This can help the wound heal more quickly:

- The gases in the air around us put pressure on the surface of our bodies. A wound vacuum device removes this pressure over the area of the wound. This can help a wound heal in several ways. It can gently pull fluid from the wound over time. This can reduce swelling, and may help clean the wound and remove bacteria. A wound VAC also helps pull the edges of the wound together. And it may stimulate the growth of new tissue that helps the wound close.

- A wound vacuum system has several parts. A foam or gauze dressing is put directly on the wound. An adhesive film covers and seals the dressing and wound. A drainage tube leads from under the adhesive film and connects to a portable vacuum pump. This pump removes air pressure over the wound. It may do this either constantly or it may do it in cycles.
- The dressing is changed every 24–72 hours. During the therapy, patient will need to carry the portable pump everywhere you go.
- The suction should not be off for longer than 2 hours daily. If the VAC suction is off for >2 hours, we must remove the VAC and cover the wound with a wet to dry gauze dressing.
    - *Need of a VAC of a wound:*
        - For a recent traumatic wound
        - For a chronic wound
        - Wounds linked to diabetes

Large wounds can take a longer time to heal.

A wound vacuum system may help your wound heal more quickly by:

- Draining excess fluid from the wound
- Reducing swelling
- Reducing bacteria in the wound
- Keeping the wound moist and warm
- Helping draw together wound edges
- Increasing blood flow to the wound
- Decreasing redness and swelling (inflammation)

Wound VAC offers some other advantages over other types of wound care. It may decrease your overall discomfort. The dressings usually need changing less often. And they may be easier to keep in place.

Indications and Contraindications for the Use of VAC

- The principal indications for the use of the mains powered VAC are:
    - Acute and traumatic wounds
    - Subacute wounds (i.e., dehisced incisions)
    - Pressure ulcers
    - Chronic open wounds (stasis ulcers and diabetic ulcers)
    - Meshed grafts
    - Flaps
- The small ambulant unit is recommended for:
    - Venous stasis ulcers
    - Lower extremity diabetic ulcers
    - Pressure ulcers
    - Lower extremity flaps
    - Dehisced incisions
    - Grafts
- Contraindications for both systems include:
    - Fistulas to organs or body cavities
    - Necrotic tissue in eschar
    - Osteomyelitis (untreated)
    - Malignancy in the wound
- Risks of VAC of a wound:
    - Bleeding (which may be severe)
    - Wound infection
    - An abnormal connection between the intestinal tract and the skin (enteric fistula)

Certain problems can increase the risk of complications, such as:

- Exposed organs or blood vessels
- High risk of bleeding from another health problem
- Wound infection
- Nearby bone infection
- Dead wound tissue
- Cancer tissue
- Fragile skin, such as from aging or longtime use of topical steroids
- Allergy to adhesive
- Very poor blood flow to your wound

Effectiveness

- A 2007 Cochrane review stated that the evidence comparing negative-pressure wound therapy (NPWT) to alternative care was flawed and required more study, but the evidence did support improved healing and called for more, better quality research to be conducted.
- A 2010 systematic review found "consistent evidence of the benefit of NPWT" in the treatment of diabetic ulcers of the feet. Results for bedsores were conflicting and research on mixed wounds was of poor quality, but promising. The review concluded "There is now sufficient evidence to show that NPWT is safe, and will accelerate healing, to justify its use in the treatment of diabetes-associated chronic leg wounds." There is also evidence, though of poor quality, to suggest that healing of other wounds may also be accelerated.

---

9. Enumerate causes of nonhealing ulcers of leg and foot. ***DNB 2017, December***

Vascular Causes

- *Peripheral arterial disease (PAD):* Poor blood supply due to narrowed or blocked arteries.
- *Chronic venous insufficiency:* Valve dysfunction in leg veins causes pooling and pressure buildup.
- *Vasculitis:* Inflammation of blood vessels can impair perfusion.
- *Thromboangiitis obliterans (Buerger's disease):* Smoking-related vascular disease.

Neuropathic Causes

- *Diabetic neuropathy:* Loss of protective sensation and pressure points lead to ulceration.
- *Leprosy:* Affects sensory nerves, predisposing to unnoticed injuries.
- *Spinal cord disorders or peripheral neuropathies:* Impaired sensation and movement.

Infectious Causes

- *Chronic or deep tissue infection:* Osteomyelitis, cellulitis.
- *Tuberculosis or fungal infections:* Especially in endemic areas.
- *Necrotizing fasciitis:* Rapidly progressive and destructive.

Metabolic and Systemic Disorders

- *Diabetes mellitus:* Poor wound healing due to microvascular disease and hyperglycemia.
- *Malnutrition:* Deficiency in protein, vitamins (especially C and zinc).
- *Renal or hepatic failure:* Impaired immune response and wound healing.
- *Immunosuppressive states:* HIV/AIDS, chemotherapy, long-term steroid use.

Pressure and Trauma

- *Pressure ulcers (decubitus ulcers):* Common in immobile patients.
- *Repetitive trauma or friction:* Ill-fitting footwear or gait abnormalities.
- Postsurgical wound dehiscence.

Malignancy

- *Marjolin's ulcer:* Squamous cell carcinoma arising in a chronic wound or scar.
- *Primary skin cancers:* Basal or squamous cell carcinoma.

Hematologic and Autoimmune Conditions

- *Sickle cell disease:* Vaso-occlusion causes ischemia.
- Antiphospholipid syndrome or other hypercoagulable states.
- *Connective tissue disorders:* e.g., Scleroderma, rheumatoid arthritis, lupus.

Iatrogenic Causes

- Radiation therapy-induced ulcers.
- Medication-related (e.g., corticosteroids, chemotherapy).
- Poor surgical technique or wound care.

10. Recent advances in the management of open wounds. Mention with special references to NPWT, ultrasound (US) therapy, and hydrotherapy. ***WBUHS 2021***

Recent Advances in the Management of Open Wounds

Scottish Intercollegiate Guidelines Network criteria selected the following 10 categories:

1. Sharp debridement and wound bed preparation with larvae or hydrotherapy
2. Wound bed preparation using antiseptics, applications, and dressing products
3. Resection of the chronic wound
4. Oxygen and other gases
5. Compression or negative pressure therapy
6. Products designed to correct aspects of wound biochemistry and cell biology associated with impaired wound healing
7. Application of cells, including platelets and stem cells
8. Bioengineered skin and skin grafts
9. Electrical, electromagnetic, lasers, shockwaves, and US
10. Other systemic therapies, which did not fit in the aforementioned categories

Negative pressure Wound Therapy in Wound Healing

- NPWT is a method of drawing out fluid and infection from a wound to help it heal. A special dressing (bandage) is sealed over the wound and a gentle vacuum pump is attached.
- Promotes wound healing at cellular level through negative pressure
- 100–120 mm Hg pressure
- Continuous or intermittent manner
- Applies mechanical forces known as macro strain (physical response) and micro strain (biological response)
- Subsequently removes exudates by an electromechanical pump
- NPWT dressings are manufacturer specified dressings used as an interface between the NPWT and the patient's wound. NPWT dressings include white or black foam, gauze, hydrocolloids, and nonwoven polyester with silicone elastomer.
- NPWT is an effective treatment method for pressure injuries, and three-dimensional wound measurement device is a usable wound assessment tool.

Ultrasound Therapy in Wound Healing

- US therapy can produce many effects and benefits other than just the potential heating effect. It increases tissue relaxation, local blood flow, scar tissue breakdown, helps in reducing local swelling and chronic inflammation, and promotes bone fracture healing.
- Low-frequency ultrasound (LFUS) is used as an adjunct (supplement) to wound care. A noncontact LFUS device is intended to provide debridement and cleansing to a wound. The device is held 0.5–1.5 cm from the wound and saline is delivered to the wound bed, which purportedly promotes healing through stimulation of cellular activity. Therapy is usually given in 3–12 minutes sessions, three times per week.

- MIST Therapy is a low energy, low intensity US delivered through a saline mist to the wound bed. The MIST Therapy system is designed to deliver therapeutic US to the wound bed without direct contact of the device to the body (noncontact).
- High-frequency (frequency: 1 MHz) mechanical vibration enhances healing at cellular level. It reduces inflammation, pain. It enhances degranulation of mast cells and subsequently collagen formation. Frequency: 1 MHz
- Recent evidence continued to support its superiority over standard of care in healing venous ulcers, but findings conflicted in terms of the effectiveness of LFUS over high-frequency ultrasound (HFUS). There are currently no standardized treatment protocols for US. Therapeutic LFUS is used to debride the wound bed, as an adjunctive topical wound treatment with standard of care, and to guide the application of other advanced therapies to chronic wounds.

Hydrotherapy in Wound Healing

- Hydrotherapy is a simple, effective, and innovative approach to the treatment of a variety of wounds, which combines the benefits of two complementary wound dressings to optimize hydration levels at all stages of the healing process.
- The discovery that a moist environment actively supports the healing response when compared with a dry environment highlights the importance of water and good hydration levels for optimal healing. The benefits of "wet" or "hyperhydrated" wound healing appear similar to those offered by moist over a dry environment.
- *Mechanical debridement:* Hydrotherapy is the use of water to remove dead and other types of unwanted tissue. The technique includes wound irrigation and therapeutic irrigation with suction, where a syringe and catheter tube is used to wash away dead tissue.
- Hydrotherapy is based on several important bioengineering principles that permit the design and development of aquatic exercise devices, techniques, and programs. These principles involve several forces (buoyancy, drag, and inertia), hydrostatic pressure, and the specific heat of water.

---

11. What are the methods of promoting soft tissue healing? ***WBUHS 2018***

Methods of Promoting Soft Tissue Healing

- Soft tissue injuries, both acute or chronic, are among the most frequent issues addressed by physical therapists, athletic trainers, and primary care physicians; however, many currently available treatment options are costly, time consuming, and potentially harmful.
- Nonsteroidal anti-inflammatory pharmacotherapies can be deleterious to soft tissue healing and harmful to the gastrointestinal and renal systems.
- Interventions such as prescription painkillers, corticosteroid injections, and platelet-rich plasma (PRP) injections can be addictive, costly, and of questionable efficacy, respectively.
- Traditional rest, time-off, and elevation therapy may not be feasible for all soft tissue injuries and patient lifestyles.
- Many use the regimen of rest, ice, compression, elevation and stabilization (RICES) to treat acute injury, but are unsure what to do if the injury becomes chronic.
- Whereas, many of these current treatment options address inflammation and pain management, therapeutic US can both manage pain and facilitate healing.
- Low-intensity therapeutic ultrasound (LITUS) is currently used in promoting healing of soft tissue injuries.
- Hyperbaric oxygen has also been used *to promote healing*. Agents such as PRP and erythropoietin (EPO) are modulators that have a positive effect on *tissue* regeneration and have been used successfully to enhance the *healing* of *wounds*.
- Stem cells of endothelial cells, originating from parts of uninjured blood vessels, develop pseudopodia and push through the ECM into the wound site to establish new blood vessels.

Growth factor	Abbreviation	Main origins	Effects
Epidermal growth factor	EGF	• Activated macrophages • Salivary glands • Keratinocytes	• Keratinocytes and fibroblast mitogen • Keratinocytes migration • Granulation tissue formation
Transforming growth factor-α	TGF-α	• Activated macrophages • T-lymphocytes • Keratinocytes	• Hepatocyte and epithelial cell proliferation • Expression of antimicrobial peptides • Expression of chemotactic cytokines
Hepatocyte growth factor	HGF	Mesenchymal cells	• Epithelial and endothelial cell proliferation • Hepatocyte motility
Vascular endothelial growth factor	VEGF	Mesenchymal cells	• Vascular permeability • Endothelial cell proliferation
Platelet-derived growth factor	PDGF	• Platelets • Macrophages • Endothelial cells • Smooth muscle cells • Keratinocytes	• Granulocyte, macrophage, fibroblast, and smooth muscle cell chemotaxis • Granulocyte, macrophage, and fibroblast activation • Fibroblast, endothelial cell, and smooth muscle cell proliferation • Matrix metalloproteinase, fibronectin, and hyaluronan production • Angiogenesis • Wound remodeling • Integrin expression regulation
Fibroblast growth factor 1 and 2	FGF-1 and 2	• Macrophages • Mast cells • T-lymphocytes • Endothelial cells • Fibroblasts	• Fibroblast chemotaxis • Fibroblast and Keratinocytes proliferation • Keratinocytes migration • Angiogenesis • Wound contraction • Matrix (collagen fibers) deposition
Transforming growth factor-β	TGF-β	• Platelets • T-lymphocytes • Macrophages • Endothelial cells • Keratinocytes • Smooth muscle cells • Fibroblasts	• Granulocyte, macrophage, lymphocyte, fibroblast, and smooth muscle cell chemotaxis • TIMP synthesis • Angiogenesis • Fibroplasia • Matrix metalloproteinase production inhibition • Keratinocytes proliferation
Keratinocytes growth factor	KGF	Keratinocytes	Keratinocytes migration, proliferation, and differentiation

12. Discuss about the role of NPWT (negative-pressure wound therapy) in the management of surgical wounds.
WBUHS 2020

The NPWT is a recent technique which facilitates wound treatment utilizing subatmospheric pressure. It consists of placing an open cell wound interface (e.g., sponge/gauze) directly on wound surface and covering it with occlusive film. Negative pressure is then applied to entire wound surface.

Contents of NPWT Dressing Pack

- Sterile open cell wound interface of small, medium, and large sizes
- Flexible vacuum tubing
- Occlusive adhesive transparent dressing
- Canister (collection chamber with connecting tubing)
- Vacuum pump.

Working Principle of NPWT

- Provides a closed and moist wound healing environment
- Decreases wound volume
- Removes excess fluids that can inhibit wound healing
- Helps remove interstitial fluid
- Promotes granulation

Indications of NPWT

- Huge, clean, and/or exudative wound while waiting for definitive wound closure
- Fixation of skin grafts (mesh grafts) and tissue flaps

Contraindications of NPWT

- Clotting disorders (risk of bleeding)
- Necrotic wound bed or eschar (barrier to new tissue growth)
- Untreated infection (due to deep extension of potential infectious focus)
- Neoplastic tissue in wound area

Technique of Application

- Cut wound interface to fit shape of wound
- Place wound interface on wound bed till flushed with edges
- Place vented end of flexible vacuum tubing
- Cover wound interface and tubing with occlusive adhesive dressing
- Ensure tight seal
- Connect open end of tubing to canister on vacuum pump
- Program prescribed amount of pressure and suction interval

Complications of NPWT

- Toxic shock syndrome
- Wound infection caused by anaerobes
- Loss of blood and fluid

Side Effects of NPWT

- Ingrowth of granulation tissue into foam
- Pain is associated with effects of suction and dressing changes
- Maceration and pressure damage to adjacent skin areas
- Reduction in perfusion caused by pressure on small vessels.

CHAPTER 12

Burns

LEARNING OBJECTIVES

- Basic Considerations
- Local and Systemic Responses to Burn Injury
- Management of Burn Patient
- Rehabilitation of Burn Patient
- Management of Burn Injury in Pregnant Patient
- Scaffold for Skin Tissue Engineering

BASIC CONSIDERATIONS

American Burn Association severity classification.

Minor	*Moderate*	*Major*
Adult <10% TBSA	Adult 10–20% TBSA	Adult >20% TBSA
Young or old <5% TBSA	Young or old 5–10% TBSA	Young or old >10% TBSA
<2% full-thickness burn	2–5% full-thickness burn	>5% full-thickness burn
	High-voltage injury	High-voltage burn
	Possible inhalation injury	Known inhalation injury
	Circumferential burn	Significant burn to face, joints, hands, or feet
	Other health problems	Associated injuries

(TBSA: total body surface area)

Classification according to depth of injury.

Burn depth	*Level of injury*	*Clinical features*	*Treatment*	*Usual result*
Superficial partial-thickness	Papillary dermis	• Blisters • Erythema • Capillary refill • Intact pain sensation	• Tetanus prophylaxis • Cleaning (e.g., with chlorhexidine gluconate) • Topical agent (e.g., 1% silver sulfadiazine) • Sterile gauze dressings • Physical therapy • Splints as necessary	• Epithelialization in 7–21 days • Hypertrophic scar rare • Return of full function
Deep partial-thickness	Reticular dermis	• Blisters • Pale white or yellow color • Absent pain sensation	• As for superficial partial-thickness burns • Early surgical excision and skin grafting an option	• Epithelialization in 21–60 days in the absence of surgery • Hypertrophic scar common • Earlier return of function with surgical therapy

Contd...

Contd...

Burn depth	*Level of injury*	*Clinical features*	*Treatment*	*Usual result*
Full thickness	Subcutaneous fat, fascia, muscle, or bone	• Blisters may be absent • Leathery, in classic, wrinkled appearance over bony prominences • No capillary refill • Thrombosed subcutaneous vessels may be visible • Absent pain sensation	• As for superficial partial-thickness burns • Wound excision and grafting at the earliest feasible time	• Functional limitations more frequent • Hypertrophic scar mainly at graft margins

Rule of nines estimation of percentage of body surface area.

		Trunk		*Extremity*		
	Head and neck	*Anterior*	*Posterior*	*Upper*	*Lower*	*Genital*
Adult	9	18	18	9	18	1
Infant	18	18	18	9	14	–

1. Burn injuries result in both local and systemic responses.

Local Response

The three zones of a burn were described by Jackson in 1947. They are:

1. *Zone of coagulation:* This occurs at the point of maximum damage. In this zone, there is irreversible tissue loss due to coagulation of the constituent proteins.
2. *Zone of stasis:* The surrounding zone of stasis is characterized by decreased tissue perfusion. The tissue in this zone is potentially salvageable. The main aim of burn resuscitation is to increase tissue perfusion and prevent any damage from becoming irreversible. Additional insults such as prolonged hypotension, infection, or edema can convert this zone into an area of complete tissue loss.
3. *Zone of hyperemia:* In this outermost zone, tissue perfusion is increased. The tissue here will invariably recover unless there is severe sepsis or prolonged hypoperfusion.

These three zones of a burn are three dimensional, and loss of tissue in the zone of stasis will lead to wound deepening as well as widening.

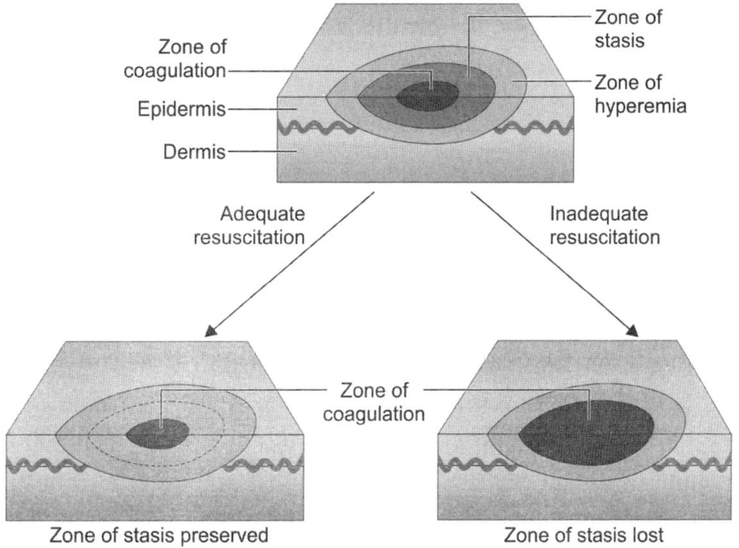

Systemic Response

- The release of cytokines and other inflammatory mediators at the site of injury has a systemic effect once the burn reaches 30% of the total body surface area.
- *Cardiovascular changes:* Capillary permeability is increased, leading to loss of intravascular proteins and fluids into the interstitial compartment. Peripheral and splanchnic vasoconstriction occurs. Myocardial contractility is decreased, possibly due to the release of tumor necrosis factor α. These changes, coupled with fluid loss from the burn wound, result in systemic hypotension and end-organ hypoperfusion.
- *Respiratory changes:* Inflammatory mediators cause bronchoconstriction, and in severe burns, adult respiratory distress syndrome can occur.
- *Metabolic changes:* The basal metabolic rate increases up to three times its original rate. This, coupled with splanchnic hypoperfusion, necessitates early and aggressive enteral feeding to decrease catabolism and maintain gut integrity.
- *Immunological changes:* Nonspecific downregulation of the immune response occurs, affecting both cell-mediated and humoral pathways.

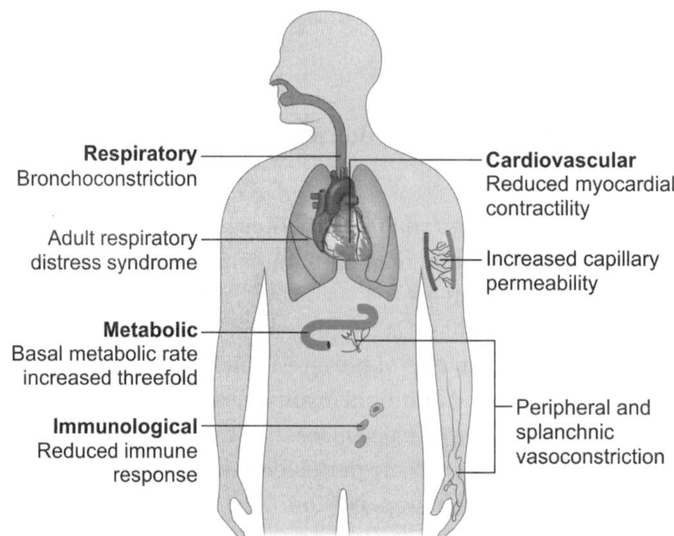

2. A 60-kg male sustained second-degree burns involving head, neck, front, and back of the chest along with smoke inhalation syndrome 8 hours ago. Briefly discuss the management and likely complications in this case. ***WBUHS 2021***

Rule of nines.

		Trunk		Extremity		
	Head and neck	*Anterior*	*Posterior*	*Upper*	*Lower*	*Genital*
Adult	9	18	18	9	18	1
Infant	18	18	18	9	14	–

As per rule of nine, the body surface area burnt is 9 + 18 + 18 = 45%.

So, the amount of fluid needed in the first 24 hours = 4 × 45 × 60 mL = 10,800 mL = 10.8 L of Ringer's lactate (RL).

As the patient came 8 hours after the accident, the whole 10.8 L of RL was to be infused in the next 16 hours.

- Check for urine output. It should be 0.5 mL–1 mL/kg body weight/h
- Colloid-containing solutions should be held for intravenous (IV) therapy until after the first 24 hours postburn.
- *Ensure adequate analgesia:* Strong opiates should be used.

- Prevent hypothermia.
- Prevent stress ulcers.
- Foley catheterization.
  As there is an inhalational injury, the patient should be kept on IV steroids.

Primary Survey

- The primary survey should follow the guidelines established by the American College of Surgeons' Advanced Trauma Life Support Course.
- Airway assessment and security are the number one priority.
- Breathing is evaluated for effort, depth of respiration, and auscultation of breath sounds.
- *Circulation:* Circulatory support in the form of aggressive and prompt fluid resuscitation is a cornerstone of early burn management.
- Remove all clothing to halt continued burn from melted synthetic compounds or chemicals and assess the full extent of body-surface involvement in the initial examination.

Analgesia and Sedation

- Severely burned patients may be restless and anxious from hypoxemia or hypovolemia rather than pain.
- IV narcotic analgesics and sedatives may be administered in small, frequent doses.

Wound Care

- Partial-thickness burns are painful when air currents pass over the burned surface. Gently covering the burn with clean linen relieves the pain and deflects air currents.
- Do not break blisters or apply an antiseptic agent.
- Any applied medication must be removed before appropriate antibacterial topical agents can be applied.
- Application of cold compresses may cause hypothermia. Do not apply cold water to a patient with extensive burns.

Antibiotics: Should be reserved for the treatment of infection.

Tetanus: Determination of immunization status is very important.

---

3. Discuss consciously the principles of management and rehabilitation in a patient with 50% mixed burn injury.
WBUHS 2022

Assessment

- The mechanism of injury
- Associated injuries
- *Patient age:* Patient age has a major effect on outcome, with infants and elderly patients being at the highest risk.
- *State of health:* Preexisting medical problems affecting the management should be noted, including allergies, medications, hypertension, and diabetes mellitus.
- Prehospital treatment
- Prehospital treatment is ascertained and recorded, including care provided by the patient and by the emergency response team. Administered fluids are documented carefully and subtracted from estimated fluid requirements for the first 24 hours of injury, a prehospital setting.

Primary Survey

- Primary survey should follow the guidelines established by the American College of Surgeons' Advanced Trauma Life Support Course.
- Airway assessment and security is the number one priority.
- Breathing is evaluated for effort, depth of respiration, and auscultation of breath sounds.

- *Circulation:* Circulatory support in the form of aggressive and prompt fluid resuscitation is a cornerstone of early burn management.
- Remove all clothing to halt continued burn from melted synthetic compounds or chemicals and assess the full extent of body-surface involvement in the initial examination.

Burn-specific Secondary Survey

Depth of burn:

- First-degree burns are limited to the epidermis.
- Second-degree burns, which are subdivided into superficial or deep partial-thickness burns, are limited to the dermal layers of the skin.
- Full-thickness (third- or fourth-degree) burns

Fluid Therapy

According to the Modified Parkland formula:

Amount of fluid needed in the first 24 hours = 4 × percentage of burn × body weight in kg

- So, the amount of RL to be given = 4 × b × 50 = 200 b mL (b = body weight)
- Patient should receive 100 b mL of RL in the first 8 hours and 100 b mL of RL in the next 16 hours.
- Check for urine output, it should be 0.5–1 mL/kg body weight/hour.
- Colloid-containing solutions should be held for IV therapy until after the first 24 hours postburn.
- *Ensure adequate analgesia:* Strong opiates should be used.
- Prevent hypothermia.
- Prevent stress ulcers.
- Foley catheterization.

Further Management

- Circulatory insufficiency caused by a circumferentially burned limb is best relieved by escharotomy. Escharotomies are usually not required within the first 6 hours of burn injury.
- *Fasciotomy:* It is seldom required but may be necessary to restore circulation for patients with associated skeletal trauma, crush injury, or burns involving tissue beneath the investing fascia.
- *Gastric tube insertion:* If there is nausea, vomiting, abdominal distention, or if >20% of the total body surface area is burnt.

Analgesia and Sedation

- Severely burned patients may be restless and anxious from hypoxemia or hypovolemia rather than pain.
- IV narcotic analgesics and sedatives may be administered in small, frequent doses.

Wound Care

- Partial-thickness burns are painful when air currents pass over the burned surface. Gently covering the burn with clean linen relieves the pain and deflects air currents.
- Blisters should not be broken.
- Any applied medication must be removed before appropriate antibacterial topical agents can be applied.
- Application of cold compresses may cause hypothermia. Do not apply cold water to a patient with extensive burns.

Antibiotics should be reserved for the treatment of infection.

Tetanus: Determination of immunization status is very important.

Full-thickness burns require excision and grafting unless they are <1 cm in diameter. Grafting is required within 3 weeks in order to minimize scarring.

After Healing

- The area of healed burns should be moisturized and massaged to reduce dryness.
- A high-factor sun cream should be used to prevent further damage and pigmentation changes.
  - Rehabilitation from a burn injury is a lengthy process, which starts on day 1 and involves a continuum of care through to scar maturation and beyond. It involves a dedicated multidisciplinary team of professionals and the full participation of the patient.
  - Goals include promotion of wound healing, scar suppression, pain reduction, and prevention of complications.

Second phase (wound care): The objective here is excision of nonviable tissue and biological closure, infection prevention, and facilitation of wound healing while ensuring adequate pain control.

Principles of Rehabilitation

- Promote adaptation.
- Emphasize abilities.
- Treat the whole person.
- Time
- Educate
- People-centered care

The Aims of Rehabilitation

- Maintaining range of movement
- Minimizing the development of contracture and the impact of scarring
- Prevention of deformity
- Maximizing psychological well-being
- Maximizing social integration
- Maximizing functional ability and recovery
- Enhancing quality of life

Stages of Rehabilitation

Postburn management can span from inception to the hospital to several months or years, depending on the severity of the injury. Stages of rehabilitation can be divided into early and later stages although there is no clear-cut time frame for each as they are both thought to overlap.

Early Stage

This is also known as the wound healing phase. Essentially, the aims of this stage are as follows:

- *Respiratory care:* Chest clearance can be achieved by raising the head and chest region. Physiotherapy techniques such as deep breathing exercises, vibrations, percussion, postural drainage, coughing, and suctioning can be employed to clear excess secretions. If the patient sustains burn injuries on the chest with no concomitant respiratory involvement, percussions and vibrations should be avoided to prevent reinjury to already traumatized tissue.
- *Prevention of edema:* It can be gained by elevating all affected limbs and must also commence on the day of injury to prevent sites of burns from deepening.
- *Prevention of contractures and stiffness:* Splinting and proper positioning will help achieve this aim. Also performing active or passive range of motion (ROM) exercises, depending on the patient's level of consciousness, is crucial in the prevention of these complications.
- Pain control is obtainable by performing therapies during wound dressing and debridement, if possible. Analgesics should also be administered prior to therapy sessions to encourage participation in movement activities. The physiotherapist can use transcutaneous electrical nerve stimulation (TENS) to enhance pain relief.

- Prevention of deep vein thrombosis can be achieved by encouraging early ambulation.
- Prevention of pressure sores

Later Stage

This stage, also known as the posthealing stage, focuses more on the following:

- An improvement in muscle strength, endurance, balance, and coordination owing to prolonged bed immobilization
- Scar management
- Ambulation with little or no assistance
- Engaging in functional activities
- Integration into society

Rehabilitation after Grafting

A period of 5–7 days is allowed so that the graft can "take" and circulation would not be impaired. This means that movement is not encouraged in the grafted areas; nevertheless, the surrounding parts of the body can still be moved.

Physiotherapy Intervention in Postburn Management

- Therapeutic exercises to maintain and improve ROM as well as enhance muscle strength.
- TENS to relieve pain and pruritus (itching)
- Hydrotherapy to encourage ROM exercises, especially when there is marked pain, and the patient is fearful to move his/her limbs.
- Paraffin wax therapy when applied to contractures in the extremities can improve ROM
- *Extracorporeal shockwave therapy (ESWT):* Low-energy ESWT along with traditional physiotherapy has been shown to relieve burn scar pain and pruritus and improve health-related quality of life. It can also be used to improve scar appearance and functional mobility in patients with severe burns.
- Scar tissue massage to improve the pliability of scars.

4. Discuss the management of 40% burns in a 22-year-old female patient of 50-kg body weight, carrying 12 weeks pregnancy.

Obstetric Management of the Pregnant Burned Woman

Total % burn	*Age of gestation*		*Management*
<30	First trimester		No obstetric interference
	Second trimester		No obstetric interference
	Third trimester	• >36 weeks • <36 weeks	• Induce labor/cesarian section • Conservative approach and monitoring of heart rate
30–50	First trimester		Fetal monitoring by ultrasound 3–4 weeks
	Second trimester		Fetal monitoring every 3–4 weeks Tocolytic therapy
	Third trimester	• >36 weeks • <36 weeks	• Deliver fetus within 48 hours • Careful fetal monitoring
50–70	First trimester		Terminate pregnancy
	Second trimester		Terminate pregnancy
	Third trimester	If baby is viable Intrauterine death	• Induce labor/cesarian section within 24 hours • No active intervention up to 4 weeks/monitoring of fetus of hemocoagulation factors
>70	First trimester		No treatment
	Second trimester		No treatment
	Third trimester		Cesarian section as an emergency procedure at the earliest

5. Discuss the design criteria and functional requirements of Scaffolds for skin tissue engineering in burn patient. ***WBUHS 2025***

Designing scaffolds for skin tissue engineering in burn patients requires addressing specific criteria and functional requirements to promote effective wound healing, tissue regeneration, and functional restoration. Burn injuries, particularly severe ones, often result in significant loss of skin layers, necessitating scaffolds that mimic the native skin's structure and support cellular growth, vascularization, and integration with host tissue. Below is a detailed discussion of the design criteria and functional requirements for such scaffolds:

Design Criteria for Scaffolds in Skin Tissue Engineering

- *Biocompatibility:*
  - The scaffold material must be nontoxic, nonimmunogenic, and compatible with the host tissue to avoid adverse reactions such as inflammation or rejection.
  - It should support cell adhesion, proliferation, and differentiation without eliciting a foreign body response.
- *Biodegradability and bioresorbability:*
  - The scaffold should degrade at a controlled rate that matches the rate of new tissue formation, ensuring that it provides temporary support without requiring surgical removal.
  - Degradation products must be non-toxic and easily metabolized or excreted by the body.
- *Porosity and pore structure:*
  - A highly porous structure (typically 80–90% porosity) with interconnected pores is essential to allow cell infiltration, nutrient diffusion, and waste removal.
  - Pore sizes should be optimized:
    - 100–200 μm for fibroblast infiltration and dermal regeneration.
    - 20–50 μm for epidermal cell growth.
  - The scaffold should mimic the extracellular matrix (ECM) of the skin to provide a suitable microenvironment.
- *Mechanical properties:*
  - The scaffold must have mechanical strength and elasticity similar to native skin to withstand physiological stresses and maintain structural integrity during healing.
  - It should be flexible to conform to the wound site and durable enough to handle surgical manipulation.
- *Surface topography and chemistry:*
  - The scaffold surface should promote cell adhesion and migration through appropriate topography (e.g., micro- or nano-scale features) and chemical cues (e.g., functionalization with bioactive molecules like growth factors or peptides).
  - Hydrophilicity is crucial to facilitate cell attachment and nutrient absorption.
- *Vascularization support:*
  - The scaffold should promote angiogenesis to ensure adequate blood supply to the regenerating tissue, especially for deep burns where vascular networks are damaged.
  - Incorporation of pro-angiogenic factors (e.g., VEGF) or channels for vascular growth is beneficial.
- *Antimicrobial properties:*
  - Burn wounds are highly susceptible to infections. Scaffolds should incorporate antimicrobial agents (e.g., silver nanoparticles, antibiotics, or natural compounds like chitosan) to prevent bacterial colonization.
  - Alternatively, the scaffold design should allow easy integration with antimicrobial dressings.
- *Customization and scalability:*
  - The scaffold should be customizable to fit the size, shape, and depth of the burn wound.
  - It should be scalable for large-scale production to meet clinical demands, with consistent quality and cost-effectiveness.
- *Ease of application and integration:*
  - The scaffold should be easy to handle during surgical application and integrate seamlessly with the surrounding healthy tissue.
  - It should support suturing or adhesion to the wound bed without causing additional trauma.

Functional Requirements for Scaffolds in Skin Tissue Engineering

- *Wound coverage and protection:*
  - The scaffold must act as a temporary barrier to protect the wound from external factors such as infection, dehydration, and mechanical trauma.
  - It should maintain a moist wound environment to promote healing and prevent desiccation.
- *Support for cellular growth and differentiation:*
  - The scaffold should provide a 3D environment that supports the growth of key skin cells, including keratinocytes (for epidermis formation), fibroblasts (for dermal matrix production), and endothelial cells (for vascularization).
  - It should facilitate the deposition of ECM components like collagen, elastin, and glycosaminoglycans.
- *Promotion of epidermal and dermal regeneration:*
  - The scaffold should have a bilayer or composite structure to mimic the epidermis and dermis:
    - *Epidermal layer:* A thin, dense layer to support keratinocyte proliferation and barrier function restoration.
    - *Dermal layer:* A thicker, porous layer to support fibroblast infiltration and collagen synthesis.
  - It should promote re-epithelialization to restore the skin's protective barrier.
- *Facilitation of angiogenesis:*
  - The scaffold must support the formation of new blood vessels to supply oxygen and nutrients to the regenerating tissue.
  - This can be achieved through the incorporation of angiogenic growth factors or by designing a porous architecture that allows vascular ingrowth.
- *Controlled delivery of bioactive molecules:*
  - The scaffold should serve as a delivery platform for growth factors (e.g., EGF, FGF, TGF-β), cytokines, or drugs to enhance tissue regeneration and reduce inflammation.
  - Controlled release mechanisms ensure sustained delivery without burst effects that could cause toxicity.
- *Infection control:*
  - The scaffold must minimize the risk of infection by either incorporating antimicrobial agents or being compatible with topical antimicrobial treatments.
  - It should also allow monitoring of the wound site for signs of infection.
- *Integration with host tissue:*
  - The scaffold should promote seamless integration with the surrounding skin to minimize scarring and contracture.
  - It should support the migration of host cells into the scaffold to facilitate tissue remodeling.
- *Regulation of inflammation:*
  - The scaffold should modulate the inflammatory response to prevent chronic inflammation, which can delay healing or lead to hypertrophic scarring.
  - Incorporation of anti-inflammatory agents or materials with immunomodulatory properties (e.g., hyaluronic acid) can be beneficial.
- *Support for long-term functional restoration:*
  - The scaffold should contribute to the restoration of skin functionality, including barrier properties, thermoregulation, and sensory functions.
  - For severe burns, it should support the regeneration of skin appendages (e.g., hair follicles, sweat glands) where possible.

Additional Considerations for Burn Patients

- *Severity of burns:*
  - For superficial burns, scaffolds may focus on rapid re-epithelialization.
  - For full-thickness burns, scaffolds must support both dermal and epidermal regeneration, often requiring a bilayer structure or combination with autografts/allografts.

- *Patient-specific factors:*
  - The scaffold design should account for patient-specific factors such as age, immune status, and comorbidities (e.g., diabetes), which can affect healing.
  - Pediatric patients may require scaffolds with higher elasticity to accommodate growth.
- *Clinical practicality:*
  - Scaffolds should be easy to store, sterilize, and transport to ensure availability in emergency settings like burn units.
  - Off-the-shelf availability is critical for acute burn management.
- *Regulatory and ethical considerations:*
  - Materials used in scaffolds (e.g., collagen, chitosan, synthetic polymers like PLGA) must comply with regulatory standards (e.g., FDA, CE marking).
  - If using biological components (e.g., allogeneic cells), ethical sourcing and safety testing are crucial.

Examples of Scaffold Materials

- *Natural polymers:*
  - *Collagen:* Mimics the native ECM, supports cell adhesion, and is biodegradable.
  - *Chitosan:* Antimicrobial and promotes wound healing.
  - *Hyaluronic acid:* Enhances hydration and modulates inflammation.
  - *Fibrin:* Supports cell migration and angiogenesis.
- *Synthetic polymers:*
  - *Poly (lactic-co-glycolic acid) (PLGA):* Tunable degradation and mechanical properties.
  - *Polyurethane:* Flexible and durable for large wounds.
  - *Polycaprolactone (PCL):* Biodegradable and supports long-term tissue integration.
- *Composite scaffolds:*
  - Combining natural and synthetic materials (e.g., collagen-PCL) to balance biocompatibility and mechanical strength.
  - Incorporation of bioactive molecules (e.g., growth factors, antimicrobial peptides) to enhance functionality.
- *Decellularized matrices:*
  - Decellularized dermal matrices (e.g., Alloderm, Integra) provide a natural ECM-like structure and are widely used in burn treatment.

CHAPTER 13

Damage Control Surgery

LEARNING OBJECTIVES

- ➢ Damage Control Resuscitation
- ➢ Damage Control Surgery

DAMAGE CONTROL RESUSCITATION

1. What is damage control surgery and damage control resuscitation? ***WBUHS 2022, DNB 2021 JUNE***

2. Discuss damage control surgery in critically injured patients. ***AIIMS, Raipur 2025; WBUHS 2017***

3. What are the indications of damage control surgery (DCS)? What are the steps of DCS? ***WBUHS 2023***

4. Describe the principles of damage control surgery and resuscitation in trauma with indications and steps involved. ***MUHS, Maharashtra 2025***

Introduction

- Hemorrhage is the leading cause of shock in trauma patients resulting in 40% of trauma-related fatalities.
- These patients typically present with acute circulatory failure, which is a direct result of severe bleeding.
- Addressing an exsanguinating patient presents a series of formidable challenges in the realm of critical care.
- First and foremost is the assessment of the physiological status, as rapid and accurate evaluation is essential to guide interventions effectively.
- Hemorrhage control becomes an immediate priority, necessitating swift measures to identify bleeding sources to stabilize the patient's condition.
- Simultaneously, healthcare providers must address ongoing resuscitation needs, which often involve replenishing lost blood and fluids.
- Damage control resuscitation (DCR) is an integral component of a major trauma patient care approach, rather than an isolated intervention.
- The primary objective is to proactively address all the hidden physiological abnormalities.
- The optimal goal is to optimize patient outcomes.
- Therefore, DCR underscores the necessity of a coordinated and multifaceted approach to ensure the provision of the best possible care and facilitate patient recovery.
- A comprehensive understanding of these DCR dynamics is imperative for healthcare professionals dedicated to improving outcomes in trauma care.
    - *Following are the components of DCR:*
        - Permissive hypotension—maintain lower blood pressure levels to avoid exam exacerbating bleeding
        - Limit isotonic crystalloids—minimize the use of balanced electrolyte solutions to prevent fluid overload

    - Balance blood product transfusion—administer a well-proportioned ratio of blood products to restore circulating volume and improve clotting function
    - Coagulopathy correction targeted interventions to address abnormal clotting parameters
- *Indications for DCR:*
    - Acute major trauma with hemorrhage risk
    - Significant injuries to the abdominal or thoracic viscera
    - Severe pelvic trauma
    - Extensive amputation
    - Multiple fractures of long bones.

Permissive Hypotension

- It is a critical component of DCR employed in the management of critically injured patients, particularly those with severe hemorrhage.
- It involves deliberately allowing controlled low blood pressure in the early phases of resuscitation, instead of aggressively attempting immediate normalization of blood pressure.
- The rationale behind permissive hypotension is to prevent the worsening of bleeding from injured blood vessels by maintaining a lower pressure, which assists in limiting blood loss.
- By prioritizing hemorrhage control and optimizing oxygen delivery to vital organs, permissive hypotension seeks to strike a balance between maintaining tissue perfusion and preventing further bleeding, ultimately enhancing survival chances for trauma patients.
- However, it requires meticulous monitoring and precise execution to ensure that the advantages of controlled hypotension are not outweighed by the risks of insufficient tissue perfusion.
- Target systolic blood pressure is 70–90 mm Hg or mean arterial pressure (MAP) approximately equal to 50 mm Hg for a patient in hemorrhagic shock and without suspected head injuries.

Limit Isotonic Colloids

- Minimization of isotonic crystalloids is a significant aspect of DCR, especially in managing promo patients with hemorrhagic shock.
- This approach aims to reduce the excessive utilization of isotonic crystalloid fluid like lactated Ringer's solutions during the initial resuscitation phase.
- Overloading patients with these fluids can result in dilution of clotting factors exacerbating bleeding and increasing the risk of complications.
- Instead, DCR advocates for the early utilization of blood products, such as packed red blood cells (RBCs) and fresh frozen plasma (FFP), to replace lost blood volume and maintain coagulation function.
- By minimizing isotonic crystalloids and emphasizing blood products, DCR optimizes the resuscitation strategy, enhancing outcomes for trauma patients by effectively addressing the underlying issues hemorrhage and coagulopathy.
- Studies have shown that patients who received delayed fluid resuscitation had a higher survival rate at discharge from the hospital compared to those who received immediate fluid resuscitation.

Balanced Blood Product Transfusion

- DCR is defined as rapid hemorrhage control through early administration of blood products in a balanced ratio (1:1:1 for units of plasma to platelets to RBCs; a ratio that is the closest approximation to reconstituted whole blood), prevention, and immediate correction of hemorrhagic shock.
- The administration of blood products consisting of FFP, packed RBCs, and platelets, the ratio of which resembles whole blood, is recommended early in the resuscitation.
- *The PROMMTT (Prospective, Observational Multicenter Major Trauma Transfusion) Study:* This study found that earlier and higher ratios of plasma and platelets were associated with decreased inhospital mortality in severely injured trauma patients. The study also suggested that a balanced transfusion strategy, including the use of plasma and platelets, may improve outcomes in trauma patients requiring massive transfusion.

- *Transfusion of Plasma, Platelets, and Red Blood Cells in a 1:1:1 versus a 1:1:2 Ratio and Mortality in Patients with Severe Trauma: The PROPPR (Pragmatic, Randomized, Optimal Platelet and Plasma Ratios) Randomized Clinical Trial:* This study suggested that a balanced transfusion strategy, including the use of plasma and platelets, may improve outcomes in trauma patients requiring massive transfusion.

Coagulopathy Correction

- Coagulopathy is a major component of the lethal triad directly exacerbating hemorrhage. Both acidosis and hypothermia can cause coagulopathy.
- In addition to the coagulopathy of the lethal triad, researchers recognize three other categories of coagulopathy related to trauma. These are acute traumatic coagulopathy (ATC) from endogenous anti-coagulation, consumptive coagulopathy, and dilutional coagulopathy.
- The first one is observed in one-third of trauma patients and is characterized by a prolongation of the prothrombin time together with prolonged clotting time in viscoelastic hemostatic assays (VHAs).
- Recently, the injury itself has been reported to cause early coagulopathy, which is known as "trauma-induced coagulopathy" or "ATC." ATC is an obvious early coagulopathy and occurs prior to significant dilution, within 30 minutes of injury, and affects a quarter of the patients with severe trauma. Patients with this coagulopathy have higher mortality than those with normal clotting function.
- Although the pathophysiology of ATC is not fully understood, it is thought to occur following injury and concomitant hypoperfusion. ATC is affected primarily through activated protein C, which causes both anticoagulant effects and fibrinolytic effects by inhibiting plasminogen activator inhibitor 1.
- These recent understandings of ATC have guided the principle and practice of DCR, which directly addresses the hemostatic dysfunction of the severely injured patient.
- Simultaneous transfusion of FFP and platelets (PLTs) along with the first units of RBCs while minimizing crystalloid infusion was recently recommended as a renewed DCR strategy.

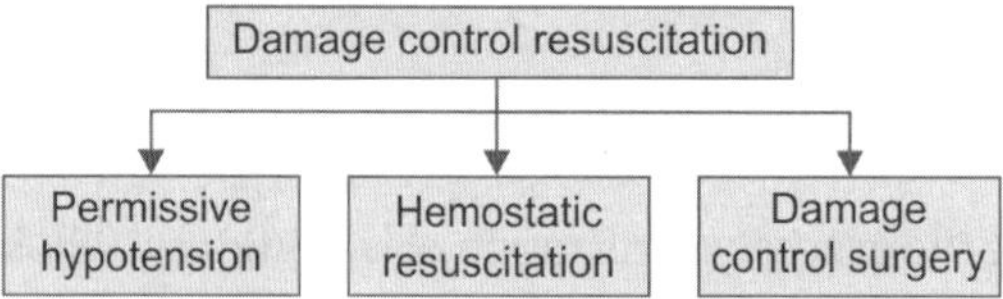

DAMAGE CONTROL SURGERY

Damage control surgery is a technique of surgery utilized to care for critically ill patients. While typically trauma surgeons are heavily involved in treating such patients, the concept has evolved to other subspecialty services. The leading cause of death among trauma patients remains uncontrolled hemorrhage and accounts for approximately 30–40% of trauma-related deaths.

Indications

- Pre- and intraoperative hypothermia (median temperature <34°C),
- Acidosis (median pH < 7.2), and/or
- Coagulopathy

DCS can be divided into the following three phases:

1. Initial laparotomy
2. Intensive care unit (ICU) resuscitation
3. Definitive reconstruction.

Each of these phases has defined timing and objectives to ensure the best outcomes. The following goes through the different phases in order to illustrate step by step how one might approach this. There are clearly different approaches throughout the country, and no one way is necessarily correct. However, the ability to evaluate objectively the differences and then choose the one phase that fits your team is important.

1. *Initial laparotomy:*
   - This is the first part of the damage control process whereby there are some clear-cut goals that the surgeons should achieve. The first is controlling hemorrhage followed by contamination control, abdominal packing, and placement of a temporary closure device.
   - Minimizing the length of time spent in this phase is essential. For groups (i.e., trauma centers) to be effective in DCS, a multidisciplinary team is critical.
   - The approach to caring for such critically ill patients is dependent on nurses, surgeons, critical care physicians, operating room staff, blood bank personnel, and administrative support. In addition to having the right team in place is having a prepared team.
   - The ability to mobilize personnel, equipment, and other resources is bolstered by preparation; however, standardized protocols ensure that team members from various entities within the healthcare system are all speaking the same language.
   - This has been seen during the implementation of complex processes such as the massive transfusion protocol (MTP).
   - Controlling hemorrhage as discussed above is the most important step in this phase.
   - Eviscerating the intra-abdominal small bowel and packing all four abdominal quadrants usually will allow surgeons to establish initial hemorrhagic control.
   - Depending on the source of hemorrhage, a number of different maneuvers might need to be performed allowing for control of aortic inflow.
   - Solid organ injury (i.e., spleen, kidney) should be dealt with by resection. When dealing with hepatic hemorrhage, a number of different options exist such as performing a Pringle maneuver that would allow for control of hepatic inflow. Surgeons can also apply manual pressure, perform hepatic packing, or even plug penetrating wounds.
   - Certain situations might require leaving the liver packed and taking the patient for angioembolization or if operating in a hybrid operating room having performed an on-table angioembolization.
   - Vessels that are able to be ligated should be considered, and one should consider shunting other vessels that do not fall into this category. This has been described by Reilly and colleagues when they shunted the superior mesenteric artery to decrease the length of time spent in the operating room.
   - Once hemorrhage control is achieved, one should quickly proceed to controlling intra-abdominal contamination from hollow-viscus organs.
   - The perception might be that one could quickly perform an anastomosis. This should not be attempted in the damage control setting.
   - The key is to simply prevent continued intra-abdominal contamination and to leave the patient in discontinuity.
   - A number of different techniques can be employed such as the utilization of staplers to come across the bowel, or primary suture closure in small perforations. Once the procedure is completed, the abdomen should be packed.
   - Many of these patients become coagulopathic and can develop diffuse oozing. It is important to not only pack areas of injury but also pack areas of surgical dissection.
   - There are various methods that can be utilized to pack the abdomen. Packing with radiopaque laparotomy pads allows for the benefit of being able to detect them via X-ray prior to definitive closure.
   - As a rule, abdomens should not be definitively closed until there has been radiologic confirmation that no retained objects are present in the abdomen.
   - The final step of this phase is applying a temporary closure device.
   - Numerous methods of temporary closure exist, with the most common technique being a negative vacuum-type device.

- Regardless of which method one decides to use, it is important that the abdominal fascia is not reapproximated.
- The ability to develop abdominal compartment syndrome is a real concern and is described by Schwab.

2. *Intensive care unit resuscitation:*
   - Upon completion of the initial phase of damage control, the key is to reverse the physiologic insult that has taken place.
   - This specifically relates to factors such as acidosis, coagulopathy, and hypothermia (lethal triad) that many of these critically ill patients will develop.
   - When developing a strategy to best care for these patients, the same principles of having a multidisciplinary team that works together in parallel for the same end result apply.
   - The intensivist is critical in working with the staff to ensure that the physiologic abnormalities are treated.
   - This typically requires close monitoring in the ICU, ventilator support, and laboratory monitoring of resuscitation parameters (i.e., lactate). In utilizing a number of different resuscitation parameters, the critical care team can have a better idea as to which direction is progressing.
   - The first 24 hours will often require a significant amount of resources (i.e., blood products) and investment of time from personnel within the critical care team. In many circumstances, especially trauma patients will require a variety of injuries to be addressed by other specialties.
   - Moving the patient early on, unless absolutely necessary, can be detrimental. Certain circumstances might require this, and the patients should continue to receive care from the critical care team during the entire transport period.
3. *Definitive reconstruction:*
   - The third step in DCS is addressing closure of the abdomen.
   - Definitive reconstruction occurs only when the patient is improving. At this point in the process, the critical care team has been able to correct the physiologic derangements.
   - The optimization will typically take 24–48 hours depending on how severe the initial insult is. Prior to being taken back to the operating room, it is paramount that the resolution of acidosis, hypothermia, and coagulopathy has occurred.
   - The first step after removing the temporary closure device is to ensure that all abdominal packs are removed.
   - Typically, the number of packs has been documented in the initial laparotomy; however, an abdominal radiograph should be taken prior to definitive closure of the fascia to ensure that no retained sponges are left in the abdomen.
   - Once the abdominal packs are removed, the next step is to re-explore the abdomen allowing for the identification of potentially missed injuries during the initial laparotomy and re-evaluating the prior injuries.
   - Attention is then turned to performing the necessary bowel anastomosis or other definitive repairs (i.e., vascular injuries).
   - An attempt should be made to close the abdominal fascia at the first take back in order to prevent complications that can result from having an open abdomen.
   - The concern for early closure of the abdomen with the development of compartment syndrome is a real one.
   - A method to pre-emptively evaluate whether fascial closure is appropriate would be to determine the difference in peak airway pressure (PAP) prior to closure and right after closure.
   - An increase of over 10 would suggest that the abdomen be left open.
   - It is important to obtain an abdominal radiograph to ensure that no retained sponges are left intra-operatively.
   - After about 1 week if the abdomen is not able to be closed, surgeons should consider placing an absorbable mesh to cover the abdominal contents.
   - This will then allow granulation to occur over a few weeks with the subsequent ability to place a split-thickness skin graft (STSG) on top for coverage.
   - These patients will clearly have a hernia that will need to be fixed 9–12 months down the line.

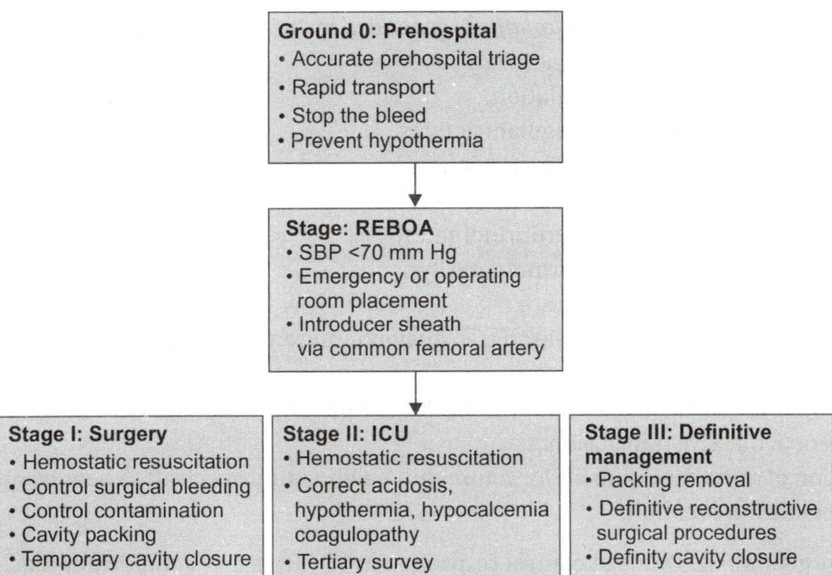

(REBOA: resuscitative endovascular balloon occlusion of the aorta; ICU: intensive care unit; SBP: spontaneous bacterial peritonitis)

5. Describe briefly the acute coagulopathy of trauma (ACoT). Rationale of damage control resuscitation (DCR) in civilian trauma. ***WBUHS 2021***

- *Acute Coagulopathy of Trauma Shock (ACoTS)* is caused by a combination of tissue injury and shock, and may occur without significant fluid administration, clotting factor depletion or hypothermia.
  - Acute coagulopathy of trauma occurs in patients with shock and is characterized by a systemic anticoagulation and hyperfibrinolysis, dilution, acidemia and consumption of coagulation proteases do not appear to be significant factors at this stage.
  - There is evidence to implicate activation of the protein C pathway in this process.
  - Diagnosis of acute coagulopathy currently relies on laboratory assessment of clotting times.
  - These tests do not fully characterize the coagulopathy and have significant limitations, which reduce their clinical utility.

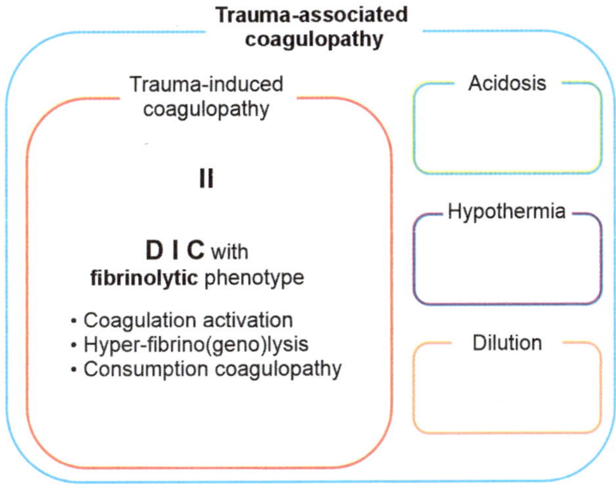

Pathophysiology of trauma-induced coagulopathy is generated by the following pathophysiological mechanisms:

- *Coagulation activation:*
  - Procoagulants in the systemic circulation
  - Impairment of endogenous anticoagulant activity
  - Thrombin generation in the systemic circulation
- *Hyperfibrino(geno)lysis:*
  - Acute release of t-PA-induced Hyperfibrino(geno)lysis
  - Coagulation activation-induced fibrino(geno)lysis
- *Consumption coagulopathy:*
  - Acute coagulopathy results in increased transfusion requirements, incidence of organ dysfunction, critical care stay and mortality.
  - Recognition of an early coagulopathic state has implications for the care of shocked patients and the management of massive transfusion.
  - Identification of novel mechanisms for traumatic coagulopathy may lead to new avenues for drug discovery and therapeutic intervention.

Damage control resuscitation: Damage control resuscitation (DCR) is a systematic approach to the management of the trauma patient with severe injuries that starts in the emergency room and continues through the operating room and the intensive care unit.

- *Components of DCR:*

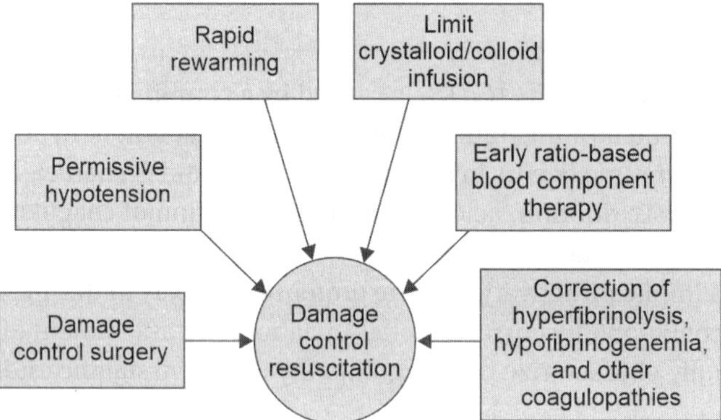

  - Coagulopathy observed in trauma patients was thought to be a resuscitation-associated phenomenon.
  - The replacement of lost and consumed coagulation factors was the mainstay in the resuscitation of hemorrhagic shock for many decades.
  - Twenty years ago, damage control surgery (DCS) was implemented to challenge the coagulopathy of trauma. It consists of three steps: abbreviated surgery to control the hemorrhage and contamination, resuscitation in the intensive care unit (ICU), and planned re-operation with definitive surgery.
  - The resuscitation strategy of DCS focused on the rapid reversal of acidosis and prevention of hypothermia through the first two steps. However, direct treatment of coagulopathy was not emphasized in DCS.
  - Recently, better understanding of the pathophysiology of coagulopathy in trauma directs that the patient should directly address this coagulopathy during major trauma resuscitation.
  - Damage control resuscitation (DCR), the strategic approach to the trauma patient who presents in extremis, consists of balanced resuscitation, hemostatic resuscitation, and prevention of acidosis, hypothermia, and hypocalcemia.
  - In balanced resuscitation, fluid administration is restricted and hypotension is allowed until definitive hemostatic measures begin.

- The administration of blood products consisting of fresh frozen plasma, packed red blood cells, and platelets, the ratio of which resembles whole blood, is recommended early in the resuscitation.
  - DCR strategy is now the most beneficial measure available to address trauma-induced coagulopathy, and it can change the treatment strategy of trauma patients.
  - DCS is now incorporated as a component of DCR. DCR as a structured intervention begins immediately after rapid initial assessment in the emergency room and progresses through the operating theater into the ICU in combination with DCS.
  - By starting from ground zero with the performance of DCS, DCR allows the trauma surgeon to correct the coagulopathy of trauma.
  - The effect of the reversal of coagulopathy in massively hemorrhagic patients may change the operative strategy with DCS.

CHAPTER 14

Daycare Surgery

LEARNING OBJECTIVE

- ➢ Daycare Surgery

DAYCARE SURGERY

1. Write in brief about daycare surgery.	***WBUHS 2008, MAMC 2022***
2. Discuss the role of day care surgery.	***KIIT University, Odisha 2025***
3. Write a note on daycare surgery.	***DY Patil Education Society, Deemed to be University 2024***
4. Discuss the principles of daycare surgery.	***Srimanta Sankaradeva University, Assam 2025***

Introduction

- In modern-day hospitals, there is an established belief in ambulating the surgical patient as early as possible.
- This philosophy has gone a step further by sending the postoperative patient home as soon as the critical period or immediate postoperative nursing needs have been met.
- This has led to the concept of daycare surgery.

History

- The first report of operations being performed under general anesthesia on an ambulatory basis in the western hemisphere was that of Dr RM Waters of Sioux City, Iowa, in 1918.
- The first successful free-standing outpatient surgery center was opened by Charles Hill and four associates called Dudley Street Ambulatory Surgical Centre in Providence, Rhode Island, in 1968.

Prerequisites

- Daycare surgery needs some degree of postoperative specialized nursing care necessitating postoperative observation for a few hours.
- All daycare surgical patients essentially come early in the morning and after the surgery is over and the postoperative observation is uneventful, the patient is discharged home the same day.
- Facilities and standards of care in the daycare surgical unit must be comparable to those provided for inpatients.
- The patient is to be formally admitted to a daycare unit, full workup and documentation are to be done, and there should be facilities to observe the patient for 12 hours with the possibility of admission.

Advantages of Daycare Surgery

Advantages to the patient		Advantages to the purchaser/hospital
• Prebooked date and less likely to be canceled • Shorter waiting lists and lesser uncertainty of a long wait • Easier domestic arrangements • Earlier mobilization • Minimal disruption of the patient's personal life • Earlier return to normal environment	• Reduced risk of cross infection • Avoidance of disruptive nights in hospital wards • Less loss of time at work • Less psychological disturbances in children • Lesser chances of cancellation due to pressures of emergency surgeries in a dedicated daycare facility	• Reduced cost • High patient satisfaction • High-volume, low-risk surgery • Lesser incidence of hospital-acquired infections • Cost-effective

Disadvantages of Daycare Surgery

- The need for a responsible person to oversee the daycare patient at home for the first 24–48 hours.
- The restriction of daycare surgery to experienced senior staff; little opportunity for junior staff to practice.
- Extra work for the general practitioner in the postoperative period; patients often ring them for advice or treatment.
- The cost-effectiveness of the unit is reduced when less complex cases are dealt with on a daily basis.

Contraindications to Daycare Surgery

- *Medical:*
  - Angina at rest, myocardial infarct in last 6 months
  - Hypertensive patients—diastolic >105 mm Hg, cardiac failure
  - Acute respiratory infection, asthma—moderate-to-severe require increased observation, chronic bronchitis, and emphysema.
  - *Gross obesity:* Body mass index >35 kg/m^2
  - Insulin-dependent diabetics
- *Psychological:* Psychologically unstable, e.g., psychosis, the concept of day surgery is unacceptable to the patient.
- *Social:*
  - Lives over 1 hour away from the center
  - No reliable person to drive patient home after surgery and look after them for the first 24–48 hours postoperatively.
  - At home, there is no access to a lift, telephone, or indoor toilet and bathroom.

Selection of Procedures

The procedures that can be undertaken as daycare surgical procedures:

Orchidopexy	Hemorrhoidectomy	Carpal tunnel decompression	Extraction of cataract with/without implant	Reduction of nasal fracture
Circumcision	Laparoscopic cholecystectomy	Excision of ganglion	Correction of squint	Operation for bat ears
Inguinal hernia repair	Varicose vein stripping or ligation	Arthroscopy	Myringotomy	Dilatation and curettage/ hysteroscopy
Excision of breast lump	Transurethral resection of bladder tumor	Bunion operations	Tonsillectomy	Laparoscopy
Anal fissure dilatation or excision	Excision of Dupuytren's contracture	Removal of metalware	Submucous resection	Termination of pregnancy

The British Association of Day Surgery (BADS) has recommended inclusion of another 50 procedures under the name of Trolley of Procedures.

Types of Daycare Surgical Centers

- James E Davis and Wallace A Reed described that daycare surgery can take place in various settings which are basically of four types in use.
  1. *Hospital integrated unit:*
     - This unit provides a designated area to which patients are admitted and from which they are discharged home and in which preoperative evaluation and preparation are carried out.
     - The hospital operating rooms and recovery rooms are used for both inpatients and daycare surgery patients.
     - There is only one advantage of this type of unit, i.e., having to make little capital investment, but the disadvantage is that it is difficult to blend inpatients and daycare surgery patients in the same operating schedule.
  2. *Hospital autonomous unit:*
     - This unit is totally self-sufficient.
     - This type of unit is located within the hospital or on the grounds of the hospital but operates totally independent of other portions of the hospital.
     - A tailor-made area is available for daycare surgery to provide the best patient care from the point of view of the physical facilities.
     - There is greater satisfaction on the part of all personnel, patients, and surgeons since everything is tailor-made.
     - The major disadvantage of this unit is loss of flexibility because if the unit is not successful or sufficiently utilized, it is unlikely that the space can be utilized for alternative services of the hospital without any additional capital investment.
  3. *Hospital satellite unit:* This is an autonomous facility which is sponsored and/or operated by the hospital but located away from the campus of the hospital.
  4. *Free-standing unit:*
     - This is an autonomous unit which is not geographically or administratively part of any other healthcare facility.
     - The advantage of this type of unit is that it meets the needs of a particular community as far as their daycare surgery requirements are concerned.
     - The disadvantages of this type of unit are that there is a possibility of an increase in the net community cost and also a greater distance from the hospital's emergency backup facilities.

Complications

- The complication rates in day surgery, resulting in unexpected readmissions, are equally divided between problems with surgery and anesthesia:
  - Hemorrhage, pain in 50%.
  - Nausea and vomiting, dizziness in 50%

Conclusion

- Daycare surgery has now come to be an accepted modality of treatment for most surgical patients and it has multiple advantages to all the stakeholders as well as the patients, besides being an economically better option for the health sector which is beleaguered with scarce resources.
- Therefore, creating more daycare centers should be in the better interest of the patients and the nation as a whole.

CHAPTER 15

Infections

LEARNING OBJECTIVES

- Coronavirus Disease 2019 (COVID-19)
- Human Immunodeficiency Virus (HIV)
- *Helicobacter pylori*
- Tetanus
- Ascariasis
- Infection and Carcinogenesis

CORONAVIRUS DISEASE 2019

1. How has the COVID-19 pandemic affected the surgical training? ***WBUHS 2021 Supplementary***

Impact on Education and Training

- As attention was diverted toward keeping hospitals afloat during the tsunami of problems washed in with the COVID-19 pandemic, education, and training suffered greatly
- Departmental/deanery teaching, courses, and conferences were canceled
- Uncertainties about fellowships, training progression
- Cancellation of elective theater lists
- Severe decline in routine emergency cases, especially in COVID exclusive hospitals

Impact on Patients

- With rising cases and deaths, patients were urged to stay at home unless absolutely required
- This was a double-edged sword as whilst this prevented services from being overwhelmed, it also meant late presentation of conditions
- Patients with cancer slowly succumbed to their disease for lack of surgery or chemoradiotherapy
- Acute conditions like appendicitis were confined to conservative managements.

Other Ways of Communication

- Telemedicine
- Online conferences
- Webinars
- Sharp increase in academic activities during period of containment

The perspective of surgical residents on current and future training in light of the COVID-19 pandemic:

- 16% saw a complete halt to their activity, 29% saw activity decline by 90%, 39% by 75%, and 9% by 50%.
- 36.5% had completely stopped consultations
- 57% of surgical residents had been recruited to work in COVID-related departments
- 23% reported having been infected by COVID-19; 67% of whom had been working in COVID-19 units when this happened

- 6% of respondents were provided continuous education
- 81% felt they were able to widen their theoretical knowledge regarding their specialty. 60% of residents felt that their surgical skills training had suffered but were able to spend more time on research and study.
- *But at the end...*
  We are doctors and we want to treat patients

HUMAN IMMUNODEFICIENCY VIRUS

2. What is postexposure prophylaxis (PEP) for HIV? How is it implemented? *WBUHS 2018*

"Postexposure prophylaxis" refers to the comprehensive management given to minimize the risk of infection following potential exposure to blood-borne pathogens [HIV, hepatitis B virus (HBV), and hepatitis C virus (HCV)].

This includes:

I. First aid
II. Counseling
III. Risk assessment
IV. Relevant laboratory investigations based on informed consent of the source and exposed person
V. Depending on the risk assessment, the provision of short-term (4 weeks) of antiretroviral drugs
VI. Follow-up and support

"Exposure" which may place one healthcare provider (HCP) at risk of blood-borne infection is defined as:

- Per cutaneous injury (e.g., needlestick or cut with a sharp instrument),
- Contact with the mucous membranes of the eye or mouth,
- Contact with nonintact skin (particularly when the exposed skin is chapped, abraded, or afflicted with dermatitis), or
- Contact with intact skin when the duration of contact is prolonged (e.g., several minutes or more) with blood or other potentially infectious body fluids.
  - *Body fluids considered being "at risk":* Blood, semen, vaginal secretions, cerebrospinal fluid, synovial, pleural, peritoneal, pericardial fluid, and amniotic fluid
  - Other body fluids contaminated with visible blood
  - *Body fluids considered being "not at risk":* Tears, sweat, saliva, urine, and feces unless these secretions are visibly contaminated with blood.

The risk of transmission of HIV via different modes of exposure is given in a tabular form:

Human immunodeficiency virus (HIV) transmission risk of different routes.

Exposure route	*HIV*
Blood transfusion	90–95%
Perinatal	20–40%
Sexual intercourse	0.1–10%
Vaginal	0.05–0.1%
Anal	0.065–0.5%
Oral	0.005–0.01%
Injecting drugs use	0.67%
Needlestick exposure	0.3%
Mucus membrane splash to eye and oronasal	0.09%

Needlestick exposure for hepatitis B virus (HBV) is 9–30% and for hepatitis C virus (HCV) is 1–10%

Step 1: Management of Exposure Site—First Aid

- For skin, if the skin is broken after a needlestick or sharp instrument:
  - Immediately wash the wound and surrounding skin with water and soap and rinse
  - Do not scrub
  - Do not use antiseptics or skin washes (bleach, chlorine, alcohol, and Betadine)
  - Do not squeeze the wound to bleed it. Do not put the pricked finger in mouth.
- After a splash of blood or body fluids:
  - *To unbroken skin:*
    - Wash the area immediately
    - Do not use antiseptics
  - *For the eye:*
    - Irrigate exposed eye immediately with water or normal saline.
    - Sit in a chair, tilt head back, and ask a colleague to gently pour water or normal saline over the eye.
    - If wearing contact lens, leave them in place while irrigating, as they form a barrier over the eye and will help protect it.
    - Once the eye is cleaned, remove the contact lens and clean them in the normal manner. This will make them safe to wear again.
    - Do not use soap or disinfectant on the eye.
  - *For mouth:*
    - Spit fluid out immediately.
    - Rinse the mouth thoroughly, using water or saline and spit again. Repeat this process several times.
    - Do not use soap or disinfectant in the mouth.
    - Consult the designated physician of the institution for management of the exposure immediately.

Step 2: Establish Eligibility for PEP

Assessment of the nature of exposure and risk of transmission:

- The HIV seroconversion rate of 0.3% after an accidental epithelial breach (AEB) (for percutaneous exposure) is an average rate.
- The real risk of transmission depends on the amount of HIV transmitted (amount of contaminated fluid and the viral load).
- A designated person/trained doctor must assess the risk of HIV transmission following an AEB. This evaluation must be made rapidly, so as to start any treatment as soon as possible after the accident (ideally within 2 hours but certainly within 72 hours).
- This assessment must be made thoroughly (because not every AEB requires prophylactic treatment).
- The first dose of PEP should be administered within the first 72 hours of exposure and the risk reevaluated as soon as possible.
- If the risk is insignificant, PEP could be discontinued, if already commenced.
- Two main factors determine the risk of infection:
  1. The nature of exposure and
  2. The status of the source patient.

The nature of exposure can be classified into three categories: mild, moderate, and severe, as shown here in a tabular form.

Categories of Exposure

Category	*Definition and example*
Mild exposure	Mucus membrane/nonintact skin with small volumes *Example:* A superficial wound (erosion of the epidermis) with a plain or low caliber needle, or contact with the eyes or mucus membranes, subcutaneous injections following small-bore needles
Moderate exposure	Mucus membrane/nonintact skin with large volumes or percutaneous superficial exposure with solid needle *Example:* A cut or needlestick injury penetrating gloves
Sever exposure	Percutaneous with large volume: *Examples:* • An accident with a high caliber (≥18 G) visibly contaminated with blood • A deep wound (hemorrhagic wound and/or very painful) • Transmission of a significant volume of blood • An accident with material that has previously been used intravenously or intra-arterially

The wearing of gloves during any of these accidents constitutes a protective factor.

Note: In case of an AFB with material such as discarded sharps/needles, contaminated for >48 hours, the risk of infection becomes negligible for HIV, but still remains significant for HBV. HBV survives longer than HIV outside the body.

Assessment of the HIV Status of the Source of Exposure

- PEP needs to be started as soon as possible after the exposure and within 72 hours.
- PEP is not effective when given >72 hours after exposure.
- A baseline rapid HIV testing should be done before starting PEP. Initiation of PEP where indicated should not be delayed while waiting for the results of HIV testing of the source of exposure.
- Informed consent should be obtained before testing of the source as per national HIV testing guidelines.

Categories of Situations Depending on Results of the Source

Source of human immuno-deficiency virus (HIV) status	*Definition of risk in source*
HIV negative	Source is not HIV infected but consider hepatitis B virus (HBV) and hepatitis C virus (HCV)
Low risk	HIV positive and clinically asymptomatic
High risk	HIV positive and clinically symptomatic
Unknown	Status of the patient is unknown, and neither the patient nor his/her blood is available for testing (example: injury during medical waste management the source patient might be unknown). The risk assessment will be based only upon the exposure (HIV prevalence in the locality can be considered)

Assessment of the Exposed HCP

- The exposed individual should have confidential counseling and assessment by an experienced physician.
- The exposed individual should be assessed for preexisting HIV infection intended for people who are HIV negative at the time of their potential exposure to HIV.
- Exposed individuals who are known or discovered to be HIV positive should not receive PEP.
- They should be offered counseling and information on prevention of transmission and referred to clinical and laboratory assessment to determine eligibility for antiretroviral therapy (ART).
- Besides the medical assessment, counseling exposed HCP is essential to allay fear and start PEP (if required) at the earliest.

Step 3: Prescribing PEP Regimen

There are two types of regimens:

1. *Basic regimen:* Two-drug combination
2. *Expanded regimen:* Three-drug combination

The decision to initiate the type of regimen depends on the type of exposure and HIV serostatus of the source person.

Human Immunodeficiency Virus Postexposure Prophylaxis Evaluation

	Status of source		
Exposure	***HIV + and asymptomatic***	***HIV + and clinically symptomatic***	***HIV status unknown***
Mild	Consider two-drug PEP	Start two-drug PEP	Usually no PEP or consider two-drug PEP
Moderate	Start two-drug PEP	Start three-drug PEP	Usually no PEP or consider two-drug PEP
Severe	Start three-drug PEP	Start three-drug PEP	Usually no PEP or consider two-drug PEP

(HIV: human immunodeficiency virus; PEP: postexposure prophylaxis)

Human immunodeficiency virus testing of the source patient should not delay the decision about whether or not to start PEP. Start two-drug first if required, then send for consultation or refer. In the case of a high risk exposure from a source patient who has been exposed to or is taking antiretroviral medications, consult an expert to choose the PEP regimen, as the risk of drug resistance is high.

Dosages of the Drugs for PEP

Medication	***Two-drug regimen***	***Three-drug regimen***
Zidovudine (AZT)	300 mg twice a day	300 mg twice a day
Stavudine (d4T)	30 mg twice a day	30 mg twice a day
Lamivudine (3TC)	150 mg twice a day	150 mg twice a day
Protease inhibitors		• *First choice:* Lopinavir/ritonavir (LPV/r) – 400/100 mg twice a day or 800/200 mg once daily with meals • *Second choice:* Nelfinavir (NLF) – 1250 mg twice a day or 750 mg thrice a day with empty stomach • *Third choice:* Indinavir (IND) – 800 mg every 8 hours and drink 8–10 glasses (>1.5 liters) of water daily
• If protease inhibitors are not available and the third drug is indicated one can consider using efavirenz (EFV 600 mg once daily) • Monitoring should be done for side effects of this drug. As for example, central nervous system (CNS) toxicity, such as nightmares and insomnia • Fixed drug combinations are preferred if available. Ritonavir requires refrigeration		

PEP Regimens to be Prescribed by Health Centers

Regimen	***Preferred***	***Alternative***
Two-drug regimen (basic PEP regimen)	*First choice:* Zidovudine (AZT) + Lamivudine (3TC)	*Second choice:* Stavudine (d4T) + Lamivudine (3TC)
Three-drug regimen (expanded PEP regimen)—consult expert opinion for starting third drug, e.g., LPV/r, NLF or IND		
Not recommended	• DdI + d4T combination • NNRTI such as nevirapine should not be used in PEP	

For Exposure During Pregnancy

- If the exposed person is pregnant, the decision to use any antiretroviral drug during pregnancy should involve discussion between the woman and her HCPs regarding the potential benefits and risks to her and her fetus.
- There is a clear contraindication for *efavirenz* (first 3 months of pregnancy) and *indinavir* (prenatal).
- In conclusion, for a female HCP considering PEP, a pregnancy test is recommended if there is any chance that she may be pregnant.
- Pregnant HCP are recommended to begin the basic two-drug regimen, and if a third drug is needed, *nelfinavir* is the drug of choice.

Notes

- Possible side effects occur mainly at the beginning of the treatment and include nausea, diarrhea, muscular pain, and headache.
- The person taking the treatment should be informed that these may occur and should be dissuaded from stopping the treatment as most side effects are mild and transient, though possibly uncomfortable.
- Anemia and/or leukopenia and/or thrombocytopenia may occur during the month of treatment.
- A complete blood count (CBC) and liver function tests (transaminases) may be performed at the beginning of treatment (as baseline) and after 4 weeks.
- It is important that side effects should be explained before initiating PEP so that the symptoms are not confused with symptoms of seroconversion to HIV.
- Adherence information is essential with psychological support.
- More than 95% adherence is important in order to maximize the efficacy of the medication in PEP.

Step 4: Laboratory Evaluation

- The reason for HIV testing soon after an occupational exposure is to establish a "baseline" against which to compare future test results.
- When offered HIV testing, the exposed person should receive standard pretest counseling according to the national HIV testing and counseling guidelines, and should give informed consent for testing.
- Confidentiality of the test result must be ensured.

Step 5: Follow-up

- Whether or not PEP prophylaxis has been started, follow-up is indicated to monitor for possible infections and provide psychological support.
- In addition, in the weeks following an AEB, the exposed person must be monitored for the eventual appearance of signs indicating an HIV seroconversion: acute fever, generalized lymphadenopathy, cutaneous eruption, pharyngitis, nonspecific flu symptoms, and ulcers of the mouth or genital area.
- These symptoms appear in 50–70% of individuals with an HIV primary (acute) infection and almost always within 3–6 weeks after exposure.
- When a primary (acute) infection is suspected, referral to an ART center or for expert opinion should be arranged rapidly.
- An exposed person should be advised to use precautions (e.g., avoid blood or tissue donations, breastfeeding, unprotected sexual relations, or pregnancy) to prevent secondary transmission, especially during the first 6–12 weeks following exposure. Condom use is essential.
- *Follow-up HIV testing:* Exposed persons should have post-PEP HIV tests.
- Testing at the completion of PEP may give an initial indication of seroconversion outcome if the available antibody test is very sensitive.
- However, testing at 4–6 weeks may not be enough as use of PEP may prolong the time to seroconversion; and there is not enough time to diagnose all persons who seroconvert.
- Therefore, testing at 3 months and again at 6 months is recommended.
- Very few cases of seroconversion after 6 months have been reported. Hence, no further testing is recommended if the HIV test at 6 months is negative.

3. Acquired immunodeficiency syndrome (AIDS) and the surgeon. ***WBUHS 2008***

4. HIV infection in healthcare workers. ***WBUHS 2011***

Introduction

- The incidence of HIV is steadily increasing in India.
- Screening of these patients by routine testing of all patients is not possible; so Universal Work Precautions take an important place to prevent transmission of HIV in the healthcare settings.
- Fundamentally this prevention can be achieved by the following means.

Barrier Precautions

- *Use of gloves:* A surgeon needs to wear gloves while doing any of the following procedures: Literature shows that two pairs of gloves afford better protection than one pair of gloves.
  - Dressing a wound
  - Starting an intravenous (IV) drip
  - Taking blood samples
  - Doing any operative procedures
  - Doing a PR, PV, or examination of the oral cavity
- Use of mask and cap.
- Use of glasses/special masks for protection of eyes.
- Use of plastic apron.
- Use of correct footwear.

I. A methodical approach to all procedures.
II. *Proper care and disposal of the sharps:* Like use of puncture proof containers in operation theater (OT).
III. Doing all the procedures in the OT in a controlled and deliberate manner.

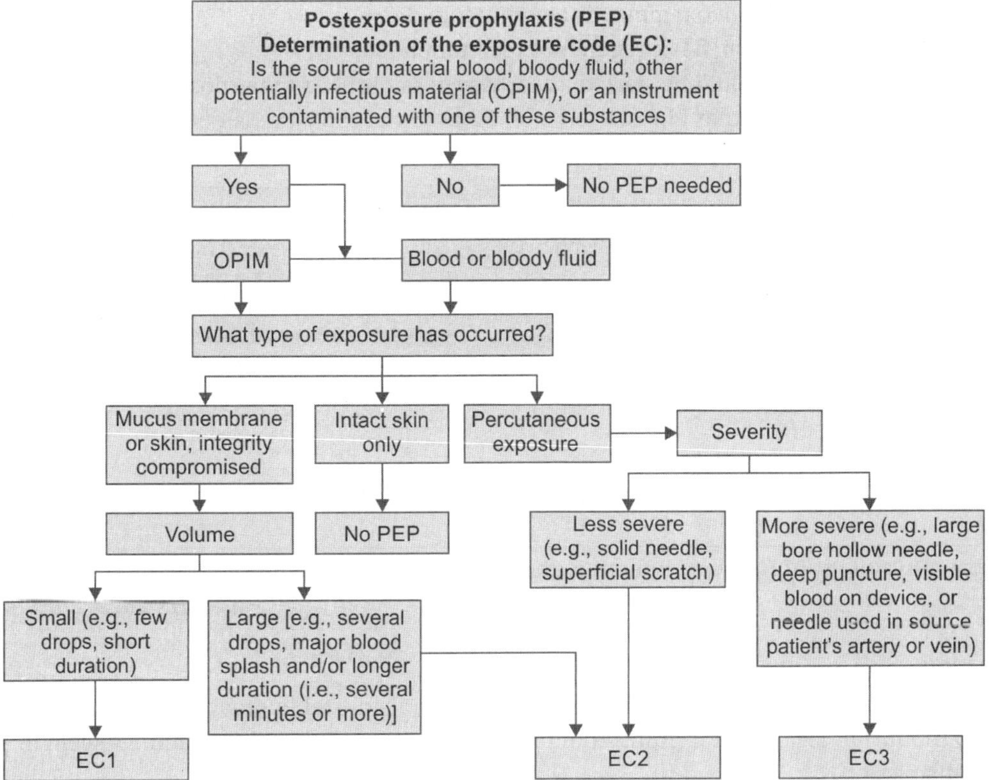

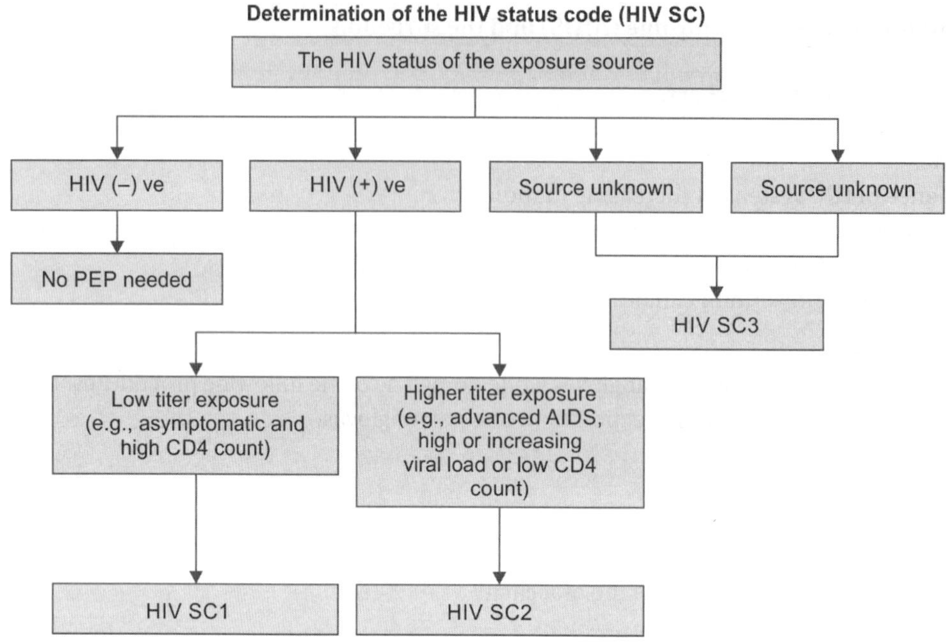

(AIDS: acquired immunodeficiency syndrome; HIV: human immunodeficiency virus; PEP: postexposure prophylaxis)

Making a Recommendation for PEP

- *EC1 + HIV SC1:* PEP is probably not required.
- *EC1 + HIV SC2:* Basic regimen should suffice.
- *EC2 + HIV SC1:* Basic regimen is recommended.
- *EC2 + HIV SC2:* Expanded regimen is recommended.
- *EC3 + HIV SC1 or SC2:* Expanded regimen is recommended.
- *EC2 or EC3 + HIV SC unknown:* Basic regimen is recommended.

Postexposure prophylaxis should be started as early as possible after the exposure. The ideal time to start PEP is <6–12 hours. It is also known that PEP started after 72 hours of exposure is not beneficial and therefore is not recommended.

Basic regimen	*Expanded regimen*
• Zidovudine (AZT)—600 mg in divided doses (300 mg twice a day or 200 mg thrice a day) for 4 weeks • Lamivudine (3TC)—150 mg twice a day for 4 weeks	• Zidovudine (AZT)—600 mg in divided doses (300 mg twice a day or 200 mg thrice a day) for 4 weeks • Lamivudine (3TC)—150 mg twice a day for 4 weeks • Indinavir—800 mg thrice daily for 4 weeks. Alternatively, in place of indinavir we can use nelfinavir in the dosage of 750 mg thrice daily

HELICOBACTER PYLORI

5. Discuss pathophysiology of *H. pylori* infection and its current management.

WBUHS 2022, 2025 Supplementary

Pathophysiology

- The most common route of *H. pylori* infection is either oral-to-oral (stomach contents are transmitted from mouth to mouth) or fecal-to-oral (from stool to mouth) contact. Parents and siblings seem to play a primary role in transmission.

- In a susceptible host, *H. pylori* results in chronic active gastritis that may lead, in turn, to duodenal and gastric ulcer disease, gastric cancer, and mucosa-associated lymphoid tissue lymphomas (MALTomas).
  - *H. pylori* infection causes chronic active gastritis, which is characterized by a striking infiltration of the gastric epithelium and the underlying lamina propria by neutrophils.
  - T and B lymphocytes, macrophages, and mast cells.
  - Mast cells, usually responsible for the immune response balance, may be important effector cells in the pathogenesis of gastritis.
  - However, *H. pylori* does not seem to invade the gastric mucosa, although evidence suggests that the mucus layer provides a niche wherein the bacterium is protected from gastric secretions.
- The release of host cytokines after direct contact of *H. pylori* with the epithelial cells of the gastric lining could recall the inflammatory cells in the infected area.
- Another hypothesis states that *H. pylori* may recall immune cells from a far because of its own molecules, such as urea or lipopolysaccharide (LPS).
- According to one hypothesis, *H. pylori* may induce the production of autoantibodies against the host's gastric lining.
- The LPS of *H. pylori* shows certain blood group antigens, such as Leb, Lex, Ley, and H-type I.
  - Such antigens are thought to represent important virulence factors involved in the adhesive process of the germ.
  - Leb constitutes an adhesin, and differences exist in the Le compositions of adherent and nonadherent bacteria.
  - This, perhaps, accounts for a relationship between adhesion and Le expression. Hage and colleagues identified the BabA protein (blood group antigen-binding adhesin) in *H. pylori* that interacts with gastric mucus binding Leb antigens, confirming the relationship.
  - As a consequence, H+ bridges may be formed, strongly anchoring the bacterium to the gastric mucosa.
  - In addition, any Le antigen shows phase variation leading to the spontaneous and random switching on and off of the expression of these antigens. For example, the H-type I antigen seems to be the result of a reversible singular nucleotidic deletion/insertion in a tract of a glycosyl transferase gene.
  - The LPS of the *H. pylori* also seems to influence tumoral proliferation of enterochromaffin-like (ECL) cells, stimulating the intracellular polyamine biosynthesis pathway and ornithine decarboxylase activity by the activation of a CD14 receptor on the ECL cell
- In 1997, Tomb and coworkers completely sequenced the *H. pylori* genome, and some differences were found in gene encoding factors that are likely to interact with the host, such as surface proteins.
  - Two of the most important genes of *H. pylori* are *VACA* and *CAGA*.
  - The *VACA* gene codes for the Vac-A cytotoxin, a vacuolating toxin.
  - Most *H. pylori* strains (60%), by unexplained causes, do not produce this protein.
  - The *CAGA* gene codes for the Cag-A protein, which seems to stimulate the production of chemotactic factors for the neutrophils by the gastric epithelium of the host.
  - A certain proportion of *H. pylori* strains (40%), by unexplained causes, does not produce this protein.
- After the exposure to CAGA-positive *H. pylori* strains, an increase in catalase, glutathione peroxidase, and superoxide dismutase activity has been reported.
  - This increase is associated with fewer deoxyribonucleic acid (DNA) adducts and reduced susceptibility of the gastric cells to the irreversible injuries from reactive oxygen species (ROS) compared with exposure to CAGA-negative *H. pylori* strains.
  - Such alterations of the ROS scavenging enzymes may partly account for the increased risk of gastric cancer in individuals with *H. pylori* infection.

Laboratory Studies

- Noninvasive diagnostic studies include the carbon 13 urea breath test (UBT), fecal antigen test, and serologic parameters (pepsinogen I and II, *H. pylori* antibody) as surrogate markers of *H. pylori* gastritis and as indicators of gastritis severity.

- Patients with new peptic ulcer disease should have a carbon 13 UBT, they should be tested for antibody titers, or they may require an investigation for stool antigens.
- *H. pylori fecal antigen test:*
  - This novel rapid test is based on monoclonal antibody immunochromatography of stool samples. The test has been reported to be very specific (98%) and sensitive (94%).
  - The results are positive in the initial stages of infection and can be used to detect eradication after treatment.
- *Carbon 13 urea breath test:*
  - The carbon 13 UBT is based on the detection of the products created when urea is split by the organism.
  - Patients are asked to drink urea (usually with a beverage) labeled with a carbon isotope (carbon 13 or carbon 14).
  - After a certain duration, the concentration of the labeled carbon is measured in the breath. The concentration is high only when urease is present in the stomach. Because the human stomach does not produce urease, such a reaction is possible only with *H. pylori* infection.
  - The breath test is expensive but is becoming increasingly more available. Other problems include false-negative results due to infection with coccoid forms of *H. pylori* that do not produce as much urease or the use of antibiotics, bismuth, histamine 2 (H2) blockers, or proton-pump inhibitors (PPIs).
- *H. pylori serology:*
  - The serology test has a high (>90%) specificity and sensitivity. It is currently based on the quantitation of immunoglobulin G antibodies against *H. pylori* by the means of an enzyme-linked immunosorbent assay.
  - It is useful for detecting a newly infected patient, but it is not a good test for follow-up of treated patients because the results do not indicate present infection with *H. pylori.*
  - The antibody titer may remain elevated for a long time after *H. pylori* eradication.
  - The number of false-positive results is age related and increases with age.
- *Antibiogram:*
  - In geographic areas with a high resistance rate against metronidazole and clarithromycin, culture for antibiotic susceptibility testing (antibiogram) seems to be useful.
  - Alternatively, metronidazole and clarithromycin should not be recommended as first-line drugs in such areas.
- *Esophagogastroduodenoscopy:*
  - In patients with prior peptic ulcer disease, an esophagogastroduodenoscopy (EGD) with biopsy and histological studies may be performed. Also, a carbon 13 UBT is helpful in these patients.
  - An EGD is often necessary in patients with symptoms of peptic ulcer disease in order to view the condition of the mucosal lining of the stomach and duodenum and to obtain biopsy specimens from the gastric antrum and corpus.
  - An echography associated with an EGD is mandatory in patients with biopsy results that are positive for gastric MALTomas in order to allow a more precise staging of the disease.
- *Histologic examination:* Biopsy sampling of both the antrum and corpus is required for histologic accuracy in the evaluation of gastritis.

Approach Considerations

- Selected 2021 American Gastroenterological Association (AGA) best practices
  - Antibiotic resistance is typically the cause of refractory *H. pylori* infection (i.e., persistent infection following attempted eradication therapy).
  - Thoroughly review prior antibiotic exposures. In the setting of any history of treatment with macrolides or fluoroquinolones, avoid clarithromycin- or levofloxacin-based regimens, respectively, owing to the greater possibility of resistance. However, consider amoxicillin, tetracycline, and rifabutin as subsequent therapies in refractory *H. pylori* infection as resistance to these antibiotics is rare.
  - Adjunct therapies, including probiotics, have been proposed, but they are considered experimental as their benefits remain unproven for treating refractory *H. pylori* infection.

- 2020 World Society of Emergency Surgery (WSES) guidelines
  - Perforated and bleeding peptic ulcer clinical practice guidelines were released in January 2020 by the WSES. Indications for antimicrobial therapy and for *H. pylori* testing in patients with bleeding peptic ulcer are as follows empirical antimicrobial therapy not recommended.
  - *H. pylori* testing in all patients. If positive for *H. pylori*, eradication therapy recommended.
  - *First-line eradication therapy:* Standard triple therapy [i.e., amoxicillin, clarithromycin, and PPI).
  - *First-line therapy, if high clarithromycin resistance detected:* 10-day sequential therapy with four drugs (i.e., amoxicillin, clarithromycin, metronidazole, and PPI).
  - *Second-line therapy if first-line failed:* 10-day levofloxacin-amoxicillin triple therapy.
  - Start standard triple therapy after 72–96 hours of IV PPI, for 14-day duration.

TETANUS

6. Tetanus prophylaxis. ***RGUHS, Karnataka 2025; WBUHS 2008***

- Tetanus is a serious illness characterized by muscle spasms and stiffness.
- Mortality is about 20% and is due to respiratory muscle spasm.
- Tetanus is a disease that can be prevented by primary vaccination and regular revaccination.
- The patient's appointment at the emergency outpatient clinic provides an ideal opportunity to examine appropriate tetanus vaccination and, if necessary, administer it.
- Primary vaccination includes a series of four toxoid injections for preschool children or three toxoid injections if started at age 7 or older.
- After the primary vaccination, children receive a booster shot at age 5, and additional booster shots every 10 years thereafter.
- Patients presenting to the emergency department with clean and minor wounds are considered adequately vaccinated if they have received a primary vaccination and received a booster within the last 10 years. If the wound is "dirty" (which includes wounds and burns contaminated with saliva, feces, or dirt), revaccination within the last 5 years is required to ensure vaccination.
- If the patient has not received primary immunization (or if the patient is unsure), provide passive immunity with tetanus immune globulin (TIG). Tetanus and diphtheria toxoid should be administered at the same time, but at different injection sites. This initiates the primary immunization, but adequate follow-up must be arranged to ensure completion of the series.
- Note that diphtheria toxoid is added to ensure adequate resistance to diphtheria in the population.
- Patients sometimes report being allergic to the toxoid. Side effects such as local pain, erythema, fever, malaise, and rash are common but should not prevent further vaccinations.
- A true anaphylactic or severe neurological reaction to the toxoid is the only contraindication to further immunization with tetanus and diphtheria toxoid.
- If the patient has had a really severe reaction in the past, they should get TIG at the emergency clinic and then following up with an allergist to assess vaccination status.

The table summarizes The Centers for Disease Control and Prevention (CDC) tetanus prevention guidelines of tetanus immunization:

For Clean and Minor Wounds

	Give patient tetanus diphtheria toxoid?	*Give patient tetanus immune globulin?*
Unknown or less than three doses of absorbed tetanus toxoid	Yes	No
More than three doses of absorbed tetanus toxoid	No (unless >10 years since last booster)	No

For All other Wounds

	Give patient tetanus diphtheria toxoid?	*Give patient tetanus immune globulin?*
Unknown or less than three doses of absorbed tetanus toxoid	Yes	Yes
More than three doses of absorbed tetanus toxoid	No (unless >5 years since last booster)	No

Tetanus Prophylaxis Guidelines

Tetanus prophylaxis for children 6 weeks through 6 years				
	Clean and minor wounds		*All other wounds*[1]	
History of adsorbed tetanus toxoid	*DTaP*[2]	*TIG*	*DTaP*[2]	*TIG*
Unknown or less than three doses	*Yes* (the primary series should be completed)	No	*Yes* (the primary series should be completed)	Yes
Three or more doses (If only three doses of fluid tetanus toxoid have been received, a fourth dose of toxoid, preferably an adsorbed toxoid, should be given)	*No* (Yes if the routine immunization schedule has lapsed)	No	*No* (Yes if the routine immunization schedule has lapsed or if it has been >5 years since the previous dose)	No
Tetanus prophylaxis for 7–9 years				
	Clean and minor wounds		*All other wounds*[1]	
History of adsorbed tetanus toxoid	*Td*	*TIG*	*Td*	*TIG*
Unknown or less than three doses	*Yes*	No	*Yes*	Yes
Three or more doses (If only three doses of fluid tetanus toxoid have been received, a fourth dose of toxoid, preferably an adsorbed toxoid, should be given)	*No* (Yes if the routine immunization schedule has lapsed)	No	*No* (Yes if it has been >5 years since the previous dose)	*No*
Tetanus prophylaxis for 10 years and older				
	Clean and minor wounds		*All other wounds*[1]	
History of adsorbed tetanus toxoid	*Tdap/Td*[3]	*TIG*	*Tdap/Td*[3]	*TIG*
Unknown or less than three doses	*Yes*	No	*Yes*	Yes
Three or more doses (If only three doses of fluid tetanus toxoid have been received, a fourth dose of toxoid, preferably an adsorbed toxoid, should be given)	*No* (Yes if it has been >10 years since the previous dose)	No	*No* (Yes if it has been >5 years since the previous dose)	*No*

[1]Including, but not limited to wounds contaminated with dirt, feces, soil or saliva; puncture wounds, avulsions; wounds resulting from missiles (gunshots), crushing, burns or frostbite.

[2]DTaP is licensed for use in children 6 weeks up through 6 years of age. Use DT only if patient has a contraindication to acellular pertussis.

[3]Tdap vaccine is the preferred vaccine for adolescents and adults who have not previously received a dose of Tdap. There are two Tdap vaccines: Boostrix is licensed for persons 10–18 years of age. ADACEL is licensed for persons 11–64 years of age. Administer Td if Tdap is not available.

(DT: diphtheria and tetanus; DTaP: diphtheria, tetanus, and pertussis; Td: tetanus and diphtheria; Tdap: tetanus, diphtheria, and pertussis; TIG: tetanus immune globulin)

ASCARIASIS

7. Ascariasis. ***WBUHS 2022***

Introduction

- Ascariasis is the most common helminthic infection.
- It is caused by *Ascaris lumbricoides*, which is the largest parasite from the class of nematodes commonly known as roundworms.
- Symptomatic ascariasis occurs during the adult worm's intestinal or larval migration phase and may manifest as growth retardation, pneumonitis, intestinal obstruction, or hepatobiliary and pancreatic injury.

Clinical Features

- Early symptoms of ascariasis during pulmonary transmission (first 10–14 days after ingestion) include cough, shortness of breath, wheezing, urticaria, bleeding, and chest pain.
- In some countries like Saudi Arabia it can be seasonal after rain.
- Returning travelers may also have Löffler syndrome and eosinophilic pneumonia, if exposed to a high-risk environment.
- Abdominal pain or abdominal pain, bloating, colic, nausea, loss of appetite, and intermittent diarrhea may be symptoms of partial or complete intestinal obstruction by adult worms in the late stages of infection 6–8 weeks after ingestion of the egg.
- Adult worms are excreted in the stool and can be seen in a stool examination.
- Jaundice, nausea, vomiting, fever, and severe or radiating abdominal pain may indicate cholangitis, pancreatitis, liver abscess, or appendicitis.

Complications

- Ascariasis complications are related to the worm burden and location of the relatively large nematode.
- These include acute abdomen, upper gastrointestinal bleeding, small bowel obstruction, volvulus and enteritis, peritonitis, biliary colic, acute cholecystitis, acute pancreatitis, acute cholangitis, and liver abscess.
- As such, ascariasis can be considered a potential cause of surgical emergency in endemic areas.

Laboratory Studies

- *Stool examination for ova and parasites:*
  - Visualization of large, brown 60 μm × 50 μm trilayered eggs is confirmatory.
  - However, stool examination may be negative for ova for up to 40 days after infection because of the time needed for migration and maturation of the worm.
  - However, it may take 40 days for eggs to appear in the stools and if only infested with male worms, there may be no eggs at all.
  - Adult *A. lumbricoides* worms can be visualized in the stool or the patient may notice them when passed.
  - Mature worms are 35 cm long (females 20–35 cm; males 15–30 cm) and 6 mm in diameter. The worms are white or pink and are tapered at both ends.
- *Sputum examination: Ascaris* larvae may be observed in microscopic wet preparations of sputum during the pulmonary migration phase.
- *CBC with differential:* Results will reveal peripheral eosinophilia during the tissue migration phase of the infection. It may take weeks to resolve, but can be masked with the administration of steroids. It is more likely in the early lung phase than the late phase.
- *Serological tests:* Serum immunoglobulin G (IgG) and immunoglobulin E (IgE) are elevated during early infection, but this finding is not clinically useful.

- *Imaging studies:*
  - *Chest radiographs/CT chest:* Images may show fleeting opacities during pulmonary migration. Bilateral, round infiltrates, or ground glass opacities with ill-defined margins with variable sizes ranging from several millimeters to centimeters may be seen in patients with high eosinophilia. Infiltrates may show migratory pattern or become confluent as the worms move in the lung tissue.
  - *Abdominal radiographs/CT abdomen/MRI:* Plain radiographs may show aggregated worms in the intestine, especially in children. A whirlpool pattern of intraluminal worms may be visible. Narrow-based air fluid levels without distended loops of bowel on upright plain films suggest partial obstruction. Wide-based air fluid levels with distended loops suggest complete obstruction. Barium swallow study may also reveal adult worms as filling defects or if ingested by worms show their alimentary canal.
  - *CT scanning or MRI* may demonstrate worms in the bowel. CT or MRI may demonstrate adult *Ascaris* worms in the liver or bile ducts in case of hepatobiliary disease. Magnetic resonance cholangiopancreatography (MRCP) may detect adult worms in bile or pancreatic ducts. Ultrasonography can also be useful for demonstration of hepatobiliary or pancreatic infestations.

Treatment Algorithm

- *Early phase:*
  - Management of pulmonary manifestations in the early phase of *Ascaris* infection consists of supportive care with inhaled bronchodilators for wheeze and cough or systemic corticosteroids for severe pneumonitis.
  - However, it is imperative to rule out *Strongyloides* by examination of sputum and stool for *Strongyloides* larvae and serologic testing due to concern of *Strongyloides* hyperinfection syndrome-associated multiorgan system dysfunction and septic shock secondary to steroid administration.
  - Anthelminthic therapy is generally not administered during the pulmonary phase and is delayed to 2 months after resolution of pulmonary symptoms, because the efficacy of drugs against larvae in the lungs is uncertain.
- *Late phase:*
  - Management of intestinal manifestations in the late phase of *Ascaris* infection include management of the individual presentation or complications such as intestinal obstruction, malnutrition, hepatobiliary involvement, and pancreatitis.
  - *Malnutrition:* Due to high parasitic burden, ascariasis results in malnutrition secondary to poor intestinal absorption of lactose, proteins, and vitamins A and C. This is seen as growth retardation and poor cognitive development in young children, with improvement seen after treatment. However, due to the demographics of the disease in areas with poor housing and sanitation, there are socioeconomic factors that confound the nutritional deficiencies as well.
- *Hepatobiliary and pancreatic involvement:*
  - Ascariasis can cause obstructive jaundice, ascending cholangitis, biliary colic, biliary strictures, liver abscesses, and bile duct perforation with peritonitis during the migration phase of the adult worms.
  - It can also cause acalculous cholecystitis due to parts of dead worms serving as a nidus for biliary stones; this results in recurrent pyogenic cholangitis if present in the bile duct or pancreatitis if obstructing the pancreatic duct. This accounts for about a third of the biliary and pancreatic disease.
- *Other manifestations:* Migration of worms outside the gastrointestinal tract may produce atypical presentation including ectopic sites such as the mouth, nose, esophagus, lungs, lacrimal ducts, umbilicus, inguinal canal, or skin. This is unusual and is seen in physiological stress associated with febrile illness, anthelmintic medications, starvation, or other acute serious illness.

INFECTION AND CARCINOGENESIS

8. Infection and carcinogenesis. ***WBUHS 2014***

Bacterial

- *Helicobacter pylori* is known to cause MALT lymphoma.
- *Salmonella typhi and cancer development:* Among the several risk factors for gallbladder cancer (cholelithiasis, obesity, and exposure to certain chemicals), chronic infection with *S. typhi* is of great importance. Chronic carriers of this pathogen have an approximately eightfold excess risk of developing gallbladder carcinoma than noncarriers and an approximately 200-fold excess risk of developing hepatobiliary carcinoma, compared with people who have had acute typhoid and have cleared the infection.
- *Chlamydia species and cancer development: C. pneumoniae* is a gram-negative bacillus and a compulsory intracellular parasite. It causes respiratory infection in >50% of adults leading to a higher incidence of pneumonia. It has been suggested that persistent *C. pneumoniae* inflammation correlates with increased risk of lung cancer. According to some data, elevated *C. pneumoniae* antibody titers have been observed in lung cancer. It has been reported that individuals with elevated IgA antibody titers to this organism have up to a twofold increased lung cancer risk.

Viral

- Many cancers originate from a viral infection; this is especially true in animals such as birds, but less so in humans.
- 12% of human cancers can be attributed to a viral infection.
- The mode of virally induced tumors can be divided into two, acutely transforming or slowly transforming.
- In acutely transforming viruses, the viral particles carry a gene that encodes for an overactive oncogene called viral-oncogene (v-onc), and the infected cell is transformed as soon as v-onc is expressed.
- In contrast, in slowly transforming viruses, the virus genome is inserted, especially as viral genome insertion is obligatory part of retroviruses, near a proto-oncogene in the host genome.
- The viral promoter or other transcription regulation elements, in turn, cause overexpression of that proto-oncogene, which, in turn, induces uncontrolled cellular proliferation.
- Because viral genome insertion is not specific to proto-oncogenes and the chance of insertion near that proto-oncogene is low, slowly transforming viruses have very long tumor latency compared to acutely transforming virus, which already carries the viral-oncogene.
- Viruses that are known to cause cancer such as human papillomavirus (HPV) (cervical cancer), hepatitis B (liver cancer), and Epstein–Barr virus (EBV) (a type of lymphoma), are all DNA viruses. It is thought that when the virus infects a cell, it inserts a part of its own DNA near the cell growth genes, causing cell division. The group of changed cells that are formed from the first cell dividing all have the same viral DNA near the cell growth genes. The group of changed cells are now special because one of the normal controls on growth has been lost.

Helminthiasis

- Certain parasitic worms are known to be carcinogenic
- *These include:*
  - *Clonorchis sinensis* (the organism causing clonorchiasis) and *Opisthorchis viverrini* (causing opisthorchiasis) are associated with cholangiocarcinoma.
  - *Schistosoma* species (the organisms causing schistosomiasis) is associated with bladder cancer.

Chronic Bacterial Infections and Carcinogenesis

Pathogens	*Main associated cancer*
Salmonella typhi	• Gallbladder carcinoma • Hepatobiliary carcinoma • Colorectal carcinoma • Carcinoma of pancreas • Carcinoma lung
Chlamydia species	
• *Chlamydia pneumoniae* • *Chlamydia trachomatis* • *Chlamydia psittaci*	• Carcinoma lung • Ovarian cancer • Ocular lymphoma
Mycobacterium tuberculosis	• Carcinoma lung • Kaposi's sarcoma
Schistosoma species	
Schistosoma haematobium	• Bladder carcinoma • Cervical carcinoma
Schistosoma mansoni	Colorectal carcinoma
Schistosoma japonicum	• Hepatocellular carcinoma • Colorectal carcinoma
Tropheryma whipplei	• Lymphoma • Gastric adenocarcinoma
Liver flukes	
• *Opisthorchis viverrini* • *Clonorchis sinensis*	• Cholangiocarcinoma • Cholangiocarcinoma
Various causative agents of chronic osteomyelitis	• Squamous cell carcinoma of the skin • Basal cell carcinoma of the skin • Fibrosarcoma • Myeloma • Angiosarcoma • Rhabdomyosarcoma
Various causative agents of hidradenitis suppurativa	• Lymphoma • Squamous cell carcinoma of the skin • Hepatocellular carcinoma

CHAPTER 16

Tuberculosis

LEARNING OBJECTIVES

- Surgical Manifestations of Abdominal Tuberculosis
- Presentation, Diagnosis, and Surgical Management of Abdominal Tuberculosis
- Tuberculous Peritonitis

1. Classify abdominal tuberculosis. Discuss the role of surgery in abdominal tuberculosis.

RGUHS, Karnataka, 2025; WBUHS 2025 Supplementary

Abdominal Tuberculosis (ATB)

Common surgical differential diagnosis in our daily practice.

Epidemiology:

- *Both gender:* Equally affected
- *Most common age:* 35–45 years

Risk factors:

- Alcoholic liver disease
- *Human immunodeficiency virus (HIV) infection:* 9% of all new tuberculosis (TB) cases are related to HIV
- Advanced age
- Low socioeconomic status

Types of abdominal tuberculosis:

- Intestinal (49%)
- Peritoneal (42%)
- Nodal (4%)
- Solid visceral (5%)

Intestinal Tuberculosis

Ulcerative type		***Hyperplastic type***
• Formation of mucosal ulcers		• Extensive inflammatory changes
– Bleeding – Perforation	• Fistula • Stricture	– Obstruction – Mass

Peritoneal Tuberculosis

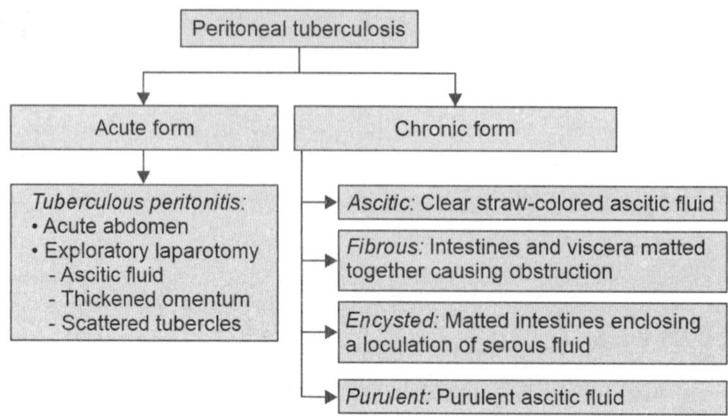

Nodal/Glandular Tuberculosis

- *Less common:* Enlargement of
  - Mesenteric lymph nodes.
  - Retroperitoneal lymph nodes
- Complications—abscess formation

Solid Visceral TB

Intra-abdominal viscera: Liver, kidney, spleen, pancreas.

Role of Surgery

- Surgery is usually reserved for patients who have developed complications, including free perforation, confined perforation with abscess or fistula, massive bleeding, complete obstruction, or obstruction not responding to medical management.
- Obstruction is the most common complication; patients with multiple and/or long strictures are less likely to respond to medical therapy.
- Obstruction may be exacerbated during anti-tuberculous therapy due to healing by cicatrization.
- The choice of surgical procedure depends on site and extent of disease, status of the remaining gut, general condition of the patient, surgeon's expertise and individual preference.
- The surgical resection should be conservative. Multiple small bowel strictures may be treated by stricturoplasty to avoid major resection.
- An alternative may be colonoscopic balloon dilation, which can be used to manage readily accessible, short and fibrous tuberculous ileal strictures causing subacute obstructive symptoms.
- In a considerable number of cases complicated with fecal peritonitis and intraabdominal sepsis, a two stage procedure with creation of a stoma (ileostomy) was preferred to primary anastomosis.
- Creation of a stoma followed by reversal of stoma in a well prepared gut after 10–12 weeks of ATD therapy reduces the risks of anastomotic leaks and septic complications.

Role of Laparoscopy in Proven Cases of Peritoneal TB

The laparoscopic appearances can be classified into three types:

1. Thickened peritoneum with miliary yellowish white tubercles with or without adhesions
2. Only thickened peritoneum with or without adhesions
3. Fibroadhesive pattern

Biopsies were avoided from fibroadhesive lesions due to risk of complications.

2. Clinical presentation and diagnosis of abdominal tuberculosis. *WBUHS 2019, RIMS-IMPHAL 2022*

Because of varied clinical manifestations, one or the other form of ATB may mimic any one of the following:

- Malignant neoplasms, e.g., lymphoma and carcinoma
- Inflammatory bowel disease
- Cirrhosis of the liver, especially peritoneal TB
- Ileocecal mass may mimic appendicular lump or malignancy cecum or other conditions.

A high degree of suspicion combined with proper use of diagnostic modalities will help in the timely diagnosis of the disease.

Type	*Clinical presentation*
Ulcerative	• Chronic diarrhea, malabsorption, intestinal perforation (occasional) • Bleeding in colorectal tuberculosis is rare but reported occasionally
Hypertrophic	Intestinal obstruction or an abdominal (ileocecal) lump
Strictures/constrictive	Recurrent subacute intestinal obstruction (e.g., vomiting, constipation, distension, and colicky pain). There may be associated gurgling sounds or the feeling of a moving ball of wind in the abdomen and visible distended intestinal loops with visible peristalsis. These symptoms get relieved with the passage of flatus/stool. Sometimes, acute intestinal obstruction may develop
Anorectal	Stricture or fistula-in-ano
Gastroduodenal	Peptic ulcer with or without gastric outlet obstruction may develop
Liver and spleen	Hepatosplenomegaly is usually a part and parcel of disseminated tuberculosis, which is accompanied by fever, night sweats, and decreased or loss of appetite. Microscopic involvement shows granulomatous hepatitis
Peritoneum	Abdominal distension and ascites, sometimes there may be a soft cystic lump due to lobulated ascites
Lymph node	As a mass or lump of matted lymph nodes in the central abdomen or as vague abdominal pain. There is associated fever, night sweats, and malaise

Diagnosis

- The isolation of acid-fast bacilli (AFB) is the gold standard for diagnosis of pulmonary TB but may not be possible for establishing the diagnosis of various forms of ATB.
- So far, the diagnosis of ATB has been made either on the histological evidence of TB in the tissue (e.g., evidence of tubercles with caseation or demonstration of AFB in a lesion) or typical operative findings suggestive of TB or animal inoculation or tissue culture yielding the growth of *M. tuberculosis.*
- Now with the advent of better radio-imaging procedures, new criteria for the diagnosis were suggested:
  - Clinical manifestations suggestive of TB
  - Imaging evidence indicative of ATB
  - Histopathological or microbiological evidence of TB
  - Therapeutic response to treatment

Investigations

- Blood examination may show varying degrees of anemia, leukopenia, and raised erythrocyte sedimentation rate (ESR).
- *Serum biochemistry:* Serum albumin level may be low. Serum transaminases are normal. A high level of serum alkaline phosphatase may be observed in hepatic TB.
- *Purified protein derivative (PPD) skin testing/Mantoux test:* This gives supportive evidence to the diagnosis of ATB in 55–70% of patients if positive; however, a negative tuberculin test may also be observed in one-third of patients.

- *Imaging techniques:*
    - *Plain X-ray of abdomen and chest:* It (erect and supine films) is useful for simple investigation. It may show the presence of multiple air-fluid levels and dilated loops of the gut in case there is subacute or acute intestinal obstruction.
    - Calcification in the abdominal lymph nodes also indicates TB.
    - *Barium studies:* The barium studies are sensitive and most useful for the diagnosis of intestinal TB.

Findings of barium meal follow-through study in intestinal TB:
Group I: Highly suggestive of intestinal TB if one or more of the following features are present:
- Deformed ileocecal valve with dilated ileum
- Contracted cecum with abnormal ileocecal or terminal ileum
- Stricture of ascending colon with shortening or involvement of ileocecal region

Group II: Suggestive of intestinal TB if one of the following features is present:
- Contracted cecum
- Ulceration or narrowing of terminal ileum
- Stricture of ascending colon
- Multiple sites of narrowing and dilatation leading to the formation of small bowel loops

Group III: Nonspecific changes
- Features of adhesions, dilatation, and mucosal thickening of small bowel loops

Group IV: Normal study
- *Ultrasonography (USG):*
    - USG is beneficial in extraintestinal (peritoneum, lymph nodes) TB.
    - The USG of the abdomen may show a mass of matted loops of small bowel with thickened walls, rolled up or diseased omentum, and loculated ascites.
    - Fine septae (complete or incomplete) and echogenic debris (seen as fine strands and particulate matter) may be seen within tubercular ascites. These septae are due to the high fibrin content of the exudative ascitic fluid.
    - However, these findings are not specific to TB as they may be observed in malignant ascites. Peritoneal thickening and nodularity are the other ultrasonographic findings of peritoneal TB.
- *Computed tomography (CT):*
    - Abdominal CT scan is better than ultrasound for detecting high-density ascites, lymphadenopathy with caseation, bowel wall thickening, and irregular soft-tissue densities in the omental area.
    - Abdominal lymphadenopathy is the most common manifestation of TB on CT. Contrast-enhanced CT (CECT) is better than plain CT and shows four patterns of contrast enhancement, i.e.,
        1. Peripheral enhancement
        2. Nonhomogeneous enhancement
        3. Homogeneous enhancement
        4. Homogeneous nonenhancement
            - Though not pathognomonic, the pattern of peripheral rim enhancement could be highly suggestive of TB.
            - A similar pattern is seen in metastatic lymphadenopathy.
            - The presence of calcification in the lymph nodes in the absence of a known primary tumor suggests tubercular lymphadenitis.
            - TB involves predominantly the omental, mesenteric, and upper para-aortic lymph nodes, while lower para-aortic lymph nodes are commonly involved in Hodgkin's and non-Hodgkin's lymphoma.
- *Magnetic resonance imaging (MRI):* MRI when compared to CT has no added advantage in the diagnosis of ATB; hence, its utility in ATB is limited.

- *Endoscopy:* This visualizes the tubercular lesion directly; hence, it is a useful tool in the diagnosis of colonic and gastroduodenal TB and helps in the confirmation of the diagnosis by obtaining histopathological evidence of TB.
- *Laparoscopy:* This examination is an effective method of diagnosing tubercular peritonitis because
  - It directly visualizes the inflamed thickened peritoneum studded with whitish-yellow miliary tubercles
  - Biopsy of the peritoneum confirms the diagnosis
  - Laparoscopy facilitates an accurate diagnosis in 80–90% of patients.
- *Ascitic tap (paracentesis):*
  - The ascitic fluid in TB is exudative (protein >3 g%) with serum-ascites albumin gradient <1.1 g%.
  - Ascitic fluid white blood cell (WBC) count is 150–4,000 cells/mm^3 and consists of predominant lymphocytes. Neutrophils may be seen in the early stages of the disease. Red blood cells (RBCs), sometimes, may also be seen.
  - Ascitic fluid reveals AFB only in <3% of the cases and culture for *Mycobacterium tuberculosis* is positive only in 20% of patients.
  - Adenosine deaminase (ADA) activity in ascitic fluid is a sensitive and specific marker for TB. Ascitic fluid to serum ADA ratio >0.985 was also found to be suggestive of TB. Falsely low levels of ADA can be found in immunocompromised individuals.
  - Interferon γ (INF-γ), an important immunoregulator, is produced by T-lymphocytes in response to stimulation with specific antigens and is capable of activating the macrophages, increasing their bactericidal activity against *M. tuberculosis*. High levels of INF-γ have been found in ascites due to TB than nontubercular.
- *Serodiagnosis:*
  - Conventional histological and microbiological methods are often inadequate for the diagnosis of ATB as it is a paucibacillary disease.
  - A number of serological tests based on the detection of antibody to a variety of mycobacterial antigens developed but all of them have a low predictive value. Polymerase chain reaction (PCR) assay for detection of *M. tuberculosis* in endoscopic biopsy specimens has shown promising results.
- *Soft-tissue biopsy and culture:* Invasive diagnostic procedures are indicated with suspected ATB. In addition to specimens of involved sites (lymph node, intestine, peritoneum, and liver biopsy), bone marrow aspiration for culture may be useful and have a good diagnostic yield in disseminated (miliary) TB, particularly in HIV-infected patients.

3. Surgical manifestations of abdominal tuberculosis. *WBUHS 2014; AIIMS, Bhopal 2023*

Common surgical differential diagnosis in our daily practice.

Epidemiology:

- *Both genders:* Equally affected
- *Most common age:* 35–45 years

Risk factors:

- Alcoholic liver disease
- *Human immunodeficiency virus (HIV) infection:* 9% of all new TB cases are related to HIV.
- Advanced age
- Low socioeconomic status

Types:

- Intestinal (49%)
- Peritoneal (42%)
- Nodal (4%)
- Solid visceral (5%)

Intestinal Tuberculosis

Ulcerative type	*Hyperplastic type*
• Formation of mucosal ulcers: – Bleeding – Perforation – Fistula – Stricture	• Extensive inflammatory changes – Obstruction – Mass

Peritoneal Tuberculosis

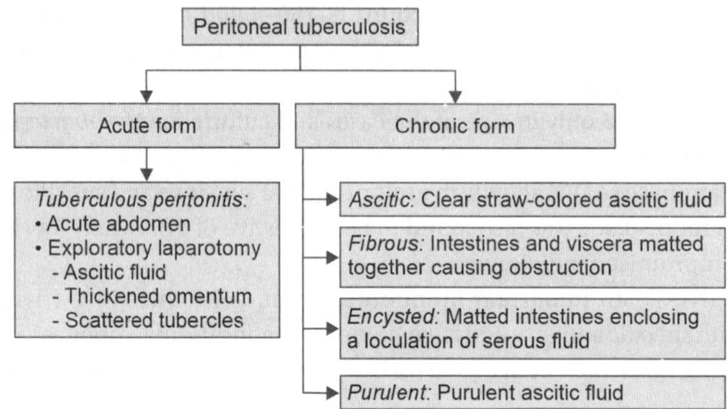

Nodal/Glandular TB

- Less common
- Enlargement of
  - Mesenteric lymph nodes
  - Retroperitoneal lymph nodes
- Complications—abscess formation

Solid Visceral TB

Intra-abdominal viscera: Liver, kidney, spleen, and pancreas.

Clinical Presentations

Acute form (41%)	*Chronic form (50%)*	*Combined form (9%)*
• Peritonitis • Intestinal obstruction • Perforation • Gastrointestinal (GI) bleeding	• Chronic pain • Ascites • Weight loss • Diarrhea and vomiting • Fever • Mass	

4. Paustian's criteria to diagnose abdominal tuberculosis. Discuss the role of surgery in ATB. ***WBUHS 2021***

- Paustian's criteria suggest that the diagnosis be established if any one of the following four criteria is observed:
  1. Histology showing tubercles with caseating necrosis, suggestive operative findings
  2. Consistent histology from mesenteric lymph nodes, animal inoculation or
  3. Culture showing growth of *M. tuberculosis*, or
  4. Histology showing AFB in the lesion
- Paustian's criteria are difficult to apply in most cases and Logan's modification of Paustian's criteria, which uses the response to antitubercular therapy (ATT), has often been used to establish the diagnosis.

- On the other hand, the appropriate time and manner of establishing an adequate response to ATT has remained unclear.
- The investigational modalities for the diagnosis of ATB include radiological, biochemical, histology, and microbiological, including molecular tests and ancillary or supportive tests.
- Certain tests like the Mantoux skin test may have ancillary value but cannot be used as a standalone diagnostic tool as it may be compromised by a false-positive (underlying Bacillus Calmette-Guérin vaccination, cross-reaction with other mycobacteria) and false-negative (disseminated TB, immunosuppression, recent infection, and extremes of age).
- Chest X-ray may be able to detect active or past evidence of pulmonary TB and thereby provide corroborative evidence of ATB; such changes may be detectable in a quarter of the patients.
- Interferon-gamma release assays (IGRA) may overcome some limitations of Mantoux testing and do not have cross-reactivity with Bacillus Calmette-Guérin or other mycobacteria; however, their positivity is consistent with *M. tuberculosis* infection but cannot be used to diagnose active disease.
- HIV testing should be performed in all patients suspected to have ATB.

Surgery

- Surgery is usually reserved for patients who have developed complications, including free perforation, confined perforation with abscess or fistula, massive bleeding, complete obstruction, or obstruction not responding to medical management.
- Obstruction is the most common complication; patients with multiple and/or long strictures are less likely to respond to medical therapy.
- Obstruction may be exacerbated during antituberculous therapy due to healing by cicatrization.
- The choice of surgical procedure depends on the site and extent of disease, status of the remaining gut, general condition of the patient, surgeon's expertise, and individual preference.
- The surgical resection should be conservative. Multiple small bowel strictures may be treated by stricturoplasty to avoid major resection.
- An alternative may be colonoscopic balloon dilation, which can be used to manage readily accessible, short, and fibrous tuberculous ileal strictures causing subacute obstructive symptoms.
- In a considerable number of cases complicated with fecal peritonitis and intra-abdominal sepsis, a two-stage procedure with creation of a stoma (ileostomy) was preferred to primary anastomosis.
- Creation of a stoma followed by reversal of the stoma in a well-prepared gut after 10–12 weeks of antitubercular drug (ATD) therapy reduces the risks of anastomotic leaks and septic complications.

Role of Laparoscopy in Proven Cases of Peritoneal TB

Laparoscopic appearances can be classified into three types:

1. Thickened peritoneum with miliary yellowish-white tubercles with or without adhesions
2. Only thickened peritoneum with or without adhesions
3. Fibroadhesive pattern

   Biopsies were avoided from fibroadhesive lesions due to the risk of complications.

TUBERCULOUS PERITONITIS

5. Tuberculous peritonitis. ***WBUHS 2012, RIMS-IMPHAL 2012***

Introduction

Peritoneal TB is an uncommon site of extra-pulmonary infection caused by *M. tuberculosis*. The risk is increased in patients with cirrhosis, HIV infection, diabetes mellitus, or underlying malignancy, following treatment with antitumor necrosis factor (anti-TNF) agents, and in patients undergoing continuous ambulatory peritoneal dialysis.

- Infection occurs most commonly following reactivation of latent TB foci in the peritoneum that were established from hematogenous spread from a primary lung focus.
- It can also occur via hematogenous spread from active pulmonary or miliary TB. Much less frequently, the organisms enter the peritoneal cavity transmurally from an infected small intestine or contiguously from tuberculous salpingitis.

As the disease progresses, the visceral and parietal peritoneum become increasingly studded with tubercles. Ascites develops secondary to "exudation" of proteinaceous fluid from the tubercles, similar to the mechanism leading to ascites in patients with peritoneal carcinomatosis.

Clinical Features

Clinical findings in peritoneal TB are indistinguishable from those in bacterial peritonitis. Fever, abdominal pain, and cloudy fluid are the most common presenting symptoms. Cell count cannot be used to differentiate peritoneal TB from other forms of peritonitis.

Investigations

- More than 60% of peritoneal TB cases have a predominance of polymorphonuclear neutrophils.
- Blood and sputum AFB cultures and PPD skin testing are often negative.
- Specialized tests, with increased accuracy but not readily available at most hospitals, include spectrophotometric analysis of adenosine deaminase levels in ascitic fluid and serum and polymerase chain reaction (PCR) assays that amplify mycobacterial 16S ribosomal RNA.
- CT scanning remains the most convenient and consistent diagnostic test with accuracy as high as 85%.
- Previous studies have also shown ultrasound-guided fine needle aspiration (FNA) of abdominal ascitic fluid for analysis to be a reliable diagnostic modality.

Treatment

- With suggestive clinical manifestations and bacteriologic proof of active TB anywhere in the patient, an operation is not mandated.
  - In the presence of features of peritonitis, and in the absence of definitive bacteriologic proof, exploratory laparotomy is indicated for diagnostic purposes.
  - Anti-TB chemotherapy is highly effective and is the treatment of choice.

Surgical Instruments and Energy Sources

LEARNING OBJECTIVES

- Staples and Staplers in Surgery
- Energy Sources/Energy Devices in Surgery, Electrosurgery, and Ultrasonic Dissection
- Laser in Surgery
- Indocyanine Green (ICG)

1. Staples in surgery.

The Tamil Nadu Dr MGR Medical University 2025; WBUHS 2015

Introduction

Surgical staples are specialized staples used in surgery in place of sutures to close skin wounds and connect or remove parts of the bowels or lungs. A more recent development, from the 1990s, uses clips instead of staples for some applications; this does not require the staple to penetrate.

- The first commercial staplers were made of stainless steel with titanium staples loaded into reloadable staple cartridges.
- Modern surgical staplers are either disposable and made of plastic, or reusable and made of stainless steel. Both types are generally loaded using disposable cartridges.

Types and Applications

- The staple line may be straight, curved, or circular.
- Circular staplers are used for end-to-end anastomosis after bowel resection or, somewhat more controversially, in esophagogastric surgery. The instruments may be used in either open or laparoscopic surgery, different instruments are used for each application.
- Laparoscopic staplers are longer, thinner, and may be articulated to allow for access from a restricted number of trocar ports.
- Some staplers incorporate a knife, to complete excision and anastomosis in a single operation.
- Staplers are used to close both internal and skin wounds. Skin staples are usually applied using a disposable stapler, and removed with a specialized staple remover. Staplers are also used in vertical banded gastroplasty surgery (popularly known as "stomach stapling").
- Vascular stapler for reducing warm ischemia in organ transplantation. With this model each stapler end can be mounted on donor and recipient by independent surgical teams without care for reciprocal orientation, being the maximal possible vascular axis torsion $\leq 30°$. Activating guidewire is connected just immediately before firing.
- While devices for circular end-to-end anastomosis of the digestive tract are widely used, despite intensive research circular staplers for vascular anastomosis never had yet significant impact on the standard hand (Carrel) suture technique.

- Apart from the different modalities of coupling of vascular (everted) in respect to digestive (inverted) stumps, the main basic reason could be that, particularly for small vessels, the manuality and precision required just for positioning on the vascular stumps and action of any device cannot be significantly inferior to that required to carry out the standard hand suture, then making of little utility the use of any device.
- An exception to that, however, could be organ transplantation where these two phases, i.e., device positioning at the vascular stumps and device action can be carried out in different times, by different surgical teams, in safe conditions when the time required does not influence donor organ preservation, i.e., at the back table in cold ischemia condition for the donor organ and after native organ removal in the recipient.

Staple Materials

- Although most surgical staples are made of titanium, stainless steel is more often used in some skin staples and clips.
- Titanium produces less reaction with the immune system and, being nonferrous, does not interfere significantly with magnetic resonance imaging (MRI) scanners, although some imaging artifacts may result.
- Synthetic absorbable (bioabsorbable) staples are also now becoming available, based on polyglycolic acid, as with many synthetic absorbable sutures.
- Titanium staples are not suspected of causing nickel reactions because nickel is rarely if ever used in titanium alloys.

2. Staplers in surgery. ***WBUHS 2020***

3. Discuss the uses and advantages of staplers in surgery. ***WBUHS 2025***

Goals of Stapler

- Close abdominal wounds
- Join internal organs to restore to normal function
- Maintain hemostasis
- Reduce tissue trauma
- Reduce contamination
- Prevent postoperative morbidity and infections

Advantages of Stapling

- Stapling anastomosis is faster than traditional suturing techniques, hence reduced operating time. Reduces tissue trauma by minimizing tissue handling.
- Prevents contamination
- The availability of staplers has fostered the development of procedures that were difficult with traditional techniques because of limited access.
- Stapled tissue and anastomoses heal as reliably and rapidly as sutured anastomosis
- Not user dependent

Use of Surgical Staplers

- *Linear staplers:*
    - Close internal organs prior to transaction
    - Close the common opening or enterotomy after the creation of an anastomosis
    - Make side-to-side or functional end-to-end anastomosis
    - Biopsy or wedge resection of the lung and closing of the bronchus and to close pulmonary vessels prior to their division
    - Resection of solid organs, such as liver and pancreas

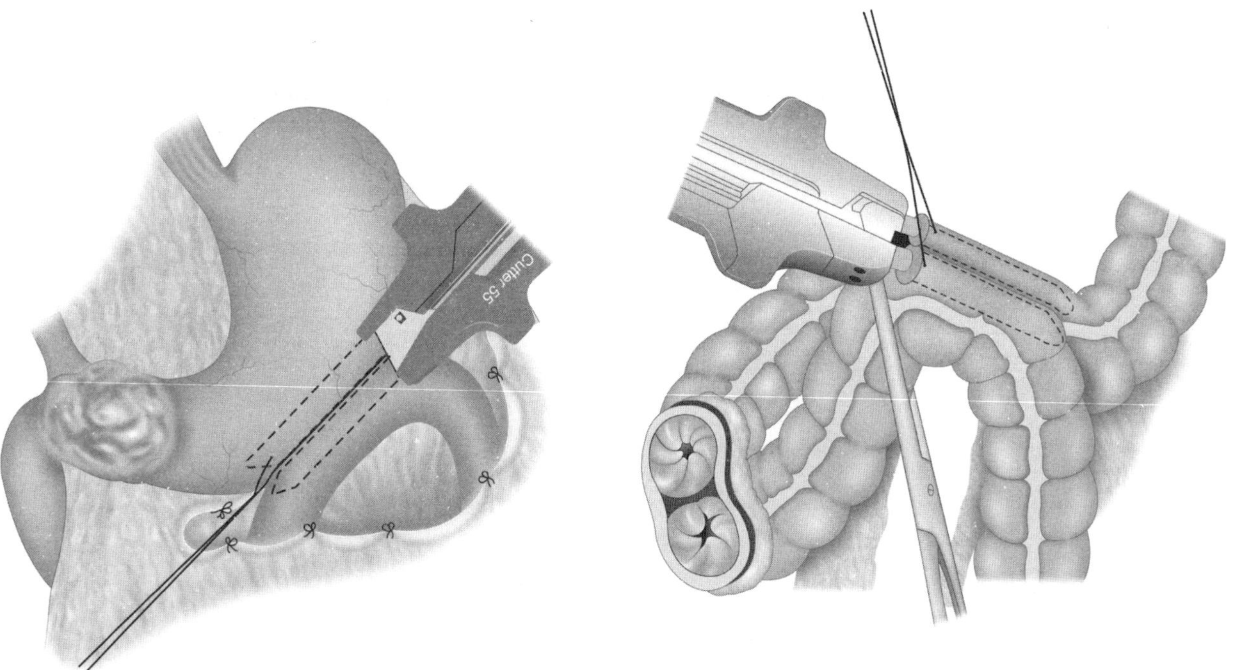

- *Circular staplers (intraluminal staplers):*
  - End-to-end anastomosis, e.g., colorectal anastomosis in low anterior resection (LAR)
  - End-to-side anastomosis, e.g., ileocolostomy after right hemicolectomy
  - Side-to-side anastomosis, e.g., side-to-side gastrojejunostomy after Billroth II gastrectomy

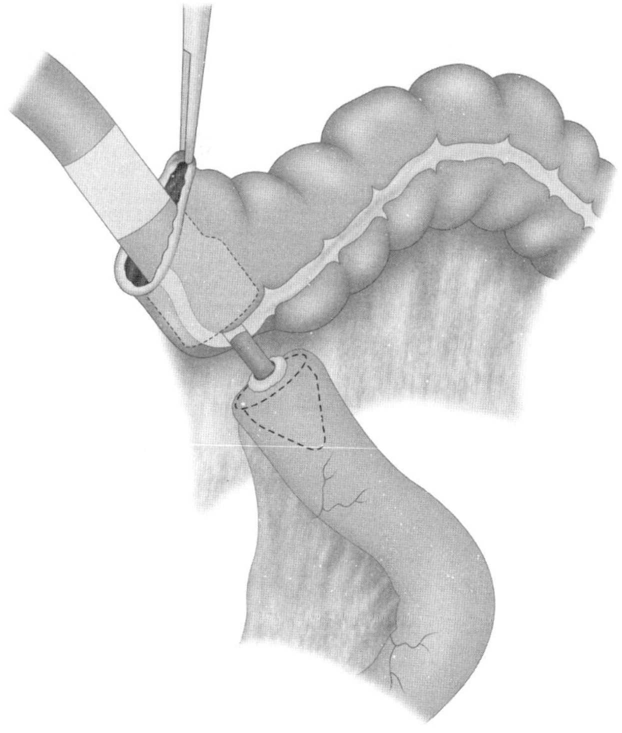

- *Curvilinear cutting staplers (contour stapler):*
  - Transabdominal proctectomy
  - Very-low-anterior resection of the rectum (as it is able to fit into the narrow confines of the pelvis)

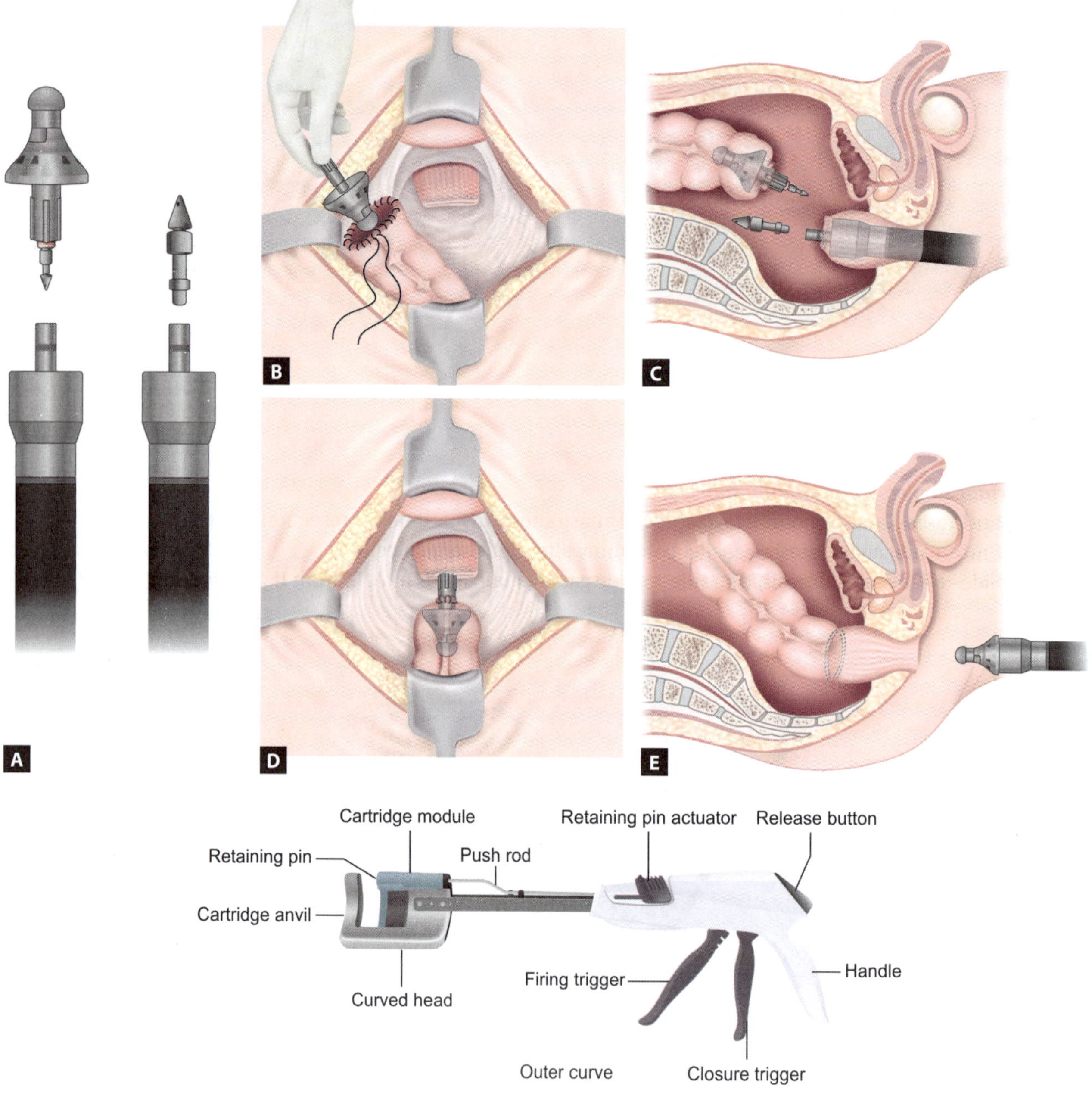

- *Procedure for prolapse and hemorrhoid (PPH) staplers:*
  - Used to excise prolapsed rectal mucosa at the top of the anal canal as a treatment for prolapsing hemorrhoids.

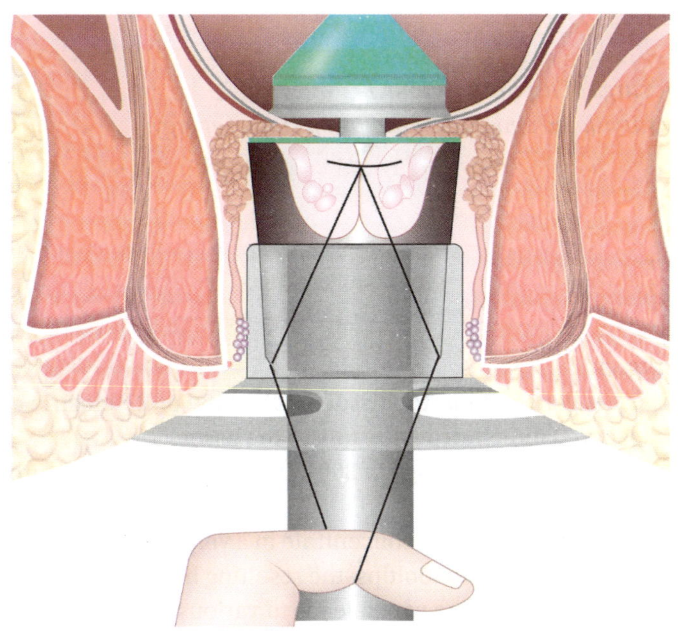

Side-to-side Anastomosis (Functional End-to-end Anastomosis)

Critical Concepts

- Nontension
- Gastrointestinal anastomosis (GIA) stapler
- Align antimesenteric sides of the bowel together
- Staggered staple lines

Anastomotic Leaks in Stapled Anastomosis

Anastomotic leaks reported may or may not involve the staple lines, dependent upon the method of surgery used.

Anastomotic Leaks

- Major/manifested leaks
- Minor leaks etiology of staple line leaks

Etiology of Staple Line Leaks

- Mechanical/tissue causes—seen in the first 2 days following the surgery.
- More commonly seen in ischemic causes—ischemic leaks that happen 5–7 days postoperatively.

4. Discuss the energy devices in the operation theater. Mention the principles of safe use of electrosurgery.
RGUHS, Karnataka 2025; WBUHS 2021 Supplementary

5. Energy sources and devices in surgery. ***KGMU, Lucknow 2025***

Most Commonly Used Energy Devices

I. *Monopolar electrocautery*

II. *Bipolar electrocautery:*
   - Bipolar diathermy
   - LigaSure
   - EnSeal
   - Gyrus Plasma Kinetics

III. *Ultrasonic energy:*
   - Harmonic scalpel
   - Cavitron *ultrasonic surgical aspirator* (CUSA)

IV. *Light amplification by stimulated emission of radiation (laser) energy:*
   - *Nd:YAG laser*
   - *Argon laser*
   - *CO_2 laser*

V. *Argon beam coagulator*

VI. *Radiofrequency (RF) ablation*

VII. *THUNDERBEAT*

- *Mechanism of electrosurgery:*
  - In electrosurgery, heat is generated in the tissue by the flow of RF electric current, unlike electrocautery where the heat is transferred directly from the tool to the tissue.
  - The use of RF current (voltage in the range of 300–500 KHz) eliminates neuromuscular stimulation, which ceases above 100 KHz.
  - When the RF electrical energy is made to concentrate in a very small area in the tissue, typically by applying the energy through pointed or hooked tooltips, the resulting high concentration of current flow in a narrow area increases the cellular temperature which leads to various effects on the tissue including, coagulation, desiccation or dehydration, and carbonization.
  - The RF energy can be applied to tissue by using either monopolar or bipolar tools. In monopolar electrosurgery, the electrical circuit is completed by the passage of current from the active electrode at the surgical site to the dispersive electrode (or the return electrode) attached to the body of the patient.
  - The active electrode can be of any form (usually a point, hook, or blade) with sharp edges and/or blunt edges.
  - The sharp edges increase the current density (the amount of current per unit area) and are used for cutting whereas the blunt edges are used for coagulation.
  - The return electrode is usually a wide pad, attached to the skin of the patient, which disperses the heat and safely leads the current out of the body.
  - In bipolar electrosurgery both active and return electrodes are located in the same tool and the electrical circuit is closed by the small area of tissues that are grasped or manipulated by the tool.
  - Bipolar tools are, thus, usually designed as grippers or forceps. Since the current only has to travel short distances in bipolar surgery, the voltage required for the surgery is low.
  - Lower voltage is better for uniform drying of the tissue which minimizes the chance of rebleeding.
  - Thus the bipolar devices are more suitable for coagulation rather than cutting.
- *The basic working principle of ultrasonic surgical instruments:*
  - Such as ultrasonically activated scalpel (UAS) is to use the low-frequency mechanical vibrations (ultrasonic energy in the range of 20–60 kHz) of the tooltips or the blades for tissue cutting and coagulation.
  - The cutting using an ultrasonic surgical instrument is achieved by two methods.
  - For tissues and muscles with high protein densities, the mechanical stretching of the tissues beyond their elastic limit due to the longitudinal motion of the sharp blades between 60 and 100 μm at 55.5 kHz is used for cutting.
  - For tissues with low protein densities, such as the liver, the cavitation effect in which intercellular water is vaporized at lower temperatures due to mechanical vibrations, thereby rupturing the cells is used for cutting.
  - In general, the cutting and coagulation in UAS depends on various factors, such as grip pressure, the shape and area of the blades in contact with the tissues, and the power settings.
  - Lasers generate heat by applying a concentrated beam of light.
  - In a laser system, electromagnetic or light waves are amplified multiple fold in an optical resonator (which contains mirrors and a gain medium) and passed out in the form of high-intensity light waves.

- The amount of amplification in the resonator determines the amount of energy transmitted by the light waves which are then absorbed by the tissue.
- This energy absorbed by the tissue then manifests itself into heat which cuts and coagulates the tissue.

- *In argon beam coagulation (ABC)*, a directed beam of argon gas from the electrode tip aids in the conduction of the RF current to the tissue by ionization.
  - Like a laser, this is a noncontact method where the argon gas—which is a good conductor of electricity acts as a means of transportation of the current from the tool to the tissue.
  - ABC performs faster than conventional coagulation systems and provides a more uniform and shallower coagulation region which results in faster dispersion thus minimizing tissue damage.
- *THUNDERBEAT* is the world's first integration of both bipolar and ultrasonic energies delivered simultaneously from a single instrument.

Principles of Safe Use of Electrosurgery

Basic Principles of Electrosurgery

- Energy in wattage (power) is the product of current and voltage. Power is the amount of current times the voltage level at a given point measured in wattage or watts (W). It corresponds to the rate of work being performed, W = V × I.
- Ohm's law, I = V/R, shows the relationship between the properties of electrosurgical energy.
- Current (I) is what flows on a wire or conductor like water flowing down a river. Current flows from negative to positive on the surface of a conductor. Current is measured in amperes (A) or amps.
- Voltage (V) is the difference in electrical potential between two points in a circuit. It is the push or pressure behind current flow through a circuit and is measured in volts (V).
- Resistance determines how much current will flow through a component. Resistors are used to control voltage and current levels. A very high resistance allows a small amount of current to flow. A very low resistance allows a large amount of current to flow. Resistance is measured in ohms (Ω).

Principles of Electrosurgery

- Modern-day electrosurgery is the utilization of alternating current at RF levels.
- In electrosurgery, the patient is included in the circuit and current enters the patient's body.

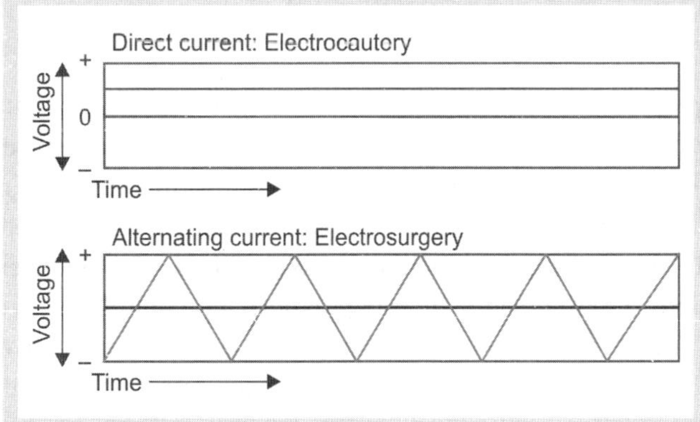

Electrical current flows when electrons from one atom move to an adjacent atom through a circuit. Heat is produced when electrons encounter resistance. For current to flow, a continuous circuit is needed. In the operating room, the circuit is composed of the patient, electrosurgical generator, active electrode, and return electrodes. The electrosurgical unit is the source of the voltage.

Electrical energy is converted to heat in tissue as the tissue resists the flow of current from the electrode.

Three tissue effects are possible with today's electrosurgical units—cutting, desiccation, and fulguration.

Achieving these effects depends on the following factors: Current density, time, electrode size, tissue conductivity, and current waveform:

- *Current density:* As expected, the greater the current that passes through an area, the greater the effect will be on the tissue.
- *Time:* The length of time a surgeon uses an active electrode determines the tissue effect. Too long an activation will produce wider and deeper tissue damage. Too short an activation will result in the absence of the desired tissue effect.
- *Electrode size:* With respect to electrode size, smaller electrodes provide a higher current density and result in a concentrated heating effect at the site of tissue contact. Following the same principle, the patient return electrode used in monopolar electrosurgery is large in relation to the active electrode in order to disperse the current returning to the electrosurgical unit and minimize heat production at this return electrode site.
- *Tissue conductivity:* Various tissue types have a different electrical resistance, which affects the rate of heating. Adipose tissue and bone have high resistance and are poor conductors of electricity, whereas muscle and skin are good conductors of electricity and have low resistance.
- *Current waveforms:* The final determinant of how tissue responds to electrosurgery is the current type. Electrosurgical units produce three different waveforms, i.e., (1) cut, (2) blend, and (3) coagulation.

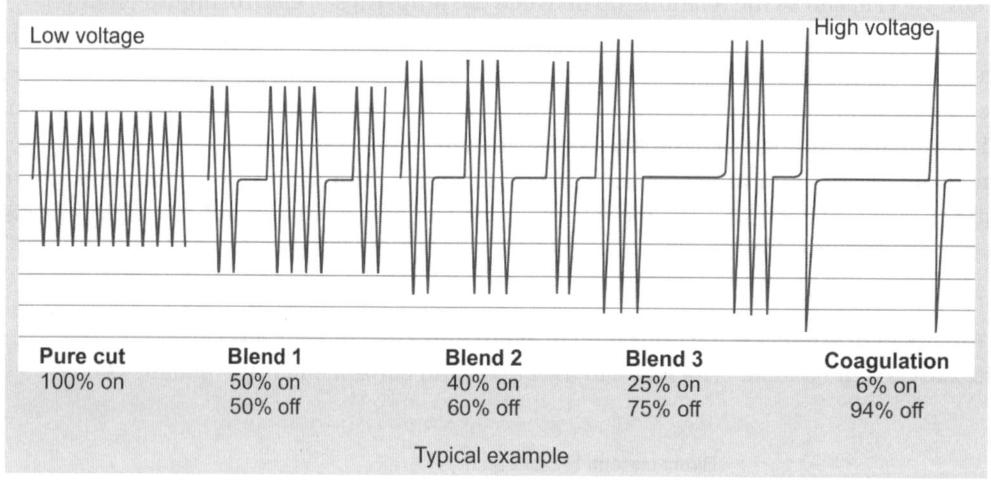

- A pure cutting (vaporization) waveform is continuous, unmodulated, and undamped. A coagulation waveform is interrupted, modulated, and damped current. A blend waveform is a modification of the cutting waveform and is used when hemostasis is needed while cutting. This waveform type consists of a combination of both cutting and coagulation waveforms. Higher blend settings translate into more time between bursts of current and greater coagulation, as seen in the following examples: Blend 1 (80% cut and 20% coagulation), blend 2 (60% cut and 40% coagulation), and blend 3 (50% cut and 50% coagulation).
- A cutting current power setting must be between 50 and 80W to be effective. Ideally, the electrode is held slightly away from the tissue to create a spark gap or steam envelope through which the current arcs to the tissue. This spark gap results from heating up the atmosphere between the electrode and the tissue. The coagulation current is effective with the power settings in the range of 30 and 50W.
- Fulguration (spray) is a noncontact coagulation that also utilizes a spark gap to mediate tissue effects, which results in heating and necrosis as well as greater thermal spread. Desiccation (deep) is another form of coagulation in which direct contact is made with the tissue, resulting in electrical energy being converted into heat within the tissue. The end result is deeper necrosis and greater thermal spread.

Comparison of tissue effects of four energy modalities.				
	Monopolar	*Traditional bipolar*	*Advanced bipolar*	*Ultrasonic*
Tissue effect	• Cutting • Coagulation	Coagulation	• Cutting • Coagulation	• Cutting • Coagulation
Power setting	50–80 W	30–50 W	Default	55,000 Hz frequency
Thermal spread	Not well assessed	2–6 mm	1–4 mm	1–4 mm
Maximum temperature	>100°C	>100°C	Not well assessed	<80°C
Vessel sealing ability	Not applicable	Not applicable	Seal vessels ≤ 7 mm	Seal vessels ≤5 mm
Technique	Not applicable	Not applicable	Tension free application	Tension free application

Electrothermal injury may result from the following situations: Direct application, direct coupling, insulation failure, capacitive coupling, and so forth.

To ensure safe use of electrosurgical devices:
- Inspect insulation carefully
- Use the lowest possible power setting
- Use a low-voltage waveform (cut)
- Use a brief intermittent activation
- Do not activate in open circuit
- Do not activate in close proximity or direct contact with another instrument

6. Outline the principles of surgical diathermy. ***WBUHS 2021 Supplementary, MAMC 2022***

7. Discuss about its use in surgery. ***MAMC 2022***

8. Principles of diathermy, effects of diathermy and complications of diathermy.
Maharashtra University of Health Sciences, 2025

Introduction
- Electrosurgical units (diathermy machines) were first introduced during the early 20th century to facilitate hemostasis and/or the cutting of tissue during surgical procedures (Meeker–Rothrock, 1999).
- This is achieved by passing normal electrical current via the diathermy machine and converting it into a high-frequency alternating current (HFAC). This HFAC produces heat within body tissues to coagulate bleeding vessels and cut through tissue.

There are two different types of electrosurgery: Monopolar and bipolar:
1. Monopolar electrosurgery is the emittance of the HFAC from the diathermy via an active electrode through the patient's body tissues and then returned back to the diathermy machine via a dispersive electrode (patient return pad).
2. Bipolar electrosurgery is the emittance of the HFAC from the diathermy machine down one prong of a bipolar forceps through the tissue that has been placed between the forceps tips and returned to the diathermy machine via the second prong. Bipolar diathermy does not require a dispersive electrode (patient return pad)

Background

Electrosurgery has three effects on body tissue:
1. Cut-generation of heat destroys tissue cell
2. Coagulation-tissue cells contract to increase normal clotting
3. Fulguration-cell walls destroyed through dehydration

Mechanism

- Molecular rotation occurs in materials containing polar molecules with an electric dipole moment placed in an electromagnetic field. When the field oscillates, as with an electromagnetic wave, these molecules rotate to constantly align with it. This is called *dipole rotation.*
- When the field changes, the molecules change direction. The rotating molecules push, pull, and collide with other molecules (through electrical forces), distributing energy to neighboring molecules and atoms in the material.
- Temperature is the average kinetic energy (energy of motion) of the atoms or molecules in a material, so mixing molecules in this way will by definition increase the temperature of the material.
- Dipole rotation is thus the mechanism by which energy in the form of electromagnetic radiation is converted into thermal energy in matter. (There are many other mechanisms for this transformation to occur).
- Dipole rotation is a mechanism often referred to as dielectric heating and is most often observed in the microwave oven where it works most effectively with liquid water and much less with fats, sugars, and frozen water.
- This is because fats and sugars are much less polar than water molecules and thus are less affected by the forces generated by fluctuating electromagnetic fields.
- *Frozen water molecules do not react for another reason:* They are pinned down and cannot spin freely, so they cannot accelerate as much in response to electromagnetic forces from electromagnetic waves.
- Electrosurgery is the application of a high-frequency (HF) electric current to biological tissue as a means to cut, coagulate, desiccate, or fulgurate tissue. Its benefits include the ability to make precise cuts with limited blood loss.
- Electrosurgical devices are frequently used during surgical operations helping to prevent blood loss in hospital operating rooms or in outpatient procedures.
- In electrosurgical procedures, the tissue is heated by an electric current. Although electrical devices may be used for the cauterization of tissue in some applications, electrosurgery is usually used to refer to a quite different method than electrocautery.
- The latter uses heat conduction from a probe heated by direct current to the temperature of an incandescent lamp (similar to a soldering iron).
- This can be achieved in a dry cell DC Pen-Lamp Type device.
- Electrosurgery, on the other hand, uses alternating current to directly heat the tissue itself. When this results in the destruction of small blood vessels and the bleeding stops, it is technically an electrocoagulation process, although "electrocautery" is sometimes used loosely and untechnically to describe it.
- Electrosurgery is often mistakenly called *diathermy*. Unlike ohmic heating by electric current passing through the conductive tissue in conventional electrosurgery, diathermy means dielectric heating, produced by the rotation of molecular dipoles in an HF alternating electric field.
- This effect is most widely used in microwave ovens which operate at gigahertz frequencies.
- Electrosurgery is commonly used in dermatological, gynecological, cardiac, plastic, ocular, spine, ear, nose, and throat (ENT), maxillofacial, orthopedic, urological, neurosurgery, and general surgical procedures as well as certain dental procedures.
- Electrosurgery is performed using an electrosurgical generator (also referred to as a power supply or waveform generator) and a handpiece including one or several electrodes, sometimes referred to as an RF knife.
- The apparatus when used for cutting or coagulation in surgery is still often referred to informally by surgeons as a "Bovie", after the inventor.

Applications:

- Cutting through tissue during surgical procedures.
- Coagulating blood vessels to stop bleeding.
- Destroying abnormal tissue

Intended Effects of Diathermy

- Surgical use:
  - Coagulation (hemostasis—stops bleeding)
  - Cutting through tissues (e.g., in electrocautery)
  - Minimal bleeding due to simultaneous cauterization
  - Sterilization of surgical site (via heat)
- Therapeutic use:
  - Pain relief (e.g., in osteoarthritis, muscle spasms)
  - Muscle relaxation
  - Increased blood flow and healing
  - Reduction of inflammation
  - Improved tissue extensibility before physiotherapy

Complications and Risks

Surgical Diathermy Complications

- Burns (commonest risk)
  - At electrode site or return pad (monopolar)
  - Due to poor grounding or malfunctioning equipment
- Electric shock
  - Rare but can occur with faulty equipment
- Fire or explosion risk
  - Especially in oxygen-rich environments (e.g., during facial surgery or in anesthetized patients)
  - Flammable agents (e.g., alcohol-based preps) can ignite
- Nerve or tissue damage
  - If heat spreads beyond intended area
- Interference with medical devices
  - Pacemakers and defibrillators can malfunction
- Smoke inhalation hazard
  - Electrosurgical smoke (plume) may contain harmful substances

Therapeutic Diathermy Complications

- Excessive heating/burns
  - Especially in areas with metal implants or poor sensation
- Tissue overheating
  - Can damage internal organs or cause fat necrosis
- Adverse effects in contraindicated conditions:
  - Pregnancy (risk to fetus)
  - Malignancy (may stimulate cancer cell growth)
  - Over areas of infection or thrombosis
  - Pacemakers/implanted electronics (can interfere)
- Skin irritation or discomfort

Contraindications to Diathermy (Surgical & Therapeutic)

- Cardiac pacemakers or neurostimulators
- Pregnancy (especially pelvic/lower back use)
- Malignant tumors
- Active infections
- Open wounds (for therapeutic diathermy)
- Metal implants (careful risk assessment required)

9. Discuss the principles of advanced energy devices. ***WBUHS 2022***

Energy Sources in Surgery

- Electrical
- Ultrasonic
- Laser
- Argon beam coagulator

Basic Principles of Electrosurgery

- In electrosurgery, alternating current (AC) is applied to the tissue to produce a thermal effect through ohmic heating, which is selectively used to destroy the tissue.
- In electrosurgery, the tissue behaves as an ohmic resistance. The frequency of the alternating current is at least 300 KHz, it is used to avoid unwanted electrolysis in the tissue (since nerve stimulation occurs at a lower frequency).
- That is why electrosurgery is also called HF surgery or RF surgery. In the process of RF electrosurgery
- Inside cells, electromagnetic energy is first converted into kinetic energy and then into heat energy.
- The desired effect of electrosurgery depends on the electrical properties of the tissue and the contact time, the area, size, and surface area of the electrode in contact with the tissue.
- The Joule effect is the basic principle of tissue heating in electrosurgery
- Current is passed between the electrodes—active and neutral
- Three electrical properties, viz., current (I), voltage (V), and impedance or resistance (R) affect tissue temperature rise. In an electronic circuit, these characteristics are related as Ohm's law.
- V (voltage) = I (current) × R (resistance) or I = V/R
- Another important electrical property that determines the relationship between current and voltage is power (P):

$$\text{Power (P)} = \text{Voltage (V)} \times \text{current (I) or } P = V^2/R$$

- Power density is proportional to the square of the current.
- When the electrode is in contact with the tissue, it heats up the most.
- The power density then decreases by the fourth power of distance as the current penetrates deeper into the tissue.
- An active electrode is a point with a small contact surface where a thermal effect occurs.
- In a monopolar system, the neutral electrode is like a plate with a larger area.
- Hence low current density is produced for thermal effect.
- In a bipolar system, both electrodes are integrated into the same instrument.
- The thermal effect depends mainly on the heating rate and the temperature reached (T), which in turn depends on the power density and contact time. For tissues, the thermal effect is classified into two categories, i.e., coagulation (slower heating T <100°C) and cutting (faster heating T >100 °C)

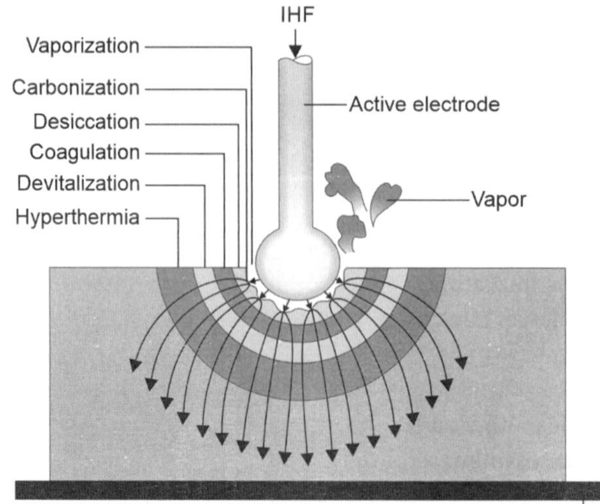

Thermal Effect on Human Tissue

Tissue temperature	Effect
<40°C	None
40-50°C	*Hyperthermia:* Changes appear as in cellular membrane and internal molecular structure, edema formation time-dependent cell death (necrosis)
60-80°C	• Coagulation (denaturation of internal proteins) • Destruction of cell membranes and coagulation of extracellular collagen • Devitalization
100°C	Evaporation of cell liquid/vaporization (depending on heating power)
>1,000°C	Carbonization

Types of Electrosurgical Systems

- Monopolar or unipolar
- Bipolar
- LigaSure vessel sealing system (LVSS)
- *Monopolar instrument:*
  - Monopolar instrument has two separate electrodes in the circuit, one of which acts as an active electrode and the other as a spreading or passive electrode, and is placed laterally between the two electrodes (for cutting or steaming, the active electrode should be made like a barbed hook, with a narrow point or edge of a blade.
  - To dry local coagulation and hemostasis, the active electrode must have a slightly large surface area, for example, on the side of the blade or in the form of tapes.
- *Bipolar instrument:*
  - In a bipolar instrument, both electrodes are placed in the same instrument.
  - The basic concept of a bidirectional system is that only part of the patient's tissue participates in the circuit. The tissue is placed between the electrodes.
- *LigaSure vessel sealing system:*
  - It is an advanced bipolar instrument used to close vessels up to 7 mm in diameter. It compacts tissue using high current at low voltage (180 V).
  - The closure phenomenon is caused by a unique combination of pressure energy and electric current.
  - It applies a high coactive pressure when the tissue temperature is generated, at this stage a hydrogen cross bond is first broken and then renatured, resulting in a high tensile strength.
  - Fused collagen and elastin provide a plastic permanent seal up to 7 mm in diameter. The average compression period is 2–4 seconds.
  - LigaSure vessel sealing system has a unique active tissue response, i.e., coagulated tissue electrical bioimpedance feedback.
  - This function monitors the power supply and automatically turns it off when the tissue closing cycle ends and the tissue does not engage the LVSS jaws.

Ultrasonic Energy Devices

- *Harmonic scalpel (HS):*
  - The harmonic scalpel is a surgical instrument that simultaneously cuts and coagulates tissue.
  - It uses ultrasonic vibrations instead of electric current to cut tissue.
  - The harmonic scalpel operates at a frequency of 55.5 KHz or 55,500 vibrations.
  - Oscillating the cell contents at such a high rate vaporizes the cytoplasm.
  - This in turn breaks down intercellular bridges and allows tissue dissection.
  - Therefore, it is also known as ultrasound. It also causes coagulation of blood vessel wall and seals the vessels up to 5-7 mm in diameter; whereas, hook and blade can achieve coagulation of only up to 2 mm in diameter

- *THUNDERBEAT:*
  - THUNDERBEAT is the only surgical energy device that combines two types of energy in a single instrument.
  - It is the integration of advanced bipolar energy and ultrasound energy. It provides ultrasonically generated frictional energy simultaneously with electronically generated bipolar energy.
  - It can be used for cutting, dissection, histological sealing, and tissue manipulation.
  - THUNDERBEAT provides fast cutting with immediate sealing of vessels up to 7 mm and minimal thermal spread around tissue

Laser

- In modern medicine, lasers are used in the treatment of several diseases (lithotripsy, treatment of various cancers, and tumor ablation) because it is less invasive.
- Laser is short for "light amplification by stimulated emission of radiation." A laser consists of a resonator (which contains the active material to make the laser).
- This resonator is placed between two parallel mirrors, one fully reflective and the other partially reflective and partially transmitting.
- The active material is excited by an excitation source (flashlight, electric current, or other laser) until the number of atoms in the excited state is greater than the number of atoms in the ground state (a phenomenon called *population inversion*).
- When the laser material is excited, it spontaneously releases photons in all directions.
- However, a small fraction of these photons travels along the centerline of the laser system.
- The laser light returns inside the mirrors, when sufficient laser light is reached inside the cavity, the shutter opens to release the light in the form of a laser beam.

Types of Laser

- *Pulsed laser:*
  - Produce light in the form of a pulse.
  - When light comes in the form of short duration.
  - Such lasers are called *pulsed laser.*
- *Continuous laser:* They are capable of producing *continuous beams.*
  - *Argon ion laser:*
    - It is a solid-state laser.
    - This laser emits blue-green light with wavelengths of 488 and 544 nm.
    - This light passes through water and clear fluid. Its thermal radiation penetration depth is up to 1 or 2 mm in most tissues. It is mainly absorbed by the brown-red pigment of chromogen hemoglobin in blood and converts it into heat.
  - *Carbon dioxide laser (CO_2 laser):*
    - CO_2 laser is a molecular gas laser.
    - It uses mixture of nitrogen (N_2), carbon dioxide (CO_2), and helium gas.
    - It emits light from midinfrared to the far infrared region of the electromagnetic spectrum (9,600 and 10,600 nm).
    - This wavelength is mainly absorbed by water and increases the water temperature of cells.
    - Thus, used to vaporize the tissue.
    - Vaporization is the conversion of solid tissue into smoke or gas.
    - It penetrates from 0.1 to 0.2 mm with minimal thermal effect on surrounding tissue.
    - A portable hand-held laser tube with a hollow needle delivers laser light in the vascular and microsurgery.
    - *Krypton laser:*
      - This laser comes in the category of gas laser. Krypton ion gas laser emits a red-yellow light with a wavelength of 476.2–647.1 nm or 0.6 µm.
      - This light is intensely absorbed by the pigment in blood and retinal epithelium. Krypton ion laser resembles with argon ion laser in its construction and uses.

- *Neodymium-doped:yttrium aluminum garnet (Nd:YAG) laser*
    - It comes in the category of solid-state laser.
    - Nd:YAG is the acronym for neodymium, yttrium, aluminum, and garnet that comprise solid-state crystal.
    - The active medium is a crystal rode of YAG with an impurity of Nd.
    - This laser operates from the near-infrared to the far-infrared region of the electromagnetic spectrum.
    - The fundamental wavelength is 1,064 nm.
    - This wavelength penetrates from 3 to 5 mm.
    - Light from Nd:YAG laser is poorly absorbed by hemoglobin or water but intensely absorbed by tissue protein.
    - Thus, the laser operates in Q-switching mode to store energy in the resonator during pumping action followed by the release of a single, short pulse of high energy.
    - The main advantage of a laser is its thermal stability to produce high-quality continuous beams at room temperature.
- *Ruby laser:*
    - It is a solid-state laser that emits red light with a wavelength of 694 nm or 0.6 μm.
    - Ruby laser is excited by the flash lamp and can be Q-switched for getting a high-quality pulsed laser beam.
    - Blood vessels and transparent fluid do not absorb this radiation. It is a pulsed laser and is capable of large fields of energy.
- *Argon plasma coagulator (APC):* APC is a device used for thermal coagulation of tissue. APC is used in open and laparoscopic surgery.
    - *Basic principle of APC:*
        - APC is an electrocoagulation device. It uses an HF monopole current to pass the tissue through ionized argon gas (argon plasma).
        - Electrons flow through an electrically activated ionized argon gas chamber and the probe reaches the target tissue.
        - The current causes coagulation on the surface of the tissue. The depth of coagulation depends on the power of the generator, the flow rate of argon gas, the duration of application, and the distance of the sensor from the target tissue.
        - A thin superficial and electrically insulating layer is produced by thermocoagulation.
        - This insulating layer increases electrical resistance in the treated area, which conducts current through another point of low-resistance tissue.

10. Ultrasonic dissection in surgery—its technique, advantages, and disadvantages. ***WBUHS 2016***

Introduction

- There are two types of ultrasonic dissectors: (1) Low-power, which break water-containing tissues by cavitation, leaving organized structures with low water content, e.g., blood vessels, bile ducts, etc.; and (2) high-power systems that cut loose areolar tissue using frictional heating and simultaneously cut and coagulate the edges.
- Therefore, low-power systems (CUSA and Selector) are used in liver surgery and they do not coagulate blood vessels.
- High-power systems are widely used, especially in fundoplication and laparoscopic colon surgery.
- It is important to remember that high-power ultrasound dissection systems can cause additional damage due to excessive heating and this is well documented in clinical practice.
- Ultrasonic surgical dissection allows coagulation and cutting with less instrument traffic (reduction in operating time), less smoke, and no electrical current.
    - Mechanical energy at 55,500 vibrations/s.
    - Disrupts hydrogen bonds and forms a coagulum

- *Temperature by harmonic scalpel:* 80–100°C
- *Temperature through Electrocoagulation:* 200–300°C
- Collateral damage
- Tissue necrosis

Harmonic Scalpel and Ultrasonic Scalpel

Ultrasonic scalpels (harmonic scalpels) are ideal for dividing small and medium-sized veins and closing them simultaneously with tamponade and heat. However, larger veins > 2 mm in diameter require additional measures (clips, ties, or clamps) to control bleeding. Other disadvantages of the harmonic scalpel are the lack of tissue selectivity and relatively high cost. Ultrasonic surgical applicators are also designed in the form of a hook, spatula, or ball coagulator.

Harmonic Scalpel

- The advantage of the cavitation ultrasound aspirator is that it removes debris and is tissue-selective, e.g., dividing the liver but sparing the bile and blood vessels. This enables safe and rapid dissection with reduced tissue damage and blood loss compared to a harmonic scalpel.
- Problems associated with its use include emptying of the pneumoperitoneum and vibration and streaming that clouds the telescope lens, requiring constant cleaning.

11. Discuss the use of energy source devices in laparoscopic surgery. ***WBUHS 2018***

Bipolar

In bipolar electrosurgery, both the active electrode and return electrode functions are performed at the site of surgery. The two tines of the forceps perform the active and return electrode functions. Only the tissue grasped is included in the electrical circuit. Because the return function is performed by one tine of the forceps, no patient return electrode is needed.

Monopolar

Monopolar is the most commonly used electrosurgical modality. This is due to its versatility and clinical effectiveness. In monopolar electrosurgery, the active electrode is in the surgical site. The patient's return electrode is somewhere else on the patient's body. The current passes through the patient as it completes the circuit from the active electrode to the patient's return electrode.

PK Gyrus Spatula Electrode—Bipolar Vaporization and Desiccation

PK Gyrus has also been used to create a spatula electrode, which almost looks like an armadillo that has multiple electrode surfaces that can be used to both desiccate and cut. This is the first evolution of bipolar electrosurgical cutting. This is a surface desiccation at a rotation 90° cut, surface rotation desiccation, rotate 90°, and cut. So, we have both bipolar PK pulsed desiccation and coagulation, as well as cutting.

EnSeal

There is another device that is very innovative and is known as EnSeal. Where now the generator has really been put in the jaws. What you have is you have a plastic that has been embedded with nickel spheres, it is temperature sensitive. When the plastic is cool, it will conduct. Then when it heats up at a certain specified temperature, it will turn into a different form called amorphous, it would not conduct anymore. Now, when it cools down, it will start to conduct again. This will happen almost in a near infinite number of times until everything is uniformly heated, and ultimately no more current can flow along these nanosphere nickel elements of the plastic jaws; that is called EnSeal, again, a low-voltage, impedance feedback modality. Here is a simple transection. It also has a mechanical arm that comes down after the desiccation and allows you to desiccate after the ligation of the tissue; and the cut, through another low-voltage impedance feedback device.

Ultrasonic energy = Mechanical energy: Ultrasonic energy is mechanical energy and ultrasonic forces are used to cut and coagulate. And in somewhat of a similar fashion, the context of how collagen works and how it is configured, and how it is manufactured by the body is that if you agitate collagen enough you can deconfigure it by breaking up the hydrogen bonds. You can denature the protein. Then if you keep rubbing tissue, just as if I kept rubbing your back, it would start to get warm, the heat starts to form steam, and the steam starts to percolate through the tissue. As the tissue gets percolated with steam, what happens is it falls apart, which is called *cutting*. So, the ultrasonic energy creates steam, which percolates through the parenchyma, breaks up the parenchyma, and tissue falls apart is called cutting.

Argon Beam Laser

- Argon gas is an inert, noncombustible, and easily ionized gas that is used in conjunction with monopolar electrosurgery to produce fulguration.
- Essentially, the electrical current ionizes the argon gas, thereby creating a more efficient pathway for that current to flow since the gas is much more conductive than air, therefore providing a bridge between your tissue and also the electrode.
- Less smoke is produced with the argon beam coagulator since there is less depth of injury.
- Despite these advantages, the argon beam coagulator suffers from one very significant drawback in laparoscopic surgery, namely, high flow infusion of argon gas to the abdominal cavity which not only boosts the intra-abdominal pressure to very damaging levels but could also lead to fatal gas embolism.

The LigaSure

- The LigaSure system (Valleylab, Boulder, and Colorado) LVSS utilizes a brand-new bipolar technology for vascular sealing having a higher current and lower voltage (180 V) than conventional electrosurgery.
- It uses a unique mixture of pressure and energy to produce vessel fusion.
- This fusion is accomplished by melting the elastin and collagen within the vessel walls and reforming it right into a permanent, plastic-like seal. It does not depend on a proximal thrombus along with classic bipolar electrocautery.
- This unique energy output leads to virtually no sticking or charring, and also the seals can withstand three times normal systolic blood pressure level.

Thunderbeat

- It is the world's first and only advanced energy system that delivers two well-established forms of energy to a tissue simultaneously
  - Ultrasonic energy for superior dissection and fast cutting
  - Advanced bipolar energy for secure hemostasis and sealing of vessels up to 7 mm in diameter.

12. Discuss the role of LASER in surgery. ***WBUHS 2017***

13. Discuss the role of LASER in surgical practice. ***WBUHS 2025 Supplementary***

- Laser surgery is a type of surgery that uses a laser (in contrast to using a scalpel) to cut the tissue.
- Examples include the use of a laser scalpel in otherwise conventional surgery, and soft-tissue laser surgery, in which the laser beam vaporizes soft tissue with high water content.
- Laser surgery is commonly used on the eye. Techniques used include laser-assisted subepithelial keratectomy (LASEK), which is used to correct near and far-sightedness in vision, and photorefractive keratectomy, a procedure that permanently reshapes the cornea using an excimer laser to remove a small amount of the human tissue.
- Types of surgical lasers include carbon dioxide (CO_2), argon, Nd:YAG laser, and potassium titanyl phosphate, from among others.

Effects

- *Photochemical effect:* Clinically referred to as photodynamic therapy. Photosensitizer (photofrin II) is administered which is taken up by the tumor tissue and later irradiated by laser light resulting in highly toxic substances with resultant necrosis of the tumor. Photodynamic therapy is used in palliation of esophageal and bronchial carcinoma and ablation of mucosal cancers of the gastrointestinal tract and urinary bladder.

- *Photoablative effect:* Used in eye surgeries such as band keratoplasty and endarterectomy of the peripheral blood vessels.
- *Photothermal effect:* This property is used for endoscopic control of bleeding, e.g., bleeding peptic ulcers and esophageal varices
- *Photomechanical effect:* Used in intraluminal lithotripsy

Equipment

- A 40W CO_2 laser used for soft-tissue laser surgery
- Surgical laser systems, sometimes called "laser scalpels," are differentiated not only by the wavelength but also by the light delivery system—flexible fiber or articulated arm and by other factors.
- CO_2 lasers were the dominant soft-tissue surgical lasers.

Applications

- *Soft tissue:* Soft-tissue laser surgery is used in a variety of applications in humans (general surgery, neurosurgery, ENT, dentistry, orthodontics, and oral and maxillofacial surgery)
- *Dermatology and plastic surgery:* Lasers are also used for laser-assisted lipectomy.
- *Eye surgery:* Various types of laser surgery are used to treat refractive error:
  - LASIK, in which a knife is used to cut a flap in the cornea, and a laser is used to reshape the layers underneath, to treat refractive error
  - Intra-LASIK, a variant in which the flap is also cut with a laser
  - Photorefractive keratectomy photorefractive keratectomy (PRK) and LASEK, in which the cornea is reshaped without first cutting a flap
  - Laser thermal keratoplasty, in which a ring of concentric burns is made in the cornea, which causes its surface to steepen, allowing better near vision

Lasers are also used to treat nonrefractive conditions, such as:

- Phototherapeutic keratectomy (PTK), in which opacities and surface irregularities are removed from the cornea
- Laser coagulation, in which a laser is used to cauterize blood vessels in the eye, to treat various conditions
- Lasers can be used to repair tears in the retina:
  - *Endovascular surgery:* Laser endarterectomy is a technique in which an entire atheromatous plaque in the artery is excised. Laser recanalization of blocked arteries. Other applications include laser-assisted angioplasties and laser-assisted vascular anastomosis.
  - *Foot and ankle surgery:* Lasers are used to treat several disorders in foot and ankle surgery. They are used to remove benign and malignant tumors, treat bunions, debride ulcers and burns, excise epidermal nevi, blue rubber bleb nevi, and keloids, and removal of hypertrophic scars and tattoos.

    A CO_2 laser is used in surgery to treat onychocryptosis (ingrown nails), onychauxis (club nails), onychogryphosis (Ram's horn nail), and onychomycosis (fungus nail).
  - *Gastrointestinal tract:*
    - Peritoneum—laser is used for adhesiolysis
    - Peptic ulcer disease and esophageal varices—laser photoablation is done
    - Coagulation of vascular malformations of the stomach, duodenum, and colon
    - Lasers can be effectively used to treat early gastric cancers provided they are <4 cm and without lymph node involvement. Lasers are also used in treating oral submucous fibrosis.
    - Palliative laser therapy is given in advanced esophageal cancers with obstruction of lumen. Recanalization of the lumen is done which allows the patient to resume a soft diet and maintain hydration.
    - Ablative laser therapy is used in advanced colorectal cancers to relieve obstruction and to control bleeding.

- Laser surgery is used in hemorrhoidectomy, and is a relatively popular and noninvasive method of hemorrhoid removal.
- Laser-assisted liver resections have been done using CO_2 and Nd:YAG lasers.
- Ablation of liver tumors can be achieved by selective photovaporization of the tumor.
- Endoscopic laser lithotripsy is a safer modality compared to electrohydraulic lithotripsy.

- *Oral and dental surgery:*
  - The CO_2 laser is used in oral and dental surgery for virtually all soft-tissue procedures, such as gingivectomies, vestibuloplasties, frenectomies, and operculectomies.
  - The CO_2 10,600 nm wavelength is safe around implants as it is reflected by titanium, and thus has been gaining popularity in the field of periodontology. The laser may also be effective in treating peri-implantitis.
- *Spine surgery:* Laser spine surgery first began seeing clinical use in the 1980s and was primarily used within discectomy to treat lumbar disc disease under the notion that heating a bulging disc vaporized enough tissue to relieve pressure on the nerves and help alleviate pain.
- *Other surgery:* The CO_2 laser is also used in gynecology, genitourinary, general and thoracic surgery, otorhinolaryngology, orthopedic, and neurosurgery.
- *Hard tissues:* Lasers are used to cut or ablate bones and teeth in dentistry.

INDOCYANINE GREEN

14. The use of indocyanine green (ICG) dye in present-day surgery. ***WBUHS 2023***

15. Describe indocyaninegreen fluorescence imaging (ICG). Mention its application in Hepatobiliary(HPB) Surgery and colorectal procedures. ***Maharashtra University of Health Sciences 2025.***

Indocyanine green (ICG) fluorescence imaging is an advanced intraoperative imaging technique used in various surgical specialties to enhance visualization of anatomical structures and assess tissue perfusion. ICG is a water-soluble, tricarbocyanine dye that binds to plasma proteins and fluoresces when exposed to near-infrared (NIR) light (around 800 nm). It is administered intravenously, and its fluorescence can be detected using specialized camera systems, providing real-time visualization during surgery.

Uses in Present-day Surgery

- To visualize the biliary tree during laparoscopic cholecystectomy.
- In patients undergoing colorectal surgeries with intestinal resection and anastomosis, to assess the perfusion of the anastomotic ends after intestinal resection.
- To assess the bowel viability in patients presenting with complicated hernia
- Oncological cases presenting for adequate clearance—the local lymph node basin can be explored to identify the sentinel node.
- In patients with peripheral arterial occlusive disease presenting with gangrene to assess the vascularity of the limb, level of amputation, and healing of stump coupled with vascular bypass interventions.
- In patients undergoing major reconstructive surgeries and local flap procedures following plastic surgical principles to predict flap uptake.

Applications in Hepatobiliary (HPB) Surgery

In HPB surgery, ICG fluorescence imaging offers several valuable applications:

- *Liver tumor detection:*
  - ICG can selectively accumulate in certain liver tumors (like hepatocellular carcinoma and some metastases), allowing surgeons to detect and delineate tumors intraoperatively with fluorescence.
  - Helps identify small or occult lesions not visible by conventional imaging or palpation.

- *Liver segment mapping:*
  - After selective injection into the portal vein branch of a liver segment, ICG can delineate anatomical segments due to segment-specific perfusion patterns.
  - Assists in anatomical liver resections by highlighting segmental borders in real time.
- *Biliary anatomy visualization:*
  - ICG is excreted via the bile, allowing fluorescence-based cholangiography.
  - Useful in identifying the biliary tree during procedures like cholecystectomy or bile duct reconstruction, reducing the risk of bile duct injury.

Applications in Colorectal Surgery

In colorectal procedures, ICG fluorescence imaging plays a critical role in:

- *Assessment of bowel perfusion:*
  - After intravenous injection, ICG highlights perfused tissues, helping surgeons assess blood flow at anastomotic sites.
  - Aims to reduce the risk of anastomotic leaks by ensuring adequate perfusion before completing the bowel connection.
- *Lymphatic mapping and sentinel lymph node detection:*
  - ICG injected around the tumor can help trace lymphatic drainage pathways.
  - Assists in identifying sentinel lymph nodes during oncologic resections, potentially improving staging and treatment planning.

CHAPTER 18

Sterilization and Disinfection

LEARNING OBJECTIVES

- Sterilization of Surgical Instruments
- Sterilization of Endoscopes
- Sterilization of Laparoscopic Instruments
- Disposal of Hospital Waste Products

1. Sterilization of surgical instruments. ***WBUHS 2009***

2. Briefly discuss the sterilization techniques of OT instruments. ***WBUHS 2025 Supplementary***

Cleaning, Sterilization, and Maintenance of Surgical Instruments

- *Rinsing:* Immediately after the surgery, wash the tools under warm (not hot) running water. Flushing should remove all blood, body fluids, and tissues.
- *Cleaning:* If not done immediately after washing, instruments must be immersed in a solution containing water and neutral pH 7 detergent.

Ultrasonic Cleaning

- Use manual cleaning for micro and sensitive instruments.
- Instruments must be treated in the cleaning agent for the full recommended cycle—usually 5–10 minutes.
- Place the instruments in the ultrasonic cleaner in the open position.
- Make sure that the "sharp" (scissors, knives, osteotomes, etc.) blades do not touch other instruments. All instruments must be completely submerged.
- Do not put different metals (stainless steel, copper, chrome, etc.) in the same cleaning program.
- Change the solution frequently—at least as often as recommended by the manufacturer.
- After ultrasonic cleaning, rinse the instruments with water to remove the ultrasonic cleaning solution.

Automatic Washer Sterilizers

Follow the manufacturer's recommendations, but make sure the instruments are lubricated after the last wash cycle and before the sterilization cycle.

Manual Cleaning

- Most instrument manufacturers recommend ultrasonic cleaning as the best and most efficient way to clean surgical instruments, especially instruments with hinges, locks, and other moving parts.
- If ultrasonic cleaning is not available, follow the steps given here:
  - Use stiff plastic cleaning brushes (nylon, etc.).
  - Do not use steel wool or wire brushes except stainless steel wire brushes specifically recommended for instruments such as bone files and stained areas of scratched handles.
  - Use only neutral pH (7) detergents, because low pH detergents will cause corrosion of the stainless protective surface and black spots if not washed properly.

- Detergent with a high pH creates a brown stain on the surface, which also prevents the smooth operation of the device.
- Brush sensitive instruments carefully and, if possible, handle them completely separately from normal instruments.
- Ensure that all instrument surfaces are visibly clean and free of stains and tissue. This is a good time to check the operation and condition of each device.

Check and ensure that:

- The blades of the scissors slide smoothly all the way to the end (they must not be open in the closed position).
- Test the scissors by cutting them into thin gauze
- Tweezers are correctly aligned with the tips
- Hemostats and needles do not show light between the jaws, are easily locked and open, and joints are not too loose
- Check the jaw surfaces of the needles for wear
- The suction tubes are clean inside. Coil devices work properly.
- Knives (they have sharp, intact blades)
  - After cleaning, rinse the instruments thoroughly under running water.
  - Open and close scissors, hemostats, needles, and other hinged instruments during flushing to ensure that hinged areas and the exterior of instruments are flushed.
  - *After cleaning:* If one intend to store the instruments, allow them to air dry and store them in a clean, dry environment.

Autoclaving

If instruments are to be reused or autoclaved:

- Lubricate all instruments with any "metal-to-metal" features, such as scissors, hemostats, needles, and self-locking retractors.
- It is better to surgical lubricants, such as instrument milk. Do not use WD-40, oil, or other industrial lubricants.
- Put instruments up for autoclaving either individually or in sets.

Individual Instruments

Disposable paper or plastic bags are ideal. For instruments with ratchet locks (e.g., needle holders and hemostats), be sure to use a bag wide enough (4" or wider) to allow the instrument to be sterilized in the open (unlocked) position.

Instrument Sets

- Open all instruments and sterilize them in the open position.
- Place heavy instruments on the bottom of the set (if two layers are required).
- Never lock the instrument while autoclaving.
- It is not sterile because steam does not penetrate metal-to-metal surfaces.
- The device develops cracks in the hinge areas due to thermal expansion during the autoclave cycle.
- Do not overload the autoclave chamber as pockets may form in the autoclave chamber preventing steam penetration.
- Place a towel on the bottom of the pan to absorb excess moisture while autoclaving.
- This will reduce the chances of getting "wet packs." Make sure the towels used in the sterilization of instruments have no detergent residue and are neutral—pH (7) if immersed in water.
- This can be a real problem as laundries frequently use inexpensive but high pH (9–13) detergents and do not properly rinse out or neutralize those detergents in the final wash/rinse cycle.
- Bleaching agents such as Clorox are also sometimes added and not neutralized.

Caution

- At the end of the autoclave cycle—before the drying cycle—open the autoclave door and open it more than a crack (about three-fourths).
- Carry out the drying cycle for the time recommended by the autoclave manufacturer. If the autoclave door is fully opened before the drying cycle, cold room air flows into the room, causing condensation on the instruments.
- This leads to water spots on the instruments and also causes wet packing.
- If the instruments show unusual stains during sterilization, please contact your local instrument representative.

Cold Sterilization

- Most cold sterilizing solutions render instruments sterile only after 10 hours of immersion.
- This prolonged chemical exposure can be more damaging to surgical instruments than a standard 20-minute autoclave cycle.
- If the instruments need to be "disinfected" only, cold sterilization is okay as disinfection will place in only 10 minutes.

Difference Between Sterile and Disinfected

- *Sterile*—an absolute term (no living organism survives)
- *Disinfected*—basically clean. Always use the proper sterilization/cleaning technique to render the instrument in the required condition for use. For instruments with Tungsten Carbide inserts (needle holders, scissors, and tissue forceps), we do not recommend the use of solutions containing benzyl ammonium chloride which will destroy the Tungsten Carbide inserts.

---

3. Sterilization of endoscopes. ***WBUHS 2010***

Introduction

The infection associated with endoscopic surgery—routine surgical site infections (SSIs) and nontuberculous mycobacteria (NTM).

Features to Consider when Purchasing a Machine

- The number of scopes that can be processed simultaneously.
- A cycle counter and fault indicator.
- A water treatment system that prevents recontamination of processed instruments during rinsing. Filtration using bacteria-retaining filters with a pore size of 0.2–0.45 micron is satisfactory.
- A reliable, effective, and simple machine disinfection system.
- An air-drying facility to expel fluids and dry the channels of the cope at the end of a cycle.
- A facility to irrigate the channels of the cope with alcohol before storage.
- A leak test facility.
- A print-out, of cycle parameters, which can be retained for quality assurance, records.

Cleaning and Disinfection—Practical Recommendations

- *At the start of the day:*
    - The instruments to be used should be checked.
    - If instruments have been thoroughly cleaned and disinfected at the end of the previous day, they should be put through an automated cleaning and disinfection process.
    - All channels be flushed with disinfectant.
    - The instrument should be fully immersed in disinfectant for the correct contact time.
    - Requires flushing manually using a 2-mL syringe and a channel adapter.
    - The valves that will be used during the list, ideally one set per case, should be disinfected in the same way.
    - After disinfection, copes and valves should be rinsed in bacteria-free water ensuring all traces of disinfectant are removed from the channels, control body, and eyepiece.

- The instrument should then be plugged into the light source and connected to the suction pump. Air should be blown through all the channels to expel excess fluid.
- The instrument should then be ready for use.

Cleaning and Disinfection of Endoscopes Between Cases

- Before detaching the instrument, the air/water channels should be flushed with water.
- After thorough flushing instrument should be checked for any leaks and other faults.
- Perform all the steps from 2 to 8 as mentioned earlier.
- All valves should be removed and cleaned individually with a cottonwood bud or small brush.
- The suction/biopsy channel should be cleaned properly prior to reinsertion.
- When the channels have been cleaned the suction and air/water ports must be cleaned.
- The instrument must be immersed in disinfectant for the correct contact time.
- The relevant work surfaces must be wiped clean.

Cleaning and Disinfection of Endoscopes after the Last Case

- Leak test the cope, clean, and disinfect with Cidex orthophthaldehyde (OPA)/2% glutaraldehyde/peracetic acid/chlorine dioxide performing steps 2–8 as mentioned.
- Copes should be stored hanging vertically in designated ventilated cupboards, not in their transit cases.
- All valves used during the list should, after disinfection and rinsing, be dried with a cotton wool bud and lubricated with silicone oil. They should not be replaced in the endoscope case for storage.

Cleaning and Disinfection of Accessories is also Essential

Disinfectants used for endoscopes:

- Orthophthaldehyde
- Formalin cabinets
- Hydrogen peroxide gas plasma method

4. Sterilization of laparoscopic instruments (LI). ***Gujarat Health University 2025; WBUHS 2014***

Introduction

- Laparoscopic surgery requires sophisticated and precisely calibrated instruments.
- The essential difference between instruments used in open surgery and people utilized for laparoscopic surgery would be that the latter are more complex in design and yet delicate in construction.
- Thus, laparoscopic instruments are more vulnerable to the lodging of bioburden (microorganisms and debris) within their crevices.
- Thus, the laparoscopic instruments are difficult to clean, sterilize adequately, and maintain as compared to their counterparts used in open surgery.
- Moreover, owing to their delicate design, the gentlest methods have to be used for cleaning in addition to sterilization.
- Also, meticulous cleaning and maintenance in addition to sterilization are necessary so as not to compromise the safety of the patient, the surgeon, or other operating room personnel.
- The rise in complexity of the laparoscopic procedures as also the emergence of resistant strains of bacteria, mycobacteria, fungi, and viruses makes it imperative to effectively clean and disinfect instruments.
- Sterilization is the absolute elimination or destruction of forms of microbial life. It may be achieved with steam, gas, or chemicals.
- However, disinfection is the relative removal of pathogenic organisms except spores.

Disinfection can be

- High level—where all life forms except the spores are destroyed
- Intermediate level—where some fungi, viruses, and spores are spared

- Low level—where fungi, viruses, spores, and mycobacteria remain undestroyed. For laparoscopic instruments ideally sterilization or at best higher-level disinfection should be used.

Cleaning and Sterilization

Optimal processing of laparoscopic instruments involves several steps that reduce the risk of transmitting infection from used instruments along with other.

They are:

- Dismantling
- Decontamination
- Precleaning
- Cleaning and rinsing
- Drying
- Sterilization
- Storage
- For proper processing, it is essential to perform the steps in the correct order.
- Most major hospitals have a Central Sterile Supplies Department (CSSD) where the instruments are transported to the operating room for processing.
- Even in hospitals or nursing homes that do not have an elaborate CSSD, the fundamental steps in processing of instruments can be followed provided a well-established protocol is in place, and designated personnel receive the responsibility for the same.
- Proper processing of instruments forms an intrinsic aspect of their care which should undoubtedly significantly help in increasing their lifetime and trouble-free service.

A method of cleaning that is growing in popularity is ultrasonic cleaning. This method is, by far, the most efficient and effective available today. Its simplicity of use and superior efficiency is quickly making ultrasonic cleaning the preferred choice. Actually, ultrasonic cleaning is 16 times better than hand cleaning. The instruments are placed in the ultrasonic unit for 10–15 minutes and use a neutral pH solution. Attention should be directed at the following points during ultrasonic cleaning:

- Before placing into the ultrasonic unit, the instruments are cleaned of all visible debris.
- It is preferable to not mix instruments made of dissimilar metals (such as aluminum and stainless) in the same cycle.
- It is important to ensure that the instruments have ample room. The ultrasonic cleaner should not be overloaded.
- As with all types of cleaning, all instruments ought to be opened so ratchets and box locks are fully subjected to the cleaning process.
- Upon completion of the cycle, the instruments are removed immediately and rinsed.

Drying

- The instruments should be dried at the end of the cleaning and rinsing cycle before they are packed for sterilization.
- This in real is ideally achieved by using an air gun that blows all the water droplets off the surfaces of instruments or by using an oven. The second, however, may be available only in CSSD units.

Sterilization

- The Centers for Disease Control and Prevention (CDC) recommends that rigid laparoscopic instruments be sterile or, in the event that is not feasible, they be high-level disinfected.
- There are three sterilization processes available to us—steam, ethylene oxide, and peracetic acid.
- Because of product knowledge and proprietary design information, the instrument manufacturer may be the just one who can provide sterilization recommendations.

Steam Sterilization

- Steam sterilization in an autoclave is among the most typical forms of sterilization used in healthcare facilities.
- Autoclaving at 121°C for 15 minutes is ideal for all reusable metal instruments. It is effective, cheap, and nontoxic.
- Laparoscopes may be sterilized by flash or vacuum steam sterilization. Before sterilization, all the instruments that are insulated, all silicone tubing, and all sorts of cords ought to be doubly covered with a cloth to prevent connection with the hot metallic container.
- They are then put into the autoclave.
- Flash sterilization is carried out at 135°C at 30 psi pressure for 60 minutes.
- This process requires postvacuum and dry cycles.
- The instruments should rest on the sterilizer rack for 45 minutes to prevent water condensation about the lens all cords should be doubly wrapped in a cloth to avoid contact with the hot metallic container.
- They are then put into the autoclave.
- Flash sterilization is completed at 135°C at 30 psi pressure for an hour.
- This method requires postvacuum and dry cycles.
- The instruments should rest on a sterilizer rack for 45 minutes to prevent water condensation about the lens.

Gas Sterilization

- Using ethylene oxide (EO) would work for all disposable instruments, insulated hand instruments and tubing employed for gas, suction, and irrigation.
- Endoscopic instruments may be sterilized with either cold or warm EO gas, with respect to the manufacturer's instructions.
- With cold gas, the temperatures are set at 85°C, and the instruments are subjected for 4 hours and 30 minutes.
- Aeration must then follow for 12 hours. Warm gas sterilization happens at 145°C for 2 hours and 30 minutes, followed by 8 hours of aeration.
- The benefits of EO are that the items are not damaged, it is noncorrosive to optics, and also it permeates porous material.
- Its main disadvantages are its cost, toxicity, the requirement for aeration, and being a longer process.

High-level Disinfection

- When sterilization is not available or feasible, high-level disinfection (HLD) is used for instrument processing. HLD eliminates bacteria, viruses, fungi, and parasites but does not reliably kill all bacterial endospores, which cause diseases, such as tetanus, gas gangrene, and atypical mycobacterial infections.
- HLD would work for items that will come in connection with broken skin or intact mucous membranes.
- The effectiveness of HLD depends on the following:
    - The amount and kind of microorganisms, organic material (blood, other fluids, and tissues), and other matter (for example, dirt) present on the instrument or other item
    - It is important to decontaminate and thoroughly clean instruments along with other items before HLD.
- Agents that are employed for HLD include 2% glutaraldehyde, 6% stabilized hydrogen peroxide, and peracetic acid (acetic acid/hydrogen peroxide).
- Proper storage temperatures and expiration date. Solutions should be replaced any time they become cloudy.
- The efficiency of glutaraldehyde is influenced by the organic load, contact time, and use pattern, concentration, physical configuration of instruments, temperature, and pH. Occupational Safety and Health Administration (OSHA)'s established maximum allowable exposure limit for glutaraldehyde is 0.2 ppm.
- Fiberoptic light cords and telescopes have to be soaked in 2% glutaraldehyde not <10 minutes.
- Soaking should not exceed twenty minutes.
- The endocamera could also disinfected by 10 minutes of submersion in 2% glutaraldehyde. Care must be taken to leave the plug end of the cord away from the solution.
- Alternately, a sterile drape over the camera and cord may be used.

- Soakage of other metallic instruments, including trocars, and hand instruments, has become recommended for an hour, to avoid infection with atypical mycobacterial infection.
- Formaldehyde, glutaraldehyde from phenolic derivatives, iodophors, hypochlorites, phenolics, and quaternary ammonium compounds are unpopular and have been condemned.
- Formaldehyde is potentially cancer-causing and very irritating to the skin, eyes, nose, and respiratory tract.
- Furthermore, its efficacy is found wanting, and for that reason, routine utilization of formaldehyde for sterilizing instruments and other items are not recommended.

Newer Methods of Sterilization

Important for hospitals with high workload is the rapid turnaround times for instruments that cannot be sterilized satisfactorily with steam or dry heat. One of the newer sterilizer systems—STERRAD—uses hydrogen peroxide vapor and low-temperature gas plasma to sterilize most devices quickly with no toxic residues. Usually, the process takes about 75 minutes to wrap and dry the instruments and devices. Within the chamber, a deep vacuum is drawn.

Storage

- Items ought to be used or properly stored soon after sterilization or HLD so they do not become contaminated.
- Proper storage is as important as proper decontamination, cleaning, sterilization, or HLD.
- If items are not stored properly, all of the effort and supplies used to properly process them will have been wasted, and the things are going to be contaminated.
- Specific instructions for proper storage rely on whether sterilization or HLD continues to be performed, the method used, and whether the items are wrapped or unwrapped.

The shelf-life of a wrapped item is suffering from numerous factors, including:

- The kind of packing material used
- The number of times those are handled
- The number of people who handle the pack
- The cleanliness, humidity, and temperature from the storage space
- Whether the packs are stored on open or closed shelves
- Whether dust covers (for example, sealed plastic bags) are utilized
  - For optimal storage, sterile packs are put in closed cabinets in areas that are not heavily trafficked, have moderate temperatures, and are dry or of low humidity.
  - Under optimal storage conditions and with minimal handling, properly wrapped items can be considered sterile as long as they remain intact and dry.
  - Storage time and the handling of sterile packs ought to be kept to a minimum because the probability of contamination increases over time and with increased handling.
  - When in doubt about the sterility of a pack, consider it to become contaminated and resterilize the item before use.

---

5. Universal precaution. ***WBUHS 2009***

Universal precautions refer to the practice, in medicine, of avoiding contact with patients' bodily fluids, by means of the wearing of nonporous articles, such as medical gloves, goggles, and face shields.

Under universal precautions, all patients are considered to be possible carriers of blood-borne pathogens. The guideline recommends wearing gloves when collecting or handling blood and body fluids contaminated with blood, wearing face shields when there is a danger of blood splashing on mucous membranes, and disposing of all needles and sharp objects in puncture-resistant containers.

Universal precautions are designed for doctors, nurses, patients, and healthcare support workers who are required to come into contact with patients or bodily fluids. This includes staff and others who may not come into direct contact with patients.

Universal precautions are typically practiced in any environment where workers are exposed to bodily fluids, such as:

• Blood • Semen • Vaginal secretions	• Synovial fluid • Amniotic fluid • Cerebrospinal fluid	• Pleural fluid • Peritoneal fluid • Pericardial fluid

Bodily fluids that do not require such precautions include:

• Feces • Nasal secretions • Urine	• Vomitus • Perspiration	• Sputum • Saliva

Universal precautions are the infection control techniques that were recommended following the acquired immunodeficiency syndrome (AIDS) outbreak in the 1980s. Every patient is treated as if infected and therefore precautions are taken to minimize risk.

Protective clothing includes but is not limited to:

- Barrier gowns
- Gloves
- Eyewear (goggles or glasses)
- Face shields
- All the patients must be regarded as potentially infected with blood-borne pathogens.
  - Strict hand washing must be practiced before and after each patient contact.
  - *The hands should be washed immediately if they are contaminated with blood or body fluids.* Gloves must be used:
    - If contamination of blood or body fluids is expected
    - To place intravenous tubes
    - Gloves must not be reused

Gowns or aprons should be used during procedures where blood or other body fluids may be splashed and when contamination with blood or body fluids is likely:

- To avoid contact with the mucous membranes of the mouth, nose and eyes, masks, and glasses (goggles) should be worn during procedures that may cause drops or splashes of blood or other body fluids.
- *Items contaminated with blood or body fluids must be removed:*
  - For single use in red bags marked "dangerous infectious waste."
  - Single-use products must be cleaned with a hospital-approved disinfectant and sent to central services for sterilization.
  - Avoid needle stick injuries. Used needles must not be closed or bent; they must be placed in a visibly marked puncture-resistant container specifically designed for such disposal. You may prefer to administer all the medications through a closed screen to avoid needle stickiness.
    - Bleeding should be cleaned immediately with a 5.25% solution of sodium hypochlorite diluted with water (1:10 with household bleach).
    - Healthcare workers with exudative lesions or weeping rash should refrain from all patient care and handling until the condition has resolved.
    - To minimize the need for mouth-to-mouth resuscitation, disposable mouthpieces, resuscitation bags, or other breathing equipment must be available.
    - Pregnant health workers must strictly follow precautions to minimize the risk of human immunodeficiency virus (HIV) infection.
    - All samples must be stored in a leak-proof plastic bag labeled "biohazard."

6. **Describe classification of hospital waste and appropriate methods of disposal.**
Ayush University Chhattisgarh 2025

7. **Types of biomedical waste and classification, impact of improper biomedical waste management.**
Rajasthan University of Health Sciences 2025

8. **Describe classification of hospital waste and appropriate methods of disposal.**
Maharshatra University of Health Sciences 2025

Hospital waste, also known as healthcare or medical waste, is classified based on its source, risk level, and disposal requirements. The classification ensures safe handling, treatment, and disposal to prevent health and environmental hazards. Below is a detailed classification of hospital waste:

General Waste

- *Description:* Nonhazardous waste similar to domestic waste, posing no significant risk to health or the environment.
- *Examples:*
  - Paper, cardboard, and packaging materials.
  - Food waste and kitchen scraps.
  - Noncontaminated plastic, glass, or office waste.
- *Management:* Disposed of like regular municipal waste through recycling, composting, or landfilling.

Infectious Waste

- *Description:* Waste contaminated with pathogens that can cause infections.
- *Examples:*
  - Used bandages, gauze, and swabs with blood or bodily fluids.
  - Cultures and stocks of infectious agents from labs.
  - Waste from isolation wards or infected patients.
- *Management:* Requires segregation in color-coded (usually yellow) containers, followed by autoclaving, incineration, or other sterilization methods.

Pathological Waste

- *Description:* Human tissues, organs, or body parts generated during medical procedures.
- *Examples:*
  - Tissues, organs, or fetuses from surgeries or autopsies.
  - Blood and bodily fluids.
- *Management:* Stored in sealed, leak-proof containers (often yellow or red) and typically incinerated or buried in designated facilities.

Sharps Waste

- *Description:* Items that can puncture or cut, posing a risk of injury or infection.
- *Examples:*
  - Needles, syringes, and scalpel blades.
  - Broken glass vials or ampoules.
  - Lancets and IV catheters.
- *Management:* Collected in puncture-resistant, leak-proof containers (often red or yellow) and incinerated or autoclaved before disposal.

Chemical Waste

- *Description:* Waste containing hazardous chemicals from medical or laboratory activities.
- *Examples:*

  - Expired or unused pharmaceuticals (e.g., drugs, vaccines).
  - Disinfectants, solvents, and laboratory reagents.
  - Heavy metals like mercury from thermometers or batteries.
- *Management:* Segregated in chemically resistant containers, neutralized or treated through specialized chemical waste disposal methods.

Pharmaceutical Waste

- *Description:* Expired, unused, or contaminated drugs and vaccines.
- *Examples:*
  - Expired medications.
  - Contaminated drug vials or IV bags.
  - Cytotoxic drugs (used in chemotherapy).
- *Management:* Collected in designated containers and disposed of via high-temperature incineration or returned to suppliers for safe disposal.

Radioactive Waste

- *Description:* Waste containing radioactive substances from diagnostic or therapeutic procedures.
- *Examples:*
  - Contaminated materials from radiotherapy (e.g., gloves, swabs).
  - Radioactive isotopes used in imaging or treatment.
- *Management:* Stored in lead-lined containers until radioactivity decays to safe levels, then disposed of per regulatory guidelines.

Genotoxic/Cytotoxic Waste

- *Description:* Waste containing substances that are mutagenic, teratogenic or carcinogenic.
- *Examples:*
  - Cytotoxic drugs used in cancer treatment.
  - Waste from chemotherapy, including contaminated gloves or tubing.
- *Management:* Handled with extreme care, stored in secure containers, and incinerated at high temperatures in specialized facilities.

Pressurized Containers

- *Description:* Waste from gas cylinders or aerosol cans that pose explosion risks.
- *Examples:* Inhalers, oxygen cylinders, or anesthetic gas containers.
- *Management:* Collected separately and disposed of through specialized recycling or destruction processes to prevent explosions.

Heavy Metal Waste

- *Description:* Waste containing heavy metals, often from medical equipment.
- *Examples:*
  - Mercury from broken thermometers or sphygmomanometers.
  - Batteries or dental amalgam.
- *Management:* Segregated and sent to specialized recycling or hazardous waste treatment facilities.

Key Notes on Management

- *Segregation:* Waste is sorted at the point of generation using color-coded bins (e.g., yellow for infectious, red for sharps, blue for recyclables) to ensure proper handling.
- *Regulations:* Classifications and disposal methods are guided by local and international regulations, such as WHO guidelines or country-specific laws (e.g., EPA in the US, Biomedical Waste Rules in India).
- *Treatment:* Common methods include incineration, autoclaving, chemical disinfection, or landfilling in secure sites, depending on the waste type.

- *Risk:* Improper handling of hazardous waste (infectious, sharps, chemical, etc.) can lead to infections, environmental pollution, or occupational hazards.

This classification helps healthcare facilities manage waste effectively, minimizing risks to staff, patients, and the environment. If you need specific details (e.g., regulations in a particular country or disposal techniques), let me know!

Improper biomedical waste management poses significant risks to public health, the environment, and occupational safety. Below is a detailed overview of its impacts:

Public Health Risks

- *Spread of infections:* Improperly disposed infectious waste (e.g., contaminated bandages, needles) can spread pathogens like HIV, hepatitis B and C, and antibiotic-resistant bacteria to healthcare workers, waste handlers, and the public.
- *Contamination of water and food:* Biomedical waste dumped in open areas or water bodies can contaminate drinking water or food chains, leading to diseases like cholera, typhoid, or gastrointestinal infections.
- *Increased disease transmission:* Scavengers or animals accessing improperly disposed waste can spread pathogens, increasing the risk of zoonotic diseases or community outbreaks.

Environmental Pollution

- *Soil and water contamination:* Chemical and pharmaceutical waste, such as expired drugs or heavy metals (e.g., mercury), can leach into soil and groundwater, disrupting ecosystems and affecting agriculture.
- *Air pollution:* Burning biomedical waste in open dumps or low-temperature incinerators releases toxic pollutants like dioxins and furans, which are carcinogenic and contribute to respiratory issues.
- *Ecosystem damage:* Radioactive or genotoxic waste can harm flora and fauna, leading to long-term ecological imbalances.

Occupational Hazards

- *Injuries and infections:* Healthcare workers, waste handlers, and sanitation staff are at risk of needle-stick injuries or exposure to infectious waste, leading to potential infections.
- *Chemical exposure:* Improper handling of chemical waste (e.g., disinfectants, cytotoxic drugs) can cause burns, respiratory problems, or chronic health issues for workers.
- *Lack of training:* Inadequate training on waste segregation and handling increases risks for hospital staff and waste management personnel.

Legal and Financial Consequences

- *Regulatory Noncompliance:* Failure to follow biomedical waste regulations (e.g., WHO guidelines, EPA rules, or country-specific laws) can result in fines, legal action, or closure of healthcare facilities.
- *Increased costs:* Mismanagement leads to higher costs for cleanup, legal penalties, or treating infections caused by improper disposal, burdening healthcare systems.

Community and Social Impacts

- *Public safety threats:* Improperly disposed sharps or infectious waste in public areas can injure community members, particularly children or scavengers.
- *Aesthetic and social issues:* Open dumping of biomedical waste creates unsightly and unhygienic conditions, lowering community trust in healthcare systems and authorities.
- *Spread to vulnerable populations:* Improper disposal near residential areas can disproportionately affect marginalized communities, exacerbating health disparities.

Long-term Global Health Risks

- *Antimicrobial resistance (AMR):* Improper disposal of pharmaceutical waste, especially antibiotics, can contribute to the development and spread of drug-resistant bacteria in the environment.

- *Persistent pollutants:* Chemicals like dioxins from improper incineration persist in the environment, accumulating in the food chain and causing long-term health issues like cancer or reproductive disorders.

Examples of Real-world Impacts

- *India (2019):* Improper disposal of biomedical waste in open dumps led to hepatitis outbreaks in some regions, with scavengers and local communities most affected.
- *Global concern:* The WHO estimates that 15% of healthcare waste is hazardous, and mismanagement contributes to millions of infections annually, especially in low-resource settings.

Mitigation Strategies

- *Proper segregation:* Use color-coded bins to separate waste at the source.
- *Training and awareness:* Educate healthcare workers and waste handlers on safe practices.
- *Advanced treatment:* Employ high-temperature incineration, autoclaving, or microwave treatment for hazardous waste.
- *Regulatory enforcement:* Strict adherence to local and international guidelines (e.g., Biomedical Waste Management Rules, 2016 in India).
- *Monitoring and auditing:* Regular inspections of waste management practices in healthcare facilities.

CHAPTER 19

Radiology

LEARNING OBJECTIVES

- USG: Breast Ultrasound and Preoperative Ultrasound
- Small Bowel Enema
- CT Scan and MRI
- Endoscopic Ultrasound
- Cholangiogram
- Nuclear Medicine and FDG-PET

ULTRASOUND (USG)

1. Breast ultrasound. *WBUHS 2010*

- Ultrasonography is used to characterize a breast lesion identified by the physical examination or mammography.
- It can determine whether a lesion is solid or cystic and can define the size, contour, or internal texture of the lesion.
- Although, it is not a useful screening modality by itself due to significant false-positive rates. When used as an adjunct with mammography, ultrasonography may improve the diagnostic sensitivity of benign findings to >90%, especially among younger patients for whom mammographic sensitivity is lower due to denser breast tissue.
- In those patients with a known cancer, ultrasound is sometimes used to detect additional suspicious lesions and/or to map the extent of disease.
- Benign breast masses usually show smooth contours, round or oval shapes, weak internal echoes, and well-defined anterior and posterior margins.
  Breast cancer characteristically has irregular walls but may have smooth margins with acoustic enhancement.
- Ultrasonography is used to guide fine-needle aspiration biopsy, core-needle biopsy, and needle localization of breast lesions. It is highly reproducible and has a high patient acceptance rate, but does not reliably detect lesions that are 1 cm or less in diameter.

Uses

- *Determining the nature of a breast abnormality:*
  - The primary use of breast ultrasound today is to help in diagnosing breast abnormalities detected during a physical examination and to characterize potential abnormalities seen on mammography or breast magnetic resonance imaging (MRI).
  - Ultrasound imaging can help to determine if an abnormality is solid (which may be a noncancerous lump of tissue or a cancerous tumor), fluid-filled (such as a benign cyst), or both cystic and solid. Ultrasound can also help show additional features of the abnormal area.
  - Doppler ultrasound is used to assess blood supply in breast lesions.

- *Supplemental breast cancer screening:* Mammography is the only screening tool for breast cancer that is known to reduce deaths due to breast cancer through early detection.
- *Screening:*
  Ultrasound can be offered as a screening tool for women who:
  - Are at high risk for breast cancer and unable to undergo an MRI examination.
  - Are pregnant or should not be exposed to X-rays (which is necessary for a mammogram).
- *Ultrasound-guided breast biopsy*

2. Preoperative ultrasound. ***WBUHS 2012***

Introduction

Ultrasound relies on high-frequency sound waves generated by a transducer containing piezoelectric material. The generated sound waves are reflected by tissue interfaces, and by ascertaining the time taken for a pulse to return and the direction of a pulse, it is possible to form an image.

- Medical ultrasound uses frequencies in the range 3–20 MHz
- Abdominal imaging uses transducers with a frequency of 3–7 MHz
- Higher-frequency transducers are used for superficial structures, such as musculoskeletal and breast ultrasound

Dedicated transducers have also been developed for endocavitary ultrasound such as transvaginal scanning and transrectal ultrasound of the prostate, allowing high-frequency scanning of organs by reducing the distance between the probe and the organ of interest

A further application of dedicated probes has been in the field of endoscopic ultrasound, allowing exquisite imaging of the wall of a hollow viscus and the adjacent organs, such as the gastric wall and the pancreas

- *Doppler ultrasound:* Reflection of an ultrasound wave from moving objects such as red blood cells cause a change in the frequency of the ultrasound wave. By measuring this frequency change, it is possible to calculate the speed and direction of the movement
- *Doppler imaging* is widely used in the assessment of arterial and venous disease, in which stenotic lesions cause an alteration in the normal velocity
- Furthermore, diffuse parenchymal diseases such as cirrhosis may cause an alteration in the normal Doppler signal of the affected organ

Uses

- It is the first-line investigation of choice for assessment of the liver, biliary tree, and renal tract.
- Ultrasound is also the *imaging method of choice in obstetric assessment and gynecological disease.*
- High-frequency transducers have made ultrasound the best imaging technique for the evaluation of thyroid and testicular disorders.
- It is also an invaluable tool for *guiding needle placement in interventional procedures* such as biopsies and drainages, allowing *direct real-time visualization* of the needle during the procedure.
- The role of preoperative ultrasound in the evaluation of cervical lymph nodes in patients with known thyroid cancer has been widely explored.
- For hepatobiliary system:
  - *Gallbladder:* The gallbladder wall should be ≤2 mm (in a distended or fasting gallbladder). Collapsed gallbladders, seen when the subject has eaten, typically appear thickened. The maximum dimension of the gallbladder is 5 × 10 cm.
  - *Common hepatic duct:* The common hepatic duct (inner wall to inner wall) is usually measured at the level of the hepatic artery. In the normal fasting state, it should be <7 mm in patients <60 years old and <10 mm in patients older than 60 years of age.
  - *Common bile duct (CBD):* The normal CBD diameter increases with age and in patients who have had a cholecystectomy. In patients in their 40s, the normal mean diameter is 4 mm. The normal mean diameter

then increases by 1 mm every decade, and authors have proposed that in elderly patients the normal upper limit of normal be set at 8.5 mm. The CBD is commonly up to 10 mm in patients who have undergone a cholecystectomy.
  - *Liver:* The span of the liver in the right mid-clavicular line should be <16 cm.
- Ligament, tendon, and muscle injuries are also probably best imaged in the first instance by ultrasound.
- *Preoperative staging of colon cancer patients:* Ultrasound can be a valuable alternative to computed tomography (CT).
- Ultrasound will demonstrate most foreign bodies in soft tissues, including those that are not radiopaque.

Disadvantages
- The disadvantages of ultrasound are that it is highly operator-dependent, and most of the information is gained during the actual process of scanning as opposed to reviewing the static images.
- Another drawback is that the ultrasound wave is highly attenuated by air and bone, and thus little information is gained with regard to tissues beyond bony or air-filled structures; alternative techniques may be required to image these areas.

Ultrasound

Strengths:
- No radiation
- Inexpensive
- Allows interaction with patients
- Superb soft-tissue resolution in the near field
- Dynamic studies can be performed
- First-line investigation for hepatic, biliary, and renal disease
- Endocavitary ultrasound for gynecological and prostatic disorders
- Excellent resolution for breast, thyroid, and testis imaging
- Good for soft tissue, including tendons and ligaments
- Excellent for cysts and foreign bodies
- Doppler studies allow assessment of blood flow

Weaknesses:
- Interpretation only possible during the examination
- Long learning curve for some areas of expertise
- Resolution dependent on the machine available
- Images cannot be reliably reviewed away from the patient.

SMALL BOWEL ENEMA

3. Small bowel enema. ***WBUHS 2009, 2010***

Small Bowel Enema or Enteroclysis

Indications
- Suspected inflammatory bowel disease, including the exclusion of small bowel disease in Crohn's colitis
- Intermittent or partial small bowel obstruction

Preparation

One day before the test—have a normal breakfast, and clear fluids only for lunch (no solid foods or dairy products). After lunch take two Dulcolax tablets. Drink one glass of clear liquid every hour until bed. At 6 pm take one bottle of Citromag followed by a glass of water. On the day of the test, have nothing to eat or drink.

Time to Perform
60–90 minutes.

Procedure
This procedure involves inserting a thin tube through the mouth, esophagus, and past the stomach to inject barium methylcellulose and water into the small bowel. This allows for better visualization of the small bowel than can be seen during a small bowel follow-through. The back of the throat is "frozen" to allow easier passage of the tube.

Problem
- Greater discomfort to the patient, a higher radiation dose, and the possibility that gastroduodenal disease may not be seen.
- The investigation requires more experienced radiologists.
- Some radiologists advocate that small bowel enema with careful fluoroscopy and vigorous manual palpation can produce acceptable results with less cost, radiation exposure, and discomfort to the patient.

COMPUTED TOMOGRAPHY SCAN

4. CT scan. ***WBUHS 2006***

- CT scanning is a combination of special X-ray equipment with computers to produce multiple sectional images or pictures of the body which can be reconstructed and examined.
- CT scans of bones, soft tissue, organs, and blood vessels provide greater clarity and resolution compared to X-ray exams.
- Using these specialized equipment and expertise to create and interpret CT scans of the body, radiologists can more easily diagnose problems in the human body.

Some Common Uses
- Examination of the chest, abdomen, and pelvis as it provides a detailed, cross-sectional view of all types of tissue.
- Often intraoperative consultation (IOC) for diagnosing malignancies, including lung, liver, and pancreatic cancer.
- CT with angiogram plays a significant role in the detection, diagnosis, and treatment of vascular diseases, pulmonary embolism, and for abdominal aortic aneurysms (AAA).
- Invaluable in diagnosing and treating spinal problems and musculoskeletal disorders, hairline fractures, etc.

For children, CT imaging is more often used to evaluate:

Lymphoma	Neuroblastoma	Congenital malformations of blood vessels	The kidneys

Computed tomography scan can also be used to:
- Identification and grading of organ/vascular trauma.
- Interventions, such as guided biopsies, abscess drainages, and minimally invasive tumor treatments
- Follow-up in surgical cases. Assess response to treatment
- Staging of malignancies, planning, and plotting radiation fields
- Measure the bone mineral density.

Benefits
- Painless, noninvasive, and accurate
- Ability to image bone, soft tissue, and blood vessels at the same time
- Detailed images of many types of tissue as well as the lungs, bones, and blood vessels, unlike X-ray
- CT examinations are fast and simple, cost-effective
- Less sensitive to patient movement than MRI
- CT can be performed if you have an implanted medical device of any kind, unlike MRI

- CT imaging provides real-time imaging, making it a good tool for interventional radiology
- A diagnosis determined by CT scanning may eliminate the need for unnecessary intervention
- No radiation remains in a patient's body after a CT examination
- No immediate side effects

Risks
- There is always a slight chance of cancer from excessive exposure to radiation. However, the benefit of an accurate diagnosis far outweighs the risk.
- The effective radiation dose for this procedure varies. CT scanning is, in general, not recommended for pregnant women unless medically necessary because of potential risk to the baby.
- Nursing mothers should wait for 24 hours after contrast material injection before resuming breast-feeding.
- The risk of serious allergic reactions to contrast materials that contain iodine is extremely rare, and radiology departments are well-equipped to deal with them.
- Because children are more sensitive to radiation, they should have a CT study only if it is essential for making a diagnosis and should not have repeated CT studies unless absolutely necessary.

Limitations
- Soft-tissue details in areas, such as the brain, internal pelvic organs, knee, and shoulder can be more readily and clearly seen with MRI. The exam is not generally indicated for pregnant women.
- A person who is very large may not fit into the opening of a conventional CT scanner or may be over the weight limit for the moving table which is usually about 450 pounds.

MAGNETIC RESONANCE IMAGING

5. MRI in cancer management.

Introduction

MRI, nuclear magnetic resonance imaging (NMRI), or magnetic resonance tomography (MRT) is a medical imaging technique used in radiology to visualize detailed internal structures. Magnetic resonance imaging makes use of the property of nuclear magnetic resonance (NMR) to image nuclei of atoms inside the body.

Magnetic resonance imaging is highly sensitive for cancer staging, problem-solving, posttreatment surveillance, and other indications.

- It can detect primary breast cancers and additional foci of cancer that are occult to standard imaging.

Magnetic resonance imaging has been shown to be useful in:
- Staging biopsy-proven primary breast carcinoma
- Detecting an occult primary breast cancer in a patient with proven axillary node involvement but negative results on mammography and ultrasonography
- Ascertaining the extent of disease after lumpectomy with positive margins or close margins
- Investigating suspected pectoralis muscle invasion
- Assessing response to chemotherapy, including preoperative chemotherapy
- Looking for suspected recurrent disease, such as in a postsurgical scar
- A compelling clinical presentation with negative or equivocal imaging results
- Problem-solving, i.e., workup of uncertain imaging findings that could not be resolved even after special mammographic and ultrasonographic techniques were used
- Needle localization and guided biopsy
- Known or suspected rupture of breast implants
- Screening patients with certain well-defined risk factors for breast cancer
    - *MRI in hepatic imaging:*
        - Detection of liver lesions and its vascularity

- MRI in tumor angiogenesis
- *Lymph node evaluation*
- MRI in suspected recurrent disease
- With the advent of powerful gradient coil systems and high-resolution surface coils, MRI has recently extended its role in the staging of rectal cancer. The crucial advantage of MRI is not that it enables exact T-staging but a precise evaluation of the topographic relationship of a tumor to the mesorectal fascia. Magnetic resonance imaging is currently the only imaging modality that is highly accurate in predicting whether or not it is likely that a tumor-free margin can be achieved and thus provides important information for planning of an effective therapeutic strategy, especially in patients with advanced rectal cancer.
- The primary indication for MRI of the prostate is the evaluation of prostate cancer.
- MRI scans can aid in diagnosis, particularly in helping to distinguish soft tissue sarcomas from benign tumors, as well as showing the extent of the tumor.
- MRIs are also used to monitor the patient after treatment to see if the tumor has recurred.

ENDOSCOPIC ULTRASOUND

6. Role of endoscopic ultrasound in diagnostic evaluation. ***WBUHS 2019***

Endoscopic ultrasound (EUS) or echoendoscopy is a procedure in which endoscopy (insertion of a probe into a hollow organ) is combined with ultrasound to obtain images of the internal organs in the chest, abdomen, and colon. It can be used to visualize the walls of these organs or to look at adjacent structures. Combined with Doppler imaging, nearby blood vessels can also be evaluated.

- *Upper digestive tract:*
  - It allows for screening for pancreatic cancer, esophageal cancer, gastric cancer, and benign tumors of the upper gastrointestinal tract.
  - It also allows for characterization and biopsy of any focal lesions found in the upper gastrointestinal tract, such as esophageal tuberculosis.
  - Less commonly this procedure is used to identify the malformations and masses in the bile ducts and pancreatic ducts.
  - Organs such as the liver, pancreas, and adrenal glands are easily biopsied, as are any abnormal lymph nodes. In addition, the gastrointestinal wall itself can be imaged to see if it is abnormally thick, suggesting inflammation or malignancy.
  - The technique is highly sensitive for the detection of pancreatic cancer (90–95% sensitivity), particularly in patients who are suspected to have a mass or present with jaundice.
  - Its role in staging patients with pancreatic cancer is limited to local metastases; however, in combination with a CT scan which provides information on regional metastases, it provides an excellent imaging modality for the diagnosis and staging of pancreatic carcinoma.
  - Endoscopic ultrasound can also be used in conjunction with endoscopic retrograde cholangiopancreatography (ERCP). The ultrasound probe is used to locate gallstones that may have migrated into the common bile duct.
- *Lower digestive tract:* Echoendoscopy can also be used for imaging of the rectum and colon, although these applications are lesser known. It is used primarily to stage newly diagnosed rectal or anal cancer. EUS-guided fine needle aspiration may be used to sample lymph nodes during this procedure. Evaluation of the integrity of the anal sphincters may also be done during lower EUS procedures.
- *Respiratory tract:* An endoscopic ultrasound probe placed in the esophagus can also be used to visualize lymph nodes in the chest surrounding the airways (bronchi), which is important for the staging of lung cancer.

7. Endoluminal ultrasound. ***WBUHS 2011***

- Diagnostic procedure of choice in evaluation of anorectal disorders.
- Best imaging modality for staging of rectal cancer.
- Invaluable in workup for fecal incontinence and suppurative anorectal conditions.
    - Introduced in 1952
    - Used in Clinical Practice since 1983
    - 3D ultrasound recently developed
    - Currently being evaluated in efficacy compared to 2D ultrasound and MRI.

Equipment and Technique

- Endocavitary probe with a rotating transducer
- 7 or 10 MHz transducer
- Latex balloon covering the probe which is filled with water to distend the rectum.
- Phosphosoda enema for bowel preparation in left lateral decubitus position
- Digital rectal examination (DRE) and proctoscopy
- Wide bore proctoscope to facilitate positioning of probe above the lesion
- Balloon is filled with 30–60 cc of water and real-time image obtained

Image Interpretation

- Five-layer model
    - *Beynon and colleagues:*
        - Three hyperechoic (white) layers separated by two hypoechoic (black) layers.
        - *First white layer:* Interface between balloon and mucosa
        - *Second black layer:* Mucosa and muscularis
        - *Third white layer:* Submucosa
        - *Fourth black layer:* Muscularis propria
        - *Fifth white layer:* Interface between muscularis propria and fat

Accuracy of ERUS

Accurate in determining the depth of invasion	Significant learning curve
Moderately accurate in the assessment of lymph node involvement	Highly operator dependent

Factors for Misinterpretation

Close proximity to the anal verge	Artifact from air or stool	Postbiopsy or surgical changes	Hemorrhage
Improper balloon inflation	Refraction artifacts		Pedunculated tumors

Postoperative Follow-up

- ERUS may improve the ability to diagnose recurrence in 30%
- Baseline ultrasound at 3 months
- Optimal interval and length of time for serial follow-up has not been determined
- Suggested every 3–4 months for first 2 years then every 6 months for 5 years

T-TUBE CHOLANGIOGRAM

8. Importance of T-tube cholangiogram in current-day surgical practice. ***WBUHS 2021 Supplementary***

Indications

- Patient must have a T-tube in situ
- Patients with possibility of residual small gallstones

- Obstructive jaundice
- Bile duct stricture

Contraindications
- Nonconsent by the patient to the procedure
- Contrast or iodine allergy
- Pregnancy
- Barium study within last 3 days

Recent Trends
- Exploration of CBD with the retrieval of common bile duct stone followed by T-tube drainage is still the standard treatment of choledocholithiasis when all other standard minimally invasive procedures like ERCP have failed. A T-tube cholangiogram is done to exclude any leftover stones.
- Repair of iatrogenic bile duct injury over a T-tube can be done in case of minimum or no segmental loss. Postoperative T-tube cholangiogram helps to assess the patency of the common bile duct.
- Indications for cholangiography after transplantation are failure of liver function tests to return to normal, a rise in bilirubin or liver function test levels, obstructive symptoms associated with clamping the T-tube, bile drainage from the tube insertion site, wound, or surgical drains, and signs and symptoms of cholangitis. In addition, routine T-tube cholangiograms are generally obtained before tube removal.

NUCLEAR MEDICINE

9. Use of nuclear medicines in surgery.

Introduction
- Nuclear medicine is a branch of medical imaging in which radioactive material in small dosages are used to diagnose or treat a variety of disorders, such as malignancies and heart diseases.
- These are noninvasive and painless.
- Radioactive materials called radiopharmaceuticals or radiotracers are used.
- The radiotracer is either injected into a vein, swallowed, or inhaled as a gas and eventually accumulates in the organ or area of concern and emits gamma rays.
- This energy is detected by a device called a gamma camera, a positron emission tomography (PET) scanner, and/or probe which together with a computer, measure the amount of radiotracer absorbed by your body and to produce special images offering details on both the structure and function of organs and tissues.
- Nuclear medicine images can be superimposed with CT or MRI to produce special views known as image fusion or coregistration which allows the information from two different imaging studies to be correlated and interpreted as one image, leading to improved accuracy and precision.
- Therapeutic procedures such as radioactive iodine (I-131), lutetium-177 (Lu-177) therapy that use radioactive material to treat malignancies of thyroid and carcinoids respectively among others.

Nuclear medicine imaging scans are performed to:
- Analyze renal function
- Used to assess myocardial perfusion
- Assess pulmonary perfusion
- Identify inflammation in the gallbladder
- Evaluate bones for fractures, tumors, and inflammatory conditions
- Staging of malignancies
- Locate occult and obscure GI bleed
- Locate the presence of infection

- Measure thyroid function to detect hypo/hyperthyroidism
- Investigate abnormalities in the brain, such as seizures, memory loss, and abnormalities in blood flow
- Assessment of lymphatics in patients with breast cancer or melanoma

In pediatrics, nuclear medicine is also used to:
- Investigate congenital abnormalities in the esophagus, kidneys, and intestines.
- Evaluate the patency of lacrimal ducts and shunts in the brain and heart.

Nuclear medicine therapies include:
- Radioactive iodine (I-131)—hyperthyroidism (overactive thyroid gland, for example, Graves' disease) and differentiated thyroid malignancies.
- Radioactive antibodies—lymphoma
- Radioactive phosphorus (P-32)—blood disorders
- Radioactive materials used to treat painful tumor metastases to the bones.
- Radioactive iodine laced with metaiodobenzylguanidine (I-131 MIBG) used to treat adrenal gland tumors in adults and neuroblastoma in children.

POSITRON EMISSION TOMOGRAPHY SCAN

10. Positron emission tomography (PET) scan. *The Tamil Nadu Dr MGR Medical University 2025; WBUHS 2008*

Positron emission tomography is a nuclear medicine imaging technique that produces a three-dimensional (3D) image of the functional processes in the body. It detects pairs of gamma rays which are indirectly emitted by a positron-emitting radionuclide (tracer), introduced into the body on a biologically active molecule.

Images of these tracer concentration in 3D or four-dimensional (4D) space (the fourth dimension being time) within the body are then reconstructed with the aid of a CT X-ray scan performed on the patient during the same session, in the same machine to produce the final image.

Most commonly chosen, biologically active molecule for PET is fluorodeoxyglucose (FDG), a glucose analog which is taken up by metabolically active tissues, the concentrations of tracer imaged then give tissue metabolic activity, in terms of regional glucose uptake.

Combination of PET with CT and MRI

Positron emission tomography scans are increasingly read alongside CT or MRI scans, the superimposed combination giving both anatomic and metabolic information because PET imaging is most useful in combination with anatomical imaging such as CT, modern PET scanners are now equipped with integrated high-end multidetector-row CT scanners; hence, the two sets of images are more-precisely registered, so that areas of abnormality on the PET imaging can be more perfectly superimposed with anatomy on the CT images. This is very useful in showing detailed views of moving organs or structures with higher anatomical variation.

PET-MRI: Only the head and brain can be imaged currently.

Radionuclides

Radionuclides used in PET scanning are typical isotopes with short half-lives, such as carbon-11 (~20 minutes), nitrogen-13 (~10 minutes), oxygen-15 (~2 minutes), and fluorine-18 (~110 minutes).

The most commonly used radionuclide in clinical PET scanning is fluorine-18 in the form of FDG. The half-life of fluorine-18 is long enough that it can be manufactured commercially at offsite locations.

Limitations

- Risk of radiation exposure, though the risk to the patient from lack of knowledge about disease progress which is usually a malignancy is much greater than the risk from the test radiation

- High costs of cyclotrons

Positron emission tomography is a valuable technique for some diseases and disorders because it is possible to target the radiochemicals used for particular bodily functions.

Oncology

- FDG-PET can be used for diagnosis, staging, and monitoring treatment of various malignancies, such as lymphomas, breast, and lung cancer
- Detects residual or recurrent disease

Neurology

- PET neuroimaging is based on the principle that areas of high radioactivity are associated with increased brain activity; hence, an early diagnosis of Alzheimer's disease can be done.
- *Neuropsychology/cognitive neuroscience:* To study links between specific psychological processes or disorders and brain activity with their locations.

Cardiology

Atherosclerosis and vascular disease and myocardial perfusion studies.

Psychiatry

- Numerous compounds that bind selectively to neuroreceptors have been radiolabeled with C-11 or F-18. Radioligands binding to dopamine receptors (D1 and D2 reuptake transporter), serotonin receptors [5-hydroxytryptamine receptor 1A (5HT1A), 5HT2A, and reuptake transporter], opioid receptors (mu), and other sites have been used successfully.
- These studies have been performed examining the state of these receptors in patients compared to healthy controls in schizophrenia, substance abuse, mood disorders, and other psychiatric conditions.

Pharmacology

In preclinical trials, it is possible to radiolabel a new drug and inject it into animals.

Pulse Shape Discrimination (PSD)

The PSD is a technique used to define which pulse is related to each crystal. Different techniques were introduced to discriminate between two types of pulses according to their shape (indeed due to the decay time).

---

11. Role of FDG-PET CT scan in gastrointestinal surgery.

18F-fluorodeoxyglucose (^{18}FDG)-PET has been widely used to evaluate various types of malignant tumors, including lung, esophageal, colorectal cancer, and lymphomas.

Colorectal Cancer

- Initial staging of colorectal cancer can be done
- Recurrent colon cancer and evaluation of response to therapy:
  - In patients treated with novel therapies such as radiofrequency ablation and a combination of cryotherapy and hepatic artery chemotherapy, FDG-PET may be more accurate than CT in distinguishing post-therapy changes from recurrent or residual tumors.
  - *Local-pelvic recurrence:* FDG-PET accurately demonstrates recurrent colorectal cancer in patients who have indeterminate findings at CT or MR imaging.

Esophageal Cancer

- FDG-PET is a robust imaging modality to diagnose and evaluate stages of esophageal cancer.
- FDG-PET has also been shown to have a prognostic value that can be applied to patient management and aid in the development of emerging therapies.

Carcinoma Stomach

It is commonly believed that 18-FDG PET-CT improves tumor, node, and metastasis (TNM) staging. Taking into consideration the primary lesion staging, different factors may influence the diagnostic accuracy, such as the histological type of the tumor, its size or location, and the physiological FDG uptake by the gastric wall.

Pancreatic Cancer

It plays a vital role in early diagnosis and accurate staging, predicts survival, and monitors therapeutic effectiveness and pancreatic cancer recurrence.

Hepatic Malignancy

It is a sensitive tool in detecting recurrent extrahepatic lesions of hepatocellular carcinoma (HCC) after hepatectomy or radiofrequency ablation, which has a diagnostic sensitivity of 90–100% for recurrent or metastatic hepatic tumors.

Gallbladder and Bile Duct Malignancies

- For gallbladder cancer, the primary aim of performing FDG-PET is to identify distant metastases and recurrence.
- It can also help to detect bile duct cancer.

CHAPTER 20

Orthopedics

LEARNING OBJECTIVES

- Osteomyelitis
- Vascular Problem of Supracondylar Fracture of Humerus
- Cervical Rib and its Effect

1. Osteomyelitis. *WBUHS 2009*

Introduction

- Acute hematogenous osteomyelitis is a disease of growing bones.
- It is common in infants and children but rare in adults unless they are immunocompromised or have diabetes.

Etiology

- *Infants: Staphylococcus aureus, Streptococcus,* and *Escherichia coli*
- *Children: S. aureus, Streptococcus,* and *Haemophilus influenzae B*
- *Adults: S. aureus*
- *Sickle cell patients: Salmonella* sp
- *Rare causes:* Brucella, tuberculosis (TB), spirochetes, and fungi

Pathological Features

- Organisms are located near the metaphysis of the growing end of a long bone.
- *The following steps usually occur:*
  - *Inflammation:* Acute inflammation with venous congestion.
  - *Humidification:* After 2–3 days a medullary pus forms, which penetrates the periosteum.
  - *Necrosis:* After 7 days, circulation is impaired, and infectious thrombosis leads to necrosis and pocket formation (a sequela) of dead tissues.
  - *Repair:* After about 10–14 days, new bone forms from the periosteal layer, from which the swelling (involucrum) has been removed.
  - *Leakage:* Defects (cloacae) can develop in the involucrum that allow pus and sequestration to break down, allowing separation. This can also be achieved by surgical release and removal.

Clinical Features

- Usually, a child with a history of trauma or infection (skin or respiratory infection).
- Fever, pain, and malaise develop after a few days.
- The child may limp or refuse to bear weight.
- Long bone tissue examination may show localized swelling or redness.
- Babies may feel sick, sleepy, or irritable.
- Newborns can develop life-threatening sepsis, in which clear inflammation of a long bone develops, or a more benign form in which symptoms develop slowly but bone changes are extensive and often multiple.

Investigations

- Plain radiographs may be normal for the first 10 days. Do not be sure!
- A technetium-99m bone scan is usually positive in the first 24–48 hours and effective in early confirmation of the diagnosis.

X-ray Features

- Soft-tissue swelling is an early sign; look for displacement of fat planes.
- Patchy lucencies develop in the metaphysis at around 10 days.
- Periosteal new bone may be seen.
- Involucrum formation is only apparent at around 3 weeks.
- Sequestrum appears radiodense compared to the surrounding bone, which is osteopenic.
- Normal bone density occurs with healing.

Laboratory Test Results

- Primary biliary cholangitis (PBC)—normally with a raised neutrophil count
- Erythrocyte sedimentation rate (ESR)—increased
- C-reactive protein (CRP)—increased
- Blood cultures are positive in 50% of cases (use to inform and adjust antibiotic therapy)
- Perform urea and creatinine, liver function tests (LFTs), and glucose.

Treatment

- Pain relief by bed rest, splintage, and analgesics.
- Give intravenous (IV) antibiotics according to the local guidelines (after blood cultures and pus swab samples are taken), e.g., flucloxacillin IV and then PO qds for up to 6 weeks dose—adjusted according to age, clindamycin if penicillin—allergic, vancomycin if MRSA (methicillin-resistant *Staphylococcus aureus*), and ampicillin for *Haemophilus.*
- Surgical drainage of mature subperiosteal abscess with debridement of all necrotic tissues, obliteration of dead spaces, adequate soft-tissue coverage, and restoration of an effective blood supply.

Complications

- Disseminated systemic infection, e.g., septicemia and cerebral abscess
- Chronic osteomyelitis
- Septic arthritis
- Deformity due to epiphyseal involvement.

Chronic Osteomyelitis

Causes

- Occasionally following acute hematogenous osteomyelitis
- Most common following contaminated trauma and open fractures
- After joint replacement surgery
- Primary chronic infections of bone
- Secondary to acute osteomyelitis.

Features

- Sinus formation due to sequestra or resistant bacteria
- Prevented by adequate treatment of the initial acute attack.

Treatment

- Conservative (simple dressings) may be appropriate (elderly). Recurrent attacks with spontaneous recovery may occur, and surgery should be reserved for cases where an abscess forms.
- Chronic abscess may require drainage, debridement of all necrotic tissue, and obliteration of dead spaces. May involve plastic surgery to achieve soft-tissue cover and restoration of an effective blood supply.

- Closed suction drainage/irrigation systems can be effective, especially if irrigation fluid contains antibiotics. The disadvantage is that early blockage of the system can occur.
- Antibiotic (gentamicin) impregnated beads or sponges deliver high local levels and may be beneficial in areas of poor blood supply; hence, systemic antibiotic penetration occurs.
- Unresolving cases may require amputation.

Secondary to Trauma (Open Fractures)

- Prevention by an early aggressive approach to compound fractures with debridement and lavage of contaminated tissue:
  - Excise all dead tissues widely and remove all devitalized bone fragments, i.e., with no soft-tissue connections.
  - Copious lavage is necessary.
  - Skeletal stabilization is mandatory.
  - IV antibiotics, e.g., IV cefuroxime ± metronidazole if anaerobes may be involved (soil).
- Treat established chronic infection as above with the removal of internal foreign bodies, e.g., metalwork, and possible application of external fixation.

Secondary to Joint Replacement Surgery

- Rare, but is often a disaster for the elective patient.
- Prevention is better than cure. Dedicated laminar flow theaters, strict theater discipline, and prophylactic IV antibiotics are mandatory.
- 50% will require surgical intervention.
  - Initial joint irrigation, debridement, and tissue sampling can be attempted if the prosthesis is still solid and not loose.
  - If grossly infected, the prosthesis must be removed, the surfaces debrided, and an antibiotic cement spacer placed on the raw bone ends to allow the soft-tissue envelope to settle.
  - Once inflammatory markers have settled (CRP is the best) and the clinical infection has resolved, second-stage replacement of the spacer with a new prosthetic joint can go ahead. This may take 12 months and may not be possible.

Chronic Osteomyelitis as an Initial Presentation

- *Brodie's abscess:*
  - An isolated well-contained chronic abscess.
  - *Treatment:* Operative drainage with excision of the abscess wall and antibiotics.
- *Tuberculosis:*
  - Usually associated with other systemic features of the disease.
  - May present acutely.
  - Muscle atrophy develops and spontaneous discharge of a cold abscess may lead to sinus formation and destruction of bone.
  - Spinal TB may cause vertebral collapse leading to acute neurology—Pott's paraplegia.
- *Syphilitic osteomyelitis:*
  - Associated with advanced, tertiary disease in adults. Features include diffuse periostitis (with sabre tibia) or localized gummata with sequestra, sinus formation, and pathological fractures. X-rays show periosteal thickening with punched-out areas in sclerotic bone.
  - Infants with congenital disease have epiphysitis and metaphysitis. X-rays show areas of sclerosis near the growth plate separated by areas of rarefaction.
- *Mycotic osteomyelitis:*
  - Typically occurs in immunocompromised patients.
  - Bone granulomas, necrosis, and suppuration present without worsening acute illness.
  - Usually occurs as spread from primary lung infections such as coccidiomycosis, cryptococcosis, blastomycosis, and histoplasmosis.
  - *Treatment:* Amphotericin B and/or surgical excision.

2. Vascular problem of supracondylar fracture of humerus. *WBUHS 2009*

Supracondylar fractures of the humerus in children remain a challenging problem.

The possibility of Volkmann's ischemic contracture is rare but devastating. The role of arteriography and indications for operative repair of the brachial artery remain controversial.

In addition, the treatment of a pink yet pulseless hand is also unclear.

- Vascular compromise occurs in about 5–20% of children with supracondylar fractures. Less than 1% will be complicated by compartment syndrome and the resulting sequelae of Volkmann's contracture.
- A median nerve palsy may mask a pending compartment syndrome (because there will be no pain).
- *Fractures* with *posterolateral* displacement of distal fragments are more susceptible to vascular injury since the medial spike of the proximal humerus can tether the brachial artery.
- Tenting of the artery from the bicipital aponeurosis.
- The bicipital aponeurosis may be involved in the anatomical etiology of arterial compromise after swelling in supracondylar fracture.

Treatment

- While the patient is being worked up, consider applying a continuous *pulse* oximeter so nurses can follow an objective measurement of perfusion.
- *Arteriography:* Fracture reduction usually restores the pulses, and therefore reduction should not be delayed by waiting for an angiographic study; arteriography is only indicated if circulation is not restored following reduction.
- If circulation is not restored by closed reduction, immediate open reduction and surgical exploration of the artery are indicated.
- Arteriography is not indicated since it provides little additional information and only delays restoration of circulation to the extremity.
- Morbidity associated with surgical exposure of the artery is low.
- Procrastination will only increase patient morbidity.
- Possible compartment syndrome will need fasciotomy.

3. Cervical rib and its effects. *WBUHS 2010*

Introduction

- Arterial compression is almost universally associated with a bony abnormality of the thoracic outlet. Cervical ribs, which occur in 0.5–1.5% of the normal population, are present in >95% of patients with arterial thoracic outlet syndrome (TOS).
- Repetitive compression and trauma to the subclavian artery lead to intimal injury/ulceration at the site of compression or poststenotic dilation/aneurysmal degeneration of the artery just distal to the point of compression.
- Mural thrombus forming at the site of the damaged intima or within an aneurysm can then embolize down the arm, leading to ischemic symptomatology.

Effects of Cervical Rib

- Patients with symptomatic arterial TOS most commonly present with symptoms of digital ischemia related to microembolization of platelet aggregates formed on intimal lesions or mural thrombus from poststenotic aneurysms.
- Early symptoms may include unilateral Raynaud's syndrome, or complaints of digital cyanosis, pallor, coldness, pain, and paresthesias. Findings are most common in the thumb and index finger because of the direct pathway of the radial artery.

- If the arterial lesion is not diagnosed and corrected, repeated embolization will lead to obliteration of the distal arterial bed, with worsening ischemia leading to digital ulceration and gangrene.
- Macroembolization to the larger arteries of the arm presents as acute limb ischemia, the severity of symptoms depending on the patency of the distal arterial tree. Even a relatively small embolus can be limb-threatening if preceded by multiple episodes of microembolization.
- Thrombotic occlusion of the subclavian artery can also occur. Physical examination may be normal or reveal signs of ischemia of varying degrees and extents.
- A supraclavicular bruit or pulsatile mass may occasionally be detected.
- Concomitant symptoms of neurogenic TOS may be present but are often overshadowed by ischemic symptomatology.
- Patients with Raynaud's symptoms or subtle signs of digital ischemia should always undergo segmental pressure testing including the digital waveforms to rule out an occlusive process.
- In the absence of a documented collagen vascular disorder or severe arteriosclerosis, the presence of a small artery (palmar/digital) occlusive disease should always lead to arteriography.
- Patients with macroemboli and no obvious cardiac source should also undergo arteriography to exclude a proximal arterial source. Arteriography should include complete views from the aortic arch to the fingertips.
- If the subclavian artery appears normal in the neutral position, a repeat view should be obtained with the arm abducted. Magnified views of the hand following vasodilator injection are helpful in distinguishing embolic occlusions from intrinsic disease.
- Arteriographic findings can be subtle, ranging from minor wall irregularities and minimal poststenotic dilation to frank aneurysms.
- Duplex scanning may be useful in patients who present with pulsatile supraclavicular masses or questionable findings on arteriography.

CHAPTER 21

Compartment Syndrome

LEARNING OBJECTIVE

➢ Compartment Syndrome

1. Write notes on compartment syndrome. ***WBUHS 2016***

Introduction

- Compartment syndrome is a painful condition that occurs when pressure within the muscles builds to dangerous levels. This pressure can decrease blood flow, which prevents nourishment and oxygen from reaching nerve and muscle cells.
- Compartment syndrome can be either acute or chronic.
- Acute compartment syndrome is a medical emergency. It is usually caused by a severe injury. Without treatment, it can lead to permanent muscle damage.
- Chronic compartment syndrome, also known as exertional compartment syndrome, is usually not a medical emergency. It is most often caused by athletic exertion.

Description

- Compartment syndrome develops when swelling or bleeding occurs within a compartment.
- Because the fascia does not stretch, this can cause increased pressure on the capillaries, nerves, and muscles in the compartment.
- Blood flow to muscle and nerve cells is disrupted. Without a steady supply of oxygen and nutrients, nerve and muscle cells can be damaged.
- In acute compartment syndrome, unless the pressure is relieved quickly, permanent disability and tissue death may result. This does not usually happen in chronic (exertional) compartment syndrome.
- Compartment syndrome most often occurs in the anterior (front) compartment of the lower leg (calf). It can also occur in other compartments in the leg, as well as in the arms, hands, feet, and buttocks.

Anatomy

- Compartments are groupings of muscles, nerves, and blood vessels in your arms and legs. Covering these tissues is a tough membrane called a fascia.
- The role of the fascia is to keep the tissues in place, and therefore the fascia does not stretch or expand easily.

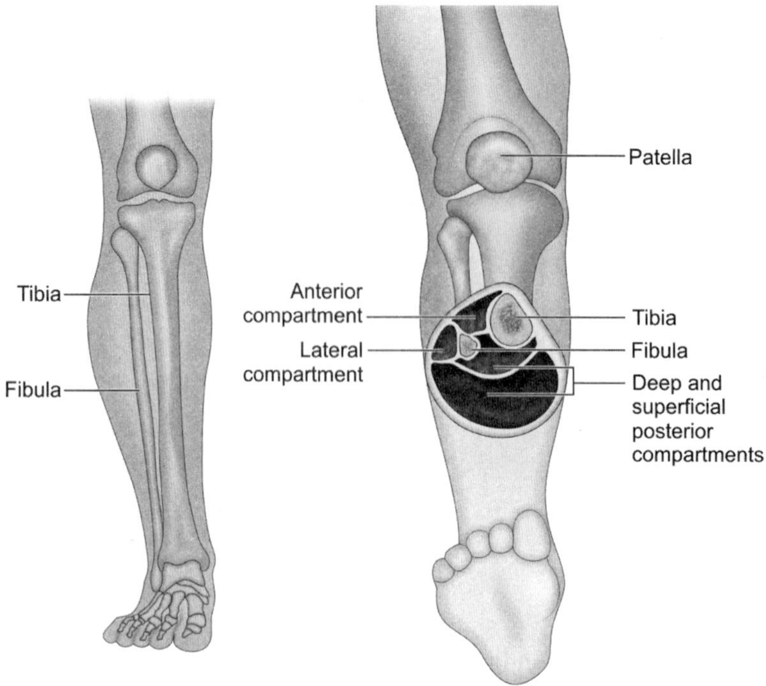

Causes

Acute Compartment Syndrome

Acute compartment syndrome usually develops after a severe injury, such as a car accident or a broken bone. Rarely, it develops after a relatively minor injury.

Conditions that may bring on acute compartment syndrome include:

- *A fracture*
- *A badly bruised muscle.* This type of injury can occur when a motorcycle falls on the leg of the rider or a football player is hit in the leg with another player's helmet.
- *Re-established blood flow after blocked circulation:*
  - This may occur after a surgeon repairs a damaged blood vessel that has been blocked for several hours.
  - A blood vessel can also be blocked during sleep.
  - Lying for too long in a position that blocks a blood vessel and then moving or waking up can cause this condition.
  - Most healthy people will naturally move when blood flow to a limb is blocked during sleep.
  - The development of compartment syndrome in this manner usually occurs in people who are neuro logically compromised.
  - This can happen after severe intoxication with alcohol or other drugs.
- *Crush injuries*
- *Anabolic steroid use:* Taking steroids is a possible factor in compartment syndrome.
- *Constricting bandages:* Casts and tight bandages may lead to compartment syndrome. If symptoms of compartment syndrome develop, remove or loosen any constricting bandages. If you have a cast, contact your doctor immediately.

Chronic (Exertional) Compartment Syndrome

- The pain and swelling of chronic compartment syndrome are caused by exercise.
- Athletes who participate in activities with repetitive motions, such as running, biking, or swimming, are more likely to develop chronic compartment syndrome.
- This is usually relieved by discontinuing the exercise and is usually not dangerous.

Symptoms

Acute Compartment Syndrome

The classic sign of acute compartment syndrome is pain, especially when the muscle within the compartment is stretched.

- The pain is more intense than what would be expected from the injury itself. Using or stretching the involved muscles increases the pain.
- There may also be tingling or burning sensations (paresthesias) in the skin.
- The muscle may feel tight or full.
- Numbness or paralysis are late signs of compartment syndrome. They usually indicate permanent tissue injury.

Chronic (Exertional) Compartment Syndrome

Chronic compartment syndrome causes pain or cramping during exercise. This pain subsides when activity stops. It most often occurs in the leg.

Symptoms may also include:

- Numbness
- Difficulty moving the foot
- Visible muscle bulging

Treatments for Compartment Syndrome

- *Acute compartment syndrome:* This must be treated in a hospital using a surgical procedure called an emergency fasciotomy.
- *Chronic compartment syndrome:*
  - Chronic compartment syndrome is not usually dangerous and can sometimes be relieved by stopping the exercise that triggers it and switching to a less strenuous activity.
  - Physiotherapy, shoe inserts (orthotics), and nonsteroidal anti-inflammatory medicines may help—speak to your general practitioner (GP) about this.
  - Surgery (see above) will only be considered if your symptoms persist despite the above measures.

---

2. Discuss the anatomy of the different compartments of the thigh and leg. Describe with diagram the different incisions to decompress the said compartments. ***WBUHS 2025***

Compartments of the Thigh

The thigh is anatomically divided into three compartments:

1. *Anterior compartment*
   - *Muscles:* Quadriceps femoris (rectus femoris, vastus lateralis, vastus medialis, vastus intermedius), sartorius, iliopsoas.
   - *Nerve supply:* Femoral nerve
   - *Blood supply:* Femoral artery
   - *Function:* Knee extension and hip flexion
2. *Medial compartment*
   - *Muscles:* Adductor longus, adductor brevis, adductor magnus (adductor part), gracilis, obturator externus
   - *Nerve supply:* Obturator nerve
   - *Blood supply:* Obturator artery
   - *Function:* Hip adduction
3. *Posterior compartment*
   - *Muscles:* Hamstrings (biceps femoris, semitendinosus, semimembranosus), part of adductor magnus (hamstring part)
   - *Nerve supply:* Tibial portion of sciatic nerve
   - *Blood supply:* Perforating branches of deep femoral artery
   - *Function:* Hip extension and knee flexion

Compartments of the Leg

The leg (below the knee) is divided into four compartments:

1. *Anterior compartment*
   - *Muscles:* Tibialis anterior, extensor hallucis longus, extensor digitorum longus, fibularis tertius
   - *Nerve supply:* Deep peroneal (fibular) nerve
   - *Blood supply:* Anterior tibial artery
   - *Function:* Dorsiflexion of foot and toe extension
2. *Lateral compartment*
   - *Muscles:* Fibularis (peroneus) longus, fibularis brevis
   - *Nerve supply:* Superficial peroneal (fibular) nerve
   - *Blood supply:* Perforating branches of fibular artery
   - *Function:* Eversion of the foot
3. *Superficial posterior compartment*
   - *Muscles:* Gastrocnemius, soleus, plantaris
   - *Nerve supply:* Tibial nerve
   - *Blood supply:* Posterior tibial artery
   - *Function:* Plantarflexion of the foot
4. *Deep posterior compartment*
   - *Muscles:* Tibialis posterior, flexor hallucis longus, flexor digitorum longus, popliteus
   - *Nerve supply:* Tibial nerve
   - *Blood supply:* Posterior tibial and fibular arteries
   - *Function:* Plantarflexion, toe flexion, foot inversion

Compartment Syndrome and Decompression (Fasciotomy)

Compartment syndrome occurs when increased pressure within a muscle compartment impairs circulation and nerve function. If untreated, it can lead to tissue necrosis.

Surgical management: Fasciotomy

Fasciotomy involves making incisions in the skin and fascia to relieve pressure.

Diagram: Fasciotomy Incisions

- *Thigh fasciotomy incision*
  - *Lateral incision* (along lateral intermuscular septum) gives access to anterior and posterior compartments.
  - *Medial incision* can be added for better access to the medial compartment.

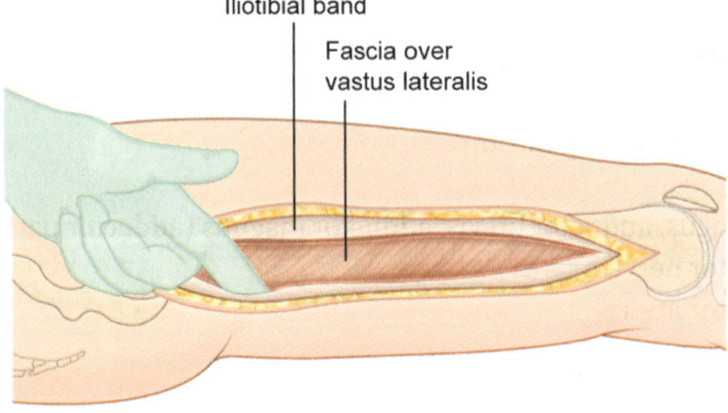

Diagram description

- A line drawn along the lateral aspect of the thigh, just anterior to the iliotibial tract.
- Medial incision along the medial thigh over the adductor compartment.

- *Leg fasciotomy incisions*
  - Two-incision, four-compartment fasciotomy is commonly used.
    1. Lateral incision (for anterior and lateral compartments)
       - Made *1 cm anterior to the fibula,* extending from just below the fibular head to just above the lateral malleolus.

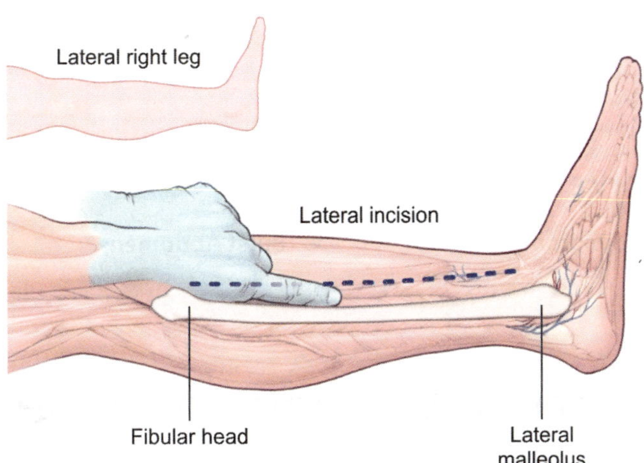

    2. Medial incision (for superficial and deep posterior compartments)
       - Made 2 cm posterior to the medial border of the tibia, extending from below the tibial tuberosity to above the medial malleolus.

Diagram Description
- *Lateral leg:* Incision anterior to fibula
- *Medial leg:* Incision posterior to tibia

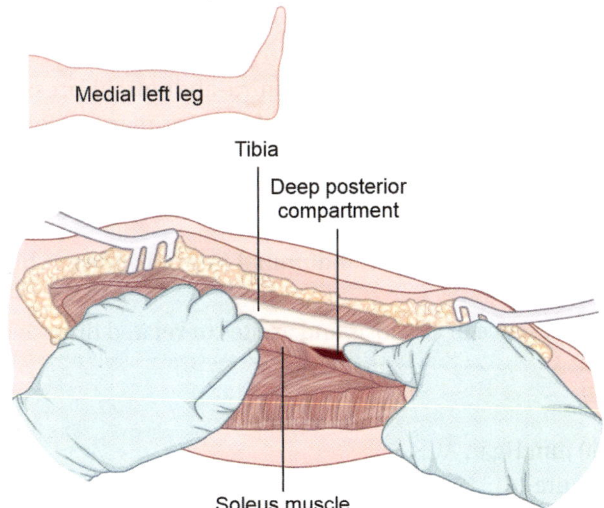

CHAPTER 22

Acute Abdomen and Abdominal Compartment Syndrome

LEARNING OBJECTIVES

- Abdominal Compartment Syndrome
- Open Abdomen
- Burst Abdomen

ABDOMINAL COMPARTMENT SYNDROME

1. What are the causes of the development of abdominal compartment syndrome (ACS)? What are its physiological consequences? Discuss the diagnosis and treatment of ACS. ***WBUHS 2022***

2. Define abdominal perfusion pressure (APP) and ACS. What are the common causes and risk factors of ACS? How does one manage ACS? ***WBUHS 2023***

3. What is abdominal compartment syndrome? Discuss the pathophysiology, evaluation and non-operative management strategies. ***WBUHS 2025***

Introduction

Abdominal compartment syndrome occurs when the intra-abdominal pressure (IAP) is too high, similar to compartment syndrome in an extremity. The three types of ACS (primary, secondary, and chronic) have different and sometimes overlapping causes:

1. Primary or acute ACS occurs when intra-abdominal pathology is directly and proximally responsible for the compartment syndrome.
2. Secondary ACS occurs when no visible intra-abdominal injury is present but injuries outside the abdomen cause fluid accumulation.
3. Chronic ACS occurs in the presence of cirrhosis and ascites or related disease states, often in the later stages of the disease.

Definitions

- APP = MAP – IAP· APP <60 mm Hg in ACS
  (MAP = mean arterial pressure)
- ACS occurs when the abdomen becomes subject to increased pressure. The specific cause of ACS is not known, although some causes can be sepsis and severe abdominal trauma. Increasing pressure reduces blood flow to abdominal organs and impairs pulmonary, cardiovascular, renal, and gastrointestinal (GI) function, causing multiple organ dysfunction syndrome and death.
- ACS is the end result of untreated intra-abdominal hypertension (IAH). ACS may result from large-volume intravenous (IV) fluid resuscitation.

- It is organ dysfunction caused by increased intracranial–abdominal pressure >12 mm Hg (IAH). Organ dysfunction is usually respiratory, cardiovascular system (CVS), or renal but can be any organ (normal IAP 2–7 mm Hg)

Primary ACS

Causes of primary (acute) ACS include the following:
- Penetrating trauma
- Intraperitoneal hemorrhage
- Pancreatitis
- External compressing forces, such as debris from a motor vehicle collision or after a large structure explosion
- Pelvic fracture
- Rupture of abdominal aortic aneurysm (AAA)
- Perforated peptic ulcer.

Secondary ACS

Secondary ACS may occur in patients without an intra-abdominal injury when fluid accumulates in volumes sufficient to cause IAH. Causes include the following:
- *Large-volume resuscitation:* The literature shows significantly increased risk with infusions >3 L.
- *Large areas of full-thickness burns:* Hobson et al., demonstrated ACS within 24 hours in burn patients who had received an average of 237 mL/kg over a 12-hour period.
- Penetrating or blunt trauma without identifiable injury
- Postoperative
- Packing and primary fascial closure, which increases incidence.
- Sepsis

Chronic ACS

Causes of chronic ACS include the following:
- Peritoneal dialysis
- Morbid obesity
- Cirrhosis
- Meigs syndrome
- Intra-abdominal mass

Physiological Consequences
- *Cardiovascular:*
  - A rise in the IAP leads to a fall in cardiac output, mainly due to compression of the inferior vena cava and reduction in venous return to the heart.
  - Cardiac output is reduced despite apparent rises in central venous pressure (CVP), pulmonary artery occlusion pressure, and systemic vascular resistance.
- *Respiratory:*
  - Raised IAP will effectively splint the diaphragm and lead to a rise in peak airway pressure and intra-thoracic pressure and subsequently a reduced venous return to the heart.
  - The increase in airway pressures may also exacerbate barotrauma and contribute to the development of acute respiratory distress syndrome.
- *Renal:*
  - An acute increase in IAP leads to oliguria and anuria probably due to compression of the renal vein and renal parenchyma.
  - Renal blood flow and glomerular filtration are decreased with a corresponding increase in renal vascular resistance.

- *Cerebral:* The rise in IAP and intrathoracic pressure leads to a rise in CVP which prevents adequate venous drainage from the brain, leading to a rise in intracranial pressure and worsening of intracerebral edema.

Diagnosis: Measuring the Pressure

- Insert a Foley catheter and clamp the tube distal to the sample port.
- Instill 5–1,000 mL of saline into the bladder so as to leave a continuous column of fluid from the bladder to the sample port on the Foley.
- Insert an 18 g catheter into the sample port and connect to a CVP transducer.
- Level the transducer at the symphysis pubis.

Diagnostic Features

Distended abdomen	Massive IV fluid requirements	Hypoxemia refractory to increase FiO_2 and PEEP	Wide pulse pressure
IAP >20 mm Hg	Oliguria to anuria not responding to volume repletion	Hypercarbia	Acidosis
Elevated peak airway pressure	Decreased cardiac output	Hypercapnia	

(IAP: intra-abdominal pressure; IV: intravenous; PEEP: positive end-expiratory pressure)

Imaging Studies

- *Abdominal computed tomography (CT) scan can reveal many subtle findings.*
  - *Round-belly sign:* Abdominal distention with an increased ratio of anteroposterior-to-transverse abdominal diameter (ratio >0.80)
  - Collapse of the vena cava
  - Bowel wall thickening with enhancement
  - Bilateral inguinal herniation
- *Plain abdominal radiographic studies are often useless in identifying ACS.* They may show evidence of free air or bowel obstruction.
- *Abdominal ultrasonography* may reveal an aortic aneurysm, particularly with large aneurysms, but bowel gas or obesity makes performing the study difficult.

The following laboratory studies may be indicated:

- Comprehensive metabolic panel (CMP)
- Complete blood cell count (CBC)
- Amylase and lipase assessment
- Prothrombin time (PT) and activated partial thromboplastin time (aPTT) if the patient is heparinized.
- Cardiac marker assays
- Urinalysis and urine drug screen
- Measurement of serum lactate levels (at many institutions, the sample must be kept on ice)
- *Arterial blood gas (ABG):* This is a quick way to measure the pH, lactate, and base deficit.

Critical Level of IAP

Burch et al., described a grading system of elevated IAP:

- Grade I (10–15 cmH_2O)
- Grade II (15–25 cmH_2O)
- Grade III (25–35 cmH_2O)
- Grade IV (>35 cmH_2O)

Points to Remember

- Most of the patients with grade III and all of the patients with grade IV elevations in IAP should undergo abdominal decompression.
- Even at lower pressures, the onset of the syndrome of ACS should prompt abdominal decompression.
- Consider a persistent elevation of IAP beyond 20–25 cmH_2O (15–19 mm Hg) as IAH and institute therapy, even in the absence of established signs of ACS.
- A recent concept is to calculate APP as the difference between MAP and IAP, with an APP of 50 mm Hg as the optimal level.

Treatment/Treatment Approaches for IAH

- If ACS is suspected, the focus of prehospital care is to immediately transport the patient to the emergency department (ED). Remove any constricting garments. Do not place anything on the patient's abdomen.
- Avoid overly aggressive fluid resuscitation, especially in extremity injuries. The over-resuscitated patient is much more likely to develop ACS, and often the prehospital setting is where this begins.
- In the ED, the first priority of the ED physician is to consider the diagnosis in any patient with the appropriate mechanisms of injury or pathology.
- Therapy should include fluid resuscitation and transfusion if needed, as well as surgical consultation.
- The first step in the evaluation of an increased IAP, especially in the presence of agitation and restlessness, is to sedate and, if necessary, chemically paralyze the patient.
- If the bladder pressures are still high and/or systemic manifestations of IAH (as described above) are evident, the appropriate treatment, in most instances, is abdominal decompression by laparotomy.
- If the abdomen was previously closed by fascial sutures, there was no previous laparotomy, or bedside decompression is not efficacious or possible, a formal operating room (OR) laparotomy should be performed.
- At laparotomy, the abdomen is decompressed, abdominal fluid and/or blood evacuated, and hemostasis obtained or ensured.
- The results of abdominal decompression are usually rather dramatic, with decreased inspiratory pressure, improved gas exchange, lessened systemic vascular resistance, and increased cardiac index and oxygen delivery.
- The gut appearance will improve, and, if measured, oxygenation of the gut can be shown to have improved. A brisk increase in urinary output occurs.
- If the abdomen is already "open," this may involve the opening of the temporary closure (mesh, plastic, or towel clips, etc.), evacuation of the abdomen of fluid and blood, removal of abdominal packs (with repacking, if necessary), and enlargement of the abdominal space to accommodate the edematous and swollen contents.
- Evacuation of hemoperitoneum by ultrasound (US)-guided paracentesis may be employed with success in patients with nonoperative management of hepatic and splenic injuries.
- Once abdominal decompression is achieved, it is the usual practice to leave the abdominal fascia and skin "open" with some type of foreign material at the skin level to prevent evisceration.
- These materials include various absorbable or nonabsorbable types of mesh, an artificial burr device, sterilized saline bags with or without a zipper (the Bogota bag), dressings with moist gauze or Vi-drapes, "vacuum-pack," etc.
- All have in common the goals of preventing evisceration, allowing enlargement of the abdominal cavity, keeping the IAP low, and preventing reoccurrence of IAH and ACS.
- Pharmacologic therapy is less effective than mechanical drainage. Pressors have a role but may not be equally effective in treating ACS.
- Inpatient care in acute ACS is directed by critical care physicians and surgeons.
- If an intensive care unit (ICU) patient experiences decompensation, ACS should be re-examined as a potential cause.
- IAH may be an ongoing process in any patient with pathology-producing intra-abdominal fluid loss. Repeat or continuous IAP measurement is indicated. The abdomen should be clear of any heavy objects.

Intra-abdominal Hypertension Assessment Algorithm

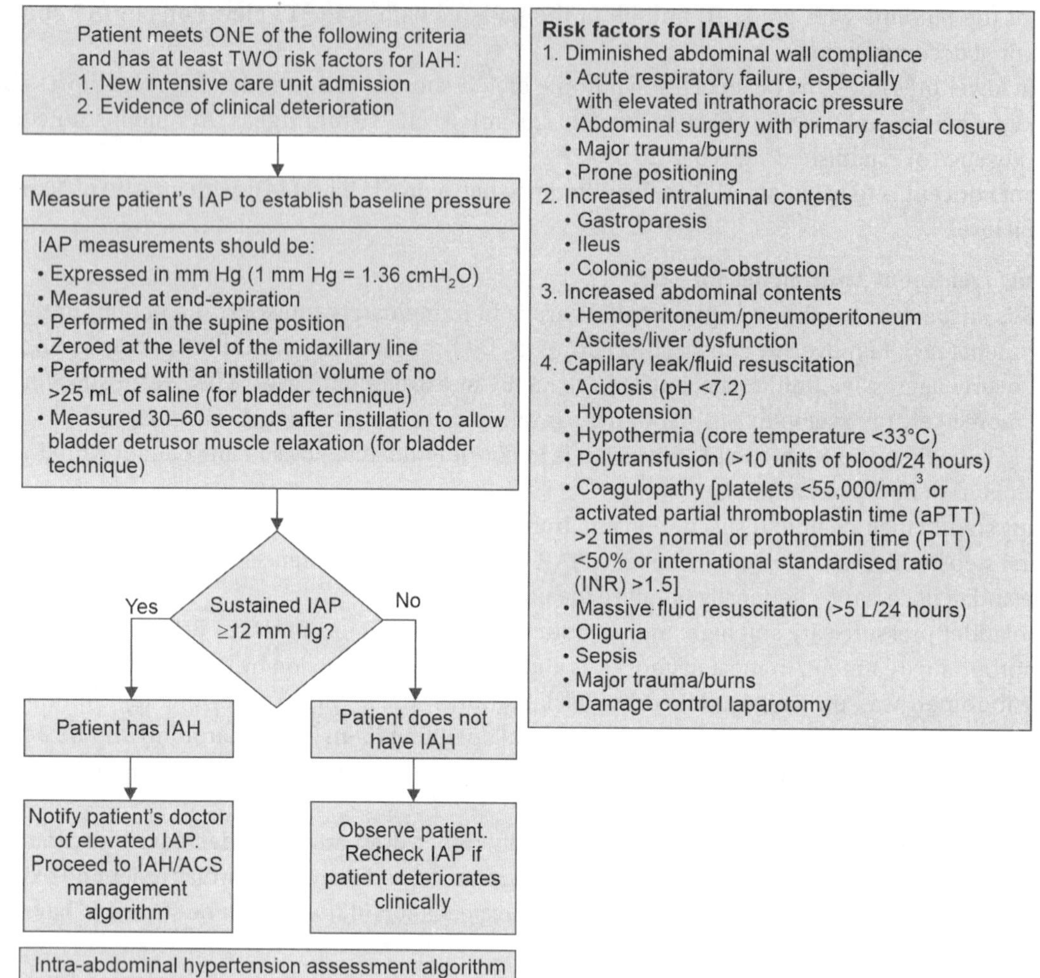

Intra-abdominal hypertension assessment algorithm

(ACS: abdominal compartment syndrome; IAH: intra-abdominal hypertension; IAP: intra-abdominal pressure)

4. What is ACS? What are the effects of it on individual organs? How do you manage the complications?

WBUHS 2014

Abdominal compartment syndrome occurs when the abdomen becomes subject to increased pressure. The specific cause of ACS is not known, although some causes can be sepsis and severe abdominal trauma. Increasing pressure reduces blood flow to abdominal organs and impairs pulmonary, cardiovascular, renal, and gastrointestinal (GI) function, causing multiple organ dysfunction syndrome and death.

Abdominal compartment syndrome is the end result of untreated IAH. It may result from large-volume intravenous fluid resuscitation.

Pathophysiology

- It occurs when tissue fluid within the peritoneal and retroperitoneal space (either edema, retroperitoneal blood, or free fluid in the abdomen) accumulates in such large volumes that the abdominal wall compliance threshold is crossed and the abdomen can no longer stretch.
- Once the abdominal wall can no longer expand, any further fluid leaking into the tissue results in fairly rapid rises in the pressure within the closed space.

- Initially, this increase in pressure does not cause organ failure but does cause organs to not work properly— this is called IAH and is defined as a pressure over 12 mm Hg in adults.
- However, if the pressure continues to rise over 20 mm Hg and organs begin to fail, the syndrome has now progressed to the end-stage highly fatal process termed abdominal compartment syndrome.
- These pressure measurements are relative. Small children get into trouble and develop compartment syndromes at much lower pressures while young previously healthy athletic individuals may tolerate an abdominal pressure of 20 mm Hg very well.
- The underlying cause of the disease process is capillary permeability caused by the systemic inflammatory response syndrome (SIRS) that occurs in every critically ill patient.
- SIRS leads to leakage of fluid out of the capillary beds into the interstitial space in the entire body with a profound amount of this fluid leaking into the gut wall, mesentery, and retroperitoneal tissue.
- Peritoneal tissue edema secondary to diffuse peritonitis and abdominal trauma.

Causes

- Fluid therapy due to massive volume resuscitation
- Retroperitoneal hematoma secondary to trauma and aortic rupture
- Peritoneal trauma secondary to emergency abdominal operations
- Reperfusion injury following bowel ischemia due to any cause
- Retroperitoneal and mesenteric inflammatory edema secondary to acute pancreatitis
- Ileus and bowel obstruction
- Intra-abdominal masses of any etiology
- Abdominal packing for control of hemorrhage
- Closure of the abdomen under undue tension
- Ascites/intra-abdominal fluid accumulation.

Risk Factors

- Large-volume resuscitation
- Massive transfusion protocol use
- Management with an open body cavity
- Core hypothermia
- Coagulopathy requiring component therapy
- Severe sepsis or septic shock
- Critical illness in the setting of cirrhosis or other liver diseases.

Grading of ACS

Grade	*Bladder pressure (mm Hg)*	*Recommendation*
I	10–15	Maintain normovolemia
II	16–25	Hypervolemic resuscitation
III	26–35	Decompression
IV		Decompression and re-exploration

Abdominal compartment syndrome clinical manifestations	
Central nervous system ↑ Intracranial pressure ↓ Cerebral perfusion pressure *Cardiac* Hypovolemia ↓ Cardiac output	*Gastrointestinal* ↓ Celiac blood flow ↓ SMA blood flow ↓ Mucosal blood flow ↓ pHi

Contd...

Contd...

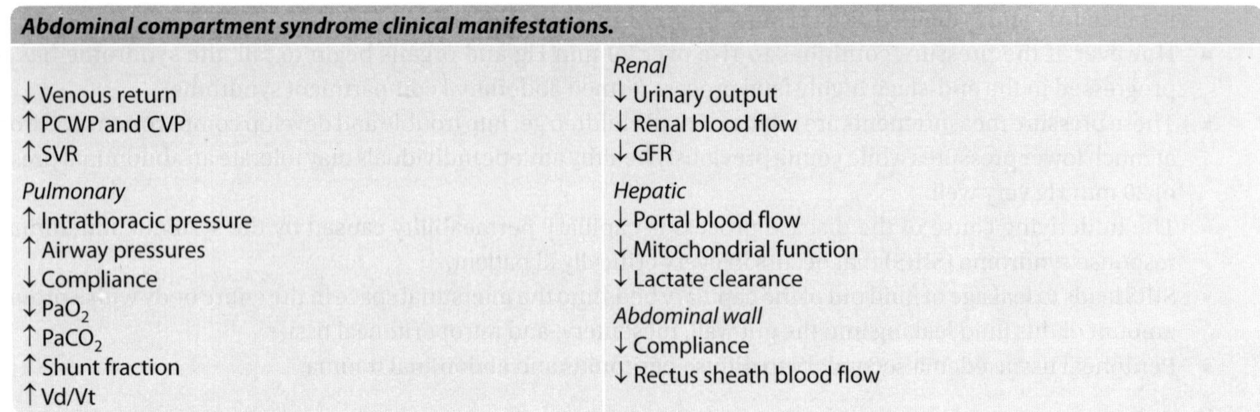

Abdominal compartment syndrome clinical manifestations.	
	Renal
↓ Venous return	↓ Urinary output
↑ PCWP and CVP	↓ Renal blood flow
↑ SVR	↓ GFR
Pulmonary	*Hepatic*
↑ Intrathoracic pressure	↓ Portal blood flow
↑ Airway pressures	↓ Mitochondrial function
↓ Compliance	↓ Lactate clearance
↓ PaO_2	*Abdominal wall*
↑ $PaCO_2$	↓ Compliance
↑ Shunt fraction	↓ Rectus sheath blood flow
↑ Vd/Vt	

(CVP: central venous pressure; GFR: glomerular filtration rate; PCWP: pulmonary capillary wedge pressure; SMA: superior mesenteric artery; SVR: systemic vascular resistance; Vd/Vt: dead space/tidal volume ratio)

Intra-abdominal Pressure Monitoring Algorithm

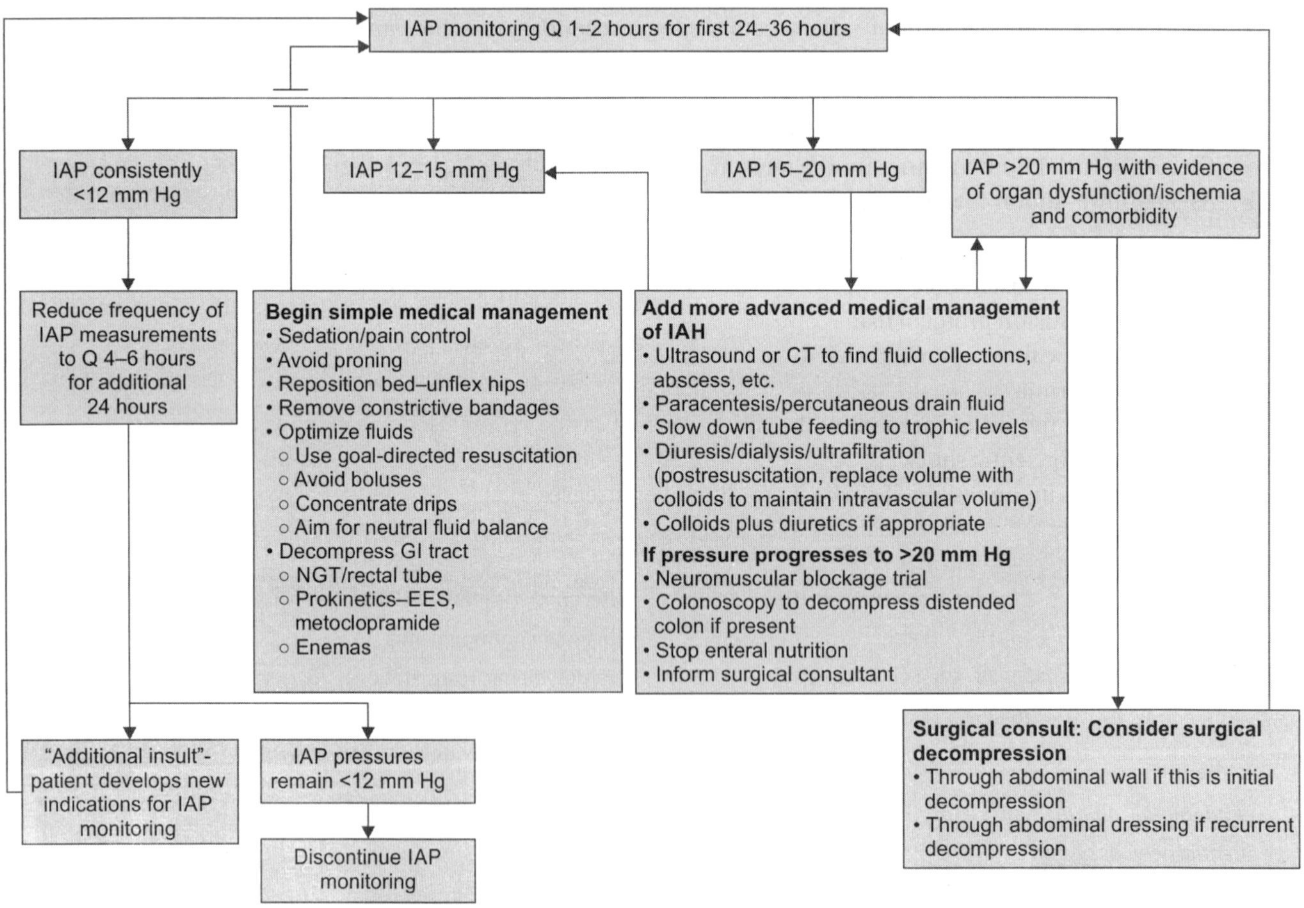

IAP monitoring Q 1–2 hours for first 24–36 hours

IAP consistently <12 mm Hg

IAP 12–15 mm Hg

IAP 15–20 mm Hg

IAP >20 mm Hg with evidence of organ dysfunction/ischemia and comorbidity

Reduce frequency of IAP measurements to Q 4–6 hours for additional 24 hours

Begin simple medical management
- Sedation/pain control
- Avoid proning
- Reposition bed–unflex hips
- Remove constrictive bandages
- Optimize fluids
  - Use goal-directed resuscitation
  - Avoid boluses
  - Concentrate drips
  - Aim for neutral fluid balance
- Decompress GI tract
  - NGT/rectal tube
  - Prokinetics–EES, metoclopramide
  - Enemas

Add more advanced medical management of IAH
- Ultrasound or CT to find fluid collections, abscess, etc.
- Paracentesis/percutaneous drain fluid
- Slow down tube feeding to trophic levels
- Diuresis/dialysis/ultrafiltration (postresuscitation, replace volume with colloids to maintain intravascular volume)
- Colloids plus diuretics if appropriate

If pressure progresses to >20 mm Hg
- Neuromuscular blockage trial
- Colonoscopy to decompress distended colon if present
- Stop enteral nutrition
- Inform surgical consultant

"Additional insult"- patient develops new indications for IAP monitoring

IAP pressures remain <12 mm Hg

Discontinue IAP monitoring

Surgical consult: Consider surgical decompression
- Through abdominal wall if this is initial decompression
- Through abdominal dressing if recurrent decompression

(EES: erythromycin ethylsuccinate; GI: gastrointestinal; IAH: intra-abdominal hypertension; IAP: intra-abdominal pressure; NGT: nasogastric tubes)

Nonoperative medical management: Early detection of elevated IAP via bladder pressure monitoring and introduction of a treatment protocol are required for optimal results.

Non-operative Management of Abdominal Compartment Syndrome (ACS)

Early Recognition and Monitoring

- *Measure intra-abdominal pressure (IAP)* regularly in at-risk patients using bladder pressure measurements.
- Monitor for *signs of organ dysfunction* (renal, respiratory, cardiovascular).

Optimize Fluid Management

- Avoid excessive fluid resuscitation (positive fluid balance ↑ IAP).
- Use goal-directed fluid therapy (based on lactate clearance, urine output, etc.).
- Consider *diuretics or fluid restriction* in stable patients with fluid overload.
- *Colloids* may reduce total fluid volume requirements.

Improve Abdominal Wall Compliance

- Ensure adequate *sedation and analgesia* to minimize muscle tension.
- Use *neuromuscular blockade (NMB)* temporarily to reduce abdominal wall tone.
- Avoid tight dressings, abdominal binders, or anything that restricts the abdominal wall.

Decompress Gastrointestinal Tract

- *Nasogastric (NG) tube* to decompress the stomach.
- *Rectal tube* to relieve colonic distention.
- Administer *prokinetic agents* (e.g., metoclopramide, erythromycin) to promote GI motility.
- Avoid constipation—use *laxatives or enemas* if appropriate.

Optimize Ventilation and Perfusion

- Adjust ventilator settings (especially in patients with ARDS) to prevent increased thoracic pressure.
- Ensure adequate *mean arterial pressure (MAP)* to maintain abdominal perfusion pressure (APP = MAP-IAP).
- Target *APP > 60 mm Hg* to ensure organ perfusion.

Medical Adjuncts

- Consider use of *vasoactive agents* to support perfusion if hypotension is present.
- *Avoid nephrotoxic drugs* in the setting of renal hypoperfusion.

Treat Underlying Causes

- Prompt management of *sepsis, pancreatitis, bowel obstruction*, or *hemorrhage* to reduce IAP.
- Evacuate *intra-abdominal fluid collections or hematomas* if accessible via percutaneous drainage.

Frequent Reassessment

- Recheck IAP every 4–6 hours (or more often) depending on clinical status.
- Watch for worsening organ dysfunction despite non-operative measures.

Indications for Transition to Surgical Decompression

If non-operative measures fail and any of the following are present:

- Sustained IAP >25 mm Hg with new organ dysfunction.
- Worsening acidosis, oliguria/anuria, or respiratory compromise.
- Refractory hypotension or multiorgan failure.

Conditions Requiring Temporary Closures

- Primary closure of the abdominal cavity cannot be accomplished
- Primary closure of the abdominal cavity should not be done
  - Stage, or "damage control" laparotomy
  - "Second-look" operation required
  - Abdominal compartment syndrome prophylaxis
- Development of abdominal compartment

Pathogenesis of Different Organ Dysfunction in ACS

Effect on Different Organs

- *Cardiovascular:*
  - A rise in the IAP leads to a fall in cardiac output, mainly due to compression of the inferior vena cava and reduction in venous return to the heart.
  - Cardiac output is reduced despite apparent rises in CVP, pulmonary artery occlusion pressure, and systemic vascular resistance.
- *Respiratory:*
  - Raised IAP will effectively splint the diaphragm and lead to a rise in peak airway pressure and intra-thoracic pressure and subsequently a reduced venous return to the heart.
  - The increase in airway pressures may also exacerbate barotrauma and contribute to the development of acute respiratory distress syndrome.
- *Renal:*
  - An acute increase in intra-abdominal pressure leads to oliguria and anuria probably due to compression of the renal vein and renal parenchyma.
  - Renal blood flow and glomerular filtration are decreased with a corresponding increase in renal vascular resistance.
- *Cerebral:*
  - The rise in IAP and intrathoracic pressure leads to a rise in CVP which prevents adequate venous drainage from the brain, leading to a rise in intracranial pressure and worsening of intracerebral edema.

When the decision is made that the abdominal cavity should not be closed, all efforts should be made to preserve the fascia for later definitive closure.

There are Several Temporary Closures of the Abdominal Cavity

A. *Endogenous*—nonfascial closure:
  - *Towel clip closure* (skin only)—2 cm from the edge and 2 cm apart, covered by an adherent plastic drape.
  - Suture closure—skin only ("the mortician closure")

B. *Closure with prosthetics:*
  - *Plastic silo*—polyvinyl plastic silo, plastic wound drape can be used for this temporary closure. Some have advocated the 3-L plastic bag, primarily used on the urologic service for irrigation. All silo material should be sewn to the skin.

C. *Mesh:*
  - *Absorbable:* Polyglactin or polyglycolic are often used when it is felt that primary closure cannot be achieved within a brief interval of days and that secondary closure by granulation tissue over the midgut will be necessary. Four stages in the use of absorbable mesh to cover the abdominal cavity are:

    Fabian Protocol

    I. Coverage of the midgut with absorbable mesh
    II. Removal of mesh after formation of granulation (2–3 weeks)
    III. Application of split-thickness skin grafts
    IV. Definitive closure in 6–12 months
  - *Nonabsorbable:* There are more permanent meshes such as polypropylene mesh or Gore-Tex patch.

D. *Zippers or Velcro devices:* The overall concept of these devices is appealing, because they allow repeated evaluations of the abdominal cavity, along with the ability to perform necessary irrigations of the contaminated field.

Open Abdomen (OA)

- There are situations when the abdominal cavity is left open for a period of time because of either early or late abdominal sepsis due to failure of the closed/semiclosed methods.

- Although the exposed bowel can be directly covered with moist gauze packs, the risk of intestinal fistula formation is still exceedingly high.

Vacuum-assisted Temporary Abdominal Closure (TAC) Device

- A thin plastic sheet, a sterile towel, closed suction drains, and a large adherent operative drape
- This dressing system permits increases in intra-abdominal volume, without a dramatic elevation in IAP.

OPEN ABDOMEN

5. Management of patients with OA. ***WBUHS 2015***

Introduction

- The term "open abdomen" refers to a defect in the abdominal wall that exposes the abdominal viscera.
- Damage control surgery (DCS) associated with trauma and ACS are the most frequent reasons for leaving an abdomen open.
- OA exposes the viscera and leads to fluid and heat loss, which can be reduced with TAC techniques until the abdomen can be closed primarily, closed functionally, or graft coverage of the exposed viscera provided.

OA

- Mortality and complication rates remain high.
- Abdominal wall/gut reconstruction after a period of open management, may be extremely technically challenging (especially in the setting of an intestinal fistula) and is best undertaken in specialist centers.

Indications for and Management of the OA

- Intestine is a highly vascularized structure with a rich network of arteries, veins, capillaries, and lymphatics.
- In pathologic states, decreased fluid clearance from the extracellular space can result in swelling of the intestinal wall several times the normal diameter, potentially interfering with bowel perfusion.
- Furthermore, the peritoneal surface is highly vascularized and possesses inflammatory cells.
- The net result is excretion of pro-inflammatory substances that increase the local inflammatory response as well as systemic absorption leading to SIRS and may progress to a multiorgan dysfunction syndrome (MODS).
- Premature closure of the abdomen can exacerbate the inflammatory response and potentially accelerate the syndrome.

Pathophysiology

OA Treatment

- The OA treatment can be defined as leaving the fascial edges of the abdominal wall intentionally unapproximated.
- *Aliases include:* Laparostomy and TAC lavage
- Nowadays, the OA procedure has been widely applied and has improved clinical outcomes.

Indications to Leave the Abdomen Open

- Major abdominal trauma
- Massive bowel edema
- Need for multiple explorations
- Extensive abdominal wall defects re-explorations
- IAH
- ACS
- *Severe abdominal sepsis:* As in secondary peritonitis, unsatisfactory source control
    - Theoretically, OA is assumed to improve drainage and increases bacterial killing (improved oxygenation). Very little evidence is there to support this technique in treating intra-abdominal infections depending on the degree of peritoneal contamination per se.

The only two sufficient indications for OA management are:
1. Intestinal edema from sepsis or resuscitation that may precipitate ACS if the abdomen is closed
2. Planned reoperation

Complications of OA Management

Ileus	Esophageal atresia (EA) fistula	Bleeding	Hernia	Heat/fluid loss
Infection	Defective ventilation	Defective ventilation	Fascial retraction	Fascial retraction

These complications can be minimized by:
- Understanding the pathophysiology found in the OA
- Using materials that minimize trauma to the abdominal contents
- Prevention of severe intra-abdominal sepsis
- Facilitation of multiple re-explorations, if needed
- Prevention of abdominal wall loss
- Tension-free fascial closure

Management of a Patient with OA
- *General management:*

Wound management	IV fluids	Heat loss control	Analgesia and sedation
Nutrition	TAC	Dressing	Definitive closure

- *IV fluid administration:*
  - The first 24 hours in an ICU after returning from OR frequently require large fluid infusions to optimize preload.
  - It can be challenging to balance this need with the restrictive resuscitation that minimizes visceral edema.
  - Literature favors early aggressive fluid resuscitation guided by goal-directed fluid therapy followed by the use of vasopressors to maintain physiological parameters.
- *Heat loss control:*
  - On arrival in the ICU, patients are frequently cold.
  - The OA will further increase heat loss.
  - Active and passive methods of rewarming may be required.
- *Analgesia and sedation:*
  - The need for analgesia is not significantly different to that after major surgery in which the abdomen is closed.
  - Pain control will go hand in hand with the management of agitation and stress of the striking sight of OA, especially if associated with enteroatmospheric fistula (EAF).
  - Established protocols involve the use of fentanyl and midazolam in combination, with expert and sympathetic psychological support.
- *Nutrition:*
  - OA may represent a source of protein/nitrogen loss (patients are inevitably severely insulin resistant and profoundly catabolic).
  - Intestinal failure develops in at least 15% of these patients.
  - Enteral nutrition (EN) should be employed whenever possible (↓ septic complications and↓ time before closure).
  - Patients with EAF usually require parenteral nutrition (PN) but may also be satisfactorily fed by "fistuloclysis."
  - Nutritional support can be optimized by consultation with specialist dieticians.
- *Temporary abdominal closure (TAC):*
  - OA is maintained by a TAC device.

- Many techniques exist; the ideal technique should fulfill the following goals:
    - Easy reaccess to the abdominal cavity (patients with OA require multiple trips to the OR, i.e., every 24–48 hours for as long as 2 or 3 weeks using staged abdominal explorations).
    - Protection of the abdominal contents
    - Prevention of (or better lowering) bacterial contamination and infection
    - Prevention of evisceration (selective tamponade)
    - Preservation of fascia
    - Prevention of fascial retraction and loss of domain
    - Quantification of the third space losses
    - Keeping the patient dry.
    - Providing abdominal support for ventilation.
    - Prevention of IAH (high-risk patients can rapidly develop high abdominal pressures secondary to bleeding, pack placement, and rapid accumulation of the third space fluid)

TAC

Vacuum Pack Technique or "Vacuum-assisted Closure" or "Negative-pressure Wound Therapy (NPWT)"

- A simple three-layer system using negative pressure for abdominal support:
    I. *Fenestrated polyurethane sheet wrap* around the bowels (prevents bowel adherence to the anterior abdominal wall and facilitates fluid drainage)
    II. *Sponge (granular foam dressing)*
    III. *Adhesive plastic sheet (applied over the sponge)*
- A uniform suction (100–150 mm Hg or lower if hemostasis is crucial) is applied to the sponge layer using sophisticated software giving specific alarms when NPWT is impaired or interrupted.

General Indications of NPWT

- Chronic wounds [e.g., methicillin-resistant *Staphylococcus aureus* (MRSA)]
- OA
- Partial-thickness burns
- Indolent ulcers [diabetes mellitus (DM), bed sores, and venous]

Mechanism of action: Continuous negative pressure applied to the wound surface helps wound healing by evoking two wound responses:

A. Physical response:
    - Approximation of wound edges
    - Removal of excess fluids
    - Reduction of tissue edema
B. Biological response:
    - Removal of exudates that may contain inhibitors of healing
    - Reduction of edema with better tissue perfusion
    - Cell-surface strain (microdeformation) by negative pressure induces cellular stretch → cells become more metabolically active → fibroblast migration, cell proliferation, extracellular matrix deposition
    - With repeated dressing, the granulation tissue gradually fills the gap allowing subsequent secondary closure.
    - Granulation tissue formation

Alternatives Include Bogota Bag or two Plastic Sheets Stuck Together with Perforations

- *Dressing:* After the decision has been made to leave the abdomen open, dressing should be available in the theater.
    - Easy to apply
    - Protecting the skin and viscera to ↓ fistula formation
    - Easy to remove for redressing

- *Definitive closure at a second-look laparotomy "delayed primary closure":*
    - Plan a strategy for closing the abdomen at almost the same time as the decision to leave it open.
    - *Timing:* In general, delayed primary closure will be possible within several days, once hemodynamic stability and visceral edema subside (IAH is avoided).
    - When the abdomen is left open for long periods, fascial retraction with loss of domain ensues. If it is not possible to close the abdomen by day 10, it may not be possible at all.
    - Delayed primary closure is more likely to be possible after DCS for surgery or hemorrhage (e.g., ruptured AAA) than for treatment of abdominal sepsis or ACS.
    - When primary closure is not possible, fascial closure rates of 60% at a second-look laparotomy have been reported although the rate of incisional hernia may be as high as 30%.
    - If so, available options may include:
        - Planned ventral hernia
        - Skin graft
        - Component separation
        - Canica abdominal reapproximation anchor (ABRA) closure system

Planned Ventral Hernia

- Collagenization of the wound converts granulation tissue into scar.
- Absorbable mesh may be used to provide some stability to the abdominal wall.
- Wound contraction will occur over 3–6 months.
- Over the succeeding months to a year, the collagen is slowly removed, and a hernia will become apparent.
- Surgical correction carries extensive risks with at least a 30% complication rate including:

Skin necrosis	Abdominal compartment syndrome	Skin grafting	Prolonged intubation	Recurrence
Bowel ischemia		Easier wound care	Wound infection	Death

Skin Graft

- Less EAF rates
- Viscera are left to granulate, and a skin graft is undertaken.
- Giant ventral hernia is inevitable but can be repaired after an interval of at least 6–12 months.

Component Separation Technique

- The abdominal wall flap is mobilized from the underlying fascia; this is done until lateral to the linea semilunaris.
- Care to be taken to maintain the abdominal wall muscle perforators to avoid devascularization of the skin
- A small incision is then made in the external oblique just lateral to the linea semilunaris
- With the aid of a hemostat, the incision is taken cephalad till the lower ribs and caudad to the pubis using cautery.
- Medial traction of the rectus muscle by the assistant helps to accomplish the procedure.
- This is done bilaterally.
- Up to 14 cm can be gained in the abdominal wall per side.
- Midline closure
- In rare circumstances, adequate skin cover is not possible despite the application of the previously described techniques.
- Complex myocutaneous flaps have been successfully used to close such defects.
- Success with anterolateral thigh and rectus abdominis flaps have been described.
- Gore-Tex Dual Mesh in the initial stage
- Subsequent stages involve serial excision-towel clamping of the mesh or resuturing of the mesh every 72 hours to 2 weeks.
- Vacuum-assisted closure (VAC) may be placed over the mesh.

- Mesh is then excised, and the fascia is reapproximated with component separation and bioprosthetic reinforcement
- Allows for primary closure in ~90% without planned ventral hernia.
- Average time to definitive closure is 46 days.

ABRA Closure System

- It restores the primary closure option for full-thickness abdominal defects by approximating the skin and fascial margins for low-tension primary closure.
- It acts by turning the "flat abdomen" with eviscerating contents to a "rounded abdomen" with a more voluminous abdominal cavity.
- All necrotic tissues, adhesions, or unhealthy granulation tissues are excised to achieve clean mobile wound margins.
- Any pre-existing abdominal closure device should be removed prior to ABRA application.
- ABRA—The abdominal reapproximation anchor system

BURST ABDOMEN

6. Management of burst abdomen. ***WBUHS 2006***

The basic treatment principle for the repair of the disrupted wound is resuturing of wound edges.

- *Nonoperative management:* It is utilized for unstable patients, or where there is no evisceration, or fascial closure is not possible because of bowel edema.
  - Abdominal binder to support disrupted abdominal wound
  - Gauge packing/covering the gut with a sterile moist occlusive dressing. This allows the abdominal wall to granulate which may be skin grafted later. A ventral develops which is treated after 6 months, when the inflammatory process subsides facilitating entry into the abdomen.
- *Operative treatment:* Heavy nonabsorbable suture such as nylon or polypropylene no. 1 is used. Wide interrupted sutures with bites of 3 cm from the edge at a distance of 3 cm or less are taken. External sutures are removed after 3 weeks.
- *Unclosable abdomen:* Sometimes, it is difficult to close the abdomen because of:
  - Gross abdominal sepsis
  - Major abdominal trauma
  - Retroperitoneal hematoma
  - Loss of abdominal wall due to necrotizing fasciitis

Various techniques of TAC are used as follows:

- *Skin-only closure:* This is done when the patient needs re-exploration within 24 hours.
- *Bogota bag:* This is made by gas-sterilized urobag which is cut in an oval shape and sutured to skin or rectus sheath. The advantages of this method of closure are easy availability, low cost, nonadherence to gut, prevention of evisceration, and ease of application.

  Disadvantages of the technique are tearing of the skin, adherence of the bowel to the abdominal wall, and no control of third space fluid loss which leaks out and produces hypothermia and hypovolemia.
- *Mesh closure:* Its advantages include the use of placement and facilitation of re-exploration. The three types of meshes in use are:
  1. *Absorbable mesh:* It is used for temporary closure and is good for infected abdomen, but incisional hernia is inevitable.
  2. *Polypropylene mesh:* It is a nonabsorbable mesh with a risk of erosion to bowel and fistula formation. It resists infection and forms dense adhesions.

3. *Polytetrafluoroethylene (PTFE):* The main advantage of PTFE is relative freedom from adhesion formation. It is soft and pliable and conforms to the defect very well. The disadvantages are poor tolerance to infection, inability to skin graft, and high cost.

- *Wittmann patch:* This allows re-exploration and facilitates closure of the abdomen with serial narrowing and trimming of mesh. The incidence of IAH and ACS is high with the Wittmann patch.
- *Vacuum pack:* it is a modification of the Bogota bag. A nonadherent polyethylene sheet with fenestrations is placed over the viscera and covered with moist towels. Two silicone drains are placed over the towels and the wound is sealed with iodoform-impregnated adhesive dressings. Continuous wall suction is applied at 100–150 mm Hg. Patients are serially re-explored at the time of change of dressings.
- *VAC therapy:* Here, primary closure of the abdominal wall can be achieved.
- *Sure-closure skin-stretching system application*
- *Delayed primary fascial closure:* This can be done within 7–10 days if the abdominal cavity can be closed without a significant rise in IAP.
- *Fabian protocol:* It provides staged care of the burst abdominal wound. The patients are then brought after 6–12 months for abdominal wall reconstruction.
    - *Stage I:* Absorbable mesh placement
    - *Stage II:* Mesh removal or allowance of granulation tissue to grow
    - *Stage III:* Split-thickness skin graft if granulation tissue is adequate
    - *Stage IV:* Definite abdominal reconstruction.

---

7. Discuss laparoscopic management of acute abdomen. ***Tripura University 2024; WBUHS 2010***

The acute abdomen is characterized by the sudden appearance of abdominal complaints that oblige the surgeon to decide promptly whether to operate immediately, to treat conservatively or to observe the patient.

Possibilities for initial diagnosis of the acute abdomen:

- Localized peritonitis
    - Acute cholecystitis
    - Acute appendicitis (right lower abdomen)
    - Acute diverticulitis

Generalized peritonitis of unknown origin:

- Peritonitis by perforation
    - Perforated gastroduodenal ulcer
    - Perforated acute diverticulitis (colon sigmoid)
    - Small intestinal perforation (typhoid, trauma)

Intestinal obstruction:

- Role of laparoscopic procedure in different causes of acute abdomen;
    - Percutaneous transhepatic cholecystostomy is a valuable and effective procedure in a high-risk group of patients with acute cholecystitis.
    - Early laparoscopic cholecystectomy is the treatment of choice in patients with acute cholecystitis with acceptable risk.
    - Helical CT or an USG will resolve the diagnosis in many patients with right iliac fossa.
    - All patients suspected of acute appendicitis should have an USG. Patients will be clinically divided in equivocal and unequivocal appendicitis.
    - Unequivocal clinical diagnosis plus positive USG will require diagnostic laparoscopy followed by laparoscopic appendicectomy.
    - Unequivocal clinical diagnosis plus negative USG will lead to clinical observation. Helical CT should be done to exclude other diagnoses. If the clinical condition worsens, a diagnostic laparoscopy should be performed.

- An equivocal clinical diagnosis will lead to clinical observation. If local peritonitis develop, a diagnostic laparoscopy should be performed.
- Diagnostic laparoscopy should be performed in all patients with signs of generalized acute abdomen in whom no clear cause is suspected after clinical, radiological and laboratory investigation. A correct diagnosis will dictate the right surgical approach.
- Laparoscopic closure of perforated duodenal ulcer, in experienced hands, confers superior short-term benefits in terms of postoperative pain and wound morbidity.
- Laparoscopic lavage and drainage in the acute management of perforated acute diverticulitis is a promising alternative to more radical procedures.
- Laparoscopy is an effective procedure for the treatment of acute small bowel obstruction with acceptable risk of morbidity and early recurrence, but conversion rates of 30–40%, should be expected.

8. Principles in USG imaging and its role in acute abdomen. ***KIIT University, Odisha 2025***

Principles of Ultrasonography (USG) Imaging

Ultrasonography (USG) is a noninvasive imaging technique that uses *high-frequency sound waves* to produce real-time images of internal organs, tissues, and blood flow. The core principles include:

- *Sound wave transmission and reflection:*
  - A *transducer* emits high-frequency sound waves (2–15 MHz) into the body.
  - These waves interact with tissues and organs and are *reflected back* to the transducer depending on tissue density and composition.
- *Echo generation:*
  - Different tissues reflect sound waves differently (based on *acoustic impedance*).
    - *Fluid-filled structures* (e.g., gallbladder, cysts) appear *anechoic* (dark).
    - *Solid organs* (e.g., liver, spleen) show varying *echogenicity*.
    - *Air* or *bone* causes high reflection or shadowing.
- *Image construction:* Reflected echoes are converted into electrical signals and processed by the machine to form a *real-time grayscale image*.
- *Doppler principles (Optional):*
  - Doppler USG assesses *blood flow* by measuring frequency shifts in the reflected waves.
  - Useful in detecting vascular abnormalities or perfusion.

Role of USG in Acute Abdomen

USG is often the *first-line imaging modality* in patients with acute abdominal pain due to its availability, speed, safety (no radiation), and diagnostic utility. It is particularly helpful in *differentiating surgical from nonsurgical causes*.

Key Roles

- *Gallbladder and biliary tract:*
  - Detects *cholelithiasis, cholecystitis* (thickened wall, pericholecystic fluid), and *biliary dilation*.
  - Can show *gallstones, CBD stones,* or *biliary sludge*.
- *Liver and spleen:*
  - Identifies *liver abscesses, trauma, hematomas,* or *splenic rupture*.
  - Evaluates for *hepatomegaly, cirrhosis,* or *portal hypertension*.
- *Appendix:*
  - Can confirm *acute appendicitis* (noncompressible tubular structure >6 mm, periappendiceal fluid).
  - Particularly useful in children and thin patients.
- *Kidneys and urinary tract:*
  - Identifies *hydronephrosis, renal stones, pyelonephritis,* or *urinary retention*.
  - Helps rule out *obstructive uropathy*.

- *Gynecological causes:*
  - Evaluates *ectopic pregnancy, ovarian torsion, ruptured ovarian cyst, or PID.*
  - *Transvaginal USG* provides higher accuracy.
- *Aorta and vascular:* Screens for *abdominal aortic aneurysm (AAA)* or *aortic dissection* in unstable patients.
- *Free fluid or gas:*
  - Can detect *free intraperitoneal fluid* (e.g., blood in trauma or ascites).
  - Limited in detecting *free air*, which is better seen on X-ray or CT.
- *Intestinal pathologies:* Can aid in diagnosing *intussusception, bowel wall thickening*, or *obstruction* (with dilated loops and peristalsis assessment).

Advantages of USG in Acute Abdomen

- Bedside capability (e.g., *FAST scan* in trauma)
- No radiation
- Safe in pregnancy and pediatric populations
- Dynamic assessment (e.g., peristalsis, tenderness)

Limitations

- Operator-dependent
- Limited by *obesity* or *bowel gas*
- Less effective for deep or complex intra-abdominal pathology compared to CT.

Esophagus and Stomach

LEARNING OBJECTIVES

- Esophageal Manometry
- Motility Disorders of Esophagus
- Benign Esophageal Stricture
- Corrosive Poisoning
- Esophageal Perforation
- GERD and Hiatus Hernia
- Barrett's Esophagus
- Esophageal Cancer
- GE Junction Tumour
- Dieulafoy's Lesion
- *H. pylori* and Peptic Ulcer Disease
- Gastric Volvulus
- Gastric Outlet Obstruction and Carcinoma Stomach
- D1 versus D2 Gastrectomy
- Roux Syndrome
- Recent Advances in the Management of Gastric Cancer
- Role of Intraperitoneal Chemotherapy and Molecular Targeted Therapy in Carcinoma Stomach

ESOPHAGEAL MANOMETRY

ZENKER'S DIVERTICULUM

1. Zenker's diverticulum and its management. ***Gujarat Health University 2025***

Zenker's Diverticulum (Pharyngoesophageal Diverticulum)

Definition

Zenker's diverticulum is a *pulsion-type false diverticulum* that occurs in the *posterior hypopharyngeal wall,* just above the *upper esophageal sphincter (cricopharyngeus muscle).*

- It involves *herniation of mucosa and submucosa* through a weak area of muscle known as *Killian's dehiscence.*
- Because only mucosa and submucosa protrude, it's a *false diverticulum* (not all layers of the wall are involved).

Location

- At the *junction of the pharynx and esophagus,* specifically:
  - Between the *thyropharyngeus* (part of inferior pharyngeal constrictor) and *cricopharyngeus* muscles.

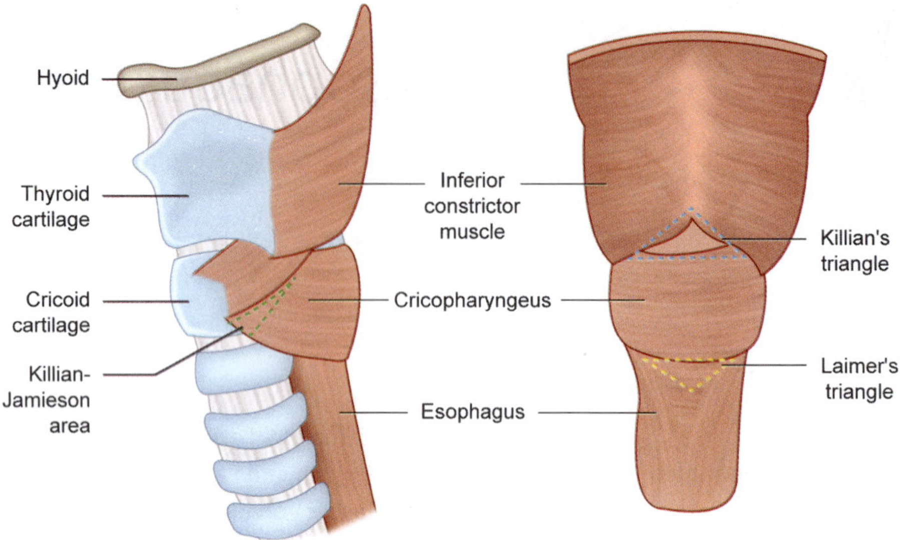

Pathophysiology (Mechanism)

- *Cricopharyngeal dysfunction* → failure of the upper esophageal sphincter to relax properly during swallowing.
- This causes *increased intraluminal pressure* during swallowing.
- The mucosa herniates posteriorly through *Killian's dehiscence* → forming the diverticulum.

Type

- *False (pseudodiverticulum)*—only mucosa and submucosa.
- *Pulsion diverticulum*—due to increased internal pressure (not traction).

Common in

- Elderly men (typically >60 years old)

Clinical Features

- *Dysphagia* (difficulty swallowing, especially solids)
- *Regurgitation* of undigested food (sometimes hours after eating)
- *Halitosis (foul breath)*—due to food retention
- *Coughing or choking* while eating
- *Aspiration pneumonia*
- *Neck mass* that may gurgle on palpation (rare, in large diverticula)
- *"Boyce's sign"*—gurgling noise in the neck on palpation

Diagnosis

- *Barium swallow (esophagogram)* → shows posterior outpouching above the esophagus.
- *Endoscopy* — may confirm diagnosis but should be done *with caution* (risk of perforation).

Treatment

Definitive treatment is surgical (relieves obstruction and eliminates the pouch).

Options

- *Endoscopic diverticulotomy (stapling or laser division)*
  - Minimally invasive
  - Divides the *common wall (septum)* between diverticulum and esophagus
  - Often done with *cricopharyngeal myotomy*
- *Open surgery (for large or complicated diverticula):* Diverticulectomy + cricopharyngeal myotomy
- *Cricopharyngeal myotomy* is essential in all cases to prevent recurrence.

Complications
- Aspiration pneumonia
- Ulceration or bleeding within the pouch
- Rarely, *carcinoma* (squamous cell carcinoma) in long-standing cases
- Perforation during endoscopy

INVESTIGATIONS

2. Esophageal manometry. ***WBUHS 2021 Supplementary***

Introduction

Esophageal manometry is a test that is used to measure the function of the lower esophageal sphincter (the valve that prevents reflux, or backward flow, of gastric acid into the esophagus) and the muscles of the esophagus.

Indications

Esophageal manometry is indicated for the following situations:
- Evaluation of noncardiac chest pain or esophageal symptoms not diagnosed by endoscopy [or after gastroesophageal reflux disease (GERD) has been excluded]
- Evaluation for achalasia or another type of nonobstructive dysphagia
- Preoperative evaluation for patients undergoing corrective surgery for GERD, particularly if an alternative diagnosis such as scleroderma or achalasia is being considered.
- Postoperative evaluation of dysphagia in patients who underwent corrective surgery for reflux or after treatment of achalasia
- Prior to esophageal pH monitoring to assess the location of the LES for proper electrode positioning
- Evaluation of esophageal motility problems associated with systemic diseases

According to the Lyon Consensus, high-resolution manometry (HRM) is not useful for the direct diagnosis of GERD but can be useful in the setting of GERD by providing adjunctive information [e.g., on esophagogastric junction (EGJ) barrier function, esophageal body motor function, contractile function, or EGJ obstruction].

Contraindications

Esophageal manometry is contraindicated in the following situations:
- Patients with altered mental status or obtundation
- Patients who cannot understand or follow instructions
- Suspected or known pharyngeal or upper esophageal obstruction (e.g., tumors)

MOTILITY DISORDERS OF ESOPHAGUS

3. Enumerate the motility disorders of esophagous. Briefly describe Achalasia cardia. ***WBUHS 2021***

Classification of Motility Disorders of Esophagus

Inadequate LES relaxation	*Uncoordinated contraction*	*Hypercontraction*	*Hypocontraction*
• Classic achalasia • Atypical disorders of LES relaxation	Diffuse esophageal spasm	• Nutcracker esophagus • Isolated hypertensive LES	Ineffective esophageal motility

(LES: lower esophageal sphincter)

Achalasia Cardia

Introduction

Achalasia is rare but is the most common primary esophageal motility disorder. Achalasia is characterized by loss of effective esophageal body peristalsis and failure of the LES to relax with swallowing, resulting in esophageal dilation.

Epidemiology

- Primary achalasia is most frequently seen in middle and late adulthood (age 30–70 years) with no gender predilection.
- Most cases are idiopathic; however, a similar appearance may occur in Chagas disease.
- Patients with Allgrove syndrome (triple A syndrome) also have achalasia which is very similar to the primary form of the disease.

Pathology

The characteristic pathology is alteration in the ganglia of Auerbach plexus.

Clinical Features

- The classic triad of presenting symptoms consists of dysphagia, regurgitation, and weight loss.
- However, heartburn, postprandial choking, and nocturnal coughing are seen commonly.
- The dysphagia that patients experience begins with liquids and progresses to solids.
- As the water builds up pressure, retrosternal chest pain is experienced and can be quite severe until the LES opens and is quickly relieving.
- Regurgitation of undigested, foul-smelling foods is common, and with progressive disease, aspiration can become life-threatening. Pneumonia, lung abscess, and bronchiectasis often result from long-standing achalasia.
- The dysphagia progresses slowly over years, and patients adapt their lifestyle to accommodate the inconveniences that accompany this disease.
- Patients often do not seek medical attention until their symptoms are quite advanced and will present with marked distension of the esophagus.

Investigations

- Diagnostic chest X-ray (CXR) often shows a fluid-filled, dilated esophagus, and absence of a gastric air bubble.
- A barium esophagogram demonstrates tapering (bird's beak) of the distal esophagus and a dilated proximal esophagus.
- Esophageal manometry is the definitive diagnostic test for achalasia.
  Characteristic manometric findings include the absence of peristalsis, mirror-image, contractions, and limited or absent relaxation of the LES with swallowing.
- Endoscopy rules out benign strictures or malignancy.
  When these symptoms are caused by malignant obstruction, the syndrome is referred to as pseudoachalasia.

Classification

It may be divided into three distinct types based on manometric patterns:

1. Type I (classic) with minimal contractility in the esophageal body
2. Type II with intermittent periods of panesophageal pressurization
3. Type III (spastic) with premature or spastic distal esophageal contractions

Treatment

- Medical treatment decreases the LES tone and includes nitrates and calcium-channel blockers.
- Surgical treatment with a modified Heller esophagomyotomy has been shown to produce excellent results in >90% of patients.

A concomitant antireflux procedure (270° or 180° fundoplication) with the esophagomyotomy helps avoid late stricture due to GERD caused by the incompetent LES:

- Peroral endoscopic myotomy (POEM) consists of endoscopically creating a submucosal tunnel; then dividing the circular muscle layer of distal esophagus, LES, and proximal stomach, keeping the mucosa intact.
- Dysphagia outcomes, postoperative pain, and symptomatic GERD are similar to laparoscopic Heller/fundoplication.
- POEM is highly effective in relieving symptoms of achalasia; patients can experience significant GERD postoperatively.

4. Etiology, different methods of diagnosis, and treatment of achalasia cardia.
The Tamil Nadu Dr MGR Medical University 2025; WBUHS 2021 Supplementary

Etiology

- There is some evidence that achalasia is an autoimmune disease.
- A European study compared immune-related deoxyribonucleic acid (DNA) in persons with achalasia with that of controls and found 33 single-nucleotide polymorphisms (SNPs) associated with achalasia. All of them were found in the major histocompatibility complex region of chromosome 6, a location associated with auto immune disorders such as multiple sclerosis, lupus, and type 1 diabetes.
- Primary achalasia is most frequently seen in middle and late adulthood (age 30–70 years) with no gender predilection.
- Most cases are idiopathic; however, a similar appearance may occur in Chagas disease.
- Patients with Allgrove syndrome (triple A syndrome) also have achalasia which is very similar to the primary form of the disease.

Diagnosis

Recommendations for the proper diagnosis of the disorder include the following:

- Performing an esophageal motility test on all patients suspected of having achalasia
- Using esophagram findings to support a diagnosis
- Using barium esophagram, as recommended for patients with equivocal motility testing
- Endoscopic assessment of the gastroesophageal junction and gastric cardia, as recommended, to rule out pseudoachalasia

Laboratory Studies are Generally Noncontributory

Esophageal pressure topography (EPT) may be the preferred assessment modality of esophageal motility over conventional line tracings (CLT).

Plain Radiograph

Chest radiograph findings include:

- Convex opacity overlapping the right mediastinum. Occasionally may present as a left convex opacity if the thoracic aorta is tortuous.
- Air-fluid level due to stasis in a thoracic esophagus filled with retained secretions and food
- Small or absent gastric bubble
- Anterior displacement and bowing of the trachea on the lateral view
- Patchy alveolar opacities, usually bilateral, may be seen. These represent acute pneumonitis or chronic aspiration pneumonia related to dysphagia.

Fluoroscopy with Barium Swallow

A barium swallow study may be used to confirm esophageal dilatation, in addition to assessing for mucosal abnormalities.

Findings

- Bird beak sign or rat tail sign
- Esophageal dilatation
- *Tram track appearance:* Central longitudinal lucency bounded by barium on both sides
- Incomplete LES relaxation that is not coordinated with esophageal contraction
- Pooling or stasis of barium in the esophagus when the esophagus has become atonic or noncontractile (a late feature in the disease)
- Uncoordinated, nonpropulsive, and tertiary contractions
- Failure of normal peristalsis to clear the esophagus of barium when the patient is in the recumbent position, with no primary waves identified.

- When the barium column is high enough (with the patient standing), the hydrostatic pressure can overcome the LES pressure, allowing passage of esophageal content.
- A hot or carbonated drink during the examination may help visualize sphincter relaxation and barium emptying

Computed Tomography (CT)

- Patients with uncomplicated achalasia demonstrate a dilated, thin-walled esophagus filled with fluid/food debris.
- Overall, CT has little role in directly assessing patients with achalasia, but is useful in assessing common complications.
- Careful assessment of the wall of the esophagus should be undertaken to identify any focal regions of thickening which may indicate malignancy.
- The lungs should be inspected for evidence of aspiration.

Esophageal Manometry

It is the criterion standard in helping to diagnose the classic findings of achalasia. These findings include the following:

- Incomplete relaxation of the LES in response to swallowing
- High resting LES pressure
- Absent esophageal peristalsis

Prolonged esophageal pH monitoring is important for the following reasons:

- To rule out GERD
- To determine if abnormal reflux is being caused by treatment

Treatment Recommendations

- Initial therapy should be either graded pneumatic dilation (PD) or laparoscopic surgical myotomy with a partial fundoplication in patients fit to undergo surgery.
- Procedures should be performed in high-volume centers of excellence.
- Initial therapy choice should be based on patient age, sex, preference, and local institutional expertise.
- Botulinum toxin therapy is recommended for patients not suited to PD or surgery.
- Pharmacologic therapy can be used for patients not undergoing PD or myotomy and who have failed botulinum toxin therapy (nitrates and calcium channel blockers most common).
- The goal of therapy for achalasia is to relieve symptoms by eliminating the outflow resistance caused by the hypertensive and nonrelaxing LES. Once the obstruction is relieved, the food bolus can travel through the aperistaltic body of the esophagus by gravity.
- Calcium channel blockers and nitrates are used to decrease LES pressure.
- Approximately, 10% of patients benefit from this treatment. This treatment is used primarily in elderly patients who have contraindications to either pneumatic dilatation or surgery.
    - Endoscopic treatment includes an intrasphincteric injection of botulinum toxin to block the release of acetylcholine at the level of the LES, thereby restoring the balance between excitatory and inhibitory neurotransmitters.
    - This treatment has limited value. Only 30% of patients treated endoscopically still have relief of dysphagia 1 year after treatment. Most patients need repeated botulinum toxin injections, with short-lasting clinical benefits.
    - Pneumatic dilatation performed by a qualified gastroenterologist is the recommended treatment in those sporadic cases in which surgery is not appropriate.
    - A laparoscopic Heller myotomy is considered by many to be the appropriate primary treatment of patients with achalasia. A Heller myotomy and a partial fundoplication performed from the chest (thoracoscopic) have a high incidence of gastroesophageal reflux.
    - Peroral endoscopic myotomy has been introduced relatively recently as a novel approach to achalasia.

5. Per oral endoscopic myotomy (POEM).

SAIMS, Indore 2025; WBUHS 2014, 2025 Supplementary; NTRUHS, Vijayawada 2025

Introduction
- Peroral endoscopic myotomy is an exciting innovation for the treatment of achalasia.
- POEM has a clinical success rate ranging from 82 to 100%, with a self-limited adverse event occurrence of <10% and no mortality.
- Key anatomic landmarks for this submucosal dissection that are important to recognize, including the aortic arch, left main bronchus, and left atrium.

Contraindications to Performing POEM
- Severe pulmonary disease
- Cirrhosis with portal hypertension
- Severe coagulopathy
- Severe esophageal submucosa fibrosis (e.g., from irradiation)

Other Advantages
- POEM has been shown to be effective in end-stage achalasia (severe sigmoid achalasia or megaesophagus) and does not preclude surgical esophagectomy if unsuccessful.
- This is the treatment of choice for patients with type III achalasia who have a high rate of problematic chest pain after both standard Heller myotomy and PD, likely owing to the relatively short length of muscular disruption limited by these two approaches to the distal esophagus.

Principles
- The targeted length of the myotomy should be ≥6 cm (beginning 2 cm in cardia), and is 8–10 cm on average.
- Longer myotomies have been performed with successful outcomes in patients with well-defined spastic esophageal disorders, including spastic achalasia (Chicago classification type III), jackhammer esophagus, and diffuse esophageal spasm.

Complications: Relatively uncommon, adverse events include bleeding, radiologic mediastinitis, peritonitis, and thoracic effusions.

BENIGN ESOPHAGEAL STRICTURE

6. Benign esophageal stricture. *WBUHS 2013*

Introduction
- Benign (noncancerous) esophageal stricture is a condition in which the diameter of the esophagus is made narrow by scar tissue.
- Even though the condition is not cancerous, it can still cause serious health issues. Narrowing of the esophagus can cause swallowing difficulty and also increases choking risk.

Causes

Benign esophageal stricture can be caused by damage to the esophagus that results in the formation of scar tissue. The most common cause is GERD.

Other Causes of the Condition
- Extended use of a nasogastric (NG) tube (a tube inserted through the nose, into the esophagus and the stomach)
- Ingestion of an acidic or corrosive substance, such as batteries or household cleaners
- Damage caused by an endoscope (a thin, lighted tube used to see images inside the body for evaluation)
- Treatment of esophageal varices (enlarged veins in the esophagus that can bleed and require repair, often with an endoscope)
- Radiation therapy to the chest or neck

Risk Factors
- Previous esophageal scarring
- GERD is the most common cause of scarring.

Symptoms
- *Dysphagia:* Difficulty swallowing or feeling that food is not passing into the stomach normally
- Painful swallowing
- Unintended weight loss
- *Regurgitation of food or liquids:* Substances from the stomach flow back into the esophagus or up into the mouth
- Heartburn

Potential Complications
- Problems with swallowing can prevent people from getting the right amount of food and fluids necessary for good nutrition, which may lead to dehydration and malnutrition.
- With the narrowing of the esophagus, denser solid foods, such as meat, can become lodged in the esophagus above the stricture, causing one to choke or have trouble breathing.
- Regurgitating foods and liquids can result in pulmonary aspiration. This could result in choking or aspiration pneumonia, a condition where the lungs and the airways leading into the lungs become inflamed.

Diagnosis
- *Barium swallow test:* In this test, a series of X-rays of the esophagus are taken during and after drinking a barium contrast material. This contrast material is a liquid that will temporarily coat the linings of esophagus to help it show up more clearly on the X-ray images.
- *Upper GI endoscopy:* In this test, an endoscope is inserted into the esophagus to allow for examination and biopsy of a stricture to determine its cause.
- *Esophageal pH monitoring:* In this test, a tube is inserted through your mouth into your esophagus to measure how much stomach acid enters your esophagus over a 24-hour period.

Treatment

Treatment will vary depending on the severity of the stricture as well as its underlying cause. Treatment options may include:
- *Esophageal dilation:* In most cases, esophageal dilation, or stretching, is the preferred option. This procedure is performed under general or local anesthesia for your comfort. An endoscope is passed through your mouth and into your esophagus, stomach, and small intestine. A small balloon on the end of the endoscope is inflated to stretch the esophagus.
  This procedure may need to be repeated after a period of time to prevent the stricture from narrowing again.
- *Esophageal stent placement:* The insertion of esophageal stents can provide relief from stricture. A stent is a thin tube that may be made of plastic, expandable metal, or flexible mesh material.
- *Diet and lifestyle:* Daily lifestyle and dietary choices can be effective in managing chronic GERD, which is the primary cause of stricture.

Recommendations
- Avoiding tight clothes
- Elevating the head of your bed to reduce backup of stomach contents
- Fasting for 3 hours before bedtime
- Losing approximately 5% of your body weight
- Stopping smoking
- Avoiding alcohol
- Choosing smaller, instead of larger, meals
- Avoiding foods that cause reflux, such as:

Spicy foods	Fatty foods	Carbonated beverages	Chocolate	Coffee and caffeinated products	Tomato-based foods	Citrus products

Drugs and Medication

Proton pump inhibitors (PPIs) are the most effective options for managing GERD.

The PPIs used to control GERD include:

- Omeprazole
- Lansoprazole
- Pantoprazole
- Esomeprazole

Other medications may also be effective in treating GERD and reducing your risk of stricture. They are:

- Antacids
- Sucralfate, which provides a barrier that lines the esophagus and stomach to protect it from acidic stomach juices.
- Medications such as ranitidine and famotidine, which decrease the secretion of acid.
  - *Surgery:* If medication and esophageal dilation are ineffective, surgery is recommended.
  - Treatment can be difficult in the rare cases where stricture is caused by a nonfunctioning esophagus. In these extreme cases, an esophageal replacement may be the only effective option.

CORROSIVE POISONING

7. Management of Corrosive Esophageal Injury. ***WBUHS 2018***

- Corrosive ingestion can be accidental or suicidal.
- It occurs most commonly in children due to accidental ingestion.
- Injury depends upon nature of substance, its viscosity, concentration, amount, and contact time.
- The injury caused by corrosive substances results from ischemia, thrombosis, and inflammation.
- Acid causes instant burning and hence lesser quantity is ingested as compared to alkali and thereby acid causes less severe injury.
- Acid also results in formation of protective eschar which prevents deeper damage but strong acid ingestion can cause transmural injury.

Initial Evaluation

- Short history to be taken regarding the nature and amount of the substance.
- Patient should be asked for symptoms of dysphagia, odynophagia, refusal to drink, chest pain, vomiting, and epigastric pain.
- Any attempt of lavage or vomiting will cause the agent to reflux into the esophagus causing further damage. Hence, lavage or NG tube insertion is avoided.
- Hoarseness of voice and stridor indicates airway injury and should be addressed urgently if present.
- Patient is kept nil per oral (NPO) and fluid resuscitation and broad-spectrum antibiotic is given.
- Available evidence suggests no benefit of PPIs.
- Abdominal and CXR is done to look for pneumoperitoneum, pneumomediastinum, and pleural effusion. Pleural effusion indicates esophageal perforation and requires chest tube drainage.

Phases of Injury

1. Phase of acute necrosis and thrombosis occurs in 1–4 days after ingestion
2. Phase of granulation and ulceration occurs in 3–12 days. Esophagus is most friable in this phase. Any manipulation such as endoscopy or dilatation should be done with great care.
3. Healing phase begins from 3 weeks after injury and usually takes 1–6 months to complete wound healing. Surgery for stricture cases unamendable to dilatation should wait beyond this period.

Upper GI Endoscopy

Early endoscopy is recommended as 30% of patients will have no injury to the esophagus and can be discharged. Endoscopy is usually done within 24–48 hours after ingestion. After that endoscopy is not advised as esophagus may enter the phase of ulceration and granulation, in which esophagus can get easily perforated.

Grades of Injury in Endoscopy and Management

- Grade I (edema and erythema) or Grade IIa (erosions and ulcers)—oral feeding should be resumed immediately and patient can be discharged after stabilization.
- Grade IIb (circumferential ulceration)—oral feeding can start once the patient can swallow saliva. 30–70% of these patients will develop stricture. Therefore, barium swallow is recommended at 3 weeks and early dilatation should be followed accordingly.
- Grade IIIa (scattered areas of necrosis)—associated with risk of perforation and stricture development in 90% of cases.
- Grade IIIb (extensive necrosis)—patient may need emergency exploration. *CT scan may be used to confirm the thickness of necrotic area.*

Grades of Injury in CT Scan

Have higher sensitivity and specificity than endoscopic score. It could provide further information regarding involvement of adjacent organs:

- Grade I—no definite swelling of esophageal wall (<3 mm)
- Grade II—edematous wall thickening (>3 mm) without periesophageal soft tissue infiltration
- Grade III—edematous wall thickening with periesophageal soft tissue infiltration
- Grade IV—edematous wall thickening with periesophageal soft tissue infiltration and blurring of tissue interface or localized fluid collection around esophagus

Feeding Jejunostomy

It should be done with grade III and above injuries on endoscopy and patients with dysphagia.

Endoscopic Esophageal Dilatation

- Early dilatation is usually done at 3 weeks after acute inflammatory phase. After 8 weeks scar tissue is completely formed and the result of dilatation is poor.
- Never try to dilate with >3 dilators of progressively increasing diameter if considerable resistance is encountered.
- Weekly or biweekly dilatation is done to obtain 40-Fr luminal competency.
- Strictures that could not be dilated to 14 mm over five sessions with biweekly interval is defined as refractory stricture.
- For refractory stricture, there are modalities such as intralesional steroid injection, mitomycin C injection, and esophageal stent.
- Most of the refractory strictures will require esophageal replacement.

Esophageal Replacement

- Rarely in isolated involvement of esophagus with sparing of stomach, gastric conduit can be used
- If both are involved then colonic conduit is used.
- If stomach and colon both are unavailable then jejunal interposition grafts are used.
- Reconstruction may be complicated due to scarring of hypopharynx, lack of stomach as conduit, peritoneal adhesions, and scarring of mesocolon. The conduit is brought up to the neck through substernal route as posterior mediastinal space is obliterated due to prior chemical injury and mediastinitis.
- Esophagectomy should be done as carcinoma can occur in about 30% of patients and it also prevents the development of mucocele. But resection is difficult due to presence of periesophageal tissue involvement and there is risk of injury to airway and thoracic duct.

Colonic Conduit

- Right colon is used with middle colic artery based as antiperistaltic loop and left colon is used with ascending branch of left colic artery as isoperistaltic loop.

- More commonly preferred one is left colon as smaller diameter of left colon matches relatively to esophagus; presence of constant and reliable blood supply of left colon and can propel solid content.

Contraindications

Primary colonic disease, inadequate blood supply, and short or fibrosed colonic mesentery.

Disadvantages

- Multiple anastomosis is required. Thus, more chances of anastomotic disruption, leak, septicemia, empyema, and mediastinitis.
- Necrosis and leak are potentially life-threatening in colon.
- Colon has got poor acid resistance unlike jejunum.
- Tendency to dilate gradually and causing redundancy is a problem.
- Extremely slow emptying time is another problem.
- Late and long-term complications are many. They are transhiatal herniation, colocutaneous/colobronchial fistula, stricture at anastomotic sites, peptic ulceration of redundant colon and bleeding, and cologastric adenocarcinoma.

8. Management of acute esophageal injuries due to corrosive ingestion. *WBUHS 2008*

Caustic Injury

- Caustic injuries of the esophagus can have devastating consequences, and the best cure for this condition is an ounce of prevention.
- In children, ingestion of caustic materials is accidental and tends to be in small quantities.
- There are both acute and chronic phases to caustic esophageal injuries.
- The acute phase is dependent on the severity and location of the injury and on the type of substance ingested (acid versus alkali), the form of the substance (liquid versus solid), the quantity and concentration of the substance ingested, the amount of residual food in the stomach, and the duration of tissue contact.

Alkali Ingestion

Alkaline substances dissolve tissues by liquefactive necrosis, deeply penetrating the tissues they touch. There are three phases of tissue injury from alkali ingestion.

I. *Phase 1:* The acute necrotic phase lasts 1–4 days after injury, during which coagulation of intracellular proteins results in cell necrosis. The surrounding tissues develop an intense inflammatory reaction.

II. *Phase 2:* The ulceration and granulation phase is next and starts 3–5 days after injury and lasts about 3–12 days. It is during this time that the tissues slough and granulation tissue begins to fill in the ulcerated base left behind. The esophagus is at its weakest point during this second phase.

III. *Phase 3:* In the third phase, cicatrization and scarring begin, and the newly formed connective tissue begins to contract, resulting in esophageal narrowing. This occurs 3 weeks after the initial injury. Adhesions form between areas of granulation resulting in bands that significantly constrict the esophagus. During this time, efforts are aimed at reducing stricture formation.

Three Phases of Tissue Injury from Alkali Ingestion

Phase	*Tissue injury*	*Onset*	*Duration*	*Inflammatory response*
I	Acute necrosis	1–4 days	1–4 days	• Coagulation of intracellular proteins • Inflammation
II	Ulceration and granulation	3–5 days	3–12 days	• Tissue sloughing • Granulation of ulcerated tissue bed
III	Cicatrization and scarring	3 weeks	1–6 months	• Adhesion formation • Scarring

Acid Ingestion

- Ingestion of acid is difficult because it gives an immediate burning in the mouth.
- When compared with lye ingestions, the quantity and concentrations are quite modest.
- Acid substances cause coagulative necrosis, forming an eschar that limits tissue penetration.
- In some cases, acid burns result in full-thickness injury, although in most, it is limited.
- Within 48 hours, the extent to which the acid will injure the esophagus is already determined.
- These injuries tend to be less severe and relatively spare the esophagus over the stomach.

Symptoms and Diagnosis

- Symptoms of caustic burns to the esophagus are determined by the severity of the burn and parallel the stages of tissue injury.
- During phase one, patients may complain of oral and substernal pain, hypersalivation, odynophagia and dysphagia, hematemesis, and vomiting.
- During stage two, these symptoms may disappear only to see dysphagia reappear as fibrosis and scarring begin to narrow the esophagus throughout stage three.
- A fever is usually an indicator that esophageal injury is present.
- Symptoms of respiratory distress, such as hoarseness, stridor, and dyspnea, suggest upper airway edema and are usually worse with acid ingestion.
- Pain in the back and chest may indicate a perforation of the mediastinal esophagus, whereas abdominal pain may indicate abdominal visceral perforation.
- Diagnosis is initiated with a physical examination specifically evaluating the mouth, airway, chest, and abdomen.
- Careful inspection of the lips, palate, pharynx, and larynx is done.
- Auscultation of the lungs is critical to determining the degree of upper airway involvement.
- The abdomen is examined for signs of perforation.
- Early endoscopy is recommended 12–24 hours after ingestion to identify the grade of the burn.
- Radiographic examination in adults is not a useful tool at initial presentation but is helpful in later stages to assess stricture formation.
- Serial chest and abdominal radiographs are indicated to follow patients with questionable chest and abdominal examinations.
- A CT scan is indicated in a patient with an equivocal endoscopic examination in whom there is a strong index of suspicion for a perforation.

Endoscopic Grading and Treatment of Corrosive Esophageal and Gastric Burns

Degree of burn	*Endoscopic evaluation*	*Treatment*
First degree	• Mucosal hyperemia • Edema	• 48-hours observation • Acid suppression
Second degree	• Limited hemorrhage • Exudates • Ulceration • Pseudomembrane formation	• Aggressive IV resuscitation • IV antibiotics • Acid suppression
Third degree	• Mucosal sloughing • Deep ulcerations • Massive hemorrhage • Complete luminal obstruction • Charring • Perforation	• Inhaled steroids • Fiberoptic intubation (if needed)

Treatment

The treatment of caustic lesions of the esophagus is determined by the extent of the injury and addresses the injuries that occur both in the acute and chronic phase.

Acute Phase

- Management of the acute phase is aimed at limiting and identifying the extent of the injury.
- It begins with neutralization of the ingested substance.
- If a patient presents within the first hour of ingestion, neutralization is attempted.
- Alkalis (including lye) are neutralized with half-strength vinegar or citrus juice. Acids are neutralized with milk, egg whites, or antacids.
- Emetics and sodium bicarbonate need to be avoided.
- Further treatment is guided by the extent of injury endoscopically identified and the patient's underlying condition.

No Evidence of Burn

- Early observation is safe in those asymptomatic patients whose physical examination and initial endoscopy are negative. Oral nutrition may be resumed when a patient can painlessly swallow saliva.
- *First-degree burn:*
  - In patients with endoscopically identified first-degree burns, 48 hours of observation is indicated.
  - Oral nutrition can be resumed when a patient can painlessly swallow saliva.
  - A repeat endoscopy and barium esophagram are done in follow-up at intervals of 1, 2, and 8 months, at which time 60%, 80%, and nearly 100% of strictures will have developed, respectively.
- Second- and third-degree burns:
  - Patients with second- and third-degree burns to the esophagus are triaged similar to burn patients.
  - Massive fluid shifts, renal failure, and sepsis can occur rapidly, and underestimation of extent of injury can lead to fatal outcomes.
  - Resuscitation is aggressively pursued.
  - The patient is monitored in the intensive care unit (ICU) and kept NPO with IV fluids. IV antibiotics and a PPI are started.
  - In patients with evidence of acute airway involvement, aerosolized steroids may be used to relieve airway obstruction.
  - Fiberoptic intubation may be needed and must be available.
  - The use of steroids to prevent stricture formation is controversial.
- The management of second- and third-degree burns of the esophagus is multifaceted and has several acceptable options:
  - Aggressive resuscitation and placement of an esophageal stent are one option.
  - Oral nutrition is resumed when a patient can painlessly swallow saliva.
  - Alternatively, a feeding tube or central venous catheter is placed, and the patient is kept NPO until oral pain subsides.
  - If the diagnosis is not secured with endoscopy, an exploratory laparoscopy (in stable patients) or laparotomy (in unstable patients) is performed.
  - A viable stomach and esophagus are left in situ, a feeding jejunostomy tube is placed, and an esophageal stent is placed endoscopically in the operating room.
  - A questionable esophagus and stomach are left in situ, and a second-look operation is planned for 36 hours.
  - Management at 36 hours is dictated by the findings at that time.
  - If full-thickness necrosis or perforation of the esophagus or stomach is found at any time, an emergent exploratory laparotomy is indicated.

- The esophagus and stomach and all affected surrounding organs and tissues are resected, an end-cervical esophagostomy is performed, and a feeding jejunostomy is placed. Postoperatively, the patient is monitored in an ICU and aggressively managed.

Management of Caustic Injury of the Esophagus

- *Acute phase:*
  - Intravenous fluids (IVF)
  - Observe
  - PPI

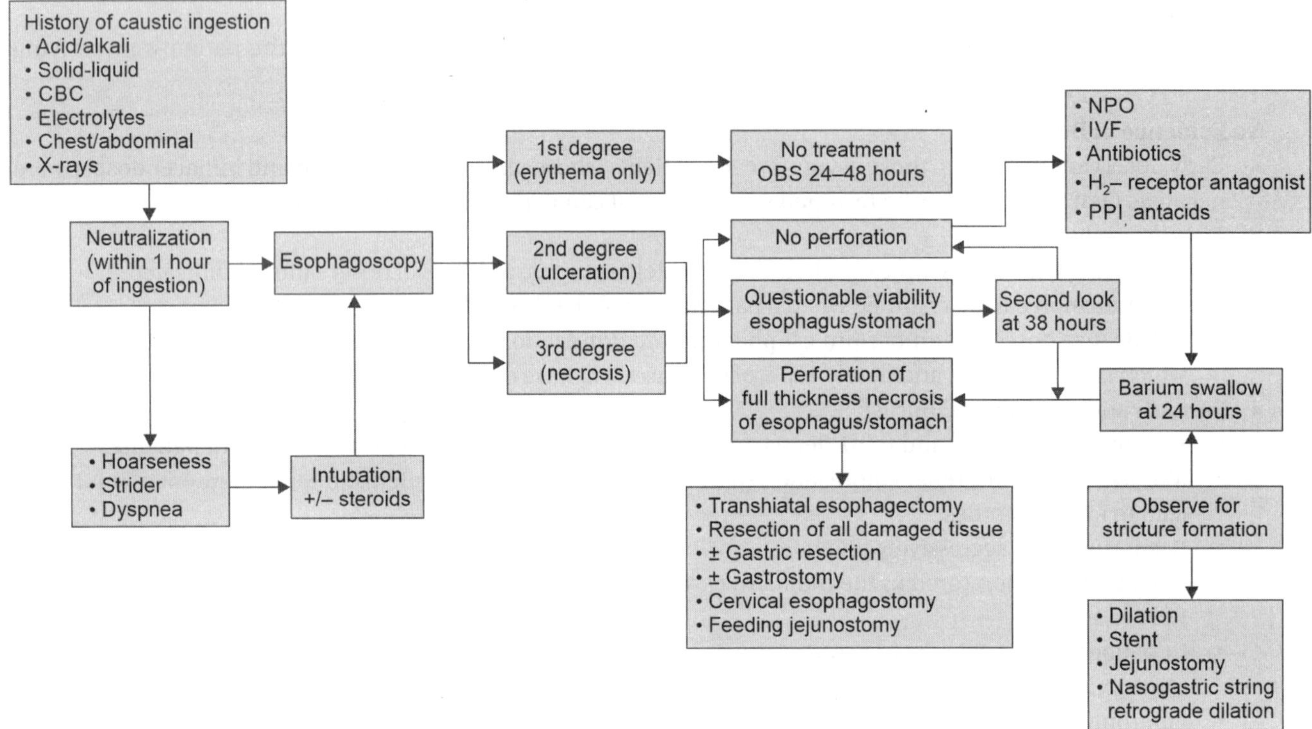

(CBC: complete blood count; NPO: nil per oral)

9. Immediate complications of corrosive acid poisoning. ***WBUHS 2010***

Common Corrosive Agents

Acids (pH < 7): Corrosives
Hydrochloride acid (pool and metal cleaners)
Hydrofluoric acid (antirust products)
Sulfuric acid (car battery fluid)

Classification of Injury

Mild-injury	
First degree	• Mucosal • Erythema/edema
Second degree	• Transmucosal • Sloughing of mucosa/ulcerations
Severe injury	
Second degree	• Transmucosal • Circumferential
Third degree	• Transmural periesophageal penetration • Dark red-black tissue exposed

Treatment Algorithm

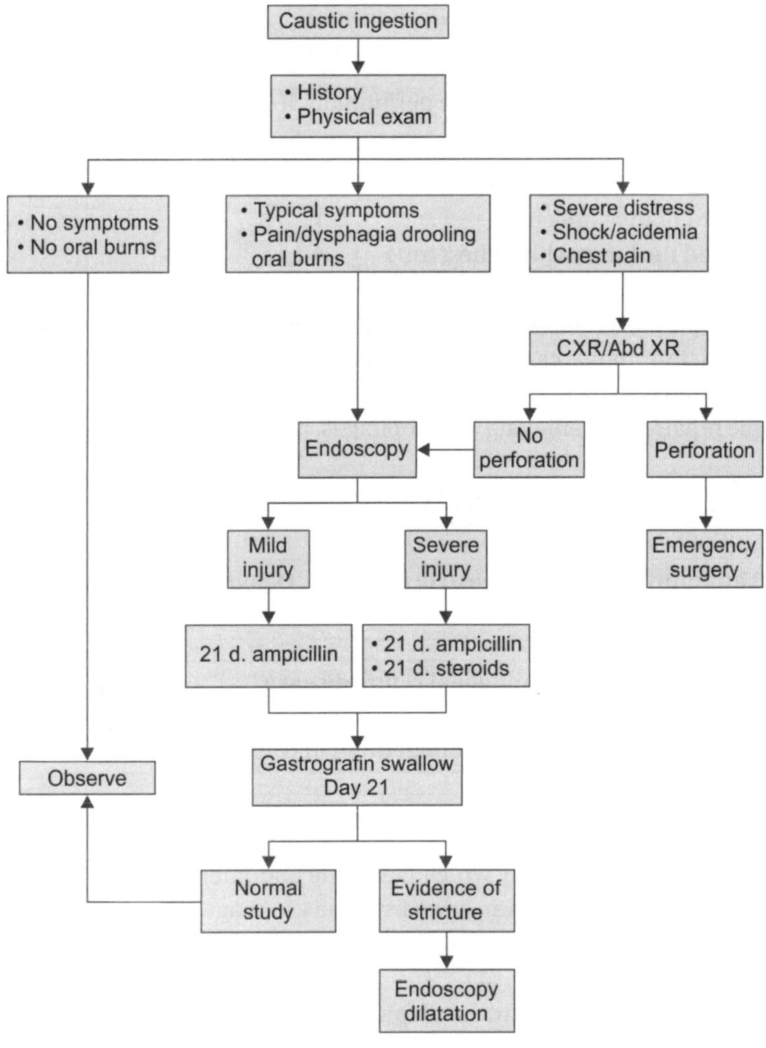

ESOPHAGEAL PERFORATION

10. What are the causes of esophageal perforation? Discuss its management. ***WBUHS 2020***

The most common cause of esophageal perforation is injury to the esophagus during another medical procedure.

Causes

- *Iatrogenic:*
  - Postinstrumentation or post-thoracic surgery (most common ~80% of cases)
  - Complication of acute radiation-induced esophagitis
- *Trauma:* Both blunt (crush-type injury) and penetrating
  - Occurs in <0.1% of blunt chest trauma
- Foreign body ingestion
- Corrosive material ingestion
- Esophageal cancer
- Spontaneous rupture postvomiting (Boerhaave syndrome)

Treatment

Surgery will depend on the location and size of the perforation. If surgery is needed, it is best done within 24 hours.

Treatment may include:

- IV fluid
- IV antibiotics to prevent or treat infection
- Draining of fluid around the lungs with a chest tube
- Mediastinoscopy
- A perforation in the uppermost (neck region) part of the esophagus may heal by itself if the patient does not eat or drink for a period of time. In this case, a stomach feeding tube is needed to provide nutrition.
- Surgery is often needed to repair a perforation in the middle or bottom portions of the esophagus. The leak may be treated by simple repair or by removing the esophagus, depending on the extent of the problem.

GASTROESOPHAGEAL REFLUX DISEASE

11. Discuss the surgical anatomy of esophagogastric junction. Discuss the investigations and management for reflux disease. ***WBUHS 2017, 2023***

12. Diagnosis and management of gastroesophageal reflux disease. ***WBUHS 2009***

13. Describe the etiology, clinical features, and management of GERD. ***KIIT University, Odisha 2025***

14. Describe evaluation and management of gastroesophageal reflux disease (GERD). ***KGMU, Lucknow 2025***

The esophagus joins the stomach at the EGJ, which lies in the abdomen just below the diaphragm. Therefore, the term "esophagogastric junction" implies a transition from the esophagus to the stomach.

The EGJ is a complex of structures, which may be defined differently by the surgeon, the anatomist, the radiologist, and the endoscopist.

- The surgeon identifies the EGJ just below the diaphragm at the upper border of the peritoneal reflection from the stomach to the distal esophagus.
- It is important to remove the gastric fat pad to accurately identify the gastroesophageal junction during a Nissen fundoplication or a Heller myotomy.

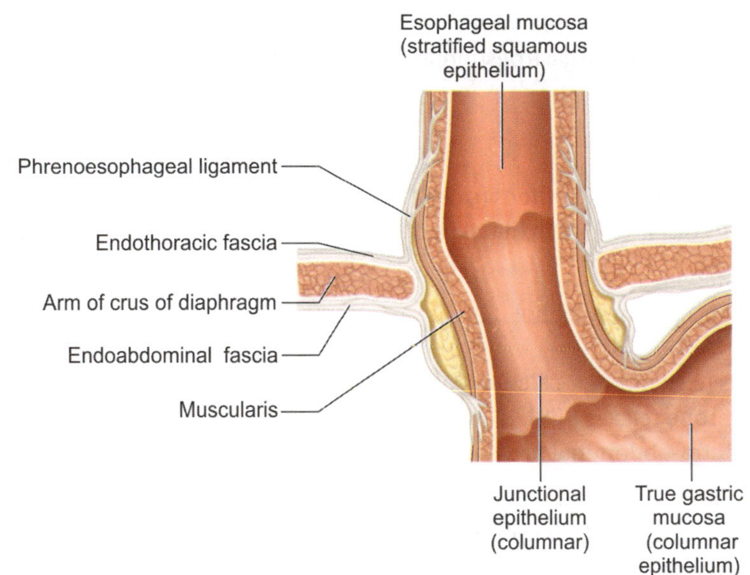

- The gross anatomist considers EGJ the termination of the tubular esophagus and the saccular stomach.
- The criteria used by microscopic anatomist to define EGJ are the distal extent of the esophageal squamous epithelium and the proximal extent of gastric oxyntic mucosa, the point beyond which no submucosal esophageal glands are found, and the change in the muscularis propria from a circular and longitudinal layer in the esophagus to a less defined muscularis propria of the stomach with a third oblique layer.
- The EGJ of the radiologist is the imaginary line of the gastric sling from the acute angle of His to the middle of the junctional mucosa at the lesser curvature, where longitudinal mucosal folds of the esophagus change to transverse folds of the stomach.
- The endoscopist defines the EGJ as the junction of the pale pink esophageal mucosa with the bright red gastric mucosa (Z line), but also considers the distal end of esophageal longitudinal mucosal veins (palisade vessels) and the proximal end of gastric longitudinal mucosal folds.
- Moreover, the muscular structure of the EGJ, forming the LES, can be evaluated by physiologic manometric methods, and EGJ can be defined as the manometric distal end of the LES.
- The external EGJ can be described as the point at which the esophageal tube becomes the gastric pouch and lies in the abdomen at the level of the 11th or 12th thoracic vertebra.
- Internally, the junction is marked by an irregular boundary between stratified squamous esophageal epithelium and columnar gastric epithelium, but this boundary may lie as far as 1–2 cm above the external junction.
- The columnar epithelium below the internal junction contains mucus-secreting glands (the cardiac glands of the histologists), and lacks the chief and parietal cells that characterize the true gastric glands of the body of the stomach.
- The term "junctional epithelium" was proposed for this area by Hayward. The external and internal junctions do not coincide.
- In addition, the loose submucosal connective tissue permits considerable sliding of the mucosa on the muscularis propria, changing the relation between them as the stomach fills with food.
- Furthermore, with damage to the distal esophagus from gastroesophageal reflux and development of a hiatal hernia, the landmarks, and relationships of structures around the junction become altered, and the identification of the precise EGJ becomes even more difficult.

Etiology (Causes) of GERD—Gastroesophageal Reflux Disease

GERD occurs when *gastric contents (acid, bile, or food)* reflux into the *esophagus* due to *failure of the normal anti-reflux barriers.*

Lower Esophageal Sphincter (LES) Dysfunction

- The *LES* is a ring of muscle at the gastroesophageal junction that normally stays *tonically contracted* to prevent reflux.
- Reflux occurs when the LES is:
  - *Hypotensive* (weak tone)
  - Experiences *transient LES relaxations* (unrelated to swallowing)
  - Or is *anatomically displaced* (as in hiatal hernia)

Causes of LES dysfunction

- Fatty foods, chocolate, caffeine, alcohol
- Smoking
- Certain medications (e.g., nitrates, calcium channel blockers, anticholinergics)
- Pregnancy (progesterone relaxes LES)
- Obesity (increased intra-abdominal pressure)

Hiatal Hernia

- The *stomach herniates through the diaphragm* into the chest, disrupting the normal pressure gradient.
- This weakens the LES and impairs clearance of refluxed material.

Impaired Esophageal Clearance

- Normally, peristalsis and saliva help clear refluxed acid.
- Conditions that impair this (e.g., *scleroderma, achalasia*, or *neuromuscular disorders*) increase reflux exposure.

Delayed Gastric Emptying

- When gastric emptying is slowed, pressure and volume in the stomach rise, promoting reflux.
- Seen in *diabetes mellitus, gastric outlet obstruction,* or after *vagotomy*.

Increased Intra-abdominal Pressure

- Common in:
  - Obesity
  - Pregnancy
  - Ascites
  - Tight clothing or belts
  - Chronic cough or straining

Mucosal Defense Impairment

Even small amounts of reflux can cause symptoms if the *esophageal mucosal barrier* (bicarbonate secretion, epithelial integrity) is compromised.

Other Contributing Factors

- *Genetic predisposition*
- *Connective tissue disorders* (e.g., scleroderma)
- *Lifestyle factors*—late-night meals, large portions, lying down after eating

Symptoms of GERD

• Heartburn	• Dysphagia for solids	• Aspiration
• Regurgitation	• Hoarseness	• Wheezing
• Abdominal pain	• Belching	• Globus
• Cough	• Bloating	

- The physical examination of patients with GERD rarely contributes to confirmation of the diagnosis.
- In patients with advanced disease, several observations may help identify the source of the patient's discomfort.
- A patient who constantly drinks water during the interview is facilitating esophageal clearance, which may be indicative of continual reflux or distal obstruction.

- Other patients with advanced disease will sit leaning forward and carry out the interview with their lungs inflated to near vital capacity. This is an attempt to keep the diaphragm flattened, the anteroposterior diameter of the hiatus narrowed, and, thus, the LES pressure elevated.
- Patients who have severe proximal reflux with regurgitation of gastric contents into their mouth may have erosion of their dentition (revealing yellow teeth due to the loss of dentin), injected oropharyngeal mucosa, or signs of chronic sinusitis.

Preoperative Evaluation

The preoperative workup in a patient being considered for operative treatment will help confirm the diagnosis, exclude other pathologic entities, and direct the operative intervention.

Endoscopy

- Endoscopy is an essential step in the evaluation of patients with GERD who are being considered for operative intervention.
- The value of the study is in its ability to exclude other diseases, especially a tumor, and to document the presence of peptic esophageal injury.
- *The degree of injury can be measured using a scoring system such as the Savary–Miller interpretation:*
  1. Indicates erythema
  2. Linear ulceration
  3. Confluent ulceration
  4. Stricture
- The extreme of mucosal injury is Barrett's esophagus. Biopsy samples are taken to confirm the metaplastic transformation and to exclude dysplasia.

Manometry

A significant amount of information about the function of the esophageal body and the LES may be obtained from stationary esophageal manometry.

- The LES is analyzed for mean resting pressure. This may be determined in two ways: A station pull-through technique and a rapid pull-through technique. The majority of laboratories reports the values recorded from the station pull-through technique.
- Normal pressures for a station pull-through at the LES range between 12 and 30 mm Hg. The sphincter generally relaxes to the pressure of the gastric baseline for several seconds when a swallow is initiated.
- Other information to be gained from the LES is the total length, the intra-abdominal length, and the location of the sphincter relative to the nares. The longer the length of the high-pressure zone and the longer the intra-abdominal component, the greater the barrier to reflux of gastric contents.
- The esophageal body is assessed to determine the effectiveness of peristalsis.
- The peristaltic activity is reported as the percentage of initiated swallows that are transmitted to each channel successfully. Normally, a patient has >80% peristalsis.
- The second characteristic of clinical importance is the amplitude of the peristaltic wave. The amplitude is simply the average of the pressures generated in the distal esophagus during effectively transmitted peristaltic waves.
- Ineffective esophageal motility (IEM) is defined as <60% peristalsis or distal esophageal amplitudes of <30 mm Hg and is often associated with significant GERD.
- It was traditionally thought that a 360° fundoplication is likely to cause an insurmountable obstruction to be swallowing and to result in dysphagia, but this idea has been challenged recently.

pH Monitoring

- The gold standard for diagnosing and quantifying acid reflux is the 24-hour pH test.
- The study is performed by placing a thin catheter containing one or more solid-state electrodes in the esophagus.
- A large amount of information may be gleaned from the study:
  - Total number of reflux episodes (pH <4)

- Longest episode of reflux
- Number of episodes lasting longer than 5 minutes
- Extent of reflux in the upright position, and extent of reflux in the supine position

- An overall score is obtained with the use of a formula that assigns a weight to each item according to its capacity to cause esophageal injury. This value, known as the De Meester score, needs to be <14.7.
- A simpler way to determine whether abnormal reflux is occurring is to estimate the total percent time, the pH is below 4 in the proximal and distal channels.
- The total percent time is calculated by dividing the time the pH was <4 by the total time of the study and multiplying by 100. In the proximal esophagus (15 cm above the LES), acid exposure normally occurs <1% of the time; in the distal esophagus (5 cm above the LES), it normally occurs <4%.

Esophagogram

- The esophagogram provides valuable information in the evaluation of patients with symptoms of GERD when an operation is contemplated or when the symptoms do not respond as expected.
- Often, spontaneous reflux during the examination will be demonstrated. Although reflux may be induced in patients who do not have the disease, the occurrence of spontaneous reflux lends support to the diagnosis of abnormal gastroesophageal reflux.
- The true value of the study is to determine the external anatomy of the esophagus and the proximal stomach. The presence and size of a hiatal hernia may be characterized. Although this neither confirms nor refutes the presence of disease, it is extremely beneficial in planning the operation.
- A mediastinal gastroesophageal junction that does not reduce into the peritoneal cavity during the study is a predictor of a more difficult operation that may require an esophageal lengthening procedure.
- Peptic esophageal strictures may also be found on an esophageal contrast study. The presence of a stricture will taint the interpretation of the 24-hour pH study, especially if it is tight enough to prevent reflux.
- Other anatomic abnormalities, such as diverticula, tumors, and unexpected paraesophageal hernias, will be discovered during an esophagogram.

Other Tests

- In unique circumstances, other diagnostic tests may be valuable.
- Occasionally, a patient will not be able to tolerate nasoesophageal intubation.
- A scintigraphic study to evaluate esophageal clearance and reflux may provide evidence of motility disorder and gastroesophageal reflux.
- Gastric distention resulting from delayed emptying may also be diagnosed with a scintigraphic study.
- Although this condition may contribute to reflux, it is not clear whether a gastric emptying procedure (pyloroplasty) needs to be added to an antireflux procedure in a patient with delayed gastric emptying.
- Some patients will have laryngeal symptoms of gastroesophageal reflux. Laryngoscopy and stroboscopic examinations will help provide objective evidence of extraesophageal reflux; findings include inflammation of laryngeal mucosa, muscle tension abnormalities, and, in severe cases, subglottic stenosis.

Treatment

- Most people will experience symptoms of reflux during their life. A smaller percentage will proceed with self-treatment.
- Lifestyle modifications are certainly helpful in avoiding gastroesophageal reflux. Cessation of smoking, decreased caffeine intake, and avoidance of large meals before lying down will help decrease transient episodes of LES relaxation.
- Elevation of the head of the bed and avoidance of constricting clothing will help prevent unfavorable pressure gradients across the gastroesophageal junction.

Medical Management

- Check for chronic anemia in such a patient and to prescribe a 6-week course of acid suppression therapy. Double dose is preferred.

- If the symptoms persist after a trial of medical therapy, a more extensive evaluation, as described earlier, would be indicated. The medications available to treat acid reflux include antacids, motility agents, histamine-2 (H_2) blockers, and PPIs.
- Pharmacologic treatment of GERD has been revolutionized by the advent of PPIs.
- Compared with H_2 blockers, PPIs are more effective at healing esophageal ulceration secondary to acid exposure.
- Long-term therapy appears to be safe even though it has been linked to gastric polyp formation. The polyps are usually hyperplastic and do not appear to be premalignant.

Surgical Therapy

- The indications for surgical therapy have changed somewhat with the advent of PPIs.
- Certainly, patients with evidence of severe esophageal injury (ulcer, stricture, or Barrett's mucosa) and incomplete resolution of symptoms or relapses while on medical therapy are appropriate to consider for operative intervention.
- Other patients with a long duration of symptoms or those in whom symptoms persist at a young age are considered for operative treatment initially. In these patients, operative therapy is considered an alternative to medical therapy rather than a treatment of last resort.
- Some patients have absolutely no response of their symptoms to the use of PPIs. They need to be scrutinized further before offering surgical treatment, as opposed to being considered medical failures who need operative treatment.
- Because the PPIs are so effective at decreasing the acid production of the stomach, the diagnosis of GERD in such patients is questioned and must be demonstrated with objective testing.
- In patients who have >10 years of life expectancy and are in need of lifelong therapy due to a mechanically defective sphincter, surgical therapy may be considered the treatment of choice.
  - *360-degree wrap (left crus approach):*
    - The technique described here is the left crus approach to a 360° wrap (Nissen fundoplication), which is the procedure of choice for most patients.
    - The left crus approach provides the advantage of a direct and early view of the short gastric vessels and the spleen.
    - After this obstacle is negotiated, there is little chance of injuring the spleen during the remainder of the procedure.
  - *Partial fundoplication:*
    - When esophageal motility is poor, a partial fundoplication may be considered to prevent obstruction to bolus propagation in the esophagus.
    - Although this was thought mandatory in all patients with IEM (peristalsis <60% or distal esophageal amplitudes <30 mm Hg), this practice has been questioned in recent years.
  - *A total fundoplication:*
    - It can be performed in most patients with IEM (except perhaps those with absent peristalsis), without an increase in development of dysphagia.
    - In fact, effective control of reflux with a total fundoplication usually improves premorbid dysphagia and often improves the esophageal motility.
    - When needed, there are many types of partial fundoplications. Regardless of the type used, the initial dissection of the esophagus is the same.
- *Anterior wrap:*
  - If an anterior wrap (e.g., Thal and Dor) is to be performed, there is no need to disrupt the posterior attachments of the esophagus.
  - The Dor and Thal fundoplications are created with the fundus folded over the anterior aspect of the esophagus.
  - They are anchored to the hiatus and esophagus as in the 360° wrap.
  - The experience with these repairs is limited in patients being treated for gastroesophageal reflux.

- They are more commonly used in patients with achalasia after an anterior myotomy has been performed.
- *Posterior wrap:*
  - If a posterior wrap (Toupet) is to be performed, the entire esophageal dissection is the same as for a 360° wrap, and the crura are reapproximated as well.
  - The reconstruction of the posterior fundoplication is initiated by passing the posterior fundus behind the esophagus from left to right.
  - The fundoplication is created by anchoring the posterior fundus to the crura and the esophagus.
  - The most cephalad sutures of the wrap incorporate all three structures (fundus, crus, and esophagus).
  - The wrap is anchored posteriorly to the crura with two or three sutures. The fundus is then sutured to the esophagus along the anterolateral aspects, creating a 220 to 250° wrap.

Endoscopic Therapy

- Recently, several endoscopic techniques have been developed for the treatment of GERD. These procedures have sparked significant interest because they each promise a mechanical treatment for reflux with less invasion than a fundoplication. These techniques attempt to augment the LES by suturing, or biocompatible polymer injection.
- There is some interest in using these endoscopic techniques in patients with recurrent GERD after antireflux surgery. Although it is tempting to avoid complicated reoperation, there is not enough experience to recommend its use at this time. Overall, it is not clear what role endoscopic treatments have in the treatment of GERD; therefore, laparoscopic antireflux surgery remains the best alternative to medical therapy.

Outcome

The results of operative intervention may be measured by relief of symptoms, improvement in acid exposure, complications, and failures.

HIATUS HERNIA

15. Hiatus hernia. ***WBUHS 2015***

Introduction

Hiatal hernias are classified according to the position of the EGJ and the existence of a true hernia sac.

Types

- Type I (sliding)
  - Leading edge of the hernia is the EGJ, which is displaced into an intrathoracic position.
  - The longitudinal axis of the stomach is aligned with the esophagus.

There is often no true hernia sac nor is there any paraesophageal component.

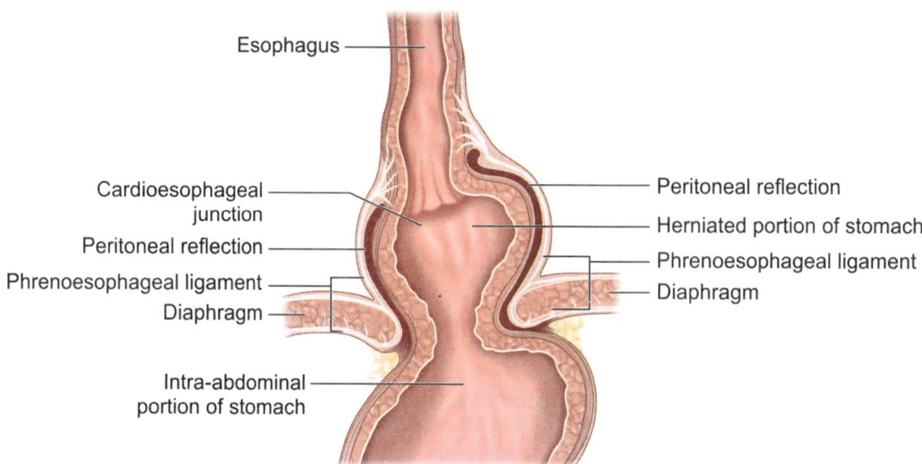

- Type II (rolling)
  - The EGJ is in its normal intra-abdominal location
  - The hernia sac (containing portions of the gastric fundus and body) develops alongside the esophagus
- Type III (combined sliding-rolling or mixed)
  - The EGJ is displaced into the thorax and like a type II, the hernia sac contains portions of the gastric fundus or body.

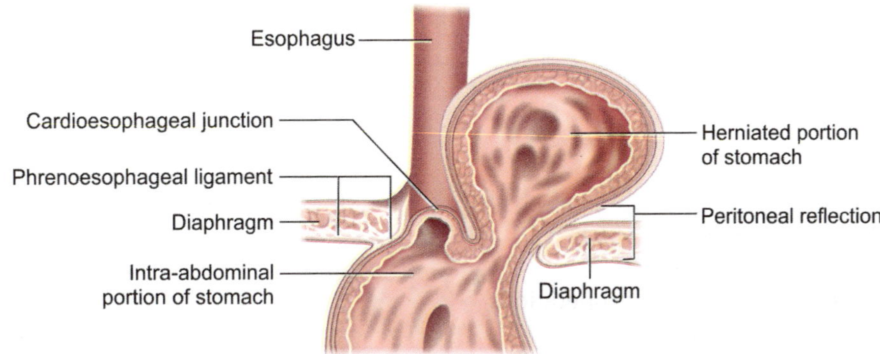

- Type IV hiatal hernia is declared in some taxonomies, when an additional organ, usually the colon, herniates as well.

The end stage of type I and type II hernias occurs when the whole stomach migrates up into the chest by rotating 180° around its longitudinal axis, with the cardia and pylorus as fixed points. In this situation, the abnormality is usually referred to as an intrathoracic stomach.

- Increasingly common with advancing age
- More often among women than men
- Symptoms are often associated with GERD

Risk Factors

Increased pressure within the abdomen caused by:

- Heavy lifting or bending over
- Frequent or hard coughing
- Hard sneezing
- Violent vomiting
- Straining
- Stress

Diagnosis

- Typical symptoms
- Suspicious CXR
- Chest CT
- Upper GI series
- In urgent situations, placement of NG tube and subsequent coiling

Management

- Evaluation
  - Endoscopy
  - Esophageal motility studies
  - Manometry and pH monitoring
    - One-third of patients will have atypical peristalsis of the esophageal body.
    - Half of symptomatic patients will have abnormal pH results.

- Indications for operation
  - Type I
  - Types II and III
    - Associated with a high-risk of complications
    - "Catastrophic" in 20–30% of patients
    - Symptoms do not predict risk
- *Findings that may prompt surgery* (even in those patients that are "not optimal")
  - Symptoms of obstruction
  - Reflux
  - Anemia
- *Trying to avoid:*
  - Further aspiration
  - Hemorrhage
  - Transfusion requirements
- *Surgical techniques:*
  - Principles similar to other hernia operations
  - Need to anchor the stomach
  - Fundoplication is controversial
  - Transthoracic versus transabdominal
- *The basic principles of operative management in hiatal hernia are:*
  - Complete reduction of the hernia and removal of the hernia sac
  - Close the hiatus
  - Restore the GEJ to an intra-abdominal location
  - Addition of an antireflux procedure

BARRETT'S ESOPHAGUS

16. Write short notes on Barrett's esophagus. ***WBUHS 2022***

Introduction

- Barrett's esophagus is a complication of chronic GERD; histologically demonstrates intestinal-type metaplasia.
- The columnar epithelium may replace the normal squamous epithelium circumferentially, or it may be asymmetric and irregular.

Prevalence

- Barrett's esophagus is diagnosed in approximately 2% of all patients undergoing esophagoscopy and in 10–15% of patients with esophagitis.
- Most patients diagnosed with Barrett esophagus are middle aged white men.

Symptoms

Symptoms of Barrett esophagus arise from chronic GERD including heartburn (50%), dysphagia (75%), and bleeding (25%).

Diagnosis

Diagnosis requires endoscopy and correlation between endoscopic and histologic appearances.

Complications

- *Esophageal ulceration and stricture* are more likely to occur in patients with Barrett esophagus than in those with GERD alone.
- *Barrett ulcers, such as gastric ulcers,* penetrate the metaplastic columnar epithelium. They occur in up to 50% of patients with Barrett esophagus.

- *A benign stricture* occurs in 30–50% of patients with Barrett's esophagus. The stricture is located at the squamocolumnar junction, which may be found proximal to the GE junction.
- The metaplastic columnar epithelium of Barrett's esophagus is prone to development of *dysplasia* detected by biopsy. Low-grade dysplasia is present in 5–10% of patients with Barrett esophagus.
- *Malignant degeneration* from benign to dysplastic to malignant epithelium occurs in Barrett esophagus.
  - *Adenocarcinomas* above the normal GE junction are characteristic of malignant degeneration in Barrett's esophagus.
  - The risk of development of adenocarcinoma in Barrett's esophagus is 50–100 times that of the general population; yet adenocarcinoma is still a rare event in a Barrett patient.
  - Approximately 0.12–0.43% per year will progress from Barrett's to adenocarcinoma.

Treatment

- Uncomplicated Barrett esophagus in *asymptomatic* patients requires endoscopic surveillance and biopsy annually or even less frequently in the absence of dysplasia.
- Uncomplicated Barrett esophagus in *symptomatic* patients should be managed like GERD patients and should have periodic endoscopic surveillance with four-quadrant biopsies. Elimination of reflux with an *antireflux procedure* may halt progression of the disease, heal ulceration, and prevent stricture formation but will not reverse the columnar metaplasia of Barrett.
- *Barrett ulcers* usually heal with medical therapy. Frequently, 8 weeks of treatment with a PPI are necessary to achieve complete healing. Ulcers that fail to heal or recur despite 4 months of medical therapy are an indication for rebiopsy and antireflux surgery.

Algorithm for Surveillance and Management of Barrett's Esophagus

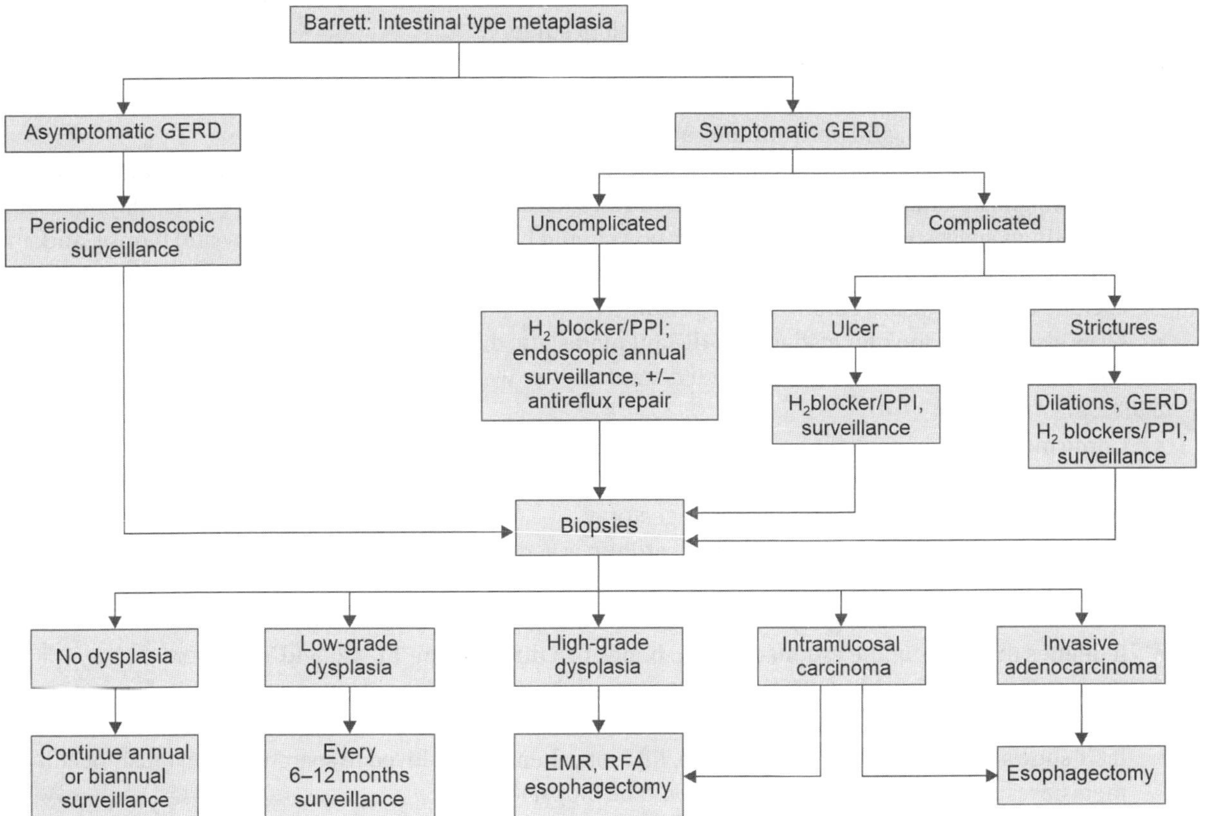

ESOPHAGEAL CANCER

17. A 65-year-old male with a lifelong history of reflux disease has been followed with routine esophagogastroduodenoscopy (EGD) which of late revealed an early esophageal cancer 3 cm proximal to GE junction in the setting of Barret's esophagus. Patient prefers for an endoscopic management. With all facilities at your disposal, how would you workup precisely stage (enumerate investigations) the disease [give the American Joint Committee on Cancer (AJCC) staging] to assess the patient's eligibility for an endoscopic management? What are the endoscopic options of management of early esophageal cancers? How would you counsel the patient? ***WBUHS 2016***

- Accurate staging of disease in patients with newly diagnosed esophageal cancer is necessary in order to instigate appropriate curative or palliative therapy.
- The following guidelines are suggested for the initial work-up of patients with newly diagnosed esophageal cancer.
- All patients should initially undergo a thorough history and physical examination, in order to detect gross evidence of metastatic disease.
- In addition, complete upper gastrointestinal endoscopy (UGIE) and/or a barium upper gastrointestinal series is indicated to assess for mucosal extent of disease.
- If these modalities show a large degree of gastric involvement, then the stomach may not be suitable for interposition at the time of esophagectomy; in such patients, a colonic interposition may be necessary.
- *CT:* A CT scan of the chest and abdomen with bolus administration of intravenous contrast should then be performed.
  - The CT is used to evaluate the primary tumor for invasion of adjacent structures (T4 disease).
  - If the CT shows findings of gross, unequivocal invasion, then surgery is not indicated. Equivocal invasion, however, requires proof before denying the patient surgery.
  - Eccentric or circumferential wall thickening >5 mm
  - An intervening fat plane between an esophageal tumor and an adjacent structure in the mediastinum (e.g., central airway, aorta, and pericardium) accurately indicates lack of invasion.
  - Lack of a fat plane does not necessarily indicate invasion, either for cachectic patients or for those with normal body weight, minimal invasion of some structures, such as pericardium or aortic adventitia, may be resectable.
  - CT findings suggesting central airway invasion should be proven via bronchoscopy and biopsy, and, in fact, all patients with an upper or middle third esophageal cancer should undergo preoperative bronchoscopy to exclude airway invasion before esophagectomy.
  - CT is also used to look for evidence of distant metastatic disease to nonregional lymph nodes (LNs), lungs, abdominal viscera, and other sites; such distant disease would preclude surgical resection.
- *EUS:*
  - Confirmation of suspected pericardial or aortic invasion is more difficult; endoscopic ultrasound (EUS) or intravascular ultrasound (IVUS) may be helpful in this regard, although most often the diagnosis is confirmed only during attempted esophagectomy.
  - Unresectable invasion of the aorta or pericardium is actually very uncommon, and care should be taken not to overdiagnose such findings.
  - It is the most accurate imaging modality for the T staging of esophageal cancer.
  - It defines the layers of the esophageal wall hence can differentiate T1, T2, and T3 tumors.
- *Positron emission tomography (PET)* imaging has been shown to be more accurate than CT in diagnosing distant metastases.
  - If CT shows apparently resectable disease, PET may then be employed to search for previously occult distant metastases; suspicious lesions at PET should be biopsied.
  - Assuming the PET study shows no evidence of distant metastatic disease, a patient may then be examined with EUS for better staging evaluation of the primary tumor (T stage) and regional LNs (N stage); suspicious LNs detected by EUS (regional or celiac axis) should undergo EUS-guided fine needle aspiration biopsy.

- At some institutions, patients with T1N0 disease at EUS and M0 disease at CT and PET proceed right to surgery.
- Those with deeper penetration of tumor and/or tumor involvement of regional LNs undergo neoadjuvant chemoradiation therapy followed by surgery.
- Patients with distant metastases (M1 disease) are usually treated nonsurgically, with chemoradiotherapy (CRT).
- Laparoscopy is performed at some centers to evaluate for occult abdominal metastases, especially for tumors arising at the gastroesophageal junction, although this is not common practice.

- *Chest radiograph:* Many indirect signs can be sought on a chest radiograph and these include:
  - Widened azygoesophageal recess with convexity toward right lung (in 30% of distal and mid-esophageal cancers)
  - Thickening of posterior tracheal stripe and right paratracheal stripe >4 mm (if tumor located in upper third of esophagus)
  - Tracheal deviation or posterior tracheal indentation/mass
  - Retrocardiac or posterior mediastinal mass
  - Esophageal air-fluid level
  - Lobulated mass extending into gastric air bubble (Kirklin sign)
  - Repeated aspiration pneumonia (with tracheoesophageal fistula)
- *Fluoroscopy/barium swallow:*
  - Irregular stricture
  - Prestricture dilatation with "hold up"
  - Shouldering of the stricture

Staging

Tumor, Node, Metastasis (TNM) Staging

- *T staging*
  - *Tx:* Primary tumor cannot be assessed
  - *T0:* No evidence of primary tumor
  - *Tis:* High-grade dysplasia
  - *T1:* Invades lamina propria, muscularis mucosae, or submucosa
    - *T1a:* Invades lamina propria or muscularis mucosae
    - *T1b:* Invades submucosa
  - *T2:* Invades muscularis propria
  - *T3:* Invades adventitia
  - *T4:* Direct extension into adjacent structures
    - *T4a:* (resectable) invades pleura, pericardium or diaphragm
    - *T4b:* (unresectable) invades other structures, e.g., aorta and trachea
- *N staging*
  - *Nx:* Regional nodes cannot be assessed
  - *N0:* No regional LN metastases
  - *N1:* 1–2 regional nodes involved
  - *N2:* 3–6 regional nodes involved
  - *N3:* >7 regional nodes involved
- *M staging*
  - *Mx:* Metastatic disease cannot be assessed.
  - *M0:* No distant metastases
  - *M1:* Distant metastases

AJCC Staging Groups

Staging is dependent on histological subtype, e.g., squamous cell carcinoma or adenocarcinoma. G refers to the grade of tumor and the location is in brackets. As with the TNM classification, X indicates inability to determine grade or location.

Squamous Cell Carcinoma

- *Stage 0:* Tis N0 M0 G1, X
- *Stage I:*
  - *Stage Ia:* T1 N0 M0 G1, X
  - *Stage Ib:*
    - T1 N0 M0 G2-3
    - T2-3 N0 M0 G1, X (lower, X)
- *Stage II:*
  - *Stage IIa:*
    - T2-3 N0 M0 G1, X (upper, middle)
    - T2-3 N0 M0 G2-3 (lower, X)
  - *Stage IIB:*
    - T2-3 N0 M0 G2-3 (upper, middle)
    - T1-2 N1 M0
- *Stage III:*
  - *Stage IIIA:*
    - T1-2 N2 M0
    - T3 N1 M0
    - T4a N0 M0

Indications for Endoscopic Treatment of Superficial Esophageal Neoplasia

- The classically accepted criteria for indication of endoscopic resection for the treatment of superficial esophageal neoplasia include:
  - In-depth involvement restricted to M1 and M2 layers (epithelium and lamina propria); maximum length of 3 cm
  - Lateral extent < three-fourths of the circumference
  - A maximum of four lesions
    - With improving techniques of endoscopic resection, especially after the advent of endoscopic submucosal dissection (ESD), these criteria tend to expand, accepting endoscopic treatment of lesions larger than 3 cm, occupying the entire circumference of the esophagus and no limit to the number of lesions, provided that all are restricted to the mucosa.

Endoscopic Treatment Modalities for Esophageal Cancer Include Resection (Mucosectomy or ESD) and Ablation Techniques

- *Endoscopic mucosal resection (EMR):* It enables accurate histological assessment of the depth of invasion of early neoplastic lesions, thus being both a diagnostic and a therapeutic intervention.
- *Endoscopic submucosal dissection:* In contrast to EMR, where large lesions may be removed piecemeal, ESD allows large lesions to be removed en bloc, as well as resection of tumors arising from the muscularis propria. ESD requires extensive training, longer procedure time and is associated with an increased risk of bleeding and perforation.
- *Radiofrequency ablation (RFA):* RFA (Medtronic) is a field ablation technique used to ablate the surface 500 μm of the gastrointestinal mucosa.
- *Argon plasma coagulation (APC):* APC uses argon gas to conduct electrical current to thermally ablate targeted tissue. APC is often used as an adjunct to alternative therapies, as it is cheap and easy to treat small areas of residual disease and has been demonstrated to significantly increase recurrence-free survival for the patients undergoing ablation after EMR compared with those having EMR alone.

Counseling of the Patient

- It can be hard to live with the idea that the cancer can come back.
- Based on what is known today, no specific way of decreasing the risk of recurrence after completion of treatment can be recommended.

- Because of the cancer itself and because of treatment, returning to normal life may not be easy for some people.
- Questions related to body image, fatigue, work, emotions, or lifestyle may arise.
- Discussing these questions with relatives, friends, or doctors may be helpful.
- However, survival rates depend on several factors, including the stage of the cancer when it is first diagnosed.
- The 5-year survival rate of people with cancer located only in the esophagus is 41%.
- The 5-year survival rate for those with disease that has spread to surrounding tissues or organs and/or the regional LNs is 23%.
- If it has spread to distant parts of the body, the survival rate is 5%.

18. Enumerate the premalignant lesions of the esophagus and discuss pathogenesis of esophageal carcinoma with reference to staging. ***WBUHS 2007***

19. Outline the treatment of carcinoma lower third of esophagus. ***RGUHS, Karnataka 2025; WBUHS 2007, 2017***

Premalignant Lesions of the Esophagus

High risk	*Intermediate risk*	*Low risk*
• Tylosis type A • Plummer-Vinson syndrome	• Reflux disease and Barrett's esophagus • Achalasia • Ectopic gastric mucosa • Previous squamous cell carcinoma of head and neck • Radiotherapy of Hodgkin's or non-Hodgkin's lymphomas	• Esophageal diverticula • Corrosive strictures • Celiac disease • Scleroderma

Pathogenesis

- There are two major forms of this disease, esophageal squamous cell carcinoma (ESSC) and adenocarcinoma.
- Other subtypes such as mucoepidermoid, adenosquamous, adenoid cystic, undifferentiated, malignant melanoma, and small cell are also seen with much less frequency.

ESSC	*Adenocarcinoma*
• Remains the most common form worldwide • ESSC is thought to originate as an epithelial dysplasia, which initially develops as a mild-to-severe dysplasia and eventually becomes invasive carcinoma • Smoking and substantial alcohol intake are the risk factors for the vast majority of ESSC cases • Only a small proportion being familial • SC is more prevalent in the upper two-thirds thoracic esophagus, and is associated with chronic mucosal injury	• The incidence of esophageal adeno carcinoma has risen remarkably over last 20 years • Adenocarcinoma is linked to chronic gastroesophageal reflux disease (GERD) which can lead to the development of metaplasia (Barrett's esophagus; 5–8% of GERD population) • Progression occurs from metaplasia to dysplasia and ultimately to adenocarcinoma in 0.5% per year • AD is usually confined to the lower esophagus, including the gastroesophageal (GE) junction

Factors Associated with Pathogenesis of Esophageal Cancer

Factor	*Squamous cell cancer*	*Adenocarcinoma*
Smoking	+++	+
Alcohol consumption	+++	–
Hot beverages	+	–
N-nitroso compounds (e.g., pickled vegetables)	+	–
Betel nut chewing	+	–
Mate drinking	+	–
Deficiencies of green vegetables and vitamins	+	–

Contd...

Contd...

Factor	Squamous cell cancer	Adenocarcinoma
Low socioeconomic class	+	–
Fungal toxin or virus	+	–
History of radiation to the mediastinum	+	+
Lye corrosive stricture	+	–
History of aerodigestive malignancy	+++	–
Plummer–Vinson syndrome	+	–
Obesity	–	++
Achalasia	+	–
Gastroesophageal reflux	–	+++
Barrett's esophagus	–	++++

American Joint Committee on Cancer (AJCC) TNM Classification for Esophageal Carcinoma				
T0	No evidence of primary tumor	Stage 0	Tis N0 M0	
T1	Invades lamina propria or submucosa			
T2	Invades muscularis propria	Stage I	T1 N0 M0	
T3	Invades adventitia			
T4	Invades adjacent structures	Stage IIA	T2 N0 M0	T3 N0 M0
N0	No regional lymph node metastasis	Stage IIB	T1 N1 M0	T2 N1 M0
N1	Regional lymph node metastasis	Stage III	T3 N1 M0	T4 any N M0
M0	No distant metastasis	Stage IV	Any T any N M1	
M1	Distant metastasis			
M1a	Invasion of celiac or cervical lymph nodes			
M1b	Other distant metastasis			

Treatment of Carcinoma Lower Third of Esophagus

Diagnosis and Pretreatment Evaluation

- A complete physical examination and directed laboratory analysis should be done in patients suspected of having carcinoma esophagus.
- Plain chest radiography is often unrewarding unless the esophagus is distended or an air fluid level is observed in the posterior mediastinum.
- Although the diagnosis of carcinoma esophagus can be suspected on a barium contrast study, endoscopy is the only modality that provides a tissue diagnosis. The diagnosis of esophageal cancer is made best from an endoscopic biopsy.

During endoscopy, it is critical to document the following:

1.	Location of the lesion (with respect to distance from the incisors)
2.	Nature of the lesion (friable, firm, and polypoid)
3.	Proximal and distal extent of the lesion
4.	Relationship of the lesion to the cricopharyngeus muscle, the GEJ, and the gastric cardia
5.	Distensibility of the stomach

- *Esophagoscopy* allows direct visualization of mucosal abnormalities and histologic diagnosis from biopsies.
- *Rigid esophagoscopy* can be helpful when the lesion is in the cervical esophagus and endoscopic examination of the upper esophageal sphincter is important.

- *Endoscopic ultrasound* combines conventional endoscopy with ultrasound technology:
  - This examination can reveal the depth of mural penetration and invasion of tumor into the periesophageal tissue.
  - The accuracy of this technique for assessing depth of tumor penetration (T status) 85–90%.
- EUS can also demonstrate extension of tumor into adjacent LNs.

Malignant LN	***Benign LN***
• Hypoechoic lymph nodes • Sharply demarcated • Larger than 5 mm	• Hyperechoic pattern • Not sharply demarcated • Have an elongated bean shape

The EUS is not always able to differentiate between benign and malignant nodes.

- *CT:*
  - Primarily used for preoperative staging
  - Local extraesophageal extension into adjacent structures such as the aorta, tracheobronchial tree, or mediastinal LNs can be detected at the time of initial presentation.
  - Approximately one-third of patients show liver metastasis or abdominal lymphadenopathy.
- *Magnetic resonance imaging (MRI):*
  - Not performed routinely and adds to the staging of esophageal cancer in few circumstances.
  - To identify involvement of vascular and neural tissues, MRI is helpful.
  - It can accurately detect T4 lesions and metastatic lesions in the liver.
  - It overstages T and N status with only 74% accuracy.
- *Positron emission tomography* allows the identification of metabolically active areas as evidence of tumor involvement. One potential advantage of PET over CT is the detection of distant metastasis. Because of the possibility of false positive findings, histological confirmation of positive PET or CT findings are often necessary.
- *Bronchoscopy* is recommended to exclude tracheal or bronchial invasion in patients with tumors proximal to the carina or in patients with symptoms suggestive of aerodigestive fistula such as recurrent pneumonia or hemoptysis.
- Surgical staging modalities such as *thoracoscopy* and *laparoscopy* have been used to define pretreatment staging but have not gained wide acceptance.

Treatment

- When a patient presents with esophageal cancer, the following variables are considered.
  - Histology, location, and local extent (depth of invasion) of the primary tumor
  - Status of the local and regional LNs
  - Presence of distant LNs or systemic disease
  - Overall condition of the patient (including nutritional status and ability to swallow)
  - Intended goal of treatment—curative or palliative
- For cancers that are limited to the abdominal esophagus or gastric cardia cancers, an abdominal–right thoracic approach as in a Lewis–Tanner esophagectomy is one option, with the proximal stomach also resected in order to gain an adequate distal resection margin.
- A left thoracoabdominal incision through the seventh or eighth rib space also gives excellent exposure of the low mediastinum and upper abdomen. A single left thoracotomy with opening up of the diaphragm is also an option. This gives reasonable exposure to the upper abdomen as well.
- However, lymphadenectomy toward the hepatoduodenal ligament is hampered.
- When a thoracotomy is not desired, opening the hiatus widely by splitting the crura laterally and the diaphragm anteriorly can gain access to the low posterior mediastinum, and distal esophagectomy can be performed with the anastomosis performed from the abdomen without the need for a thoracic incision.

- The anastomosis is made easier with a mechanical stapler. When the proximal stomach is involved by tumor, a total gastrectomy with Roux-en-Y reconstruction is preferred by many.
- From an oncological standpoint, the philosophy toward lymphadenectomy dictates the surgical approach.

Transthoracic versus Transhiatal Resection

Transthoracic	*Transhiatal*
More thorough lymphadenectomy through a thoracotomy merely improves staging, but does not affect prognosis	• The operating time is shorter and postoperative morbidity is less with the transhiatal approach • Transhiatal resection more suitable for lower esophageal tumors for which much of the mobilization can be performed under vision

Minimally Invasive Surgery

- Various combinations of minimally invasive approaches including thoracoscopy, laparoscopy, mediastinoscopy, hand-assisted laparoscopy, and open laparotomy and thoracotomy have been explored. The myriad of surgical methods tried implies a lack of consensus on which is superior.
- Potentially serious intraoperative complications can occur. These include bleeding from the azygos vein and from intercostal vessel, and injury to the aorta, tracheobronchial tree, and recurrent laryngeal nerve. The lack of tactile control is probably a contributory factor.

Extent of Resection: Axial and Lateral Margin

- An R_0 resection is consistently identified as the most important prognostic factor for long-term survival. An R_0 resection results in total removal of the tumor mass (primary and LNs) with clear proximal, distal, and lateral margins.
- Chance of a histologically positive margin reduces with increasing distance at which the esophagus is transected away from the tumor edge, and that the frequency of anastomotic recurrence is a function of the length of proximal resection margin attained.
- Taking into account shrinkage of the specimen after resection, as a guide to surgery, an in-situ margin of 10 cm (fresh contracted specimen of approximately 5 cm) should be the goal, to allow a <5% chance of anastomotic recurrence.

Note

- Intraoperative frozen section is one method to ensure a negative margin.
- Histologically involved resection margin does not necessarily lead to definite anastomotic recurrence, and a negative margin does not preclude anastomotic recurrence.
- The occurrence of skip lesions or submucosal spread can be missed, so margins may be falsely negative.
- Extramucosal recurrence with infiltration back to the anastomosis may also be indistinguishable from true anastomotic recurrence.
- Patients who have positive histologic margin are those likely to have more advanced disease, and early recurrence at more distal sites.
- Microscopic involvement of the lateral margin (macroscopically clear) results in increased chance of local recurrence and worse survival.
- Obtaining a clear lateral margin is difficult with esophageal cancer because of its anatomic position and adjacent indispensable structures.

Extent of Resection: Lymphadenectomy

- For early cancers (m1–m2 tumors involving tissue up to the lamina propria), the prevalence of lymphatic spread is negligible and thus LN dissection is not indicated. Instead, these are readily treated by EMR.
- For m3 tumors that have penetrated the lamina muscularis mucosa, and cancers that have infiltrated further into the esophagus (sm1 and deeper), the chance of lymphatic spread increases substantially, and lymphadenectomy is indicated.

- Conventional transthoracic resection usually involves a "standard two-field" lymphadenectomy, which entails removing the nodes and periesophageal tissue below the level of the carina, and the LN stations around the celiac trifurcation.
- When superior mediastinal LN dissection is performed, it is sometimes known as "extended two-field lymphadenectomy". "Three-field" lymphadenectomy involves additional bilateral cervical LN clearance.
- The rationale for extensive lymphadenectomy is that LN spread occurs widely in esophageal cancer.
- When preoperative endoscopic injection of technetium-labeled rhenium colloid into the thoracic esophageal wall is performed, radioactivity can be detected to drain via lymphatics to all three fields.
- However, there is preferential lymphatic flow from the upper and middle esophagus to the neck and upper mediastinum and from the lower esophagus to the abdomen.
- For Barrett's adenocarcinomas of the lower esophagus, presumably with less chance of superior mediastinal and cervical LN spread, radical lymphadenectomy mostly involves a standard infracarinal and upper abdominal node dissection.
- Removing positive LNs in the neck may not be clinically significant.
- Poor prognostic factors include:
  - When all three fields have metastatic nodes.
  - When a lower-third tumor has positive cervical nodes.
  - When five or more LNs are involved.
- These situations indicate advanced metastatic disease and three-field lymphadenectomy may not be justified.
- Replacing three-field lymphadenectomy with neoadjuvant, adjuvant, or intraoperative radiotherapy is alternatives, but their roles remain controversial.

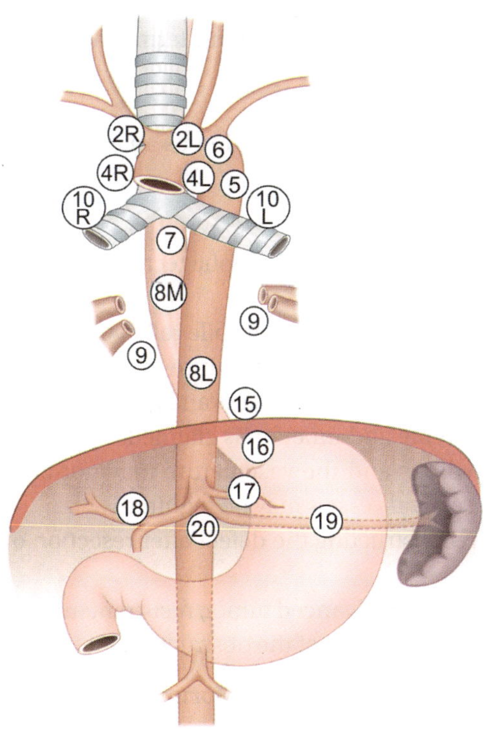

Reconstruction after esophagectomy

- The reconstruction phase of an esophagectomy determines to a significant extent the postoperative morbidity and long-term quality of life.

Gastric Conduit

- The most commonly used conduit is the gastric tube, and of the many configurations attempted, a tailored isoperistaltic tube based on the greater curvature with preservation of the right gastric and right gastroepiploic vessels is most reliable.
- Disadvantages of the gastric conduit are:
  - Postprandial discomfort due to intrathoracic stomach
  - Early satiety due to loss of normal gastric function
  - Patients may also suffer from acid reflux, possible gastric ulceration, and dysfunctional propulsion.
  - Barrett's esophagus has been reported to develop in the esophageal remnant.
  - Patients who have a low intrathoracic anastomosis tend to have more severe reflux and esophagitis compared with the high intrathoracic or cervical anastomosis.
- Preserving a longer length of esophagus, on the other hand, theoretically may enhance swallowing function, although no conclusive data are available on this point.
- Inadequate gastric emptying can also be a problem.

Colonic Conduit

- There are instances when the stomach cannot be used, such as after previous gastric resection, or tumor involvement of a substantial part of the stomach dictating its removal. In these situations, use of the colon is preferred.
- For most, colonic interposition remains an infrequently performed procedure and has the potential for more complications.
- Bowel preparation is required; mobilization of the loop is more complex; its blood supply is less reliable than that of the gastric conduit; three anastomoses are required; and when the colon becomes ischemic, the choice of alternative conduit is restricted.
- A colon conduit is more durable, and the supposed long-term functional benefits of colon interposition make it the preferred esophageal substitute.
- A colonic conduit seems to have active peristalsis
- This is cited as an explanation for its superior function as an esophageal substitute compared with a passive gastric conduit.

Jejunal Conduit

- The jejunum is used most frequently after distal esophagectomy and total gastrectomy for cancer of the lower esophagus and gastric cardia.
- A Roux-en-Y configuration seems best, as it prevents bile reflux to the esophagus.
- A jejunal loop used in a modified Merendino procedure to interpose between the esophagus and proximal stomach after limited resection of the distal esophagus and gastroesophageal junction has also been advocated.
- Excellent postoperative quality of life and function is claimed. A long jejunal loop is sometimes used to reach the neck, but preparation is tedious and the vasculature may not be reliable, and "supercharge" involving microvascular anastomosis to cervical vessels may be required.
- A free jejunal graft is used for reconstructing the defect after resection of the pharyngoesophageal segment in the neck.

When palliative resection is carried out for advanced tumor, recurrent tumor could infiltrate into the conduit placed in the posterior mediastinum. However, the site of the obstruction that produced dysphagia was not clearly stated.

Perioperative Care and Postoperative Morbidity and Mortality

- With adequate preoperative work-up, serious cardiac events such as myocardial infarction should be rare. Atrial arrhythmia is common, affecting about 20% of patients.
- In itself, atrial fibrillation is benign, but it serves as a marker for more serious underlying pulmonary and septic surgical complications.
- Occurrence of atrial arrhythmia should prompt a thorough search for a more ominous underlying cause.

- Pulmonary complications remain the most common and serious form of postoperative morbidity.
- Predictive factors include advanced age, supracarinal tumor location, and lengthened operating time.
- Neoadjuvant therapy did not lead to increased morbidity.
- Measures to improve respiratory outcome include cessation of smoking preoperatively, chest physiotherapy, avoidance of recurrent laryngeal nerve injury, cautious fluid administration to avoid fluid overload, use of a smaller chest tube, early ambulation, regular bronchoscopy, and early tracheostomy for sputum retention. Epidural analgesia is invaluable in postoperative pain relief and has been shown to improve outcome.
- Surgical complications:
  - The most common surgical complication after esophagectomy is still anastomotic leak, and the incidence can reach 30%.
  - Stapled anastomosis is popular for intrathoracic anastomosis, while the hand-sewn technique is preferred in the neck.
  - The clinical presentation of postoperative anastomotic leak ranges from an asymptomatic radiographic finding to a florid thoracic infection.
  - Early detection of anastomotic leaks is important so that timely intervention can be instituted; sometimes a high index of suspicion is important when other seemingly unrelated complications develop.
  - Treatment principles dictate adequate drainage, whether by radiological, endoscopic, or surgical means.
  - Maintenance of nutritional status is important, preferably via the enteral route, either by a fine-bore nasoduodenal tube placed endoscopically or by feeding jejunostomy.
  - The mortality of leaks remains high, in spite of recent improvements in perioperative care and intensive care support.
  - Improvements in the management of leak-related sepsis would likely lead to a decrease in morbidity and mortality.
- Other surgical complications such as:
  - Chylothorax
  - Herniation of bowel through the diaphragmatic hiatus are rare.

Combined Multimodal Treatment Strategies

- Additional treatments for esophageal cancer
- The rationale is based on the suboptimal long-term results of surgery or radiotherapy.
- Both the spatial and synergistic actions of chemotherapeutic agents and radiotherapy are explored in multimodality treatments.
- How surgical resection and these new combinations should be integrated into treatment programs is an active area of research.

Neoadjuvant Radiotherapy

- Trials of neoadjuvant radiotherapy have failed to show increased resection rate or improved survival compared with surgery alone.
- The European Organization for Research and Treatment of Cancer study suggested improved local disease control but no better long-term outcome.
- A Cochrane meta-analysis showed that if preoperative radiotherapy regimens do improve survival, then the effect is likely to be modest, with an absolute improvement in 5-year survival of around 3–4%.

Adjuvant Radiotherapy

- Postoperative radiotherapy was studied in three randomized trials, and all three demonstrated improved local disease control.
- From these studies it seems reasonable to give postoperative radiotherapy to subgroups of patients, especially those who had palliative resections, to enhance local disease control. Suitable meta-analysis should be carried out to further test the statistical validity of the conclusions.

Neoadjuvant Chemotherapy

Neoadjuvant therapy was found not to alter the rate of resection, rate of complete resection, or postoperative complications.

Adjuvant Chemotherapy

Addition of postoperative cisplatin and 5-fluorouracil (5-FU) showed good result.

Neoadjuvant Chemoradiation

Several groups have explored chemoradiation as neoadjuvant therapy. The radiation dose ranged from 20 Gy to 45.6 Gy.

Endoscopic Palliation

Endoscopic palliative treatments for more advanced tumors include:

- Placement of an esophageal prosthesis
- LASER therapy
- Intralesional injection of various substances
- Photodynamic therapy (PDT)

The two most commonly employed techniques are insertion of a prosthesis and LASER therapy. Insertion of self-expanding metallic stents (SEMS) has become the preferred method in many institutions.

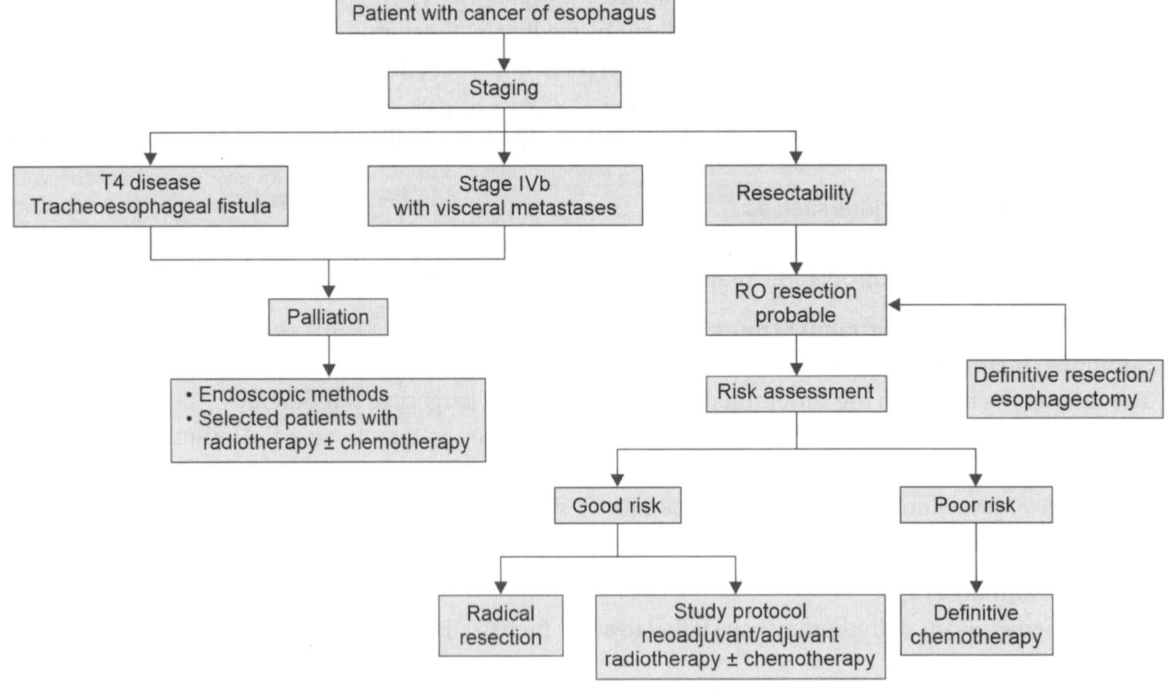

20. Discuss the current status of diagnosis and management of esophageal carcinoma. ***WBUHS 2006***

21. Describe staging of esophageal cancer. Discuss principles of management.

Srimanta Sankaradeva University, Assam 2025

Diagnosis and Pretreatment Evaluation

- A complete physical examination and directed laboratory analysis should be part of the workup of patients suspected of having CE.
- Plain chest radiography is often unrewarding unless the esophagus is distended or an air fluid level is observed in the posterior mediastinum.

- Although the diagnosis of CE can be suspected on a barium contrast study, endoscopy is the only modality that provides a tissue diagnosis.
- Esophagoscopy allows direct visualization of mucosal abnormalities and histologic diagnosis from biopsies. It will also determine if there are changes consistent with BE, because this may impact the extent of subsequent esophageal resection.
- Rigid esophagoscopy can be helpful when the lesion is in the cervical esophagus and endoscopic examination of the upper esophageal sphincter is important.
- Endoscopic ultrasound combines conventional endoscopy with ultrasound technology.
  - Esophageal carcinoma presents as a hypoechoic mass that disrupts the normal anatomy of the esophagus on endoluminal sonography.
  - This examination can reveal the depth of mural penetration and invasion of tumor into the periesophageal tissue.
  - The reported accuracy of this technique for assessing depth of tumor penetration (T status) ranges from 85 to 90%.
  - The EUS can also demonstrate extension of tumor into adjacent LNs. Hypoechoic LNs sharply demarcated and larger than 5 mm are more likely malignant, whereas LNs that are not sharply demarcated and have an elongated bean shape with hyperechoic pattern are more likely benign.
  - The EUS is not always able to differentiate between benign and malignant nodes, and the overall N staging accuracy is approximately 77%. EUS-guided fine needle aspiration of periesophageal LNs has a positive predictive value of 92% and a negative predictive value of 89% and an overall accuracy of 91%.
  - CT is primarily used for preoperative staging. The overall accuracy of CT in staging esophageal cancer is approximately 80–90%. Local extraesophageal extension into adjacent structures such as the aorta, tracheobronchial tree, or mediastinal LNs is detected in 76–86% of cases at the time of initial presentation. Approximately one-third of patients show liver metastasis or abdominal lymphadenopathy.
  - Positron emission tomography allows the identification of metabolically active areas as evidence of tumor involvement. One potential advantage of PET over CT is the detection of distant metastasis.
  - Bronchoscopy is recommended to exclude tracheal or bronchial invasion in patients with tumors proximal to the carina or in patients with symptoms suggestive of aerodigestive fistula such as recurrent pneumonia or hemoptysis. Surgical staging modalities such as thoracoscopy and laparoscopy have been used to define pretreatment staging but have not gained wide acceptance.

The esophageal cancer staging system is based on the AJCC TNM system.

American Joint Committee on Cancer TNM Classification for Esophageal Carcinoma

T0	No evidence of primary tumor	
T1	Invades lamina propria or submucosa	
T2	Invades muscularis propria	
T3	Invades adventitia	
T4	Invades adjacent structures	
N0	No regional lymph node metastasis	
N1	Regional lymph node metastasis	
M0	No distant metastasis	
M1	Distant metastasis	
M1a	Invasion of celiac or cervical lymph nodes	
M1b	Other distant metastasis	
Stage 0	Tis N0 M0	
Stage I	T1 N0 M0	
Stage IIA	T2 N0 M0	T3 N0 M0
Stage IIB	T1 N1 M0	T2 N1 M0
Stage III	T3 N1 M0	T4 any N M0
Stage IV	Any T any N M1	

Diagnosis

Imaging: Several different imaging modalities are used to stage newly diagnosed esophageal cancer.

- A barium study or an EGD may initially raise suspicion of esophageal cancer, the definitive histologic diagnosis is made with EGD and biopsy.
- Chromoendoscopy can help highlight the area of the esophagus to be biopsied and determine the extent of disease.
- Many new endoscopic techniques are being studied with the advent of increased adenocarcinoma prevalence and increased understanding of Barrett's esophagus.
- These new techniques may help diagnose early disease and include trimodality endoscopy providing high-resolution white-light endoscopy, autofluorescence and narrow-band imaging, confocal fluorescence microscopy, elastic scattering spectroscopy, and optical coherence tomography.
- Once the diagnosis is made, EUS is the modality of choice to stage local disease, that is, depth of tumor invasion, and presence of regional LNs.
- A biopsy or fine-needle aspirate of regional LNs, as well as of ascites and regional liver or adrenal metastases, can also be performed at the time of EUS.
- Lymph nodes can be pathologically staged by using EUS with fine-needle aspiration.
- Similarly, distal esophageal tumors with evidence of high mediastinal or paratracheal nodes, although regional according to the new AJCC staging, may represent metastatic disease, which would not be treated with primary surgical intervention or radiotherapy.
- Endoscopic ultrasound has consistently proved superior to CT scanning, MRI, and PET scanning in providing regional TNM staging.
- With a stenosing tumor that does not allow passage of the endoscope (around 30% of cases), the role of EUS is limited. However, in these cases the tumor is likely to be at least T3, and CT or PET scanning can be used to assess the presence of regional or distant nodal disease.
- There is currently no consensus on the role of staging laparoscopy or thoracoscopy in the era of EUS and PET scanning.
- Noninvasive staging with PET and EUS—fine-needle aspirate has become the preferred algorithm.
- Preoperative bronchoscopy is reserved for patients with potentially resectable disease located above the carina, usually squamous cancers, to rule out airway invasion.

Treatment Option Overview

- The prevalence of Barrett metaplasia in adenocarcinoma of the esophagus suggests that Barrett esophagus is a premalignant condition.
- Strong consideration should be given to resection in patients with high-grade dysplasia in the setting of Barrett metaplasia.
- Endoscopic surveillance of patients with Barrett metaplasia may detect adenocarcinoma at an earlier stage more amenable to curative resection.
- The survival rate of patients with esophageal cancer is poor.
- Asymptomatic small tumors confined to the esophageal mucosa or submucosa are detected only by chance.
- Surgery is the treatment of choice for these small tumors.
- Once symptoms are present (e.g., dysphagia, in most cases), esophageal cancers have usually invaded the muscularis propria or beyond and may have metastasized to LNs or other organs.
- In the presence of complete esophageal obstruction without clinical evidence of systemic metastasis, surgical excision of the tumor with mobilization of the stomach to replace the esophagus has been the traditional means of relieving the dysphagia.
- The optimal surgical procedure is controversial.
  - One approach advocates transhiatal esophagectomy with anastomosis of the stomach to the cervical esophagus.
  - A second approach advocates abdominal mobilization of the stomach and transthoracic excision of the esophagus with anastomosis of the stomach to the upper thoracic esophagus or the cervical esophagus.

- Surgical treatment of resectable esophageal cancers results in 5-year survival rates of 5–30%, with higher survival rates in patients with early-stage cancers. This is associated with a <10% operative mortality rate.
  - Stage 0 squamous esophageal cancer is rarely seen, but surgery has been used for this stage of cancer.
    - *Stage 0:* A stage 0 tumor is not true cancer.
    - It contains abnormal cells called high-grade dysplasia *and is really* a type of precancer.
    - The abnormal cells look like cancer cells, but they are only found in the inner layer of cells lining of the esophagus (the epithelium).
    - They have not grown into deeper layers of the esophagus.
    - This stage is often diagnosed when a routine biopsy is done in someone with Barrett's esophagus.
    - Options for treatment may include endoscopic treatments such as PDT, RFA, or EMR. Still, many doctors feel that surgery to remove the esophagus remains the standard treatment.
  - Stage I esophageal cancer—standard treatment option: Surgery.
    - *Stage I:* In this stage, the cancer has grown into some of the deeper layers of the esophagus (past the innermost layer of cells) but has not reached the LNs or other organs.
    - Some very early stage I cancers that involve only a small area of the mucosa and haven't grown into the submucosa may be treated with EMR. This may be followed by some type of endoscopic procedure to destroy any remaining abnormal areas in the esophagus lining.
    - But most patients who are healthy enough have surgery (esophagectomy) to remove the part of their esophagus that contains the cancer.
    - If the cancer is in the upper part of the esophagus (in the neck), chemoradiation may be recommended as the main treatment instead of surgery. This may cure the cancer in some patients. Close follow-up with endoscopy is very important to look for possible signs of cancer returning.
    - Patients who cannot have surgery because they have other serious health problems may be treated with chemotherapy, radiation therapy, or both together.
  - *Stage II esophageal cancer:*
    - *Standard treatment options:*
      - Surgery
      - Chemoradiation
  - Stage II includes cancers that have grown into the main muscle layer of the esophagus or through the muscle layer and into the connective tissue on the outside of the esophagus.
  - This stage also includes some cancers that have spread to 1 or 2 nearby LNs.
  - For people who are healthy enough, treatment options for this stage include surgery, chemotherapy followed by surgery, or chemoradiation followed by surgery.
  - Patients with adenocarcinoma at the place where the stomach and esophagus meet (the gastro-esophageal junction) are often treated with chemotherapy (possibly including the targeted drug Herceptin) followed by surgery.
  - If surgery is the initial treatment, chemoradiation may be recommended afterward, especially if the cancer is an adenocarcinoma or if there are signs that some cancer may have been left behind.
  - In some instances (especially for cancers in the upper part of the esophagus), chemoradiation may be recommended as the main treatment instead of surgery.
  - Patients who do not have surgery need close follow-up with endoscopy to look for possible signs of remaining cancer.
  - Patients who cannot have surgery because they have other serious health problems are usually treated with chemotherapy and radiation therapy.
  - *Stage III esophageal cancer:*
    - *Standard treatment options:*
      - Surgical resection of T3 lesions
      - Chemoradiation

- Stage III includes some cancers that have grown through the wall of the esophagus to the outer layer, as well as cancers that have grown into nearby organs or tissues. It also includes most cancers that have spread to nearby LNs.
- These cancers are treated much like stage II cancers.
- For people who are healthy enough, treatment options for this stage may include surgery, chemotherapy followed by surgery, or chemoradiation followed by surgery.
- Patients with adenocarcinoma at the place where the stomach and esophagus meet (the gastro-esophageal junction) are often treated with chemotherapy (possibly including the targeted drug Herceptin) followed by surgery.
- If surgery is the initial treatment, chemoradiation may be recommended afterward, especially if the cancer is an adenocarcinoma or if there are signs that some cancer may have been left behind.
- In some instances (especially for cancers in the upper part of the esophagus), chemoradiation may be recommended as the main treatment instead of surgery.
- Patients who do not have surgery need close follow-up with endoscopy to look for possible signs of remaining cancer. Unfortunately, even when cancer cannot be seen, it can still be present below the inner lining of the esophagus, so close follow-up is very important.
- Patients who cannot have surgery because they have other serious health problems are usually treated with chemotherapy and radiation therapy.

- *Stage IV esophageal cancer:*
  - At diagnosis, approximately 50% of patients with esophageal cancer will have metastatic disease and will be candidates for palliative therapy.
  - Standard treatment options:
    - Endoscopic-placed stents to provide palliation of dysphagia
    - Radiation therapy with or without intraluminal intubation and dilation
    - Intraluminal brachytherapy to provide palliation of dysphagia
    - Neodymium-doped yttrium aluminum garnet (Nd:YAG) endoluminal tumor destruction or electrocoagulation
    - Chemotherapy has provided partial responses for patients with metastatic distal esophageal adenocarcinomas.
  - Stage IV esophageal cancer has spread to distant LNs or to other distant organs.
  - Treatment is used mainly to help keep the cancer under control for as long as possible and to relieve any symptoms it is causing.
  - Chemotherapy may be given to try to help patients feel better and live longer, but the benefit of giving chemotherapy is not clear.
  - Radiation therapy or other treatments may be used to help with pain or trouble swallowing.

22. What are the causes of dysphagia? How do you propose to investigate a patient with this problem? Briefly discuss the therapeutic options of a case of squamous cell carcinoma of the esophagus. ***WBUHS 2009***

Causes of Dysphagia

Onset in younger age	*Onset in middle age*		*Onset in late age*
1	*2*		*3*
Esophageal web 2 Esophageal ring 1, 2	Achalasia	Myopathy 2, 3	Multiple sclerosis 2, 3 Systemic sclerosis 2
Cardiomegaly 3	Corrosive esophagitis 1, 2	Medications 1, 2, 3	Radiation therapy 2, 3
Diverticulum 3 (Zenker's–direct compression)	Cerebellar stroke 3	Upper esophageal sphincter dysfunction 3	*Candida* esophagitis 2, 3

Contd...

Contd...

Onset in younger age	*Onset in middle age*		*Onset in late age*
1	*2*		*3*
Peptic stricture 1, 2, 3	Brainstem stroke 3 Bulbar and pseudobulbar palsy	Myasthenia gravis 1, 2	Amyotrophic lateral sclerosis 2
Esophageal cancer 3	Mass brain lesion 2, 3	Peptic esophagitis 1, 2, 3	External esophageal compression 1, 2, 3
Diffuse esophageal spasm 2	Esophageal obstruction by a foreign body 2, 3	Lead poisoning 2, 3	Rabies 2, 3 Tetanus 1, 2, 3
Plummer-Vinson syndrome 2	Extrinsic laryngeal carcinoma 3	Oral cavity tumor 3	Systemic lupus erythematous 2

Investigations

- The first investigation is upper GI endoscopy with biopsy from the lesion.
- *Chest X-ray:* To exclude bronchial carcinoma.
- *Barium swallow and meal:* To look at mucosal lining and detect achalasia.
- Esophageal manometry is indicated in various clinical situations. Manometry is indicated in the evaluation of patients with dysphagia after a structural obstruction has been excluded.
- Endoluminal ultrasound scan to assess depth of invasion in case of carcinoma esophagus.
- CT scanning to evaluate local invasion, locoregional lymphadenopathy.
- The gold standard for diagnosing oropharyngeal dysphagia is Modified Barium Swallow Study or Videofluoroscopic Swallow Study (fluoroscopy). This is a lateral video X-ray that provides objective information on bolus transport, safest consistency of bolus (honey, nectar, thin, pudding, puree, and regular), and possible head positioning and/or maneuvers that may facilitate swallow function depending on each individual's anatomy and physiology.

Therapeutic Options for Squamous Cell Carcinoma—Esophagus

American Joint Committee on Cancer TNM Classification for Esophageal Carcinoma

T0	No evidence of primary tumor	
T1	Invades lamina propria or submucosa	
T2	Invades muscularis propria	
T3	Invades adventitia	
T4	Invades adjacent structures	
N0	No regional lymph node metastasis	
N1	Regional lymph node metastasis	
M0	No distant metastasis	
M1	Distant metastasis	
M1a	Invasion of celiac or cervical lymph nodes	
M1b	Other distant metastasis	
Stage 0	Tis N0 M0	
Stage I	T1 N0 M0	
Stage IIA	T2 N0 M0	T3 N0 M0
Stage IIB	T1 N1 M0	T2 N1 M0
Stage III	T3 N1 M0	T4 any N M0
Stage IV	Any T any N M1	

Treatment of Esophageal Carcinoma

Management General approaches:

- The treatment is determined by the cellular type of cancer (adenocarcinoma or squamous cell carcinoma versus other types), the stage of the disease, the general condition of the patient, and other diseases present. Adequate nutrition needs to be assured, and adequate dental care is vital.
- If the patient cannot swallow at all, a stent may be inserted to keep the esophagus patent; stents may also assist in occluding fistulas. A NG tube may be necessary to continue feeding while treatment for the tumor is given, and some patients require a gastrostomy. The latter two are especially important if the patient tends to aspirate food or saliva into the airways, predisposing for aspiration pneumonia.
- *Esophagectomy:* It is the removal of a segment of the esophagus; as this shortens the length of the remaining esophagus, some other segment of the digestive tract (typically the stomach or part of the colon or jejunum) is pulled up to the chest cavity and interposed. If the tumor is unresectable or the patient is not fit for surgery, palliative esophageal stenting can allow the patient to tolerate soft diet.

Types of Esophagectomy

- Thoracoabdominal approach which opens the abdominal and thoracic cavities together.
- Two-stage Ivor Lewis (also called Lewis–Tanner) approach with an initial laparotomy and construction of a gastric tube, followed by a right thoracotomy to excise the tumor and create an esophagogastric anastomosis.
- Three-stage McKeown approach, where a third incision in the neck is made to complete the cervical anastomosis.
    - *Endoscopic therapy for localized disease:* The candidates for endoscopic therapy are stage 1 patients with tumors invading into the lamina propria (T1 mucosal) or submucosa (T1 submucosal) that do not have regional or distant metastasis.
    - Patients with carcinoma in-situ or high-grade dysplasia can also be treated with endoscopic therapy.
    - Submucosal cancers with increased risk of nodal metastases may not be as amenable to curative therapy.
        - The two forms of endoscopic therapy that have been used for stage 0 and I disease are EMR and mucosal ablation using PDT, Nd-YAG laser, or APC.
        - EMR has been advocated for early cancers. This technique can be attempted in patients, without evidence of nodal or distant metastases, with differentiated tumors that are slightly raised and <2 cm in diameter, or in differentiated tumors that are ulcerated and <1 cm in diameter.
        - LASER therapy is the use of high-intensity light to destroy tumor cells; it affects only the treated area. This is typically done if the cancer cannot be removed by surgery. PDT, a type of laser therapy, involves the use of drugs that are absorbed by cancer cells; when exposed to a special light, the drugs become active and destroy the cancer cells.
        - Chemotherapy depends on the tumor type, but tends to be cisplatin-based (or carboplatin or oxaliplatin) every 3 weeks with 5-FU either continuously or every 3 weeks. In more recent studies, addition of epirubicin [epirubicin, cisplatin, 5-fluorouracil (ECF)] was better than other comparable regimens in advanced nonresectable cancer. Chemotherapy may be given after surgery (adjuvant, i.e., to reduce risk of recurrence), before surgery (neoadjuvant) or if surgery is not possible, in this case, cisplatin and 5-FU are used.
        - Radiotherapy is given before, during or after chemotherapy or surgery, and sometimes on its own to control symptoms. In patients with localized disease but contraindications to surgery, "radical radiotherapy" may be used with curative intent.

Follow-up

Patients are followed up frequently after a treatment regimen has been completed. Frequently, other treatments are necessary to improve symptoms and maximize nutrition.

23. Merits and demerits of gastric versus colonic conduit for esophageal replacement. ***WBUHS 2022***

	Gastric pull-up	*Colon interposition*	*Jejunal interposition*
Advantages	Fast and safe procedure; stomach easily prepared; sufficient length to reach the neck; standardized technique; one single anastomosis; dependable vascularization low rate of necrosis; minimally-invasive surgery	Long and short colon; gastric reservoir; best functional results and quality of life; reduced delayed gastric emptying; reduced reflux; generous resection margins of distal tumors; outside the field of irradiation for distal tumors (preoperative radiotherapy)	Anterograde segmental contraction; sterile environment; low leakage rate
Disadvantages	Significant loss of capacity of the gastric reservoir; reflux esophagitis (30–50%); Barrett esophagus in the remnant esophagus; shorter distal margin for distal esophageal cancer or GEJ tumor; within field of radiation therapy for distal tumors (preoperative radiotherapy)	Complex procedure, longer operative time; limits; (1) aortic aneurysm; (2) previous abdominal or colic surgery; and (3) colonic disease (inflammatory bowel disease); preoperative bowel preparation needed; higher rate of necrosis, morbidity, and mortality; 3 or 4 anastomoses; redundancy	Technically extremely complex; supercharged (microvascular anastomosis); experienced center; limitation in the length; exceptional indications

GE JUNCTION TUMOUR

24. Treatment of GE junction tumor. ***Rajasthan University of Health Sciences 2025***

A GE junction tumor refers to a *tumor located at the gastroesophageal (GE) junction,* which is the area where the *esophagus* meets the *stomach.* This region is clinically important because tumors here can behave like *esophageal cancers, gastric cancers,* or a mix of both—and the *treatment approach* depends on the *tumor's exact location and type.*

Types and Classification

GE junction tumors are commonly classified using the *Siewert classification* system:

Type	*Location (center of tumor)*	*Typical origin*	*Treatment approach*
Type I	1–5 cm above the GE junction	Distal esophagus (often Barrett's esophagus–related adenocarcinoma)	Treated like *esophageal cancer*
Type II	1 cm above to 2 cm below the GE junction	True *cardia carcinoma* (tumor of the GE junction itself)	Borderline—may need *combined approach*
Type III	2–5 cm below the GE junction	*Subcardial stomach* (upper stomach cancer invading the GE junction)	Treated like *gastric cancer*

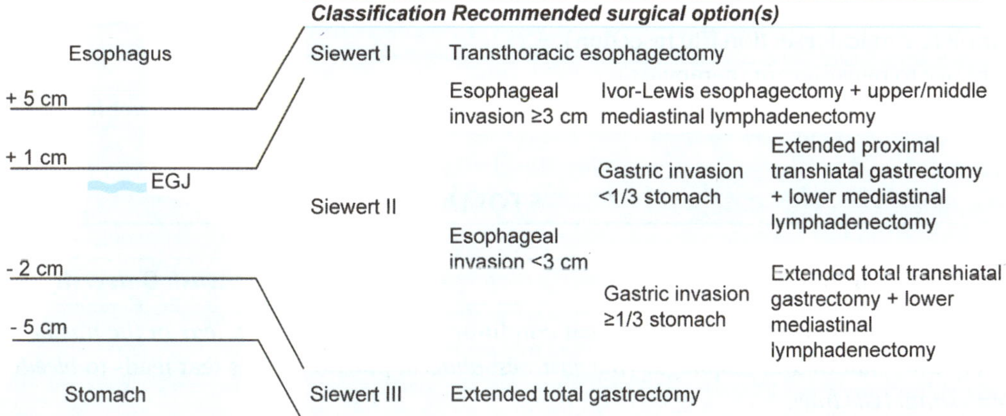

Histologic Types

Most GE junction tumors are *adenocarcinomas*, though *squamous cell carcinoma* can occur in tumors extending from the esophagus.

Risk factors for *adenocarcinoma* include:

- Gastroesophageal reflux disease (GERD)
- Barrett's esophagus
- Obesity
- Smoking
- Male sex
- High-fat, low-fiber diet

Symptoms

Common presentations include:

- Difficulty swallowing *(dysphagia)*
- Painful swallowing *(odynophagia)*
- Weight loss
- Chest or upper abdominal pain
- Regurgitation or vomiting
- Anemia from occult bleeding

Diagnosis

- *Endoscopy with biopsy* (to confirm histology and location)
- *Endoscopic ultrasound (EUS)* (to assess local invasion)
- *CT scan or PET-CT* (to check for metastases)
- *Staging laparoscopy* (for locally advanced disease)

Treatment

Depends on tumor stage and type:

- *Early stage:* Endoscopic resection (in situ or T1a)
- *Locally advanced:* Combination of *Chemotherapy and/or radiation* plus *surgery*
    - *Type I:* Esophagectomy
    - *Type III:* Gastrectomy
    - *Type II:* Individualized — may involve either approach
- *Metastatic:* Systemic therapy (chemotherapy, targeted therapy, or immunotherapy)

Prognosis

Prognosis depends on:

- Stage at diagnosis (depth of invasion, nodal involvement)
- Complete surgical resection (R0 resection)
- Response to neoadjuvant therapy

Generally, *5-year survival* ranges from *20 to 40%* for localized disease but is much lower for metastatic disease.

STOMACH

25. Mallory-Weiss syndrome. ***Ayush University, Chhattisgarh 2025***

Mallory-Weiss syndrome (MWS) is a medical condition characterized by a *tear in the mucous membrane at the junction of the stomach and esophagus (the gastroesophageal junction)*. This tear leads to *bleeding from the upper gastrointestinal (GI) tract.*

Pathophysiology

- The tear typically occurs in the *mucosa (not full thickness)* due to a *sudden rise in intra-abdominal pressure.*
- Common triggers:
  - Severe or repeated vomiting/retching
  - Coughing
  - Seizures
  - Straining (as in lifting or defecation)
- The tear is usually *longitudinal* and located at the *gastroesophageal junction* or *proximal stomach.*

Risk Factors

- *Alcohol use* (most common association)
- *Hiatal hernia*
- *Bulimia nervosa* or eating disorders with recurrent vomiting
- *Gastroenteritis*
- *Severe hiccups*
- *Pregnancy (hyperemesis gravidarum)*

Clinical Features

- *Hematemesis* (vomiting of bright red blood or coffee-ground material)
- *Melena* (black, tarry stools)
- *Epigastric or back pain* (less common)
- *History of forceful vomiting or retching* prior to bleeding

Diagnosis

- *Upper GI endoscopy* is the *gold standard:*
  - Visualizes a *linear tear* near the gastroesophageal junction
  - Confirms the *source of bleeding*
- *Laboratory tests:*
  - CBC (to assess anemia)
  - Coagulation profile
  - Liver function tests (to rule out variceal bleeding in alcoholics)

Management

Most cases *resolve spontaneously.*

- **Initial management**
  - *Stabilize the patient:*
    - Airway, breathing, circulation (ABC)
    - IV fluids if hypotensive
    - Blood transfusion if necessary
  - *Proton pump inhibitors (PPIs):* Reduce acid and promote healing
  - *Antiemetics:* Prevent further vomiting
- *Endoscopic therapy* (if bleeding persists):
  - Epinephrine injection
  - Thermal coagulation
  - Hemoclips or band ligation
- *Surgery or angiographic embolization:* Rare, reserved for refractory bleeding.

Prognosis

- *Excellent*—most tears heal within *48–72 hours.*
- *Rebleeding is rare.*
- Mortality is low unless the patient has *comorbid conditions* (e.g., cirrhosis, coagulopathy).

26. Dieulafoy's lesion. ***WBUHS 2008***

- Dieulafoy's lesions are vascular malformations found primarily along the lesser curve of the stomach within 6 cm of the gastroesophageal junction, although they can occur elsewhere in the GI tract.
- They represent rupture of unusually large vessels (1–3 mm) that are found in the gastric submucosa.
- Erosion of the gastric mucosa overlying these vessels leads to hemorrhage. The mucosal defect is usually small (2–5 mm) and may be difficult to identify. Given the large size of the underlying artery, bleeding from a Dieulafoy's lesion can be massive.
- Initial attempts at endoscopic control are often successful.
- Application of thermal or sclerosant therapy is effective in 80–100% of cases.
- In cases that fail endoscopic therapy, angiographic coil embolization can be successful.
- If these approaches fail, surgical intervention may be necessary; owing to difficulties in visualization and palpation of these lesions, prior endoscopic tattooing can facilitate the procedure.
- A gastrotomy is performed, and attempts are made at identifying the bleeding source. The lesion can then be oversewn.
- In cases in which the bleeding point is not identified, a partial gastrectomy may be necessary.

27. *Helicobacter pylori*. ***WBUHS 2011***

Introduction

Helicobacter pylori is a gram-negative, microaerophilic bacterium found in the stomach. It was identified in 1982 by Barry Marshall and Robin Warren, who found that it was present in patients with chronic gastritis and gastric ulcers, conditions that were not previously believed to have a microbial cause. It is also linked to the development of duodenal ulcers and stomach cancer.

Signs and Symptoms

- Most people (over 80%) infected with *H. pylori* show no symptoms.
- Acute infection may appear as an acute gastritis with abdominal pain (stomach ache) or nausea.
- Where this develops into chronic gastritis, the symptoms, if present, are often those of nonulcer dyspepsia: stomach pains, nausea, bloating, belching, and sometimes vomiting.
- Individuals infected with *H. pylori* have a 10–20% lifetime risk of developing peptic ulcers and a 1–2% risk of acquiring stomach cancer.
- Inflammation of the pyloric antrum is more likely to lead to duodenal ulcers, while inflammation of the corpus (body of the stomach) is more likely to lead to gastric ulcers and gastric carcinoma.
- *H. pylori* infection as an important cause of gastric malignancy.
- *H. pylori* causes chronic antigenic stimulation to stomach mucosa, B lymphocytic proliferation, and mucosa-associated lymphoid tissue (MALT) lymphoma.

Prevention

- *H. pylori* is a major cause of diseases of the upper gastrointestinal tract.
- Eradication of the infection improves symptoms including dyspepsia, gastritis, and peptic ulcers, and may prevent gastric cancer (GC).
- Rising antibiotic resistance increases the need for a prevention strategy for the bacteria.

Treatment

- Once *H. pylori* is detected in patients with a peptic ulcer, the normal procedure is to eradicate it and allow the ulcer to heal.
- The standard first-line therapy is a one week "triple therapy" consisting of PPIs such as omeprazole, lansoprazole, and the antibiotics clarithromycin and amoxicillin.
- Variations of the triple therapy have been developed over the years, such as using a different PPI, as with pantoprazole or rabeprazole, or replacing amoxicillin with metronidazole for people who are allergic to penicillin.

- Such a therapy has revolutionized the treatment of peptic ulcers, and has made a cure to the disease possible; previously, the only option was symptom control using antacids, H_2-antagonists, or PPIs alone.
- An increasing number of infected individuals is found to harbor antibiotic-resistant bacteria.
- This results in initial treatment failure and requires additional rounds of antibiotic therapy or alternative strategies, such as a quadruple therapy, which adds a bismuth colloid, such as bismuth subsalicylate.
- For the treatment of clarithromycin-resistant strains of *H. pylori*, the use of levofloxacin as part of the therapy has been suggested.

Prognosis

- *H. pylori* colonizes the stomach and induces chronic gastritis, a long-lasting inflammation of the stomach. The bacterium persists in the stomach for decades in most people.
- Most individuals infected by *H. pylori* will never experience clinical symptoms despite having chronic gastritis.
- Approximately 10–20% of those colonized by *H. pylori* will ultimately develop gastric and duodenal ulcers. *H. pylori* infection is also associated with a 1–2% lifetime risk of stomach cancer and a <1% risk of gastric MALT lymphoma.
- In the absence of treatment, *H. pylori* infection—once established in its gastric niche—is widely believed to persist for life.
- In the elderly, however, it is likely infection can disappear as the stomach's mucosa becomes increasingly atrophic and inhospitable to colonization.
- The proportion of acute infections that persist is not known, but several studies that followed the natural history in populations have reported apparent spontaneous elimination.
- The incidence of acid reflux disease, Barrett's esophagus, and esophageal cancer has been rising dramatically.
- *H. pylori* accounts for the recent increase in incidence of several diseases, including type 2 diabetes, obesity, and asthma.

PEPTIC ULCER DISEASE

28. Investigations of peptic ulcer syndrome. ***WBUHS 2006***

Introduction

- History and physical examination are probably of limited value in distinguishing between gastric and duodenal ulceration. Routine laboratory studies include a complete blood count, liver chemistries, serum creatinine, and calcium levels.
- A serum gastrin level should also be obtained in patients with ulcers that are refractory to medical therapy or require surgery.
- An upright chest radiograph is usually performed when ruling out perforation.
- The two principal means of diagnosing peptic ulcers are upper GI radiography and fiberoptic endoscopy.
- Contrast radiography is less expensive, and most (90%) can be diagnosed accurately. However, about 5% of ulcers that appear radiographically benign are malignant. *H. pylori* testing should also be done in all patients with suspected peptic ulcer disease (PUD).

***H. pylori* Testing**

- *Serology:*
  - *H. pylori* infection elicits a local as well as a systemic immunoglobulin G (IgG)-mediated immune response, so serology can be used to diagnose *H. pylori*.
  - Serology is the diagnostic test of choice when endoscopy is not indicated and has about 90% sensitivity and specificity associated with it.
  - *Limitations of serology testing*:
    - Antibody titers can remain high for a year or more.
    - This test cannot be used to assess eradication after therapy.

- *Urea breath test:*
  - This test is based on the ability of *H. pylori* to hydrolyze urea.
  - Its sensitivity and specificity are both >95%.
  - The urea breath test is less expensive than endoscopy and samples the entire stomach.
  - False-negative results can occur if the test is done too soon after treatment, so it is usually best to test 4 weeks after therapy is finished.
  - The urea breath test is the method of choice to document eradication.
- *Rapid urease assay:*
  - The method of choice to diagnosis *H. pylori* if endoscopy is employed is the rapid urease test.
  - This is another test based on the ability of *H. pylori* to hydrolyze urea.
  - The enzyme urease catalyzes degradation of urea to ammonia and bicarbonate, creating an alkaline environment that can be detected by a pH indicator.
  - Consequently, endoscopy is performed and gastric mucosal tissue biopsied.
  - Mucosal biopsy samples are placed into a liquid or solid medium containing urea and a pH indicator.
  - Sensitivity is about 90% and specificity 98%, and the results are available within hours.
- *Histology:*
  - Endoscopy can also be performed with biopsy samples of gastric mucosa followed by histologic visualization of *H. pylori.*
  - This test is widely available and affords the clinician the ability to assess the severity of gastritis as well as to confirm the presence or absence of the organism.
- *Culture:*
  - Culturing of gastric mucosa obtained at endoscopy can also be performed to diagnosis *H. pylori.*
  - The sensitivity is about 80% and specificity 100%.
  - It requires laboratory expertise, it is not widely available, it is relatively expensive, and diagnosis requires up to 3–5 days until a diagnosis is made.

Upper Gastrointestinal Radiography

- Diagnosis of peptic ulcer by upper GI radiography requires the demonstration of barium within the ulcer crater, which is usually round or oval, and may or may not be surrounded by edema.
- This study is useful to determine the location and the depth of penetration of the ulcer as well as the extent of deformation from chronic fibrosis.
- With single-contrast radiographic techniques, as many as 50% of duodenal ulcers may be missed, whereas with double-contrast studies, 80–90% of ulcer craters can be detected.
- The location of a gastric ulcer is of little predictive value in establishing malignancy as benign, and malignant ulcers can occur anywhere in the stomach.
- The size of the gastric ulcer may have some predictive value in that larger lesions are more likely to be malignant than smaller ones.
- In addition, the finding of an ulcer with an associated mass; interrupted, fused, or nodular mucosal folds approaching the margin of the crater; or an ulcer with irregular filling defects in the ulcer crater is suggestive of a malignancy.
- *Fiberoptic endoscopy:*
  - Endoscopy is the most reliable method of diagnosing a gastric ulcer.
  - When multiple biopsies and brushings for cytology are performed, the probability of diagnosing a malignancy is in excess of 90%.
  - In general, benign ulcers have smoother, more regular, rounded edges with a flat, and smooth ulcer base.
  - Malignancy is more often associated with a mass that may protrude into the lumen or has folds surrounding the ulcer crater that are nodular, clubbed, fused, or stop short of the ulcer margin.
  - Multiple biopsy specimens are necessary for any of these ulcers because ruling out a malignancy is mandatory.

- In addition to providing diagnostic abilities, endoscopy provides the ability to sample tissue for *H. pylori* testing and may also be used for therapeutic purposes in the setting of GI bleeding.

29. Gastric outlet obstruction in adults. *WBUHS 2012*

30. Describe etiology, clinical features, and management of gastric outlet obstruction. *Gujarat Health University 2025*

31. Surgical anatomy of gastric outlet. Metabolic derangement in gastric outlet obstruction. Management of benign gastric outlet obstruction. *KGMU, Lucknow 2025*

32. How would you manage a patient of gastric malignancy with outlet obstruction? *WBUHS 2018, RIMS, Imphal 2022*

33. Metabolic changes and its management in gastric outlet obstruction. *WBUHS 2013, 2019*

34. Discuss the pathophysiological basis of fluid and electrolyte abnormalities in gastric outlet obstruction. How do you prepare a patient of such a condition before surgery? *WBUHS 2008*

Surgical Anatomy of Gastric Outlet

Introduction

The *surgical anatomy of the gastric outlet* is centered around the *distal part of the stomach*, the *pyloric canal*, and the *duodenum*. It's a key region for understanding operations such as *pyloromyotomy, antrectomy*, and *vagotomy*, as well as for recognizing conditions like *gastric outlet obstruction* and *pyloric stenosis*.

The *gastric outlet* refers to the *distal portion of the stomach that leads into the duodenum*—primarily the *pyloric antrum, pyloric canal*, and *pylorus* (the muscular sphincter controlling gastric emptying).

Anatomical Divisions of the Stomach (Relevant to Outlet)

From proximal to distal:

- *Cardia*—near gastroesophageal junction
- *Fundus*—dome-shaped part above the cardia
- *Body (Corpus)*—main part of the stomach
- *Antrum (Pyloric antrum)*—distal, funnel-shaped part leading to the pyloric canal
- *Pyloric canal*—short, narrow segment leading to the *pylorus*

Pylorus

- *Definition:* A *muscular sphincter* that regulates passage of gastric contents into the duodenum.
- *Length:* ~1–2 cm
- *Structure:*
  - *Pyloric sphincter muscle:* Thickened circular layer of smooth muscle.
  - *Pyloric ring:* Palpable landmark during surgery.
- *Location (Surface Anatomy):*
  - Lies on the transpyloric plane (L1 vertebral level).
  - Midway between the jugular notch and the pubic symphysis.
  - On the right side of midline, ~2.5 cm from it.

Blood Supply

Structure	*Arterial supply*	*Venous drainage*
Pylorus and Antrum	• *Right gastric artery* (branch of proper hepatic artery) • *Right gastroepiploic artery* (branch of gastroduodenal artery) • *Left gastric artery* (minor contribution)	Corresponding veins drain into *portal vein* (directly or via splenic/SMA branches)

Lymphatic Drainage

- *Right gastric nodes* and *right gastroepiploic nodes*
- Drain into *celiac lymph nodes*
- Important in *gastrectomy and cancer spread*

Nerve Supply

Component	Function
Parasympathetic (Vagus nerve)	• Stimulates gastric motility and secretion • Controls pyloric relaxation
Sympathetic (T6–T9 via celiac plexus)	• Inhibits motility • Contracts pyloric sphincter

Surgical relevance: Vagotomy (cutting vagal branches) reduces acid secretion but can delay gastric emptying unless combined with drainage procedure (e.g., *pyloroplasty*).

Relations

Relation	Structures
Anterior	Left lobe of liver, anterior abdominal wall, gallbladder (sometimes)
Posterior	Pancreas (head), gastroduodenal artery, bile duct, portal vein
Superior	Liver
Inferior	First part of duodenum

Surgical Relevance

- *Pyloromyotomy (Ramstedt's procedure):* For congenital hypertrophic pyloric stenosis — incision through the pyloric muscle to relieve obstruction.
- *Pyloroplasty:* Widening of the pyloric canal, often with truncal vagotomy.
- *Antrectomy:* Removal of the distal stomach (including pylorus and antrum).
- *Gastric outlet obstruction:* Often due to peptic ulcer disease, carcinoma, or scarring—knowledge of blood and nerve supply is vital for management.

Definition of Gastric Outlet Obstruction

It is a clinical condition of the pylorus or pyloric canal of the stomach that causes blocks the entry of food particles from the stomach to the duodenum (first section of the small intestine). Pyloric canal is a narrow tubular passage that forms an opening between the stomach and small intestine. It is generally not considered as a separate clinical entity and is usually a physiological consequence of other abdominal disorders.

This condition is also abbreviated as GOO.

Causes

Benign causes	Malignant causes
• PUD • Gastric polyps • Ingestion of caustics • Pyloric stenosis • Congenital duodenal webs • Gallstone obstruction (Bouveret syndrome) • Pancreatic pseudocysts • Bezoars • Gastric TB • Gastric Crohn's	• Pancreatic cancer • Carcinoma gallbladder • Ampullary cancer • Duodenal cancer • Cholangiocarcinoma • Gastric cancer • Lymphoma • Metastases to the gastric outlet

Symptoms

- *Projectile vomiting:* Patients are found to forcibly eject the contents of the stomach through the mouth, owing to pyloric obstruction.
- *Constipation:* While emptying the bowels, patients may face difficulties and acute discomfort that usually occur infrequently. In this condition, hard, dry, and small stools are passed. Eliminating these can be quite painful.
- *Weight loss:* Loss of fluids and reduced appetite may result in sudden decrease in weight.
- *Epigastric pain:* It is one of the most common symptoms of this stomach disorder. It is generally associated with acute pain arising in the upper middle part of the abdomen.
- *Dehydration:* Persistent vomiting may lead to significant loss of body fluids, primarily causing excessive water deficiency.
- *Electrolyte imbalance:* Hypochloremia, a deficiency of chloride ion in bloodstream due to prolonged vomiting, is a common symptom observed during this condition. Excessive loss of potassium (hypokalemia) and hydrochloric acid (metabolic alkalosis), which occurs as a consequence of dehydration, highly contributes to this sudden reduction in body chlorides.
- *Wasting:* Continuous degeneration of the body muscle and fat tissues may occur in the affected individuals, owing to low intake and high loss of nutrients (especially that of proteins). Malignant conditions of the stomach could be the primary factor, causing this gradual deterioration of the muscle tissues.

Metabolic Changes and its Management in Gastric Outlet Obstruction

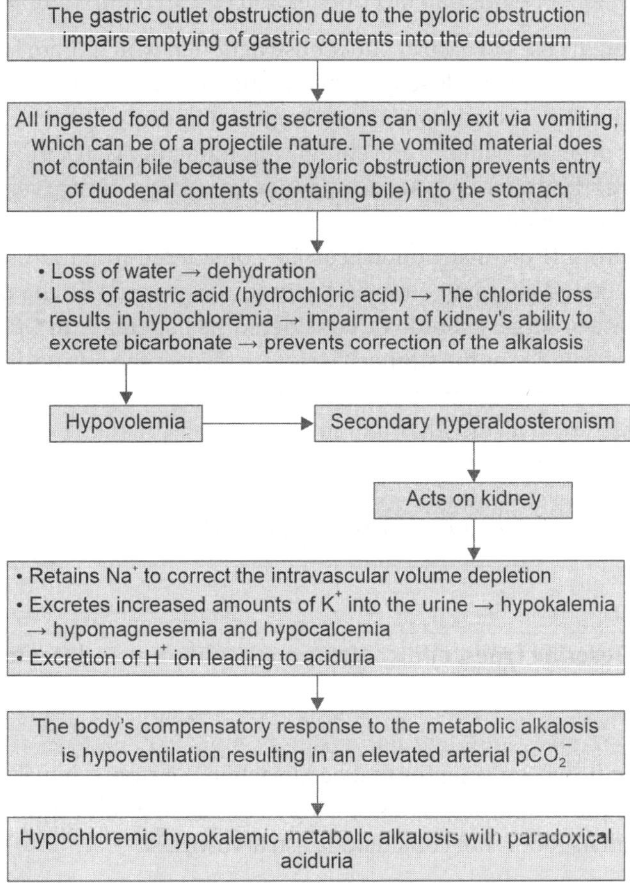

Management of the Patient

- Rehydration with IV isotonic saline with potassium supplementation. Replacing the sodium chloride and water allows the kidney to correct the acid–base abnormality.

- Following rehydration, it may become obvious that the patient is also anemic, the hemoglobin being spuriously high on presentation.
- The stomach should be emptied using a wide-bore gastric tube. Pass an orogastric tube and lavage the stomach until it is completely emptied.
- Then endoscopy and contrast radiology
- Biopsy of the area around the pylorus is essential to exclude malignancy.
- The patient should also have an antisecretory agent, initially given intravenously to ensure absorption.
- Build up nutrition

Preoperative Management

- First and foremost is hydration and correction of electrolyte imbalances.
- *Sodium chloride solution:* Initial IV fluid of choice
- Potassium deficits must be corrected.
- *NG tube:* To decompress stomach
- Nutrition should be maintained, if needed TPN.
- For malignant lesions, anemia should be corrected—Hb% should be at least 8 g%.
- To investigate for finding out the actual cause.

Definitive Management to be done After Diagnosing the cause of GOO.

In most patients with peptic ulcer disease, the edema will usually settle with conservative management with nasogastric suction, replacement of fluids and electrolytes and proton pump inhibitors.

Surgical: Surgery is indicated in cases of gastric outlet obstruction in which there is significant obstruction and in cases where medical therapy has failed. Endoscopic balloon therapy may be attempted as an alternative to surgery, with balloon dilation reporting success rates of 76% after repeat dilatons.

Surgery forms the final option for patients presenting with refractory GOO. Most common surgeries for peptic strictures include vagotomy and antrectomy, vagotomy and pyloroplasty, truncal vagotomy and gastrojejunostomy, pyloroplasty and laparoscopic variants.

Gastrojejunostomy (Billroth II reconstruction) can be considered in patients with preserved anatomy like peptic GOO, however with altered anatomy, Rouxen-Y jejunostomy would be the preferred option. Placement of a jejunostomy tube at the time of surgery should be considered, as patients with GOO are already malnourished.

Also in chronically dilated conditions the stomach is slow to recover the normal rate of emptying. In peptic GOO, gastrojejunostomy can be combined with truncal vagotomy and antrectomy. Laparoscopic gastrojejunostomy for the relief of GOO is associated with a smoother and more rapid postoperative recovery and shorter hospital stay compared with open surgery and should become the new gold standard.

GASTRIC VOLVULUS

35. Gastric volvulus. ***WBUHS 2021***

36. What is gastric volvulus? Describe types, clinical features, evaluation and treatment for patients with Gastric Volvulus disease. ***WBUHS 2025***

Introduction

- Gastric volvulus is a specific type of volvulus that occurs when the stomach twists on its mesentery.
- It should be at least 180° and causes bowel obstruction to be called gastric volvulus.
- Merely gastric rotation on its root is not considered gastric volvulus.

Epidemiology

- Organoaxial volvulus is more common in adults, responsible for 60% of presentations.
- Mesenteroaxial volvulus is more common in children.

Clinical Presentation: Patients may Present with the Classic Triad of Borchardt

- Severe sudden epigastric pain
- Intractable retching without vomiting
- Inability to pass a NG tube
- Chronic symptoms are more common in patients with mesenteroaxial volvulus.

Differential Diagnosis

- Epiphrenic diverticulum
- Postoperative state of the stomach
- Hiatal hernia

Pathology

Subtypes

- *Organoaxial volvulus*
  - More common of the two types in adults (two-thirds of cases)
  - Commonly occurs in the setting of trauma or paraesophageal hernia.
  - Stomach is rotated along its long axis (along the cardiopyloric line, which is drawn between the cardia and the pylorus).
  - Mirror image of normal anatomy can occur with reversal of the greater and lesser curves.
  - Antrum rotates anterosuperiorly.
  - Fundus rotates posteroinferiorly.
  - Complete (>180°) present with obstruction or ischemia
  - Incomplete rotation (<180°) also called organoaxial position of the stomach, usually asymptomatic
- *Mesenteroaxial volvulus*
  - Less common in adults, but is more common than organoaxial volvulus in the pediatric population (59% of gastric volvulus).
  - Rotation around short axis from the lesser to greater curvature (i.e., perpendicular to the cardiopyloric line)
  - Usually incomplete, <180° displacement of antrum above gastroesophageal junction; stomach appears upside-down with the antrum and pylorus superior to the fundus and proximal body.
  - Coincides with the axis of mesenteric attachment and is associated with severe obstruction and strangulation.
  - Less associated with diaphragmatic defect
  - Plain films may show an intrathoracic stomach with two air fluid levels.

Associations

- Wandering spleen
- Congenital diaphragmatic hernia
- Diaphragmatic eventration
- Laparoscopic adjustable gastric banding

Radiographic Features

Plain Radiograph

- *Chest Radiograph*
  - Intrathoracic; upside-down stomach
  - Mediastinal or retrocardiac air-fluid level
  - Abdominal radiograph, when performed with the patient upright
  - Unexpected location of the gastric bubble
  - Double air-fluid level
  - Large, distended stomach
  - Collapsed small bowel

Fluoroscopy

- *Upper GI:*
  - Distended stomach in left upper quadrant extending into thorax
  - Inversion of stomach
  - Volvulus with >180° twist causes luminal obstruction
  - Incomplete or absent entrance of contrast material into and/or out of stomach is indicative of acute obstructive volvulus—"beaking" may be demonstrated at point of twist.
  - *Mesenteroaxial:* Antrum and pylorus lie above gastric fundus.

CT

- The appearance depends on points of torsion, extent of gastric herniation, and final positioning of stomach.
- Distended stomach with antropyloric transition point, located at the level of or superior to the fundus
- Linear septum may be visible within the gastric lumen which corresponds to the site of torsion.
- Entire stomach may be herniated.
- *Both can result in:*
  - Volvulus
  - Obstruction
  - *Ischemia:* Ischemia seen as lack of contrast enhancement of gastric wall, with or without pneumatosis.

Treatment and Prognosis

- Surgical repair, including stomach detorsion and gastropexy, is the main treatment modality for gastric volvulus.
- Detorsion may be performed open or laparoscopically. If the stomach is strangulated or necrotic, gastric resection may be required.

CARCINOMA STOMACH

37. Discuss the blood supply and lymphatic drainage of stomach and outline rationale of D2 gastrectomy in carcinoma stomach. Mention different types of reconstructions following such procedure.
WBUHS 2007; Rajasthan Health University 2025; KIIT University, Odisha 2025

38. Discuss the etiopathology, types, clinical features and management of carcinoma stomach. ***WBUHS 2016***

39. Describe the pathology and staging of carcinoma stomach. ***RIMS, Imphal 2012***

40. Give the anatomical description of the different lymph nodal stations draining mainly stomach with a schematic diagram and discuss the role of sentinel lymph node biopsy in the setting of gastric cancers.
WBUHS 2017

41. Describe the lymph node status in relation to spread of carcinoma stomach. Discuss in detail the different types of gastric carcinoma and prognosis in respect to lymph node harvest. ***WBUHS 2015***

42. D2 gastrectomy. ***WBUHS 2011***

43. Write down the different clinical presentation of carcinoma stomach. Discuss the merits and demerits of D2 gastrectomy. ***WBUHS 2025 Supplementary***

Arterial Supply and Venous Drainage of Stomach

Arterial Supply

- The large majority of the gastric blood supply is from the celiac axis via four named arteries.

- The left and right gastric arteries form an anastomotic arcade along the lesser curvature, and the right and left gastroepiploic arteries form an arcade along the greater gastric curvature.
- The consistently largest artery to the stomach is the left gastric artery, which usually arises directly from the celiac trunk and divides into an ascending and descending branch along the lesser gastric curvature.
- Approximately 15% of the time, the left gastric artery supplies an aberrant vessel which travels in the gastrohepatic ligament (lesser omentum) to the left side of the liver.
- Rarely, this is the only arterial blood supply to this part of the liver, and inadvertent ligation may lead to clinically significant hepatic ischemia.
- The second largest artery to the stomach is usually the right gastroepiploic artery, which arises fairly consistently from the gastroduodenal artery behind the first portion of the duodenum.
- The left gastroepiploic artery arises from the splenic artery, and together with the right gastroepiploic artery, forms the rich gastroepiploic arcade along the greater curvature.
- The right gastric artery usually arises from the hepatic artery near the pylorus and hepatoduodenal ligament, and runs proximally along the distal stomach.
- In the fundus along the proximal greater curvature, the short gastric arteries and veins arise from the splenic circulation.
- There also may be vascular branches to the proximal stomach from the phrenic circulation.

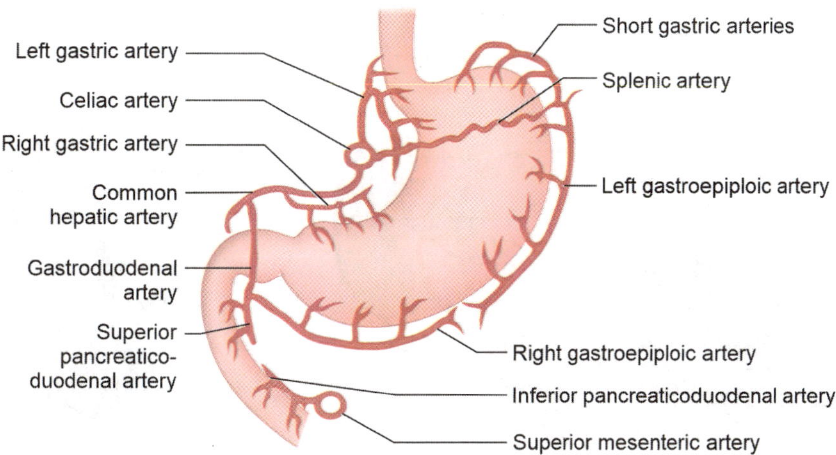

Venous Drainage

Veins draining stomach accompany arteries along the greater and lesser curvatures:

- Right and left gastric veins in portal vein
- Short and left gastroepiploic veins into splenic veins
- Right gastroepiploic vein into superior mesenteric vein
- Prepyloric vein into right gastric vein

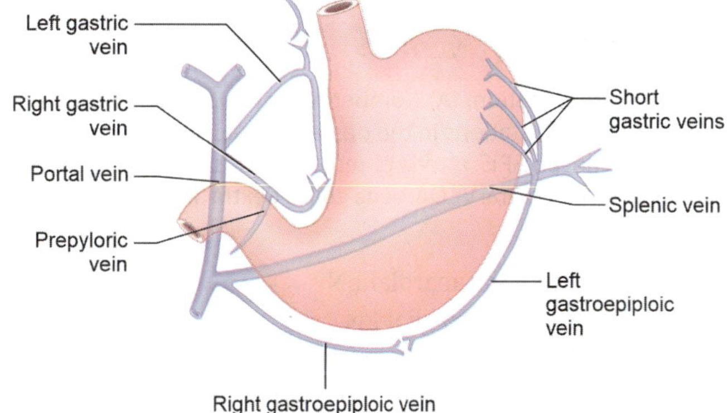

The Lymph Node Stations According to Japanese Classification

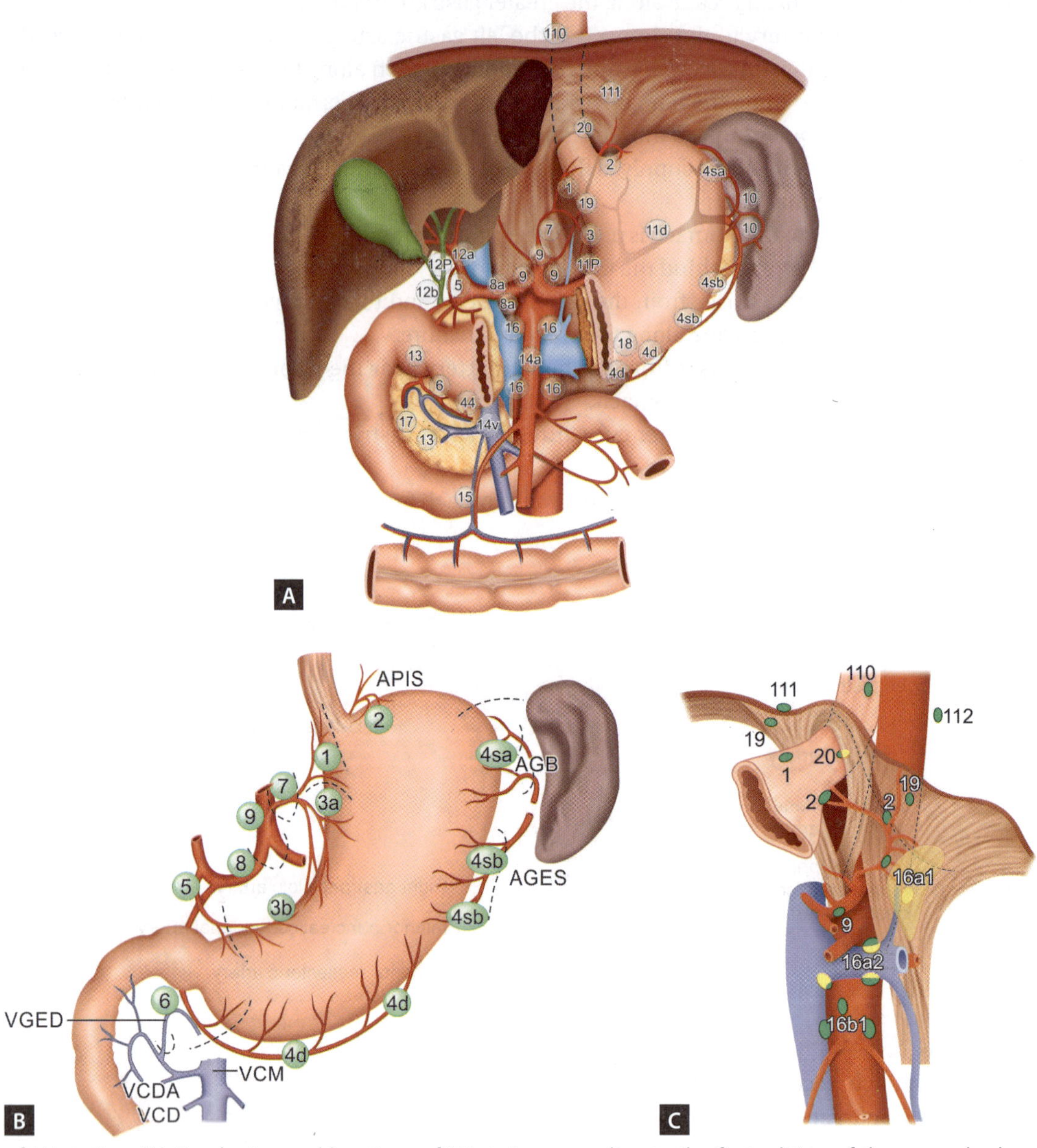

Locations of LN station. (A) Numbering and locations of LN station according to the first edition of the general rules of the JRSGC; (B) Location of LN stations in the posterior area; and (C) Location of LN stations in subphrenic area. (JRSGC: Japanese Research Society for Gastric Cancer; APIS: arteria phrenic inferior sinistra; AGB: arteriae gastricae breves; AGES: arteria gastroepiploica sinistra; VGED: vena gastroepiploica dextra; VCDA: vena colica dextra accessoria; VCM: vena colica media; VCD: vena colica dextra)

No. 1—Right paracardial LN
No. 2—Left paracardial LN
No. 3—LN along the lesser curvature
No. 4sa—LN along the short gastric vessels
No. 4sb—LN along the left gastroepiploic vessels
No. 4d—LN along the right gastroepiploic vessels
No. 5—Suprapyloric LN

No. 6—Infrapyloric LN
No. 7—LN along the left gastric artery
No. 8a—LN along the common hepatic artery (anterosuperior group)
No. 8p—LN along the common hepatic artery (posterior group)
No. 9—LN around the celiac artery No. 10—LN at the splenic hilum
No. 11p—LN along the proximal splenic artery
No. 11d—LN along the distal splenic artery
No. 12a—LN in the hepatoduodenal ligament (along the hepatic artery)
No. 12b—LN in the hepatoduodenal ligament (along the bile duct)
No. 12p—LN in the hepatoduodenal ligament (behind the portal vein)
No. 13—LN on the posterior surface of the pancreatic head
No. 14v—LN along the superior mesenteric vein
No. 14a—LN along the superior mesenteric artery (SMA)
No. 15—LN along the middle colic vessels
No. 16a1—LN in the aortic hiatus
No. 16a2—LN around the abdominal aorta (from the upper margin of the celiac trunk to the lower margin of the left renal vein)
No. 16b1—LN around the abdominal aorta (from the lower margin of the left renal vein to the upper margin of the inferior mesenteric artery)
No. 16b2—LN around the abdominal aorta (from the upper margin of the inferior mesenteric artery to the aortic bifurcation)
No. 17—LN on the anterior surface of the pancreatic head
No. 18—LN along the inferior margin of the pancreas
No. 19—Infradiaphragmatic LN
No. 20—LN in the esophageal hiatus of the diaphragm
No. 110—Paraesophageal LN in the lower thorax
No. 111—Supradiaphragmatic LN
No. 112—Posterior mediastinal LN

Grouping of Regional Lymph Nodes (Groups 1-3) by Location of Primary Tumor According to the Japanese Classification of Gastric Carcinoma

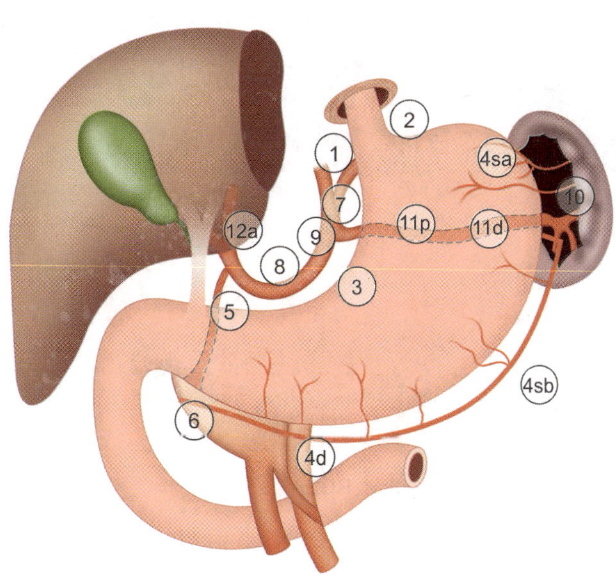

Lymph node station (no.)	Description	Location of primary tumor in stomach		
		Upper third	Middle third	Lower third
1	Right paracardial	1	1	2
2	Left paracardial	1	3	M
3	Lesser curvature	1	1	1
4sa	Short gastric	1	3	M
4sb	Left gastroepiploic	1	1	3
4d	Right gastroepiploic	2	1	1
5	Suprapyloric	3	1	1
6	Infrapyloric	3	1	1
7	Left gastric artery	2	2	2
8a	Anterior comm. hepatic	2	2	2
8p	Posterior comm. hepatic	3	3	3
9	Celiac artery	2	2	2
10	Splenic hilum	2	3	M
11p	Proximal splenic	2	2	2
11d	Distal splenic	2	3	M
12a	Left hepatoduodenal	3	2	2
12b,p	Posterior hepatoduodenal	3	3	3
13	Retropancreatic	M	3	3
14v	Superior mesenteric vein	M	3	2
14a	Superior mesenteric artery	M	M	M
15	Middle colic	M	M	M
16al	Aortic hiatus	3	M	M
16a2,b1	Para-aortic, middle	M	3	3
16b2	Para-aortic, caudal	M	M	M

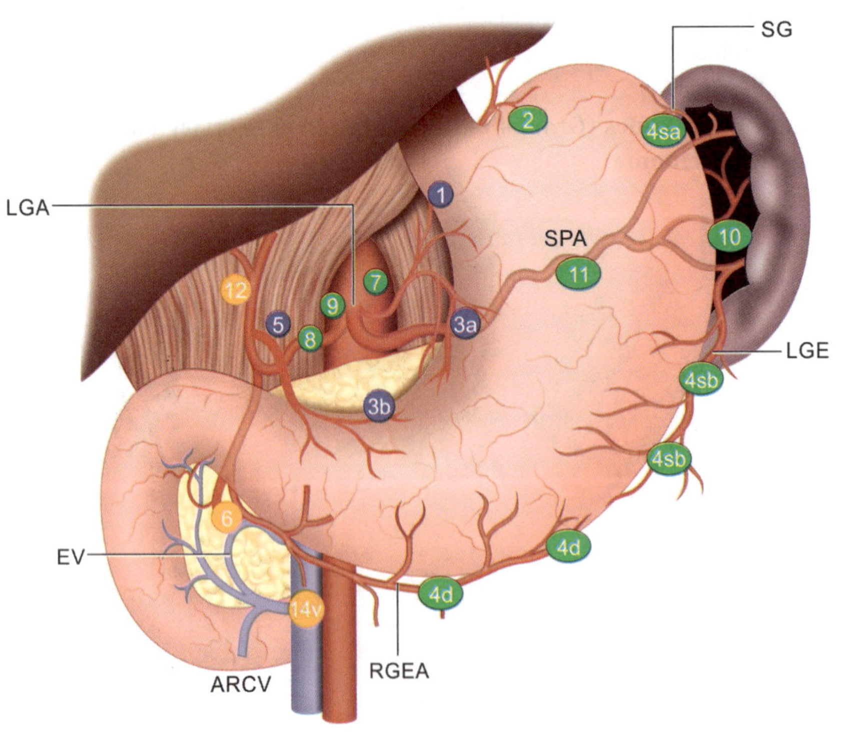

Station type	Station no.	Station location
Regional (perigastric)	1	Right paracardial region
	2	Left paracardial region
	3	Lesser curvature
	4	Greater curvature
	5	Suprapyloric region
	6	Infrapyloric region
Other regional	7	Left gastric artery trunk
	8	Common hepatic artery
	9	Celiac artery
	10	Splenic hilar region
	11	Splenic artery
12	12	HDL
Distant	13	Posterior surface of pancreatic head
	14v	Superior mesenteric vein
	15	Middle colic region
	16	Para-aortic region
	17	Anterior surface of pancreatic head beneath pancreatic sheath
	18	Inferior border of pancreatic body
	19	Infradiaphragmatic lymph nodes along subphrenic artery
	20	Paraesophageal lymph nodes in diaphragmatic hiatus
	110	Paraesophageal lymph nodes in lower thorax
	111	Supradiaphragmatic region
	112	Posterior mediastinal region

The Japanese Introduced the Concept of Tiers (Level) with Lymphatic Spread. Nodal Stations Defined as Level (Tier) N1, N2, and N3 Vary Depending on Location of Tumor

- Level (tier) N1 LNs are generally perigastric nodes within 3 cm of primary tumor.
- Level (tier) N2 LNs are distant perigastric node and along the main arteries supplying stomach (hepatic and splenic arteries).
- Level (tier) N3 LNs are distal most nodes outside normal lymphatic pathway of stomach.

Carcinoma Stomach

Etiopathology

- *Predisposing factors:*
  - Diet rich in nitrosamines (smoked or fresh fish, pickled fruit)
  - Chronic atrophic gastritis (CAG)
  - Blood group A
  - Chronic gastric ulceration related to *H. pylori*
- *Epidemiology:*
  - Gastric cancer is the 14th most common cancer in the world, the incidence of which has been decreasing over the past 70 years.
  - Twice as common in men as it is in women, and the incidence is higher among black men than white men.
  - The incidence also increases with age, peaking in the seventh decade.
  - Studies of migrant populations from areas of high incidence to areas of low incidence suggest that environmental exposure as well as other cultural or genetic factors influence the predisposition to GC.

- There has been a noticeable shift in the site of GC from the distal stomach to the more proximal stomach over the past several decades.
- The incidence of adenocarcinoma of the gastric cardia has increased steadily, whereas the incidence of cancer in other anatomic subsites has decreased.
- The increase was most noticeable for white men and is possibly linked to a history of smoking or heavy alcohol use.

Factors Associated with Increased Risk for Developing Stomach Cancer

Nutritional	*Environmental*	*Social*	*Medical*
• Low fat or protein consumption • Salted meat or fish • High nitrate consumption • High complex-carbohydrate consumption	• Poor food preparation (smoked and salted) • Lack of refrigeration • Poor drinking water (well water) • Smoking	• Low social class	• Prior gastric surgery • *Helicobacter pylori* infection • Gastric atrophy and gastritis • Adenomatous polyps • Male gender

Types

World Health Organization Histologic Typing of Gastric Cancer
• Adenocarcinoma – Papillary adenocarcinoma – Tubular adenocarcinoma – Mucinous adenocarcinoma – Signet-ring cell carcinoma • Adenosquamous carcinoma • Squamous cell carcinoma • Small cell carcinoma • Undifferentiated carcinoma • Others

Lauren Classification System

Intestinal	*Diffuse*
Environmental	Familial
Gastric atrophy, intestinal metaplasia	Blood type A
Men > women	Women > men
Increasing incidence with age	Younger age group
Gland formation	Poorly differentiated, signet ring cells
Hematogenous spread	Transmural/lymphatic spread
Microsatellite instability APC gene mutations	Decreased E-cadherin
p53, p16 inactivation	p53, p16 inactivation

(APC: adenomatous polyposis coli)

Staging:

- The pathologic staging system currently in use worldwide is the AJCC TNM staging system.
- The TNM system can adequately stratify patients into distinct groups with different risks for tumor-related death.
- In the current staging system, a minimum of 15 nodes must be evaluated for accurate staging.
- Nodal staging is then determined by the number of positive nodes, with pN1 reflecting 1–6 positive nodes, pN2 designating 7–15 positive nodes, and pN3 > 15 positive nodes.

- Some data suggest location of the primary (cardia compared with distal tumors) may independently predict survival. However, the current AJCC staging system does not reflect the poorer prognosis for proximal gastric tumors noted in some studies.
  - R0 describes a microscopically margin-negative resection, in which no gross or microscopic tumor remains in the tumor bed.
  - R1 indicates removal of all macroscopic disease, but microscopic margins are positive for tumor.
  - R2 indicates gross residual disease.
- Long-term survival can be expected only after an R0 resection; therefore, a significant effort should be made to avoid R1 or R2 resection.

TNM Classification of Carcinoma of the Stomach

Category	*Criteria*
Primary tumor (T)	
TX	Primary tumor cannot be assessed
T0	No evidence of primary tumor
Tis	Carcinoma in situ: Intraepithelial tumor without invasion of the lamina propria
T1	Tumor invades lamina propria or submucosa
T2	Tumor invades muscularis propria or subserosa
T2a	Tumor invades muscularis propria
T2b	Tumor invades subserosa
T3	Tumor penetrates serosa (visceral peritoneum) without invasion of adjacent structures
T4	Tumor invades adjacent structures
Regional lymph nodes (N)	
NX	Regional lymph node(s) cannot be assessed
N0	No regional lymph node metastasis
N1	Metastasis in 1–6 regional lymph nodes
N2	Metastasis in 7–15 regional lymph nodes
N3	Metastasis in >15 regional lymph nodes
Distant metastasis (M)	
MX	Distant metastasis cannot be assessed
M0	No distant metastasis
M1	Distant metastasis

Preoperative Evaluation

- When GC is suspected based on history and physical examination, flexible upper endoscopy is the diagnostic modality of choice.
- During endoscopy, multiple biopsy samples (seven or more) should be obtained around the ulcer crater to facilitate histologic diagnosis.
- The addition of direct brush cytology to multiple biopsy specimens may increase the diagnostic accuracy of the study.
- Additionally, the size, location, and morphology of the tumor should be noted and other mucosal abnormalities carefully evaluated.

- In select patients with advanced disease, EUS can gauge the extent of gastric wall invasion as well as evaluate local nodal status.
- EUS cannot reliably distinguish tumor from fibrosis; therefore, it is not a good modality for evaluating response to therapy.
- When the diagnosis of GC is confirmed, further studies should include a complete blood count, serum chemistries to include liver function tests, coagulation studies, CXR, and CT scan of the abdomen.
- In women, a pelvic CT scan or ultrasound is also recommended. CT of the chest may be needed for proximal GCs. CT can readily detect the presence of visceral metastatic disease as well as malignant ascites. The major limitations of CT are in the evaluation of early gastric primaries and in the detection of small (<5 mm) metastases in the liver or on peritoneal surfaces.
- Because of the inaccuracy of CT and other modalities for the detection of macrometastases <5 mm on the peritoneal surface or liver, laparoscopy is recommended as the next step in the evaluation of patients with locoregional disease.
- The addition of laparoscopic ultrasonography may increase the sensitivity of laparoscopic staging in GC as it has in other abdominal malignancies.
- Cytologic analysis of peritoneal fluid or of fluid obtained by peritoneal lavage may reveal the presence of free intraperitoneal GC cells, identifying patients with otherwise occult carcinomatosis.
- Patients with positive findings on peritoneal cytology have a poor prognosis, similar to that of patients with macroscopic stage IV disease.
- False-positive results can be obtained, and not all studies confirm the prognostic significance of positive findings.
- More sensitive methods of detecting free intraperitoneal GC cells, such as immunostaining and reverse-transcriptase polymerase chain reaction for carcinoembryonic antigen (CEA) messenger RNA, are under investigation.

Surgical Treatment

- The optimal surgical management of GC must be tailored to the extent and location of disease.
- In the absence of distant metastatic spread, aggressive surgical resection of the gastric tumor is justified.
- The extent of gastric resection is determined by the need to obtain a resection margin free of microscopic disease.
- At least 6 cm from the tumor mass is necessary to ensure a low rate of anastomotic recurrence. The appropriate surgical procedure should be determined by the location of the tumor and the known pattern of spread.
- Tumors of the cardia and proximal stomach account for 35–50% of all gastric adenocarcinomas.
- In general, proximal tumors are more advanced at presentation than more distant tumors, so curative resections are rare.
- For proximal lesions, either total gastrectomy or proximal gastric resection is necessary to remove the tumor.
- Japanese surgeons perform splenectomy and partial pancreatectomy during D2 resections for primaries, whose drainage includes these echelons.
- Because of the increased morbidity in the patients receiving these adjunctive resections, Western surgeons do not typically resect the spleen or pancreas unless involved by direct extension from a T4 tumor.
- Splenectomy is no longer advocated as a routine adjunctive procedure to gastrectomy for cancer. Local organ resection, especially of the spleen, pancreas, or transverse colon, should be performed only when needed to accomplish an R0 resection.
  - D1 dissection—if a dissection removes N1 nodes (perigastric nodes along the left and right pericardial nodes, lesser and greater curvature, suprapyloric, and infrapyloric)
  - D0 dissection—anything < a D1
  - D2 dissection—D1 plus removal of nodes along the left gastric artery, common hepatic artery, celiac trunk, and splenic artery
  - D3 dissection—D2 plus removal of nodes along the hepatoduodenal ligament and root of the mesentery

- D4 dissection—D3 plus removal of para-aortic and paracolic LNs
- These terminologies for LN dissection are for GCs in general and are not meant only for early GC. D1 dissection is classified as conservative LN dissection (CLND) and D2 to D4 dissections are considered extended LN dissections (ELND).

D2 Gastrectomy

In D2 Gastrectomy, level (tier) N2, i.e., distant perigastric node and nodes along the main arteries supplying stomach (hepatic and splenic arteries) are removed.

- D2 lymphadenectomy can be performed with low morbidity-mortality, and a 5-year survival of >50%. The procedure offers benefit in terms of survival for a certain percentage of patients with positive level N2 LNs.
- The rationale for extended lymphadenectomy has been enhanced local control. The clearance of the possible metastatic nodes in the region outside of the perigastric nodes is presumed to impact on overall patient survival rates.
- The proponents of systemic LND point to numerous anatomical/lymphographic studies, histopathologic analyses, statistical analyses of LN metastases, clinical prognostic observations, and advances in surgical techniques to support their argument that ELND is the most effective procedure to treat the lymphatic spread to GC.

Steps

- Abdomen is opened from the bilateral subcostal incision or midline incision.
- Omni retractor, Thomson's or similar retractor is used to lift up the rib cage. There should be good exposure of the stomach, lesser omentum, greater omentum, and duodenum.
- Abdominal cavity is explored for metastasis especially liver, pouch of Douglas, ovaries, base of mesentery, mesocolon, and pelvis.
- Note the site of tumor, extent, and depth of the malignancy, is there involvement of any adjacent structure
- Bring down the hepatic flexure of colon and do a wide Kocher's maneuver.
- Omentum is now taken down from the transverse colon with the anterior layer of mesocolon.
- The dissection goes toward the right toward right gastroepiploic artery and sweeping the sub pyloric group of LNs up.
- The hepatoduodenal ligament is cleared preserving the accessory left hepatic artery if present.
- Dissection in the porta might be done but not required because for D2 gastrectomy the other LNs that need removal are hepatic artery, left gastric artery, splenic artery, and celiac artery group.
- Right gastric artery is ligated and duodenum cut and stapled and oversewn.
- Transected part of stomach and duodenum is now lifted up and tissue inferior to the common hepatic artery with the pancreatic capsule is taken off. Celiac trunk will now need to be exposed.
- Splenic hilum will now be approached from below and all the lymphatic tissue will now need to be swept towards the left gastric artery.
- In the Dutch trial, D2 dissection did not improve long-term survival or decrease the risk of relapse. However, the D1 and D2 groups were not well balanced.
- Resection of the spleen was an independent risk factor for reduced survival but splenectomy and pancreatectomy was significantly more often performed in the D2 than the D1 group.

Contraindications of Proceeding with a D2 Gastrectomy

- Liver secondaries
- Serosal deposits
- Positive cancer cells in peritoneal fluid
- LNs in para-aortic region or base of mesocolon

Different Reconstruction after D2 Gastrectomy

- *Subtotal gastrectomy:* Billroth I procedure—digestive tract reconstruction

- *Subtotal gastrectomy* with Billroth I or Billroth II
- *Total gastrectomy* with jejunal interposition or Roux-en-Y reconstruction
- *Total gastrectomy, Roux-en-Y Procedure:* Digestive tract reconstruction

(A) Subtotal gastrectomy with a Billroth II anastomosis. (B) Total gastrectomy with a Roux-en-Y anastomosis.

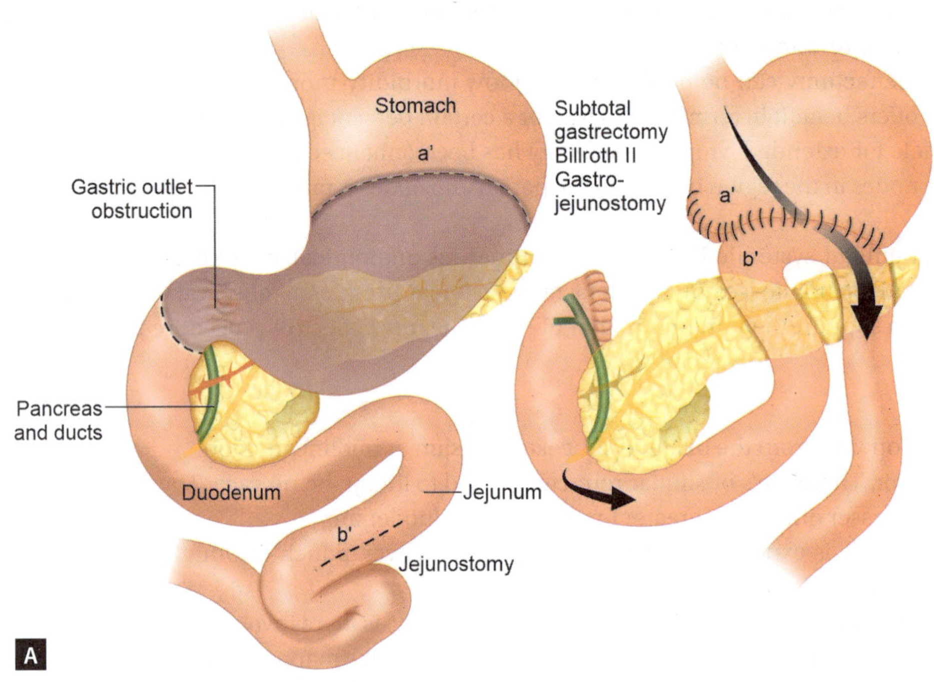

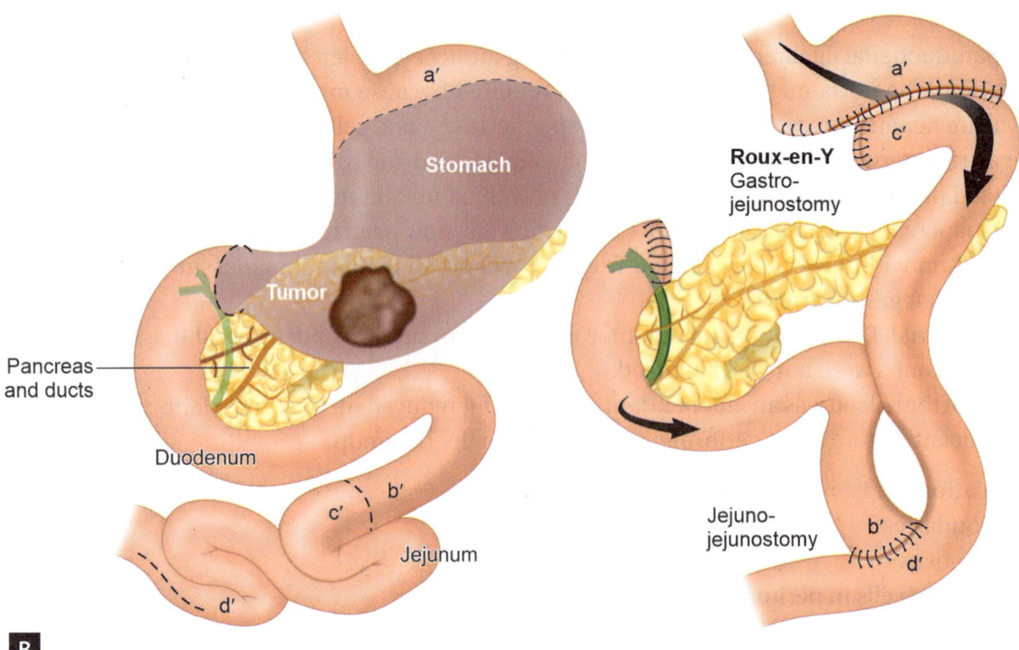

Roux–en–y gastrojejunostomy

- There is abundant evidence that proximal gastric resection results in higher morbidity and mortality than total gastrectomy.
- Total gastrectomy should be considered the procedure of choice for proximal gastric lesions.
- Distal tumors account for about 35% of all GCs.
- Recent studies have indicated no difference in 5-year survival between patients undergoing potentially curative subtotal versus total gastrectomy, subtotal gastrectomy is appropriate for patients in whom a negative margin resection can be performed.
- A luminal margin of 5–6 cm is recommended with frozen section analysis when a subtotal gastric resection is performed for adenocarcinoma.

Merits and Demerits of D2 Gastrectomy

Merits of D2 Gastrectomy

Merit	*Explanation*
1. Better oncological clearance	Removes more lymph nodes, improving local control and staging accuracy
2. Improved survival	Associated with better long-term survival in *stage II and III gastric cancers* (especially in high-volume centers)
3. Accurate staging	Allows for more precise pathological staging (≥15 lymph nodes examined)
4. Reduced recurrence	Lower risk of locoregional recurrence compared to less extensive lymphadenectomy
5. Standard of care in many countries	Widely accepted and recommended in *Japan, South Korea*, and increasingly globally

Demerits of D2 Gastrectomy

Demerit	*Explanation*
1. Increased operative time and complexity	More technically demanding than D1 gastrectomy
2. Higher morbidity (in inexperienced hands)	Risk of complications such as *pancreatic fistula, splenic injury*, or *bleeding*
3. Higher mortality in low-volume centers	Poorer outcomes when done without adequate surgical expertise or support
4. Risk of nutritional deficiencies	Due to total/subtotal gastrectomy and loss of gastric functions
5. Not always beneficial in early-stage cancer	May not significantly improve outcomes in early-stage tumors (T1N0, etc.)

Palliative Treatment

- Because 20–30% of GC patients present with stage IV disease, clinicians must be familiar with different methods of palliative treatment. The goal of palliative treatment is the relief of symptoms with minimal morbidity.
- Surgical palliation of advanced GC may include resection or bypass alone or in conjunction with percutaneous, endoscopic, or radiotherapy techniques.
- Complete staging is necessary to determine the appropriate method of palliation for individual patients.
- In the presence of peritoneal disease, hepatic metastases, diffuse nodal metastases, or ascites, palliation of bleeding or proximal gastric obstruction would preferably be obtained nonoperatively.
- Nonoperative therapies include laser recanalization and endoscopic dilation with or without stent placement.
- Patients who undergo stent placement for gastric outlet obstruction are frequently able to tolerate solid foods and may not require additional interventions.

Adjuvant Therapy

- Two cycles of 5-FU and leucovorin with subsequent concurrent CRT, using the same chemotherapeutic agents, as adjuncts following an R0 resection of gastric adenocarcinoma can be used.
- More recently, a British MRC randomized trial (MAGIC) demonstrated improved overall and disease-free survival in patients treated with preoperative or postoperative chemotherapy (ECF).

Neoadjuvant Therapy

- Neoadjuvant chemotherapy is currently under investigation and has yielded some promising results.
- Currently, NCCN guidelines recommend adjuvant chemoradiation with a 5-FU-based regimen following complete surgical resection for patients with T3, T4, or node-positive cancers.
- Additionally, patients with microscopically positive resection margins should also have adjuvant therapy.

Role of Sentinel Lymph Node Biopsy in Gastric Cancer

- SLN biopsy using a radioisotope in patients with GC is a technically feasible and accurate technique, and it is a minimally invasive approach in the assessment of patient nodal status.
- The concept of SLN characterization is of great interest to many surgical oncologists because it may be a guideline to the determination of the extent of cancer surgery. The clinical implications of SLN biopsy, however, in GC remain controversial.
- Maruyama et al. asserted that SLN biopsy in GC could not be used for reducing the extent of lymphadenectomy because of the complicated lymphatic streams from the stomach and the presence of frequent skip metastases.
- Tsuburaya et al. reported that the sensitivity of SLN biopsy performed by exploring the adjacent basin would be very low, especially for the lesions in the lesser curvature and posterior wall.
- However, Kitagawa et al. recently claimed that SLN mapping during laparoscopic surgery, and during laparotomy, is a sensitive and feasible intraoperative technique for identifying LN metastasis in patients with GC.
- SLN mapping and biopsy in patients with GC using ^{99m}Tc-tin colloid proved satisfactory.
- Unlike breast cancer and malignant melanoma, a preoperative lymphoscintigraphy in cases of SLN biopsy for GC may be not available.
- The skip metastasis in GC has been considered an obstacle to the utilization of the SLN concept.
- Skip metastasis in GC, however, is not an obstacle in the use of SLN concept because a SLN biopsy can localize and identify such metastasis.
- Micrometastasis in GC using antibodies to cytokeratin was found in 4–6.3% of cases in other studies.
- In conclusion, SLN biopsy in GC using a radioisotope proved technically feasible for the detection of SLN located at level II or I and accurately predicted metastasis in the regional LNs in each patient. This technique may be of a great benefit to surgeons for the determination of the extent of lymphadenectomy in GC. A multicenter validation study of SLN biopsy should establish standard guidelines for deciding the extent of lymphadenectomy in GC.

44. Roux syndrome following gastrectomy. ***WBUHS 2015***

Introduction

- Controversial—real entity or consequence of vagal denervation
- Incidence—as high as 30% in some reports, others have not found it to be clinically significant.

Symptoms

- Postprandial epigastric fullness
- Nausea and intermittent vomiting
- Often weight loss

Cause for Symptoms

- Thought to be the result of an atonic roux limb that serves to impede gastric emptying.

- Some believe it is a result of the loss of duodenal pacemaker.
  - Pace setter potentials are fastest in the duodenum, spread distally to the terminal ileum.

Studies have demonstrated that when the jejunum is transected, the frequency of the pace setter potentials is decreased and ectopic pacemakers appear, driving potentials retrograde toward the stomach

- Dysmotility occurs in all patients, symptoms appear in some
- Miedema et al. found that although transit was universally slowed in the Roux limb, there was no transit difference between asymptomatic and symptomatic patients.
- It seems to be more common in patients with a large gastric remnant and after truncal vagotomy.

Diagnosis

- Difficult to diagnose
- UGIE can be interpreted as normal or complete GOO.
- EGD usually reveals a widely patent anastomosis.
- True syndrome generally a late complication
- Usually in women

Treatment

- *Medical:* Prokinetic agents
- *Surgical:*
  - Aggressive gastric resection with R-Y reconstruction is the mainstay of treatment.
  - Extent of gastric resection is debated.
  - Others advocate gastric resection if gastric motility seems to be the problem and resection of the Roux limb if it appears unusually dilated or flaccid, with R-Y, Billroth II, or the uncut roux as reconstruction.

45. Discuss the evidence-based comparison of D1 and D2 dissections for carcinoma of stomach. ***WBUHS 2010***

- *Depending on extent of lymphadenectomy there are three types of curative gastric resection:*
  1. D1 limited lymphadenectomy—all N1 tier LNs are removed en bloc with stomach.
  2. D2 systemic lymphadenectomy—all level N1 and N2 nodes removed with stomach, if any N2 tier node not removed, then represented as D1/D2 resection.
  3. D3 extended lymphadenectomy—more radical en bloc resection including third tier nodes.

The standard D2 gastrectomy removes the peritoneal layer over pancreas and anterior mesocolon, along with nodes along hepatic and splenic arteries and crural nodes, in addition to the tissue removed in D1 resection.

The ideal lymphadenectomy for GC should accurately stage the extent of disease and predict prognosis.

- It should have the potential to improve survival by selectively and completely removing all metastatic LNs, with minimal morbidity and mortality.
- Optimal extent of LN dissection (LND) for GC has not been determined and is certainly not standardized.
- At the time of resection, the macroscopic assessment of nodal metastases is notoriously unreliable, and the intraoperative assessment of microscopic LN metastases is costly and impractical.
- Furthermore, the pattern of LN involvement depends on numerous factors, including location of the primary tumor and depth of tumor invasion.
- Opinion over the optimum resection for patients with GC remains divided, and the literature polarized.

Comparison

- The impressive outcomes after D2 gastrectomy published in large retrospective series from Japan (Soga et al. 1979; Maruyama et al. 1987) have not been reproduced in randomized comparative studies from Europe (Bonenkamp et al. 1995–1999; Cuschieri et al. 1996–1999).
- The two largest randomized studies both report significantly greater operative morbidity and mortality associated with an extended D2 lymphadenectomy when compared with the less aggressive D1 lymphadenectomy, and have failed to demonstrate any survival advantage for a D2 resection.

- Many of the serious complications associated with D2 resections were associated with resections of the pancreas and spleen (Bonenkamp et al. 1995; Cuschieri et al. 1996), and the best long-term survival was observed in patients undergoing D2 gastrectomy without pancreaticosplenectomy (Cuschieri et al. 1999). Although this latter report concluded than a classical D2 resection offered no survival advantage over a D1 resection, the possibility that a modified D2 resection, preserving pancreas and spleen, might be better than a D1 resection was not dismissed (Cuschieri et al. 1999).
- Poor outcomes after surgery for GC in Britain are due to the greater age, comorbidity, advanced stages of disease, and greater body mass indices of Western patients when compared with their Japanese counterparts.
- Most esophago-GC surgery in Britain and much of the West, has by tradition, been performed by general surgeons. Radical lymphadenectomy is a painstaking, technically demanding procedure, which has usually remained within the province of small numbers of specialist upper gastrointestinal surgeons.
- D1 perigastric lymphadenectomy remains the most commonly performed operation for GC in the West.
- Both MRC ST01 and the Dutch trial have received criticism over the relative inexperience of many different surgeons performing D2 lymphadenectomy.
- Furthermore, the existence of a relationship between caseload and operative mortality remains controversial. The specialist surgical unit in Leeds has described a long learning curve during the adoption of D2 gastrectomy, with 10 years elapsing before operative mortality fell to 5%.
- D2 lymphadenectomy can be performed with low morbidity-mortality, and a 5-year survival of >50%. The procedure offers benefit in terms of survival for a certain percentage of patients with positive level N2 LNs.
- The rationale for extended lymphadenectomy has been enhanced local control. The clearance of the possible metastatic nodes in the region outside of the perigastric nodes is presumed to impact on overall patient survival rates.
- The proponents of systemic LND point to numerous anatomical/lymphographic studies, histopathologic analyses, statistical analyses of LN metastases, clinical prognostic observations, and advances in surgical techniques to support their argument that ELND is the most effective procedure to treat the lymphatic spread to GC.
- Japanese surgeons have been actively performing extended lymphadenectomy (D2, removal of perigastric nodes and nodes along the left gastric, common hepatic, celiac, and splenic arteries; or D3, D2 plus removal of nodes in the hepatoduodenal ligament, in the retropancreatic space and along the vessels of the transverse mesocolon).
- In recent years, interest has expanded to superextended lymphadenectomy (D4) of nodes around abdominal aorta (para-aortic LNs from aortic hiatus to aortic bifurcation).
- Because the therapeutic value of this D4 procedure remains controversial, Maeta et al. initiated a prospective study to compare D3 and D4 lymphadenectomy.
- Surgical treatment of microscopic disease in grossly normal para-aortic LNs may generate occasional long-term survivors. Selecting appropriate candidates who might benefit from D4 resections needs to be refined.
- In the recently published Dutch trial, the cumulative risk of relapse was lower in patients with spleen preservation than in those with splenectomy, but the aim of the study was to compare D1 and D2 resections.
- The description D dissection for the determination of extent of LN dissection arises from the Japanese classification (JRSGC).
  - D1–D4 dissection correspondences to the anatomical site of dissection of levels N1–N4.
  - The rationale for ELND is that it achieves a R0 resection due to clearance of the metastatic extraperigastric LNs that cannot be removed with a limited D1 node dissection.
  - Thus, it increases the curative resection rate, reduces the locoregional recurrence rate, and may improve survival.
  - This hypothesis for improvement of both local control and survival after D2 dissection is supported by a large number of Japanese observational studies that based on historical comparisons.

- Furthermore, several prospective but nonrandomized studies and other observational Western series have shown encouraging long-term results with D2 dissection.
- However, many surgeons in the West argue against the therapeutic value of D2 dissection and are clearly against the routine use of D2 dissection for Western patients.
- In their opinion, D2 dissection increases postoperative morbidity and mortality rates and does not improve long-term survival.
- This argument has been based on retrospective studies, which have failed to demonstrate any survival benefit in favor of D2 dissection.
- In the Dutch trial, D2 dissection did not improve long-term survival or decrease the risk of relapse. However, the D1 and D2 groups were not well balanced.
- Resection of the spleen was an independent risk factor for reduced survival but splenectomy and pancreatectomy were significantly more often performed in the D2 than the D1 group.

---

46. Define early gastric cancer. Diagnosis and management of early gastric carcinoma.

Srimanta Sankaradeva University, Assam 2025

Definition

Early GC (EGC) is defined as being confined to the mucosa or the submucosa, regardless of the presence or absence of regional LN metastasis.

The Japanese Gastric Cancer Association classification has good correlation with the T staging as described in the TNM staging. T1 disease corresponds to M or SM according to Japanese classification, T2 disease with MP or SS, T3 with SE, and T4 disease with SI.

- *TX:* Primary tumor cannot be assessed.
- *T1:* Tumor invasion of mucosa and/or muscularis mucosa (M) or submucosa (SM)
- *T2:* Tumor invasion of muscularis propria (MP) or subserosa (SS)
- *T3:* Tumor penetration of serosa (SE)
- *T4:* Tumor invasion of adjacent structures (SI)

By definition, early GC is T1 disease according to TNM staging or M/SM disease as per the Japanese classification.

The depth of invasion (M, SM1, and SM2) is determined and recorded only when the vertical margin (VM) is negative (SM1): Submucosal invasion < 0.5 mm, SM2; invasion > 0.5 mm).

This further subdivision of SM into SM1 and SM2 has been considered because SM2 disease has a significantly greater rate of lymph nodal involvement than SM1 disease.

Investigations

- CT remains the modality of choice for staging of GC. The sensitivity of a CT scan to determine nodal status ranges from 50 to 95% and specificity from 40 to 99%. For assessing depth of invasion, EUS remains the primary choice for determining T staging.
- *Endoscopy:* Conventional endoscopy is the standard investigation for GC. To detect early GCs, chromoendoscopy has more role than conventional endoscopy.
- Lateral extent of the tumor must be identified for endoscopic resection and this is well seen by chromoendoscopy.

Tumor size, location, or depth of tumor does not affect the clarity of the images. Chromoendoscopy clarified the border in a significantly higher percentage of differentiated adenocarcinomas.

Staging

- The current AJCC TNM staging classification remains the best prognostic system for assessing survival from gastric adenocarcinoma.
- At least 15 LNs are required for proper staging.
- Metastatic lymph node ratio (MLR) is the ratio between metastatic LNs and total evaluated LNs as opposed to the total number of positive nodes and is valuable in cases of inadequate LN evaluation.

Management

- *Surgery:* Proximal subtotal gastrectomy, total gastrectomy, and Roux-en-Y reconstruction with or without jejunal 'J' pouch and distal radical gastrectomy are the commonly performed surgeries for proximal and distal GCs, respectively. Most of these surgeries are performed for more advanced GCs but are also often appropriate for early GCs.
- *Laparoscopic surgery:* In the revised Japanese Gastric Cancer Treatment Guidelines, laparoscopy-assisted gastrectomy is classified as an investigational procedure eligible for stage IA and IB cancers only.
- *Endoscopic mucosal resection:* Also known as "Strip biopsy". EMR are indicated in well-differentiated adenocarcinoma, tumor ≤20 mm in elevated type, ≤10 mm in depressed type, not associated with peptic ulcer and invasion limited to the mucosa.
    - *Advantages*—minimal invasion, low cost, patient tolerance, and better patient quality of life after the operation.
    - *Disadvantages*—larger-sized lesions cannot be resected completely by EMR at one time. Thus, the entire pathologic specimen cannot be submitted for proper analysis.
    - *Types*—EMR-precut, EMR-cap, and EMR-ligation
- *Endoscopic submucosal dissection:*
    - It was developed for en bloc resection of large lesions among the intramucosal GCs.
    - ESD used the technique of improved needle-knife under endoscopy to strip the tumors directly from the submucosal layer.
    - ESD had a relatively higher incidence rate of complications such as bleeding and perforation.
    - More operating time was needed in the ESD group than in the EMR group.
    - Higher en bloc resection rate and higher histologically complete resection rate in ESD compared to EMR (even for tumors <20 mm).
    - Lower recurrence rate in ESD than EMR
    - Perforation was more common in ESD but bleeding was similar in both procedures.
    - Tumor location in the upper and middle portions of the gastric body, ulceration, unskillful operation, and blind hemostasis and lesion size >3 cm are all considered as risk factors of perforation.
    - If this occurs, it is repaired by metal clips and majority do not require surgical operations.
- *Elective lymph node dissection:*
  The degree of LN dissection was traditionally based on the Japanese staging system in which nodal stations were assigned into groups N1, N2, or N3.
    - D1 dissection—if a dissection removes N1 nodes (perigastric nodes along the left and right pericardial nodes, lesser and greater curvature, suprapyloric, and infrapyloric)
    - D0 dissection—anything less than a D1
    - D2 dissection—D1 plus removal of nodes along the left gastric artery, common hepatic artery, celiac trunk, and splenic artery.
    - D3 dissection—D2 plus removal of nodes along the hepatoduodenal ligament and root of the mesentery.
    - D4 dissection—D3 plus removal of para-aortic and paracolic LNs.
    - These terminologies for LN dissection are for GCs in general and are not meant only for early GC. D1 dissection is classified as CLND and D2 to D4 dissections are considered ELND.
    - Dutch trial and the Medical Research Council (MRC trial) showed no benefit when comparing D1 and D2 dissection and increased morbidity and mortality in D2 group.
    - These trials have serious limitations and a final view about the benefits of D2 dissection cannot be made at present.
    - Lymph node dissection may be avoided in intramucosal disease (M) and superficial submucosal invasion (SM1).
    - However, the risk of LN metastasis is significant in EGC with deeper submucosal invasion (SM2) and D2 lymphadenectomy is probably an appropriate surgery for SM2 group of early GC and for the other advanced but resectable GCs.

47. Recent advances in the management of gastric cancer. ***WBUHS 2022***

48. Recent advances in management of early gastric cancer. ***WBUHS 2021, 2025; RIMS, Imphal 2022***

For Early GC

- *Basic considerations:*
  - Up to 10% of GCs are missed at upper endoscopy; focus should be on quality improvement in UGIE.
  - Chronic atrophic gastritis and gastric intestinal metaplasia (GIM) are both precursors to GC and warrant ongoing cancer surveillance if changes are extensive.
  - High-definition endoscopy with image enhancement is preferred over high-definition white light endoscopy alone for the recognition of gastric premalignant conditions.
  - Where endoscopic appearances suggest CAG and/or GIM, staging biopsies should be taken from at least two areas of the stomach (antrum and corpus and lesser and greater curve for each).
  - Where enhanced imaging is available and with the appropriate expertise, targeted biopsies to visible mucosal abnormalities should also be taken for staging purposes.
  - Early GC should be managed by referral centers with expertise in endoscopic resection. Lesions that meet standard criteria should be treated with ESD.
- *Establishing the diagnosis and assessment of extent of local disease:*
  - *Upper GI Endoscopy and guided biopsy*—location and extent
  - *EUS*—most sensitive for T staging, also enables assessment of regional LNs (N status) and fine needle aspiration cytology (FNAC) of suspicious nodes
  - *Magnifying endoscopy, chromoendoscopy*
- *Gastric biopsy mapping*
  - *Nontargeted biopsy:*
  - Distal antrum, lesser curvature, 3–5 cm of pylorus
  - Same in greater curvature
  - Lesser curvature incisura
  - Proximal corpus lesser curvature
  - Proximal corpus greater curvature
  - *Targeted biopsy*
- *Staging:*
  - *T Stage*
    - *Endoscopy:*
      - *Mucosal disease:* Smooth surface protrusion or depression, slight marginal elevation, and smooth tapering of converging folds.
      - *Submucosal disease:* Irregular surface, marginal elevation and clubbing, abrupt cutting, and fusion of converging folds
    - *EUS:* Accuracy 67%
    - *Endoscopic resection:* ESD/EMR
  - *N Stage*
    - *ESD:* Staging and treatment for EGC
    - *EMR:* Like variceal ligation, abnormal area is identified, suctioned in a cap, band applied, and removed with snare

Lymph node:

- Metastasis seen in large tumor, undifferentiated, ulcer, lymphovascular invasion (LVI), and submucosal invasion.
- *EUS:* Detect enlarged LN, FNA can be done. It can differentiate regional and metastatic LN (pancreatoduodenal, retropanc, SMA, Middle colic, paraaortic, RP)

The standard indication for endoscopic resection of gastric dysplasia and invasive cancer includes the following criteria:

- Low-grade dysplasia
- High-grade dysplasia
- Well or moderately differentiated intramucosal adenocarcinoma, irrespective of size and without ulceration.
- Well or moderately differentiated intramucosal adenocarcinoma, <3.0 cm in size if ulcerated.
- Well or moderately differentiated submucosal adenocarcinoma, <3.0 cm in size, with superficial submucosal invasion (Sm1; <500 μm submucosal invasion as measured in a vertical line from the deepest fiber of the muscularis mucosae).
- Poorly differentiated intramucosal adenocarcinoma, ≤2.0 cm in size

Lesions endoscopically resected with these pathological features should be considered to have been curatively treated.

Treatment of Metastatic and Unresectable Gastric Cancer

- Several cytotoxic agents are active in advanced GC, including fluoropyrimidines, platinum, taxanes, and irinotecan.
- The choice of treatment depends on patient performance status and medical comorbidities as well as the toxicity profile of the regimen.
- Combination regimens offer higher response rates and improved survival compared with single-agent therapy.
- Treatment goals are typically palliative in intent and are aimed at controlling symptoms, controlling disease, and extending life.
- A fluoropyrimidine and platinum doublet is typically the preferred backbone regimen for most patients.
- Oxaliplatin is considered to be as effective as cisplatin and is the choice platinum in most modern regimens.
- In very fit patients who are willing to sacrifice toxicity for higher response rates and potentially longer progression-free survival (PFS), a triplet regimen combining a fluoropyrimidine, oxaliplatin, and docetaxel can be considered.
- In patients with overexpression or amplification of human epidermal growth factor receptor 2 (HER2) (also known as *ERBB2*), trastuzumab should be added to cytotoxic first-line chemotherapy, as reviewed in detail below.
- In patients with a programmed cell death ligand 1 (PD-L1) combined positive score (CPS) ≥5, nivolumab should be added to first-line chemotherapy.
- In the second-line treatment for metastatic GC, cytotoxic chemotherapy agents not already used in the first line can be attempted.
- Several years ago, ramucirumab was added.
- Ramucirumab is a monoclonal antibody that binds to vascular endothelial growth factor receptor 2 (VEGFR-2), blocking receptor activation.
- The oral cytotoxic agent trifluridine-tipiracil, combining an antimetabolite trifluridine with a thymidine phosphorylase inhibitor (tipiracil), has been shown to have a survival benefit over placebo
- Immunotherapy

Immunotherapy in Gastric Cancer

High Microsatellite Instability/Mismatch Repair-Deficient Tumors

- The Cancer Genome Atlas (TCGA) Research Network performed a comprehensive molecular characterization of 295 untreated gastric adenocarcinomas and categorized GC into four subtypes: MSI-H tumors, EBV-positive tumors, tumors exhibiting chromosomal instability (CIN), and genomically stable tumors.
- Mismatch repair (MMR) genes are responsible for fixing errors that occur during DNA replication.
- Immune checkpoint therapies and an additional anti-HER-2 targeted agent have been approved. Immune checkpoint therapy in the front-line setting has become relevant in advanced GAC through phase 3 trials of nivolumab, pembrolizumab, and sintilimab.

49. Discuss the role of adjuvant chemoradiotherapy in stomach carcinoma as per current available evidence. What are the advantages of neoadjuvant chemotherapy in nonmetastatic cancer?

WBUHS 2021 Supplementary

Adjuvant Chemoradiotherapy in Stomach Carcinoma

- *US INT-0116 trial*
  - The landmark INT0116 trial published in 2001 demonstrated the efficacy of adjuvant CRT compared with surgery alone for the treatment of locally advanced gastric cancer (LAGC).
  - In this multicenter PHASE III randomized trial, 556 patients with resected adenocarcinoma of the stomach or gastroesophageal junction were randomly assigned to surgery followed by postoperative CRT or surgery-alone groups, and most of them were staged T3/T4 (69%) and N^+ (85%) with high risk of recurrence. In the adjuvant treatment group, patients received three cycles of 5-FU-based chemotherapy periradiation, and radiation was delivered with a total dose of 45 Gy in 25 fractions.
  - After a median follow-up of 5 years, the adjuvant CRT group showed a significant improvement in OS (40% *vs.* 22%) and a decrease in the local recurrence rate (19% *vs.* 29%) compared with the surgery-alone group.
- *ARTIST trial*
  - Effect of addition of RT to adjuvant CT after D2 lymphadenectomy
  - No significant difference
  - Subgroup analysis—survival advantage in subjects with LN metastasis
- *MAGIC trial*
  - Evaluated patients with resectable gastric, esophagogastric, and lower esophageal cancers
  - Surgery alone versus surgery with perioperative chemotherapy (three preoperative and three postoperative cycles of ECF)
  - Treatment group had significantly better pathologic results (downstaging) and long-term outcome
  - Drawback—inadequate staging and inadequate LN dissection
- *FRENCH trial*
  - Combined neoadjuvant and adjuvant chemotherapy
  - 5-FU and cisplatin
  - Better outcome with perioperative chemotherapy (CT)
- *CLASSIC trial*
  - D2 gastrectomy versus D2 gastrectomy + adjuvant CT (eight 3-week cycles of capecitabine and oxaliplatin)
  - Significantly higher rates of disease-free survival and OS with adjuvant CT
- *CRITICS trial*
  - Chemoradiotherapy after induction CT in GC
  - Comparing perioperative ECF versus adjuvant CRT
  - Ongoing trial in Holland; results awaited

Benefits of a Neoadjuvant Approach have been Demonstrated in the Management of Gastrointestinal Malignancies

- Neoadjuvant therapy is probably underutilized in the management of gastric carcinoma. The morbidity associated with gastric resection precludes timely adjuvant therapy in a subset of patients and multimodality therapy has proven efficacy.
- Neoadjuvant therapy allows for an assessment of response to therapy, may improve treatment compliance and can inform selection of patients for surgical resection.
- A European randomized trial demonstrated survival benefit when patients were treated with three cycles of preoperative chemotherapy (ECF) followed by surgery and then three cycles of postoperative chemotherapy compared with surgery alone.
- The benefit was comparable to that obtained with postoperative chemoradiation in a US trial. However, the Gastric Chemotherapy Group for Japan did not demonstrate a significant survival benefit with neoadjuvant chemotherapy.

- A meta-analysis of 15 randomized controlled trials concluded that the addition of neoadjuvant chemotherapy to surgery reduces overall mortality at 3 and 5 years in patients with advanced GC [relative risk (RR) = 0.74 and 0.82, respectively] and reduces overall mortality at 1, 2, 3, and 5 years in patients with esophago-GC (RR = 0.79, 0.83, 0.84, and 0.91 respectively).
- In patients with esophago-GC, neoadjuvant therapy reduces the overall recurrence rate (RR = 0.80).
- However, neoadjuvant therapy does not influence morbidity and perioperative mortality rates in either gastric or esophago-GC.

50. Role of intraperitoneal therapy in the treatment of adjuvant therapy of resectable gastric cancer.

- Intraperitoneal chemotherapy is a promising and feasible option for GC with chance of peritoneal dissemination. There were several cases with long-term prognosis where conversion surgery was achieved.
- Numerous randomized clinical trials (RCTs) have compared surgery alone with adjuvant chemotherapy, but definitive evidence is lacking.
- There are different regimens, including monochemotherapy; combined chemotherapy with 5-FU derivatives, mitomycin C, and other therapies but no anthracyclines; combined chemotherapy with 5-FU derivatives, mitomycin C, and anthracyclines.
- Possible treatments include neoadjuvant systemic chemotherapy (NAC), neoadjuvant intraperitoneal and systemic chemotherapy (NIPS), cytoreductive surgery (CRS), and perioperative chemotherapy which may include hyperthermic intraperitoneal chemotherapy (HIPEC) and/or early postoperative intraperitoneal chemotherapy (EPIC).
- Surgical treatment failure with resection site and intra-abdominal tumors are the most common sites of first recurrence in GC after potentially curative resection.
- Sources of recurrence after curative resection are:
  - Spontaneous spreading from the primary tumor
  - Surgical trauma causing scattering of cancer cells during the surgical procedure.
- If serosal surface invasion has occurred within the primary tumor, then spontaneous dissemination is more common and patients are frequently found to have viable intraperitoneal cancer cells (positive cytology).
- Tumor cells can also seed the intra-abdominal cavity during surgery according to the tumor cell entrapment hypothesis.

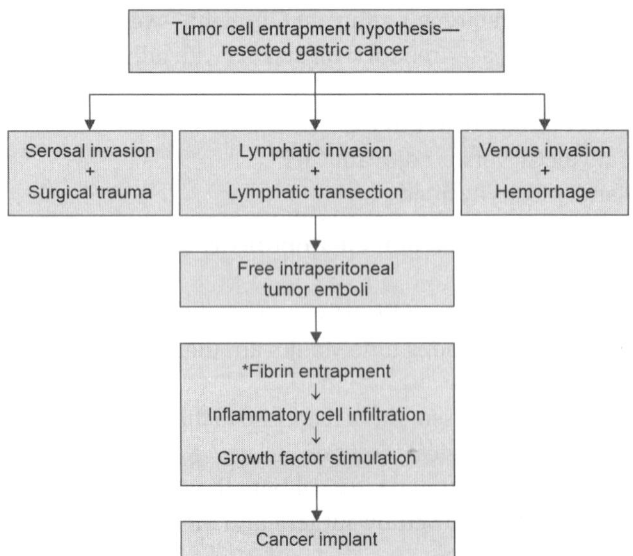

*Occurs at resection site, on abraded bowel surfaces, and beneath abdominal incision.

- Perioperative or intraoperative chemotherapy can eliminate progression of peritoneal implantation after curative surgery; however, it cannot treat residual disease within LNs.
- Therefore, an adequate lymphadenectomy is essential.
- Intraperitoneal chemotherapy enters the peritoneal nodule by simple diffusion so it only penetrates to 1 or 2 mm. It is not effective in LNs.
- Approximately 40–50% of patients had a first site of recurrence in their peritoneal cavity and the development of local-regional recurrence had a negative impact on overall survival.
- The potential role of adjuvant treatments for GC remains to be clarified. The survival results of the MRC adjuvant gastric infusion chemotherapy (MAGIC) trial suggested that patients with operable GC may benefit from perioperative regimen of ECF.
- The role of perioperative intraperitoneal chemotherapy may be regarded as complimentary to adjuvant systemic treatment.
- The fundamental goal of intraperitoneal chemotherapy administration is to maximize the total amount of drug delivered into the peritoneal surface, while minimizing that delivered to the systemic circulation.
- The rationales for adjuvant intraperitoneal chemotherapy are to eradicate residual disease by direct cytotoxic effects, generated by high drug concentrations in the peritoneal cavity and to reduce systemic toxicity.
- However, intraperitoneal chemotherapy has several foreseeable shortcomings in the management of GC.
  - Firstly, the depth of drug concentration by simple diffusion was limited to 1 or 2 mm.
    - Therefore, in patients with macroscopic peritoneal carcinomatosis, the efficacy of this intraperitoneal delivery is questionable.
    - Several centers have utilized peritonectomy procedures to remove all macroscopic disease, followed by intraperitoneal chemotherapy.
    - This approach is associated with relatively higher morbidity and cost, and therefore should be restricted to selected patients in experienced peritonectomy centers.
  - Secondly, GC spreads not only by the transcoelomic route, but also via lymphatic and hematogenous dissemination.
    - The containment of disease with targeted local-regional therapy alone, in high-risk patients, may not be adequate.
  - Thirdly, relatively higher complication rates associated with intraperitoneal chemotherapy should be recognized.

Role of Molecular Therapy in the Treatment of Adjuvant Therapy of Resectable GC

- In the recent few decades, the development of molecular targeted agents has advanced explosively. Based on the ToGA trial, trastuzumab, a monoclonal antibody against HER2, was used as one of the standard options for HER2-positive gastric and EGJ adenocarcinoma in the unresectable or metastatic condition.
- Thereafter, the efficacy of ramucirumab, a monoclonal antibody VEGFR-2 antagonist, for gastric and EGJ adenocarcinoma was demonstrated by the REGARD and RAINBOW trials.
- Recently, the ONO-4538-12/ATTRACTION-2 trial indicated that nivolumab, a monoclonal antibody inhibitor of PD-1, prolonged the OS of patients with unresectable advanced or recurrent gastric and EGJ adenocarcinoma.
- The ST03 trial was designed to assess the usefulness of the addition of bevacizumab, a monoclonal antibody against VEGF in the treatment for patients with resectable gastric and EGJ adenocarcinoma.
- Pembrolizumab, a humanized antibody that binds to the PD-1 receptor was suggested to be effective for advanced GC.

CHAPTER 24

Bariatric and Metabolic Surgery

LEARNING OBJECTIVES

- Definition and Classification of Obesity
- Indications and Contraindications for Bariatric Surgery
- Preoperative Workup of a Patient for "Bariatric Surgery"
- Different Types of Bariatric Surgery
- Merits and Demerits of Various Surgical Procedures in Treatment of Morbid Obesity
- Endoscopic Bariatric Procedure
- Risk Associated with "Metabolic Surgery" Procedure
- Compare Minigastric Bypass with Roux-en-Y Gastric Bypass

---

1. Define obesity and outline its classification. Define metabolic surgery. Discuss the indications and contraindications for bariatric surgery. ***WBUHS 2021 Supplementary***

---

2. What is morbid obesity? Discuss the ill effects of this condition. What are the surgical options for this condition? ***WBUHS 2009***

---

3. Mention the different morbidity of obesity. What is morbidly obese? Discuss the management of morbid obesity. ***WBUHS 2007***

---

4. Define morbid obesity and outline the various surgical options and their rationale. ***WBUHS 2008***

---

5. A 40-year-old patient with morbid obesity is being evaluated for bariatric surgery. Discuss current surgical options and advances in metabolic surgery. ***Maharashtra University of Health Sciences 2025***

---

6. Discuss the current status of different types of bariatric surgery. ***WBUHS 2010***

---

7. What are the various metabolic surgeries? ***KIIT University, Odisha 2025***

---

8. Merits and demerits of various surgical procedures in treatment of morbid obesity. ***RIMS, Imphal 2012, 2022***

---

9. What are the different types of metabolic surgery and how do they influence metabolism? ***WBUHS 2023, Tripura University 2024***

---

10. Briefly discuss the nutritional consequences of weight loss surgery. ***WBUHS 2025***

11. Define metabolic surgery. Describe its physiological basis and risk associated with metabolic surgical procedure. ***WBUHS 2024***

12. Overview of bariatric surgery and write indications and principles of any one bariatric procedure. ***RGUHS, Karnataka 2025***

13. Discuss about preoperative workup of a patient for "bariatric surgery". ***WBUHS 2022, 2023***

14. Write in brief on preoperative evaluation, selection of patient and complications of bariatric surgery. ***WBUHS 2025 Supplementary***

15. Discuss the risk associated with "metabolic surgery" procedure. ***WBUHS 2020***

16. Briefly discuss the criteria for patient selection, various surgical options and postoperative complications of bariatric surgery. ***DNB, June 2019***

17. Bariatric surgery patient selection. ***Gujarat Health University 2025***

Definition of Obesity

- Body mass index (BMI) is a calculation that takes a person's weight and height into account to measure body size.
- In adults, obesity is defined as having a *BMI* of 30 or more according to the Centers for Disease Control and Prevention (CDC).

Classification of Obesity

BMI	*Class*
185 or under	Underweight
185 to <25.0	Normal weight
25.0 to <30.0	Overweight
30.0 to <35.0	Class 1 obesity
35.0 to <40.0	Class 2 obesity
40.0 or over	Class 3 obesity (also known as morbid, extreme, or severe obesity)

Some modifications to the World Health Organization (WHO) definitions have been made by particular organizations. The surgical literature breaks down class II and III or only class III obesity into further categories whose exact values are still disputed.

- Any BMI ≥35 or 40 kg/m^2 is severe obesity.
- A BMI of ≥35 kg/m^2 and experiencing obesity-related health conditions or ≥40 or 45 kg/m^2 is morbid obesity.
- A BMI of ≥45 or 50 kg/m^2 is super obesity.

Definition of Morbid Obesity

Morbid obesity is defined as being either 100 pounds above ideal body weight, or twice ideal body weight, or having a BM > 40 in Western population and >37.5 in Asian population.

Ill Effects of Morbid Obesity

Medical	*Psychological*	*Economic*	*Social*
Coronary heart disease Prevalence 6 times higher	Depression	Cost of futile weight loss treatment	Social isolation
			Daily prejudice
Noninsulin-dependent diabetes mellitus—twice as high	Insomnia	Cost of treating various medical conditions	Verbal abuse
Dyslipidemias			Physical abuse
Hypertension		Inability to obtain insurance coverage or increased premium	Sexual abuse
Gastroesophageal reflux disorder	Suicide		Limitations in performing daily activities
Gallstones			Difficulty with hygiene
Osteoarthritis	Neurotic disorders	Cost of special clothing	Clothing limitations
Sleep apnea		Difficulty obtaining good job or promotion	Limited mobility
Malignancy	Self-hate and feeling of guilt		Limited access to seats, passageways, etc.

Complications of Morbid Obesity

- *Cardiac*
  - Hypertension
  - Sudden cardiac death (myocardial infarction)
  - Coronary artery disease
  - Deep venous thrombosis
  - Heart failure
  - Venous stasis
- *Pulmonary*
  - Obesity hypoventilation syndrome
  - Asthma
  - Obstructive sleep apnea
- *Metabolic*
  - Type II diabetes
  - Hyperlipidemia
  - Hypercholesterolemia
  - Nonalcoholic steatohepatitis
- *Musculoskeletal*
  - Degenerative joint disease
  - Lumbar disc disease
  - Osteoarthritis
  - Ventral hernias
- *Gastrointestinal*
  - Cholelithiasis
  - Gastroesophageal reflux disease
- *Genitourinary/gynecologic*
  - Stress incontinence
  - Polycystic ovarian syndrome
  - Menstrual irregularities
- *Infectious*
  - Fungal infections
  - Necrotizing soft tissue infections

- *Neurologic*
  - Pseudotumor cerebri
  - Stroke

Definition of Bariatric Surgery

Bariatric surgery, from the Greek "baros" meaning "weight," is synonymous with weight loss surgery. Bariatric surgery indicates a variety of gastrointestinal (GI) surgical procedures originally designed to induce weight reduction in morbidly obese patients.

Mechanisms of Weight Loss

Bariatric surgery typically achieves weight loss through three primary mechanisms:

- *Restriction:* Reduces the amount of food the stomach can hold, leading to early satiety (feeling of fullness after consuming less food).
- *Malabsorption:* Alters the way the body absorbs nutrients, leading to decreased absorption of calories, fats, and sugars.
- *Hormonal changes:* Affects hormones involved in hunger, satiety, and metabolism.

Indications for Bariatric Surgery

Indications

Essentials:

- Bariatric surgery may be considered for a severely overweight patient to support lifestyle changes and to improve the permanence of the results of weight reduction. Criteria include:
  - BMI exceeding 40 kg/m^2
  - BMI exceeding 35 kg/m^2 plus a related disease or a risk factor for such a disease
  - BMI 30–35 kg/m^2 in a person with type 2 diabetes, if conservative treatment of obesity and diabetes has not produced adequate results.
- The patient must have undergone about 6 months of conservative treatment leading to lifestyle changes and to a weight loss of about 5%. Such treatment should primarily be provided in primary healthcare before referring the patient to specialized care.
- The long-term results of bariatric surgery are usually significantly better than those achieved with conventional management.
- The greatest benefits offered by bariatric surgery include a reduction in obesity-related diseases and easier management of such diseases, as well as perceived improvement in the quality of life.
- The most common methods are gastric bypass and sleeve gastrectomy.
- After bariatric surgery, all patients need permanent vitamin and trace element replacement.

Criteria for Surgery

- The patient's age is between 18 and 65 years. In exceptional cases, surgery may be considered in patients of 13–17 years.
- Prior to surgery, the patient has participated successfully (weight loss about 5%) in a weight management program offered by a healthcare unit (group, individual or internet-based 6-month treatment) but the result has not been sufficient in relation to the weight loss target or has not been maintained after treatment.
- It is essential that the patient has been shown to be able to make lifestyle changes and that the results were not achieved with a very low-calorie diet (VLCD), alone.
- BMI
  - Exceeding 40 kg/m^2
  - Exceeding 35 kg/m^2 in a patient with a related disease or a risk factor for such a disease, such as:
    - Type 2 diabetes or its preliminary stage
    - Sleep apnea requiring continuous positive airway pressure (CPAP) therapy

- Hypertension requiring medication
- Osteoarthritis of weight-bearing joints (or other severe disease of the musculoskeletal system)
- Dyslipidemia
- Asthma
- Polycystic ovary syndrome (PCOS)
- Infertility

- 30–35 kg/m^2 in a person with type 2 diabetes, if conservative treatment of obesity and diabetes has not produced adequate results.

- The patient must be able to change his/her eating habits as required by the surgery (small portions evenly spaced and slow eating), to commit to permanent vitamin and trace element replacement and to adapt mentally to the new, altered self-image. The patient must have a realistic understanding of the impacts of the procedure.
- General suitability for surgery

Contraindications

- Severe eating disorder requiring treatment, in which case the patient should be referred for psychiatric consultation.
- Excessive use of alcohol
- Severe mental health problem requiring treatment, in which case the patient should be referred for psychiatric consultation.
- Severe systemic diseases (e.g., liver cirrhosis or serious heart disease)
- Disease affecting the upper digestive tract and requiring follow-up by endoscopies
- Need for continuous use of nonsteroidal anti-inflammatory drugs
- The patient has been unable to lose any weight, even temporarily, with conservative treatment.

Things to be Evaluated

Gastrointestinal evaluation	*Birth control counseling*	*Cardiac risk assessment*	*Pulmonary evaluation*	*Endocrine evaluation*
• Endoscopy • Ulcers (*Helicobacter pylori*) • Esophageal disorders • Irritable bowel syndrome • Crohn's disease	• Absence of pregnancy • Birth control • Risky pregnancy in the early postoperative period (1–2 years) • Weight loss may improve fertility	• Stress testing • Echocardiogram • Medication adjustment • Cardiac clearance	• Obstructive sleep apnea (testing and treatment) • Asthma • Smokers	• Diabetes management • Diabetes education • Thyroid disease

Preparation

The preoperative evaluation should be holistic, integral, and includes an assessment by an interprofessional team encompassing endocrinologists, dieticians, psychologists, anesthesiologists, nurses, cardiologists, and the surgeon.

Psychological Evaluation

- Patients should be psychologically fit to undergo bariatric surgery. A psychological clearance is one of the first steps in the preoperative workup of the patient.
- Patients should undergo evaluation for a history of mental disorder, depression, eating disorders, prior weight loss attempts, compliance with therapy, and substance misuse.
- Patients identified to have alcohol dependence need a referral for rehabilitation and detoxification before the procedure.

- The patient should achieve at least 1-year abstinence prior to surgery, solidly documented.
- Smoking cessation should be encouraged and documented before proceeding with the operation; cessation of smoking has demonstrated improved outcomes and reduced postoperative complications.
- The support system available for the patient should also be evaluated. Studies have shown that patients with strong family and community support are more likely to have better outcomes.

Nutritional Evaluation

- Nutritional assessment and patient education will help guide the patient toward dietary modifications that are necessary after surgery.
- Education regarding patient expectations should also be included to ensure clear objectives regarding weight loss.
- As a general rule, a patient undergoing sleeve gastrectomy should expect to lose about 60–65% of excess body weight in 2 years, and a patient undergoing gastric bypass should expect a weight loss of 70–75% of excess body weight in the same period.
- Weight maintenance strategies should be a topic of discussion with the patient.
- Glycemic control in the diabetic patient undergoing bariatric surgery is of extreme importance and should be encouraged and monitored.
- A licensed dietician typically performs the nutritional evaluation.

Weight Loss Plan

- A guided weight loss plan is necessary. A documented weight loss program can improve outcomes after surgery and does not preclude the patient from undergoing weight loss surgery in most cases.
- The weight loss plan should include nutritional assessment and a guided exercise plan.
- Weight loss goals should be delineated and monitored during every visit of the patient during the preoperative period.
- Failure to lose weight due to lack of adherence to the plan and diet can be a predictor of how reliable the patient will be with lifestyle modifications needed in the postoperative period.
- A failure to lose weight even after following the plan should also be documented so that more aggressive support can be provided before and after the bariatric procedure.

Medical Clearance

- A complete evaluation is necessary before the patient is cleared to undergo bariatric surgery.
- This evaluation should include a detailed history and physical, review of past medical and surgical history, a review of psychosocial factors that could influence weight loss (employment, housing, and family core), laboratory workup, and anthropometric measurement.
- Functional status should be documented as it directly correlates with perioperative outcomes.
- The patient should also complete screening for cardiac disease and obstructive sleep apnea (OSA). Patients with OSA symptoms should be referred for a sleep study.
- Laboratory workup should include a comprehensive metabolic panel, complete blood count, levels of iron, vitamins, and folate, type and screen, hemoglobin A1C, and a coagulation panel.

Preoperative Imaging

- There is no consensus regarding the imaging modalities that should be obtained before a bariatric procedure.
- This also depends on whether the patient had previous bariatric surgery or any type of surgery that may have affected the anatomy of the GI tract.
- Such imaging can be used to guide the surgeon determine what type of bariatric surgery to offer the patient.
- An abdominal ultrasound is necessary for patients undergoing gastric bypass to identify possible liver pathology and cholelithiasis.

Other Preoperative Considerations

- Esophagogastroduodenoscopy (EGD) is not routinely a recommended procedure in the workup for bariatric surgery.
- The American Society of Metabolic and Bariatric Surgery advises the use of endoscopy only for those patients with significant GI symptoms.

Anesthetic Preoperative Considerations

- Anesthesiological evaluations are of fundamental importance as obesity correlates with various comorbidities that can make intraoperative management difficult and complicate the postoperative course.
- Obesity-related conditions include heart disease, hypertension, stroke, type 2 diabetes, gastroesophageal reflux disease (GERD), and among others.
- The evaluation of history and clinical-instrumental assessment are important to assess the degree of functional impairment and can help the clinician determine which of the disorders can be corrected or improved (e.g., improvement of blood glucose and blood pressure).
- Furthermore, a careful drug history is necessary, as several agents such as diet drugs and appetite suppressors can impact the anesthetic management by inducing cardiopulmonary and GI problems.

Evaluation of the cardiorespiratory status: Enrolled patients should be evaluated for ischemic heart disease, systemic and pulmonary hypertension, right or left ventricular failure signs, and sleep-disordered breathing. OSA is usually investigated through the 8-item STOP-Bang Questionnaire (S = Snoring; T = Tired; O = Observed) and includes the following:

- Has anyone observed the patient stop breathing or choking/gasping during sleep?'
- P = Pressure
- B = BMI over 35
- A = Age older than 50
- N = Neck size
- G = Gender—male greater than female

In addition to the standard ECG that may demonstrate signs of right ventricular hypertrophy, further cardiac evaluation may include stress echocardiography and cardiopulmonary exercise testing.

Airway management:

- Airway management can represent a severe challenge for anesthesiologists. Difficult or failed intubation, indeed, is more common in patients with obesity than in the nonobese population.
- Obesity correlates with a 30% greater chance of difficult or failed intubation. Thus, preoperative identification of patients at high risk for airway management problems is mandatory.
- Predictive scores of difficult intubation such as thyromental distance and neck circumference as well as the range of motion of the neck and larynx must have a careful evaluation.
- The Mallampati score is the most important parameter. It evaluates the visibility of the base of the uvula, faucial pillars, and soft palate; and classifies patients into four classes.

Other Anesthetic Considerations

- There is also a concern for venous access in patients with obesity; thus, before anesthesia, one should closely examine the extremities for good veins or consider inserting of a central line.
- IV access is vital for induction of anesthesia, administration of medications, and hydrating the patient.
- At the same time, the pharmacist should recommend the appropriate dose of medications based on body weight.

Bariatric surgery is an elective procedure, and it is essential to optimize the patient's functional and health status prior to surgery.

Medical Therapy for Severe Obesity

- *Medical therapy* for severe obesity has limited short-term success and almost nonexistent long-term success.
- Once severely obese, the likelihood that a person will lose enough weight by dietary means alone and remain at a BMI below 35 kg/m^2 is estimated at 3% or less.
- A 10% weight loss attained over a period of months at a rate of 0.5–2 lb/week is the initial goal of medical therapy.
- *Very low-calorie diets fall into two categories:* Those that primarily restrict fat intake and those that primarily restrict carbohydrate intake.
- Both diets produce weight loss that is insufficient to affect any major change in health status.
- Two medications are used:
  - Sibutramine blocks presynaptic receptor uptake of both norepinephrine and serotonin, thereby potentiating their anorexic effect in the central nervous system.
  - Orlistat inhibits pancreatic lipase and thereby reduces absorption of up to 30% of ingested dietary fat.
  - A maximum weight loss of up to 10% of body weight has been noted in unselected individuals taking either or both drugs; however, weight is regained within 12–18 months.
  - For a severely obese individual, neither drug has proved to be effective therapy alone.

Types of Metabolic Surgery

Restrictive	*Largely restrictive/mildly malabsorptive*	*Largely malabsorptive/mildly restrictive*	*Other procedures*
Vertical banded gastroplasty (VBG) (historic purposes only)	Roux-en-Y gastric bypass (RYGB)	Biliopancreatic diversion (BPD)	Endoluminal sleeve
Laparoscopic adjustable gastric banding (LAGB)		Duodenal switch (DS)	Jejunoileal bypass

- Restrictive procedures that limit the amount of food intake by reducing the size of the stomach.
- Malabsorptive procedures that interfere with absorption of food from the digestive tract.
- Combined restrictive and malabsorptive procedures
  - The two most commonly performed operations for weight loss in the United States are the RYGB and the adjustable gastric band (AGB).
  - Both procedures could be done laparoscopically with smaller incisions than those required for traditional open approach (laparotomy).

Vertical Banded Gastroplasty

This procedure has now largely been abandoned.

Causes

- Poor long-term weight loss
- A high rate of late stenosis of the gastric outlet
- A tendency for patients to adopt a high-calorie liquid diet, thereby leading to regain of weight.
- Weight regain several years after surgery is typically due to a breakdown of the vertical staple line and patients report new dietary freedom. Revisional surgery and conversion to a gastric bypass usually result in durable weight loss but can be associated with a higher rate of perioperative complications.

Adjustable Gastric Banding

- The AGB procedure may be performed with any of three types of adjustable bands.
- They all work on the principle of restriction of oral intake by limiting the volume of the proximal part of the stomach.
- Their advantage over the traditional VBG is adjustability.
- Gastric banding is a least-invasive operation with 50–60% EWL over 5 years but long-term results are unknown and the complication rate may be cumulative.

Roux-en-Y Gastric Bypass

Essential components of Roux-en-Y gastric bypass:

- Small proximal gastric pouch
- Gastric pouch constructed from the cardia of the stomach to prevent dilation and minimize acid production
- Gastric pouch divided from the distal part of the stomach
- Roux limb at least 75 cm in length
- Enteroenterostomy constructed to avoid stenosis or obstruction
- Closure of all potential spaces for internal hernias

Results of Roux-en-Y gastric bypass:

- RYGB has an established track record longer than that of any other operation. Its recovery after RYGB is improved after a laparoscopic approach.
- This improvement is largely related to the decrease in postoperative pain experienced by patients after laparoscopic RYGB versus open RYGB.
- Weight loss with both approaches was comparable (68% loss of excess weight for laparoscopic RYGB vs. 62% loss of excess weight for open RYGB).
- Another important advantage of the laparoscopic approach for RYGB is a decrease in the incidence of wound complications and incisional hernia seen after RYGB.
- There is no difference in the rate resolution of comorbid conditions or weight loss between the two procedures after RYGB.
- Resolution of comorbid conditions after open and laparoscopic RYGB has generally been excellent.
- Rate of resolution and improvement of diabetes, hypertension, and obstructive sleep apnea is significant.
- Metabolic syndrome is cured or ameliorated with gastric bypass.
- Hyperlipidemia, hypercholesterolemia, and hypertriglyceridemia have been improved significantly in patients undergoing RYGB.
- RYGB has also been shown to resolve the symptoms of pseudotumor cerebri, as well as cure the difficult problem of venous stasis ulcers.
- Immediate resolution of symptoms of GERD occurs in >90% of cases.

Biliopancreatic Diversion

- BPD produces weight loss based primarily on malabsorption, but it does have a mild restrictive component.
- The intestinal tract is reconstructed to allow only a short so-called common channel of the distal 50 cm of terminal ileum for absorption of fat and protein.
- The alimentary tract beyond the proximal part of the stomach is rearranged to include only the distal 200 cm of ileum, including the common channel.
- The proximal end of this ileum is anastomosed to the proximal end of the stomach after performing a distal hemigastrectomy.
- The ileum proximal to the end that is anastomosed to the stomach is in turn anastomosed to the terminal ileum within the 50–100 cm distance from the ileocecal valve, depending on the surgeon's preference and the patient's size.

Duodenal Switch

- This modification was developed to help lessen the high incidence of marginal ulcers after BPD.
- The mechanism of weight loss is similar to that of BPD.
- An appendectomy is followed by measurement of the terminal ileum. Notably in the DS procedure, the common channel is 100 cm and the entire alimentary tract is 250 cm.
- However, the major difference between DS and BPD is the gastrectomy and the proximal anatomy. Instead of a distal hemigastrectomy, a sleeve gastrectomy of the greater curvature of the stomach is performed.

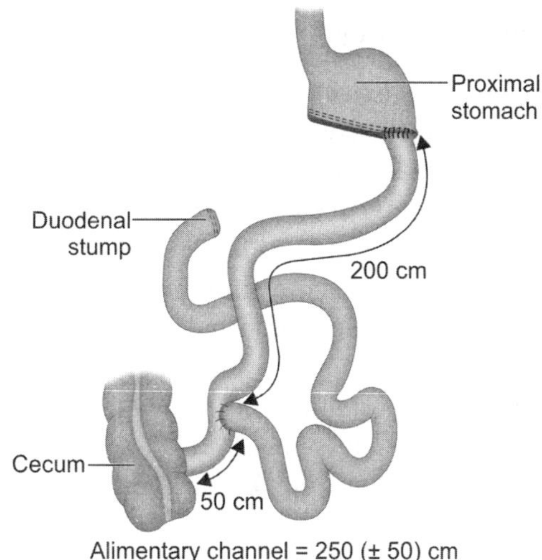

Schematic diagram of biliopancreatic diversion.

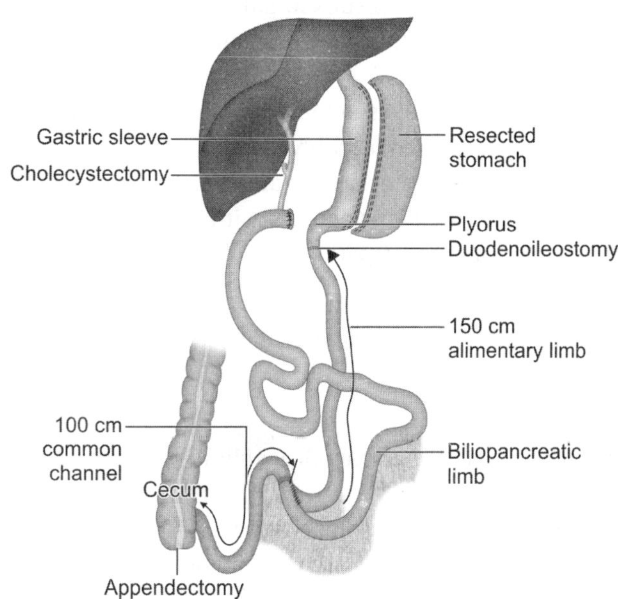

Schematic diagram of duodenal switch.

- This procedure is done as the initial part of the operation because if the patient exhibits any intraoperative instability, the operation can be discontinued after the sleeve gastrectomy alone.
- A two-stage DS has been used in patients who have an extremely high BMI and are high operative risks.
- The goal is to produce a lesser curvature gastric sleeve with a volume of 150–200 mL.
- After sleeve gastrectomy, or preceding it in smaller patients, the duodenum is divided with the stapler approximately 2 cm beyond the pylorus.
- The distal connections are performed as for BPD. The distal anastomosis is created at the 100-cm point proximal to the ileocecal valve.

- The proximal anastomosis is created between the proximal end of the 250 cm of terminal ileum and the first portion of the duodenum. The duodenoileostomy is an antecolic end-to-side duodenoenterostomy.

Results of biliopancreatic diversion/duodenal switch:
- Excess weight loss after BPD/DS is the highest of all the bariatric operations
- In a recent study comparing morbidly obese patients with a BMI > 50 kg/m^2, there was significantly more EWL at 12, 18, and 24 months postoperatively after DS than after RYGB.
- Thus, some surgeons argue that superobese patients fare better and maintain weight loss better in the long-term after undergoing DS than after other bariatric operations.
- BPD/DS has also been highly effective in treating comorbid conditions, including hypertension, diabetes, lipid disorders, and OSA.
- Lipid disorders and type 2 diabetes are almost uniformly resolved after BPD/DS.
- Hypertension is cured in 83.4% and OSA resolves in 91.9% of patients.
- After BPD, patients typically have between two and four bowel movements per day. Excessive flatulence and foul-smelling stools are the rule.
- Relatively selective malabsorption of starch and fat provides the major mechanism of weight loss, although the partial gastric resection does contribute a restrictive component to the operation.
- When protein malnutrition does occur, the common channel may need to be lengthened with a reoperation.
- Major considerations for achieving excellent results in patients offered BPD/DS include the ability to reliably monitor these patients, as well as confirm that they are being compliant with the recommendations to take appropriate vitamin supplements.
- Supplements include multivitamins, as well as at least 2 g of oral calcium per day. Supplemental fat-soluble vitamins, including D, K, and A, are indicated monthly as well.
- Because of a high incidence of morbidity and mortality in patients with a BMI > 60 kg/m^2 undergoing laparoscopic DS, surgeons developed the two-stage DS, with sleeve gastrectomy alone performed as the first stage to decrease morbidity in this superobese patient population.

Other Procedures
- Endoluminal sleeve
- Jejunoileal bypass

Comments
- Cultural factors, surgeon, and patient preference drive choice of operation which should be based on the balance of risk and benefit.
- Bariatric surgery pays for itself within 3–4 years after surgery.
- Bariatric surgery patients have better long-term survival than obese controls.
- Several surgeons have proposed a two-stage procedure for a superobese patient, who often has a large liver that precludes safe retraction for gastric bypass, because of the recognition that the DS procedure has been associated with much higher mortality and morbidity rates in the superobese (BMI > 60 kg/m^2).
- Now, reports of vertical sleeve gastrectomy (VSG) alone suggest that weight loss is sufficient to preclude conversion to gastric bypass or DS.
- Gastric pacing has been performed in several trials but has not gained widespread acceptance. The concept is to stimulate gastric smooth muscle by implanting a pacemaker in the body of the stomach to induce early satiety, which reduces caloric intake and therefore results in weight loss.
- Increasingly, surgeons are observing effects of bariatric operations not just on the physical reduction of caloric intake or malabsorption. Alteration in comorbid conditions caused by metabolic processes may prove equally as important. For example, bariatric operations may have important metabolic components that alter the hormonal/cytokine/metabolic rate of patients.

Types of Bariatric Surgery and their Physiological Effects

Different types of bariatric surgery have varying effects on the digestive system. The most common types include:

Gastric Bypass (Roux-en-Y)

- *Restriction:* The stomach is divided into a small upper pouch that holds about 20–30 mL of food, significantly limiting food intake.
- *Malabsorption:* The small intestine is rerouted, bypassing a portion of the duodenum and jejunum, which reduces the absorption of calories and nutrients.
- *Hormonal changes:* Gastric bypass surgery has significant effects on gastrointestinal hormones, such as—
  - *Increased levels of GLP-1 (glucagon-like peptide-1):* GLP-1 is a hormone that enhances insulin secretion, promotes satiety, and reduces food intake. Higher levels of GLP-1 contribute to improved glucose metabolism and appetite control.
  - *Decreased nightline:* Ghrelin is known as the "hunger hormone" and is significantly reduced after gastric bypass, leading to a reduced sensation of hunger.
  - *Alterations in leptin:* Leptin, a hormone related to energy balance and fat storage, may also change post-surgery, contributing to a reduction in hunger signals.

Sleeve Gastrectomy

- *Restriction:* A large portion of the stomach (about 75–85%) is removed, leaving a tubular structure resembling a sleeve. This reduces the stomach's capacity to hold food, thus limiting caloric intake.
- *Hormoal changes:*
  - Similar to gastric bypass, sleeve gastrectomy significantly reduces ghrelin levels, leading to reduced hunger.
  - Increases in GLP-1 levels help promote satiety and enhance insulin sensitivity.

Adjustable Gastric Banding (Lap-Band)

- *Restriction:* An adjustable band is placed around the upper part of the stomach to create a small pouch. This limits food intake by inducing early satiety.
- *Hormonal effects:* Unlike gastric bypass or sleeve gastrectomy, gastric banding tends to have less impact on gut hormones and may result in slower and more gradual weight loss.

Biliopancreatic Diversion with Duodenal Switch (BPD/DS)

- *Combination of restriction and malabsorption:* This procedure combines a sleeve gastrectomy with a more extensive rerouting of the small intestine, causing both reduced stomach size and significant malabsorption of nutrients.
- *Significant malabsorption:* BPD/DS leads to a dramatic decrease in the absorption of calories and fats, contributing to substantial weight loss.
- *Hormonal changes:* Similar to other surgeries, BPD/DS increases GLP-1 and reduces ghrelin, contributing to improved satiety and metabolic control.

Gut Hormonal Changes

The gut is a crucial player in regulating appetite, energy balance, and metabolism. Bariatric surgery has profound effects on several gut hormones, which influence weight loss and metabolic health.

- *Ghrelin:* Produced in the stomach, ghrelin is a major regulator of appetite and food intake. It stimulates hunger and increases food consumption. After bariatric surgery, especially gastric bypass and sleeve gastrectomy, ghrelin levels decrease significantly, leading to reduced hunger and appetite.
- *GLP-1 (Glucagon-Like Peptide-1):* GLP-1 is released from the intestines in response to food intake and promotes insulin secretion, slows gastric emptying, and enhances satiety. Bariatric surgeries like gastric bypass and sleeve gastrectomy lead to elevated levels of GLP-1, contributing to improved glucose control and reduced hunger.
- *PYY (Peptide YY):* PYY is a hormone secreted by the intestines that reduces appetite and slows gastric motility. Increased levels of PYY after bariatric surgery promote satiety and a feeling of fullness after eating smaller amounts of food.

- *Insulin sensitivity:* Bariatric surgery, especially gastric bypass, leads to improved insulin sensitivity and reduced insulin resistance. This is partly due to the changes in gut hormones like GLP-1 and PYY, which enhance insulin secretion and glucose metabolism. Many patients experience improvements in type 2 diabetes following surgery.

Metabolic Effects

Bariatric surgery has significant effects on metabolism, particularly in relation to glucose and lipid metabolism:

- *Improved glucose metabolism:* Bariatric surgery leads to improved insulin sensitivity and decreased insulin resistance, contributing to better control of blood glucose. This can result in remission of type 2 diabetes in many patients.
- *Changes in lipid profile:* There are also improvements in lipid metabolism, with decreases in triglycerides, LDL cholesterol, and increases in HDL cholesterol.
- *Reduction in inflammation:* Obesity is associated with chronic low-grade inflammation, which contributes to many obesity-related diseases. Bariatric surgery helps to reduce systemic inflammation, leading to improvements in cardiovascular health and other comorbidities.

Effects on Appetite and Satiety

- Bariatric surgery often leads to a significant reduction in appetite and an increase in feelings of fullness, partly due to changes in gut hormones and altered food processing.
- Patients report reduced cravings for high-calorie foods, and they often find it easier to adhere to a healthy diet post-surgery due to the physical restriction and hormonal changes that influence appetite and satiety.

Long-term Physiological Effects

- *Nutrient deficiencies:* Over time, some patients may develop nutrient deficiencies, particularly in vitamins and minerals (e.g., vitamin B_{12}, iron, calcium), especially if there is significant malabsorption (as in gastric bypass or BPD/DS).
- *Changes in gut microbiome:* Bariatric surgery can alter the gut microbiome, which may play a role in the changes to metabolism and weight loss. Some studies suggest that the microbial community in the intestines may be a contributing factor to the improved metabolic function seen after surgery.
- *Weight regain:* While bariatric surgery leads to significant initial weight loss, some patients may experience weight regain over time. This can be influenced by changes in eating behaviors, hormonal adaptations, and lifestyle factors.

Impact on Comorbidities

Bariatric surgery has profound effects on many obesity-related comorbidities, including:

- *Type 2 diabetes:* Significant improvements or remission in type 2 diabetes are common after bariatric surgery due to better insulin sensitivity and glucose control.
- *Hypertension:* Blood pressure often improves after weight loss, as a result of reduced body fat and improved metabolic function.
- *Sleep apnea:* Many patients experience improvement or resolution of obstructive sleep apnea after significant weight loss.
- *Joint pain and mobility:* Reduced weight can alleviate strain on joints and improve mobility, which is especially important for patients with osteoarthritis or other musculoskeletal issues.

Risks

Metabolic surgical procedures, including various types of bariatric surgery, can lead to significant weight loss and improvements in metabolic health. However, they also carry risks and potential complications. Here's an overview of the main risks associated with these surgical procedures:

Surgical Risks

- *Anesthesia complications:* Risks associated with general anesthesia, including respiratory issues or allergic reactions.

- *Intraoperative risks:* Potential for bleeding, injury to surrounding organs, or complications related to the surgical technique.

Postoperative Complications

- *Infection:* Surgical site infections can occur, requiring treatment and potentially further interventions.
- *Blood clots:* Increased risk of deep vein thrombosis (DVT) and pulmonary embolism (PE), especially in patients with limited mobility postsurgery.
- *Leaks:* An anastomotic leak (leakage from a surgical connection) can occur, leading to serious complications like peritonitis.

Nutritional Deficiencies

- *Malabsorption:* Procedures like gastric bypass or biliopancreatic diversion can lead to inadequate absorption of vitamins and minerals, resulting in deficiencies such as:
  - Vitamin B_{12}
  - Iron
  - Calcium
  - Vitamin D
- *Protein deficiency:* Insufficient protein intake can lead to muscle wasting and other health issues.

Gastrointestinal Issues

- *Dumping syndrome:* Rapid gastric emptying can cause nausea, vomiting, and diarrhea after eating high-sugar or high-fat foods.
- *Gallstones:* Rapid weight loss can increase the risk of gallstone formation, which may require surgical intervention.

Psychological Effects

- *Mental health issues:* Some patients may experience anxiety, depression, or changes in body image post-surgery. Ongoing psychological support may be necessary.
- *Eating disorders:* In some cases, there may be a development of new or exacerbated eating disorders.

Weight Regain

Long-term maintenance: Some patients may experience weight regain due to changes in eating behavior, lack of adherence to dietary guidelines, or metabolic adaptations.

Specific Risks by Procedure Type

- *Gastric bypass:* Risk of complications such as bowel obstruction or strictures at the connection site.
- *Sleeve gastrectomy:* Potential for leakage at the staple line or narrowing of the stomach (stricture).
- *Adjustable gastric banding:* Risks include band slippage, erosion, or port-related complications.
- *Biliopancreatic diversion:* Higher risk of nutritional deficiencies and complications due to the extensive malabsorption.

Benefits and Risks of Weight-loss Surgery

Benefits of weight-loss surgery:

- *Weight loss:* Most patients begin to lose weight right away. Some gain some of the weight back, but most are able to keep the weight off for long periods.
  - In general, combined restrictive and malabsorptive procedures (like gastric bypass) are more successful than restrictive procedures (like AGB) at promoting weight loss.
    - Gastric bypass is the most successful procedure. In the first 2 years after gastric bypass, average weight loss is 65% of excess weight. On the other hand, average weight loss with AGB is 35% of excess weight.
    - With gastric bypass, no band is introduced into the body. Also, it is a good operation for a sweet eater because eating sugar makes the patient feel ill (referred to as "dumping").

- The lap-band system has the advantages of being less invasive, providing a faster recovery, and avoiding alteration of anatomy of the GI tract. It is adjustable and reversible with normal stomach restoration. No opening of the stomach or intestines occurs that could cause a leak.
- People who undergo one of these procedures are much more likely to reach their goal and keep weight off if they also adopt a plan of healthy eating and regular exercise.
- *Improved health:* Most obesity-related medical conditions improve drastically after surgery, especially diabetes, sleep apnea, and hypertension.
    - After surgery mortality rate is reduced and improvements are seen in many of the health risks associated with obesity.
    - Overall, quality of life, self-image, and mobility are reported to be better.

Risks of weight-loss surgery:

- Disadvantages of gastric bypass—a patient who has gastric bypass may develop the following complications:
    - "Dumping syndrome"—patients experience nausea, abdominal cramping, and diarrhea after eating sugar. Other symptoms include weakness or faintness.
    - Narrowing or ulcer formation or leak at the stomach to intestine connection, these may require reoperation.
    - *Incisional hernia:* This is more common in open bariatric surgery.
    - *Blood clot in the leg:* This may migrate to the lung.
    - In addition to surgical complications, long-term consequences of the malabsorption arise if patients with gastric bypass do not take supplemental vitamins, iron, and calcium. These nutritional deficiencies include the following:
        - Vitamin deficiencies (A, B_{12}, D, E, and K)—deficiencies of vitamin B_{12}, folate, and iron can cause anemia.
        - Mineral deficiencies (calcium, iron, and folic acid)—calcium deficiency is a concern because it may lead to osteoporosis and other bone disorders.
- Disadvantages of AGB
    - The lap-band system is not the operation of choice in sweet eaters or patients with severe GERD.
    - There is a low possibility of port leak or infection, as well as slippage, erosion, or migration of the band. This may require reoperation. High conversion rates of band to gastric bypass have been reported in American studies and may reflect patient selection.

In experienced hands, the benefits of surgery are typically viewed to outweigh the risks. The immediate operative mortality rate for both AGB and RYGB is about 1%.

Weight regain after bariatric surgery: Some patients may regain weight after bariatric surgery. This may be due to many factors, among them the following:

- Noncompliance with postoperative diet
- Noncompliance with postoperative exercise
- Stretching of the stomach pouch
- Communication between the pouch and the rest of the stomach
- Band problems

Risk associated with metabolic surgery:

- Dumping syndrome
- Low blood sugar
- Malnutrition
- GERD
- Cholelithiasis
- Vomiting
- Ulcers
- Bowel obstruction

- Anastomotic leaks
- Hernias

AGB:
- *Benefits:* No risk of leak, low risk of metabolic disturbance due to no changes in GI tract anatomy.
- *Risks:* Band slippage, band erosion, leakage or kinking of tubing, increased reflux

Laparoscopic Sleeve Gastrectomy
- *Benefits:* Technical simplicity, pylorus preservation leads to no risk of dumping syndrome, low-risk metabolic disturbances.
- *Risks:* Leak from gastric staple line, reflux, gastric outlet obstruction due to stenosis, and increased reflux.

Roux-en-Y Gastric Bypass
- *Benefits:* Increased weight loss versus restrictive procedures and improved gastric reflux.
- *Risks:* GJ stenosis, malabsorption leading to nutritional deficiencies (primarily iron and B_{12} deficiencies), marginal ulcer risk, internal limb obstruction, and anastomotic leak.

Biliopancreatic Diversion
- *Benefits:* Improved percentage of EWL and improved maintenance over RYGB, excellent resolution of obesity-related comorbidities
- *Risks:* Difficult procedure, marginal ulcer risk, anastomotic leak, and malabsorption leading to high risk for vitamin and protein deficiencies.

Duodenal Switch
- *Benefits:* Improved percentage of EWL and improved maintenance over RYGB, excellent resolution of obesity-related comorbidities, pylorus preserved leading to low risk of ulcers.
- *Risks:* Difficult procedure, anastomotic leak, and malabsorption leading to high risk for vitamin and protein deficiencies.

18. Describe various "Endoscopic Bariatric Procedure". ***WBUHS 2022***

- Available surgical procedures include laparoscopic and open RYGB, sleeve gastrectomy, AGB, VBG, DS, and BPD.
- Endoscopic modalities in the treatment of obesity can be categorized into the following: Restrictive procedures, malabsorptive procedures, gastric function/emptying regulation, and gastric aspiration.

Endoscopic Bariatric Procedures
- *Endoluminal restrictive procedures:*
  - *EndoCinch:* Suturing device (suction chamber) pleats using tagged suture
  - *Transoral gastroplasty system (TOGA):* 18-mm metallic device placed in stomach. A set of guided staplers staple pouch created along lesser curvature (8 cm long tube from GE junction)
  - *POSE (Primary obesity surgery endoluminal):* Suturing gastric folds mainly in fundus (aim is to reduce the size and capacity of stomach)
- *Space-occupying devices:*
  - *Bioenterics intragastric balloon (ORBERA):*
    - Induces early satiety
    - Feeling of fullness
    - Slow gastric emptying
- *Malabsorptive devices:*
  - *Duodenojejunal bypass:*
    - *Endobarrier:* 60 cm long impermeable plastic sleeve anchored in duodenal bulb, extends up to proximal jejunum, creates barrier and delays absorption.

- There is a low possibility of port leak or infection, as well as slippage, erosion, or migration of the band. This may require reoperation. High conversion rates of band to gastric bypass have been reported in American studies and may reflect patient selection.

In experienced hands, the benefits of surgery are typically viewed to outweigh the risks. The immediate operative mortality rate for both AGB and RYGB is about 1%.

Weight Regain after Bariatric Surgery

Some patients may regain weight after bariatric surgery. This may be due to many factors, among them the following:

- Noncompliance with postoperative diet
- Noncompliance with postoperative exercise
- Stretching of the stomach pouch
- Communication between the pouch and the rest of the stomach
- Band problem

19. Compare minigastric bypass with Roux-en-Y gastric bypass. ***WBUHS 2019***

- Minigastric bypass (MGB) is considered safer than traditional gastric bypass. The former involves only one connection called anastomosis. On the other hand, the RYGB involves multiple rerouting.
- There is a smaller chance of a leak or an internal hernia as a consequence of the MGB
- MGB is also able to provide rapid weight loss and control type 2 diabetes before weight loss takes place.
- MGB can be reversed in some circumstances.
- MGB has shorter operating time and shorter hospital stay as compared to RNYGB.
- Some studies indicated that MGB had a higher type 2 diabetes mellitus remission rate and similar hyper- tension remission rate compared with RYGB.
- GERD is more with MGB.
- The excellent safety of the MGB procedure may be explained by its simplicity, short operation time, and less anastomotic leaks.

Small Intestine

LEARNING OBJECTIVES

- Gut Rotation
- Narrow Band Imaging in GIT Lesions
- Duodenum: Duodenal Stump Blow Out, Duodenal Fistula, and Superior Mesenteric Artery (SMA) Syndrome
- Gastrointestinal (GI) Hormones
- Premalignant bowel lesions
- Carcinoid Tumor and Carcinoid Syndrome
- Gastrointestinal Stromal Tumor (GIST)
- Inflammatory Bowel Disease (IBD) and Pouch Surgery
- Mesenteric Ischemia
- Intestinal Fistula
- Enterocutaneous Fistula (ECF)
- Small Bowel Syndrome
- Intestinal Failure
- Acute Intestinal Obstruction

STAGES OF GUT ROTATION

1. Describe the stages of gut rotation and its applied significance. ***Ayush University Chhattisgarh 2025***

Gut Rotation: Stages and Applied Significance

Introduction

- The *midgut* undergoes *physiological herniation, rotation,* and *return* into the abdominal cavity during embryonic development.
- *Purpose:* Proper positioning of the intestines, fixation of the mesentery, and formation of the adult gut configuration.
- *Timeline:* Occurs between the *5th and 12th weeks of intrauterine life.*

Stages of Midgut Rotation

- *Stage 1—Physiological Herniation and Initial Rotation (5th–6th week)*
  - The *midgut loop* elongates rapidly, outgrowing the abdominal cavity.
  - It *herniates into the umbilical cord* (physiological herniation).
  - The *midgut loop* has:
    - *Cranial limb* → forms most of small intestine (jejunum, upper ileum).
    - *Caudal limb* → forms distal ileum, cecum, ascending colon, and proximal 2/3 of transverse colon.
  - *Rotation:* The midgut rotates *90° counterclockwise* around the *axis of the superior mesenteric artery (SMA).*
    - Cranial limb moves to the *right.*
    - Caudal limb moves to the *left.*
- *Stage 2—Return to the Abdominal Cavity and Further Rotation (10th–11th week)*
  - The midgut returns to the abdominal cavity as it enlarges.
  - The *cranial limb* re-enters *first* and lies *centrally and inferiorly* (forming small intestine loops).

- The *caudal limb* returns *later* and lies *superiorly and to the right.*
- During this return, the midgut undergoes an *additional 180° counterclockwise rotation,* making a *total of 270°* rotation.

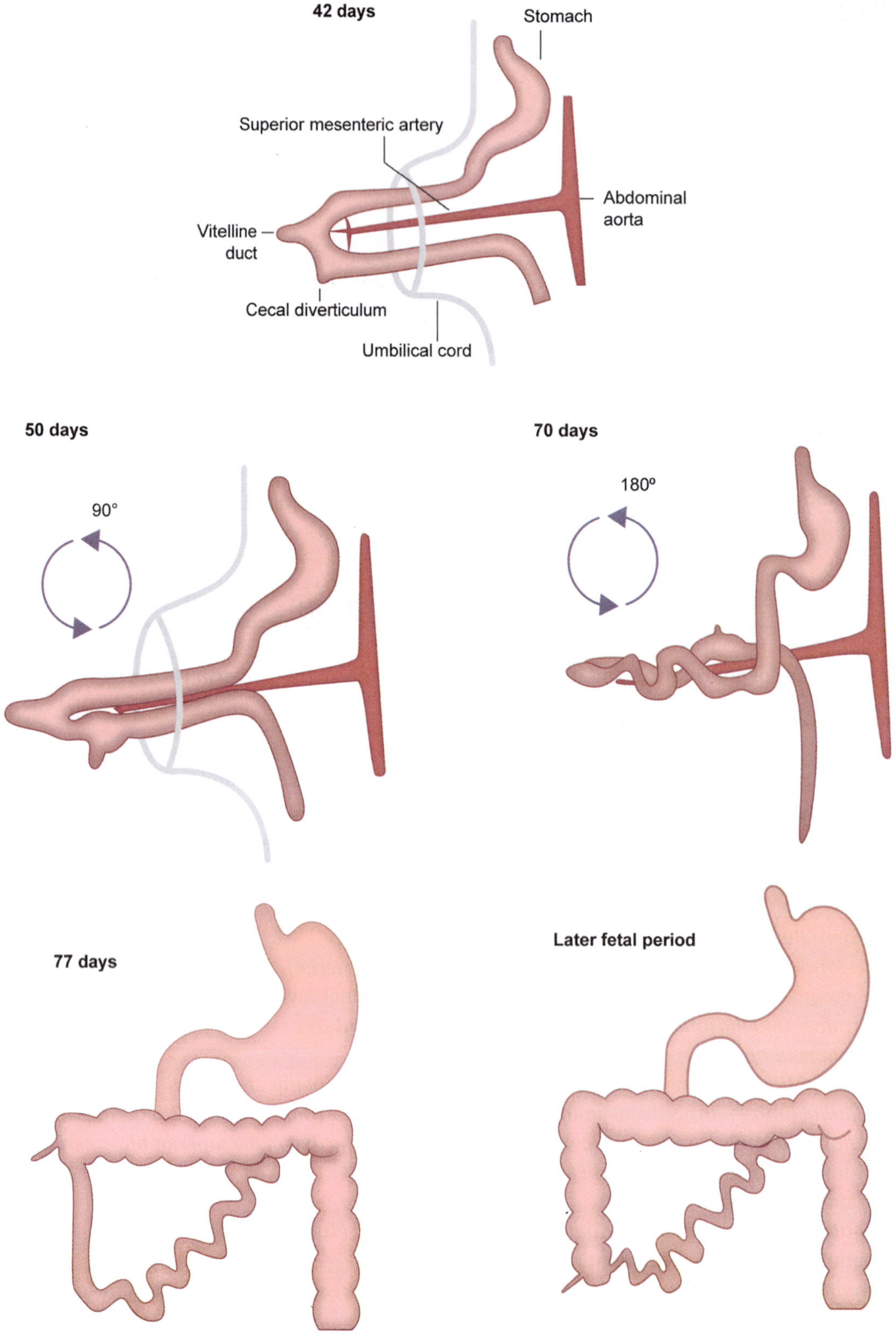

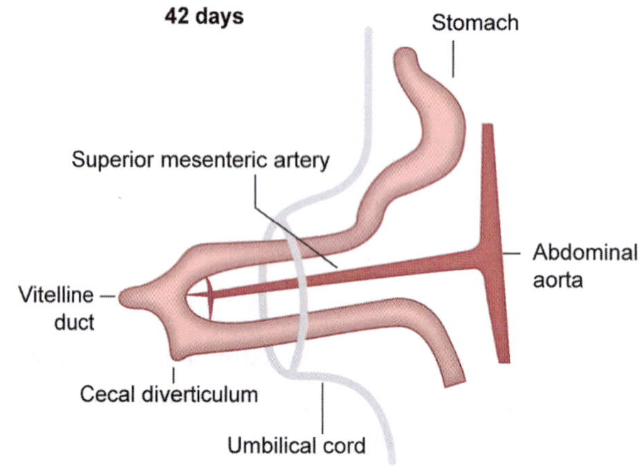

50 days

90°

70 days

180º

77 days

Later fetal period

  - This places:
    - *Jejunum and ileum* → central and left regions.
    - *Cecum and ascending colon* → initially near right upper quadrant, later descending to right iliac fossa.
- *Stage 3—Fixation of the Mesentery (11th–12th week)*
  - The intestines become *fixed* to the posterior abdominal wall.
  - The *mesenteries fuse* with the peritoneum of the posterior abdominal wall, leading to *retroperitoneal* positioning of:
    - Duodenum (except 1st part)
    - Ascending colon
    - Descending colon
  - The *mesentery of the small intestine* remains intraperitoneal and mobile.

Between the 5th and 10th weeks of gestation, the midgut loop elongates by herniating into the umbilical cord. The midgut communicates with the yolk sac by the vitellointestinal duct (Vitellius duct).

First, the midgut rotates 90° counterclockwise around the superior mesenteric artery. Then, it re-enters in the abdominal cavity, undergoing another 180° counterclockwise rotation.

After complex 270° counterclockwise rotation (90°+180°), the cecum is in the right upper quadrant of the abdominal cavity. Thereafter, the enlargement of the colon pushes the cecum down to its final position.

Summary of Total Rotation

Stage	Timing	Event	Degree of Rotation	Final Result
1	5–6 weeks	Physiological herniation	90° counterclockwise	Cranial limb right, caudal left
2	10–11 weeks	Return to abdomen	+180° counterclockwise	Total 270°; intestines in final order
3	11–12 weeks	Fixation	—	Retroperitoneal positioning of some parts

Applied (Clinical) Significance

- *Malrotation:*
  - *Cause:* Incomplete or abnormal rotation of the midgut.
  - *Types:*
    - *Nonrotation (only 90°):* Small intestine on right, large intestine on left.
    - *Reversed rotation (clockwise):* Colon lies *behind SMA* → possible obstruction.
  - *Clinical presentation:* Volvulus (twisting), obstruction, bilious vomiting in neonates.
- *Midgut volvulus:*
  - *Cause:* Mobile, unfixed small bowel twists around SMA → vascular compromise.
  - *Effect:* Intestinal ischemia and necrosis.
  - *Presentation:* Sudden onset bilious vomiting in newborn, abdominal distension, shock.
  - *Management:* Emergency surgery (Ladd's procedure).
- *Subhepatic cecum and appendix:*
  - *Cause:* Cecum fails to descend to right iliac fossa.
  - *Clinical importance:* May lead to *atypical location of appendicitis pain* (right upper quadrant).
- *Internal hernias:* Due to abnormal peritoneal folds or mesenteric fixation defects → small bowel trapped → obstruction.
- *Omphalocele: Failure of return* of herniated midgut → bowel remains in umbilical cord, covered by peritoneum and amnion.
- *Meckel's Diverticulum:*
  - *Persistence of vitelline duct,* often associated with midgut rotation area.
  - May present with bleeding, inflammation, or obstruction.

NARROW BAND IMAGING IN GIT LESIONS

2. Use of narrow band imaging in GIT lesions. ***RGUHS Karnataka 2025.***

Narrow Band Imaging (NBI) in GIT Lesions

Principle

- *NBI* is an *optical image enhancement* technology used in endoscopy (developed by Olympus)
- It uses *filtered light of specific narrow wavelengths* instead of white light:
  - *Blue light (415 nm)* → absorbed by *superficial capillaries* (shows surface patterns)
  - *Green light (540 nm)* → penetrates deeper and highlights *subepithelial vessels*

These wavelengths correspond to *hemoglobin absorption peaks*, making blood vessels appear dark and enhancing the *mucosal microvascular architecture.*

Mechanism

Feature	*Description*
Light source	Narrow-band blue and green light filters (no dyes needed)
Effect	Enhances contrast between blood vessels and surrounding mucosa
Result	Improves visualization of mucosal surface and capillary pattern, helping identify early neoplastic changes

Uses of NBI in Gastrointestinal Tract

Esophagus

- *Barrett's esophagus:*
  - Detects *intestinal metaplasia* and *dysplasia* by revealing abnormal mucosal and vascular patterns.
  - Helps target *biopsies* instead of random sampling.
  - *Pit and vascular pattern classification* can predict dysplasia.
- *Early esophageal carcinoma:*
  - Distinguishes *squamous cell carcinoma* or *adenocarcinoma* from inflammation.
  - Detects *intrapapillary capillary loop (IPCL)* changes:
    - Irregular, dilated, or tortuous loops → suggest carcinoma in situ or early invasive cancer.

Stomach

- *Chronic Gastritis and Intestinal Metaplasia*
  - Enhances mucosal patterns to identify *atrophy* or *intestinal metaplasia* (light blue crest sign).
- *Early Gastric Cancer*
  - Differentiates *benign vs malignant* lesions by assessing *microvascular (MV)* and *microsurface (MS)* patterns.
  - NBI magnification allows *real-time optical biopsy*, sometimes replacing dye-based chromoendoscopy.

Duodenum

- Improves detection of *ampullary lesions* and *adenomas* in familial adenomatous polyposis.
- Differentiates between *adenoma* and *normal mucosa.*

Small Intestine

- Limited role due to reach; used with *enteroscopy* to detect *angioectasias* and *small bowel tumors.*

Colon and Rectum

- *Colorectal Polyps*
  - Characterizes polyp histology *in vivo*:
    - NICE (NBI International Colorectal Endoscopic) classification:

Type	Appearance	Likely diagnosis
1	Pale, indistinct vessels	Hyperplastic
2	Brown, regular vessels/pattern	Adenomatous
3	Dark, irregular vessels, amorphous surface	Cancerous

- Helps decide whether to *resect or leave* diminutive polyps ("resect and discard" policy).

- *Early Colorectal Cancer*
  - Delineates tumor margins and depth of invasion (useful before endoscopic mucosal resection or ESD).

Inflammatory Bowel Disease (IBD)
- Detects *dysplasia* in long-standing *ulcerative colitis* or *Crohn's colitis.*
- Evaluates mucosal healing and microvascular restoration in response to therapy.

Advantages
- Non-invasive (no dyes).
- Enhances early detection of *neoplasia and dysplasia.*
- Allows *targeted biopsies* → fewer samples, higher diagnostic yield.
- Real-time "*optical biopsy*" capability.
- Useful for guiding *endoscopic resection margins.*

Limitations
- Requires *training* and *experience* for accurate interpretation.
- Reduced visibility in *bleeding, inflammation, or poor preparation.*
- Limited depth of visualization (surface only).
- Availability and cost of high-end equipment.

Applied clinical significance:

Region	NBI Use	Clinical benefit
Esophagus	Barrett's, early cancer	Detect dysplasia early
Stomach	Gastritis, metaplasia, early gastric cancer	Targeted biopsy, staging
Colon	Polyps, cancer	Optical biopsy, resection planning
IBD	Dysplasia surveillance	Early neoplastic change detection

DUODENUM

3. Discuss about duodenal stump blow out. ***WBUHS 2021***

Introduction
- Duodenal stump blow-out is the leakage of the blind end of the duodenum.
- It occurs between second and fifth postoperative days.

Causes
- Technical failure
- Postoperative pancreatitis
- Attempt to close a severely diseased and scarred, edematous duodenal stump
- Blood clots in the duodenal bed leading to infection
- Excessive use of sutures at the stump leading to necrosis

Etiopathology
- It occurs as a complication of Billroth II gastrectomy.
- It can also happen after duodenal switch operation.

- It can also occur after radiation in gastrectomy patients.
- Usually occurs on the fourth or fifth day after surgery.
- It is due to improper closure of duodenal stump, especially when the duodenum is inflamed and edematous.
- Duodenal leak occurred after gastric surgery in 1–3% of patients

Clinical Features

- The patient who was previously convalescing satisfactorily may suddenly present with severe abdominal pain, fever, and shock-like state.
- Jaundice may develop within 48 hours owing to the absorption of bile from peritoneal cavity.
- If the abdomen is drained, bile-stained fluid may be seen emerging at the drain site.

Diagnosis

The diagnosis of duodenal stump leak is challenging.

- Because of antegrade peristalsis of the pancreaticobiliary limb, the ingested oral contrast usually does not reach the duodenal stump, and the direct signs such as contrast extravasation are not usually present in duodenal stump leak.
- Indirect signs such as extraluminal air bubbles or fluid collection adjacent to the stump should raise the suspicion of the stump leakage.
- It is an important complication because of the pancreaticobiliary content of secretions.

Investigations

- *Blood investigations:* Complete hemogram, liver function test (LFT), serum electrolytes, urea, and creatinine
- *Imaging studies:* Straight X-ray abdomen, ultrasonography (USG)—whole abdomen, and contrast-enhanced computed tomography (CECT)—whole abdomen
- *Analysis of abdominal secretions in drain*

Treatment

- Intravenous fluids should be started.
- Adequate surgical drainage should be provided.
- Surgery is indicated when there is peritonitis, unresponsive fistula, or distal obstruction.
- Fluoroscopy-guided percutaneous catheter placement can be considered as a safe and effective treatment option for postgastrectomy duodenal stump leakage in patients with gastric cancer.
- Once the life-threatening phase is over, the priority should be to give adequate nutrition.
- Total parenteral nutrition (TPN) can be administered.
- If the patient's clinical condition worsens, surgery becomes mandatory and duodenostomy appears to be the most effective surgical procedure.
- Surgical loop connection relieves the obstruction distally.

4. Duodenal fistula.

Definition

An opening through the duodenal wall and into the peritoneal cavity, into another organ, or through the abdominal wall.

Causes

- Surgical repair of perforated duodenal ulcer may be followed by external duodenal fistula (EDF).
- Blunt abdominal trauma—duodenal injury.
- Accidental trauma during—biliary surgery, right hemicolectomy, nephrectomy, etc.
- Leakage from duodenal stump from gastric resection.

Contributing Factors

- Infection
- Hematoma formation

- Impaired blood supply
- Poor nutrition
- Improperly placed drains

Types
- End type
- Lateral type.

Classification
- *Internal*
- *External:*
    - *Low output:* <200 mL/day
    - *Intermediate output:* 200–500 mL/day
    - *High output:* >500 mL/day

Effects
- This condition is associated with electrolyte imbalance, iron malabsorption, and malnutrition
- Exposure of tissues to copious amount of enzymes-rich secretions resulting in skin excoriation and sepsis.

Diagnosis
- If drain is placed—see the drain fluid—if there is any suspicion (bile)—give methylene blue dye orally—see the color of drain fluid
- USG—intra-abdominal collection
- CT scan—site and extent

Treatment
- Surgery in such patients, who are often malnourished and hypercatabolic, is associated with high morbidity and mortality rates.
- Fistula output of >500 mL/day was defined as a high-output fistula. Fistula sites were managed using a variable combination of techniques, including continuous slow suction, ileostomy bag, wound manager, and silver paint.
- Serum electrolytes, serum protein, and hemoglobin were monitored.
- All patients should undergo abdominal USG to look for any intra-abdominal collection. If collections were found, they should be managed by ultrasound-guided pigtail drainage/aspiration or drainage at laparotomy.
- Blood and fluid cultures were obtained and broad-spectrum antibiotics administered according to sensitivity profile of the organisms grown.
- The patients who were initially managed with nonoperative treatment must be followed by surgery, if required, for failure of fistula closure by conservative treatment.
- Peritonitis or failure to introduce the Ryle's tube into the jejunum for enteral feeding prompted early surgery.
- TPN.
- Conservative treatment followed by late surgery achieved healing/control of fistula in all patients.
- An enteral feeding line should be established at the earliest.
- Failure to establish nasojejunal feeding or peritonitis warrants early surgery.

Surgery
- The surgical approaches in the management of duodenal fistula include exteriorization, exclusion, closure, or excision of fistula, i.e., Billroth II gastrectomy. The exteriorization procedure converts an uncontrolled duodenal leak into a controlled EDF.
- Pyloric exclusion, which diverts gastric juice away from the fistula, is indicated in large perforations that are difficult to close.
- Jejunal serosal patch or Roux-en-Y anastomosis may be other options in these difficult situations.
- Cholecystoduodenoplasty has also been claimed to be a successful technique in high-output duodenal fistula.
- Use of rectus abdominis muscle flap to close large duodenal fistula and have reported good results.

- Gastrectomy (Billroth II) may be recommended in large perforations with or without accompanying bleed in young patients with early peritonitis, however, it is associated with high mortality in the presence of sepsis.

5. Superior mesenteric artery syndrome. ***WBUHS 2014***

Introduction

Superior mesenteric artery (SMA) syndrome (also known as *Wilkie's syndrome*) is a rare acquired vascular compression disorder in which acute angulation of SMA results in compression of the third part of the duodenum leading to obstruction.

Epidemiology

- It is an uncommon but well-recognized clinical entity.
- About 400 cases have been described in English literature.
- Is seen more commonly in females than in males.
- It usually occurs in older children and adolescents.

Clinical Presentation

- Patients with SMA syndrome may present acutely, with chronic insidious symptomatology, or with an acute exacerbation of chronic symptoms
- Acute presentation is usually characterized by signs and symptoms of duodenal obstruction
- Chronic cases may present with long-standing vague abdominal symptoms, early satiety and anorexia, or recurrent episodes of abdominal pain, associated with vomiting

Pathophysiology

Normally, fat and lymphatic tissues around the SMA provide protection to the duodenum against compression. Under conditions of severe weight loss, this cushion around the SMA is diminished, causing angulation and reduction in the distance between the aorta and the SMA. This is usually associated with conditions causing significant weight loss such as:

- Anorexia nervosa
- Malabsorption
- Hypercatabolic states (burns, major surgery, and malignancy)
- Severe congestive heart failure causing cachexia

Other Conditions which may also Precipitate this Syndrome

- Increased spinal lordosis
- Application of a body cast
- Short ligament of Treitz
- Unusually low origin of SMA

Radiographic Features

The diagnosis of SMA syndrome is based on clinical symptoms and radiologic evidence of obstruction.

- *Plain film:* Plain radiograph demonstrates a dilated, fluid- and gas-filled stomach
- *Fluoroscopy:* Barium radiography shows dilatation of the first and second part of the duodenum, extrinsic compression of the third part, and a collapsed small bowel distal to the crossing of the SMA
- *CTA/MRA:* CT-angiography or magnetic resonance angiography (MRA) enable visualization of vascular compression of the duodenum and measurement of aortomesenteric distance precisely.
    - Normally, the aortomesenteric angle and aortomesenteric distance is 25–60° and 10–28 mm, respectively
    - In SMA syndrome, both parameters are reduced, with values of 6–15° and 2–8 mm.

Treatment and Prognosis

Traditionally, treatment has consisted of conservative measures such as:

- Nasogastric decompression and hyperalimentation followed by oral feeding with frequent small meals
- Posturing maneuvers during meals and motility agents may be helpful in some patients

Surgery may be Considered if Conservative Treatment Fails

- Duodenojejunostomy is effective in the majority of patients
- Laparoscopic duodenojejunostomy offers a new minimally invasive therapeutic approach to SMA syndrome
- Laparoscopic surgery involving lysis of the ligament of Treitz with mobilization of the duodenum is another minimally invasive approach.

GASTROINTESTINAL HORMONES

6. Write notes on gastrointestinal hormones. ***WBUHS 2014, 2016***

7. Gastrointestinal hormones and their uses.

Introduction

- The gastrointestinal hormones (or gut hormones) constitute a group of hormones secreted by entero- endocrine cells in the stomach, pancreas, and small intestine that control various functions of the digestive organs.
- Enteroendocrine cells do not form endocrine glands but are spread throughout the digestive tract. They exert their autocrine and paracrine actions that integrate all of gastrointestinal function.
- *Cholecystokinin (CCK):*
  - It is produced by duodenal and jejunal cells and enteric nerves in response to intraluminal amino acids and fats.
  - CCK induces gallbladder contraction, pancreatic enzyme secretion, and relaxation of the sphincter of Oddi.
- *Enteroglucagon:*
  - It is secreted from ileal and colonic L cells is produced in response to intraluminal fat and bile acids.
  - Inflammatory processes, such as Crohn's disease (CD) and celiac sprue, can dramatically increase enteroglucagon secretion.
- *Gastric inhibitory peptide (GIP):*
  - It is secreted by duodenal and jejunal K cells in response to active transport of monosaccharides, long-chain fatty acids, and amino acids
  - It inhibits gastric acid and pepsinogen secretion and gastric emptying and stimulates insulin release.
- *Gastrin:*
  - It is secreted by duodenal G cells in response to vagal stimulation and intraluminal peptides.
  - Gastrin stimulates acid secretion by the gastric fundus and body and increase gastric mucosal blood flow.
- *Motilin:*
  - It is produced by duodenal and jejunal M cells in response to duodenal acid, vagal stimulation, and gastrin-releasing peptide.
  - Motilin initiates phase III of the migrating motor complex (MMC) during the fasting state.
  - Erythromycin is useful as a promotility agent due to its action as a motilin agonist.
- *Secretin:*
  - Duodenal and jejunal S cells release secretin in response to acid, bile salts, and fatty acids in the duodenum.
  - Secretin increases bicarbonate and water secretion from pancreatic ducts.
  - It inhibits gastric acid secretion and gastric motility.
- *Somatostatin:*
  - Intestinal D cells and enteric neurons secrete somatostatin in response to intraluminal fat, protein, and acid.
  - It broadly inhibits gut exocrine and endocrine function.
  - Somatostatin and its analog, octreotide, are often used to decrease the volume of intestinal secretions in patients with enterocutaneous fistulas (ECFs).
- *Vasoactive intestinal peptide (VIP):*
  - It is secreted throughout the small intestine in response to vagal stimulation.
  - VIP increases mesenteric blood flow, intestinal motility, and pancreatic and intestinal secretions.

8. Write in short on premalignant bowel lesion. ***WBUHS 2024***

Premalignant bowel lesions refer to abnormal growths or changes in the bowel that have the potential to develop into cancer if left untreated. These lesions are not cancerous at the time of detection, but they carry a higher risk of progressing to malignancy over time. Common premalignant lesions include:

- *Adenomas (Colorectal Polyps):*
  - *Description:* These are growths on the inner lining of the colon or rectum. Adenomas are the most well-known premalignant lesions.
  - *Risk:* The risk of malignancy increases with factors such as size, histologic type (tubular, villous, or tubulovillous), and degree of dysplasia (cellular abnormalities).
  - *Management:* Regular screening through colonoscopy is recommended for early detection and removal to prevent progression to colorectal cancer.
- *Inflammatory Bowel Disease (IBD):*
  - *Description:* Chronic inflammatory conditions such as ulcerative colitis and Crohn's disease can cause persistent inflammation in the bowel, which increases the risk of developing dysplasia and subsequently colorectal cancer.
  - *Risk:* The longer the duration and extent of the disease, the higher the risk of developing premalignant changes.
  - *Management:* Surveillance colonoscopies and biopsies are recommended for early detection of dysplasia.
- *Sessile Serrated Adenomas/Polyps (SSA/Ps)*
  - *Description:* These polyps are more difficult to detect and may be flat or slightly elevated. They are particularly associated with the serrated pathway of colorectal cancer development.
  - *Risk:* SSA/Ps have a higher risk of becoming cancerous, especially in the right colon.
  - *Management:* Regular surveillance is recommended due to their potential for malignant transformation.
- *Familial Syndromes:*
  - *Hereditary nonpolyposis colorectal cancer (HNPCC) or lynch syndrome:* A genetic predisposition that leads to an increased risk of developing colorectal cancer due to mutations in mismatch repair genes.
  - *Familial adenomatous polyposis (FAP):* A genetic disorder where numerous polyps develop in the colon at an early age, and these have a very high likelihood of turning malignant if not removed.

Management: Individuals with genetic predispositions require closer monitoring and earlier screening.

CARCINOID

9. Write in brief about carcinoid tumor. ***WBUHS 2015***

Introduction

- Carcinoid tumors, because of their neuroendocrine origin, have neurosecretory capabilities and hence the ability to secrete a variety of peptides and bioactive amines.
- Chief among these are 5-hydroxytryptamine (5-HT) or serotonin, histamine, norepinephrine, adrenocorticotropic hormone (ACTH), etc.
- They arise from cells of diffuse neuroendocrine system. These cells are found throughout the GI tract and bronchopulmonary system.
- Carcinoid tumors occur most frequently in the GI tract, in bronchopulmonary system, and other locations such as ovary, gallbladder, thymus, testis, cervix, and breast.

Pathology

- Grossly carcinoid tumors appear as solid and yellow-tan lesions. They are usually solitary, except in stomach and ileum where they may be multicentric.

- They are often submucosal and they may cause ulceration. There is intense desmoplasia within and surrounding the tumor.
- Histologically they appear as uniform, small, and round cells with rare mitotic figures. Foregut and hindgut carcinoid are typically argyrophil and midgut (serotonin secreting) carcinoids are argentaffin.
- Immunohistochemical stains like chromogranins A, B, and C are reliable serum markers for detection of neuroendocrine tumors (NETs). About 80% of carcinoids will have elevated levels of chromogranin A. A high level of chromogranin A is a poor prognostic indicator in individuals with metastatic disease.

Clinical Presentation

- Carcinoid tumors are often discovered incidentally during surgery, endoscopic procedures, or imaging studies.
- They may also present either by causing symptoms due to mass effect or due to their secretory products.
- Mass effect may occasionally cause pain but more commonly causes luminal obstruction (due to tumor growth or scarring).
- Symptoms are often nonspecific, consisting of malaise, vague abdominal pain, or weight loss.
- Carcinoid syndrome is an unusual presentation of GI carcinoids.
- The classic product serotonin may produce diarrhea. ACTH producing tumors will cause Cushing's syndrome, while gastrin producing tumors may cause Zollinger–Ellison (ZE) syndrome.

Classification

- *Carcinoid tumors have been classified according to their embryologic region of origin:* Foregut, midgut, and hind gut.
- Foregut carcinoids include those arising in esophagus, stomach, pancreas, and duodenum.
- Midgut carcinoids comprise of those arising in the distribution of SMA distribution, including appendix and ileum.
- Hind gut carcinoids include those arising in the distribution of inferior mesenteric artery (IMA) distribution including the rectum.

Esophagus

- Esophageal carcinoids are extremely rare. Dysphagia is the most common presentation.
- Mostly treated by esophagogastrectomy.

Stomach

- Stomach is the most common foregut location for carcinoid tumors.
- Pernicious anemia and chronic atrophic gastritis are risk factors for the development of gastric enterochromaffin-like (ECL) cell tumor. This may be secondary to the hypergastrinemia caused by the absence of significant acid output in such patients.
- They are much more common in those patients with MEN-type 1.
- The average age of presentation of patients with gastric carcinoid tumors is 62 years.
- Patients are often asymptomatic, carcinoids often found incidentally during upper GI endoscopy.
- When symptoms occur, they are usually dyspeptic.
- Endoscopic ultrasonography (EUS) can be helpful in defining the depth of invasion and providing deep submucosal biopsy specimen.
- CT and MRI may be helpful in finding hepatic metastasis. All patients with gastric carcinoids have elevations of chromogranin A levels.
- Management of gastric carcinoid tumors is controversial.
- Carcinoids secondary to pernicious anemia/atrophic gastritis and MEN-1 tend to have a more benign course, with occasional spontaneous regression.

Pancreas

- The differentiation between pancreatic carcinoids and other NETs of pancreas is primarily a matter of definition.

- Pancreatic carcinoids have been defined as a tumor with the histologic features of a NET and with obviously increased serotonin metabolism.
- Pancreatic carcinoids tend to present late. Abdominal pain, diarrhea, and weight loss are the most common presenting symptoms.
- Most patients presents with metastasis. Treatment is by surgical resection.
- Pancreaticoduodenectomy is often required.
- It has better survival rates than those of other pancreatic malignancies but worse than those of carcinoids in other sites.

Duodenum

- Carcinoids of duodenum represent approximately 2% of carcinoids.
- Duodenal carcinoids most commonly discovered during endoscopy.
- They rarely produce serotonin and therefore virtually no association with carcinoid syndrome. Half of the cases produce gastrin.
- Ampullary carcinoids frequently present with jaundice. Approximately 25% of patients with periampullary carcinoids have von Recklinghausen's disease.
- The risk of metastasis increases with increased size of the primary tumor.
- The treatment of duodenal and ampullary carcinoid tumor is by resection.

Small Intestine

- Ileum is the most common site for carcinoid tumors, accounting for almost 30% of all carcinoids.
- Carcinoids form approximately 28–38% of all small bowel cancers.
- Average age of presentation is 62–65 years. Small bowel carcinoids are multifocal in 25% of cases.
- They present as vague abdominal pain, intermittent intestinal obstruction, and infarction of small bowel due to SMA occlusion.
- Overt carcinoid syndrome is uncommon as an initial presentation.
- Carcinoid syndrome usually indicates hepatic or retroperitoneal metastasis and signifies an unfavorable outcome.
- If found early, primary tumor and the associated lymphatics should be resected surgically.

Appendix

- It is a less common site of GI carcinoids.
- The proportion of appendiceal tumors that are carcinoids is high.
- Majority are <1 cm in size.
- Frequency of distant metastasis increases with the size of the tumor.
- They cause symptoms early due to appendiceal luminal obstruction with consequent appendicitis. Have a favorable prognosis.
- Simple appendicectomy is indicated for tumors <1 cm size and a right hemicolectomy for tumors >2 cm size.

Colon

- Colonic carcinoids account for <10% of carcinoid tumors.
- They occur more commonly on right side, about two-thirds involving ascending or proximal transverse colon.
- They tend to present as larger lesions than most other carcinoids, averaging around 5 cm.
- Symptoms are usually due to bulky advanced lesions.
- Advanced lesions may cause pain or colonic obstruction.
- Surgical resection and lymph node clearance should be performed. No adjuvant treatment is effective. 5-year survival is worst.

Rectum

- Constitutes 19% of all carcinoids.
- More than 80% are still localized at the time of diagnosis.

- Appear as local nodules.
- Tumors may produce symptoms as bleeding, pain, or decreased stool caliber; weight loss and changing bowel habits may be detected incidentally.
- Carcinoid syndrome is distinctly uncommon due to rectal lesions.
- Rectal carcinoids have been treated endoscopically, by local excision, (lesions <2 cm) and by radical excision with either a low anterior resection or APR (lesions >2 cm).

10. Pathophysiology of carcinoid tumor. ***WBUHS 2019***

11. Clinical features of abdominal small bowel carcinoid tumor. ***WBUHS 2021 Supplementary***

Pathophysiology

- Carcinoid tumors produce several vasoactive substances, most prominently serotonin. It is commonly thought that serotonin is the cause of the flushing, but this is only partially correct.
- The flushing also results from secretion of kallikrein, the enzyme that catalyzes the conversion of kininogen to lysyl-bradykinin.
- The latter is further converted to bradykinin, one of the most powerful vasodilators known.
- Other components of the carcinoid syndrome are:
    - Diarrhea (probably caused by the increased serotonin, which greatly increases peristalsis, leaving less time for fluid absorption)
    - A pellagra-like syndrome (probably caused by diversion of large amounts of tryptophan from synthesis of the vitamin B_3 niacin, which is needed for NAD production, to the synthesis of serotonin and other 5-hydroxyindoles)
    - Fibrotic lesions of the endocardium, particularly on the right side of the heart resulting in insufficiency of the tricuspid, valve and less frequently, the pulmonary valve and, uncommonly, bronchoconstriction.
        - The pathogenesis of the cardiac lesions and the bronchoconstriction is unknown, but the former probably involves activation of serotonin 5-HT2B receptors by serotonin.
        - When the primary tumor is in the gastrointestinal tract, as it is in the great majority of cases, the serotonin and kallikrein are inactivated in the liver; manifestations of carcinoid syndrome do not occur until there are metastases to the liver or when the cancer is accompanied by liver failure (cirrhosis).
        - Carcinoid tumors arising in the bronchi may be associated with manifestations of carcinoid syndrome without liver metastases because their biologically active products reach the systemic circulation before passing through the liver and being metabolized.
    - In most patients, there is an increased urinary excretion of 5-HIAA (5-hydroxyindoleacetic acid), a degradation product of serotonin. The biology of these tumors differs from many other tumor types.

Clinical Features

- Carcinoid tumors are often discovered incidentally during surgery, endoscopic procedures, or imaging studies.
- Diarrhea is the most common and earliest symptom.
- They may also present either by causing symptoms due to mass effect or due to their secretory products.
- Mass effect may occasionally cause pain but more commonly causes luminal obstruction (due to tumor growth or scarring).
- Symptoms are often nonspecific consisting of malaise, vague abdominal pain, or weight loss.
- They can present as intermittent intestinal obstruction, infarction of small bowel due to SMA occlusion.
- *Carcinoid syndrome is an unusual presentation of GI carcinoids:* The classic product serotonin may produce diarrhea. ACTH producing tumors will cause Cushing's syndrome, while gastrin producing tumors may cause ZE syndrome.

12. What is carcinoid syndrome? Discuss the management of gastrointestinal carcinoids. *WBUHS 2017*

Carcinoid syndrome is a paraneoplastic syndrome comprising the signs and symptoms that occur secondary to carcinoid tumors. The syndrome includes flushing and diarrhea, and less frequently, heart failure, emesis and bronchoconstriction. It is caused by endogenous secretion of mainly serotonin and kallikrein.

Management

Diagnosis: With a certain degree of clinical suspicion, the most useful initial test is the 24-hour urine levels of 5-HIAA, the end product of serotonin metabolism. Patients with carcinoid syndrome usually excrete >25 mg of 5-HIAA per day.

Imaging

- For localization of both primary lesions and metastasis, the initial imaging method is Octreoscan, where indium-111 labeled somatostatin analogs (octreotide) are used in scintigraphy for detecting tumors expressing somatostatin receptors.
- Median detection rates with Octreoscan are about 89%, in contrast to other imaging techniques such as CT scan and MRI with detection rates of about 80%.
- Gallium-68 labeled somatostatin analogs such as ^{68}Ga-DOTA-Octreotate (DOTATATE), performed on a positron emission tomography (PET)/CT scanner is superior to conventional Octreoscan.
- Usually, on a CT scan, a spider-like/crab-like change is visible in the mesentery due to the fibrosis from the release of serotonin. ^{18}F-fluorodeoxyglucose (^{18}F-FDG) PET/CT, which evaluate for increased metabolism of glucose, may also aid in localizing the carcinoid lesion or evaluating for metastases.
- Chromogranin A and platelets serotonin are increased.

Localization of Tumor

- Tumor localization may be extremely difficult.
- Barium swallow and follow-up examination of the intestine may occasionally show the tumor.
- Capsule video endoscopy has recently been used to localize the tumor. Often laparotomy is the definitive way to localize the tumor.
- Another form of localizing a tumor is the Octreoscan. A tracer agent of indium-111 is injected into a vein where then the tumors absorb the radionuclide indium-111 and become visible on the scanner. Only the tumors absorb the somatostatin agent indium-111 making the scan highly effective.
- ^{123}I-metaiodobenzylguanidine (^{123}I-MIBG) will also concentrate in carcinoid tumors, including the low percentage (~15%) that are negative with ^{111}In-octreotide

Treatment

For Symptomatic Relief of Carcinoid Syndrome

- Octreotide [a somatostatin analog which decreases the secretion of serotonin by the tumor and, secondarily, decreases the breakdown product of serotonin (5-HIAA)]
- Telotristat ethyl (Xermelo) along with a somatostatin analog in patients not responding to somatostatin analog monotherapy is a tryptophan hydroxylase inhibitor and reduces the production of serotonin.
- Peptide receptor radionuclide therapy (PRRT) with lutetium-177, yttrium-90, or indium-111 labeled to octreotate is highly effective.
- Methysergide maleate (antiserotonin agent but not used because of the serious side effect of retroperitoneal fibrosis)
- Cyproheptadine (an antihistamine drug with antiserotonergic effects)

Alternative Treatment for Qualifying Candidates

- Surgical resection of tumor and chemotherapy [5-fluorouracil (5-FU) and doxorubicin]

- Endovascular, chemoembolization, and targeted chemotherapy directly delivered to the liver through special catheters mixed with embolic beads (particles that block blood vessels), used for patients with liver metastases.

13. Write in brief about carcinoid syndrome. ***WBUHS 2009***

Carcinoid syndrome is a paraneoplastic syndrome comprising the signs and symptoms that occur secondary to carcinoid tumors. The syndrome includes flushing and diarrhea, and less frequently, heart failure, emesis, and bronchoconstriction. It is caused by endogenous secretion of mainly serotonin and kallikrein.

Typical Carcinoid Syndrome

- Most common clinical pattern, caused by metastatic midgut carcinoids. Serotonin is released into circulation. It is then converted into 5-HIAA, which is excreted in urine.
- Patients with typical carcinoid syndrome have elevated plasma and platelet serotonin and increased 5-HIAA in urine.
- Clinically it is characterized by flushing, diarrhea, nonspecific abdominal pain, bronchospasm, pellagra-like skin lesions, and progressive right heart failure.

Atypical Carcinoid Syndrome

- Most often associated with foregut carcinoid tumors. It presents with a different pattern of flushing, it occurs again in head and neck region but it appears patchier. It also shows central clearing and increased pruritus.
- Asthma and/or signs of peptic ulceration are occasional presentations due to increased systemic levels of histamine. Patients have high plasma levels of 5-HTP and normal levels of serotonin.
- Urinary levels of 5-HIAA are typically normal to slightly elevated.

Diagnosis

Based on typical clinical history, 24-hour urinary 5-HIAA levels.

Carcinoid Crisis

- Acute exacerbation of carcinoid syndrome may occur in a number of situations but most commonly in the setting of surgical or anesthetic stresses.
- Patients with known carcinoid tumors should receive somatostatin analogs before surgery to suppress mediator release.
- Symptoms such as hyperglycemia, hypertension, and bronchospasm are treated by routine medical means.

Imaging Studies

- Visualization of primary carcinoid tumor is more difficult than identification of metastatic disease.
- CT scan and MRI are nonspecific and often nonlocalizing. They are useful when lesions are >1 cm in size. May be used to identify metastatic disease.
- Somatostatin receptor scanning using radiolabeled somatostatin analogs (indium-111 labeled pentetreotide I^{123} labeled tyrosine) is helpful in localizing primary occult tumors and in staging of patients with known metastatic disease.

Treatment of Metastatic Disease/Carcinoid Syndrome

Majority of such patients are not the candidates for curative treatment. The focus of therapy is palliation of symptoms.

- *Surgery:* For hepatic metastasis—
  - Resection
  - Orthotropic liver transplantation (OLT)
  - Cytoreductive therapy
  - Hepatic artery embolization
  - Chemoembolization
- *Immunotherapy:* Interferon (controversial)

- *Chemotherapy:* Marginal benefit
- *Pharmacologic therapy:* Mainstay of palliative therapy
  - *Somatostatin analogs:* Octreotide and lanreotide (long acting)
  - *Serotonin receptor blockers:* Methysergide, cyproheptadine, ketanserin, and ondansetron
  - *Inhibitor of serotonin synthesis:* Para-chlorophenylalanine
- *Radiotherapy:* For palliation of metastasis to bone and central nervous system

GASTROINTESTINAL STROMAL TUMOR

14. Gastrointestinal stromal tumors. ***WBUHS 2007; KNRUHS Telengana 2025***

15. Define GIST. Discuss the pathogenesis and characteristics of GIST. Discuss the treatment modalities of GIST. ***WBUHS 2012, 2015; Rims, Imphal 2022***

16. Enumerate current management and prognostic features of gastrointestinal stromal tumors. ***DY Patil Educational Society, Deemed to be University 2024***

17. Enumerate the sites of GIST and explain the principles of management of GIST. ***RGUHS, Karnataka 2025***

18. Management of aggressive GIST. ***WBUHS 2010***

Introduction

Gastrointestinal stromal tumors (GISTs) are rare malignancies. Although they are the most common sarcoma of the gastrointestinal (GI) tract, they represent only 0.2% of all GI tumors.

Definition

GISTs are the most common mesenchymal tumors of the GI tract. They are defined as KIT (CD117, stem cell factor receptor-positive mesenchymal spindle cell or epithelioid neoplasms primary in the GI tract, omentum, and mesentery. GISTs typically present in older individuals and are most common in the stomach (60–70%), followed by small intestine (20–25%), colon and rectum (5%), and esophagus (<5%).

Pathology

- GISTs are tumors of connective tissue, i.e., sarcomas; unlike most gastrointestinal tumors, they are nonepithelial.
- About 70% occur in the stomach, 20% in the small intestine and <10% in the esophagus. Small tumors are generally benign, especially when cell division rate is slow, but large tumors disseminate to the liver, omentum, and peritoneal cavity. They rarely occur in other abdominal organs.
- Some tumors of the stomach and small bowel, referred to as leiomyosarcomas (malignant tumor of smooth muscle), would most likely be reclassified as GISTs today on the basis of immunohistochemical staining.
- GIST exhibit heterogeneous histologic features, and are most often composed of long fascicles of bland spindle cells with pale to eosinophilic cytoplasm and rare nuclear pleomorphism.
- GIST occasionally exhibit epithelioid characteristics, including sheets of round to oval-shaped cells with abundant eosinophilic cytoplasm and nuclear atypia.
- Based upon their histologic and immunohistochemical features, GIST are thought to arise from the interstitial cells of Cajal (ICC), which are components of the intestinal autonomic nervous system that serve as pacemakers regulating intestinal peristalsis.
- Mutations of the KIT proto-oncogene in the vast majority of GIST. KIT is a receptor tyrosine kinase that is activated when bound to a ligand known as steel factor or stem cell factor. KIT is important in the development and maintenance of components of hematopoiesis, gametogenesis, and intestinal pacemaker cells.

- GIST are now identified by the near universal expression of the CD117 antigen (~95%), part of the KIT receptor, in the appropriate histopathologic context. CD117 expression is characteristic of most GIST, but not of other gastrointestinal smooth muscle tumors, which are more likely to express high levels of desmin and smooth muscle actin.

Molecular Biology of Gastrointestinal Stromal Tumors

- These tumors are nearly universally characterized by the expression of KIT, a transmembrane receptor tyrosine kinase encoded by the c-kit proto-oncogene and recognized by the immunohistochemical stain for CD117.
- The *c-kit* gene is a cellular homologue of the v-kit oncogene found in the genome of the feline sarcoma virus. Stem cell factor is the natural ligand for KIT, and under normal physiologic conditions, two molecules of KIT form a dimer by binding to two molecules of the ligand, with the resulting dimerization leading to activation of the intracellular tyrosine kinase. Ligand independent activation of the KIT kinase leads to signal transduction abnormalities favoring proliferation and enhancement of cell survival mechanisms.
- The gain-of-function kinase activity results in ligand-independent KIT autophosphorylation and constitutive activation and is probably a hyperproliferative transforming event. The mutations are often physically located within 11 amino acids (Lys-550 to Val-560) in the juxtamembrane domain (exon 11) and can be characterized as either deletions, point mutations, or insertions. In the unusual event that these mutations occur in a germ cell line, the family lineage is characterized by instances of multiple GISTs.
- Further compelling evidence for KIT mutation in the pathogenesis of GIST has been substantiated by transfection experiments of mutated KIT leading to cellular clonal transformation of the transfectant.

Genetics

- Although some families with hereditary GISTs have been described, most cases are sporadic.
- In GIST cells, the *c-kit* gene is mutated approximately 85–90% of the time. 35% of the GIST cells with wild-type (i.e., not mutated) *c-kit* instead have a mutation in another gene, platelet-derived growth factor receptor alpha (PDGFR-α), which is a related tyrosine kinase.
- Mutations in the exons 11, 9 and rarely 13 and 17 of the *c-kit* gene are known to occur in GIST. D816V point mutations in c-kit exon 17 are responsible for resistance to targeted therapy drugs like imatinib mesylate, a tyrosine kinase inhibitor.
- Mutations in c-kit and PDGFRA are mutually exclusive.

Classification of primary gastrointestinal stromal tumors by risk of metastasis.

Risk category	***Size***	***Mitotic count***
Very low	<2 cm	<5 per 50 HPFs
Low	2–5 cm	<5 per 50 HPFs
Intermediate	• <5 cm • 5–10 cm	• 6–10 per 50 HPFs • <5 per 50 HPFs
High	• >5 cm • >10 cm • Any size	• >5 per 50 HPFs • Any mitotic rate • >10 per 50 HPFs

(HPF: high-power field)

Characteristics of GIST

- GIST is most commonly diagnosed in adults 50–80 years of age, with a mean age of 60.
- The male-to-female ratio is approximately 1:1.
- The majority of patients with GIST are symptomatic, with the most common symptoms being abdominal pain, early satiety, and bloating related to the presence of a space-occupying mass.
- GI bleeding and anemia are frequently noted and are due to erosion of mucosa by the tumor.

- The most common location is the stomach (60–70%), followed by the small bowel (20–25%), colorectum (5%), and esophagus (5%). Rarely, cases of GIST originating within the retroperitoneum, omentum, appendix, gallbladder, pancreas, and mesentery have been described.
- Approximately 20% of GISTs are asymptomatic and discovered incidentally by radiographic imaging or endoscopy, or they may be an unexpected surgical finding. These incidental tumors are often asymptomatic, noncystic submucosal masses most commonly found during endoscopy.
- Although some GISTs are small submucosal solid tumors found incidentally, the majority are larger than 5 cm and are symptomatic because they are a space-occupying abdominal mass.
- The tumor can directly invade adjacent structures in the abdomen. The most common site of spread is to the liver.
- Spread to the peritoneum may be seen.
- In distinction to gastric adenocarcinoma or gastric/small bowel lymphoma, malignant lymphadenopathy is uncommon (<10%).
- GI bleeding and the insidious anemia of chronic blood loss are not uncommon with large necrotic GISTs.

Signs and Symptoms

Patients present with:

- Difficulty in swallowing
- Gastrointestinal hemorrhage or metastases (mainly in the liver)
- Intestinal obstruction is rare, due to the tumor's outward pattern of growth
- Often, there is a history of vague abdominal pain or discomfort, and the tumor has become rather large by time the diagnosis is made

(Generally, the definitive diagnosis is made with a biopsy, which can be obtained endoscopically, percutaneously with CT or ultrasound guidance or at the time of surgery)

Diagnosis

- *HPE:* The characteristics of GISTs (spindle cells in 70–80%, epithelioid aspect in 20–30%). Smaller tumors can usually be found to the muscularis propria layer of the intestinal wall. Large ones grow, mainly outward, from the bowel wall until the point where they outstrip their blood supply and necrosis (die) on the inside, forming a cavity that may eventually come to communicate with the bowel lumen.
- *Immunohistochemistry (IHC):* Use IHC (specific antibodies that stain the molecule CD117). 95% of all GISTs are CD117-positive (other possible markers include CD34, DOG-1, desmin, vimentin and others). Other cells that show CD117 positivity are mast cells.

If the CD117 stain is negative and suspicion remains that the tumor is a GIST, the newer antibody DOG-1 (discovered on GIST-1) can be used. Also sequencing of KIT and PDGFRA can be used to prove the diagnosis.

Radiology

Imaging and Diagnostic Studies

- *Endoscopy:*
  - The endoscopic appearance of a primary GIST is that of a submucosal lesion, with or without ulceration, present in the upper or lower GI tract. These lesions are visually indistinguishable from other GI tumors of smooth muscle origin.
  - Because of their submucosal location, fine-needle aspiration (FNA) or core biopsy with endoscopic ultrasound guidance is commonly required to obtain tissue for diagnosis.
- *CT scan:*
  - CT scans are critical to determine the anatomic extent of a GIST and to assist with operative planning. The CT findings vary with the size of the lesions.

    - Small GIST have sharp margins, an intraluminal growth pattern, and are of homogenous density on both unenhanced and contrast-enhanced scans.
    - In contrast, larger lesions have irregular margins, extraluminal growth patterns, and inhomogeneous density.
    - Radiographic signs corresponding to aggressive malignant GIST include calcification, ulceration, necrosis, cystic areas, fistula formation, metastasis, ascites, and signs of infiltration of local tissues.
    - CT is unable to differentiate between inflammatory adhesions and malignant involvement of adjoining organs.
    - It is also unlikely to identify any peritoneal metastasis smaller than 2 cm in diameter.
- Endoscopic examination of primary gastric GIST is helpful.
- GIST commonly present as submucosal tumors in the wall of the GI tract. Central necrosis of high-risk tumors or erosion into blood vessels can produce local inflammation or significant GI bleeding.
- *PET scan:*
    - PET is a useful adjunct to CT for evaluating GIST, particularly as a means of assessing response to chemotherapy.
    - Metabolically active GIST accumulates ^{18}F-FDG, and blockade of the KIT receptor results in a rapid suppression of this activity.
- Functional blockade of KIT activation is produced by specific inhibitors of KIT tyrosine kinase activity, such as imatinib mesylate.
- Barium fluoroscopic examinations (upper GI series and small bowel series) and CT are commonly used to evaluate the patient with upper abdominal pain.

  Both are adequate to make the diagnosis of GIST, although small tumors may be missed, especially in cases of a suboptimal examination.

  Small GISTs appear as intramural masses. When large (>5 cm), they most commonly grow outward from the bowel.

Treatment

- Tumor size, mitotic rate, and location can be used to predict the risk of recurrence in GIST patients. Tumors <2 cm with a mitotic rate of <5/50 high-power field (HPF) have been shown to have lower risk of recurrence than larger or more aggressive tumors.
- Nevertheless, all GIST tumors should be considered to have malignant potential.
- Surgery is the mainstay of therapy for nonmetastatic GISTs.
- The goal of surgery in the management of primary GIST is complete gross resection with an intact pseudo-capsule. At laparotomy the abdomen should be carefully explored for any evidence of metastatic disease on the peritoneal surfaces or in the liver. GISTs should be handled gently and with care to avoid rupture.
- Segmental resection of the stomach or intestine can be performed with the intent of negative margins. Partial or wedge gastrectomy is a viable option because GIST cells do not manifest submucosal spread, as is common with adenocarcinoma.
- Lymph node metastases are rare, and routine removal of lymph nodes is typically not necessary.
- Laparoscopic surgery, has been shown to be effective for removal of these tumors without needing large incisions.

Gastrointestinal stromal tumors were notorious for being resistant to chemotherapy, with a success rate of <5%.

- Recently, the c-kit tyrosine kinase inhibitor imatinib (Glivec/Gleevec), a drug initially marketed for chronic myelogenous leukemia, was found to be useful in treating GISTs, leading to a 40–70% response rate in metastatic or inoperable cases.
- The 2-year survival of patients with advanced disease has risen to 75–80% following imatinib treatment.
- Patients who develop resistance to imatinib may respond to the multiple tyrosine kinase inhibitor sunitinib.
- The effectiveness of imatinib and sunitinib depend on the genotype.

Management of Primary Localized GIST

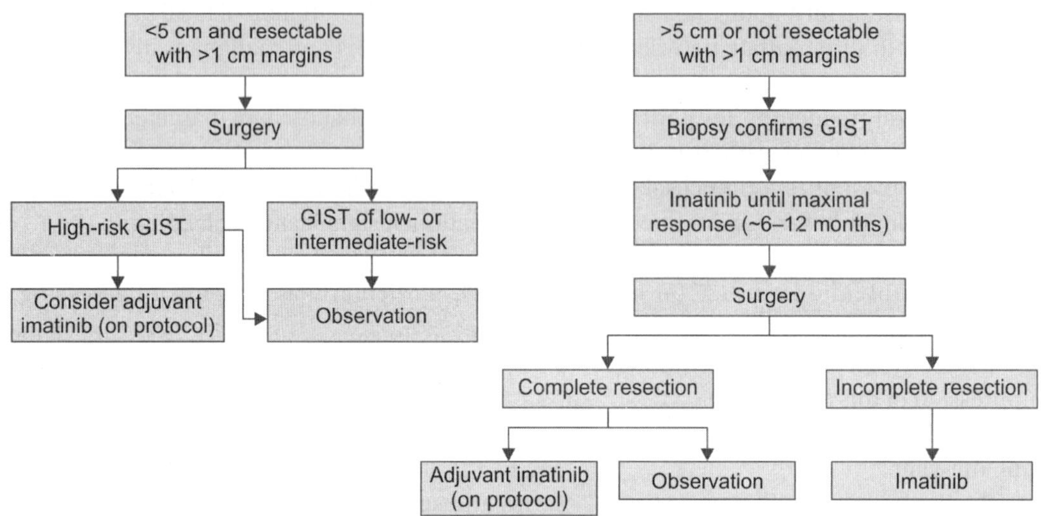

(GIST: gastrointestinal stromal tumor)

Management of Metastatic GIST

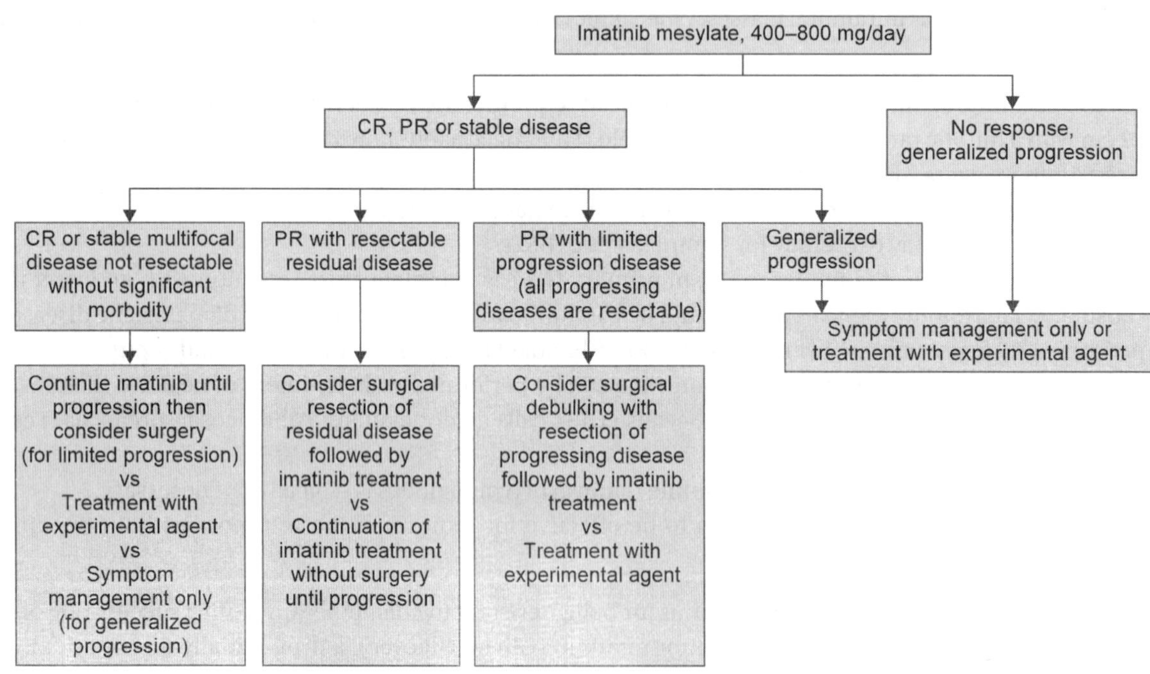

(CR: complete response; GIST: gastrointestinal stromal tumor; PR: partial response)

Management of Aggressive GIST

Surgical Management of Localized Primary Disease

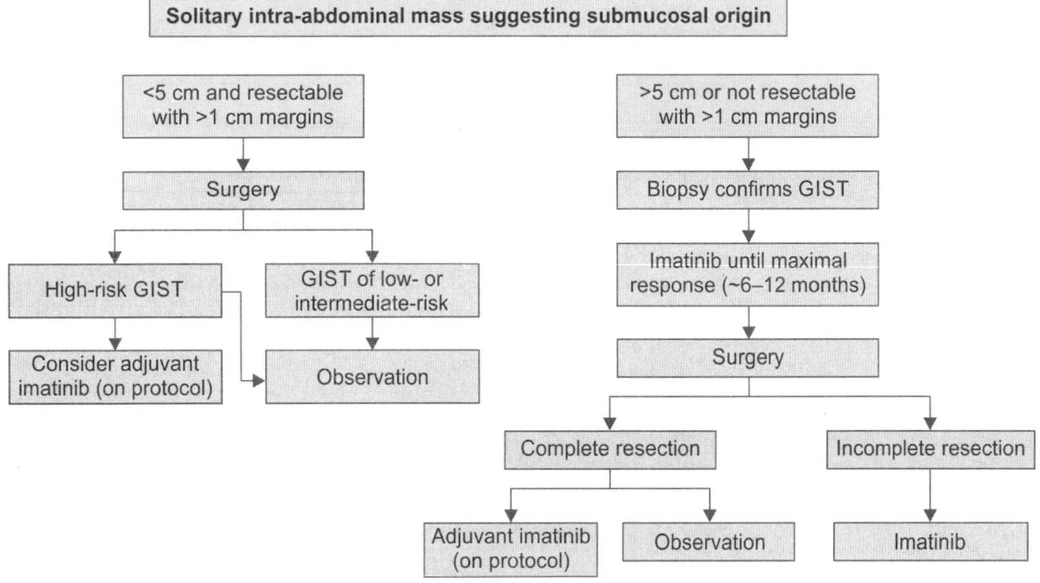

(GIST: gastrointestinal stromal tumor)

Postsurgical Follow-up

- The typical sites of tumor recurrence following resection of a GIST with curative intent are the local resection bed, the liver, and the peritoneum.
- Pulmonary metastases are uncommon. In general, the time to recurrence reflects the original growth pattern of the tumor, and recurrences as early as 3 months following resection have been observed.
- Most centers use abdominal/pelvic CT scanning for posttreatment follow-up, with PET scanning or MRI reserved for clarification of equivocal CT findings.
- Because more recurrences occur within the first 5 years after surgery, imaging intervals of 3 to 6 months are standard for patients in the first 5 years of post-treatment follow-up, with annual evaluation thereafter.
- At present there are no specific serum-based markers for the detection of recurrent GIST.

Adjuvant Therapy

- For patients with localized GIST treated with surgery alone, the reported recurrence rate at 5 years varies considerably, with recurrent disease developing in 2–15% of those with low-risk and 70–90% of those with high-risk primary tumors.
- In the absence of adjuvant therapy, approximately 50% of patients receiving potentially curative surgery will develop either locally recurrent or metastatic disease within 5 years, yielding 5-year survival rates of 40–55%.
- The effectiveness of imatinib in managing metastatic disease has led to combined modality treatment of high-risk localized tumors.

Use of Imatinib in Unresectable Primary Disease

- The success of imatinib in managing metastatic disease led to its use as a means of improving the resectability of technically inoperable primary tumors.
- Surgery is performed when tumor size has decreased to the point at which resection is technically possible, and/or when successive CT scans show no further tumor shrinkage.
- Generally, this occurs from 9 to 12 months following initiation of chemotherapy. Following surgery, these high-risk patients are routinely maintained on imatinib indefinitely, as long as drug-related toxicity is minimal.

Management of Metastatic GIST

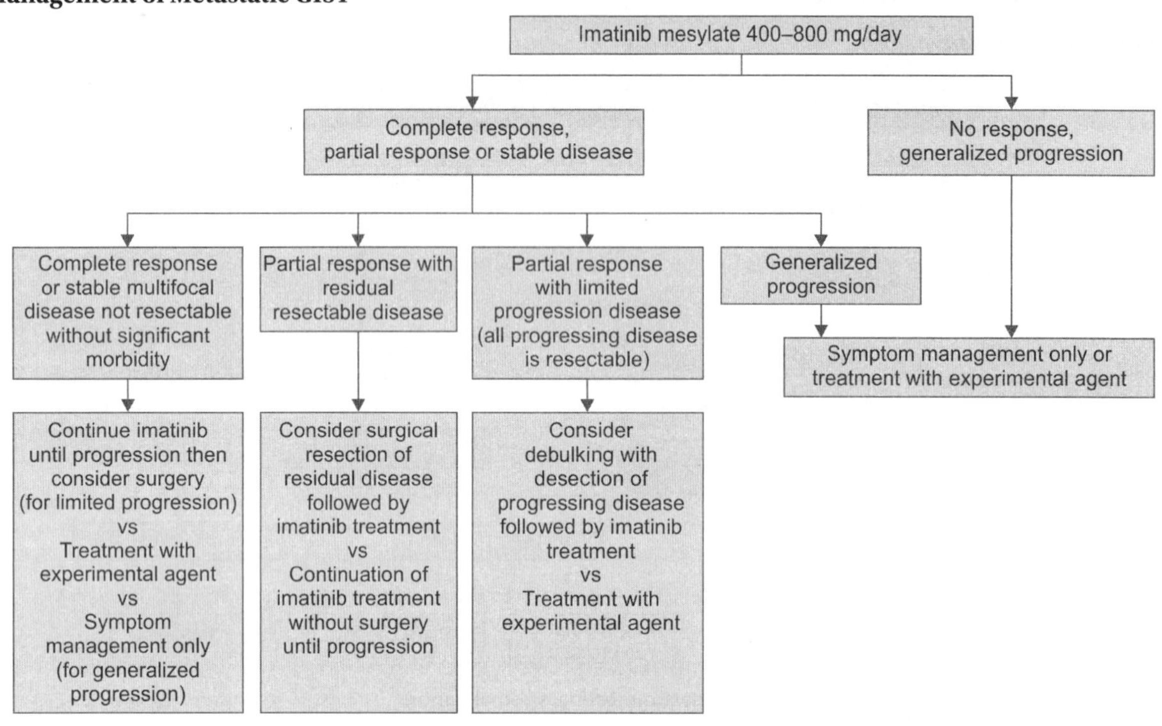

(GIST: gastrointestinal stromal tumor)

New Therapies for Management of Primary and Secondary Drug Resistance

- A number of different agents are currently under investigation in clinical trials to determine their utility as second-line drugs for the management of imatinib-resistant GIST.
- These agents have been selected based upon their ability to disrupt KIT tyrosine kinase activity, or to inhibit targets that are downstream of KIT or PDGFRA.
- At least one of these, sunitinib, has shown some efficacy in phase II studies. Sunitinib is a tyrosine kinase inhibitor with activity against KIT, PDGFR, FLT3, and VEGFR.
- Lymphadenectomy is unnecessary because lymph node metastases are rare.

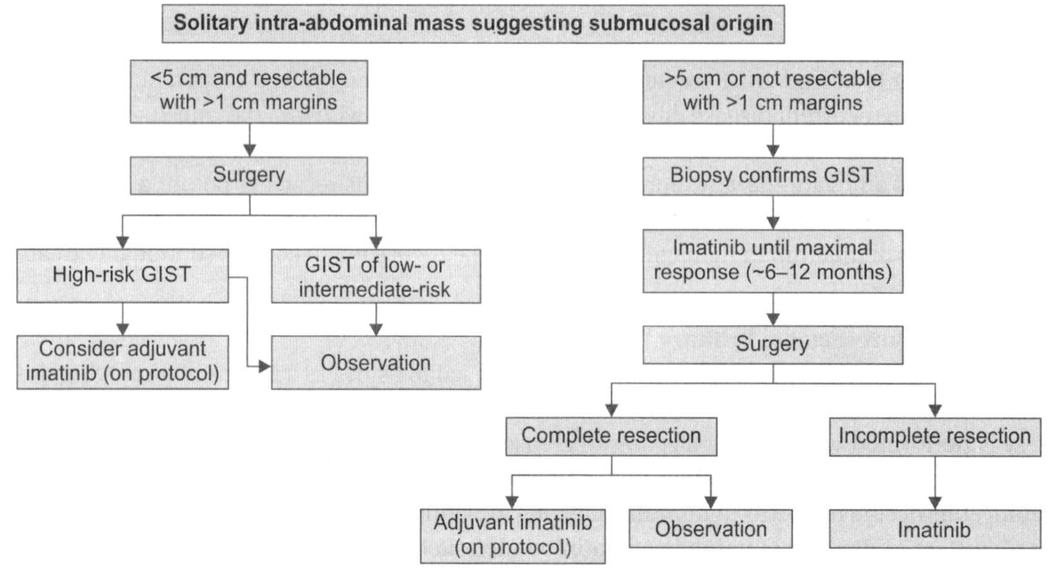

(GIST: gastrointestinal stromal tumor)

19. Write about scope of neoadjuvant tyrosine kinase receptor inhibitor therapy of GIST.

- Imatinib, sunitinib, and regorafenib are standards of care in advanced and metastatic GISTs.
  - *Imatinib:* First-line treatment in advanced/metastatic GISTs
  - *Sunitinib:* Second-line treatment in patients with GIST after failure of or intolerance to imatinib
  - *Regorafenib:* A recent standard of care for GISTs
- Based on the high rate of responses observed with imatinib in patients with metastatic GIST, preoperative use of imatinib aims to reduce tumor bulk to facilitate complete surgical resection or increase the likelihood of organ preservation of initially unresectable or borderline resectable disease.
- The initial dose of imatinib of 400 mg/day is considered to be reasonable as a standard dose.
- There is not enough evidence about the appropriate treatment period of neoadjuvant imatinib therapy for advanced GIST.
- The pharmacological effect of imatinib therapy is promptly expressed, but it takes time to decrease tumor size because imatinib works as a cytostatic agent. Therefore, imatinib needs to be administered for longer periods than the usual neoadjuvant chemotherapies for carcinoma.
- GIST often shows expansive development, and is often diagnosed after experiencing an increase in size without defined subjective symptoms such as obstruction, bleeding and pain. Therefore, the range of organ resection may be enlarged or multiple organ involvement may be necessary for resection of large tumors. For this reason, preoperative treatment is also expected to be favored from the viewpoint of organ/function preservation by tumor shrinkage.
- The importance of neoadjuvant treatment lies in its feasibility and its survival outcome. The feasibility of neoadjuvant imatinib therapy seems to be well established from the results of clinical trials. However, proof of the survival effectiveness of neoadjuvant-setting imatinib therapy has not been sufficiently demonstrated.
- It is expected that the long-term results of phase II study for large gastric GIST in Japan and South Korea will prove the survival benefit of neoadjuvant imatinib therapy.
- The benefits of neoadjuvant therapy with other tyrosine kinase inhibitors against imatinib resistant GIST are also controversial. Since GIST is a rare disease and cases are limited, neoadjuvant therapy should be registered in nationwide or worldwide clinical trials/databases to compile meaningful bodies of evidence.

INFLAMMATORY BOWEL DISEASE

20. Describe the types of ulcerative colitis. Its complications and indications of surgery.
Maharashtra University of Health Sciences 2025

21. Surgical management of ulcerative colitis (UC). ***WBUHS 2010***

Types of Ulcerative Colitis

Ulcerative colitis (UC) is a *chronic idiopathic inflammatory bowel disease* affecting the *colon and rectum,* characterized by *continuous mucosal inflammation* starting from the *rectum* and extending proximally for a variable distance.

Classification by Extent of Involvement (Anatomic Types)

Type	*Area involved*	*Features/Clinical notes*
Ulcerative proctitis	Rectum only (distal 15 cm)	• Mildest form • Tenesmus, urgency, rectal bleeding • No systemic features
Proctosigmoiditis	Rectum + Sigmoid colon	• Common form of distal UC • Mucus and blood in stool, urgency, cramping

Contd...

Contd...

Type	Area involved	Features/Clinical notes
Left-sided colitis (Distal colitis)	Rectum → Descending colon up to splenic flexure	• Continuous inflammation from rectum • Left lower quadrant pain, bloody diarrhea
Extensive colitis	Extends beyond splenic flexure but not entire colon	• More severe symptoms, weight loss, systemic features
Pancolitis (Total colitis)	Entire colon (rectum to cecum)	• Severe diarrhea, bleeding, systemic toxicity • Increased risk of *colorectal carcinoma* • May cause backwash ileitis (mild inflammation of terminal ileum)

Classification by Severity (Truelove and Witts Criteria)

Severity	Stools/ day	Blood in stool	Fever (degree C)	Pulse (per minute)	Hb (g/dL)	ESR (mm/h)	Clinical features
Mild	<4	Small amount	<37.5	<90	>11	<30	Mild pain, no systemic toxicity
Moderate	4–6	Variable	<37.8	<100	10–11	30–50	Moderate pain, minimal toxicity
Severe	>6	Frequent, with visible blood	≥37.8	≥100	<10	<50	Systemic toxicity, weight loss
Fulminant (Toxic)	>10	Continuous bleeding	≥37.8	>100	<10	>50	Severe pain, abdominal distension, risk of toxic megacolon perforation

Classification by Clinical Course

Type	Description
Acute self-limited	Single attack, complete remission after treatment
Chronic intermittent (Relapsing-remitting)	Most common pattern—periods of remission and exacerbations
Chronic continuous	Persistent active disease without remission
Fulminant (Toxic colitis)	Rapidly progressive, severe inflammation → risk of toxic megacolon and perforation

Endoscopic Appearance by Type

- *Mild UC:* Erythema, fine granularity, loss of vascular pattern
- *Moderate UC:* Marked erythema, friability, erosions, contact bleeding
- *Severe UC:* Ulceration, spontaneous bleeding, pseudopolyps

Applied Clinical Significance

- *Extent* determines:
  - Disease *severity and symptoms*
  - *Therapeutic approach* (topical vs systemic therapy)
  - *Surveillance colonoscopy* intervals (especially for pancolitis)
- *Pancolitis* → highest risk of *colorectal carcinoma*
- *Distal UC* (proctitis, left-sided) → may be managed with *topical mesalamine (5-ASA)* alone.

Indications for Surgery in Ulcerative Colitis

- Intractability
- Dysplasia-carcinoma
- Massive colonic bleeding
- Toxic megacolon

Fulminant Colitis and Toxic Megacolon

- Patients with fulminant colitis typically present with high fever, severe abdominal pain, tenderness, tachycardia, and leukocytosis.

- These patients require hospitalization with intravenous hydration, nasogastric decompression, high-dose intravenous steroids if the patient is steroid dependent, and broad-spectrum antibiotics.
- Intravenous hyperalimentation may be useful.
- Patients should be closely monitored with serial abdominal exams and leukocyte counts.
- Deterioration or lack of improvement within 24–48 hours of the initiation of medical treatment warrants an urgent procedure because the mortality rate is increased four-fold in patients with colonic perforation.
- Restorative proctocolectomy with ileal pouch–anal anastomosis (IPAA) as a single-staged procedure has been reported for toxic megacolon.
- Proctectomy and anastomosis are generally not done in the acutely ill patient with an unprepared bowel.
- A total abdominal colectomy with ileostomy and preservation of the rectum is therefore the preferred operation for this condition. This procedure can be expeditiously performed with relatively low morbidity and mortality.
- Even in the emergency setting a transverse colostomy or ileostomy can be done. After recovery from the acute illness (usually over a period of several months), the patient could then be treated with restorative proctocolectomy with IPAA, or total proctocolectomy, depending on the circumstances.

Massive Bleeding

- Massive hemorrhage from UC is an uncommon event, occurring in <5% of patients requiring operation.
- Patients obviously require resuscitation and stabilization before surgery, with replenishment of extracellular volume and transfusions as needed.
- Subtotal colectomy is the procedure of choice and will usually suffice.
- However, if bleeding continues from the remaining rectal mucosa, emergency proctectomy may be required.

Intractability

- Colitis with debilitating symptoms refractory to medical therapy is the most common indication for operative therapy. It has been demonstrated that patients' quality of life after surgery for UC is improved, regardless of the procedure performed.
- Complications of long-term steroid therapy, such as diabetes mellitus, avascular necrosis of the femoral head, cataracts, psychiatric problems, osteoporosis, and weight gain, are a frequent indication for surgical resection, even though the patient's symptoms may be controlled while on steroids.
- Elective surgery should also be considered in patients with significant extracolonic manifestations refractory to nonoperative measures.

Dysplasia or Carcinoma

The finding of dysplastic changes in the colon or carcinoma is an indication for surgical intervention as discussed previously.

Operations

Elective surgical options for UC include total proctocolectomy with ileostomy, restorative proctocolectomy with IPAA, and total proctocolectomy with a continent ileal reservoir (Kock pouch).

Total Proctocolectomy with End Ileostomy

- Total proctocolectomy has the advantage of removing all diseased mucosa, thereby preventing further inflammation or the potential for progression to dysplasia or carcinoma.
- The major disadvantage of this procedure is the need for a permanent ileostomy.
- In addition, despite improvements in bowel preparation, antibiotics, and surgical technique, total proctocolectomy still has a fairly high morbidity rate.
- Most of the morbidity is related to perineal wound healing, adhesions, the ileostomy, and complications of pelvic dissection.

Total Proctocolectomy with Continent Ileostomy

- The continent ileostomy was introduced by Kock.
- The major problem with the Kock pouch is the high complication rate necessitating reoperation in up to half of patients.

- Since the introduction of restorative proctocolectomy and IPAA, the popularity of the continent ileostomy has declined, and it is seldom used.
- Currently, the most common surgery related to continent ileostomies is revisional surgery.
- The Kock procedure should not be performed in obese patients, debilitated patients, or any patient with physical or mental handicap that would prohibit safe catheterization of the reservoir.
- The procedure is contraindicated in patients with CD because of the high incidence of recurrence of Crohn's causing failure of the pouch.

Total Proctocolectomy with Ileal Pouch–Anal Anastomosis

- Restorative proctocolectomy with IPAA has become the most common definitive operation for the surgical treatment of UC.
- The procedure involves a near-total proctocolectomy with preservation of the anal sphincter complex.
- A single-chambered pouch is fashioned from the distal 30 cm of the ileum and sutured to the anus using a double-stapled technique.
- Alternatively, a hand-sewn anastomosis may be fashioned between the pouch and the anus after stripping the distal rectal mucosa from the internal anal sphincter (mucosectomy).
- Patients who undergo total proctocolectomy and IPAA typically have between five and seven bowel movements in a 24-hour period. Function continues to improve with time, with numerous studies demonstrating a decrease in the number of daily bowel movements during the ensuing 3–24 months after reestablishment of continuity.
- Restorative proctocolectomy and IPAA are associated with both early and late complications. A common complication is small bowel obstruction. Bowel obstruction after IPAA tends to be severe and requires surgery in almost half of cases. Another significant complication is pelvic sepsis.
- Anastomotic and pouch suture line leaks are devastating complications that can lead to pelvic abscess and seriously threaten the integrity and functionality of the pouch. Treatment of pelvic sepsis secondary to pouch leaks usually requires a diverting ileostomy and drainage of any abscesses. Delayed ileostomy closure after resolution of IPAA complications has no deleterious functional effects. A pouch-vaginal fistula is a specific form of pelvic sepsis that is difficult to manage and occurs in up to 7% of women.
- Inflammation of the mucosa of the ileal pouch, or pouchitis, occurs in 7–33% of patients with UC treated by IPAA.

A suggested algorithm for elective operations for patients with intractable mucosal UC is presented here:

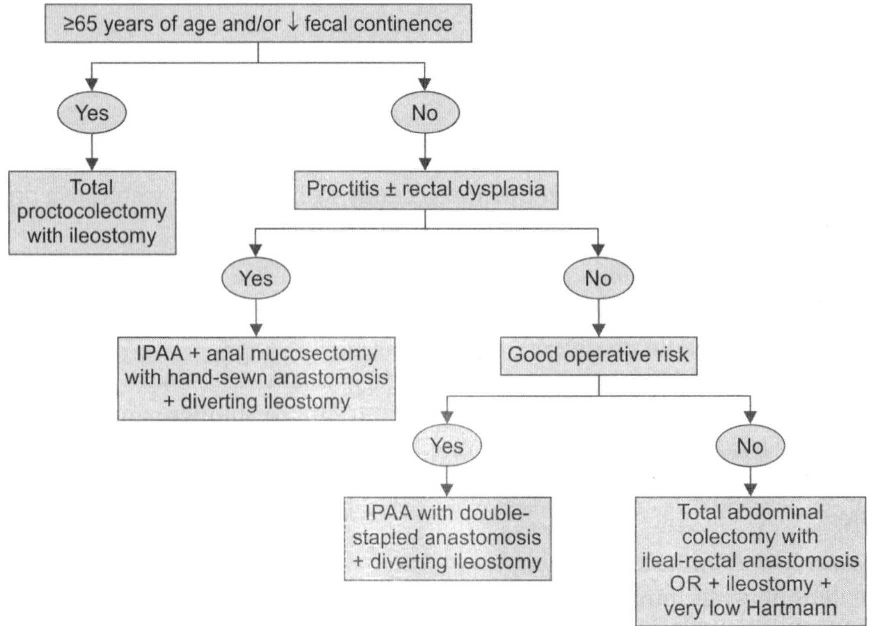

(IPPA: ileal pouch–anal anastomosis)

Postoperative Care

- Nasogastric tubes are usually removed at the completion of the procedure, and liquid diets are offered to patients in the early recovery period. Diet is advanced with return of bowel function as evidenced by ileostomy function.
- If a pelvic drain is used, it is typically removed after 48–72 hours.
- Bladder catheters are typically left in place for 3–4 days depending on the difficulty of pelvic dissection.
- A water-soluble contrast enema is performed about 10 weeks postoperatively to ensure an intact IPAA. If the enema shows a leak, the contrast examination is repeated in 6 weeks; close to 95% of anastomotic leaks heal in the absence of pelvic sepsis. If the radiograph shows no leak, the diverting ileostomy is closed.

Complications of Ulcerative Colitis

Intestinal (Local) Complications

- *Hemorrhage*
  - *Cause:* Erosion of mucosa and ulceration.
  - *Features:*
    - Common, usually mild → chronic anemia.
    - Occasionally *massive bleeding* → life-threatening (rare).
  - *Management:* Blood transfusion, control of disease activity, surgery if refractory.
- *Toxic Megacolon*
  - *Definition:* Acute dilatation of the colon (>6 cm, usually transverse colon) with severe inflammation and systemic toxicity.
  - *Pathophysiology:* Loss of colonic muscle tone due to inflammation and nitric oxide-mediated paralysis.
  - *Clinical Features:* Abdominal distension, pain, fever, tachycardia, leukocytosis.
  - *Complications:* Perforation, sepsis, death.
  - *Management:*
    - Bowel rest, IV steroids, IV fluids, antibiotics.
    - *Urgent colectomy* if no improvement within 24–48 hours or signs of perforation.
- *Perforation*
  - *Cause:* Deep ulceration and transmural necrosis (often in toxic megacolon).
  - *Consequences:* Peritonitis, sepsis.
  - *Management:* Emergency colectomy.
- *Strictures*
  - *Cause:* Long-standing chronic inflammation → fibrosis and scarring.
  - *Common sites:* Sigmoid or rectosigmoid region.
  - *Clinical concern:* May mimic or hide *colorectal carcinoma* → biopsy essential.
  - *Management:* Surgical resection if obstructive or malignant suspicion.
- *Colorectal Carcinoma*
  - *Risk factors:*
    - Duration >8–10 years.
    - *Extent* of disease (↑ risk with pancolitis).
    - *Severity* of inflammation.
    - Associated *primary sclerosing cholangitis (PSC).*
  - *Pathogenesis:* Dysplasia → carcinoma sequence.
  - *Surveillance:*
    - Colonoscopy every 1–2 years after 8 years of pancolitis.
    - Random biopsies or chromoendoscopy to detect dysplasia.
  - *Management:* Colectomy if high-grade dysplasia or carcinoma found.
- *Pseudopolyps*
  - *Cause:* Regenerating mucosa between ulcers.
  - *Significance:* Benign but may cause bleeding or confusion with neoplasia.

- *Backwash Ileitis*
  - *Definition:* Mild inflammation of terminal ileum in severe pancolitis due to reflux of inflammatory contents.
  - *Usually asymptomatic* and resolves with treatment of colitis.
- *Malnutrition and Electrolyte Imbalance*
  - Due to chronic diarrhea and poor intake:
    - *Dehydration*
    - *Hypokalemia*
    - *Hypoalbuminemia*
    - *Weight loss*

Extra-Intestinal Complications

Inflammation may extend beyond the colon, often *immune-mediated* and sometimes *parallel disease activity*.

System	***Complication***	***Notes***
Musculoskeletal	Peripheral arthritis (type 1 & 2), ankylosing spondylitis, sacroiliitis	Type 1 parallels bowel disease activity
Hepatobiliary	Primary sclerosing cholangitis (PSC), fatty liver, autoimmune hepatitis, gallstones	PSC may progress to cholangiocarcinoma
Skin	Erythema nodosum, pyoderma gangrenosum	Erythema nodosum parallels disease; pyoderma may persist independently
Eye	Episcleritis, uveitis, iritis	Uveitis may cause visual loss if untreated
Hematologic	Anemia (iron deficiency, chronic disease), thrombocytosis, venous thromboembolism	Hypercoagulable state common in active disease
Renal	Nephrolithiasis (uric acid or oxalate stones), amyloidosis	Rare
Others	Oral aphthous ulcers	Often with active colitis

Complications of Treatment

Drug	***Possible complications***
Corticosteroids	Cushingoid features, osteoporosis, infections, glucose intolerance
Azathioprine/6-MP	Bone marrow suppression, hepatotoxicity, pancreatitis
Sulfasalazine/Mesalamine	Allergic rash, infertility (in men), hemolysis in G6PD deficiency
Biologics (anti-TNF)	Opportunistic infections, reactivation of TB or hepatitis B

22. Biologic therapy for inflammatory bowel disease. *WBUHS 2007*

Rationale for Biological Therapy

Cytokines involved in inflammatory bowel disease (IBD)

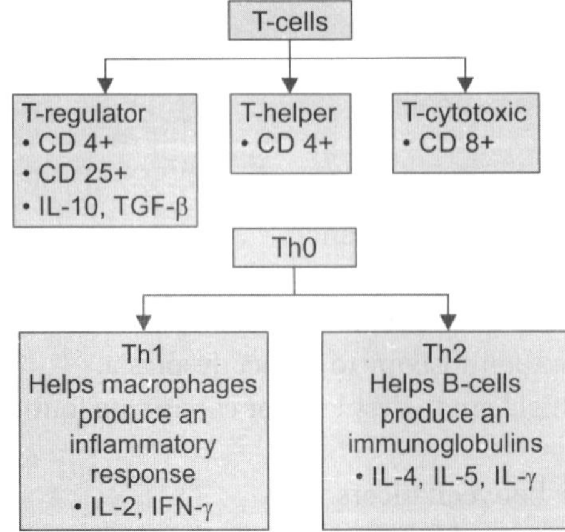

(IL: Interleukin; TGF: transforming growth factor; Th1: T helper cell type 1; Th2: T helper cell type 2)

Basic science research showed that there were many cytokines that were elevated in both CD and UC.

- In CD, cytokines are of the type 1 (Th1) cytokines which include Tumor necrosis factor-α (TNF-α), interleukin-2, and interferon γ.
- UC was less conclusively linked to the production of Th2 cytokines.

Biologic Therapy for Crohn's Disease

- *Infliximab:*
    - Infliximab monoclonal antibody infliximab is a mouse-human chimeric antibody to TNF-α. It first was used in the treatment of rheumatoid arthritis, and was the first biological agent used in the treatment of IBD. It is also used in the treatment of psoriasis and ankylosing spondylitis.
    - Infliximab has shown significant success in treating CD.
- *Other monoclonal antibodies:*
    - These include etanercept (which is the soluble receptor for TNF.
    - Adalimumab (which is a humanized recombinant antibody to TNF) showed effectiveness in patients with moderate-to-severe CD, but less than that of infliximab. It however conveys an advantage in that it is given by subcutaneous injection as opposed to infliximab, which is given by intravenous infusion.
    - Two other recombinant medications were reported to have benefit in moderate-to-severe CD.
        1. Certolizumab is a Fab fragment of a humanized anti-TNF alpha monoclonal antibody that is attached to polyethylene glycol to increase its half-life in circulation.
        2. Natalizumab is an anti-integrin monoclonal antibody that shown utility as induction and maintenance treatment for moderate-to-severe CD. However, it has been associated with progressive multifocal leukoencephalopathy.

Biologic Therapy for UC

A range of biological drugs have been evaluated recently for their therapeutic effect in treating patients with UC. Positive clinical trials include anti-TNF-α antibodies, anti-CD3 antibodies, and anti-adhesion molecules.

- *Infliximab:* Infliximab, a chimeric monoclonal antibody to TNF-α, has been used for the treatment of UC. Infliximab has a proven role in patients with acute severe UC.
- *Adalimumab:* Adalimumab is a humanized anti-TNF agent administered subcutaneously. Current trials are in progress to evaluate the efficacy in the treatment of UC.
- *Visilizumab (anti-CD3 antibody):* Visilizumab is a humanized immunoglobulin G2 monoclonal antibody that binds specifically to human CD3 expressed on T cells, thereby inducing T-cell apoptosis. Visilizumab demonstrated clinical benefit in patients with severe UC refractory to intravenous steroids.
- *Alpha-4-integrin blockade:*
    - Alpha-4 integrins facilitate leukocyte migration across vascular endothelium at the sites of inflammation. The development of monoclonal antibodies that inhibit or block alpha-4 integrins permitted the targeting of lymphocyte trafficking into the intestine as a novel therapeutic intervention.
        - Natalizumab is available for use under a restricted license in the US, for patients with CD who are resistant to other therapies.
        - A more gut-selective humanized antibody to the alpha-4 beta-7 integrin has been evaluated in a multicenter, double-blind, and placebo-controlled trial.
- *Anti-interleukin IL-2 receptor antibody (daclizumab):* An uncontrolled pilot study demonstrated that daclizumab, a humanized monoclonal antibody to the IL-2 receptor (CD25), may be effective for the treatment of active UC.

23. Management of complications of Crohn's disease. ***KGMU Lucknow 2025***

Management of complications of *Crohn's disease (CD)* involves both *medical* and *surgical* strategies, depending on the type and severity of the complication. Crohn's can affect any part of the GI tract and often leads to *inflammatory, fibrostenotic,* or *penetrating* complications.

Intestinal Complications

Strictures (Fibrostenotic Disease)

Presentation: Obstruction, abdominal pain, distension, vomiting, constipation.

Management:

- *Acute partial obstruction:*
  - Bowel rest (NPO), IV fluids, nasogastric decompression.
  - IV corticosteroids if active inflammation suspected.
- *Chronic or fibrotic strictures:*
  - *Endoscopic balloon dilatation* (for short, accessible strictures <5 cm).
  - *Surgical resection or stricturoplasty* for long/multiple strictures or failed dilation.
- *Prevent recurrence:* Optimize medical therapy (e.g., biologics).

Fistulas

Types: Entero-enteric, entero-vesical, entero-cutaneous, entero-vaginal, perianal.

Management:

- *Initial:* Control sepsis (abscess drainage, antibiotics such as ciprofloxacin/metronidazole).
- *Medical:*
  - Anti-TNF agents (e.g., infliximab, adalimumab).
  - Immunomodulators (azathioprine, 6-MP) for maintenance.
- *Surgical:*
  - Resection of diseased bowel and repair of fistula when conservative therapy fails or for complex fistulas.
  - Perianal fistulas often need *seton placement* + medical therapy.

Abscesses

Presentation: Fever, localized tenderness, leukocytosis.

Management:

- *Imaging:* CT or MRI pelvis.
- *Drainage:*
  - Percutaneous under radiologic guidance (preferred).
  - Surgical drainage if not accessible percutaneously.
- *Antibiotics:* Broad-spectrum (e.g., ceftriaxone + metronidazole).
- *After control of infection:* Initiate or optimize immunosuppressive therapy.

Massive Hemorrhage

Management:

- Supportive (IV fluids, blood transfusion).
- Localization via colonoscopy, angiography, or CT angiogram.
- Endoscopic or angiographic embolization.
- Surgical resection if persistent or severe bleeding.

Perforation

Management:

- Emergency *surgery* (resection of perforated segment, exteriorization or primary anastomosis depending on condition).
- IV fluids, antibiotics, and supportive care.

Extra-intestinal Complications

Nutritional Deficiencies

- *Causes:* Malabsorption, resection, chronic diarrhea.

- *Management:*
  - Vitamin B_{12}, folate, iron, vitamin D, calcium, zinc supplementation.
  - Enteral nutrition preferred; parenteral if severe.

Osteoporosis/Osteopenia
- *Prevention:* Calcium + vitamin D, minimize corticosteroid use.
- *Treatment:* Bisphosphonates if indicated.

Gallstones/Nephrolithiasis
- *Due to:* Bile salt malabsorption or oxalate absorption.
- *Management:* Hydration, low-fat and low-oxalate diet, bile acid binders (cholestyramine).

Extra-intestinal Manifestations
- *Arthritis/Ankylosing spondylitis:* NSAIDs (with caution), biologics.
- *Erythema nodosum/Pyoderma gangrenosum:* Corticosteroids, biologics.
- *Uveitis:* Ophthalmologic care, systemic steroids.

Surgical Complications and Recurrence
- *Postoperative recurrence* is common (especially at anastomotic site).
- *Prevention:*
  - Smoking cessation.
  - Postoperative prophylaxis with biologics or immunomodulators.

24. Discuss clinical features and management of Crohn's disease. ***KIIT University Odisha 2025.***

Crohn's Disease: Clinical Features and Management

Overview
- *Crohn's disease (CD)* is a *chronic, relapsing inflammatory bowel disease (IBD)* that can involve *any part of the gastrointestinal tract* from *mouth to anus,* most commonly the *terminal ileum and proximal colon.*
- *Key pathological features:*
  - *Transmural inflammation* (involves full wall thickness)
  - *Skip lesions* (normal mucosa between diseased segments)
  - *Granulomatous inflammation* (non-caseating granulomas on biopsy)
  - *Fibrostenotic and fistulizing complications*

Clinical Features

General Presentation
- Usually *chronic and relapsing* course with *periods of remission and exacerbation.*

Gastrointestinal Features

Feature	***Description***
Abdominal pain	Typically in *right lower quadrant* (terminal ileum). Crampy; may mimic appendicitis
Chronic diarrhea	May be watery or steatorrheic; sometimes with blood or mucus (less than UC)
Weight loss and anorexia	Due to malabsorption and chronic inflammation
Low-grade fever, malaise	Common during active disease
Growth failure	In children/adolescents due to malnutrition and inflammation
Perianal disease	Fissures, fistulas, abscesses, skin tags—*common and characteristic* of Crohn's
Mass in right iliac fossa	Thickened loops or abscess formation
Oral lesions	Aphthous ulcers, "cobblestone" mucosa

Extra-intestinal Manifestations

System	*Manifestations*
Musculoskeletal	Peripheral arthritis, ankylosing spondylitis, sacroiliitis
Skin	Erythema nodosum, pyoderma gangrenosum
Eye	Uveitis, episcleritis
Hepatobiliary	Fatty liver, primary sclerosing cholangitis, gallstones
Renal	Oxalate stones, amyloidosis
Others	Oral aphthae, clubbing, thromboembolic phenomena

Complications

- *Local (Intestinal):*
  - Strictures → obstruction
  - Fistulas (enterovesical, entero-enteric, perianal, etc.)
  - Abscesses
  - Malabsorption
  - Perforation (rare)
  - Increased risk of small bowel carcinoma
- *Systemic:*
  - Nutritional deficiencies (B_{12}, folate, iron, vitamin D, zinc, protein)

Diagnosis (Brief Overview)

Investigation	*Findings / Purpose*
Blood tests	Anemia, ↑ ESR/CRP, low albumin, B_{12} deficiency
Stool tests	Rule out infection (*C. difficile*, parasites)
Endoscopy (Ileocolonoscopy)	Skip lesions, aphthous ulcers, cobblestone mucosa, rectal sparing
Biopsy	Transmural inflammation, non-caseating granulomas
Imaging (CT/MR enterography)	Bowel wall thickening, strictures, fistulas, abscesses ("string sign of Kantor" on barium study)

Management

Management depends on *disease severity*, *site*, and *complications*.

Goals:

- Induce and maintain remission
- Prevent complications
- Improve nutrition and quality of life

General Measures

- *Nutrition:*
  - High-calorie, high-protein diet.
  - Vitamin and mineral supplementation (iron, B_{12}, folate, vitamin D, calcium, zinc).
  - Enteral nutrition may induce remission, especially in children.
- *Smoking cessation:* strongly recommended (smoking worsens Crohn's).
- *Avoid NSAIDs* (may exacerbate disease).

Pharmacological Therapy

- *Induction of Remission*

Disease severity	**Drugs used**
Mild–Moderate (Ileocolic disease)	Oral or topical *5-ASA (mesalamine)*; sometimes *budesonide* (controlled-release steroid)
Moderate–Severe	*Systemic corticosteroids* (prednisolone 40–60 mg/day)
Severe/Refractory	*Biologics* (anti-TNF: infliximab, adalimumab; anti-integrin: vedolizumab; anti-IL-12/23: ustekinumab)
Associated infection	Antibiotics (ciprofloxacin, metronidazole) — especially for perianal or fistulizing disease

- *Maintenance of Remission*

Drug class	**Examples**	**Notes**
Immunomodulators	Azathioprine, 6-mercaptopurine, methotrexate	For long-term maintenance; steroid-sparing
Biologics	Infliximab, adalimumab, vedolizumab, ustekinumab	For moderate–severe or refractory disease
5-ASA	Limited benefit for small bowel disease; used in colonic Crohn's	
Corticosteroids	*Not for maintenance* (used only for induction)	

Management of Complications

Complication	**Management**
Stricture	Endoscopic balloon dilatation (short), surgical resection/stricturoplasty (long)
Fistula/Abscess	Drain abscess, antibiotics (ciprofloxacin + metronidazole), biologics (anti-TNF), surgery if refractory
Obstruction/Perforation	Surgical resection
Nutritional deficiency	Replace B_{12}, iron, folate, vitamin D, calcium
Perianal disease	Sitz baths, antibiotics, seton drainage, anti-TNF therapy

Surgical Management

- *Indications:*
  - Failure of medical therapy
  - Obstruction due to strictures
  - Fistula or abscess not responding to drugs
  - Perforation or massive hemorrhage
  - Malignancy or dysplasia
- *Principles:*
  - *Conservative, limited resection* (disease often recurs at anastomosis).
  - Procedures include:
    - Segmental resection
    - Stricturoplasty (preserves bowel length)
    - Drainage of abscesses
    - Seton for perianal fistulas

Follow-up

- Regular monitoring for recurrence and nutritional status.
- Colonoscopic surveillance for cancer (in long-standing colonic disease).
- Vaccinations (especially before biologic therapy: influenza, pneumococcal, hepatitis B).

25. Surgical considerations during pregnancy and delivery with Crohn's disease. *WBUHS 2021 Supplementary*

- Fertility remains a topic of concern among many patients with IBD. Female patients whose IBD is under control and who have not previously undergone pelvic surgery have fertility rates comparable with those of women of the same age who do not have IBD. Disease remission does not only improves fertility rates.
- Patients with IBD, whether CD or UC, tend to have pregnancy outcomes worse than those of women without IBD. Studies have further shown that the chances of a poor pregnancy outcome in patients with CD are higher than those in patients with UC.
- In most female patients with IBD who conceive while their disease is in remission, the IBD tends to remain in remission throughout the pregnancy and in the postpartum period. Patients with IBD who conceive when their disease is active, 66% continue to have active disease or experience worsening of their IBD. In up to 45% of patients with UC who conceive while their disease is active, the colitis worsens during pregnancy; in 24%, the colitis continues to be active but stable, and in the remainder of patients, the disease goes back into remission.
- Among patients with CD who conceive while their disease is active, the disease goes into remission in one-third, remains stably active in one-third, and worsens in one-third.
- The European Crohn's and Colitis Organization's guidelines recommend surgery in pregnant women with IBD for the same indications as in non-pregnant patients (obstruction, perforation, abscess, hemorrhage, or active disease refractory to medical treatment). A temporary stoma might be preferred over primary anastomosis to prevent postoperative complications.

  With respect to the timing of surgery during pregnancy, some small series have reported a higher risk of miscarriage in the first trimester and of preterm delivery in the third trimester. However, urgent surgery should not be delayed, as even higher complications should be expected otherwise.

  It is already known that steroids, thiopurines, and anti-TNF agents are safe during pregnancy and in the offspring. In recent years, new drugs such as vedolizumab, ustekinumab, and tofacitinib have become part of the therapeutic armamentarium for patients with IBD.
- Taking into consideration the morbidity and mortality associated with surgery in pregnant IBD patients, medical options and percutaneous drainage of abscesses should be tried before referring patients for surgery.
- Nevertheless, the risk of active IBD should be weighed against the risk of surgery, as sustained illness is associated with higher morbidity for the mother and the fetus. When the indication for surgery is finally established, the interventions should be carried out by referral teams involving gastroenterologists, colorectal surgeons, obstetricians and neonatal specialists in a multidisciplinary manner within a single unit in order to perform the procedure with the greatest probability of success.

Key Points

- Women with CD have an overall lower rate of fecundity than healthy women.
- A collaborative multidisciplinary approach between gastroenterologists, surgeons, and obstetricians is important to manage pregnancy and delivery issues in women with CD.
- Disease control of the mother preconception is likely to ensure the best outcome for the baby.
- Knowledge of those CD-related medications which are teratogenic or otherwise contraindicated during pregnancy is essential.
- Most pregnant women with CD can undergo vaginal delivery with satisfactory outcomes.
- However, there is a higher rate of CS in pregnant women with CD, particularly those with perianal CD.
- Women with CD should be offered CS for the same indications as other women.
- Women with active perianal CD should consider elective CS.

26. Pouch Surgery. ***WBUHS 2009, 2025 Supplementary***

27. What are the commonly created types of pouches after total colectomy? Discuss the merits and demerits of pouch creation. ***WBUHS 2016***

Introduction

- The IPAA, also known as an ileoanal pouch, restorative proctocolectomy, ileal-anal pull-through, or sometimes referred to as a J-pouch, S-pouch, W-pouch, or an internal pouch, is an internal reservoir; usually situated where the rectum would normally be. It is formed by folding loops of small intestine (the ileum) back on themselves and stitching or stapling them together. The internal walls are then removed thus forming a reservoir. The reservoir is then stitched or stapled into the perineum where the rectum was.
- Ileoanal pouches are constructed for people who have had their large intestine surgically removed due to disease or injury.

Indications

Diseases and conditions of the large intestine which may require surgical removal include:

- UC
- CD
- Familial adenomatous polyposis
- Colon cancer
- Toxic megacolon

Types of Pouches

- *J-pouch:*
    - The "J-pouch" may be used to treat people with UC or familial polyposis who need to have and most of the rectum surgically removed
    - A J-pouch may also be called the following names:
        - Ileoanal reservoir
        - Ileoanal anastomosis
        - Pull-through
        - Endorectal pull-through
        - Pelvic pouch
        - IPAA

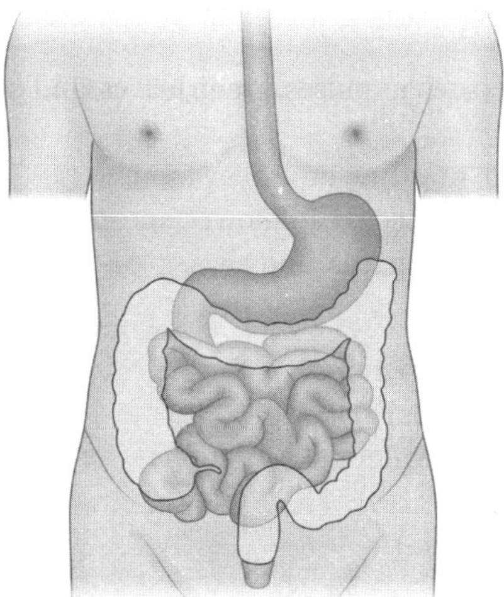

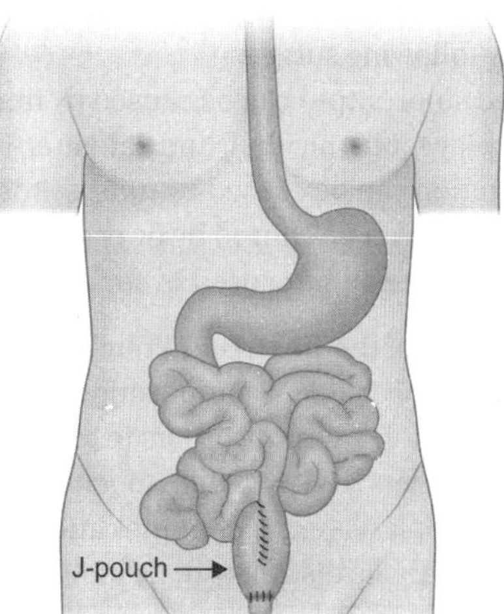

When the large intestine and rectum are removed due to colorectal disease, another pathway must be devised for solid waste to exit the body. A J-pouch, a surgically created "J"-shaped reservoir, is an alternate way to store and pass stool.

- *K-pouch:*
  - The K-pouch is an option for people with poor anal sphincter function and those who have had their sphincters previously removed and have a traditional ostomy but wish to avoid the encumbrance of an external appliance
  - *A K-pouch may also be referred to as:*
    1. Koch pouch
    2. Continent ileostomy

Pouch Failure and Pouch Repair:
Occasionally, a pouch will fail to work properly due to complications like leakage or inflammation. When pouch failure occurs, surgical options may include pouch revision, creation of a redo pouch, or neo-pouch creation. In some circumstances, the conversion of a J-pouch into a K-pouch may be considered to preserve continence and improve patients' quality of life.

Pouch Behavior

- Immediately after the surgery is complete, the patient tends to pass liquid stool with frequent urgency, and he or she may have 8 to 15 bowel movements per day, but this eventually decreases with time.
- Because the ileoanal pouch is considerably smaller a reservoir than the colon, patients tend to have more frequent bowel motions; typically six to eight times a day.
- Also because the ileum does not absorb as much water as the colon, the stools tend to be less formed, and sometimes fluid.
- Because the ileum does not absorb as much of the gastric acid produced by the stomach as the colon did, pouch output also tends to burn the anal region slightly, and many patients find it helpful to wash the area regularly, sometimes using protective barrier cream.

Diet

- Because more water is lost through pouch output, patients can get dehydrated easily and can also suffer salt deficiency. For this reason, some are encouraged to add extra salt to meals.
- Persistent dehydration is often supplemented with an electrolyte mix drink.
- Immediately after surgery, patients are encouraged to eat low fiber, high protein/carbohydrate meals, but after the pouch function has settled, most are able to reintroduce a fully varied diet. There are some foods that are known to irritate the pouch, however, and though they may be introduced carefully, are best avoided immediately following surgery:
  i. Increased stool output can be caused by fibrous foods (such as pulses, green leaves, and raw vegetables) and also by spicy foods, alcohol, and caffeine.
  ii. Anal irritation can be caused by nuts, seeds, citric acid, raw fruit, and spicy food.
  iii. Increased gas can be caused by fizzy drinks, milk, beer, broccoli, cauliflower, sprouts, cabbage, etc.
  iv. Increased odor can be caused by foods such as fish, onions, garlic, and eggs.

Diseases/Disorders of the Ileal Anal Pouch

- Surgery related/mechanical complications (e.g., fistulas and strictures)
- Inflammatory or infections disorders (e.g., pouchitis and cuffitis)
- Functional disorders (e.g., irritable pouch syndrome and pelvic floor dysfunction)
- Dysplasia or neoplasia (e.g., adenomas and cancers)
- Systemic or metabolic disorders (e.g., malnutrition and anemia).

Merits of Pouch

- Acts as a reservoir
- Overcomes the difficulty of hand-sewn anastomosis
- Keeps the functional volume of intestine
- Overcomes the postoperative hazards of stoma

Demerits of Pouch

Pouchitis

Pouchitis is inflammation of the ileal pouch, which is created in the management of patients with UC, indeterminate colitis, or rarely, other colitis.

- Patients with pouchitis typically present with bloody diarrhea, urgency in passing stools, or discomfort while passing stools. The loss of blood and/or dehydration resulting from the frequent stools will frequently result in nausea. In fewer cases, pain can occur with pouchitis.
- Endoscopy in patients with pouchitis usually reveals erythematous pouch mucosa, loss of pseudocolonic vasculature or other architecture, and friability of the mucosa. Biopsies show evidence of inflammatory cells or red blood cells in the lamina propria.
- Pouchitis is usually treated with antibiotics and specifically usually with ciprofloxacin and metronidazole. In refractory cases, probiotics such as VSL-3 and Bio-K$^+$ may be useful.

Complications of Pouch

Complication	*Functional manifestation*	*Other manifestations*	*Investigation*
Pouchitis	Liquid stool, blood, and urgency	Abdominal pain, and fever	Proctoscopy and biopsy
Chronic intestinal obstruction	Liquid stool	Abdominal pain and distension	Plain or contrast radiology, CT
Evacuation disorder: • Ileoanal stenosis • Long distal segment	 • Frequent, small volume stool • Frequent, small volume stool. May need to intubate		 • Digital examination, pouchogram • Pouchogram
'Functional' • Low capacitance reservoir • Functional frequency	 • Frequent, small volume stool. Urgency • Phasic frequency		 • Pouchogram • Ambulant pressure monitoring

MESENTERIC ISCHEMIA

28. Define bowel ischemia. What are the sequelae of acute and chronic bowel ischemia? Discuss the principle of management of such patients. ***WBUHS 2018***

- Ischemic bowel disease encompasses a heterogeneous group of disorders caused by acute or chronic processes, arising from occlusive or nonocclusive etiologies, which result in decreased blood flow to the gastrointestinal tract.
- The clinical course may range from transient and reversible to fulminant.
- The clinical course may range from transient and intestinal ischemia can be classified into three types: (1) Acute mesenteric ischemia, (2) Chronic mesenteric ischemia, and (3) Colonic ischemia.
- Acute mesenteric ischemia may also be further subdivided into embolic mesenteric ischemia, thrombotic mesenteric ischemia, and venous mesenteric ischemia.

Acute Ischemia

Presentation

Early	**Late**
Prominent symptoms of GI emptying (nausea, vomiting, diarrhea)	• Bloody diarrhea • Abdominal distension • Features of peritonitis: – Fever – Shock – Tachycardia

Early diagnosis requires high index of suspicion

Sequelae

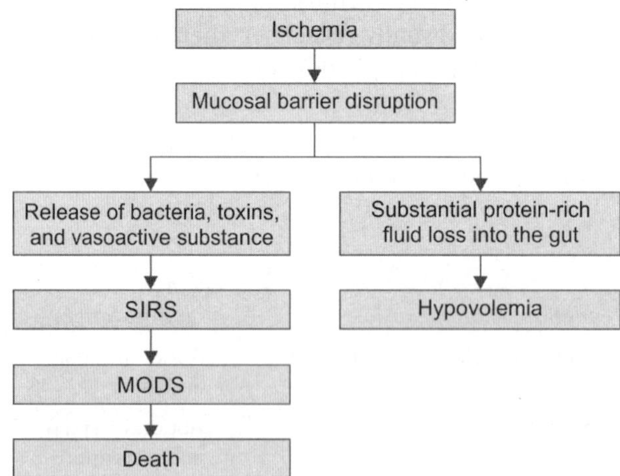

(GI: gastrointestinal; MODS: multiple organ dysfunction syndrome; SIRS: systemic inflammatory response syndrome)

Principle of Management in Acute Ischemia

Definitive surgical exploration:

- Assessment of bowel viability
- Determination of underlying cause
- *Determination of underlying pathology:* Thrombosis or Embolism?

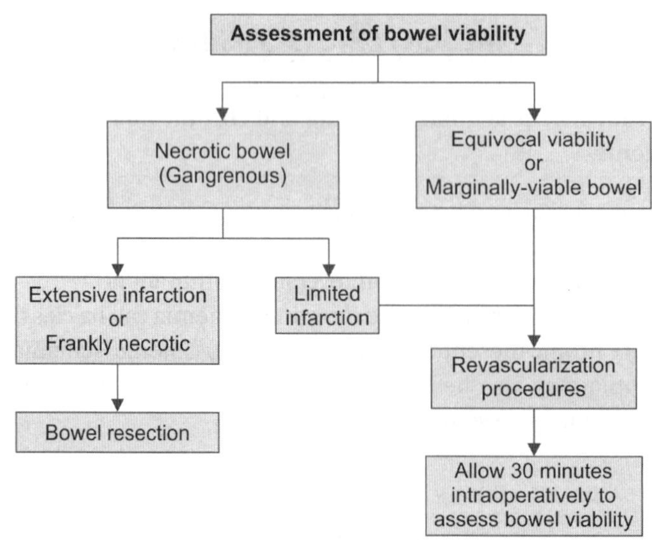

- Mesenteric revascularization
- Resection of necrotic bowel
- Second look laparotomy

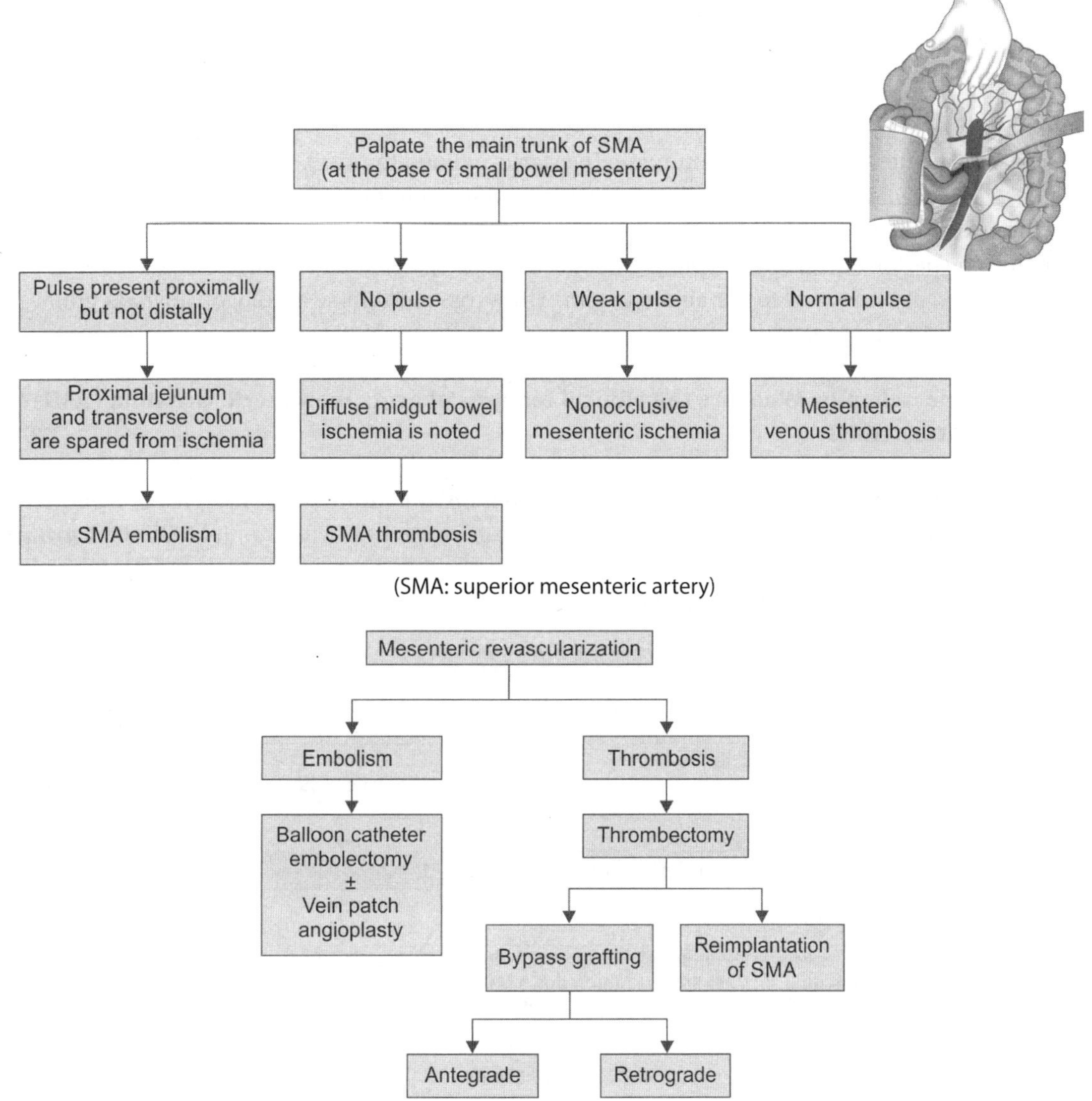

(SMA: superior mesenteric artery)

(SMA: superior mesenteric artery)

Chronic mesenteric ischemia is a condition in which plaque builds up in the major arteries including the celiac and superior mesenteric arteries that supply blood to the small intestine or small bowel.

These blood clots in the small intestine and bowels can lead to:

- Weight loss
- Pain with eating

Chronic mesenteric ischemia is often multifactorial in etiology. The most common cause is atherosclerosis involving the proximal portions of the coeliac artery, SMA, or IMA.

Less common etiologies include:

- Dissection
- Vasculitis
- Fibromuscular dysplasia

- Radiation
- Cocaine abuse

Chronicity of the symptoms is caused by the gradual decrease in blood flow to the intestines. The normal vascular supply to the bowel is from the coeliac artery, superior mesenteric, and inferior mesenteric arteries. Extensive collateralization can occur between the vascular territories of these vessels. Because of this collateral circulation, patients may experience symptoms, not until two or three major mesenteric vessels are involved.

Treatment

- Anticoagulant medications, such as Coumadin (warfarin, a blood thinner), to reduce the risk of blood clots.
- *Angioplasty and stenting:* A balloon catheter is used to attempt to open the artery and a small stent is placed inside the artery to keep it open.
- Surgery may be performed to remove plaque (endarterectomy), bypass the blocked vessel to restore blood flow to the intestines, or remove or repair an aneurysm. The surgeon may use autologous bypass grafts or artificial grafts during the bypass procedure.

29. Classify mesenteric ischemia. What are the clinical features of acute mesenteric ischemia (AMI)? How will you diagnose and treat AMI? ***WBUHS 2023***

30. Describe the etiology and pathogenesis of mesenteric ischemia. Outline the principles of treatment of acute mesenteric artery occlusion. ***RGUHS, Karnataka 2025***

31. Write in brief about acute mesenteric ischemia. ***WBUHS 2015***

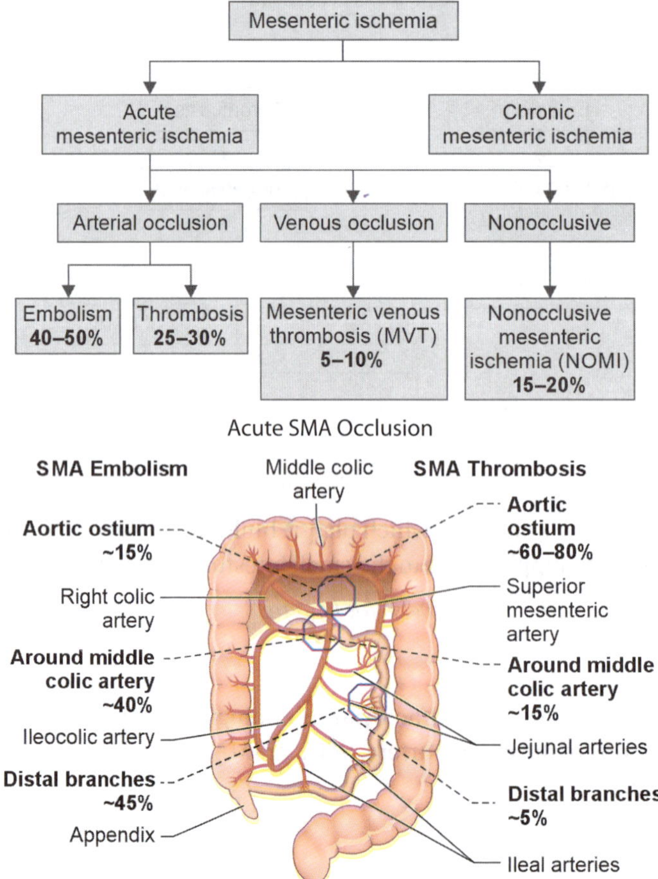

Presentation

- The classic description of patients who present with embolic disease of the mesenteric vessels is of sudden-onset midabdominal pain described as pain out of proportion to physical examination findings and is associated with immediate bowel evacuation.
- However, only approximately one-third of patients present with the triad of abdominal pain, fever, and heme-positive stools.
- A recent history of a myocardial infarction, atrial fibrillation, mural thrombus, mitral valve disease, left ventricular aneurysm, or embolic disease should suggest the diagnosis.
- If the etiology of the acute mesenteric ischemia is secondary to thrombotic occlusive disease, before the acute presentation, these patients typically describe symptoms of chronic abdominal pain following meals and will usually have experienced significant weight loss.
- These patients typically have other manifestations of diffuse atherosclerotic disease, such as coronary artery disease, peripheral artery disease, and carotid stenosis.
- Patients who present with nonocclusive mesenteric ischemia (NOMI) present in a manner slightly different from patients with embolic or thrombotic etiologies.
- It usually occurs during severe low-flow states and represents extreme mesenteric vasoconstriction.
- It is much more common among severely ill patients in an intensive care setting who require vasopressors.
- The symptoms are typically less acute and more diffuse and may wax and wane throughout its course.

Diagnosis

- Once suspected by history and physical examination results, noninvasive or invasive studies can confirm the diagnosis of mesenteric ischemia. Abdominal plain X-ray films are nondiagnostic. They may reveal edematous bowel with thumbprinting. In severe cases, the X-ray films may reveal gas in the bowel wall and the portal vein. However, more commonly plain films reveal a pattern consistent with an ileus or are completely unremarkable.
- CT and MRA are the most commonly used noninvasive studies to confirm the diagnosis of mesenteric ischemia. Traditional CT scan technology could evaluate arterial patency, anatomy, calcifications, and aneurysms. Furthermore, it could evaluate the status of the bowel and help identify other causes of abdominal pain.
- Helical CT scan technology and the more recently developed multislice, multiarray helical CT scan technology with maximum intensity projection (MIP) could visualize visceral arterial anatomy with three-dimensional spatial resolution. The origin of the celiac artery and the SMA can be well visualized.
    - With helical CT scan secondary, tertiary, and smaller branches are less well defined. For this, contrast-enhanced angiography remains the gold standard.
    - CT scan technology also tends to overestimate the degree of critical stenosis compared to conventional angiography. However, with the advent of multiarray or multidetector technology, this limitation appears to be less of an issue because the images obtained are more sensitive for the detection of arterial stenotic lesions.
    - Finally, the amount of calcification present at the origin of the vessel can make it difficult to determine the true degree of stenosis with CT scan technology.
- Recent advances in magnetic resonance technology with contrast-enhanced three-dimensional MRA have made MRA imaging of visceral vessels much more practical than earlier studies.
- One benefit of MRA technology over CT scan is the use of gadolinium. Gadolinium is significantly less nephrotoxic compared to the intravenous contrast used for CT scans. A well-known limitation of MRA technology, similar to CT scan, is that it will adequately assess the distal branches of the mesenteric vessels.
- Contrast angiography has long been considered the gold standard for imaging of the visceral vessels. It is performed in a transfemoral manner using the Seldinger technique.
- Arteriography should include both anteroposterior and lateral views of the celiac artery, the SMA, and the IMA. The origins of the celiac artery and the SMA are best visualized on the lateral view, whereas the middle and distal SMA and IMA are best visualized on the anteroposterior view. Delayed views are useful to evaluate for NOMI.
    - A classic angiographic pattern is associated with mesenteric ischemia of embolic versus thrombotic disease.

- Of all three mesenteric vessels, emboli typically lodge in the SMA given the less acute angle of the origin of this vessel from the main axis of the aorta.
- The celiac artery and IMA arise off the aorta at more perpendicular angles.
- When emboli lodge in the SMA, they usually lodge distal to the middle colic branch and the jejunal branch.
- With thrombotic disease, the thrombus usually forms at the atherosclerotic plaque. For most patients, this region is usually at the origin of the mesenteric vessel.
- Therefore the angiogram typically demonstrates complete absence of flow in the mesenteric vessel, often making it difficult to ascertain the location of the origin of the mesenteric vessel.

In addition to the superior image quality of contrast-enhanced angiography, another benefit of angiography is the ability to perform selective injections of each mesenteric vessel. Furthermore, with NOMI, the SMA can be selectively catheterized to instill papaverine.

In the case of chronic mesenteric ischemia with stenotic lesions of the mesenteric vessels, this would allow for percutaneous balloon angioplasty and/or stent placement.

Therefore not only is angiography the gold standard for diagnostic imaging, but it also provides important therapeutic options.

Intraoperative Evaluation

Often, the diagnosis of mesenteric ischemia is considered in the operating room when a patient is explored for abdominal pain and necrotic bowel is encountered.

In this case, the root of the mesentery should be palpated for a pulse.

Alternatively, a handheld Doppler can be used to listen to the quality and character of the arterial signal.

Intraoperative angiography can also be performed.

Assessment of Bowel Viability

- Multiple techniques have been described to assess bowel viability intraoperatively following revascularization.
- After restoration of flow, the bowel may contain frankly necrotic segments in need of resection, areas of normal bowel, and areas of marginally perfused bowel.
- It is this latter category that often provides a challenge to the surgeon.
- Many diagnostic options are available to the clinician.
- These range from determination of the pulse quality and character, use of a handheld intraoperative Doppler, intravenous fluorescein, and transcutaneous oxygen measurements (TCO_2) to a second-look exploratory laparotomy.
- All of these methods are relatively simple to perform, but each has its limitations. Obviously, clearly necrotic or nonviable bowel must be resected at the time of the operation.
- Determination of the viability of marginally perfused bowel is more difficult.
- Intraoperatively, the color, motility, and integrity of the bowel should be evaluated.
- The appearance of ischemic intestine includes loss of the normal sheen, dull-gray discoloration, and lack of peristalsis.
- Determination of the character and quality of the pulsation in the antimesenteric border and the mesenteric arcades may help determine which bowel will remain viable once revascularization has been performed.
- Intraoperative Doppler assessment of the perfusion of the bowel can be performed using a sterilized, continuous-wave Doppler ultrasound flow detector.
- The probe is placed on the antimesenteric border of the intestine to detect pulsatile Doppler signals. However, even in the best of hands, this technique remains unreliable in predicting which bowel will remain viable.
- *Second-look laparotomy* is essential in the management of acute mesenteric ischemia. No matter which adjunctive method is used intraoperatively to assess bowel perfusion and viability, second-look laparotomy is the most reliable means of determining viability of marginally perfused bowel once revascularization has been performed. The decision to perform a second-look laparotomy should be determined during the first operation and adhered to no matter what the condition of the patient is 24–48 hours later.

Management

- Once the diagnosis of acute mesenteric ischemia has been suspected or proven, prompt therapeutic intervention is necessary, regardless of the etiology of the mesenteric ischemia.
- The patient should be placed on appropriate cardiac monitors, and intravenous lines should be instituted for aggressive fluid resuscitation.
- Acidosis should be corrected. Pain should be controlled with analgesics.
- Intravenous heparinization and antibiotics should be administered promptly.
- A Foley catheter is inserted to monitor urine output.
- Any precipitating event should be sought out and corrected.

Nonocclusive Mesenteric Ischemia

- Management of NOMI is largely nonoperative. Once the diagnosis has been established with angiography, the treatment of the underlying precipitating cause is the most important therapeutic intervention.
- Methods such as optimizing fluid resuscitation, improving cardiac output, and eliminating vasopressor agents will have the greatest impact on outcome.
- An adjunctive therapy is selective catheterization of the SMA with direct intra-arterial infusion of papaverine (30–60 mg/h).
- The infusion is continued for at least 24 hours. Repeated angiography at regular intervals is required to determine the effectiveness of this therapy. If the patient presents with peritoneal signs on physical examination, an exploratory laparotomy will be required to resect frankly necrotic or gangrenous bowel.
- If an intra-arterial infusion of papaverine has been initiated, it is important to continue this throughout the exploratory laparotomy. It is also imperative to perform a second-look laparotomy in this cohort of patients given the waxing and waning of this disease process.

Mesenteric Embolic Disease

- The goal in the surgical treatment of acute mesenteric ischemia is to restore normal pulsatile flow to the SMA and resect nonviable intestine.
- In general, revascularization precedes resection.
- Depending on the etiology, the therapeutic approach varies. For embolic disease of the SMA, a surgical embolectomy is performed.
- Percutaneous interventional treatment of acute SMA occlusion has been described in the literature. However, its application is limited because most patients present with symptoms that warrant an exploratory laparotomy to evaluate intestinal viability.
- Even if thrombolytic therapy could restore blood flow to the ischemic intestine, most patients will experience pain sufficient to necessitate exploration.
- Furthermore, physical examination alone is not adequate to predict the extent and degree of intestinal ischemia.

Mesenteric Thrombotic Disease

- Acute mesenteric ischemia secondary to thrombotic disease occurs in patients with longstanding atherosclerotic disease of the mesenteric vessels. When this occurs, usually the entire midgut is involved.
- Surgical treatment consists of a surgical bypass, either in an antegrade or a retrograde manner. The conduit of choice for the treatment of acute mesenteric ischemia is autologous greater saphenous vein in a reversed fashion. Synthetic graft material should be avoided in the setting of acute bowel ischemia, given the high risk of transmural bowel infarction and perforation.
- During acute mesenteric ischemia in which time is of the essence and prompt revascularization of the bowel is required, it is often more simple to perform a retrograde bypass from the infrarenal aorta or iliac artery because the exposure is much more simple.
- Although the management of acute mesenteric ischemia is initially surgical, the morbidity and mortality from this disease process are due to the ischemia/reperfusion insult and remain difficult to manage.

INTESTINAL FISTULA

32. Discuss about metabolic changes in high output fistula.

Fluid losses: The effect of fistula output is best appreciated by an analysis of daily gastrointestinal secretions.

Source	*Amount of secretion per day*
• The salivary and gastric glands	• 1.5 L
• Pancreas	• 1 L
• Bile	• 1 L
• Duodenal Brunner's glands	• 200 mL
• Small intestine	• 1.8 L

- Therefore, 8–10 L of fluid flows through the jejunum each day, depending on the oral intake. In the intact functioning intestine 98% of this fluid is (re)absorbed; leaving only 100–200 mL of fluid to be excreted in the stool. Most (7–8 L) of this absorption occurs proximal to the ileocecal valve.
- In the case of proximal fistulae there is a potential for serious compromise of fluid balance even when there is a reasonable extent of more distal intact small intestine, in that large fluid volumes may exit through the fistula rather than proceeding distally to allow absorption to occur.
- Enzymes and electrolytes (especially sodium and magnesium) inevitably accompany fluid, as do essential nutrients.
- The nutritional and fluid balance issues are less with distal fistulae, as small intestinal absorption leaves less fluid and fewer nutrients to be lost as long as the small bowel proximal to the fistula is in good functional condition.
- Reduction of gastrointestinal tract fluid secretion is an integral part of fistula treatment, as discussed in the following.

Metabolic Derangements

- It is not only the volume that is critical with high-output fistulae but also the composition of the secretions at various levels of the gastrointestinal tract.
- *Gastric juice* contains hydrogen, chloride, sodium, and potassium ions, the concentrations differing significantly between the fasting and fed states. Feeding increases the hydrogen ion concentration from about 50 mM to up to 100 mM, increases chloride from 90 to 120 mM, but decreases sodium from 40 to about 25 mm
- *Duodenal fistulae* consequently lead to loss of fluid rich in hydrogen and chloride ions, especially after eating, culminating in hypochloremic, and hypokalemic metabolic alkalosis together with hypovolemia.
- The combination of *Brunner's gland secretions, bile, and pancreatic secretions* serve to neutralize gastric acid secretion.
- The main electrolytes in bile are sodium and chloride, whereas bicarbonate and sodium make up most of the pancreatic juice.
- The sodium concentration of about 140 mM is independent of the activity state of the pancreas, but the bicarbonate concentration increases from 40 to up to 145 mM following stimulation.
- Fistulous discharge at the level of the upper jejunum is therefore associated with significant losses of sodium, chloride, and bicarbonate ions.

Enzymes and Skin

- By the time the gastric contents have reached the jejunum, an array of enzymes has been released and activated within the gut lumen.
- Salivary amylase and gastric pepsin, together with potent pancreatic proteolytic enzymes including trypsin, chymotrypsin, and carboxypeptidases, commence carbohydrate, and protein digestion.
- Other pancreatic enzymes including lipase, amylase, phospholipase, and cholesterol esterase are also activated and are found in the effluent from high-output fistulae.

- These enzymes contribute to delay in wound closure and can lead to major excoriation of previously normal skin.

The Role of Gut Hormones

- Gastric acid secretion is accompanied by the release of gastrin, histamine, somatostatin, and CCK.
- Gastrin and histamine exert a paracrine and endocrine effect to activate the acid-secreting parietal cell and the somatostatin-secreting D cell. CCK is released from duodenal and upper jejunal mucosa.
- CCK is a potent gastrin stimulus and serves to perpetuate gastric acid secretion. It also stimulates the release of gastric somatostatin. Both of these actions are mediated in an endocrine manner.
- Somatostatin, on the other hand, is a potent inhibitory hormone and switches off gastric acid secretion by direct action on the parietal and ECL cells and indirectly by inhibiting gastrin secretion. Somatostatin thus mediates its actions in endocrine, paracrine, and neurocrine manners to regulate gastrointestinal motility and secretion.
- Glucagon-like peptide 2 (GLP2) has attracted considerable attention as a therapeutic agent for intestinal injury since its identification as a potent stimulator of mucosal epithelial proliferation.
- Preliminary trials in patients with short bowel syndrome (SBS) have yielded improvements in intestinal absorption of both fluids and nutrients. A GLP2-induced reduction of gastric acid secretion and gastric motility is perhaps particularly relevant in terms of its potential as a therapeutic agent for patients with ECF. As yet there are no studies specifically examining the effects of GLP2 on high-output fistulae.

Associated Short Bowel Features

- Fistulae related to intestinal surgery, IBD, and radiation enteritis are often accompanied by SBS, which may occur because the residual bowel is actually short, because it is functionally impaired, or because the dominance of effluent from a proximal fistula precludes reabsorption from distal (otherwise intact) intestine.
- Problems with fluid balance and reduced absorptive capacity for nutrients are then to be expected. Early recognition of these complicating factors is crucial to a good outcome.

33. Discuss about management of intestinal fistula. ***WBUHS 2019; Rims, Imphal 2022***

Laboratory Studies

- Although laboratory tests do not help diagnose or confirm the presence of intestinal fistulas, they are important for defining the patient's clinical condition and guiding treatment.
- A complete blood count (CBC) should be obtained. An elevated white blood cell (WBC) count suggests associated infection.
- Abscesses, soft-tissue infection adjacent to an ECF, bacteremia, or bloodstream infection may be present.
- Elderly patients or those who are severely nutritionally depleted may not manifest an elevated WBC count as an indicator of infection.
- An electrolyte panel is helpful. Electrolyte imbalances and dehydration are common in patients with high-output ECFs because of intestinal fluid loss.
- Hypokalemia, hypochloremia, and metabolic alkalosis are observed in patients with high-output gastric fistulas.
- Patients with pancreatic and small bowel fistulas have associated hyponatremia, hypokalemia, and metabolic acidosis.
- Nephroenteric fistulas are often associated with decreased renal function, which manifests as elevated creatinine and blood urea nitrogen (BUN) and a reduced glomerular filtration rate (GFR).
- Serum albumin levels are used to predict fistula closure and mortality. In one study, a serum albumin level higher than 3.5 mg/dL was associated with no mortality, whereas a level below 2.5 mg/dL was associated with a mortality of 42%.
- Higher levels of short-turnover proteins (e.g., serum transferrin, prealbumin, and retinol-binding protein) are used to predict fistula closure. A serum transferrin level higher than 200 mg/dL is associated with a higher rate of fistula closure and a lower mortality and vice versa.

Imaging Studies

- CT allows identification as well as guided drainage of associated abscesses or fluid collection. CT with oral contrast can also identify the site of the fistula.
- Gastric, duodenal, and proximal small bowel fistulas can be readily identified. The presence or absence of distal bowel obstruction can be revealed; if intraluminal contrast passes distal to the fistula site, then distal obstruction is unlikely.
- Passage of the oral contrast, as well as the early presence of contrast within the colonic lumen, can demonstrate the gastrocolic fistula tract.
- The presence of periaortic inflammation, air collection, or fluid collection characterizes aortoenteric fistulas.
- Fistulography is performed to confirm and define the location of an ECF. Closed-suction drainage catheters are placed under radiologic guidance to drain abscesses or fluid collections. If the drainage contents are clearly enteric, the area is allowed to drain adequately for 7–10 days. This period allows a tract to form.
- The patient is stabilized with correction of electrolyte imbalances and administration of antibiotics. Water-soluble contrast is injected via the drainage catheter under fluoroscopy or during CT. Intraluminal passage of contrast confirms the presence and defines the origin of the fistula. A complete contrast study of the GI tract should follow fistulography.
- Small bowel follow through contrast radiography often identifies enteroenteric fistulas in patients with CD and chronic radiation enteritis.

Medical Therapy

Initial treatment of intestinal fistulas is medical, including resuscitation, control of sepsis, local control of fistula output, nutritional support, pharmacologic management, and radiologic investigations. The final therapeutic step, if necessary, is definitive surgery to restore GI tract continuity.

Early surgery is infrequently required but may be necessary in the following circumstances:

- Sepsis or abscess formation not amenable to percutaneous drainage
- Complete distal intestinal obstruction
- Uncontrolled bleeding from fistula
- Removal of mesh or other foreign bodies
- Inability to control the fistula without surgical drainage
- Aortoenteric fistulas (definitively managed by means of emergency surgery as soon as the diagnosis is made)

Delayed surgery is most commonly indicated in patients whose fistulas have not healed after several (typically 4–8) weeks of comprehensive conservative treatment. Specific indications include the following:

- Continued high output from fistula after patient has been given nothing by mouth and started on parenteral nutrition (PN)
- Continued signs of infection after institution of adequate antibiotic therapy and drainage of associated abscesses
- Uncontrolled bleeding

Surgical Therapy

The surgical procedure for intestinal fistula treatment depends on the structures involved. The basic surgical principles for treatment of all intestinal fistulas include the following:

- The procedure involves resection of the intestinal segment, fistula tract, and the adjacent part of the involved structure
- In the absence of extensive infection or inflammation, primary anastomosis of the divided intestinal segments is done to reestablish GI continuity and repair of the involved structure to maintain function
- In the presence of extensive infection or inflammation, the divided intestinal segments are exteriorized and the surgical procedure is modulated to allow replacement or maximal preservation of function
- A staged procedure is performed after the infection and inflammation subsides to reestablish GI continuity and reconstruction of the affected structure

ENTEROCUTANEOUS FISTULA

34. What are the causes of enterocutaneous fistula? Classify them and give an outline of their management. ***WBUHS 2009, 2015***

35. Nutritional management in enterocutaneous fistula. ***AIIMS, Raipur 2025***

36. Discuss the guideline in management of postoperative enterocutaneous fistula. ***Tripura University 2025***

Enterocutaneous fistula is one in which there is communication between the intestinal tract and the skin.

- Enterocutaneous fistulas result from several processes:
  i. Diseased bowel extending to surrounding structures;
  ii. Extraintestinal disease involving otherwise normal bowel;
  iii. Trauma to normal bowel including inadvertent or missed enterotomies; or
  iv. Anastomotic disruption following surgery for a variety of conditions.

Causes	*Risk factors*
Inflammatory processes, such as infection or inflammatory bowel disease (most often Crohn's disease)	History of radiation
Radiation to the abdomen (most often given as part of cancer treatment)	Poor nutrition and old age
Trauma, especially penetrating wounds such as those due to a stabbing or gunshot	Malignancy

Fistulas between the alimentary tract and skin may be classified as postoperative or spontaneous.

Anatomical Classification

- *External fistulas:* Fistulas which communicate with the skin.
- *Internal fistulas:* Fistulas which communicate with intraperitoneal or intrathoracic organs.

Internal fistulas that bypass only short segments of bowel may not be symptomatic; however, internal fistulas of bowel that bypass significant length of bowel or that communicate with either the bladder or vagina typically cause symptoms and become clinically evident.

Internal fistulas may be:

- Oral, pharyngeal, and esophageal fistulas
- Gastric fistulas
- Small bowel fistulas
- Colonic fistulas

Physiologic Classification

Fistulas may be divided into:

- High output (>500 mL per day),
- Moderate output (200–500 mL/day), and
- Low output (<200 mL/day) groups.

Predictive factors for spontaneous closure and/or mortality.

Factor	*Favorable*	*Unfavorable*
Organ of origin	• Oropharyngeal • Esophageal • Duodenal stump • Pancreaticobiliary • Jejunal • Colonic	• Gastric • Lateral duodenal • Ligament of Treitz • Ileal

Contd...

Contd...

Factor	Favorable	Unfavorable
Etiology	• Postoperative • Appendicitis • Diverticulitis	• Malignancy • Inflammatory bowel disease
Output	Low (<200–500 mL/day)	High (>500 mL/day)
Nutritional status	• Well-nourished • Transferrin >200 mg/dL	• Malnourished • Transferrin <200 mg/dL
Sepsis	Absent	Present
State of bowel	• Healthy adjacent tissue • Intestinal continuity • Absence of obstruction	• Diseased adjacent bowel • Distal obstruction • Large abscess • Bowel discontinuity • Previous irradiation
Fistula characteristics	• Tract >2 cm • Bowel wall defect <1 cm^2	• Tract <1 cm • Defect >1 cm^2 • Epithelialization • Foreign body
Miscellaneous	Original operation performed at same institution	Referred from outside institution

Prevention

Proper preoperative patient preparation and meticulous surgical technique will lessen the risk of postoperative fistula formation. In the elective setting, operation may be delayed to allow for normalization of nutritional parameters, thus optimizing wound healing and immune function. Several nutritional characteristics have been suggested to increase the risk of anastomotic breakdown:

- Weight loss of 10–15% of total body weight over 3–4 months;
- Serum albumin <3 mg/dL;
- Serum transferrin <220 mg/dL;
- Anergy to recall antigens; or
- Inability to perform activities of daily living due to weakness or fatigue.

Management phases of fistula		
Phase	**Goals**	**Time course**
Recognition/stabilization	• Resuscitation with crystalloid, colloid, or blood • Control of sepsis with percutaneous or open drainage and antibiotics • Electrolyte repletion • Provision of nutrition • Control of fistula drainage • Commencement of local skin care and protection	24–48 hours
Investigation	• Fistulogram to define anatomy and characteristics of fistula • CECT is also helpful	7–10 days
Decision	• Evaluate the likelihood of spontaneous closure • Decide duration of trial of nonoperative management	10 days to 6 weeks

Contd...

Contd...

Phase	Goals	Time course
Definitive management	• Plan operative approach • Refunctionalization of entire bowel • Resection of fistula with end-to-end anastomosis • Secure abdominal closure • Gastrostomy and jejunostomy	When closure unlikely or after 4–6 weeks
Healing	• Continue nutritional support until full oral nutrition achieved • Zinc supplementation • Psychological and emotional support	5–10 days after closure until full oral nutrition

(CECT: contrast-enhanced computed tomography)

SMALL BOWEL SYNDROME

37. Write an overview of short bowel syndrome. ***WBUHS 2010, 2021***

38. What are the adaptive changes in the retained bowel in small bowel syndrome? What are the factors deciding the outcome of short bowel syndrome? Discuss the treatment of short bowel syndrome. ***WBUHS 2017***

39. What is short gut syndrome? How do you manage such patients? ***RGUHS, Karnataka 2025***

40. Define short bowel syndrome. What are its causes? How do you manage a patient with short bowel syndrome?

Short Bowel Syndrome

It is a malabsorptive state and symptom complex that follows massive small bowel resection. In adults, the normal length of the small intestine (SI) varies from 300 to 600 cm and correlates directly with body surface area. The length of combined jejunum and ileum that increases the risk for developing SBS in adults is <200 cm of functional bowel or <30% of the initial SI length with the presence of the terminal ileum. SBS may be seen with greater lengths of SI if an underlying disease, such as Crohn's or radiation enteritis, is present.

In the adult, the length of the small bowel varies from 300 to 600 cm and correlates directly with body surface area. Several factors determine the severity of SBS, including the extent of resection, the portion of the GI tract removed, the type of disease necessitating the resection, the presence of coexistent disease in the remaining bowel, and the adaptability of the remaining bowel.

Children tend to develop SBS when only 30% or less of normal SI length for age is left, and infants may survive resection of up to 85% of their bowel because of enhanced adaptation and growth.

Generally, resection resulting in <120 cm of intact bowel leads to SBS (<150 cm if ending in an ileostomy, <75 cm if colon remains). SBS may not develop until <75 cm or 1 mg/kg of SI remains.

Introduction

Infants may survive resection of up to 85% of bowel owing to the enhanced ability of the bowel to adapt and grow with the child. Because of its specialized absorptive function, resection of the ileum is usually not well tolerated. However, the entire jejunum can be resected without serious adverse nutritional sequela.

Etiology

- SBS is characterized by dehydration, electrolyte derangements, acidic diarrhea, steatorrhea, malnutrition, and weight loss.

- Congenital anomalies leading to SBS include intestinal atresia, midgut volvulus with intestinal necrosis, and necrotizing enterocolitis.
- In children, the most common etiologies for SBS include necrotizing enterocolitis, congenital intestinal atresia, midgut volvulus, and gastroschisis.
- In middle-aged adults, IBD, and trauma are the leading causes of massive intestinal resection.
- In the elderly, prominent causes include mesenteric ischemia and strangulated hernia.
- The leading causes of massive intestinal resection in adults and elderly patients are mesenteric ischemia, trauma, IBD, strangulated hernia, SI or mesenteric neoplasms, volvulus, and portal vein thrombosis.

Pathophysiology

Short bowel syndrome is characterized by diarrhea, dehydration, electrolyte disturbances, steatorrhea, malnutrition, and weight loss.

Adaptive Changes in the Small Bowel Following Extensive Resection

- Increased bowel circumference
- Increased bowel wall thickness
- Increased bowel length
- Increased villus height
- Increased crypt depth
- Increased cell proliferation and migration to villus tip

The adaptation phase has the following characteristics:

- Begins within 48 hours of resection and lasts up to 1–2 years
- Approximately 90% of the bowel adaptation takes place during this phase
- Enterocyte hyperplasia, villous hyperplasia, and increased crypt depth occur, resulting in increased surface area; intestinal dilatation and lengthening also occur
- Luminal nutrition is essential for adaptation and should be initiated as early as possible; PN is also essential throughout this period.

Adaptation

- The SI undergoes several adaptive changes in response to massive SI resection in an attempt to counteract the development of SBS.
- Structural adaptations, including greater bowel caliber, increased villus height, deeper crypts, and enhanced enterocyte proliferation and apoptosis, act to increase the absorptive surface area and nutrient transport of the bowel.
- Slower transit and increased nutrient absorption occurs through functional adaptations such as temporary hypergastrinemia, increased gastric acid secretion, slower gastric emptying (especially if colon present), substantially increased colonic absorption of water and electrolytes, and colonocyte degradation of carbohydrates into short-chain fatty acids (SCFA), which increases caloric uptake up to 50%.
- With resection of the jejunum, the distal small intestine has the greatest adaptive potential and can assume many of the absorptive properties of the proximal GI tract. Cellular hyperplasia and bowel hypertrophy occur over a 2- to 3-year period, increasing the absorptive surface area. Fat absorption is the metabolic process most likely to be permanently impaired; other functions adjust and normalize fairly well.
- *Fluid and electrolyte response:* Of the 7–10 L of fluid presented daily to the SI, only 1–2 L are delivered into the colon.
- Significant quantities of electrolytes are absorbed in this process. With SBS, this physiology is altered. Fortunately, the right colon can absorb a significant amount of the increased fluid it encounters with SBS.

Factors Determining the Outcome of Short Bowel Syndrome

- SBS has a highly variable prognosis depending on the type and extent of surgical resection. The bowel generally gains absorptive capacity with time, a process called intestinal adaptation.

- Approximately 50% of patients are able to be weaned from PN within 2 years.
- Prognosis is directly related to length of bowel and dependency on PN. The highest-risk patients are those with <50 cm of remaining bowel, those with proximal jejunostomies, and those with mesenteric thrombosis or radiation enteritis as an underlying etiology.
- Some patients have lived up to 35 years or more; 5-year survival rate in patients with no malignancy is approximately 85%.

Adults

- *Limited small bowel resection:* Patients with >100 cm of residual bowel and an intact small bowel-colonic anastomosis have an excellent prognosis. Intestinal adaptation and dietary instruction allows these patients to eventually live normal lives with relatively little morbidity or mortality.
- *Terminal ileum resection:* Intestinal adaptation cannot replace the terminal ileum's role in bile salt and vitamin B_{12} absorption. While prognosis is still excellent, lifelong management of bile salt and vitamin malabsorption is required.
- *Extensive bowel resection:* Weaning from PN is more difficult in patients with 100 cm or less of residual small bowel, particularly in those who lack a colon or colonic anastomosis.
- *Intestinal transplantation:* Mortality and morbidity rates are significant, but are improving due to an increase in surgical experience and improved immunosuppression regimens. Short-term survival approaches 90% (similar to liver transplantation), but 5-year survival is closer to 50%. The prognosis becomes much worse if patients remain PN dependent.

Children

Children usually acquire SBS because of a congenital abnormality or a catastrophic event such as midgut volvulus. It remains one of the most morbid conditions of infancy and childhood, with survival rates from 73 to 89%. Younger children may have a more adaptable intestine than adults; there are anecdotal reports of children living independent of PN with as little as 10 cm of residual small intestine. However, if children become dependent on PN, the risk of liver failure is much greater than in adults.

Treatment

- Nutritional support
- Medications
- Surgery
- Intestinal transplant

Malabsorption and Malnutrition

- *Gastric hypersecretion:* It is seen early in the postoperative period and can persist for prolonged periods. Increased acid load may injure distal bowel mucosa, leading to hypermotility and impaired absorption. The severity of hypersecretion correlates directly with the extent of bowel resection. This generally is more pronounced after jejunal than after ileal resection. Loss of an intestinal inhibitory hormone has been implicated.
- *Cholelithiasis:* Altered bilirubin metabolism after ileal resection increases the risk of gallstones secondary to a decreased bile salt pool, which causes a shift in the cholesterol saturation index. Chronic TPN also increases risk of cholelithiasis.
- *Hyperoxaluria and nephrolithiasis:* Excessive fatty acids within the colonic lumen bind intraluminal calcium. Unbound oxalate, normally made insoluble by calcium binding and excreted in the feces, thus is absorbed readily, resulting in hyperoxaluria and calcium oxalate urinary stone formation.
- *Diarrhea and steatorrhea:* Rapid intestinal transit, presence of hyperosmolar enteric contents in the distal bowel, disruption of the enterohepatic bile acid circulation, and bacterial overgrowth all promote diarrhea and steatorrhea. Fat absorption is most severely impaired by ileal resection. The delivery of bile acids into the colon produces a reactive watery diarrhea that may be severe. Unabsorbed fats in the colon further inhibit absorption and stimulate secretion of water and electrolytes.

- *Intestinal microflora:* Loss of the ileocecal valve permits reflux of colonic bacteria into the small bowel. Intestinal dysmotility further promotes bacterial colonization. Bacterial overgrowth and changes in the indigenous microbial population result in pH alteration and deconjugation of bile salts, with resultant malabsorption, fluid loss, and decreased vitamin B_{12} absorption. Infectious diarrhea (bacterial or viral) is a major cause of morbidity.

Acute Phase Treatment

- The primary goal in the acute phase (initial 4 weeks) is to stabilize the metabolic, respiratory, and cardiovascular parameters related to the fluid shifts and sepsis that frequently accompany massive small bowel resection. TPN, strict intake and output records, and close monitoring of serum electrolytes are critical in the early management of patients with SBS.
- Prolonged ileus may result from deranged motility patterns and changes in intraluminal milieu. PN should be provided until GI function resumes. If the ileus is unusually persistent, underlying mechanical obstruction or sepsis should be suspected and investigated.
- Gastric hypersecretion requires H_2-receptor antagonists or proton-pump inhibitors to reduce the hypersecretory response and protect against peptic ulceration. Antacids take effect immediately and should be administered routinely in patients with SBS.
- Nutritional support should be instituted early to maintain a positive nitrogen balance and to promote wound healing and adaptation of the remaining bowel. Enteral nutrition has a positive trophic effect on the bowel mucosa, stimulates the remaining intestine, and should be started as soon as possible, even if caloric goals are not met. Initial feeds should be gradual, continuous low volume, low fat, and isosmotic. Isotonic salt-glucose solutions are useful.

Maintenance Phase Treatment

Maintenance therapy in SBS focuses on long-term nutritional goals, support of adaptation that takes place over the first 1–2 years, and addressing various clinical issues that arise.

- Nutritional support with supplemental vitamins, trace elements and minerals (zinc, selenium, and iron), and essential fatty acids (linoleic acid) should be given parenterally until adequate enteral absorption is achieved.
- Absorption of the fat-soluble vitamins A, D, E, and K is especially prone to compromise. Vitamin B_{12} and calcium uptake are also affected by altered fat absorption and should be supplemented.
- Potassium and magnesium losses should be closely monitored as well.
- Growth hormone and glutamine have been used with some success to treat inadequate adaptation and TPN dependence.
- Diarrhea is often multifactorial in SBS, and dietary modifications can improve symptoms. H_2-receptor blockers reduce gastric acid production and secretory volume. Chelating resins like cholestyramine reduce intraluminal bile salts and resultant diarrhea but affect the systemic bile salt pool.
- Antisecretory medications, such as loperamide or somatostatin analogs, may be beneficial, although octreotide can inhibit the adaptation. Low-dose narcotics [diphenoxylate hydrochloride and atropine (Lomotil), codeine, or tincture of opium] are efficacious but addictive.
- Bacterial overgrowth should be evaluated by stool culture and antimicrobials, such as metronidazole or tetracycline, administered as needed.
- Late complications are common and include nephrolithiasis, cholelithiasis, nutritional deficiencies (e.g., anemia, bone disease, and coagulopathy), liver dysfunction, TPN-related difficulties, and central venous catheter-related issues like thrombosis or sepsis.
- Anastomotic leaks, fistulas, strictures, and late bowel obstructions can also occur well beyond the early postoperative period and commonly require reoperation.

Chronic Treatment

- Diarrhea has many causes in SBS. Frequently, dietary modification improves symptoms. H_2-receptor antagonists reduce acid production and the volume of enteric contents. Chelating resins, such as cholestyramine, reduce intraluminal bile salts, and subsequent diarrhea but affect the available systemic bile salt pools.
- Antisecretory medications, such as loperamide and somatostatin analog, may be beneficial.
- Low-dose oral narcotics, such as diphenoxylate hydrochloride and atropine (Lomotil) or codeine, are efficacious but addictive.
- Bacterial overgrowth should be evaluated by stool culture and prophylactic antimicrobials administered as needed.
- Nutritional support with supplemental vitamins, trace elements and minerals, and essential fatty acids should be given parenterally until adequate enteral absorption is established.
- The absorption of fat-soluble vitamins A, D, E, and K is especially likely to be compromised. Vitamin B12 and calcium absorption are also affected by altered fat absorption and should be supplemented.
- If required, chronic TPN can be administered nightly to permit normal daytime activities.

Late complications, mostly secondary to metabolic derangements, are common. Problems include nephrolithiasis, cholelithiasis, nutritional deficiency (e.g., anemia, bone disease, and coagulopathy), liver dysfunction, TPN-related complications, and central venous catheter–related problems, e.g., sepsis or thrombosis. Anastomotic leak, fistula, stricture, and obstruction can also occur well beyond the early postoperative period. Late obstruction (partial or complete) is fairly common, and reoperative rates are high.

Medical Therapy of Short Bowel Syndrome

Standard management	
Clinical issue	***Medical therapy***
Hypergastrinemia/gastric hypersecretion	H_2 blocker or proton pump inhibitor
Diarrhea	• *First line of therapy:* Loperamide and diphenoxylate • *Second line of therapy:* Codeine and DTO • Avoid octreotide
Bile salt-induced diarrhea	Cholestyramine (if colon is in continuity and <100 cm ileum)
Electrolyte losses (e.g., K^+, Mg^{++}, and Ca^{++})	Replete as needed (may need to give IV if increase in diarrhea with oral repletion)
Vitamin deficiency (e.g., A, D, E, K, and B_{12})	• Monitor and replete as necessary; may require chronic administration • Liquid vitamins may be better absorbed than pill form
Mineral deficiency (e.g., zinc, selenium, and iron)	• Monitor and replete as necessary; may require chronic administration • Liquid minerals (in a combined multivitamin/mineral preparation) may be better absorbed than pill form
	Specialized treatment
Bacterial overgrowth	Metronidazole and tetracycline
Large electrolyte and fluid loss not controlled with standard management	Octreotide
Inadequate adaptive response and TPN dependence despite standard management	Consider growth hormone and glutamine

(DTO: deodorized tincture of opium; IV: intravenous; TPN: total parenteral nutrition)

Recommended Diet for Short Bowel Syndrome

Standard management		
	Colon in continuity	*No colon in continuity*
Protein	20–30% of caloric intake	20–30% of caloric intake
Fat	20–30% of caloric intake	30–40% of caloric intake
Carbohydrate	50–60% of caloric intake	30–40% of caloric intake
Fluid	Isotonic or hypoosmolar	Isotonic and high-sodium oral rehydration solution
Oxalate	Restrict intake	No restrictions
Specialized treatment		
	Colon in continuity	No colon in continuity
Soluble fiber	5–10 g/day if stool output >3 L	5–10 g/day if stool output >3 L

Surgical Therapy

- Various surgical procedures have been described for the management of SBS, but have not been widely adopted. The most commonly used intestinal lengthening procedures for patients with SBS are serial transverse enteroplasty (STEP) and the Bianchi procedure that similarly have been shown to decrease TPN dependence, increase oral caloric intake, and reverse liver disease.
- The Bianchi isolates the dual blood supply of the SI by separating the mesenteric borders, longitudinally divides the intestine, and creates an isoperistaltic end-to-end, hand-sewn anastomosis.
- Isolated small bowel transplants or multivisceral transplantations (including the liver for patients with severe cholestatic cirrhosis from chronic TPN) are additional options for SBS. Prevention of complications and minimizing the extent of initial bowel resection that lead to SBS is extremely important.
- Intestinal transplantation has improved with the introduction of the new immunosuppressive agent tacrolimus (FK506). Intestinal transplantation procedures have included primarily isolated small intestinal grafts and combined liver–small intestinal grafts with a few more extensive cluster grafts in a large series reported from the International Intestinal Transplant Registry.
- An alternative to intestinal transplantation is mucosal stem cell transplantation, which involves transplanting enterocytes onto a biomatrix and achieving regeneration of intestinal mucosa. This procedure is, at best, preliminary but has shown some promise in experimental studies.

One has to Tailor Treatment to the Severity of the Patient's Disease

- Treatment for mild SBS involves eating small, frequent meals; drinking fluid; taking nutritional supplements; and using medications to treat diarrhea.
- Treatment for moderate SBS is similar to that for mild SBS, with the addition of PN as needed.
- Treatment for severe SBS involves use of PN and oral rehydration solutions. Patients may receive enteral nutrition or continue normal eating, even though most of the nutrients are not absorbed. Both enteral nutrition and normal eating stimulate the remaining intestine to work better and may allow patients to discontinue PN.
- Some patients with severe SBS require PN indefinitely or surgery.

41. Pathophysiology of short bowel syndrome. ***WBUHS 2015***

Physiologic derangements in SBS are the result of the loss of large amounts of intestinal absorptive surface area. The sequelae of this loss include malabsorption of water, electrolytes, macronutrients (i.e., proteins, carbohydrates, and fats), and micronutrients (i.e., vitamins, minerals, and trace elements).

- The GI tract is a vital locus for water and electrolyte absorption and transport. In addition to managing exogenously obtained sources of these nutrients, such as daily water intake and the electrolytes found in liquid and solid foods, the GI tract must deal with its own considerable daily secretions.

- GI tract processes 8,000–9,000 mL of fluid per day, with the vast majority of this derived from endogenous secretions. Fluid reabsorption by the healthy GI tract is efficient (98%), and only 100–200 mL are lost in fecal matter each day. The great majority (80%) of this reabsorption occurs in the small intestine.
- Disturbances in the major determinants of intestinal fluid absorption negatively impact the ability to reabsorb this large fluid load. The major determinants include intestinal mucosal surface area, the health or integrity of the mucosa, the status of small bowel motility, and the osmolarity of solutes in the intestinal lumen.
- Clinically, these disturbances can manifest as major components of SBS, namely diarrhea, dehydration, and electrolyte imbalance. Thus, SBS can be produced by clinical entities that result in critical loss of mucosal surface area (e.g., massive small bowel resection) or degrade mucosal integrity (e.g., radiation enteritis).
- Macronutrients and micronutrients are absorbed along the length of the small intestine. However, the jejunum has taller villi, deeper crypts, and greater enzyme activity than the ileum. Therefore, under normal conditions, about 90% of digestion and absorption of significant macronutrients and micronutrients are accomplished in the proximal 100–150 cm of the jejunum. This includes absorption of proteins; carbohydrates; fats; vitamins B, C, and folic acid; and the fat-soluble vitamins A, D, E, and K.
- However, if a significant portion or all of the jejunum is resected, the absorption of proteins, carbohydrates, and most vitamins and minerals can be unaffected because of adaptation in the ileum. Unfortunately, enzymatic digestion suffers because of the irreplaceable loss of enteric hormones produced by the jejunum. Biliary and pancreatic secretions decrease. Gastrin levels rise, causing gastric hypersecretion. The resultant high acid output from the stomach may injure the small bowel mucosa.
- Additionally, the low intraluminal pH creates unfavorable conditions for optimal activity of the pancreatic enzymes that are present. Diarrhea may then result if a large osmotically active solute load of unabsorbed nutrients is delivered to the ileum and colon.
- Ileal resection severely decreases the capacity to absorb water and electrolytes. In addition, the terminal ileum is the site of absorption of bile salts and vitamin B_{12}. Loss of significant lengths of ileum almost invariably results in diarrhea. Continued loss of bile salts following resection of the terminal ileum leads to fat malabsorption, steatorrhea, and loss of fat-soluble vitamins.
- Retention of the ileocecal valve plays a pivotal role in massive small bowel resection. If the ileocecal valve can be preserved, intestinal transit is slowed, allowing more time for absorption. If the ileocecal valve is lost, transit time is faster, and loss of fluid and nutrients is greater. Furthermore, colonic bacteria can colonize the small bowel, worsening diarrhea and nutrient loss.
- Preservation of the colon has positive and negative attributes. Philips and Giller demonstrated that colonic water absorption could be increased to as much as five times its normal capacity following small bowel resection.
- Also, by virtue of its resident bacteria, the colon has the inherent capacity to metabolize undigested carbohydrates into short-chain fatty acids, such as butyrate, propionate, and acetate. These are a preferred fuel source for the colon. Interestingly, work by Pomare and colleagues and Halverstad demonstrated that the colon can absorb up to 500 kcal daily of these metabolites, which then can be transported via the portal vein to be used as a somatic fuel source.
- In contrast, maintenance of the colon increases the incidence of urinary calcium oxalate stone formation. Oxalate is normally bound by calcium in the small bowel and thus is insoluble when it reaches the colon. After massive enterectomy, much of this calcium is bound by free intraluminal fats. Free oxalate is delivered to the colon, where it is absorbed. This can eventually lead to saturation of the urine with calcium oxalate crystals and result in stone formation. Retention of the colon in the absence of a competent ileocecal valve can lead to small intestinal bacterial overgrowth.

The physiologic changes and adaptation of patients with SBS can be viewed in three phases.

1. The acute phase occurs immediately after massive bowel resection and may last up to 3–4 months. It is associated with malnutrition and fluid and electrolyte loss through the GI tract. Fluid and electrolyte loss through the GI tract may be as high as 6–8 L/day. Patients will have abnormal LFT results and transient hyperbilirubinemia.

Enteral feedings may also be initiated, but it should be relatively slow. Patients with <100 cm of small intestine will require TPN. The presence of ileocecal valve or colon may play a significant role in the outcome of these patients.

2. The adaptation phase generally begins 2–4 days after bowel resection and may last up to 12–18 months. During this second phase, up to 90% of the bowel adaptation may occur. Villous hyperplasia, increased crypt depth, and intestinal dilatation occur. Early continuous feedings with a high viscosity elemental diet may reduce the duration of TPN.
3. In the maintenance phase, the absorptive capacity of the GI tract is at its maximum. Some patients may still require TPN. In other patients, nutritional and metabolic homeostasis can be achieved by small meals and supplemental nutritional support for life. These patients will also require vitamins and mineral supplements, including vitamins A, B_{12}, and D, magnesium, and zinc.

To summarize, the acute phase has the following characteristics:

- Starts immediately after bowel resection and lasts 1–3 months
- Ostomy output of >5 L/day
- Life-threatening dehydration and electrolyte imbalances
- Extremely poor absorption of all nutrients
- Development of hypergastrinemia and hyperbilirubinemia

The adaptation phase has the following characteristics:

- Begins within 48 hours of resection and lasts up to 1–2 years
- Approximately 90% of the bowel adaptation takes place during this phase
- Enterocyte hyperplasia, villous hyperplasia, and increased crypt depth occur, resulting in increased surface area; intestinal dilatation; and lengthening also occur
- Luminal nutrition is essential for adaptation and should be initiated as early as possible; PN is also essential throughout this period

The maintenance phase has the following characteristics:

- The absorptive capacity of the intestine is at its maximum
- Nutritional and metabolic homeostasis can be achieved by oral feeding, or patients are committed to receiving supplemental or complete nutritional support for life.

---

42. Complications of short bowel syndrome. Role of intestinal transplant in short bowel syndrome.

WBUHS 2021 Supplementary

Complications of Short Bowel Syndrome

- *Gastric hypersecretion:* It is seen early in the postoperative period and can persist for prolonged periods. Increased acid load may injure distal bowel mucosa, leading to hypermotility and impaired absorption. The severity of hypersecretion correlates directly with the extent of bowel resection. This generally is more pronounced after jejunal than after ileal resection. Loss of an intestinal inhibitory hormone has been implicated.
- *Cholelithiasis:* Altered bilirubin metabolism after ileal resection increases the risk of gallstones secondary to a decreased bile salt pool, which causes a shift in the cholesterol saturation index. Chronic TPN also increases risk of cholelithiasis.
- *Hyperoxaluria and nephrolithiasis:* Excessive fatty acids within the colonic lumen bind intraluminal calcium. Unbound oxalate, normally made insoluble by calcium binding and excreted in the feces, thus is absorbed readily, resulting in hyperoxaluria and calcium oxalate urinary stone formation.
- *Diarrhea and steatorrhea:* Rapid intestinal transit, presence of hyperosmolar enteric contents in the distal bowel, disruption of the enterohepatic bile acid circulation, and bacterial overgrowth all promote diarrhea and steatorrhea. Fat absorption is most severely impaired by ileal resection. The delivery of bile acids into the colon

produces a reactive watery diarrhea that may be severe. Unabsorbed fats in the colon further inhibit absorption and stimulate secretion of water and electrolytes.

- *Intestinal microflora:* Loss of the ileocecal valve permits reflux of colonic bacteria into the small bowel. Intestinal dysmotility further promotes bacterial colonization. Bacterial overgrowth and changes in the indigenous microbial population result in pH alteration and deconjugation of bile salts, with resultant malabsorption, fluid loss, and decreased vitamin B_{12} absorption. Infectious diarrhea (bacterial or viral) is a major cause of morbidity.

Intestinal transplantation has improved with the introduction of the new immunosuppressive agent tacrolimus (FK506). Intestinal transplantation procedures have included primarily isolated small intestinal grafts and combined liver–small intestinal grafts with a few more extensive cluster grafts in a large series reported from the International Intestinal Transplant Registry.

An alternative to intestinal transplantation is mucosal stem cell transplantation, which involves trans- planting enterocytes onto a biomatrix and achieving regeneration of intestinal mucosa. This procedure is, at best, preliminary but has shown some promise in experimental studies.

Indications for Intestinal Transplantation in Small Bowel Syndrome

- Severe SBS [gastrostomy, duodenostomy, and residual small bowel (<10 cm in infants and <20 cm in adults)]
- Intestinal failure with frequent hospitalizations, narcotic dependency, or pseudo-obstruction Intestine transplantation may be performed in isolation, with liver transplant, or as part of a multivisceral transplant including any combination of liver, stomach, pancreas, and/or colon. There are notable differences in patient and transplant outcomes for intestine transplants with and without liver.

Intestinal transplantation should be recommended for patients on TPN with associated problems as follows:

- Impending or overt liver failure secondary to intestinal failure-associated liver disease (IFALD)
- Thrombosis of two or more central veins
- Two or more episodes per year of systemic sepsis secondary to line infections, or a single episode of fungal sepsis
- Frequent episodes of severe dehydration

Additional indications for intestinal transplantation include the following:

- Severe SBS [gastrostomy, duodenostomy, and residual small bowel (<10 cm in infants and <20 cm in adults)]
- Intestinal failure with frequent hospitalizations, narcotic dependency, or pseudo-obstruction Patient unwillingness or inability to resume long-term PN.
- In highly selected patients, multivisceral organ transplantation may have a role in the treatment of slow-growing abdominal cancers that are deemed nonresectable.

43. Mention the biochemical, immunological, and nutritional derangements in short bowel syndrome.
WBUHS 2018

Metabolic Changes in Short Bowel Syndrome

- SBS is characterized by dehydration, electrolyte derangements, acidic diarrhea, steatorrhea, malnutrition, and weight loss.
- Congenital anomalies leading to SBS include intestinal atresia, midgut volvulus with intestinal necrosis, and necrotizing enterocolitis.
- In middle-aged adults, IBD and trauma are the leading causes of massive intestinal resection.
- In the elderly, prominent causes include mesenteric ischemia and strangulated hernia.

Adaptation

The distal small intestine has the greatest adaptive potential and can assume many of the absorptive properties of the proximal GI tract. Cellular hyperplasia and bowel hypertrophy occur over a 2- to 3-year period, increasing the absorptive surface area. Fat absorption is the metabolic process most likely to be permanently impaired; other functions adjust and normalize fairly well. Fluid and electrolyte response. Of the 8–10 L of fluid presented daily to the small intestine, only 1–2 L are delivered into the colon. Significant quantities of electrolytes are absorbed in this process. With SBS, this physiology is altered. Strict intake and output records and close monitoring of serum electrolytes are critical in the early management of patients with SBS.

Malabsorption and Malnutrition

- *Gastric hypersecretion:* It is seen early in the postoperative period and can persist for prolonged periods. Increased acid load may injure distal bowel mucosa, leading to hypermotility and impaired absorption. The severity of hypersecretion correlates directly with the extent of bowel resection. This generally is more pronounced after jejunal than after ileal resection. Loss of an intestinal inhibitory hormone has been implicated.
- *Cholelithiasis:* Altered bilirubin metabolism after ileal resection increases the risk of gallstones secondary to a decreased bile salt pool, which causes a shift in the cholesterol saturation index. Chronic TPN also increases risk of cholelithiasis.
- *Hyperoxaluria and nephrolithiasis:* Excessive fatty acids within the colonic lumen bind intraluminal calcium. Unbound oxalate, normally made insoluble by calcium binding and excreted in the feces, thus is absorbed readily, resulting in hyperoxaluria and calcium oxalate urinary stone formation.
- *Diarrhea and steatorrhea:* Rapid intestinal transit, presence of hyperosmolar enteric contents in the distal bowel, disruption of the enterohepatic bile acid circulation, and bacterial overgrowth all promote diarrhea and steatorrhea. Fat absorption is most severely impaired by ileal resection. The delivery of bile acids into the colon produces a reactive watery diarrhea that may be severe. Unabsorbed fats in the colon further inhibit absorption and stimulate secretion of water and electrolytes.
- *Intestinal microflora*: Loss of the ileocecal valve permits reflux of colonic bacteria into the small bowel. Intestinal dysmotility further promotes bacterial colonization. Bacterial overgrowth and changes in the indigenous microbial population result in pH alteration and deconjugation of bile salts, with resultant malabsorption, fluid loss, and decreased vitamin B_{12} absorption. Infectious diarrhea (bacterial or viral) is a major cause of morbidity.

INTESTINAL FAILURE

44. Define intestinal failure. What are the types of intestinal failure? Describe their causes and outline management. ***WBUHS 2015, 2019***

45. Recent advances in the management of type 3 intestinal failure. ***WBUHS 2019***

46. What is type 3 intestinal failure? Discuss the management policy. ***WBUHS 2016***

Introduction

Intestinal failure occurs when a person's intestines cannot digest food and absorb the fluids, electrolytes and nutrients essential to life and normal development. Patients must then receive TPN, which provides liquid nutrition through a catheter or needle inserted into a vein in the arm, groin, neck, or chest.

Definition of Intestinal Failure

The term intestinal failure encompasses multiple days of inadequate GIT length/function that prevent adequate nutrient absorption. SBS refers to loss of bowel length usually >75%.

It results from obstruction, dysmotility, surgical resection, congenital defect, and loss of absorption.

Types—Hope Hospital Classification

- Type I
- Type II
- Type III

Type I

- Short-term
- Common
- *Causes:*
  - Acute intestinal inflammation—IBD, RT, and CT
  - Ileus—postoperative (MC), trauma, sepsis, acute pancreatitis, pancreatitis, and multiple organ dysfunction syndrome (MODS)
  - Intestinal obstruction/pseudo-obstruction
- Self-limiting
- Nutritional support <14 days

Type II

- Weeks–months (>28 days)
- After major bowel resection
- Associated with sepsis, nutritional, and metabolic complications
- Require PN

Type III

- Long-term >6 months
- MC causes SBS
- Irreversible
- Home PN
- Candidate for autologous reconstruction or transplant

Types: Intestinal failure can be categorized into three types:

1. *Type 1:* This type of intestinal failure is short term, self-limiting, and often perioperative in nature. This type is common and these patients are managed successfully in a multitude of healthcare settings, especially surgical wards, including all units which perform major, particularly abdominal surgery. Some patients on high-dependency units (HDUs) or intensive care units (ICUs) will also fall into this category.
2. *Type 2:* This occurs in metabolically unstable patients in hospital and requires prolonged PN over periods of weeks or months. It is often associated with sepsis, and may be associated with renal impairment. These patients often need the facilities of an intensive care or HDU for some or much of their stay in hospital. This type of intestinal failure is rare and needs to be managed by a multiprofessional specialist intestinal failure team. Poor management of type 2 intestinal failure increases mortality and is expected to increase the likelihood of later development of type 3 intestinal failure.
3. *Type 3:* This is a chronic condition requiring long term parenteral feeding. The patient is characteristically metabolically stable but cannot maintain his or her nutrition adequately by absorbing food or nutrients via the intestinal tract. These are, in the main, the group of patients for which HPN or electrolyte (HPE) are indicated.

Causes of Intestinal Failure

The most common cause of intestinal failure is SBS where at least half or more of the small intestine has been removed. SBS is typically a postsurgical condition for treatment of conditions such as trauma or necrotizing enterocolitis.

Pediatric versus Adult Causes

Intestinal failure may also be caused by functional disorders such as CD, a digestive disorder, or chronic idiopathic intestinal pseudo-obstruction syndrome. The conditions leading to intestinal failure are age-dependent. That is, some conditions are more closely associated with pediatric intestinal failure while others are more common with intestinal failure in adults.

- *Pediatric conditions causing intestinal failure:*
  - Congenital malformations such as small bowel atresia, gastroschisis, and aganglionosis

- Infections of the gastrointestinal tract such as necrotizing enterocolitis
- SBS following extensive bowel surgeries secondary to mesenteric ischemia (e.g., midgut volvulus)
- Absorptive impairment (e.g., intestinal pseudo-obstruction, and microvillus inclusion disease)

- *Adult conditions causing intestinal failure:*
  - SBS following extensive surgeries secondary to mesenteric ischemia (following thrombosis, embolism, volvulus, or trauma)
  - IBD such as CD
  - Small bowel tumors such as Gardner's syndrome (familial colorectal polyposis)
  - Tumors of the mesenteric root and retroperitoneum (desmoid tumor)

Treatment

- The clinical features of intestinal failure include intractable diarrhea or a high-output stoma, weight loss, dehydration, vitamin and mineral deficiency, and malnutrition.
- Acute intestinal failure is usually temporary and often attributable to infection or perioperative complications.
- Chronic intestinal failure results from intestinal resection(s), gastrointestinal disease, or small bowel dysfunction.

Management

- Specific management depends on the amount, type, and integrity of the remaining bowel, as the presence of even part of the large bowel can significantly increase absorption.
- The aim is to maximize gastrointestinal function and, where necessary, supplement fluid and nutrient intake by the least invasive means, thus providing the individual with the best possible quality of life.

Maximizing Gastrointestinal Function

- There are a number of sites in the gastrointestinal tract that affect the rate of gastric emptying and thus influence gastrointestinal motility.
- These sites (or brakes) occur in the stomach, the proximal small bowel, the distal small bowel, and the colon and rectum.
- Absence of any or all of these sites will lead to decreased intestinal transit time, high intestinal fluid loss and reduced absorption of fluid and nutrients. (Intestinal transit time refers to the time that food and fluids remain in the gastrointestinal tract).
- Increasing intestinal transit time is therefore an important consideration in optimizing gastrointestinal function as it will increase fluid and nutrient absorption and decrease intestinal losses.
- Medication antidiarrheal medications such as loperamide and codeine phosphate are commonly used to reduce motility and enhance absorption.
- To maximize their effectiveness they should be taken half an hour before food. An additional dose before bedtime can be of enormous psychological benefit by reducing the fear of incontinence or leakage from a stoma.
- Antisecretory medications such as histamine 2 (H_2)-receptor antagonists or proton pump inhibitors can lead to a reduction in output from the gastrointestinal tract by reducing the secretion of gastric acid.
- Large doses of both antidiarrheal and antisecretory medications may be necessary to compensate for the decreased intestinal transit time and impaired absorption.

Nutritional Support in Intestinal Failure

- Reducing the intake of hypotonic fluids is arguably the most important intervention in maximizing gastrointestinal function is to reduce the amount of hypotonic fluid (such as water, tea, coffee, and squash) entering the intestine, as this will significantly reduce the amount of fluid the intestine has to assimilate.
- The sodium concentration in the jejunum is maintained at 90 mmol/L. Drinking hypotonic fluid dilutes the sodium concentration causing a net efflux of sodium from the plasma in order to restore the concentration to 90 mmol/L.
- *Facilitating small bowel adaptation:* A final consideration in maximizing intestinal function is facilitating small bowel adaptation. Following intestinal resection the remaining bowel undergoes structural and functional

changes. The small bowel dilates and lengthens and there is a reduction in motility. These changes result in increased intestinal function. The controlling mechanisms behind adaptation are not yet fully understood, but it is believed that the presence of nutrients within the intestine is an important factor.

- Patients with intestinal failure are encouraged to eat for a number of reasons. In addition to being important in small bowel adaptation, the presence of nutrients within the intestine is also important in maintaining normal gastrointestinal flora and the gut barrier function, e.g., preventing infection factors that can impact on intestinal function.
- *Supplementing fluid/nutrient intake:* The small intestine transports between 7 and 9 L of fluid a day, absorbing about 80% of this so that only about 1–2 L enters the colon.
- The colon absorbs fluid, so that only 100–200 mL is actually excreted each day. Although there will be alteration in fluid and nutrient absorption in all patients with intestinal failure, the most significant will occur in those in whom there has been a significant loss of intestine.
- A reduction in absorptive area, such as in someone with a proximal small bowel stoma or ECF, will result in a greater volume of fluid excreted and subsequent fluid and electrolyte imbalance and a degree of malabsorption.
- The need for fluid and nutrient replacement is determined by a number of factors, namely, the amount of available intestine, the volume of daily intestinal losses, and the ability to maintain a satisfactory weight. Individuals with <75 cm of jejunum, an intestinal output of >2,500 mL/day, and absorption below about one-third of all energy taken orally will usually be dependent on long-term PN.
- Those with 75–100 cm of jejunum, and average daily outputs of about 1,200–2,500 mL/day, may require parenteral supplementation of fluid while being able to maintain their nutritional status with an enteral regime including food and/or supplemental enteral nutrition.
- While long-term parenteral supplementation of fluids and nutrients will help prevent dehydration and malnutrition, it imposes restrictions on an individual's daily life. Large fluid volumes usually mean infusion times of at least 12 hours, and while cyclical infusion overnight permits freedom from the infusion pump during the day, the patient may suffer disrupted sleep due to the need to pass urine frequently during the night.
- It is important to note that even though a patient may be dependent on PN or fluid, this does not mean that other aspects of their treatment regimen can be relaxed. Fluid and nutrient needs are determined by a patient's average daily fluid balance and if there is a significant shift in this, e.g., by drinking excessive amounts of hypotonic fluid or not taking medication, they will still become dehydrated.

New Therapeutic Agents

- Growth hormone has received approval from the US Food and Drug Administration (FDA) for the management of SBS. Various treatment strategies with growth hormone and other agents are being tried in patients with SBS. In one randomized controlled trial, a combination of an adequate diet plus growth hormone plus glutamine produced results that were superior to dietary therapy alone.
- Another hormone, GLP-2, may have a role in stimulating intestinal mucosal adaptation in patients with SBS, although its mechanism of action is not completely clear. This agent is now undergoing evaluation in a phase 3 trial.

Intestinal Failure and Transplantation

- An intestinal transplant is a last-resort treatment option for patients with intestinal failure who develop life-threatening complications from TPN. Long-term TPN can result in complications including bone disorders, catheter-related infections, and liver failure. Over an extended period of time, TPN also can damage veins used to administer the nutrition via the catheter.
- An intestinal transplant is a complex procedure requiring a highly skilled multidisciplinary transplant team. An isolated intestinal transplant surgery takes approximately 3–4 hours to complete whereas a multivisceral (multiorgan) transplant operation can take up to 12 hours.

There are three major types of intestinal transplants:

1. *Isolated intestinal (small bowel) transplantation:*
   - In an isolated intestinal transplant, the diseased portion of the small intestine is removed and replaced with a healthy small intestine from a donor.
   - In an isolated intestinal transplant, the disease limited to the small bowel only without liver failure.
   - This procedure can be lifesaving for patients with irreversible intestinal failure that has become life-threatening.
2. *Combined liver and intestinal transplantation:*
   - Combined liver and intestine transplantation is done for patients with both liver and intestinal failure.
   - In this procedure, the diseased liver and intestine are removed and replaced with a healthy liver and intestine from an organ donor.
   - Complications of intravenous nutrition (TPN) are the main cause of liver failure attendant to intestinal failure.
   - Without a transplant, patients with intestinal and liver failure have an expected median survival of 6–12 months while continued on TPN.
3. *Multivisceral transplantation:*
   - Multivisceral transplantation is performed where two or more intra-abdominal organs (including the intestines) are failing.
   - The transplanted organs may include the stomach, duodenum, pancreas, intestine, and liver.
   - This complex procedure can be life-saving for patients with combined abdominal organ failure resulting diseases such as Gardner's syndrome (familial colorectal polyposis), a premalignant colorectal condition and intestinal pseudo-obstruction (decreased ability of the intestines to push food through).

Evaluation for Intestinal Transplantation

During the evaluation process, a detailed medical history is taken and numerous studies (tests) are performed to determine whether an intestinal transplant is likely to benefit the patient including:

- Abdominal CT scan
- Barium enema
- Blood tests for liver function, electrolytes, kidney function, and antibodies to certain viruses
- Colonoscopy
- Electrocardiogram (ECG) and echocardiogram
- Endoscopy
- Motility studies
- Ultrasound of the circulatory system
- Upper gastrointestinal and small bowel X-ray series

Intestinal Transplant Procedure

In an Intestinal transplant, the small intestine (small bowel) is surgically removed (along with any other diseased organs such as the liver), and replaced with healthy organ(s). Initially, the blood vessels of the patient and donor are connected to establish a blood supply to the transplanted intestine. The donor's intestine is then connected to the patient's gastrointestinal tract.

An ileostomy is then performed. An ileostomy is a surgically created opening through which the ileum, a section of the patient's small intestine, is brought up through the abdominal wall. This opening allows body waste to pass directly out of the body and empty into a pouch. The ileostomy also allows the transplant team to assess the health of the patient's transplanted intestine. In time, most patients are able to have the ileostomy closed. A feeding tube is also placed into the stomach to help the patient transition to an oral diet.

Management of Type 3 Intestinal Failure

- Aim—maintain adequate nutrition, fluid electrolyte balance—PN
- Mortality more with >60 years, <50 cm bowel, and jejunostomy

Type of SBS	Length of remnant bowel
1 (jejunostomy)	<100–150 cm
2 (jejunocolic)	<60 cm
3 (jejunoileocolic)	<35 cm

(SBS: short bowel syndrome)

Medical Options

GLP-2 Analogs

- Teduglutide—improve intestinal adaptation and absorption
  - Crypt proliferation
  - Villous height
  - Expression of glucose transporter

Surgical Options

Autologous Reconstruction

Autologous GI reconstruction (AUGIR) aims to optimize absorptive surface and function of residual bowel.

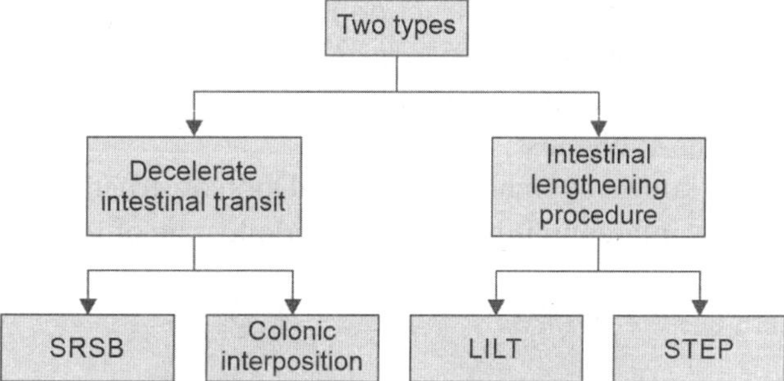

- Segmental reversal of small bowel (SRSB) a segment of 10–12 cm of jejunum is reversed and reanastomosed
- Longitudinal intestinal lengthening and tailoring (LILT)—intestine divided longitudinally, 2 halves refashioned in tubes, and anastomosed
- Serial transverse enteroplasty (STEP) serial transverse division of intestine on alternate sides

Small Bowel Transplantation

Radical treatment is the last option.

Indications

- Hepatic failure secondary to PN
- Thrombosis >2 central veins
- Frequent severe dehydration despite intravenous fluid
- Single episode of septic shock/acute respiratory distress syndrome (ARDS)

Graft-Cadaveric Donors

Types:

- Isolated intestinal transplant
- Combined liver and intestinal transplant
- Multivisceral transplant (SI, stomach, spleen, and liver)
- Modified multivisceral transplant that exclude liver

Survival rate:

- 1 year—80%
- 5 years—60%

Intestinal tissue engineering:
- Acellular dermal matrix
- Small intestinal submucosa

ACUTE INTESTINAL OBSTRUCTION

47. Closed loop obstruction. ***WBUHS 2008***

48. Discuss the causes, pathophysiological changes, complications and management of Closed loop intestinal obstruction. ***WBUHS 2025***

Introduction

A *closed loop obstruction* is a specific type of bowel obstruction in which two points along the course of a bowel are obstructed, usually but not always with the transition points adjacent to each other at a single location. The closed loop refers to a segment of bowel without proximal or distal outlets for decompression.

Definition

Closed loop obstruction is a specific type of obstruction in which two points along the course of a bowel are obstructed at a single location thus forming a closed loop.

- Usually this is due to adhesions, a twist of the mesentery or internal herniation.
- In the large bowel it is known as a volvulus.
- In the small bowel it is simply known as small bowel closed loop obstruction. Especially in the small bowel the risk of strangulation and bowel infarction is high with a mortality rate of 10–35%.

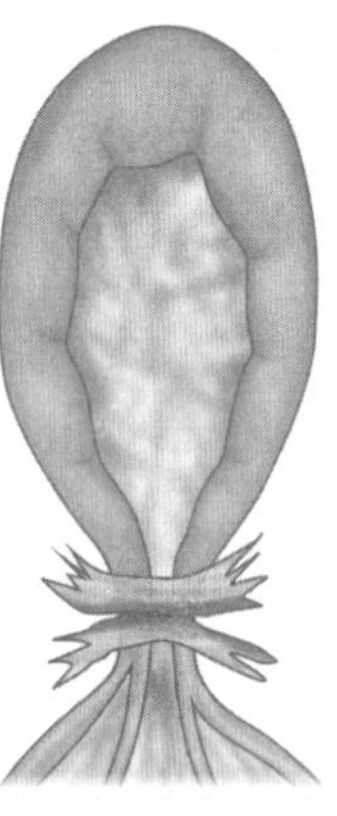
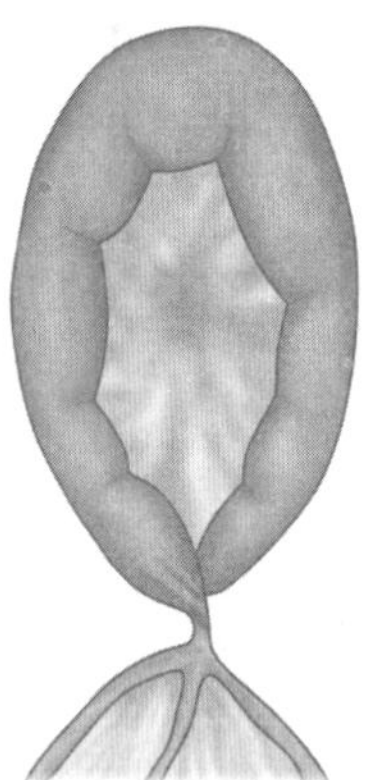

Clinical Presentation

Patients present with signs and symptoms of bowel obstruction, including crampy abdominal pain, vomiting, abdominal distension, and high pitched or absent bowel sounds.

Complications

Closed loop obstructions are at higher risk than nonclosed loop obstructions for strangulation (compromised blood supply) or distension-related ischemia, resulting in intestinal necrosis, and perforation.

Pathology

- Closed loop small bowel obstructions are usually secondary to adhesions, volvulus, or hernia. A similar related pathology is the large bowel volvulus (either sigmoid or cecal)
- Large bowel obstructions occurring at a single point combined with a competent ileocecal valve, which occurs in 75% of patients, also create closed loop physiology with risk of cecal perforation.

- Some publications describe two separate components of the obstruction:
  1. *Closed loop syndrome:*
     - Incarcerated loop (closed loop) continues to secrete fluid and distends, inducing parietal vascular constraints (normally it does contains very little or no gas with the exception of when it involves the colon (fermentation gases).
     - Induced extravasation of blood and plasma from venous stasis both in the excluded loop and in the adjacent mesentery, increasing the intestinal distension.
  2. *Supralesional syndrome:*
     - Segment of intestine upstream from proximal point of obstruction progressively distends to the stomach.
     - Slower than in case of an incarcerated segment.

Associations

- *Internal hernias or congenital or iatrogenic defects in the mesentery or omentum:* May serve to trap a segment of the bowel leading to a closed-loop obstruction a result of surgically created rents in the mesentery
- Those with a Roux-en-Y gastric bypass are also at increased risk for closed-loop obstruction

Radiographic Features

Computed Tomography

Computed tomography findings of a closed-loop obstruction depend in part on the orientation of the loop relative to the plane of imaging. Some or all of the following signs may be demonstrated on CT:

- *Marked distension of a segment of small bowel:* >3 cm is the generally accepted caliber for distended small bowel (see the 3-6-9 rule)
- Radially distributed, C- or U-shaped small bowel loops
- *"Double beak sign":* Tapering bowel loops at the point of obstruction
- "Whirl sign" of the tightly twisted mesentery
- Two adjacent collapsed loops of bowel
- If strangulation is present, signs of bowel ischemia

Treatment and Prognosis

Risk of strangulation leads to high morbidity and mortality in closed loop bowel obstructions. Immediate surgical intervention is required.

49. Write in brief about Strangulated hernia. ***WBUHS 2008***

50. Clinical features and management of strangulated inguinal hernia. ***WBUHS 2019; Rims, Imphal 2022***

Introduction

Strangulated hernias refer to hernias that have their blood supply cut off. When this occurs, any tissue in the hernia, such as intestines, can become ischemic and die quickly. This means that quick surgery is imperative to save the herniated tissue.

Symptoms

- They are irreducible and are always painful
- Extreme tenderness and redness in the area of the bulge
- Sudden pain that worsens in a short period of time
- Fever
- Tachycardia
- Vomiting and nausea
- Severe infection
- Also, the affected person may feel ill in general

Management

Diagnosis should be done on the basis of history and clinical examination. Straight X-ray abdomen can help in the diagnosis.

Emergency Management

- Resuscitation:
  - Establish IV access. Consider giving crystalloid fluid if there is a suspicion of a complicated hernia.
  - Catheterize and place on a fluid balance chart if hypotensive.
  - Blood for full blood count (FBC) [hemoglobin (Hb) and white cell count (WCC)], urea, creatinine, and electrolytes (Na and K)

Definitive Management

- Surgery:
  - Opening up the sac—examination of bowel—if color is changed—apply 100% oxygen and hot mop— if color changes to normal with return of peristalsis—reduction of hernia content with repair of hernia.
  - If viability of gut is not restored—resection anastomosis and repair of hernia.

Appendix, Colon, Rectum, and Anal Canal

LEARNING OBJECTIVES

- ➢ Appendix: Alvarado Score, Ochsner–Sherren Regime
- ➢ Volvulus
- ➢ Stoma
- ➢ FAP, HNPCC, Adenoma-carcinoma Sequence
- ➢ Colorectal Cancer: Prognostic Factors, Follow-up
- ➢ TME, TEM, TAMIS
- ➢ Locally Recurrent Rectal Cancer
- ➢ Colorectal Liver Metastasis
- ➢ Solitary Rectal Ulcer Syndrome
- ➢ Rectal Prolapse
- ➢ Pilonidal Sinus
- ➢ Surgical Anatomy of Rectum and Anal Canal, Anal Incontinence
- ➢ Fistula in Ano
- ➢ Hemorrhoids
- ➢ Fissure in Ano
- ➢ Anal Malignancy

APPENDIX

1. Alvarado score. ***WBUHS 2012***

Introduction

The Alvarado score is a clinical scoring system used in the diagnosis of appendicitis. The score has six clinical items and two laboratory measurements with a total 10 points.

- *The score:* Elements from the patient's history, the physical examination, and from laboratory tests:
  - Abdominal pain that migrates to the right iliac fossa.
  - Anorexia (loss of appetite) or ketones in the urine
  - Nausea or vomiting
  - Pain on pressure in the right iliac fossa
  - Rebound tenderness
  - Fever of 37.3°C or more
  - Leukocytosis, or >10,000 white blood cells per microliter in the serum
  - Neutrophilia, or an increase in the percentage of neutrophils in the serum white blood cell count.
- The two most important factors, tenderness in the right lower quadrant and leukocytosis, are assigned two points, and the six other factors are assigned one point each, for a possible total score of 10 points.
- A score of 5 or 6 is compatible with the diagnosis of acute appendicitis. A score of 7 or 8 indicates a probable appendicitis, and a score of 9 or 10 indicates a very probable acute appendicitis.
- A popular mnemonic used to remember the Alvarado score factors is MANTRELS—migration to the right iliac fossa, anorexia, nausea/vomiting, tenderness in the right iliac fossa, rebound pain, elevated temperature (fever), leukocytosis, and shift of leukocytes to the left (factors listed in the same order as presented above). Due to the popularity of this mnemonic, the Alvarado score is sometimes referred to as the MANTRELS score.

Alvarado Score

Feature	*Score*
Migration of pain	1
Anorexia	1
Nausea	1
Tenderness in right lower quadrant	2
Rebound tenderness	1
Elevated temperature	1
Leukocytosis	2
Shift of white blood cell count to the left	1
Total	**10**

Complementary Value

The original Alvarado score describes a possible total of 10 points, but those medical facilities that are unable to perform a differential white blood cell count, are using a modified Alvarado Score with a total of 9 points which could be not as accurate as the original score. The high diagnostic value of the score has been confirmed in a number of studies across the world. The consensus is that the Alvarado score is a noninvasive, safe, diagnostic method, which is simple, reliable and repeatable, and able to guide the clinician in the management of the case.

2. Ochsner–Sherren regime.

Ochsner–Sherren Regime

Traditionally, it was believed that surgery during the phase of acute appendicitis with a mass was potentially dangerous and could lead to life-threatening complications because of edema and the fragility of important structures such as the terminal ileum and caecum.

The essential components are now as follows:

- Nursing the patient in a popped-up position encouraging gravitational flow of any exudates toward the pelvis.
- Nothing is to be given by mouth for an initial 24–48 hours while the patient is kept on intravenous fluids.
- Intravenous antibiotics are administered with regular monitoring of vital sign a as well as measurement of the size of the mass.
- If the patient's general condition improves, the size of the mass reduces and the fever and anorexia subside, the patient is usually allowed liquids orally and then diet. If this is tolerated discharge home is considered. After 6 weeks an interval appendectomy is performed.
- On the other hand, if the condition of the patient deteriorates, the size of the mass increases, pulse rate increases or general peritonitis develops, or the patient becomes septic then the conservative management is curtailed and the patient is considered for operation.

It is argued that interval appendectomy is unnecessary after successful conservative management of an appendicular lump.

This approach can be applied in selected patients who do not develop recurrent symptoms.

3. Discuss in brief on controversies in management of acute appendicitis. ***WBUHS 2024***

The management of acute appendicitis has been a subject of debate and controversy due to varying treatment approaches, differing clinical opinions, and evolving evidence. Some of the key areas of controversy include:

Antibiotic Therapy vs. Surgery

- *Conservative management:* Some studies have shown that antibiotics alone can effectively treat uncomplicated acute appendicitis, especially in certain patient populations (e.g., older adults, high surgical risk). This has led to debates on whether routine appendectomy (surgical removal of the appendix) is always necessary.

- *Surgical management:* Traditional treatment for appendicitis has been immediate appendectomy, and many surgeons advocate for surgery as the gold standard to prevent complications such as perforation or abscess formation.

Controversy: The key debate lies in whether antibiotics alone are sufficient, especially for uncomplicated cases. Proponents argue that conservative management can reduce surgical risks and hospital costs, while opponents emphasize the risk of recurrence or missed diagnoses (e.g., cancer).

Laparoscopic vs. Open Appendectomy

- *Laparoscopic surgery:* This minimally invasive technique has become increasingly popular due to its advantages, such as smaller incisions, shorter recovery time, and reduced risk of wound infection.
- *Open appendectomy:* Traditional open surgery, often involving a larger incision, is still used, particularly in cases where laparoscopic surgery is not feasible or when the appendix is difficult to reach (e.g., in obese patients).

Controversy: The debate centers on whether laparoscopic appendectomy truly offers significant benefits over open surgery in terms of long-term outcomes, costs, and recovery. While many studies favor laparoscopic surgery, there is still a belief that in some situations (e.g., complicated appendicitis or extreme obesity), open surgery may be more appropriate.

Timing of Surgery

- *Early surgery:* Most guidelines recommend early appendectomy within 24 hours of diagnosis to reduce the risk of complications like perforation.
- *Delayed surgery:* Some studies suggest that delaying surgery for a few days could help reduce complications or allow inflammation to subside, making the surgery technically easier.

Controversy: While early surgery is generally accepted as best practice, the benefit of delaying surgery in certain situations, such as in cases of complicated appendicitis (e.g., abscess), remains contentious.

Management of Perforated Appendicitis

- *Drain placement and delayed surgery:* In cases of perforated appendicitis, some practitioners prefer placing a drain and postponing surgery to allow the infection to settle, followed by a later appendectomy.
- *Immediate surgery:* Others argue for an immediate appendectomy, even in the case of perforation, to remove the source of infection as quickly as possible.

Controversy: The timing of surgery in perforated appendicitis and whether initial drainage or immediate surgery is preferable is still debated. While some studies support staged management (drain placement first), others favor a single-stage surgery approach.

Role of Imaging in Diagnosis

- *Routine imaging:* While ultrasound and CT scans are commonly used to confirm the diagnosis of appendicitis, their routine use is controversial due to concerns over cost, radiation exposure (in the case of CT), and potential for misdiagnosis.
- *Clinical diagnosis:* Some experts advocate for a clinical diagnosis of appendicitis without the need for imaging, especially in high-probability cases.

Controversy: The use of imaging in appendicitis diagnosis remains debated, with concerns about unnecessary radiation exposure and the accuracy of imaging techniques.

---

4. Discuss the recent concepts in the management of acute appendicitis. ***KGMU, Lucknow 2025***

Diagnosis and Risk-stratification

Key Points

- Many recent guidelines emphasize *structured scoring systems* [e.g., Appendicitis Inflammatory Response (AIR) score] in addition to clinical + laboratory findings. For example the 2025 Swedish National Guideline recommends use of the AIR score for all ages.

- *Imaging remains central:* Ultrasound as first line (especially children/pregnant), CT (or MRI) if unclear. The guidelines stress combining clinical score + imaging rather than relying purely on one.
- There is emphasis on avoiding unnecessary surgery ("negative appendectomy") by optimizing diagnosis; the Swedish guideline emphasizes uniform care, quality indicators.

What's New/Evolving

- More rigorous grading of evidence for appendicitis management in national guidelines (e.g., the Swedish guideline uses GRADE).
- Some new scoring systems and research on tools to help decision making (e.g., a 2025 BMC surgery article on a "scoring system for emergency surgery in acute appendicitis" from China) though these are still early.
- Better delineation of *uncomplicated* vs *complicated* appendicitis in diagnostic algorithms, rather than a "one size fits all" approach. The shifting understanding is that these may be quasi-different disease entities.

Implications for Practice

- Use a validated clinical score (e.g., AIR) plus labs + imaging to stratify patients.
- In settings where CT is limited (as in many parts of India), an algorithm combining score + ultrasound may help reduce misdiagnosis.
- Recognize that the decision for surgery vs conservative may depend on careful risk stratification

Nonoperative (Antibiotic) Management for *Uncomplicated* Appendicitis

What the Evidence Shows

Several recent reviews/meta-analyses (both in adults and children) have examined antibiotic-only treatment for uncomplicated appendicitis (i.e., no perforation, no abscess, no faecalith in many studies).

For example:

- *In children:* A JAMA Pediatrics meta-analysis found in 7 RCTs (1,480 children) that nonoperative management (NOM) had *significantly higher failure rate at 1 year, lower* success, and *higher major complications* compared to appendectomy.
- *In adults:* A comprehensive review noted that although antibiotics are an option, appendectomy remains gold-standard given higher efficacy and lower complication rate.

Recent Guideline Stance

- The 2025 Swedish guideline treats nonoperative management with caution; it emphasizes appendectomy remains standard in many cases, especially given higher recurrence and risk of missed pathology.
- The 2024/25 review article (for adults) suggests that NOM is an emerging option for selected patients (mild disease, no appendicolith, good access to follow-up) but not yet replacement for surgery.

What's New/Nuanced

- *Importance of patient selection:* Factors such as presence of appendicolith, higher WBC, longer duration of symptoms increase risk of failure of antibiotics. For example, a recent US cohort (2021–24) found that presence of an appendicolith increased risk of needing surgery after initial antibiotics (OR ~3.2).
- *Recognition of recurrence risk:* Even when initial antibiotic treatment works, recurrence rates are substantial (e.g., in children ~18 events/100 observations in 1 year in meta-analysis) and major complications can occur.
- *Shared-decision making:* Because antibiotic-only management gives a modest faster return to daily life (e.g., in children ~1.3 days earlier return to school) but trade-offs in recurrence, this emphasizes discussing risks/benefits with patient/family.
- Cost/health-system implications: Some evidence of increasing uptake of antibiotic approach (e.g., in US cohort the rate of appendectomy dropped from ~85% to ~77% between 2016 and 2022).

Practical Guidance

- *Candidates for antibiotic-first:* Uncomplicated appendicitis (no perforation, no abscess, no fecalith or high-risk features), good follow-up access, patient willing to accept risk of recurrence.

- For other patients (children/adults) especially with risk features, appendectomy remains preferred.
- Important to counsel about recurrence and need for possible later surgery, and to have robust follow-up.
- In resource-limited settings, antibiotic strategy might be attractive, but infrastructure for follow-up must exist—and local microbial/antibiotic resistance patterns need to be considered.

Operative Management—Timing, Approach and in Complicated Cases

Timing and Approach

- Laparoscopic appendectomy remains standard in most centers for uncomplicated appendicitis. The US data 2016–22 show ~92% laparoscopic vs ~8 % open; robotic use increasing but still small.
- *Regarding timing:* Older teaching was "appendectomy as soon as possible to avoid perforation". Recent guidelines suggest that immediate vs delayed (within say 12–24 hours) may both be acceptable depending on logistic/patient factors. For example, the SAGES guideline notes a "conditional recommendation" for immediate vs delayed (>12 hours) appendectomy depending on circumstances.
- Minimally invasive approaches and enhanced recovery pathways are more firmly embedded now.

Complicated appendicitis (perforation, abscess/phlegmon)

- The management of complicated cases is evolving:
  - If there is an established abscess or phlegmon, many centers now favour initial percutaneous drainage + antibiotics, delayed interval appendectomy if needed, rather than urgent surgery in all cases.
  - The guideline from SAGES mentions higher rate of neoplasm in interval appendectomy specimens (especially >40 years) so interval appendectomy may be advisable in some.
- *Postoperative antibiotics:* Recent evidence suggests shorter antibiotic courses (3–5 days) in complicated appendicitis are sufficient, avoiding unnecessarily long antibiotic exposure.

Recent Guideline Updates

- The 2025 Swedish guideline covers both uncomplicated and complicated cases, addresses nursing care, follow-up, quality registers.
- The focus is shifting more to *tailoring* the operative plan based on individual risk, disease severity, patient factors, rather than a one-size approach.

Practical Implications

- *For a patient with suspected uncomplicated appendicitis:* Laparoscopic appendectomy is still mainstay unless good candidate for antibiotic approach.
- In complicated cases: Assess for abscess/phlegmon on imaging. If present, drainage + antibiotics may avoid emergent surgery; but careful follow-up and consideration for interval appendectomy (especially in older patients) is important.
- *Adhere to established perioperative protocols:* Minimize delays, use prophylactic antibiotics appropriately, shorten postoperative antibiotic duration when safe.

Ancillary Concepts: Quality of care, follow-up, patient-centeredness

- The 2025 Swedish guideline emphasizes *quality indicators* and uniform care across centers (reducing variation) in diagnosis, treatment, follow-up of appendicitis.
- There is increasing recognition of *patient choice* (especially relating to antibiotic vs surgery) and discussing trade-offs (speed of recovery vs risk of recurrence).
- There is also more attention to protocols to reduce postoperative infections, checklists (as per a 2025 article on "surgeon's checklist" for postappendectomy infections) indicating that beyond "what to do" we are also asking "how to do it well".
- *In research/technology:* Machine learning/ultrasound-based models are being explored for diagnosis (though still early stage) to possibly refine decision-making.

Specific Considerations Relevant to India/Developing-World Settings

- In India/South Asia, delayed presentations, limited access to advanced imaging (CT), and variable surgical infrastructure are realities. So:
  - Use of ultrasound + clinical scoring may be especially valuable.
  - Antibiotic-first strategies may be appealing where surgical capacity is constrained—but only if safe follow-up and selection criteria are met.
  - Access to minimally invasive surgery (laparoscopy) may be variable; open appendectomy still has a role but where laparoscopy exists it should be standard for better recovery.
  - Local antibiotic resistance patterns matter when choosing antibiotic regimens.
  - Cost, patient preferences, work-return issues may lean toward minimally invasive or nonoperative approaches—but always balanced against recurrence risk, etc.

---

5. Appendicitis in pregnancy. *Ayush University, Chhattisgarh 2025*

Introduction

- *Acute appendicitis* remains the *most common nonobstetric surgical emergency* in pregnancy, occurring in about 1 in *1,000–2,000 pregnancies.*
- *Diagnosis is often delayed* because of physiological and anatomical changes in pregnancy, leading to *higher rates of perforation (20–40%)* and fetal loss if not promptly treated.
- Recent literature (2023–2025) continues to refine diagnostic *algorithms, imaging choices, and surgical approaches* for this unique group.

Pathophysiology and Anatomical Considerations

- The *gravid uterus displaces the appendix upward and laterally,* especially after 20 weeks' gestation—pain may localize to the *right upper quadrant or flank* rather than the right lower quadrant.
- *Leukocytosis and mild tachycardia* are normal in pregnancy, making diagnosis less specific.
- Perforation risk is higher in late pregnancy due to delayed diagnosis and reduced peritoneal defense mechanisms.

Diagnosis—Current Approach

- Clinical assessment
  - Still the first step, but unreliable alone. Classical signs (McBurney's, Rovsing's) often absent.
  - *Right upper quadrant or flank tenderness,* nausea, and vomiting may predominate.
- Laboratory investigations
  - *Leukocytosis >16,000/mm^3* or *neutrophilia* may support diagnosis but are not definitive.
  - *CRP elevation* adds diagnostic value but lacks specificity.
- Imaging

Current (2024–25) Consensus Recommendations

Imaging modality	*Role*	*Key points*
Ultrasound (USG)	1st-line	Noninvasive, safe; sensitivity ~70–80%. Visualization decreases with gestational age
MRI (without gadolinium)	2nd-line if USG equivocal	High sensitivity (~95%) and specificity (~98%); preferred over CT to avoid radiation
CT scan (low-dose)	Only if MRI unavailable and diagnosis uncertain	Associated fetal radiation dose <50 mGy, considered acceptable if necessary for maternal health

Recent Trend (2023–2025)

- Greater use of *MRI as standard second-line test.*
- Use of *point-of-care ultrasound (POCUS)* for rapid screening in emergency settings.

Management—Updated Evidence

- Surgical management remains the gold standard
    - *Appendectomy* is still the *definitive treatment*; delay >24 hours increases perforation risk and adverse fetal outcomes.
    - *Negative appendectomy* (removal of a normal appendix) is less harmful than missed perforation in pregnancy.
- Laparoscopic vs. open appendectomy

Aspect	*Laparoscopic appendectomy*	*Open appendectomy*
Current trend	Preferred in most centers; supported by SAGES, EAES, and ACOG (2024 updates)	Still used where laparoscopy unavailable or patient unstable
Benefits	Less pain, faster recovery, shorter hospital stay, fewer wound infections	Avoids pneumoperitoneum risks
Safety	Generally safe in all trimesters with precautions (CO_2 <12 mm Hg, left-lateral tilt, minimal Trendelenburg)	Safe but larger incision, more pain
Evidence	Recent meta-analyses show comparable fetal outcomes to open surgery when performed by experienced surgeons	—

Precautions During Laparoscopy

- Use *open (Hasson) entry* to avoid uterine injury.
- Maintain *intra-abdominal pressure ≤12 mm Hg.*
- Ensure *maternal end-tidal CO_2 monitoring.*
- *Left lateral tilt* to avoid aortocaval compression.

- Antibiotic therapy
    - Broad-spectrum antibiotics covering *gram-negative and anaerobes* (e.g., *cephalosporin + metronidazole*).
    - Avoid tetracyclines, fluoroquinolones, and aminoglycosides unless no alternatives.
- Nonoperative (Antibiotic-only) management
    - Not routinely recommended in pregnancy.
    - Limited data (e.g., small 2022–24 series) suggest higher recurrence and risk of perforation; therefore surgery remains standard.
    - Can be *temporarily* considered in early gestation if surgery unavailable and diagnosis uncertain—with close follow-up and imaging.

Maternal and Fetal Outcomes

Parameter	*Nonperforated appendicitis*	*Perforated appendicitis*
Fetal loss	<2–5%	20–35%
Preterm labor	<10%	up to 40%
Maternal mortality	<1%	2–5%

Key message: *Prompt diagnosis and timely surgery markedly reduce both maternal and fetal morbidity.*

Perioperative and Obstetric Considerations

- *Obstetric consult* for fetal assessment before and after surgery.
- *Fetal monitoring (*Doppler or cardiotocography) for ≥24 weeks gestation.
- *Tocolytics* (e.g., nifedipine) only if uterine irritability occurs postoperative.
- *Thromboprophylaxis* if immobilized or in later pregnancy.
- Early ambulation and hydration to prevent preterm contractions.

Postoperative Care

- Standard postoperative antibiotics (24 hours for uncomplicated, 3–5 days if perforated).
- Continue fetal monitoring.
- Avoid NSAIDs in the third trimester; use paracetamol or opioids (short-term).
- Resume obstetric follow-up.

VOLVULUS

6. Sigmoid volvulus. *WBUHS 2022*

Introduction

Sigmoid volvulus is a cause of large bowel obstruction and occurs when the sigmoid colon twists on the sigmoid mesocolon.

Epidemiology

Large bowel volvulus accounts for ~5% of all large bowel obstructions, with ~60% of intestinal volvulus involving the sigmoid colon. It is more common in the elderly.

Clinical Presentation

Symptoms are that of a large bowel obstruction: Constipation, abdominal bloating, nausea, and/or vomiting. Onset may be acute or chronic.

Pathology

Etiology

There is a wide range of causes; some are region-specific:

- Chronic constipation and/or laxative abuse
- Fiber-rich diet (especially in Africa)
- Chagas disease (especially in South America)

Associations

Chronic neurological conditions (e.g., Parkinson disease, multiple sclerosis, and pseudobulbar palsy). Medications from chronic psychiatric conditions (e.g., chronic schizophrenia).

Radiographic Features

Sigmoid volvulus is differentiated from a cecal volvulus by its ahaustral wall and the lower end pointing to the pelvis.

Abdominal Radiograph

Abdominal radiographs will show a large, dilated loop of the colon, often with a few air-fluid levels.

Specific signs include:

- Coffee bean sign
- Frimann Dahl's sign—three dense lines converge toward site of obstruction
- Absent rectal gas

CT

- *Whirl sign:* Twisting of the mesentery and mesenteric vessels
- *Bird's beak sign:* If rectal contrast has been administered.
- *X-marks-the-spot sign:* Crossing loops of bowel at the site of the transition
- *Split wall sign:* Mesenteric fat seen indenting or invaginating the wall of the bowel.

Treatment

- Once, the diagnosis of sigmoid volvulus is confirmed, treatment must be immediate, as delay means more likelihood of bowel wall death and gangrene.

- Up to 80% of people with this condition die from gangrene if intervention is delayed.
- There are two approaches to treatment. The first step is to free the acute obstruction, and then to fix the redundant part of the bowel in a bid to reduce or defer reoccurrence.
- In the UK, a rigid sigmoidoscope is often passed into the sigmoid colon through the anus under direct vision.
- Once the junction between the rectum and sigmoid is negotiated and passed, it could open up the obstruction, letting off the trapped wind in the twisted bowel.
- This is followed by spontaneous unwinding of the obstruction, with massive explosion of feces to the exterior. A flatus tube is then left in place.
- The patient may need fluid replacement, and resuscitation if severely dehydrated, if signs of infection have set in.
- If there is evidence suggestive of perforation, then the abdomen is opened and dealt with.
- In up to 90% of patients with sigmoid volvulus, the condition reoccurs after untwisting, without a definitive operation. For this reason, anyone with a sigmoid volvulus would need to be operated during the same admission if fit enough, to fix down the excessive bowel length.
- Sigmoidectomy with end-to-end anastomosis or Hartmann's procedure is done.

STOMA

7. Describe the preoperative preparation, operative steps, and complications of transverse colostomy.

WBUHS 2008

Indications of Transverse Loop Colostomy

- Obstruction of the distal (left) colon or rectum where primary resection and anastomosis of the obstructing lesion are unsafe or impossible.
- To protect a low anastomosis of the rectum.

Preoperative Preparation

In obstructed patients, fluid and electrolyte imbalances should be corrected to the extent possible in an expeditious manner prior to surgery.

- The amount of time available to do this depends on factors such as:
- Degree of dilation of the proximal colon
- Risk of perforation

In general, it is desirable to verify the presence of mechanical obstruction and the site of obstruction using CT scanning with rectal contrast, water-soluble contrast enema, or endoscopy.

- A site for the colostomy should be chosen over the rectus sheath and away from all bony prominences to allow for placement of the ostomy base plate.
- Preoperative prophylactic antibiotics *(cefuroxime + metrogyl)* are given 30 minutes prior to incision.
- Deep venous thrombosis prophylaxis with sequential compression devices or subcutaneous heparin is employed according to the patient's risk factors.

Procedure

Step 1: The patient is positioned supine and general anesthesia is used to allow for adequate exploration. Draping exposes the area from xiphoid to umbilicus and just lateral to rectus sheath edges.

Step 2: A midline incision can be made or a transverse incision over the right rectus muscle. If the colostomy is intended to be permanent, placement of the stoma in the left transverse colon through a midline or left rectus incision may help to prevent subsequent prolapse. The incision in any case must be large enough to permit safe manipulation and delivery of the dilated colon segment.

Step 3: The dilated transverse colon is identified by following the omentum down to its colonic attachment and the omentum and dilated segment of colon are delivered through the abdominal wall up into the operative field.

Step 4: The omentum is separated from the colon over a short distance by sharp or cautery dissection through the avascular plane and the omentum then transected at right angles to the colon between clamps, allowing it to remain attached to the colon but fall back into the peritoneal cavity out of the way.

Step 5: If the colon is extremely tense or difficult to handle, it is possible to decompress it with an aspirating needle and close the opening with a suture, incorporating the hole into the site of the eventual colostomy.

Step 6: A short segment on the mesenteric border of the colon is cleared to allow passage of a small Penrose drain. The Penrose is then used as a handle to pull up the colon segment. It is important to bring enough colon out of the abdominal cavity to eliminate tension once the bridge has been placed under the loop.

Step 7: The fascia is closed with 0 absorbable suture loosely enough to allow for easy passage of a finger between the colon and the fascia. A few of the epiploic fat attachments and/or the colon serosa are tacked to the fascia with Vicryl suture to prevent herniation.

Step 8: The subcutaneous layer is closed with 3-0 absorbable suture and the skin with 3-0 simple sutures. The skin closure should extend close to the colon but be loose enough to allow passage of a finger around the edge of the wound next to the colon.

Step 9: The Penrose drain is withdrawn while simultaneously replacing it with a supporting rod or bridge. The rod is fastened to the skin with nylon suture. The exact nature of fixation to the skin will vary between different devices.

Step 10: The colon loop is opened along one of the teniae coli for approximately one-third of its length, incorporating any previous decompression site. The edges of the opened bowel are everted and gently approximated to the dermis, except at the point where the rod or bridge pass behind the loop, or the opening may be left alone to evert overtime.

Step 11: An opening is fashioned in the ostomy disc just large enough to fit around the ostomy flush against the surface, and the disc is placed on the skin.

Postoperative Care

- The ostomy can be expected to become edematous while the rod is in place.
- The absorbable sutures in the derma should be removed at about 10 days if they have not dissolved.
- The initial size of the opening in the colon should take this into account to allow for function in spite of the edema. The rod or bridge is left in place 6–10 days and then removed, allowing for shrinkage of the stoma and a reduction in the size of the base plate opening.
- The wound and surrounding skin should be checked for any signs of infection as part of the follow-up care.
- A good seal is mandatory each time the bag is changed, although this can be hard to accomplish until the bridge is removed.
- The absorbable sutures in the derma should be removed at about 10 days.

Complications

Early

- Bleeding may occur from the stoma site.
- Retraction of stoma
- Necrosis of the stoma may occur if it is brought up under too much tension.

Late

- Either the proximal or distal end of the stoma may prolapse.
- Herniation of small bowel through the incision opening may occur if the fascial closure is not snug enough.

Follow-up

- In time, the size of the bag is decreased gradually to fit the smaller stoma.
- The patient should in general be referred to an enterostomal therapist if they did not see one preoperatively.
- Closure of the ostomy is planned when the reason for its initiation is no longer in existence.
- Contrast studies through the stoma and through the rectum are performed prior to colostomy closure.

8. Colostomy and stoma care. ***WBUHS 2011***

A colostomy is a surgical procedure in which a stoma is formed by drawing the healthy end of the large intestine or colon through an incision in the anterior abdominal wall and suturing it into place. This opening, in conjunction with the attached stoma appliance, provides an alternative channel for feces to leave the body. It may be reversible or irreversible depending on the circumstances.

Indications

- A section of the colon has been removed, e.g., due to colon cancer requiring a total mesorectal excision (TME), diverticulitis, injury, etc., so that it is no longer possible for feces to exit via the anus.
- A portion of the colon (or large intestine) has been operated upon and needs to be "rested" until it is healed. In this case, the colostomy is often temporary and is usually reversed at a later date, leaving the patient with a small scar in place of the stoma. Children undergoing surgery for extensive pelvic tumors commonly are given a colostomy in preparation for surgery to remove the tumor, followed by reversal of the colostomy.

Types

- *Loop colostomy:* This type of colostomy is usually used in emergencies and is a temporary and large stoma. A loop of the bowel is pulled out onto the abdomen and held in place with an external device. The bowel is then sutured to the abdomen and two openings are created in the one stoma: One for stool and the other for mucus.
- *End colostomy:* A stoma is created from one end of the bowel. The other portion of the bowel is either removed or sewn shut (Hartmann's pouch).
- *Double barrel colostomy:* The bowel is severed and both ends are brought out onto the abdomen. Only the proximal stoma is functioning.

Colostomy surgery that is preplanned usually has a higher rate of long-term success than surgery performed in an emergency situation.

- *Colostomy with irrigation:* People with colostomies who have ostomies of the *sigmoid colon* or *descending colon* may have the option of irrigation, which allows for the person to not wear a pouch, but rather just a gauze cap over the stoma, and to schedule irrigation for times that are convenient.
- *Colostomy without irrigation:* Colostomies are not viewed positively due to the misconception that it is difficult to hide the pouch and the smell of feces, or to keep the pouch securely attached. However, modern colostomy pouches are well-designed, odor-proof, and allow stoma patients to continue normal activities.

Latex-free tape is available for ensuring a secure attachment. People with colostomies must wear an *ostomy pouching system* to collect intestinal waste. Ordinarily, the pouch must be emptied or changed several times a day depending on the frequency of activity; in general the further from the *anus* (i.e., the further "up" the intestinal tract) the ostomy is located the greater the output and more frequent the need to empty or change the pouch.

Alternatives

The preferred option by the surgical community, wherever possible, is now an internal coloanal pouch which eliminates the need for an external pouch. In place of an external appliance, an internal ileo-anal pouch is constructed using a portion of the patient's lower intestine, to act as a new rectum to replace the removed original.

Stoma Care

- Stoma care is the first thing that a stoma patient learns even before the surgical procedure itself.
- Explain the patient about the stoma and its need.
- There are three main types of stoma, indicating the three areas in which a stoma operation could be the solution: Ileostomy, colostomy, and urostomy.
- The ileostomy stoma is introduced when the patient is suffering from Crohn's disease, ulcerative colitis, or any sort of upper digestive tract cancer.
- The colostomy stoma is used when colon or anus cancer is wreaking havoc on the patients' body.
- The urostomy stoma comes in handy when the bladder has a problem.

Stoma Pictures

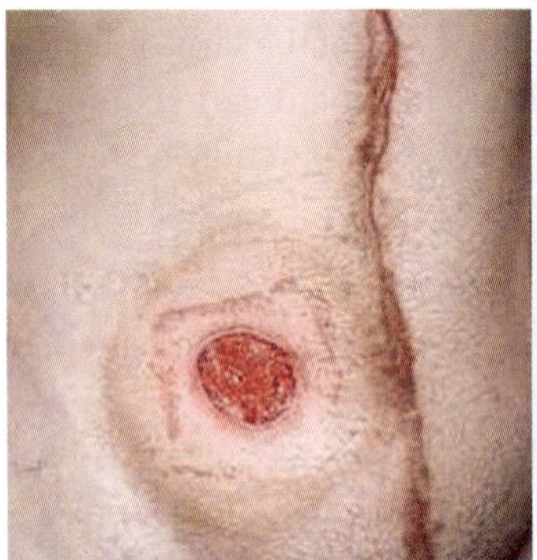
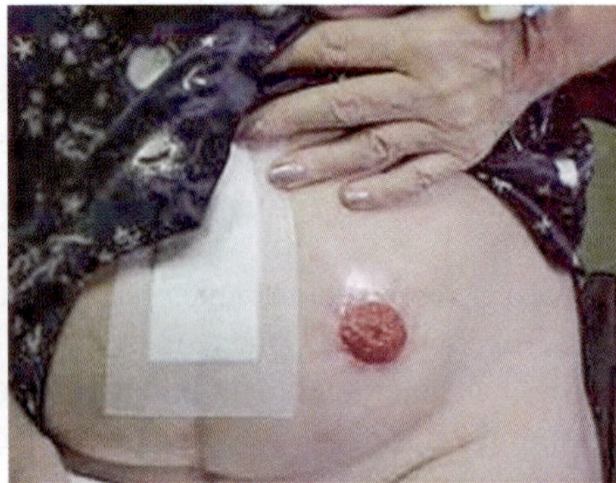
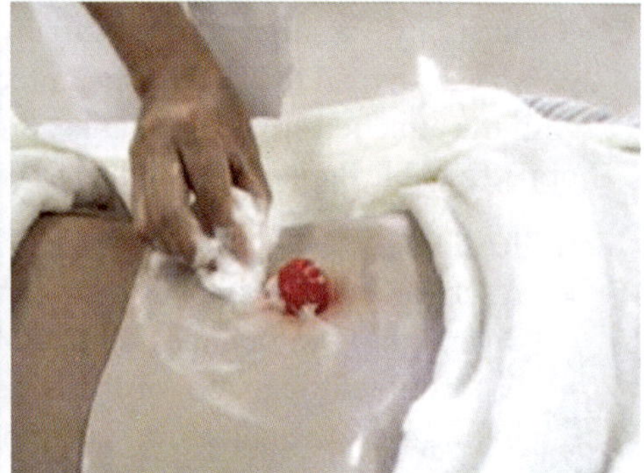

- *Stoma care begins before the surgery itself. The first step toward stoma care is the psychological counseling:* The patient must be made aware that the stoma will change his or her life for the better and it will probably prolong his or her life with decades. Also, the sufferer must understand that their life will continue as planned, that the fact that they have a stoma is not a hindrance.
- *The second step in the stoma care program is the presurgery treatment:* A special diet, some physical exercises, and vitamins and minerals are all included. The diet is meant to make the digestion process easier than usual, the physical exercises are meant to strengthen patient's body and the vitamins and minerals should energize your organism.
- However, only after the surgery begins the real stoma care. In the first few weeks after the surgery, patient will not be allowed to leave the hospital. The physician needs to keep an eye on the patient and the nurses need to teach you how to take care of the stoma. Several stoma complications can be avoided by remaining hospitalized: Infection, fever, bleeding, and skin rashes. The surgeon also monitors the healing process of the surgery and advocates when the patient will start routine works and normal life.

After being released from the hospital, patient will need some help for another few weeks. Afterward he or she can take manage his or her stoma care all on your own. There are a few things that you must respect, no matter the situation, when talking about the stoma care:

- *Monitor stoma bag carefully:* In the first few months, need to monitor to avoid any leakage or bursting.
- Change the stoma bag as often as it is necessary, but not more often than one should—changing the bag more often than necessary will lead to the loosening of the stoma, to leakage, and to skin problems.
- *Watch for any skin damage signs:* The skin surrounding the stoma is the perfect barometer.

9. Describe present day approach for creation and care of intestinal stoma. ***WBUHS 2020***

Introduction

An ostomy is named according to the part of intestine used to construct it. A colostomy is the creation of a stoma from part of the colon (large bowel), where the intestine is brought through the abdominal wall and attached to the skin, diverting normal intestinal fecal matter through the stoma instead of the anus. An ileostomy is created from the ileum (small bowel), which is brought through the abdominal wall and used to create a stoma. A urostomy or ileal conduit is a stoma created using a piece of the intestine to divert urine to the outside of the body. Creation of stoma:

There are certain key aspects to creating an ideal end ileostomy or colostomy.

Among the Principles

- Excise a circular skin disc approximately 2.5 cm in diameter at the previously marked site.

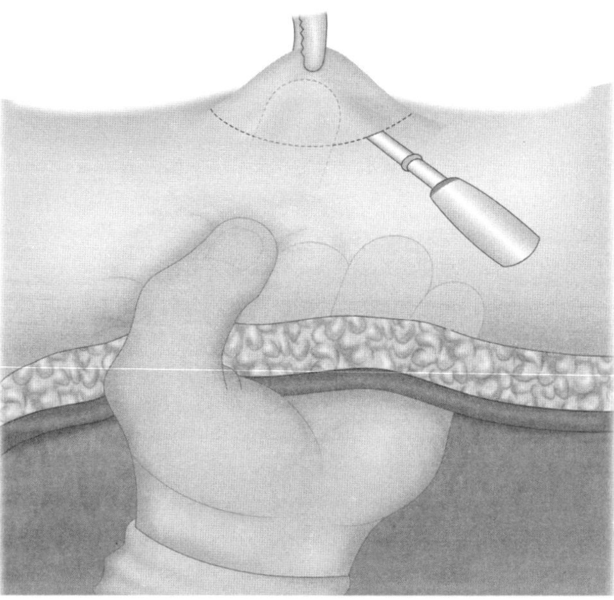

Excision of skin disc at stoma site.

- Divide the subcutaneous tissue with small retractors until the anterior rectus sheath is exposed. Do not excise or "core-out" subcutaneous tissues.
- Make a vertical incision in the anterior rectus sheath approximately 3 cm in length. At the midpoint of the incision, make a perpendicular 1-cm incision laterally. The lateral counter incision keeps the stoma opening away from the midline incision.

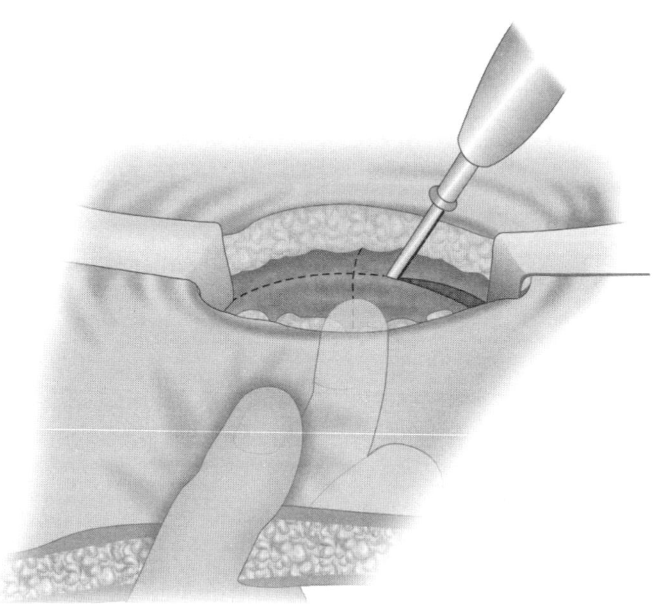

Cruciate incision in anterior fascia.

- Split the rectus abdominis muscle in the direction of its fibers.

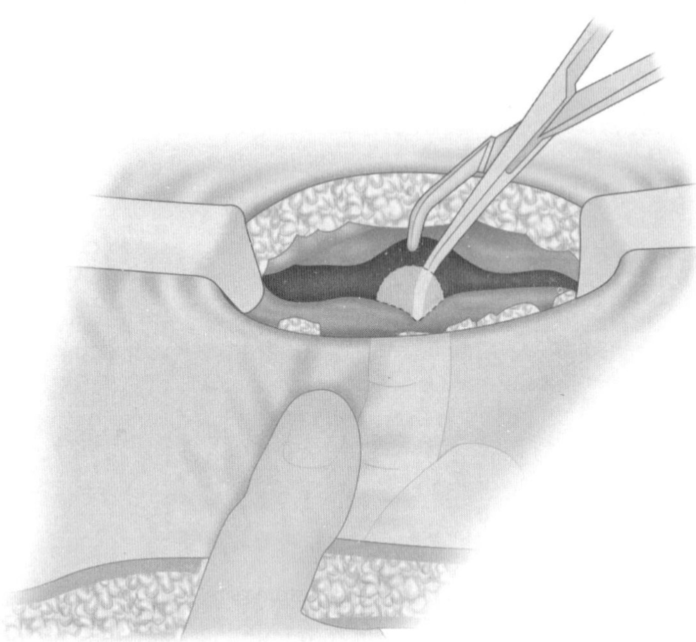

Splitting of rectus muscle in direction of fibers.

- Create a vertical incision in the posterior rectus sheath.

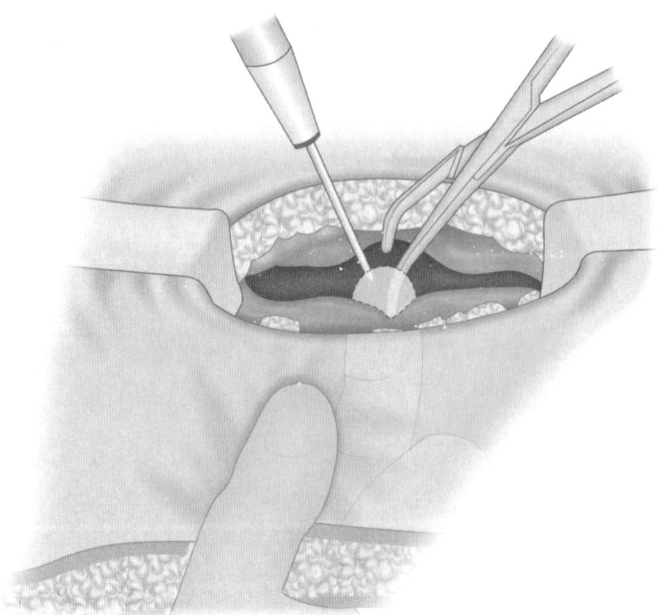

Incision of posterior rectus sheath.

- Deliver the previously divided bowel through the abdominal wall without twisting it. "Pushing" from within the abdominal cavity is preferred to "pulling" when exteriorizing the bowel.

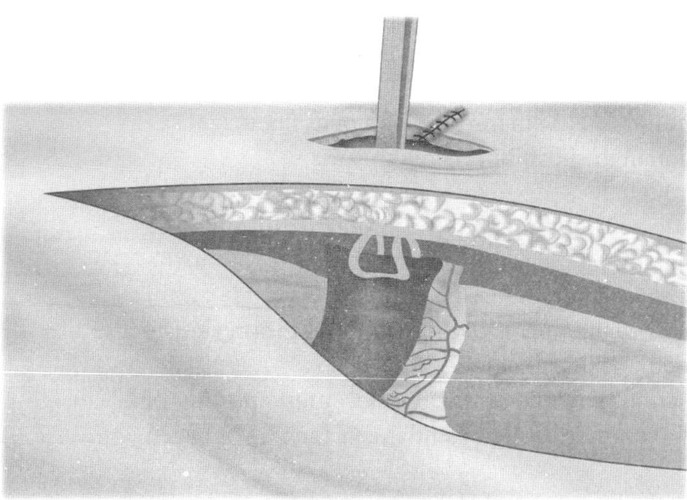

Delivery of bowel through stoma site.

- Again, confirm that the bowel is viable and not twisted.
- For a colostomy, the colon should extend 2 cm above the skin surface. For an ileostomy 5 cm of bowel should be pulled through. The matured colostomy should protrude 0.5–1 cm above the skin. The matured ileostomy should protrude 2–2.5 cm.
- Excise the staple line at end of the bowel cleanly with a no. 10 scalpel blade. Ileostomies must be everted. Eversion of a colostomy is optional and should ideally be dictated by the stomal therapist who will be working with the patient long term. The abdominal incision should be closed before this step. However, if there is concern that the stoma is under too much tension or has questionable viability, the abdomen can be closed after stoma maturation.
- Perform the enterocutaneous anastomosis with interrupted absorbable sutures that take full-thickness bites of the end of the colon and the dermal layer of the skin.
- Colostomies may be matured flush or can be everted similar to ileostomies.
- Ileostomies are everted by placing "triplicate" sutures. First, the suture is placed through the dermis, followed by a seromuscular bite 4–5 cm from the proximal to the distal end of the ileum. The final bite is passed full-thickness through the cut end of the bowel. Three everting sutures, away from the mesentery, will often evert the stoma effectively. Gaps can be closed with standard sutures between the triplicate sutures.

Loop Ileostomy Creation

When simple fecal diversion is required, a loop ileostomy is most often the procedure of choice. The purpose of a diverting stoma is most commonly to prevent fecal material from reaching a distal portion of the bowel, either because of fear of anastomotic leak or to treat a leak or injury. Loop ileostomies are created using the following technique:

- Identify an appropriate loop terminal ileum that will protrude easily at the stoma site. A segment at least 20 cm from the ileocecal junction will facilitate subsequent stoma reversal. Any closer to the cecum may make a stapled anastomosis at the time of reversal more difficult. It is also important to confirm and mark the distal bowel with a suture or marker to ensure proper orientation.
- Make a circular skin incision that is slightly larger than that required for an end stoma at the previously marked site and excise the skin.
- Part the subcutaneous tissue with small retractors until the anterior rectus sheath is exposed. Do not excise this tissue.

- Make a vertical incision in the anterior rectus sheath approximately 2 cm in length. At the midpoint of the incision, make a perpendicular 1-cm incision laterally. This will keep the stoma opening away from the midline incision.
- Split the rectus abdominis muscle in the direction of its fibers.
- Make a vertical incision in the posterior rectus sheath.
- Deliver the bowel through the abdominal wall.
- Placement of a plastic self-retaining wound protector through the stoma trephine will facilitate passage of the bowel through the subcutaneous tissue, especially in obese individuals.
- Confirm that the bowel is viable and not twisted by using the previously placed suture or mark in the distal segment.
- Transect 80% of the circumference of the antimesenteric portion of the bowel wall just above where the distal end meets the skin between two Allis clamps.
- Peel back the edges of the bowel to reveal the two openings. Exchange the catheter for the stoma bridge, if desired. The proximal limb should still protrude approximately 2.5 cm, but the distal limb can be matured flush with the skin.

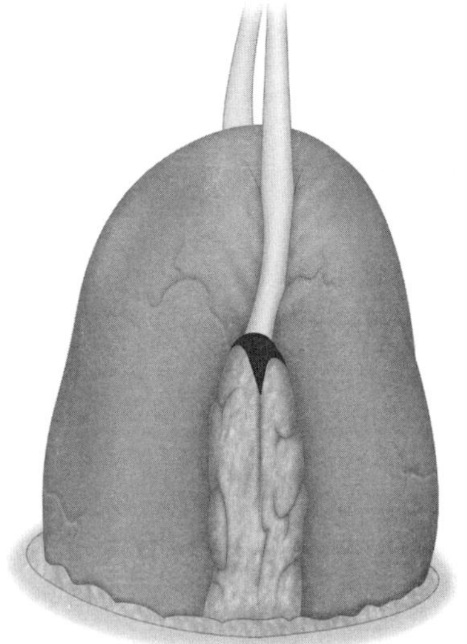
Loop ileostomy creation. Ileum is elevated through stoma site with a Penrose drain. Care is taken to avoid twisting.

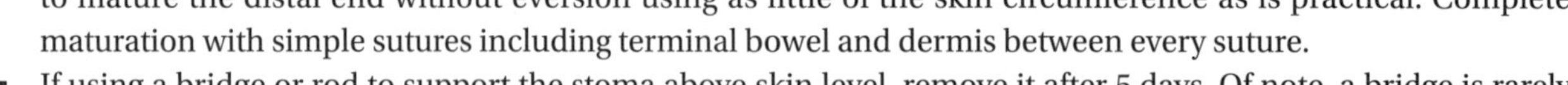

- Mature the stoma (proximal end of the bowel) by eversion with standard "triplicate" sutures on either side of the mesentery and the antimesenteric border with interrupted absorbable sutures. It is best to mature the distal end without eversion using as little of the skin circumference as is practical. Complete maturation with simple sutures including terminal bowel and dermis between every suture.

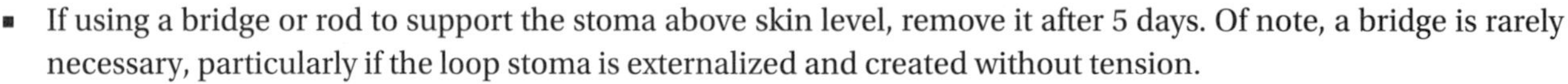

- If using a bridge or rod to support the stoma above skin level, remove it after 5 days. Of note, a bridge is rarely necessary, particularly if the loop stoma is externalized and created without tension.

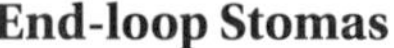

End-loop Stomas

- When creating a temporary stoma, it is always preferable, if possible, to bring the proximal and distal bowel loops through the same trephine in the abdominal wall. Among other advantages, this eases eventual stoma reversal by avoiding formal laparotomy.
- With standard loop stomas, this occurs by definition, but in other circumstances, it only occurs through proper technique and advanced planning.
- End-loop stomas can be created with remote intestinal segments following bowel resection. They consist of end-loop ileoileostomy, ileocolostomy, or colocolostomy. For example, it may be unsafe to perform a primary anastomosis after a right colectomy for trauma. An end-loop ileocolostomy (terminal ileum and transverse colon exiting through the same stoma site) is a viable alternative to an end ileostomy.
- Hartmann's pouch, which would require a formal laparotomy for reversal in the future.
- Similar stomas can be performed following small bowel or left colon resections.

Whether using adjacent or remote intestinal segments, the technique for creating an end-loop stoma is similar:

- The stapled proximal end is passed through the preselected stoma site.
- Only the antimesenteric border of the stapled distal end is then advanced through the same trephine. The antimesenteric corner of the staple line is cut off and the small open segment of the distal bowel is matured flush to the skin using as little of the stoma circumference as possible.
- The proximal end is then matured in the standard fashion.
- A full thickness stitch between the proximal and distal ends completes the procedure.
- An end-loop sigmoid colostomy is an ideal stoma for distal fecal diversion for incontinence or in association with complex anorectal procedures.

- A stoma created with this technique will be easily reversible but will also function well should reversal be contraindicated.

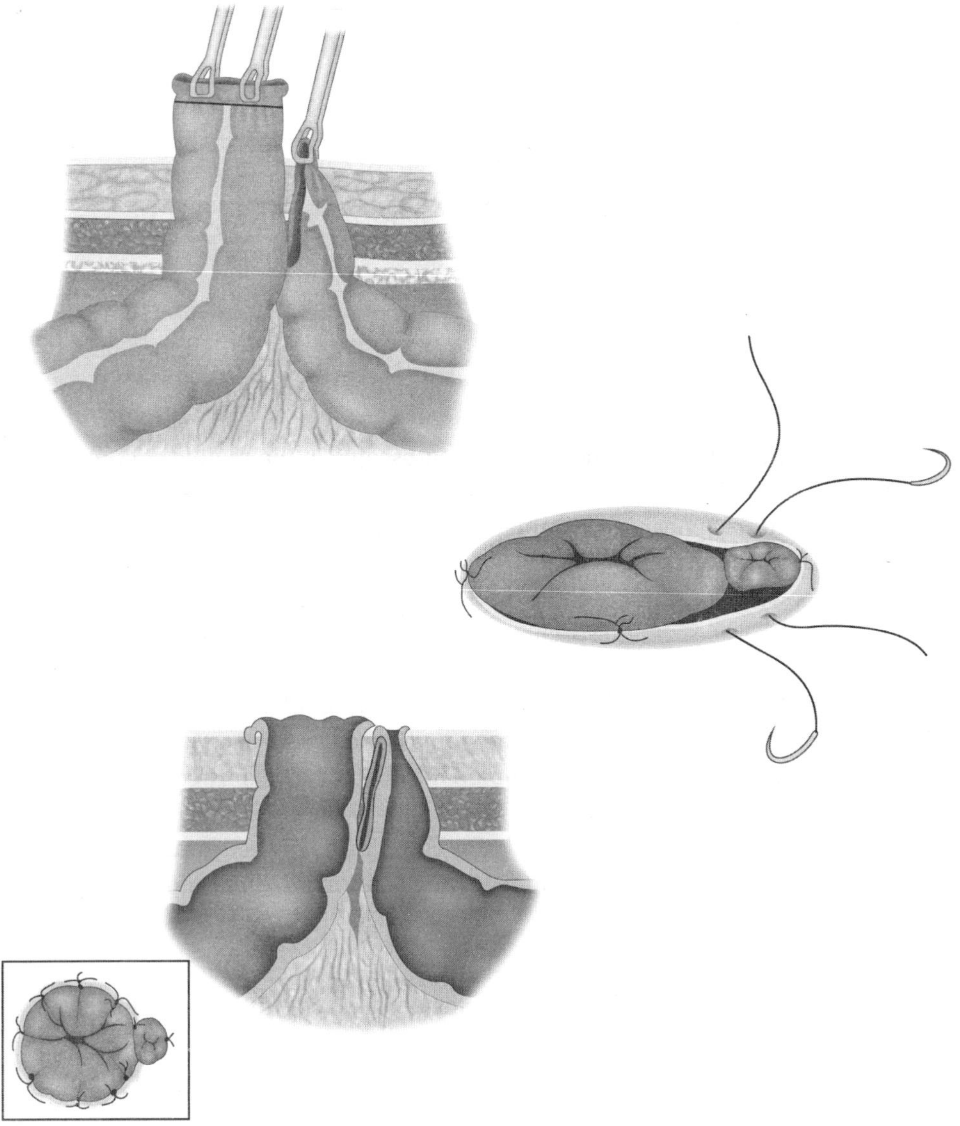

End-loop colostomy creation.

Laparoscopic Stoma Creation

- Fecal diversion for unresectable cancers, severe perineal disease, or trauma is a fairly common procedure. Laparoscopic colostomy or ileostomy creation is an attractive alternative to a formal laparotomy, especially when ostomy creation is the sole purpose of the operation.
- As with any laparoscopic procedure, preoperative planning and patient positioning are key to success.
- Use of Trendelenburg positioning and right or left patient rotation, depending on the ostomy to be performed, will help expose the bowel segment targeted for stoma creation.
- Port placement depends upon the type of stoma undergoing creation. Using the future stoma site as a trocar site may be advantageous.
- Laparoscopic technique for stoma creation is detailed as follows.

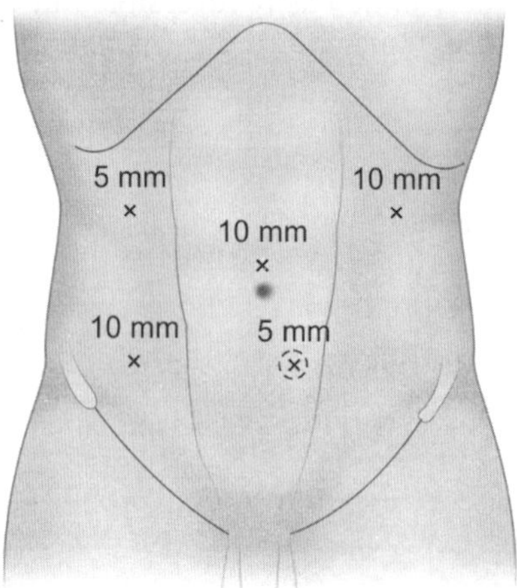

Potential port locations for laparoscopic ostomy creation.

- Place the first trocar, which will accommodate the laparoscope, in the middle abdomen on the side opposite the future stoma.
- If the previously marked site appears acceptable once the laparoscope is inserted, place a 5-mm port through the future stoma site.
- Pass an atraumatic bowel clamp through this port, and grasp the needed segment of bowel and assess for mobility. If the desired bowel segment reaches without tension, enlarge the port site into a standard stoma trephine.
- Marking the distal bowel prior to exteriorization with the felt tip of a marker held in a laparoscopic grasper facilitates proper orientation of the bowel once the stoma is matured.
- If the bowel requires mobilization, which is common in sigmoid colostomy creation, place additional ports as necessary, and mobilize along the white line of Toldt.
- Enlarge the fascial defect as needed and deliver the bowel through the stoma site without twisting. Prior to maturing the stoma, reestablish pneumoperitoneum and confirm proximal and distal orientation of the bowel.
- Mature the stoma in the standard fashion.

Pouching Systems (Ostomy Appliances)

- Individuals with colostomies, ileostomies, or urostomies have no control or sensation of frequency or output of the stoma.
- Patients with ostomies must wear a pouching system to collect the effluent from the stoma and protect the skin from irritation.
- The pouching system must be completely sealed to prevent leaking of the effluent and to protect the surrounding peristomal skin.
- The disposable pouching systems can be either a one-piece or a two-piece flexible system consisting of a plastic bag and a flange (skin barrier) that sit against the patient's skin.
- The flange may be flat or convex.
- The ostomy pouch and flange come together to form one integrated, leakproof unit.
- The pouch has an open end to allow effluent to be drained, and may be closed using a plastic clip or Velcro strip.
- There are many different types of pouching systems to meet different needs.

Depending on the patient, a surgical procedure may be performed to create an internal pouch to collect feces or urine, which eliminates the need for an external pouch:

- The continent ileostomy is made from part of the ileum and is flushed a number of times each day to clean out the effluent.

- An ileoanal ostomy is a pouch created above the anal sphincter and is also created from a portion of the ileum.
- Two types of internal urinary diversions may be created from part of the intestine. The first is an orthotopic neobladder, where a bladder is created and placed in the body at a normal bladder position; over time, with continent training, the patient can learn to void normally. The second type is a continent urinary reservoir, where a pouch is created from part of the intestine, and a catheter is inserted a number of times during the day to remove the urine.

Physical and Emotional Assessment

- Patients may have comorbidities that affect their ability to manage their ostomy care.
- Conditions such as arthritis, vision changes, Parkinson's disease, or poststroke complications may hinder a patient's coordination and function to manage the ostomy.
- In addition, the emotional burden of coping with an ostomy may be devastating for some patients and may affect their self-esteem, body image, quality of life, and ability to be intimate.
- It is common for ostomy patients to struggle with body image and an altered pattern of elimination. Ensure the patient has the appropriate referrals to the wound and ostomy nurse and social workers, as well as access to support groups or online support groups.
- As a health care provider, be very aware of nonverbal cues: Take care not to show disgust at the ostomy or at odor that may be present when changing an appliance or pouching system.

Safety Considerations

- Pouching system should be changed every 4–7 days, depending on the patient and type of pouch.
- Always consult a wound care specialist or equivalent if there is skin breakdown, if the pouch leaks, or if there are other concerns related to the pouching system.
- Patients should participate in the care of their ostomy, and healthcare providers should promote patient and family involvement.
- Encourage the patient to empty the pouch when it is one-quarter to one-half full of urine, gas, or feces.
- Ostomy product choices are based on the patient's needs and preference.
- Follow all postoperative assessments for new ostomies according to agency policy.
- Medications and diet may need adjusting for new ileostomies/colostomies.
- An ostomy belt may be used to help hold the ostomy pouch in place.
- Factors that affect the pouching system include sweating, high heat, moist or oily skin, and physical exercise.
- Always treat minor skin irritations right away. Skin that is sore, wet, or red is difficult to seal with a flange for a proper leakproof fit.

Caring for a Colostomy

- Use the right size pouch and skin barrier opening.
- Pouching system must be changed regularly to avoid leaks and skin irritation.
- Be careful when pulling the pouching system away from the skin and don't remove it more than once a day unless there's a problem.
- Skin around the stoma should be cleaned with water.

---

10. Current management of diverticulitis. ***KGMU, Lucknow 2025***

- "Uncomplicated diverticulitis" – Localized colonic inflammation (e.g., wall thickening, pericolic fat stranding) without abscess, perforation with diffuse peritonitis, fistula, obstruction, or large bleeding.
- "Complicated diverticulitis" = One or more of abscess, obstruction, fistula, free or contained perforation, significant bleeding, etc.
- Imaging (especially CT scan) is very useful in differentiating uncomplicated vs complicated and guiding management.

Initial Evaluation and Diagnosis

- *Clinical suspicion:* Left lower quadrant pain, fever, leukocytosis, changes in bowel habits; however many other abdominal pathologies must be considered.
- In the presence of diagnostic uncertainty (first episode, atypical features, higher risk of complications) abdominal/pelvic CT scan with contrast is recommended.
- If CT is unavailable, ultrasound or MRI may be alternatives, but CT remains the standard.
- Laboratory workup includes CBC, CRP/ESR, renal function, etc. Imaging is particularly important if signs suggest complications (e.g., peritonitis, sepsis, abscess).

Management of Uncomplicated Diverticulitis

For patients who are stable, with no signs of complication, and no major comorbidities:

Outpatient vs. Inpatient

- Many patients with uncomplicated disease can be managed as outpatients—e.g., able to take oral fluids, tolerate diet, have adequate social support, no signs of systemic infection.
- Hospitalization reserved for: inability to tolerate oral intake, immunocompromised, suspected complications, significant comorbidities.

Diet/Bowel Rest

- Traditionally, bowel rest/clear liquids → then gradual progression. Newer data show that many patients may tolerate an unrestricted diet early if they are stable.
- Once acute inflammation improves, advance diet as tolerated; longer term, a high-fiber diet is recommended to reduce recurrence risk.

Antibiotics

- A major shift: In immunocompetent patients with mild uncomplicated diverticulitis, selective (rather than routine) use of antibiotics is recommended. Several guidelines note that antibiotics do not significantly alter outcomes (time to recovery, rupture, surgery) compared to supportive care alone, in selected patients.
- However, antibiotics are still indicated if: signs of systemic infection (fever, tachycardia, leukocytosis), immunocompromised state, comorbidities, evidence of larger segment of inflammation/abscess on imaging, or failure to improve.

Example: The American College of Physicians (ACP) guideline (2022) suggests initially managing select patients without antibiotics.

Follow-up and Monitoring

- Patients managed outpatient should have close monitoring (clinical reassessment within a few days) to detect worsening or complications.
- *Education on lifestyle:* Maintain healthy weight, exercise, high-fiber diet, avoid smoking, minimize regular use of NSAIDs (non-aspirin) because of risk of diverticular complications.

Treatment Principles for Complicated Diverticulitis of the Colon

The management of complicated diverticulitis depends on the specific complication, the patient's clinical condition, and the severity of the disease. General treatment principles include:

- *Antibiotic therapy:*
  - Administer broad-spectrum intravenous antibiotics to cover gram-negative and anaerobic bacteria (e.g., piperacillin-tazobactam, ceftriaxone plus metronidazole).
  - Tailor antibiotics based on culture results and clinical response.
- *Abscess management:*
  - For small abscesses (<4 cm), conservative treatment with antibiotics may suffice.

- For larger abscesses (>4 cm), perform percutaneous drainage under imaging guidance (e.g., CT-guided drainage) alongside antibiotics.
- Surgical intervention may be required if drainage is not feasible or fails.

- *Surgical intervention*
  - *Emergency surgery:* Indicated for perforation, generalized peritonitis, sepsis, or uncontrolled infection. Procedures include Hartmann's procedure (sigmoid resection with end colostomy) or primary resection with anastomosis in select cases.
  - *Elective surgery:* Considered for recurrent episodes, fistula formation, strictures, or persistent symptoms after initial treatment. Options include resection of the affected colon segment with or without anastomosis.
  - Laparoscopic surgery may be preferred in stable patients to reduce recovery time.
- *Supportive care:*
  - Bowel rest (nothing by mouth) for severe cases, with gradual reintroduction of diet as symptoms improve.
  - Intravenous fluids and electrolyte management to maintain hydration and correct imbalances.
  - Pain management with appropriate analgesics, avoiding NSAIDs due to risk of worsening inflammation.
- *Management of specific complications:*
  - *Fistula:* Surgical repair (e.g., resection of the affected colon and closure of the fistula) is often required.
  - *Obstruction/stricture:* Endoscopic stenting may be used temporarily, but surgical resection is often necessary for long-term relief.
  - *Peritonitis/sepsis:* Urgent surgery (e.g., exploratory laparotomy) and aggressive antibiotic therapy are critical.
  - *Hemorrhage:* Endoscopic or angiographic interventions may control bleeding; surgery is reserved for refractory cases.
- *Monitoring and Follow-up:*
  - Close monitoring in a hospital setting for severe cases, with imaging (e.g., CT scan) to assess response to treatment.
  - Colonoscopy or imaging after recovery (typically 6–8 weeks) to evaluate the colon and rule out malignancy or other pathology.
  - Lifestyle modifications (e.g., high-fiber diet, weight management) to prevent recurrence.
- *Multidisciplinary approach:*
  - Involve gastroenterologists, surgeons, infectious disease specialists, and radiologists as needed.
  - Nutritional support and counseling for patients with prolonged recovery or complications.

Treatment is tailored to the patient's overall health, the severity of complications, and response to initial therapy. Early recognition and intervention are critical to prevent life-threatening outcomes.

---

11. Enumerate complications of diverticulitis of colon. Write down the treatment principle of complicated diverticulitis of colon. ***WBUHS 2025***

Complications of Diverticulitis of the Colon

Diverticulitis, an inflammation or infection of diverticula (small pouches in the colon wall), can lead to several complications, including:

- *Abscess formation:* A localized collection of pus due to infection, often requiring drainage.
- *Perforation:* A tear in the colon wall, leading to leakage of intestinal contents into the abdominal cavity.
- *Peritonitis:* Inflammation of the peritoneal cavity, often secondary to perforation, causing severe infection.
- *Fistula formation:* Abnormal connections between the colon and other organs (e.g., bladder, small intestine, or skin), such as colovesical or colovaginal fistulas.
- *Intestinal obstruction:* Partial or complete blockage of the colon due to inflammation, scarring, or strictures.
- *Sepsis:* A life-threatening systemic infection resulting from untreated or severe diverticulitis.
- *Colonic stricture:* Narrowing of the colon due to chronic inflammation or scarring, leading to bowel obstruction.

- *Hemorrhage:* Severe bleeding from diverticula, though more common in diverticulosis than diverticulitis.
- *Intra-abdominal adhesions:* Scar tissue bands forming in the abdomen, potentially causing pain or obstruction.

Treatment Principles for Complicated Diverticulitis of the Colon

The management of complicated diverticulitis depends on the specific complication, the patient's clinical condition, and the severity of the disease. General treatment principles include:

- *Antibiotic therapy:*
  - Administer broad-spectrum intravenous antibiotics to cover gram-negative and anaerobic bacteria (e.g., piperacillin-tazobactam, ceftriaxone plus metronidazole).
  - Tailor antibiotics based on culture results and clinical response.
- *Abscess management:*
  - For small abscesses (<4 cm), conservative treatment with antibiotics may suffice.
  - For larger abscesses (>4 cm), perform percutaneous drainage under imaging guidance (e.g., CT-guided drainage) alongside antibiotics.
  - Surgical intervention may be required if drainage is not feasible or fails.
- *Surgical intervention:*
  - *Emergency surgery:* Indicated for perforation, generalized peritonitis, sepsis, or uncontrolled infection. Procedures include Hartmann's procedure (sigmoid resection with end colostomy) or primary resection with anastomosis in select cases.
  - *Elective surgery:* Considered for recurrent episodes, fistula formation, strictures, or persistent symptoms after initial treatment. Options include resection of the affected colon segment with or without anastomosis.
  - Laparoscopic surgery may be preferred in stable patients to reduce recovery time.
- *Supportive care:*
  - Bowel rest (nothing by mouth) for severe cases, with gradual reintroduction of diet as symptoms improve.
  - Intravenous fluids and electrolyte management to maintain hydration and correct imbalances.
  - Pain management with appropriate analgesics, avoiding NSAIDs due to risk of worsening inflammation.
- *Management of specific complications:*
  - *Fistula:* Surgical repair (e.g., resection of the affected colon and closure of the fistula) is often required.
  - *Obstruction/stricture:* Endoscopic stenting may be used temporarily, but surgical resection is often necessary for long-term relief.
  - *Peritonitis/sepsis:* Urgent surgery (e.g., exploratory laparotomy) and aggressive antibiotic therapy are critical.
  - *Hemorrhage:* Endoscopic or angiographic interventions may control bleeding; surgery is reserved for refractory cases.
- *Monitoring and follow-up:*
  - Close monitoring in a hospital setting for severe cases, with imaging (e.g., CT scan) to assess response to treatment.
  - Colonoscopy or imaging after recovery (typically 6–8 weeks) to evaluate the colon and rule out malignancy or other pathology.
  - Lifestyle modifications (e.g., high-fiber diet, weight management) to prevent recurrence.
- *Multidisciplinary approach:*
  - Involve gastroenterologists, surgeons, infectious disease specialists, and radiologists as needed.
  - Nutritional support and counseling for patients with prolonged recovery or complications.

Treatment is tailored to the patient's overall health, the severity of complications, and response to initial therapy. Early recognition and intervention are critical to prevent life-threatening outcomes.

POLYPOSIS AND ADENOMA-CARCINOMA SEQUENCE

12. Polyposis coli. ***WBUHS 2009***

Hereditary Cancer Syndromes/Polyposis Coli

	Hereditary adenomatous polyposis syndromes		***Hereditary hamartomatous polyposis syndromes***			***Ruvalcaba-Myhre-Smith Syndrome (Bannayan-Zonana syndrome)***
Hereditary nonpolyposis colon cancer	***Familial adenomatous polyposis/Gardner's syndrome***	***Turcot's syndrome***	***Cowden's disease***	***Familial juvenile polyposis***	***Peutz-Jeghers syndrome***	
GI features						
Small number of colorectal polyps	Hundreds to thousands of colorectal polyps; duodenal adenomas and gastric polyps, usually fundic gland	Colorectal polyps, which may be few or resemble classic familial adenomatous polyposis	Polyps most commonly of colon and stomach	Juvenile polyps mostly in the colon but throughout GI tract Defined by ≥10 juvenile polyps	Small number of polyps throughout GI tract but most common in small intestine	Hamartomatous GI polyps, usually lipomas, hemangiomas, or lymphangiomas
Other clinical features						
Muir-Torre variant: Sebaceous adenomas, keratoacanthomas, sebaceous epitheliomas, and basal cell epitheliomas	Osteomas, desmoid tumors, epidermoid cysts, and congenital hypertrophy of retinal epithelium	Brain tumors, including cerebellar medullo-blastoma and glioblastomas	Mucocutaneous lesions, thyroid adenomas, and goiter and fibroadenomas and fibrocystic disease of the breast, uterine leiomyomas, and macrocephaly	Congenital abnormalities in at least 20%, including malrotation, hydrocephalus, cardiac lesions, Meckel's diverticulum, and mesenteric lymphangioma	Pigmented lesions of skin; benign and malignant genital tumors	Dysmorphic facial features, macrocephaly, seizures, intellectual impairment, and pigmented macules of shaft and glans of penis
Malignancy risk						
70–80% lifetime risk for colorectal cancer; 30-60% lifetime risk for endometrial cancer; ↑ risk for ovarian cancer, gastric carcinoma, transitional cell carcinoma of the ureters and renal pelvis, small bowel cancer, and sebaceous carcinomas	Colorectal cancer risk approaches 100%; ↑ risk for periampullary malignancy, thyroid carcinoma, central nervous system tumors, and hepatoblastoma	Colorectal carcinoma and brain tumors	10% risk for thyroid cancer and up to 50% risk for adenocarcinoma of breast in affected women	9–25% risk for colorectal cancer; ↑ risk for gastric, duodenal, and pancreatic cancer	↑ risk for GI malignancy and pancreatic cancer and adenoma malignum of cervix; unknown risk for breast cancer	Malignant GI tumors identified but lifetime risk for malignancy unknown

Contd...

Contd...

	Hereditary adenomatous polyposis syndromes			***Hereditary hamartomatous polyposis syndromes***		***Ruvalcaba-Myhre-Smith***
Hereditary nonpolyposis colon cancer	***Familial adenomatous polyposis/ Gardner's syndrome***	***Turcot's syndrome***	***Cowden's disease***	***Familial juvenile polyposis***	***Peutz-Jeghers syndrome***	***Syndrome (Bannayan-Zonana syndrome)***
Screening recommendations						
• Colonoscopy at age 20–25 years; repeat every 1–3 years • Transvaginal ultrasound or endometrial aspirate at age 20–25 years; repeat annually (expert opinion only)	• Flexible procto-sigmoidoscopy at age 10–12 years; repeat every 1–2 year until age 35; after age 35 repeat every 3 years • Upper GI endoscopy every 1–3 years starting when polyps first identified	• Same as for familial adenomatous polyposis • Also consider imaging of the brain	• Annual physical exam with special attention to thyroid • Mammography at age 30 or 5 years before earliest breast cancer case in the family • Routine colon cancer surveillance (expert opinion only)	• Screening by age 12 years if symptoms have not yet arisen • Colonoscopy with multiple random biopsies every several years (expert opinion only)	Upper GI endoscopy, small bowel radiography, and colonoscopy every 2 years; pancreatic ultrasound and hemoglobin levels annually; gynecologic examination, cervical smear, and pelvic ultrasound annually; clinical breast exam and mammography at age 25 years; clinical testicular exam and testicular ultrasound in males with feminizing features (expert opinion only)	No known published recommendations
Genetic basis						
AD	AD	AD	AD	AD inheritance in some families	AD	AD
• MLH1 (chromosome 3p) • MSH2 (chromosome 2p) • MSH6/GTMP (chromosome 2p)	APC (chromosome 5q)	APC mutations identified predominantly in families with cerebellar medullo-blastoma	PTEN (chromosome 10q)	Subset of families with mutation in SMAD4 (DRC4) (chromosome 10q)	STK11 (chromosome 19p)	PTEN (chromosome 10q)
• PMS1 (chromosome 2q) • PMS2 (chromosome 7q)		MLH1, PMS2 mutations identified in families with predominance of glioblastomas				

Contd...

Contd...

	Hereditary adenomatous polyposis syndromes		*Hereditary hamartomatous polyposis syndromes*			*Ruvalcaba-Myhre-Smith*
Hereditary nonpolyposis colon cancer	***Familial adenomatous polyposis/Gardner's syndrome***	***Turcot's syndrome***	***Cowden's disease***	***Familial juvenile polyposis***	***Peutz-Jeghers syndrome***	***Syndrome (Bannayan-Zonana syndrome)***
Genetic testing						
Clinical testing of MLH1 and MSH2 genes available	Clinical testing of APC gene available	Clinical testing of APC and MLH1 genes available	Research testing of PTE N gene available	Families being collected for research studies only	Research testing of STK11 gene available	Research testing of PTEN gene available

(AD: autosomal dominant; GI: gastrointestinal; ↑: increased).

Surgical Management

- Surgical treatment of patients with familial adenomatous polyposis (FAP) is directed at removal of all affected colonic and rectal mucosa. Restorative proctocolectomy with ileal pouch-anal anastomosis (IPAA) has become the most commonly recommended operation.
- An alternative approach, total abdominal colectomy with ileorectal anastomosis, was used extensively before the development of the technique of IPAA and has certain advantages.

Surveillance

- The management of patients with HNPCC is somewhat controversial, but the need for close surveillance in patients known to carry the mutation is obvious.
- It is usually recommended that a program of surveillance colonoscopy should begin at the age of 20 years.
- Colonoscopy is repeated every 2 years until the age of 35 years, and then annually thereafter.
- In women, periodic vacuum curettage is begun at age 25 years, as are pelvic ultrasound and CA-125 levels.
- Annual tests for occult blood in the urine should also be obtained because of the risk for ureteral and renal pelvic cancer.

13. Discuss the pathology and management of familial adenomatous polyposis. ***WBUHS 2021***

14. FAP

Pathology

Familial adenomatous polyposis syndrome is characterized by the presence of hundreds or thousands of colonic adenomatous polyps, usually tubular or tubulovillous. The rectum is occasionally spared. Less commonly they affect the small bowel and stomach.

Genetics

- Familial adenomatous polyposis syndrome results from mutation of the tumor suppressor adenomatous polyposis coli (APC) gene located on chromosome 5q21-2. Around one-third of cases are thought to be sporadic (i.e., no family history) and two-thirds thought to be familial.
- *MUTYH* gene has been associated with APC-negative FAPS; this has an autosomal recessive inheritance 6 and this is often called MUTYH-associated polyposis (MAP).

Variants

There are three variants of FAPS:

1. Gardner syndrome
2. Attenuated FAP
3. Familial polyposis coli

Management

Investigations

- Sigmoidoscopy.
- Colonoscopy
- Esophagogastroduodenoscopy (EGD) and side-viewing duodenoscopy
- CT or MRI—imaging of the abdomen and pelvis may be used, especially to evaluate desmoid tumors.

Medical Care

- Medical care is mainly based on endoscopic surveillance to detect the onset of polyposis.
- Consequently, surgery would prevent the development of colon cancer.
- However, in view of the increased risk for the development of other cancers, continued medical follow-up is required with a number of surveillance tests, as colectomy would only address the potential risk of colon cancer.
- A number of drugs (e.g., celecoxib and sulindac) have been used successfully to reduce the number and the size of polyps in patients with FAP. However, they are insufficient as a primary modality of therapy.

Endoscopic Surveillance

- Flexible sigmoidoscopy should be performed every 1–2 years starting at age 10–12 years in patients with FAP to document the onset of polyposis.
- Sigmoidoscopic surveillance and ablation of any polyps in the retained rectum or ileal pouch should be performed every 3–6 months in patients with FAP who have undergone colonic (total or subtotal) resection.
- There is an increased risk for adenomas and carcinomas in the ileal pouch, as there is increased epithelial cell proliferation at this site as compared to the afferent ileal loop.
- Once polyps are detected, colonoscopic surveillance is recommended to remove large polyps in patients who have not had an operation.
- This is important because surgery (colectomy) is usually deferred until an appropriate psychological age is reached (usually late teenaged years to early twenties).
- However, if the polyps have advanced histologic features, then early surgery is recommended.
- Front- and side-view EGD should be performed every 1–3 years once the diagnosis is made and after surgical therapy.
- The front-view EGD allows for the detection of gastric and duodenal polyps. The side-view duodenoscope allows for the examination of the ampulla of Vater.
- Capsule endoscopy is useful for the surveillance of jejunal-ileal polyps in selected patients but is not recommended for duodenal or ampullary surveillance.
- Some patients who are at high risk may benefit from screening with endoscopic ultrasound for periampullary and ampullary tumors.

Treatment

- Drugs used in the treatment of FAP include sulindac and celecoxib—these drugs have no primary role as sole therapy for patients with FAP who have not had surgical therapy. However, in patients with FAP who have had colectomy with ileoanal anastomosis, sulindac or celecoxib may be beneficial in reducing the size and the number of adenomatous polyps in the remaining rectum.
- Screening of family members of patients with FAP should begin by age 12 years. Flexible sigmoidoscopy every 1–2 years until the patient is aged 35 years is adequate, then every 3 years thereafter. Genetic testing may eliminate the need for surveillance in some family members.
- Desmoid tumors (intra-abdominal) may respond to antiestrogen therapy (tamoxifen) and sulindac because estrogen appears to promote their growth.
- Chemotherapy with doxorubicin and dacarbazine may be attempted if no response is observed with other therapies.

Surgical Care

- Colectomy with mucosal proctectomy and ileoanal pouch pull-through (proctocolectomy with IPAA) is the procedure of choice at many centers. This procedure allows retention of the rectal function. Other options include subtotal colectomy with ileoanal anastomosis and total proctocolectomy with ileostomy.
- If medical therapy and endoscopic therapy do not control polyp growth, rectal resection may be needed in patients who have a retained rectum (such as in subtotal colectomy). Desmoid tumors may be resected with adequate margins. This generally is reserved for patients with ureteral or intestinal obstruction.

Dietary Considerations

Patients with colectomy often have a change in bowel habits, for which changes in diet can lead to vitamin-mineral deficiencies. Vitamin B_{12} deficiency occurs from rapid intestinal transit, ileal resection, and ascending bacterial overgrowth.

15. What is adenoma-carcinoma sequence in colorectal cancers? *WBUHS 2018*

The adenoma-carcinoma sequence in sporadic and hereditary colorectal cancer.

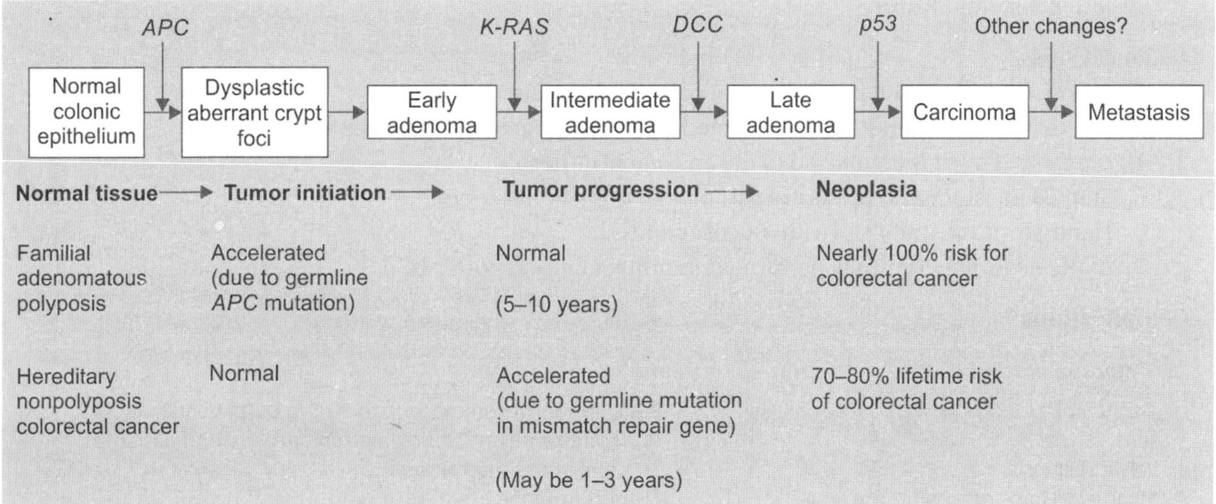

16. Discuss the indications, steps and complications of restorative proctocolectomy. *AIIMS, Bhubaneswar 2024*

Restorative Proctocolectomy

Commonly involving the ileal pouch-anal anastomosis (IPAA)—is a surgical procedure performed primarily for patients with ulcerative colitis (UC) or familial adenomatous polyposis (FAP). It involves the removal of the colon and rectum, with the creation of a neorectum (usually a J-pouch) from the terminal ileum that is anastomosed to the anal canal, allowing for the preservation of continence.

Indications

- *Ulcerative colitis (UC):*
  - Medically refractory UC.
  - UC with dysplasia or carcinoma.
  - Complications such as perforation, massive bleeding, or toxic megacolon.
  - Elective surgery in patients seeking definitive treatment to avoid lifelong immunosuppressive therapy.
- *Familial adenomatous polyposis (FAP):*
  - Presence of hundreds to thousands of adenomatous polyps.
  - High risk or presence of colorectal carcinoma.
  - Prophylactic surgery in adolescents or young adults.

- *Other indications (less common):*
  - Certain cases of indeterminate colitis (with caution).
  - Rare hereditary colorectal cancer syndromes.

Surgical Steps

The operation can be done in one, two, or three stages depending on the patient's condition:

One-stage procedure (less common)

1. *Total proctocolectomy with IPAA and no temporary ileostomy.*

Two-stage procedure (most common)

1. *Stage 1:* Total proctocolectomy + IPAA + loop ileostomy.
2. *Stage 2:* Ileostomy closure (after 6–12 weeks when healing is confirmed).

Three-stage procedure (used in critically ill or high-risk patients)

1. *Stage 1:* Subtotal colectomy + end ileostomy (rectum left in place).
2. *Stage 2:* Proctectomy + IPAA + loop ileostomy.
3. *Stage 3:* Ileostomy closure.

Technical Steps

1. *Total Proctocolectomy:* Removal of entire colon and rectum.
2. *Pouch creation:* Typically a J-pouch formed from 30–40 cm of terminal ileum.
3. *Anastomosis:* Pouch is connected to the anal canal either:
   - Stapled anastomosis (preserves part of anal transitional zone).
   - Hand-sewn anastomosis (with mucosectomy).
4. *Diverting Ileostomy:* Typically performed to protect the anastomosis.

Complications

Early (postoperative)	*Late*
• *Anastomotic leak (4–10%):* May lead to pelvic sepsis • Pelvic abscess • Small bowel obstruction • Wound infection • Ileus • Bleeding	• Pouchitis (most common, up to 50% in UC patients) – Treated with antibiotics (metronidazole, ciprofloxacin) • Stricture at the anastomosis • Fistula formation • Pouch failure (requiring excision or permanent ileostomy) • *Fertility issues:* Especially in women; pelvic dissection can affect fallopian tubes • Incontinence or poor function – Increased stool frequency (~4–6/day), especially early on – Nighttime soiling or urgency in some patients

COLORECTAL CANCER

17. Mention the prognostic factors for colorectal cancers. What is the follow-up protocol for such cancers?

WBUHS 2018

Prognostic and Predictive Factors for Colorectal Cancer

- *Stage:* Stage is the most important prognostic factor for colorectal cancer. The lower the stage at diagnosis, the better the outcome. Tumors without distant metastasis have more favorable prognosis than those that have distant metastases.

- *Surgical margins:* The prognosis is better if there are no cancer cells in the tissue removed with the tumor than if there are cancer cells in the tissue (called positive surgical margins).
- *Cancer cells in lymph and blood vessels:* Cancer cells can move or grow into nearby lymph vessels and blood vessels called lymphovascular invasion. Tumors that don't have lymphovascular invasion have a better prognosis than tumors that have lymphovascular invasion.
- *Carcinoembryonic antigen (CEA) levels:* The lower the CEA level before surgery, the more favorable the prognosis.
- *Bowel obstruction or perforation:* Patients who have a bowel obstruction or perforation at diagnosis have a less favorable prognosis.
- *Grade:* High-grade colorectal cancer means that the cancer cells are poorly differentiated or undifferentiated. High-grade cancers have a poorer prognosis than low-grade cancers.
- *Type of tumor:* Mucinous adenocarcinoma, signet ring cell carcinoma, and small cell carcinoma have a less favorable prognosis than other types of colorectal tumors.
- *Microsatellite instability (MSI):* MSI is a change to the genetic material, or DNA, in a cell. Some colorectal cancer cells show MSI. Tumors that have cells with high MSI (MSI-H) have a more favorable prognosis than tumors without MSI (called microsatellite stable or MSS).
- *Gene changes:* The following genes are linked with colorectal cancer and affect prognosis.
  - *DCC* gene is found at chromosome 18q. It is a tumor suppressor gene that normally controls cell growth and death. Part of chromosome 18q, along with the *DCC* gene, are often missing in colorectal cancer cells. When the *DCC* gene is missing, cell growth, division, and death may be uncontrolled. Missing the *DCC* gene is also linked with metastases and resistance to chemotherapy. Colorectal tumors with cancer cells that are missing part of chromosome 18q and the *DCC* gene may have a poor prognosis.
  - *KRAS* gene can be mutated, or changed, in some colorectal cancer cells. KRAS gene mutations mean that the cancer cells are unlikely to respond to targeted therapy drugs such as cetuximab and panitumumab. People with colorectal cancer cells that test positive for the KRAS gene mutation have a less favorable prognosis because targeted therapy drugs will not work on the tumor.
  - *BRAF* gene mutations mean that the cancer cells may be more aggressive. As a result, people with cancer cells that have the BRAF gene mutation have a worse prognosis.

Follow-up care recommendations for colorectal cancer by years after treatment.

Follow-up care recommendations	***Year 1***	***Year 2***	***Year 3***	***Years 4 and 5***
Doctor's visit	Every 3–6 months	Every 6 months	Every 6 months	Every 6 months
CEA test	Every 3 months	Every 3 months	Every 3 months	As determined by your doctor
CT scan (chest and abdomen)	Every year, if recommended by your doctor	Every year, if recommended by your doctor	Every year, if recommended by your doctor	As determined by your doctor
CT scan (pelvis) (rectal cancer only)	Every year, if recommended by your doctor	Every year, if recommended by your doctor	Every year, if recommended by your doctor	As determined by your doctor
Colonoscopy	Once		At 3 years	
Proctosigmoidoscopy (rectal cancer only)	Every 6 months for 5 years			

18. CME and CVL in colon cancer surgery. ***AIIMS, Raipur 2025; Rajasthan University of Health Sciences 2025***

CME and CVL Concepts were Introduced to Standardize Oncologic Quality

Concept	*Definition/Principle*	*Analogy*
CME (Complete Mesocolic Excision)	Sharp dissection along the embryological planes to remove the *entire mesocolon intact,* enveloped by its visceral fascia, with minimal violation of the mesocolic surface	Similar to *TME* in rectal cancer
CVL (Central Vascular Ligation)	Division (ligation) of the *feeding vessels at their origin* from the superior or inferior mesenteric arteries, ensuring maximal lymph node harvest along the main vascular trunks	Equivalent to *high tie* of the mesenteric vessels

Together, CME + CVL aim for an *"en bloc" removal* of the colon segment, mesocolon, and associated lymphatic drainage up to the root of supplying vessels.

Surgical Anatomy

- The *mesocolon* is a fascial envelope containing lymphatics, vessels, and fat.
- Dissection along the *mesofascial plane* (between visceral and parietal fascia) preserves this integrity.
- CVL ensures clearance of D3 nodes (central lymph nodes at vascular origin).

Colon segment	*Vessel ligated (CVL)*	*Main nodal basin cleared*
Right colon	Ileocolic, right colic, right branch of middle colic—at SMA origin	D1–D3 along SMA
Transverse colon	Middle colic at SMA	D3 at root of SMA
Left/sigmoid colon	Inferior mesenteric artery (IMA) at origin or left colic	D3 along IMA

Key Principles of CME + CVL Technique

- *Sharp dissection along embryological planes* (between mesocolon and retroperitoneum).
- *Preserve the visceral mesocolic fascia*—specimen surface should be smooth and intact.
- *Central vascular ligation* at the root of the feeding artery/vein (SMA/SMV or IMA/IMV).
- *Adequate longitudinal margins* (≥10 cm proximally and distally).
- *Mobilization of the entire mesocolon* to the vascular origin.
- *En bloc resection* of involved adjacent structures if T4.

ME vs Conventional Colectomy—Key Differences

Feature	*Conventional colectomy*	*CME + CVL*
Plane of dissection	Often random; may violate mesocolon	Along embryological mesofascial plane
Mesocolic envelope	Frequently disrupted	Intact (visceral fascia preserved)
Vascular ligation	Intermediate (D2)	Central (D3)
Nodal yield	~12–15 nodes	20–35 nodes
Local recurrence	Higher (~6–10%)	Lower (~3–5%)
5-year survival	Slightly lower	Improved (esp. stage II–III)

Minimally Invasive CME (Lap/Robotic)

Recent Developments

- Laparoscopic CME + CVL is now *standard* in expert centers.
- *Robotic CME* gaining traction due to enhanced dexterity and 3D visualization, especially for CVL near SMA/SMV.
- Ongoing trials (e.g., *CME-ROBO 2024, JCOG1905*) are comparing robotic vs laparoscopic CME outcomes.

Safety
- When done in experienced hands, *no increase in morbidity* or 30-day mortality vs conventional colectomy.
- Conversion rates <10%.
- Similar anastomotic leak rates (~2–3%).

Pathologic Assessment

Pathology now evaluates CME specimens similar to TME:
- *Plane of surgery* (mesocolic, intramesocolic, muscularis propria).
- *Mesocolic surface integrity* (smooth vs torn).
- *Length of vascular pedicle and number of nodes retrieved* (>12 minimum; ≥20 ideal).
- *R0 margin status.*

Grading systems are used to audit CME quality.

Complications and Concerns

Potential issue	Comment/mitigation
Vascular injury (SMA/SMV/IMA)	Use 3D mapping, fluorescence imaging; meticulous dissection
Prolonged operative time	Reduces with experience
Increased lymphatic leak/chyle leak	Controlled by meticulous ligation
Autonomic nerve injury (esp. IMA dissection)	Stay within fascial planes; avoid excessive traction
Learning curve	~30–50 cases for proficiency; structured training recommended

CME + CVL in Guidelines (as of 2024–25)

Guideline	Recommendation
European Society of Coloproctology (ESCP 2024)	CME recommended for all curative colon resections where expertise available
NCCN (2025)	Encourages high ligation (D3) and intact mesocolic resection; recognizes CME as standard in specialized centers
Japanese JSCCR (2024)	Classifies D3 lymphadenectomy as standard for T2–T4 colon cancers
SAGES/EAES (2024)	Endorses minimally invasive CME as oncologically equivalent to open CME when performed by trained surgeons

19. A 50-year-old lady presenting with bright red blood per rectum was sent for colonoscopy which revealed an apple–core lesion at 12 cm from the anal verge. The biopsy revealed moderately differentiated adenocarcinoma. CT scan of abdomen/pelvis demonstrated a large mass in rectum measuring 5 × 4 cm with no liver metastatic liver or adenopathy. MRI of pelvis revealed a rectal mass with excessive mesorectal lymphadenopathy.

Give a precise tumor-node-metastasis (TNM) stage of her disease (AJCC 7th Edition, 2010) along with the staging system. Mention few selected pathologic prognostic factors for the disease and precise management protocol for the lady in detail with references to the evidences. ***WBUHS 2016***

Rectal Cancer Staging

TNM Staging

Primary Tumor Staging (T):
- *Tx:* Primary tumor cannot be assessed
- *T0:* No evidence of primary tumor
- *Tis:* Carcinoma in situ: Intraepithelial or invasion of lamina propria
- *T1:* Tumor invades submucosa

- *T2:* Tumor invades muscularis propria
- *T3:* Tumor invades through the muscularis propria into the subserosa or into nonperitonealized perirectal tissues
  - *T3a:* Tumor extends <1 mm beyond muscularis propria
  - *T3b:* Tumor extends 1–5 mm beyond muscularis propria
  - *T3c:* Tumor extends 5–15 mm beyond muscularis propria
  - *T3d:* Tumor extends 15 mm beyond muscularis propria
- *T4:* Tumor invades directly into other organs or structures and/or perforates visceral peritoneum
  - *T4a:* Tumor penetrates to the surface of the visceral peritoneum
  - *T4b:* Tumor directly invades or is adherent to other organs or structures

Regional Lymph Nodes (N)

The size cut off for mesorectal nodes is usually taken at 5 mm.

- *Nx:* Regional nodes not assessed
- *N0:* No regional lymph nodes
- *N1:* Metastasis in 1–3 regional (perirectal) lymph nodes
  - *N1a:* Metastasis in one regional lymph node
  - *N1b:* Metastasis in 2–3 regional lymph nodes
  - *N1c:* Tumor deposit(s) in the subserosa, mesentery, or nonperitonealized pericolic or perirectal tissues without regional nodal metastasis
- *N2:* Metastasis in 4 or more regional lymph nodes
  - *N2a:* Metastasis in 4–6 regional lymph nodes
  - *N2b:* Metastasis in 7 or more regional lymph nodes

Metastases

- *Mx:* Cannot be assessed
- *M0:* No distant metastasis
- *M1:* Distant metastasis
  - *M1a:* Metastasis confined to one organ or site (for example, liver, lung, ovary, and nonregional node)
  - *M1b:* Metastases in more than one organ/site or the peritoneum

Stage Groupings

- *Stage 0:* Tis N0 M0
- *Stage I:* T1-2, N0 M0
- *Stage II:*
  - *IIa:* T3, N0, M0
  - *IIb:* T4a, N0, M0
  - *IIc:* T:4b, No, Mo
- *Stage III:*
  - *IIIa:* T1-2, N1, M0
  - *IIIb:* T3-4, N1, M0
  - *IIIc:* T3-4b, N2, M0
- *Stage IV:* Any T, any N M1

TNM Staging of this Lesion is T3c N2b M0—Stage is IIIc

Prognostic Pathological Factors

- Local extent of tumor assessed pathologically
- Regional lymph node metastasis assessed pathologically
- Blood or lymphatic vessel invasion
- Preoperative CEA elevation
- Histologic grade
- Radial margin (specimens with nonperitonealized surfaces)
- Histologic type
- Tumor classification after neoadjuvant therapy
- *Histologic features associated with MSI-H:* Host lymphoid response to tumor and medullary or mucinous histologic type

- High degree of MSI
- *Histologic type:* Medullary carcinoma and mucinous carcinoma
- Loss of heterozygosity at 18q and allelic loss of deleted in colon cancer gene
- Tumor border configuration

Management Protocol

- Following surgical removal of rectal cancer, the cancer is referred to as stage III rectal cancer if the final pathology report shows that the cancer has invaded any of the local lymph nodes, but cannot be detected in other locations in the body.
- A variety of factors ultimately influence a patient's decision to receive treatment of cancer. The purpose of receiving cancer treatment may be to improve symptoms through local control of the cancer, increase a patient's chance of cure, or prolong a patient's survival. The potential benefits of receiving cancer treatment must be carefully balanced with the potential risks of receiving cancer treatment.
- The following is a general overview of the treatment of stage III rectal cancer. Circumstances unique to your situation and prognostic factors of your cancer may ultimately influence how these general treatment principles are applied. The information on this website is intended to help educate you about your treatment options and to facilitate a mutual or shared decision-making process with your treating cancer physician.
- Most new treatments are developed in clinical trials. Clinical trials are studies that evaluate the effectiveness of new drugs or treatment strategies. The development of more effective cancer treatments requires that new and innovative therapies be evaluated with cancer patients. Participation in a clinical trial may offer access to better treatments and advance the existing knowledge about treatment of this cancer. Clinical trials are available for most stages of cancer. Patients who are interested in participating in a clinical trial should discuss the risks and benefits of clinical trials with their physician. To ensure that you are receiving the optimal treatment of your cancer, it is important to stay informed and follow the cancer news in order to learn about new treatments and the results of clinical trials.

Neoadjuvant Therapy

Neoadjuvant therapy refers to treatment given prior to surgery. Many patients with Stage III rectal cancer receive neoadjuvant chemotherapy and radiation therapy; the goals are to reduce the risk of cancer recurrence and to shrink the cancer prior to surgery. If patients are in poor health and unable to tolerate chemotherapy and/or radiation therapy, surgery may be the initial treatment.

Surgical Treatment

- The standard surgical procedures used to remove stage III rectal cancer include low anterior resection (LAR) or abdominoperineal resection (APR). The choice of operation depends on the location of the rectal cancer.
- If the cancer is very low in the rectum (near the anus), a patient may need to have an APR. This involves an incision in the abdomen and an incision around the anus. Because both the rectum and the anus are removed, an APR requires a permanent colostomy.

Laparoscopic Surgery

- Laparoscopic surgery is used for many types of surgery with the short-term advantages of less pain, fewer wound complications, quicker postoperative recovery, and shorter hospital stays.
- Laparoscopic-assisted surgery appears to be about as likely to be curative as the standard approach for earlier-stage cancers.

Adjuvant Therapy

The goal of providing additional treatment after surgery (adjuvant therapy) is to reduce the risk of cancer recurrence by eliminating any remaining cancer. For patients who received neoadjuvant (before-surgery) chemotherapy and radiation therapy, additional chemotherapy is often given after surgery. If patients did not receive neoadjuvant therapy, they may be treated with both chemotherapy and radiation therapy after surgery.

Strategies to Improve Treatment

Improved Approaches to Radiation Therapy

- Advances have been made in the ability of physicians to precisely target the area of the cancer. The goal is to deliver effective doses of radiation to the cancer while sparing healthy tissue to the extent possible.
- One newer approach to delivering radiation therapy is intensity-modulated radiation therapy (IMRT). IMRT starts with a three-dimensional image of the cancer, and allows to deliver different doses of radiation to different areas. The potential advantages for patients include both better tumor control and fewer side effects.

Targeted Therapies

- Targeted therapies are anticancer drugs that interfere with specific pathways involved in cancer cell growth or survival.
- Some targeted therapies block growth signals from reaching cancer cells; others reduce the blood supply to cancer cells; and still others stimulate the immune system to recognize and attack the cancer cell.
- Depending on the specific "target", targeted therapies may slow cancer cell growth or increase cancer cell death.
- Targeted therapies may be used in combination with other cancer treatments such as conventional chemotherapy.
- Targeted therapies that have shown a benefit for selected patients with advanced rectal cancer include bevacizumab, cetuximab, and panitumumab.

20. Role of radiotherapy in colorectal cancer. ***WBUHS 2006***

Colorectal cancer is the third most common malignancy in the United States. Worldwide, there were approximately 1 million new cases and 500,000 deaths secondary to colorectal cancer. Approximately 80% of patients with colorectal cancer present with localized disease; however, despite surgery with curative intent, patients still face a significant risk of local and distant recurrence and cancer-related mortality.

Surgical resection of the primary tumor with acceptable margins and concurrent, en bloc lymph node dissection remains the standard of care for patients who present with localized disease and remains the most effective modality of cure of colorectal cancer. The likelihood of cure is directly related to the depth of tumor penetration through the bowel wall and lymph node metastasis. While patients with lymph node involvement can be cured with surgery alone, up to 40–60% of these patients will have recurrence or will die of metastatic disease.

Rationale for Adjuvant Therapy

Patients with colorectal cancer who undergo surgery with curative intent, in whom no gross postoperative disease is detectable, may still develop either local recurrence or distant metastasis. This is due to the existence of micrometastatic disease present at the time of surgery that remains in the tumor bed after resection or by tumor cells that spread by lymphatic or blood vessels to distant sites. The main goal of adjuvant therapy is to eliminate these micrometastases. This goal should be achieved while maintaining the best possible quality of life for the patient without compromising the ability to cure the malignancy. The identification of patients with a sufficiently high risk of recurrence to warrant the risks of adjuvant chemotherapy and possible radiation therapy depends on appropriate staging.

The treatment of rectal cancer has changed significantly during the past 20 years, and there is considerable controversy today concerning the precise role of surgery, radiation therapy, and chemotherapy, and the ideal timing of each modality with relation to the others. Although information from clinical trials has provided data supporting the multimodality treatment of rectal cancer, the criteria for patient selection remains controversial. However, some generalities can be made at the present time.

Radiation therapy offers significant benefit to many patients with rectal cancer, and preoperative radiation is superior to postoperative radiation. Until recently, preoperative radiation (combined with chemotherapy) has generally been reserved for locally advanced distal rectal cancers (within 10 cm of the anal verge, stage II or higher), but a recent analysis based on a cooperative 7-year trial of the National Research Council (NRC) of the United Kingdom and the National Cancer Institute of Canada (NCIC) has shown that short-term preoperative radiation (25 Gy over 5 days) results in a significant reduction in the local recurrence rate and improved disease-free survival for all stages of rectal cancer.

Stage I	*No adjuvant therapy*
Stage II or III	Neoadjuvant chemoradiation for 5 weeks
Low/mid lesion	• 5-FU-based chemotherapy with XRT (180 cGy 5 days/week x 5 weeks) • Rest for 6 weeks • Total mesorectal excision • Rest for 4 weeks • Continue 5-FU–based chemotherapy for 8 weeks
High lesion	• Preoperative or postoperative chemotherapy • Total mesorectal excision
Stage IV	• LAR or APR for palliation/prevention of obstruction or bleeding • Adjuvant chemotherapy • 5-FU + leucovorin ± irinotecan or oxaliplatin with individualized XRT

(APR: abdominoperineal resection; 5-FU: 5-fluorouracil; LAR: low anterior resection; XRT: external-beam radiation therapy)

21. What would be the precise roll of PET-CT scan in the evaluation of colorectal cancer? Discuss the measures to improve the resectability of nonresectable CRC liver metastasis. ***WBUHS 2017***

Role of PET-CT

Positron emission tomography (PET) is considered particularly effective in identifying whether cancer is present or not, if it has spread, if it is responding to treatment, and if a person is cancer free after treatment. Cancers for which PET is considered particularly effective include lung, head and neck, colorectal, esophageal, lymphoma, melanoma, breast, thyroid, cervical, pancreatic, and brain as well as other less-frequently-occurring cancers.

- *Early detection:* Because PET images biochemical activity, it can accurately characterize a tumor as benign or malignant, thereby avoiding surgical biopsy when the PET scan is negative. Conversely, because a PET scan images the entire body, confirmation of distant metastasis can alter treatment plans in certain cases from surgical intervention to chemotherapy.
- *Staging of cancer:* PET is extremely sensitive in determining the full extent of disease, especially in lymphoma, malignant melanoma, breast, lung, colon, and cervical cancers. Confirmation of metastatic disease allows the physician and patient to more accurately decide how to proceed with the patient's management.
- *Checking for recurrences:* According to the literature (see "Sources"), PET is currently considered to be the most accurate diagnostic procedure to differentiate tumor recurrences from radiation necrosis or postsurgical changes. Such an approach allows for the development of a more rational treatment plan for the patient.
- *Assessing the effectiveness of chemotherapy:* The level of tumor metabolism is compared on PET scans taken before and after a chemotherapy cycle. A successful response seen on a PET scan frequently precedes alterations in anatomy and would, therefore, be an earlier indicator of tumor response than that seen with other diagnostic modalities.

Colorectal Cancer and PET

- As with all types of cancer, early diagnosis of colorectal cancer is key to its cure. Colorectal cancers probably develop slowly over a period of several years. Before a true cancer develops, there are often earlier changes in the lining of the colon or rectum. If found early, before it has metastasized, the disease is considered curable. However, as the tumor spreads to lymph nodes, a patient's chance of living at least five years drops to 40–60%. If the cancer has already spread to distant organs, the long-term survival may be lower. As it relates to the diagnosis of early colorectal cancer, a study found that PET was capable of noninvasively detecting an early colon cancer as small as 16 mm as well as other cancers in the whole body and considered it to be a suitable screening examination.
- Before PET, it was extremely difficult to monitor patients for suspected recurrence of colorectal cancer. The other techniques available for staging and assessment of potential recurrences may lack sensitivity and precision and frequently result in diagnostic and therapeutic delays. One study found that the sensitivity

and specificity of PET/CT to colon cancer recurrence in patients after resection were 96.5% and 82.1%, respectively.

- In many colorectal cancer patients, pelvic CT could demonstrate a suspicious mass, but cannot distinguish mass tumor recurrence from postoperative or postradiation scar or is a recurrent cancer that must be treated. Further evaluation usually involves a biopsy. A positive biopsy is highly predictive of recurrence but because it is impossible to sample the entire mass, a negative biopsy cannot exclude recurrence.
- Imaging with PET is critical in looking for the return of the cancer. In many patients with colorectal cancer, a mass may develop in the pelvis. A PET scan can identify whether the mass is suspicious of being cancerous because it will pick up the radioactive glucose and be seen on the scan results. If, however, the mass is scarring caused by the radiation treatments, no glucose uptake will be seen in the area of the mass. Reports in the scientific literature find that, in some tumors, PET correctly identifies detected lesions up to 95% of the time; however, the final word will of course rest with the pathology if a biopsy is performed.
- PET can be used to image tumor response to therapy and to detect recurrence in successfully treated lesions. After surgery and other treatments, PET is an extremely important tool in monitoring whether any cancer cells have returned and if treatment should be restarted.
- PET can find with near 100% certainty after a single course of chemotherapy if a patient with metastatic colorectal cancer is not responding positively to treatment.
- PET is capable of showing the extent of the disease (called staging) of colorectal cancer. For patients whose cancer is newly diagnosed, it is important to determine if the cancer has spread to other parts of the body so that appropriate treatment can be commenced, while avoiding unnecessary therapies at the same time. Colorectal cancer is less likely to recur after 5 years of there being no evidence of the disease; thus, most patients who live 5 years without recurrence are considered cured. In the interim, however, ensuring that PET is a part of regular follow-up testing is important according to researchers.
- In colorectal cancer, if the lymph nodes near the tumor or if a distant organ such as the liver has become involved by the cancer, they will take up more of the radioactive glucose. Whether or not distant organs are involved is a critical factor in deciding what the surgical and medical treatment will be. Some studies have shown that even if the cancer has spread in a limited fashion outside the colon, surgery combined with chemotherapy can be done to remove these other tumors and reduce the chance of recurrence.

The benefits of PET include:

- It often replaces multiple medical testing procedures with a single examination, while producing imaging information of superior quality.
- It may validate and/or alter patient management and care.
- It may reduce or eliminate ineffective and unnecessary surgical or other medical treatments and hospitalization.
- It may reduce significantly overall healthcare costs and avoids needless pain to the patient.
- It is done in approximately 2 hours and provides interpretation virtually immediately.
- It may show the progress of disease and how the body responds to treatment.
- It may diagnose disease before it shows up on other tests.

TME, Transanal Endoscopic Microsurgery (TEM), and Transanal Minimally Invasive Surgery (TAMIS)

22. Discuss the role of TME and TEM in colorectal cancer. ***WBUHS 2018***

Role of TME in Colorectal Cancer

Introduction

- The concept of TME is proposed by Heald over 20 years ago.
- The mesocolon and retroperitoneum are separated by two mesothelial layers with a connective tissue layer between them corresponding to the TME plane of dissection (the “holy” embryological plane).
- The colonic mesentery contains the blood and lymphatic vessels and nodes emanating from and going to the corresponding colonic segments.

- Central vascular ligation (CVL) is the cornerstone of radical excision principles.
- The goal of CVL is to remove as much lymph nodes and associated vascular structures in a vertical or ascending direction potentially removing lymph node metastases, as well as vascular and neural invasion of the regional drainage area.

Significance and benefits of TME

- TME (which can be defined as complete excision of visceral mesorectum to the level of the levator, with the preservation of the pelvic nerves) is the gold standard for the treatment of rectal cancers and the middle lower third of the rectum.
- Local recurrence arises mainly as a result of incomplete surgical resection. Mesorectal tissue seems to be an ideal substrate for the spreading of tumor. In rectal cancer, local recurrence is present in the absence of distant metastases.
- Macroscopic examination of the mesorectal surface helps us evaluate the quality of the surgical specimen.
- Mesorectal defects are classified into three categories:
  1. *Complete:* Mesorectum is intact, smooth with only minor irregularities without defect 15 mm.
  2. *Moderate:* Moderate bulk to mesorectum but irregularity of the mesorectal surface; muscularis propria is not visible with the exception of the area of insertion of levator muscles,
  3. *Incomplete:* Little bulk to mesorectum with defects down into muscularis propria.
- Several studies have proved that TME has reduced the local recurrence rates.
- TME can eradicate lymphatic spread in high-grade carcinomas (>5 cm above the dentate line), but it cannot achieve complete removal of the lymphatic spread of lower rectal neoplasms (<5 cm from the dentate line).
- Wide mesorectum excision (WME), which keeps the distal rectum and improves the postoperative anal function. Thus, the rule is that TME for all tumors is 8 cm or less from the anterior anal edge, for tumors above 8 cm, WME should be performed.
- TME can result in a 20% improvement in the 4-year survival rate, and the Norwegian Rectal Cancer Group showed a greater improvement.

Quirke, West, and collaborators have developed a grading system based on the grading system used in the MRC CR07 trial for rectal cancer:

- *Mesocolic plane of resection:* "Good" surgery, performed along mesofascial interface; producing intact, inviolate mesocolon with a smooth peritoneal surface.
- *Intramesocolic plane of resection:* "Moderate" characterized by irregular breaches in the mesocolon, none reaching the muscularis propria of the colon.
- *Muscularis propria plane of resection:* "Poor" characterized by disruption of the mesocolon, with breaches the visceral muscularis propria.

The quality of mesorectum excision according to procare criteria:

The quality of mesorectum excision in TME samples proposed by PROCARE guide. Samples and whole (fresh) and transverse cross-sections (after fixation) should be examined to adequately evaluate mesorectum excision.	
Smooth, regular	• Intact mesorectum with only minor irregularities on a smooth mesorectum surface • No defect deeper than 5 mm • There is no cone at the distal margin of the sample • Smooth circumferential resection limit on the incision
Slightly irregular	• Moderate volume of mesorectum, but irregularity of the mesorectum surface • Moderate coning of the sample • Muscularis propria is not visible at all places, with the exception of the levator insertion
Very irregular	A small volume of mesorectum with defects down to muscularis propria and/or very irregular circumferential resection margin on the incision

- The elements of the pathology report consist of completeness of mesorectum, the circumferential resection margin (CRM), type and grade of the carcinoma, the number of positive lymph nodes, and vascular invasion.
- The newer MRI techniques may play a role in determining preoperatively mesorectum and the CRM in order to select patients with a high risk of CRM involvement and for those patients preoperative radiochemotherapy is the treatment of choice.
- PET scanning may have a role in determining locally advanced tumor response to neoadjuvant chemotherapy.

Role of TEM in Colorectal Cancer

Introduction

- Transanal endoscopic microsurgery was developed by Professor Gerhard Buess
- TEM utilizes a closed proctoscopic system whereby endoluminal surgery is accomplished with high-definition magnification, constant CO_2 insufflation, and long-shafted instruments.
- TEM offers several advantages over conventional transanal excision. It provides better exposure, visualization, and access to reach lesions higher in the rectum than standard transanal excision.
- It is associated with less morbidity and quicker recovery time than a radical transabdominal approach.
- A combined multifunctional endosurgical unit regulates suction, irrigation, intrarectal pressure, and gas insufflation. Suction removes fluid, blood, waste, and smoke.
- Irrigation helps to maintain a relatively clean operative field and can rinse the end of the scope. CO_2 insufflation maintains distention of the rectum throughout the procedure and flow can be increased as high as 6 L/min. The intrarectal pressure is set at a desired level (usually 10–15 cmH_2O) and the four functions mentioned above are regulated to achieve a constant steady state at that level.

TEM can be used as:

- In selected patients with rectal cancer of lesions smaller than 3 cm.
- Anatomically accessible lesions localized to the bowel wall (T1N0)
- Lesions confined to the extraperitoneal region of the rectum
- Lesions occupying <40% of the circumference of the bowel lumen; Well-differentiated or moderately differentiated lesions
- Lesions not associated with lymphovascular invasion
- Mobile lesions
- Polypoidal lesions
  - Operating time, blood loss, length of hospital stay, and analgesic requirement associated with TEM were significantly less than those associated with abdominal resection. The recurrence rates of tumors following TEM have been reported to range from 2.4 to 16%.
  - The use of TEM as palliative surgery for advanced rectal lesions is also acceptable for patients with comorbid conditions and disseminated disease who are otherwise unfit for more radical surgery.

Contraindications for TEM include the following:

- Positive lymph nodes
- Distant metastasis
- Ulcerated tumor
- Large tumor extending into muscularis propria (contraindicated owing to the increased risk of lymph node invasion)
- Poorly differentiated tumor
- Lymphovascular invasion
- TEM excision of favorable pT1 cancers is safe as sole therapy, outcome is not necessarily compromised if prompt radical surgery is performed after TEM, TEM alone is not appropriate for T2 or greater lesions, and most patients who experience recurrence after TEM can be salvaged with radical surgery.

23. Give the detailed anatomy of pararectal endopelvic fascia with the related autonomic nerves in reference to proper execution of TME. Describe the different local excision procedures for early rectal cancers. ***WBUHS 2013***

24. Evaluate the place of pathological evaluation in colorectal cancer with special reference to TME. ***WBUHS 2008***

25. Describe the principles and steps of TME for carcinoma rectum. ***WBUHS 2015***

26. Discuss the role of TME for rectal cancers. ***RIMS, Imphal 2022***

27. A 45-year-old male is diagnosed with rectal cancer. Outline the algorithm for diagnosis, the role of total mesorectal excision (TME) and neoadjuvant therapy. ***Maharashtra University of Health Sciences 2025***

Algorithm for Diagnosis of Rectal Cancer

Clinical Evaluation

- *Symptoms:*
  - Rectal bleeding
  - Altered bowel habits
  - Tenesmus, mucus discharge
  - Pain or obstruction (advanced disease)
  - Weight loss, anemia
- *History and examination:*
  - *Digital rectal examination (DRE):* Location, mobility, fixation, sphincter tone
  - General examination for metastatic signs (hepatomegaly, lymph nodes)

Initial Diagnostic Investigation

Colonoscopic Evaluation

- Colonoscopy
  - Visualizes entire colon and rectum
  - Biopsy → *Histopathological confirmation* (adenocarcinoma, etc.)
  - Rule out synchronous lesions

Local Staging (Pelvic Assessment)

After biopsy confirms *rectal adenocarcinoma*, proceed to *local staging*:

Investigation	*Purpose*
MRI pelvis (high-resolution)	Gold standard for local staging → assesses T stage, mesorectal fascia (CRM), nodal status, extramural vascular invasion (EMVI)
Endorectal ultrasound (ERUS)	Useful for early T1–T2 lesions; defines depth of invasion
Rigid/flexible sigmoidoscopy	Confirms exact distance from anal verge and morphology

Distant Staging (Metastatic Workup)

Investigation	*Purpose*
CT chest, abdomen, pelvis	Detects liver, lung, nodal, or peritoneal metastases
CEA (carcinoembryonic antigen)	Baseline tumor marker for prognosis and follow-up
PET-CT (optional)	If equivocal CT findings or suspicion of occult metastasis

Multidisciplinary Team (MDT) Discussion

- Combine clinical, radiologic, and pathologic findings
- Define stage (using AJCC TNM staging)
- Decide treatment plan:
  - Early-stage → surgery
  - Locally advanced → neoadjuvant therapy
  - Metastatic → systemic therapy ± surgery

Endopelvic Fascia

Meshwork of smooth muscle, ligaments, blood vessels, and connective tissue lying between the parietal and visceral fascia, sometimes condensing to form fibrous fascial septa which separate and suspend the organs.

- Anatomists use the name subserous fascia whereas surgeons refer to this layer of retroperitoneal fascia as endopelvic fascia.
- Hypogastric sheath separates retropubic space from presacral space; conduit for vessels and nerves
- Transverse cervical (cardinal) ligaments—part of hypogastric sheath; run from lateral pelvic wall to uterine cervix and vagina; transmits uterine artery and provides passive support for the uterus
- Vesicovaginal septum
- Rectovesical septum
- Rectovaginal septum

Endopelvic Fascia—Ligaments

- *Female:* Pubovesical ligaments attach bladder to pubic symphysis.
- *Male:* Puboprostatic ligaments attach bladder to pubic symphysis.
- Sacrogenital—these are thickenings of the fascia, not specific ligaments
- Uterosacral ligaments attach upper vagina, upper portion of cervix, and uterus to the third sacral vertebra.
- Cardinal ligaments (aka Mackenrodt's) attach upper vagina, cervix, and uterus to the side walls of the pelvis
- Round ligaments attach uterus to mons pubis.
- Broad ligaments attach uterus to medial aspect of the ilium.
- Urachus ligament attaches bladder to umbilicus (formed from the remnants of the umbilical vein).

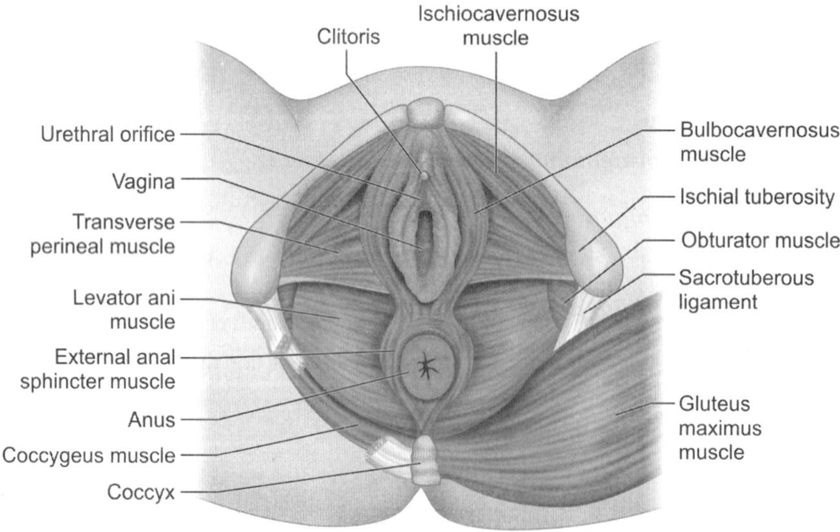

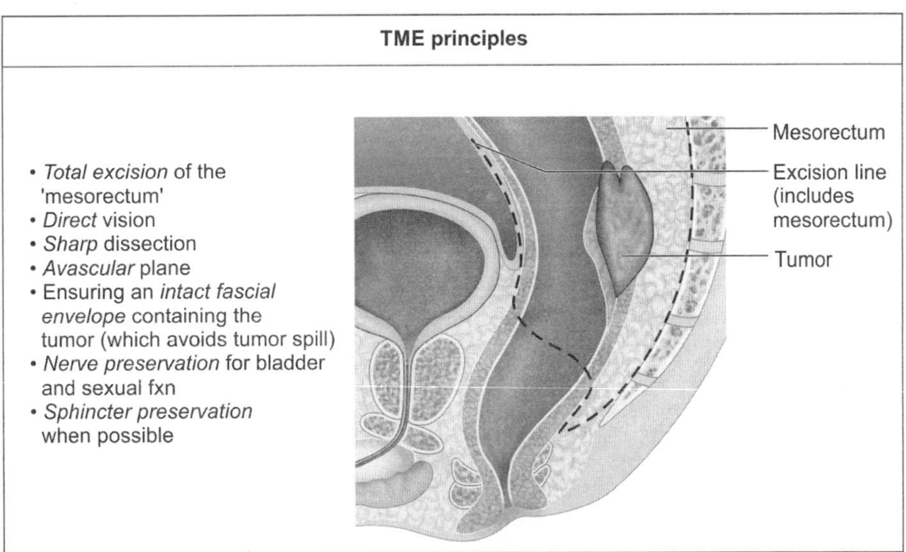

Schematic Diagram of Abdominal Autonomic Nervous System

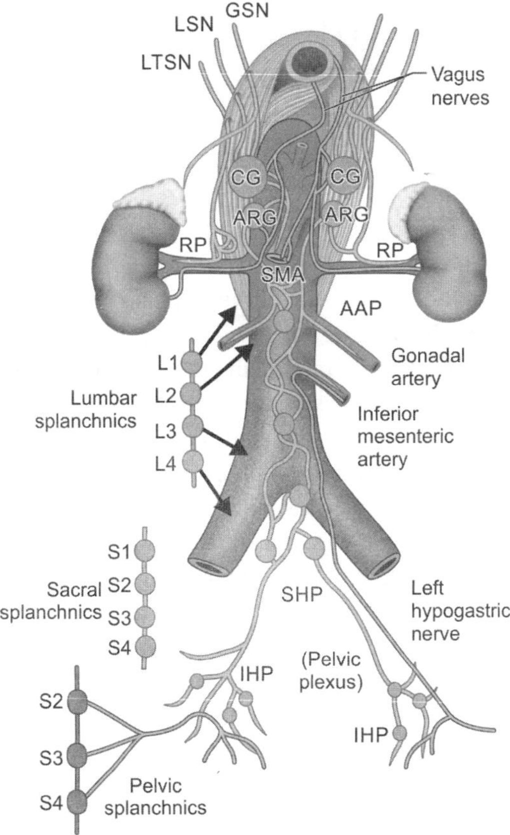

Schematic diagram of autonomic (sympathetic and parasympathetic) innervations of rectum and anal canal.

[AAP: abdominal aortic plexus; RP: renal plexus; CG: coeliac ganglion; GSN: greater splanchnic nerve (T5-9); IHP: inferior hypogastric plexus; LSN: lesser splanchnic nerve (T10-11); LSN: least splanchnic nerve (T12); SHP: superior hypogastric plexus; lumbar splanchnics (L1-4); sacral splanchnics (S1-4)]

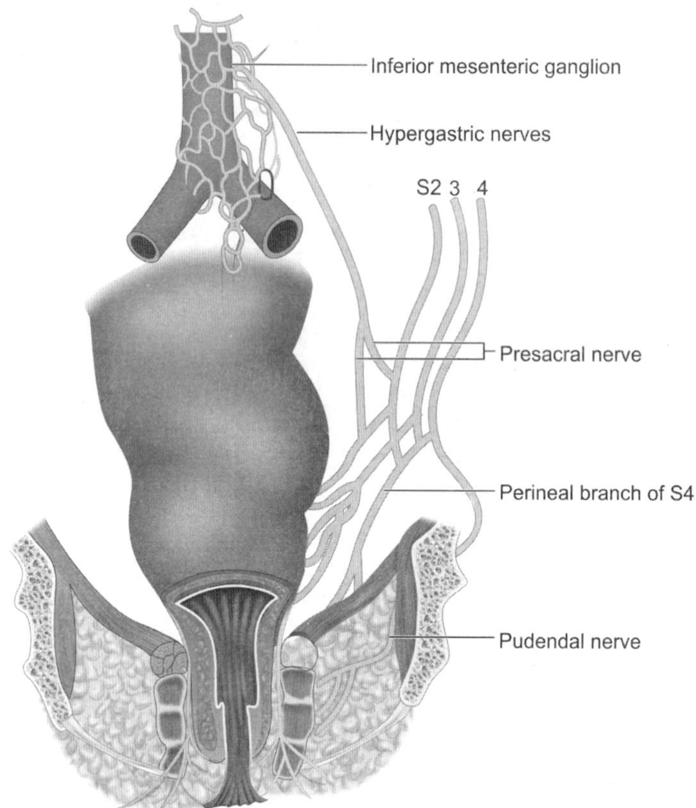

Steps:

- *Extent and technique of TME:* The sigmoidal vessels are isolated. There is a clear space on either side of the vessels. Care is taken to preserve the hypogastric nerves. The sigmoid is divided. The point of vessel ligation is at the level of the left colic artery. The colon is divided and packed cephalad, out of the field. The left colon is mobilized by incising the white line of Toldt and freeing the splenic flexure attachments.
- TME begins by pulling the rectum up and incising the peritoneum on both sides down to meet anteriorly at the deepest point in the cul-de-sac. By retracting the rectum anteriorly, a loose areolar plane of avascular tissue is visible. Dissection in this plane prevents entry into presacral veins. The nerves are visible and kept posterior to the plane of dissection. Both ureters should be visualized and retracted laterally. The tumor should be removed en bloc to include organs directly involved with tumor extension, such as the ovaries, uterus, bladder wall, and vagina. The presacral fascia is incised down to the rectosacral (Waldeyer's) fascia, a thickened band attaching the rectum to the endopelvic fascia at the S4 level. Divide this fascia and continue dissection to the coccyx.
- Continue the dissection laterally down to the lateral ligaments or "stalks," which may contain the middle rectal vessels. In fact, only 25% of patients have distinct branches of the middle rectal vessels in these ligaments. The lateral dissection ends at the levator muscles, the caudad boundary of the pelvic cavity.
- The anterior dissection is the most difficult because the planes are less distinct and the fat of the mesorectum is thin. This dissection is continued parallel to the plane of Denonvilliers' fascia between the rectum and the posterior wall of the vagina or the seminal vesicles. These structures are elevated anteriorly. Small vessels that traverse this area have a propensity for nuisance bleeding. The entire mesorectum should be contained within the fascia propria of the extraperitoneal rectum.
- The point of transection is chosen distal to the tumor. Multiple studies comparing distal cancer spread have shown that a 2-cm margin is necessary for low rectal excisions to perform an adequate oncologic resection.
- Less than 2–4% of tumors will have intraluminal implantation beyond 2 cm distally. Rigid sigmoidoscopy may be used to identify a point at least 2 cm distal to the carcinoma.

- Depending on the depth of the pelvis and therefore the diameter of the pelvis, a linear stapler of 30-, 45-, or 60-mm length is used for the first staple line in the double-stapling technique.
- The bowel is clamped just proximal to this point, the stapler is fired, and the rectum sharply transected and handed off the field. The operating field is secondarily isolated with towels while the open colon is manipulated.
- The proximal end of the colon is prepared by resecting off residual fat where the anastomosis is to be constructed. The staple line is sharply excised.
- A purse-string suture of 2-0 or 3-0 polypropylene is placed using full-thickness bites at 2-mm intervals.
- The anvil of the selected circular stapling device is inserted and the purse-string suture is tied around the shaft.
- The stapler is inserted transanally up to the previous staple line where the rectum was cut across.
- The trocar is introduced through or adjacent to the staple line. The anvil and the stapler are joined.
- The colon is inspected to verify that no adjacent tissue is entrapped and that the bowel is not twisted. The stapler is fired, opened slightly, and then removed. This is the second staple line in the double-stapling technique.
- The tissue removed in the stapler is checked to see that the tissue from the proximal and distal bowel is intact in two rings, the so-called "doughnuts."
- Check the anastomosis by clamping the bowel proximally, filling the pelvis with saline, and insufflating air under direct vision with a rigid proctoscope to see if bubbles can be detected coming through the anastomosis from the abdominal view.
- The rigid proctoscope permits assessment of the anastomosis for bleeding or saline entering the lumen from the abdomen.
- For the low coloanal anastomosis and for the preoperatively radiated pelvis, we routinely perform a diverting loop ileostomy at a premarked site.
- The site is kept away from bony prominences, the umbilicus, scars, and creases and is determined with the patient sitting, standing, and lying supine.
- This can usually be closed within 12 weeks of surgery.
- A 2 cm in diameter skin opening is made; dissection is carried down to the anterior rectus sheath.
- The fascial sheath is opened in a cruciate fashion, the muscle split bluntly, and the posterior peritoneum opened.
- The ileum is brought through the rectus muscle, identifying which end is proximal. The ostomy is matured following skin closure and dressing placement.
- The ileum is incised transversely 1 cm above the skin on the distal limb of the loop.
- As these cut edges of the ileum are sewn to the skin, the proximal ileum is everted to create an elevated tip.

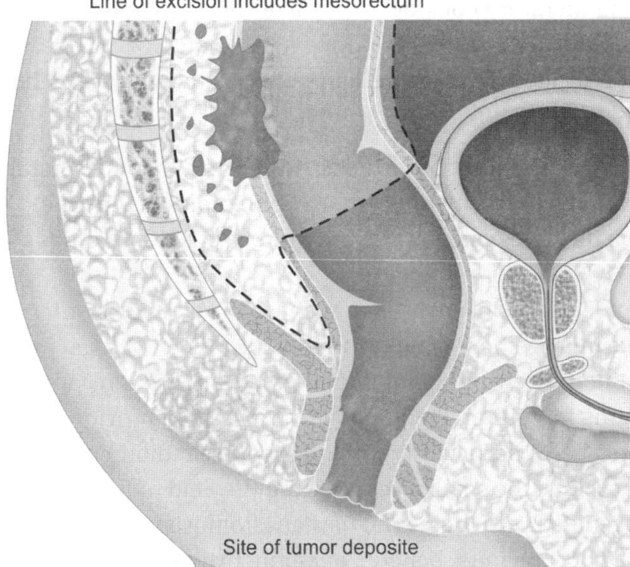

Macroscopic examination of the mesorectal surface helps us evaluate the quality of the surgical specimen.

Mesorectal defects are classified into three categories:

1. *Complete:* Mesorectum is intact, smooth with only minor irregularities without defect >5 mm;
2. *Moderate:* Moderate bulk to mesorectum but irregularity of the mesorectal surface; muscularis propria is not visible with the exception of the area of insertion of levator muscles, and
3. *Incomplete:* Little bulk to mesorectum with defects down into muscularis propria.

Circumferential Resection Margin

- After the introduction of TME, the CRM on the nonperitonealized surface of the resected rectal specimen is one of the most important predictors of local recurrence. Quirke et al. were the first to show that the radial or CRM is an important factor for local recurrence. The CRM can be involved by the tumor in various ways, such as direct spread, by tumor emboli in veins, lymphatics, or lymph nodes or by tumor deposits discontinuous from the main growth.
- The rectum is covered anteriorly by peritoneum and only in the area below the peritoneal reflection is there a risk of the CRM being involved. The posterior area, which continues up to the sigmoid mesocolon, is at risk of being involved by the tumor not only by direct spread but also with metastatic deposits in lymph nodes. The mesorectum is thinner anteriorly than posteriorly and the risk of a positive resection margin is higher for anteriorly located tumors than in posterior ones.
- Microscopic tumor nodules can be observed in the mesorectum. Studies have shown that the presence of widespread microscopic nodules in the mesorectum was present in up to 38.7%.
- Other studies proved that lymph nodes <5 mm in diameter are more often involved by the tumor than bigger ones. Such findings pinpoint the importance of TME.
- The pathologist must differentiate the peritonealized from nonperitonealized one. If a tumor is detected on the nonperitonealized surface, adjuvant radiotherapy may be appropriate without the dimensions of the tumor to be considered.
    - The macroscopic CRM is measured with a ruler; the microscopic CRM measurement is done better by using a sheet of graph paper that is photocopied onto a sheet of acetate and cut to size than to using the Vernier scale
    - The CRM is divided into two categories—(1) An involved (positive) CRM when the tumor extends to within 1 mm of the circumferential margin and (2) An uninvolved (negative) CRM when the distance between the tumor and CRM is >1 mm.
    - All the studies in the literature consider a positive CRM to be a distance between tumor and margin of <1 mm.
    - Several studies also indicated that the frequency of a positive CRM is higher in APR than in LAR.

TME with or without Radiotherapy

- The initial report by Heald expounded the virtue of TME as an adjunctive therapy in its own right but shied away from suggesting TME as a replacement for chemoradiotherapies of the time.
- Adjunctive combination therapies came to the fore with the positive findings of Krook and colleagues published in 1991.
- A National Institutes of Health consensus statement followed shortly afterward, which cemented the acute change in postoperative management of rectal tumors.
- Now patients were routinely receiving chemoradiotherapy, and trials regarding preoperative timing of adjuvant radiotherapy were coming to fruition. Preoperative radiotherapy provides a number of potential benefits—the disease may be "down-staged" (particularly with long-course radiotherapy), small extramural deposits may be cleared, techniques to exclude the small intestine from the field of therapy are more effective, the field should be relatively better oxygenated, and there is no new anastomosis.
- Intuitively, the oncologic locoregional benefits of adjunctive radiotherapy would marry well with augmented clearance by TME. The combination of techniques would be expected to convey low local failure rates.

The pathological assessment of mesorectal excision:

- Careful macroscopic evaluation of the resection specimen should be standardized. This may be supplemented by stain marking after postoperative filling the inferior mesenteric or superior rectal artery with ink or methylene blue solution. Photodocumentation is highly desirable. The pathological assessment of adequacy of mesorectal excision should be taken into account in selection for adjuvant radiotherapy.
- Objective macro- and microscopic assessment of mesorectal excision by pathologists is essential for quality management throughout patient care and in clinical trials.

Local excision procedures are: Local options for surgical management include transanal local excision, trans-sacral excision (Kraske approach), trans-sphincteric resection (Bevan or York-Mason approach), TEM, and electrocoagulation.

Transanal local excision should be performed as a full-thickness excision where the perirectal fat serves as the deep plane of dissection.

The Kraske excision is used for lesions too large or proximal for transanal local excision, and allows for removal of some perirectal lymph nodes. A perineal incision is made just above the anus, the coccyx is removed, and the fascia is divided. The rectum is mobilized through this incision, and a wide local excision or sleeve resection can be performed.

The trans-sphincteric procedure is identical to the Kraske procedure, except that the anal sphincter is divided posteriorly in the midline. The anus is reconstructed at completion of the operation, with little risk of functional impairment.

Transanal Endoscopic Microsurgery

Indications

- Lesion <3 cm
- Mobile
- Polypoid in shape
- Anatomically accessible localized to bowel wall (T1N0)
- Confined to extraperitoneal region of the rectum
- Occupies <40% of the circumference of bowel lumen
- Well or moderately differentiated
- Absence of lymphovascular invasion.

In TEM, an operating rectoscope is used to perform a full-thickness disc excision of the rectum, with primary closure. Fulguration is completed in multiple steps with the patient under general or regional anesthesia, and involves charring of the tumor, then scraping with a curette. There is a 10–20% risk of delayed hemorrhage due to sloughing of the scar at 7–10 days.

Full-thickness local excision is preferred overdestructive approaches because the complete specimen is available for assessment of depth of invasion, margins, and pathologic features known to be prognostic for lymph node involvement.

28. Discuss in brief about indications and modalities in neoadjuvant therapy of rectal cancer. How will you manage a case of clinical complete response to neoadjuvant therapy in rectal cancer? ***Tripura University 2024***

Neoadjuvant Therapy in Rectal Cancer

Indications

Neoadjuvant (preoperative) therapy is given *before surgery* to downstage the tumor, improve resectability, and reduce local recurrence.

Main indications:

- Locally advanced rectal cancer (LARC):
    - *T3–T4* tumors (tumor extends beyond muscularis propria)
    - *Node-positive (N1–N2)* disease

- *Threatened or involved mesorectal fascia (MRF)* on MRI→ Predicts positive circumferential resection margin (CRM)
- *Low rectal tumors* where sphincter preservation is desired
- *Fixed or bulky tumors* not amenable to immediate resection

Modalities of Neoadjuvant Therapy

- *Long-course chemoradiotherapy (LCCRT)*
  - *Radiation:* 45–50.4 Gy in 25–28 fractions (5–6 weeks)
  - *Concurrent chemotherapy:*
    - 5-Fluorouracil (continuous infusion) or
    - Capecitabine (oral)
  - *Advantages:* Higher rate of pathological complete response (pCR), better downstaging
  - *Surgery:* Typically 6–8 weeks after completion
- *Short-course radiotherapy (SCRT):*
  - *Radiation:* 25 Gy in 5 fractions (1 week)
  - *Surgery:* Either immediate (within 1 week) or delayed (after 6–8 weeks for downstaging)
  - *Advantages:* Shorter duration; suitable for fit patients with resectable tumors
- *Total neoadjuvant therapy (TNT):*
  - Incorporates systemic chemotherapy (FOLFOX, CAPOX) before or after chemoradiation
  - Aims to control micrometastases early and improve compliance
  - Increasingly favored in locally advanced and high-risk cases

Management of Clinical Complete Response (cCR)

Definition

Clinical Complete Response (cCR)—No residual tumor detected clinically, endoscopically, or radiologically after neoadjuvant therapy.

Assessment

- *Digital rectal examination (DRE):* Smooth, pliable scar; no palpable mass
- *Endoscopy:* Whitening, telangiectasia, or scar; no ulcer/mass
- *MRI:* Fibrosis without residual signal intensity (mrTRG 1–2)
- *Biopsy:* Negative or nondiagnostic for residual disease
- *CEA:* Normalized

Management Options

- Watch-and-Wait ("Non-Operative Management")
  - For *carefully selected patients* with confirmed cCR
  - *Close surveillance protocol:*
    - DRE + proctoscopy + CEA every 3 months for 2 years, then every 6 months
    - MRI pelvis every 6 months for 2 years
    - CT chest/abdomen annually
  - *Rationale:* Many cCR patients remain disease-free; avoids morbidity of rectal surgery (esp. permanent colostomy)
- Radical surgery (TME)
  - *Total mesorectal excision (TME)* remains the standard of care
  - Indicated when:
    - Response is *incomplete or uncertain*
    - *High-risk* features (e.g., initial T4, threatened MRF)
    - Patient prefers definitive surgery

- *Local Excision (in selected cases)*
  - For small residual lesions confined to bowel wall after good response
  - Transanal endoscopic microsurgery (TEMS) or transanal minimally invasive surgery (TAMIS)

If Local Regrowth Occurs After Watch-and-Wait

- Occurs in ~20–30% within first 2 years
- Usually *locoregional and salvageable* with timely surgery (TME)
- Hence, *strict surveillance* is essential

29. Evaluate the place of pathological evaluation in colorectal cancer with special reference to TME.

WBUHS 2008

Introduction

TME is a standard technique for treatment of colorectal cancer, devised some 20 years ago by Professor Bill Heald at the UK's Basingstoke District Hospital for patients with advanced rectal cancers, surgery that includes TME often provides the best possible patient outcomes and survival.

- The mesorectum is a fatty tissue directly adjacent to the rectum that contains blood vessels and lymph nodes. When rectal cancers recur, it is often in these lymph nodes.
- Patients who have rectal cancer that is confined to the lower two-thirds of the rectum are generally considered good candidates for TME surgery.

Principles of TME

Although TME has been modified over time, the basic principle of excising tumor and the mesorectum en bloc remains its foundation. This principle is based on the original observations of Moynihan19 in 1908 regarding potential pathways for lymphatic spread and also on the hypothesis of Heald that the mesorectum represents embryological advantages conferring protection against tumor dissemination until the terminal stages. Lymphoscintigraphy further demonstrated this in an anatomical study of the lymphatics that drain the rectum.

There are some operative factors that are likely to affect outcomes. These predominately center on a fastidious approach to the technique, involving specimen-oriented surgery and allowing for additional time as needed.

Operative factors associated with compromised outcome.

Factor	*Outcome*
Disruption of "tumor–mesorectal package"	Scrupulous, unhurried, and sharp dissection technique
Contamination of field by viable tumor	• Seal transected bowel • Hypotonic or antiseptic washout
Dissection along embryological plane	• Meticulous knowledge of anatomy • Meticulous anastomosis • Adequately informed assistant
Increased anastomotic leak rate	Low threshold for defunctioning stoma, particularly in male
Urinary and sexual dysfunction	Identification and preservation of relevant autonomic nerves

- The principle holds that specimen-oriented surgery must be accompanied by specimen-oriented histopathology, which is essential for appropriate staging and audit. It also emphasizes careful evaluation of circumferential margins since macroscopic evaluation by the operating surgeon is not reliable.
- A Quirke-based detailed histopathological approach as an audit method for surgeons. This not only provides objective data that may be extrapolated to define competence, but also may provide an immediate stimulus to surgeons regarding their technique.
- Although perhaps controversial, the advent of TME has highlighted the previously disregarded inter-surgeon and inter-institution variability noted in locoregional recurrence following curative rectal cancer surgery, even when institutional selection bias is taken into account. Such inherent variability would not be tolerated in the realm of medical and radiological oncology.

The Pathological Assessment of Mesorectal Excision

- Careful macroscopic evaluation of the resection specimen should be standardized. This may be supplemented by stain marking after postoperative filling the inferior mesenteric or superior rectal artery with ink or methylene blue solution. Photodocumentation is highly desirable. The pathological assessment of adequacy of mesorectal excision should be taken into account in selection for adjuvant radiotherapy.
- Objective macro- and microscopic assessment of mesorectal excision by pathologists is essential for quality management throughout patient care and in clinical trials.

30. Laparoscopic total mesorectal excision for rectal cancer. *WBUHS 2012*

TME is a common procedure used in the treatment of colorectal cancer in which a significant length of the bowel around the tumor is removed. TME addresses earlier treatment concerns regarding adequate local control of rectal cancer while performing an anterior resection.

The term TME strictly applies when performing an LAR for tumors of the middle and the lower rectum, wherein it is essential to remove the rectum along with the mesorectum up to the level of the levators. The principles of TME (sharp mesorectal excision) are also applied during an abdominoperineal excision of the rectum and for tumors of the upper rectum, although these are considered distinct from standard TME. In an abdominoperineal excision of the rectum where the tumor exists below the level of the levators, the lateral margins of the tumor are inferior to the mesorectum and the benefits of TME do not apply. Anterior resections involving the upper rectum may be completed with mobilization of the rectum to beyond 5 cm of the lower margin of the tumor, and which is often above the level of the levator and is sometimes referred to as *partial mesorectal excision*.

The treatment of rectal cancers is multimodal with adjuvant radiotherapy and chemotherapy having benefits in some settings. In addition, accurate preoperative staging is dependent on good radiological support. It is therefore necessary to subject all rectal cancers to multidepartment conference and to design individualized treatment plans based on a well-defined protocol. This serves the dual purpose of maintaining a consistent evidence-based approach as well as creating a dataset for prospective analysis and feedback.

Indications

Total mesorectal excision is indicated as a part of LAR for patients with adenocarcinoma of the middle and lower rectum. TME is now considered the gold standard for tumors of the middle and the lower rectum.

Outcomes

Circumferential resection margin positivity rate is about 5% or less for LARs with TME, whereas it is between 10% and 25% for abdominoperineal excision of the rectum. There is understandably a higher local recurrence rate following abdominoperineal excision of the rectum. Five-year survival and disease-free survival rates are significantly lower with TME.

Laparoscopic TME is a feasible but technically demanding procedure (12% conversion rate). Excellence of surgical technique is of particular relevance in the treatment of rectal cancer. Routine excision of the intact mesorectum during resection of cancers of the middle and lower rectum has resulted in the lowest incidence of local recurrences ever reported.

Patients with tumors located in the low and middle rectum can be selected for laparoscopic TME based on the following criteria—elective surgery, absence of occlusion, and American Society of Anesthesiologists (ASA) status I to III. Neither morbid obesity nor prior pelvic surgery is considered a contraindication to laparoscopic TME. When the neoplasm at digital examination reached the anatomic anal canal or was fixed to the pelvic floor, the patient is not a good candidate for laparoscopic TME.

Preoperative work-up consists of clinical evaluation, total colonoscopy, CT scan, upper abdominal ultrasound, and endoscopic ultrasound. Patients preoperatively staged T3 or T4 without distant metastases are treated by preoperative radiochemotherapy (45 Gy during 4 weeks together with systemic 5-fluouracil intravenous infusion) and are evaluated with clinical examination and CT scan 21 days after the completion of the treatment. Definitive inclusion in this study was decided at this point, excluding locally advanced tumor (i.e., T4 in the TNM classification).

Patients are followed up with physical examination, digital examination, serum CEA assay, ultrasound of the liver, CT scan, chest radiograph, and colonoscopy. Every case of suspected local recurrence is histologically confirmed.

Laparoscopic TME is feasible and safe. The laparoscopic approach to the surgical treatment of operable rectal cancer does not seem to entail any oncologic disadvantages. Laparoscopic TME with preservation of anal sphincter is a safe and minimally invasive technique with less postoperative pain and rapid recovery, and importantly, it has preserved the function of the sphincter.

Laparoscopic TME and sphincter preservation have the following advantages:

- It helps surgeons identify accurately the interspace of loose connective tissue between visceral and parietal pelvic fascia, and select operative access by amplifying inner image on the monitors.
- 25° or 30° laparoscope, the third eye of the surgeon, can reach the narrow lesser pelvis and magnify the local vision.
- It is more definite to identify and protect the pelvic autonomic nerve fiber and plexus due to its magnifying function.
- Hemostatic benefit was owed to minimally invasive sharp dissection with minimal blood loss under laparoscopic view.

However, the laparoscopic technique has its disadvantages, such as long operative time, short of direct hand feeling, technical constraints of the narrow pelvis, difficulty in assessing adequate surgical margins and in ultralow rectal cross clamping, and a long learning course for surgeons.

---

31. What is transanal minimal invasive surgery? Give outline of its indications, contraindications, advantages, and limitations. How is TAMIS different from transanal endoscopic microsurgery?

WBUHS 2021 Supplementary, WBUHS 2023, DNB, June 2019

Introduction

Transanal minimally invasive surgery (TAMIS) is a technique that was originally devised as a hybrid between TEM and single-site laparoscopy for resection of rectal lesions.

Transanal minimally invasive surgery (TAMIS) was developed in 2009 as a method to locally excise premalignant and select malignant lesions of the rectum with curative intent. The technique is an extrapolation of single-port laparoscopy.

Characteristics of Tumors Amenable to Local Excision

- T1N0 or T2N0 lesion
- <4 cm in diameter
- <40% circumference of the lumen
- <10 cm from dentate line
- Well- to moderately differentiated histology
- No evidence of lymphatic or vascular invasion on biopsy
- Patients with extensive metastatic disease and poor prognosis who require local control.
- Adjuvant treatment for patients with lymphatic invasion, T1 with poor prognosis features, T2 lesions.
- The indications for TAMIS are similar to TEM and standard transanal resection for benign and malignant lesions determined by EUS or MRI.
    - For malignant masses, TAMIS is generally appropriate for patients with early rectal cancer, which is defined as invasive adenocarcinoma confined to the submucosal layer, or T1.
    - This can be further categorized into low-risk T1 adenocarcinomas of the rectum, which are characterized as small (<4 cm), well-differentiated tumors without lymphatic, vascular, or perineural involvement.
    - For patients with poor histologic features (lymphovascular or perineural invasion, poor differentiation, and tumor budding), discussion at a multidisciplinary tumor board should ensue to reach a consensus on subsequent treatment.
    - T1 cancers with deeper submucosal invasion (sm2 or sm3) as determined by the Kikuchi classification of sessile lesions may confer metastatic potential to lymph nodes and should essentially be treated as a T2 lesion.

- For indeterminate T1 versus T2 lesions with no evidence of nodal disease, a TAMIS resection can serve as definitive biopsy confirming T stage and guiding further treatment with the final pathology.
- In a study by Dudek in 2008, the most favorable outcomes were in those pT2 lesions resected with negative margins that went on to receive adjuvant radiotherapy; all 12 of the patients were disease-free after a median follow-up of 3 years. Conversely, patients with uT2 lesions may be down staged with preoperative chemotherapy and radiation prior to TAMIS resection.
- Advanced lesions (T3) can be considered for TAMIS resection when patients are deemed medically unfit to have a more radical surgery. Patients found to have nodal disease or distant metastases should be evaluated by a multidisciplinary tumor board where available and considered for chemotherapy and radiation prior to surgical resection.
- The indications for TAMIS can also be broadened to include local excision of clinical T0 (cT0) lesions in patients with locally advanced rectal cancer after neoadjuvant therapy for the purpose of confirming mural complete pathologic response.
- Though there are limited data evaluating the effectiveness of TAMIS for resection of carcinoid tumors, it seems a likely alternative for removing small rectal carcinoids either primarily or after incomplete endoscopic removal.

Contraindications for TAMIS

- Positive lymph nodes
- Distant metastasis
- Ulcerated tumor
- Large tumor extending into muscularis propria (contraindicated owing to the increased risk of lymph node invasion)
- Poorly differentiated tumor
- Lymphovascular invasion

Advantages of TAMIS

- A clear visualization of the operating field when compared to other transanal approach techniques especially in the mid to upper rectum, and thus is a safe and feasible option of treatment of rectal pathologies in various locations of the rectum.
- The primary difference between the two techniques is that a resterilized, reusable port is used for TEM, while a disposable port is used for TAMIS.
- Transanal endoscopic microsurgery offers several advantages over conventional transanal excision. It provides better exposure, visualization, and access to reach lesions higher in the rectum than standard transanal excision. It is associated with less morbidity and quicker recovery time than a radical transabdominal approach. The major limitations of TEM are that it requires expensive, highly specialized equipment and has a steep learning curve. Accordingly, it should be performed only by skilled and experienced surgeons.
- In a meta-analysis comparing TEM with endoscopic submucosal dissection (ESD) for the treatment of rectal tumors, the two procedures were found to be similar with regard to the rates of resection, adverse events, and recurrence; however, both the procedure time and the duration of hospitalization were shorter with ESD.
- It offers several benefits over TEM. It requires minimal setup time, and the use of existing laparoscopic cameras and instruments offers a lower-cost alternative to TEM. Nonetheless, the learning curve appears to be generally comparable.
- A comparison of patients who underwent TEM (n = 53) or TAMIS (n = 68) for resection of intraluminal rectal tumors showed that although median operating time was significantly shorter for TAMIS (45 vs. 65 minutes), blood loss was negligible in both groups. Resection margins, lesion grade, and invasion depth were comparable for the two approaches; however, the postoperative readmission rate was significantly higher in the TEM group (17% vs. 4.4%).

Limitations of TAMIS

- Despite these advantages, there are still a few challenges commonly encountered with TAMIS. First, lesions behind a valve of Houston are difficult to excise on a TAMIS platform.
- TAMIS is challenging in obese patients with abundant adiposity in the gluteal region.
- TAMIS requires a camera assistant, and therefore needs synchrony and communication between the surgeon and the assistant.

LOCALLY RECURRENT RECTAL CANCER

32. Describe the presentation and diagnosis of locally recurrent rectal cancer. Discuss the management strategy of locally recurrent rectal cancer. ***WBUHS 2014***

Recurrent Rectal Cancer

Local recurrence of rectal adenocarcinoma is seen in up to 30% of patients. Although recurrence may be seen at the distal margin of the anastomosis, most develop from residual cancer on the pelvic wall. The time course for recurrences to present through the anastomosis is approximately 18 months.

These tumors are fixed to the pelvic wall and surrounding viscera.

- *They cause significant symptoms, such as:*
  - Intractable pelvic pain
  - Bleeding
  - Cramping or constipation
  - Urinary tract dysfunction
  - Chronic pelvic sepsis

Diagnosis

- When patients present with these symptoms or with a rising CEA level, a workup including CT scan of the abdomen and pelvis, ERUS, MRI of the pelvis, and PET scan may be helpful.
- A careful pelvic examination is mandatory.
- A biopsy, either via sigmoidoscopy or CT-guided, should be used to confirm the diagnosis pathologically.
- If external radiation has not been used before, it should be considered.
- The surgeon should review the imaging studies and determine which organs are involved, such as the vagina, uterus, prostate, bladder, sacrum, and small intestine, which will require en bloc resection.
- Urology consult should be obtained if there is any question of prostate or bladder involvement; ureteral stents should be placed preoperatively. Removal of the rectum and urinary bladder with surrounding lymphatic tissue results in a permanent colostomy and ileal conduit.

Treatment

Intraoperative Radiation Therapy

- Intraoperative radiation therapy (IORT) may be considered in patients with pelvic sidewall recurrence. This is performed in an operating room–radiation therapy suite.
- Resection with negative microscopic margins and absence of vascular invasion independently predicts improved local control and survival after resection and IORT.
- The major morbidities of IORT include peripheral neuropathy and ureteral stenosis.

Palliation

- These tumors are difficult to palliate.
- Surgical resection combined with aggressive multimodality therapy is advocated to avert the morbidity of pelvic disease and to prolong survival in a subset of patients, with survival rates up to 30%.
- Most patients, however, will not be offered curative surgery on the basis of comorbidities, poor performance status, distant metastases, or locally unresectable disease on preoperative imaging. These patients may be offered palliative intervention.

Chemoradiation

- Patients with rectal cancer who undergo surgery with intention to cure and without evidence of gross disease postoperatively may still develop local recurrence or distant metastases.
- Up to 10% of patients who undergo TME with tumor-free radial and distal margins may develop local failure.
- The goal of adjuvant therapy is to eliminate the micrometastatic disease present at the time of surgery.
  - *Adjuvant chemoradiation:* In 1990, the National Institutes of Health consensus statement concluded that "combined postoperative chemotherapy and radiotherapy improves local control and survival in stages II and III patients and is recommended."
    - Most of the information regarding chemotherapy for colorectal cancer comes from trials of colon cancer rather than for rectal cancer.
    - The NSABP C-04 (National Surgical Adjuvant Breast and Bowel Project C-04) trial studied stages II and III colon cancer patients and demonstrated that 5-fluorouracil (5-FU) and leucovorin (LV) treatment had a significantly better 5-year survival rate compared with 5-FU and levamisole.
    - Several trials have suggested a benefit for adjuvant chemoradiation for rectal cancer in patients with resected stage II–III cancers.
    - The GITSG (Gastrointestinal Tumor Study Group) trial demonstrated that combined chemoradiation resulted in an improvement in overall survival as well as a decrease in local recurrence.
    - NCCTG (North Central Cancer Treatment Group) trial demonstrated that the addition of chemotherapy to radiation reduced both local recurrence and distant metastases and improved survival.
  - *Radiation therapy used alone* as adjuvant therapy may improve local recurrence and survival rates. A theoretical reason to use postoperative radiation therapy is that more appropriate patient selection can be achieved because pathologic staging is performed prior to radiation.
    - Disadvantages include radiating the neorectum and small bowel and a lower tendency of patients to complete their radiation.
  - *Neoadjuvant chemoradiation:* There are a number of potential advantages for using neoadjuvant chemoradiation.
    - They include the ability to deliver higher doses of chemotherapy with radiation.
    - Another advantage is not only to downstage the tumor, which has been noted in 60–80% of patients, but also to achieve a pathologic complete response, which occurs in 15–30% of patients.
    - The ability to "shrink" the tumor facilitates surgical resection, thereby allowing one to achieve negative margins and perform an operation in patients who otherwise would require an APR.
    - Additional advantages include radiating tissues with a greater oxygen supply, not radiating the anastomosis, and decreased likelihood of developing radiation enteritis because small bowel is less likely to enter the pelvis.
    - Finally, patients are more likely to complete the course of radiation therapy because it precedes their surgical resection.
    - A meta-analysis concluded that preoperative radiation therapy plus surgery compared with surgery alone significantly reduced the 5-year overall mortality rate, cancer-related mortality rate, and local recurrence rate.
    - Current practice is to recommend preoperative staging with ERUS or MRI to all patients with rectal adenocarcinoma and then to offer chemoradiation to medically fit patients with curative intent who have T3–T4 or N-positive rectal carcinoma. Some patients with bulky T2 lesions near the sphincters should also be considered for neoadjuvant chemoradiotherapy in order to improve sphincter preservation.
    - Neoadjuvant therapy then is followed by TME with APR or TME with an end-to-side or colonic J-pouch reconstruction. Postoperatively, patients who have had involved lymph nodes either by preoperative staging or on the final pathology report are encouraged to have additional postoperative chemotherapy.
    - Postoperative chemotherapy in node-negative patients or patients who have had a complete response is determined on a case-by-case basis.

33. How do you assess the resectability in a case of rectal carcinoma as per latest NCCN guidelines?
WBUHS 2023

Assessment of resectability in case of rectal cancer as per latest NCCN guidelines:

- Unresectable rectal cancer is defined as a primary or locally recurrent tumor involving or abutting adjacent organs or structures (cT4) or palpably fixed cT3 lesion.
- All rectal cancers must be tested for mismatch repair (MMR)/MSI status.
- Treatment algorithms for clinical stage II, III, and IV rectal cancers are now stratified by MMR/MSI status, recognizing the role of immunotherapy.
- The option of surgery only for T3N0 low-risk, upper rectal cancer. MRI is recommended to identify location.
- For patients who did not receive neoadjuvant therapy, no postsurgery RT for pT1-3, N1, and pT3N0 cases (adjuvant chemo only).
- Neoadjuvant therapy is the only option for clinical stage II/III rectal cancer.
- FOLFIRINOX is added as a standard option in the neoadjuvant setting (and is preferred over FOLFOXIRI) for clinical stage II/III DNA MMR (dMMR)/MSI-H cancers, the "preferred" neoadjuvant therapy is checkpoint inhibitor immunotherapy.
- *Metastatic rectal cancer patients:*
    - Consider PET-CT in addition to standard imaging for potentially resectable metastatic rectal cancer
    - All metastatic RC patients are recommended to receive chemotherapy prior to surgery (exception of surgery to relieve symptomatic obstruction in selected cases).

Patients with the following may be candidates for local excision:

- Lesions located in low rectum (within 8–10 cm)
- Lesions occupying less than one-third of the rectal circumference
- Mobile exophytic or polypoid lesions
- Lesions <3 cm in size
- T1 lesions
- Low-grade tumor (well or moderately differentiated)
- Negative nodal status (clinical and radiographic)

Low anterior resection—performed for upper rectal tumors and the final anastomosis was below the level of peritoneal reflection. Ultra-LAR (ULAR)—performed for mid and low rectal tumors. A resection is said to be ultralow if the colorectal anastomosis was within 2 cm from the anorectal junction.

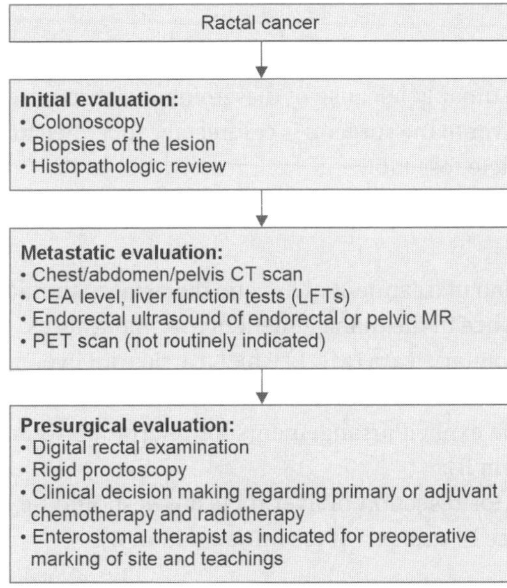

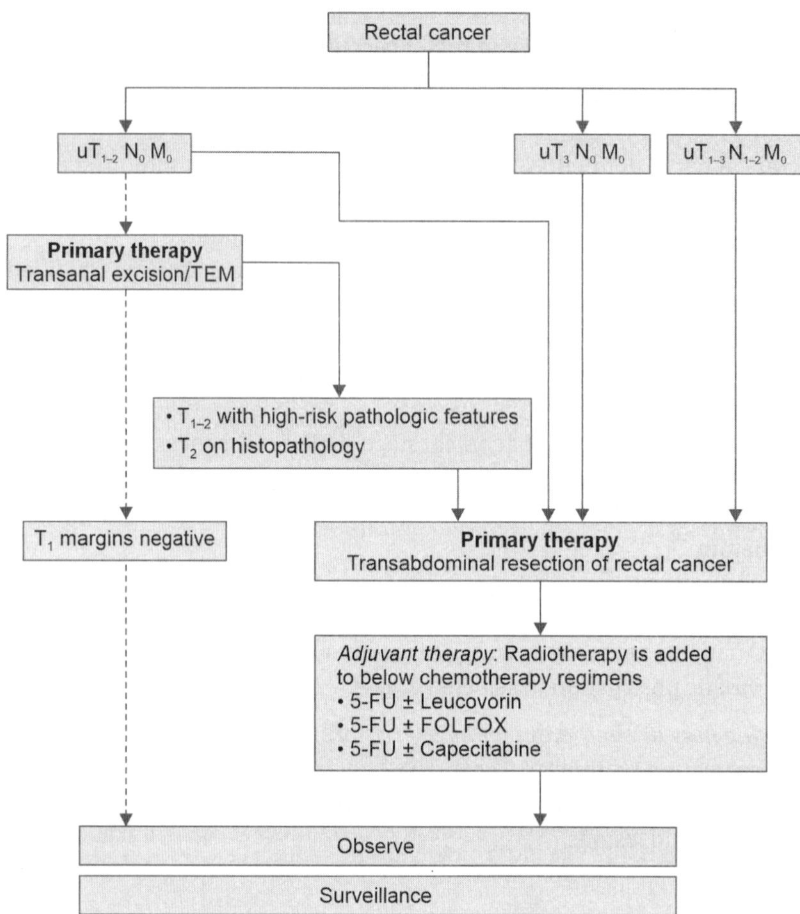

COLORECTAL LIVER METASTASIS

34. What are the guidelines for considering liver resection in colorectal liver metastasis? Describe colorectal liver metastasis management protocol.

Introduction

The most common malignant tumors of the liver are metastatic lesions. The liver is a common site of metastases from gastrointestinal tumors presumably because of dissemination through the portal venous system. The most relevant metastatic tumor of the liver to the surgeon is colorectal cancer because of the well-documented potential for long-term survival after complete resection.

Guidelines

- *General:*
  - Patients under consideration of treatment of hepatic metastases should be discussed at a multidisciplinary meeting which has experience in the management of liver metastases.
  - A hepatobiliary multidisciplinary team (MDT) which carries out liver resection should be based in a cancer center serving a population of at least two million. When two or three networks cooperate to create a single joint team, there should be explicit arrangements for referral between networks (category of evidence II; strength of recommendation B).
  - Consideration of patients for resection of liver metastases should be carried out at a single high-volume center (category of evidence II; strength of recommendation B).

- *At time of presentation of primary colorectal cancer:*
  - Patients with primary colorectal cancer should have a CT scan of the abdomen and pelvis performed with intravenous contrast and ideally a maximum collimation of 5 mm. This should be performed preoperatively or, in the case of an emergency, as soon as practical thereafter (category of evidence II; strength of recommendation B).
  - A chest CT is ideal to assess the presence of pulmonary metastases but a chest *X*-ray is considered satisfactory (category of evidence III; strength of recommendation C).
  - The whole of the colon should be visualized to ensure a "clean colon" (category of evidence II; strength of recommendation B).
  - A baseline measurement of CEA should be performed (category of evidence III; strength of recommendation C).
- *Following curative resection of primary colorectal cancer:*
  - Following treatment of the primary disease, some patients will prove to be unfit or unwilling to have further treatment and in such cases follow up is inappropriate.
  - Other patients will prove to have metastatic disease at presentation. Some of these will have isolated liver metastases and should be managed as described in these guidelines.
  - Patients undergoing R0 colorectal resection may be candidates for adjuvant chemotherapy and a further abdominal contrast enhanced CT (or MRI) should be performed following completion of chemotherapy (category of evidence III; strength of recommendation C).
  - *Where possible patients over the age of 50 years should be considered for randomization to the FACS trial, the UK NCRN trial of follow up strategies.*
    If the patient is ineligible for trial inclusion, does not wish to participate in the randomized trial, or if the unit is not recruiting to the trial, the following follow-up schedule is appropriate:
  - CT scan of the abdomen and pelvis should be undertaken as a minimum in the 2 years following completion of treatment of the primary disease (category of evidence III; strength of recommendation C).
  - Colonoscopy repeated after 5 years.
  - The case for routine serial CEA measurements is unproven (category of evidence III; strength of recommendation C).
- *Further staging investigation to detect extrahepatic involvement in patients with colorectal liver metastases:*
  - For a patient discovered to have isolated liver metastases, CT of the chest, abdomen, and pelvis should be performed by the liver surgery unit or using protocols agreed with that unit. The liver surgery center will also often perform liver specific imaging by local protocol.
  - Biopsy of hepatic lesions should not be performed without discussion with the regional hepatobiliary unit (category of evidence III; strength of recommendation C).
  - Patients with "high-risk" primary disease [T4 (perforated); C2 (apical node)] should have careful preoperative investigations that might include PET and laparoscopy (category of evidence III; strength of recommendation C).

35. What are the indications of neoadjuvant therapy in carcinoma rectum? How do you manage a case of rectal carcinoma with hepatic metastasis? ***WBUHS 2025***

Indications for Neoadjuvant Therapy in Carcinoma Rectum

Neoadjuvant therapy, typically involving chemotherapy, radiotherapy, or a combination (chemoradiotherapy), is used in rectal carcinoma to improve outcomes. Indications include:

- *Locally advanced rectal cancer (T3/T4 or Node-Positive Disease):*
  - Tumors staged as T3 (invading through the muscularis propria) or T4 (invading adjacent structures) on MRI or endorectal ultrasound.
  - Presence of regional lymph node involvement (N1/N2).

- *Aim:* Downstage the tumor to improve resectability, reduce local recurrence, and increase sphincter preservation.

- *Tumors threatening the circumferential resection margin (CRM):*
  - MRI showing tumor within 1 mm of the mesorectal fascia or involvement of the CRM.
  - *Aim:* Shrink the tumor to achieve a clear surgical margin (R0 resection).
- *Mid or low rectal tumors:*
  - Tumors located in the middle or lower third of the rectum (within 12 cm from the anal verge), where sphincter preservation is a goal.
  - *Aim:* Reduce tumor size to allow sphincter-sparing surgery (e.g., low anterior resection) instead of abdominoperineal resection.
- *High-risk features:*
  - Extramural venous invasion (EMVI) or lymphovascular invasion identified on imaging.
  - Poorly differentiated tumors or mucinous histology.
  - *Aim:* Improve local control and reduce systemic spread.
- *Selected cases of early-stage disease:*
  - T2 tumors in the low rectum where neoadjuvant therapy may facilitate sphincter preservation.
  - *Aim:* Avoid permanent colostomy in select patients.
- *Specific scenarios:*
  - Fixed or bulky tumors that are borderline resectable.
  - Patients with high surgical risk where tumor shrinkage may reduce operative morbidity.
  - *Aim:* Optimize surgical outcomes and reduce complications.

Common Neoadjuvant Regimens

- *Short-course radiotherapy:* 25 Gy in 5 fractions over 1 week, followed by surgery within 1–2 weeks.
- *Long-course chemoradiotherapy:* 45–50.4 Gy over 5–6 weeks with concurrent 5-fluorouracil (5-FU) or capecitabine, followed by surgery after 6–8 weeks.
- *Total neoadjuvant therapy (TNT):* Chemotherapy (e.g., FOLFOX or CAPOX) followed by chemoradiotherapy to maximize tumor response and treat micrometastases.

Management of Rectal Carcinoma with Hepatic Metastasis

Rectal carcinoma with hepatic metastasis is considered stage IV disease and requires a multidisciplinary approach. Management depends on the extent of the primary tumor, the resectability of metastases, and the patient's performance status. The following principles guide treatment:

Initial Assessment:

- *Staging:* Perform a full workup including:
  - Colonoscopy with biopsy to confirm rectal adenocarcinoma.
  - MRI pelvis to assess the primary tumor (T/N stage, CRM involvement).
  - CT chest/abdomen/pelvis to evaluate metastases.
  - PET-CT (if available) to detect additional metastatic sites.
  - CEA levels for baseline and monitoring.
- *Liver metastasis evaluation:*
  - Assess number, size, location, and resectability of liver lesions (e.g., using the Fong score).
  - Classify as resectable, potentially resectable (after conversion therapy), or unresectable.
- *Multidisciplinary team (MDT):* Involve oncologists, surgeons, radiologists, and hepatobiliary specialists.

Treatment Principles

- *Goal:* Achieve local control of the rectal tumor, manage metastatic disease, and optimize survival or palliation.
- *Approach:* Treatment is individualized based on resectability of metastases, primary tumor characteristics, and patient factors.

Resectable Liver Metastases

- *Systemic chemotherapy:*
  - Administer neoadjuvant chemotherapy (e.g., FOLFOX, FOLFIRI, or CAPOX) ± targeted agents (e.g., bevacizumab for RAS wild-type, cetuximab/panitumumab for KRAS/NRAS wild-type) for 2–3 months to reduce tumor burden and assess biology.
  - Reassess resectability with imaging after chemotherapy.
- *Local treatment for rectal tumor:*
  - Neoadjuvant chemoradiotherapy (long-course, 45–50.4 Gy with 5-FU/capecitabine) to downstage the primary tumor and improve local control.
  - Surgery for the rectal tumor (e.g., low anterior resection or abdominoperineal resection) after 6–8 weeks.
- *Liver-directed therapy:*
  - Synchronous or staged resection of liver metastases (e.g., segmentectomy, wedge resection, or hemihepatectomy).
  - Consider perioperative chemotherapy (3 months pre- and postliver surgery) to reduce recurrence risk.
- *Sequence:*
  - *Options include:*
    - Simultaneous resection of rectal tumor and liver metastases in fit patients with limited metastatic disease.
    - *Staged approach:* Address the primary tumor first (if symptomatic, e.g., obstruction/bleeding) or liver metastases first (if rectal tumor is asymptomatic).
- *Adjuvant therapy:* Postsurgical chemotherapy to complete 6 months of total therapy.

Potentially Resectable Liver Metastases

- *Conversion therapy:*
  - Use intensive chemotherapy regimens (e.g., FOLFOXIRI ± bevacizumab or cetuximab) to shrink metastases and convert to resectable status.
  - Reassess resectability every 2–3 months with imaging.
- *Rectal tumor management:*
  - Neoadjuvant chemoradiotherapy or total neoadjuvant therapy to control the primary tumor.
  - Surgery for the rectal tumor if resectable, followed by liver-directed therapy (resection, ablation, or combination).
- *Liver-directed therapies:*
  - If resection becomes feasible, proceed with surgery.
  - If still unresectable, consider radiofrequency ablation (RFA), microwave ablation, or transarterial chemoembolization (TACE) for select lesions.

Unresectable Liver Metastases

- *Palliative systemic therapy:*
  - Chemotherapy (e.g., FOLFOX, FOLFIRI, or CAPOX) ± targeted agents (bevacizumab, cetuximab, or panitumumab based on molecular profile).
  - Continue until disease progression or intolerance, with second-line options (e.g., irinotecan-based regimens).
- *Local control of rectal tumor:*
  - Chemoradiotherapy to prevent local complications (e.g., obstruction, bleeding, or fistula).
  - Consider palliative surgery (e.g., diverting colostomy) for symptomatic relief if the tumor is unresectable.
- *Liver-directed palliative therapies:*
  - Selective internal radiation therapy (SIRT) or TACE for liver-dominant disease.
  - Palliative ablation for symptom relief in select cases.
- *Supportive care:*
  - Pain management, nutritional support, and psychosocial care.
  - Manage complications (e.g., biliary obstruction, ascites) with stents or drainage.

Additional Considerations

- *Molecular profiling:* Test for KRAS/NRAS/BRAF mutations and microsatellite instability (MSI) to guide targeted therapy and immunotherapy (e.g., pembrolizumab for MSI-high tumors).
- *Symptom management:* Address symptoms like bleeding, obstruction, or tenesmus with endoscopic stenting, radiotherapy, or surgery as needed.
- *Follow-up:* Regular imaging (every 3 months initially), CEA monitoring, and MDT review to assess treatment response and adjust plans.
- *Clinical trials:* Enroll patients in trials for novel therapies (e.g., immunotherapy, targeted agents) if standard options are exhausted.

Prognosis

- *Resectable metastases:* 5-year survival rates of 30–50% with curative-intent surgery and chemotherapy.
- *Unresectable metastases:* Median survival of 2–3 years with modern systemic therapies, depending on response and patient factors.

36. Management of colorectal liver metastasis. ***WBUHS 2023***

37. Discuss the current trends of management of colorectal liver metastasis. ***WBUHS 2016; RIMS, Imphal 2022***

Introduction

- Colorectal cancer (CRC) is the second-most common cause of cancer death in western countries. The liver is the most frequent and often unique site of metastasis in CRC, both at the time of diagnosis (20–25% of cases) or after an apparently radical surgery on the primary tumor (40% of cases).
- The liver is the most common site of metastases for tumor sites that drain initially via the portal circulation. Metastatic liver disease is found in 10–25% of patients having surgery for primary colorectal cancer.
- As the chemotherapeutic regimens in the adjuvant and metastatic settings currently differ, patients who are not candidates for resection usually require a tissue diagnosis or definitive imaging before beginning chemotherapy.
- In this setting, percutaneous biopsy may be appropriate. The presence of a new mass lesion, increasing levels of CEA, and a history of colorectal cancer should provide enough evidence of disease to justify treatment. Biopsy carries risk for tumor dissemination (which should be enough to discourage unwarranted biopsies) as well as minor risks for bleeding and pneumothorax.
- Goals for management of metastatic colorectal cancer are to provide the patient with an optimum quality of live for the longest duration possible. Resection of hepatic metastases is now associated with long-term survival and low mortality such that patients who would have been denied surgical treatment in previous eras are now routinely offered locally aggressive treatment options.

Presentation and Diagnosis

- Presentation of liver metastases may be either synchronous or metachronous. Synchronous disease, commonly defined as liver metastasis occurring within 12 months of the colon or rectal primary, represents 13–25% of newly diagnosed colorectal liver metastases.
- Disease is found primarily on preoperative imaging or intraoperative exploration. In these patients, the original presentation is often related to the primary neoplasm, whereas liver metastases are incidental findings.
- Common presenting symptoms generally include fever, fatigue, weight loss, and anorexia. Patients may also describe a sense of abdominal fullness or even upper abdominal and right flank pain.
- Physical examination may reveal a palpable liver mass or hepatomegaly, jaundice, and ascites. More commonly, the physical examination is unremarkable.
- The optimal timing for synchronous liver metastases is controversial. Although a staged approach with initial resection of the primary lesion followed by hepatic resection 3 months later has been practiced, an increasing number of hepatic surgeons are utilizing a simultaneous, collaborative approach with the colorectal surgeon during the initial operation.
    - Metachronous disease develops in 20–25% of patients.

- The presentation of metachronous hepatic metastases varies according to the method by which they are detected. In unscreened populations, hepatic metastases can be detected only if the patient is having symptoms referable to the metastatic process.
- Other more commonly used methods of early detection in patients who previously had curative treatment for primary colorectal cancer include serial serum CEA determination and serial surveillance with cross-sectional imaging and/or ultrasonography.
- Presently, most metachronous presentations are not amenable to resection because of the late presentation or detection. Thus, dedicated, systematic follow-up for patients with a resected colorectal primary would lead to identification of patients who would benefit from hepatic resection.

Diagnostic tests for hepatic colorectal metastases include serum CEA levels, CT, MRI, PET, ultrasonography, and laparoscopy.

CEA

- CEA level has a sensitivity of ~75% and a specificity of 90–95% in detecting hepatic recurrence. CEA levels also have prognostic significance in patients undergoing evaluation for hepatic metastasectomy.
- Patients with a preoperative CEA level <200 ng/mL had a median survival of 38 months, and those with a level >200 ng/mL had a median survival of 24 months.
- PET is an appropriate second test in patients with increasing levels of CEA and no clear abnormalities on CT of the chest, abdomen, or pelvis. Combined CT-PET devices have also been developed that provide both physiologic and anatomical detail in the same setting.

USG

- The most important use of ultrasonography is during surgery. Intraoperative ultrasonography can detect occult colorectal metastases not seen on CT or transabdominal ultrasonography and has an overall sensitivity of 96%.
- Intraoperative ultrasonography is also useful in demonstrating segmental hepatic anatomy. This is particularly important when the tumor is in proximity to the inflow or outflow vessels. The value of intraoperative ultrasonography is operator dependent but in well-trained hands has been shown to alter the preoperative surgical plan in nearly 20% of patients.

CT scan: This test identifies the tumor(s) and pinpoints their size and location in the liver, as well as their relation to the vascular/biliary structures.

MRI: This test identifies the tumor(s) and pinpoints their size and location in the liver, as well as their relation to the vascular/biliary structures. It also helps the doctor to determine the overall health of the liver.

PET scan: This is a whole-body scan that looks for evidence of active cancer throughout the body.

Liver Biopsy

Diagnostic Laparoscopy

Diagnostic laparoscopy is useful prior to planned hepatic resection for colorectal metastases. It can aid in identifying lesions that may have been missed on preoperative cross-sectional imaging studies. Performance of laparoscopy does add time, expense, and its unique morbidities and has, therefore, not been universally practiced. A clinical risk score (CRS) has been described to clarify the role of preresectional laparoscopy yield.

Treatment

- *Systemic chemotherapy:*
  - With ~80% of patients with colorectal hepatic metastases presenting with nonresectable disease, systemic chemotherapy represents the main if not the only form of therapy for many patients. Chemotherapy may also play a role in transforming a portion of patients with unresectable disease into resection candidates.
  - Systemic agents have been introduced that may elicit a better response than standard 5-FU-LV–based treatment for advanced disease. Irinotecan (IR) and oxaliplatin (OX) combined with FU-LV appear to have a higher response rate than FU-LV alone.

- IR has also been shown to facilitate resectability in patients initially deemed unresectable.
- Addition of the monoclonal antibody against vascular endothelial growth factor (VEGF), bevacizumab, to the combination chemotherapy has been shown to improve survival significantly.
- The success of the modern chemotherapeutic agents for metastatic colorectal cancer is creating new opportunities for long-term survival in nonresectable patients. The application of neoadjuvant therapy for resectable disease also warrants investigation in clinical trials.

Targeted Therapy

- *Bevacizumab:* It binds to a protein called VEGF. VEGF is involved in the development of a blood supply within a growing cancer; this blood supply is essential for the tumor to grow and spread. Bevacizumab enhances the antitumor effect of other chemotherapy drugs. Bevacizumab is not effective when given by itself, but is generally given in combination with other drugs, such as FU (or capecitabine), OX, and IR.
- *Ramucirumab:* It is a protein that binds to a receptor for VEGF (VEGFR2), thus targeting signaling through the same pathway that bevacizumab does. Like bevacizumab, ramucirumab enhances the antitumor effect of other chemotherapy drugs.
- *Aflibercept:* Intravenous aflibercept represents another method of interfering with a tumor's blood supply; it is a fusion protein that acts by "trapping" VEGF and preventing it from activating its receptors on the tumor cells.
- *Regorafenib:* It is a pill form of a drug that blocks several VEGF receptors as well as other proteins referred to as kinases.
- *Cetuximab:* It targets a different protein, the epidermal growth factor receptor (EGFR), which is found in about 80% of colorectal cancers. It is effective even if EGFR is not found in an individual tumor. It does not work for all patients. It depends on whether or not the tumor has specific genetic abnormalities (a mutation in a set of genes called RAS genes or in a separate gene called BRAF). If the tumor has a *RAS* or a *BRAF* gene mutation, cetuximab does not work.
- *Panitumumab:* Like cetuximab, panitumumab also targets the EGFR. Like cetuximab, it is effective only for tumors that do not have a specific mutation in one of the RAS genes or in BRAF.
- *Trifluridine-tipiracil:* It is an oral agent that contains two components, trifluridine and tipiracil, each of which have different properties. In the United States, trifluridine-tipiracil is approved for the treatment of patients who have been previously treated with fluoropyrimidine-, OX-, and IR-containing chemotherapy regimens as well as other targeted therapies.
- *Operative management:*
  - Hepatic resection is currently the most effective form of therapy for colorectal metastases confined to the liver. It is important to have a definition of resectability to maintain a standard for evaluation. Resectability is defined as complete gross resection while retaining a sufficient liver remnant with intact biliary drainage and vasculature.
  - One of the more frequently used systems (CRS, "Fong" score) includes variables such as:
    - Node-negative primary
    - Single hepatic metastasis
    - Hepatic metastasis size <5 cm
    - CEA <200 ng/mL
    - Disease-free interval >1 year

  These variables suggest a better metastasectomy disease-free survival:
  - With nearly 80% of hepatic parenchyma being safe to remove, hepatic resection should be considered in many patients. It is equally important to identify patients who have conditions and/or factors that would preclude a resectional strategy.
  - Accepted contraindications to metastasectomy include poor overall health, inadequate liver reserve, inability to achieve margin-negative resection, and the presence of extrahepatic disease.
  - Anatomic or segmental resections are currently favored over large wedge resections, although there are currently scant data on this subject. The oncologic principle of getting an adequate negative margin should

be applied. Anatomic resections offer the best chance for achieving negative margins while maintaining maximum liver parenchyma.
- The resection margin is also critical in trying to achieve a cure. A positive histologic margin has been shown to be associated with poor long-term survival. The optimal surgical margin width, however, remains debatable. There have been no definitive studies showing that 1 cm or greater is favorable to a grossly negative margin. Thus, the importance of achieving a negative margin favors anatomic resections over wedge resections. It is likely, however, that a wedge resection is oncologically equivalent in the event that a negative margin can be reliably obtained.
- The success of resection of hepatic colorectal metastases has resulted in looking for ways to extend resectability. One technique is through preoperative portal vein embolization (PVE). The procedure is based on the physiologic phenomenon of liver atrophy of the embolized lobe and liver hypertrophy of the contralateral lobe. This augments the volume of the remaining liver and allows safe large-volume resectional strategies. The portal vein is usually reached through a percutaneous transhepatic route under ultrasound and fluoroscopic guidance.

Ablative Options

Ablative therapies are also available for patients with unresectable disease who do not have apparent extrahepatic metastases. Patients with inadequate hepatic reserve despite technically resectable lesions are also candidates. Local ablative techniques such as radiofrequency ablation (RFA) and cryoablation treat tumors in situ, effecting tumor killing by thermal mechanisms.

RFA

- RFA can be employed through percutaneous, laparoscopic, thoracoscopic, and open procedures.
- Size and location of the tumor dictate choice of treatment. Ultrasound guidance facilitates accurate and safe probe placement.
- Small lesions (<3 cm) located on the periphery are best suited for percutaneous approach.
- The laparoscopic approach with intraoperative ultrasonography has higher accuracy for detecting hepatic lesions than transcutaneous ultrasonography and is safer for mobilizing and ablating tumors that are close to or in contact with surrounding organs.
- A thoracoscopic approach is useful for tumors situated on the dome of the liver that are difficult to reach percutaneously or laparoscopically.
- When a question of efficacy or safety arises, an open approach should be used.
- *Portal vein embolization:* PVE is another modality used preoperatively for patients where the extent of liver resection is expected to result in less than the optimal functional liver volume of 25–40%, necessary to prevent postoperative liver failure.
- *Hepatic arterial infusion:*
  - The use of hepatic arterial infusion pump (HAIP) placement and administration of chemotherapy is based on the observation that hepatic tumors derive their blood supply primarily from the hepatic artery, in contrast to normal hepatic parenchyma, which is principally supplied by the portal vein. Therefore, infusion of chemotherapeutic agents through the hepatic arterial circulation should lead to high concentrations of the agents within tumor cells while sparing the normal hepatic parenchyma.
  - In addition, several agents are efficiently extracted within the liver such that systemic concentrations and concomitant toxicities are further reduced. Fluorodeoxyuridine is the most common agent administered by the intra-arterial route, although FU-LV has also been delivered in this fashion.

38. Liver metastasis from colorectal cancer—improving resectability.

Introduction

- 25% of patients diagnosed with colorectal cancer will have liver metastasis at presentation.
- Another 50% of patients will have recurrent diseases developed within liver.

- 85% of tumor recurrences are detected within 2.5 years after resection of the primary colorectal cancer and the remaining 15% are detected within the next 2.5 years.
- Death in colorectal cancer is often a result of liver metastasis.
- Surgical resection of distant metastasis can produce long-term survival and cure in some patients.

Improved 5-year Survival

- During the past two decades the 5-year survival rates for hepatic colorectal metastases patients have almost doubled, from 30 to 60%.
- The introduction of new chemotherapeutic agents and the shift in the criteria of surgical resection were the main factors in this progress.
- Previous absolute or relative contraindications to resection included the presence of extrahepatic disease, involvement of hepatic pedicle lymph nodes, and an inadequate resection margin of <1 cm.
- All above contraindications for hepatic resection have been challenged and have already lost their importance in patient selection for hepatectomy.

Current Criteria

- It focuses on what should be left after hepatic resection.
- Previous criteria for resection, such as the size, location, number of intrahepatic metastases, and the presence of bilobar or extrahepatic disease have been largely abandoned.
- Nowadays, the definition of resectability includes a complete resection with tumor-free surgical margins (R0 resection), sparing at least two liver segments having an independent inflow, outflow, and biliary drainage.
- The amount of the liver remnant after resection should not be <20% and 30% of the total liver volume in normal and cirrhotic patients, respectively.
- This can be accurately predicted by CT or MRI during preoperative evaluation.

Prognostic Variables for Liver Metastasis

- Age >70
- Primary tumor stage
- Primary tumor location (colon > rectum)
- Clinical presentation suggestive of metastasis (sign/symptoms and laboratory abnormalities)
- Synchronous metastasis
- Size of metastatic lesion(s)
- Extent of liver involvement
- Interval between primary diagnosis and appearance of metachronous metastasis (diagnostic interval ≤1 year)
- Multiple metastasis
- Presence of satellite lesions
- Presence of extrahepatic disease

Preoperative investigations before resection of colorectal liver metastases are focused on:

- Determining the diagnosis
- Anatomically defining the lesion in the liver parenchyma for surgical planning
- Meticulous staging to rule out extrahepatic disease

Preoperative work up for candidates for resection of metastasis:

- Detailed history and physical examination
- Laboratory investigations including complete blood count (CBC) and liver function tests (LFTs)
- Chest X-ray
- CT or MRI of abdomen/pelvis
- Colonoscopy (if not done within 6 months)
- PET scan

Patient Selection for Resection

- *Criteria for absolute unfit for surgery:*
  - Nontreatable extrahepatic disease, unresectability
  - Involvement of >70% of the liver or six *v* segments
  - Radiographic evidence of involvement of the hepatic artery, major bile ducts, main portal vein, or celiac/paraaortic lymph nodes.
  - Modern multidisciplinary consensus defines resectable
  - CRC liver metastases simply as tumors that can be resected completely, leaving an adequate liver remnant
- *Criteria for resectability:*
  - General criteria for fitness. Good performance status.
  - Absence of extra hepatic disease.
  - Specific criteria that decide the outcome:
    - Risk of recurrence.
    - Clinical risk score
  - Anatomical criteria for respectability:
    - Number of metastases
    - Precise location
    - Relationship with the portal pedicle and the hepatic veins
- *Clinical risk score:*
  - Five clinical criteria each assigned 1 point:
  - Node-positive primary
  - 12-month disease-free interval
  - More than one liver tumors
  - Largest tumor >5 cm, CEA >200 ng/mL
  - *Principles of resection in colorectal liver metastases:* An R0 resection of both the intra- and extrahepatic disease sites must be feasible. At least two adjacent liver segments need to be spared. Vascular inflow and outflow, as well as biliary drainage to the remaining segments, must be preserved. The volume of the liver remaining after resection (i.e., the future liver remnant) must be adequate
- *Preoperative patient evaluation:*
  - Colonoscopy, chest/abdominal/pelvic CT
  - CBC, platelets
  - CEA
  - Determination of tumor K-RAS status
  - Needle biopsy—if clinically indicated PET-CT only if potentially surgically curable M1 disease. Conversion therapy for initially unresectable metastases. Induction chemotherapy in patients with isolated but initially unresectable CRC liver metastases.

39. Liver resection for colorectal liver metastasis. ***WBUHS 2020***

Introduction

- Hepatic resection of metastatic colorectal cancer has become the treatment of choice for selected patients after resection of the primary colorectal cancer.
- Despite variability in criteria for patient selection, survival outcomes have ranged consistently from 25 to 45%.

Liver Resection for Colorectal Metastases

- The aim of liver resection (resectability) is to remove all macroscopic disease with clear (negative) margins and leave sufficient functioning liver.
- Patients with solitary, multiple, and bilobar disease who have had radical treatment of the primary colorectal cancer are candidates for liver resection.

- The ability to achieve clear margins (R0 resection) should be determined by the radiologist and surgeon in the regional hepatobiliary unit.
- The surgeon should define the acceptable residual functioning volume, approximately one-third of the standard liver volume, or the equivalent of a minimum of two segments.
- The liver surgeon and anesthetist should take the clinical decision regarding fitness for surgery.
- If deemed medically unfit for surgery, patients should be considered for ablative therapy.
- Patients with extrahepatic disease that should be considered for liver resection include:
    - Resectable/ablatable pulmonary metastases
    - Resectable/ablatable isolated extrahepatic sites—for example, spleen, adrenal, or respectable local recurrence
    - Local direct extension of liver metastases to, for example, diaphragm/adrenal that can be resected.
- Normal contraindications to liver resection would include uncontrollable extrahepatic disease such as:
    - Nontreatable primary tumor
    - Widespread pulmonary disease
    - Locoregional recurrence
    - Peritoneal disease
    - Extensive nodal disease, such as retroperitoneal, mediastinal, or portal nodes
    - Bone or CNS metastases

Tumors Borderline for Resection

- Those patients with tumors thought to be borderline for resection may have resectable or ablatable disease and should be referred for discussion with the regional hepatobiliary unit before chemotherapy.
- Resectability may be achieved by PVE or two-stage hepatectomy to increase hepatic functional reserve and also by combinations of surgery and ablation.

SOLITARY RECTAL ULCER SYNDROME

40. Solitary rectal ulcer syndrome. ***WBUHS 2007, 2015***

Introduction

Solitary rectal ulcer syndrome can cause rectal bleeding with straining when you pass bowel movements.

Solitary rectal ulcer syndrome most commonly involves one ulcer, but sometimes more than one rectal ulcer can occur or polyp-like masses may form. Solitary rectal ulcer syndrome is a rare and poorly understood disorder that occurs in people with chronic constipation.

Treatments for solitary rectal ulcer syndrome range from changing your diet and fluid intake to surgery.

Definition

Solitary rectal ulcer syndrome is a condition that occurs when a sore (ulcer) develops in the rectum. The rectum is a muscular tube that's connected to the end of your colon. Stool passes through the rectum on its way out of the body. Signs and symptoms of solitary rectal ulcer syndrome include:

- Constipation
- A feeling of incomplete passing of stool
- Pain or a feeling of fullness in your pelvis
- Passing mucus from your rectum
- Rectal pain or anal sphincter spasms
- Rectal bleeding
- Straining during bowel movements
- However, some people with solitary rectal ulcer syndrome may experience no symptoms

Causes

It is not always clear what causes solitary rectal ulcer syndrome. Doctors believe stress or injury to the rectum may cause rectal ulcers to form.

Examples of situations that could injure the rectum include:

- Attempts to manually remove impacted stool
- Constipation or impacted stool
- Intussusception, which occurs when part of the intestine slides inside another part
- Radiation therapy used to treat cancer in the abdomen or pelvis
- Rectal prolapse, which occurs when the rectum protrudes from the anus
- Straining during bowel movements
- Use of ergotamine suppositories, an antimigraine treatment
- Uncoordinated tightening of the pelvic floor muscles that slow blood flow to the rectum

Tests and procedures used to diagnose rectal ulcers include:

- Sigmoidoscopy
- USG
- *An X-ray of the rectum*—defecation proctography

Treatments

- Treatment for solitary rectal ulcer syndrome depends on the severity of condition.
- People with mild signs and symptoms may find relief by making lifestyle changes to control chronic constipation.
- People with more severe signs and symptoms may require treatments such as behavior therapy and surgery.
- Behavior therapy to stop straining during bowel movements.

Some people strain during bowel movements out of habit. Behavior therapy can help one learn to relax the pelvic muscles and avoid straining during bowel movements. In one technique called biofeedback, a specialist teaches the patient to control certain involuntary body responses, such as tightening of anus or pelvic floor muscles during defecation. Biofeedback may make the patient more aware of straining and help to control it.

Surgery

Surgical procedures used to treat rectal ulcer include:

- *Surgery to remove the rectum:* An operation to remove the rectum may be an option for people with severe rectal ulcer signs and symptoms. Colostomy may be done.
- *Rectopexy (when there is associated rectal prolapse):* Rectopexy corrects rectal prolapse by using stitches to secure the rectum in its anatomically correct position.

RECTAL PROLAPSE

41. Pathophysiology and treatment of rectal prolapse. ***WBUHS 2017***

42. Prolapsed rectum—etiology and treatment.

Rajiv Gandhi Institute of Health Sciences, 2019, Gujarat University 2024

The pathophysiology of rectal prolapse is not completely understood or agreed upon. There are two main theories, which essentially are different ways of expressing the same idea.

- The first theory postulates that rectal prolapse is a sliding hernia through a defect in the pelvic fascia.
- The second theory holds that rectal prolapse starts as a circumferential internal intussusception of the rectum beginning 6–8 cm proximal to the anal verge. With time and straining, this progresses to full-thickness rectal prolapse, though some patients never progress beyond this stage.

The pathophysiology and etiology of mucosal prolapse most likely differ from those of full-thickness rectal prolapse and internal intussusception. Mucosal prolapse occurs when the connective tissue attachments of the rectal mucosa are loosened and stretched, thus allowing the tissue to prolapse through the anus. This often occurs as a continuation of long-standing hemorrhoidal disease and is treated as such.

Often, prolapse begins with an internal prolapse of the anterior rectal wall and progresses to full prolapse.

Etiology

The precise cause of rectal prolapse is not defined; however, a number of associated abnormalities have been found. As many as 50% of prolapse cases are caused by chronic straining with defecation and constipation.

Other predisposing conditions include the following:

- Pregnancy
- Previous surgery
- Diarrhea
- Benign prostatic hypertrophy
- Chronic obstructive pulmonary disease (COPD)
- Cystic fibrosis
- Pertussis (i.e., whooping cough)
- Pelvic floor dysfunction
- Parasitic infections—amebiasis and schistosomiasis
- Neurologic disorders—previous lower back or pelvic trauma/lumbar disc disease, cauda equina syndrome, spinal tumors, and multiple sclerosis
- Disordered defecation (e.g., stool withholding)

Treatment

Nonoperative Management

- Generally, a prolapsed rectum can be reduced with gentle digital pressure; an incarcerated rectal prolapse is rare.
- Although no medical treatment is available for rectal prolapse, internal prolapse should always be first treated medically with bulking agents, stool softeners, and suppositories or enemas. Biofeedback may be helpful if paradoxical pelvic floor contraction also exists.
- Contributing factors, such as constipation and diarrhea, should be addressed and eliminated if possible. Supportive care should be provided according to the clinical picture, particularly in the presence of an irreducible prolapse and with gangrene or rupture of the rectal mucosa. Obtain a prompt surgical evaluation if anal incontinence is present.
- If the prolapse cannot be reduced and the viability of the bowel is in question, emergency resection is required. Rupture of the rectum also constitutes a surgical emergency.

Surgical Options

Contraindications for surgical correction of rectal prolapse are based on the patient's comorbidities and his or her ability to tolerate surgery. Surgical treatments can be divided into two categories according to the approach used to repair the rectal prolapse: Abdominal procedures and perineal procedures. The choice between an abdominal procedure and a perineal procedure is mainly dictated by the patient's age and comorbidities.

Abdominal Surgical Procedures

- Abdominal repairs are typically performed in younger, healthier patients, whose life expectancy is longer. For these patients, procedures with lower recurrence rates but higher morbidities are most appropriate. The choice of abdominal procedure is often dictated by the extent of the associated constipation and by the surgeon's preference.

- Laparoscopic surgical rectopexy procedures have been developed that have outcomes as good as those of open abdominal procedures but are associated with shorter hospital stays and greater patient comfort.
  - *Anterior resection:*
    - Patients with rectal prolapse and constipation often have a redundant colon, and some surgeons believe that resection of this alleviates constipation and decreases recurrence of rectal prolapse.
    - In an anterior resection for rectal prolapse, the rectum is mobilized to the level of the lateral ligaments, and the redundant colon (sigmoid) is resected. The left colon is then anastomosed to the top of the rectum.
  - *Marlex rectopexy:* In a Marlex rectopexy (Ripstein procedure), the entire rectum is mobilized down to the coccyx posteriorly, the lateral ligaments laterally, and the anterior cul-de-sac anteriorly (see the image below). A nonabsorbable material (e.g., Marlex mesh or an Ivalon sponge) is fixed to the presacral fascia. The rectum is placed on tension, and the material is partially wrapped around the rectum to keep it in position.

Perineal Surgical Procedures

- Perineal procedures have higher recurrence rates but lower morbidities and are often performed in elderly persons or in patients for whom general anesthesia is contraindicated.
  - *Anal encirclement:*
    - With anal encirclement (Thiersch wire), a nonabsorbable band is placed subcutaneously around the anus.
    - The purpose of this procedure is to keep the rectum from prolapsing by restricting the size of the anal lumen. Anal encirclement is effective in mechanically preventing the rectum from prolapsing, but it does not treat the underlying disorder.
    - Complications from this procedure include obstruction with fecal impaction and erosion of the wire with infection.
    - Anal encirclement is no longer commonly performed; it is usually reserved for only the most debilitated patients and for patients with the highest surgical risks, in whom palliation is the goal. Anal encirclement carries a very high risk of fecal impaction.
  - *Delorme mucosal sleeve resection:* In a Delorme mucosal sleeve resection, a circumferential incision is made through the mucosa of the prolapsed rectum near the dentate line; with the electrocautery, the mucosa is stripped from the rectum to the apex of the prolapse and excised. The denuded prolapsed muscle is then pleated with a suture and reefed up like an accordion, and the transected edges of the mucosa are sutured together. This procedure is often used for small prolapses but may also be used for large ones.
  - *Altemeier procedure:* The Altemeier procedure (perineal rectosigmoidectomy) for rectal prolapse provided excellent results across all age groups with minimal morbidity, allowing for short hospital stays and periods of convalescence.

---

43. Compare the surgical treatment options for procidentia of rectum. **WBUHS 2018**

Abdominal Surgical Procedures

Abdominal repairs are typically performed in younger, healthier patients, whose life expectancy is longer. For these patients, procedures with lower recurrence rates but higher morbidities are most appropriate. The choice of abdominal procedure is often dictated by the extent of the associated constipation and by the surgeon's preference.

Laparoscopic surgical rectopexy procedures have been developed that have outcomes as good as those of open abdominal procedures but are associated with shorter hospital stays and greater patient comfort.

Anterior Resection

- Patients with rectal prolapse and constipation often have a redundant colon, and some surgeons believe that resection of this alleviates constipation and decreases recurrence of rectal prolapse.
- In an anterior resection for rectal prolapse, the rectum is mobilized to the level of the lateral ligaments, and the redundant colon (sigmoid) is resected. The left colon is then anastomosed to the top of the rectum.

- This anastomosis is performed without laxity in the colon so that the rectum is held in place and can no longer prolapse.
- It is not thought to address anatomic abnormalities such as poor rectal fixation.

Marlex Rectopexy

- In a Marlex rectopexy (Ripstein procedure), the entire rectum is mobilized down to the coccyx posteriorly, the lateral ligaments laterally, and the anterior cul-de-sac anteriorly (see the image below).
- A nonabsorbable material (e.g., Marlex mesh or an Ivalon sponge) is fixed to the presacral fascia. The rectum is placed on tension, and the material is partially wrapped around the rectum to keep it in position. To prevent a circumferential obstruction, the anterior rectal wall is not covered with the sponge or mesh.
- The peritoneal reflections are then closed to cover the foreign body. The Marlex mesh or sponge causes an intense inflammatory reaction that scars and fixes the rectum into place. This procedure should not be performed on patients who have a large component of constipation or a very redundant sigmoid colon, because the symptoms are likely to worsen. If the rectum is inadvertently entered during mobilization, the foreign material should not be implanted, because of the risk of infection.
- Although the rate of Marlex erosion into the rectum is low, management is extremely difficult, and for this reason, many surgeons prefer resection with suture rectopexy to Marlex fixation.

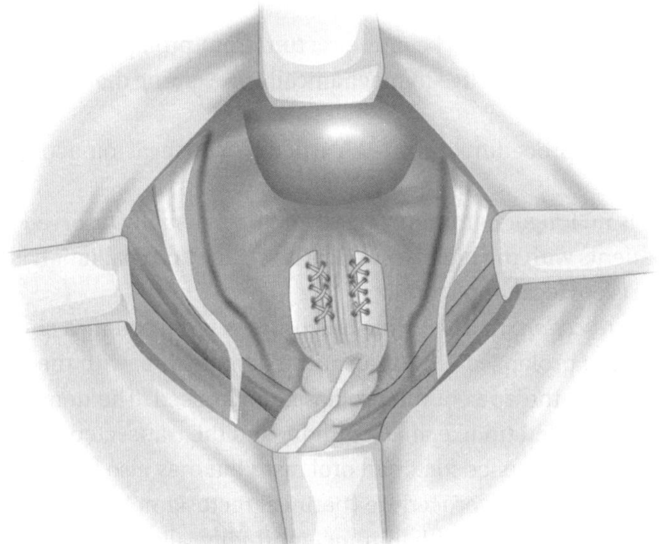

Marlex rectopexy for rectal prolapse

Suture Rectopexy

A suture rectopexy is essentially the same as a Marlex rectopexy, except that the rectum is fixed to the presacral fascia with suture material rather than mesh or an Ivalon sponge.

Resection Rectopexy

- A resection with rectopexy (Frykman–Goldberg procedure) is a combination of an anterior resection and a Marlex rectopexy; it is a good option for patients with a significant component of constipation. The rectum is completely mobilized to the coccyx posteriorly, to the lateral ligaments laterally (some surgeons divide the lateral ligaments), and to the cul-de-sac anteriorly.
- The redundant sigmoid colon is then resected, and the remaining colon is anastomosed to the top of the rectum. The lateral ligaments (or the rectal fascia) are then sutured to the presacral fascia with the rectum on tension, which keeps the rectum in place and prevents further rectal prolapse.
- The rectopexy is accomplished with suture instead of nonabsorbable mesh because the bowel is opened for the anastomosis and the mesh may become contaminated.

Perineal Surgical Procedures

Perineal procedures have higher recurrence rates but lower morbidities and are often performed in elderly persons or in patients for whom general anesthesia is contraindicated.

Anal Encirclement

- With anal encirclement (Thiersch wire), a nonabsorbable band is placed subcutaneously around the anus. The purpose of this procedure is to keep the rectum from prolapsing by restricting the size of the anal lumen.
- Anal encirclement is effective in mechanically preventing the rectum from prolapsing, but it does not treat the underlying disorder.
- Complications from this procedure include obstruction with fecal impaction and erosion of the wire with infection.
- Anal encirclement is no longer commonly performed; it is usually reserved for only the most debilitated patients and for patients with the highest surgical risks, in whom palliation is the goal. Anal encirclement carries a very high risk of fecal impaction.

Delorme Mucosal Sleeve Resection

- In a Delorme mucosal sleeve resection, a circumferential incision is made through the mucosa of the prolapsed rectum near the dentate line; with the electrocautery, the mucosa is stripped from the rectum to the apex of the prolapse and excised.
- The denuded prolapsed muscle is then pleated with a suture and reefed up like an accordion, and the transected edges of the mucosa are sutured together.
- This procedure is often used for small prolapses but may also be used for large ones.

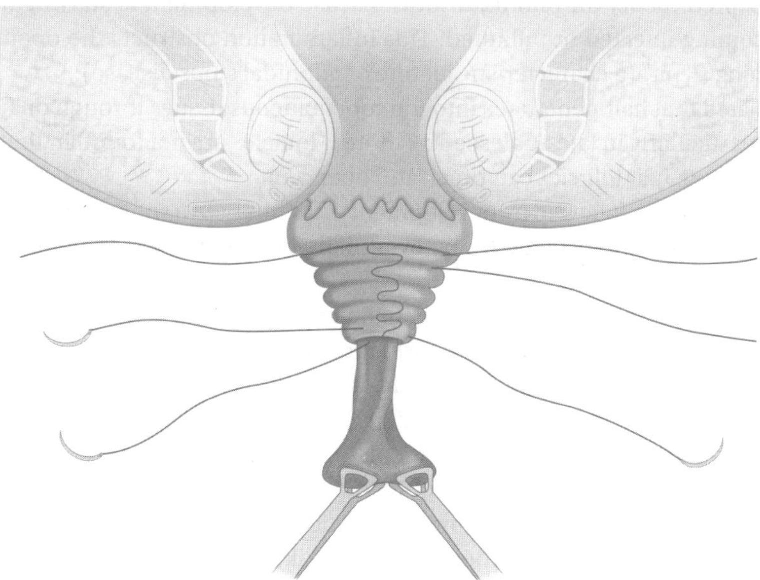

Delorme mucosal sleeve resection for rectal prolapse.

Altemeier Perineal Rectosigmoidectomy

- In an Altemeier perineal rectosigmoidectomy, a full-thickness circumferential incision is made in the prolapsed rectum about 1–2 cm from the dentate line.
- The hernia sac is entered, and the prolapse is delivered. The mesentery of the prolapsed bowel is serially ligated until no further redundant bowel can be pulled down.
- The bowel is transected and either hand-sewn to the distal anal canal or stapled with a circular stapler.
- Before anastomosis, some surgeons plicate the levator ani muscles anteriorly, which may help improve continence.

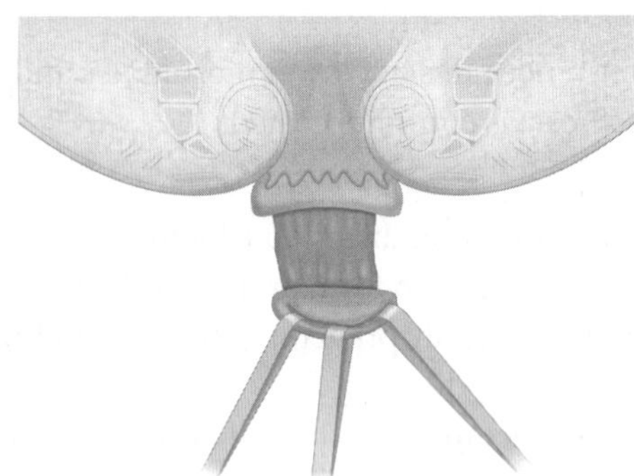

Altemeier perineal rectosigmoidectomy for rectal prolapse.

Hemorrhoidectomy: Mucosal prolapse is treated with a hemorrhoidectomy.

Perineal stapled prolapse resection: Although the procedure is fast and safe, the long-term functional outcome was poor, and the recurrence rate was 44%.

PILONIDAL SINUS

44. What are the most widely accepted theories in the causation of the pilonidal sinus? Discuss the minimal invasive operative treatment of pilonidal sinus. ***WBUHS 2021 Supplementary***

The most widely accepted theory for pilonidal sinus disease development is starting from a hair follicle in the intergluteal cleft becoming infected or inflamed. This inflammation obstructs the opening of the follicle, which extends inward, forming a "pit" (a characteristic feature of pilonidal sinus disease).

- It has been postulated that hair penetrates into the subcutaneous tissues through dilated hair follicles, which is thought to occur particularly in late adolescence, though follicles are not found in the walls of cysts.
- Upon sitting or bending, hair follicles can break and open a pit.
- Debris may collect in this pit, followed by development of a sinus with a short tract, with a not clearly understood suction mechanism involving local anatomy, eventually leading to further penetration of the hair into the subcutaneous tissue.
- This sinus tends to extend cephalad, likely owing to mechanical forces involved in sitting or bending.
- A foreign body-type reaction may then lead to formation of an abscess.
    - If given the opportunity to drain spontaneously, this may act as a portal of further invasion and eventually formation of a foreign body granuloma. Infection may result in abscess formation.
- Microscopically, the sinus where the hair enters is lined with stratified squamous epithelium with slight cornification. Additional sinuses are frequent. Cyst cavities are lined with chronic granulation tissue and may contain hair, epithelial debris, and young granulation tissue. Cutaneous appendages are not seen in the wall of cysts, meaning the cysts lack epithelial lining, unlike the sinus. Cellular infiltration consists of PMNs, lymphocytes, and plasma cells in varying proportions. Foreign body giant cells in association with dead hairs are a frequent finding.
- In summary, three pieces are instrumental in this process:
    1. The invader, hair
    2. The force, causing hair penetration
    3. The vulnerability of the skin

Minimally Invasive Treatments for Pilonidal Sinus

- Minimally invasive treatments for pilonidal sinus consist of circumferential incision of the pilonidal orifices avoiding wide cutaneous margins and a selective subcutaneous extirpation of the sinus without closure of the wound (sinusectomy).

- *Endoscopic approach:*
  - Video-assisted ablation of pilonidal sinus (VAAPS)
  - *Endoscopic pilonidal sinus treatment (EPSiT):* Both VAAPS and EPSiT use a "fistuloscope", which is inserted into the external opening of the pilonidal sinus—the diagnostic phase identifies the anatomy of the pilonidal sinus and any secondary tracts or abscess cavities by direct vision.

SURGICAL ANATOMY OF RECTUM AND ANAL CANAL WITH ANAL INCONTINENCE

45. Describe the surgical anatomy of rectum and anal canal. Write about etiology and management of anal incontinence? ***WBUHS 2011; RIMS, Imphal 2012; AIIMS, Patna 2025***

46. Describe the anatomy of anal sphincter. What is its importance while managing a case of rectal cancer? ***WBUHS 2023***

47. Write down the anal musculature of and physiology of anal canal in respect of fecal incontinence. ***WBUHS 2024***

48. Describe the anatomy of anal sphincter. How do you evaluate its function? ***WBUHS 2016***

- The rectum normally lies attached to its mesorectum within the curve of the sacrum with limited mobility. The junction of the rectosigmoid is most consistently found at the sacral promontory and descends only 2 or 3 cm during a Valsalva maneuver.
- The rectum exits the pelvis anteriorly surrounded by a sling of muscle from the pubis through a slit in the pelvic floor. The sling is created by the puborectalis muscle that circles around behind the rectum and reinserts on the pubis anteriorly.
- The anal canal itself measures 3–4 cm and is a funnel-shaped extension of the pelvic floor musculature. The pressure generated by this voluntary muscle prevents egress of rectal contents. The internal sphincter muscle is a continuation of the thickened circular muscle of the rectum. As such, it is an autonomic muscle and has no voluntary control.

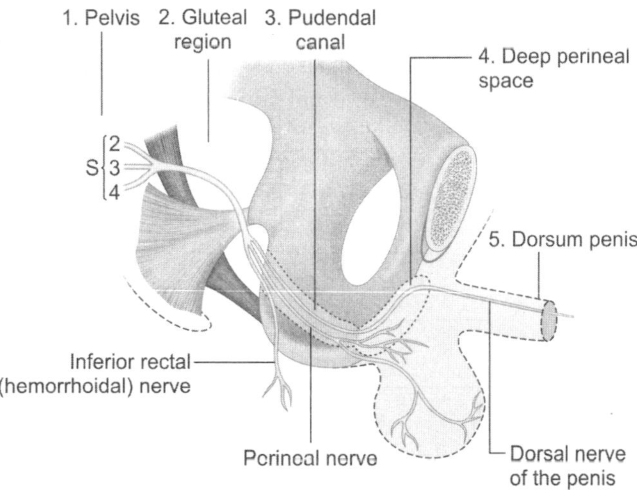

- *The anorectum receives both sympathetic and parasympathetic nerves.* The sympathetic nerves originate from thoracolumbar segments, and unite below the inferior mesenteric artery to form the inferior mesenteric plexus. These fibers then descend to the superior hypogastric plexus located just inferior to the aortic bifurcation. These purely sympathetic fibers bifurcate and descend as the hypogastric nerves. Parasympathetic fibers from

S2, S3, and S4 (the nervi erigentes) join the hypogastric nerves anterolateral to the rectum to form the inferior hypogastric plexuses. Mixed fibers from the plexuses innervate the prostate, rectum, bladder, penis, and internal anal sphincter. The sympathetic innervation of the internal sphincter is motor, while the parasympathetic innervation is inhibitory.

- The innervation of the voluntary muscles of the pelvic floor is via direct fibers from S2, S3, and S4 in the pelvis from the sacrum. The nerves of the external sphincter are derived from S2, S3, and S4 nerve roots from the sacral plexus and arrive at the external sphincter via the pudendal nerve around the ischial spine at Alcock's canal.
- It is useful to consider the anus and surrounding structures as a single unit, the anorectum. The anorectum includes the perianal skin, the anal canal, the anal sphincters, and the distal rectum. The three main anatomic points of reference are the anal verge, the dentate line, and the anorectal ring. The distal external boundary of the anal canal is the anal verge, which is also the junction between the anal and perianal skin. Anal epithelium (anoderm) is devoid of the hair follicles, sebaceous glands, and apocrine glands that are present in the perianal skin, a fact worth remembering when attempting to distinguish between hidradenitis (inflammation of the apocrine glands in the perianal skin) and cryptoglandular anal disease.
- The cephalad border of the anal canal is a true mucocutaneous junction, the dentate line. This union of the embryonic ectoderm with the endodermal gut resides approximately 1.0–1.5 cm above the anal verge. In a transitional zone of 6–12 mm in length, the columnar epithelium of the rectum changes to cuboidal epithelium which joins the squamous epithelium at the dentate line.
- The upper border of the anal sphincteric complex is the anorectal ring. It may be palpated by digital examination about 1.0–1.5 cm above the dentate line.
- Anatomists consider the anal canal to begin at the dentate line and end at the anal verge. However, most surgeons consider the anal canal to start at the anorectal ring and terminate at the anal verge.
- Just above the dentate line, the rectal mucosa forms from 8 to 14 longitudinal folds known as the rectal columns. Between each two columns at the dentate line is a small pocket termed an anal crypt. The glands may extend through the internal sphincter as far as the intersphincteric plane, but they do not extend into the external sphincter.
- Below the dentate line, cutaneous sensations of heat, cold, touch, and pain are conveyed by afferent fibers in the inferior rectal nerves. Cephalad to the dentate line, poorly defined dull sensations, elicited when the mucosa is pinched, or internal hemorrhoids are ligated, are probably carried by parasympathetic fibers.
- *Blood supply:* The superior rectal artery, the terminal branch of the inferior mesenteric artery, descends to the upper rectum where it divides into lateral branches. Subsequent smaller divisions penetrate the rectal wall. The middle rectal arteries arise from the internal iliac arteries and supply the distal rectum and upper anal canal. The inferior rectal arteries, branches from the internal pudendal arteries, cross the ischiorectal fossae to supply the anal sphincters.

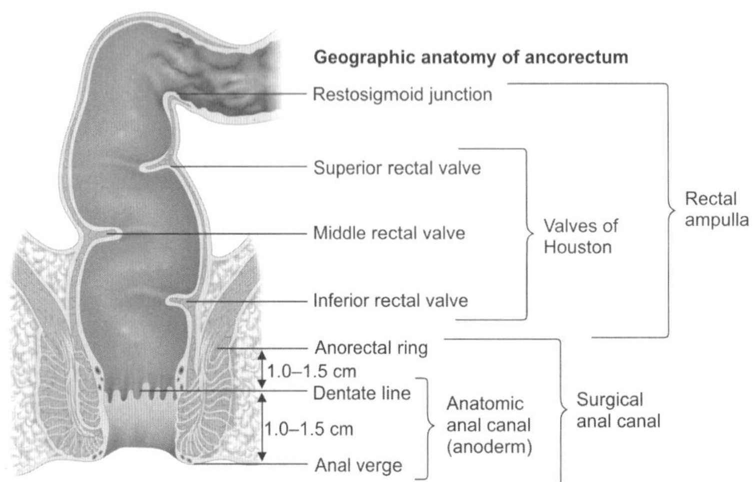

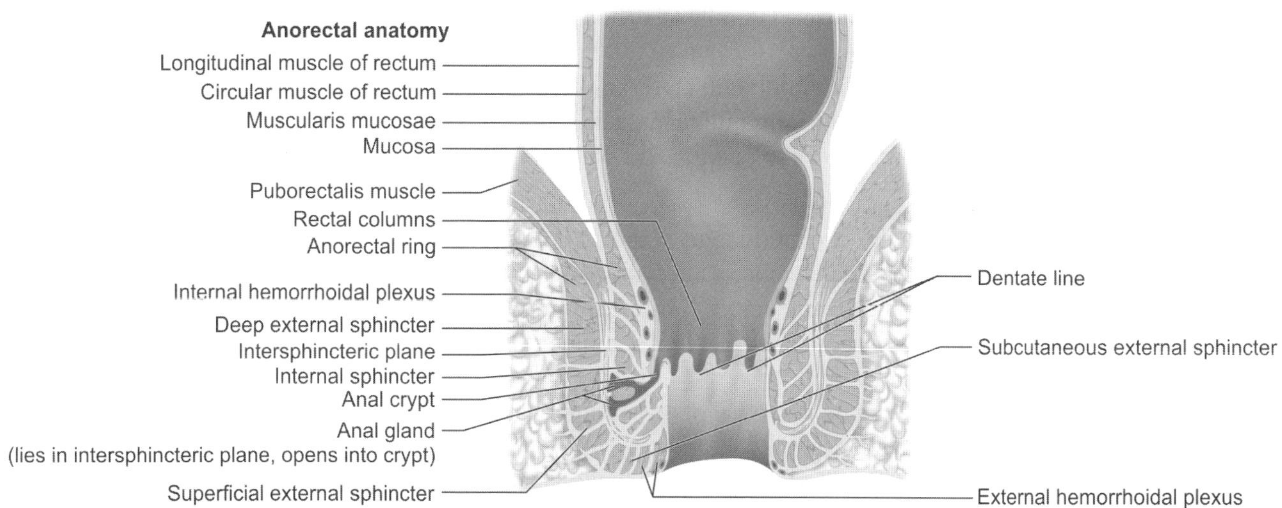

- *Venous drainage:*
  - There are two paths for venous blood return from the anorectum.
  - Above the dentate line, venous blood flows into the portal system through the superior rectal vein and inferior mesenteric vein.
  - Below the dentate line, the external hemorrhoidal plexus drains into the internal iliac vein via the middle rectal vein or via the pudendal vein, which receives blood from the inferior rectal vein.

Surgical Anatomy of Anal Canal and Evaluation of Function of Anal Sphincter

The anal canal commences at the level where the rectum passes through the pelvic diaphragm and ends at the anal verge. The muscular junction between the rectum and anal canal can be felt with the finger as a thickened ridge—the anorectal "bundle" or "ring".

Anal Canal Anatomy

The Anorectal Ring

- The anorectal ring marks the junction between the rectum and the anal canal.
- It is formed by the joining of the puborectalis muscle, the deep external sphincter, conjoined longitudinal muscle, and the highest part of the internal sphincter.
- The anorectal ring can be clearly felt digitally, especially on its posterior and lateral aspects.

The Puborectalis Muscle

- Puborectalis, part of the funnel-shaped muscular pelvic diaphragm, maintains the angle between the anal canal, and rectum and hence is an important component in the continence mechanism.
- The muscle derives its nerve supply from the sacral somatic nerves, and is functionally indistinct from the external anal sphincter.
- The position and length of the anal canal, as well as the angle of the anorectal junction, depend to a major extent on the integrity and strength of the puborectalis muscle sling.
- It gives off fibers that contribute to the longitudinal muscle layer.

The External Sphincter

- The external sphincter forms the bulk of the anal sphincter complex and, although traditionally it has been subdivided into deep, superficial, and subcutaneous portions, it is a single muscle (Goligher), which is variably divided by lateral extensions from the longitudinal muscle layer.
- Some of its fibers are attached posteriorly to the coccyx, whereas anteriorly they fuse with the perineal muscles. Being a somatic voluntary muscle, the external sphincter is red in color and is innervated by the pudendal nerve.

The Intersphincteric Plane

- Between the external sphincter muscle laterally and the longitudinal muscle medially exists a potential space, the intersphincteric plane.
- This plane is important as it contains intersphincteric anal glands and is also a route for the spread of pus, which occurs along the extensions from the longitudinal muscle layer.
- The plane can be opened up surgically to provide access for operations on the sphincter muscles.

The Longitudinal Muscle

- The longitudinal muscle is a direct continuation of the smooth muscle of the outer muscle coat of the rectum, augmented in its upper part by striated muscle fibers originating from the medial components of the pelvic floor.
- Most of the muscle continues caudally before splitting into multiple terminal septa that surround the muscle bundles of the subcutaneous portion of the external sphincter to insert into the skin of the lowermost part of the anal canal and adjacent perianal skin.
- Milligan and Morgan named the most medial of these septa, passing around the inferior border of the internal sphincter, the "anal intermuscular septum".
- As it descends, however, it gives off fibers that pass medially across the internal sphincter to reach the submucosal space, and laterally across the external sphincter and ischiorectal space to reach the fascia of the pelvic side walls.
- As well as providing a supportive mesh for the anal canal and other muscular components, its ramifications provide potential pathways for the spread of infection.
- During defecation, its contraction widens the anal lumen, flattens the anal cushions, shortens the anal canal, and everts the anal margin; subsequent relaxation allows the anal cushions to distend and thus contribute to an airtight seal.

The Internal Sphincter

- The internal sphincter is the thickened (2–5 mm) distal continuation of the circular muscle coat of the rectum, which has developed special properties and which is in a tonic state of contraction.
- This involuntary muscle commences where the rectum passes through the pelvic diaphragm and ends above the anal orifice, its lower border palpable at the intersphincteric groove, below which lie the most medial fibers of the subcutaneous external sphincter, and separated from it by the anal intermuscular septum.
- When exposed during life, it is pearly-white in color and its circumferentially placed fibers can be seen clearly.
- Although innervated by the autonomic nervous system, it receives intrinsic nonadrenergic and noncholinergic (NANC) fibers, stimulation of which causes release of the neurotransmitter nitric oxide, which induces internal sphincter relaxation.

The Epithelium and Subepithelial Structures

- The pink columnar epithelium lining the rectum extends through the anorectal ring into the surgical anal canal. Passing downward the mucous membrane becomes cuboidal and redder in color whereas above the anal valves it is plum colored.
- Just below the level of the anal valves, there is an abrupt, albeit wavy, transition to stratified squamous epithelium, which is parchment colored.
- This wavy junction constitutes the dentate line.
- The dentate line is a most important landmark both morphologically and surgically, representing the site of fusion of the proctodeum and postallantoic gut, and being the site of the crypts of Morgagni (synonym: anal crypts, sinuses).
- The latter are small pockets between the inferior extremities of the columns of Morgagni through which anal ducts that communicate with deeper placed anal glands open into the anal lumen.
- The squamous epithelium lining the lower anal canal is thin and shiny and is known as the anoderm; it differs from the true skin in that it has no epidermal appendages, i.e., hair and sweat glands. At the dentate line, the anoderm is attached more firmly to deeper structures.

- The mucosa and submucosa above the dentate line are uneven and thrown into folds, the so called anal cushions.
- There are variations in the numbers and positions of these cushions but there are usually three, corresponding to those seen in later life.
- These are described classically as occupying the left lateral, right posterior, and right anterior positions, and they continue proximally as the primary rectal foldings.
- Secondary foldings (the rectal columns of Morgagni) lie both over and between the primary folds. This area is the caudal limit of the so called epithelial transitional zone, below which the stratified squamous epithelium is richly innervated by sensory nerve endings serving several modalities including touch, pain, and temperature.
- The bulk of the anal cushions themselves, situated in the upper part of the anal canal, receive only visceral afferent innervation and, although there is perception of stretching, sensitivity to noxious stimuli is much more blunted than distally.
- Between the epithelial layer and the internal sphincter lies the submucosa, consisting of vascular, muscular, and connective tissue supportive elements.
- From the longitudinal muscle, medial extensions cross the internal anal sphincter and form part of the supporting meshwork of the submucosa, blending with the true submucosal smooth muscle layer, and thereby supporting the mucosa itself.
- Parks described the increased density of fibers that insert into the mucosa of the anal crypts at the level of the dentate line, termed the "mucosal suspensory ligament".
- One feature of this structure is that it separates the superior (portal) and inferior (systemic) hemorrhoidal plexuses, another is that the mucosa is more firmly tethered to underlying tissues at this level than above.
- It is important to appreciate that the meshwork of supporting tissues (muscle fibers and connective tissue) within the subepithelial space is intimately linked to deeper structures within the anal sphincter complex, including the internal sphincter, longitudinal muscle layer and external anal sphincter, and indeed structures beyond the sphincter complex.
- With age, the smooth muscle component of this mesh is reduced and muscle fibers are gradually replaced with fibroelastic connective tissue, which in turn becomes fragmented.

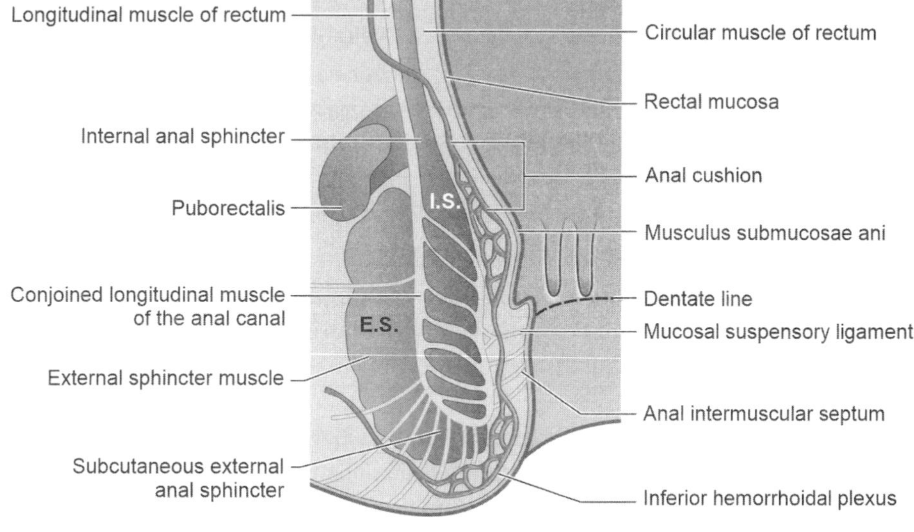

Relevant anatomy of the anus.

Blood Supply

- In addition to the meshwork support of the lining of the anal canal, the subepithelial space contains venous dilatations supported by the same fibroelastic connective tissue and smooth muscle scaffolding.

- Venous dilatations are seen in the submucosa both above and below the level of the dentate line; they are much more numerous above although tend to be larger below.
- The divisions of the superior rectal artery were not constant and that, furthermore, the anal submucosa may sometimes receive blood supply from the middle and inferior rectal arteries.
- There is also presence of free communications between tributaries of the superior, middle, and inferior rectal veins, as well as tiny direct arteriovenous communications with the submucosal venous dilatations.
- These communications have been shown both histologically and radiologically, and the oxygen tension of the blood contained within the venous dilatations (as well as the color) is more arterial than venous.

Venous Drainage

- The anal veins are distributed in a similar fashion to the arterial supply.
- The upper half of the anal canal is drained by the superior rectal veins, tributaries of the inferior mesenteric vein and thus the portomesenteric venous system, and the middle rectal veins, which drain into the internal iliac veins.
- The inferior rectal veins drain the lower half of the anal canal and the subcutaneous perianal plexus of veins: they eventually join the internal iliac vein on each side.

Lymphatic Drainage

- Lymph from the upper half of the anal canal flows upward to drain into the postrectal lymph nodes and from there goes to the para-aortic nodes via the inferior mesenteric chain.
- Lymph from the lower half of the anal canal drains on each side first into the superficial and then into the deep inguinal group of lymph glands.
- However, if the normal flow is blocked, e.g., by tumor, the lymph can be diverted into the alternative route.

Anal Incontinence

Anal Incontinence etiology.

Mechanical	***Neurogenic***	***Idiopathic***
Obstetric injury	Pudendal nerve stretch	No clear etiology
Fistula disease	Strain	Medical illness
Trauma	Prolonged labor	Irradiation
Iatrogenic	Trauma	Irritable bowel syndrome
Systemic disease		Multiple sclerosis, diabetes mellitus, and scleroderma
Diarrheal states		

The normal continence mechanism has several components:

- Rectal capacitance and compliance are essential. The rectum normally holds between 200 and 250 mL. It distends readily with filling and has limited muscular activity intrinsically.
- The sampling reflex is a function of rectal distension allowing anal sphincter relaxation via an intramural reflex to the internal sphincter.
- The rectal contents can then be sensed in the sensory nerve-rich transitional zone and anoderm to discriminate the true nature of the rectal contents. This sampling reflex occurs frequently throughout the day to provide continence and also serves to initiate the defecation process.
- The voluntary external sphincter muscle contraction in response to this sampling reflex provides the final active component of anal continence. The subconscious voluntary contraction of the external sphincter, puborectalis, and pelvic floor muscles provide complete control of rectal contents.
- The pelvic floor muscles maintain continual activity, even during sleep, to provide anal continence. This also seems to be a learned response since infants and children require 1–2 years to achieve control.

- It is important to realize that the degree of incontinence affects the lifestyle of the patient. The frequency of incontinence may vary and the loss of control may involve solid stool, liquid stool, or gas only.
- Frequent episodes of incontinence of gas only may be as incapacitating as infrequent episodes of solid stool. It is essential to document the exact type of incontinence before planning treatment. It is especially important to clearly define the incontinence before attempting to report a series of patients who undergo a specific treatment. There is no universally accepted grading scale to assess severity and impact of fecal incontinence.
- The American Society of Colon and Rectal Surgeons validated a fecal incontinence severity index and a fecal incontinence quality of life index to help standardize the assessment of anal incontinence.

Diagnosis and Evaluation

- Signs of anal incontinence in the office include a thin perineal body with scarring between the vagina and the anal canal and a poor squeeze on command.
- There is controversy regarding the adequacy of digital assessment of the anal sphincter mechanism. It is possible that an experienced examiner may be able to determine the adequacy of resting tone, but it is difficult to quantify and accurately evaluate the voluntary squeeze pressure generated by an anal sphincter mechanism. It is also essential to rule out the presence of a rectovaginal fistula in the setting of an anterior sphincter injury.

Examination of the Anus

- Careful clinical examination will be diagnostic in the vast majority of patients complaining of anal symptoms but it requires a relaxed patient who is informed of what the examination will entail, a private environment, a chaperone (for the security of both parties), and good light.
- Most commonly, the patient is examined in the left lateral (Sims) position with the buttocks overlying the edge of the examination couch and with the axis of the torso crossing, rather than parallel with, the edge of the couch.
- Alternatively, in younger patients, the prone jack-knife or knee-elbow positions may be used. The examining couch should be of sufficient height to allow easy inspection and access for any necessary maneuvers. A protective glove should be worn.

Inspection

- Look for presence of any skin lesions and whether they are confined to the perineum or evident elsewhere on general examination, e.g., psoriasis, lichen planus, or on genital examination, e.g., warts, candidiasis, lichen sclerosus et atrophicus, and the vesicles of herpes simplex virus (HSV); evidence of anal leakage; whether the anus is closed or patulous; and the position of the anus and perineum at rest and on bearing down (the latter may reveal prolapse of hemorrhoids or even the rectum).
- Pain on parting the buttocks, perhaps together with the presence of a sentinel tag, may indicate the presence of an underlying fissure, but may also prompt the need for examination under anesthesia (EUA) to exclude more suspicious pathology, for example squamous cell carcinoma of the anal canal.

Digital Examination with the Index Finger

- At the apex of the canal, the sling of puborectalis is felt posteriorly; supralevator induration feels bony hard and is more easily appreciated if unilateral.
- The posterior surface of the prostate gland with its median sulcus can be palpated anteriorly in male patients; in female patients, the uterine cervix can be palpated.
- The presence of any distal intrarectal, intra-anal, or extraluminal mass is recorded. Sphincter length, resting tone and voluntary squeeze are assessed. On withdrawal the examining finger is inspected for the presence of mucus, blood, or pus and to identify stool color.

Proctoscopy

- Proctoscopy, performed with the patient in the same position, allows a detailed inspection of the distal rectum and anal canal.

- Minor procedures can also be carried out through this instrument, e.g., treatment of hemorrhoids by injection or banding (see below) and biopsy. Asking the patient to bear down on slow withdrawal of the proctoscope may reveal a descending intussusceptions.

Sigmoidoscopy

- It should always be carried out even when an anal lesion has been confirmed. Rectal pathology, e.g., colitis or carcinoma, is frequently associated with an anal lesion, e.g., fissure or hemorrhoids.
- Sometimes rectal pathology is found that is independent of the anal lesion and which requires treatment.

Physiological aspects of the anal sphincters and pelvic floor, and special investigations:

- Anal continence and defecation are highly complex processes that necessitate the structural and functional integrity of the cerebral, autonomic, and enteric nervous systems, the gastrointestinal tract (especially the rectum) and the pelvic floor and anal sphincter complex, any of which may be compromised and lead to disturbances of function of varying severity.
- The sphincter mechanism provides the ultimate barrier to leakage and its integrity can be assessed fairly simply and objectively in the physiology laboratory (Swash and Henry). Perineal position and degree of descent on straining (markers of pelvic floor and pudendal nerve function) can be quantified, and functional anal canal length, resting tone (reflective predominantly of internal sphincter activity) and squeeze increment (reflective of external sphincter function) can be measured by a variety of simple manometric techniques.
- The structural integrity of the sphincters can be visualized with endoluminal ultrasound, and neuromuscular function can be measured by assessment of conduction velocity along the pudendal nerve on each side, or, more painfully, by needle electromyogram (EMG) studies.
- In the elderly especially, but also in younger patients, disorders relating to rectal sensorimotor dysfunction can lead to "overflow" of rectal contents through what may be an otherwise normal sphincter.
- The dynamics of defecation can also be assessed radiologically by evacuation proctography, in which radio-opaque pseudo stool is inserted into the rectum and the patient asked to rest, squeeze, and then bear down to evacuate the rectal contents under real-time imaging.
- Proctography can be combined with synchronous EMG and pressure studies (Williams) to yield more information about possible reasons [mechanical (rectocele, intussusception) or functional (anismus, lack of effort)] for disordered defecation in an individual. Results of all physiological tests have to be compared with a normal range and within the context of the patient's symptoms, and are used to guide rational rather than empirical treatment strategies.

Anal Manometry

- It is useful to document reduced resting and squeeze pressures as well as sphincter length in individual sphincter quadrants.
- Normal resting pressure is at least 40 mm Hg, normal squeeze pressure is 80 mm Hg, which is usually double the resting pressure, and sphincter length is >3 cm.
- Normal sensation should allow detection of a balloon inflated with 10–20 mL of air. Maximal tolerable volume is usually over 100 mL of air-filled balloon distention.

Electromyography

- Single fiber density determination is not routinely performed.
- Pudendal nerve terminal motor latency determination measures the conduction velocity of the nerve action potential through the terminal 4 cm of the pudendal nerve between Alcock's canal and the external sphincter.
- A delay in conduction reflects injury to the fast-conducting fibers of the nerve. This injury usually is the result of stretch, direct trauma, or systemic disease.
- The normal terminal motor latency is 2.2 ± 0.2 ms.
- Any delay in conduction velocity greater than this indicates nerve injury.

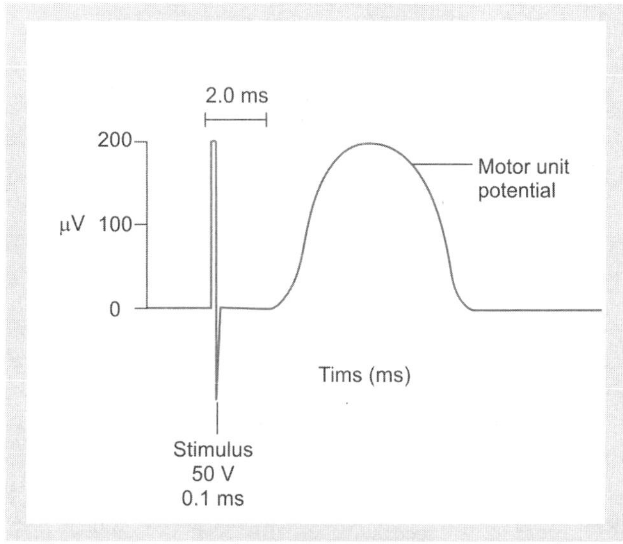

Terminal motor latency

Transrectal Ultrasound

- The most sensitive method for documenting sphincter injury may be the anal ultrasound using a 360° rotating 10-MHz transducer.
- The focal length of the anal probe is approximately 1–2 cm and allows evaluation of the anal sphincter muscles in three dimensions as the probe is withdrawn from the rectum. Scarring at the site of an injury is usually easily seen by endoanal ultrasound.
- A rectovaginal fistula can also be detected.

MRI

- High-resolution MRI with an endoanal coil is a newer diagnostic modality that can detect sphincter defects similarly to endoanal ultrasound.
- Endoanal coil MRI may also show sphincter atrophy or thinning not detectable by endoanal ultrasound that may have an impact on the success of surgical repair.

An algorithm for the Evaluation and Management of Anal Incontinence can be Produced using these Diagnostic Techniques

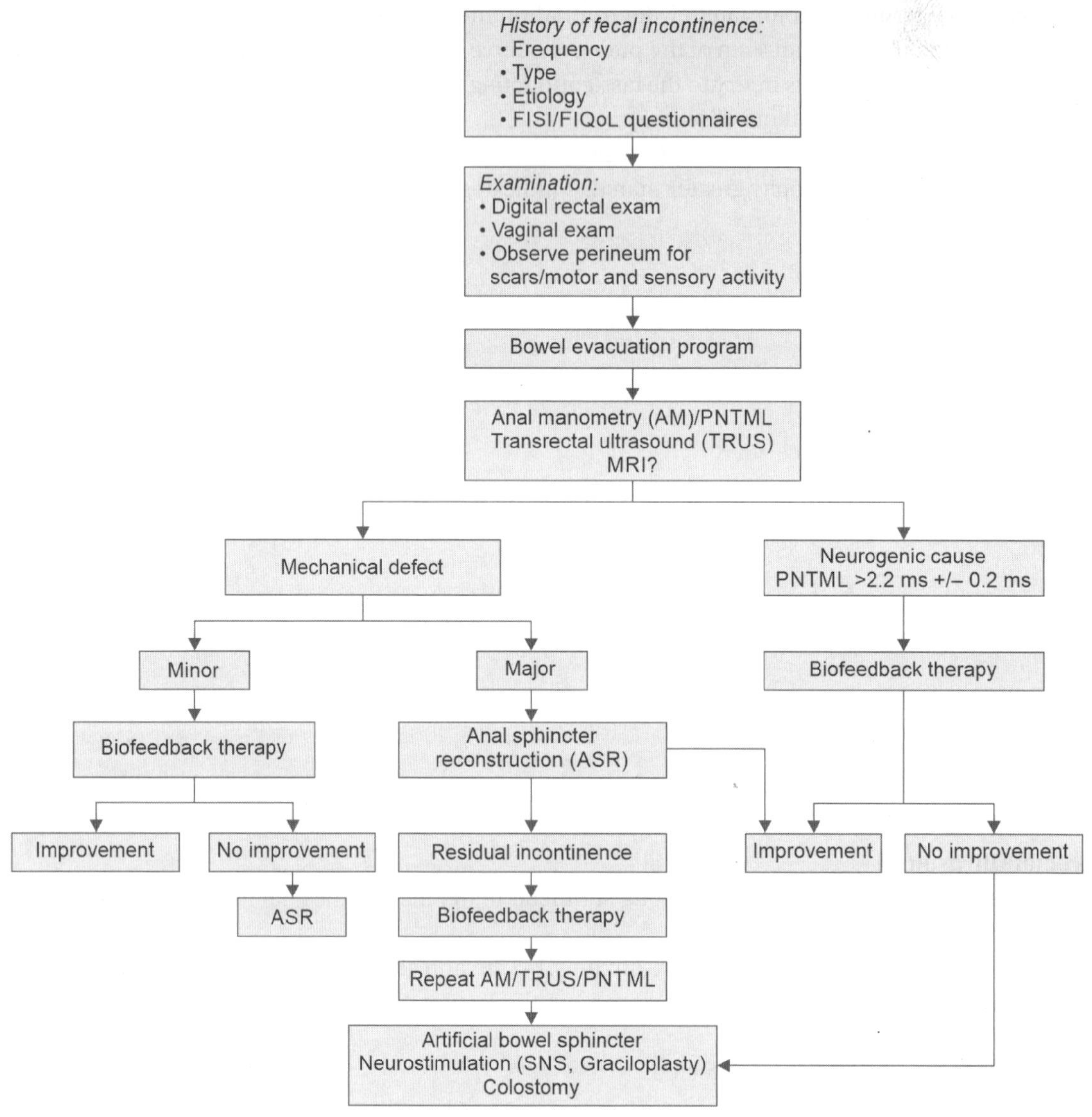

Treatment

Anal Sphincter Reconstruction

- Anal sphincter repair can be performed successfully in most patients who have an isolated mechanical sphincter defect.
- The patient requires a complete bowel preparation in order to avoid a colostomy at the time of the procedure.
- The ends of the injured sphincter are identified in the anterior perineum in patients with obstetric injury, and they are overlapped and secured or reefed in the midline to reconstruct the circular muscle.
- Control of solid and liquid stool will be adequate in 90% of patients after this type of repair. However, complete continence is usually only achieved in 75–90% of patients and the long-term results may even be less satisfactory.
- Leakage of liquid, mucus, and gas may continue to affect patients after repair. Improvement in squeeze pressures has been shown to correlate best with functional outcome.
- The presence of at least one normal pudendal nerve is necessary for an improvement after sphincter reconstruction.

- Complications of wound infection, fistula formation, and breakdown of the sphincter repair are reduced by leaving a drain in the perineal body after the repair.
- A repeat procedure is usually successful in those cases in whom the sphincter repair is disrupted.

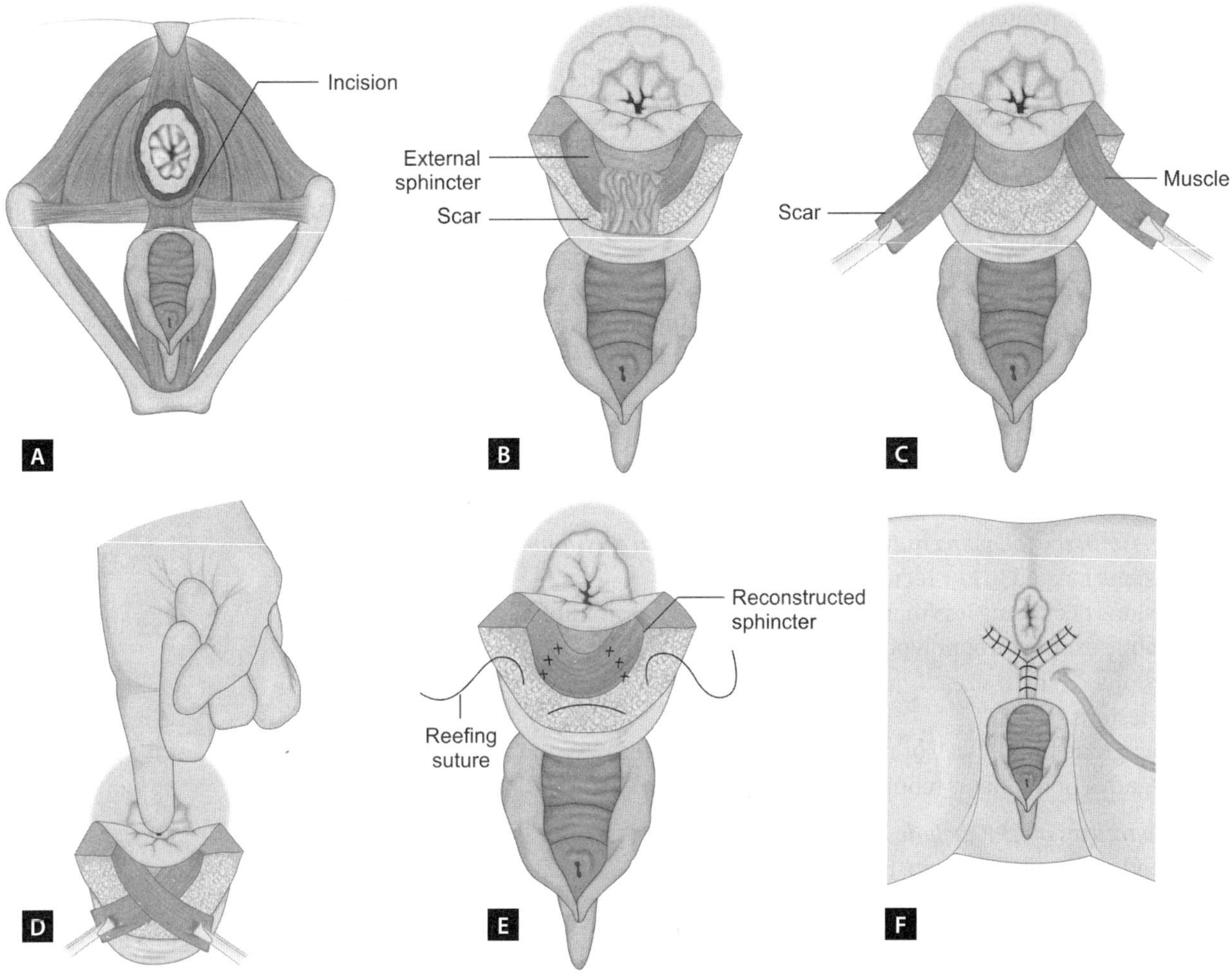

Anal sphincter overlapping muscle repair. (A) Anterior incision and perineal view of muscles; (B) Rectal flap is created and sphincter muscles are isolated; (C) Muscle flaps are fully mobilized; (D) Muscle flaps are overlapped around a 15-mm rubber dilator or fingertip; (E) Muscle flaps are sutured in place and the perineal body repaired; (F) A drain is placed behind the vaginal wall and the wall closed.

Muscle Sensory Retraining or Biofeedback

- Operant conditioning using manometric and balloon sensation techniques is possible in patients with a mechanical sphincter defect.
- Electromyographic anal plugs also provide biofeedback for conditioning. Pre- and postoperative biofeedback may aid in functional improvement.
- Patients with extremely poor pudendal nerve function or complete disruption of the anal sphincter will not benefit at all.

Other Treatments and New Modalities

- New techniques have been developed, including implantation of an artificial sphincter of silicone or a neurostimulator that provides constant activity in a muscle transferred to the anal canal (i.e., dynamic graciloplasty).
- "Pacemakers" implanted in the pelvis for sacral nerve stimulation of the anus have also been used.

- These techniques are indicated for severe, idiopathic fecal incontinence when all else has failed. They are expensive procedures, and some have a high risk of complications, but patients with severe neuromuscular damage and even those who have had the sphincter mechanism removed may benefit from reconstruction of the anal sphincter.
- The Parks posterior sphincter repair has been shown to yield poor results in patients with severe anal incontinence.

Preservation of both anal and rectal reservoir function in treatment of rectal cancer is highly preferred by patients. Sphincter-saving procedures for rectal cancer are now considered the standard of care.

Factors influencing sphincter and organ preservation in patients with rectal cancer can be described as follows:

- Surgeon training
- Surgeon volume
- Use of neoadjuvant chemoradiotherapy

The following factors are associated with difficult sphincter preservation:

- Male sex
- Morbid obesity
- Preoperative incontinence
- Direct involvement of anal sphincter muscles with carcinoma
- Bulky tumors within 5 cm from the anal verge

Patients with the following may be candidates for local excision:

- Lesions located in low rectum (within 8–10 cm)
- Lesions occupying less than one-third of the rectal circumference
- Mobile exophytic or polypoid lesions
- Lesions <3 cm in size
- T1 lesions
- Low-grade tumor (well or moderately differentiated)
- Negative nodal status (clinical and radiographic)

Disadvantages of APR include the following:

- Need for permanent colostomy
- Significantly higher short-term morbidity and mortality
- Significantly higher long-term morbidities
- Higher rate of sexual and urinary dysfunction

Recommendations

- It is currently recommended in patients with stage II and III rectal cancer to convert to a sphincter-preserving operation using preoperative combined chemoradiation therapy, since it has been shown to reduce the risk of local recurrence and to increase survival.
- The technique of intersphincteric resection permits the surgeon to achieve conservative surgery in patients with a tumor close to or in the anal canal without compromising local control and survival. Tumor distance from the anal verge is no longer a limit for sphincter-saving resection.

HEMORRHOIDS

49. Stapled hemorrhoidectomy. ***WBUHS 2008***

Introduction

Severe cases of hemorrhoidal prolapse, third and fourth degree, will normally require surgery. Traditional hemorrhoidectomy is notorious for the level of post operative pain the patient must endure, coupled with a long recuperation period.

Newer surgical procedures include stapled transanal rectal resection (STARR) and procedure for prolapse and hemorrhoids (PPH). Both STARR and PPH are contraindicated in persons with either enterocele or anismus.

Procedure for Prolapse and Hemorrhoids

PPH uses a circular stapler to reduce the degree of prolapse. The procedure avoids the need for wounds in the sensitive perianal area thus reducing postoperative pain considerably, and facilitates a speedier return to normal activities.

Development

- This procedure was first described by an Italian surgeon Dr Antonio Longo, Department of Surgery, University of Palermo in 1993 and since then has been widely adopted through Europe.
- This procedure avoids the need for wounds in the sensitive perianal area and, as a result, has the advantage of significantly reducing the patient's post operative pain. Follow-up on relief of symptoms indicate a similar success rate to that achieved by conventional hemorrhoidectomy.
- Since PPH was first introduced it has been the subject of numerous clinical trials and in 2003 the National Institute of Clinical Evidence (NICE) in the UK issued full guidance on the procedure stating it was safe and efficacious.

Working Principle

Prolapse

- PPH employs a unique circular stapler which reduces the degree of prolapse by excising a circumferential strip of mucosa from the proximal anal canal.
- This has the effect of pulling the hemorrhoidal cushions back up into their normal anatomical position.

Bleeding

- In addition to correcting the symptoms associated with the prolapse, problems with bleeding from the piles are also resolved by this excision.
- Although the cushions may be totally or partially preserved, the blood supply in interrupted or venous drainage is improved by the repositioning.
- Any external component which remains will usually regress over a period of 3–6 months.
- Prominent skin tags may, on occasion, be removed during the operation, but this has not been associated with any significant increase in pain.

Indications

The PPH is generally indicated for the more severe cases of hemorrhoidal prolapse (third and fourth degree) where surgery would normally be indicated. It may also be indicated for patients with minor degree hemorrhoids who have failed to respond to conservative treatments. The procedure may be contraindicated when only one cushion is prolapsed or in severe cases of fibrotic piles which cannot be physically repositioned.

- *The procedure:* Usually, the patient will be under general anesthetic, but only for 20–30 minutes. Many cases have been successfully performed under local or regional anesthesia and the procedure is suited to day case treatment.
- *Postoperative course:* Due to the low level of postoperative pain and reduced analgesic use, patients will usually be discharged either the same day or on the day following surgery.
  Most patients can resume normal activities after a few days when they should be fit for work. The first bowel motion is usually on day two and should not cause any great discomfort. Staples may be passed from time to time during defecation. This is normal and should not be a cause for concern.
- *Postoperative complications:* Urinary retention in the immediate postoperative period appears to be the most common complication.

A condition called post-PPH syndrome is also possible. This occurs when the staples are placed slightly low and it can cause the internal sphincter muscle to become inflamed. Treatment includes anti-inflammatory oral medications and suppositories.

50. Modern surgical management of hemorrhoids. ***WBUHS 2013, RIMS, Imphal 2022***

- Scalpel surgery is now rarely needed.
- The treatment choices for internal hemorrhoids include infrared coagulation, radiofrequency coagulation, direct current coagulation, rubber band ligation, sclerotherapy, cryosurgery, scalpel surgery, and laser surgery.
- Scalpel surgery is generally reserved for advanced fourth-degree hemorrhoids and is most often done on inpatients. Laser surgery is said to be less painful, but this has proved difficult to verify.
- Sclerotherapy is usually indicated only in first- and second-degree lesions.
- Cryotherapy is also little used because of the profuse and prolonged discharge, the complications such as excessive sloughing and sphincter injury, and the poor results.
- The least expensive and possibly the most widely used equipment is a rubber band ligator. This is suitable for first- to third-degree hemorrhoids. The bands are easy to apply, but the drawback is that two people are needed, one to hold the anoscope and the other to apply the bands. The treatment can cause severe pain if the bands are placed too low, and there is a small risk of perineal sepsis, which can, very rarely, be fatal.
- The infrared coagulator is gaining rapid acceptance for outpatient treatment of internal first- and second-degree hemorrhoids and some third-degree ones.
- *LigaSure and Harmonic Scalpel hemorrhoidectomy:* Both LigaSure (Valleylab, Covidien) and Harmonic Scalpel (Ethicon Endo-Surgery) have been used more recently for hemorrhoidectomy due to their ability to coagulate and cut tissue.
- LigaSure is a bipolar electrothermal device, while Harmonic Scalpel relies on ultrasonic waves that have their effect locally with reduced lateral thermal effect; the theoretical advantage of using such devices being a reduction in tissue damage adjacent to the excised hemorrhoidal tissue.
- Results from trials comparing Harmonic Scalpel with more traditional methods of hemorrhoidectomy have generated differing conclusions.

Doppler-guided, transanal hemorrhoidal dearterialization is a minimally invasive treatment using an ultrasound Doppler to accurately locate the arterial blood inflow. These arteries are then "tied off" and the prolapsed tissue is sutured back to its normal position. It has a slightly higher recurrence rate, but fewer complications compared to a hemorrhoidectomy.

Stapled hemorrhoidectomy, also known as stapled hemorrhoidopexy (procedure for PPH). It involves the removal of much of the abnormally enlarged hemorrhoidal tissue, followed by a repositioning of the remaining hemorrhoidal tissue back to its normal anatomical position. It is generally less painful and is associated with faster healing compared to complete removal of hemorrhoids. However, the chance of symptomatic hemorrhoids returning is greater than for conventional hemorrhoidectomy so it is typically only recommended for grade 2 or 3 disease.

51. Write a note on surgical management of hemorrhoids. ***WBUHS 2025 Supplementary***

Surgical Management of Hemorrhoids

Hemorrhoids, also known as piles, are swollen and inflamed vascular structures in the anal canal, which may cause bleeding, pain, and prolapse. While conservative treatments are often effective for mild cases, surgical management is indicated in severe, recurrent, or complicated hemorrhoids, particularly Grade III and IV.

Indications for Surgery

- Persistent symptoms despite conservative treatment
- Prolapsed hemorrhoids that do not reduce
- Recurrent thrombosis
- Significant bleeding causing anemia
- External hemorrhoids with complications (e.g., thrombosis, ulceration)

Common Surgical Procedures

- *Hemorrhoidectomy (Excisional)*
  - *Types:*
    - *Open (Milligan-Morgan)*—wound left open to heal by secondary intention
    - *Closed (Ferguson)*—wound is sutured closed
  - *Indications:* Large external hemorrhoids, mixed hemorrhoids, or those with complications.
  - *Advantages:* Low recurrence rate.
  - *Disadvantages*: Postoperative pain, longer recovery time.
- *Stapled Hemorrhoidopexy (PPH*—Procedure for Prolapse and Hemorrhoids)
  - Uses a circular stapling device to excise a ring of rectal mucosa and reposition hemorrhoidal tissue.
  - *Indications:* Circumferential prolapsing hemorrhoids (Grade III/IV).
  - *Advantages:* Less postoperative pain, quicker recovery.
  - *Disadvantages:* Higher recurrence rate, risk of serious complications (e.g., rectal perforation, sepsis).
- *Doppler-Guided Hemorrhoidal Artery Ligation (DG-HAL)*
  - Identifies and ligates hemorrhoidal arteries using a Doppler probe, often combined with mucopexy.
  - *Advantages:* Minimally invasive, less pain, outpatient procedure.
  - *Disadvantages:* May be less effective for large prolapsed hemorrhoids.

Postoperative Care

- Pain management (NSAIDs, local anesthetics)
- Sitz baths
- High-fiber diet and stool softeners

Monitoring for complications (bleeding, infection, urinary retention)

FISTULA-IN-ANO

52. Fistula-in-ano. *WBUHS 2008, Rajiv Gandhi Institute of Health Sciences 2019*

53. Write short notes on types and management of fistula-in-ano. *WBUHS 2020*

54. Classify fistula-in-ano. Discuss the principle of management.
WBUHS 2025; Srimanta Sankaradeva University, Assam 2025

55. Recent methods of surgical management of fistulae in ano. *WBUHS 2015, RIMS, Imphal 2022*

56. Describe the classification, diagnosis and treatment of perianal fistula.
Maharashtra University of Health Sciences 2025

A fistula is an abnormal connection of two epithelial surfaces and the two surfaces joined in fistula-in-ano are the anorectal lining and the perineal or vaginal skin. Very common, especially in otherwise fit young adults. May occur in the presence of Crohn's disease. Minor association with obesity and diabetes mellitus. Very rarely due to trauma or ulceration of anorectal tumors.

A fistula-in-ano, or anal fistula, is a chronic abnormal communication, usually lined to some degree by granulation tissue, which runs outward from the anorectal lumen (the internal opening) to an external opening on the skin of the perineum or buttock (or rarely, in women, to the vagina).

Causes of Fistula-in-Ano

Persistent cryptoglandular sepsis	*Malignancy:* Anal and rectal	Foreign body	Pilonidal disease
Anal fissure	Leukemia or lymphoma	Inflammatory bowel disease	Lymphogranuloma venereum
Trauma	Other pelvic malignancy	Diverticulitis	Osteomyelitis
Assault	Radiation injury	Actinomycosis	Urethroperineal fistula
Iatrogenic	Anal intercourse	Hidradenitis suppurativa	AIDS

The most common cause is sepsis arising in an anal gland that forces its way out through the anal tissues to appear in the perianal or, in women, vaginal skin (cryptoglandular theory of fistula-in-ano). Often presents initially as an acute perianal abscess. The tissues through which the track pushes determines the classification of fistulas.

Classification of Anorectal Fistulas

- *Intersphincteric (the most common):* The fistula track is confined to the intersphincteric plane.
- *Trans-sphincteric:* The fistula connects the intersphincteric plane with the ischiorectal fossa by perforating the external sphincter.
- *Suprasphincteric:* Similar to trans-sphincteric, but the track loops over the external sphincter and perforates the levator ani.
- *Extrasphincteric:* The track passes from the rectum to perineal skin, completely external to the sphincteric complex.

Clinical Features

- *Acute perianal abscess:* Rapid onset of severe perianal or perineal pain. Swelling and erythema of the perianal skin with fever and tachycardia.
- *Recurrent perianal sepsis:* Recurrent intermittent sepsis typified by gradual build-up of pressure sensation and swelling in the perianal skin and eventual discharge of blood-stained purulent fluid.
- *Chronic perianal discharge:* Persistent low-grade sepsis of the track with chronic discharge of seropurulent fluid via a punctum that is usually clearly identified by the patient.

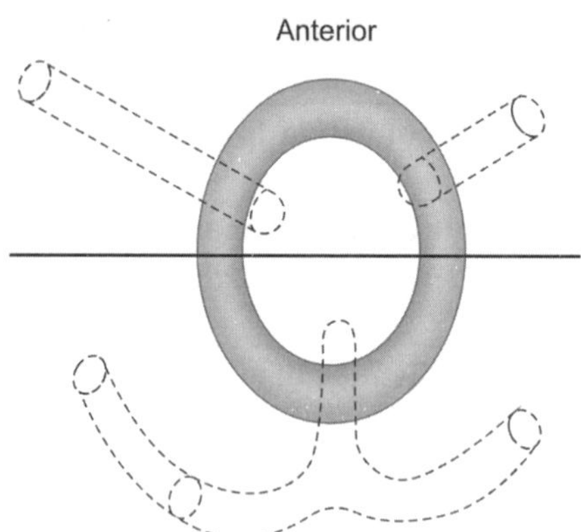

Clinical Assessment

- A full medical (including obstetric, gastrointestinal, anal surgical, and continence) history and proctosigmoidoscopy are necessary to gain information about sphincter strength and to exclude associated conditions.
- Determine the site of the internal opening; the site of the external opening(s); the course of the primary track; the presence of secondary extensions; and the presence of other conditions complicating the fistula.

Diagnosis and Investigations

Diagnosis and investigation should aim to confirm the presence of a fistula and identify the course of the track to determine the type of fistula.

- Examination of the perineum and rectal examination may reveal a palpable fibrous track.
- EUA with probing of any external opening to aid identification of the course of the track.
- Endoanal ultrasound (sometimes with hydrogen peroxide injected into the track) identifies the course of the track.
- MRI scanning is probably the most sensitive method of determining the course of the track and identifying any occult perianal or pelvic sepsis.
- Flexible sigmoidoscopy if associated colorectal disease, e.g., Crohn's disease, is suspected.

Goodsall described a means of predicting the offending crypt and internal opening based on the location of the external opening. In brief, an external opening posterior to an imaginary coronal plane bisecting the anus would have an internal opening at the posterior midline, whereas an external opening anterior to this plane would have an internal opening radially directed straight to the nearest anal gland. Goodsall's rule has been shown to be more accurate for women than men and more accurate for posterior than anterior openings. Goodsall's rule has been shown to be misleading for external openings >3 cm from the anal verge.

Treatment

Principles of Management

- *Closure of the internal opening:* This is crucial for preventing recurrence by addressing the source of the infection.
- *Drainage of infection:* Any pus or infected tissue must be effectively drained to allow the tract to heal properly.
- *Eradication of the fistulous tract:* The entire channel connecting the anal canal to the skin must be removed or obliterated.
- *Sphincter preservation:* The goal is to maintain fecal continence, which may require sphincter-saving procedures for fistulas involving the anal sphincter muscles.

Medical Treatment

- Antibiotics may reduce symptoms from recurrent sepsis but cannot treat the underlying fistula.
- Medical treatment of inflammatory bowel disease may dramatically reduce symptoms from associated fistulas.

Surgical Treatment

Fistulotomy: • Single stage • Multiple stage	*Seton:* • Cutting • Noncutting • Draining (Crohn's disease)	York-Mason posterior trans-sphincteric approach
Anorectal mucosal advancement flap	Fibrin glue filling of tract	Remicade (Crohn's disease)
Dermal island advancement flap		Fistulectomy

Surgical Management

- *Fistulotomy:*
  - This is the standard treatment for low simple anal fistulas, submucosal, and low intersphincteric fistulas.
  - The indications are low cryptoglandular fistulas, low chronic fistulas, and simple fistulas where 30–50% of the tracts pass through the sphincter, which is not anterior in female, single tract, nonrecurrent, continent, and nonchronic.
  - Fistulotomy is usually a single stage procedure but in complex procedures it can be used as a staged procedure with adjuvant seton or glue therapy. The incontinence rate varies from 0 to 40% in intersphincteric fistulas.
- *Radiation ablation* of tract is another improvement in techniques of fistulectomy. It is known to have decreased gas continence as radiation frequency ablation causes minimal damage to surrounding tissue.
- *LASER surgery:* LASER ablation is limited to the lumen of fistulas making the technique sphincter saving.
- *Ultrasound dissection* of the fistulous tract is a future advancement. The recurrence rate of fistulotomy is 7–16% after 2 years follow-up. This recurrence rate increases to 40% after 6 years.
- *Fistulectomy:* Studies have shown that the fistulectomy does not offer any additional advantage over the fistulotomy procedure.

Newer Modalities

- *Fibrin glue:* It is a mixture of fibrinogen, thrombin, and calcium ions which when combined form a soluble clot due to cleavage of fibrinogen to fibrin. This clot seals the fistula tract in 30–60 seconds. Between days 7 and 14 the tract is replaced by synthesized collagen. The advantages of this procedure are that it is a simple procedure without any learning curve. There is no decrease in level of continence and also other treatment options remain open in case of a failure.
- *Fibrin plug:* The plug is made up of lyophilized porcine small intestinal submucosa shaped in a conical fashion which increases the mechanical stability thus avoiding dislodgement during straining. The reasons for failure of the plug are improper securing of the plug to the primary opening leading to dislodgement. Multiple fistula tracts have been associated with higher failure rates.
- *Adipose-derived stem cells (ASCs)* have been used in the treatment of complex anal fistulas.
- *Mucosal advancement flap:* This is a sphincter-sparing procedure where endorectal/endoanal flaps are advanced to close the internal ring with or without closure of the tract.
- *VAAFT* (video-assisted anal fistula treatment)
- *LIFT procedure:* It is ligation of the intersphincteric fistula tract.

Principles of surgical treatment are as follow:

- Drainage of any acute sepsis if present.
- Prevention of recurrent sepsis usually by insertion of a loose seton suture, e.g., silastic sling.
- Low fistula-in-ano. Lay open track, remove all chronic granulation tissue, and allow to heal spontaneously (fistulotomy). Little risk of impairment of continence due to minimal division of sphincter tissues.
- *High fistula-in-ano:*
    - Remove fistula track and close the internal opening (core fistulectomy and endorectal flap advancement).
    - Slowly divide the sphincter tissue between the fistula and the perianal skin (cutting seton): Low risk of incontinence.
    - Fill the fistula with fibrin glue.

57. Narrate the new treatment strategies for crypto-glandular fistula-in-ano. ***WBUHS 2021, RIMS, Imphal 2022***

58. Classification of new treatments for anal fistula.

59. Recent advances in treatment of fistula in ano. ***NTRUHS, Vijayawada 2024***

Novel Biomaterials

Autograft

- *Autograft- ASC:* ASC were used either on its own or along with fibrin glue.
- *Autograft-platelet rich plasma:* A pilot study explored the use of autologous platelet-rich plasma as an adjunct to the staged mucosal advancement flap.

Allograft

- *Allograft-acellular dermal matrix (ADM):*
    - Human ADM is a commercially available allogenic tissue graft. It is derived from donated human skin containing intact collagen fibers, elastin filaments, and glycosaminoglycans.
    - It lacks cellular components that may contribute to tissue rejection.
- *Acellular extracellular matrix (AEM)*

Xenograft

- *Xenograft-Permacol™ solid implant/suspension—porcine dermal cross-linked collagen:* Xenograft may be derived from numerous tissue and animal sources.
- *Xenograft-ADM:* Newly developed biomaterial ADM

- *Xenograft-AEM/porcine intestinal submucosal collagen:* It can be used in low anorectal fistula.

Energy Devices

Fistula LASER closure/FiLAC: This sphincter-preserving technique uses diode laser source and radial emitting laser probe, which works by destroying the lining of the fistula and simultaneously obliterating the remaining track by shrinking the tissue around the probe.

New Types of Seton Suture

- *Comfort drain:*
  - A significant proportion of patients are treated with the placement of long-term seton within the tract.
  - The Comfort Drain consists of a metal probe, a silicone drain, and a polypropylene closure mechanism.
- *Cable tie:*
  - A self-locking cable tie was used as a seton.
  - Patients were followed up in the clinic where it was tightened, if found to be loose, without any analgesia.

Hybrid Techniques

- *BioLIFT:*
  - Ligation of inter-sphincteric fistula tract (LIFT) was first described by Rojanasakul in 2007 with reported healing rates of up to 94%.
  - Identification of the fistula tract in the intersphincteric plane and secured ligation of the tract followed by removal of infected tissue and fistula tract. Any defect in the external sphincter muscle is then repaired with sutures.
  - An attempt has been made to reinforce this repair further by insertion of a bioprosthetic graft in the inter-sphincteric plane e BioLIFT, although the technique was initially described in rectovaginal fistula repairs
- *LIFT-plug (ADM):* A further modification of the LIFT procedure used human ADM as a bioprosthetic plug.
- *Collagen matrix and rectal flap/Permacol injection and advancement flap:* Permacol™ has been proposed as infill biomaterial to treat fistulas.

Others

- *Over the scope clip/the OTSC Proctology clip system:* The OTSC™ Proctology system (Ovesco Endoscopy AG, Tuebingen, Germany) consists of a clip and applicator and is a modification of the endoscopic OTSC™ clip, which is made of a super elastic shape memory alloy (Nitinol).
- *Video-assisted anal fistula treatment:*
  - VAAFT has been described in one report.
  - This technique utilizes a fistuloscope, an obturator, a unipolar electrode, an endobrush, and cyanoacrylate glue.
  - Diagnostic fistuloscopy under irrigation is followed by an operative phase of fulguration of the fistula tract, closure of the internal opening using stapler or mucocutaneous flap and a further reinforcement with cyanoacrylate glue.

The ideal treatment for anal fistula remains elusive despite technological advances in treatment and increasing cost of treatments.

---

60. Recent methods of surgical management of fistula-in-ano. ***WBUHS 2015***

Surgical Management

- *Fistulotomy:*
  - This is the standard treatment for low simple anal fistulas, submucosal, and low intersphincteric fistulas.
  - The indications are low cryptoglandular fistulas, low chronic fistulas, and simple fistulas where 30–50% of the tracts pass through the sphincter, which is not anterior in female, single tract, nonrecurrent, continent, and nonchronic.

- Fistulotomy is usually a single stage procedure but in complex procedures it can be used as a staged procedure with adjuvant seton or glue therapy. The incontinence rate varies from 0 to 40% in intersphincteric fistulas.

- *Radiation ablation* of tract is another improvement in techniques of fistulectomy. It is known to have decreased gas continence as radiation frequency ablation causes minimal damage to surrounding tissue.
- *Ultrasound dissection* of the fistulous tract is a future advancement. The recurrence rate of fistulotomy is 7–16% after 2 years follow-up. This recurrence rate increases to 40% after 6 years.
- *Fistulectomy:* Studies have shown that the fistulectomy does not offer any additional advantage over the Fistulotomy procedure.

Newer Modalities

- *Fibrin glue:* It is a mixture of fibrinogen, thrombin, and calcium ions which when combined form a soluble clot due to cleavage of fibrinogen to fibrin. This clot seals the fistula tract in 30–60 seconds. Between days 7 and 14 the tract is replaced by synthesized collagen. The advantages of this procedure are that it is a simple procedure without any learning curve. There is no decrease in level of continence and also other treatment options remain open in case of a failure.
- *Fibrin Plug:* The plug is made up of lyophilized porcine small intestinal submucosa shaped in a conical fashion which increases the mechanical stability thus avoiding dislodgement during straining. The reasons for failure of the plug are improper securing of the plug to the primary opening leading to dislodgement. Multiple fistula tracts have been associated with higher failure rates.
- *Adipose-derived stem cells* have been used in the treatment of complex anal fistulas.
- *Mucosal advancement flap:* This is a sphincter-sparing procedure where endorectal/endoanal flaps are advanced to close the internal ring with or without closure of the tract.
- *LIFT procedure:* It is ligation of the intersphincteric fistula tract.

---

61. Management of fissure-in-ano. ***Gujarat University 2025***

Anal fissure is a linear ulcer in the anoderm distal to the dentate line, usually in the *posterior midline* (90%) due to high resting anal tone and ischemia.

- *Acute fissure:* <6 weeks duration, fresh edges, minimal fibrosis.
- *Chronic fissure:* >6 weeks, indurated edges, sentinel pile, hypertrophied anal papilla, exposed internal sphincter fibers.

Goals of Management

- Relieve pain and spasm.
- Promote healing by improving blood flow and relaxing internal sphincter.
- Prevent recurrence.
- Avoid incontinence.

Pathophysiology—Key to Management

- Cycle of pain → spasm → ischemia → nonhealing ulcer.
- High resting pressure o*f internal anal sphincter (IAS)* reduces anodermal perfusion, preventing healing.
- Hence, *therapy aims to reduce IAS tone,* either chemically (medical) or surgically.

Diagnosis

- *Clinical diagnosis:* Visual inspection, gentle separation of buttocks.
- *Digital rectal examination/anoscopy* avoided in acute phase due to pain.
- *Rule out secondary causes:* Crohn's disease, tuberculosis, carcinoma, HIV, syphilis (especially if atypical or lateral fissure).

Management

Stage	Approach	Goal
Acute fissure	Conservative + medical	Relieve spasm, heal fissure
Chronic fissure/recurrence	Medical ± minimally invasive procedure	Sphincter relaxation
Refractory/complicated	Surgical (LIS or alternatives)	Definitive healing

Conservative and Medical Management

General Measures

- *High-fiber diet* (20–30 g/day), fluids >2 L/day.
- *Bulk laxatives* (psyllium, isabgol, methylcellulose).
- *Warm sitz baths* 2–3× daily for 10–15 minutes
- *Analgesics/topical local anesthetic* (lidocaine 2%).
- *Avoid straining and constipation.*

These measures alone heal up to *50–60% of acute fissures.*

Topical Pharmacologic Therapy ("Chemical Sphincterotomy")

Aim → Relax IAS and improve blood flow.

Drug	Mechanism	Healing rate	Adverse effects/notes
Topical Nitroglycerin (0.2–0.4%)	NO donor → relaxes IAS	60–70%	Headache (30–40%), hypotension
Topical calcium channel blockers (Diltiazem 2%, Nifedipine 0.2–0.3%)	Inhibit smooth muscle contraction	65–90%	Minimal side effects (preferred first line)
Topical 2% Lidocaine + Diltiazem combo	Symptom + healing benefit	Increasingly popular (2024 studies)	Safe and well tolerated
Topical Bethanechol/Sildenafil (experimental)	Smooth muscle relaxants	Early studies	Under evaluation

Recent trend (2024): Topical calcium channel blockers (CCBs) are now preferred over nitroglycerin due to better tolerability and comparable efficacy (Cochrane review, 2023).

Botulinum Toxin (Botox) Injection

- *Mechanism:* Chemical denervation → temporary sphincter relaxation (~2–3 months).
- *Dose:* 20–40 units injected into IAS (1–2 sites lateral to fissure).
- *Healing rate:* 70–90%.
- *Recurrence:* ~15–25%.
- *Side effects:* Transient flatus incontinence (<5%).

Surgical Management

Indicated when:

- No healing after 6–8 weeks of optimal medical therapy.
- Chronic fissure with fibrosis/sentinel pile.
- Recurrent fissure.
- Fissure with high resting anal pressure.

Lateral Internal Sphincterotomy (LIS)—Gold Standard

Technique:

- Open or closed method; partial division of IAS (to level of fissure base).
- Relieves spasm permanently.

Outcomes

Parameter	Result
Healing rate	90–98%
Recurrence	<5%
Minor flatus incontinence	3–8%
Major incontinence	<1% (if proper technique)

Guideline Updates (ASCRS 2023, ESCP 2024)

- *Tailored LIS* (division up to fissure apex only) is recommended to minimize incontinence risk.
- Avoid full-length LIS, especially in multiparous women or low-pressure sphincters.

Advancement Flap Procedures

- Indicated when LIS contraindicated (e.g., low-pressure sphincter, obstetric injury, Crohn's disease).
- *Procedure:* Sliding/mucosal or V-Y advancement flap covers the fissure → promotes healing by blood supply restoration.
- Healing: 80–90%, minimal incontinence risk.

Fissurectomy ± Botulinum Injection/Advancement Flap

- *Fissurectomy:* Excision of fibrotic edges, preserving IAS; used with Botox or flap for chronic fissure.
- Recent RCTs show comparable healing to LIS when combined with Botox or flap, with minimal incontinence.

Recent Concepts (2024–25)

Concept	Summary
Tailored LIS	Limits sphincter division to fissure apex; equal healing, less incontinence
Botulinum + Fissurectomy	Effective alternative for high-risk patients (women, elderly)
Topical CCBs first-line	Diltiazem/nifedipine outperform GTN with fewer side effects
Laser fissure ablation (experimental)	Early data show faster pain relief, minimal sphincter trauma (needs validation)
Pelvic floor physiotherapy/biofeedback	Helpful adjunct in recurrent or functional fissure cases

Stepwise Management Algorithm

Step 1: Acute fissure → Conservative + Topical CCB or GTN (Heal 60–80% in 4–6 weeks)
Step 2: Persistent/chronic → Botulinum toxin ± Fissurectomy (if available)
Step 3: Refractory/recurrent → Tailored LIS (gold standard)
Step 4: Special cases (low sphincter tone, obstetric injury, Crohn's) → Advancement flap/fissurectomy + Botox.

62. Discuss the role of chemotherapy/radiotherapy in management of anorectal malignancies. ***WBUHS 2018***

63. Novel radiotherapy techniques for the treatment of anal cancer. ***WBUHS 2021***

Role of chemotherapy/radiotherapy in rectal cancer:

- *Intraoperative radiation therapy:* It may be considered in patients with pelvic sidewall recurrence. This is performed in an operating room-radiation therapy suite. Resection with negative microscopic margins and absence of vascular invasion independently predicts improved local control and survival after resection and IORT. The major morbidities of IORT include peripheral neuropathy and ureteral stenosis.
- *Adjuvant chemotherapy* has become a standard treatment of advanced rectal cancer: Adjuvant therapy for rectal cancer should routinely be considered to reduce local recurrence and possibly improve overall survival.

The drugs most commonly used are:

- Fluorouracil often given with folinic acid
- Capecitabine
- Oxaliplatin
- Irinotecan
- Trifluridine and tipiracil

Preoperative chemoradiotherapy followed by TME and postoperative chemotherapy with fluorouracil and OX is standard treatment for stage II to stage III locally advanced rectal cancer.

Current recommendations for chemoradiation in rectal cancer patients after radical resection	
Stage I	No adjuvant therapy
Stage II or III	Neoadjuvant chemoradiation for 5 weeks
Low/mid lesion	• 5-FU-based chemotherapy with XRT (180 cGy 5 days/week × 5 weeks) • Rest for 6 weeks • Total mesorectal excision • Rest for 4 weeks • Continue 5-FU–based chemotherapy for 8 weeks
High lesion	Preoperative or postoperative chemotherapy
	Total mesorectal excision
Stage IV	• LAR or APR for palliation/prevention of obstruction or bleeding • Adjuvant chemotherapy • 5-FU + leucovorin ± irinotecan or oxaliplatin with individualized XRT

(APR: abdominoperineal resection; 5-FU: 5-fluorouracil; LAR: low anterior resection; XRT: external-beam radiation therapy)

Neoadjuvant chemoradiation, including chemotherapy with a 5-FU–based regimen, results in a modest survival benefit and decreased local recurrence over radiation therapy alone. It is generally reserved for patients with large, bulky tumors, or evidence of nodal metastases (stage II/III, especially T4 lesions) in mid and low rectal tumors.

Role of chemotherapy/radiotherapy for anal canal cancer:

- Chemotherapy is particularly effective for treating anal cancer when given in combination with radiation therapy, as discussed above. The combined treatment allows the use of lower radiation doses and improves the likelihood of completely destroying the tumor.
  - Chemoradiotherapy is the first treatment for most anal cancers. This can often cure the cancer without the need for surgery.
  - Given along with radiation after surgery to try to kill any cancer cells that may have been left behind. This is called *adjuvant therapy*. It's done to lower the chance of the cancer coming back.
  - Used if anal cancer has spread to distant parts of the body, such as the liver or lungs. This can help keep the cancer under control or relieve symptoms it's causing.

In most cases, two or more drugs are used at the same time because one drug can boost the effect of the other.

- The main drug combination used to treat anal cancer is 5-FU and mitomycin.
- The combination of 5-FU and cisplatin is also used, especially in people who can't get mitomycin or for advanced anal cancer.

In these treatments, the 5-FU is a liquid given into a vein 24 hours a day for 4 or 5 days. The other drugs are given more quickly on certain other days in the treatment cycle. And radiation is given 5 days a week for at least 5 weeks.

Novel Radiotherapy Techniques for the Treatment of Anal Cancer

Cancers of the anal canal are rare, comprising approximately 10% of malignancies in the anorectal region, although its incidence has been increasing over the past several decades. While the traditional approach to treatment was with APR, this has evolved in the modern era to concurrent chemoradiation as organ-preserving treatment.

Radiotherapy Techniques

- *Interstitial radiotherapy (brachytherapy):* This technique is usually reserved for accessible, small tumors often in the mouth or oropharynx
- External beam radiotherapy (EBRT)
- Immobilization
- 3-D conformal and stereotactic radiotherapy
- Intensity-modulated radiotherapy (IMRT)
- *EBRT:*
    - With EBRT local control for primary tumors <4 cm is 90% at 10 years, whereas it is 65% for primary tumors >4 cm.
    - Probability of local control was related to the T stage. Overall, 74% of patients maintained a functional anus.
    - Techniques associated with radiation therapy have evolved with the utilization of IMRT.
    - This inverse planning method of EBRT increases the therapeutic ratio by increasing conformal dose to the target structures while reducing dose to surrounding normal tissue.
    - IMRT is clinically associated with decreased acute toxicity. It is important to note that quality control and technical aspects of IMRT are challenging and conformal radiation therapy requires training in target volume contouring as demonstrated in RTOG 0529 by the number of plans failing central review.
    - Radiation therapy for anal cancer has historically involved two- or three-dimensional conformal (3DCRT techniques, but IMRT has become the most widely utilized radiation therapy technique for anal cancer, with 3DCRT used in a very small minority of patients. The NCCN currently recommends IMRT over 3DCRT for radiation therapy in anal cancer.
    - Compared with non-IMRT radiation therapy, IMRT delivers significantly less radiation to normal tissue, leading to reduced rates of toxicity-related treatment interruption.

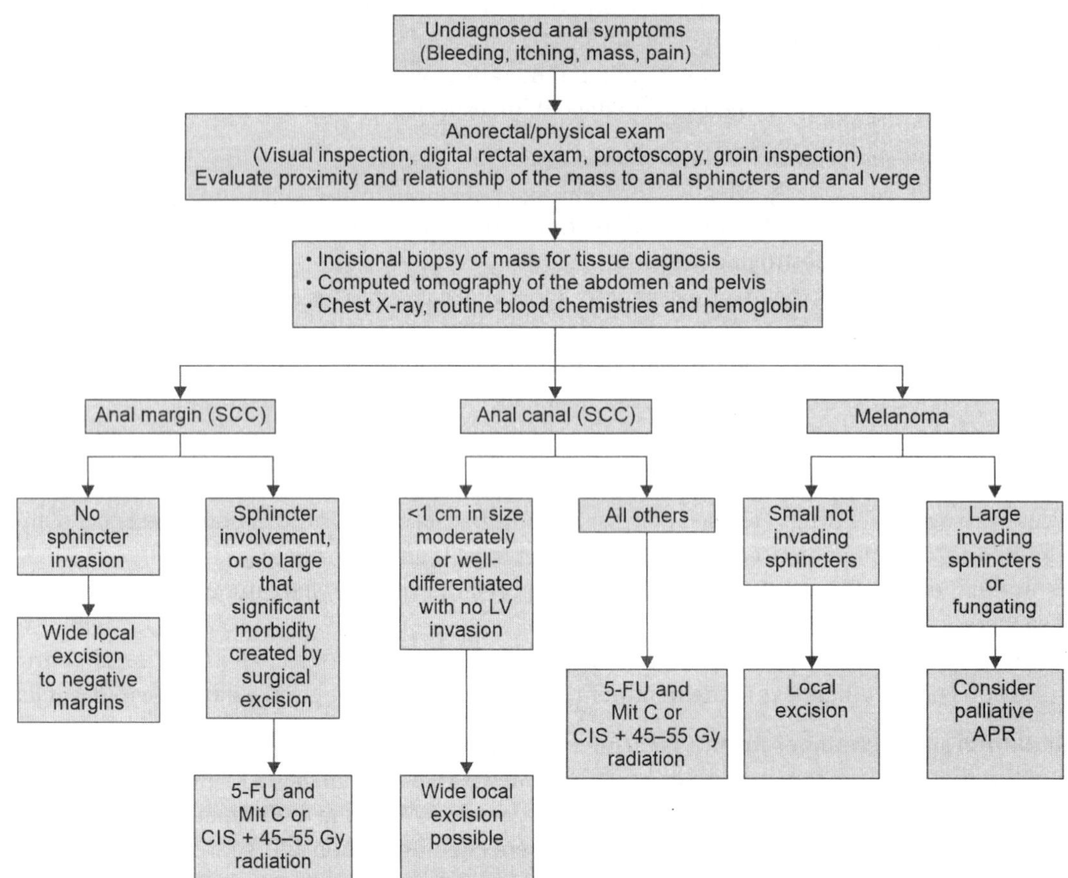

CHAPTER 27

Umbilicus

LEARNING OBJECTIVES

- Weeping Umbilicus
- Disease of Umbilicus
- Umbilical Fistula

WEEPING UMBILICUS

1. What are the causes of weeping umbilicus? Discuss the problem related to vitellointestinal duct and their remedy.

2. Discharging lesions of umbilicus. **WBUHS 2013**

Causes of Weeping Umbilicus

Urachal abnormalities	*Vitellointestinal duct abnormalities*	*Inflammatory and related disorders*
• Urachal sinus • Urachal diverticulum • Urachal cyst • Vesicoumbilical fistula • Alternating sinus	• Umbilical adenoma/polyp • Vitelline sinus • Umbilical fistula	• Umbilical granuloma • Omphalitis

The vitelline duct is a connection between the midgut and yolk sac.

Usually, involutes in 7–9 weeks.

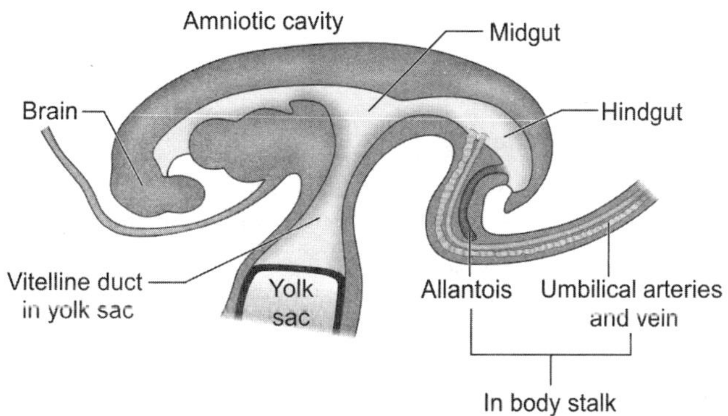

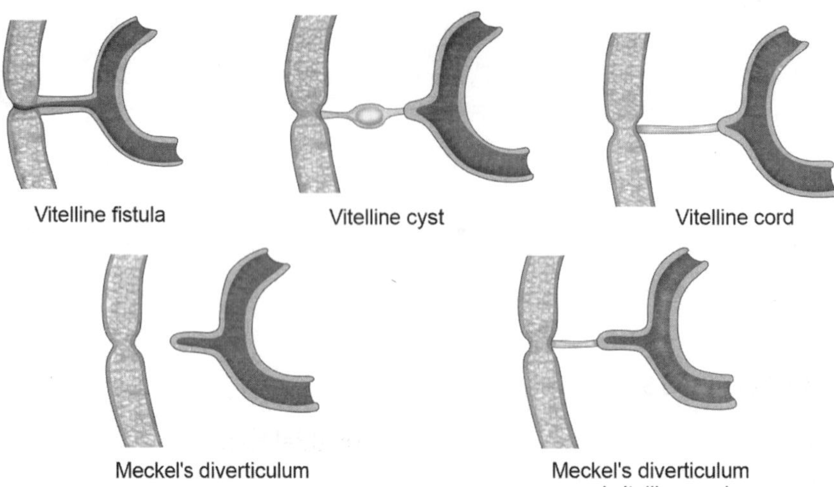

Vitelline duct abnormalities.

Treatment

- Symptomatic children with vitellointestinal or omphalomesenteric duct remnants should be resuscitated before intervention.
- Those with significant hemorrhage should be transfused.
- Patients with obstructive symptoms should be resuscitated as rapidly as possible to obviate the need for ischemic bowel resection.
- The incision chosen varies with the symptoms and the age of the patient.
- Children with feculent umbilical drainage or prolapse of the omphalomesenteric duct remnant can be explored by a small infraumbilical incision.
- When connected to the ileum, a patent vitellointestinal duct may have a wide lumen or be a high-output fistula.
- This may lead to fluid and electrolyte deficits, especially in neonates, and treatment should be expeditious.
- The treatment of a patent vitellointestinal is wedge or segmental resection.
- Children with Meckel's diverticulitis or a bleeding Meckel's diverticulum are operated on by using a transverse appendectomy incision with medial extension if necessary. Patients with suspected intestinal obstruction should be explored through a generous laparotomy incision.

DISEASE OF UMBILICUS

3. What are the diseases of the umbilicus?

Diseases of umbilicus

Condition	*Etiology*
A. Single umbilical artery	• Isolated (more common) • Associated with congenital anomalies
B. Urachal abnormalities – Urachal sirus – Urachal diverticulum – Urachal cyst – Vesicoumbilical fistula – Alternating sinus	• Congenital • Distally patent urachus • Proximally patent urachus • Patent midportion of urachus • Complete patency of urachus • Cyst communicating with both umbilicus and bladder

Contd...

Contd...

Condition	***Etiology***
C. Vitellointestinal duct (VID) abnormalities – Umbilical adenoma/polyp – Vitelline sinus – Meckel's diverticulum – Vitelline cyst – Umbilical fistula – Fibrous bands	 • Congenital distal VID remnant • Distally patent VID • Proximally patent VID • Patent midportion of VID • Complete patency of VID • Fibrous remnants of VID
D. Umbilical ring abnormalities – Umbilical hernia – Gastroschisis – Exomphalos – Omphalocele	• Acquired (A) or congenital (C) • Failure of closure of the umbilical ring after cord separation (A) • Paraumbilical muscular defect in anterior abdominal wall (C) • Failure of midgut to retract from the umbilical cord into the abdomen (C) • Defect of anterior abdominal wall due to incomplete closure of umbilical ring (C)
E. Round ligament of liver – Recanalization of the portal vein	 Portal hypertension
F. Extraperitoneal paravesical spaces – Fluid collections	 Several
G. Inflammatory and related disorders – Umbilical granuloma – Omphalitis – Necrotizing fasciitis – Leukocyte adhesion deficiency	• Inflammatory process • Overgrowth of granulation tissue and low-grade infection • Simple infection • Polymicrobial infection • Neutrophil chemotaxis disorder
H. Neoplastic disorders	Primary and secondary

Umbilical Abnormalities

- *Urachal abnormalities:*

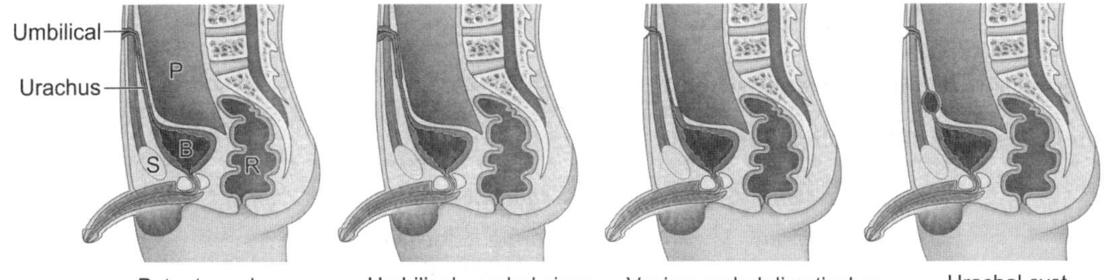

Patent urachus   Umbilical-urachal sinus   Vesicourachal diverticulum   Urachal cyst

  - Patent urachus (50%)
  - Urachal cyst (30%)
  - Urachal sinus (15%)
  - Vesicourachal diverticulum (5%)

- *Vitelline duct abnormalities:*

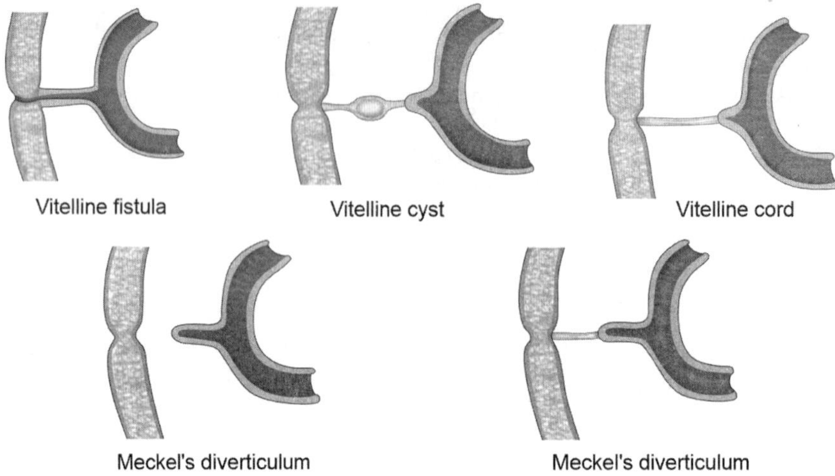

- Umbilical hernia
- Omphalitis
- Delayed cord separation

UMBILICAL FISTULA

4. Umbilical fistula. ***WBUHS 2012***

Introduction

It is an abnormal passage from the umbilicus to the intestine or, more frequently, to the remnant of the canal in the median umbilical ligament that connects the fetal bladder with the allantois.

Vitelline Umbilical Fistula

- May present as an umbilical polyp.
- May drain enteric contents.
- Fistulogram shows communication with the bowel.

Differential Diagnosis of Umbilical Fistula

Etiology	*Presenting age*	*Diagnostic dues*
Omphalitis	Newborn	• Purulent discharge • Periumbilical edema and erythema
Umbilical granuloma	Newborn	• Homogenous gray mass • Resolves with topical silver nitrate
Patent omphalomesenteric duct	Newborn	• Feculent or bilious discharge • Presence of second lumen in umbilical cord
Patent urachus	Newborn	• Urine in discharge • Presence of second lumen in umbilical cord
Urachal cyst	Older children/ adolescent	• Purulent discharge • Tender mass
Urachal carcinoma	Adult (40–70 years)	• Clinically silent • Nontender mass
Umbilical hernia ulceration	Any age	Skin breakdown and purulent discharge +/-feculent material
Abdominal abscess	Any age	Often more lateral to the umbilicus

Embryologic precursor of the urachus and omphalomesenteric duct. The urachus forms from the involution of the allantoic duct.

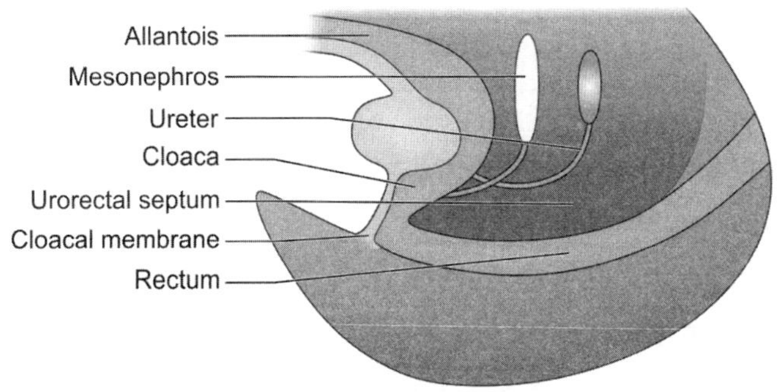

Imaging Studies

- Barium enema
- Fistulogram
- Ultrasonogram (USG)
- Computed tomography (CT) scan

Treatment

Surgical excision of the fistulous tract.

CHAPTER 28

Peritoneum, Omentum, and Mesentery

LEARNING OBJECTIVES

- Omentum
- Peritonitis
- Pseudomyxoma Peritonei
- HIPEC
- Mesenteric Cyst
- Mesenteric Ischemia
- Retroperitoneum
- Retroperitoneal Hematoma
- Chylous Ascites

1. Discuss anatomy of omentum. Enumerate surgical uses of omentum. ***NTRUHS, Vijayawada 2025***

Anatomy of the Omentum

The *omentum* is a fold of *peritoneum* that extends from the stomach and proximal duodenum to adjacent abdominal organs. It is richly vascularized and plays important roles in *immunity, fat storage, infection control,* and *tissue healing.*

Types of Omentum

- *Greater omentum:*
  - A large, apron-like peritoneal fold that hangs down from the *greater curvature of the stomach* and *first part of the duodenum.*
  - Drapes over the *transverse colon* and *small intestines.*
  - Composed of *four layers of peritoneum* (formed by the fusion of two double layers).
  - Contains *fat, lymphatics, blood vessels, and immune cells.*
  - Mobile and can migrate to areas of infection or inflammation (hence called the *"policeman of the abdomen"*).

Attachments: From the greater curvature of the stomach → down over intestines → then turns posteriorly to attach to the *transverse colon.*

- *Lesser omentum:*
  - A smaller peritoneal fold stretching from the *lesser curvature of the stomach and proximal duodenum* to the *liver.*

Forms the anterior wall of the *lesser sac (omental bursa).*

Divided into:

- *Hepatogastric ligament*—between liver and stomach
- *Hepatoduodenal ligament*—between liver and duodenum; contains the *portal triad:*
  - Hepatic artery proper
  - Portal vein
  - Common bile duct

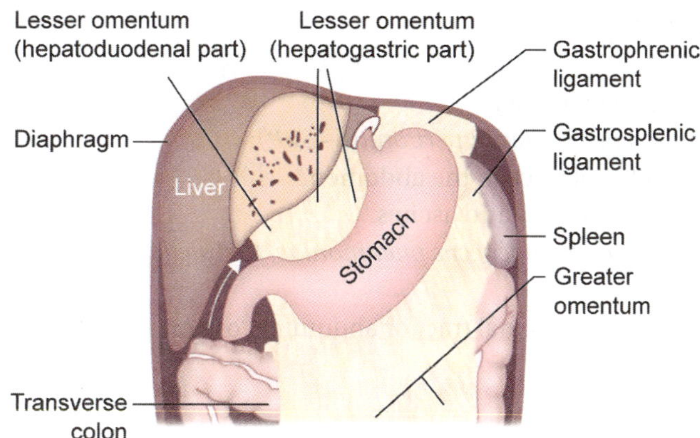

Functions of the Omentum

- *Immune defense:* Contains macrophages and lymphocytes
- *Infection control:* Moves toward and adheres to inflamed or perforated areas (e.g., perforated appendix)
- *Fat storage*
- *Angiogenesis and tissue repair*
- *Prevents adhesion formation* postsurgery

Surgical Uses of the Omentum

Owing to its vascularity, mobility, and immune properties, the omentum is used in various surgical procedures:

- *Omental patch (graham's patch):*
  - *Indication:* Perforated peptic ulcer
  - A tongue of omentum is used to plug the perforation and sutured over it.
- *Flap coverage in reconstructive surgery:*
  - Used as a *vascularized flap* to fill defects or protect grafts in:
    - Mediastinal wounds after cardiac surgery
    - Chest wall or sternal defects
    - Pelvic or perineal wounds
    - Brain or spinal surgeries (e.g., for CSF leak sealing)
- *Reinforcement of anastomoses:*
  - Omentum wrapped around GI anastomosis sites to:
    - Reduce leak risk
    - Promote healing
- *Coverage of vascular grafts:* Prevents infection and supports healing of grafts (e.g., aortic grafts)
- *Control of infection:* Omental "plugging" of abscess cavities or infected spaces
- *Bladder or ureteric repair:* Used to cover or support urinary tract repairs
- *Hernia repair:* Occasionally used in complex or recurrent hernia repairs as a filler
- *Transposition in ischemic diseases:* Omental transfer to ischemic organs (like heart or brain) has been tried experimentally due to its angiogenic properties

2. Define peritonitis. Describe the aetiopathogenesis, clinical features, investigations, management, complications, and prognosis of peritonitis. ***Maharashtra University of Health Sciences 2025***

Definition

Peritonitis is *inflammation of the peritoneum*, the serous membrane lining the abdominal cavity and covering the visceral organs. It can be *localized or generalized, infectious or sterile*, and is typically a medical emergency.

Etiopathogenesis of Peritonitis

Aetiology

Peritonitis can be classified based on cause:

- *Primary peritonitis (spontaneous bacterial peritonitis—SBP):*
  - Infection without an evident source in the abdomen.
  - Common in patients with cirrhosis and ascites.
  - *Common organisms: E. coli, Streptococcus pneumoniae, Klebsiella.*
- *Secondary peritonitis:*
  - Due to a breach in the gastrointestinal tract or abdominal organ.
  - Causes include:
    - Perforated peptic ulcer
    - Ruptured appendix
    - Diverticulitis
    - Bowel ischemia or infarction
    - Trauma
    - Postoperative anastomotic leak
- *Tertiary peritonitis:*
  - Persistent or recurrent peritonitis after adequate treatment of secondary peritonitis.
  - Often due to hospital-acquired, resistant organisms.

Pathogenesis

- Bacteria or chemical irritants (e.g., bile, gastric contents) enter the sterile peritoneal cavity.
- Trigger an acute inflammatory response.
- Leads to:
  - Vasodilation
  - Increased capillary permeability
  - Exudation of fluid into peritoneal cavity
  - Paralytic ileus
  - Hypovolemia
  - Sepsis and possibly multiorgan failure if untreated

Clinical Features

Symptoms	*Signs*
• Severe abdominal pain (often sudden and generalized) • Fever and chills • Nausea and vomiting • Abdominal distension • Constipation or obstipation • Anorexia • Altered mental status (especially in elderly or septic patients)	• Tender, rigid abdomen ("board-like") • Rebound tenderness • Guarding • Reduced or absent bowel sounds • Hypotension, tachycardia, tachypnea (in sepsis) • Signs of shock in advanced cases

Investigations

- *Blood tests:*
  - *CBC:* ↑ WBC (leukocytosis)
  - *CRP and ESR:* Elevated
  - Blood cultures
  - Electrolytes, renal and liver function tests
  - Serum amylase/lipase (to rule out pancreatitis)

- *Imaging:*
  - *X-ray abdomen (erect):* Free air under diaphragm in perforation
  - *Ultrasound:* Fluid collection, source of infection
  - *CT abdomen (with contrast):* Identifies perforation, abscesses, inflammation
- *Diagnostic paracentesis:*
  - Especially in suspected SBP
  - Ascitic fluid analysis:
    - WBC >250 cells/mm^3 (mainly neutrophils)
    - Positive culture
    - Low glucose, high LDH

Management

General Principles

- Hospital admission (often ICU)
- NPO (nil per os)—no oral intake
- IV fluid resuscitation
- Correction of electrolyte imbalance
- *Broad-spectrum IV antibiotics:* E.g., Piperacillin-tazobactam or a combination of 3rd-generation cephalosporin + metronidazole
- Analgesia and antipyretics

Specific Management

- *Primary peritonitis:*
  - Antibiotics alone often sufficient (e.g., cefotaxime for SBP)
  - Treat underlying liver disease or consider TIPS
- *Secondary peritonitis:*
  - *Surgical intervention required:*
    - Laparotomy or laparoscopy
    - Repair of perforation, appendectomy, drainage of abscess
  - *Peritoneal lavage* to remove contaminated fluid
- *Tertiary peritonitis:*
  - Prolonged antibiotic therapy
  - Repeat surgical exploration may be necessary
  - Manage underlying immunosuppression or hospital-acquired infections

Complications

- Sepsis and septic shock
- Multiorgan failure
- Abscess formation (e.g., subphrenic, pelvic)
- Adhesions → bowel obstruction
- Paralytic ileus
- Death (if untreated or delayed treatment)

Prognosis

- Depends on:
  - Cause and extent of peritonitis
  - Time to diagnosis and treatment
  - Patient comorbidities (e.g., diabetes, cirrhosis)
  - Organism virulence and antibiotic resistance

- *Primary peritonitis* has a better prognosis with early antibiotics.
- *Secondary peritonitis* has a higher mortality, especially with delayed surgery.
- *Tertiary peritonitis* carries a guarded prognosis due to complexity and resistance.

3. Pseudomyxoma peritonei. ***WBUHS 2021, Gujarat Health University 2024***

Introduction

- *Pseudomyxoma peritonei* refers to syndrome of progressive intraperitoneal accumulation of mucinous ascites related to a mucin-producing neoplasm. It is most commonly caused by a mucinous tumor of the appendix.
- Much less commonly, mucinous tumors of colon, rectum, stomach, pancreas, and urachus are implicated. There is some ongoing contention as to whether primary ovarian tumors are a frequent source in their own right or whether in these cases, the appendix is the primary site and the ovarian lesion is metastatic.

Terminology

- The terminology regarding pseudomyxoma peritonei can be a bit confusing and continues to evolve over time. In 2016, a consensus group, the Peritoneal Surface Oncology Group International, published guidelines for classification for mucinous appendiceal tumors and associated peritoneal disease (An "appendiceal mucocele" is a descriptive term which refers to the appearance of a dilated mucin-filled appendix.
- Although this is the imaging manifestation of appendiceal mucinous tumors, appendiceal mucoceles may also represent non-neoplastic etiologies such as mucosal hyperplasia or retention cyst related to luminal obstruction.

Pathology

- Pseudomyxoma peritonei (of appendiceal origin) is due to invasion or rupture of the appendix from a mucin-secreting appendiceal tumor.
- The characteristic mucinous ascites is composed of acellular mucin and a variable amount of neoplastic epithelial cells. Indeed, pseudomyxoma peritonei is not a histologic diagnosis—the label merely implies grossly mucinous intraperitoneal deposits.
- The remarkable feature of pseudomyxoma peritonei is that this neoplastic, progressive process often arises from a seemingly benign or well-differentiated primary tumor.
- However once there is intraperitoneal spread, the mucinous deposits tend to follow routes of normal peritoneal fluid flow, spreading along the pelvis, paracolic gutters, liver capsule, and omentum while often sparing mobile organs, for example, small bowel.
- Pseudomyxoma peritonei may be divided into two pathological subtypes which have etiological and prognostic significance:
- *Peritoneal adenomucinosis:*
  - A peritoneal neoplasm composed largely of mucin associated with fibrosis with minimal cytological atypia and mitoses.
  - The primary tumor is generally an adenoma.
- *Peritoneal mucinous carcinoma:*
  - Characterized by proliferative epithelium, glands, nests, or individual cells with marked cytologic atypia
  - The primary is a mucinous adenocarcinoma.

Radiographic Features

- Pseudomyxoma peritonei is characterized by loculated collections of fluid which accumulate along peritoneal surfaces, classically resulting in a scalloped appearance of coated abdominal organs and omental caking. An appendiceal mucocele (representing a mucinous appendiceal tumor) may be visualized.
- Since appendiceal tumors are most common etiology, early peritoneal disease may be limited to the right lower quadrant abdomen.
- Deposits tend to localize to site of physiologic lymphatic absorption of ascites (omentum, underneath right hemidiaphragm) and dependent areas (e.g., paracolic gutters, right retrohepatic space, and lower pelvis).

- Deposits tend to spare the more mobile small bowel until later in disease, when it eventually causes bowel obstruction.
- *Plain radiograph:* May show evidence of ascites with centrally displaced small bowel loops and scattered punctate or curvilinear calcifications
- *Ultrasound (US):*
  - Echogenic peritoneal masses or ascites with echogenic particles which (unlike other forms of particulate ascites such as hemoperitoneum or pus in the peritoneum) do not move.
  - Small bowel loops displaced medially
  - May show scalloping of the liver, spleen, and at times other organs
- *Computed tomography (CT):*
  - Simple or loculated low attenuation fluid throughout intraperitoneal spaces, omentum, and mesentery
  - Scalloping of visceral surfaces, particularly the liver
  - Often with scattered (curvilinear or punctate) calcifications
  - Tends to remain localized to peritoneal cavity—thoracic and nodal lesions metastases uncommon
- *Magnetic resonance imaging (MRI):*
  - *Reported signal characteristics of the collections include:*
    - *T1:* Typically low signal
    - *T2:* Typically high signal
    - *T1 C+ (Gd):* May show enhancement

Treatment and Prognosis

- This is a progressive and often fatal disease.
- Recurrent bowel obstructions are commonly due to the fibrosis and adhesions in advanced disease.
- Treatment is surgical debulking followed by infusion of intraperitoneal chemotherapy.
- Aggressive surgical treatment has been considered based on the calculation of the peritoneal cancer index (PCI), which is a prognostic indicator based on the amount of tumor found at laparoscopy. This index has been performed using CT or MRI.

---

4. What is hyperthermic intraperitoneal chemotherapy (HIPEC)? Indications for HIPEC. Complications of HIPEC. ***WBUHS 2021***

---

5. What is HIPEC? Write its use in gastrointestinal tract cancers and its cefficacy. ***Srimanta Sankaradeva University, Assam 2025***

Introduction

- *Hyperthermic intraperitoneal chemotherapy* (often abbreviated as *HIPEC*) is a form of chemotherapy used for the treatment of peritoneal involvement with malignancy.
- It usually involves the instillation of heated (to around 41–43°C) chemotherapy agents directly into the abdominopelvic cavity immediately after surgery.
- It delivers a high dose directly to the site of potential residual microscopic cancer cells while minimizing systemic toxicity.
- Heating to this temperature is thought to increase drug penetration and cytotoxicity.

Stages

- Cytoreductive surgery is the first stage of HIPEC surgery.
- The second stage is the HIPEC procedure.

HIPEC has Several Advantages Over Standard Chemotherapy

- It is a single treatment done in the operating room, instead of multiple treatments over several weeks.
- 90% of the drug stays within the abdominal cavity, decreasing toxic effects on the rest of the body.
- It allows for a more intense dose of chemotherapy.

Indications

The most common cancers treated with HIPEC	
• Adrenal cancer • Appendix cancer • Colon and rectal cancer • Gastric (stomach) cancer • Liver cancer	• Mesothelioma • Ovarian cancer—for patients with newly diagnosed stage III primary epithelial ovarian or fallopian tube carcinoma • Pancreatic cancer • Peritoneal cancer—primary peritoneal carcinoma

Side effects of HIPEC surgery			
• Pain • Nausea	• Vomiting • Diarrhea	• Constipation • Bloating	• Weight loss • Difficulty sleeping

6. Define peritoneal carcinomatosis. How will you assess such case? Discuss the role of cytoreductive surgery and HIPEC in CP. ***Rajasthan University of Health Sciences, 2025; WBUHS 2024***

7. Peritoneal carcinomatosis. ***Tamil Nadu Health Medical Univesrity 2024.***

Peritoneal carcinomatosis (PC) is intraperitoneal dissemination (carcinosis) of any form of cancer that does not originate from the peritoneum itself.

Peritoneal carcinomatosis (PC) refers to the spread of cancer to the peritoneum, the lining of the abdominal cavity, often originating from cancers of the digestive tract or female reproductive organs.

Assessing a case of peritoneal carcinomatosis involves a combination of clinical evaluation, imaging studies, and sometimes diagnostic procedures. Here's how the assessment generally unfolds:

Clinical Evaluation

- *History:* Detailed patient history is crucial. Look for symptoms such as—
  - Abdominal pain or discomfort
  - Abdominal distension or bloating
  - Unexplained weight loss
  - Loss of appetite (anorexia)
  - Nausea or vomiting
  - Changes in bowel habits (e.g., constipation)
  - Ascites (fluid accumulation in the abdomen)
  - Fatigue or weakness
- *Physical examination:* The physical examination may reveal—
  - Abdominal tenderness or masses
  - Ascites (which could be detected by abdominal examination, fluid wave, or percussion)
  - Palpable masses or organ enlargement (like hepatomegaly if liver involvement)
  - Signs of malnutrition

Imaging Studies

- *Abdominal ultrasound:* Often the first imaging test to assess ascites, identify masses, or detect fluid accumulation in the abdomen.
- *CT scan (Contrast-enhanced):* The gold standard imaging modality to assess peritoneal carcinomatosis. It can reveal:
  - Peritoneal thickening or nodularity
  - Presence of peritoneal implants or metastases
  - Ascites
  - The extent and location of tumor spread (important for staging)
- *MRI:* Sometimes used for more detailed soft tissue contrast, especially if evaluating the mesentery or peritoneal surface.
- *PET scan:* Can be helpful for detecting metabolic activity of tumors and identifying metastatic disease.

Diagnostic Procedures

- *Paracentesis:* If ascites is present, fluid can be aspirated for analysis. The fluid is analyzed for:
  - *Cytology:* To check for malignant cells (peritoneal carcinomatosis is often confirmed if cancer cells are found).
  - *Biochemistry:* To assess protein and lactate dehydrogenase (LDH) levels, which can suggest malignancy.
  - *Microbiology:* To rule out infections or other causes of ascites.
- *Laparoscopy:* A minimally invasive procedure where a camera is inserted into the abdomen to directly visualize peritoneal implants or masses. Biopsies can also be taken for histological examination to confirm cancer.

Laboratory Tests

- *Tumor markers:* Common markers include—
  - CA-125 (especially useful in ovarian cancer, which commonly causes peritoneal carcinomatosis)
  - CEA (Carcinoembryonic antigen)
  - CA 19-9 (particularly in pancreatic, gastric, or colon cancers)
- *Complete blood count (CBC):* To assess for anemia or infection.
- *Liver function tests:* To assess liver involvement or metastasis.
- *Renal function tests:* To evaluate kidney function if ascites or malignancy affects renal circulation.

Histopathological Confirmation

A biopsy (often obtained during laparoscopy or paracentesis) is necessary for definitive diagnosis. Histopathological examination will confirm if the peritoneal implants are malignant and, if so, identify the origin of the cancer (e.g., primary gastrointestinal, ovarian, or other sources).

Staging

- Once peritoneal carcinomatosis is diagnosed, further workup for staging is important:
  - *TNM Staging:* The peritoneum is part of the "M" (metastasis) staging in various cancers.
  - *Ascitic Fluid Analysis:* To determine the cancer type and if the ascites is malignant or benign.
- For example, in ovarian cancer, peritoneal carcinomatosis is often considered part of the disease's advanced stage.

Multidisciplinary Approach

The management of peritoneal carcinomatosis is complex and usually involves a multidisciplinary team including oncologists, surgeons, radiologists, and pathologists. Based on the assessment, treatment options such as chemotherapy (systemic or intraperitoneal), surgery, or palliative care may be considered.

Cytoreductive surgery (CRS) and HIPEC are critical components in the management of peritoneal carcinomatosis, a condition where cancer cells spread to the peritoneal surfaces. This condition is most commonly associated with cancers like colorectal, ovarian, gastric, and appendiceal malignancies.

Cytoreductive Surgery (CRS)

Cytoreductive surgery refers to the surgical removal of as much visible tumor as possible from the peritoneal cavity. The goal of CRS is to reduce the tumor burden in the peritoneal cavity to as low a level as possible, ideally to leave no visible disease or less than 2.5 mm of residual tumor, which is known as a complete cytoreduction (CC0). The extent of resection depends on the number, size, and location of the tumors. This procedure often involves:

- Removal of involved organs or parts of organs (e.g., bowel, omentum, spleen, or peritoneum).
- Excision of peritoneal nodules.
- Management of complications, like bowel obstructions, caused by tumor masses.

The role of CRS is to achieve a complete or nearly complete resection of peritoneal disease, which can significantly improve patient survival rates and quality of life in selected patients. The success of CRS is influenced by the tumor type, the extent of spread, the patient's overall health, and the skill of the surgical team.

Hyperthermic Intraperitoneal Chemotherapy (HIPEC)

After the CRS procedure, HIPEC is often employed to address microscopic disease that may remain in the peritoneal cavity. HIPEC involves the intraoperative administration of heated chemotherapy directly into the peritoneal cavity. The key components of HIPEC are:

- *Chemotherapy agents:* Typically, agents like cisplatin or mitomycin C are used.
- *Hyperthermia:* The chemotherapy solution is heated to a temperature of around 41–42°C (105.8–107.6°F) to enhance the cytotoxic effects of the drugs, as heat can increase the penetration of chemotherapy agents into tumor cells, making them more effective.

HIPEC offers several advantages in treating peritoneal carcinomatosis, including:

- *Direct delivery of chemotherapy:* It allows for a high concentration of chemotherapy to be delivered directly to the site of disease, which increases the drug's efficacy while minimizing systemic toxicity.
- *Improved drug penetration:* The heat increases the permeability of the tumor cells, improving the chemotherapy's ability to penetrate the tissue and target residual microscopic disease.
- *Increased cytotoxicity:* Hyperthermia can directly kill tumor cells and sensitize them to the effects of chemotherapy.

Combining CRS and HIPEC

The combination of CRS and HIPEC has shown significant promise in improving outcomes for patients with peritoneal carcinomatosis. Studies have demonstrated that this approach can lead to long-term survival in patients who would otherwise have a poor prognosis, especially in cancers like colorectal cancer with peritoneal metastasis or pseudomyxoma peritonei (a rare condition usually due to appendiceal cancer).

Key benefits of CRS plus HIPEC include:

- *Improved survival rates:* When performed together, these treatments can offer long-term survival benefits, especially when CC0 is achieved.
- *Reduced recurrence:* By removing macroscopic disease and treating microscopic disease with heated chemotherapy, the chances of recurrence can be reduced.
- *Symptom management:* CRS and HIPEC can also help manage symptoms caused by the spread of cancer, like bowel obstructions, peritoneal irritation, and ascites.

However, the combination is not suitable for all patients. The decision to use CRS and HIPEC depends on several factors:

- The patient's performance status and ability to withstand major surgery.
- The extent of the peritoneal spread (e.g., the Peritoneal Cancer Index, or PCI, is often used to guide the decision-making).
- The histological type of cancer.
- The response to prior treatments (e.g., chemotherapy or radiotherapy).

Challenges and Considerations

While CRS and HIPEC can be highly effective, there are also challenges:

- *Complexity and risk of complications:* These are major surgeries with significant risks, including infection, organ dysfunction, and complications from the chemotherapy.
- *Selection of patients:* Not all patients are candidates for CRS and HIPEC. Factors such as the extent of the peritoneal disease, general health, and the potential for complete cytoreduction are important considerations.
- *Recurrence:* Despite aggressive treatment, recurrence remains a significant issue in peritoneal carcinomatosis, and additional treatments, including systemic chemotherapy or repeat CRS/HIPEC, may be required.

Conclusion

Cytoreductive surgery combined with hyperthermic intraperitoneal chemotherapy is a promising treatment modality for peritoneal carcinomatosis. While it has shown to improve survival and quality of life for many patients, the approach requires careful patient selection, skilled surgical teams, and multidisciplinary management. It remains a cutting-edge treatment for advanced malignancies that involve the peritoneal cavity, offering hope for patients with otherwise limited treatment options.

8. Mesenteric cyst. ***WBUHS 2010***

Introduction

- Cysts of the mesentery are benign lesions.
- Incidence is less than one in 100,000.
- The etiology of such cysts remains unknown, but several theories regarding their development exist, including degeneration of the mesenteric lymphatics or simply arising as a congenital anomaly.

Classification

- *Cysts of lymphatic origin:*
  - Simple lymphatic cyst
  - Lymphangiomas
- *Cysts of mesothelial origin:*
  - Simple mesothelial cyst
  - Benign cystic mesotheliomas
  - Malignant cystic mesotheliomas
- *Cysts of enteric origin:*
  - Enteric duplication cyst
  - Enteric cysts
- *Cysts of urogenital origin*
- *Matures cystic teratomas (dermoid cysts)*
- *Nonpancreatic pseudocysts*
  - Cysts of traumatic origin
  - Cysts of infectious origin
- *Chylolymphatic (most common)*—arises in congenitally misplaced lymphatic tissue that has no efferent communication with the lymphatic system; it arises most frequently in the mesentery of the ileum. It is almost invariably solitary. A chylolymphatic cyst has an independent blood supply. Enucleation is possible without resecting gut.
- *Simple (mesothelial)*
- *Enterogenous*—derived either from a diverticulum of the mesenteric border of the intestine due to sequestration from the intestinal canal during embryonic life or from a duplication of the intestine. The muscle in the wall of an enteric duplication cyst and the bowel with which it is in contact have a common blood supply; removal of the cyst always entails resection of the related portion of intestine.
- *Urogenital remnant*
- *Dermoid (teratomatous cyst)*

Clinical Features

- Found more often in the second decade of life
- Mesenteric cysts may be asymptomatic or cause symptoms of a mass lesion.
- Symptoms can be acute or chronic.
- Acute abdominal pain caused by a mesenteric cyst is usually caused by rupture or torsion of the cyst or acute bleeding into the cyst. It could be an infection.
- Mesenteric cysts can also cause chronic intermittent abdominal pain secondary to compression of adjacent structures or spontaneous torsion followed by twisting of the cyst.
- Mesenteric cysts can cause nonspecific symptoms such as anorexia, nausea, vomiting, fatigue, and weight loss.
- Physical examination may reveal a mass lesion that moves only from the patient's right to left or from left to right (Tillaux sign), i.e., in a plane at right angles to the mesenteric attachments. Variable swelling around the cyst
- There is a resonant zone around the cyst.

Imaging Studies

- CT, abdominal US, and MRI have been used to evaluate patients with mesenteric cysts. All of the above-mentioned imaging modalities show a cystic structure without a solid component in the midgut.
- They are usually single-eyed, but sometimes they can be or multi-eyed.
- Regardless of the imaging modality used, it can be difficult to distinguish these cystic masses from rare solid mesenteric tumors with cystic components such as cystic stromal tumor or mesothelioma.
- Cystic lymphangioma of the mesentery can appear as multiple, often large cysts in the background of abdominal pain. They can be difficult to treat and almost always recur after surgery.

Diagnosis

All conventional methods of diagnosing abdominal tumors should be used for diagnosis, with US and CT, and especially nuclear magnetic resonance, providing most of the tumor size and location.

Maintenance

- Total cystectomy is the treatment of choice. An open approach was recommended, although there are already reports of successful laparoscopic cystectomy in the literature.
- Intraoperative differentiation of lymphocyst and lymphangioma is extremely important and can only be achieved by pathohistological examination of the cyst wall. If an intraoperative biopsy is not possible or the finding is inconclusive, each cyst must be removed in its entirety due to the aforementioned risk associated with cystic lymphangioma.

---

9. Classify mesenteric ischemia. What are the clinical features of acute mesenteric ischemia (AMI)? How will you diagnose and treat AMI? ***WBUHS 2023***

---

10. Describe the etiology and pathogenesis of mesenteric ischemia. Outline the principles of treatment of acute mesenteric artery occlusion. ***RGUHS, Karnataka 2025***

---

11. Describe the diagnosis and management of Superior Mesenteric Vascular thrombosis. ***Gujarat Health University 2024***

Introduction

- AMI is a catastrophic abdominal emergency characterized by sudden critical interruption to the intestinal blood flow which commonly leads to bowel infarction and death.
- It is an uncommon but life-threatening disease.
- Incidence ~1 in every 1,000 hospital admissions
- Mortality remains as high as 60–80%.
- Prognosis is poor.

Classification of Mesenteric Ischemia

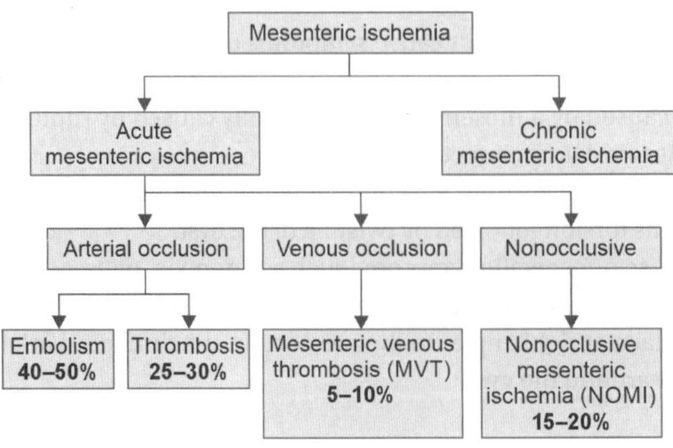

Acute SMA Occlusion

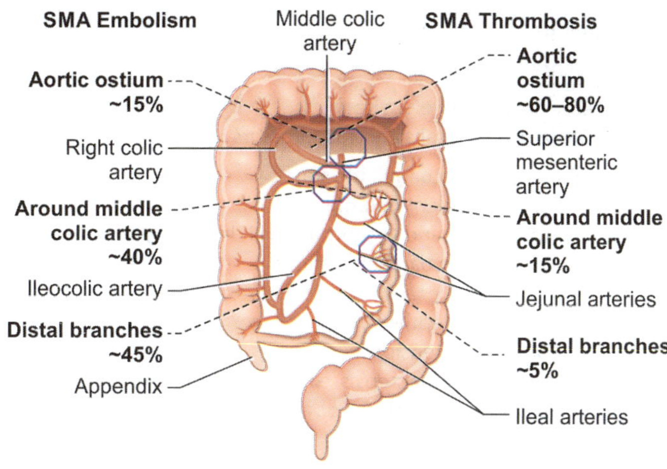

(SMA: superior mesenteric artery)

AMI due to Embolism

- Embolism—most common cause of AMI.
- Majority of emboli arise from the heart, most commonly the left atrium in patients of atrial fibrillation.
- Superior mesenteric artery (SMA) is most commonly affected—acute angle of origin from abdominal aorta.

AMI due to Thrombosis

- Commonly involves the aortic ostium
- Thrombosis occurs on top of atherosclerosis.
- Prognosis—worse than embolic ischemia
- Often previous history of:
  - Intestinal angina
  - Sitophobia—fear of eating
  - Significant weight loss

AMI due to Nonocclusive Disease

- Results from systemic hypoperfusion or low flow states—carotid-cavernous fistula (CCF), shock, and in critically ill patients following surgery
- Causes—intense vasospasm and sympathetic-induced vasoconstriction
- Most lethal--because once arterial vasospasm is initiated, it may persist even after correction of the initiating event
- Prognosis is very poor.

AMI due to Venous Thrombosis

- Least common
- Typically affects superior mesenteric vein and rarely inferior mesenteric vein

Cause	*Etiology*	*Incidence (%)*
Embolism	• Cardiac – Atrial fibrillation – Mural thrombus following myocardial infarction – Left atrial myxoma – Prosthetic heart valves • Proximal aortic disease, e.g., aneurysm and atheromas • Iatrogenic, e.g., arteriography	Most common (40–50%)

Contd...

Contd...

Cause	*Etiology*	*Incidence (%)*
Thrombosis	Mesenteric atherosclerosis	25–30%
Nonocclusive mesenteric ischemia	• Low-flow states, e.g., shock • Drugs, e.g., digitalis and vasopressors	15–20%
Mesenteric vein thrombosis	• Inherited hypercoagulable states – Factor V Leiden mutation – Protein C, S, and antithrombin III deficiency • Acquired hypercoagulable states – Malignancy – Oral contraceptives – Portal hypertension – Intra-abdominal sepsis, e.g., acute pancreatitis – Postoperative states, e.g., abdominal surgery	Least common (5–10%)

Clinical Features of AMI

- *Classical description of early symptom:* Severe abdominal pain that is out of proportion to physical findings in 95% cases
- *Early:* Prominent symptoms of gastrointestinal (GI) emptying (nausea, vomiting, and diarrhea)
- *Late:*
  - Bloody diarrhea
  - Abdominal distension
  - *Features of peritonitis:*
    - Fever
    - Shock
    - Tachycardia

Investigations

Blood Test

Most common laboratory abnormalities are:

- Hemoconcentration
- Leukocytosis (neutrophilic)
- Metabolic acidosis
- Lactic acidosis (in more advanced case)

Other Serum Markers Raised

- Amylase
- Alkaline phosphatase (ALP)

Imaging Studies

- *Straight X-ray abdomen in erect posture:* Dilated bowel loops
- *Doppler ultrasonography (USG):*
  - Able to identify severe stenosis or total or partial occlusion and velocity of blood flowing through the vessels
  - *Unable to detect:*
    - Emboli beyond the proximal main vessel
    - Nonobstructive mesenteric ischemia
- *Contrast-enhanced CT (CECT) abdomen:*
  - Gas in bowel wall (pneumatosis intestinalis)
  - Gas in mesenteric vein
  - May be excessive portal venous gas
  - Bowel wall edema

- May show SMA occlusion with embolus
- May show SMA thrombus
- May show pneumoperitoneum
- *Angiography:* Gold standard
  - *Noninvasive:*
    - CT-angiography
    - Magnetic resonance angiography (MRA)
- Invasive
  - Catheter (conventional method)
    - *Findings on angiography:*
      - Filling defects
      - Stenosis or blockage

Management

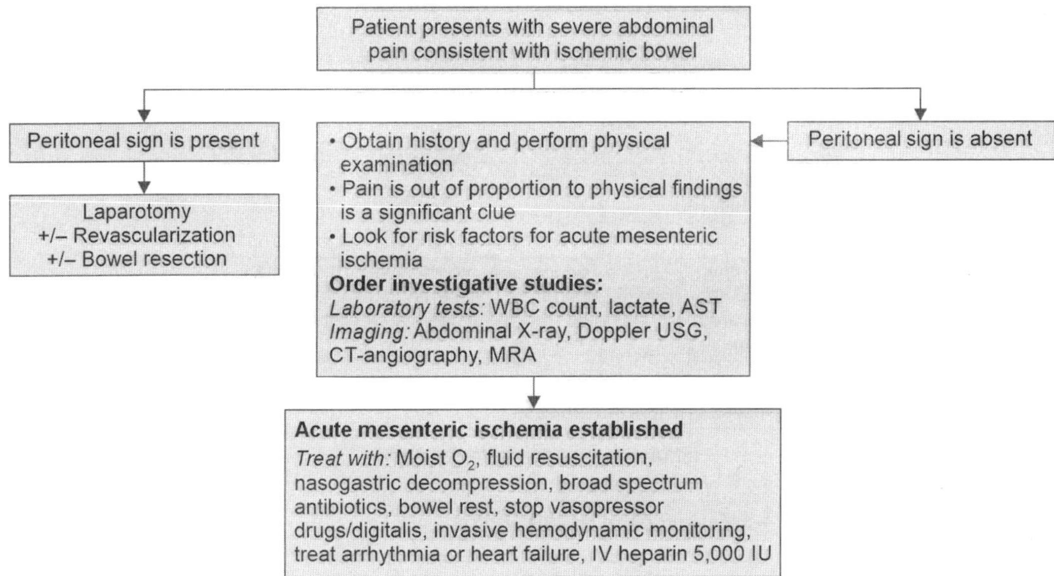

(AST: aspartate aminotransferase; CT: computed tomography; IV: intravenous; MRA: magnetic resonance angiography; USG: ultrasonography; WBC: white blood cell)

Definitive Surgical Exploration

- *Midline laparotomy:*
  - Assessment of bowel viability
  - Determination of underlying cause
  - Mesenteric revascularization
  - Resection of necrotic bowel
  - Second-look laparotomy

Assessment of bowel viability.

Clinical judgment	*Doppler ultrasonography (USG)*	*Fluorescein*
• Pink serosa • Visible peristalsis • Positive pulsations • Bleeding from cut edges	Handheld Doppler (detects antimesenteric blood flow)	Injection of intravenous (IV) sodium fluorescein (1 g) and inspection under Wood's lamp (Viable bowel has smooth, uniform fluorescence)

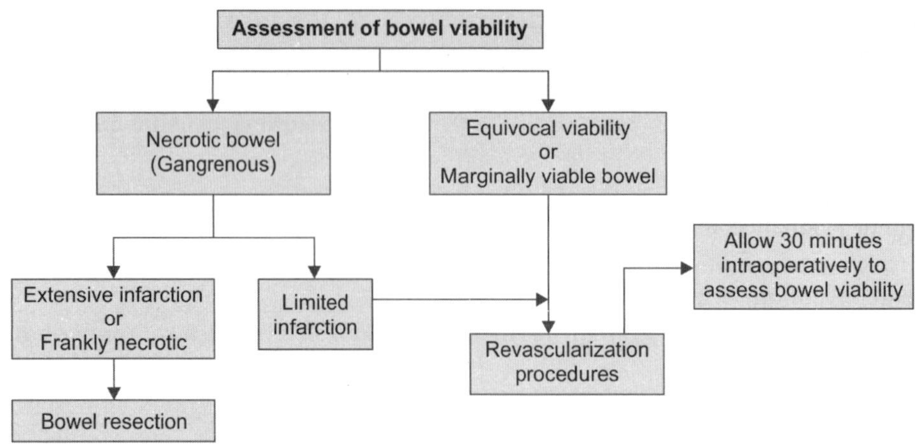

Determination of Underlying Pathology: Thrombosis or Embolism?

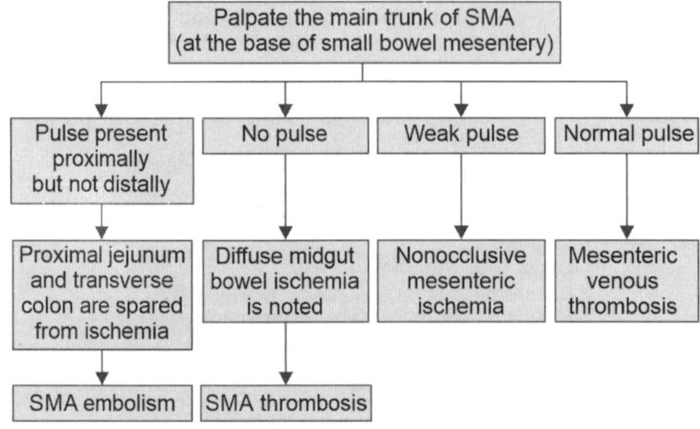

(SMA: superior mesenteric artery)

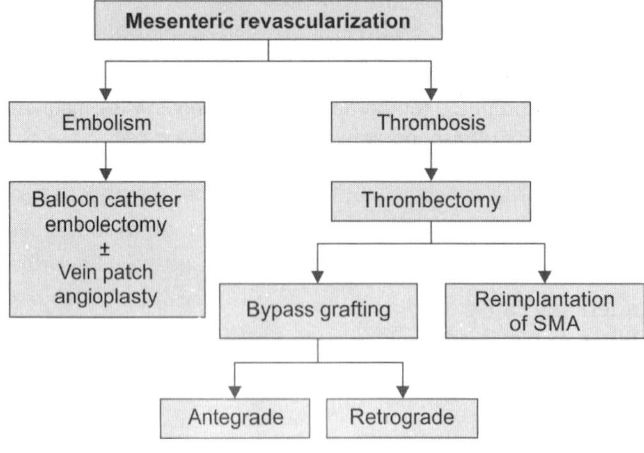

(SMA: superior mesenteric artery)

Resection of Necrotic Bowel

- Frankly necrotic bowel segments—resection
  Marginal viable bowel (equivocal viability):
  - May improve over hours
  - Consider second-look laparotomy

Second-look Laparotomy

- Some advocate routine second-look laparotomy at 24–48 hours—claimed reduced mortality rate
- A selective approach and perform a second laparotomy when patient deteriorates clinically
- Can avoid unnecessary second operation if patient remains well

After Revascularization (Embolectomy or Bypass)

Consider postrevascularization papaverine (arterial spasm may persist even after embolectomy or thrombectomy)

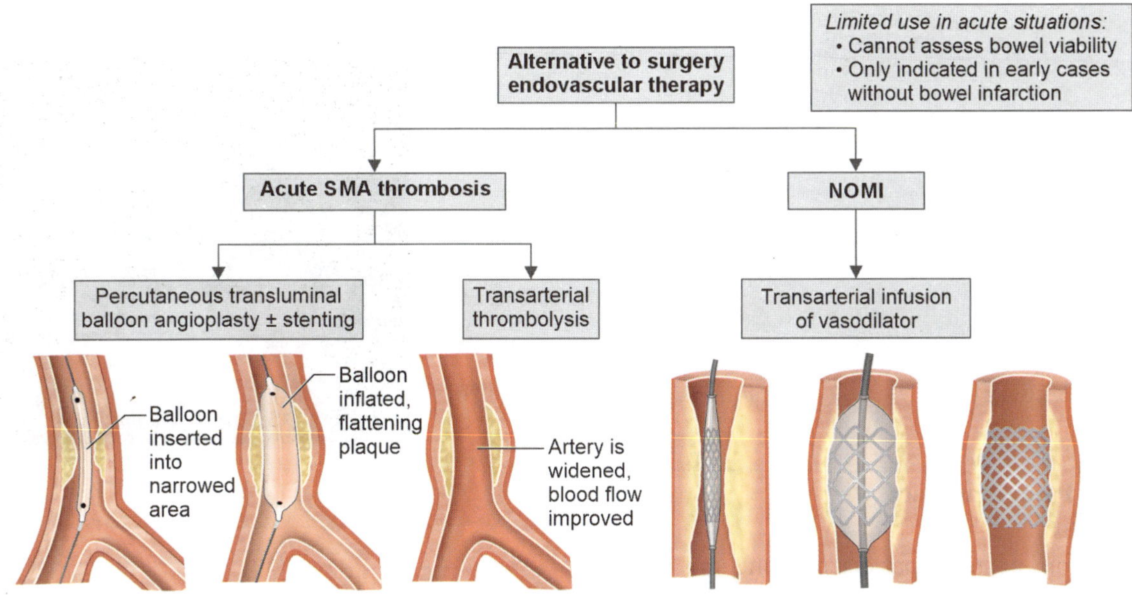

(NOMI: nonocclusive mesenteric ischemia; SMA: superior mesenteric artery)

Management of Nonocclusive Mesenteric Ischemia

- Correct underlying condition
- Optimize fluid status, improve cardiac output, and eliminate vasopressors (alpha-blocker)
- Consider catheter-directed intra-arterial infusion of vasodilator (papaverine 30–60 mg/h)
- Laparotomy if peritoneal signs develop

Management of Mesenteric Venous Thrombosis

- Anticoagulation with heparin is mainstay of treatment.
- Workup for hypercoagulability
- Laparotomy if peritoneal signs develop

Summary

- AMI is an abdominal emergency in both if physical signs are present or absent.
- We have very less time for investigation, so assessing clinically is important.
- Every minute wasted is equal to every centimeter of small bowel we lose.
- Angiography is diagnostic as well as therapeutic.
- Preoperative heparin infusion and postoperative papaverine infusion are must.
- Still prognosis is poor and mortality is as high as 80%.

12. Describe boundaries of retroperitoneum and give a short account of management of retroperitoneal hemorrhage. ***WBUHS 2016***

13. Discuss the management of retroperitoneal hematoma. ***WBUHS 2025 Supplementary***

Boundaries of Retroperitoneal Space

- Anterior—posterior parietal peritoneum and posterior—transversalis fascia
- Superior—diaphragmatic fascia and inferior—pelvic brim
- *Major compartments:* Anterior pararenal space and posterior pararenal space Perirenal space—the largest of all three compartments.

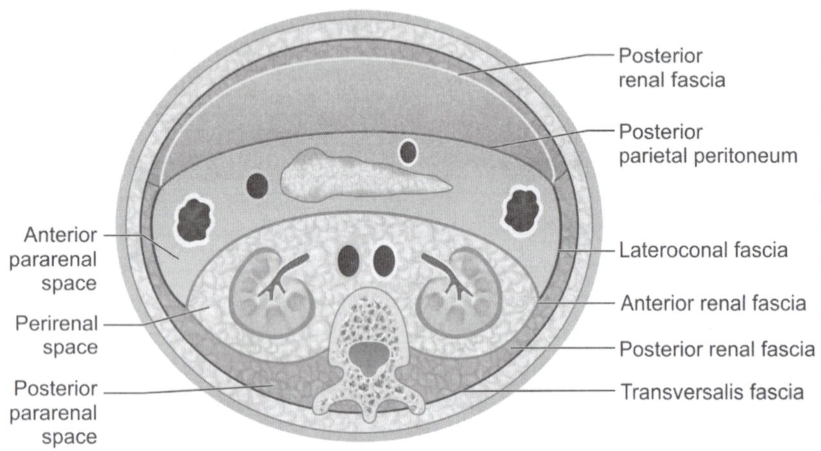

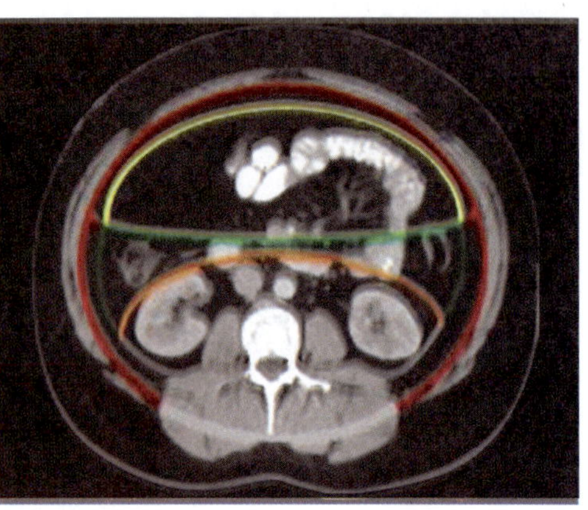

Anterior Pararenal Space

Boundaries

- Anterior—posterior parietal peritoneum
- Posterior—anterior renal fascia (Gerota's fascia)
- Lateral—lateroconal fascia

This space is continuous across the midline. But pathologies remain to one side.

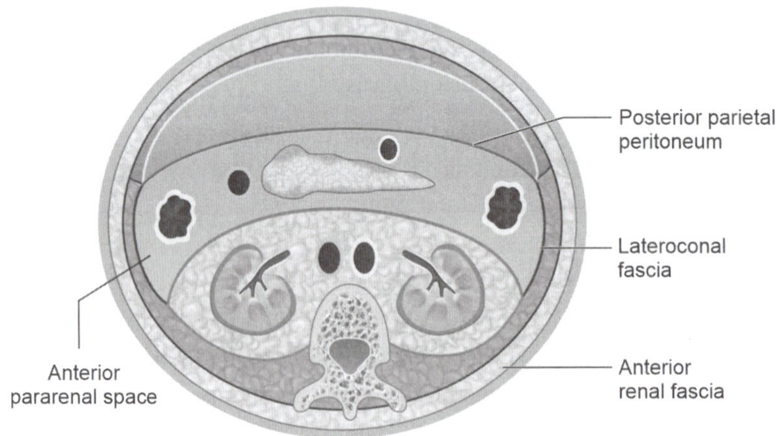

Posterior Pararenal Space

Posterior pararenal space is a thin compartment.

Boundaries

- Anteromedial—the posterior renal fascia (Zuckerkandl fascia) and lateroconal fascia
- Posterolateral—the transversalis fascia

- Medial—margin of the psoas muscle and quadratus lumborum muscles opens laterally toward the flank and inferiorly toward the pelvis.

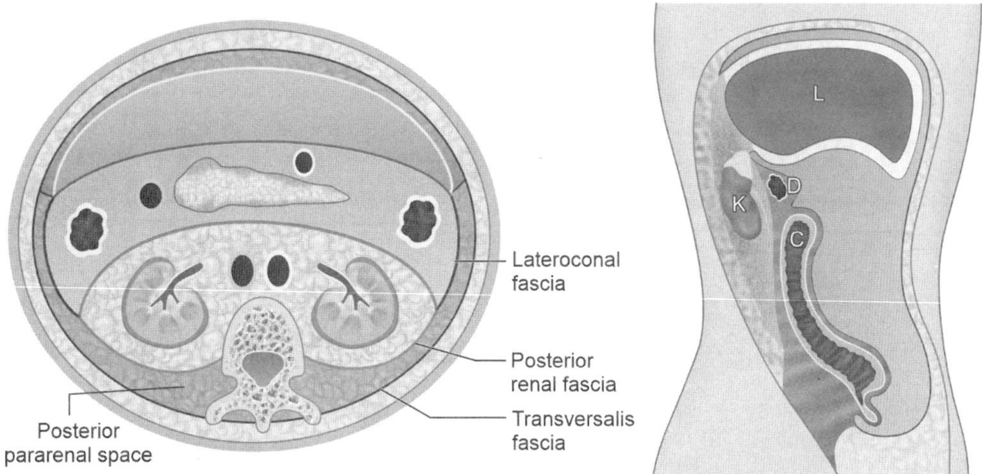

This space is closely related to the posterior surfaces of the ascending and descending colon; therefore, inflammatory processes originating in these colonic segments easily extend into this space.

The posterior pararenal fat is also adjacent to the junction of the anterior and posterior renal fasciae, so fluid collections coursing within these pathways can track into the posterior pararenal space.

Perirenal Space (Gerota's Space)

Perirenal space lies in the central compartment of the retroperitoneum, lateral to the lumbar spine. Inverted cone-shaped with superolateral-to-inferomedial orientation.

Boundaries

- Anterior—anterior renal fascia (Gerota's fascia)
- Posterior—posterior renal fascia (fascia of Zuckerkandl)
- Superior—it opens into bare area of liver and the mediastinum.
- Medial—blends with the connective tissue surrounding the great vessels
- Lateral—lateroconal fascia
    - Laterally, the anterior and the posterior renal fascia blend and the posterior layer of the posterior renal fascia continues anterior laterally to form the lateroconal fascia.
    - Lateroconal fascia continues anterolaterally behind the colon to blend with the parietal peritoneum.

Midline Communication

There is evidence of potential communication across the midline between the two perirenal spaces anterior to the lower aorta and inferior vena cava and posterior to the anterior renal fascia at the level of lower lumbar vertebrae (L3–5).

Open Inferior Ends

Inferiorly, this space blends loosely with the iliac fascia and periureteric connective tissue, having its inferior apex open toward the upper margins of the psoas muscles, ureter, iliac vessels, and to the prevesical and presacral spaces.

At this level, the perirenal spaces do not communicate.

Thoracic Communication

The perirenal space communicates superiorly with the mediastinum through splanchnic foramina of the diaphragmatic crura and small transdiaphragmatic perforations and lymphatic vessels, providing conduits of potential disease spread between the thorax and the abdomen.

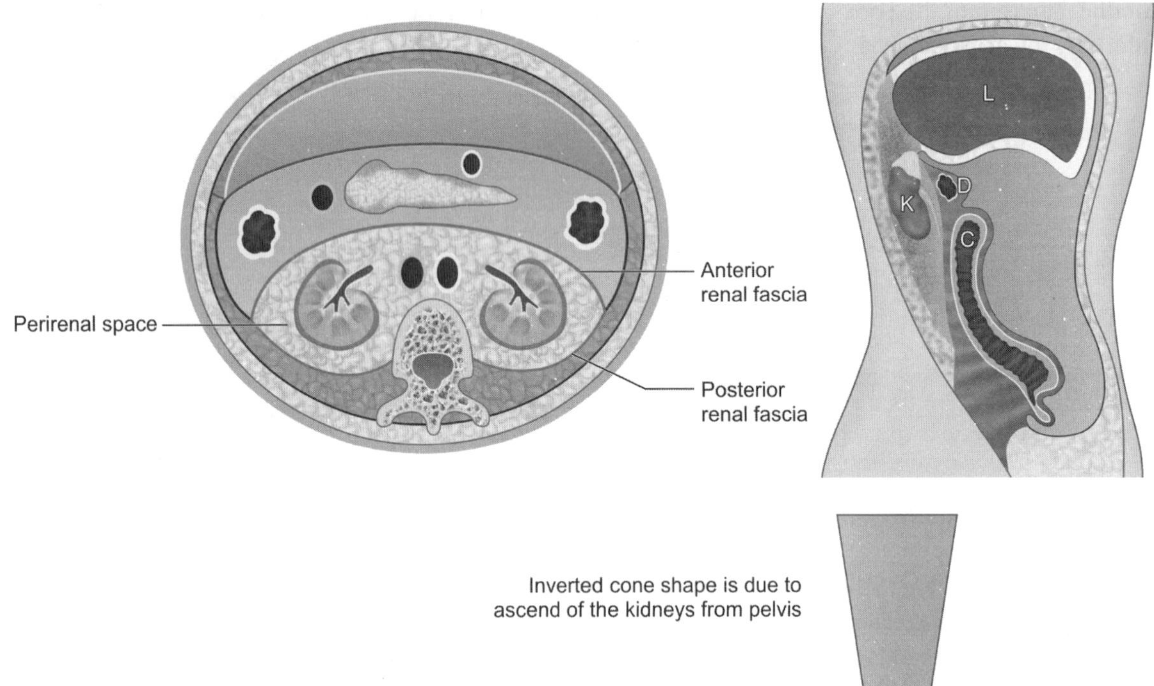

Management of Retroperitoneal Hemorrhage

Radiographic Features

The radiographic features can be variable depending on the stage of the hematoma.

Plain Film—Abdominal Radiograph

Nonspecific but may show:

- Displaced bowel loops
- In case of an aortic aneurysm as the cause, there may be calcification of aortic aneurysm giving obliteration of psoas muscle outline.
- A clue toward the cause in the correct clinical context

US

- Spillage of hemorrhage into the peritoneal cavity can be picked up.
- A large hematoma in the retroperitoneum may be seen.
- May show indirect evidence of displacement of retroperitoneal structures
- The presence of an abdominal aortic aneurysm with periaortic hemorrhage could favor a ruptured aortic aneurysm as the cause.

CT

Retroperitoneal structures have a hazy margin with fluid tracking through the retroperitoneum.

- *Noncontrast:*
  - Acute and subacute hematomas—heterogeneous high attenuation
  - Chronic hematomas—low attenuation
- *CECT*—without dedicated angiography: Well-defined margin in case of a formed hematoma and absence of contrast enhancement

CT Angiography

On angiography, an active bleeding point or the breach in the wall of aneurysm (if it is an underlying cause) may be identified.

MRI–MRA

On MRI, a retroperitoneal hematoma has a variable appearance depending on the stage of the blood. It helps in better assessment as it can distinguish between blood and a neoplasm:

- Acute and subacute stages—hyperintense on T1- and T2-weighted image
- Chronic stage—hypointense is present on T1- and T2-weighted images

Treatment

Management is based on the overall clinical context and vital signs of the patient, the cause, and stage of the hemorrhage.

Medical

Initial medical management involves:

- Correction of coagulation disorders
- Reversal of any anticlotting therapies (e.g., octaplex for warfarin)
- Intravenous fluid resuscitation
- Blood transfusion
- Admission to appropriate level of care [e.g., high dependency unit (HDU) for significant bleeds]

Although no consensus guidelines exist for retroperitoneal hemorrhage, it is accepted that patients with small hematomas or without ongoing bleeding can be managed conservatively.

Interventional Radiology

It was previously thought that spontaneous retroperitoneal hemorrhage is related to microvascular causes which cannot be treated endovascularly. However, endovascular treatments now have a proven role in management, including:

- Stent graft placement
- Arterial embolization
- Chronic hematomas can become infected and are evacuated by percutaneous drainage or surgery. It has a better prognosis compared to that of the acute type.
- Spontaneous retroperitoneal hemorrhage occurs in critically ill patients who are taking anticoagulant or antiplatelet medications, or both.
- Femoral vascular access common etiology of clinically silent, large retroperitoneal hematoma formation
- Traumatic retroperitoneal hematoma can occur after either blunt or penetrating trauma.

Traumatic retroperitoneal hematomas are divided into three anatomic zones:

- *Zone 1:* Centrally located, associated with pancreaticoduodenal injuries or major abdominal vascular injury
- *Zone 2:* Flank or perinephric regions, associated with injuries to the genitourinary system or colon
- *Zone 3:* Pelvic location, frequently associated with pelvic fractures or ileal–femoral vascular injury

Surgery

- Inappropriate surgical evacuation can exacerbate hemorrhage by relieving hematoma-induced tamponade.
- However, active retroperitoneal hemorrhage giving a large intra-abdominal hemoperitoneum can be fatal and can require emergency surgery.

---

14. Retroperitoneal zones in relation to trauma. ***KGMU, Lucknow 2025***

Retroperitoneal Zones in Relation to Trauma

In trauma surgery, especially in *penetrating or blunt abdominal trauma,* the retroperitoneal space is divided into *three anatomical zones* to guide *diagnosis and surgical management.* This classification helps determine *whether exploration is required,* particularly during *laparotomy* for trauma.

What is the Retroperitoneum? The *retroperitoneum* is the space in the abdomen behind the peritoneal cavity. It contains:

- *Vascular structures* (aorta, IVC)
- *Organs:* Kidneys, pancreas, adrenal glands, parts of the duodenum, ascending and descending colon
- *Ureters and lymphatics*

Retroperitoneal Zones

Zone	*Location*	*Contents*	*Clinical relevance*
Zone 1	*Central* (midline) from the diaphragm to the sacrum	Aorta, IVC, pancreas, duodenum (2nd–4th parts), para-aortic lymph nodes	*Always explored* if hematoma is present (due to major vascular injury risk)
Zone 2	*Flanks* (lateral to kidneys, perinephric region)	Kidneys, ureters, colon (ascending and descending), adrenal glands	*Exploration is selective,* depends on stability and mechanism (usually not explored in blunt trauma if stable)
Zone 3	*Pelvis*	Iliac vessels, rectum, pelvic organs, bladder	*Usually not explored* surgically due to difficulty in controlling bleeding and risk of disrupting tamponade—*managed conservatively or with interventional radiology (e.g., embolization)*

Management Principles in Trauma

Zone	*Blunt trauma*	*Penetrating trauma*
Zone 1	Explore	Explore
Zone 2	*No exploration* unless expanding hematoma or signs of renal injury	Selective exploration
Zone 3	*No exploration*—manage with *pelvic binder,* angiographic embolization	Rarely explored—same as blunt

15. Retroperitoneal fibrosis (RPF).

Introduction

- *RPF* (Ormond disease) is a condition that has previously been described as chronic periaortitis. It is an uncommon fibrotic reaction in the retroperitoneum that typically presents with ureteral obstruction.
- The disease is part of a spectrum of entities that have a common pathogenetic process, consisting an inflammatory response to advanced atherosclerosis of the abdominal aorta, combined with autoimmunologic factors:
  - Idiopathic retroperitoneal fibrosis (IRF)
  - Perianeurysmal RPF
  - *Isolated periaortitis:* Corresponds to a nonaneurysmal form of chronic periaortitis
  - Inflammatory abdominal aortic aneurysm (IAAA)

Epidemiology

- RPF is an uncommon condition with a reported estimated incidence of 1.38 cases per 100,000 people.
- The mean age is approximately 64 years with a male-to-female ratio of 3:1.

Etiology

- *Idiopathic:* Ormond disease (70% benign)
- Radiation
- Medication
  - Methyldopa
  - Ergotamine
  - Methysergide (discontinued migraine medication)
- *Inflammation:* Pancreatitis and pyelonephritis
- *Malignant:* Desmoplastic reaction and lymphoma

- Prolonged exposure to asbestos
- Retroperitoneal bleeding, e.g., after trauma or medical procedure

Radiographic Features

- Contrast-enhancing fibrosis involving retroperitoneal structures causing obstruction and displacement of urinary tract and blood vessels.
- *Fluoroscopy: Intravenous urogram (IVU)*—the ureters are classically deviated medially, giving a clear path that deviates from its normal course.
- *CT:* RPF appears as soft tissue and has a similar density to soft tissue. It is usually located around the aorta and/or iliac artery. The lesion does not extend into the arterial or excretory phase and does not invade the ureters or arteries. In almost all cases, there is no growth behind the aorta and the aorta is not displaced. If there is a transition, lymphoma is more likely.
- *MRI:* T1W is usually dark on MRI and T2W unless there is active inflammation, which can make T2W images hyperintense. Pelvic widening and medial deviation of the ureters are common features.
- *Fluorodeoxyglucose (FDG)-positron emission tomography (PET):* Uptake is seen in active inflammation and absent in metabolically inactive disease. Treatment and prognosis.
- RPF can lead to ureteral obstruction and subsequent renal failure. In some cases, perforation of the ureter as a result of obstructions has been described.

Differential Diagnosis: Retroperitoneal lymphoma.

Treatment and Prognosis

- RPF may lead to ureteric obstruction and consequent renal failure.
- In some cases, a blowout of the ureter is described as a result of the obstruction.

16. Describe the pathology, clinical features and treatment of idiopathic retroperitoneal fibrosis. ***WBUHS 2024***

Idiopathic Retroperitoneal Fibrosis (IRF), also known as Ormond's disease, is a rare condition characterized by the presence of fibrous tissue in the retroperitoneum. This fibrous tissue can encase and obstruct surrounding structures, particularly the ureters, leading to a variety of clinical manifestations.

Pathology

- *Fibrosis:* The hallmark of IRF is the deposition of dense, collagenous fibrous tissue within the retroperitoneum. This tissue often encases the abdominal aorta, inferior vena cava, and the ureters. The fibrous tissue may lead to fibrosis-induced obstruction or compression of vital structures.
- *Inflammatory component:* Although the disease is termed "idiopathic," it has been suggested that a chronic inflammatory response plays a role in its development. However, no clear infectious or autoimmune etiology has been identified. In some cases, the fibrotic tissue might have a granulomatous component.
- *Focal vs. diffuse:* In some cases, the fibrosis may be localized to specific areas of the retroperitoneum (such as around the iliac vessels), while in other cases, it may be more diffuse.

Clinical Features

Symptoms of IRF arise primarily from the compression or obstruction of surrounding structures, and they can vary depending on the extent and location of the fibrous tissue.

Renal Symptoms

- *Hydronephrosis:* The most common and significant clinical feature is hydronephrosis, which results from ureteral obstruction. This can lead to flank pain, dull aching in the abdomen, or renal failure if left untreated.
- *Renal dysfunction:* Due to ureteral obstruction or renal parenchymal involvement, patients may develop impaired kidney function or even kidney failure in severe cases.

Pain

- *Abdominal or flank pain:* A frequent presenting symptom, often secondary to obstruction or inflammation.
- *Back pain:* Can be a result of the fibrous tissue impinging on the structures in the lower back and retroperitoneum.

Systemic Symptoms

- *Fatigue, malaise, and weight loss:* These general symptoms can occur due to chronic inflammation or the systemic effects of the disease.
- *Fever:* Some individuals may present with low-grade fever.

Other Manifestations:

- *Vascular compression:* Involvement of the aorta or inferior vena cava can lead to signs of vascular obstruction, including lower limb edema or deep vein thrombosis.
- *Other Organ involvement:* Occasionally, other organs such as the pancreas or bile ducts may be involved due to encroachment by the fibrosis, though this is less common.

Diagnosis:

Imaging:

- *CT scan or MRI:* These are essential for diagnosing IRF. They can identify the characteristic retroperitoneal mass with a fibrous, soft tissue appearance and demonstrate the degree of ureteral obstruction and hydronephrosis.
- *Ultrasound:* May be useful in detecting hydronephrosis but lacks the specificity to confirm fibrosis.

Biopsy: In some cases, a biopsy of the fibrous tissue may be required to rule out other causes of retroperitoneal fibrosis, such as malignancies or infections. Histopathologically, IRF shows dense fibrosis with lymphocytic infiltration and sometimes granulomas.

Laboratory Tests:

- *Kidney function tests:* Elevated creatinine and blood urea nitrogen (BUN) levels may indicate renal impairment.
- *Markers of inflammation:* Elevated ESR (erythrocyte sedimentation rate) and CRP (C-reactive protein) levels may be noted, though these are nonspecific.

Treatment

Treatment of IRF aims to reduce the fibrotic tissue, manage complications, and prevent further organ damage, especially kidney function impairment.

Medical Treatment

- *Corticosteroids:* Prednisone or other corticosteroids are the mainstay of treatment, as they can reduce inflammation and fibrosis. High doses are typically used initially, followed by a gradual taper.
- *Immunosuppressive drugs:* If steroids are ineffective or if there is recurrence, other immunosuppressive agents such as methotrexate, azathioprine, or mycophenolate mofetil may be used.
- *Tamoxifen:* Some studies have suggested that tamoxifen, a selective estrogen receptor modulator, may help reduce the fibrosis in some cases, though it is not a first-line treatment.

Surgical Treatment

- *Ureteral stenting:* To relieve obstruction, ureteral stents or nephrostomy tubes may be placed to bypass the blocked ureters, allowing for drainage of the kidneys and relief of hydronephrosis.
- *Surgical decompression:* In cases where there is significant ureteral or vascular obstruction, surgical intervention may be required to remove the fibrous tissue or relieve the compression.

Management of Complications

- *Kidney failure:* If the patient presents with significant kidney dysfunction or failure, dialysis may be required temporarily until the condition improves with treatment.
- *Renal transplantation:* In rare cases where there is irreversible kidney damage, renal transplantation may be considered.

Monitoring and Follow-up

- Regular follow-up with imaging studies and kidney function tests is essential to monitor for recurrence or progression of the disease.
- Long-term therapy may be necessary to prevent relapse of fibrosis.

---

17. Write a note on chylous ascites. *WBUHS 2023*

---

18. Discuss the etiopathology, diagnosis and treatment of chylous ascites. *WBUHS 2024*

Chylous Ascites: Etiopathology, Diagnosis, and Treatment

Chylous ascites (CA) refers to the accumulation of chyle (a milky fluid containing lymph and emulsified fat) in the peritoneal cavity. This condition arises due to disruption or obstruction of the lymphatic system, leading to leakage of chyle into the abdomen. Chylous ascites is relatively rare but can occur in association with various underlying conditions.

Definition: True chylous ascites is defined as the presence of ascitic fluid with high fat (triglyceride) content, usually higher than 110 mg/dL.

Pathophysiology

Chylous ascites is an uncommon clinical condition that occurs as a result of disruption of the abdominal lymphatics. Multiple causes have been described, including the following:

- Abdominal surgery
- Blunt abdominal trauma
- *Malignant neoplasms:* Hepatoma, small bowel lymphoma, small bowel angiosarcoma, and retroperitoneal lymphoma
- Spontaneous bacterial peritonitis
- *Cirrhosis:* Up to 0.5% of patients with ascites from cirrhosis may have chylous ascites.
- Pelvic irradiation
- Peritoneal dialysis
- Abdominal tuberculosis
- Carcinoid syndrome
- Congenital defects of lacteal formation

Milky ascites is subdivided into three groups as follows:

1. *True chylous ascites:* Fluid with high triglyceride content
2. *Chyliform ascites:* Fluid with a lecithin-globulin complex due to fatty degeneration of cells
3. *Pseudochylous ascites:* Fluid that is milky in appearance due to the presence of pus

Etiopathology of Chylous Ascites

The pathogenesis of chylous ascites revolves around the leakage of chyle into the peritoneal cavity. This can result from various etiologies that affect the lymphatic system. The causes can be broadly classified into *congenital, acquired,* and *miscellaneous* factors:

A. Congenital Causes

- *Congenital lymphatic malformations:*
  - *Milroy disease* and other congenital lymphatic anomalies can lead to defective lymphatic drainage, causing chylous leakage.
  - *Chylous cysts* or *lymphangiomas* can sometimes rupture, leading to chylous ascites.

B. Acquired Causes

- *Trauma:*
  - *Surgical trauma:* Surgery involving the abdomen (especially in the context of cancer resections or lymph node dissections, such as in abdominal, pelvic, or retroperitoneal surgeries) can damage lymphatic vessels and lead to chylous leakage.
  - *Blunt trauma:* Trauma to the abdomen can also rupture lymphatic vessels or the thoracic duct, causing chyle to spill into the abdominal cavity.
- *Infections:*
  - *Tuberculosis (TB):* Abdominal tuberculosis can damage the lymphatic system, particularly in the peritoneum, leading to chylous ascites.
  - *Filariasis:* In tropical regions, *Wuchereria bancrofti* infection leads to lymphatic filariasis, which can cause obstructive chylous ascites due to damage to the lymphatic vessels.
- *Neoplastic diseases:*
  - *Lymphoma* (Hodgkin and non-Hodgkin) is one of the most common cancers associated with chylous ascites.
  - *Gastrointestinal cancers* such as *pancreatic cancer, gastric cancer*, or *colon cancer* can infiltrate the lymphatics and block lymphatic drainage, leading to chylous ascites.
  - *Mesothelioma:* A rare cause associated with pleural or peritoneal malignancies.
- *Lymphatic obstruction or compression:*
  - *Right-sided heart failure, cirrhosis* (especially with portal hypertension), and *renal failure* can increase pressure in the lymphatic system and cause leakage of chyle into the abdominal cavity.
- *Inflammatory or autoimmune disorders:*
  - Conditions like *sarcoidosis* or *systemic lupus erythematosus* (SLE) can cause inflammation and fibrosis of lymphatic vessels, leading to chylous ascites.
- *Idiopathic causes:* In some cases, the cause of chylous ascites cannot be identified despite extensive investigation.

Diagnosis of Chylous Ascites

The diagnosis of chylous ascites is based on clinical suspicion and specific diagnostic tests.

A. Clinical Features

- *Symptoms:*
  - Abdominal distension (due to ascitic fluid accumulation).
  - Weight loss.
  - Fatigue.
  - Mild to moderate hypoproteinemia (due to loss of proteins in the chyle).
- *Complications:*
  - Sepsis is the most common complication, and sudden death has been reported in patients with chylous ascites.
  - The prognosis in adult patients with chylous ascites is poor due to its association with malignancy and severe liver disease.
  - However, pediatric patients and adult patients with postsurgical and posttraumatic chylous ascites have a favorable prognosis.
- *Physical examination:*
  - Abdominal tenderness and signs of peritoneal irritation if there is infection.
  - Fluid wave or shifting dullness suggestive of ascites.

B. Laboratory Tests

- *Ascitic fluid analysis:*

- *Milky appearance* of the fluid is a hallmark of chylous ascites.
- *Triglyceride levels:* The ascitic fluid triglyceride concentration is typically greater than 110 mg/dL (this is a key diagnostic criterion for chylous ascites).
- *Chylomicrons:* The presence of chylomicrons in the ascitic fluid can confirm the diagnosis of chylous ascites.
- *Cell count and culture:* Exclude infection, and check for white blood cell count to assess inflammation (e.g., in cases of TB or bacterial infections).

- *Other ascites tests include the following:*
  - Specific gravity is 1.010–1.054.
  - Total fat content is 4–40 g/L.
  - Glucose and amylase levels usually are normal.
  - Cholesterol level usually is low.
  - Leukocyte count generally is high, from 232 to 2560 cells/mm^3, usually with a marked lymphocytic predominance.
  - Total protein content varies from 1.4–6.4 g/dL, with a mean of 3.7 g/dL.
  - This variation reflects changes in serum proteins and dietary habits.
  - Microbiologic cultures usually are negative
- *Serum triglycerides:* Serum triglycerides may also be elevated but are generally less useful than ascitic fluid analysis.
- *Lymphoscintigraphy:* This imaging technique can be used to track the flow of lymphatic fluid and identify the site of leakage or obstruction in the lymphatic system.
- *CT/MRI Imaging:*
  - *Abdominal CT* or *MRI* may reveal underlying causes, such as lymphatic obstruction, tumors, or lymphatic malformations.
  - *MRI lymphangiography* or *contrast-enhanced CT* can help locate lymphatic leakage or blockage.
- *Thoracic duct catheterization:* A diagnostic technique used to directly visualize and sample lymphatic fluid from the thoracic duct to confirm the source of the chyle.

TREATMENT OF CHYLOUS ASCITES

Treatment of chylous ascites is focused on addressing the underlying cause and managing the chyle leak. The approach can be conservative or surgical, depending on the severity and the cause of the condition.

A. Conservative Management

- *Dietary modifications:*
  - *Medium-chain triglyceride (MCT) diet:* MCTs are absorbed directly into the portal circulation, bypassing the lymphatic system. This diet is often the first-line therapy for managing chylous ascites, especially in cases associated with lymphatic disruption.
  - *Fat restriction:* A low-fat diet may help reduce the volume of chyle produced and ease the burden on the lymphatic system.
- *Drainage:*
  - *Paracentesis:* For symptomatic relief of ascites, especially if fluid accumulation is significant. However, repeated paracentesis is not a long term solution.
- *Octreotide: Somatostatin analogs* (like octreotide) may be used in some cases to reduce lymphatic fluid production, though their efficacy in chylous ascites remains variable.
- *Nutritional support:* Adequate nutritional support is critical in managing chylous ascites, as it can lead to malnutrition due to the loss of protein and fat. Total parenteral nutrition (TPN) may be required in refractory cases.

B. Surgical Treatment

- *Lymphatic fistula repair:*
  - If the underlying cause is a surgically correctable abnormality, such as a lymphatic duct injury or fistula, surgical repair may be required.
  - *Ligation or embolization* of the leaking lymphatic vessels or thoracic duct can be effective, especially in cases due to trauma or surgical injury.
- *Lymphatic bypass or bowel resection:* In cases where there is extensive lymphatic obstruction or malformation, surgical bypass of the obstructed lymphatic system may be necessary.
- *Peritoneovenous shunt:* In cases where the ascites is refractory to treatment and the cause cannot be corrected, peritoneovenous shunting may be used to drain ascitic fluid into the venous circulation.
- *Thoracic duct embolization:* In cases related to a leak in the thoracic duct, thoracic duct embolization using materials like coils or glue may be performed.

CHAPTER 29

Lymphoma

LEARNING OBJECTIVES

- Staging Laparotomy in Lymphomas
- Gastric Lymphoma
- Non-Hodgkin's lymphoma

1. Current status of staging laparotomy in lymphomas. *WBUHS 2011*

Introduction

- Advances in the treatment of Hodgkin's disease have transformed a once-fatal disease into a highly curable one.
- Disease stage remains the principal determinant of therapy, with early-stage patients (I–II) treated primarily with radiotherapy and advanced-stage patients (III–IV) receiving combination chemotherapy or combined-modality therapy.

Ann Arbor Staging for Lymphoma

Stage I:

Either of the following means the disease is stage I:

- The lymphoma is in only one lymph node area or lymphoid organ, such as the thymus (I).
- The cancer is found only in 1 area of a single organ outside of the lymph system (IE).

Stage II:

Either of the following means the disease is stage II:

- The lymphoma is in two or more groups of lymph nodes on the same side of (above or below) the diaphragm (the thin band of muscle that separates the chest and abdomen), for example, this might include nodes in the underarm and neck area but not the combination of underarm and groin nodes (II).
- The lymphoma extends from a single group of lymph node(s) into a nearby organ (IIE). It may also affect other groups of lymph nodes on the same side of the diaphragm.

Stage III:

Either of the following means the disease is stage III:

- The lymphoma is found in lymph node areas on both sides of (above and below) the diaphragm.
- The cancer may also have spread into an area or organ next to the lymph nodes (IIIE), into the spleen (IIIS), or both (IIISE).

Stage IV:

Either of the following means the disease is stage IV:

- The lymphoma has spread outside of the lymph system into an organ that is not right next to an involved node.
- The lymphoma has spread to the bone marrow, liver, brain or spinal cord, or the pleura (thin lining of the lungs).

The Role of Staging Laparotomy in Lymphoma

Staging laparotomy remains the gold standard for evaluating microscopic disease in the abdomen, including the spleen and liver.

- From its introduction, staging laparotomy was intended only for patients in whom radiation therapy (RT) potentially could be the sole therapeutic modality.
- Surgical staging allows treatment to be chosen with specific knowledge regarding the extent of the disease.
- Patients who prove to have pathologic early-stage disease in the absence of bulky mediastinal lymphadenopathy may be treated safely with radiation alone with an anticipated disease-free survival (DFS) of >75% for pathologic stage IA and IIA (PS IA-IIA) disease.
- Furthermore, pathologic staging may permit the use of smaller radiation fields. In a group of patients with pathologic early-stage disease and other favorable prognostic factors (such as young age and nodular sclerosis or lymphocyte-predominant histology), mantle field irradiation alone may be sufficient. In those patients who still require subdiaphragmatic irradiation after laparotomy, splenectomy allows delivery of a smaller dose to the abdomen without jeopardizing the left kidney and lung base.
- Despite these attractive advantages, compelling reasons exist to avoid surgical staging. A laparotomy delays by at least 2–3 weeks the implementation of therapy, as the patient recuperates after a 5–7-day hospitalization. While laparoscopic splenectomy may shorten the recuperative period, this procedure does not afford the full nodal examination that can be obtained with the open procedure.
- Staging laparotomy has associated morbidity and mortality. Published mortality rates range from 0.3 to 1%, but should not represent a major concern at most centers.
    - Morbidity poses the greater threat. Major complications include cardiac arrest, wound infection or dehiscence, postoperative hemorrhage, subphrenic abscess, pulmonary embolism, pneumonia, sepsis, and small bowel obstruction from adhesions.
    - Minor complications include postoperative atelectasis, urinary tract infections, urinary retention, and prolonged ileus.

---

2. Gastric lymphoma.

Introduction

- About 30% of the patients with non-Hodgkin lymphoma (NHL) present as extranodal disease
- Gastrointestinal (Gl) tract is the most common site of presentation
- Within the GI tract, the stomach is the most common site (65%), small intestine (18%), and colon and rectum (15%)
- The liver, gallbladder, and pancreas collectively account for only 2%.
- The overall survival with treatment for extranodal NHL, Including NHL of the Gl tract, is similar to that for nodal NHL
- 90% of primary gastrointestinal non-Hodgkin's lymphoma (PGINHL) is of B-cell lineage
- Diffuse large B cell lymphoma (DLBCL) comprises approximately 60% of PGINHL
- Mucosa-associated lymphoid tissue (MALT) lymphoma, primarily occurring in the stomach compromises 30%
- Only T-cell PGINHL of significance—enteropathy-associated T-cell lymphoma (ETL) (5%)

Risk Factors

- *Helicobacter pylori* infection
- Immunosuppression after solid organ transplantation
- Celiac disease
- Epstein–Barr viral infection
- Inflammatory bowel disease
- Human immunodeficiency virus (HIV) infection

Diffuse Large B-cell Lymphoma

- Most common histologic subtype of PGINHL
- 50% of primary gastric lymphomas
- 30–50% of primary gastric DLBCLs have components of MALT lymphoma
- Germ-center subtypes:
  - *BCL2* gene (114,181) and amplification of REL/chromosome 2p
  - Down-regulation of NF-κB
- *Activated B-cell subtypes:* Upregulation of NF-κB
- DLBCL is frequently the result of a mutation in *BCL6*
  - Associated with longer disease-free survival
  - The neoplastic cells are of B-cell phenotype, expressing pan B-cell antigens (CD19, CD20, CD22, and CD79a)
  - The typical immunophenotype is $CD20^{+}$, $CD45^{+}$, and CD_3^{-}

Mucosa-associated Lymphoid Tissue Lymphoma

- 50% of all primary lymphomas of the stomach
- *H. pylori* infection—90% in patients with MALT lymphoma
- Divided into *H. pylori* positive or negative
- *H. pylori*-negative MALT lymphomas have a higher positive rate for t(11;18)(q21;q21) translocation t(11;18)—aggressive behavior

Enteropathy-associated T-cell Lymphoma

- 5% of PGINHL
- Most often in the jejunum but may affect multiple segments of small intestine refractory celiac disease (not responding >12 months)
- Refractory celiac disease (RCD) presents as an exacerbation with abdominal pain, diarrhea, and weight loss
- De novo—presents acutely as Gl perforation, obstruction, or hemorrhage
- ETL has a poor prognosis (<30% of patients alive at a 2-year follow-up)
- ETL that occurs in the setting of RCD has a worse prognosis
- DRCD—classified based on intraepithelial lymphocyte (IEL)
- *Type II:*
  - Involves a clonal expansion of abnormal IELs
  - Evolves into ETL in 60–80% of the cases

Role of Surgery

- Acute obstruction, intussusception, Gl bleed, or perforation as the presenting symptom of a GI lymphoma
- It is not necessary to achieve microscopically negative margins.
- As an unexpected finding
- Establishing diagnosis
- Rare instance of bleeding or perforation in a patient receiving antineoplastic therapy

Clinical Workup

- Immunophenotyping with a panel of immunohistochemical (IHC) stains including CD20, CD3, CD5, CD10, CD45, BCL2, BCL6, Ki-67, IRF/MUM1, and MYC with or without cell surface marker CD45, CD3, CD5, CD19, CD10, and CD20 for suspected DLBCL.
- For suspected MALT lymphoma, IHC for CD21 or CD23 and for cyclin D1 (CCND1) should be added.
- If a diagnosis of lymphoma is suspected clinically and/or on a frozen section of surgical biopsy but is not definitively established, fresh and nonfixed tissue is set aside.
- Hepatitis B surface antigen (HBsAg) testing (rituximab reactivates)
- Multigated acquisition (MUGA) scan or echocardiogram: If an anthracycline-based chemotherapy regimen is needed.

Staging

Lugano Staging System for Gastric Lymphoma

Stage	Description
I	Tumor confined to GI tract
IE1	Involvement of mucosa +/– submucosa
IE2	Involvement of muscularis propria +/– serosa
II	Tumor extension into the abdomen
II1	Involvement of local nodes (paragastric for gastric lymphoma)
II2	Involvement of local nodes (paraaortic, paracaval, pelvic, or inguinal)
IIE	Serosa penetration involves adjacent organs/tissues
IV	Disseminated extranodal involvement or supradiaphragmatic nodal involvement

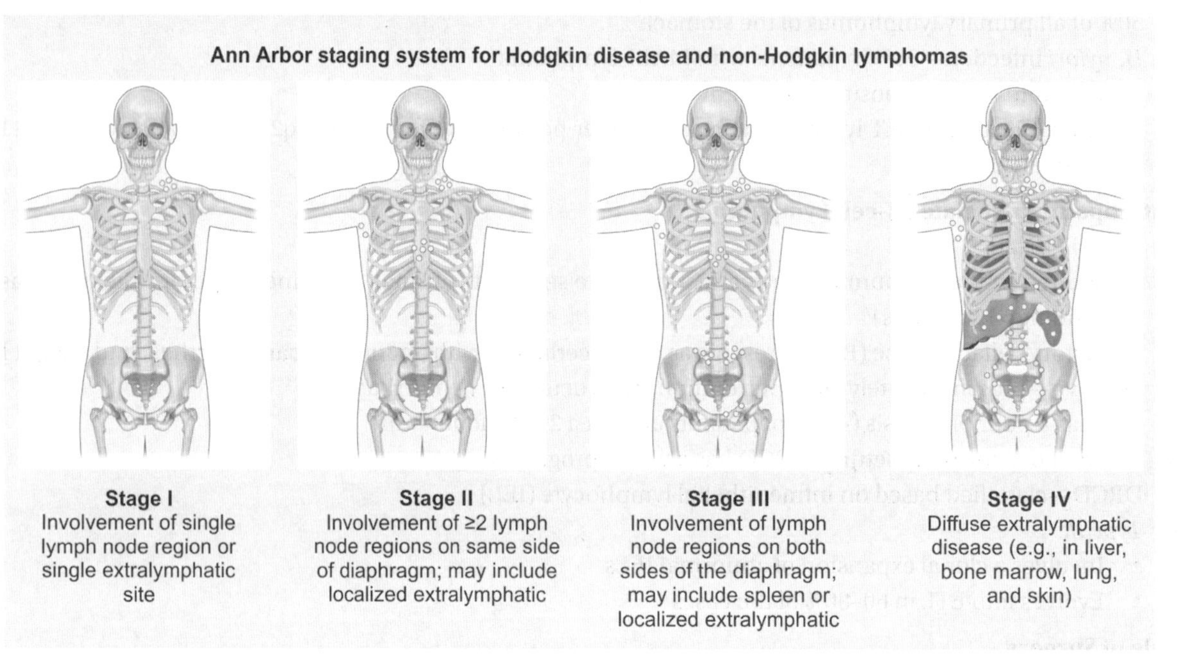

Treatment—MALT Lymphoma

- MALT lymphoma of GI or pulmonary origin had inferior survival compared to MALT lymphoma arising in ocular, cutaneous, or endocrine sites a molecular analysis for t(11:18) by fluorescence in situ hybridization (FISH) or polymerase chain reaction (PCR) is recommended—does not respond to *H. pylori* treatment, aggressive
  - *IE1, IE2, or IIE in patients who are H. pylori positive: H. pylori* eradication and endoscopy at 3 months
  - *H. pylori-negative and lymphoma-free at 3 months:* Continue observation
  - *H. pylori* persists second-line antibiotic treatment is given
  - *H. pylori is eradicated but lymphoma persists:* No clinical symptoms, observation can continue with repeat endoscopy in 3 months
  - Progressive or symptomatic disease: RT [30 gray (Gy)] along with second-line antibiotic treatment if *H. pylori* persists
  - *H. pylori*-positive but also t(11:18) positive:
    - Symptomatic-antibiotic therapy for eradication of infection and involved site radiation therapy (ISRT) or rituximab if ISRT is contraindicated
    - IE disease and asymptomatic: Initial trial of antibiotic therapy only and close

Follow-up

- IE or IIE who are *H. pylori*-negative:
  - ISRT (or rituximab if ISRT is contraindicated)
  - Follow-up endoscopy 3 months after RT with rebiopsy
- *Stage IV disease requiring treatment:* Rituximab cyclophosphamide, doxorubicin, vincristine, and prednisone (RCHOP)
- *Nongastric MALT lymphoma:* ISRT
- MALT lymphoma with concurrent large cell transformation principles for DLBCL

Treatment—DLBCL

- Ann Arbor stages I or II disease:
  - Standard first-line therapy is six cycles of RCHOP
  - Addition of ISRT for bulky disease (defined as >7.5 cm in maximal diameter)
- *Nonbulky:* Three cycles of RCHOP plus RT or six cycles of RCHOP without radiation
- *Double-hit DLBCL (MYC rearrangement in addition to BCL2 or BCL6 rearrangement):*
  - Inferior outcomes with RCHOP
  - More intense regimens, such as dose-adjusted etoposide, prednisone, vincristine, cyclophosphamide, doxorubicin, and rituximab (DA-EPOCH-R)
- *Higher-stage disease (Ann Arbor III and IV):* Clinical trial or high-dose therapy with autologous stem cell rescue

Evolving Therapies

- Ibrutinib—an irreversible inhibitor of Bruton tyrosine kinase, an important constituent of the B-cell receptor pathway (BCRP)
- Idelalisib (BCRP)
- Obinutuzumab—anti-CD20
- Pidilizumab, pembrolizumab, and nivolumab—anti-programmed cell death ligand 1 (anti-PDL1)

---

3. Discuss clinical features, staging and management of Non-Hodgkin's lymphoma. ***WBUHS 2011***

Clinical Features

- The clinical manifestations of non-Hodgkin lymphoma (NHL) vary with such factors as the location of the lymphomatous process, the rate of tumor growth, and the function of the organ being compromised or displaced by the malignant process.
- The Working Formulation classification groups the subtypes of NHL by clinical behavior—that is, low-grade, intermediate-grade, and high-grade.

Low-grade lymphomas:

- Peripheral adenopathy that is painless and slowly progressive is the most common clinical presentation in these patients.
- Spontaneous regression of enlarged lymph nodes can occur in low-grade lymphoma, potentially causing confusion with an infectious condition.
- Primary extranodal involvement and B symptoms (i.e., temperature >38°C, night sweats, weight loss >10% from baseline within 6 months) are not common at presentation, but they are common in patients with advanced, malignant transformation (i.e., evolution from a low-grade to an intermediate- or high-grade lymphoma) or end-stage disease.
- Bone marrow is frequently involved and may be associated with cytopenia.
- Fatigue and weakness are more common in patients with advanced-stage disease.

Intermediate- and high-grade lymphomas:

- These types of lymphomas cause a more varied clinical presentation.

- Most patients present with adenopathy.
- More than one third of patients present with extranodal involvement; the most common sites are the gastrointestinal (GI) tract (including the Waldeyer ring), skin, bone marrow, sinuses, genitourinary (GU) tract, thyroid, and central nervous system (CNS).
- B-symptoms are more common, occurring in approximately 30–40% of patients.
- Lymphoblastic lymphoma, a high-grade lymphoma, often manifests with an anterior superior mediastinal mass, superior vena cava (SVC) syndrome, and leptomeningeal disease with cranial nerve palsies.
- Patients with Burkitt lymphoma (occurring in the United States) often present with a large abdominal mass and symptoms of bowel obstruction. Obstructive hydronephrosis secondary to bulky retroperitoneal lymphadenopathy obstructing the ureters can also be observed in these patients.
- Primary CNS lymphomas are high-grade neoplasms of B-cell origin. Most lymphomas originating in the CNS are large cell lymphomas or immunoblastomas, and they account for 1% of all intracranial neoplasms. These lymphomas are more commonly observed in patients who are immunodeficient because of conditions such as Wiskott-Aldrich syndrome, transplantation, or AIDS.
    - Cotswolds-modified Ann Arbor classification:
        - *Stage I:* One nodal group or lymphoid organ (e.g., Spleen or thymus)
            - *Stage IE:* One extranodal site
        - *Stage II:* Two or more nodal groups, same side of diaphragm
            - *Stage IIE:* localized extranodal site with stage II criteria, both on the same side of the diaphragm
        - *Stage III:* Nodal groups on both sides of the diaphragm
            - *Stage IIIS (1):* With splenic involvement
            - *Stage IIIE (2):* With localized extranodal site
            - *Stage IIISE:* Both
        - *Stage IV:* Disseminated involvement of one or more extralymphatic organ (e.g. Lung, bone) +/– any nodal involvement

Additional Staging Variables

- *A:* Asymptomatic
- *B:* Presence of B symptoms (fever, night sweats and weight loss)
- *X:* Bulky nodal disease—nodal mass >1/3rd of intrathoracic diameter or 10 cm in dimension

Treatment

The treatment of non-Hodgkin lymphoma (NHL) varies greatly, depending on the following factors:

- Tumor stage
- Phenotype (B-cell, T-cell or natural killer [NK] cell/null-cell)
- Histology (i.e., low-, intermediate-, or high-grade)
- Symptoms
- Performance status
- Patient age
- Comorbidities
    - Most of the chemotherapy for NHL, whether combination or single-drug, can be administered in an outpatient setting, at an infusion clinic.
    - Growth factor support (e.g., granulocyte-colony stimulating factor [GCSF], granulocyte macrophage–colony stimulating factor [GM-CSF], erythropoietin) is also administered in an outpatient treatment setting.
    - Infusional chemotherapy (e.g., infusional cyclophosphamide, doxorubicin, and etoposide [CDE], which should be administered continuously for 4 days) should be administered as inpatient treatment.
    - High-dose chemotherapy and bone marrow and/or stem cell transplantation are administered in an inpatient setting of a tertiary hospital with an approved transplant center.

- For the initial treatment of patients with intermediate- or high-grade lymphoma and patients with bulky disease, an inpatient setting is recommended in order to monitor for tumor lysis syndrome and to manage appropriately.
- Admit patients with NHL for complications of disease progression (e.g., pain control for intractable pain) or adverse effects from chemotherapy (e.g., dehydration secondary to diarrhea, vomiting requiring IV hydration, severe mucositis).
- Patients with fever during neutropenia should be admitted for broad-spectrum antibiotic therapy.

Treatment Options

Many effective treatment options exist for NHL patients, including:

- Active surveillance (also known as watchful waiting)
- Chemotherapy
- Radiation therapy
- Stem cell transplantation
- Novel targeted agents
- Newer versions of established agents
  - The form of treatment chosen depends on the type of lymphoma and the stage of disease, as well as other factors including age, prior therapies received and the patient's overall health.
  - Some patients may relapse (disease returns after treatment) or become refractory (disease does not respond to treatment).
  - However, numerous treatment options exist for patients with relapsed or refractory NHL, which are often referred to as secondary therapies.
  - Many of the novel therapeutic agents that have been approved by the United States Food and Drug Administration, as well as those being investigated in clinical trials, focus specifically on those with relapsed or refractory disease.

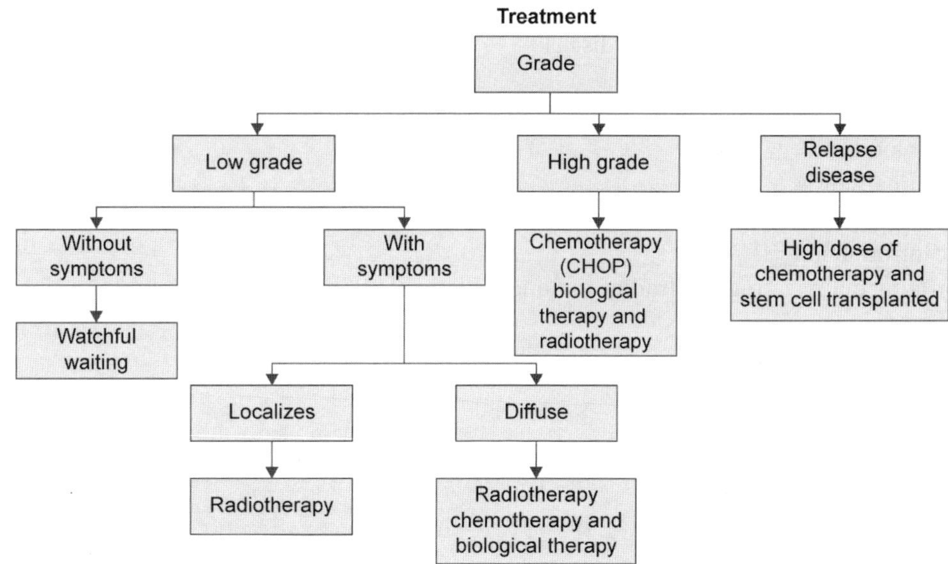

Surgical Diseases of Liver

LEARNING OBJECTIVES

- Pyogenic Liver Abscess and Amebic Liver Abscess
- Hydatid Disease of Liver
- Hepatic Segments and Liver Resection
- Primary and Secondary Hepatic Malignancies
- Space-occupying Lesions (SOLs) Liver

LIVER ABSCESS

1. Pyogenic liver abscess trend of management. ***WBUHS 2021***

Causes

- Biliary disease (most common)
  e.g., stones and cholangiocarcinoma
- Colonic disease
  e.g., diverticulitis, appendicitis, Crohn's disease
- Cryptogenic disease
- Pancreatitis
- Infection of blood
- Intra-abdominal sepsis
- Infection of biliary system
- Traumatic introduction
  e.g., penetrating injury, iatrogenic [radiofrequency ablation (RFA)]

Common Bacterial Causes

- *Streptococcus milleri*
- *Escherichia coli (E. coli)*
- *Streptococcus faecalis*
- Klebsiella pneumonia
- *Proteus vulgaris*
- *Bacteroides*
- Opportunistic pathogens (*Staphylococcus*)

Diagnosis

- Blood ceruloplasmin (CP) (no leukocytosis)
- Hemoglobin estimation (anemia)
- Serum albumin levels (falls rapidly)
- Ultrasonography (USG) and computed tomography (CT) scanning
- Guided aspiration to confirm the diagnosis

Treatment

- An untreated hepatic abscess is nearly uniformly fatal as a result of complications that include sepsis, empyema, or peritonitis from rupture into the pleural or peritoneal spaces and retroperitoneal extension.
- Treatment should include drainage—either percutaneous or surgical.

Medical Care

- Antibiotic therapy as a sole treatment modality is not routinely advocated, though it has been successful in a few reported cases.
- Antimicrobial treatment is a common adjunct to percutaneous or surgical drainage.

Surgical Treatment

- Surgical drainage was the standard of care until the introduction of percutaneous drainage. With the refinement of image-guided techniques, percutaneous drainage and aspiration have become the standard of care.
- Current indications for the surgical treatment of pyogenic liver abscess are for the treatment of:
  - Underlying intra-abdominal processes, including signs of peritonitis
  - Existence of a known abdominal surgical pathology (e.g., diverticular abscess); failure of previous drainage attempts
  - The presence of a complicated, multiloculated, thick-walled abscess with viscous pus
  - Shock with multisystem organ failure is a contraindication for surgery.

Open surgery can be performed by either of the following two approaches:

- A transperitoneal approach allows for abscess drainage and abdominal exploration to identify previously undetected abscesses and the location of an etiologic source.
- For high posterior lesions, a posterior transpleural approach can be used; although this affords easier access to the abscess, the identification of multiple lesions or a concurrent intra-abdominal pathology is lost.

A laparoscopic approach is also commonly used in select cases. This minimally invasive approach affords the opportunity to explore the entire abdomen and to significantly reduce patient morbidity.
Postoperative complications are not uncommon and include recurrent pyogenic liver abscess, intra-abdominal abscess, hepatic or renal failure, and wound infection.

---

2. Amebic liver abscess. ***DNB, June 2018***

Introduction

Amebic liver abscess is caused by the parasitic protozoan *Entamoeba histolytica (E. histolytica).*

Etiology

- Two species of ameba infect humans. *Entamoeba dispar (E. dispar)* is associated with an asymptomatic carrier state.
- *E. histolytica* is not only responsible for all forms of invasive disease.
- The life cycle involves cysts, invasive trophozoites, and fecally contaminated food or water to initiate the infection.
- Fecal-oral transmission occurs; the cyst passes through the stomach into the intestine unscathed, and then pancreatic enzymes start to digest the outer cyst wall.
- The trophozoite is then released into the intestine and multiplies there.
- Normally, no invasion occurs and the patient develops amebic dysentery alone or becomes an asymptomatic carrier.
- In a small number of cases, the trophozoite invades through the intestinal mucosa, travels through the mesenteric lymphatics and veins, and begins to accumulate in the hepatic parenchyma, forming an abscess cavity.
- Liquefied hepatic parenchyma with blood and debris gives a characteristic "anchovy paste" appearance to the abscess.

Symptoms
• Pain • Fever • Nausea and vomiting • Anorexia • Weight loss • Malaise • Diarrhea • Cough or pleurisy • Pruritus
Signs
• Hepatomegaly • Right upper quadrant tenderness • Pleural effusion or rub • Right upper quadrant mass • Ascites • Jaundice
Laboratory data
• Increased alkaline phosphatase • WBC count >10,000/mm^3 • Hematocrit <36% • Albumin <3 g/dL • Bilirubin >2 mg/dL

Diagnosis

- Blood culture
- Hemoglobin estimation
- Stool examination (trophozoites and cysts)
- Radiography
- Aspiration
- USG and CT scan
- Sigmoidoscopy
- Liver function tests
- Serological tests

Distinguishing Clinical Characteristics of Patients with Hepatic Abscesses

Amebic	***Pyogenic***
Age <50 years	Age >50 years
Male:female ratio 10:1	Male:female ratio 1:1
Hispanic descent	No ethnic predisposition
Recent travel to endemic area	Malignancy
Pulmonary dysfunction	High fevers
Abdominal pain	Pruritus
Diarrhea	Jaundice
Abdominal tenderness	Septic shock
Hepatomegaly	Palpable mass

Management

- Metronidazole 800 mg TDS for 5–10 days
- Aspiration
- Repeated imaging of liver

Complications

- Complications from amoebic abscesses occur secondary to rupture of the abscess into the peritoneum, pleural cavity, or pericardium.
- Extrahepatic sites also have been described in the lung, brain, skin, and genitourinary tract, presumably from hematogenous spread.
- Ruptured amoebic liver abscesses are associated with mortality rates up to 50%.

HYDATID DISEASE OF LIVER

3. Hydatid cyst of the liver. ***AIIMS, Patna 2025; NTRUHS, Vijayawada 2025***

4. Discuss the clinical features, diagnosis and treatment for hepatic hydatid disease. ***WBUHS 2016***

5. Discuss diagnosis and management of hydatid cyst in liver. ***RIMS, Imphal 2022***

6. Write down the management of hydatid cyst in liver. ***WBUHS 2009, 2023***

Introduction

Hydatid disease is a zoonotic parasitic disease most frequently caused by *Echinococcus granulosus* and the liver is the most commonly involved organ in two thirds of patients.

Clinical Features

- After infection with *Echinococcus granulosus*, humans are usually asymptomatic for a long time.
- The growth of the cyst in the liver is variable, ranging from 1–5 mm in diameter per year.
- Most primary infections consist of a single cyst, but up to 20–40% of infected people have multiple cysts.
- The symptoms depend not only on the size and number of cysts but also on the mass effect within the organ and upon surrounding structures.

Noncomplicated Cysts

- Hydatid cyst of the liver is frequently silent and only diagnosed incidentally during abdominal investigation for other pathology.
- The clinical signs appear gradually with the increase volume of the cyst.
- The most common symptom, when it occurs, is right upper quadrant or epigastric pain and the most common findings on examination are an enlarged liver and a palpable mass.
- Pressure effects are initially vague. They may include nonspecific pain, cough, low-grade fever, and the sensation of abdominal fullness.
- As the mass grows, the symptoms become more specific because the mass impinges on or obstructs specific organs.

Complicated Cysts

- Patients may also present with complications of the cyst such as biliary communication, intraperitoneal rupture (spontaneous or post-traumatic) and, rarely, intrathoracic or intrapericardial rupture.
- Cyst rupture can be associated with anaphylaxis secondary to the highly antigenic content of the cyst fluid or may be silent and present with multiple intraperitoneal cysts.
- With secondary infection, tender hepatomegaly, chills, and spiking temperatures occur.
- Urticaria and erythema occur in cases of generalized anaphylactic reaction.
- With biliary rupture, the classic triad of jaundice, biliary colic, and urticaria occurs.

Diagnosis

It is based on careful history, imaging and serology, and a high index of suspicion in at-risk population.

Laboratory Tests

- Alkaline phosphatase (ALP) and gamma-glutamyl transferase (GGT) can be mildly elevated in one third of patients.
- Elevated bilirubin (>1 mg/dL) and increased ALP are symptoms of cystobiliary communication.
- WBC are elevated only if cyst has become secondarily infected.
- Serum immunoglobulin (I g) levels are elevated in 31% of patients.

Imaging

- USG and CT are standard investigation for diagnosis, percutaneous treatment, and post-treatment follow-up of hydatid cysts
  - USG is the preferred first-line imaging followed by CT which gives more precise information regarding morphology of cyst, including size, location, number and relationship to adjacent structures.
  - Hydatid cysts appear as well-defined, circumscribed cystic lesions with clear membrane
  - Cysts are staged according to content patterns
  - The *World Health Organization (WHO)* introduced a standardized classification of USG images of cystic echinococcosis to obtain comparable results in patients worldwide and to link disease status with each morphological type of hydatid cysts:

Cyst type	*Status*	*USG features*
CL	Active	Signs not pathognomonic, unilocular, no cyst wall
CE1	Active	Cyst wall, hydatid sand
CE2	Active	Multivesicular, cyst wall, rosette-like
CE3	Transitional	Detached laminated membrane, water lily sign
CE4	Inactive	Heterogenous, hypo/hyperechoic contents
CE5	Inactive	Thick, calcified wall, no daughter cysts

Gharbi Classification on USG Features of Hydatid Cyst

Type	*USG appearance*
I	Pure fluid collection
II	Fluid collection with split wall (detached membrane)
III	Fluid collection with septa and/or daughter cysts
IV	Heterogenous echo pattern (hyperechoic with high internal echoes)
V	Reflecting walls (cyst with reflecting calcified thick wall)

- *CT scan:*
  - Multidetector row CT has the highest sensitivity of imaging of the cyst (100%).
  - It is the best mode to detect the number, size, and location of the cysts. It may provide clues to presence of complications such as infection and intrabiliary ruptures.
  - It is also helpful in identifying exogenous cysts and the volume of the cyst can be estimated.
  - CT is an important investigation when there is a diagnostic uncertainty on ultrasound (type I and IV of Gharbi), when planning surgical intervention or when recurrent disease is diagnosed.
  - In case of peritoneal hydatidosis, CT scan is indicated before surgery to assess the number and the exact localizations of the cysts. In case of ruptures in the thorax, the CT scan allows a better study of the lung parenchyma and ensures a percutaneous drainage of the pleural collection.

- *Magnetic resonance imaging (MRI):*
  - MRI delineates the cyst capsule better than CT scan as a low intensity on both T1- and T2-weighted images.
  - However, CT scan is better in demonstrating mural calcifications; cysts <3 cm may not show any specific features and small peritoneal cysts may be missed.
- *Endoscopic retrograde cholangiopancreatography (ERCP):*
  - *ERCP* remains an important tool in cases where a rupture into the biliary tree has occurred, allowing both the diagnosis of major biliary communication and clearance of the common bile duct (CBD) prior to surgery or intervention by the means of sphincterotomy.
- *Direct cholangiography:*
  - Intraoperative cholangiography is performed through a cystic drain or a T Tube in a suspected intrabiliary rupture and bile duct obstruction.
  - This method is used to detect postoperative complications following surgery.

Serology is used for:

- Differential diagnosis of a cystic liver mass
- Epidemiological surveillance
- Post-treatment follow-up

The sensitivity and specificity of tests depend on quality of antigens.

Immunoelectrophoresis

The diagnostic value ranges from 91 to 94% for hepatic cysts. It is used for post-treatment follow-up.

Enzyme-linked Immunosorbent Assay (ELISA)

- Sensitivities range from 64 to 100% depending on antigens used.
- IgG remains positive for 4 years after treatment, so it is not suitable for follow-up.
- IgM has been reported to be negative after 6 months of treatment.

Blotting

- Allows molecular weight analysis of antigens detected by patient's serum.
- Western blotting used in diagnosis and post-treatment follow-up.

Treatment Options

- Surgery
- Percutaneous aspiration
- Medical treatment
- *Conservative management:* Asymptomatic and small (<5 cm) cysts can be followed-up with wait-and-see policy. Also, densely calcified hydatid cysts are accepted as dead cysts and can be monitored without any specific therapy.

Surgical Treatment

- *Types:*
  - *Conservative:* Involves inactivation of protoscolices and removal of cyst contents—cystectomy
  - *Radical:* Includes total excision of cyst and pericyst layers along with portion of surrounding liver—pericystectomy/liver resection
  - The rapid development of laparoscopic techniques has encouraged surgeons to replicate principles of conventional hydatid surgery using a minimally invasive approach.

  The criteria to exclude laparoscopic treatment of hydatid cyst of liver are:

  - Rupture of the cyst in biliary tract
  - Central localization of the cyst
  - Cysts dimension >15 cm

- Number of cysts >3
- Thickened or calcified walls
- Opening of bile ducts that leak bile

- *The principles of liver hydatid surgery include:*
  - Inactivation of protoscolices within cyst fluid
  - Evacuation of cyst contents
  - Prevention of spillage of cyst contents
  - Secure closure of any cystobiliary communication
  - Management of residual cyst cavity
- *Postoperative complications:*
  - Biliary fistula
  - Biliary stricture
  - Recurrence

Percutaneous Aspiration

- *Indications:*
  - Univesicular cysts
  - Univesicular cysts with detached membrane
  - Some multiple cysts
- *Contraindications:*
  - Inaccessible to puncture
  - Cysts in which puncture may damage important vascular structures
  - Peripheral cysts that do not have sufficient layer of hepatic tissue to promote safe transhepatic puncture
  - Cysts that have ruptured into bile duct, peritoneum, or pleural space
- *Techniques:*
  - PAIR (puncture, aspiration, injection, and reaspiration)
  - Catheterization technique
  - PEVAC (percutaneous evacuation of cyst content)

Chemotherapy

There are four objectives of medical treatment:

- Definite cure
- Reduction in cyst viability
- Preoperative treatment
- Perioperative prophylaxis
  - Perioperative prophylaxis should start 1 week before the procedure.
  - Post-treatment prophylaxis—3–8 weeks for uncomplicated cases and 3–6 months for complicated cases
  - Treatment is usually administered in 3–4 courses lasting 4 weeks, separated by 2-week interval.
  - Albendazole is the drug of choice.

Endoscopic Management of Hydatid Cyst

- The ERCP is effective in diagnosing biliary tree involvement from the cyst.
- The endoscopic management is useful in presence of intrabiliary rupture, which requires exploration and drainage of the biliary tract and also after surgery in presence of residual hydatid material (membranes and daughter cyst) left in biliary tree.
- During the endoscopic exploration, the biliary tree is cleared of any hydatid material with a balloon catheter or a dormia basket.
- The endoscopic sphincterotomy is also performed to facilitate drainage of the CBD.

7. Percutaneous treatment of hydatid cyst.

8. PAIR therapy for hydatid cyst. ***WBUHS 2007***

Techniques

- PAIR
- Catheterization technique
- PEVAC
- *PAIR* is a percutaneous treatment technique for hydatid disease.

Indications for PAIR	*Contraindications to PAIR*	*Complications of PAIR*
• Refusal of surgery • Inoperable cases • Type I, II, and III cysts • Cystic lesion ≥5 cm in diameter • Multiple cysts ≥5 cm in diameter in different liver segments • Relapse postsurgery • Lack of response to chemotherapy • Children over 3 years • Pregnant women	• Noncooperative patients • Inaccessible or risky location of the liver cyst • Cyst in spine, brain, and/or heart • Inactive or calcified lesion • Cyst communicating with the biliary tree • Patients should be followed clinically after PAIR treatment. Recurrence is increased in more complicated cysts, including those with multiple daughter cysts	• Urticaria • Anaphylaxis • Subcapsùlar hematoma • Fever • Biliary fistula • Secondary infection of cyst cavity • Hypotension/hypotensive shock

- *Catheter drainage* and injection of sclerosing agents, as well as a modified catheter technique (MoCaT), have been used for treatment of hydatid disease of liver.

9. Complications and medical treatment of hydatid cyst.

Introduction

- Echinococcosis (hydatid disease) is a zoonosis caused by the larval stage of *Echinococcus granulosus* (also known as *Taenia echinococcus*).
- Humans are accidental intermediate hosts, whereas animals can be both intermediate and definitive hosts.
- The two main types of hydatid disease are caused by *E. granulosus* and *E. multilocularis.*
- Infection with echinococcal organisms is the most common cause of liver cysts in the world.

Medical Treatment

- *Medical therapy* for echinococcosis is limited to the benzimidazoles (mebendazole and albendazole) and used alone is only 30% successful.
- Albendazole is readily absorbed from the intestine and metabolized by the liver to an active form.
- Mebendazole is poorly absorbed and is inactivated by the liver.
- Albendazole is thus the drug of choice for medical therapy.
- Greater success rates may be seen in extrahepatic manifestations of the disease and with the alveolar form caused by *E. multilocularis.*
- Given for at least 3 months preoperatively, albendazole reduces the recurrence rate when cyst spillage, partial cyst removal, or biliary rupture has occurred. Duration of therapy in these instances is at least 1 month.

Complications

Complications from hydatid cysts are seen in one third of patients:

- Most commonly, the cyst ruptures internally or externally, followed by secondary infection, anaphylactic shock, and liver replacement, in order of decreasing frequency.
- Viable hydatid cysts are space-occupying lesions with a tendency to grow.
- In confined areas such as the central nervous system, even small cysts can cause severe symptoms.
- In less confined areas, symptoms depend on the site and size of the cyst. Symptoms result from direct pressure or distortion of neighboring structures or viscera.

- Compressive atrophy of the surrounding hepatocytes and fibrosis occurs and these cysts may grow to such an enormous size that they replace an entire lobe.
- As the cysts enlarge, they may also rupture. If rupture of only the endocyst occurs, the content is retained within the pericyst.
- A communicating rupture is a rupture into the biliary or bronchial tree.
- Frank intrabiliary rupture is the most common complication of hydatid cysts and is reported in 5–25% of cases.
- A free rupture occurs when hydatid contents rupture throughout the peritoneal, pleural, or pericardial cavity.
- Acute symptomatic rupture into the peritoneal cavity occurs in 1–4% of patients and may precipitate anaphylactic shock.

SEGMENTS OF LIVER AND HEPATECTOMY

10. Hepatic segments. ***WBUHS 2012***

11. Surgical anatomy of liver and its importance in liver resection. ***WBUHS 2007, WBUHS 2025 Supplementary***

12. Surgical anatomy of liver. ***KGMU, Lucknow 2025; Ayush University, Chhattisgarh 2025***

13. Segmental anatomy of the liver and various types of liver resection. ***DNB 2017, December***

- Historically, the liver was divided into left and right lobes by the obvious external landmark of the falciform ligament.
- The liver was divided into right and left lobes, determined by portal and hepatic vein branches.
- Briefly, a plane without any surface markings running from the gallbladder to the left side of the inferior vena cava (IVC) (known as the portal fissure or Cantlie's line) divided the liver into right and left lobes.
- The right lobe was further divided into anterior and posterior segments.
- The left lobe was divided into a medial segment (also known as the quadrate lobe) that lies to the right of the falciform ligament and umbilical fissure and a lateral segment lying to the left.
- This system, although anatomically more correct, is only sufficient for mobilization of the liver and simple hepatic procedures.
- It does not describe the more intricate and functional segmental anatomy that is essential to understand before pursuing complex hepatobiliary surgery.
- The functional anatomy of the liver is composed of eight segments, each of which is supplied by a single portal triad (also called a pedicle) composed of a portal vein, hepatic artery, and bile duct.
- These segments are further organized into four sectors that are separated by scissurae, containing the three main hepatic veins.

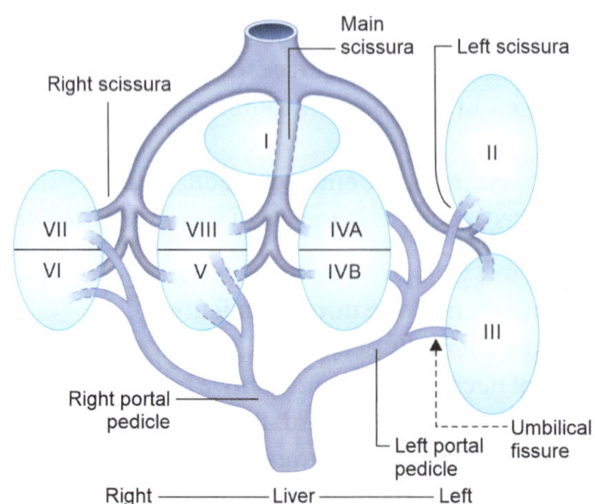

A schematic demonstration of the segmental anatomy of the liver.

- The four sectors are even further organized into the right and left liver (the phrase right and left liver is preferable to right and left lobe because there is no external mark that allows the identification of the right and left liver).
- This system was originally described in 1957 by Woodsmith and Goldburne as well as Couinaud and defines hepatic anatomy as it is the most relevant to surgery of the liver.
- Each segment receives its own portal pedicle (triad of portal vein, hepatic artery, and bile duct).
- The eight segments are illustrated and the four sectors, divided by the three main hepatic veins running in scissurae, are shown.
- The umbilical fissure is shown to contain the left portal pedicle.

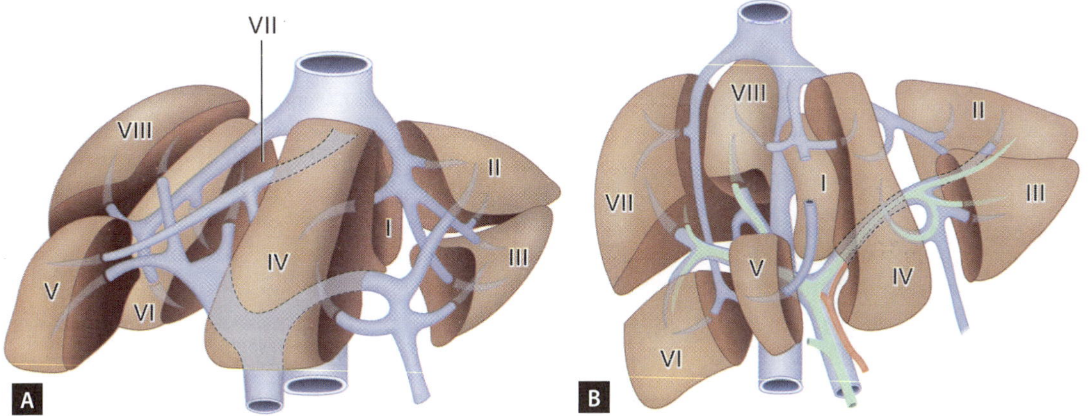

(A) Segmental anatomy of the liver as seen at laparotomy in the anatomic position and (B) In the ex vivo position.

- The main scissura contains the middle hepatic vein, which runs in an anteroposterior direction from the gallbladder fossa to the left side of the vena cava and divides the liver into right and left hemilivers.
- The line of the main scissura is also known as Cantlie's line.
- The right liver is divided into anterior (segments V and VIII) and posterior (segments VI and VII) sectors by the right scissura, which contains the right hepatic vein.
- The right portal pedicle, composed of the right hepatic artery, portal vein, and bile duct, splits into right anterior and posterior pedicles that supply the segments of the anterior and posterior sectors.
- The left liver has a visible fissure along its inferior surface called the umbilical fissure.
- The ligamentum teres (containing the remnant of the umbilical vein) runs into this fissure.
- The falciform ligament is contiguous with the umbilical fissure and ligamentum teres.
- The umbilical fissure is not a scissura, does not contain a hepatic vein, and in fact, contains the left portal pedicle (triad containing the left portal vein, hepatic artery, and bile duct), which runs in this fissure, branching to feed the left liver.
- The left scissura runs posterior to the ligamentum teres and contains the left hepatic vein. The left liver is split into an anterior (segments III and IV) and posterior (segment II—the only sector composed of a single segment) sector by the left scissura.
- At the hilum of the liver, the right portal triad has a short extrahepatic course of about 1–1.5 cm before entering the substance of the liver and branching into anterior and posterior sectoral branches.
- The left portal triad, however, has a long extrahepatic course of up to 3 or 4 cm and runs transversely along the base of segment IV in a peritoneal sheath that is the upper end of the lesser omentum.
- The left portal triad, as it runs along the base of segment IV, is separated from the liver substance by connective tissue known as the hilar plate.
- The continuation of the left portal triad runs anteriorly and caudally in the umbilical fissure and gives branches to segments II and III and recurrent branches to segment IV.

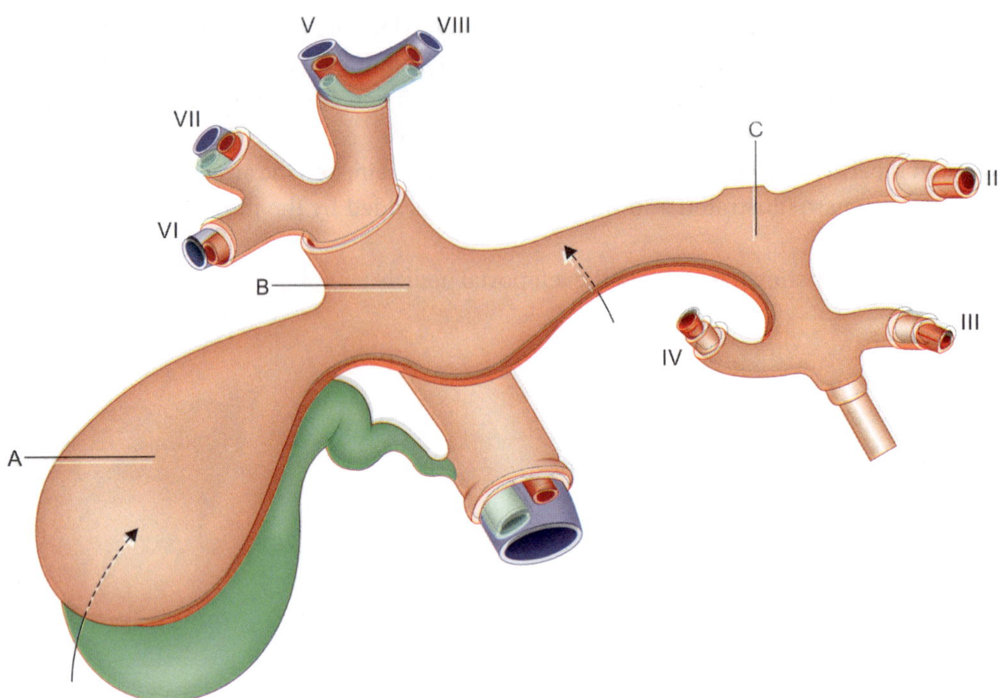

The plate system is illustrated. (A) The cystic plate between the gallbladder and the liver; (B) The hilar plate at the biliary confluence at the base of segment IV; (C) The umbilical plate above the umbilical portion of the portal vein. The arrows show the plane of dissection of the cystic plate for cholecystectomy and the hilar plate for exposure of the hepatic duct confluence and the main left hepatic duct.

- The caudate lobe (segment I) is the dorsal portion of the liver and embraces the IVC on its posterior surface and lies posterior to the left portal triad inferiorly and the left and middle hepatic veins superiorly.
- The main bulk of the caudate lobe is to the left of the IVC, but inferiorly, it traverses between the IVC and left portal triad, where it fuses to the right liver (segments VI and VII).
- This part of the caudate lobe is known as the right portion or the caudate process.
- The left portion of the caudate lobe lies in the lesser omental bursa and is covered anteriorly by the gastro-hepatic ligament (lesser omentum) that separates it from segments II and III anteriorly.
- The gastrohepatic ligament attaches to the ligamentum venosum (sinus venosus remnant) along the left side of the left portal triad.
- The vascular inflow and biliary drainage to the caudate lobe comes from both the right and left systems.
- The right side of the caudate (the caudate process) largely derives its portal venous supply from the right portal vein or the bifurcation of the main portal vein, whereas the left portion of the caudate derives its portal venous inflow from the left main portal vein.
- The arterial supply and the biliary drainage of the right portion are generally through the right posterior sectoral system and the left portion through the left main vessels.
- The hepatic venous drainage of the caudate is unique in that multiple small veins drain posteriorly directly into the IVC.
- The posterior edge of the left side of the caudate terminates into a fibrous component that attaches to the crura of the diaphragm and also runs posteriorly, wrapping behind the IVC and attaching to segment VII of the right liver.
- Up to 50% of the time, this fibrous component is composed either partially or completely of liver parenchyma, and thus liver tissue may completely encircle the IVC.
- This important structure is known as the IVC ligament and is important when mobilizing the right liver or the caudate lobe off of the vena cava.

- Anomalous development of the liver is uncommonly encountered. Complete absence of the left liver has been reported. A tongue of tissue extending inferiorly off of the right liver has been described (Riedel's lobe).
- Rare cases of supradiaphragmatic liver in the absence of a hernia sac have been noted.

Nomenclature for Most Common Major Anatomic Hepatic Resections

Segments	*Couinaud, 1957*	*Goldsmith and Woodburne, 1957 Brisbane, 2000*	
V–VIII	Right hepatectomy	Right hepatic lobectomy	Right hemihepatectomy
IV–VIII	Right lobectomy	Extended right hepatic lobectomy	Right trisectionectomy
II–IV	Left hepatectomy	Left hepatic lobectomy	Left hemihepatectomy
II, III	Left lobectomy	Left lateral segmentectomy	Left lateral sectionectomy
II–V, VIII	Extended left hepatectomy	Extended left lobectomy	Left trisectionectomy

14. Liver resection: Indications, brief steps, and results. ***WBUHS 2011***

Indications

Most hepatectomies are performed for the treatment of hepatic neoplasms, both benign and malignant.

- Benign neoplasms include hepatocellular adenoma, hepatic hemangioma, and focal nodular hyperplasia.
- The most common malignant neoplasms (cancers) of the liver are metastases; those arising from colorectal cancer are among the most common and most amenable to surgical resection. The most common primary malignant tumor of the liver is the hepatocellular carcinoma (HCC).
- Hepatectomy may also be the procedure of choice to treat intrahepatic gallstones or parasitic cysts of the liver.
- Partial hepatectomies are also performed to remove a portion of a liver from a live donor for transplantation.

Nomenclature for Most Common Major Anatomic Hepatic Resections

Segments	*Couinaud, 1957*	*Goldsmith and Woodburne, 1957 Brisbane, 2000*	
V–VIII	Right hepatectomy	Right hepatic lobectomy	Right hemihepatectomy
IV–VIII	Right lobectomy	Extended right hepatic lobectomy	Right trisectionectomy
II–IV	Left hepatectomy	Left hepatic lobectomy	Left hemihepatectomy
II, III	Left lobectomy	Left lateral segmentectomy	Left lateral sectionectomy
II–V, VIII	Extended left hepatectomy	Extended left lobectomy	Left trisectionectomy

Techniques

- A hepatectomy is considered a major surgery done under general anesthesia.
- Access is accomplished by laparotomy, typically by a bilateral subcostal ("chevron") incision, possibly with midline extension (Calne or "Mercedes-Benz" incision).
- Hepatectomies may be anatomic, i.e., the lines of resection match the limits of one or more functional segments of the liver as defined by the Couinaud classification or they may be nonanatomic, irregular, or "wedge" hepatectomies.
- Anatomic resections are generally preferred because of the smaller risk of bleeding and biliary fistula; however, nonanatomic resections can be performed safely as well in selected cases. For details on the variety of anatomic hepatectomies and the specific nomenclature, cf. the International Hepato-Pancreato-Biliary Association (IHPBA) Terminology for Liver Resections.
- The maneuver is usually performed during a hepatectomy to minimize blood loss; however, this can lead to reperfusion injury in the liver due to ischemia.
- A liver resection must consider the disease to be treated and the goals of the operation, whether a margin-negative resection of a malignancy or the removal of benign tissue to alleviate symptoms.
- The most basic steps can be distilled down to inflow (portal vein, hepatic artery, and bile duct) control, outflow (hepatic veins) control, and parenchymal transection with preservation of a liver remnant of adequate size with intact inflow, biliary drainage, and venous outflow.

- The most common approach to an anatomic resection, in the most common order, is mobilization of the liver to be resected, dissection of inflow and outflow structures, division of the inflow, division of the outflow, and parenchymal transection.
- Mobilization of the liver involves division of the right or left triangular ligaments, freeing up the liver from the diaphragm.
- Often, the liver must be mobilized completely off of the vena cava (which it straddles) and this requires careful dissection and division of multiple retrohepatic caval venous branches.
- For major resections, the hepatic vein of the resected portion of liver is often encircled before the resection.
- There are a variety of techniques to dissect, control, and divide inflow vessels. Classic inflow control is obtained by a dissection of the liver hilum with control of the portal vein and hepatic artery to the hemiliver to be resected. These can be suture ligated or can be divided with vascular staplers.
- Unless tumor proximity mandates, we advocate dividing the bile duct within the liver substance to absolutely minimize contralateral biliary injuries related to anatomic anomalies.
- Inflow control can also be obtained by dissection of the intrahepatic inflow pedicle to the anatomic section of liver to be resected.
- Recall that the inflow structures invaginate peritoneum at the hepatic hilus and run intrahepatically as an invested pedicle of the three inflow structures.
- The inflow pedicle can be encircled by making flanking hepatotomies or by splitting parenchyma down to the pedicle of interest.
- The pedicle can usually be divided with a vascular stapler, but suture ligation is sometimes necessary.
- Classically, the hepatic vein is divided in its extrahepatic position and can also usually be done with a vascular stapler.
- The hepatic vein can also be divided within the substance of the liver during parenchymal transection.
- There are numerous methods of parenchymal transection, ranging from complex ultrasonic irrigators to radiofrequency energy coagulators to a simple clamp-crushing technique.
- All of these, in experienced hands, can be used effectively to minimize blood loss and it is important to develop a specific technique that you are comfortable with.
- Ultimately, parenchymal transection is about dissecting intrahepatic anatomy, controlling vascular and biliary structures, minimizing blood loss, and avoiding injury to the future liver remnant.

Complications

- Bleeding is the most feared technical complication and may be grounds for urgent reoperation.
- Biliary fistula is also a possible complication, albeit one more amenable to nonsurgical management.
- Pulmonary complications such as atelectasis and pleural effusion are commonplace and dangerous in patients with underlying lung disease. Infection is relatively rare.
- Liver failure poses a significant hazard to patients with underlying hepatic disease; this is a major deterrent in the surgical resection of HCC in patients with cirrhosis.
- It is also a problem, to a lesser degree, in patients with previous hepatectomies (e.g., repeat resections for reincident colorectal cancer metastases).

15. Staged hepatectomy procedures. *WBUHS 2021*

Introduction

A two-stage hepatectomy procedure consists in combining two sequential liver resections when it is impossible to resect all liver metastases in a single procedure while preserving at least 30% of the functional liver volume to avoid postoperative lethal liver failure.

Two-stage Hepatectomy

- The preoperative evaluation includes liver ultrasound, a spiral CT scan of the chest, abdomen, and pelvis, and bone scintigraphy.

- Local recurrence of the primary is excluded by colonoscopy.
- At the laparotomy for resection, the abdomen is carefully explored for any extrahepatic tumor deposit, with fresh-frozen biopsy of any suspicious lymph node.
- The objective of the first hepatectomy is to make the second hepatectomy potentially curative.
- The liver tumors are precisely mapped, using manual palpation and intraoperative ultrasound.
- Mapping permits the surgeon to achieve this by resecting the highest possible number of liver tumors (the majority of patients) or by clearing tumor tissue from the less-invaded hepatic lobe, leaving the other to be further resected after regeneration.
- During the first-stage hepatectomy, a minimum amount of dissection is performed on the liver that will be dissected in the second stage.
- We avoid dividing the corresponding triangular ligament and the ipsilateral vascular structures to prevent further fibrous adhesions.
- Postoperative chemotherapy is given to control tumor growth, beginning 3 weeks after liver resection so that it does not interfere with initial liver regeneration.
- The timing of the second hepatectomy is selected as a function of liver regeneration, control of remnant liver tumor by chemotherapy, and the probability that the second hepatectomy can be curative.
- The same preoperative evaluation and laparotomy protocols are used as in the first stage, with the exception of a larger dissection of the remnant liver.
- The median interval between the two stages was 4 months.
- Nonsurgical treatments were combined with chemotherapy to increase the feasibility of the two-stage hepatectomy.
- Cryosurgery was used in one patient for two liver metastases that were unlikely to be resectable at the second hepatectomy.
- Portal embolization of the liver to be resected was used in six patients in whom the extent of the expected second-stage resection exceeded 60% of the total parenchymal volume.
- Portal embolization was also used before the first-stage hepatectomy in one patient.
- Postoperative follow-up patients are followed up by serum tumor markers [carcinoembryonic antigen CEA), CA 19-9], liver ultrasound, and spiral CT scans of the chest, abdomen, and pelvis at 3-month intervals.
- If the overall procedure has been complete, as confirmed by histology margins and return to normal levels of tumor markers and there is no sign of tumor recurrence, chemotherapy is discontinued after eight courses.
- In case of a new recurrence, chemotherapy is restarted.

16. Write in brief about hepatic adenoma. *DNB 2017, December*

Introduction

Hepatic adenoma (also called hepatocellular adenoma) is a rare, benign liver tumor that typically arises from hepatocytes. It has important clinical implications due to risks of bleeding, malignant transformation, and rupture.

Key Features

Epidemiology	• Most common in women of childbearing age (15–45 years) • Strongly associated with oral contraceptive use • Rare in men, but riskier when present
Etiology/Risk Factors	• Oral contraceptives (estrogen-based) • Anabolic steroids (in men) • Glycogen storage diseases (esp. type I and III) • Obesity and metabolic syndrome
Clinical Presentation	• Often asymptomatic, incidental finding • May cause right upper quadrant pain • Sudden pain and hypotension if rupture with hemorrhage occurs
Complications	• Hemorrhage (esp. tumors >5 cm) • Malignant transformation (to hepatocellular carcinoma, esp. β-catenin subtype)

Imaging and Diagnosis

Modality	*Findings*
Ultrasound	Well-defined, hyperechoic or mixed lesion
CT Scan	Hypervascular lesion with arterial phase enhancement, possibly heterogenous due to hemorrhage
MRI	Useful for characterizing fat, hemorrhage, or distinguishing from focal nodular hyperplasia
Biopsy	Usually avoided unless diagnosis is uncertain or malignancy is suspected

Subtypes (Molecular Classification)

- *HNF1α-mutated:* Common in women, fatty changes, low malignant potential
- *Inflammatory:* Most common, associated with obesity, high bleeding risk
- *β-catenin activated:* Higher risk of malignant transformation
- *Unclassified:* Lacks the features of the other types

Management

Situation	*Recommended Action*
<5 cm and asymptomatic	Stop OCPs, monitor with imaging
>5 cm or symptomatic	Surgical resection (due to risk of bleeding or malignancy)
Men with adenoma	Resection generally advised (higher cancer risk)
Rupture or hemorrhage	Emergency management: embolization or surgery

Prognosis

- Generally good with appropriate management.
- Recurrence is rare after resection.
- Monitoring is needed if managed conservatively.

17. Discuss the clinical features, investigations, and management of primary liver carcinoma. *WBUHS 2014*

Clinical Presentation

- Most commonly, patients presenting with HCC are men 50–60 years of age who complain of right upper quadrant abdominal pain and weight loss and have a palpable mass.
- In countries endemic for hepatitis B virus (HBV), presentation at a younger age is common and probably related to childhood infection.
- Unfortunately, in unscreened populations, HCC tends to present at a later stage because of the lack of symptoms in early stages.
- Presentation at an advanced stage is often with vague right upper quadrant abdominal pain that sometimes radiates to the right shoulder.
- Nonspecific symptoms of advanced malignancy such as anorexia, nausea, lethargy, and weight loss are also common.
- Another common presentation of HCC is hepatic decompensation in a patient with known mild cirrhosis or even in patients with unrecognized cirrhosis.
- HCC can rarely present as a rupture, with the sudden onset of abdominal pain followed by hypovolemic shock secondary to intraperitoneal bleeding.

Other Rare Presentations

- Hepatic vein occlusion (Budd-Chiari syndrome)
- Obstructive jaundice
- Hemobilia
- Fever of unknown origin

- Less than 1% of cases of HCC present with a paraneoplastic syndrome, usually
- Hypercalcemia, hypoglycemia, and erythrocytosis
- Small incidentally detected tumors have become a more common presentation because of the knowledge of specific risk factors
- Screening programs for diagnosed HBV or hepatitis C virus (HCV) infection
- Increasing use of high-quality abdominal imaging

For Patients Suspected of Suffering from HCC, the Aims of Diagnostic Investigations

- Verification of diagnosis
- Determine extent of disease
- Determine functional liver reserve
- Assess biologic determinants that are predictors of long-term prognosis

Diagnosis

- Diagnosis is often confirmed with a biopsy.
- Diagnosis can sometimes be confirmed with blood or imaging tests.
- Physical examination
- Blood test for alpha-fetoprotein (AFP); 50–70% of people with primary liver cancer have elevated levels.
- Ultrasound of the abdomen
- CT or computed axial tomography (CAT) scan
- MRI
- Angiogram
- Laparoscopy
- Radiologic investigation is a critical part of the diagnosis of HCC
  - *Ultrasound plays* a significant role in screening and early detection of HCC, but definitive diagnosis and treatment planning rely on CT and/or MRI.
  - *Contrast-enhanced CT (CECT)* and *MRI* protocols aimed at diagnosing HCC take advantage of the hypervascularity of these tumors and arterial phase images are critical to assess the extent of disease adequately.
  - CT and MRI also evaluate the extent of disease in terms of peritoneal metastases, nodal metastases, and extent of vascular and biliary involvement.
  - Detection of bland or tumor thrombus in the portal or hepatic venous system is also important and can be diagnosed with any of these modalities.
  - AFP measurements can be helpful in the diagnosis of HCC.
    - An AFP level >20 ng/mL is noted in approximately 75% of documented cases of HCC.
    - False-positive elevations of serum AFP levels can be seen in inflammatory disorders of the liver, such as chronic active viral hepatitis.
    - The specificity and positive-predictive values of AFP improve with higher cutoff levels (e.g.,400 ng/mL) but at the cost of sensitivity.
    - With improvements in imaging technology and the ability to detect smaller tumors, AFP is largely used as an adjunctive test in patients with liver masses.
    - AFP levels are particularly useful in monitoring treated patients for recurrence after normalization of levels.
  - If atypical features appear on imaging, a biopsy should be obtained for histologic diagnosis.
  - For hepatic nodules larger than 2 cm, a triple-phase CT or MRI scan is required if typical features of HCC are identified in combination with an AFP level >200 ng/mL.
  - If typical features appear on imaging, the diagnosis of HCC is confirmed.
  - If atypical features are seen, then biopsy is required to confirm the histologic diagnosis.

- At present, the diagnosis of HCC can be made according to the guidelines of the Barcelona-2000 European Association for the Study of the Liver (EASL) Conference and to successive modifications of guidelines from the American Association for the Study of Liver Disease (AASLD).
- Pathologic diagnoses of HCC are made according to the International Working Party criteria. For hepatic nodules from 1–2 cm in size, a triple-phase CT and MRI scan must show typical features of HCC—arterially enhancing mass with washout of contrast in delayed phases—to confirm the diagnosis.

Treatment

- There are a large number of treatment options for patients with HCC, reflecting the heterogeneity of this disease and the lack of a proven superior treatment, except complete resection.
- Selection of the appropriate patient for resection is critical and must take into account the condition of the liver and extent of disease.
- Patients with Child–Pugh class B or C cirrhosis or portal hypertension do not tolerate resection.

Treatment Options for HCC

- *Surgical:*
  - Resection
  - Orthotopic liver transplantation
- *Ablative:*
  - Ethanol (EtOH) injection
  - Acetic acid injection
  - Thermal ablation (cryotherapy, RFA, and microwave)
- *Transarterial embolization:*
  - Chemoembolization
  - Radiotherapy
- *Combination of transarterial and ablative*
- *External beam radiation*
- *Systemic:*
  - Chemotherapy
  - Hormonal
  - Immunotherapy

Pugh's Modification of Child's Grading of Cirrhosis

Measurements	*1 point*	*2 points*	*3 points*
Bilirubin (mg/dL)	1–1.9	2–2.9	>2.9
Prothrombin time prolongation (seconds)	1–3	4–6	>6
Albumin (g/dL)	>3.5	2.8–3.4	<2.8
Ascites	None	Mild	Moderate-to-severe

Child's A: 5–6 points; B: 7–9 points; and C: 10–15 points

Cancer of the Liver Italian Group Score

Clinical parameters	*Cutoff values*	*Points*
Child–Pugh class	A	0
	B	1
	C	2

Contd...

Contd...

Clinical parameters	Cutoff values	Points
Tumor morphology	Uninodular, <50% extension	0
	Multinodular, <50% extension	1
	Massive or extension, >50%	2
AFP (ng/dL)	<400	0
	>400	1
Portal vein thrombosis	No	0
	Yes	1

Score ranges from 0 to 6; a score of 4 to 6 is generally considered advanced disease, whereas a score of 0 to 3 has the potential for long-term survival.

Cancer Treatment

Surgery

- Most successful in patients with small tumors (smaller than 5 cm) and with good liver function
- *Hepatectomy:* Portion of the liver is removed when the cancer is limited to one part of the liver.
- *Liver transplantation:* Used to treat cancer confined to the liver if a suitable donor is found. Must fulfill strict criteria
- A variety of prognostic factors predictive of survival after resection have been identified, but none are universally agreed on.
- The most commonly cited negative prognostic factors are tumor size, cirrhosis, infiltrative growth pattern, vascular invasion, intrahepatic metastases, multifocal tumors, lymph node metastases, margin less than 1 cm, and lack of a capsule.
- The best outcomes are found in patients with single small tumors, but size alone should not contraindicate resection.
- Multifocal tumors and major vascular invasion are generally associated with a poor outcome but some groups advocate resection in highly select patients.

Ablation of Liver Tumor

- Percutaneous
- Laparoscopy
- Open method

Percutaneous Technique is Best Choice for Early-stage Liver Tumor Who are not Surgical Candidates

Selection Criteria

- Single tumor <5 cm
- Multiple tumors <3 nodule and <3 cm
- No evidence of vascular invasion
- No extrahepatic spread
- Performance status test—0
- Cirrhosis with Child-Pugh class A or B

Percutaneous Methods

Chemical ablation	Thermal ablation
Ethanol injection Acetic acid injection	• Radiofrequency ablation (RFA) • Microwave • Laser ablation • Cryoablation

Cancer Treatment

Radiation Therapy

- The use of high-energy X-rays to destroy cancer cells
- The use of high energy X-rays or other particles to destroy cancer cells
- *Internal beam:* The use of implants inside the body. Radioactive beads may be inserted into the artery that supplies the tumor with blood.
- *External beam:* Outside the body—rarely used for HCC
- Side effects can include fatigue, mild skin reactions, upset stomach, and loose bowel movements.

Chemotherapy

- Use of drugs to kill cancer cells
- One or a combination of drugs may be used.
- Side effects may include nausea and vomiting, loss of appetite, diarrhea, fatigue, and risk of infection.
- Side effects often go away after treatment is finished.

Targeted Therapy

- Targets faulty genes or proteins that contribute to cancer growth and development
- Sorafenib (Nexavar), an antiangiogenic and antiproliferative drug (starves the tumor by disrupting its blood supply), may be used to treat tumors that cannot be removed with surgery.

18. Discuss the treatment options for primary and secondary hepatic malignancies. *WBUHS 2018*

Treatment

Surgical	*Ablative*	*Transarterial embolization*	*Combination: Trans-arterial and ablative*	*Radiotherapy*	*Systemic*
• Resection • Orthotopic liver transplantation	• Ethanol (EtOH) injection • Acetic acid injection • Thermal ablation (cryotherapy, radiofrequency ablation, microwave)	• Chemoembolization • Radiotherapy		External beam radiation	• Chemotherapy • Hormonal • Immunotherapy

- *Surgery:*
  - Most successful in patients with small tumors (smaller than 5 cm) and with good liver function
  - *Hepatectomy:* Portion of the liver is removed when the cancer is limited to one part of the liver.
  - *Liver transplantation:* Used to treat cancer confined to the liver if a suitable donor is found. Must fulfill strict criteria
- *Ablation of liver tumors:*
  - Routes
    - Percutaneous
    - Laparoscopy
    - Open method

Percutaneous technique is best choice for early-stage liver tumor who are not surgical candidates.

Selection Criteria

- Single tumor <5 cm
- Multiple tumors <3 nodule and <3 cm
- No evidence of vascular invasion

- No extrahepatic spread
- Performance status test—0
- Cirrhosis with Child-Pugh class A or B

Percutaneous Methods

- *Chemical ablation:*
    - Ethanol injection
    - Two percent acetic acid injection
- *Thermal ablation:*
    - *RFA*
    - *Microwave*
    - *Laser ablation*
    - *IV cryoablation*

RFA

- RFA uses electrical current, passed through a small needle placed directly into a liver tumor, to destroy cancer cells with heat
- As the temperature within the tissue becomes elevated beyond 60°C, necrosis happens. RFA can be performed by percutaneous, surgical, or laparoscopic approaches.

Management of Secondary Liver Malignancies

Liver metastasis is cancer that starts in another part of the body and spread to the liver. It is sometimes called secondary liver cancer or metastatic liver disease. Liver metastasis is not the same as cancer that starts in the liver (called primary liver cancer). Liver metastasis is much more common than primary liver cancer.

Some kinds of cancer are more likely to spread to the liver than others. The most common types of cancer that spread to the liver are:

- Colorectal
- Lung
- Breast
- Pancreatic
- Stomach
- Melanoma
- Neuroendocrine

Investigations

- *Blood tests:*
    - Blood tests are usually done to check your general health and find out how well the liver is working.
    - The most common blood tests used to help diagnose liver metastases are liver function tests.
    - Other blood tests that may be abnormal include a complete blood count (CBC), and blood glucose (sugar) and blood clotting tests.
    - Sometimes tumor marker tests are done.
        - CEA is a tumor marker measured in the blood.
        - It is usually checked during follow-up after treatment for colorectal cancer.
        - An increase in CEA levels over time could mean the cancer has come back and it may have spread to the liver.

Imaging Tests

Imaging tests are an important part of diagnosing liver metastases. It is common for people to have one or more imaging tests when the doctor thinks the cancer may have spread to the liver. The imaging tests used to diagnose liver metastases include the following:

- CECT scan is a common imaging test to check for liver metastases. It can also check for metastases in organs and tissues around the liver.
- Ultrasound is used to check for an enlarged liver or changes in its shape or texture. It is also used to guide a biopsy needle or laparoscope to a specific area of the liver.
- MRI may be used to find small metastatic tumors in the liver. It is usually used when doctors are not certain about the results of other imaging tests such as CT scan or ultrasound.
- Positron emission tomography (PET) scan may be used to check for metastases in organs and tissues around the liver. It is often used when there is a history of colorectal or stomach cancer.

Biopsy

- A biopsy is the removal of cells or tissues so they can be examined under a microscope.
- It may be needed to diagnose liver metastases.
- A biopsy may also be done to check tumor markers that help guide treatment.
- A percutaneous needle biopsy or endoscopic biopsy during laparoscopy may be used.

Other Tests

If liver metastases are found before the primary cancer is diagnosed, some tests to be done. These tests may include:

- CT scan of the chest to check for lung cancer
- Colonoscopy to check for colorectal cancer
- Laparoscopy to examine organs in the abdomen and pelvis

Treatments and Supportive Therapies

- *Chemotherapy:*
  - Chemotherapy is the most common treatment for liver metastases. It is used to help stop or slow the growth of cancer and relieve symptoms.
  - Chemotherapy may also be used to shrink the cancer so surgery can be done or it may be given after surgery to lower the risk of the cancer coming back.
  - Chemotherapy is sometimes used along with other treatments such as targeted therapy.
  - *Systemic chemotherapy* means that the drugs circulate throughout the body to destroy cancer cells.
  - Hepatic arterial infusion (HAI) is a procedure that delivers chemotherapy directly to liver tumors. The chemotherapy is supplied through a pump to the main artery of the liver (called the hepatic artery). Floxuridine (FUDR) is the most common chemotherapy drug used in HAI.
- *Chemoembolization, or transarterial chemoembolization (TACE),* is a procedure that delivers chemotherapy directly to liver tumors.
- Chemoembolization may be used to stop or slow the growth of liver metastases when the cancer has only spread to the liver.
- *Targeted therapy:*

  Targeted therapy may be used to control the growth of liver metastases from some types of cancer, such as:
  - Bevacizumab or cetuximab is used for colorectal cancer
  - Erlotinib is used for pancreatic cancer

  Targeted therapy is given intravenously (through a needle into a vein) or orally (as a pill by mouth). It is most often used along with chemotherapy.
- *Surgery:*
  - Surgery may be used to treat liver metastasis when only cancer are found in one area or a few areas. It is most often used for colorectal cancer that has spread to the liver.

- *Ablation therapy:*
  The following ablation therapies may be used to treat liver metastases. Side effects will depend mainly on the procedure done and how much of the liver is treated.
  - *RFA* uses electrical currents to create heat that destroys cancer cells.
  - *Cryotherapy* uses extreme cold to freeze and destroy abnormal and cancerous cells or tissue. It is also called cryosurgery or cryoablation.
  - Percutaneous ethanol injection
- *Radiation therapy* is not used that often to treat liver metastases. This is because radiation can damage the liver (called radiation-induced liver disease). In rare cases, external beam radiation may be given to the whole liver to relieve symptoms (called palliative treatment).
  Newer radiation therapy techniques can deliver more targeted doses of radiation to the liver tumors and lower the risk of liver damage.
- *Radioembolization*, or *selective internal radiation therapy*, is a procedure that delivers radiation directly to liver tumors.
  Radioembolization may be used to slow the growth of liver metastases and relieve symptoms when other treatments cannot be used.
- *Stereotactic body radiation therapy* may be used when there are 1–3 small liver metastases.
- *Hormonal therapy:*
  - Hormonal therapy is a treatment that adds, blocks, or removes certain hormones to slow or stop the growth of cancer cells that need hormones to grow.
  - Hormonal therapy may be used to help slow the growth of tumors in the liver and relieve symptoms. It is given for some types of cancer that have spread to the liver, especially breast cancer.
  - Side effects of hormone therapy will depend mainly on the type of hormonal therapy. Common side effects of many types of hormonal therapy are hot flashes, weight gain, and less interest in sex.
- *Pain medicines:*
  - Pain medicines can be given different ways. They are usually given orally or intravenously. The most common pain medicines used for liver metastases are:
    - Opioids such as morphine and codeine
    - Corticosteroids such as dexamethasone
    - Nonsteroidal anti-inflammatory drugs (NSAIDs) such as ibuprofen

  Living with liver metastases: In many cases, liver metastasis is a *chronic condition*. Adjusting to life with liver metastases often takes time.

19. Approach to diagnosis of liver SOL. ***WBUHS 2019***

Evaluation

History	Clinical examination	Laboratory tests—complete hemogram, liver function test (LFT), albumin, international normalized ratio (INR)	Tumor markers—AFP, CEA, CA 19-9

Presentation

- Asymptomatic
- Nodule on screening in cirrhotic patients
- Presenting with pain and fever
- SOL in a known patient of extrahepatic malignancy

Algorithm for Solitary SOL of Liver in USG

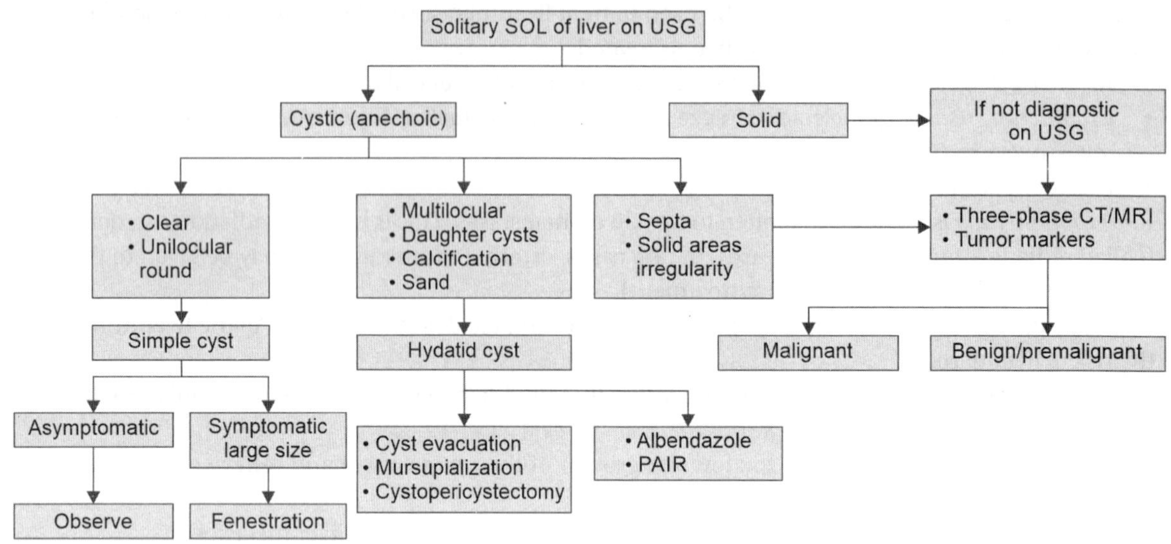

(CT: computed tomography; MRI: magnetic resonance imaging; PAIR: puncture, aspiration, injection, and reaspiration; SOL: space-occupying lesions; USG: ultrasonography)

Algorithm on Solid Lesions on USG

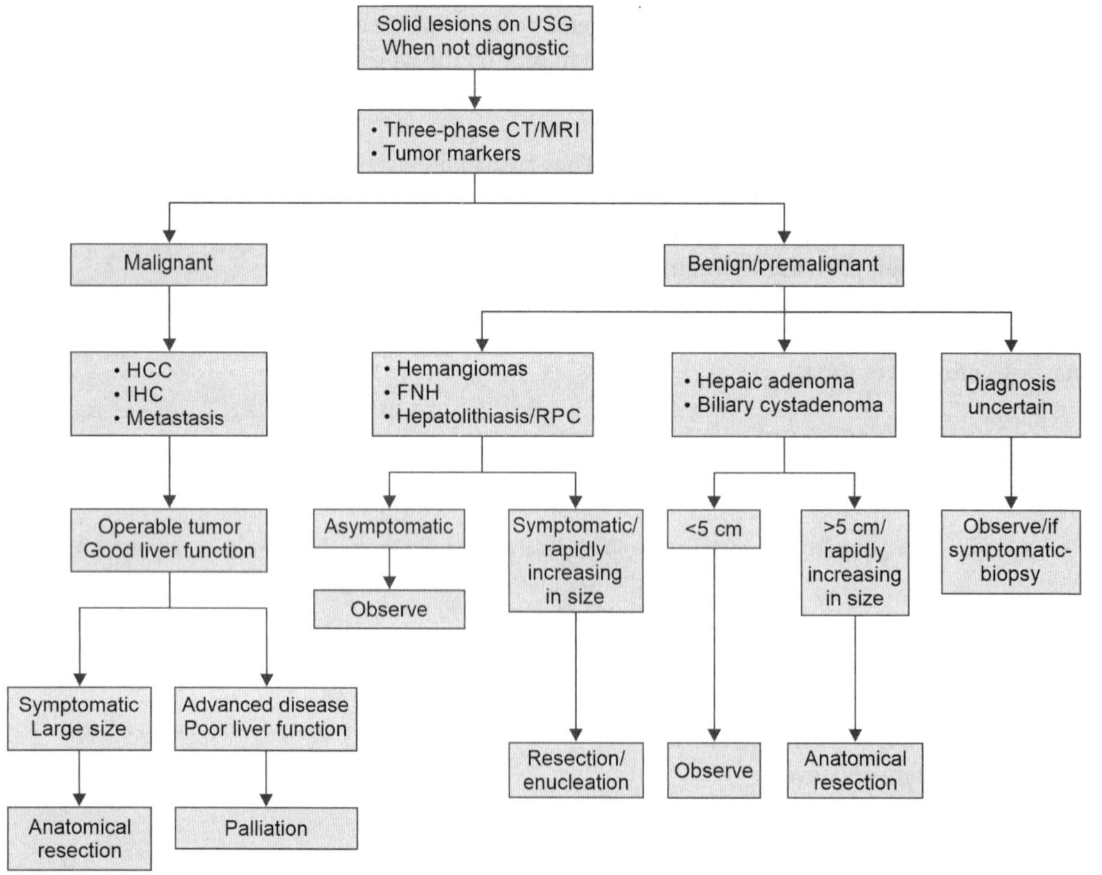

(CT: computed tomography; FNH: focal nodular hyperplasia; HCC: hepatocellular carcinoma; IHC: intrahepatic cholangiocarcinoma; MRI: magnetic resonance imaging; RPC: recurrent pyogenic cholangitis; USG: ultrasonography)

Algorithm for Multiple Liver SOL on USG

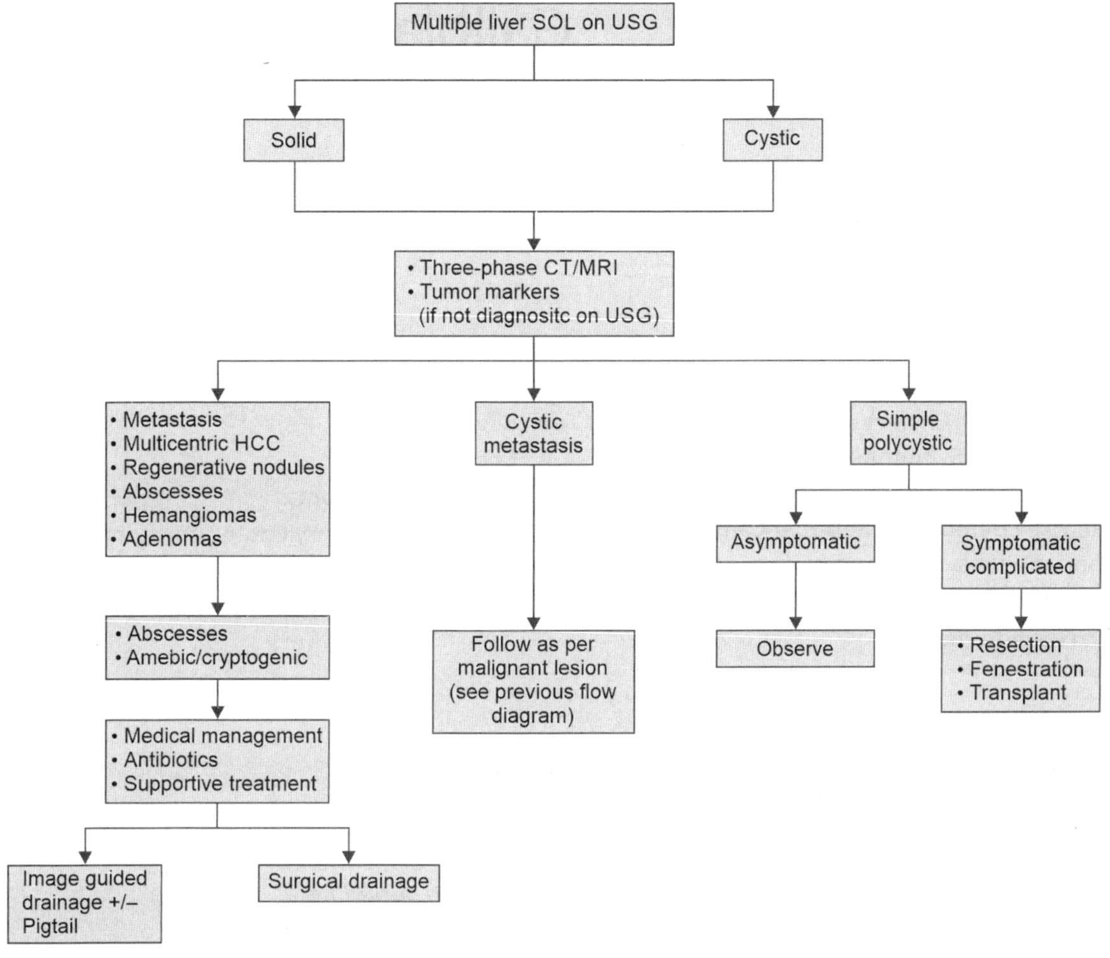

(CT: computed tomography; FNH: focal nodular hyperplasia; HCC: hepatocellular carcinoma; MRI: magnetic resonance imaging; SOL: space-occupying lesions; USG: ultrasonography)

CHAPTER 31

Gallbladder and Bile Duct

LEARNING OBJECTIVES

- Bilirubin Metabolism
- Acute Acalculous Cholecystitis, Silent Gallstones, Management of Symptomatic Gallstone in Pregnancy
- Incidentally Detected Gallbladder Cancer, Advanced Gallbladder Cancer
- Hemobilia
- Mirizzi's Syndrome
- Recurrent Pyogenic Cholangitis
- Bile Duct Injury
- Choledochal Cyst
- Cholangiocarcinoma
- Evaluation of Biliary Enteric Anastomosis for Benign Biliary Disorder
- Approach to or Evaluation of Obstructive Jaundice

BILIRUBIN METABOLISM

1. Write an overview of bilirubin metabolism. ***WBUHS 2021***

Normal bilirubin metabolism can be summarized as a series of steps, including:

- Production
- Uptake by the hepatocyte
- Conjugation
- Excretion into bile ducts
- Delivery to the intestine

Physiology

- In adults, 250–350 mg of bilirubin is produced each day. Approximately 80–85% of this bilirubin is derived from the destruction of senescent red blood cells by the reticuloendothelial system.
- The remaining 15–20% comes from the breakdown of nonhemoglobin proteins, such as myoglobin and the cytochromes.
- In reticuloendothelial cells, the microsomal enzyme heme oxygenase cleaves heme into biliverdin.
- Biliverdin is reduced to bilirubin by the cytosolic enzyme biliverdin reductase before being released into the circulation.
- In this unconjugated form, bilirubin is water insoluble and is transported to the liver tightly bound to albumin.
- The liver removes unconjugated bilirubin and other organic anions bound to albumin from plasma.
- When the bilirubin–albumin complex enters the sinusoidal circulation of the liver, three distinct metabolic phases are recognized:
  1. Hepatocyte uptake
  2. Conjugation
  3. Excretion into bile

- Unconjugated bilirubin is transported across the sinusoidal membrane of the hepatocyte into the cytoplasm.
- Inside the hepatocyte, unconjugated bilirubin is bound by a cytoplasmic protein, in this case glutathione S-transferase.
- The microsomal enzyme uridine diphosphate–glucuronyl transferase then conjugates the insoluble unconjugated bilirubin with glucuronic acid to form the water-soluble conjugated forms, bilirubin monoglucuronide (15%) and bilirubin diglucuronide (85%).
- Conjugated bilirubin is excreted from the hepatocyte into the bile canaliculus by an active transport mechanism.
- Excretion into bile is the rate-limiting step in bilirubin metabolism.
- After excretion, bile flows through the biliary ductal collecting system, may or may not be stored in the gallbladder (GB) and enters the duodenum.
- In the terminal ileum and colon, bilirubin is converted by bacterial enzymes into urobilinogen.
- About 10–20% of the urobilinogen is reabsorbed from the intestine into the portal circulation, creating an enterohepatic circulation.
- This recycled urobilinogen may be re-excreted into the bile by the liver or into urine by the kidney.
- The remaining urobilinogen in the intestine is converted to stercobilinogen, which gives stool its characteristic brown color.

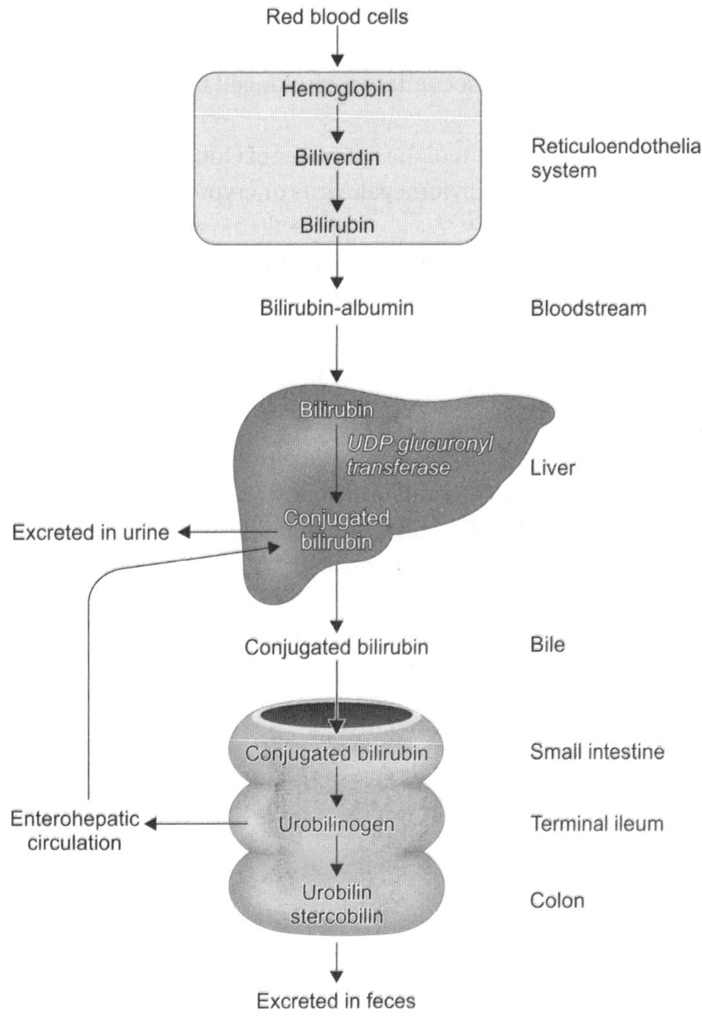

GALLBLADDER—CHOLECYSTITIS

2. Write short note on acute acalculous cholecystitis (AAC). ***WBUHS, 2010***

Introduction

Acute acalculous cholecystitis often complicates the course of intensive care unit (ICU) patients and those recovering from trauma or nonbiliary tract surgery. This disorder has a more fulminant course and is often associated with gangrene, perforation, and empyema. If left untreated, it has a mortality rate as high as 70%.

Signs/Symptoms

- Classic signs and symptoms of abdominal pain, right upper quadrant pain, and fever may be missing in critically ill patients.
- Laboratory tests such as bilirubin and leukocytosis may be elevated for different reasons. Unexplained fever and sepsis may be the only manifestation of acalculous cholecystitis.

Risk Factors for AAC

- Previous surgery and trauma
- Visceral hypoperfusion
- Mechanical ventilation
- Biliary stasis and gallbladder dysmotility secondary to prolonged fasting
- Total parenteral nutrition (TPN)
- Narcotics may play a role by causing spasm of the sphincter of Oddi.
- The AAC can be caused by infection with cytomegalovirus or cryptosporidium in patients infected with human immunodeficiency virus.
- Ischemia/hypoperfusion may play a role also in pathogenesis of AAC.
- Studies have shown a significant association between the duration of cardiopulmonary bypass and the incidence of AAC.

Diagnosis

There are various diagnostic modalities available.

- Radionuclide cholescintigraphy with intravenous morphine cholescintigraphy (RC/MC) has the highest sensitivity (90%), followed by CT scan (67%) and ultrasound (29%).
- If the suspicion for biliary sepsis and AAC is high, the initial test should be RC/MC and follow-up with CT to look at the remainder of the abdomen if RC/MC is normal. CT abnormalities include a dilated gallbladder with thickened walls, sludge in the gallbladder, and pericholecystic fluid outside of the gallbladder.
- If suspicion for AAC is low, CT is used to search for abdominal pathology. If CT is suggestive of AAC, follow with RC/MC.

Algorithm for Evaluation of Patients for Suspected AAC

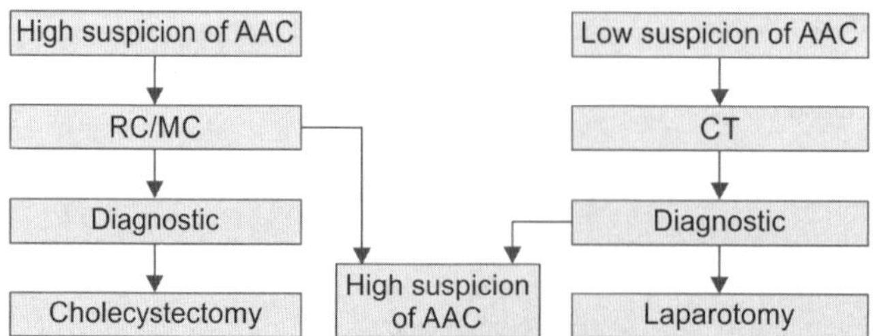

(AAC: acute acalculous cholecystitis; CT: computed tomography; MC: morphine cholescintigraphy; RC: radionuclide cholescintigraphy)

Treatment

- Treatment is open or laparoscopic cholecystectomy. In critically ill patients, ultrasound-guided percutaneous cholecystotomy tube placement can provide temporary relief. The usual organisms include gram-negative bacteria.
- Antibiotics are used pending the result of cultures. Adequate coverage can be provided with ampicillin and gentamicin, ticarcillin/clavulanate, piperacillin/tazobactam, or ampicillin/sulbactam. If the patient is penicillin allergic, a combination of cefotetan or cefoxitin with another antibiotic that covers pseudomonas and anaerobes is adequate.

3. Mucocele of gallbladder. ***NTRUHS, Vijayawada 2025***

Mucocele of the Gallbladder

A mucocele of the gallbladder refers to an overdistended gallbladder filled with mucus or mucoid secretions, rather than bile. It is an uncommon condition and is usually a result of chronic obstruction of the cystic duct, typically due to gallstones or rarely, a tumor or stricture.

Pathophysiology

- Obstruction of the cystic duct → gallbladder continues to secrete mucus → bile is reabsorbed → gallbladder gradually fills with mucinous fluid.
- No communication with the biliary tree due to the obstruction.
- Over time, the gallbladder becomes *distended, thin-walled, and filled with clear or mucinous fluid.*

Etiology (Causes)

- *Gallstones* (most common cause)
- Chronic cholecystitis
- Cystic duct stricture
- Gallbladder carcinoma (rare)
- Compression from adjacent structures (e.g., tumors or inflammation)

Clinical Features

Often *asymptomatic,* but when symptoms occur:

- Right upper quadrant abdominal pain
- Palpable, non-tender mass (Courvoisier's law if it's a painless enlargement with jaundice—more likely malignancy)
- Nausea, vomiting (if complicated)
- Symptoms of cholecystitis if infection occurs

Differential Diagnosis

- Gallbladder hydrops
- Empyema of the gallbladder
- Gallbladder carcinoma
- Biliary cyst
- Choledochal cyst

Investigations

- *Ultrasound:* First-line imaging
  - Enlarged, distended gallbladder
  - Clear, anechoic fluid (no internal echoes if not infected)
  - Absence of gallstones (or presence, depending on cause)
- *CT scan/MRI:* For further anatomical detail
- *MRCP:* If biliary tract involvement needs to be assessed

Complications

- Secondary infection → *Empyema*
- Gallbladder rupture → *Peritonitis*
- Pressure atrophy of gallbladder wall
- Gallbladder carcinoma (if chronic and untreated)

Treatment

- *Cholecystectomy* (surgical removal of gallbladder) is the treatment of choice.
  - Laparoscopic approach is often feasible.
  - Open surgery may be required in complicated or suspicious cases (e.g., possible malignancy).
- *If infection is suspected:* Preoperative antibiotics

---

4. Silent gallstones. ***WBUHS 2013***

Introduction

- Cholelithiasis is common (10–25%) in the general population, with the majority (70–80%) being asymptomatic at the time of diagnosis, and only few (10–20%) produce symptoms or complications in lifetime. Cholecystectomy, either open or laparoscopic, is straightforward for symptomatic gallstones, unlike the controversies in asymptomatic or silent gallstones.
- Asymptomatic gallstones may be defined as those having caused no symptoms or the ones detected incidentally during investigations in the absence of gallstone-related symptoms (biliary colic) or complications (cholecystitis, cholangitis, and pancreatitis).
- Vague or nonspecific abdominal symptoms, e.g., dyspepsia, epigastric discomfort, flatulence, or nausea, are not considered gallstone related as they are common in the general population with or without other gastrointestinal problems.

Asymptomatic Gallstone and the Risk of Gallbladder Carcinoma

- Since 80% of gallbladder carcinoma patients show presence of gallstone, gallstone is definitely a precancerous condition.
- The risk of carcinoma is higher in patients with gallstone >3 cm in diameter and in women than in men.

Asymptomatic Gallstone

Symptoms and/or Complications

- The risk of biliary pain is 10% at 5.
- The vast majority of gallstones (80%) do not cause any symptoms over few decades.
- More than 90% of patients will have symptoms before any complications (acute cholecystitis, obstructive jaundice, and acute pancreatitis) occur.
- The risk of complication is 3% at 10 years.

Treatment of Asymptomatic Gallstones

- Surgical treatment of asymptomatic gallstones without medically complicating diseases is discouraged.
- The risk of complications arising from interventions is higher than the risk of symptomatic disease.
- Approximately 25% of patients with asymptomatic gallstones develop symptoms within 10 years.

Persons with diabetes and women who are pregnant should have close follow-up to determine if they become symptomatic or develop complications.

However, cholecystectomy for asymptomatic gallstones may be indicated in the following patients:

- Patients with large gallstones >2 cm in diameter
- Patients with nonfunctional or calcified (porcelain) gallbladder observed on imaging studies and who are at high risk of gallbladder carcinoma

- Patients with spinal cord injuries or sensory neuropathies affecting the abdomen
- Patients with sickle cell anemia in whom the distinction between painful crisis and cholecystitis may be difficult.

Patients with risk factors for complications of gallstones may be offered elective cholecystectomy, even if they have asymptomatic gallstones. These groups include persons with the following conditions and demographics:
- Cirrhosis
- Portal hypertension
- Children
- Transplant candidates
- Diabetes with minor symptoms

Patients with a calcified or porcelain gallbladder should consider elective cholecystectomy due to the possibly increased risk of carcinoma (25%). Refer to a surgeon for removal as an outpatient procedure.

Medical Dissolution of Gallstones

Ursodeoxycholic acid (ursodiol) is a gallstone dissolution agent. In humans, long-term administration of ursodeoxycholic acid reduces cholesterol saturation of bile, both by reducing liver cholesterol secretion and by reducing the detergent effect of bile salts in the gallbladder (thereby preserving vesicles that have a high cholesterol carrying capacity). Desaturation of bile prevents crystals from forming and, in fact, may allow gradual extraction of cholesterol from existing stones.

In patients with established cholesterol gallstones, treatment with ursodeoxycholic acid at a dose of 8–10 mg/kg/day PO divided bid/tid may result in gradual gallstone dissolution. This intervention typically requires 6–18 months and is successful only with small, purely cholesterol stones. Patients remain at risk for gallstone complications until dissolution is completed. The recurrence rate is 50% within 5 years. Moreover, after discontinuation of treatment, most patients form new gallstones over the subsequent 5–10 years.

5. Describe management of symptomatic gallstone in pregnancy. ***WBUHS 2019***

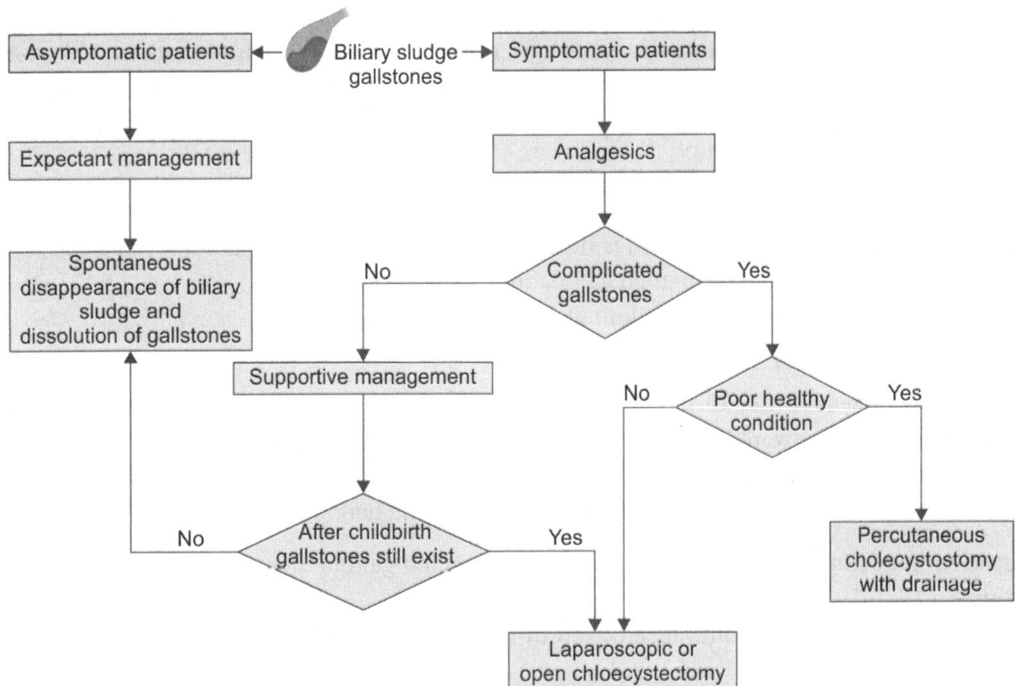

Flowchart depicting the standard therapy of biliary sludge and gallstones during pregnancy.

Treatment Considerations

- Biliary sludge and gallstones should be considered similar in almost all respects.
- Surgery generally is reserved for pregnant women with recurrent or unrelenting biliary pain refractory to medical management or with complications related to gallstones, including obstructive jaundice, acute cholecystitis, gallstone pancreatitis, or suspected peritonitis.
- For its safety, laparoscopic or elective cholecystectomy is one of the most common treatments for gallbladder gallstones in pregnant women, but it is recommended after the second trimester in order to reduce the rate of spontaneous abortion and preterm labor.
- If cholecystectomy is required during pregnancy, laparoscopic surgery is first recommended because of its relative safety.
- Of special note is that the timing of surgery is important.
- The effect of laparoscopic surgery on a developing fetus in the first trimester is unknown and surgery is more difficult in the third trimester with uterine enlargement.
- The second trimester, therefore, is believed to be the optimal time for cholecystectomy.
- A supportive management is highly recommended if possible, delaying more definitive treatment until childbirth.

GALLBLADDER CANCER

6. Explain management strategy for incidentally detected carcinoma gallbladder.

WBUHS 2023, 2025 Supplementary

7. Discuss the management of incidental carcinoma of gallbladder.

Srimanta Sankaradeva University, Assam 2025; Gujarat Health University 2024

Introduction

- Surgical resection is the only potentially curative treatment for gallbladder carcinoma.
- Only 10–30% of gallbladder carcinoma patients have resectable disease on presentation.
- Radical cholecystectomy is the standard surgical procedure performed for gallbladder carcinoma.
- The management of gallbladder carcinoma including incidentally detected gallbladder carcinoma depends on the T stage (depth of invasion).

Definition

- Incidental gallbladder carcinoma (IGBC) is defined as GBC found in histopathology analysis after removal of gallbladder tissue for symptomatic benign gallbladder disease.
- 70% of all GBC cases are discovered incidentally by the pathologist.

Key Facts

- Because of the increased use of laparoscopic cholecystectomy (LC) and difficulty in diagnosis of GBC preoperatively, IGBC discovered during and after LC has become more frequent.
- There is usually early cancer confined to the gallbladder and difficult to diagnose on ultrasonography.
- They preferentially metastasize to the regional lymph node and liver parenchyma.

For management guidelines, patients with incidentally detected gallbladder carcinoma can be divided into two clinical groups:

1. Those with gallbladder carcinoma discovered during laparoscopic or open cholecystectomy for assumed benign disease.
2. Patients with gallbladder carcinoma diagnosed histopathologically after simple cholecystectomy (open/laparoscopic) for benign gallbladder disease.

Algorithmic approach for incidentally detected gallbladder carcinoma discovered during cholecystectomy for gallstone disease:

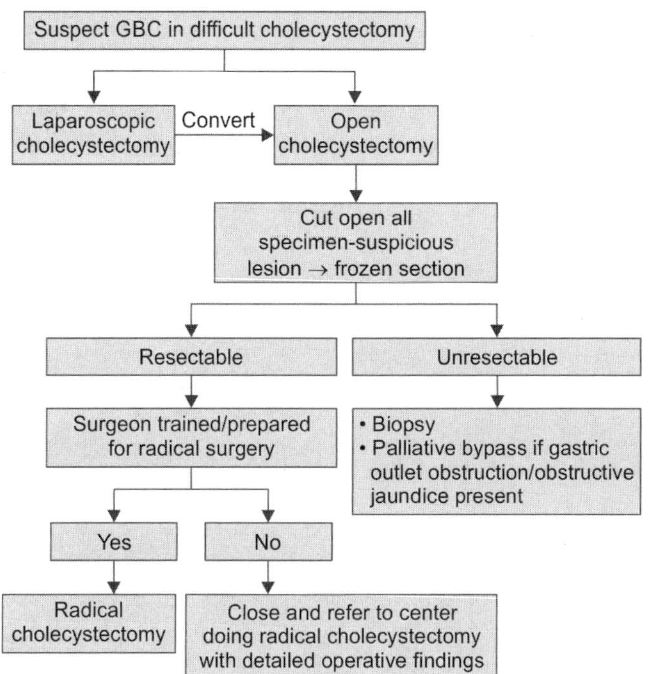

Management of incidentally discovered carcinoma gallbladder on pathologic examination:

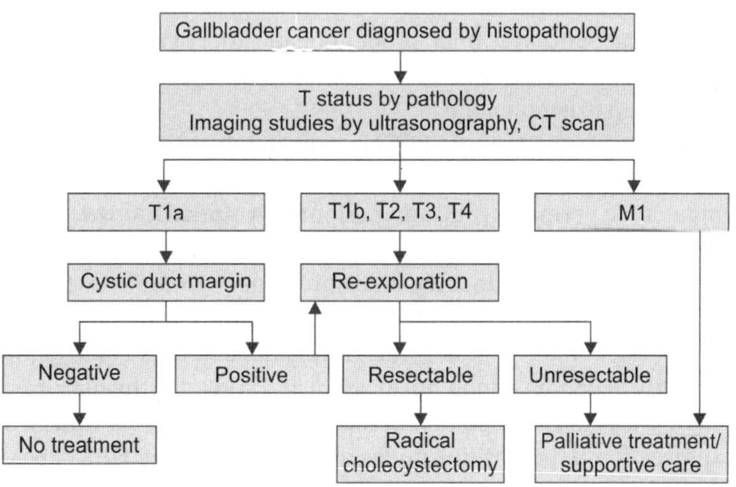

8. Write about surgery for advanced gallbladder cancer. ***WBUHS 2012***

Gallbladder cancer is the most common cancer of the biliary tract worldwide. In majority of cases, the outcome of patients with advanced gallbladder cancer is not good. It has been historically considered as an incurable malignancy. Often gallbladder cancer presents in advanced stage with invasion of the contagious adjacent organs, e.g., liver, duodenum, colon, or bile duct.

Advanced Gallbladder Cancer

T3/N1 or any T and disease between II and III TNM.

TNM Staging for Gallbladder Cancer

T1	Tumor invades lamina propria (T1a) or muscular (T1b) layer
T2	Tumor invades perimuscular connective tissue, no extension beyond the serosa or into the liver
T3	Tumor perforates the serosa (visceral peritoneum) and/or directly invades into liver and/or one other adjacent organ or structure such as the stomach, duodenum, colon, pancreas, omentum, or extrahepatic bile ducts
T4	Tumor invades main portal vein or hepatic artery or invades multiple extrahepatic organs and/or structures
N0	No lymph node metastases
N1	Regional lymph node metastases
M0	No distant metastases
M1	Distant metastases
Stage	***Stage grouping***
IA	T1 N0 M0
IB	T2 N0 M0
IIA	T3 N0 M0
IIB	T1 N1 M0
	T2 N1 M0
	T3 N1 M0
III	T4 any N M0
IV	Any T any N M1

N1: Cystic duct, pericholedochal, periportal, hilar, proper hepatic artery group of lymph node
N2: Posterosuperior and posteroinferior pancreaticoduodenal artery, common hepatic artery, celiac artery, and superior mesenteric artery group of lymph node:

- Contrast-enhanced computed tomography (CECT) is more helpful in demonstrating a mass in the GB or lymph node (LN) in the hepatoduodenal ligament (HDL) and peripancreatic region. Endoscopic ultrasound (EUS) is helpful for examination of the peripancreatic and periportal lymphadenopathy. Levels of tumor markers CEA, CA19-9, and CA242 may be raised in GB cancer.
- Curative resection of the tumor and its locoregional spread provide the only hope of long-term survival. The extent of resection may range from an extended cholecystectomy with a 2-cm nonanatomic wedge of liver in the gallbladder bed in segments IVB plus V and lymphadenectomy to an extended right hepatectomy and pancreaticoduodenectomy depending upon the location and spread of the tumor.
- Lymph node evaluation is a critical component of radical surgery. Patients with N1 disease achieve long-term survival with radical resection if the positive nodes are confined to the HDL. Positive nodes in more distant groups are associated with poor outcome.
- The risk of (+)ve regional LN in patients with T3 or T4 disease can be estimated in individual cases by pre-operative sampling of the key nodes by EUS and frozen section.
- The probability of LN metastasis in patients with T3 or T4 disease is as high as 64%. However, the risk of lymphatic spread is minimal if N12b (pericholedochal), N12c (cystic duct), and N13a (peripancreatic posterosuperior).
- Routine resection of bile duct is not advisable unless it is involved primarily by a T or pericholedochal node.
- If the tumor has invaded organs such as duodenum, stomach, or colon then limited resection (wedge/sleeve) should be considered instead of formal organ resection.
- Once porta hepatis has been involved and patient presents with jaundice, curative resection is unlikely.
- Planned cytoreduction or debulking surgery should not be done.

COMMON BILE DUCT

9. Describe hemobilia. *WBUHS 2012*

Introduction

Hemobilia implies bleeding into biliary tree. It can present as acute upper gastrointestinal (UGI) bleeding. It should be considered in upper abdominal pain presenting with UGI bleeding especially when there is a history of liver injury or instrumentation.

Hemobilia occurs when there is a fistula between a vessel of the splanchnic circulation and the intrahepatic or extrahepatic biliary system.

Causes

- Trauma, accidental or iatrogenic, e.g., due to procedures like cholecystectomy
- Instrumentation, e.g., after endoscopic retrograde cholangiopancreatography (ERCP)
- Gallstone
- Inflammatory conditions ranging from ascariasis to polyarteritis nodosa (PAN)
- Vascular malformation
- Tumor
- Coagulopathy
- Liver biopsy

Clinical Features

- Clinical feature "Quincke's" triad of upper abdominal pain, upper gastrointestinal hemorrhage, and jaundice is classical but only present in 22% cases.
- It can be immediately life threatening in major bleeding.
- However, in minor hemobilia, patient is hemodynamically stable despite significant blood loss being apparent.

Investigation

- Combination of OGD, CT scan, and angiography depending on clinical situation, bearing in mind that hemobilia may present many days after injury.
- Cholangiography is performed if there is a percutaneous access or if ERCP is undertaken.

Management

- Most bleeding from instrumentation is minor and would settle spontaneously.
- When indicated, management is directed toward stopping bleeding and relieving obstruction if present, which is achieved either by surgical ligation of hepatic artery or by endoscopic embolization.
- Endoscopic transarterial embolization (TAE) is preferred initially because of high success rate and less complication. TAE involves the selective catheterization of a hepatic artery followed by embolic occlusion.
- Surgery is indicated when TAE has failed or sepsis present in biliary tree or drainage has failed.

10. Mirizzi's syndrome. *NTRUHS, Vijayawada 2025*

Definition

Mirizzi's syndrome is a *rare complication of gallstone disease* in which a *gallstone becomes impacted in the cystic duct or Hartmann's pouch* of the gallbladder, leading to *external compression or erosion into the common hepatic duct (CHD) or common bile duct (CBD)*, causing *obstructive jaundice*.

Pathophysiology

- A gallstone gets *impacted in the cystic duct or Hartmann's pouch.*
- This leads to:
  - *Extrinsic compression* of the common hepatic duct (early stages).

- *Chronic inflammation*, leading to:
  - *Fibrosis*
  - *Erosion into CHD or CBD*
  - Formation of a *cholecystocholedochal fistula* (in advanced stages).

Classification (Csendes Classification)

Type	*Description*
Type I	External compression of CHD by stone in Hartmann's pouch or cystic duct
Type II	Cholecystocholedochal fistula involving <1/3rd of CBD circumference
Type III	Fistula involving 1/3rd to 2/3rds of CBD
Type IV	Fistula involving >2/3rds or complete CBD wall destruction
Type V	Presence of cholecystoenteric fistula (e.g., to duodenum or colon), with or without gallstone ileus

Clinical Features

Symptom	*Notes*
Jaundice	Painless or mild, due to bile duct obstruction
Right upper quadrant pain	Due to cholecystitis or inflammation
Fever	If cholangitis develops
Murphy's sign	May be positive (inflammation of gallbladder)

Investigations

Test	*Findings*
Ultrasound	Gallstones, dilated intrahepatic ducts, possible mass near CHD
MRCP	Noninvasive, shows compression or fistula
ERCP	Gold standard for diagnosis; can also be therapeutic
CT scan	Shows inflammation, gallbladder mass, or fistula
LFTs	Elevated bilirubin, ALP, GGT (cholestatic pattern)

Differential Diagnosis

- Cholangiocarcinoma (Klatskin tumor)
- Gallbladder cancer
- Primary sclerosing cholangitis
- Biliary strictures
- Choledocholithiasis

Mirizzi syndrome can mimic cholangiocarcinoma—hence called a *"pseudotumor"* of the bile duct.

Management

Type	*Treatment*
Type I	*Cholecystectomy* (laparoscopic or open depending on inflammation)
Type II–IV	Complex surgery: • *Cholecystectomy + biliary reconstruction* • *T-tube drainage*, or • *Roux-en-Y hepaticojejunostomy* (for major CBD defects) |
Type V	Also requires repair of *enteric fistula* or management of *gallstone ileus preoperative biliary drainage*—Via *ERCP stenting* if jaundice or cholangitis is present

11. Discuss the etiology, presentation, and management of recurrent pyogenic cholangitis. ***WBUHS 2018***

Introduction

- The underlying mechanism of recurrent pyogenic cholangitis (RPC) is unclear.
- Most experts believe that RPC is initiated by helminthic infection of the bile ducts and/or sludge/stone formation from deficient glucuronidation as a consequence of profound malnutrition.
- Hepatolithiasis is associated with clonorchis sinensis and ascaris lumbricoides infestation of the liver.
- The initial insult(s) to the bile ducts precipitates a cycle of biliary stone formation and infection that results in recurrent episodes of pyogenic cholangitis.

Clinical Features

- An acute attack of cholangitis
- A history of recurrent attacks of cholangitis typified by fevers and right upper quadrant (RUQ) abdominal pain
- Complications of pyogenic cholangitis
- As the disease progresses, patients may develop cholangiocarcinoma and present with constitutional symptoms, including weight loss, easy fatigability, and jaundice.
- Presentation can be atypical with no pain or fever especially in the elderly population.

Investigations and Diagnosis

Laboratory Investigations

- *Complete blood count:* A leukocytosis with a left shift is typical in patients with pyogenic cholangitis.
- *Liver function tests:* Aminotransferases, serum bilirubin, and alkaline phosphatase typically are elevated in patients with RPC.
- *Prothrombin time:* This may become prolonged if persistent cholestasis with consequent fat malabsorption and vitamin K deficiency is present. This is important to exclude because hypoprothrombinemia can impact the safety of invasive procedures and is easily correctible with parenteral vitamin K in this setting.
- *Blood cultures:* These are mandatory because many patients are bacteremic. The blood culture results often help to guide antibiotic choice.
- *Ova and parasites:* Clonorchis infection frequently is associated with RPC and should be sought and treated when present.

Imaging Studies

- *Noninvasive imaging studies:* Noninvasive imaging studies include transabdominal ultrasonography, computed tomography (CT) scanning, and magnetic resonance cholangiopancreatography (MRCP).
- Ultrasonography is the preferred initial test during the primary workup. This imaging modality may demonstrate segmental biliary dilatation, hepatolithiasis, and liver abscesses, if present.
- CT scanning may demonstrate centrally dilated bile ducts with peripheral tapering. Cholangiohepatitis has a predilection for the left lobe of the liver, and predominantly left-sided findings should prompt consideration of this diagnosis in patients from endemic areas. Other potential findings on CT scans include bile duct stones and pyogenic liver abscesses.
- The role of MRCP in the investigation of biliary disease continues to evolve in spite of the poor availability of magnetic resonance imaging (MRI) facilities in many regions of the world where RPC is endemic. MRI produces axial images and can be performed to evaluate the portal and hepatic venous system.
- MR cholangiography may quickly replace endoscopic retrograde cholangiopancreatography or percutaneous transhepatic cholangiography as the imaging modality of choice for delineating the biliary tree.

Invasive Techniques

- The choice of endoscopic (i.e., ERCP) versus percutaneous cholangiography hinges on the patient's anatomy and general health status and on the availability of local expertise.
- Very often, a combination of both techniques is necessary to achieve complete ductal clearance of stones and to ensure that drainage of the biliary tree has been optimized.

Treatment

- Patients must be treated with a multidisciplinary approach by multiple subspecialists. Preferably, care should be rendered by individuals who are regional experts in interventional endoscopy, radiology, and hepatobiliary surgery.
- Medical care generally involves parenteral antibiotics, avoidance, and/or prompt recognition and treatment of complications. Patients who are malnourished require nutritional rehabilitation.
- A biliary drainage procedure is necessary to achieve resolution of the initial infection and to pursue the ultimate goal of preventing further attacks of recurrent cholangitis. The choice of biliary drainage procedure should hinge on patient presentation, comorbidities, cholangiographic findings, and local expertise.
- Initial biliary decompression is achieved at ERCP, which also allows for the delineation of the biliary tree, an essential step in the planning of the definitive decompressive procedure. Sphincterotomy, stricture dilatation, and placement of a biliary endoprosthesis (stent) often are necessary to achieve biliary decom- pression and, when appropriate, to alleviate stasis or luminal compromise in the biliary tree, thus preventing further episodes of pyogenic cholangitis. The results of endotherapy appear to be durable in well-selected patients.
- In some patients, initial medical management may fail and patients may require emergency surgery. These patients often have acute suppurative cholecystitis and require emergent cholecystectomy or percutaneous cholecystotomy (as a temporizing measure). Definitive surgery is directed toward optimizing biliary outflow and is determined by the anatomical extent of involvement.
- Surgery is necessary in patients who have concomitant cholelithiasis or complex hepatolithiasis.
- The surgical approach is based on the appearance at cholangiography and on axial imaging or MRCP.
- The usual surgical approach includes the following:
  - Cholecystectomy
  - Intraoperative stone clearance by ERCP
  - Percutaneous cholangiography
  - Lithotripsy (i.e., mechanical, laser, and electrohydraulic)
  - A definitive biliary drainage procedure
- Definitive drainage procedures include operative sphincteroplasty and appropriate biliodigestive bypass.
- Many surgeons favor performing a Roux-en-Y choledochojejunostomy. Access to the Roux limb for reintervention (if necessary) is achieved percutaneously or endoscopically.

BILE DUCT INJURY

12. Describe the management of iatrogenic bile duct injury. ***WBUHS 2011***

13. Management of benign biliary stricture. ***KGMU, Lucknow 2025***

Introduction

- Most benign strictures follow iatrogenic bile duct injury, most commonly during laparoscopic cholecystectomy.
- Most injuries are recognized intraoperatively or during the early postoperative period, and with appropriate management, the long-term results are acceptable.
- Long-term sequelae of unrecognized or inappropriately managed biliary strictures may lead to recurrent cholangitis, secondary biliary cirrhosis, and portal hypertension.

Pathogenesis

A number of factors may be involved in the occurrence of bile duct injuries during laparoscopic cholecystectomy.

These include:

- Acute or chronic inflammation, obesity, anatomic variations, and bleeding
- Surgical technique with inadequate exposure and failure to identify structures before ligating or dividing them are the most common cause of significant biliary injury.

- The bile duct injury rate is increased in patients with complications of gallstones, including acute cholecystitis, pancreatitis, cholangitis, and obstructive jaundice.
- Surgeon training and experience were recognized as factors in early reports of laparoscopic bile duct injuries. As surgeon experience increases beyond 20 cases, the bile duct injury rate decreases.
- Aberrant biliary anatomy is often cited as a factor in biliary injuries:
  - The bile duct may be narrow and can be mistaken for the cystic duct.
  - The cystic duct may travel parallel to the common bile duct (CBD) before joining it, misleading the surgeon to the wrong place. Also, the cystic duct may enter the right hepatic duct, and the right hepatic duct may run aberrantly, coursing through the triangle of Calot and entering the common hepatic duct (CHD).
- A number of other technical factors have been implicated in biliary injuries:
  - The classic injury occurs when excessive cephalad retraction of the gallbladder may align the cystic duct with the common bile duct, allowing the latter to be mistaken for the cystic duct.
  - Careless use of electrocautery may lead to thermal injury.
  - Dissection deep into the liver parenchyma may cause injury to intrahepatic ducts.
  - Poor clip placement close to the hilar area or to structures not well visualized can result in a clip across the bile duct.

Presentation

- Patients with bile duct injuries can present intraoperatively, in the early postoperative period, or months, or years after the initial injury.
- About 25% of major ductal injuries are recognized intraoperatively because of bile leakage, an abnormal cholangiogram, or late recognition of the anatomy.
- The most common presentation of a complete occlusion of the common hepatic or bile duct is jaundice with or without abdominal pain.
- Patients may also present months or years after prior surgery with cholangitis or cirrhosis secondary to a biliary tract injury.

Diagnosis and Management

- The management of bile duct injury is dependent on the timing of diagnosis and extent and level of injury. Inappropriate management of biliary strictures may result in significant morbidity.
- Isolated, small, noncautery-based partial lateral bile duct injury recognized at time of cholecystectomy can be managed with placement of a T tube. The T tube can be placed at the site of the injury if this is similar in size to a choledochotomy.
- However, if the biliary injury is more extensive, or if there is significant thermal damage owing to cautery-based trauma, or if the injury involves >50% of the circumference of the bile duct wall, an end-to-side choledochojejunostomy with a Roux-en-Y loop of jejunum should be performed.
- Similarly, major bile duct injuries, including transections of the common bile or common hepatic duct, can be repaired if recognized at the time of cholecystectomy.
- Isolated hepatic ducts <3 mm or those draining a single hepatic segment can be safely ligated.
- Ducts >3 mm are more likely to drain several segments or an entire lobe and need to be reimplanted.
- If one is uncertain or underexperienced, and no colleague with sufficient expertise is immediately available, placing a drain followed by referral to an experienced center is the most appropriate course of action.

Management of the bile duct injury recognized after cholecystectomy: Most large series report the incidence of ductal injury after laparoscopic cholecystectomy to be 0.3–0.85%. In general, patients with a bile leak will present early, whereas patients with postoperative biliary strictures alone often present with jaundice or cholangitis months to years after the initial injury.

Diagnosis

- Abdominal imaging with ultrasonography or CT should be performed in patients with signs of abdominal pain or peritonitis, sepsis, or any other clinical suspicion of biloma.

- Such patients must be stabilized with immediate parenteral antibiotics and image-guided percutaneous drainage of any fluid collections.
- Patients with signs and symptoms of cholangitis should undergo urgent cholangiogram with bile duct drainage.
- Cholangiography should be performed to establish the presence of ductal stricture, identify the level of the stricture, and identify the nature of the injury when necessary.
- ERCP may be easier to obtain in a patient with a biliary stricture and cholangitis who requires urgent cholangiography and biliary decompression.
  - However, this is only useful in patients with bile duct continuity.
  - Cystic duct leaks or small tangential injuries can be treated with endoscopic stenting. In situations in which the biliary stricture is too tight to pass with ERCP.
  - Percutaneous transhepatic cholangiography (PTC) may be performed for proximal biliary decompression.
- CT arteriography should be considered in the preoperative evaluation of patients with benign biliary strictures:
  - Unrecognized injury to the hepatic artery or a portal vein branch occurs with a frequency of 12–47% concomitant with a bile duct injury.
  - If significant bleeding required urgent control at the time of the original operation, a vascular injury should be considered.
  - The presence of a right hepatic artery disruption should not affect the surgical repair of a bile duct injury. In patients presenting with late strictures with evidence of liver dysfunction, a CT arteriogram should be performed to evaluate for evidence of portal hypertension.

Intraoperative Considerations

The management of postoperative biliary strictures following ductal injury depends on:

- The degree of injury, the presence of stricture-induced complications
- The operative risk of the patient

After recognition of a bile duct injury or stricture, a multidisciplinary team consisting of experienced inter- ventional radiologists, endoscopists, and surgeons, coordinated by an experienced hepatobiliary surgeon, should plan the following specific goals:

- Control the infection (abscess or cholangitis)
- Drain the biloma
- Complete the cholangiography
- Provide definitive therapy with controlled reconstruction or stenting

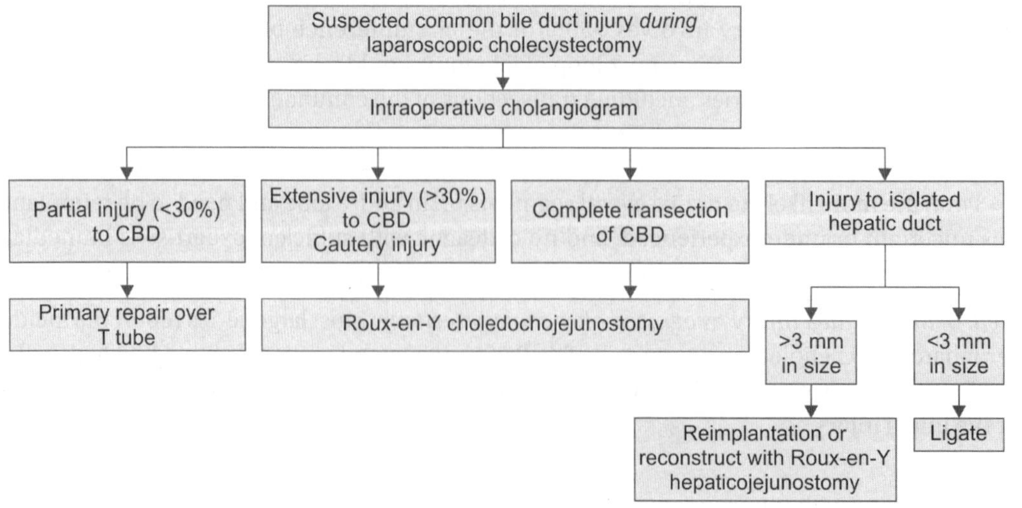

(CBD: common bile duct)

14. Classification and management algorithm of post laparoscopic cholecystectomy bile duct injury.

WBUHS 2015, 2016, 2018

15. Describe the Strasberg classification of bile duct injury and outline the management.

WBUHS 2025 Supplementary

Laparoscopic cholecystectomy (LC) has been associated with a higher incidence of IA bile duct injuries:

- *LC:* 0.4–0.8%
- *Traditional open cholecystectomy (OC):* 0.1–0.3%

Association

- Increased mortality and morbidity
- Reduced long-term survival
- Reduced quality of life
- *Infrequent*—but among the leading sources of malpractice claims against surgeons
- Between 34 and 49% of surgeons are expected to cause such an injury during their career.
- Awareness and preventative methods are of clinical importance to surgeons.

Risk Factors

Anatomical

- Anatomical variations (biliary and vasculature)
- Bleeding, scarring, and obesity

Laparoscopic: Lack of depth perception, tactile feedback, and full manual maneuverability

Improper surgical approach:

- Improper lateral retraction (insufficient or excessive)
- 0° scope
- Approach plane too deep

Lack of Conversion to OC during Difficult Cases

Mechanism of Injury

- *Initially:* Surgeon's learning curve—steady
- *Anatomical misidentification:* Excision, incision, or transection of biliary anatomy
- *Injuries:* Common bile duct, common hepatic duct, right and left hepatic ducts, right hepatic artery, and ducts draining hepatic segments
- *Anatomical variations (biliary and vasculature)*
- *Electrocautery, thermal injury:* Stricture of CBD or hepatic ducts, bile leak
- *Mechanical trauma:* Stricture of the biliary ducts, bile leaks
- Improper surgical approach

Thermal Injuries

- Inappropriate use of electrocautery near biliary ducts
- May lead to stricture and/or bile leaks
- Mechanical trauma can have similar effects

Strasberg Classification

- *Type A:* Cystic duct leaks or leaks from small ducts in the liver bed
- *Type B:* Occlusion of a part of the biliary tree, almost invariably the aberrant right hepatic ducts
- *Type C:* Transection without ligation of the aberrant right hepatic ducts
- *Type D:* Lateral injuries to major bile ducts
- *Type E:* Subdivided as per Bismuth classification into E1 to E5

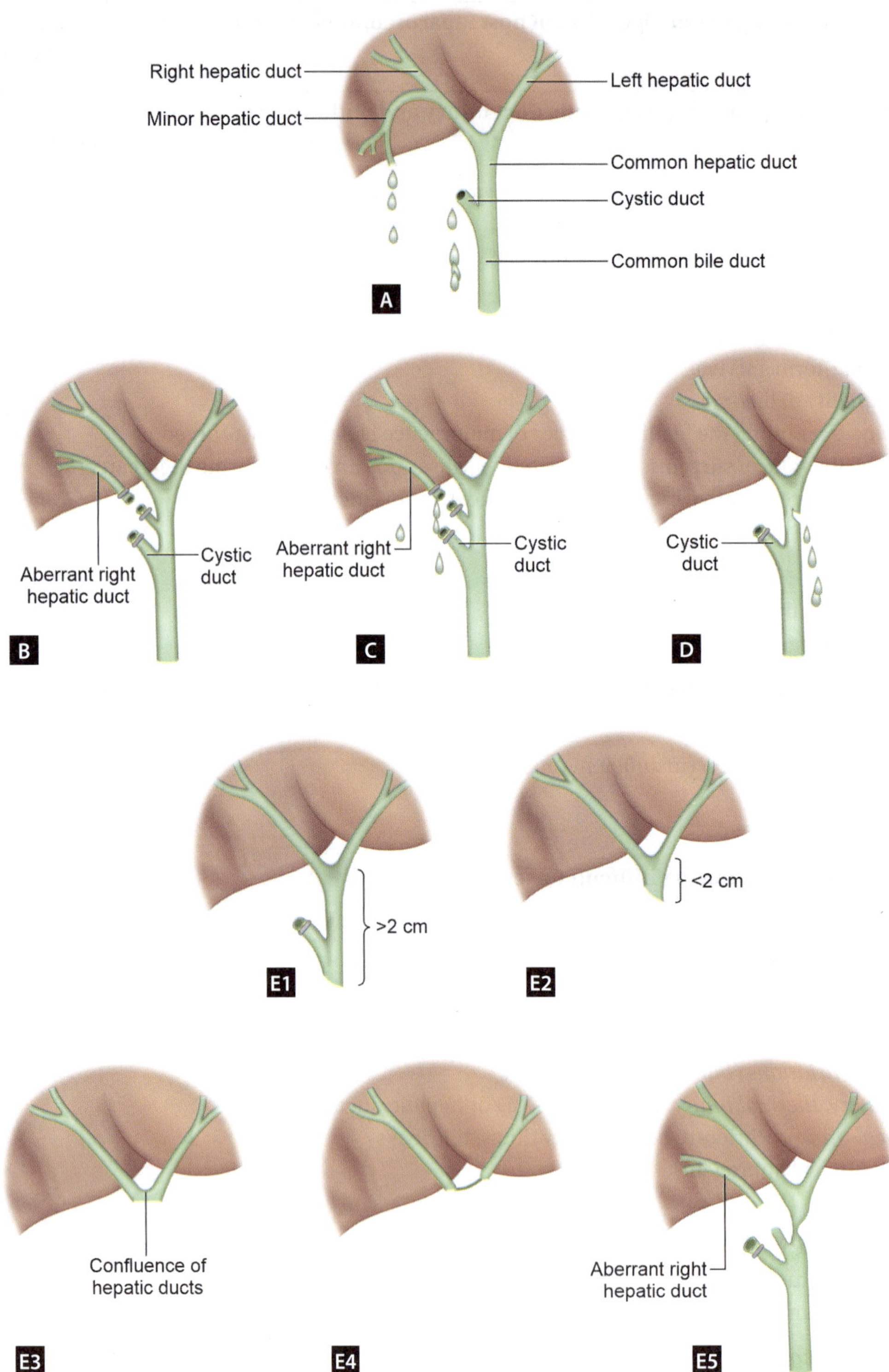

E: injury to main duct (Bismuth):

- *E1:* Transection >2 cm from confluence
- *E2:* Transection <2 cm from confluence
- *E3:* Transection in hilum

- *E4:* Separation of major ducts in hilum
- *E5:* Type C plus injury in hilum

Lau classification (2007):

- *Type 1:* Leaks from cystic duct stump or small ducts in liver bed
- *Type 2:* Partial CBD/CHD wall injuries without (2A) or with (2B) tissue loss
- *Type 3:* CBD/CHD transection without (3A) or with (3B) tissue loss
- *Type 4:* Right/left hepatic duct or sectoral duct injuries without (4A) or with (4B) tissue loss
- *Type 5:* Bile duct injuries associated with vascular injuries

Mechanism of common bile duct injury (Stewart–Way classification).	
Class I	CBD mistaken for cystic duct, but recognized cholangiogram incision in cystic duct extended into CBD
Class II	Lateral damage to the CHD from cautery or clips placed on duct-associated bleeding, poor visibility
Class III	CBD mistaken for cystic duct, not recognized CBD, CHD, RL hepatic ducts transected and/or resected
Class IV	RI ID mistaken for cystic duct. RHA mistaken for cystic artery, RHD and RHA transected Lateral damage to the RHD from cautery or clips placed on duct

(CBD: common bile duct; CHD: common hepatic duct; RHA: right hepatic artery; RHD: right hepatic duct)

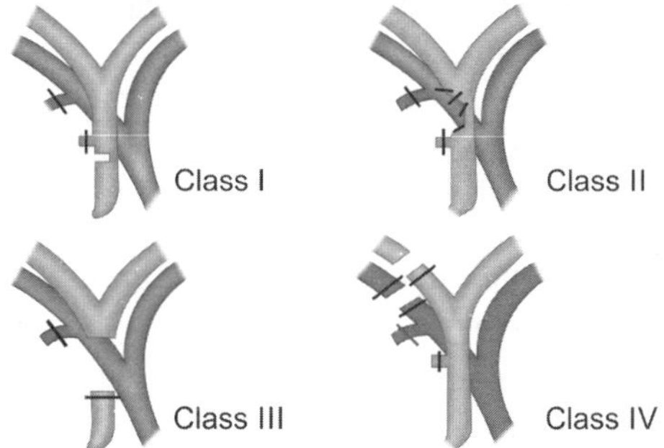

Stewart–Way classification laparoscopic bile duct injuries.

Goals of therapy in iatrogenic bile duct injury:

- Control of infection limiting inflammation:
    - Parenteral antibiotics
    - Percutaneous drainage of periportal fluid collections
- Clear and thorough delineation of entire biliary anatomy:
    - MR CP/PTC
    - ERCP (especially if cystic duct stump leak suspected)
- Re-establishment of biliary enteric continuity:
    - Tension-free, mucosa-to-mucosa anastomosis
    - Roux-en-Y hepaticojejunostomy
    - Long-term transanastomotic stents if involving bifurcation or higher

Management

- Only 25–33% of injures are recognized intraoperatively
- If experienced, convert to open procedure and perform cholangiography (determine extent of injury)
- If not experienced, perform the cholangiogram laparoscopically with intent of referring patient (placement of drains)
- Consult an experienced hepatobiliary surgeon
- *Acute management:*
    - Biliary catheter for decompression of biliary tract and control of bile leaks
    - Percutaneous drainage of intraperitoneal bile collection

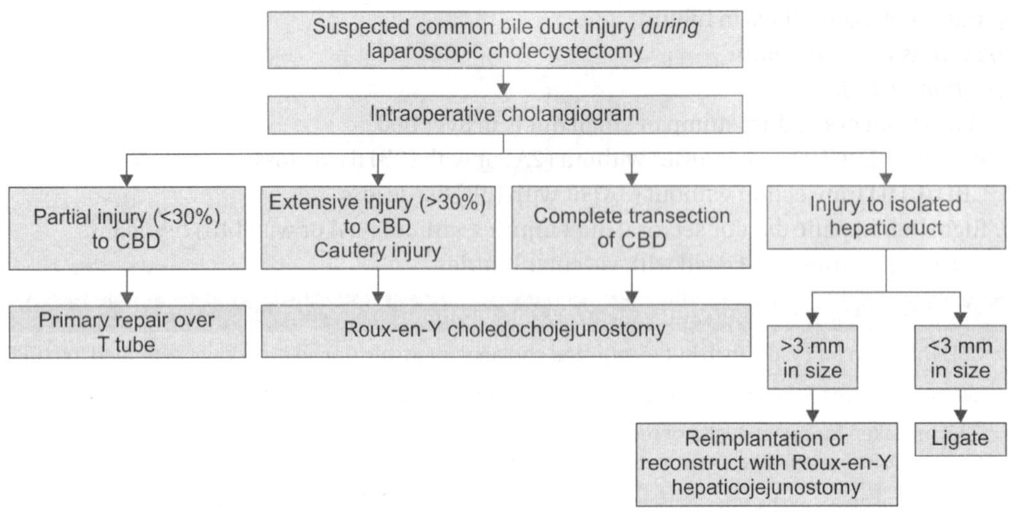

(CBD: common bile duct)

16. Factors responsible for bile duct injury. How bile duct injury can be graded? Classify postoperative bile duct injury. ***WBUHS 2021 Supplementary***

17. Discuss the types and management of biliary ductal injury. ***WBUHS 2024***

Introduction

Most benign strictures follow iatrogenic bile duct injury, most commonly during laparoscopic cholecystectomy. Most injuries are recognized intraoperatively or during the early postoperative period, and with appropriate management, the long-term results are acceptable. Long-term sequelae of unrecognized or inappropriately managed biliary strictures may lead to recurrent cholangitis, secondary biliary cirrhosis, and portal hypertension.

Pathogenesis

A number of factors may be involved in the occurrence of bile duct injuries during cholecystectomy.

These include:

- Acute or chronic inflammation, obesity, anatomic variations, and bleeding
- Surgical technique with inadequate exposure and failure to identify structures before ligating or dividing them are the most common cause of significant biliary injury.
- The bile duct injury rate is increased in patients with complications of gallstones, including acute cholecystitis, pancreatitis, cholangitis, and obstructive jaundice.
- Surgeon training and experience were recognized as factors in early reports of laparoscopic bile duct injuries. As surgeon experience increases beyond 20 cases, the bile duct injury rate decreases.
- Aberrant biliary anatomy is often cited as a factor in biliary injuries:
  - The bile duct may be narrow and can be mistaken for the cystic duct.
  - The cystic duct may travel parallel to the common bile duct before joining it, misleading the surgeon to the wrong place. Also, the cystic duct may enter the right hepatic duct, and the right hepatic duct may run aberrantly, coursing through the triangle of Calot and entering the common hepatic duct.
- A number of other technical factors have been implicated in biliary injuries:
  - The classic injury occurs when excessive cephalad retraction of the gallbladder may align the cystic duct with the common bile duct, allowing the latter to be mistaken for the cystic duct.
  - Careless use of electrocautery may lead to thermal injury.
  - Dissection deep into the liver parenchyma may cause injury to intrahepatic ducts.
- Poor clip placement close to the hilar area or to structures not well visualized can result in a clip across the bile duct.

Bismuth Classification of Benign Bile Duct Strictures

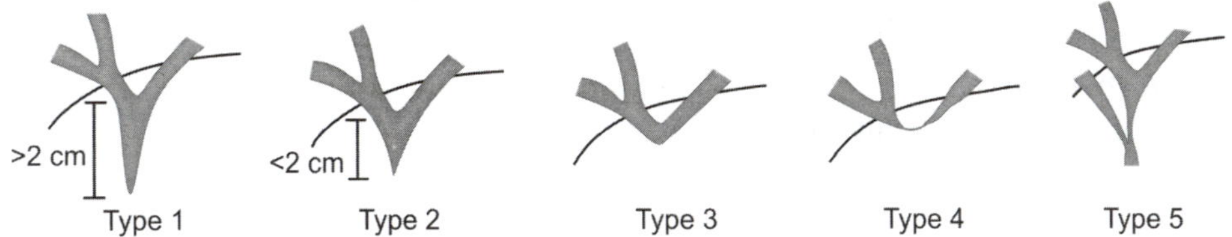

Strasberg Classification

- *Type A:* Cystic duct leaks or leaks from small ducts in the liver bed
- *Type B:* Occlusion of a part of the biliary tree, almost invariably the aberrant right hepatic ducts
- *Type C:* Transection without ligation of the aberrant right hepatic ducts
- *Type D:* Lateral injuries to major bile ducts
- *Type E:* Subdivided as per Bismuth classification into E1 to E5

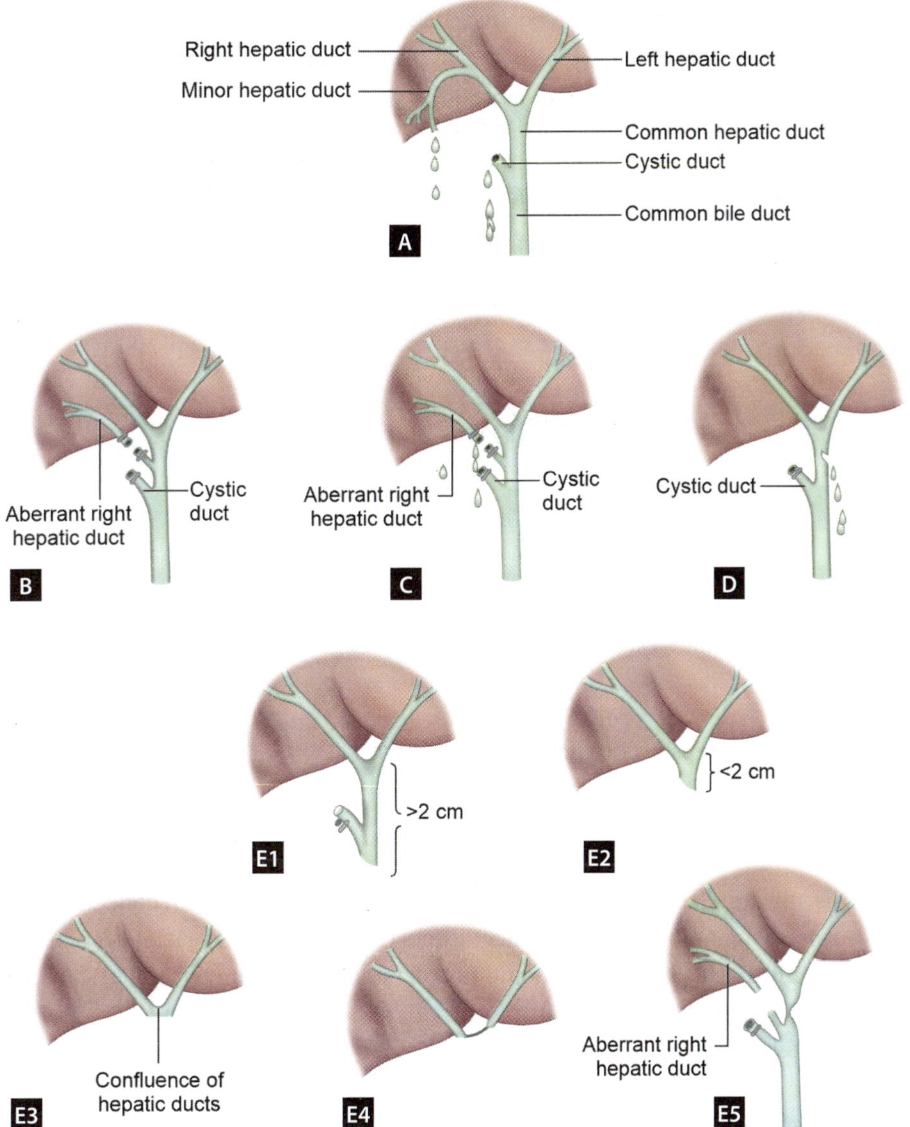

E: injury to main duct (Bismuth):

- *E1:* Transection >2 cm from confluence
- *E2:* Transection <2 cm from confluence
- *E3:* Transection in hilum
- *E4:* Separation of major ducts in hilum
- *E5:* Type C plus injury in hilum

Lau classification (2007):

- *Type 1:* Leaks from cystic duct stump or small ducts in liver bed
- *Type 2:* Partial CBD/CHD wall injuries without (2A) or with (2B) tissue loss
- *Type 3:* CBD/CHD transection without (3A) or with (3B) tissue loss
- *Type 4:* Right/left hepatic duct or sectoral duct injuries without (4A) or with (4B) tissue loss
- *Type 5:* Bile duct injuries associated with vascular injuries

Mechanism of Common Bile Duct Injury (Stewart-Way Classification).	
Class I	CBD mistaken for cystic duct, but recognized cholangiogram incision in cystic duct extended into CBD
Class II	Lateral damage to the CHD from cautery or clips placed on duct-associated bleeding, poor visibility
Class III	CBD mistaken for cystic duct, not recognized CBD, CHD, R. L hepatic ducts transected and/or resected
Class IV	RI ID mistaken for cystic duct. RHA mistaken for cystic artery, RHD and RHA transected Lateral damage to the RHD from cautery or clips placed on duct

(CBD: common bile duct; CHD: common hepatic duct; RHA: right hepatic artery; RHD: right hepatic duct)

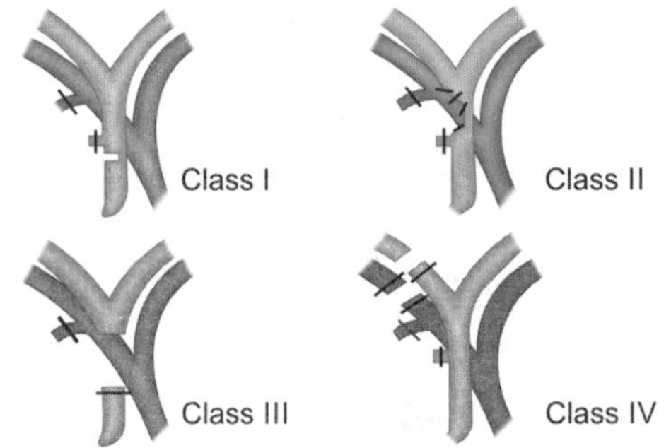

Stewart–Way classification laparoscopic bile duct injuries

Management

- *Treat/relieve complications:* Sepsis, obstruction, and fistula
- Characterize bile duct injury
- Treat injury
- Follow-up
- If pain, fever, sepsis, no jaundice (i.e., likely A)—US or CT to evaluate and drain collection.
- If bile is found—can use hepatobiliary iminodiacetic acid (HIDA) scan to see if leak is active.
- If leak is active, then ERCP will characterize it and treat it (stent and sphincterotomy).
- If jaundice—start with ERCP ± US.
- ERCP will not characterize proximal biliary tree
- PTC is invaluable
- May be difficult if no dilation

- Can drain effectively—temporize
- If already draining bile—fistulogram

When to Operate

- Intraoperatively, C, D, or E injuries are seen
- If recognized, need to convert to open
- Ideally, intraoperatively at first operation or ASAP
- Otherwise, if no experience—drain and refer
- If injury took place >72 hours, try to temporize at least 8 weeks, ideally 12 weeks.
- Let inflammation settle and thermal/devascularization injury to manifest itself fully.
- If uncontrolled sepsis—then no delay

Type A

Endoscopic internal stenting:

- Reduces pressure gradient
- Procedure of choice for treating bile duct leaks
- 7- and 10-Fr stents can be inserted without sphincterotomy
- Prompt therapeutic response seen
- Cessation of bile extravasation in 70–95% of cases within a period of 1–7 days

Type B

Most asymptomatic:

- Usually present late or discovered incidentally
- If affected segment small—no treatment
- If large and cholangitis—consider hepaticojejunostomy versus segmental resection

Type C

- Oversew if duct is <2 mm
- Otherwise, enteric anastomosis

Type D

Some can be treated with stent:

- Repair over a T tube
- Intubate or separate stab drain

Type E

Hepaticoduodenostomy—usually avoided—too much tension

Hepaticojejunostomy:

- End-to-end:
- If no loss of length and clean cut higher incidence of stricture
- Some do not recommend due to ischemia of CBD

Principle of repair:

- Tension free
- Mucosa to mucosa
- Adequate diameter

Follow-up:

- Liver function test (LFT)
- USG
- HIDA
- MRCP

18. Discuss the common anatomical variations of the extra-hepatic biliary tract. Discuss the principles of management of a case with Class III (Stewart–Way classification) bile duct injury.

Srimanta Sankaradeva University, Assam 2025

Common Anatomical Variations of the Extrahepatic Biliary Tract

The *extra-hepatic biliary tract* includes the structures *outside the liver* that transport bile from the liver to the duodenum.

These are:

- Right and left hepatic ducts
- Common hepatic duct (CHD)
- Cystic duct
- Common bile duct (CBD)

Anatomical variations in this system are *common*, occurring in *25–50%* of individuals, and are *clinically significant*, especially during hepatobiliary surgeries (e.g., cholecystectomy, liver transplantation). Failure to recognize them can result in *bile duct injury*.

Cystic Duct Variations

Variation	*Description*
Low insertion of cystic duct	Cystic duct joins the *lower part of CHD or upper CBD* (near duodenum)
High insertion of cystic duct	Cystic duct joins CHD near the confluence of the hepatic ducts
Medial insertion	Cystic duct joins CHD from the *left (medial) side* instead of right
Parallel course	Cystic duct runs *parallel and closely adherent* to CHD for some distance before joining
Spiral insertion	Cystic duct spirals around CHD before joining
Short or absent cystic duct	Cystic duct is very short or seems absent, making dissection difficult during surgery
Accessory cystic duct	An extra duct draining into CHD or CBD—rare but dangerous if missed

Hepatic Duct Variations

Variation	*Description*
Trifurcation	Right anterior, right posterior, and left hepatic ducts all meet at a common point—no proper right hepatic duct
Right posterior duct drains into left hepatic duct	Common variation (up to 15%)—can be mistaken for an accessory duct
Right anterior or posterior draining directly into CHD or cystic duct	May lead to bile leak if injured during surgery
Accessory hepatic ducts	Extra ducts draining segments of the liver directly into extrahepatic ducts (e.g., duct of Luschka)—risk of postoperative bile leak

Common Bile Duct (CBD) Variations

Variation	*Description*
Retroduodenal course	Normally the CBD passes behind the duodenum, but its course can vary
Pancreaticobiliary maljunction	The bile and pancreatic ducts join *outside* the duodenal wall—associated with higher risk of *cholangiocarcinoma* or *pancreatitis*

Gallbladder Variations (Related)

Though not part of the biliary ducts per se, gallbladder variations often impact surgery:

Variation	Description
Intrahepatic gallbladder	Gallbladder partially or completely embedded in the liver
Phrygian cap	Folded fundus of the gallbladder
Double gallbladder	Two gallbladders—very rare

Mechanism of Common Bile Duct Injury (Stewart–Way Classification).	
Class I	CBD mistaken for cystic duct, but recognized cholangiogram incision in cystic duct extended into CBD
Class II	Lateral damage to the CHD from cautery or clips placed on duct-associated bleeding, poor visibility
Class III	CBD mistaken for cystic duct, not recognized CBD, CHD, RL hepatic ducts transected and/or resected
Class IV	RI ID mistaken for cystic duct. RHA mistaken for cystic artery, RHD and RHA transected Lateral damage to the RHD from cautery or clips placed on duct

(CBD: common bile duct; CHD: common hepatic duct; RHA: right hepatic artery; RHD: right hepatic duct)

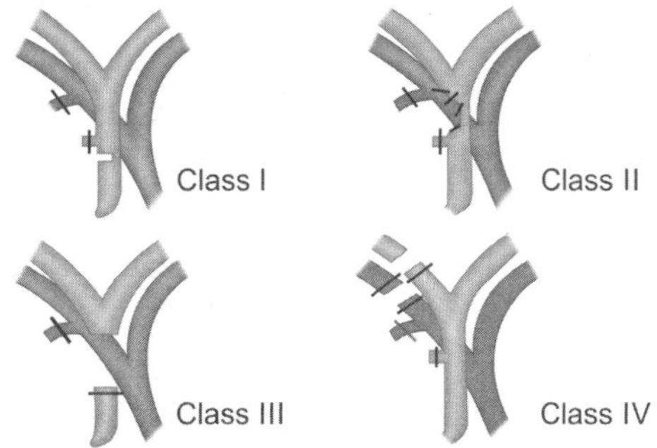

Stewart–Way classification laparoscopic bile duct injuries

Description of Class III Bile Duct Injury

Class III injuries are the most common type, accounting for approximately 60% of BDIs. They involve complete transection of the main bile duct (typically the CHD or CBD), invariably including the cystic duct-CHD junction, with excision of a variable portion of the proximal duct. This results from misidentifying the CBD as the cystic duct during dissection, leading to division and partial removal of the bile duct along with the gallbladder. Subdivisions include:

- *IIIa:* Remnant of CHD preserved.
- *IIIb:* Transection at the cystic duct-CHD junction.
- *IIIc:* Excision including the biliary confluence.
- *IIId:* Transection above a lobar or secondary duct.

These injuries disrupt biliary continuity, causing bile leakage, potential peritonitis, and risks of strictures if untreated. Associated vascular injuries (e.g., right hepatic artery) occur in some cases but are less common than in Class IV.

Principles of Management

Management of Class III BDIs prioritizes early recognition, sepsis control, multidisciplinary input, and referral to high-volume hepatobiliary (HPB) centers, as outcomes are significantly better with expert intervention. The approach varies by timing of diagnosis (intraoperative, early postoperative [<6 weeks], or delayed [>6 weeks]), patient stability, and injury extent. Key principles include stabilizing the patient, draining collections, and planning definitive reconstruction while avoiding attempts by inexperienced surgeons, which succeed in only about 21% of cases.

Diagnosis

- *Intraoperative recognition:* Occurs in <25–30% of cases and is ideal. Use intraoperative cholangiography (IOC) or indocyanine green fluorescence cholangiography to confirm anatomy and injury extent. If unrecognized, place drains and refer immediately.
- *Postoperative presentation:* Suspect BDI with persistent pain, bile in drains, fever, jaundice, elevated liver enzymes, or peritonitis signs. Initial imaging includes abdominal ultrasound for collections or dilation, followed by CT for fluid assessment and vascular evaluation. Magnetic resonance cholangiopancreatography (MRCP) is the gold standard for delineating biliary integrity and leak sites. Hepatobiliary iminodiacetic acid (HIDA) scans confirm active leaks but lack precise localization. Endoscopic retrograde cholangiopancreatography (ERCP) aids in leak level assessment and therapeutic stenting.
- *Additional steps:* Percutaneously drain any collections under imaging guidance to control sepsis and inflammation. For delayed diagnosis, allow 2–3 months for stabilization before repair.

Initial Management and Stabilization

- *Control bile leak and infection:* Use broad-spectrum antibiotics (e.g., piperacillin/tazobactam) for 5–7 days post-source control, adding antifungals if needed. Provide nutritional support and manage peritonitis with urgent lavage if diffuse.
- *Temporary measures:* ERCP with sphincterotomy and stenting, or percutaneous transhepatic biliary drainage (PTBD), to decompress the system and bridge to surgery. In friable tissues, a pedicled omental patch may serve as interim repair.
- *Referral:* Immediate transfer to an HPB center if local expertise is lacking, as this reduces complications like strictures (odds ratio 0.28).

Definitive Surgical Repair

- *Preferred approach:* Roux-en-Y hepaticojejunostomy is the standard for Class III due to tissue loss and tension risks, achieving 80–90% long-term success. Use a T-tube or internal Y-drain for protection.
- *Alternatives:* End-to-end anastomosis only if tension-free and no significant loss (rare in Class III); protect with a T-tube. Laparoscopic or robotic-assisted techniques offer minimally invasive options with comparable outcomes.
- *Timing considerations:* Intraoperative repair by experts; otherwise, delay until inflammation resolves (e.g., ≥3 weeks poststabilization) to lower morbidity (14% vs. 39% for immediate). Avoid repair in active infection.
- *Associated injuries:* Manage vascular issues (e.g., hepatic artery) with angioembolization or resection if ischemic; do not routinely repair isolated right hepatic artery injuries.

Outcomes and Follow-up

Successful repair yields high patency rates, but complications occur in 36% of cases, including bile leaks (11%), strictures (30%), wound infections, or dehiscence. Mortality is around 2%. Long-term risks include cholangitis, cirrhosis, portal hypertension, or need for redo surgery/transplant if delayed or mismanaged. Quality of life is impaired compared to uncomplicated cases, with high litigation rates. Follow-up involves monitoring for strictures via imaging and liver function tests, with interventions like stenting or redo hepaticojejunostomy if needed. Early expert management and referral are critical for optimal results.

---

19. Explain the pathophysiological changes occurring following bile duct injury. Discuss role of various imaging modalities. Compare early versus delayed repair strategies. ***WBUHS 2025***

Pathophysiological Changes Following Bile Duct Injury (BDI)

Bile duct injury, often occurring during laparoscopic cholecystectomy or other hepatobiliary surgeries, triggers a cascade of pathophysiological changes that can lead to significant morbidity. These changes depend on the type, severity, and timing of the injury.

1. **Immediate consequences**:
   - *Bile leakage:* Injury to the bile duct (e.g., laceration, transection, or clip misplacement) leads to bile extravasation into the peritoneal cavity or localized collections (bilomas). This causes chemical peritonitis, leading to abdominal pain, fever, and potential sepsis.
   - *Obstruction:* Partial or complete transection may obstruct bile flow, causing upstream biliary dilatation, cholestasis, and elevated liver enzymes (e.g., bilirubin, alkaline phosphatase, gamma-glutamyl transferase).
   - *Inflammatory Response:* Bile in the peritoneal cavity triggers an inflammatory reaction, recruiting cytokines and immune cells, which may lead to adhesions, abscess formation, or systemic inflammatory response syndrome (SIRS).
2. **Short-term pathophysiology**:
   - *Infection:* Stagnant bile or bilomas are prone to bacterial contamination, leading to cholangitis, intra-abdominal abscesses, or sepsis.
   - *Hepatic dysfunction:* Prolonged bile leakage or obstruction impairs hepatocyte function, causing jaundice, pruritus, and malabsorption of fat-soluble vitamins due to reduced bile delivery to the intestine.
   - *Vascular compromise:* Concomitant injury to the right hepatic artery (seen in ~20% of BDIs) may cause ischemia to the bile duct or liver, exacerbating tissue damage and complicating repair.
3. **Long-term pathophysiology**:
   - *Stricture Formation:* Chronic inflammation and fibrosis at the injury site lead to bile duct strictures, causing recurrent cholangitis, secondary biliary cirrhosis, and portal hypertension over time.
   - *Liver Damage:* Persistent obstruction or recurrent infections may progress to liver fibrosis, cirrhosis, or end-stage liver disease.
   - *Biliary Fistula:* Uncontrolled bile leaks may form fistulae (e.g., biliocutaneous or bilioenteric), leading to chronic bile loss, electrolyte imbalances, and malnutrition.
4. **Systemic effects**:
   - *Sepsis and multiorgan failure:* Severe infections from untreated bile leaks or abscesses can lead to systemic sepsis, acute kidney injury, or acute respiratory distress syndrome.
   - *Metabolic disturbances:* Chronic cholestasis impairs fat and vitamin absorption, leading to deficiencies (e.g., vitamins A, D, E, K) and coagulopathy.

Role of Imaging Modalities in Bile Duct Injury

Imaging plays a critical role in diagnosing BDI, assessing its extent, and guiding management. The choice of modality depends on clinical presentation and suspected injury type.

1. **Ultrasound (US)**:
   - *Role:* First-line imaging to detect fluid collections (bilomas), biliary dilatation, or abscesses. Doppler US can assess hepatic artery patency.
   - *Advantages:* Non-invasive, widely available, no radiation, cost-effective.
   - *Limitations:* Operator-dependent, limited in visualizing specific ductal injuries or deep structures.
   - *Use case:* Initial screening for bile leaks or obstruction in patients with post-cholecystectomy pain or jaundice.
2. **Computed Tomography (CT):**
   - *Role:* Identifies intra-abdominal fluid collections, bilomas, abscesses, or associated vascular injuries. CT with IV contrast can assess liver perfusion and vascular complications.
   - *Advantages:* High-resolution imaging, detects associated injuries (e.g., liver ischemia), widely available.
   - *Limitations:* Radiation exposure, limited specificity for precise ductal anatomy.
   - *Use case:* Suspected biloma, abscess, or complex injuries; often used when US is inconclusive.
3. **Magnetic Resonance Cholangiopancreatography (MRCP):**
   - *Role:* Non-invasive visualization of the biliary tree to identify strictures, leaks, or obstructions. Gadolinium-enhanced MRCP can assess bile extravasation.
   - *Advantages:* No radiation, excellent ductal visualization, non-invasive.

- *Limitations:* Expensive, less effective for detecting small leaks, contraindicated in patients with certain implants or renal impairment.
- *Use case:* Mapping biliary anatomy in suspected strictures or planning surgical repair.

4. **Endoscopic Retrograde Cholangiopancreatography (ERCP):**
   - *Role:* Diagnostic and therapeutic; visualizes bile ducts, identifies leaks or strictures, and allows interventions like stent placement or sphincterotomy.
   - *Advantages:* Direct visualization, therapeutic capability (e.g., stenting for leaks), high sensitivity for ductal injuries.
   - *Limitations:* Invasive, risk of pancreatitis (~5%), requires expertise.
   - *Use case:* Managing bile leaks or strictures, particularly in Strasberg Type A or D injuries.
5. **Percutaneous Transhepatic Cholangiography (PTC):**
   - *Role:* Visualizes proximal bile ducts in cases of complete obstruction or when ERCP is not feasible. Can facilitate biliary drainage.
   - *Advantages:* Effective for proximal injuries, allows therapeutic drainage.
   - *Limitations:* Invasive, risks include bleeding, infection, and bile leak.
   - *Use case:* High-grade obstructions or failed ERCP in complex injuries.
6. **Hepatobiliary Iminodiacetic Acid (HIDA) Scan:**
   - *Role:* Detects bile leaks by tracking radiolabeled tracer excretion into the biliary system and extravasation sites.
   - *Advantages:* Highly sensitive for bile leaks, non-invasive.
   - *Limitations:* Limited anatomical detail, cannot assess strictures or vascular injuries.
   - *Use case:* Confirming bile leaks when other imaging is equivocal.
7. **Intraoperative Cholangiography (IOC):**
   - *Role:* Performed during surgery to identify BDI at the time of cholecystectomy or repair.
   - *Advantages:* Real-time visualization, guides immediate repair.
   - *Limitations:* Requires surgical expertise, not always feasible intraoperatively.
   - *Use case:* Routine use during cholecystectomy to detect or prevent BDI.

Comparison of Early vs. Delayed Repair Strategies

The timing of bile duct injury repair depends on the injury type (e.g., Strasberg classification), patient condition, and surgical expertise. Both early and delayed repair strategies have distinct advantages and challenges.

Early Repair (Within Days to 1–2 Weeks Post-Injury)

- *Definition:* Repair performed immediately (intraoperatively) or within days to 1–2 weeks of injury, often for injuries identified during or shortly after surgery.
- *Indications:*
  - Intraoperative recognition of BDI (e.g., transection or major leak).
  - Stable patient with no significant infection or inflammation.
  - Availability of hepatobiliary surgical expertise.
  - Strasberg Type B, C, D, or E injuries requiring surgical reconstruction.
- *Advantages:*
  - Prevents complications like biloma, sepsis, or fistula formation.
  - Reduces hospital stay and overall morbidity in appropriately selected cases.
  - Avoids tissue fibrosis, which complicates delayed repairs.
- *Disadvantages:*
  - Inflammation or edema may obscure tissue planes, increasing technical difficulty.
  - Risk of missing associated injuries (e.g., vascular damage) if not fully evaluated.
  - Requires immediate availability of skilled hepatobiliary surgeons, which may not be feasible in non-specialized centers.

- *Techniques:*
  - Minor injuries (e.g., Type A): Endoscopic stenting or drainage.
  - Major injuries (e.g., Type E): Primary repair over T-tube or Roux-en-Y hepaticojejunostomy.
- *Outcomes:*
  - Success rates high (~90%) with experienced surgeons and minor injuries.
  - Risk of anastomotic leakage or stricture if tissues are inflamed or ischemic.

Delayed Repair (6–12 Weeks Post-Injury)

- *Definition:* Repair performed after a period of stabilization (typically 6–12 weeks), allowing inflammation and infection to resolve.
- *Indications:*
  - Late diagnosis of BDI (e.g., postoperative strictures or chronic leaks).
  - Presence of sepsis, biloma, or significant inflammation requiring initial non-surgical management.
  - Complex injuries (e.g., Type E with vascular compromise) needing preoperative optimization.
  - Lack of immediate hepatobiliary expertise.
- *Advantages:*
  - Reduced inflammation and edema improve tissue quality, facilitating precise anastomosis.
  - Allows time for preoperative imaging (e.g., MRCP, PTC) to fully delineate injury and plan reconstruction.
  - Initial non-surgical management (e.g., ERCP stenting, percutaneous drainage) stabilizes patient, reducing perioperative risks.
- *Disadvantages:*
  - Prolonged morbidity (e.g., recurrent cholangitis, jaundice, or fistula).
  - Risk of stricture formation or secondary biliary cirrhosis if repair is excessively delayed.
  - Requires multiple interventions (e.g., drains, stents) before definitive repair.
- *Techniques:*
  - Roux-en-Y hepaticojejunostomy for major injuries (Type E).
  - Stricture dilatation or stenting for less severe cases.
  - Liver resection or transplantation in rare cases of extensive liver damage.
- *Outcomes:*
  - Success rates ~85–95% in tertiary centers with experienced surgeons.
  - Lower risk of anastomotic complications due to healthier tissues, but long-term stricture rates may be similar to early repair.

Comparison Summary

Aspect	*Early repair*	*Delayed repair*
Timing	Within days to 1–2 weeks	6–12 weeks post-injury
Indications	Intraoperative detection, stable patient	Late diagnosis, sepsis, complex injuries
Advantages	Prevents complications, shorter morbidity	Better tissue quality, precise planning
Disadvantages	Inflammation, limited expertise availability	Prolonged morbidity, interim interventions
Success Rate	~90% with expertise	~85–95% in specialized centers
Preferred Injuries	Strasberg B, C, D, E (minor or major)	Strasberg E, strictures, complex cases

Clinical Considerations

- *Early repair:* Preferred when BDI is recognized intraoperatively, and a hepatobiliary surgeon is available. Immediate repair (e.g., hepaticojejunostomy) is effective for complete transections if tissues are viable.
- *Delayed repair:* Preferred for late-presenting injuries, patients with sepsis, or when preoperative optimization is needed. Temporary measures (e.g., ERCP stenting, percutaneous drainage) bridge to definitive surgery.

- *Hybrid approach:* Some cases involve initial endoscopic or percutaneous management (e.g., for bile leaks) followed by delayed surgical repair for persistent strictures.

Expertise: Outcomes are significantly better in high-volume hepatobiliary centers, regardless of timing. Transfer to such centers is recommended for complex injuries.

CHOLEDOCHAL CYST

20. Describe the etiopathology, types, clinical features, and management of choledochal cyst. ***WBUHS 2006***

21. Classify choledochal cysts. Briefly describe the clinical presentation, diagnosis and management of choledochal cyst. ***RGUHS, Karnataka 2025***

22. Choledochal cyst. ***Rajiv Gandhi Institute of Health Sciences 2019, Rajasthan University of Health Sciences 2025***

Introduction

- Cystic dilatation of the common bile duct is known as choledochal cyst (now termed as bile duct cyst), is a fairly uncommon anomaly of the biliary tract.
- Todani et al. classified this anomaly into five types. Subsequent subtypes are based on cholangiographic findings.
- Intrahepatic cholangiocarcinoma (IHCC) is the second most common primary liver cancer, and the incidence is increasing. There is a significant association between the presence of congenital choledochal cysts and the development of hepatobiliary malignancies, including IHCC.

Etiopathology

The exact cause of choledochal cyst remains obscure. Approximately 20% cases are found in adults.

- The most commonly accepted theory is an *anomalous pancreatic duct-biliary duct junction (APBDJ)*. A high common bile duct-pancreatic duct junction creates a *long common channel (longer than 15 mm)*. This results in reflux of pancreatic fluid into the distal common hepatic duct and results in mucosal injury, chronic inflammation, and weakening of the bile duct wall. This proposed mechanism is supported by elevated levels of amylase in choledochal cysts.
- More recently, abnormal function of the sphincter of Oddi has been reported to predispose to pancreatic reflux into the biliary tree and is, therefore, associated with choledochal cysts.

Types

Todani modified Alonso-Lej classification for bile duct cysts with the respective frequencies:

- *Type I (50–85%):* Cystic or fusiform dilatation of the bile duct without affecting intrahepatic bile duct.
  - *Type IA:* Cystic dilatation of the common bile duct, as well as part of the hepatic common duct and some portions from the right and left hepatic duct
  - *Type IB:* Segmental/focal dilatation of the extrahepatic common bile duct
  - *Type IC:* Fusiform dilatation of the extrahepatic biliary tree
  - *Type ID:* Cystic dilatation of the common and cystic duct
- *Type II (2%):* Real diverticulum of the extrahepatic bile duct
- *Type III (1–5%):* Choledococeles
  - *Type IIIA:* The common bile duct and the pancreatic duct enter in the cyst, which connects to duodenum through another orifice.
  - *Type IIIB:* An intra-ampullary common bile duct diverticulum.
- *Type IV (15–35%):* Presence of multiple intrahepatic and extrahepatic cysts, or only the extrahepatic ones.
  - *Type IVA:* Intra- and extrahepatic dilatations
  - *Type IVB:* Multiple dilatations in the extrahepatic bile ducts only

- *Type V (20%):* One or more cystic dilatations of the intrahepatic biliary tract (without involvement of extrahepatic biliary duct)
- *Type VI (rare):* Isolated dilatation of the cystic duct

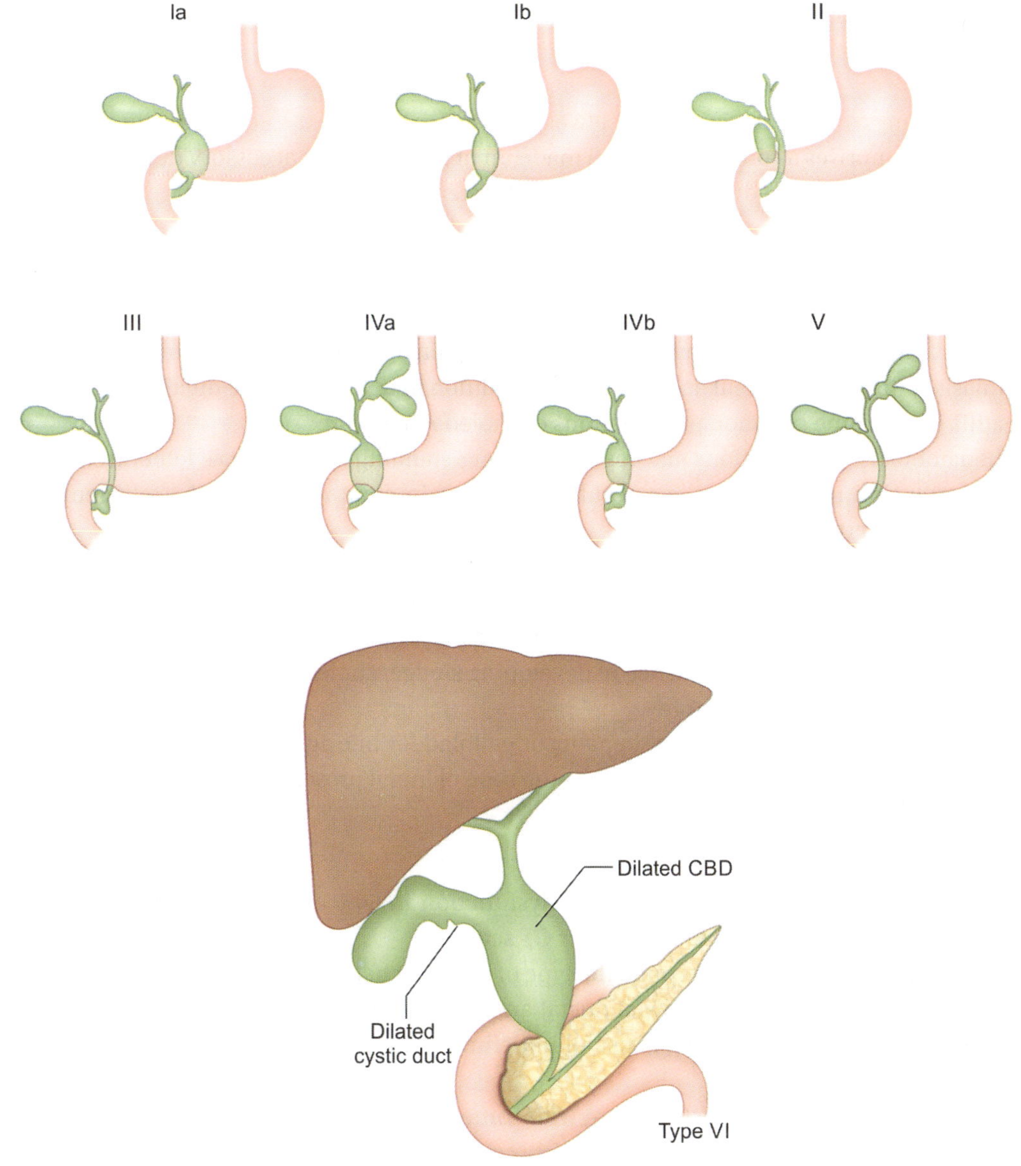

(CBD: common bile duct)

Komi classification of bile duct cysts divides anomalous union of the pancreatico-bile ducts (AUPBD) into three types based on the angle of union of the ducts.

Classification

- *Type I:* Union of the ducts at a right angle to each other
  - *Type Ia:* Without dilatation
  - *Type Ib:* With dilatation of the common channel

- *Type II:* Union of the ducts with an acute angle between them
  - *Type IIa:* Without dilatation
  - *Type IIb:* With dilatation of the common channel
- *Type III:* Comprises complex patterns of accessory pancreatic ducts, with or without intricate duct networks
  - *Type IIIa:* Is similar to the classic pancreas divisum with biliary dilatation?
  - *Type IIIb:* Characterized by the absence of the Wirsung's duct
- *Type IIIc:*
  - *Type IIIc1:* Tiny communication exists between the main duct and the accessory ducts
  - *Type IIIc2:* Comprises a common channel made up of common and accessory ducts of equal caliber
  - *Type IIIc3:* Total or partial dilatation of the ductal system

Clinical Features

- The classic clinical triad associated with choledochal cysts includes right upper quadrant pain, jaundice, and an abdominal mass. Only 10% of patients present with this triad.
- Adults have a slightly different presentation (abdominal pain and jaundice) than children.
- Cystolithiasis is the most frequent accompanying condition in adults with bile duct cysts.
- Pancreatitis is one of the common presentations of choledochal cysts.
- Severe hepatobiliary complications may result from long-standing biliary cysts if left untreated.
- Portal hypertension may develop as a result of portal vein compression by the adjacent cyst or cirrhosis secondary to long-term biliary obstruction.
- Some patients may present with variceal hemorrhage as an initial manifestation.
- Very rarely, patients may present with bilious ascites and peritonitis as a result of rupture of a choledochal cyst, and pseudocysts may appear surrounding the common bile duct.
- Those patients also have a high incidence of developing sludge, cholelithiasis, or choledocholithiasis and have commonly had a prior cholecystectomy.
- The incidence of carcinoma (bile duct, hepatic, or gallbladder in origin) in the choledochal cyst ranges from 2.5 to 26%. Many patients have biliary cancer at the time of initial presentation.

Management

Diagnosis

- Laboratory evaluation may demonstrate liver dysfunction in 60% of adult patients but is not specific. The diagnosis can be established with ultrasound or CT scan.
- Cholangiography is required to determine the type of choledochal cyst and plan operative treatment.
- ERCP is more useful in defining the distal ductal anatomy and the presence of anomalous pancreaticobiliary duct junction (APBDJ), whereas PTC is useful in defining the proximal ductal anatomy and the presence of intrahepatic disease.
- Most patients with choledochal cysts present with some nonspecific abdominal pain, particularly in the older age groups.
- The very youngest children often have jaundice, and attention is drawn right away to the biliary system. Occasionally, a mass can be palpated in the right upper quadrant.
- Pancreatitis is also a presenting sign in some patients.
- The older patients can have very mild abdominal pain and digestive complaints in the absence of jaundice, which may make a diagnosis difficult, particularly if there is not massive cystic dilation easily identified by CT or ultrasound.

Treatment

The goals of management are to relieve symptoms and prevent long-term complications of biliary cysts such as cholangitis, portal hypertension, cirrhosis, and potential carcinoma.

Treatment Options for Choledochal Cysts

Type 1	*Type IVa*
Cyst excision with Roux-en-Y hepaticojejunostomy	Extrahepatic cyst
If excision is impossible: Choledochojejunostomy and sphincteroplasty or endoscopic sphincterotomy	Excision and Roux-en-Y hepaticojejunostomy
	Lobectomy for localized disease
	Liver transplant for diffuse disease
Type II	*Type IVb*
Excision	Excision and Roux-en-Y hepaticojejunostomy
Primary closure with T-tube placement or Roux-en-Y hepaticojejunostomy	
Type III	*Type V*
Excision	Hepatic resection for localized disease
Sphincteroplasty or endoscopic retrograde cholangiopancreatography + sphincterotomy	Diffuse disease liver transplant

Follow-up

- Postoperatively, patients have problems mainly with recurrent cholangitis. There is a small but real potential problem of stenosis of the hepaticojejunostomy, and these patients should be followed for life with serial enzyme determinations and ultrasound.
- If partial obstruction occurs, elevation of alkaline phosphatase may be the only sign for the patient who is otherwise asymptomatic, leading to risk of biliary cirrhosis. Percutaneous or endoscopic dilation of the anastomosis or reoperation would be indicated in this case.
- Recurrent pancreatitis is also a possibility due to inadequate drainage of the pancreatic duct; endoscopic stenting is probably the best choice in these cases if anatomically possible.
- If patients have a choledochocele in the duodenum or pancreas and it is incompletely excised, follow-up is necessary to exclude malignancy.
- In the patient with type IV choledochal cysts, the intrahepatic ducts usually shrink down to near-normal size in the early postoperative period. If the ducts remain significantly cystic, particularly those with multiple cysts, careful periodic observation with multiple imaging modalities is indicated to exclude development of malignancy. Treatment with prophylactic antibiotics and ursodiol (Actigall) may be indicated depending on the clinical course.
- In all of these patients, follow-up with serum liver enzymes on an annual basis is indicated to avoid missing development of partial obstruction, which may lead to permanent liver damage.

CHOLANGIOCARCINOMA

23. Discuss the pathology, diagnosis, and treatment of cholangiocarcinoma. ***WBUHS 2010***

Introduction

- Most cholangiocarcinomas occur without an apparent underlying etiology or risk factor.
- Rare patients will have a bile duct adenoma or papillomatosis as a premalignant precursor of bile duct carcinoma.
- More commonly, chronic inflammation of the bile ducts is implicated as a predisposition for the development of cholangiocarcinoma.

Underlying causes of the ductal irritation include:

- *Infection:* Bacterial infection (*Salmonella typhi* carrier), parasitic infestation (*Opisthorchis viverrini* and Clonorchis sinensis in Asia)

- Anatomic anomalies of the biliary tree (choledochal cysts)
- Radiation [thorium dioxide (thorotrast) exposure]
- Idiopathic causes (primary sclerosing cholangitis).

As with other gastrointestinal cancers, mutations in several proto-oncogenes (K-*ras*, c-*myc*, c-*neu*, c-erb-2, and c-*met*), tumor-suppressor genes (p53, p16, DPC4, and bcl-2) and mismatch repair genes have all been implicated in multiple-step molecular processes leading to malignant transformation.

Pathology

Greater than 90% of bile duct cancers are adenocarcinomas.

Adenocarcinomas of the bile duct are classified as:

Sclerosing	*Nodular*	*Papillary*
Sclerosing (scirrhous) tumors, which comprise over 80% of cholangiocarcinomas, are associated with an intense desmoplastic reaction, tend to be highly invasive, and are associated with low resectability rates	Nodular tumors have the appearance of constricting annular lesions and are also associated with low resectability rates	• Papillary tumors are rare and present as bulky masses that project into the bile duct lumen • Because these lesions tend to cause symptomatic obstructive jaundice relatively early in their progression, they are associated with higher resectability rates than sclerosing or nodular tumors

Other cancer types include:

- Squamous cell carcinoma
- Small cell carcinoma
- Sarcoma

Diagnosis

- The majority of extrahepatic bile duct cancer patients present with painless jaundice. Intrahepatic cholangiocarcinomas do not usually cause hyperbilirubinemia.
- Constitutional symptoms (weight loss, anorexia, fatigue, and malaise) and abdominal pain are generally indicators of advanced cancer.
- Serum levels of bilirubin, alkaline phosphatase, and gamma-glutamyl transferase are significantly elevated, whereas serum aminotransferase levels are minimally affected. The glycoprotein marker CA19-9 has been used to diagnose bile duct cancers but lacks complete sensitivity and specificity, as do other serum tumor markers.

Investigations

- *USG:*
  - Abdominal ultrasonography is usually the first imaging modality done in a patient presenting with jaundice
  - The bile ducts proximal to the cancer will be dilated, with only intrahepatic dilation with hilar cancer and intrahepatic and extrahepatic distension with distal bile duct cancers.
  - Ultrasonography often will not visualize the primary bile duct tumor, but the site of ductal obstruction and the lack of common duct stones often suggest the diagnosis of cholangiocarcinoma.
  - Evidence of vascular involvement by hilar cholangiocarcinomas, including encasement, stenosis, and thrombosis can be detected with duplex ultrasonography.
  - Intrahepatic cholangiocarcinomas appear as malignant solid masses of the liver with no distinguishing features.
  - If the bile duct cancer is unresectable or the patient is not considered an operative candidate due to comorbidities, percutaneous or endoscopic needle biopsy or cytology should be obtained.
- *CT:*
  - For intrahepatic tumors and distal malignant bile duct obstruction, a spiral, thin-cut computerized tomography with intravenous contrast is the imaging study of choice to assess for the extent of the primary tumor, regional nodal involvement, and distant intra-abdominal metastasis.

- In a patient with suspected hilar cholangiocarcinoma, the proximal extent of ductal tumor spread, involvement of hilar blood vessels, and assessment of the parenchyma of both halves of the liver need to be determined.

- *Magnetic resonance imaging and magnetic resonance cholangiopancreatography* can offer additional information on local invasion, particularly into the porta hepatis. These tests are used selectively if CT findings are equivocal.
- *MR angiography:* It is an adjunctive for noninvasive evaluation of blood vessels. It can be used for the evaluation of portal vein system.
- *EUS:* It is useful for diagnosing T stage and taking biopsy.
- *Spyglass cholangioscopy:*
    - Direct examination of the bile ducts using a small caliber scope
    - The spyglass scope can be inserted into the bile duct or pancreatic duct to enable direct visualization during ERCP.
    - It helps to obtain biopsy specimens.

Cholangiocarcinoma is best classified anatomically into three broad groups:

1. Intrahepatic
2. Perihilar
3. Distal

American Joint Commission on Cancer (AJCC) Staging System of Extrahepatic Bile Duct Cancers

Primary tumor (T)	
TX	Primary tumor cannot be assessed
T0	No evidence of primary tumor
Tis	Carcinoma in situ
T1	Tumor confined to the bile duct histologically
T2	Tumor invades beyond the wall of the bile duct
T3	Tumor invades the liver, gallbladder, pancreas, and/or unilateral branches of the portal vein (right or left) or hepatic artery (right or left)
T4	Tumor invades any of the following: Main portal vein or its branches bilaterally, common hepatic artery, or other adjacent structures, such as the colon, stomach, duodenum, or abdominal wall
Regional lymph nodes (N)	
NX	Regional lymph nodes cannot be assessed
N0	No regional lymph node metastasis
N1	Regional lymph node metastasis (e.g., hilar, celiac, periduodenal, peripancreatic, and superior mesenteric)
Distant metastasis (M)	
MX	Distant metastasis cannot be assessed
M0	No distant metastasis
M1	Distant metastasis

Stage grouping			
Stage	***T***	***N***	***M***
Stage 0	Tis	N0	M0
Stage IA	T1	N0	M0
Stage IB	T2	N0	M0
Stage IIA	T3	N0	M0
Stage IIB	T1–3	N1	M0
Stage III	T4	Any	M0
Stage IV	Any	Any	M1

Classification of perihilar bile duct cancers according to anatomic location *(The Bismuth-Corlette classification of perihilar cholangiocarcinomas):*

Classification of perihilar bile duct cancers according to anatomic location:

- *Type I:* Tumors below the confluence of the left and right hepatic ducts
- *Type II:* Tumors reaching the confluence
- *Type IIIa/IIIb:* Tumors involving common hepatic duct and either the right or the left hepatic duct, respectively
- *Type IV:* Tumors that are multicentric or involve the confluence and both the right and left hepatic ducts

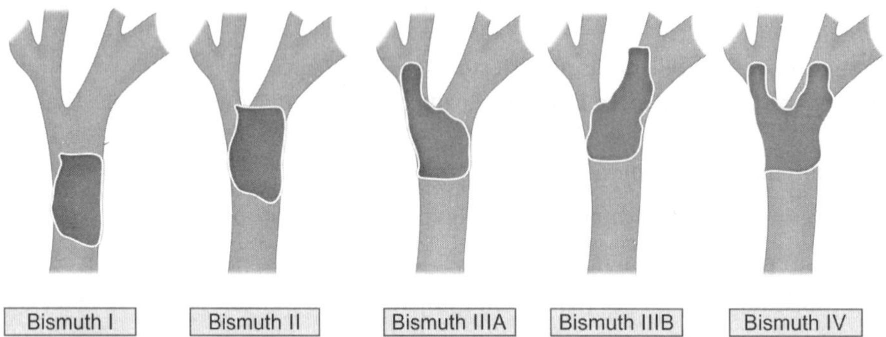

Preoperative Preparation

- The evaluation and correction of concurrent medical problems should be done.
- Clinically jaundiced patients will have reduced stores of fat-soluble vitamins, most importantly for the surgeon, vitamin K. Even if the prothrombin time is normal, a parenteral dose of vitamin K (10 mg) should be administered preoperatively to reduce the risk of perioperative hemorrhage.
- Hepatic insufficiency is one of the most common causes of postoperative morbidity and mortality in patients operated on for a bile duct cancer. There is no indication for preoperative biliary decompression for patients with distal extrahepatic bile duct cancers.
- Despite this risk, when the total bilirubin is >15 mg/dL and a major hepatic resection is planned for a perihilar bile duct cancer, many surgeons recommend transhepatic drainage of the remnant liver to allow for an improvement in hepatic function. When the projected hepatic remnant appears inadequate for a safe recovery, preoperative portal vein embolization of the tumor-involved side of the liver usually induces sufficient contralateral hepatic hypertrophy to reduce the incidence of postoperative liver insufficiency.

Radiologic Criteria to Suggest Unresectability of Cholangiocarcinoma

Bilateral hepatic duct involvement up to secondary radicals	Atrophy of one hepatic lobe with contralateral biliary radical involvement
Bilateral hepatic artery involvement	Distant metastasis
Encasement of the portal vein proximal to its bifurcation	

Operative Approach

Surgical exploration should be undertaken in good-risk patients with no evidence of metastatic or locally unresectable disease	Selective use of laparoscopy in patients with locally advanced but potentially resectable perihilar cholangiocarcinoma may avoid laparotomy in some patients with metastatic disease	In patients who are found to have extensive metastatic disease, the preoperatively placed biliary stents should be left in place
Intraoperatively, more than half of these patients are found to have either *peritoneal* or *hepatic metastases* or *locally unresectable disease*	In patients with locally advanced unresectable perihilar tumors, several operative approaches are available for palliation, including a Roux-en-Y hepaticojejunostomy to segment III or V	A cholecystectomy should be performed to avoid the risk of acute cholecystitis, which occurs in patients with long-term indwelling biliary stents

Distal cholangiocarcinoma	*Intrahepatic cholangiocarcinoma*	*Perihilar cholangiocarcinoma*
• Usually treated with pancreaticoduodenectomy • A pylorus-preserving operation is preferable • 5-year survival rates averaging 15–25%, but can be as high as 54% in selected patients who undergo complete resection for node-negative disease • If resection is not possible due to vascular encasement, cholecystectomy, Roux-en-Y hepaticojejunostomy proximal to the tumor, and a gastrojejunostomy to prevent gastric outlet obstruction should be performed	• Treated by hepatic resection, and outcomes depend on disease stage (particularly the status of the lymph nodes) and the ability to achieve negative margins • There is a broad range of long-term outcomes in patients undergoing complete resection (3-year survival rates of 22–66%)	• Bile duct resection alone leads to high local recurrence rates due to early involvement of the confluence of the hepatic ducts and the caudate lobe branches. The addition of a modified hepatic resection has improved resectability rates • Surgical treatment depends on the Bismuth–Corlette classification. For type I and II lesions, the procedure is en bloc resection of the extrahepatic bile ducts and gallbladder with 5- to 10-mm bile duct margins, and regional lymphadenectomy with Roux-en-Y hepaticojejunostomy. In addition to the above operations, type II tumors may require hepatic lobectomy • Because type II and III lesions often involve the ducts of the caudate lobe, many surgeons recommend routine caudate lobectomy. Type III and IV tumors are amenable to potentially curative resection in centers with expertise in these procedures. *Aggressive techniques such as hepatectomy and portal vein resection to achieve negative margins are now routine in specialized centers*

Palliative Therapy

- Patients with cholangiocarcinoma are at high risk for mortality secondary to hepatic failure from chronic biliary obstruction and biliary sepsis, once the bile ducts have been intubated.
- For patients with metastatic or locally advanced tumors not amenable to complete resection, the primary goals of palliation are to:
  - Provide biliary drainage to the maximal amount of functioning parenchyma
  - Prevent cholangitis
- External beam irradiation and catheter-delivered brachytherapy radiation have been recommended for patients with locally advanced, unresectable bile duct cancers.
- At present, there is no recognized efficacious chemotherapy for cholangiocarcinoma.
- For perihilar cholangiocarcinomas, nonoperative biliary decompression is best accomplished with bilateral percutaneous transhepatic catheters placed through the tumor obstruction. Atrophic portions of the liver should not be drained unless they have become infected by prior manipulation.
- Metastatic distal bile duct cancer patients are generally best managed nonoperatively with an endoscopic biliary stent.
- For patients found to have unresectable bile duct cancer at the time of celiotomy, surgical biliary bypass should be undertaken, if this can be achieved without significant morbidity.
- Distal bile duct cancers are usually readily bypassed with a loop or Roux-en-Y choledochojejunostomy or hepaticojejunostomy.
- For perihilar cholangiocarcinomas, the surgical options include a Roux-en-Y cholangiojejunostomy to the segment III duct (this procedure only decompresses the left liver with tumors that have obstructed the hepatic duct confluence) and palliative resection of the tumor with right and left hepaticojejunostomies.
- Because of an infiltrative growth pattern proximally along the bile ducts, approximately 20% of hilar cholangiocarcinoma resections undertaken with curative intent, even when including a hepatectomy, will not achieve microscopic tumor clearance, most commonly on the proximal duct margin(s).
- Transhepatic drains should be left in position in these patients and postoperative radiation treatment, with or without chemotherapy as a radiosensitizer, considered. If the liver has been adequately decompressed preoperatively, relying on transhepatic catheter drainage is also a reasonable palliative care option.

Adjuvant Therapy

- Bile duct cancers are generally radiosensitive, but the risk of toxicity from excessive exposure to radiosensitive organs, especially the liver and bowel, limits its efficacy. Multiple chemotherapy drugs, including 5-fluorouracil, mitomycin-C, doxorubicin, cisplatin, and etoposide, have shown modest response rates in bile duct cancer patients, but none of the results has generated interest for a major controlled trial of a specific chemotherapy regimen.
- Some recommend external beam radiation therapy with 5-fluorouracil following curative pancreaticoduodenectomy for distal bile duct tumors, because this treatment is commonly used for other periampullary malignancies. External beam, intraoperative radiation therapy, and brachytherapy delivered by transhepatic catheters have all been evaluated in the management of perihilar cancers.
- No adjuvant therapy is usually recommended for intrahepatic cholangiocarcinomas.

24. Discuss the radiological evaluation and preoperative assessment of resectability of hilar cholangiocarcinoma. ***WBUHS 2021***

- CT—most frequently used imaging modality to assess HCC resectability with a good sensitivity and specificity. Cholangiography is necessary to determine proximal extent.
- MRI—comparable with that of CT and can be used as an alternative imaging technique.
- Positron emission tomography (PET)/CT—best technique in detecting lymph node and distant metastasis in HCC but has no clear role in helping to evaluate issues of local resectability.
- Combining diagnostic information from these modalities can add diagnostic certainty and also prove beneficial for an optimized and individualized treatment plan.

USG

- First investigation
- Sensitive for detecting biliary ductal dilation
- Less sensitive for localization of the exact anatomic site of obstruction, hepatic masses and presence of peritoneal disease
- Duplex ultrasound—degree of vascular involvement by the tumor, degree of portal venous invasion

Endoscopic Ultrasound

- Improves the diagnosis between malignant and benign strictures relative to MRCP and CT
- Variable reported sensitivities of 25–91% and specificities of 89–100%
- Fine needle aspiration cytology (FNAC) can be taken

Triphasic Multidetector Computed Tomography (MDCT)

- Most frequently used
- Accurate depiction of a thickened bile duct wall and tumor spread into liver parenchyma or hilar vessels
- *Sensitivity:* 89%; specificity: 92%—*portal vein involvement*
- *Sensitivity:* 83%; specificity: 93%—*hepatic artery involvement*
- Underestimate LN status and peritoneal spread and hepatic metastasis <1 cm

MRI with MRCP

- Accurate map of the biliary tree even in the undrained segment
- Clearer delineation of intrahepatic extension
- Sensitivity of 94 and specificity of 71%
- Vascular invasion—inferior to MDCT
- Lymph node metastasis is less feasible—low spatial resolution

PET CT

- Combines a full-ring detector clinical PET scanner MDCT
- Both metabolic and anatomic imaging data
- Valuable than CT and MRI in detecting lymph node and distant metastases
- Sensitivity—84%; specificity—79.3%
- Sensitivity low for sclerosing variant

Intraductal Ultrasound

- Sensitivity 89–95%, specificity 86–91%

Optical Coherence Tomography

- Analogous to ultrasound
- Infrared light rather than acoustic energy
- Axial resolution of 10 μm, i.e., 10-fold better than that of high-frequency ultrasound
- Depth penetration –1 mm versus 10 mm for a 20 MHz ultrasound probe

Unresectability Criteria

- *Patient factor:*
  - Medically unfit/unable to tolerate a major operation
  - Hepatic cirrhosis with portal hypertension
- *Local tumor-related factor:*
  - Tumor extension to secondary biliary radicles bilaterally
  - Encasement or occlusion of the main portal vein proximal to its bifurcation
  - Atrophy of one hepatic lobe with contralateral portal vein branch encasement or occlusion
  - Atrophy of one hepatic lobe with contralateral tumor extension to secondary biliary radicles
  - Unilateral tumor extension to secondary biliary radicles with contralateral portal vein branch encasement or occlusion
- *Metastatic disease:*
  - Histologically proven metastases to lymph nodes outside the hepatoduodenal ligament
  - Lung, liver, peritoneal, or other distant organ metastases

25. Discuss evaluation of biliary enteric anastomosis for benign biliary disorder. ***WBUHS 2015***

The ability to achieve steady, long-term results confirms hepaticojejunostomy as the best procedure in the treatment of benign biliary strictures, even if endoscopic procedures are gaining a new role in the treatment of a greater number of patients.

Standard surgical techniques offer a good chance of cure for the majority of patients affected by extrahepatic benign biliary stricture. Nevertheless, operative repair has a long-term recurrence rate of stricture in 10–30% of patients. Advances in endoscopic procedures have provided alternative options of relieving biliary obstructions, but prolonged length of treatment and rehospitalization have to be considered if endoscopy is performed. The purpose of this study was to compare the effectiveness of endoscopic and surgical treatments of benign stenosis of the bile duct.

Because a recurrent stricture, mostly occurring in the first 5 years, can arise at any time after primary treatment, 8 10 years of follow-up is needed to determine whether repair has been successful. Our analysis was focused on patients with a length of follow-up longer than 60 months. Long-term results following both endoscopic procedures and surgical treatment were compared. The long-term outcome in our series is as good as that of other reports, which confirm that >80% of patients can be treated successfully with endoscopic or surgical procedures.

Complications after biliary enteric anastomosis for a benign disease:

Complications		
• Local – Wound infection – Biliary leak – Cholangitis/persistent jaundice – Delayed gastric emptying – Pancreatic fistula – Hemorrhage – Pancreatitis	• Systemic – Chest infection – Pulmonary edema – Acute myocardial infarction – Systemic sepsis – Renal failure	• Mortality

- Methods of evaluating a biliary-enteric bypass for obstruction or other postoperative complications include:
  - Hepatobiliary scintigraphy
  - Ultrasonography
  - Cross-sectional imaging
  - Endoscopic retrograde cholangiopancreatography
  - Percutaneous transhepatic cholangiography
- ERCP and PTC are used to define the anatomy of the biliary tree and when the need for possible intervention is anticipated.
- The use of ultrasound as a noninvasive technique for detection of biliary-enteric bypass obstruction is limited by two factors:
  1. First, the presence of gas within the bowel or the biliary tree following surgery creates difficulties in the assessment of biliary duct size.
  2. Second, if the size of the biliary ducts can be measured, ductal dilatation does not necessarily indicate an obstructive pattern in this population as dilatation may persist after surgical relief of obstruction.
- Hepatobiliary scintigraphy (HBS) using technetium-99 attached to iminodiacetic acid is a physiological imaging method that is useful for detecting biliary obstruction.

Laboratory Test

Following parameters are also evaluated:

- Bilirubin, mg/dL, median (range)
- AST, U/L, median (range)
- ALT, U/L, median (range)
- ALP, U/L, median (range)
- GGT, U/L, median (range)
- Change of bile duct size
- Stricture on the cholangiogram

A biliary-enteric anastomosis is taken as successful if after 5 years of operations the LFT values of the patient are normal with normal result in imaging studies.

26. Discuss evaluation of a patient of obstructive jaundice. ***WBUHS 2019***

27. Describe approach to obstructive jaundice. ***WBUHS 2007***

Causes of Obstructive Jaundice

Benign	Malignant
Biliary atresia	Carcinoma of head and periampullary region of the pancreas
Choledochal cyst	Cholangiocarcinoma
• CBD stones • Chronic pancreatitis	Klatskin tumor (carcinoma at the confluence of hepatic ducts above the level of the cystic duct and so will cause hydrohepatosis without GB enlargement)
Ascending cholangitis	Extrinsic compression of CBD by lymph nodes or tumors
• Biliary strictures • Parasitic infestations	Carcinoma gallbladder

(CBD: common bile duct; GB: gallbladder)

History

Common aspects overlooked in the clinical history of jaundiced patients:

- Family history of blood disorders
- Recent travel to foreign parts and work (exposure to infective agents)
- Recent drugs or changes in medications
- Recent surgery or anesthesia
- History of gallstones
- Alcohol intake, cholangitis (pain, fever, and rigors), and carcinoma, especially the head of the pancreas

History and Clinical Features Suggestive of Obstructive Jaundice

• Dark-colored urine • *Pale stools* • Yellow coloration of skin and eyes • *Itchy skin*	• *Fever, chills,* and *rigors* • Episodic right upper abdominal pain • *Weight loss* • *Diarrhea*	• Steatorrhea • Smelly stools—difficult to flush away due to fat malabsorption • *Excessive bleeding* • *Bruising*	• Enlarged liver (tender mass under right rib cage) • Enlarged spleen (tender mass under left side of rib cage) • *Night sweats* • *Anorexia, malaise*

Investigations

Blood Tests

Basic tests:

- Reticulocytosis, abnormal blood film (hemolysis), and prothrombin time
- Hepatitis screen [viral titers for hepatitis A, B, C, cytomegalovirus (CMV), Epstein–Barr virus (EBV)]
- Immunology [antismooth muscle antibodies (chronic active hepatitis) and antimitochondrial antibodies (primary biliary cirrhosis)]
- LFT

Liver Function Tests in Jaundice

	Hemolytic	Hepatocellular	Obstructive
Unconjugated bilirubin	Increased	Increased	Normal
Alkaline phosphatase	Normal	Normal	Much increased
Gamma glutaryl transferase or GGT	Normal	Increased	Much increased
Transaminases	Normal	Increased	Normal
Lactate dehydrogenase	Normal	Increased	Normal

- Patients with pancreatic head lesions frequently have elevated bilirubin and alkaline phosphatase levels suggestive of obstructive jaundice.
- Other routine laboratory studies are usually normal.
- Hemoglobin may be low.
- The two most widely used pancreatic cancer serum markers are the CEA and the Lewis blood group carbohydrate antigen CA19-9. Both are frequently elevated in patients with advanced disease. Extremely high levels of either CA19-9 or CEA usually indicate unresectable or metastatic disease.

Imaging Studies

- The main imaging modalities used for patients with suspected pancreatic neoplasms include right upper quadrant ultrasonography, CT, MRI with or without magnetic resonance cholangiopancreatography, endoscopic retrograde cholangiopancreatography, and percutaneous transhepatic cholangiography.
- Right upper quadrant ultrasonography is a commonly used initial test. It can detect gallstones, dilatation of the biliary tree, and pericholecystic fluid. This imaging modality can also pick up hepatic metastases, pancreatic masses, peripancreatic and hilar lymphadenopathy, and ascites.

- The investigation of choice in the work-up of patients suspected of a pancreatic cancer is a multidetector spiral CT and is probably the single most useful diagnostic and staging modality.
  - CT provides more complete and accurate imaging of the pancreatic head and surrounding structures.
  - It gives very important information about the immediately adjacent vascular structures such as the portal, superior mesenteric, and splenic veins, as well as the superior mesenteric artery and celiac axis.
  - The involvement of periampullary lymph nodes and retroperitoneal structures may be demonstrated.
  - Additionally, information about distant metastatic disease can be gleaned if metastatic deposits are seen in the liver or in the peritoneal cavity.
  - The presence of ascites is usually an ominous sign.
- MRCP is now being utilized to image the biliary tree and the pancreatic duct. It has the advantage of being completely noninvasive.
  - The vascular structures can also be visualized with the use of the contrast agent gadolinium and the performance of a magnetic resonance angiogram (MRA).
  - Thus, a single (long) session in a scanner can provide information about tumor size and extent (MRI), the intraductal anatomy of the biliary and pancreatic system (MRCP), and the status of the nearby vasculature (MRA).
  - The resulting scan has the potential to provide information about tumor size and extent, biliary and pancreatic ductal anatomy, and vascular involvement through a single, noninvasive procedure.
- ERCP sometimes is required to solidify the diagnosis of pancreatic cancer:
  - The classic findings of a long, irregular stricture in a pancreatic duct with distal dilation or a "double duct sign" in which there is cutoff of both the pancreatic duct and distal bile duct at the level of the genu of the pancreatic duct are pathognomonic
  - ERCP may be of benefit in patients with biliary obstruction and cholangitis whereupon an endoscopic stent can be placed for decompression.
  - ERCP is most useful when there is pancreatic duct obstruction, but no mass is evident on either CT or MRI. In this situation, it is necessary to try to distinguish chronic pancreatitis from pancreatic cancer.
- Endoscopic ultrasound is one of the most common imaging procedures used to diagnose pancreatic cancer.
  - It is often the best procedure to obtain samples of a tumor to make a definitive diagnosis of pancreatic cancer.
  - EUS may be able to find small pancreatic masses that have not been detected by computed tomography or magnetic resonance imaging scans but suspected by the doctor as a result of symptoms and/or blood test results.
  - Studies show that EUS is equal to or better than CT scans for detection of early pancreatic cancer.
- *Biopsy:* Biopsy to confirm the presence and identify the type of cancer is usually required before chemo- radiation therapy of unresectable pancreatic tumors or neoadjuvant treatment of resectable tumors. Percutaneous biopsy, performed with either CT or ultrasound guidance, or transduodenal biopsy, performed with endoscopic ultrasound guidance, is routinely employed in these situations.

Complications of Obstructive Jaundice

- *Renal failure (hepatorenal syndrome):* Caused by a combination of infection, dehydration, and a direct effect of high levels of bilirubin and other toxic products of metabolism on the kidney. Mortality is highest in patient of age 65 with an elevated blood urea—prevented by adequate fluid supplementation.
- *Biliary infection (cholangitis):* Most common in obstructive jaundice or with previously damaged biliary tree. Commonly due to Gram-negative bacteria (e.g., *Escherichia coli, Pseudomonas*)—broad-spectrum antibiotics to be instituted.
- *Disordered coagulation:* Due to decreased synthesis of vitamin K-dependent clotting factors (III, VII, IX, and X) and impaired platelet function—corrected by vitamin K injection and/or fresh frozen plasma (FFP)
- *Relative immunosuppression:* Predisposes to systemic infections (e.g., chest infection) and reduces wound healing due to combinations of jaundice, infection, and reduced protein synthesis—adequate nutrition should be prevented.

Algorithm to Approach a Patient of Obstructive Jaundice

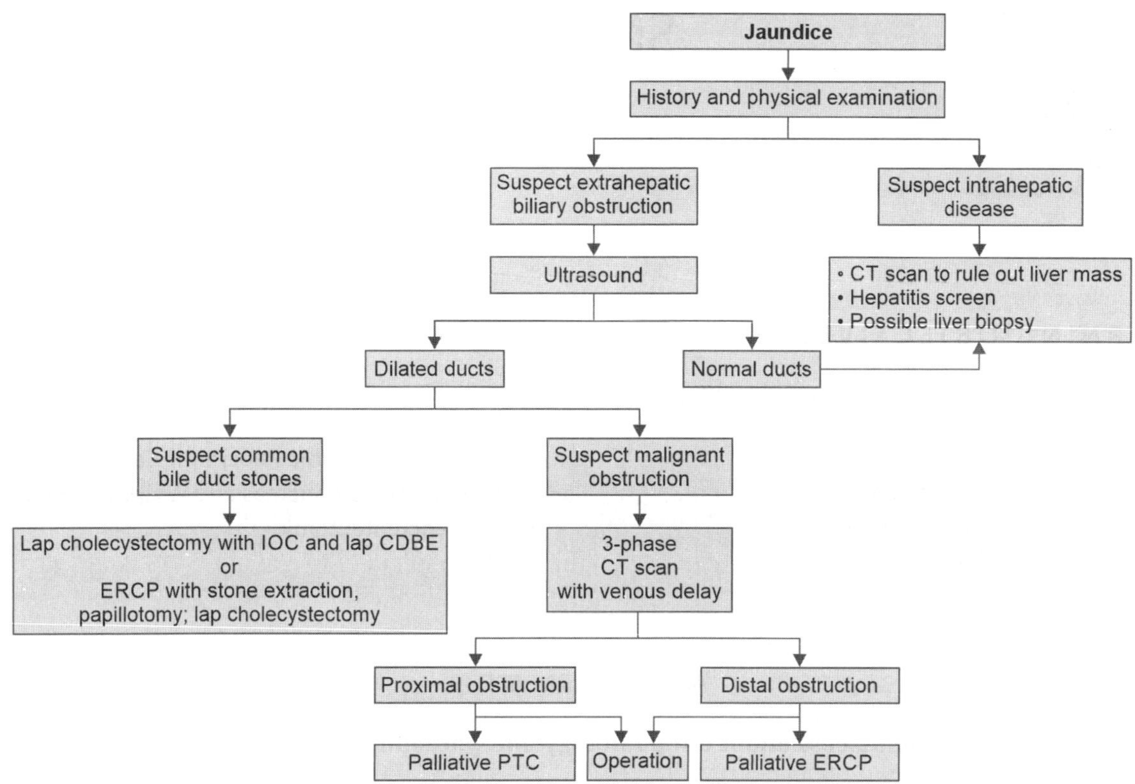

(CT: computed tomography; CDBE: common bile duct injury; IOC: intraoperative cholangiogram; ERCP: endoscopic retrograde cholangiopancreatography; PTC: percutaneous transhepatic cholangiography)

Surgical Diseases of Pancreas

LEARNING OBJECTIVES

- Acute Pancreatitis: Causes, Pathophysiology, Diagnosis, and Management
- Pancreatic Necrosis
- Role of CT Scan in Pancreatic Diseases
- Surgical Anatomy of the Pancreas
- Cystic Lesions of the Pancreas
- Chronic Pancreatitis
- Pancreatic Fistula
- Borderline Resectable Pancreatic Carcinoma
- Carcinoma Head Pancreas and Whipple's Procedure
- Distal Pancreatectomy

ACUTE PANCREATITIS

1. Enumerate causes, and discuss about etiopathology and pathophysiology of acute biliary pancreatitis. ***WBUHS 2019***

2. Write in brief the etiopathogenesis of acute pancreatitis. ***RIMS, Imphal, 2012***

3. Discuss about diagnosis of acute pancreatitis and treatment. What are the complications of acute pancreatitis?

4. Discuss the recent trends in management of acute pancreatitis. ***WBUHS 2007; RIMS, Imphal 2022***

5. Describe about the investigations used for acute pancreatitis and role of imaging in the same. ***RGUHS, Karnataka 2024***

6. Describe the aetiology of acute pancreatitis and indications of surgery in acute pancreatitis. ***Srimanta Sankaradeva University, Assam 2025***

7. What are the indications of operative intervention? ***WBUHS 2016***

Acute pancreatitis (AP) includes a wide spectrum of diseases, from one with mild self-limiting symptoms to fulminant processes with multiorgan failure and high mortality.

Etiologic Factors in Acute Pancreatitis

Metabolic	*Mechanical*	*Vascular*	*Infection*
• Alcohol • Hyperlipoproteinemia • Hypercalcemia • Drugs • Genetic • Scorpion venom	• Cholelithiasis • Postoperative • Pancreas divisum • Post-traumatic • Retrograde pancreatography • *Pancreatic duct obstruction:* Pancreatic tumor and *Ascaris* infestation • Pancreatic ductal bleeding duodenal obstruction	• Postoperative (cardiopulmonary bypass) • Periarteritis nodosa • Atheroembolism	• Mumps • Coxsackie • *Cytomegalovirus* • *Cryptococcus*

- Pancreatitis is characterized by a nonbacterial inflammation of the pancreas.
- This inflammation is caused by the activation, interstitial liberation, and digestion of the pancreas by its own digestive enzymes.
- During mild attacks, morphologic changes include pancreatic and peripancreatic edema and fat necrosis.
- In its severe form, pancreatitis is characterized by pancreatic parenchymal necrosis, extensive pancreatic and peripancreatic fat necrosis, and hemorrhage into and around the pancreas.

Acute pancreatitis has been attributed to a wide range of etiologic factors.

- Intra-acinar activation of trypsinogen, with subsequent activation of other pancreatic enzymes, is thought to play a central role in the pathogenesis of the disease.
- Furthermore, ischemia-reperfusion injury is believed to be critical to disease progression.
- A local inflammatory response in the pancreas is associated with the liberation of oxygen-derived free radicals and cytokines including interleukin 1 (IL-1), IL-6, and IL-8; tumor necrosis factor α (TNF-α); and platelet-activating factor; these mediators play an important role in the transformation from a local inflammatory response to a systemic illness.

Pathogenesis of acute pancreatitis

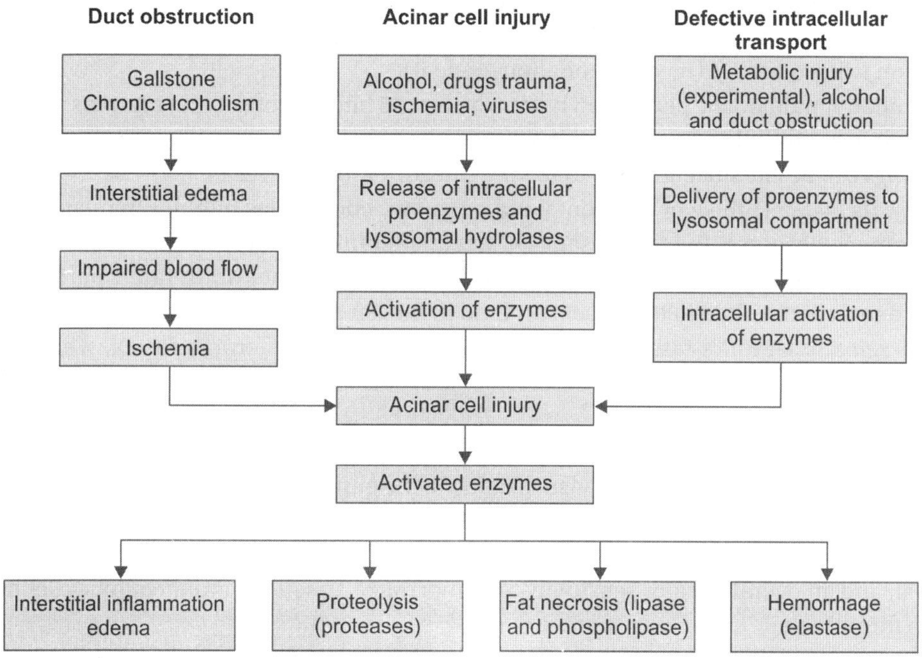

Duct obstruction
Gallstone
Chronic alcoholism
→ Interstitial edema → Impaired blood flow → Ischemia → Acinar cell injury

Acinar cell injury
Alcohol, drugs trauma, ischemia, viruses
→ Release of intracellular proenzymes and lysosomal hydrolases → Activation of enzymes → Acinar cell injury

Defective intracellular transport
Metabolic injury (experimental), alcohol and duct obstruction
→ Delivery of proenzymes to lysosomal compartment → Intracellular activation of enzymes → Acinar cell injury

Acinar cell injury → Activated enzymes → Interstitial inflammation edema; Proteolysis (proteases); Fat necrosis (lipase and phospholipase); Hemorrhage (elastase)

Effect of acute pancreatitis on other organ system:

- *Lung:* Pleural effusion, acute lung injury
- *Kidney:* Acute renal failure
- *Common bile duct:* Obstructive jaundice
- *Colon:* Colonic ischemia
- Systemic inflammatory response syndrome (SIRS)
- Multiple organ dysfunction syndrome (MODS)

Investigations and Diagnosis

Blood Investigations

Full blood count, renal function tests, liver function, serum calcium, serum amylase and lipase, and arterial blood gas analysis.

- *Amylase and lipase:*
  - Elevated serum amylase and lipase levels, in combination with severe abdominal pain, often trigger the initial diagnosis of acute pancreatitis. Serum lipase rises 4–8 hours from the onset of symptoms and normalizes within 7–14 days after treatment. Serum amylase may be normal (in 10% of cases) for cases of acute or chronic pancreatitis (CP) (depleted acinar cell mass) and hypertriglyceridemia.
  - Reasons for false positive elevated serum amylase include salivary gland disease (elevated salivary amylase) and macroamylasemia.
  - If the lipase level is about 2.5–3 times that of amylase, it is an indication of pancreatitis due to alcohol.

  Imaging

  Chest X-ray (for exclusion of perforated viscus), abdominal X-rays (for detection of "sentinel loop" dilated duodenum sign, and gallstones which are radiopaque in 10%), and computed tomography (CT) abdomen
- *Computed tomography:*
  - *Regarding the need for CT, the practice guidelines state:* "Many patients with acute pancreatitis do not require a CT scan at admission or at any time during the hospitalization, for example, a CT scan is usually not essential in patients with recurrent mild pancreatitis caused by alcohol. A reasonable indication for a CT scan at admission [but not necessarily a CT with intravenous (IV) contrast] is to distinguish acute pancreatitis from another serious intraabdominal condition, such as a perforated ulcer."
  - Patients with persisting organ failure, signs of sepsis, or deterioration in clinical status 6–10 days after admission will require CT (recommendation grade B).
  - CT abdomen should not be performed before the first 48 hours of onset of symptoms as early CT (<48 hours) may result in equivocal or normal findings.
  - *CT findings* can be classified into the following categories for easy recall:
    - *Intrapancreatic:* Diffuse or segmental enlargement, edema, gas bubbles, pancreatic pseudocysts, and phlegmons/abscesses (which present 4–6 weeks after initial onset)
    - *Peripancreatic/extrapancreatic:* Irregular pancreatic outline, obliterated peripancreatic fat, retroperitoneal edema, fluid in the lesser sac, fluid in the left anterior pararenal space
    - *Locoregional:* Gerota's fascia sign (thickening of inflamed Gerota's fascia, which becomes visible), pancreatic ascites, pleural effusion (seen on basal cuts of the pleural cavity), adynamic ileus, etc.
- *Magnetic resonance imaging (MRI):*
  - While CT is considered the gold standard in diagnostic imaging for acute pancreatitis, MRI has become increasingly valuable as a tool for the visualization of the pancreas, particularly of pancreatic fluid collections and necrotized debris.
  - Additional utility of an MRI includes its indication for imaging of patients with an allergy to CT's contrast material, and an overall greater sensitivity to hemorrhage, vascular complications, pseudoaneurysms, and venous thrombosis.
  - Another advantage of MRI is its utilization of magnetic resonance cholangiopancreatography (MRCP) sequences.
  - MRCP provides useful information regarding the etiology of acute pancreatitis, i.e., the presence of tiny biliary stones (choledocholithiasis or cholelithiasis) and duct anomalies.

Classification by Severity

Severity of AP according to the 2012 revision of the Atlanta criteria.

Severity	*Characteristics*
Mild	• No organ failure • No local or systemic complications
Moderately severe	Transient organ failure (<48 hours). Local or systemic complications without persistent organ failure
Severe	Persistent organ failure

Organ failure as defined by the Marshall criteria.	
Organ system	***Criteria for failure***
Pulmonary	PaO_2/FiO_2 ratio <300
Renal	Serum creatinine >1.9 (if normal at baseline)
Cardiovascular	SBP <90 mm Hg, not responsive to fluids

(FiO_2: fraction of inspiratory oxygen concentration; PaO_2: partial pressure of oxygen in arterial blood; SBP: systolic blood pressure)

Prognostic Indices

In predicting the prognosis, there are several scoring indices that have been used as predictors of survival.

Two such scoring systems are the (1) Ranson criteria and (2) acute physiology, age, and chronic health evaluation (APACHE II) indices.

Most, but not all studies report that the Apache score may be more accurate.

Practice guidelines state: "The two tests that are most helpful at admission in distinguishing mild from severe acute pancreatitis are APACHE II score and serum hematocrit. It is recommended that APACHE II scores be generated during the first 3 days of hospitalization and thereafter as needed to help in this distinction. It is also recommended that serum hematocrit be obtained at admission, 12 hours after admission, and 24 hours after admission to help gauge the adequacy of fluid resuscitation."

"Immediate assessment should include clinical evaluation, particularly of any cardiovascular, respiratory, and renal compromise, body mass index, chest X-ray, and APACHE II score."

Ranson criteria is a clinical prediction rule for predicting the severity of acute pancreatitis. Organ failure as defined by the Marshall criteria.	
At admission	***At 48 hours***
• Age in years >55 years • White blood cell count >16,000 cells/mm^3 • Blood glucose >10 mmol/L (>200 mg/dL) • Serum AST >250 IU/L • Serum LDH >700 IU/L	• Calcium (serum calcium <2.0 mmol/L (<8.0 mg/dL) • Hematocrit fall >10% • Oxygen (hypoxemia pO_2 <60 mm Hg) • BUN increased by 1.8 or more mmol/L (five or more mg/dL) after IV fluid hydration • Base deficit (negative base excess) >4 mEq/L • Sequestration of fluids >6 L

(AST: aspartate aminotransferase; BUN: blood urea nitrogen; LDH: lactate dehydrogenase)

The criteria for point assignment is that a certain breakpoint be met at any time during that 48-hour period so that in some situations it can be calculated shortly after admission. It applies to both gallstone and alcoholic pancreatitis.

Alternatively, pancreatitis can be diagnosed by meeting any of the following:

APACHE II Score

- Apache score of ≥8 organ failure substantial pancreatic necrosis (at least 30% glandular necrosis according to contrast-enhanced CT)
- Interpretation if the score ≥3, severe pancreatitis is likely. If the score <3, severe pancreatitis is unlikely, or when the score is 0–2: mortality is rare. When the score is 7–8: mortality is near about 100%
- APACHE II score >8 points predicts 11–18% mortality

Balthazar Scoring

Developed in the early 1990s by Emil J Balthazar et al., the computed tomography severity index (CTSI) is a grading system used to determine the severity of acute pancreatitis. The numerical CTSI has a maximum of 10 points, and is the sum of the Balthazar grade points and pancreatic necrosis grade points:

Balthazar Grade

Balthazar grade	*Appearance on CT*	*CT grade points*
Grade A	Normal CT	0 point
Grade B	Focal or diffuse enlargement of the pancreas	1 point
Grade C	Pancreatic gland abnormalities and peripancreatic inflammation	2 points
Grade D	Fluid collection in a single location	3 points
Grade E	Two or more fluid collections and/or gas bubbles in or adjacent to the pancreas	0 point

Necrosis Score

Necrosis percentage	*Points*
No necrosis	0 point
0–30% necrosis	2 points
30–50% necrosis	4 points
Over 50% necrosis	6 points

Computed tomography severity index's staging of acute pancreatitis severity has been shown by a number of studies to provide a more accurate assessment than APACHE II, Ranson, and C-reactive protein (CRP) level. However, a few studies indicate that CTSI is not significantly associated with the prognosis of hospitalization in patients with pancreatic necrosis, nor is it an accurate predictor of AP severity.

Glasgow–Imrie Criteria

Three or more positive criteria within 48 hours of admission = severe attack

- Age >55 years
- WCC >15000
- Glucose >7 mmol/L
- Blood urea >7 mmol/L
- Albumin <35 g/L
- Corrected calcium <2 mmol/L
- PaO_2 <10 kPa

Treatment

Principles of Management

Fluid resuscitation
Nutritional support
Symptomatic treatment
Management of metabolic complications
Prophylactic antibiotic coverage
Monitoring and reassessment
Role of endoscopic retrograde cholangiopancreatography (ERCP)
Role of surgery

- *Fluid therapy:* Ringer's lactate is recommended for initial fluid resuscitation in acute pancreatitis (grade 1B, strong agreement):
  - Goal-directed intravenous fluid therapy with 5–10 mL/kg/h should be used initially until resuscitation goals (see Q10b) are reached (grade 1B and weak agreement)

- The preferred approach to assessing the response to fluid resuscitation should be based on one or more of the following:
  - Noninvasive clinical targets of heart rate <120/min, mean arterial pressure between 65 and 85 mm Hg (8.7e11.3 kPa), and urinary output >0.5–1 mL/kg/h
  - Invasive clinical targets of stroke volume variation, and intrathoracic blood volume determination
  - Biochemical targets of hematocrit 35–44% (grade 2B, weak agreement)

Intensive Care Management

- Management in, or referral to, a specialist center is necessary for patients with severe acute pancreatitis and for those who may need interventional radiologic, endoscopic, or surgical intervention (grade 1C, strong agreement)
- A specialist center in the management of acute pancreatitis is defined as a high-volume center with up-to-date intensive care facilities including options for organ replacement therapy, and with daily (i.e., 7 days/week) access to interventional radiology, interventional endoscopy with endoscopic ultrasound (EUS) and endoscopic retrograde cholangiopancreatography (ERCP) assistance as well as surgical expertise in managing necrotizing pancreatitis. Patients should be enrolled in prospective audits for quality control issues and into clinical trials whenever possible (grade 2C, weak agreement).
- Early fluid resuscitation within the first 24 hours of admission for acute pancreatitis is associated with decreased rates of persistent SIRS and organ failure (grade 1C, strong agreement).
- Invasive treatment should only be used after multidisciplinary discussion in patients with sustained intra-abdominal pressure (IAP) >25 mm Hg with new-onset organ failure refractory to medical therapy and nasogastric/rectal decompression. Invasive treatment options include percutaneous catheter drainage of ascites, midline laparostomy, bilateral subcostal laparostomy, or subcutaneous linea alba fasciotomy. In the case of surgical decompression, the retroperitoneal cavity and the omental bursa should be left intact to reduce the risk of infecting peripancreatic and pancreatic necrosis (grade 2C, strong agreement).

Preventing Infectious Complications

Intravenous antibiotic prophylaxis is not recommended for the prevention of infectious complications in acute pancreatitis (grade 1B, strong agreement).

Indications

- Infective necrosis
- Sterile necrosis >50%
- Extrapancreatic infections

Preferred Antibiotics

- Carbapenem (Imipenem + cilastatin)
- Quinolones
- Metronidazole
- Third-generation cephalosporins

Probiotic prophylaxis is not recommended for the prevention of infectious complications in acute pancreatitis (grade 1B, strong agreement)

Nutritional Support

- Oral feeding in predicted mild pancreatitis can be restarted once abdominal pain is decreasing and inflammatory markers are improving (grade 2B, strong agreement)
- Enteral tube feeding should be the primary therapy in patients with predicted severe acute pancreatitis who require nutritional support (grade 1B, strong agreement)
- Either elemental or polymeric enteral nutrition formulations can be used in acute pancreatitis (grade 2B, strong agreement).

- Enteral nutrition in acute pancreatitis can be administered via either the nasojejunal or nasogastric route (grade 2A, strong agreement)
- Parenteral nutrition can be administered in acute pancreatitis as second-line therapy if nasojejunal tube feeding is not tolerated and nutritional support is required (grade 2C, strong agreement)

Biliary Tract Management

- ERCP is not indicated in predicted mild biliary pancreatitis without cholangitis (grade 1A, strong agreement). Endoscopic retrograde cholangiopancreatography is probably not indicated in predicted severe biliary pancreatitis without cholangitis (Grade 1B, strong agreement).
- ERCP is probably indicated in biliary pancreatitis with common bile duct obstruction (grade 1C, strong agreement) ERCP is indicated in patients with biliary pancreatitis and cholangitis (grade 1B, strong agreement)
- Urgent ERCP (<24 hours) is required in patients with acute cholangitis. Currently, there is no evidence regarding the optimal timing of ERCP in patients with biliary pancreatitis without cholangitis (grade 2C, strong agreement)
- MRCP and EUS may prevent a proportion of ERCPs that would otherwise be performed for suspected common bile duct stones in patients with biliary pancreatitis who do not have cholangitis, without influencing the clinical course. Endoscopic ultrasound is superior to MRCP in excluding the presence of small (<5 mm) gallstones.
- *Indications:* The indications for early ERCP are as follows:
  - Clinical deterioration or lack of improvement after 24 hours
  - Detection of common bile duct stones or dilated intrahepatic or extrahepatic ducts on CT abdomen
- *The disadvantages of ERCP are as follows:*
  - ERCP precipitates pancreatitis and can introduce infection to sterile pancreatitis
  - The inherent risks of ERCP, i.e., bleeding
  - It is worth noting that ERCP itself can be a cause of pancreatitis.

Indications for Intervention in Necrotizing Pancreatitis

Common indications for intervention (either radiological, endoscopical, or surgical) in necrotizing pancreatitis are:

- Clinical suspicion of, or documented infected necrotizing pancreatitis with clinical deterioration, preferably when the necrosis has become walled-off
- In the absence of documented infected necrotizing pancreatitis, ongoing organ failure for several weeks after the onset of acute pancreatitis, preferably when the necrosis has become walled-off (grade 1C, strong agreement)
- Routine percutaneous fine needle aspiration of peripancreatic collections to detect bacteria is not indicated, because clinical signs (i.e., persistent fever and increasing inflammatory markers) and imaging signs (i.e., gas in peripancreatic collections) are accurate predictors of infected necrosis in the majority of patients.
- Although the diagnosis of infection can be confirmed by fine needle aspiration (FNA), there is a risk of false-negative results (grade 1C, strong agreement)

Indications for intervention (either radiological, endoscopical, or surgical) in sterile necrotizing pancreatitis are:

- Ongoing gastric outlet, intestinal, or biliary obstruction due to mass effect of walled-off necrosis (i.e., arbitrarily >4–8 weeks after onset of acute pancreatitis)
- Persistent symptoms (e.g., pain, "persistent unwellness") in patients with walled-off necrosis without signs of infection (i.e., arbitrarily >8 weeks after onset of acute pancreatitis)
- Disconnected duct syndrome (i.e., full transection of the pancreatic duct in the presence of pancreatic necrosis) with persisting symptomatic (e.g., pain and obstruction) collection(s) with necrosis without signs of infections (i.e., arbitrarily >8 weeks after onset of acute pancreatitis) (grade 2C, strong agreement)

Timing of Intervention in Necrotizing Pancreatitis

- For patients with proven or suspected infected necrotizing pancreatitis, invasive intervention (i.e., percutaneous catheter drainage, endoscopic transluminal drainage/necrosectomy, minimally invasive or open necrosectomy) should be delayed where possible until at least 4 weeks after initial presentation to allow the collection to become "walled-off" (grade 1C, strong agreement).

- The best available evidence suggests that surgical necrosectomy should ideally be delayed until collections have become walled-off, typically 4 weeks after the onset of pancreatitis, in all patients with complications of necrosis. No subgroups have been identified that might benefit from earlier or delayed intervention (grade 1C, strong agreement)

Timing of Cholecystectomy (or Endoscopic Sphincterotomy)

- Cholecystectomy during index admission for mild biliary pancreatitis appears safe and is recommended. Interval cholecystectomy after mild biliary pancreatitis is associated with a substantial risk of readmission for recurrent biliary events, especially recurrent biliary pancreatitis (grade 1C, strong agreement).
- Cholecystectomy should be delayed in patients with peripancreatic collections until the collections either resolve or if they persist beyond 6 weeks, at which time cholecystectomy can be performed safely (grade 2C, strong agreement)
- In patients with biliary pancreatitis who have undergone sphincterotomy and are fit for surgery, cholecystectomy is advised, because ERCP and sphincterotomy prevent recurrence of biliary pancreatitis but not gallstone-related gallbladder disease, i.e., biliary colic and cholecystitis (grade 2B, strong agreement)

Surgery

Surgery is indicated for:

- Infected pancreatic necrosis
- Diagnostic uncertainty
- Complications

The most common cause of death in acute pancreatitis is secondary infection.

Infection is diagnosed based on two criteria:

1. Gas bubbles on CT scan (present in 20–50% of infected necrosis)
2. Positive bacterial culture on (FNA usually CT, or US-guided) of the pancreas.

Surgical options for infected necrosis include:

- Minimally invasive management—necrosectomy through a small incision in the skin (left flank) or stomach
- Conventional management—necrosectomy with simple drainage
- Closed management—necrosectomy with closed continuous postoperative lavage
- Open management—necrosectomy with planned staged reoperations at definite intervals (up to 20 plus reoperations in some cases)
- *Other measures:*
    - Pancreatic enzyme inhibitors are not proven to work
    - The use of octreotide has not been shown to improve outcomes.

The complications of acute pancreatitis.

Local	*Regional*	*Systemic*
• Fluid collections • Pancreatic ascites/pleural effusion • Pancreatic pseudocyst • Pancreatic necrosis • Infected pancreatic abscess • Hemorrhage/pseudoaneurysm	• Venous thrombosis • Paralytic ileus • Intestinal obstruction • Intestinal ischemia/necrosis • Cholestasis	• Systemic inflammatory response syndrome • Multiple organ dysfunction syndrome • Acute respiratory distress syndrome (ARDS)/ pulmonary failure • Renal failure • Cardiovascular complications • Hypocalcemia • Hyperglycemia • Disseminated intravascular coagulopathy • Protein calorie malnutrition • Encephalopathy

Complications are Treated Accordingly

A management algorithm for both mild and severe pancreatitis.

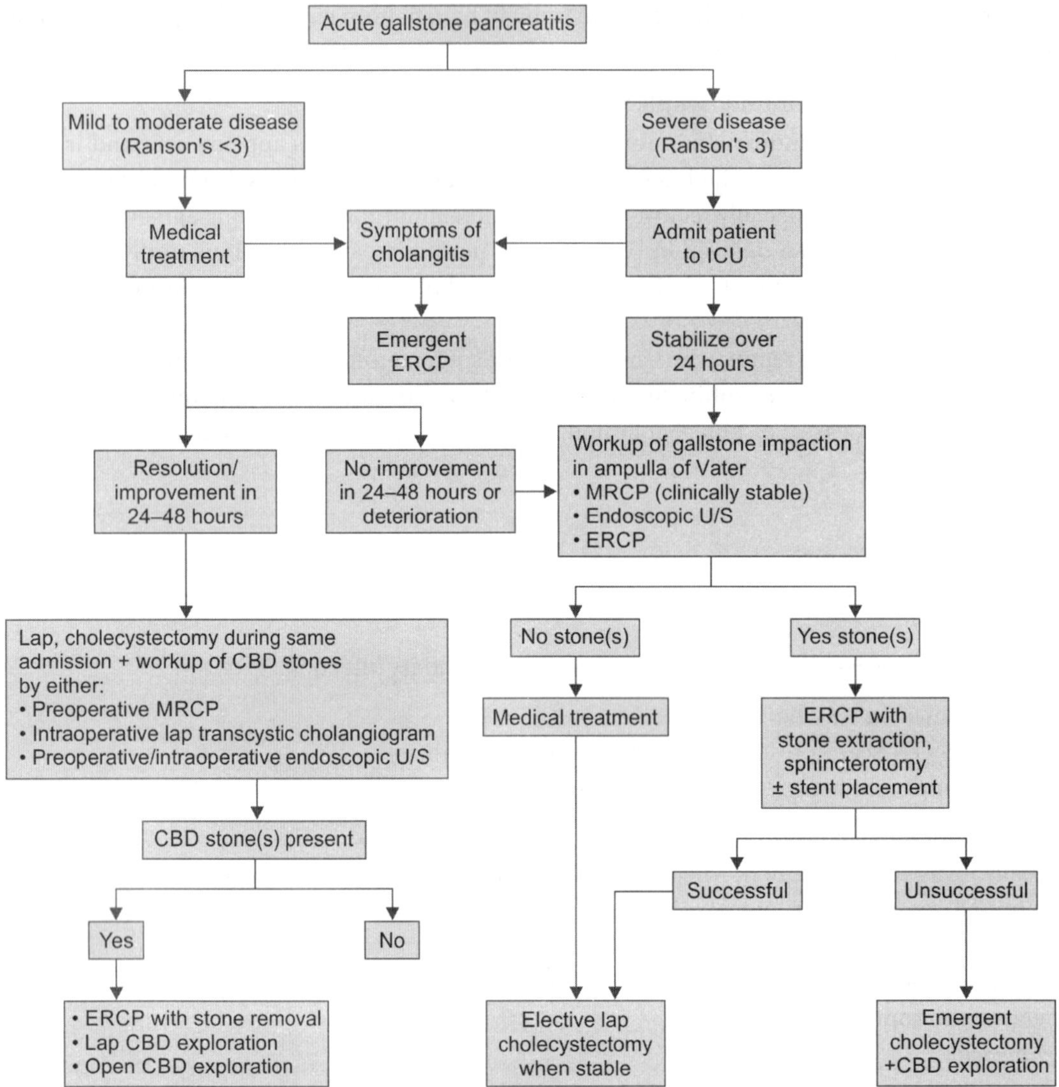

(CBD: common bile duct; ERCP: endoscopic retrograde cholangiopancreatography; ICU: intensive care unit; MRCP: magnetic resonance cholangiopancreatography)

8. Classification and modalities of management of iatrogenic duodenal perforation from ERCP. Marshal score vis-a-vis sequential organ failure assessment (SOFA) score—morbidity mortality indicators in severe acute pancreatitis. ***WBUHS 2016***

There are two proposed classifications of ERCP-related perforations:

1. In 1999, Howard et al. classified perforations into three distinct types:
   1. *Type I:* Guidewire perforation
   2. *Type II:* Periampullary perforation
   3. *Type III:* Duodenal perforation remote from the papilla
2. In 2000, Stapfer et al. classified ERCP-related perforations into four types, based on the mechanism, anatomical location, and severity of injury, which may predict the need for surgery. The Stapfer classification is the most commonly used and it divides perforations into:

i. *Type I:* Lateral or medial wall duodenal perforation
ii. *Type II:* Perivaterian injuries
iii. *Type III:* Distal bile duct injuries related to guidewire-basket instrumentation
iv. *Type IV:* Retroperitoneal air alone

Type IV is questionable and it is not a true perforation. Due to the excess compression of air in the duodenum, air bubbles can leak through the sphincterotomy area outside the duodenal lumen, into the retroperitoneal space.

Algorithm for the management of iatrogenic perforations (types II, III, and IV according to Stapfer et al. related to ERCP.

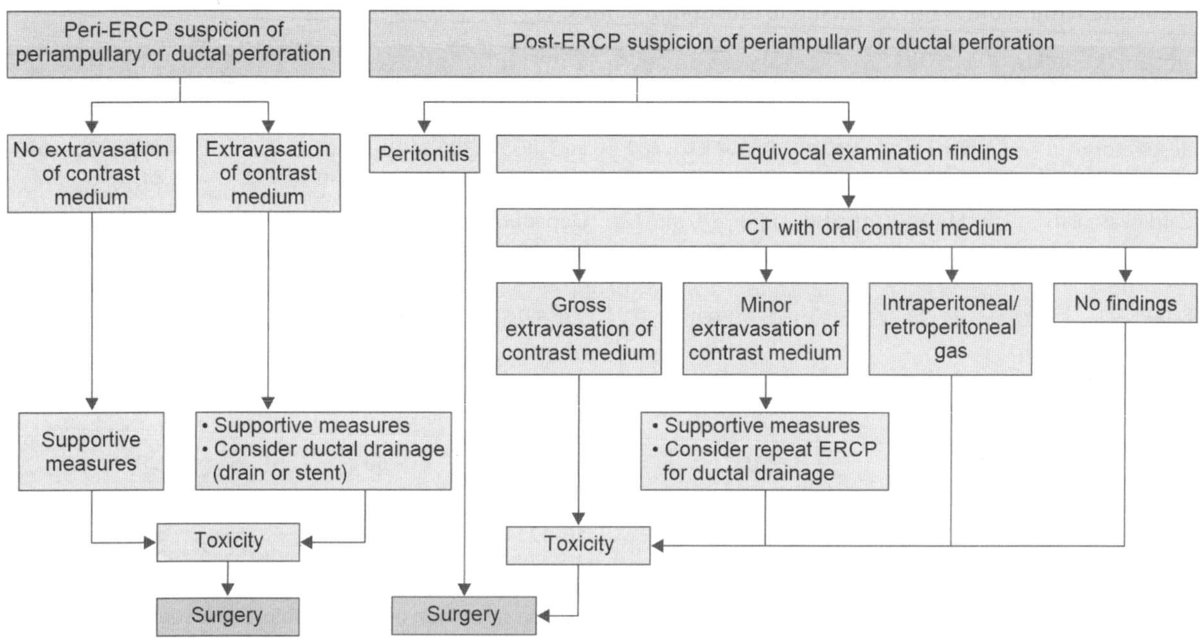

(CT: computed tomography; ERCP: endoscopic retrograde cholangiopancreatography)

Endoscope-related perforations (type I) should be referred for immediate surgery unless endoscopic closure can be achieved. Endoscopic closure using fibrin glue, endoloops, and endoclips or an over-the-scope clipping device has been described.

Mortality and Morbidity Indicators of Severe Acute Pancreatitis

- Individual components of the bedside index for severity in acute pancreatitis (BISAP) scoring system:
  - Blood urea nitrogen (BUN) > 25 mg/dL
  - SIRS: *SIRS is defined as two or more of the following:*
    - Temperature of <36 or >38°C
    - Respiratory rate >20 breaths/min of $PaCO_2$ < 32 mm Hg
    - Pulse >90/min
    - Leukocyte count >12,000 or <4,000/µL or over 10% immature forms or bands
      - Age >60 years
      - Pleural effusion detected on imaging

One point is assigned for each variable within 24 hours of presentation and added for a composite score of 0–5.

Criteria for Organ Failure Based on the Marshall Scoring System

Organ system	*Criteria for failure*
Pulmonary	PaO_2/FiO_2 ratio <300
Renal	Serum creatinine >1.9 (if normal at baseline)
Cardiovascular	SBP <90 mm Hg, not responsive to fluids

- The SOFA score is a mortality prediction score that is based on the degree of dysfunction of the six organ systems.
- The score is calculated on admission and every 24 hours until discharge using the worst parameters measured during the prior 24 hours.
- The scores can be used in a number of ways:
  - As individual scores for each organ to determine the progression of organ dysfunction
  - As the sum of scores on one single intensive care unit (ICU) day
  - As the sum of the worst scores during the ICU stay
- It is believed to provide a better stratification of the mortality risk in ICU patients given that the data used to calculate the score is not restricted to admission values.

SOFA score

Variables	*0*	*1*	*2*	*3*	*4*
Respiratory	PaO_2/FiO_2; >400 SpO_2/FiO_2: >302	PaO_2/FiO_2 <400 SpO_2/FiO_2: <302	PaO_2/FiO_2:<300 SpO_2/FiO_2:<221	PaO_2/FiO_2: <200 SpO_2/FiO_2: <142	PaO_2/FiO_2: <100 SpO_2/FiO_2:<67
Cardiovascular (doses in μg/kg/min)	MAP ≥70 mm Hg	MAP ≥70 mm Hg	Dopamine ≤5 Or any dobutamine	Dopamine >5 Norepinephrines ≤0.1 Phenylephrine ≤0.8	Dopamine >15 Or Norepinephrine >0.1 Phenylephrine >0.8
Liver (bilirubin, mg/dL)	<1 .2	1.2–1.9	2.0–5.9	6.0–11.9	>12
Renal (creatinine, mg/dL)	<1.2	1.2–1.9	2.0–3.4	3.5–4.9	>5.0
Coagulation (platelets × $10^3/mm^3$)	≥150	<150	<100	<50	<20
Neurologic (GCS score)	15	13–14	10–12	6–9	<6

(PaO_2: partial pressure of oxygen in arterial blood; SpO_2: arterial oxygen saturation of hemoglobin; SOFA: sequential organ failure assessment)

9. Paradigm shift in the fluid management of acute pancreatitis. ***WBUHS 2021***

Introduction

- Acute pancreatitis is an acute inflammation of the pancreas caused by activation, interstitial liberation, and autodigestion of pancreatic parenchyma.
- High morbidity and mortality rates
- Ranges from self-limiting mild illness to rapidly progressing severe illness ending in multiorgan failure
- 10–20% of patients develop severe form acute pancreatitis which has a 10–50% of mortality rate
- Overall case fatality rate roughly <5%

Treatment

- Multidisciplinary diagnosis and treatment should be adopted
- The early treatment of acute pancreatitis mainly includes fluid resuscitation, analgesia, and nutritional support as well as the treatment of etiology and early complications.

Fluid Resuscitation (Aggressive vs Controlled)

- Fluid therapy is the current cornerstone
- But little consensus on its application
- Recommendations in various reviews advocating vigorous fluid therapy
- *Tenner et al. (2004):* 250–500 mL/h or more for first 48 hours
- *Whitcomb et al. (2006):* 250–500 mL/h

- *Otsuki et al. (2006):* 60–160 mL/kg/day
- *Naser et al. (2011):* 20 mL/kg in emergency, then 150–300 mL/h for 24 hours

  Although aggressive fluid therapy is the cornerstone but few recent studies have suggested that controlled therapy may be better in reducing mortality and outcomes.

Summary of available studies on controlled fluid therapy:

- *Mao et al. (2010):* Rapid hemodilution increases sepsis and mortality
- *Madaria et al:* Administration of >4 L fluid/day associated with more local or systemic complications
- *Eckerwall et al:* 4 L or more fluid in 24 hours developed more respiratory complications

  Goal of fluid resuscitation is to correct hypovolemia, improve organ dysfunction, and prevent further necrosis. Excessive fluid increases tissue edema and impairs lung and cardiac functions, increasing the risk of cardiac failure.

Initial Assessment and Risk Stratification

Hemodynamic status should be assessed immediately upon presentation and resuscitative measures should began as needed:

- Assessment of tissue perfusion and O_2 delivery:
  - *Conventional:* Pulse, respiratory rate (RR), temperature, BP, and SpO_2
  - *Physiological:* White blood cell (WBC), H^+, base deficit, lactate, central venous (CV) saturation, and urine output (UO).

SIRS ≥ 2 of the following:

i. *Temperature:* >38 or <36°F.
ii. *Heart rate:* >90/min
iii. *RR:* >20/min, partial pressure of carbon dioxide (pCO_2) < 32 mm Hg.
iv. *WBC:* >12,000 or <4,000 mm^3/or >10% immature forms

Risk assessment to stratify patients into high and low-risk categories to assist triage, such as admission to an ICU

- *Rapid recognition of organ dysfunction:*
  - *Respiratory:* SpO_2 <95%
  - *Renal:* Creatinine >2 mg%/BUN ≥ 20 mg% (N = 7–20), UO < 0.5 mL/kg/h
  - *Cardiovascular system:* Mean arterial pressure (MAP) < 70 (N = 70–100) mm Hg or requires vasopressors
  - *Hematological:* Platelets $<120 \times 10^3$
  - *Neurological:* Glasgow Coma Scale (GCS) <15
  - *Hepatic:* Bilirubin >1.2 mg%
  - SIRS on admission (>2 criteria) = risk of multiple organ failure (MOF)
- CRP (peaks at 72 hours) is the only clinically used marker of disease severity; values >150 mg% after 72 hours are suggestive of SAP.

Fluid resuscitation is the mainstay of early management.

Lack of consensus on: Type of fluid (crystalloids vs. colloids), optimal administration (aggressive vs. nonaggressive), monitoring, and end points of adequate resuscitation.

- Colloids → volume overload, hyperoncotic renal impairment, coagulopathy, and anaphylactic reaction.
- Large amounts of crystalloids → pulmonary edema
- Patients with LC need more fluid

Preexisting renal or cardiac dysfunction: Restrict fluid infusion.

- Evidences show aggressive hydration within first 24 hours of onset ("therapeutic interventional window") ↓morbidity/mortality; after 48 hours it has no effect on the patient's outcome.

  Reversing hypoperfusion (maintaining MAP) and UO > 0.5 mL/kg→ averts SIRS/MODS and a cascade of events leading to PN.

Fluid Administration

- Controlled fluid resuscitation *@3 mL/kg/h* (3.0–4.0 L/24 h) × 24–48 hours with pH-balanced lactated Ringer's after a bolus infusion of 20 mL/kg (≈1,000 mL over 1 hour): limits or prevents PN in those with severe volume depletion.
- Total infusion in first 24 hours ≈3–4 L with reassessment every 8 hours for the first 24 hours.

(Monitoring: BP, pulse, urine output > 0.5 mL/kg/h, ↓ hematocrit, ↓ BUN/creatinine, central venous pressure (CVP): 8–12 cmH_2O).

- Persistent hemoconcentration (hematocrit >44–47%) at 24 hours postadmission = "inadequate fluid resuscitation."
- If the BUN remained unchanged or ↑ from its previous value 8–12 hours post start of resuscitation = "refractory" [one of causes being intra-abdominal hypertension (IAH)], i.e., IAP > 12 mm Hg.

Aggressive Fluid Resuscitation

- *Early aggressive fluid resuscitation:* Ringer's lactate (RL) @250–500 mL/h for the first 24 hours
- Similar aggressive fluid replacement after 48 hours has no effect on the outcome.
- *Within first 24 hours:* Urine output > 0.5 mL/kg/h, ↓ hematocrit/BUN are indicators of good prognosis

(no numeric goals)

Recent guidelines by the American Gastroenterological Institute on Fluid Management of Acute Pancreatitis, 2018:

- In patients with acute pancreatitis, the American Gastroenterological Association (AGA) suggests using goal-directed therapy for fluid management.
- The AGA makes no recommendation on whether normal saline or Ringer's lactate is used.

Goal-directed therapy utilizes several types of invasive [CVP, stroke volume (SV), and stroke volume index (SVI)] or noninvasive (BUN, hematocrit, urine/output, and pulse) techniques to direct the further need of fluid.

There are multiple recommendations for the rate of fluid administration. Most recommended is a bolus infusion of 20 mL/kg RL in the first hour and then an infusion of 3–4 L of RL/24 hours.

PANCREATIC NECROSIS

10. New approach to pancreatic necrosis. ***WBUHS 2019***

Diagnosis of Pancreatic Necrosis

- Blood—amylase, lipase, CRP—diagnostic and prognostic
- Contrast-enhanced computed tomography (CECT) of the abdomen:
    - After 72 hours
    - Percentage of necrosis—CT severity score

Modified CT Severity Index

- Pancreatic inflammation
    - 0—Normal pancreas
    - 2—Pancreatic changes with or without peripancreatic inflammation
    - 4—Peripancreatic fluid collection/fat necrosis
- Pancreatic necrosis:
    - 0—None
    - 2—30% or less
    - 4— >30%

Extrapancreatic Complication

- 2—One or more of pleural effusion, ascites, vascular or gastrointestinal (GI) involvement
- *Total score:*
    - *0–2:* Mild
    - *4–6:* Moderate
    - *8–10:* Severe

Treatment

- *General measures:*
  - High risk—shift to CCU/HDU
  - Respiratory support—most O_2/positive pressure ventilation/intubation
  - Hemodynamic stability:
    - IVF–NS/RL
    - Aggressive fluid therapy—first 12–24 hours—250–500 mL/h (decrease BUN)
- *Antibiotics:*
  - Not recommended routinely as prophylaxis
  - Recommended in:
    - Infected necrosis
    - No improvement after conservative treatment for 7–10 days
    - Extrapancreatic infection—cholangitis and pneumonia Recommended antibiotics—imipenem, imidazole, and quinolone
- *Routine prophylactic ERCP*—not improve the outcome
- *Analgesic—narcotic*
- *Nutrition:*
  - Enteral—recommended
  - Parenteral nutrition (PN)
- *Specific measure:*
  - All necrosis need not to be drained
  - Infected necrosis-surgical necrosectomy, if:
    - Air in necrosis—suspected
    - USG/CT-guided FNAC + Gram stain—proved
- *Necrosectomy:*
  - *Surgical necrosectomy:* Step up treatment—recommended
  - Endoscopic treatment—currently first line of management

Endoscopic transmural drainage with:

- Larger tract dilatation
- Placcmcnt of multiple stents
- Insertion of NCC (nasocystic catheter)
- FCSEMS
  - Direct debridement of solid necrotic tissue
  - Percutaneous drainage
  - Video-assisted retroperitoneal access
  - *Open necrosectomy:* When all fail

11. Pancreatic necrosectomy. ***WBUHS 2015***

Introduction

Pancreatic necrosis is a serious infection usually associated with acute pancreatitis. During recurring attacks of pancreatitis, tissue within the pancreas may die (necrotize) and later become infected. This condition is called acute necrotizing pancreatitis.

Rationale of Necrosectomy

- Infected and necrotic pancreatic tissue serves as nidus for proinflammatory factors to be released in large amounts both locally and systemically.
- This elicits a severe inflammatory reaction thereby exacerbating or amplifying features of SIRS.

- Persistence of these effects eventually leads to septicemia and multiple organ dysfunction syndrome (MODS), eventually terminating to death.
- Therefore, removal of this infected necrotic debris undoubtedly reduces the quantum of proinflammatory factors released into the system thereby reducing the systemic inflammatory response.
- A single sitting of necrosectomy may not always offer a complete eradication of the source. In most of the cases, multiple sittings may be required to ensure complete eradication of the infected source.

Therapeutic Options

Open Surgical Necrosectomy

Through a midline incision the entire abdominal cavity is assessed. A diverting ileostomy is performed in those cases wherein the retrocolic area is also involved. Once the focus of necrosis is exposed, blunt necrosectomy is performed, which ensures atraumatic removal of necrotic tissue without damaging the residual pancreatic tissue. This is followed by one of the four techniques:

1. *Open packing:* The cavity is irrigated vigorously with saline and is packed with a nonadherent dressing. The patient needs to be brought to the operating room every 48 hours for further debridement and repacking until the process of necrosis is halted and no necrotic tissue debris are seen. The abdomen is closed over drains.
2. *Planned staged re-laparotomies with repeated lavage:* This method involves planned reoperations after primary necrosectomy on every alternate day until all devitalized tissue has been removed, growth of granulation tissue has commenced and there is substantial evidence that the necrotic process has been brought under control. Repeated opening of the peritoneal cavity may be cumbersome and cause irreversible damage to the abdominal wall leading to significant morbidity. This can be eased by using a zipper being attached to the incised edges. Peritoneal drains also help in the drainage of infected material.
3. *Continuous lavage of the lesser sac and retroperitoneum:* It is a very effective method of cleaning all the necrotic residual debris. After primary necrosectomy multiple tube drains, usually four, are kept in the retroperitoneal area in juxtaposition to the pancreatic remnant. Continuous irrigation with dialysis fluid or even normal saline measuring approximately 35 L/day may help reduce the septic process significantly. The endpoint of lavage is clear effluent from the drains.
4. *Closed packing:* After primary necrosectomy the cavity is irrigated and packed with large gauze mops. Drains are also kept. Drains are removed after 7 days along with the removal of the packs.

Minimally Invasive Approach

- Minimally invasive techniques confirm significant advantage with respect to surgical outcome; however, the technique has its limitations and is best utilized if the pancreatic necrosis is <30% with massive fluid collections in the left retroperitoneal space.
- The advantages of laparoscopy are reduced inflammatory response to intervention, considerably reduced incidence of bacteremia, reduced rate of development of multiorgan failure, reduced rate of wound complications, shorter stay in ICU, and fast recovery.
- The limitations of this method are availability of expertise and lack of evidence to substantiate a statistical advantage of this methodology over the open technique.

Step-up Approach

- This consists of percutaneous drainage followed by minimally invasive retroperitoneal necrosectomy.
- The first step is percutaneous or endoscopic drainage of the collection of infected fluid to reduce sepsis.
- This may postpone the need for surgical necrosectomy during the acute phase of systemic inflammatory response (SIRS). If the drainage is still inadequate, the next step is minimally invasive retroperitoneal necrosectomy. The main factor that limits the use of this methodology is the blockage of the drainage tube before complete drainage has been achieved, thereby necessitating early necrosectomy by either a minimal access approach or an open method.

Endoscopic Methods

- The transgastric endoscopic approach which has evolved recently is an alternative approach to drain an infected pancreatic necrosis. Endoscopic necrosectomy has a similarity to natural orifice transluminal endoscopic surgery (NOTES).
- The main disadvantage of this technique is significant bleeding which can in quite few cases prove to be fatal as it is difficult to control.

12. Describe the etiopathogenesis and treatment of acute necrotizing pancreatitis. ***WBUHS 2025 Supplementary***

Acute necrotizing pancreatitis (ANP) is a severe and potentially life-threatening form of acute pancreatitis characterized by *pancreatic parenchymal and/or peripancreatic fat necrosis.* It involves complex inflammatory and necrotic processes, often leading to systemic complications.

Etiopathogenesis

- Etiology (common causes)
    - Gallstones (most common cause worldwide)
    - Alcohol abuse
    - Hypertriglyceridemia
    - Post-ERCP (Endoscopic Retrograde Cholangiopancreatography)
    - Drugs (e.g., azathioprine, thiazides)
    - Trauma
    - Infections
    - Genetic mutations (PRSS1, SPINK1, CFTR)
    - Idiopathic (~10–20% cases)
- Pathogenesis
    - *Initiation of pancreatic injury*
        - Trigger (e.g., gallstone) leads to *premature activation of trypsinogen* to trypsin *within pancreatic acinar cells*
        - This leads to *autodigestion* of pancreatic tissue
    - *Inflammatory cascade*
        - Activation of *inflammatory mediators* (TNF-α, IL-1, IL-6)
        - Recruitment of neutrophils, macrophages
        - Damage spreads to surrounding fat and tissues
    - *Pancreatic necrosis formation*
        - Ongoing ischemia and inflammation cause *tissue necrosis*
        - Can involve:
            - *Pancreatic parenchyma*
            - *Peripancreatic fat* (fat necrosis)
- Complications
    - Systemic inflammatory response syndrome (SIRS)
    - Sepsis, organ failure
    - Infected necrosis (superimposed bacterial infection)
    - Pancreatic abscess, pseudocysts

Treatment of Acute Necrotizing Pancreatitis

Initial Supportive Management (Mainstay in early phase)

- *Hospitalization*—usually ICU-level care
- *Fluid resuscitation:*
    - Aggressive IV fluids (e.g., Ringer's lactate)
    - Monitor hemodynamics, urine output, lactate

- *Pain control:* IV opioids (e.g., fentanyl, morphine)
- *Nutritional support:* Early enteral feeding (via nasojejunal or nasogastric route)
  - Avoid prolonged NPO status
  - Parenteral nutrition only if enteral route fails
- *Monitoring for complications:*
  - Organ dysfunction (renal, respiratory, cardiovascular)
  - *Daily labs:* Amylase, lipase, CRP, electrolytes, renal and liver function.

Management of Pancreatic Necrosis

- Sterile necrosis
  - Conservative treatment preferred
  - Continue supportive care
  - Monitor for signs of infection or organ failure
- Infected necrosis
  - *Suspected if:*
    - Fever, worsening clinical status
    - Gas in necrotic area on CT
  - *Confirmed with:* CT-guided fine needle aspiration (FNA) or imaging

  Management:
  - *Antibiotics* (only if infection confirmed/suspected)
    - Carbapenems, quinolones, or metronidazole—penetrate pancreatic tissue well
  - *Drainage*
    - Step-up approach:
      - *Percutaneous or endoscopic drainage* first
      - Followed by *minimally invasive necrosectomy* if needed
  - *Surgery*
    - Indicated if minimally invasive methods fail
    - Delayed until after 3–4 weeks if possible (to allow “walled-off” necrosis)

Other Supportive Measures

- Respiratory support (oxygen, mechanical ventilation if ARDS)
- Renal support (dialysis for acute kidney injury)
- Thromboprophylaxis
- Glycemic control

  Imaging and Monitoring
  - Contrast-enhanced CT scan (best for identifying necrosis)
    - Typically done 48–72 hours after onset
  - MRI or EUS as alternatives in certain cases

13. Write in brief about groove pancreatitis. ***DNB, October 2024***

Groove pancreatitis is a rare and distinct form of *chronic pancreatitis* that affects the anatomical “groove” between the *head of the pancreas*, the *duodenum*, and the *common bile duct*. It can mimic pancreatic cancer both clinically and radiologically, which makes accurate diagnosis important but sometimes challenging.

Pathology

There are two main forms:

1. *Pure form*—limited to the groove area.
2. *Segmental form*—involves both the groove and the adjacent part of the pancreatic head.

Causes and Risk Factors

- Chronic alcohol use (strongest association)
- Smoking
- Functional obstruction of the minor papilla
- Peptic ulcer disease
- Pancreas divisum (anatomic variation)
- Heterotopic pancreas in the duodenum

Symptoms

- Upper abdominal pain
- Postprandial nausea/vomiting
- Weight loss
- Sometimes mild jaundice
- Symptoms may be chronic or relapsing

Imaging Features

Imaging Modalities

- CT scan
- MRI/MRCP
- Endoscopic ultrasound (EUS)

Typical Findings

- Sheet-like mass in the groove region
- Cystic changes in the duodenal wall
- Duodenal wall thickening
- Fibrotic or scar-like changes near the minor papilla
- Preservation of the pancreatic duct (helps distinguish from cancer)

Laboratory Investigations

- May show mildly elevated pancreatic enzymes
- Tumor markers like CA 19-9 usually normal or mildly elevated (helps differentiate from pancreatic adenocarcinoma)

Differential Diagnosis

- Pancreatic head carcinoma
- Duodenal carcinoma
- Ampullary carcinoma
- Autoimmune pancreatitis

Management

- Conservative treatment (first line)
  - Alcohol and smoking cessation
  - Pain management
  - Nutritional support
  - Pancreatic enzyme supplementation
- Interventional or surgical
  - Considered in cases refractory to conservative management or if malignancy cannot be excluded:
    - Pancreaticoduodenectomy (Whipple procedure)—if cancer cannot be ruled out
    - Endoscopic drainage of cysts if symptomatic

COMPUTED TOMOGRAPHY SCAN IN PANCREATIC DISORDERS

14. Outline the role of CT scan in the diagnosis and management of pancreatic pathologies.

WBUHS 2018, WBUHS 2025 Supplementary

Role of CT scan in the diagnosis and management of pancreatic pathologies:

Acute Pancreatitis

- *Role of CT scan in diagnosis:* CECT is the standard imaging modality for the evaluation of acute pancreatitis and its complications. Using non-CECT, clinicians can establish the diagnosis and demonstrate fluid collections but cannot evaluate for pancreatic necrosis or vascular complications.
- Role of CT scan in assessing severity
- CT severity index and modified CTSI

CT severity index (Balthazar, 1990)		*Modified CT severity index (Mortele, 2004)*	
Prognostic indicator	***Points***	***Prognostic indicator***	***Points***
Pancreatic inflammation		Pancreatic inflammation	
Normal pancreas	0	Normal pancreas	0
Enlarged pancreas	1	Intrinsic pancreatic abnormalities with or without peripancreatic inflammation	2
Pancreatic abnormalities with peripancreatic inflammation	2	Pancreatic Or peripancreatic fluid collection/fat necrosis	4
Single fluid collection	3		
Two or more collection or gas	4		
Pancreatic necrosis		Pancreatic necrosis	
None	0	None	0
<30%	2	<30%	2
30–50%	4	>30%	4
>50%	6	Extrapancreatic complications	2

Chronic Pancreatitis

Computed tomography features of chronic pancreatitis include:

- Dilatation of the main pancreatic duct
- Pancreatic calcification
- Changes in pancreatic size (i.e., atrophy), shape, and contour
- Pancreatic pseudocysts

Pseudocyst Pancreas

- CT scan helps in the diagnosis and evaluation
- Pseudocysts appear as well-circumscribed, usually round, or oval peripancreatic fluid collections of homogeneously low attenuation that are usually surrounded by a well-defined enhancing wall.

Cystic Neoplasms of the Pancreas

- *Mucinous cystadenoma:*
  - The tumor contour tends to be rounded or ovoid although this is not an absolutely specific feature
  - Associated calcification when present tends to be more peripheral
  - Contents of the lesion may be heterogenous is attenuation
  - Internal septations may be present and tend to be linear or curvilinear

- *Serous cystadenoma:*
  - CT scan helps in the diagnosis:
    - Typically demonstrates a multicystic, lobulated mass in the pancreatic head sometimes described as "a bunch of grapes"
    - The individual cysts are typically <20 mm in size and >6 in number (except for the oligocystic variety
    - A characteristic enhancing central scar may be present which can show associated stellate calcification (present in ~20% of the cases)
- Intraductal papillary mucinous neoplasms or tumors [intraductal papillary mucinous neoplasms (IPMNs) or intraductal papillary-mucinous tumors (IMPTs)] are cystic tumors of the pancreas.
  - In some cases, the tumor is very localized and appears cystic. It can, therefore, be difficult to distinguish from peripheral mucinous cystadenoma/cystadenocarcinoma unless convincing communication with the duct system can be demonstrated. They do not calcify.
- *Main duct IPMN (with dilatation of the main duct >5 mm):*
  - Either segment of the pancreatic duct (or the entire duct) are dilated and filled with low-density (mucin thus water density) material
  - Overlying pancreatic parenchyma may be thinned
  - If proximal, the distal pancreatic duct may be dilated without direct involvement (cystic neoplasms can have a similar appearance)
  - Solid mural nodules are concerning for malignant transformation, and appear as hyperdense nodules protruding into the mucin-filled dilated ducts
  - Enhancing nodules following administration of contrast are very concerning
  - Occasionally mucinous material can be seen to bulge out of a dilated ampulla of Vater (uncommon but essentially pathognomonic)
- *Branch duct IPMN:*
  - The majority of the gland is normal in appearance, except for a single or multiple side branches demonstrating marked dilatation
  - Cystic mass-like appearance which often mimics cystic tumors of the pancreas
  - Its appearance has been termed a bunch of grapes due to its appearance
  - Microcystic variety has appearances similar to serous cystadenomas, but again communication with the main pancreatic duct is the key to correct diagnosis

Pancreatic Malignancy

- CT is the work-horse of pancreatic imaging
- Typically, ductal adenocarcinomas appear as poorly defined masses with extensive surrounding desmoplastic reaction.
- They enhance poorly compared to adjacent normal pancreatic tissue and thus appear hypodense on arterial phase scans in 75–90% of cases, but may become isodense on delayed scans (thus the need for multiple phase scanning when pancreatic cancer is the clinical question).
- Double duct sign may be seen.
- CT correlates well with surgical findings in predicting unresectability (positive predictive value of 89–100%).
- The most important feature to assess locally is the relationship of the tumor to surrounding vessels [superior mesenteric artery (SMA) and coeliac axis (CA)].
- If the tumor surrounds a vessel by >180°, then it is deemed T4 disease and is unresectable.

SURGICAL ANATOMY OF PANCREAS AND CYSTS OF PANCREAS

15. Describe the surgical anatomy of pancreas. Give a brief account of cysts in relation to the pancreas.

WBUHS 2006

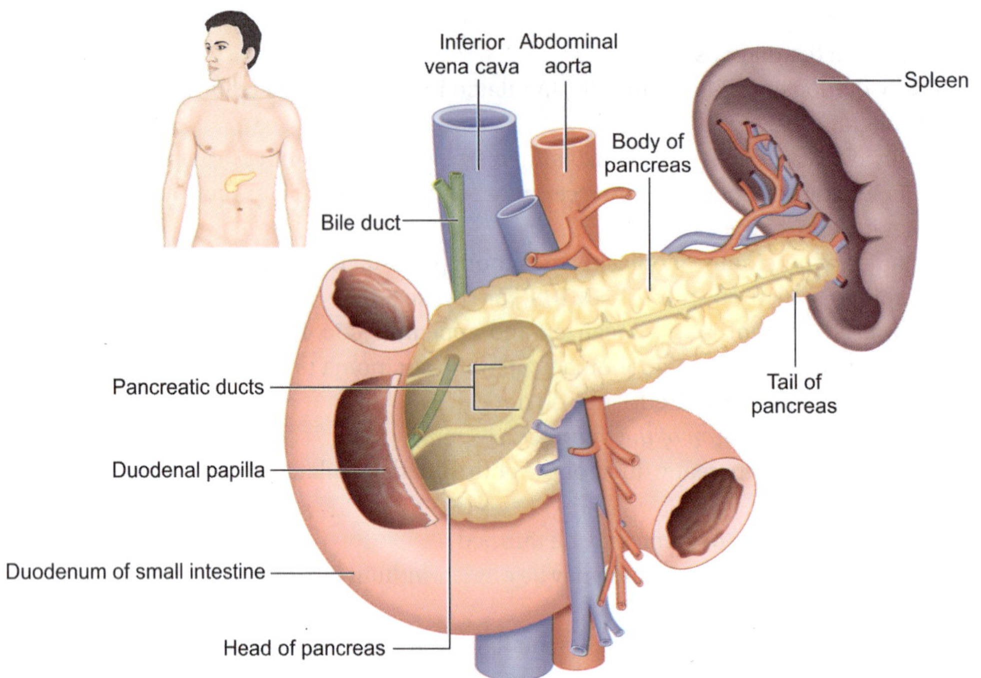

- The pancreas lies across the upper abdomen. It extends from the inside of the C loop of the duodenum to the hilum of the spleen. It lies behind the stomach and the peritoneum (the thin lining of the abdominal cavity). The head of the pancreas lies in the C-shaped duodenal curve while the tail of the pancreas lies toward the spleen. The body of the pancreas lies between the head and the tail.
- The blood supply comes from branches of the celiac, superior mesenteric, and splenic artery.

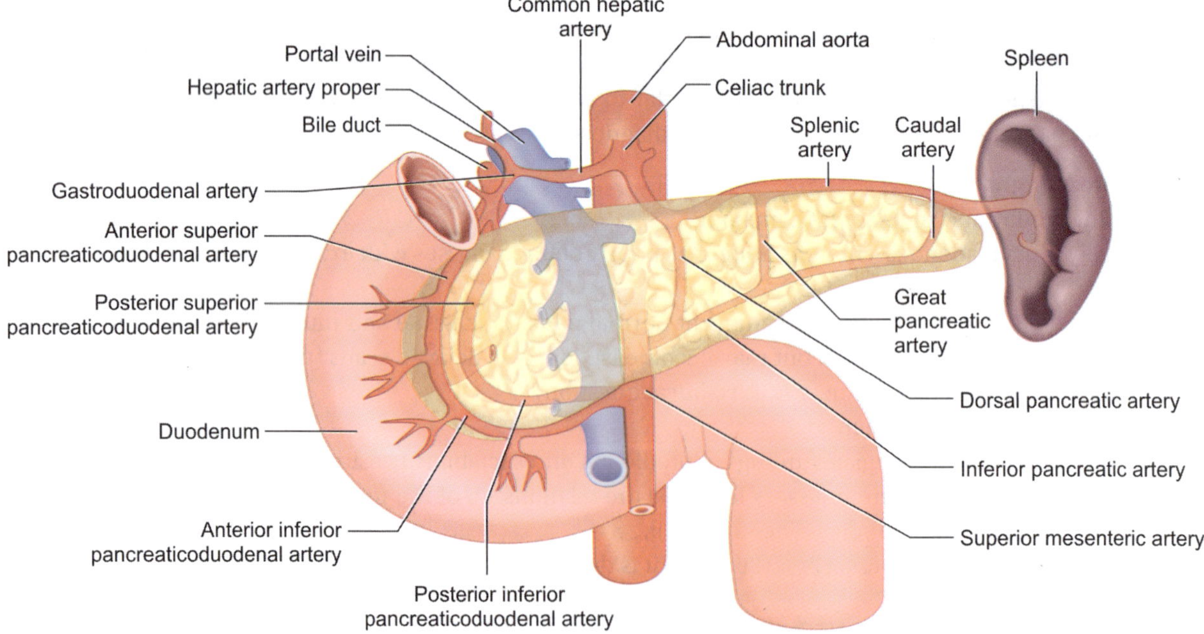

Arterial Supply to the Pancreas

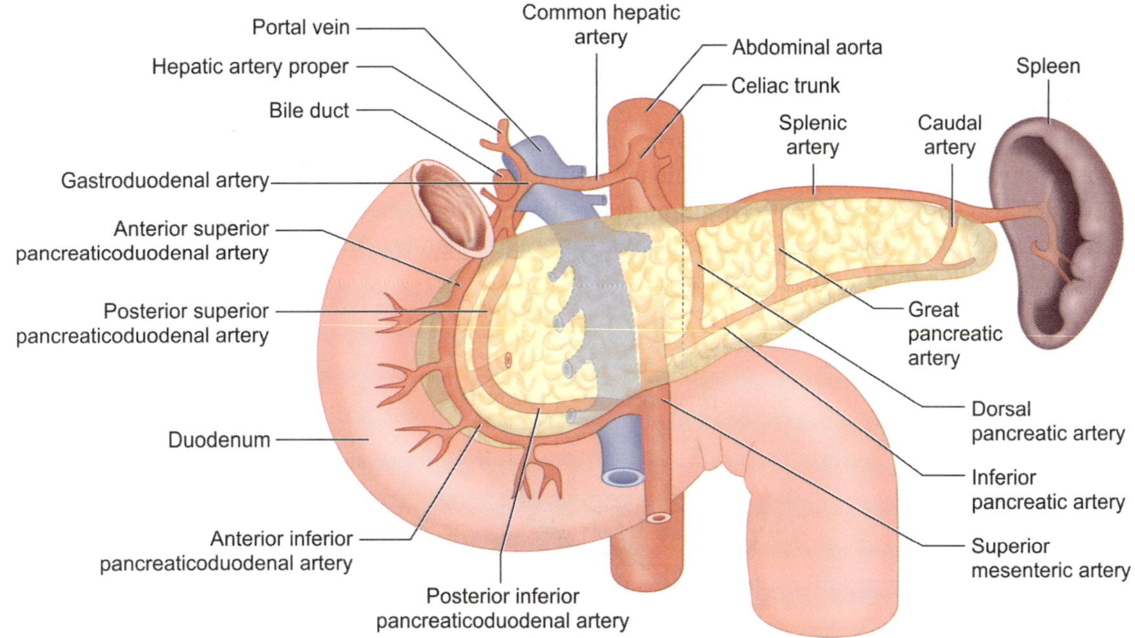

- *Arterial supply to the pancreas:* Multiple arcades in the head and body of the pancreas provide a rich blood supply. The head of the pancreas cannot be resected without devascularizing the duodenum unless a rim of pancreas containing the pancreaticoduodenal arcade is preserved.
- Blood drains by veins to the large portal vein (PV) that drains into the liver.

Venous Drainage from the Pancreas

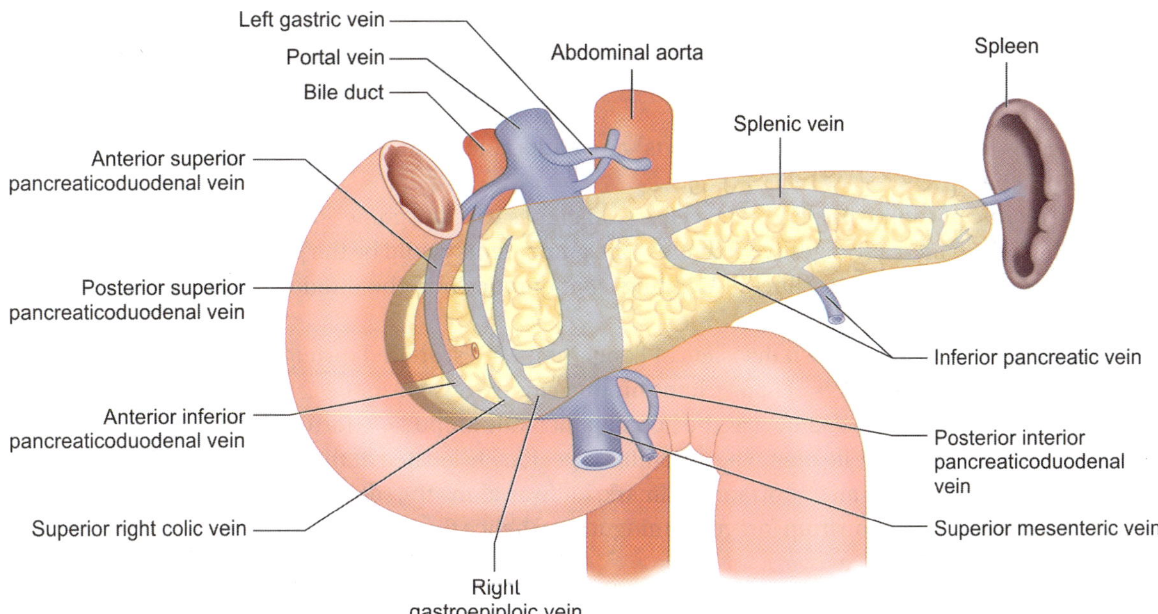

- *Venous drainage from the pancreas:* The venous drainage of the pancreas follows a pattern similar to the arterial supply, with the veins usually superficial to the arteries. Venous branches draining the pancreatic head and uncinate process enter along the right lateral and posterior sides of the portal vein. There are usually no anterior venous tributaries, and a plane can usually be developed between the neck of the pancreas and the portal and superior mesenteric veins (SMVs).
- *The lymph nodes that come from the pancreas are plentiful and follow the major arteries and veins:* Lymphatic supply to the pancreas. The lymphatic drainage from the pancreas is diffuse and widespread. The pancreatic lymphatics also communicate with lymph nodes in the transverse mesocolon and mesentery of the proximal jejunum. Tumors in the body and tail of the pancreas are often unresectable because they metastasize to these lymph nodes and to the hilum of the spleen.

Lymphatic Supply to the Pancreas

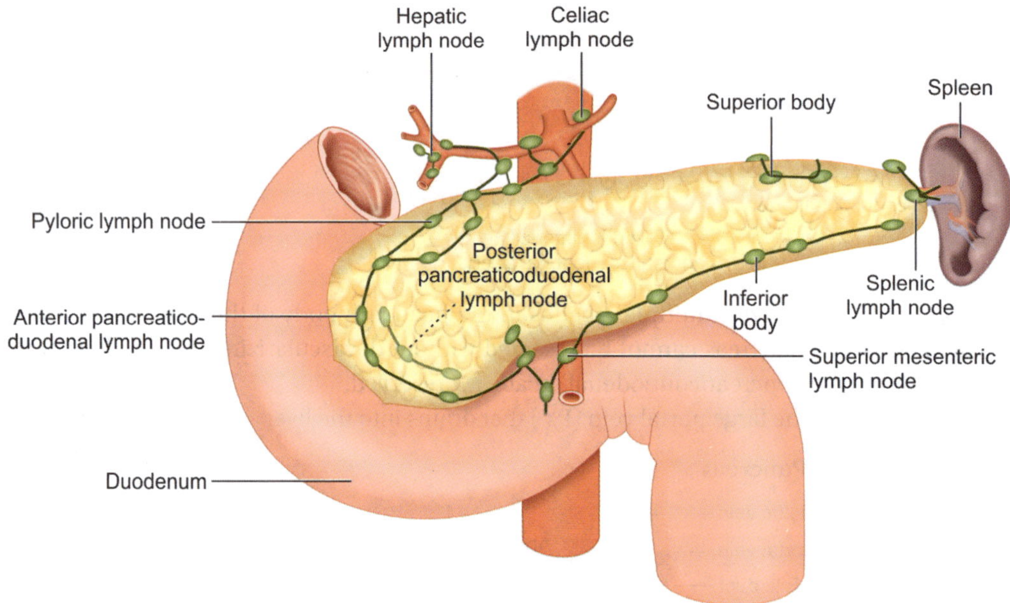

- The pancreas has both exocrine (having ducts) and endocrine (without ducts) histology (tissue as seen under the microscope)
  - The exocrine portion is analogous to a cluster of grapes with the grapes representing the secreting unit that produces the pancreatic digestive enzymes. The grape stems would be the pancreatic ducts coming together to form a single large duct (duct of Wirsung) that empties into the duodenum at a small raised area, the ampulla of Vater
  - The endocrine portion, called the islets of Langerhans, are scattered throughout the pancreas. The various cells that make up the islets of Langerhans produce numerous hormones.
  - The ampulla of Vater, also known as the hepatopancreatic ampulla, is formed by the union of the pancreatic duct and the common bile duct. The ampulla is specifically located at the major duodenal papilla.
  - The ampulla of Vater is an important landmark, halfway along the second part of the duodenum, that marks the anatomical transition from foregut to midgut (and hence the point where the celiac trunk stops supplying the gut and the SMA takes over).

Functions

- Various smooth muscle sphincters regulate the flow of bile and pancreatic juice through the ampulla— the sphincter of the pancreatic duct, the sphincter of the bile duct, and the hepatopancreatic sphincter (Sphincter of Oddi).

- The sphincter of Oddi controls the introduction of bile and pancreatic secretions into the duodenum, as well as preventing the entry of duodenal contents into the ampulla.

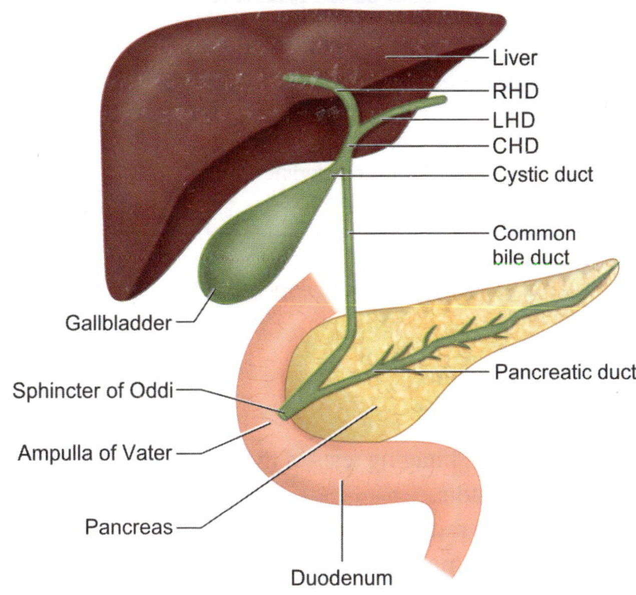

(CHD: common hepatic duct; LHD: left hepatic duct; RHD: right hepatic duct)

- Pancreatic cysts are abnormal, sac-like pockets of fluid on or within your pancreas; though, it may be alarming to learn you have a pancreatic cyst, the good news is that most pancreatic cysts are not cancerous—and many do not even cause symptoms.
- In fact, many pancreatic cysts are not technically cysts at all, called pseudocysts.
- But because some pancreatic cysts can be cancerous.

Cysts of Pancreas

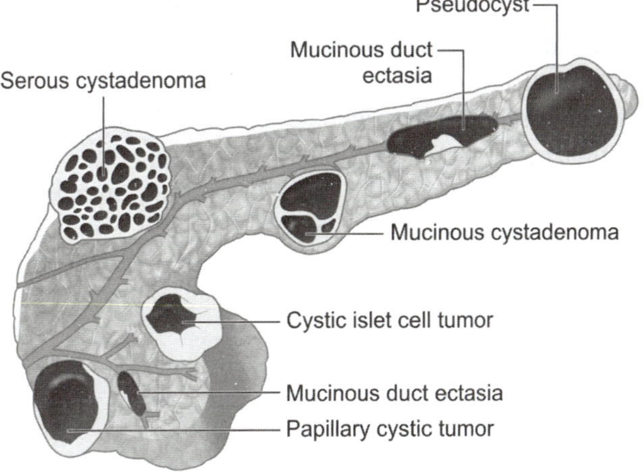

Pathologic classification of cystic neoplasms of the pancreas: The WHO international classification of tumors, 2000.

- Serous cystic neoplasm (SCN):
  - Microcystic adenoma
  - Oligocystic adenoma
- Mucinous cystic neoplasm (MCN):
  - Mucinous cystadenoma
  - Mucinous cystic tumor–borderline
  - Mucinous cystadenocarcinoma
    - Noninvasive (carcinoma in situ)
    - Invasive
- Intraductal papillary mucinous neoplasm (IPMN):
  - Adenoma
  - Borderline
  - Carcinoma in situ
  - Invasive carcinoma

Pancreatic cysts are often discovered when imaging tests of the abdomen are done for another reason. When signs or symptoms do occur, they typically include:

- Persistent abdominal pain, which may radiate to your back
- A mass you can feel in your upper abdomen, where your pancreas is located
- Nausea and vomiting
- Cysts can become infected; patient will be feverish and have persistent abdominal pain.
  - A ruptured pseudocyst is a medical emergency. When a cyst ruptures, the released fluid can damage nearby blood vessels and cause massive bleeding. It may also cause infection of the abdominal cavity (peritonitis). Seek emergency medical treatment if one has signs or symptoms of internal bleeding and shock, including:
    - Fainting
    - Severe abdominal pain
    - Decreased consciousness
    - Weak and rapid heartbeat
    - Vomiting blood

Causes

- In many cases, the cause of a particular pancreatic cyst is unknown.
- Genetic mutations can lead to cancerous cysts.
- Some cysts are associated with rare illnesses—such as von Hippel–Lindau disease, which is a genetic disorder that can affect the brain, retina, adrenal glands, kidneys, and pancreas.
- Pseudocysts often follow a bout of pancreatitis, a painful condition in which the pancreas digestive enzymes become prematurely active and digest some of the pancreas itself.
- Pseudocysts can also result from blunt trauma to the abdomen, such as during a car accident.

Risk Factors

- Heavy alcohol use
- Gallstones

Tests and Diagnosis

The biggest challenge of the diagnostic process is determining whether the pancreatic cyst is cancerous or not. The following tests are often used to help with diagnosis and to help plan treatment:

- *Medical history:* A previous history of pancreatitis or abdominal injury typically is an indication of a pseudocyst.
- *CT scan:* A CT scan can give detailed information about the structure of a pancreatic cyst. It can sometimes help differentiate cancerous cysts from noncancerous ones.

- *MRI scan:* An MRI scan can highlight subtle details of a pancreatic cyst structure, including whether there are any solid components to the cyst.
- *Endoscopic ultrasound:* One of the useful modalities.
- *Cyst fluid evaluation:* Fluid taken from a cyst is examined in a laboratory for possible signs of cancer. One such sign, or marker, is a substance called carcinoembryonic antigen (CEA). Elevated levels of CEA in the fluid sample are suggestive of cancer.

In some cases, the characteristics and location of the cyst in your pancreas—along with your age and sex—can help to pinpoint the type of cyst.

- *Serous cystadenoma:* This growth can become large enough to displace nearby organs, causing such symptoms as abdominal pain and a feeling of fullness. Serous cystadenomas occur most frequently in middle-aged women and become cancerous only rarely.
- *Mucinous cystadenoma:* This type of cyst is usually located in the body or tail of the pancreas and occurs most often in middle-aged women. It is precancerous and may already be cancerous when discovered. Larger cysts are more likely to be cancerous.
- *Mucinous duct ectasia:* More common in men, this type of cyst consists of dilated ductal segments, usually within the head of the pancreas. Also known as an intraductal papillary mucinous tumor, this type of growth is usually precancerous or cancerous.
- *Papillary cystic tumor:* A papillary cystic tumor—also known as a papillary cystic neoplasm, or solid and pseudopapillary neoplasm—occurs most often in young women and is usually located in the body or tail of the pancreas. It is usually cancerous.
- *Cystic islet cell tumor:* This type of pancreatic tumor is mostly solid but can have cyst-like components. It may be confused with other pancreatic cysts.

Treatment

Treatment differs depending on the type of cyst and whether it causes symptoms. Sometimes, no treatment is necessary.

- *Watchful waiting:* A benign pseudocyst—even a large one—can be left alone, because a serous cystadenoma so rarely evolves into cancer, it also can be left alone unless it causes symptoms or enlarges.
- *Drainage:* A pseudocyst that is causing bothersome symptoms or growing larger may be drained with a needle, often with the use of an endoscope. The endoscope can be equipped with a needle to drain the cyst.
- *Surgery:*
  - An enlarged pseudocyst or serous cystadenoma that is causing pain or other symptoms can be surgically removed; however, a pseudocyst that is removed may recur.
  - Treatment for most other types of lesions in the pancreas is generally surgical removal, because of the risk of cancer. Surgery is very effective, with little chance of recurrence.

---

16. Discuss the role of EU in evaluation of cystic lesions of pancreas and IPMN. Give the novel therapeutic options of EUS. ***WBUHS 2017***

Cystic Lesions of Pancreas

- *Unilocular*
  - Pancreatic pseudocyst
  - IPMN
  - Serous cystadenoma uncommonly uni/multilocular
  - Pancreatic cysts occur in association with:
    - Von Hippel Lindau syndrome
    - Autosomal dominant polycystic kidney disease (ADPKD)
    - Cystic fibrosis

- *Macrocystic: Multilocular*
  - Mucinous cystic neoplasm(s) of pancreas—usually body and tail
  - IPMN
  - Serous cystadenoma uncommonly uni/multilocular
  - Acinar cell cystadenocarcinoma
- *Microcystic:* Serous cystadenoma—usually head; 30% have a central scar
- *Cystic with a solid component:*
  - Macrocystic tumors can also have a solid component
  - Solid pseudopapillary tumor of pancreas
  - Primary ductal pancreatic tumor with cystic degeneration
  - Cystic degeneration of islet cell tumors
    - Insulinoma
    - Glucagonoma
      - Cystic teratoma
      - Metastases to pancreas

Retroperitoneal lesions, extrinsic to the pancreas, can of course mimic pancreatic cystic lesions, when close to the gland, for example, include:
- Cystic lymphadenopathy (e.g., necrotic)
- Duodenal diverticulum

Endoscopic Ultrasound
- Endoscopic ultrasound is an excellent imaging technique for detecting signs predictive of malignancy or aggressiveness in cystic pancreatic lesions. Such signs include internal septations, mural nodules, solid masses, vascular invasion, and lymphatic metastasis.
- An additional benefit is its capability for sampling fluid and solid components and depicting debris and wall thickness.
- Endoscopic ultrasound also shows the details of the pancreatic parenchyma and the pancreatic duct.
- Endoscopic ultrasound is invasive and operator-dependent
- Currently, endoscopic ultrasound with or without aspiration is used in the following instances:
  - Indeterminate multidetector computed tomography (MDCT) or MRCP findings; care of patients at high surgical risk owing to comorbid conditions or advanced age, which precludes them from undergoing extensive surgery; and confirmation of the malignant status of a cystic lesion before it is resected.
  - Endoscopic ultrasound-guided cyst fluid aspiration is often performed in conjunction with endoscopic ultrasound for definitive diagnosis.

WHO classification of pancreatic cystic neoplasms:
- *Serous cystic neoplasms:*
  - Serous cystadenoma
  - Serous microcystic adenoma
  - Serous oligocystic adenoma
  - Serous cystadenocarcinoma
- *Mucinous cystic neoplasm:*
  - Mucinous cystadenoma
  - Mucinous cystic neoplasm with moderate dysplasia
  - Mucinous cystadenocarcinoma
    - Noninvasive
    - Invasive

- *Intraductal papillary mucinous neoplasm:*
  - Intraductal papillary mucinous adenoma
  - Intraductal papillary mucinous neoplasm with moderate dysplasia
  - Intraductal papillary mucinous carcinoma
    - Noninvasive
    - Invasive
- *Solid pseudopapillary neoplasm:* In patients with suspected IPMNs, preoperative evaluation attempts to define the presence or absence of malignancy. Involvement of the main duct and/or side branches, and the longitudinal extent of involvement within the pancreas.

EUS: Detect communication with pancreatic duct and detect mural nodules. Sample cystic fluid and biopsy.

Therapeutic role of EUS:

- *EUS-guided drainage of intra-abdominal collections:* Drainage of peripancreatic fluid collections.
  - *Gallbladder drainage:* Cholecystectomy is the treatment of choice in patients with acute cholecystitis; however, in certain group of patients, this is not an option due to multiple comorbidities.
  - *EUS-guided biliary drainage:* The three options include:
    1. EUS-guided biliary drainage—transduodenal—for distal biliary strictures.
    2. EUS-guided biliary drainage—transgastric—for proximal biliary strictures, accessed through the left lobe of the liver.
    3. EUS-guided rendezvous—for patients who have diverticulum or the ampulla is not clearly visible.
- EUS-guided celiac plexus neurolysis/block.
- *EUS-guided treatment of tumors:*
  - EUS allows accurate targeting for the delivery of various substances directly into pancreas, liver, or subepithelial lesions.
  - *EUS-guided FNI has been reported for the treatment of:*
    - GI stromal tumors and insulinomas
    - Hepatic metastases
    - Esophageal cancer
    - Cystic neoplasms of the pancreas
    - Pancreatic adenocarcinoma
  - Various biological antitumor agents have been introduced into pancreatic and esophageal cancers under EUS-guided FNI for control of locally advanced disease.
- CyberKnife stereotactic radiotherapy has been used to treat lung, mediastinal and pancreatic tumors. The radiographic markers are placed around the tumor either surgically or using transabdominal ultrasound; however, EUS-guided judicial placement for locally advanced or recurrent pancreatic cancer seems to be a successful alternative.
- *EUS in the management of GI bleeding*: Upper GI bleeding is a common medical emergency with a mortality of 10%, and therapeutic endoscopy is the main modality of treatment. In clinical practice, it is sometimes difficult to achieve hemostasis, especially in gastric variceal bleeds. If endoscopy fails, then they are often referred for transjugular intrahepatic portosystemic shunt. It is contraindicated in patients with encephalopathy and right heart failure. Endoscopic ultrasound may be used as an alternative to achieve hemostasis in this group of patients.
- *EUS-guided tissue ablation*: There is accumulating data on the EUS-guided ablation of cystic and solid pancreatic tumors.
- *Other indications*: The other indications for interventional EUS, which are in very preliminary stages, include:
  - EUS-guided fine-needle tattoo injection for small tumor
  - EUS-guided angiography, EUS-guided Botox injection
  - EUS-guided gastroenterostomy

17. Classify cystic lesions of pancreas. Discuss the clinical features, diagnosis, complications and management of Mucinous cyst adenoma of pancreas. ***WBUHS 2025***

Classification of Cystic Lesions of the Pancreas

Cystic lesions of the pancreas are broadly classified based on their etiology, histopathological features, and malignant potential. The main categories are:

- *Non-neoplastic cysts:*
  - *Pseudocysts:* Most common, resulting from pancreatitis or trauma; no epithelial lining, filled with pancreatic fluid and debris.
  - *Congenital Cysts:* Rare, include simple cysts or those associated with syndromes like von Hippel-Lindau or polycystic kidney disease.
  - *Retention Cysts:* Caused by ductal obstruction, often small and benign.
- *Neoplastic cysts:*
  - *Mucinous Cystic Neoplasms (MCNs):*
    - *Mucinous Cystadenoma:* Benign but with malignant potential.
    - *Mucinous Cystadenocarcinoma:* Malignant counterpart.
  - *Intraductal Papillary Mucinous Neoplasms (IPMNs):*
    - Main-duct, branch-duct, or mixed-type; range from benign to malignant.
  - *Serous Cystic Neoplasms (SCNs):*
    - *Serous Cystadenoma:* Typically benign, microcystic or macrocystic.
    - *Serous Cystadenocarcinoma:* Extremely rare.
  - *Solid Pseudopapillary Neoplasms (SPNs):* Low-grade malignant potential, more common in young females.
  - *Cystic Pancreatic Neuroendocrine Tumors (cNETs):* Rare, may be functional or non-functional.
- *Inflammatory/Infectious Cysts:* Associated with chronic pancreatitis or infections (e.g., echinococcal cysts).
- *Rare cystic lesions:* Lymphoepithelial cysts, acinar cell cystadenomas, or metastatic cystic lesions.

Mucinous Cystadenoma of the Pancreas

Definition: Mucinous cystadenoma is a benign cystic neoplasm of the pancreas with mucin-producing epithelial lining and malignant potential, primarily affecting women (90% female predominance).

Clinical Features

- *Demographics:* Typically occurs in women aged 40–60 years ("mother" tumor).
- *Location:* Predominantly in the body or tail of the pancreas (95%).
- *Symptoms:*
  - Often asymptomatic, discovered incidentally on imaging.
  - Symptomatic cases may present with:
    - Abdominal pain or discomfort (due to mass effect).
    - Palpable mass in large lesions.
    - Nausea, vomiting, or early satiety if compressing adjacent structures.
    - Rarely, jaundice if near the pancreatic head.
- *Associated features:* May be associated with weight loss or fatigue if large or progressing toward malignancy.

Diagnosis

- *Imaging modalities:*
  - *Ultrasound (US):* Initial detection of cystic lesion; may show a unilocular or multilocular cyst with thick walls.
  - *Computed tomography (CT):* Preferred for characterizing cyst size, location, septations, calcifications, and mural nodules. MCNs often appear as well-defined, macrocystic lesions in the body/tail.

- *Magnetic resonance imaging (MRI)/MRCP:* Superior for assessing communication with the pancreatic duct (MCNs typically lack ductal communication, unlike IPMNs). Shows thick-walled cysts with mucin content.
- *Endoscopic ultrasound (EUS):* Gold standard for detailed evaluation; allows visualization of cyst architecture (septations, nodules) and fine-needle aspiration (FNA) for fluid analysis.

- *Cyst fluid analysis (via EUS-FNA):*
  - *Mucin:* Thick, viscous fluid, positive for mucin staining.
  - *CEA levels:* Elevated (>192 ng/mL suggests mucinous lesion, distinguishes from serous cysts).
  - *Amylase levels:* Low (unlike pseudocysts, which have high amylase).
  - *Cytology:* May show mucin-producing epithelial cells; atypical cells suggest progression to malignancy.
- *Histopathology (postresection):*
  - Confirms diagnosis with mucin-producing epithelium and ovarian-type stroma (hallmark of MCN).
  - Absence of ductal communication differentiates from IPMN.
- *Key diagnostic features:*
  - Solitary, thick-walled cyst in the body/tail.
  - No pancreatic duct communication.
  - Presence of ovarian-type stroma on histology.
  - High CEA in cyst fluid.

Complications

- *Malignant transformation:* 10–20% risk of progression to mucinous cystadenocarcinoma, especially in larger cysts (>3 cm), those with mural nodules, or in older patients.
- *Mass effect:* Compression of adjacent structures (e.g., stomach, duodenum, bile duct) causing pain, obstruction, or jaundice.
- *Infection:* Rare, but cysts can become infected, leading to abscess formation.
- *Rupture:* Rare, but can cause peritonitis or pseudocyst formation.
- *Recurrence:* Possible if incomplete resection occurs or if malignant transformation is missed.

Management

The management of mucinous cystadenoma is guided by its malignant potential, size, symptoms, and patient factors. Due to the risk of malignancy, surgical resection is often recommended.

- *Indications for surgery:*
  - All confirmed or suspected MCNs, regardless of size, due to malignant potential (unlike serous cystadenomas, which can often be observed).
  - Symptomatic lesions (e.g., pain, obstruction).
  - Cysts >3 cm, those with high-risk features (mural nodules, thick walls, or rapid growth), or elevated CEA/cytological atypia on EUS-FNA.
- *Surgical options:*
  - *Distal pancreatectomy:* Most common for MCNs in the body/tail, often with splenectomy (though spleen-preserving techniques are preferred when feasible).
  - *Enucleation:* Rarely used, only for small, well-defined lesions to avoid extensive resection.
  - *Laparoscopic approach:* Preferred for benign MCNs to minimize morbidity.
  - *Whipple procedure:* Rarely needed unless the lesion is in the pancreatic head (uncommon for MCNs).
- *Non-surgical management:*
  - *Observation:* Rarely considered, only in asymptomatic patients with small (<2 cm), low-risk lesions (no mural nodules or atypia) and significant comorbidities precluding surgery. Requires regular imaging (MRI/MRCP every 6–12 months).
  - *EUS surveillance:* For indeterminate cysts, repeated EUS-FNA may guide decision-making.
- *Postoperative care:*
  - Monitor for complications like pancreatic fistula, infection, or diabetes (if significant pancreatic tissue is resected).

- Long-term follow-up with imaging to detect recurrence, especially if margins were close or atypia was present.
- *Management of malignant transformation (mucinous cystadenocarcinoma):*
  - Aggressive resection with lymphadenectomy.
  - Adjuvant chemotherapy (e.g., gemcitabine-based regimens) for invasive carcinoma.
  - Prognosis depends on stage; early-stage cancers have a 5-year survival of ~50–60%, while advanced cases have poorer outcomes.

Key Management Guidelines (Based on Consensus, e.g., AGA, Fukuoka Guidelines):

- Resect all MCNs unless contraindicated by patient frailty or comorbidities.
- High-risk features (mural nodules, symptoms, size >3 cm, or rapid growth) mandate resection.
- Observation with imaging surveillance is reserved for low-risk, small lesions in poor surgical candidates, with shared decision-making.

---

18. A 40-year-old male treated earlier for acute pancreatitis presents with lump in center abdomen. Write differential diagnosis of this case and ways of management of this condition.

Ayush University, Chhattisgarh 2025

Diagnosis is pseudocyst pancreas

Differential Diagnoses of Pancreatic Pseudocyst

- *Pancreatic cystic neoplasms:* These are important to differentiate because they may require surgical management.
  - *Serous cystadenoma:*
    - Usually benign.
    - Microcystic appearance on imaging.
    - Central scar may be seen.
  - *Mucinous cystic neoplasm (MCN):*
    - Premalignant or malignant.
    - Typically occurs in middle-aged women.
    - Often in the body or tail of the pancreas.
  - *Intraductal papillary mucinous neoplasm (IPMN)*
    - Communicates with the pancreatic duct.
    - Can be main duct, branch duct, or mixed type.
    - Mucin secretion may be evident.
  - *Solid pseudopapillary neoplasm:*
    - Rare.
    - Young women.
    - Mixed solid and cystic components.
- *Pancreatic abscess:*
  - Infectious collection associated with necrotizing pancreatitis.
  - Contains pus rather than just fluid.
  - Usually associated with systemic signs of infection (fever, leukocytosis).
- *Walled-off pancreatic necrosis (WON):*
  - Has both fluid and necrotic tissue.
  - Seen in the late phase (>4 weeks) of *necrotizing pancreatitis.*
  - Often confused with pseudocyst, but contents are more heterogeneous.
- *Duodenal diverticulum or duplication cyst:*
  - Located near the pancreas or pancreatic head.
  - Can be mistaken for a cystic pancreatic lesion on imaging.

- *Mesenteric or omental cyst:*
  - Cystic lesions arising from the mesentery or omentum.
  - Usually separate from the pancreas but can be adjacent.
- *Cystic degeneration of a solid pancreatic tumor:*
  - Pancreatic ductal adenocarcinoma may undergo cystic degeneration.
  - Suggestive if there are solid enhancing components or ductal obstruction.
- *Choledochal cyst:*
  - Cystic dilation of the bile ducts.
  - May be confused with a pseudocyst, especially if near the pancreas.

19. Management of pseudopancreatic cyst. *DNB, 2018 June*

A *pancreatic pseudocyst* is a fluid-filled sac in the abdomen, typically arising after *acute pancreatitis,* chronic pancreatitis, or pancreatic trauma. Unlike true cysts, pseudocysts *lack an epithelial lining* and are surrounded by fibrous or granulation tissue.

Indications for Intervention

Most pseudocysts resolve spontaneously. However, *intervention is needed when*:

Indication	*Description*
Size >5–6 cm	Large cysts persisting beyond 4–6 weeks
Symptoms	Abdominal pain, nausea, vomiting, early satiety
Infection	Infected pseudocyst (fever, leukocytosis, sepsis)
Bleeding	Hemorrhage into the cyst
Obstruction	Biliary or gastric outlet obstruction
Compression	Vascular compression or splenic vein thrombosis
Persistent (>6 weeks)	Especially if no sign of reduction

Management Options

- *Conservative (observation):*
  - Indicated for asymptomatic, small (<5 cm) pseudocysts without complications.
  - Regular imaging (CT or MRI) to monitor cyst size and features.
  - *Supportive care:* Pain control, pancreatic rest (NPO), nutritional support.
- *Endoscopic drainage:*
  - *Endoscopic ultrasound (EUS)-guided cystogastrostomy or cystoduodenostomy*
    - *Preferred first-line* approach for symptomatic pseudocysts near the stomach/duodenum.
    - Involves placement of *plastic stents* or *lumen-apposing metal stents (LAMS).*
    - *Advantages:* Minimally invasive, lower complication rate than surgery.
  - *Transpapillary drainage (via ERCP):*
    - Used if cyst communicates with the pancreatic duct.
    - Especially useful in chronic pancreatitis.
- *Percutaneous drainage:*
  - CT-guided catheter drainage through the abdominal wall.
  - Often used if endoscopy fails or the pseudocyst is located in the tail of the pancreas or retroperitoneal space.
  - May lead to *external pancreatic fistulas*—less preferred than endoscopy.

Surgical Drainage

- *Indicated when:*
  - Endoscopic and percutaneous methods fail.

- Complications such as necrosis, hemorrhage, or rupture occur.
- Suspicion of neoplasm (e.g., mucinous cystic neoplasm).

- *Common surgical procedures:*
  - *Cystogastrostomy:* Cyst drains into the stomach.
  - *Cystojejunostomy:* Cyst drains into the jejunum.
  - *Cystoduodenostomy:* Cyst drains into the duodenum.
  - *Pancreatectomy:* If cyst is within a non-viable part of the pancreas.
- *Diagnostic evaluation before management*
  - *CT scan or MRI:* For localization, size, wall maturity, and complications.
  - *EUS:* For better characterization and biopsy (rule out neoplasm).
  - *Amylase/lipase levels:* In cyst fluid (usually elevated).
  - *CEA level:* Low in pseudocysts; high may indicate mucinous neoplasm.
- *Follow-up and prognosis*
  - After drainage, follow-up imaging ensures resolution.
  - Monitor for complications *like infection, recurrence, bleeding,* or *stricture.*
  - Prognosis is usually good if treated appropriately.

20. What are the complications of pseudocyst of pancreas? ***WBUHS 2011***

Complications of pseudocysts include infection, leakage, and bleeding. By mass effect, a pseudocyst also can produce early satiety (stomach), stenosis (duodenum), cholestasis (bile duct), and thrombosis (portal, superior mesenteric, and splenic veins) leading to portal or segmental hypertension and varices.

- Infection of the pancreas can take several forms. Sterile, organized pancreatic necrosis may appear as a mature pseudocyst on CT scan but be predominantly solid. These differences relate to the origin (isolated duct damage versus pancreatic necrosis) and to the amount of solid material contained within the collection.
- The rupture of a pseudocyst can occur by erosion into the adjacent gastrointestinal tract, which may resolve the pseudocyst or leave a cystoenteric fistula.
- Rupture into the peritoneum leads to pancreatic ascites and can be a dramatic presentation with acute abdominal pain and rigidity from chemical peritonitis.
- Bleeding associated with a pancreatic pseudocyst is a life-threatening complication. There are several causes of bleeding.
  - Bleeding may occur secondary to erosion of the gut mucosa with the impending development of a cystoenteric fistula.
  - This may produce hematemesis and melena. More ominous is the direct erosion of a significant visceral vessel, including the splenic, gastroduodenal, and middle colic vessels.
  - The action of pancreatic enzymes (especially elastase) on the vessel wall can lead to thinning of the vessel wall and aneurysm and pseudoaneurysm formation. This situation carries a high mortality.
  - The risk of bleeding is increased in the presence of local infection.

CHRONIC PANCREATITIS

21. Discuss the etiopathology, diagnosis, and management of chronic pancreatitis. ***WBUHS 2008***

22. Discuss the etiopathology, clinical features and management of chronic pancreatitis.
SAIMS, Indore 2025; KTRUHS, Telangana 2025

23. Discuss the etiopathology, clinical features, investigations, and management of tropical chronic pancreatitis.
RGUHS, Karnataka 2025

Etiopathology of Chronic Pancreatitis

Etiologic risk factors associated with chronic pancreatitis: TIGAR-O classification system

Toxic-metabolic

- Alcoholic
- Tobacco smoking
- Hypercalcemia
- Hyperparathyroidism
- Hyperlipidemia (rare and controversial)
- Chronic renal failure
- Medications
- Phenacetin abuse (possibly from chronic renal insufficiency)
- *Toxins:* Organotin compounds (e.g., DBTC)

Idiopathic

- Early onset
- Late onset
- Tropical
- Tropical calcific pancreatitis
- Fibrocalculous pancreatic diabetes
- Other

Genetic

- Autosomal dominant
- Cationic trypsinogen (codon 29 and 122 mutations)
- Autosomal recessive/modifier genes
- Cystic fibrosis transmembrane conductance regulator (*CFTR*) mutations
- SPINK1 mutations
- Cationic trypsinogen (codon 16, 22, and 23 mutations)
- Alpha-1 antitrypsin deficiency (possible)

Autoimmune

- Isolated autoimmune chronic pancreatitis
- Syndromic autoimmune chronic pancreatitis
- Sjögren's syndrome—associated chronic pancreatitis
- Inflammatory bowel disease—associated chronic pancreatitis
- Primary biliary cirrhosis-associated chronic pancreatitis
- Recurrent and severe acute pancreatitis
- Postnecrotic (severe acute pancreatitis)

Recurrent acute pancreatitis

- Vascular diseases/ischemic
- Postirradiation

Obstructive

- Pancreatic divisum
- Sphincter of Oddi disorders (controversial)
- Duct obstruction (e.g., tumor)
- Preampullary duodenal wall cysts
- Post-traumatic pancreatic duct scars

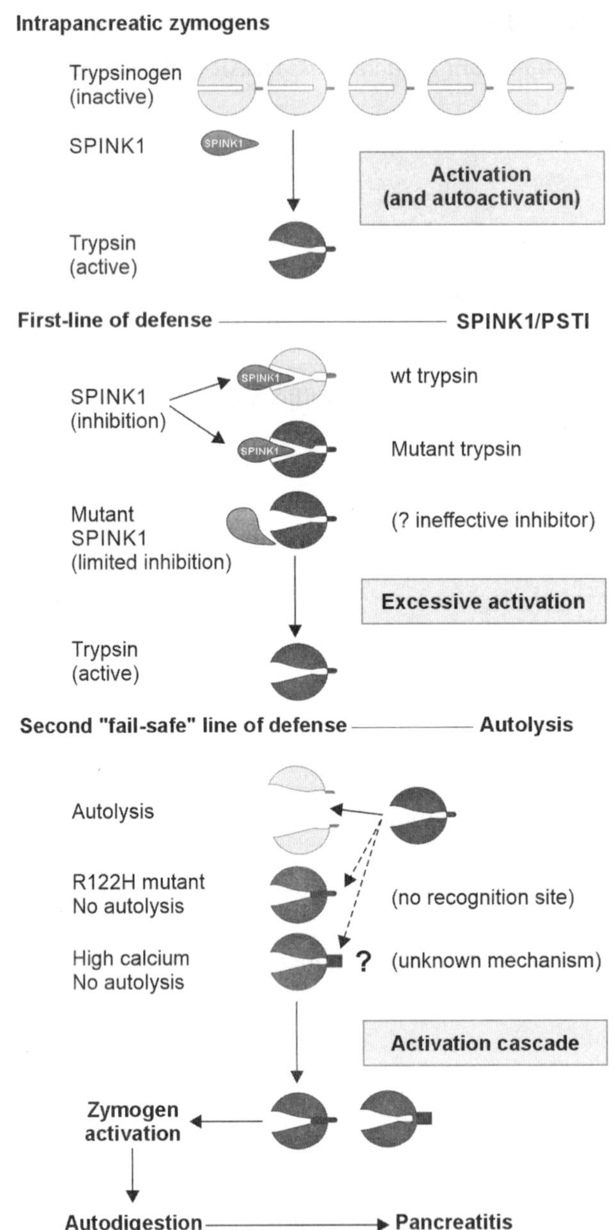

Pathology

- Initially the exocrine pancreas is affected.
- Acinar cells are lost and ductal cells are eliminated. The remaining ductal elements are buried in connective tissue.
- Islets can be seen disconnected from acinar tissue and are also surrounded by fibrosis.
- The fibrosis that is present includes collagen fibers, fibroblasts, and myofibroblasts.
- Pancreatic stellate cells in the normal pancreas reside at the base of acinar cells and harbor vitamin A-containing lipid droplets. They represent the main source of extracellular matrix and collagen in chronic pancreatitis. Ethanol can directly activate stellate cells and may also work through tumor growth factor (TGF)-beta and other proinflammatory cytokines.
- Patients with long-standing chronic pancreatitis demonstrate numerous nerves running throughout the fibrotic tissue. These nerves have lost their protective perineurium, which make them more sensitive to various

nociceptive substances. Often local inflammatory cells are seen near these nerves, which may be partially responsible for the significant pain.

Diagnosis of Chronic Pancreatitis

There has been considerable confusion concerning the clinical distinction between chronic and acute pancreatitis.

History and Clinical Feature

- Patients with chronic pancreatitis may describe prior episodes of pancreatic-type abdominal pain, and 60–0% of patients have a long history of alcohol abuse.
- There may be a family history of pancreatitis suggestive of the presence of hereditary pancreatitis or a history of autoimmune diseases, including primary sclerosing cholangitis and Sjögren's syndrome that raise suspicion of pancreatitis on an autoimmune basis.
- Diabetes mellitus or a history suggestive of malabsorption (i.e., steatorrhea) indicates that significant pancreatic endocrine or exocrine function has been lost, and this is the most compatible with the diagnosis of chronic pancreatitis.
- Typically, patients with chronic pancreatitis have upper abdominal pain radiating to the back. It can be constant or episodic and triggered by drinking alcohol or eating.
- Repeated use of heating pads or hot water bottles to treat chronic pain may result in skin lesions (*erythema ab igne*) that define the distribution of the pain.
- Some patients experience no pain.

Imaging Studies

- Radiographs or CT scans showing pancreatic calcifications are diagnostic of chronic pancreatitis. Those calcifications reflect the deposition of calcium carbonate in the intraductal protein plugs that frequently, but not invariably, occur in chronic pancreatitis.
- ERCP, CT cholangiopancreatography, or magnetic resonance cholangiopancreatography may be particularly valuable in the diagnosis of chronic pancreatitis.
- Chronic pancreatitis is characterized by irregularities of the pancreatic ducts, ductal strictures, and areas of duct dilation. The major as well as the side-branch ducts may be involved.
- Some patients with chronic pancreatitis develop dilated main pancreatic ducts (large duct disease), whereas others retain ducts of normal or even smaller than normal caliber (small duct disease).
- Some patients with chronic pancreatitis can be shown to have major ducts that have the appearance of a *"chain of lakes"* or a *"string of pearls"* that is the result of segments of dilated duct separated by areas of ductal stricture.
- Transcutaneous and endoscopic ultrasound can also be used to diagnose chronic pancreatitis if duct dilation, calcifications, pseudocysts, or parenchymal fibrosis are seen.
- Ultrasound examination is more operator-dependent and perhaps less sensitive than either CT or MRI.

Endoscopic ultrasound features of chronic pancreatitis.

Endoscopic ultrasound feature	***Implications***
Ductal changes	
• Duct size >3 mm • Tortuous pancreatic duct • Intraductal echogenic foci • Echogenic duct wall • Side-branch ectasia	• Ductal dilation • Ductal irregularity • Stones or calcification • Ductal fibrosis • Periductal fibrosis
Parenchymal changes	
• Inhomogeneous echo pattern • Reduced echogenic foci (1–3 mm) • Enhanced echogenic foci • Prominent interlobular septae • Lobular outer gland margin • Large, echo-poor cavities (>5 mm)	• Edema • Edema • Calcifications • Fibrosis • Fibrosis and glandular atrophy • Pseudocyst

Cambridge classification of chronic pancreatitis by endoscopic retrograde cholangiopancreatography.		
Grade	***Main pancreatic duct***	***Side branches***
Normal	Normal	Normal
Suggestive	Normal	<3 abnormal
Mild	Normal	3 abnormal
Moderate	Abnormal	>3 abnormal
Severe	Abnormal plus at least one of the following: • Large cavity • Duct obstruction • Dilation or duct irregularity • Intraductal filling defects	

Pancreatic function tests.

Tubeless tests:
- Fecal tests:
  - Fat stain
  - 72-hour fat content
  - Chymotrypsin, trypsin, and elastase content

Indirect tests:
- Bentiromide test
- Pancreolauryl test
- Breath tests

Tube tests:
- Lundh test meal
- Secretin or cholecystokinin test

Treatment

The treatment of chronic pancreatitis requires an interdisciplinary approach. The most common symptom in a patient with chronic pancreatitis is abdominal pain. The etiology of the pain is multifactorial and, in general, is not well understood.

- *Procedures available to the endoscopist for the treatment of pain include:*
  - Pancreatic sphincterotomy
  - Pancreatic ductal stenting
  - Extracorporeal shock wave lithotripsy (ESWL) of pancreatic stones
  - Endoscopic drainage of pancreatic pseudocysts
  - Endoscopic celiac nerve block
- *Management of other problems:*
  - In addition to pain, patients may present with exocrine or endocrine dysfunction which are managed medically.
  - Diabetes usually requires insulin and dietary restrictions.
  - Malabsorption is treated with pancreatic enzyme replacement in sufficient amounts to provide at least 30,000 units of lipase with each meal.
  - Antacid secretory medications also may be useful in patients with acid hypersecretion to avoid denaturation of the replacement enzymes.
  - Rarely, fat intake must also be limited to decrease the bothersome diarrhea that accompanies excessive steatorrhea.
  - Other reasons that a patient may present to a physician for care include various intra-abdominal complications of pancreatitis (e.g., bile duct, colonic or duodenal obstruction, and pseudocyst), and the concern for pancreatic cancer.

Indications for Surgery in Chronic Pancreatitis

- Intractable pain
- Pancreatic ductal stenosis
- Biliary obstruction (Wadsworth syndrome)
- Duodenal obstruction
- Left-sided portal hypertension from splenic vein thrombosis
- Colonic obstruction
- Pseudocyst
- Pancreatic ascites
- Pancreatic fistula
- Pancreatic carcinoma

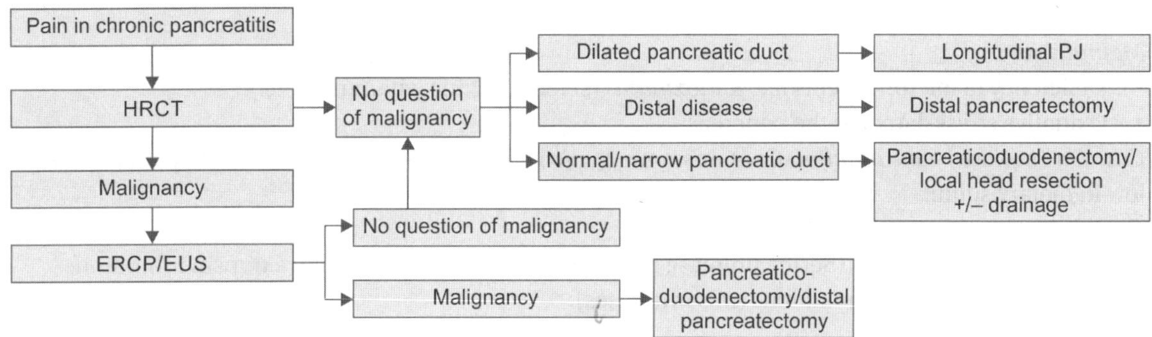

(ERCP: endoscopic retrograde cholangiopancreatography; EUS: endosonography; HRCT: high-resolution computed tomography)

- The type of operation depends on the anatomy of the pancreatic ductal system, and whether or not the pancreas is diffusely involved with the disease or it involves one part of the gland more than the others.
- Operations to relieve pain in these patients are designed to either:
  - Drain a dilated pancreatic ductal system Or
  - Resect diseased pancreatic tissue if the duct is not enlarged
- The main pancreatic duct normally measures 4–5 mm in the head, 3–4 mm in the body, and 2–3 mm in the tail of the pancreas.
- The duct is considered dilated when it is at least 7 mm in diameter in the body of the gland.
- Thus, patients with a dilated pancreatic duct (>7 mm in the body of the gland) are candidates for a drainage operation that decompresses the duct [longitudinal pancreaticojejunostomy (PJ) and Puestow procedure].
- Those with a duct that is of normal caliber will probably require resection of a part of the pancreas, usually the head of the gland (pancreaticoduodenectomy), Frey or Beger procedure.

Choice of surgical procedures for treatment of pain in chronic pancreatitis.

- Duct drainage procedure
- Lateral pancreaticojejunostomy (Partington–Rochelle modification of Puestow procedure)
- Combined duct drainage-resection procedures
- Pancreaticoduodenectomy (Kausch–Whipple)
- Longitudinal pancreaticojejunostomy with local head resection (Frey)
- Duodenum—preserving resection of the head of the pancreas (Beger)
- Pure resection procedure
- Total pancreatectomy with islet autotransplantation
- Neuroablative procedure
- Thoracic splanchnicectomy

Tropical chronic pancreatitis (TCP) is a distinct form of chronic pancreatitis seen predominantly in tropical developing countries. It has unique clinical, radiological, and etiological features compared to other types of chronic pancreatitis.

Definition

Tropical chronic pancreatitis is a *non-alcoholic*, progressive form of chronic pancreatitis that occurs *mainly in tropical regions*, particularly *South and Southeast Asia*, and *sub-Saharan Africa*. It typically presents in *childhood or early adolescence* with *abdominal pain, malnutrition*, and *diabetes mellitus*.

Epidemiology

- Common in countries like *India (especially Kerala, Tamil Nadu), Bangladesh, Indonesia,* and *Nigeria*
- *Onset:* Typically *before age 30*
- Slight male predominance
- Strong association with *malnutrition, low socioeconomic status,* and *dietary factors*

Etiology and Risk Factors

Exact cause is unknown, but multiple factors contribute:

- *Malnutrition:*
  - Deficiency of micronutrients like *antioxidants* (selenium, zinc, vitamin C, etc.)
  - Oxidative stress damages the pancreas.
- *Cassava (tapioca) consumption:* Contains *cyanogenic glycosides* → cyanide → toxic to pancreas, especially if low in dietary sulfur.
- *Genetic factors:*
  - *SPINK1 gene mutations* (Serine protease inhibitor Kazal-type 1) → defective trypsin inhibition.
  - Also PRSS1 and CFTR mutations (in some cases).
- *Other hypotheses:*
  - Autoimmunity
  - Recurrent childhood infections
  - Environmental toxins

Pathophysiology

- Repeated pancreatic injury → chronic inflammation → *fibrosis, ductal strictures*, and *calcification.*
- Leads to *exocrine and endocrine insufficiency.*

Clinical Features

Feature	***Description***
Abdominal pain	Recurrent, epigastric, radiating to the back
Diabetes mellitus	Often insulin-dependent but *without ketosis* (known as *fibrocalculous pancreatic diabetes* or FCPD)
Steatorrhea	Due to exocrine insufficiency (late finding)
Malnutrition	Common at presentation
Pancreatic calcifications	Early and prominent

Imaging Findings

X-ray Abdomen (KUB)

- Large, dense *pancreatic ductal calcifications* (seen in ~90%).

Ultrasound/CT Scan

- Dilated pancreatic duct with *intraductal calculi*
- Shrunken, fibrotic pancreas

MRCP/ERCP

- Irregular, dilated main pancreatic duct
- Side branch ectasia
- Intraductal stones

Laboratory Findings

Test	*Findings*
Blood glucose	Elevated (diabetes)
Fecal elastase	↓ in exocrine insufficiency
Pancreatic enzymes (amylase/lipase)	Often normal or low in chronic disease
Nutritional markers	Low in malnutrition

Diagnostic Criteria of TCP (Simplified)

- Young age of onset (usually <30 years)
- No history of alcohol use
- Evidence of pancreatic ductal stones/calcifications
- Exocrine and/or endocrine pancreatic insufficiency
- Tropical origin or residence

Complications

- Fibrocalculous pancreatic diabetes (FCPD)—a unique form of diabetes without ketosis
- Pancreatic pseudocyst
- Biliary obstruction
- Pancreatic carcinoma—increased risk (esp. after long-standing disease)

Management

- Medical treatment
    - *Pain control:* Analgesics, nerve blocks (celiac plexus)
    - *Pancreatic enzyme supplementation*
    - *Insulin therapy* (for diabetes)
    - *Nutritional support:*
        - High-protein, high-calorie diet
        - Vitamin and mineral supplements (esp. antioxidants)
- Surgical/endoscopic
    - Endoscopic stone extraction or ductal stenting
    - Lateral pancreaticojejunostomy (Puestow procedure)—for ductal decompression
    - Total pancreatectomy with islet cell autotransplantation (rare)

24. Compare the role of endoscopic versus open surgical treatment for chronic pancreatitis. Discuss the current recommendations for pain management of chronic pancreatitis. ***WBUHS 2018***

Endoscopic versus open surgical treatment for chronic pancreatitis:

- *Uncombined endoscopic pancreatic stone removal:* Good candidates for uncombined endoscopic pancreatic stone removal are as follows:
    - Those with three or fewer stones
    - Those with stones at the pancreatic head or body
    - Those free of pancreatic duct stricture closer to the duodenum than the pancreatic stones
    - Those with pancreatic stones 5 mm or smaller without impaction
- *Endoscopic pancreatic stone removal combined with extracorporeal shock wave lithotripsy:* If extracorporeal shock wave lithotripsy is performed before endoscopy treatment—
    - Multiple stones
    - Large stones (5 mm or bigger)
    - Stones located within the stricture site
    - Impacted stones can also be removed endoscopically

The success rate of endoscopic pancreatic stone removal without extracorporeal shock wave lithotripsy is reportedly <10%.

Endoscopic pancreatic stone removal combined with extracorporeal shock wave lithotripsy is recommended for patients with relapsing chronic pancreatitis with pancreatic stones. However, depending on the size and number of stones, even uncombined endoscopic pancreatic stone removal or uncombined extracorporeal shock wave lithotripsy also allows for a safe treatment.

Treatment of Pancreatic Stricture with Plastic Stent

Problems: The treatment goal for intense pancreatic duct stricture associated with chronic pancreatitis is to dilate the stenotic site sufficiently so that the impaired pancreatic juice outflow can be alleviated. However, advancing the guidewire beyond the stenotic area is sometimes difficult because of conditions such as tortuous or curved pancreatic duct, and pancreatic stone impaction, thus requiring this procedure to be combined with extracorporeal shock wave lithotripsy in many patients. Furthermore, pancreatic duct stricture and pancreatic cancer should be distinguished from each other.

Plastic Stent Types/Insertion Methods

Plastic stents with varying diameters (5, 7, 8.5, and 10 French) and sizes have been supplied by manufacturers. The PS is either straight or S-shaped. A stent appropriate for a given case is selected according to the intensity/location of the pancreatic duct stricture, pancreatic duct form, and the approach used (major or minor papillary approach). Recently, a type of plastic stent for the pancreatic duct made of a stent combined with a pusher as a single unit has been marketed and utilized in the prevention of stent migration. The plastic stent is kept inserted either as a single stent or as multiple stents.

Duration of Plastic Stent Placement

The mean plastic stent patency period is 2–12 months. Once the plastic stent becomes obstructed, acute pancreatitis (suppurative pancreatic ductitis in some cases) can develop as a complication; hence, during long- term insertion, the plastic stent needs to be renewed appropriately. If the stricture is alleviated, plastic stent withdrawal is possible, but complete alleviation of stricture is observed in 10% of all the cases or fewer.

Timing for Plastic Stent Removal

In a study on plastic stent withdrawal upon confirmation of alleviated stricture through pancreatography, the median total plastic stent insertion period for the withdrawn cases was 23 months and the percentage of cases that required plastic stent reinsertion for pain relapse within 1 year after withdrawal was 30%. In a study on periodical renewal of the plastic stent at intervals of 2 months and withdrawal of the plastic stent at 6 months after first insertion, the pain relapse rate at one year after plastic stent withdrawal was 48%.

Treatment of Pancreatic Duct Stricture with Multiple Plastic Stents

Plastic stent-related complications occurred in 6–39% of all cases, with mild pancreatitis being the major complication. Stent migration and pancreatic abscesses were also reported.

Treatment of Pancreatic Duct Stricture by Using a Metallic Stent

Recently, the use of metallic stents has expanded to include cases of pancreatic duct stricture, such as benign bile duct stricture.

Treatment using Endoscopic Ultrasound

- *Endoscopic ultrasound-guided drainage of the main pancreatic duct:* In cases for which transpapillary pancreatic duct stenting is not possible for reasons such as intense stricture, postoperative state, divisum, and large stones, puncture drainage of the pancreatic duct with a dilated caudal segment via the digestive tract is performed under endoscopic ultrasonography guidance.
    - Transpapillary Rendezvous approach
    - Transluminal approach

Results

- The symptom disappearance rate with this approach is 69%
- Perforation, bleeding, pancreatitis, fever, and pain were observed as complications. Migration and stent obstruction occurred at a high incidence (20–55%).

25. Endoscopic versus surgical drainage of the pancreatic duct in patients with chronic pancreatitis.

Current Status

- Because surgery has been reported to involve a high incidence of complications (18–53%) and high mortality rate (0–5%) and because patients tend to select noninvasive treatment, surgical pancreatic duct drainage for treatment of relapsing obstructive chronic pancreatitis is often selected for patients who fail to respond to endoscopic treatment.
- It is indicated for symptomatic cases where pancreatic duct stricture is intense or the presence of large pancreatic stones makes endoscopic treatment difficult. The operative procedure usually used for this purpose is side-to-side pancreatojejunostomy.

Surgical Procedures to Treat Pain in Chronic Pancreatitis

- Puestow procedure or longitudinal side-to-side pancreaticojejunostomy
- Duodenum-preserving pancreatic head resection (DPPHR)
- Frey procedure
- *Beger's procedure:*
    - A Cochrane review of endoscopic or surgical intervention for painful chronic pancreatitis pooled the data of both randomized trials. The pooled data showed that there was a higher proportion of patients with pain relief in the surgical group compared to the endoscopic group.
    - One study revealed that in the long-term, symptomatic patients with advanced chronic pancreatitis who underwent surgery as the initial treatment for pancreatic duct obstruction had more relief from pain, with fewer procedures, than patients who were treated endoscopically. Importantly, almost half of the patients who were treated with endoscopy eventually underwent surgery.
    - In patients with chronic intractable pain secondary to CP, evidence now supports proceeding to surgery earlier over endoscopy due to superiority in success rate, pain relief, and quality of life. Surgery may need to be considered at an earlier phase than it is now, preferably within 3 years of symptomatic CP.
    - Surgical therapy over endoscopic therapy for chronic pancreatitis and pancreatic duct obstruction.
    - In recent years, new treatment modalities for pancreatic stones have been developed. Extracorporeal shock wave lithotripsy, endoscopic therapy, and longitudinal pancreaticojejunostomy (LPJ) are effective for stone removal from large pancreatic ducts, especially the main pancreatic duct (MPD), and for rapid, long-term pain relief.

Pain Management in Chronic Pancreatitis

- For pain relief, current guidelines recommend a simple stepwise escalation of analgesic drugs with increasing potency until pain relief is obtained.
- Abstinence from alcohol and smoking should be strongly advised. Pancreatic enzyme therapy and antioxidants may be helpful as initial treatment.
- Endoscopic treatment can be used in patients with evidence of ductal obstruction and may be combined with extracorporeal shock wave lithotripsy. The best candidates are those with distal obstruction of the main pancreatic duct and in early stage of disease.
- Behavioral interventions should be part of the multidisciplinary approach to chronic pain management particularly when psychological impact is experienced.
- Surgery should be considered early and after a maximum of five endoscopic interventions. The type of surgery depends on morphological changes of the pancreas. Long-term effects are variable, but high success rates have been reported in open studies and when compared with endoscopic treatment.
- Finally, neurolytical interventions and neuromodulation can be considered in difficult patients.

PANCREATIC FISTULA

26. Causes, classification and management of postoperative pancreatic fistula (POPF). ***WBUHS 2016***

27. Describe the management of pancreatic fistula. ***RIMS, Imphal, 2012***

Introduction

A pancreatic fistula is an abnormal communication between the pancreas and other organs due to leakage of pancreatic secretions from damaged pancreatic ducts. An external pancreatic fistula is one that communicates with the skin, and is also known as a pancreaticocutaneous fistula, whereas an internal pancreatic fistula communicates with other internal organs or spaces. Pancreatic fistulas can be caused by pancreatic disease, trauma, or surgery.

External Pancreatic Fistulas

- An external pancreatic fistula is an abnormal communication between the pancreas (actually pancreatic duct) and the exterior of the body via the abdominal wall.
- Loss of bicarbonate-rich pancreatic fluid via a pancreatic fistula can result in a hyperchloremic or normal anion gap metabolic acidosis. Loss of a small volume of fluid will not cause a problem but acidosis is common if the volume of pancreatic fluid lost from the body is large.

Internal Pancreatic Fistulas

Internal pancreatic fistulas can result in pancreatic ascites, mediastinal pseudocysts, enzymatic mediastinitis, or pancreatic pleural effusions, depending on the flow of pancreatic secretions from a disrupted pancreatic duct or leakage from a pseudocyst.

Four final definitions summarizing the current pancreatic fistula concept according to the literature:

1. Output >10 mL/day of amylase-rich fluid postoperative (postoperation) day 5 or for >5 days
2. Output >10 mL/day of amylase-rich fluid after postoperative day 8 or for >8 days
3. Output between 25 and 100 mL/day of amylase-rich fluid after postoperative day 8 or for >8 days
4. Output >50 mL/day of amylase-rich fluid after postoperative day 11 or for >11 days

ISGPF Definition

"Output *via* an operatively placed drain (or a subsequently placed percutaneous drain) of any measurable volume of drain fluid on or after postoperative day 3, with an amylase content greater than three times the upper normal serum value".

Postoperative pancreatic fistula commonly occurs following either pancreaticoduodenectomy or distal pancreatectomy (DP).

Risk Factors for POPF

Risk factors can be classified as the following:

- Patient factors
- Disease-related factors

Patient Factors

- Though male sex is seen to be associated with increased risk for POPF, no specific reason has been found for this phenomenon. Similarly, age >70 years is associated with increased risk for POPF.
- Other risk factors for POPF that have been evaluated in various studies include duration of jaundice, creatinine clearance, and intraoperative blood loss; but none of these are found to have a definitive relation with POPF.

Disease-related Factors

- Pancreatic texture, pancreatic pathology, high pancreatic juice output, pancreatic duct size, and biochemical parameters are factors seen to contribute toward POPF.
- *Pancreatic texture:* The texture of pancreas is usually related to the underlying disease process. It is widely accepted that a fibrotic pancreatic remnant in chronic pancreatitis holds the pancreatic anastomosis well, while a soft friable pancreas found in pancreatic or periampullary cancer usually betrays.

- *High-pancreatic juice output:* In the setting of a nondilated duct in a soft textured pancreas, a high-pancreatic juice output has been considered as an important factor contributing to POPF.
- *Size of the pancreatic duct:* A small-sized pancreatic duct has been suggested as a risk factor for POPF.
- *Biochemical parameters:* Various biochemical parameters such as serum bilirubin, serum albumin, BUN, serum amylase and N-benzoyl-L-tyrosyl-p-aminobenzoic acid (BT-PABA) excretion test values have been evaluated as risk factors for POPF. A normal preoperative BT-PABA test value has been suggested as a risk factor for POPF.

Grading system to assess the severity of POPF:

Grade	***A***	***B***	***C***
Clinical conditions	Well	Often well	Ill appearing/bad
Specific treatment	No	Yes/No	Yes
Ultrasonography/computed tomography	Negative	Negative/Positive	Positive
Persistent drainage	No	Usually yes	Yes
Reoperation	No	No	Yes
Death related to POPF	No	No	Possibly yes
Signs of infections	No	Yes	Yes
Sepsis	No	No	Yes
Readmission	No	Yes/No	Yes/No

Grade A	"Transient fistula"	No clinical impact	No peripancreatic collections on CT scan; little/no change in management	Clinically well, no sepsis, no prolongation of hospital stay, and slow removal of operatively placed drains
Grade B		Clinical impact	Peripancreatic drains in place or repositioned to drain collections; change in management	Clinically fairly well, degree of infection requiring specific treatment, prolongation of hospital stay, and patients often discharged with drains in situ and observed in an outpatient setting
Grade C		Severe clinical impact	Worrisome peripancreatic collections that require percutaneous drains; major change in management usually in ICU setting; possible resurgery to salvage a difficult situation (completion pancreatectomy, etc.)	Clinically unwell; associated sepsis requiring aggressive antibiotics, octreotide, and other intensive care support; major prolongation of hospital stay; associated complications and possibility of mortality

Classification scheme for grading complications arising after PD applicable to all complications arising from PD and not just POPF:

Grade	***Definition***
I	Any deviation from the normal postoperative course without pharmacologic treatment or surgical, endoscopic, and radiological interventions. Allowed therapeutic regimens are drugs, such as antiemetics, antipyretics, analgesics, diuretics, electrolytes, and physiotherapy. This grade also includes wound infections opened at the bed side
II	Requiring pharmacologic treatment with drugs other than ones allowed for grade 1 complications. Blood transfusion and total parenteral nutrition are also included
III	Requiring surgical, endoscopic, or radiologic intervention
IIIa	Intervention not under general anesthesia
IIIb	Intervention under general anesthesia
IV	Life-threatening complication requiring intermediate care/intensive care unit management
IVa IVb	Single-organ dysfunction Multiorgan dysfunction
V	Death of a patient

Pathogenesis

- Internal pancreatic fistulas are most commonly caused by disruption of the pancreatic duct due to chronic pancreatitis.
- The chronic pancreatitis is usually alcoholic in origin in adults, and traumatic in origin in children. They may also be caused by leakage from a pancreatic pseudocyst.
- Anterior disruption of a pseudocyst or a pancreatic duct leads to leakage of pancreatic secretions into the free peritoneal cavity, leading to pancreatic ascites.
- If the duct is disrupted posteriorly, the secretions leak through the retroperitoneum into the mediastinum via the aortic or esophageal hiatus. Once in the mediastinum, the secretions can either be contained in a mediastinal pseudocyst, lead to enzymatic mediastinitis or, more commonly, leak through the pleura to enter the chest and form a chronic pancreatic pleural effusion.

Clinical Characteristics

Marked recent weight loss is a major clinical manifestation, and unresponsiveness of the ascites to diuretics is an additional diagnostic clue.

Diagnosis

Pleural or ascitic fluid should be sent for analysis. An elevated amylase level, usually >1,000 IU/L, with protein levels over 3.0 g/dL is diagnostic. Serum amylase is often elevated as well, due to enzyme diffusion across the peritoneal or pleural surface. Contrast-enhanced computed tomography and ERCP may also assist in diagnosis, with the latter an essential component of treatment.

Appropriate management of the pancreatic remnant has been one of the core issues regarding prevention of POPF. Some of the recommended methods for the management of pancreatic remnant include:

- Pancreatic duct ligation.
- Pancreatic duct obliteration.
- Pancreaticojejunostomy
- Pancreaticogastrostomy (PG)

Prevention of POPF

The measures recommended to prevent POPF following PD can be considered under the following categories:

- Pharmacological measures
- Preoperative irradiation
- Modifications in operative techniques

Pharmacological Measures

A high pancreatic juice output in a soft pancreas is an important risk factor for POPF; hence, it appears rational to hypothesize that inhibition of exocrine pancreatic secretion in the postoperative period may reduce the incidence of POPF. Somatostatin and its octapeptide analog have been used by various groups to reduce the pancreatic juice secretion and thereby prevent POPF.

Preoperative Irradiation

Preoperative irradiation of the pancreas reduces the exocrine function, as the pancreatic acinar cells are very sensitive. This forms the basis for the concept of preoperative irradiation to reduce the incidence of POPF.

Technical Modifications to Prevent POPF

- Pancreatic duct stent or drainage
- Fistulation method

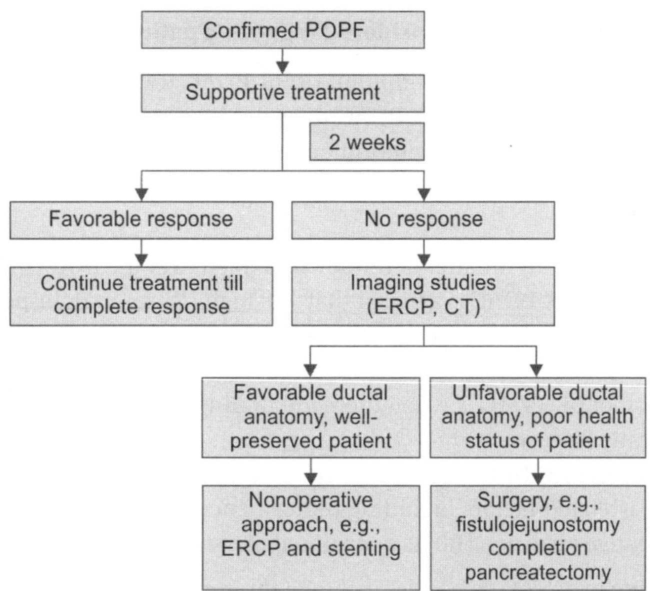

(CT: computed tomography; ERCP: endoscopic retrograde cholangiopancreatography; POPF: postoperative pancreatic fistulae)

Treatment

- Control of sepsis
- Maintenance of fluid and electrolyte balance and nutrition
- Skin protection
- Somatostatin analogues
- Percutaneous treatment
- ERCP
- Fistulojejunostomy
- Surgical options
  - Completion pancreatectomy
  - Drainage of the anastomosis
  - Reconstruction of anastomosis

The production of pancreatic enzymes is suppressed by restricting the patient's oral intake of food patient in conjunction with the use of long-acting somatostatin analogues. The patient's nutrition is maintained by total parenteral nutrition. This treatment is continued for 2–3 weeks, and the patient is observed for improvement. If no improvement is seen, the patient may be receiving endoscopic or surgical treatment. If surgical treatment is followed, an ERCP is needed to identify the site of the leak.

BORDERLINE RESECTABLE PANCREATIC CARCINOMA

28. (a) Which objective criteria should be used preoperatively to identify patients with borderline resectable pancreatic cancer?

(b) Is there enough evidence for operative exploration and resection in the presence of mesenteric-portal axis or arterial involvement?

(c) How should the pathologic specimen be examined and which definition of tumor-free resection margins should be used?

(d) Which prognostic markers should be considered regarding patient selection? ***WBUHS 2015***

(a) The consensus view was that a broader definition of BR-PDAC was required than those in current use. This is because the anatomical definition of BR-PDAC does not take into account the biology of the tumor or the physiology of the host, both of which are determinants of resectability.

The approach that is presented is derived from the "ABC" method, which was developed at the MD Anderson Cancer Centre.

The following statement captures this broader definition as agreed to at the IAP symposium:

- The anatomical definition of BR-PDAC is a tumor that is at high risk for margin-positive resection (R1, R2) when surgery is used as an initial treatment strategy. Neoadjuvant chemotherapy and/or radiotherapy is considered to increase the chance of a R0 resection and should be considered in patients with BR-PDAC.
- The biological definition of BR-PDAC is when there are findings that raise the possibility (but not certainty) of extrapancreatic metastatic disease.
- The conditional definition of BR-PDAC is when the patient has a high risk for morbidity or mortality after surgery because of host-related factors including performance status and comorbidities. These criteria apply even when margin-negative resection (R0) is considered likely following a surgery-first strategy.

The MD Anderson borderline resectable categories included three patient subsets as defined by the following clinical and radiographic characteristics:

1. *Type A:* Patients with borderline resectable tumor anatomy as defined on CT images to include one or more of the following findings: Tumor abutment (180° of the circumference of the vessel) of the SMA or CA; tumor abutment or encasement (180° of the circumference of the vessel) of a short segment of the hepatic artery, typically at the origin of the gastroduodenal artery; or short-segment occlusion of the SMV, PV, or SMV–PV confluence that was amenable to vascular resection and reconstruction because of a patent SMV and PV below and above the area of tumor-related occlusion.
2. *Type B:* Patients with borderline resectable disease owing to a concern for possible extrapancreatic metastatic disease. This subgroup of borderline resectable patients included those with CT findings suspicious for, but not diagnostic of, metastatic disease and those with known N1 disease from either prereferral laparotomy or endoscopic ultrasonography-guided fine-needle aspiration. Type B patients may have had a technically resectable, or a borderline resectable primary tumor as defined on CT images.
3. *Type C:* Patients with borderline resectable disease owing to a marginal performance status, or those with a better performance status and severe preexisting medical comorbidity thought to require protracted evaluation that precluded immediate operation. By definition, type C patients with a marginal performance status were thought to have reversible causes of their current symptoms (such as hyperbilirubinemia- induced anorexia and fatigue). Type C patients may have a radiologically resectable or a borderline resectable primary tumor.

International consensus of classification of BR-PDAC based on anatomical definition using CT imaging including coronal and sagittal sections.

Resectable: R:

- *SMV/PV:* No tumor contacts or unilateral narrowing
- *SMA, CA, CHA:* No tumor contact

Borderline resectable: BR subclassified according to SMV/PV involvement alone or arterial invasion.

- *BR-PV (SMV/PV involvement alone):*
  - *SMV/PV:* Tumor contact 180° or greater or bilateral narrowing/occlusion, not exceeding the inferior border of the duodenum
  - *SMA, CA, common hepatic artery (CHA):* No tumor contact/invasion
- *BR-A (arterial involvement):*
  - *SMA, CA:* Tumor contact of <180° without showing deformity/stenosis.
  - *CHA:* Tumor contact without showing tumor contact of the PHA and/or CA.

(The involvement of the aorta is categorized as unresectable. Presence of variant arterial anatomy is not taken into consideration)

Unresectable: UR subclassified according to the status of distant metastasis

- *Locally advanced:* LA:
  - *SMV/PV:* Bilateral narrowing/occlusion, exceeding the inferior border of the duodenum.
  - *SMA, CA:* Tumor contact/invasion of 180° or more[#]
  - *CHA:* Tumor contact/invasion showing tumor contact/invasion of the PHA and/or CA.
  - *AO:* Tumor contact or invasion
- *Metastatic (M):* Distant metastasis[$]

(CA: celiac artery; CHA: common hepatic artery; PV: portal vein; PHA: proper hepatic artery; SMA: superior mesenteric artery; SMV: superior mesenteric vein)

[#]In the cases with CA invasion of 180° or more without the involvement of the aorta and with intact and uninvolved gastroduodenal artery thereby permitting a distal pancreatectomy with en bloc celiac axis resection (DP-CAR), some members prefer this criteria to be in the BR-A category,[$] including macroscopic para-aortic and extra-abdominal lymph node metastasis.

Comparison of radiographic differences in common definitions for borderline resectable pancreatic cancer.

Effected vessel	*AHPBA/SSAT/SSO/NCCN*	*MD Anderson*	*Alliance*
SMV/PV	Abutment, impingement, encasement of the SMV PV or short-segment venous	Occlusion	Tumor-vessel interface ≥180° of vessel wall circumference, and/or reconstructable
	Occlusion		Occlusion
SMA	Abutment	Abutment	Tumor-vessel interface <180° of vessel wall circumference
HA	Abutment or short segment encasement	Abutment or short segment encasement	Reconstructable short segment interface of any degree between tumor and vessel wall
CA	Uninvolved	Abutment	Tumor-vessel interface <180° of vessel wall circumference

(AHPBA/SSAT/SSO/NCCN: Americas Hepato-Pancreato-Biliary Association/Society for Surgery of the Alimentary Tract/Society of Surgical Oncology National Comprehensive Cancer Network; CA: celiac artery; HA: hepatic artery; SMA: superior mesenteric artery; SMV PV: superior mesenteric vein portal vein)

Borderline Resectable Disease

- No extrapancreatic disease
- The following possible tumor-vessel relationships: an SMV-PV confluence that can be reconstructed even is short segment venous occlusion is present (i.e., a suitable portal vein above, and a suitable SMV below the area of occlusion); tumor abutment of the SMA of <180°; or short-segment encasement of the hepatic artery amenable to resection and reconstruction (this is usually at the origin of the gastroduodenal artery and reconstruction may or may not require interposition grafting with a short segment of reversed saphenous vein).

Definition of Respectability

Borderline resectable	NCCN version 2.2012
SMA, celiac	<180° abutment
Hepatic artery (HA)	• Gastroduodenal artery encasement up to the hepatic artery Or • Direct abutment of hepatic artery without extension to celiac axis
SMV/PV	• Impingement and narrowing of the lumen • Encasement or short-segment venous occlusion

(b) Locally advanced pancreatic cancer is described as Tumor invaded locally adjacent structures such as major blood vessels, lymph nodes, bowel, and the bile duct, without evidence of distant metastatic disease. Involvement of para-aortic LN is considered as metastasis and surgically contraindicated.
Locally advanced pancreatic cancer may or may not be resectable and would include T3 and T4, whereas T1 and T2 are considered resectable tumors.

Borderline Resectable Pancreatic Cancer

It is defined by two groups:

1. MD Anderson Cancer Center (MDACC)
2. Americas Hepato-Pancreato-Biliary Association (AHPBA)/Society of Surgical Oncology (SSO)/Society for Surgery of the Alimentary Tract (SSAT).

- MDACC group describes any venous involvement as resectable disease and only occlusion of the SMV or PV (with the possibility of reconstruction) as borderline.

Comparison of definition of borderline resectable pancreatic cancer.

	AHBPA/SSAT/SSO	*MD Anderson*	*NCCN 2012*
SMV-PV	Abutment, encasement, or occlusion	Occlusion	Abutment with impingement
SMA	Abutment	Abutment	Abutment
CHA	Abutment or short-segment encasement	Abut merit or short-segment encasement	Abutment or short-segment encasement
Celiac trunk	No abutment or encasement	Abutment	No abutment or encasement

(SMV-PV: superior mesenteric vein-portal vẹin; SMA; superior mesenteric artery. CHA: common hepatic artery)

National Comprehensive Cancer Network (NCCN) guidelines for pancreatic cancer treatment:

- *Pancreatic cancers classified into:*
  - Resectable
  - Borderline resectable
  - Unresectable

Resectable

- *Arterial:* Clear fat planes around the CA, SMA, and HA
- *Venous:* The SMV or PV abutment but no distortion of the vessels.

Borderline Resectable

Arterial

Pancreatic head/uncinate process:

- Solid tumor contact with CHA without extension to CA or hepatic artery bifurcation
- Solid tumor contact with the SMA of ≤180°
- Presence of variant arterial anatomy (for example, accessory right hepatic artery, replaced right hepatic artery, replaced CHA) and the presence and degree of tumor contact should be noted if present as it may affect surgical planning

Pancreatic body/tail:

- Solid tumor contact with the CA of ≤180°.
- Solid tumor contact with the CA of >180° without involvement of the aorta and with intact and uninvolved gastroduodenal artery.

Venous

Venous involvement of the SMV or PV with distortion or narrowing of the vein or occlusion of the vein with suitable vessel proximal and distal, allowing for safe resection and replacement.

Unresectable

- *Arterial:*
  - *Arterial (head of pancreas):* Greater than 180° encasement of the circumference of the SMA or any CA abutment.
  - *Arterial (body/tail of pancreas):* SMA or CA encasement >180°
  - *Arterial (any part of the pancreas):* Aortic invasion or encasement
- *Venous:* Unreconstructable SMV and/or PV
- *Nodal status:* Metastases to lymph nodes beyond the field of resection should be considered unresectable.

Grading system proposed by Lu et al. for predicting vascular invasion by tumor based on the degree of tumor contiguity with a vessel:

Grade	*Description*	*Comment*
Grade 0	No contiguity of tumor with a vessel	Vascular invasion in 0% of cases
Grade 1	Tumor is encasing <25% of the circumference of a vessel	0%
Grade 2	25–50% of the circumference of a vessel	57%
Grade 3	50–75% of the circumference of a vessel	88%
Grade 4	>75% of the circumference of a vessel or any vessel constriction	All cases

Grading system proposed, by Loyer et al. for predicting vascular invasion by tumor.

Grade	*Description*	*Comment*
Type A	Fat plane separates the tumor and the normal pancreatic parenchyma from adjacent vessels	Overall resection rate: 100%
Type B	Normal parenchyma separates the tumor from adjacent vessels	Overall resection rate: 100%
Type C	Tumor is inseparable from adjacent vessels, and the points of contact form a convexity against the vessels	Overall resection rate: 89%
Type D	The points of contact form a concavity against the vessels or partially encircle the vessels	Overall resection rate: 47%
Type E	Tumor encircles adjacent vessels, and no fat plane is identified between the tumor and the vessels	Overall resection rate: 0%
Type F	Tumor occludes the vessels	Overall resection rate: 0%

The increased resectability and improvement in long-term survival for patients with pancreatic cancer, extensive surgical procedures have been developed, mainly involving *vascular reconstruction techniques.*

- Birkmeyer et al. first reported aggressive surgery for borderline resectable pancreatic cancer with the first SMV resection and reconstruction in 1951.
- In 1973, Fortner first described the regional pancreatectomy. This involved a total pancreatectomy, radical lymph node clearance, combined PV resection (type 1), and/or combined arterial resection and reconstruction (type 2).

Venous Resection

- Venous involvement is not considered a contraindication to surgical resection.
- Pancreatic resection requiring venous reconstruction is technically challenging and may be associated with a higher morbidity.
- *Lygidakis et al. compared en bloc splenopancreatic and venous resection versus palliative gastrobiliary bypass and reported 2-year survival rates of 81.8 and 0%, respectively.*
- *Randomized controlled trial by Doi et al. in 2008 was closed early when interim analysis showed a clear survival benefit for PDVR with chemoradiotherapy (CRT) compared with CRT with or without a surgical bypass*

Arterial Resection

- In 2007, Hirano et al. reported their long-term follow-up for patients undergoing distal pancreatectomy with en bloc CA resection (DP-CAR)
- They reported 1-year and 5-year survival rates of 71 and 42%, respectively, and concluded that DP-CAR offers a high resectability rate and may potentially achieve complete local control in selected patients.
- Bachellier et al., in 2011, matched a group of patients undergoing *pancreatectomy with arterial resection to conventional pancreatectomy and* demonstrated similar 3-year survival rates.
- Bockhorn et al. reported one of the largest series on *pancreatectomy with simultaneous arterial resection (n = 29) and* concluded that there was *no overall difference in disease-specific survival* for patients who underwent arterial reconstruction versus those patients who underwent pancreatectomy alone.

(c) *Pathologic assessment of the surgical specimen:*

- The modifications to the TNM staging system in the current edition of the AJCC Cancer Staging Manual allow the accurate staging of patients even if they do not undergo pancreatic resection. The T4 (and Stage III) designation is reserved for locally advanced unresectable primary tumors in the absence of distant metastases.
- In addition to TNM staging, when the pancreaticoduodenectomy specimen is evaluated pathologically, the retroperitoneal margin (the soft tissue margin directly adjacent to the proximal 3–4 cm of the SMA) must be evaluated on permanent sections by inking the margin and sectioning the tumor perpendicular to the margin.
- It is critical that the surgeon identify this margin at the time of resection because it cannot be assessed retrospectively and many pathologists cannot accurately identify the retroperitoneal margin on a pancreaticoduodenectomy specimen.
- The surgeon and pathologist should classify the retroperitoneal margin after integrating the operative findings and the histologic assessment of this margin. All pancreatic resections should be classified according to residual disease status (termed "R" factor): R0, no gross or microscopic residual disease; R1, microscopic residual disease (microscopically positive surgical margins with no gross residual disease); and R2, grossly evident residual disease.
- The pathologist cannot usually differentiate an R1 (microscopically positive) from an R2 (grossly positive) retroperitoneal margin in the absence of information regarding the retroperitoneal dissection, which should be included in the operative note. The R designation should appear in the final pathology report if possible and should always be listed in the dictated operative note.
- The difficulty in differentiating R1 from R2 resections has significant implications for the conduct of clinical trials examining the potential advantage of nonsurgical therapies, especially in patients with borderline resectable tumors.

Standardized pathologic evaluation of the surgical specimen was performed as previously described. The SMA margin was defined as the soft tissue margin directly adjacent to the proximal 3–4 cm of the SMA. In all patients, the SMA margin was evaluated according to the AJCC Cancer Staging Manual guidelines:

- This margin was identified and inked by the surgeon and pathologist immediately on specimen removal and was evaluated by permanent-section microscopic examination; when tumor extended to the inked margin, the margin was considered positive.
- The technique for assessment of the SMA margin was the same regardless of whether vascular resection was performed.
- The pancreatic transection margin and the common bile/hepatic duct transection margins were evaluated by examining a complete en-face section of each margin. At the discretion of the surgeon, these two margins were usually evaluated intraoperatively using frozen-section analysis, and if positive, additional bile duct or pancreatic parenchyma was usually resected.

- An operation was designated R0 if all final margins were negative (no tumor cells were identified at any of the three resection margins) and R1 if any of the final margins were microscopically positive (tumor cells were present at one or more of the margins).

Tumor size was calculated by the pathologist by measuring the maximum gross transverse diameter of the tumor after resection. This measurement was difficult to determine in some patients after preoperative therapy because the tumor was often hard to distinguish from uninvolved adjacent pancreatic parenchyma by gross examination. The grade of neoadjuvant treatment effect was assessed on permanent sections by a faculty gastrointestinal pathologist and scored using a previously published grading system.

- A minimal pathologic response was defined as a treatment effect score of either grade I (90% or more viable tumor cells remaining after induction therapy) or IIa (50–89% remaining viable tumor cells). A partial pathologic response was defined as a treatment effect score of IIb (10–49% remaining viable tumor cells) or III (<10% remaining viable tumor cells).
- A treatment effect score of IV, indicating no remaining viable tumor cells, was used to designate a complete pathologic response.

(d) The importance of pretreatment staging to define the extent of disease as a necessary component of the conduct of clinical trials and outcome reporting evaluation of the potential value of nonsurgical therapies (chemotherapy and radiation therapy) in improving local disease control and survival of patients with pancreatic cancer requires accurate pretreatment staging (to define the study population) and a standardized system for the pathologic evaluation of surgical specimens (to determine the completeness of resection).

Prognostic Markers

- Age
- Sex
- Tumor size
- Performance status
- Regional lymph node
- Distant metastasis
- CA19-9
- Back pain

Prognostic and predictive markers in pancreatic adenocarcinoma—Science Direct.

Author	*Year chemotherapy*	*Prognostic markers*	*Number of patients*
Ueno et al.	2000 fluorouracil based, gemcitabine, cisplatin, docetaxel, epirubicin, and irinotecan	CEP, CA 19-9. ECOG PS, and albumin	103
Glen et al.	2006 N/A	CEP and albumin	187
Marechal et al.	2007 gemcitabine-based	KPS score, weight loss (10%), and AST	99
Yi et al.	2011 gemcitabine-based	CRP, albumin, liver metastasis, and ascites dissemination	298
Hamada et al.	2014 gemcitabine-based	Age, sex, ECOG PS, tumor size, lymph node metastasis, and distant metastasis	531
Xue et al.	2015 gemcitabine-based, 5-1	ECOG PS, Ca 19-9, and CEP	118

(AST: aspartate aminotransferase; CEP: C-reactive protein; CA 19-9: carbohydrate antigen 19-9; ECOC-PS: Eastern Cooperative Oncology Group Performance Status; KPS: Karnofsky Performance Status)

29. Significance of circulating tumour cells in carcinoma pancreas. ***KGMU, Lucknow 2025.***

30. Methods for increasing resectability for pancreatic cancer. ***WBUHS 2017***

Neoadjuvant therapy to be a reasonable alternative to upfront surgery followed by adjuvant therapy in patients who appear to have potentially resectable tumors, especially if there is any radiographic interface between the tumor and the mesenteric vasculature, as long as performance status and comorbidity are sufficient to tolerate treatment. Before recommending this approach over upfront surgery, we await additional data to clarify which patients might benefit the most from preoperative therapy as opposed to those for whom it is best to undertake upfront resection followed by adjuvant therapy.

Rationale and Benefit Over Initial Resection

- Improved selection of patients for whom resection will not offer a survival benefit (i.e., those who rapidly progress to metastatic disease during preoperative therapy)
- Higher rates of margin-negative resection, which is the major goal of surgery
- Early treatment of micrometastases, which are presumed to be present even without evidence of distant metastases on initial imaging, and responsible for poor long-term outcomes from initial surgical treatment of apparently localized disease.
- Greater chance of receiving effective perioperative chemotherapy, given that prolonged recovery from upfront resection prevents the delivery of postoperative adjuvant chemotherapy in approximately one-fourth of patients.

Important pretreatment considerations for individuals who will be treated initially with chemotherapy include the following:

- A tissue diagnosis should be established before initiation of therapy. This differs from a surgery-first strategy, in which preoperative tissue diagnosis may not be needed.
- For patients who present with obstructive jaundice, delivery of neoadjuvant therapy necessitates durable biliary decompression for as many as six months. This can usually be accomplished through placement of a biliary stent. This subject, which includes a discussion of different types of stents, is provided elsewhere.

Choice of Neoadjuvant Strategy

If it is chosen, the best regimen for neoadjuvant therapy is not currently defined; there are few comparator trials. For most patients who are able to tolerate it, we suggest therapy with the multiagent modified FOLFIRINOX [oxaliplatin plus irinotecan with leucovorin and short-term infusional fluorouracil (FU) regimen], followed by CRT in the absence of distant metastases, rather than a gemcitabine-based regimen.

- A neoadjuvant approach to borderline resectable PDA identifies patients who are most likely to benefit from pancreatic resection. Preoperative capecitabine-based chemoradiation is an effective, well-tolerated treatment for these patients. Neoadjuvant therapy for borderline resectable PDA warrants further investigation using treatment schedules that can safely intensify irradiation dose.
- The management of borderline resectable pancreatic adenocarcinomas (BRPCs) has seen the emergence of adjuvant regimes in the 'neoadjuvant' or 'induction therapy' role with FOLFIRINOX and nab-paclitaxel with gemcitabine. There is no robust data to suggest the survival benefit of these protocols so far; however, there has been demonstrable tolerability and increased resection rates.
- Another concept is the use of targeted agents (erlotinib or sorafenib) or immunotherapy (algenpantucel-L) in combination with gemcitabine. However, to date, none of these agents have shown any favorable survival outcome *vs* the use of gemcitabine (GEM) alone.

Chemotherapy plus Chemoradiotherapy

Although early reports of preoperative radiation therapy (RT) with or without concurrent FU demonstrated that this approach did not worsen perioperative morbidity and mortality, there was no obvious improvement in either resectability or OS. A possible limitation of these initial studies is that most used single-agent bolus FU. Subsequent studies have focused on improving the treatment regimen by optimizing chemotherapy. Two specific approaches are FOLFIRINOX plus FU-based CRT, and gemcitabine-based CRT.

FOLFIRINOX Plus Chemoradiotherapy

There are no dedicated trials examining the benefit of neoadjuvant FOLFIRINOX plus CRT that are limited to individuals with potentially resectable tumors. The following data are available to inform this issue:

In the setting of borderline resectable pancreatic cancer, neoadjuvant therapy using FOLFIRINOX in conjunction with CRT results in a high rate of R0 resection and prolonged median progression-free survival and OS compared with historical controls.

Optimal Regimen

SWOG S1505 directly compared perioperative (12 weeks preoperative and 12 weeks postoperative) treatment with FOLFIRINOX versus GEM plus nab-paclitaxel (GEM/nab) in 102 patients with potentially resectable pancreatic cancer. Resectability rates were high with both regimens (73% vs. 70%), although more patients receiving GEM/nab had a complete or major pathologic response (42% vs. 25%). A 2-year OS, the primary endpoint, was 47% with FOLFIRINOX, and 48% with GEM/nab, and neither arm met the prespecified endpoint (58% of 2-year survival). Interpretation of these results is limited by the high rate of ineligibility after central radiologic review (44 of the 147 enrolled patients). Additional information is expected from the Dutch PREOPANC-2 trial comparing neoadjuvant FOLFIRINOX to gemcitabine-based CRT for borderline and potentially resectable pancreatic cancer; accrual was completed in January 2021, and the data are maturing.

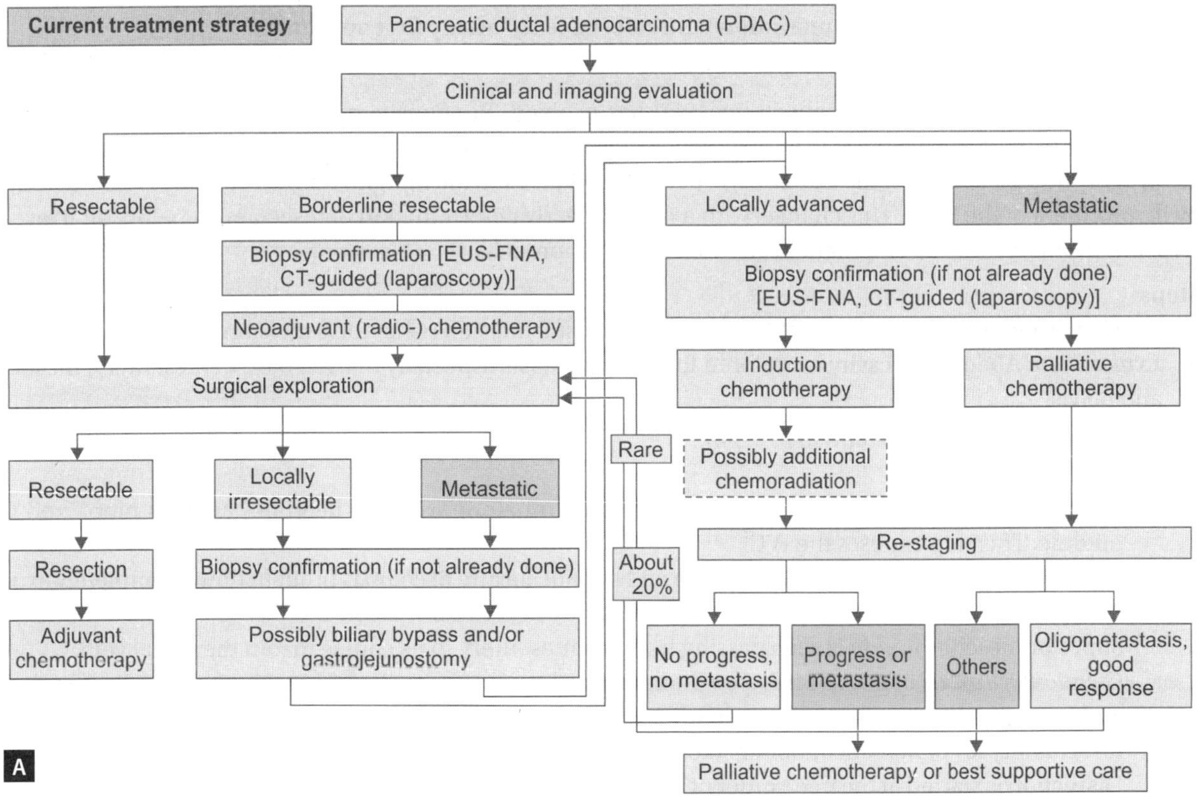

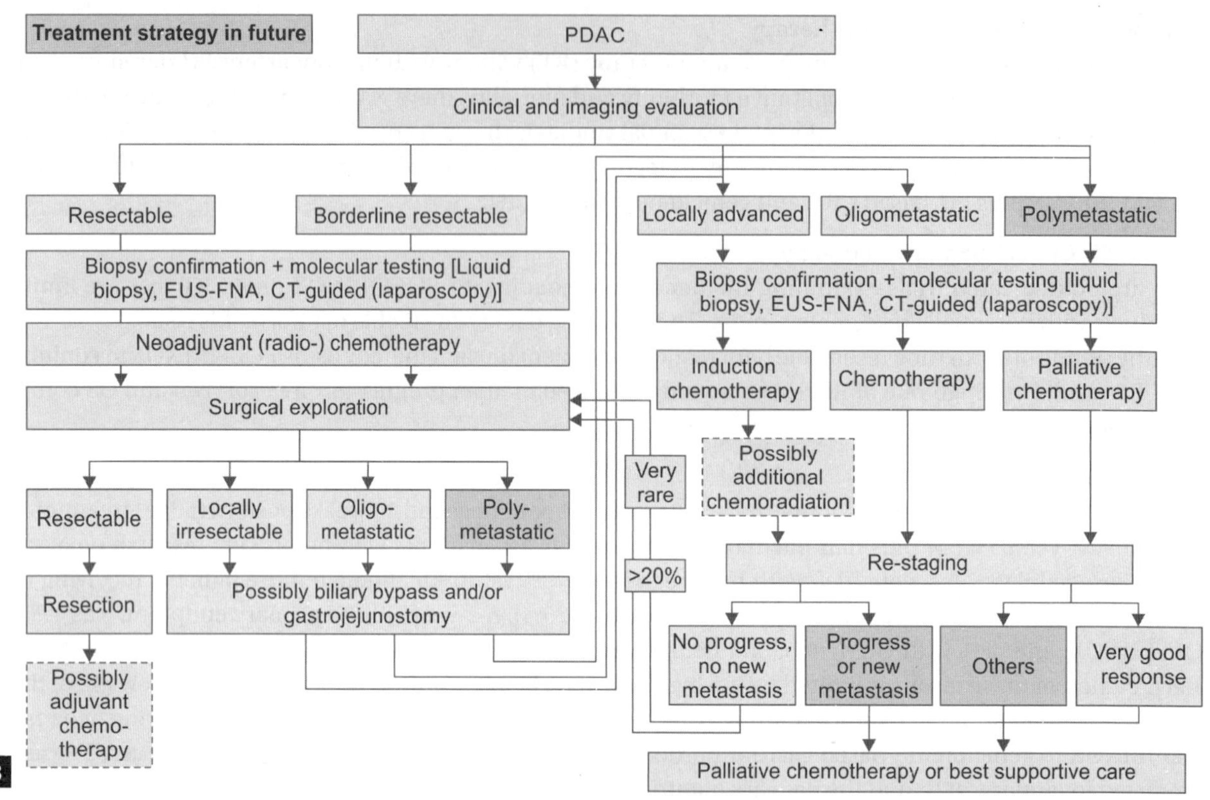

31. Enumerate the steps of Whipple operation with reference to "artery first approach."

WBUHS 2017; RIMS, Imphal 2022

The technique of pancreatoduodenectomy (PD) has evolved. Previously, nonresectability was determined by involvement of the portal vein–SMV because venous resection can be achieved safely and with greater awareness of the prognostic significance of the status of the posteromedial resection margin, nonresectability is now determined by involvement of the SMA. This change, with a need for early determination of resectability before an irreversible step, has promoted the development of an "artery-first" approach.

Steps

- *Incision:* Abdomen is opened from the bilateral subcostal incision (Chevron's incision).
- *Exploration:* Abdominal cavity is explored for the metastasis especially in liver, base of mesentery, mesocolon, and pelvis.

Now the actual Whipple procedure steps begin:

- Dissection
  - Kocher's maneuver is performed and the duodenum along with the head of pancreas mobilized to the midline. This step exposes the IVC.
  - Cattell–Braasch maneuver is the next step and hepatic flexure of colon is brought down completely exposing the retroperitoneum and separating hepatic flexure of colon from the liver.
  - Superior mesenteric vein is seen passing from the mesentery to its course to join the portal vein.
  - *Creation of Tunnel of love:* At this step attempt may be made to try and create the tunnel between the SMV and pancreas but if it is problematic it may be attempted at the later stage. It is at this crucial time the resectability for pancreaticoduodenectomy is decided.
  - Dissection is started at the free border of the lesser sac and common bile duct, right hepatic artery and portal vein are identified. At this step special care is taken to identify and safeguard accessory or replaced right hepatic artery. This artery is easily found posterolateral to the portal vein.

- Gall bladder is dissected from the liver bed and followed onto the cystic duct, the common bile duct is divided at the junction with the cystic duct. The right hepatic artery is traced back and just above the duodenum gastroduodenal artery is tied off.
- The hepatoduodenal ligament is dissected easily as it is avascular and next after clearing the lesser curve of stomach and greater curve, stomach is usually transected.
- The portal vein is now seen clearly and the tunnel between it and pancreas is fashioned.
- The pancreas is now cut and separated from the portal vein.
- Pancreaticojejunostomy can be done duct to mucosa
- *Hepaticojejunostomy is next:* Done in single layer and can be performed in an interrupted or continuous fashion.
- Gastrojejunostomy is the final step of reconstruction.
- Drains may or may not be placed depending on surgeon's experience and abdomen is closed.

Summary of indications, advantages, and disadvantages of various artery-first approaches.

Approach	*Indication(S)*	*Advantages*	*Disadvantages*
Posterior	• Posteromedial tumor in head/neck, especially involving PV-SMV • Periampullary tumor extending from body to head	• Early identification of SMA involvement • Identification of replaced RHA • Enables adequate retropancreatic lymphadenectomy • Early identification of SMV involvement and facilitates en bloc resection	Difficult in patients with peripancreatic inflammation and adhesions around head of pancreas
Medial uncinate	Malignant tumors of uncinate process	• Early identification of SMA involvement at uncinate • Early ligation of IPDA minimizes bleeding • Useful approach in peripancreatic inflammation with difficulty tunneling above PV • Useful approach for total pancreatectomy as mobilization can be achieved without transecting gland	Late identification of replaced RHA
Inferior infracolic (mesenteric)	• Locally advanced tumors with questionable infiltration of SMA at its origin from aorta • Malignant tumors of uncinate and ventral pancreas	• Early identification of replaced RHA • Allows better exposure and dissection of region posterior to SMA • Early ligation of IPDA minimizes bleeding	• Difficult in morbidly obese patients • Difficult exposure in patients with high origin of SMA
Left posterior	Tumors along uncinate and ventral pancreas	• Facilitates skeletonization of SMA in retroperitoneum without kocherization of duodenum • Early ligation of IPDA	Extensive dissection of SMA requiring antidiarrheals
Inferior supracolic (anterior)	Tumors along inferior border of pancreas	• Facilitates better retroperitoneal dissection, especially with locally advanced tumors with neoadjuvant treatment • "No-touch" technique with en bloc kocherization theoretically prevents tumor cell dissemination	Early division of stomach and neck of pancreas
Superior	Malignant tumors of superior border of pancreas	Early identification of CHA, coliac, and SMA involvement	Difficult exposure in patients with low origin of SMA

(CHA: common hepatic artery; IPDA: inferior pancreatoduodenal artery; PV: portal vein; RHA: right hepatic artery; SMV: superior mesenteric vein; SMA: superior mesenteric artery)

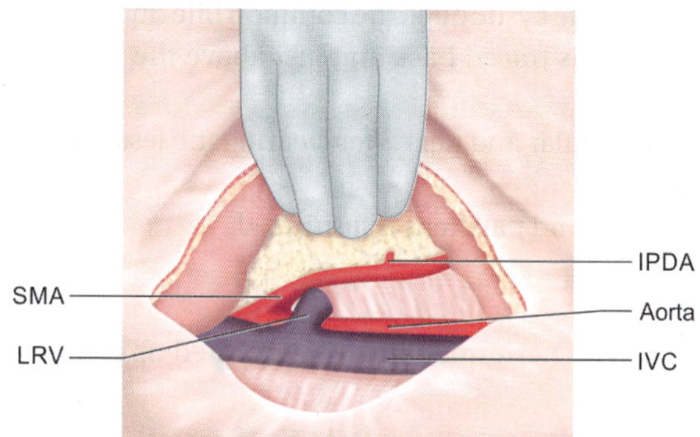

Posterior approach, exposing the origin of superior mesenteric artery (SMA) in front of the left renal vein after kocherization. For clarity the SMA has been made more apparent. (IPDA: inferior pancreatoduodenal artery; LRV: left renal vein; IVC: inferior vena cava)

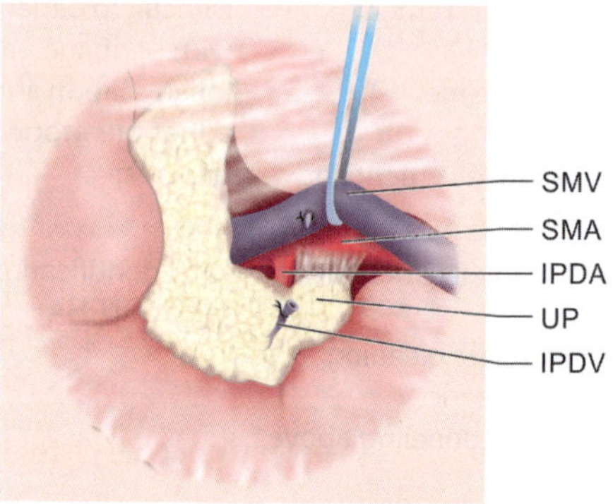

Medial uncinate approach, demonstrating the uncinate process (UP), inferior pancreatoduodenal artery (IPDA) and vein (IPDV), superior mesenteric artery (SMA) and vein (SMV) after kocherization and mobilization of the duodenojejunal flexure.

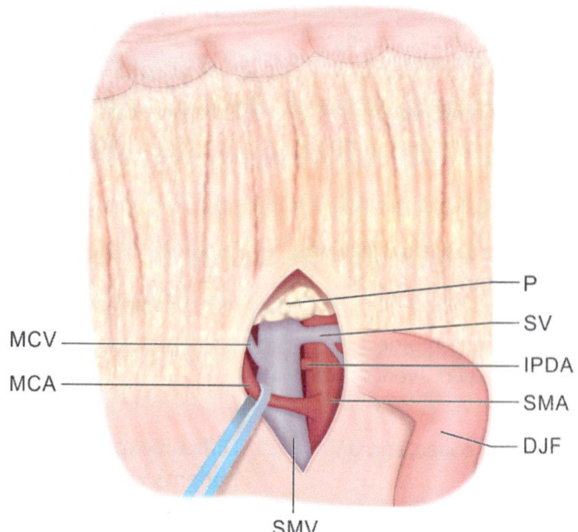

Inferior infracolic approach (mesenteric approach) exposing the superior mesenteric artery (SMA) and vein (SMV) and branches after dividing the peritoneum to the right of the duodenojejunal flexure (DJF) in the transverse mesocolon. (P: pancreas; SV: splenic vein; MCV: middle colic vein; IPDA: inferior pancreatoduodenal artery; MCA: middle colic artery)

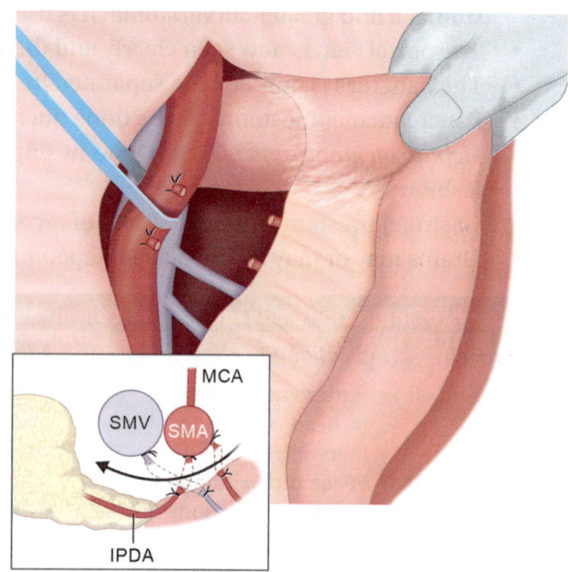

Left posterior approach, exposing the first and second jejunal arteries at their origin on the superior mesenteric artery (SMA) in the transverse mesocolon. Further traction on the proximal jejunum produces a counterclockwise rotation to the SMA that allows identification and division of the inferior pancreatoduodenal artery (IPDA) arising from the posterior surface of the SMA (inset). (MCA: middle colic artery; SMV: superior mesenteric vein)

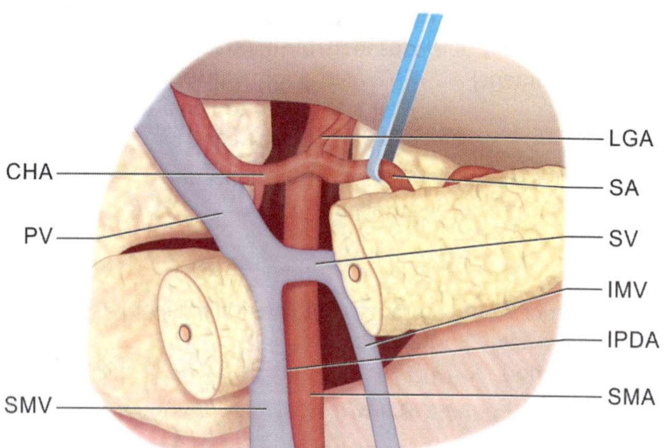

Inferior supracolic approach (anterior approach), demonstrating the superior mesenteric artery (SMA) and vein (SMV), splenic vein (SV) and celiac axis and its branches after division of the neck of the pancreas. (LGA: left gastric artery; CHA: common hepatic artery; SA: splenic artery; PV: portal vein; IMV: inferior mesenteric vein; IPDA: inferior pancreatoduodenal artery)

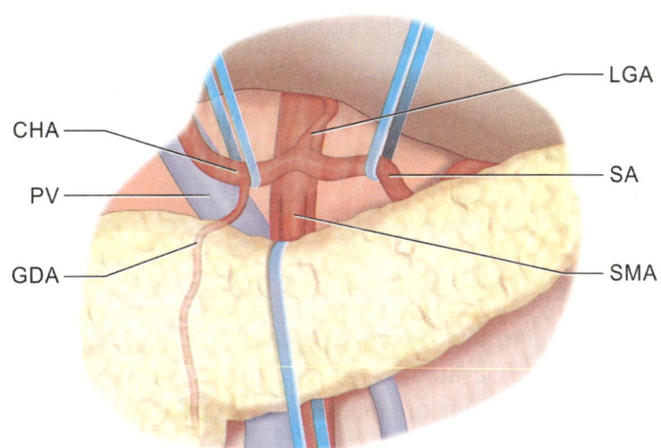

Superior approach demonstrating the celiac axis and its branches and the superior mesenteric artery (SMA) in the lesser sac above the neck of the pancreas. (LGA: left gastric artery; CHA: common hepatic artery; SA: splenic artery; PV: portal vein; GDA: gastroduodenal artery)

32. What is the clinical presentation of carcinoma head of pancreas? Discuss the preoperative evaluation and optimization of this patient. Describe briefly the surgical steps planned for this condition with appropriate illustration. ***KGMU, Lucknow 2025***

33. Describe in detail the principles, steps and complications of Whipple's procedure (pancreatoduodenectomy) in carcinoma head of pancreas. ***KIIT University, Odisha 2025***

34. Pylorus preserving pancreaticoduodenectomy. ***Rajasthan University of Health Sciences 2025***

Clinical Presentation

Carcinoma of the *head of the pancreas* typically presents with symptoms due to *biliary obstruction, duodenal involvement*, or *mass effect*. Since the head is near the *common bile duct, duodenum*, and *ampulla of Vater*, early signs often arise.

Common Clinical Features

Symptom	*Description*
Painless progressive jaundice	Most common presentation; due to bile duct compression
Dark urine and pale stools	Due to conjugated hyperbilirubinemia
Generalized pruritus	Bile salt deposition in skin
Weight loss	Due to anorexia, malabsorption, and cancer cachexia
Anorexia	Common systemic symptom
Dull upper abdominal pain or back pain	Less common early; may suggest local invasion
Palpable gallbladder (Courvoisier's sign)	Enlarged, non tender gallbladder due to obstruction
Diabetes mellitus (new-onset)	May precede diagnosis in some cases
Steatorrhea	From exocrine insufficiency or biliary obstruction
Occult GI bleeding or anemia	From duodenal invasion (rare)

Preoperative Evaluation and Optimization

The goal is to:

- Confirm diagnosis
- Assess *resectability*
- Evaluate *fitness for surgery*
- Rule out *metastasis*
- Relieve biliary obstruction if needed

A. Diagnostic Evaluation

- *Laboratory tests:*
  - *Liver function tests:* Elevated bilirubin (direct), ALP, GGT
  - *CA 19-9:* Tumor marker (may be elevated)
  - *CBC, RFT, coagulation profile:* Baseline preoperative workup
- *Imaging studies:*
  - *Ultrasound abdomen:* First step; shows biliary dilatation
  - *Contrast-enhanced CT scan (CECT): Gold standard* for assessing tumor size, vessel involvement, lymph nodes, liver metastasis
  - *MRI/MRCP:* For detailed biliary and pancreatic duct anatomy
  - *EUS (Endoscopic ultrasound) ± FNA:* If diagnosis uncertain
  - *PET-CT:* In select cases to detect occult metastases
- *Endoscopic retrograde cholangiopancreatography (ERCP):*
  - Used if biliary drainage is needed (e.g., stenting before surgery)

B. Assessing Resectability:

CT or MRI evaluates:

Factor	***Unresectable if...***
Vascular invasion	SMA, celiac trunk, or portal vein encasement
Distant metastases	Liver, peritoneum, lungs
Lymph nodes	Distant (celiac, para-aortic) involvement

Optimization for surgery:

Area	***Considerations***
Nutritional status	Often malnourished; correct hypoalbuminemia, vitamin deficiencies
Biliary drainage	Indicated if bilirubin >15–20 mg/dL, cholangitis, or delayed surgery; use ERCP with stenting
Glycemic control	Address if diabetic
Cardiopulmonary assessment	Especially in elderly or high-risk patients
Correction of coagulopathy	If present due to vitamin K deficiency
Infection screening	Urine, respiratory tract, etc.

Surgical Procedure—Whipple's Pancreaticoduodenectomy

This is the *standard surgical treatment* for resectable carcinoma head of pancreas.

Basic Concept

- Remove the *tumor* with surrounding involved structures.
- Restore *continuity* of GI and biliary tracts.

Surgical Steps (Classical Whipple's)

- *Exploration*
  - Check for liver/peritoneal metastasis.
  - Assess local invasion, lymph nodes.
- *Resection*
  - En bloc removal of:
    - *Pancreatic head*
    - *Duodenum*
    - *Distal bile duct*
    - *Gallbladder*
    - *Antrum of stomach* (in classical Whipple; pylorus is preserved in modified Whipple)
    - *Proximal jejunum*
    - Regional lymph nodes
- *Reconstruction (in 3 anastomoses):*

Step	Purpose
Pancreaticojejunostomy (PJ)	Attach remaining pancreas to jejunum
Hepaticojejunostomy (HJ)	Connect hepatic duct to jejunum
Gastrojejunostomy (GJ)	Reconnect stomach (or pylorus) to jejunum

Variants

- *Pylorus-preserving pancreaticoduodenectomy (PPPD):* Preserves gastric emptying
- *Vascular resection and reconstruction:* May be done if portal vein is partially involved

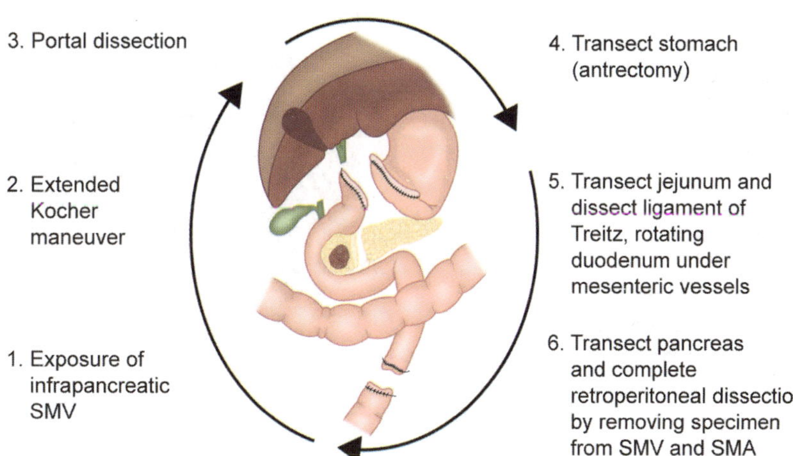

Fig. 1: The Whipple's operation is divided into six clearly defined steps to allow safe removal of the pancreatic head, distal stomach, duodenum, bile duct and gallbladder.

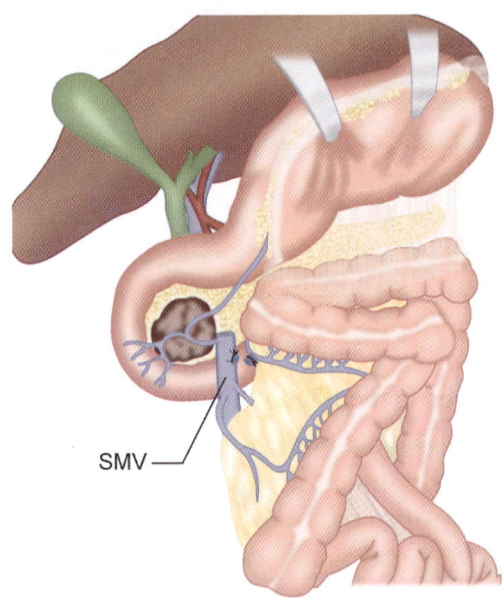

Fig. 2: Step 1. The lesser sac is entered, and the hepatic flexure of the colon is taken down. The inferior body of the pancreas is identified at the level of the proximal body of the gland. The superior mesenteric vein (SMV) is exposed at the inferior border of the neck of the pancreas adjacent to the uncinate process. When dealing with a reoperative situation (previous unsuccessful attempt at resection) or with tumor extending into the root of mesentery, we may not identify the SMV early in the operation and expose this vessel after pancreatic transection by following the anterior surface of the portal vein.

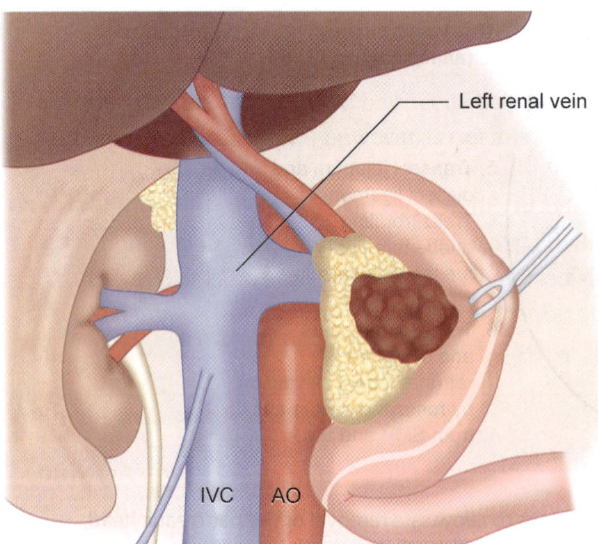

Fig. 3: Illustration of step 2. A Kocher maneuver has been performed by first identifying the inferior vena cava (IVC) at the level of the proximal portion of the transverse segment of the duodenum (D3). One can then mobilize the duodenum and pancreatic head off of the IVC in a cephalad direction thereby removing all soft tissue anterior to the IVC. Note that the Kocher maneuver is continued to the left lateral border of the aorta (AO).

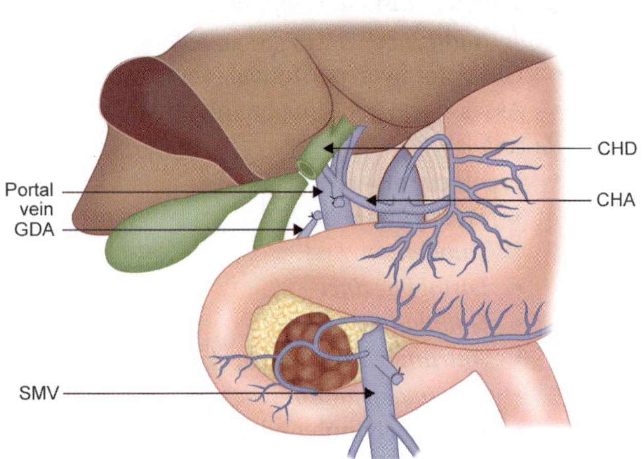

Fig. 4: Illustration of step 3. Dissection of the porta hepatis begins with identification of the common hepatic artery (CHA), by removal of the large lymph node which commonly sits anterior to this vessel. The CHA is then followed distally to allow identification and division of the right gastric artery (not shown) and the gastroduodenal artery (GDA). This allows the CHA-proper hepatic artery to be mobilized off of the underlying anterior surface of the portal vein (PV). The PV is always identified prior to division of the common hepatic duct (CHD).

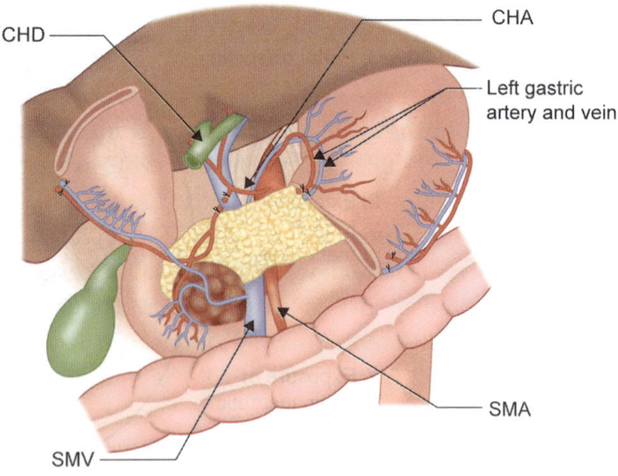

Fig. 5: Illustration of step 4. The antrum of the stomach is resected with the main specimen by dividing the stomach at the level of the third or fourth transverse vein on the lesser curvature. CHA, common hepatic artery; CHD, common hepatic duct; SMA, superior mesenteric artery; SMV, superior mesenteric vein. Sometimes the entire stomach is preserved; when this is done, the operation is called a pylorus preserving Whipple (or pancreaticoduodenectomy).

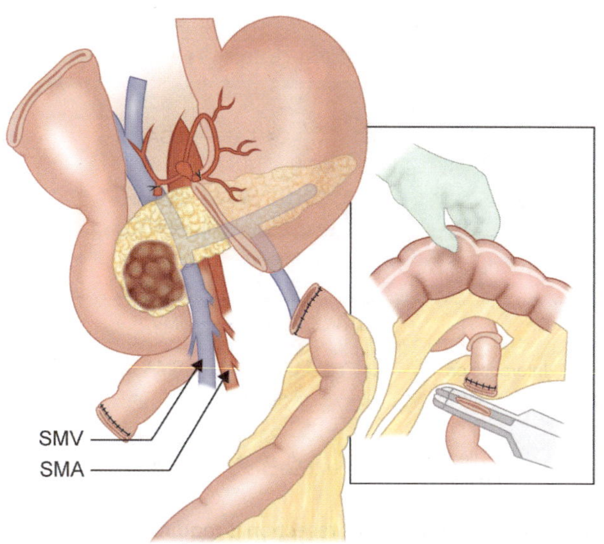

Fig. 6: Illustration of step 5. Transection of the jejunum is followed by ligation and division of its mesentery. The loose attachments of the ligament of Treitz are taken down, and the fourth and third portions of the duodenum are mobilized by dividing their short mesenteric vessels. The duodenum and jejunum are then reflected underneath the mesenteric vessels in preparation for the final and most important part of pancreaticoduodenectomy.

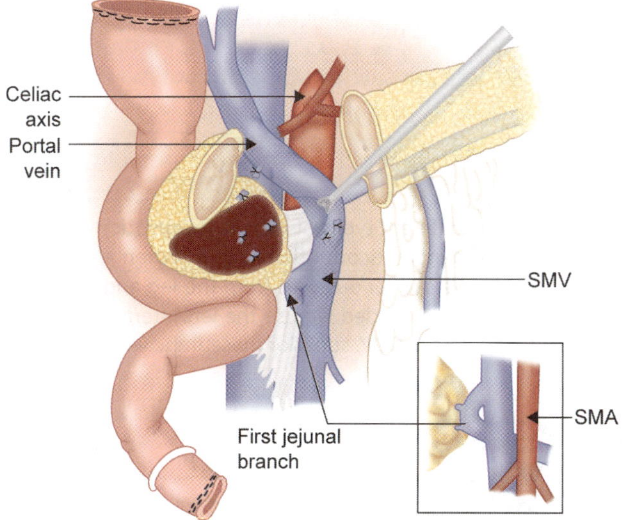

Fig. 7: Illustration of step 6. The pancreatic head and uncinate process are separated from the superior mesenteric-portal vein confluence. The pancreas has been transected at the level of the portal vein and the pancreatic head is reflected laterally, allowing identification of small venous tributaries from the portal vein and superior mesenteric vein (SMV). These tributaries are ligated and divided. CHA, common hepatic artery.

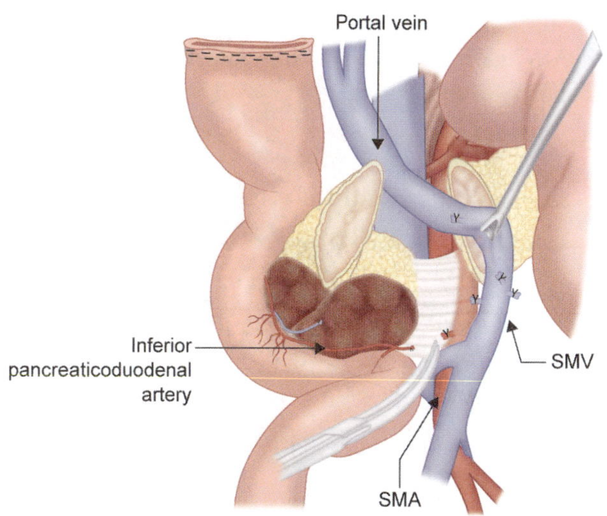

Fig. 8: Illustration of the continuation of step 6, and the final step in resection of the tumor. Medial retraction of the superior mesenteric-portal vein confluence facilitates dissection of the soft tissues adjacent to the lateral wall of the proximal superior mesenteric artery (SMA). This is the most important step in the operation from an oncologic perspective.

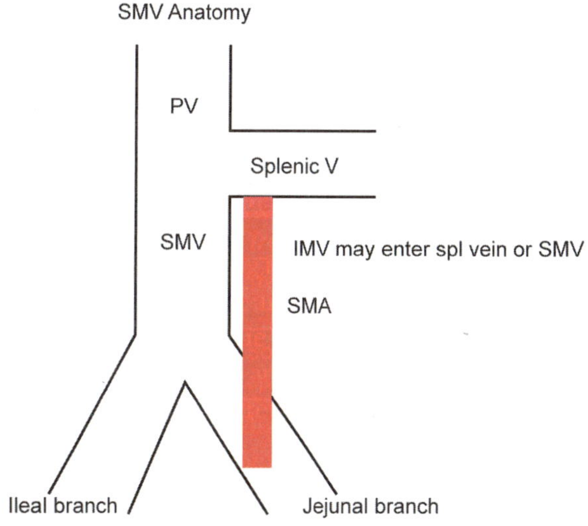

Fig. 9: Illustration of the important surgical anatomy of the superior mesenteric vein (SMV). The SMV usually bifurcates into two main branches, one to the ileum and one to the jejunum. Adequate venous return from the small bowel requires that one or the other of these two main SMV-tributaries is intact. The jejunal branch of the SMV (often referred to as the first jejunal branch) drains the proximal jejunum, travels posterior to the superior mesenteric artery (SMA), and enters the SMV along its posterolateral wall. Very rarely the jejunal branch will travel anterior to the SMA.

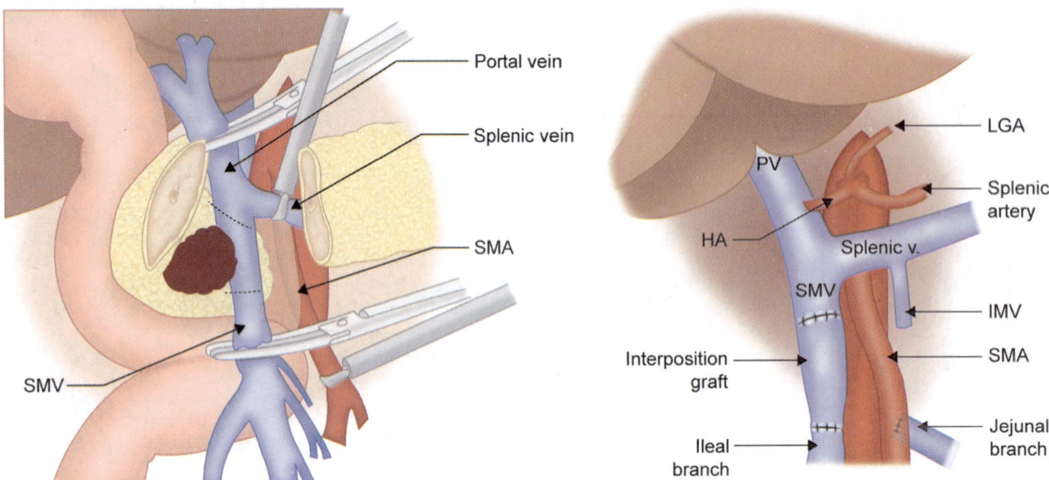

Figs. 10 and 11: Illustration of the final step in pancreaticoduodenectomy when segmental venous resection is required and the splenic vein is preserved. The intact splenic vein tethers the portal vein, making a primary anastomosis impossible in most cases. An interposition graft is used to repair the segment of vein which is removed; the left internal jugular vein from the neck is used for the graft in most cases.

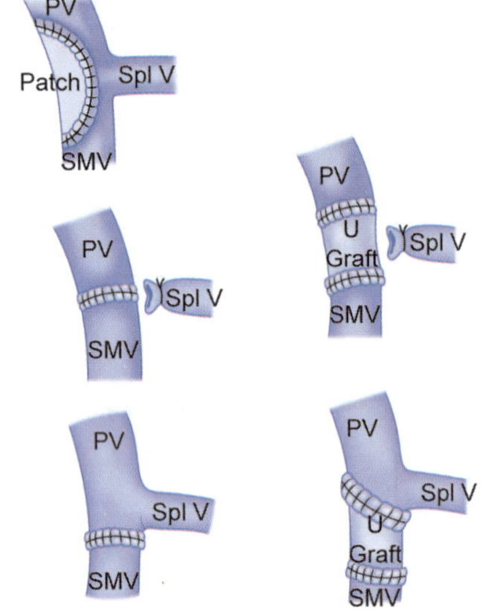

Fig. 12: Illustration of the different types of venous reconstruction used at the time of pancreaticoduodenectomy. When a patch is needed we use the saphenous vein from the leg and when an interposition graft is needed we use the left internal jugular (IJ) vein. PV, portal vein; SMV, superior mesenteric vein; Spl V, splenic vein.

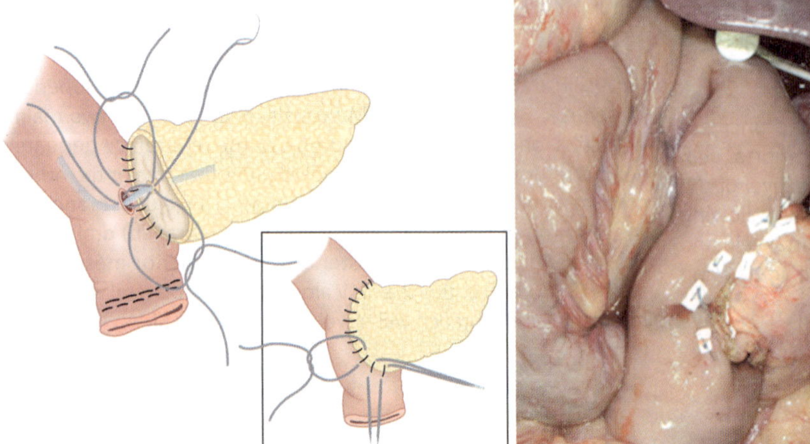

Figs. 13 and 14: Illustration of pancreaticojejunostomy. A two-layer, end-to-side, duct-to-mucosa retrocolic pancreaticojejunostomy is performed with (when the pancreatic duct is not dilated) or without a small stent. When used, the stent (4–5 cm long) is sewn to the pancreatic duct with a single absorbable monofilament suture.

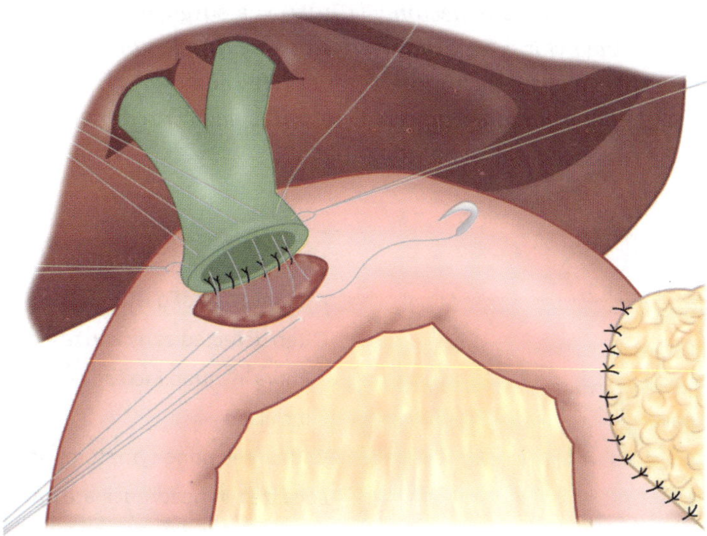

Fig. 15: Illustration of hepaticojejunostomy. A one-layer, end-to-side hepaticojejunostomy is performed with 4-0 or 5-0 absorbable monofilament sutures distal to the pancreaticojejunostomy. A stent is rarely placed in this anastomosis.

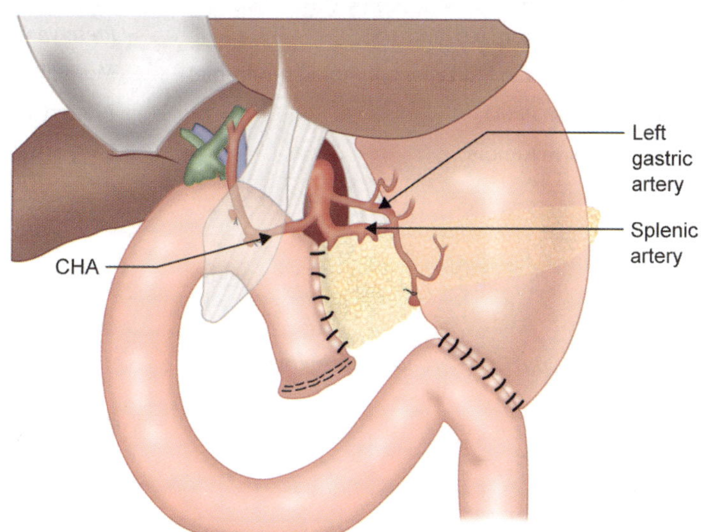

Fig. 16: Illustration of the completed reconstruction after pancreaticoduodenectomy. The falciform ligament, mobilized upon opening the abdomen, is placed over the hepatic artery to cover the stump of the gastroduodenal artery, thereby separating the hepatic artery from the afferent jejunal limb. CHA, common hepatic artery.

Closure and Postoperative Care

Following reconstruction, closed suction drains are placed near the pancreatic and biliary anastomoses to monitor postoperative drainage. The decision to place a feeding jejunostomy is based on the surgeon's preference. The abdominal closure is performed in layers.

A nasogastric tube is used overnight to decompress the stomach and is typically removed the following morning unless there is excessive output. The use of a nasogastric tube is not mandatory. On postoperative days 1 and 3, the abdominal drain contents are evaluated for amylase levels. Elevated amylase (more than 3 times the upper limit of normal serum values) may indicate a pancreatic leak, requiring management based on the leak's volume, drain content, and the patient's clinical status.

Drains are gradually removed once output is minimal, there is no evidence of a pancreatic fistula, and the patient can tolerate a regular diet.

The Pylorus-Preserving Pancreaticoduodenectomy (PPPD) is a surgical modification of the *classical Whipple procedure* designed to *preserve the pylorus and the first part of the duodenum,* while still removing the *pancreatic head* and surrounding structures involved by tumors or other pathologies.

It is commonly used to treat *periampullary tumors, pancreatic head carcinoma,* and some benign or low-grade malignant conditions.

Indications

Condition	*Notes*
Carcinoma head of pancreas	If no invasion of gastric antrum or pylorus
Ampullary carcinoma	Often detected early and resectable
Distal cholangiocarcinoma	Tumors in intrapancreatic bile duct
Duodenal carcinoma (2nd part)	If localized
Chronic pancreatitis	With unrelenting symptoms and mass effect
Neuroendocrine tumors	Localized to head/uncinate process

Key Differences: PPPD vs Classical Whipple

Feature	*Classical Whipple*	*PPPD*
Gastric resection	Removes distal stomach (antrum)	*Preserves pylorus* and antrum
Gastric emptying	Potentially better in PPPD (less dumping syndrome)	More physiologic
Anatomical continuity	More natural in PPPD	Altered in Whipple
Indications	More extensive tumors	Early stage/periampullary tumors

Structures Removed in PPPD

Resection includes:

- Head of pancreas
- Uncinate process
- Duodenum (2nd and 3rd part) *(1st part preserved with pylorus)*
- Common bile duct (CBD)
- Gallbladder
- Proximal jejunum
- Regional lymph nodes

Pylorus and proximal duodenum are preserved

Surgical Steps of PPPD

I. Exploration
   - Midline laparotomy or laparoscopic access
   - Rule out metastases (liver, peritoneum)

II. Mobilization
   - *Kocher maneuver* to mobilize duodenum and head of pancreas
   - Identify and preserve *pylorus* and *right gastric artery*

III. Dissection
   - Transect:
     - *CBD*
     - *Neck of pancreas*
     - *Proximal jejunum*
   - Ligate *gastroduodenal artery* and dissect *portal vein* area

IV. Removal of specimen
- *Remove en bloc:* Pancreatic head, uncinate process, duodenum (except 1st part), CBD, gallbladder

V. Reconstruction (Three anastomoses)

Anastomosis	*Purpose*
Pancreaticojejunostomy (PJ)	Reconnect pancreatic duct to jejunum
Hepaticojejunostomy (HJ)	Bile duct to jejunum
Duodenojejunostomy	Connect preserved pylorus to jejunum

In some variants, a *gastrojejunostomy* is done instead.

Postoperative Complications

Complication	*Notes*
Delayed gastric emptying (DGE)	Common (10–30%), even in PPPD
Pancreatic fistula	From PJ leak; major source of morbidity
Intra-abdominal abscess or sepsis	Related to leaks or infection
Hemorrhage	Early (intra-op) or late (erosion of vessels)
Nutritional deficiencies	Especially fat-soluble vitamins
Diabetes mellitus	If significant pancreatic tissue removed

- Types of distal pancreatectomy. Gujrat Health University 2024.

Distal Pancreatectomy—Overview

A *distal pancreatectomy* is a surgical procedure involving the *removal of the body and tail of the pancreas,* and often the *spleen* as well. It is performed primarily for lesions located in the *left (distal) part* of the pancreas.

Indications for Distal Pancreatectomy

Indication	*Examples*
Malignant tumors	• Pancreatic ductal adenocarcinoma (PDAC) • Pancreatic neuroendocrine tumors (PNETs) • Metastatic tumors (e.g., RCC)
Benign/mucinous neoplasms	• Mucinous cystic neoplasm (MCN) • Solid pseudopapillary neoplasm (SPN)
Cystic lesions	Serous cystadenoma (if symptomatic or large)
Chronic pancreatitis	With intractable pain or suspicion of malignancy
Trauma	Grade III or higher pancreatic injury involving body/tail

Types of Distal Pancreatectomy

Type	*Description*
With splenectomy	Most common; spleen removed along with pancreas
Spleen-preserving	Preserves immune function; used in benign conditions
Open vs. Laparoscopic/Robotic	Minimally invasive approaches are increasingly used for small or benign lesions

Surgical Steps (Distal Pancreatectomy with Splenectomy)

I. *Access and exposure*
- Midline or left subcostal incision (open) or laparoscopic ports
- Retract stomach to expose pancreas

II. *Mobilization*
- Divide *gastrocolic ligament* to enter lesser sac
- Mobilize pancreas from retroperitoneum
- Identify and preserve or ligate splenic artery and vein

III. *Dissection*
- Dissect the pancreas from *medial to lateral*
- Transect pancreas (usually with stapler)
- Control branches of *splenic vessels*

IV. *Splenectomy*

Remove spleen along with pancreatic tail and body

V. *Drain placement*

Closed suction drain may be placed near pancreatic stump

Spleen-Preserving Techniques

Used for *benign* or *low-grade malignant* lesions:
- *Warshaw technique:* Sacrifices splenic artery and vein, preserves short gastric vessels
- *Kimura technique:* Preserves splenic artery and vein (technically more challenging)

Postoperative Complications

Complication	*Description*
Pancreatic fistula	Most common; leak from transected pancreatic duct
Intra-abdominal abscess	Secondary to fistula or contamination
Post-splenectomy sepsis (OPSI)	Risk if spleen removed; pneumococcal, H. influenzae, meningococcal infections
Diabetes mellitus	If significant pancreas removed
Bleeding	From major vessels (splenic artery/vein)

Pre- and Postoperative Considerations

Preoperative:
- *Vaccination* (if splenectomy planned):
  - Pneumococcal
  - *Haemophilus influenzae* type B
  - Meningococcal
- *Imaging:* CT or MRI to localize lesion and assess resectability
- Nutritional and diabetic evaluation if needed

Postoperative:
- Monitor for *fistula* (check drain fluid amylase)
- Manage diabetes or enzyme insufficiency if needed
- Lifelong infection risk precautions (if spleen removed)

CHAPTER 33

Spleen and Portal Hypertension

LEARNING OBJECTIVES

- Subphrenic Spaces, Intraperitoneal Spaces, Subphrenic Abscess
- Anatomy and Physiology of Spleen
- Splenic Abscess
- Splenectomy, Splenic Preservation
- Esophageal and Gastric Varices
- TIPS
- Surgical Treatment of Ascites
- Gastrointestinal Hemorrhage—Upper GI, Lower GI, Obscure GI Bleeding
- EHPVO and Portal Biliopathy
- Left-sided Portal Hypertension

1. Describe intraperitoneal spaces. How to manage a case Subphrenic abscess?

WBUHS 2025; Srimanta Sankaradeva University, Assam 2025

The intraperitoneal spaces are regions within the peritoneal cavity where organs are suspended by mesenteries and surrounded by peritoneal fluid. These spaces allow organ mobility and are clinically significant for understanding fluid collection, abscess formation, or disease spread. Below is a concise description of the key intraperitoneal spaces:

Major Intraperitoneal Spaces

- *Supracolic compartment (above the transverse mesocolon):*
  - *Right subphrenic space:* Located between the diaphragm and the liver's right lobe. It's a common site for abscesses post-surgery.
  - *Left subphrenic space:* Between the diaphragm and the left lobe of the liver, spleen, and stomach. Subdivided into:
    - *Subphrenic space proper:* Anterior to the stomach.
    - *Perisplenic space:* Around the spleen, prone to fluid collection in trauma.
  - *Subhepatic space:* Below the liver, includes the Morison's Pouch (hepatorenal recess), the most dependent part in the supine position, where fluid often collects.
  - *Lesser sac (Omental Bursa):* Posterior to the stomach, communicates with the greater peritoneal cavity via the epiploic foramen (of Winslow). It's a potential site for pancreatic pseudocyst or abscess.
- *Infracolic compartment (below the transverse mesocolon):*
  - *Right paracolic gutter:* Lateral to the ascending colon, channels fluid from the pelvis to the subhepatic or subphrenic spaces.
  - *Left paracolic gutter:* Lateral to the descending colon, less prone to fluid flow due to the phrenicocolic ligament.
  - *Right and left infracolic spaces:* Medial to the ascending and descending colons, respectively, divided by the small bowel mesentery root. These are potential sites for abscesses or tumor spread.

- *Pelvic cavity:*
  - *Rectouterine pouch (Pouch of douglas):* In females, the most dependent part of the peritoneal cavity, located between the rectum and uterus. Common site for fluid accumulation or ectopic pregnancy.
  - *Vesicouterine pouch:* In females, between the bladder and uterus.
  - *Rectovesical pouch:* In males, between the rectum and bladder, the lowest point in the male pelvis.

Management of Subphrenic Abscess

Managing a subphrenic abscess, a localized collection of pus in the subphrenic space (between the diaphragm and liver or spleen), requires a systematic approach involving diagnosis, medical management, and often interventional procedures.

Diagnosis

- *Clinical presentation*
  - *Symptoms:* Fever, chills, upper abdominal pain (right or left depending on location), shoulder pain (referred due to diaphragmatic irritation), nausea, or hiccups.
  - *Signs:* Tachycardia, tenderness in the upper abdomen, reduced breath sounds if pleural effusion is present.
- *Imaging*
  - *Ultrasound:* First-line to detect fluid collections; cost-effective and non-invasive.
  - *CT scan:* Gold standard for precise localization, size, and extent of the abscess. Contrast-enhanced CT helps differentiate abscess from other fluid collections.
  - *Chest X-ray:* May show elevated hemidiaphragm, pleural effusion, or air-fluid levels.
- *Laboratory tests:*
  - Elevated white blood cell count (leukocytosis), C-reactive protein (CRP), and erythrocyte sedimentation rate (ESR).
  - Blood cultures to identify causative organisms.
  - Aspiration (if performed) for culture and sensitivity to guide antibiotic therapy.

Management

- *Antibiotic therapy*
  - *Empiric antibiotics:* Start broad-spectrum antibiotics to cover likely pathogens (e.g., gram-negative *bacilli*, anaerobes, and gram-positive cocci). Common regimens include:
    - Piperacillin-tazobactam (4.5 g IV every 6 hours) or
    - Ceftriaxone (1–2 g IV daily) plus metronidazole (500 mg IV every 8 hours).
  - Adjust antibiotics based on culture and sensitivity results.
  - *Duration:* Typically 4–6 weeks, with at least 2 weeks of IV therapy, followed by oral antibiotics if drainage is successful.
- *Drainage:*
  - *Percutaneous drainage:* Preferred for accessible abscesses.
    - Performed under ultrasound or CT guidance by an interventional radiologist.
    - A catheter is placed to drain the abscess, with follow-up imaging to confirm resolution.
    - *Indications:* Well-defined, unilocular abscesses with safe access.
  - *Surgical drainage: Indicated if:*
    - Percutaneous drainage fails or is not feasible (e.g., multiloculated abscess, difficult access).
    - Underlying source (e.g., perforated viscus) requires surgical correction.
    - *Approaches:* Laparotomy or laparoscopic drainage, depending on patient stability and surgeon expertise.
  - *Monitoring:* Regular imaging to assess drainage efficacy and catheter patency.
- *Source control:*
  - Identify and treat the underlying cause (e.g., perforated peptic ulcer, appendicitis, or postoperative complication).
  - May require additional procedures like bowel resection or repair of a perforation.

- *Supportive care*
  - *Pain management:* Analgesics (e.g., acetaminophen or opioids cautiously) for pain relief.
  - *Nutritional support:* Parenteral or enteral nutrition if oral intake is poor.
  - *Monitor complications:* Watch for sepsis, pleural effusion, or fistula formation.

Follow-up

- *Clinical monitoring:* Track fever, pain, and inflammatory markers (WBC, CRP).
- *Imaging:* Repeat CT or ultrasound to confirm abscess resolution.
- *Antibiotic adjustment:* Tailor therapy based on clinical response and culture results.
- *Address complications:* Persistent fever or worsening symptoms may indicate inadequate drainage or recurrence.

Special Considerations

- *Right vs. Left subphrenic abscess:*
  - *Right-sided:* More common, often related to liver or biliary pathology.
  - *Left-sided:* Associated with gastric or splenic issues; may involve the lesser sac.
  - *Immunocompromised patients:* Broader antibiotic coverage and lower threshold for intervention.
  - *Postoperative abscesses:* Higher suspicion in patients with recent abdominal surgery.

Prevention

- Early treatment of intra-abdominal infections (e.g., appendicitis, diverticulitis).
- Proper surgical technique to minimize postoperative leaks or contamination.
- Prophylactic antibiotics in high-risk surgeries.

2. Define and discuss subphrenic spaces and their surgical importance. ***WBUHS 2020***

3. Describe subphrenic spaces and its importance in surgery. ***WBUHS 2025***

Introduction

The complicated arrangement of the peritoneum results in the formation of four intraperitoneal spaces in which pus may collect.

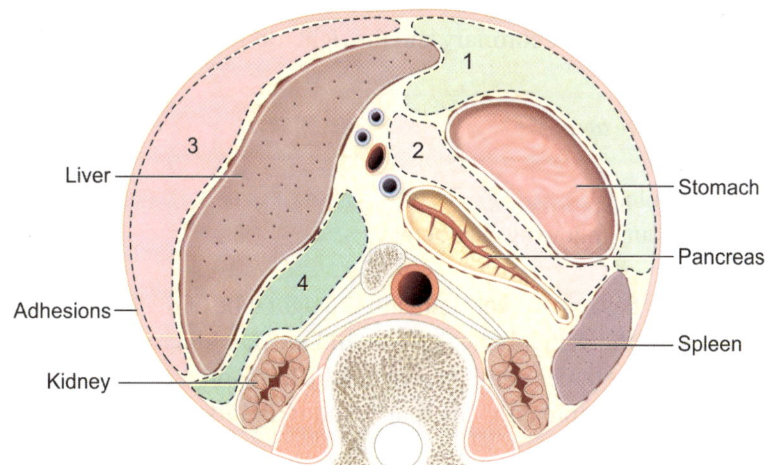

Intraperitoneal spaces on transverse section.

(1) The left subphrenic space; (2) Left subhepatic space/lesser sac; (3) Right subphrenic space; and (4) Right subhepatic space.

- *Left subphrenic space:* This is bounded above by the diaphragm and behind by the left triangular ligament and the left lobe of the liver, the gastrohepatic omentum, and the anterior surface of the stomach. To the right is the falciform ligament and to the left the spleen, gastrosplenic omentum, and diaphragm.

- *The common cause of an abscess here is an operation on:*
    - The stomach
    - The tail of the pancreas
    - The spleen
    - The splenic flexure of the colon

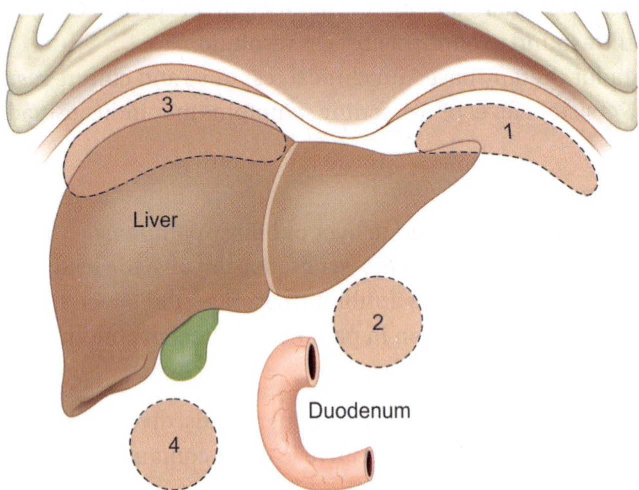

Intraperitoneal spaces on sagittal section.
(1) Left subphrenic; (2) Left subhepatic/lesser sac; (3) Right subphrenic; and (4) Right subhepatic space.

- *Left subhepatic space/lesser sac:*
    - The most common cause of infection here is complicated acute pancreatitis.
    - In practice, a perforated gastric ulcer rarely causes a collection here because the potential space is obliterated by adhesions.
- *Right subphrenic space:* This space lies between the right lobe of the liver and the diaphragm. It is limited posteriorly by the anterior layer of the coronary and the right triangular ligaments and to the left by the falciform ligament.

    Common causes of abscess here are:
    - Perforating cholecystitis
    - A perforated duodenal ulcer
    - A duodenal cap "blow-out" following gastrectomy
    - Appendicitis
- *Right subhepatic space:* This lies transversely beneath the right lobe of the liver in Rutherford Morison's pouch. It is bounded on the right by the right lobe of the liver and the diaphragm. To the left is situated the foramen of Winslow and below this lies the duodenum. In front are the liver and the gall bladder and behind are the upper part of the right kidney and the diaphragm. The space is bounded above by the liver and below by the transverse colon and hepatic flexure.
    It is the deepest space of the four and the most common site of a subphrenic abscess.
    - *Abscess usually arises from:*
        - Appendicitis
        - Cholecystitis
        - A perforated duodenal ulcer
        - Following upper abdominal surgery

Clinical Features

The symptoms and signs of subphrenic infection are frequently nonspecific.

- *Symptoms:*
  - A common history is that, when some infective focus in the abdominal cavity has been dealt with, the condition of the patient improves temporarily but, after an interval of a few days or weeks, symptoms of toxemia reappear.
    - The condition of the patient steadily, and often rapidly, deteriorates.
    - Sweating, wasting, and anorexia are present.
  - There is sometimes epigastric fullness and pain, or pain in the shoulder on the affected side, because of irritation of sensory fibers in the phrenic nerve, referred along the descending branches of the cervical plexus.
  - Persistent hiccoughs may be a presenting symptom.
- *Signs:*
  - A swinging pyrexia is usually present.
  - If the abscess is anterior, abdominal examination will reveal some tenderness, rigidity or even a palpable swelling.
  - Sometimes the liver is displaced downwards but more often it is fixed by adhesions.
  - Examination of the chest is important and, in the majority of cases, collapse of the lung or evidence of basal effusion or even an empyema is found.

Investigations

- Blood tests usually show a leukocytosis and raised C-reactive protein.
- A plain radiograph sometimes demonstrates the presence of gas or a pleural effusion. On screening, the diaphragm is often seen to be elevated (so called "tented" diaphragm) and its movements impaired.
- Ultrasound (US) or computed tomography (CT) scanning is the investigation of choice and permits early detection of subphrenic collections.
- Radiolabeled white cell scanning may occasionally prove helpful when other imaging techniques have failed.

Differential Diagnosis

- Pyelonephritis
- Amoebic abscess
- Pulmonary collapse
- Pleural empyema

Treatment

- The clinical course of suspected cases is monitored, and blood tests and imaging investigations are carried out at suitable intervals.
- If suppuration seems probable, intervention is indicated.
- Percutaneous drainage tube under US or CT control. The same tube can be used to instill antibiotic solutions or irrigate the abscess cavity.
- If an operative approach is necessary and a swelling can be detected in the subcostal region or in the loin, an incision is made over the site of maximum tenderness or over any area where edema or redness is discovered.
- If no swelling is apparent, the subphrenic spaces should be explored by either an anterior subcostal approach or from behind after removal of the outer part of the 12th rib according to the position of the abscess on imaging.

---

4. Anatomy and physiology of spleen. ***WBUHS 2007***

---

5. Describe the anatomy and physiology of spleen. What are the postsplenectomy problems?

WBUHS 2025, WBUHS 2013

6. Describe the physiology and function of spleen. ***RIMS, IMPHAL 2012***

Anatomy of Spleen

- The spleen develops from mesenchymal cells in the dorsal mesogastrium during the 5th week of gestation. The spleen is located in the posterior left upper quadrant of the abdomen.
- The convex smooth surface of the spleen faces superiorly, posteriorly, and to the left in relation to the abdominal surface of the diaphragm.
- The diaphragm separates the spleen from the pleura, the left lower lobe of the lung, and the adjacent 9th, 10th, and 11th ribs.
- The costodiaphragmatic recess of the pleura extends down as far as the inferior border of the normal-sized spleen.
- The normal size and weight vary somewhat; in adults, the approximate size of the spleen is 12 cm in length, 7 cm in width, and 3–4 cm in thickness.
- The average spleen weight in an adult is 150 g, with a range of 80–300 g.
- The visceral relationships of the spleen are with the proximal greater curvature of the stomach, the tail of the pancreas, the left kidney, and the splenic flexure of the colon.
- The parietal peritoneum adheres firmly to the splenic capsule, except at the splenic hilum.
- The peritoneum extends superiorly, laterally, and inferiorly, creating folds, which form the suspensory ligaments of the spleen.
- The splenophrenic and splenocolic ligaments are usually relatively avascular.
- The splenorenal ligament extends from the anterior left kidney to the hilum of the spleen as a two-layered fold in which the splenic vessels and the tail of the pancreas are invested.
- These two layers continue anteriorly and superiorly to the greater curvature of the stomach to form the two leaves of the gastrosplenic ligament through which the short gastric arteries and veins course.
- A fibroelastic capsule commonly known as the splenic capsule invests the organ, and from its trabeculae pass into the parenchyma, branching to form a trabecular network that subdivides the organ into small compartments.
- The splenic artery is a tortuous vessel that arises from the celiac trunk; it courses along the superior border of the pancreas.
- The branches of the splenic artery include the numerous pancreatic branches, the short gastric arteries, the left gastroepiploic artery, and the terminal splenic branches.
- The splenic artery divides into several branches within the splenorenal ligament before entering the splenic hilum, where they branch again into these trabeculae as they enter the splenic pulp.
- Small arteriolar branches leave the trabeculae, and their adventitial coat becomes replaced by a sheath of lymphatic tissue that accompanies the vessels and their branches until they divide into capillaries.
- It is these lymphatic sheaths that make up the white pulp of the spleen and that are interspersed along the arteriolar vessels as lymphatic follicles.
- The interface between the white pulp and the red pulp is known as the marginal zone.
- As the arterioles lose their sheaths of lymphatic tissue, they traverse the marginal zone and enter the red pulp, which is composed of large branching, thin-walled blood vessels called splenic sinuses and sinusoids, and thin plates of cellular tissue composing the splenic cords.
- The venous sinusoids empty into the veins of the red pulp, and these veins drain back along the trabecular veins that empty into at least five major tributaries, ultimately joining to form the splenic vein in the splenorenal ligament.
- The splenic vein runs inferior to the artery and posterior to the pancreatic tail and body. It receives several short tributaries from the pancreas.
- The splenic vein joins the superior mesenteric vein (SMV) at a right angle behind the neck of the pancreas to form the portal vein.

- The inferior mesenteric vein (IMV) often empties into the splenic vein; it may also empty into the SMV at or near the confluence of the splenic vein and SMV.

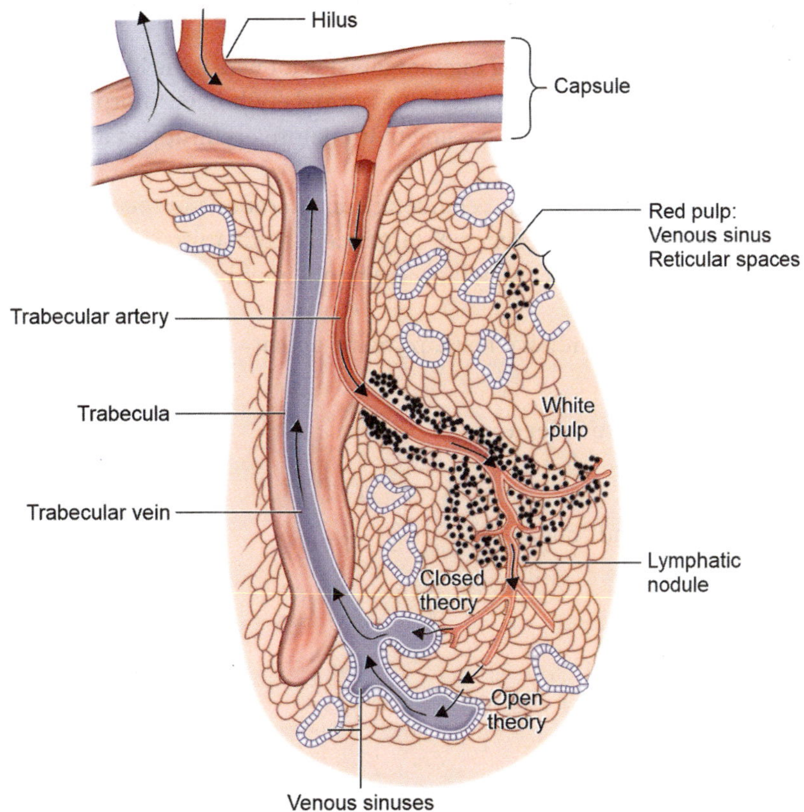

Splenic Function

Hematopoietic Functions

- The spleen has important hematopoietic functions during early fetal development, with both red and white blood cell production.
- Under certain pathologic conditions, such as myelodysplasia, the spleen can reacquire its hematopoietic function.
- Removal of the spleen does not usually result in anemia or leukopenia in an otherwise healthy person.
- Although the hematopoietic function is usually lost during fetal development, the spleen continues to function as a sophisticated filter because of the unique circulatory system and lymphoid organization, and it has blood cell monitoring and management functions as well as important immune functions throughout life.
- The functions of the spleen are closely linked to splenic structure and its unique circulatory system. The arteries flow through the white pulp (lymphoid tissues), after which part of the blood flow goes directly through endothelial cell-lined capillaries into the venous system ("closed" theory).
- Most of the blood flow, however, enters the macrophage-lined reticular meshwork, and the blood flows slowly back to the venous circulation through the venous sinuses ("open" theory). The formed blood elements must pass through slits in the lining of the venous sinuses; if they cannot pass, they are trapped in the spleen and ingested by splenic phagocytes. Removal of the spleen results in loss of both the immunologic and filtering functions.

Filtration

- The most important function of the spleen is probably its mechanical filtration, which removes senescent erythrocytes and likely contributes to control of infection.

- The spleen is important in clearing circulating pathogens that reside within erythrocytes, for example, malarial parasites, or bacteria such as *Bartonella* species.
- Mechanical filtration by the spleen may also be important for removal of unopsonized, noningested bacteria from the circulation.
- It may be particularly important for clearing microorganisms for which the host has no specific antibody.
- Splenic filtering function is important for maintaining normal erythrocyte morphology and function.
- The spleen is an important site for the processing of immature erythrocytes and for repair or destruction of deformed or aged erythrocytes.
- In the asplenic condition, there are several characteristic alterations in the morphologic appearance of the peripheral red blood cells, with the presence of target cells (immature cells), Howell–Jolly bodies (nuclear remnant), Heinz bodies (denatured hemoglobin), Pappenheimer bodies (iron granules), stippling, and spur cells.
- Aged red blood cells (120 days) that have lost enzymatic activity and membrane plasticity are trapped and destroyed in the spleen.

Biologic Substances Removed by the Spleen

- *Normal subjects:*
  - Red blood cell membrane
  - Red blood cell surface pits and craters
  - Howell–Jolly bodies
  - Heinz bodies
  - Pappenheimer bodies
  - Acanthocytes
  - Senescent red blood cells
  - Particulate antigen
- *Patients with disease:*
  - Spherocytes (hereditary-spherocytosis)
  - Sickle cells, hemoglobin C cells
  - Antibody-coated red blood cells
  - Antibody-coated platelets
  - Antibody-coated white blood cells
- The filtering function of the spleen is also an important factor in anemic conditions associated with abnormal red blood cell morphology.
- Abnormal erythrocytes that result from hereditary spherocytosis, sickle cell anemia, thalassemia, or pyruvate kinase deficiency are trapped by the splenic filtering mechanism, resulting in worsening anemia, symptomatic splenomegaly, and occasionally splenic infarction.
- In autoimmune hemolytic anemia, immunoglobulin G (IgG) bound to the cell membrane targets the red blood cells for splenic destruction by splenic macrophages.
- A similar IgG-dependent mechanism is involved in splenic platelet destruction in immune thrombocytopenic purpura (ITP).

Immune Functions

- Another major function of the spleen is the maintenance of normal immune function and host defenses against certain types of infectious agents.
- It is well established that people lacking a spleen are at a significantly higher risk for overwhelming postsplenectomy infection (OPSI) with fulminant bacteremia, pneumonia, or meningitis, as compared with those with normal splenic function.
- Asplenic subjects have defective activation of complement by the alternative pathway, leaving them more susceptible to infection.

- The spleen, with its specialized circulatory system and large supply of macrophages that are capable of ingestion of organisms not optimally opsonized with antibody, greatly enhances their clearance.
- Asplenic subjects have been found to have subnormal IgM levels, and their peripheral blood mononuclear cells exhibit a suppressed immunoglobulin response.
- The spleen is a major site of production for the opsonins properdin and tuftsin, and removal of the spleen results in decreased serum levels of these factors.
  - Properdin can initiate the alternative pathway of complement activation to produce destruction of bacteria as well as foreign and abnormal cells.
  - Tuftsin is a tetrapeptide that enhances the phagocytic activity of both polymorphonuclear leukocytes and mononuclear phagocytes.
  - The spleen is the major site of cleavage of tuftsin from the heavy chain of IgG, and circulating levels of tuftsin are suppressed in asplenic subjects.
- Neutrophil function is decreased in asplenic patients, and the defect appears to result from the absence of a circulating mediator.

7. Splenic abscess. ***WBUHS 2022***

Introduction

Splenic abscesses are rare, but potentially lethal if not accurately diagnosed and treated.

Etiology

Two-thirds arise from seeding of the spleen by a distant site, most commonly endocarditis and urinary tract infections.

Clinical Features

- Pain left upper abdomen and lower chest
- Fever

Investigations

- Abdominal CT and/or US imaging are the diagnostic modalities of choice. CT images reveal a low intensity lesion that does not enhance with contrast.
- The most common organisms are aerobic microbes (streptococci and *Escherichia coli*), but other microorganisms have also been isolated (*Mycobacterium tuberculosis* and *Salmonella typhi*).

Treatment

- Treatment includes broad-spectrum antibiotics for 14 days.
- Splenectomy is the operation of choice, but percutaneous and open drainage are options for patients who cannot tolerate splenectomy.

8. Splenectomy: Indications, complications, and immunization. ***WBUHS 2022***

9. Postsplenectomy problems. ***WBUHS 2009, 2013***

10. List the indications for splenectomy. Describe the complications of the procedure. ***RGUHS, Karnataka 2025***

Indications for Splenectomy

- *Trauma:*
  - Accidental
  - Operative
- *Oncological:*
  - Part of en bloc resection

  - Diagnostic
  - Therapeutic
- *Hematological:*
  - Spherocytosis
  - Purpura (ITP)
  - Hypersplenism
- *Portal hypertension:* Variceal surgery

The common indications for splenectomy are:

- Trauma resulting from an accident or during a surgical procedure, as for example during mobilization of the esophagus, stomach, distal pancreas, or splenic flexure of the colon
- Removal *en bloc* with the stomach as part of a radical gastrectomy, or with the pancreas as part of a distal or total pancreatectomy
- To reduce anemia or thrombocytopenia in spherocytosis, idiopathic thrombocytopenic purpura, or hypersplenism
- In association with shunt or variceal surgery for portal hypertension

Postoperative complications following splenectomy.

Bleeding complications	*Pulmonary complications*	*Septic complications*	*Others*	
Intraoperative bleeding (requiring transfusion)	Atelectasis	Wound infection	Deep venous thrombosis	Postoperative ileus
Postoperative bleeding	Pneumonia and upper respiratory tract infection	Deep line sepsis	Gout flare	Hypophyseal insufficiency
Abdominal wall hematoma	Pulmonary embolus	Urinary tract infection	Myocardial infarction	Gastric stasis
Hemothorax	Pneumothorax		Vocal cord damage	Pancreatic tail injury

Postoperative Complications

- Immediate complications specific to splenectomy include hemorrhage resulting from a slipped ligature.
- Hematemesis from gastric mucosal damage and gastric dilatation is uncommon.
- Left basal atelectasis is common, and a pleural effusion may be present.
- Injury to adjacent structures:
  - Adjacent structures at risk during the procedure include the stomach and pancreas. A fistula may result from damage to the greater curvature of the stomach during ligation of the short gastric vessels.
  - Damage to the tail of the pancreas may result in pancreatitis, a localized abscess, or a pancreatic fistula.
- Postoperative thrombocytosis may arise and, if the blood platelet count exceeds 1×10^6/mL, prophylactic aspirin is recommended. Long-term surveillance programs have emphasized an increased risk of deep vein thrombosis and pulmonary embolism. The relative risk and benefit of thromboprophylaxis in this setting has not been assessed adequately.
- Postsplenectomy septicemia may result from *Streptococcus pneumoniae, Neisseria meningitides, Haemophilus influenzae,* and *E. coli.* Long-term surveillance programs have suggested that the risk of pneumonia, meningitis and major sepsis following splenectomy is increased threefold.
  - However, the risk is greater in the young patient, in splenectomized patients treated with chemoradiotherapy and in patients who have undergone splenectomy for thalassemia, sickle cell disease and autoimmune anemia, or thrombocytopenia.
  - Overwhelming/opportunistic a major concern. Published guidelines emphasize that most infections after splenectomy could be avoided through measures that include offering patients appropriate and timely immunization, antibiotic prophylaxis, education, and prompt treatment of infection.

Immunization

The benefit of prophylactic antibiotics in this setting remains controversial.

- It is thought that children who have undergone splenectomy before the age of 5 years should be treated with a daily dose of penicillin until the age of 10 years.
- Prophylaxis in older children should be continued at least until the age of 16 years, but its use is less well defined in adults.
- Furthermore, compliance is problematic in the long term but, as the risk of overwhelming sepsis is greatest within the first 2–3 years after splenectomy, it seems reasonable to give prophylaxis during this time. However, all patients with compromised immune function should receive prophylaxis.
- Satisfactory oral prophylaxis can be obtained with penicillin, erythromycin, amoxicillin, or coamoxiclav. Suspected infection can be treated intravenously with these same antibiotics and cefotaxime or ceftriaxone, or chloramphenicol in patients allergic to penicillin and cephalosporins.
- If elective splenectomy is planned, consideration should be given to vaccinating against pneumococcus, meningococcus C (both repeated every 5 years), and *H. influenzae* type B (Hib) (repeated every 10 years). The latter two vaccines are commonly delivered as a combined preparation.
- Yearly influenza vaccination has been recommended, as there is some evidence that it may reduce the risk of secondary bacterial infection. Such vaccinations should be administered at least 2 weeks before elective surgery or as soon as possible after recovery from surgery but before discharge from hospital.
- Pneumococcal vaccination is recommended in those patients aged over 2 years. Hib vaccination is recommended irrespective of age.
- Asplenic patients should carry a medical alert and an up-to-date vaccination card. They require specific advice regarding travel and animal handling.
- Patients who have undergone splenectomy and are travelling to countries where malaria is present are strongly advised to use all physical antimosquito barriers as well as antimalarial therapy since they are at increased risk of severe malaria.
- Overwhelming postsplenectomy sepsis due to *Capnocytophaga canimorsus* may result from dog, cat, or other animal bites.
- In the trauma victim, vaccination can be given in the postoperative period, and the resulting antibody levels will be protective in the majority of cases. Antibody levels are, however, <50% of those achieved if vaccination is given in the presence of an intact spleen. Protection following vaccination is not always guaranteed.

Overwhelming Postsplenectomy Infection

- Overwhelming systemic sepsis (opportunistic post splenectomy infection) usually associated with gram-positive encapsulated bacteria such as *Streptococcus*.
- The incidence of overwhelming postsplenectomy sepsis is highest in children and has been reported as high as 4%.
- The mortality rate from overwhelming postsplenectomy sepsis is approximately 50%.
- Increasing the incidence in adults are those who have undergone splenectomy for an associated malignancy or as an incidental procedure.
- In children, those most at risk are those who have undergone splenectomy for either congenital or acquired anemias.
- The most common etiologic organisms are *S. pneumoniae, H. influenzae*, and *Neisseria meningitis*.
- As a result, vaccination against these organisms has been advocated.
- The timing of these vaccinations has been debated; however, most data would suggest that preoperative (typically 2 weeks) vaccination is best.
- Currently, the standard of care for postsplenectomy patients includes immunization with polyvalent pneumococcal vaccine (PPV23), Hib conjugate, and meningococcal polysaccharide vaccine within 2 weeks of splenectomy.
- Even with vaccination, the development of a protective level of antibody against pneumococci is only about 50%.
- Currently available vaccines elicit a T-cell–independent response and do not produce a sustained increase in antibody titers.

- Subsequently, there is a lack of evidence that indicates a substantial increase in protection in most revaccinated persons.
- Therefore, routine revaccination of immunocompetent persons who were previously vaccinated with PPV23 is not recommended by the Centers for Disease Control and Prevention (CDC).
- Revaccination is, however, recommended in high-risk individuals. Candidates for revaccination with PPV23 include the following:
  - Persons who received the 14-valent vaccine who are at highest risk for fatal pneumococcal infection (e.g., asplenic patients).
  - Adults at highest risk who received the 23-valent vaccine 6 years prior.
  - Adults at highest risk who have shown a rapid decline in pneumococcal antibody levels (e.g., patients with nephrotic syndrome, those with renal failure, and transplant recipients).
  - Children at highest risk (asplenia, nephritic syndrome, and sickle cell anemia) who would be 10 years old at revaccination.

11. Splenic preservation. *WBUHS 2009; RIMS, Imphal 2012*

An Algorithm for the Diagnostic Imaging of Patients with Suspected Blunt Splenic Trauma

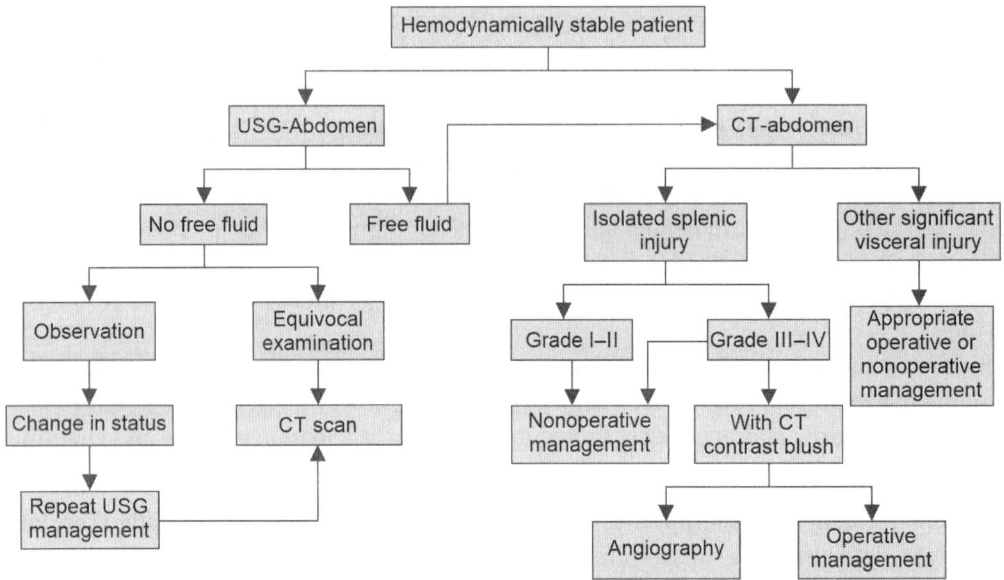

- All hemodynamically normal patients are candidates for nonoperative management.
- In addition, those patients who are initially hemodynamically labile but respond to crystalloid without further episodes of instability may also be considered for nonoperative management.
- The only true contraindication to nonoperative management in properly monitored patients is hemodynamic instability, or another indication mandating laparotomy.
- Nonoperative management should not be entertained at hospitals where surgeons, operative capabilities, and intensive care resources are not immediately available at all times.

Criteria for nonoperative management of splenic injury.

- No indications for laparotomy (physical examination signs/symptoms or other injuries)
- Hemodynamically normal after resuscitation with crystalloid
- No injuries that preclude physical examination of the abdomen [e.g., closed head injury (CHI) and spinal cord injury]
- No transfusion requirements (PRBC)
- Constant availability of surgical and critical care resources

Criteria for failure of nonoperative management.

- Increasing fluid requirements to maintain normal hemodynamic status
- Failed angioembolization of arteriovenous (AV) fistulae/pseudoaneurysm
- Transfusion requirements to maintain Hct/Hgb and normal hemodynamic status
- Increasing hemoperitoneum associated with hemodynamic liability
- Peritoneal signs/rebound tenderness

- Splenectomy should be considered in all adult patients with grades IV and V injuries. Lesser injury grades can often be managed with splenorrhaphy.
- Pediatric patients should have every attempt at splenic salvage.

Techniques for splenorrhaphy/splenic conservation surgery.

- *Topical agents:*
  - Absorbable gelatin sponge
  - Oxidized regenerated cellulose
  - Microfibrillar collagen
  - Fibrin sealant
- *Coagulation:*
  - Electrocautery
  - Argon beam coagulator
- *Mesh:*
  - Polyglactin
  - Polyglycolic acid
- *Partial/hemisplenectomy:*
  - Segmental vessel ligation, resection, mattress sutures
  - Stapler
  - Ultrasonic surgical aspirator

ESOPHAGEAL AND GASTRIC VARICES AND PORTAL HYPERTENSION

12. Causes of portal hypertension. Discuss about surgical treatment of portal hypertension. *WBUHS 2007*

Causes of portal hypertension.

Increased resistance to flow:

- Prehepatic (portal vein obstruction)
  - Congenital atresia or stenosis
  - Thrombosis of portal vein
  - Thrombosis of splenic vein
  - Extrinsic compression (e.g., tumors)
- Hepatic
  - Cirrhosis
    - Portal cirrhosis (nutritional, alcoholic, and Laënnec)
    - Postnecrotic cirrhosis
    - Biliary cirrhosis
    - Others (Wilson disease and hemochromatosis)
  - Acute alcoholic liver disease
    Chronic active hepatitis
  - Congenital hepatic fibrosis
  - Idiopathic portal hypertension (hepatoportal sclerosis)
  - Schistosomiasis
  - Sarcoidosis

Contd...

Contd...

Causes of portal hypertension.

- Posthepatic
  - Budd–Chiari syndrome (hepatic vein thrombosis)
  - Veno-occlusive disease
  - Cardiac disease
    - Constrictive pericarditis
    - Valvular heart disease
    - Right heart failure

Increased portal blood flow:

- Arterial-portal venous fistula
- Increased splenic flow
  - Banti syndrome
  - Splenomegaly (e.g., tropical splenomegaly and myeloid metaplasia)

Surgical procedures for esophageal varices.

Direct variceal obliteration:

- Variceal suture ligation
  - Transthoracic
  - Transabdominal
- Esophageal transection and reanastomosis
  - Suture technique
  - Staple technique
- Variceal sclerosis
  - Esophagoscopic
  - Transhepatic
- Variceal resection
  - Esophagogastrectomy
  - Subtotal esophagectomy

Reduction of variceal blood flow and pressure:

- Portosystemic shunts
  - End-to-side
  - Side-to-side
    - Side-to-side portacaval
    - Mesocaval
    - Central splenorenal
    - Renosplenic
- Selective shunts
  - Distal splenorenal (Warren)
  - Left gastric vena caval (Inokuchi)
- Reduction of portal blood flow
  - Splenectomy
  - Splenic artery ligation
- Reduction of proximal gastric blood flow
  - Esophagogastric devascularization
  - Gastric transection and reanastomosis (Tanner)
- Stimulation of additional portosystemic venous collaterals
  - Omentopexy
  - Splenic transposition
- *Measures to preserve hepatic blood flow after portacaval shunt*
  - Arterialization of portal vein stump

Liver Transplantation

- Any relatively young patient with cirrhosis who has survived an episode of variceal hemorrhage should be considered a candidate for liver transplantation, since any other form of therapy carries a much higher (about 80%) mortality rate within the subsequent 1–2 years as a result of repeat bleeding or complications of hepatic failure.

- Good transplantation candidates, however, should not be subjected to portosystemic shunts or other procedures if it appears that they will come to transplantation in the near future.
- In general, Child-Pugh A patients are candidates for portal decompression; Child-Pugh C patients are candidates for a transplant.
- A transjugular intrahepatic shunt is an excellent way to control bleeding while the patient is being prepared for a transplant.

Portosystemic Shunts

- Portosystemic shunts can be grouped into those that shunt the entire portal system (total shunts) and those that selectively shunt blood from the gastrosplenic region while preserving the pressure-flow relationships in the rest of the portal bed (selective shunts).
- All of the shunt operations commonly used today reduce the incidence of rebleeding to <10%, compared with about 75% in unshunted patients.
- The choice of shunt has been the subject of much debate and several randomized trials. The principal question in recent years has been whether encephalopathy and survival are better with a selective shunt (e.g., a distal splenorenal shunt) than with a total shunt (e.g., a mesocaval or an end-to-side portacaval shunt).

Severity of Hepatic Disease and Operative Risk

- The immediate death rate of an elective shunt procedure can be predicted from the patient's hepatic function as reflected by the Child-Pugh classification.
- In addition to operative death rate, the figures also correlate with the death rate in the first post shunt year.
- Thereafter, survival curves of the different risk classes become reasonably parallel.
- The severity of histopathologic changes in liver biopsies correlates with the immediate surgical death rate, the most ominous findings being hepatocellular necrosis, polymorphonuclear leukocyte infiltration, and the presence of Mallory bodies.
- The extent of histologic change also correlates with the more easily obtained data in the Child-Pugh classification (i.e., severe changes occur in class C patients), so results of biopsies have no independent predictive value.

Types of Portosystemic Shunts

Total Shunts

- The end-to-side shunt completely disconnects the liver from the portal system. The portal vein (PV) is transected near its bifurcation in the liver hilum and anastomosed to the side of the inferior vena cava. The hepatic stump of the vein is oversewn.
- Postoperatively, the wedged hepatic venous pressure (WHVP) (sinusoidal pressure) drops slightly, reflecting the inability of the hepatic artery to compensate fully for the loss of portal inflow.
- The side-to-side portacaval, mesocaval, mesorenal, and central splenorenal shunts are all physiologically similar, since the shunt preserves continuity between the hepatic limb of the portal vein, the portal system, and the anastomosis. Flow through the hepatic limb of the standard side-to-side shunt is nearly always away from the liver and toward the anastomosis.
- The end-to-side portacaval shunt gives immediate and permanent protection from variceal bleeding and is somewhat easier to perform than a side-to-side portacaval or central splenorenal shunt.
- Encephalopathy may be slightly more common after side-to-side than end-to-side portacaval shunts. Side-to-side shunts are required in patients with Budd–Chiari syndrome or refractory ascites (when the latter is treated by a portosystemic shunt).
- *The mesocaval shunt* interposes a segment of prosthetic graft or internal jugular vein between the inferior vena cava (IVC) and the SMV where the latter passes in front of the uncinate process of the pancreas.
- The mesocaval shunt is particularly useful in the presence of severe scarring in the right upper quadrant or PV thrombosis, and in some cases it may be technically easier than a conventional side-to-side portacaval shunt if a side-to-side type of shunt is necessary. In most cases, portal flow to the liver is lost after this shunt.

Selective Shunts

- Selective shunts lower pressure in the gastroesophageal venous plexus while preserving blood flow through the liver via the portal vein.
- *The distal splenorenal (Warren) shunt* involves anastomosing the distal (splenic) end of the transected splenic vein to the side of the left renal vein, plus ligation of the major collaterals between the remaining portal and isolated gastrosplenic venous system.
- In contrast to total shunts, the Warren shunt does not improve ascites and should not be performed in patients whose ascites has been difficult to control.
- Preoperative angiography should be performed to determine if the splenic vein and left renal vein are large enough and close enough together for performance of this shunt.
- Recent pancreatitis may preclude safe dissection of the splenic vein from the undersurface of the pancreas.
- *Another type of selective shunt (Inokuchi shunt)* consists of joining the left gastric vein to the IVC by a short segment of autogenous saphenous vein. The procedure has not become popular, perhaps because of its technical complexity.

Choice of Shunt

A reasonable approach to shunt selection is as follows:

- The *distal splenorenal shunt is the first choice* for *elective portal decompression.*
- If *ascites* is present or the anatomy is unfavorable, an *end-to-side portacaval shunt* is preferred.
- *Side-to-side shunts* would be done for patients with *severe ascites or Budd–Chiari syndrome.*
- *The H-mesocaval and central splenorenal* shunts are reserved for special anatomic situations in which the above operations are unsuitable. An end-to-side shunt or H-mesocaval shunt is performed for *emergency decompression.*
- *Portacaval and distal splenorenal shunts* (DSRS) are often followed by a rise in platelet count in patients with secondary hypersplenism. The response is unpredictable, however, and hypersplenism need not necessarily dictate the type of shunt since it rarely produces clinical manifestations.
- *A central splenorenal shunt,* in which *splenectomy* is performed, should not be considered preferable to other kinds of shunt just because the patient has a low platelet count.

Devascularization Operations

The objective of devascularization is to destroy the venous collaterals that transport blood from the high-pressure portal system into the veins in the submucosa of the esophagus.

Miscellaneous Operations

- Attempts have also been made to decrease portal pressure by decreasing splanchnic inflow through splenectomy or splenic artery ligation.
- Diseases characterized by marked splenomegaly may rarely be associated with portal hypertension as a consequence of increased splenic blood flow, which has been known to reach levels as high as 1,000 mL/min.
- Splenic blood flow may occasionally be increased enough in patients with cirrhosis to contribute significantly to the portal hypertension.
- However, splenectomy or splenic artery ligation in cirrhosis most often gives only a transient decrease in portal pressure, and over half of patients having these operations bleed again.
- Some workers have suggested that the absolute size of the splenic artery (a crude index of splenic flow) correlates with the clinical effectiveness of splenic artery ligation, a good result being predictable if the diameter of the artery is 1 cm or greater.

13. Management of esophageal variceal bleeding. ***WBUHS 2019***

The goals of treatment are to:

- Prevent more liver damage
- Prevent varices from bleeding
- Control bleeding if it occurs.

Preventing Liver Damage

- Avoid alcoholic beverages of any kind.
- Limit use of household cleaners and chemicals.
- Eat a healthier diet that is low in fat and high in fruits and vegetables, whole grains, and lean proteins.
- Maintain a healthy body weight (excess body fat puts stress on the liver).

Preventing Bleeding

- Medications to reduce blood pressure in the PV can reduce the risk of bleeding.
- The most commonly used medications are beta-blockers.
- These include propranolol, nadolol, and carvedilol.
- Patients with a high risk of bleeding may undergo preventive treatment with the same techniques that are used to stop bleeding. The most commonly used technique is variceal ligation.

Controlling Bleeding

- Bleeding from esophageal varices is an emergency that requires immediate treatment.
- Two different, nonsurgical treatments are available to stop variceal bleeding—variceal ligation performed through an endoscope, and transjugular intrahepatic portosystemic shunt (TIPS) done by a radiologist using X-ray.
    - *Variceal ligation:* In this procedure, tiny elastic bands are wrapped around the varices to cut off blood flow through the varices.
    - *Transjugular intrahepatic portal-systemic shunting:* This is a procedure to reduce portal blood pressure that can be used in patients who have esophageal varices that bleed due to severe cirrhosis.

Treatment of Acute Variceal Hemorrhage

- Titrate fluid resuscitation to a systolic blood pressure of 80–90 mm Hg only
- Endotracheal intubation in patients with grade III–IV encephalopathy to protect airway
- Prophylactic antibiotics increases short term survival in cirrhotic patients with acute variceal hemorrhage.
- Terlipressin, somatostatin, and octreotide control bleeding in approximately 80%–90%
- Variceal ligation appears to be equally as effective as sclerotherapy in controlling acute variceal hemorrhage.
- Balloon tamponade has a high complication rate, its use should be restricted to patients with massive bleeding not controlled by initial therapy.
- TIPS is the treatment of choice in patients unresponsive to endoscopic management.

Prevention of Rebleeding

- Beta-blockers indicated in all patients after variceal bleed.
- Overall beta-blockers reduce the risk of rebleeding by about 40% and mortality by 20%.
- Reduced incidence of rebleeding and death if beta-blockers combined with endoscopic eradication of varices
- Variceal ligation requires fewer sessions to obliterate varices and results in fewer complications compared with sclerotherapy.
- Sclerotherapy may be necessary after successful ligation therapy to eradicate small residual varices and prevent recurrence of varices.
- Liver transplantation is the definitive treatment for patients with advanced liver disease who have bled and should be considered in all such patients.

Investigations and Surgical Management of Portal Hypertension

Evaluation

- Assessment of the liver function
- Assessment of the portal circulation
- Upper GI endoscopy

Investigations

Assessment of Liver Function

- Hypoalbuminemia
- Alanine aminotransferase (ALT) and aspartate aminotransferase (AST) are moderately raised
- Prothrombin time (PT) and international normalized ratio (INR) are disturbed.
  Blood picture→ anemia, leukopenia, thrombocytopenia, or pancytopenia.

Assessment of Portal Circulation

- Duplex scan or Doppler ultrasound:
  - To assess the hepatic artery, hepatic vein, and portal vein
  - Patency of portal vein
- Upper GI Endoscopy or EGD:
  - To detect gastroesophageal varices
  - Gold standard for diagnosing variceal bleeding

Diagnosis of the etiology of liver disease is performed by:

- Immunological tests for hepatitis markers
- Other specific serological markers are alpha-foetoprotein, ceruloplasmin, alpha-1 antitrypsin, antimitochondrial antibodies, and iron studies.
- Liver biopsy
- CT/MR angiography—to map the hepatic vasculature
- Model for End-stage Liver Disease (MELD) score:
  - *Score = 0.957 × loge creatinine (mg/dL) + 0.378 × loge bilirubin (mg/dL) + 1.120 loge INR*
  - *Child–Pugh classification*

Child–Pugh classification.

	Points		
	1	***2***	***3***
Bilirubin (mg/dL)	<2	2″3	>3
Albumin (g/dL)	>3–5	2.8–3.5	<2.8
Prothrombin time (seconds)	1–3	4–6	>6
Ascites	None	Slight	Moderate
Encephalopathy	None	Minimal	Advanced

Grade A: 5–6 points; Grade B: 7–9 points; Grade C: 10–15 points

Resuscitation and Medical Measures

- Admit patient in intensive care unit (ICU)
- Fluids and blood products judiciously administered
- Somatostatin or its analogs octreotide or terlipressin administered and continued for 3–5 days
- Nonselective beta-blockers such as propanol or nadolol
- Current recommendation is to administer an antibiotic prophylaxis up to 7 days, specifically a fluoroquinolones.

Surgery for Portal Hypertension

Decompressive Shunts

Transjugular intrahepatic portosystemic shunt is a procedure that involves the creation of an artificial anastomosis between the hepatic and portal veins under fluoroscopic guidance with the use of a covered stent, shunting away blood from the hepatic sinusoids and relieving portal pressure.

Indications for TIPSS:

- Refractory bleeding
- Prior to transplant
- Child C
- Refractory ascites

Types of surgical procedure:

- Portosystemic shunts
- Nonshunt surgery—devascularization
- Liver transplantation

Portosystemic Shunts

Classification

Nonselective shunts:

- *Total shunts:*
  - Portacaval
  - Mesocaval
  - Proximal splenorenal
- *Partial shunts:* Small diameter portacaval (Sarfeh)
- *Selective shunts:* Distal splenorenal shunt

Portacaval shunt:

- Portal blood is completely redirected into IVC below the liver.
- *Two types:* End-to-side and side-to-side.
- *Side-to-side shunt is useful in preventing portal hypertension in Budd-Chiari syndrome.*

Mesocaval shunt:

- Anastomosis of the side of the SMV to the proximal end of the divided IVC, for control of portal hypertension
- The incidence of thrombosis is high.

Proximal splenorenal shunt:

- *Indication:* Extrahepatic portal venous obstruction (EHPVO)
- *Advantage:* The incidence of encephalopathy is less than after portacaval shunt.

Disadvantages:

- Less effective in rebleeding.
- If the splenic vein is <1 cm the anastomosis is liable to thrombosis.

A small diameter interposition (8–10 mm) portacaval shunt

Advantages:
- Partially decompress the portal venous system
- Hepatic portal flow is preserved

Drawbacks:
- Increased incidence of thrombosis
- Recurrence of bleeding

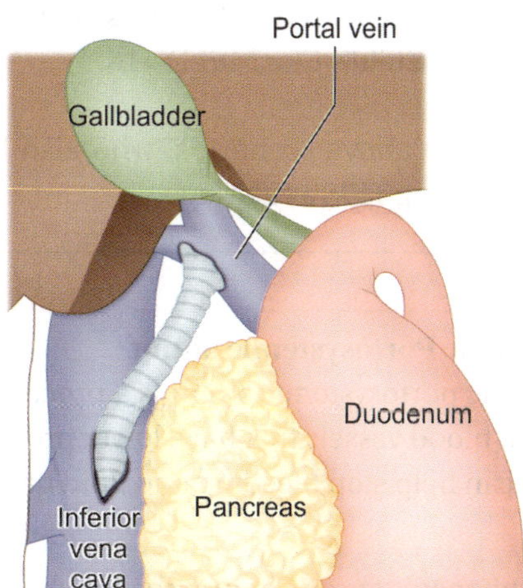

Selective shunts.

Types

- The distal splenorenal shunt (Dean Warren shunt)
- Inokuchi splenocaval shunt (IMV to IVC)
- Interposition shunts with the left gastric vein to IVC

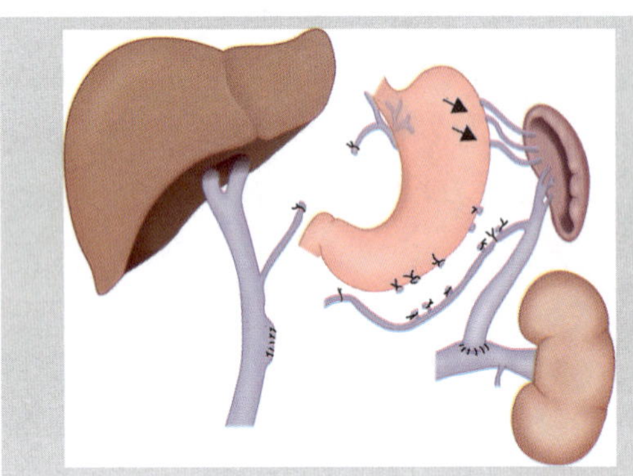

Distal splenorenal shunt:

An anastomosis of the splenic vein and the left renal vein, created to lower portal hypertension

Merits:

- The incidence of encephalopathy is low
- Liver functions remain normal

Nonshunt surgery.

Devascularization

Aim: Direct disconnection between the portal and azygos vein done by disconnecting the varices from their bleeding vessels.

Components

- Splenectomy
- Gastric and esophageal devascularization
- Esophageal transection

Ultimately Liver Transplantation is the Option

Prevention of Rebleeding

- Good-risk patients—Child's A patients or MELD <10.
  - Pharmacotherapy ± Banding
  - If they rebleed or have failure to obliterate their varices banding, they may be a candidate for decompression with TIPS or DSRS.
- Indeterminate patients—Child's B or MELD 10–16
  - Majority of patients
  - Initial treatment is with endoscopic banding and a beta-blocker
  - Subsequent treatment depends on the course of their liver disease
- End-stage liver disease—Child's C or MELD >16.
  - Liver transplantation

Patients with any of the above scenarios, who also have advanced liver disease, are candidates for liver transplantation, possibly using TIPS as a bridge.

14. TIPS. ***WBUHS 2008***

Transjugular Intrahepatic Portosystemic Shunt

Transjugular intrahepatic portosystemic shunt is a procedure that involves inserting a stent (tube) to connect the portal veins to adjacent blood vessels that have lower pressure. This relieves the pressure of blood flowing through the diseased liver and can help stop bleeding and fluid back up.

Indications for TIPS

- Patients with esophageal varices hemorrhage who are refractory to conventional medical therapy (i.e., medications administered to reduce portal pressure).

- Patients who have had maximized endoscopic banding and continue to bleed.
- Intractable ascites refractory to medical therapy
- Patients who are not surgical candidates for conventional portosystemic shunts.
- A bridge to hepatic transplantation
- Patients with recurrent hydrothorax due to cirrhosis; and
- Patients with portal hypertension due to Budd–Chiari syndrome. The application of TIPS in patients with portal hypertensive gastropathy and hepatorenal syndrome remains controversial.

Contraindications to the TIPS

- Patients with advanced hepatic encephalopathy
- Patients with significant cardiac disease (e.g., patients with marked valvular insufficiency, global cardiac dysfunction, significant pulmonary hypertension, and constrictive pericarditis)
- Patients with any polycystic liver disease in which the path of the shunt would traverse liver cysts
- Patients with active infection (peritoneal, intrahepatic, systemic, etc.)
- Patients with hypervascular primary or metastatic hepatic tumors in the path of the proposed TIPS

Relative Contraindications to TIPS

- Those patients with PV occlusion (in this setting, aggressive percutaneous interventional therapy may result in successful recanalization of the portal vein; such procedures may require percutaneous angioplasty and stenting of the PV prior to creation of TIPS)
- Patients with impending liver failure

Technique of TIPS

- Prior to the TIPS procedure, diagnostic imaging to confirm patency of the PV and to define hepatic configuration is essential.
- Portal vein patency may be assessed using color-flow Doppler US, CT with intravenous contrast, or magnetic resonance imaging (MRI)
- Patients with advanced liver disease may be hypovolemic due to:
  - Recent life-threatening variceal hemorrhage
  - Aggressive medical treatment (e.g., diuretic therapy) used for managing ascites
  - Hypovolemia due to large-volume paracenteses
- Preprocedure planning and noninvasive imaging are important for determining the approach (e.g., creating the TIPS from the right hepatic to right portal veins or middle hepatic to left portal veins).
- For the standard TIPS procedure, percutaneous puncture into the right internal jugular vein is made.
- A straight intravascular sheath is advanced to the level of the superior vena cava-right atrial junction.
- A multipurpose catheter (usually 6–7 Fr) and a standard angiographic guidewire are advanced through the sheath and used to selectively catheterize a hepatic vein.
- Free and wedged hepatic venography is generally performed, and the largest hepatic vein with the most favorable angle to the PV is selected. Often this is the right hepatic vein.
- Contrast injected with the catheter wedged in a peripheral hepatic vein may document patency of the PV and demonstrate hepatofugal flow. Carbon dioxide may also be used.
- With the hepatic vein selected, the multipurpose catheter is exchanged for an angled 9F guiding catheter.
- Through this, a 16-gauge angulated needle is directed in a manner similar to that used for transjugular liver biopsies.
- Technique modifications have included the development of smaller-gauge needles to probe through the cirrhotic liver.
- The transjugular hepatic biopsy needle is advanced through the angulated sheath.
- With the tip of the sheath in the orifice of the hepatic vein, the needle exits the distal end of the sheath, and is directed into the hepatic vein wall.

- A puncture through the hepatic vein wall and hepatic parenchyma is made and the needle is advanced toward the PV (avoiding the bifurcation).
- Needle passes are generally "blind", although some interventional radiologists monitor needle passes under imaging guidance (e.g., real-time US).
- If the PV has been entered, venous blood is aspirated. Contrast is injected to confirm PV entry.
- When the needle enters a main right or left PV branch and position is confirmed by contrast injection, a floppy-tipped guidewire is directed through the needle into the main portal vein.
- The 9F sheath is advanced through the tract.
- The needle is removed, and a catheter is directed over the guidewire into the portal vein.
- The guidewire is removed, and direct portal pressures are measured and recorded.
- The right atrial pressure is also recorded through the jugular vein sheath. The gradient between the PV and right atrium (i.e., central venous pressure) is calculated.
- A portal venogram using iodinated contrast, or alternatively carbon dioxide, is performed to define anatomy.
- A stiff guidewire is reintroduced through the 5F catheter and an angioplasty balloon is used to dilate the vein walls and parenchymal tract (i.e., between hepatic vein and portal vein).
- During dilation, a waist on the balloon is typically identified at the hepatic vein and PV entry sites.
- After complete tract dilation, the angioplasty balloon is removed over the guidewire.
- Unless a stent is placed in the newly created parenchymal tract, the tract will close.
- Therefore, it is essential that the entire course of the parenchymal tract be paved with stent material.
- If necessary, stents are overlapped to prevent gaps in coverage.
- Once the self-expanding metallic stents are deployed, repeat balloon dilation further expands the stent.
- The stent's struts are embedded in parenchymal tissue and the stent maintains patency of the percutaneously created tract between hepatic and portal veins.
- Care is taken to avoid placing the stents into the IVC or main PV because this may jeopardize possible future hepatic transplantation.
- Pressure measurements are obtained after the TIPS procedure, and the shunt is dilated again, if necessary, to increase its diameter and further reduce the gradient.
- The recommended reduction in pressure gradient remains controversial; however, most investigators attempt to reduce the gradient to approximately 10 mm Hg (this is based on retrospective data analysis in patients with portal hypertension undergoing surgically created portosystemic shunts).
- In such patients, the relationship between the presence of bleeding esophageal varices and the portal-hepatic vein gradient was evaluated.
- When the indication for the TIPS procedure is active bleeding from esophageal varices, the left gastric vein (i.e., coronary vein) may be occluded using transcatheter embolotherapy techniques.
- Gelfoam, Gianturco occlusion spring coils, and/or sclerosing agents may be used to occlude the left gastric (coronary) vein and its varicoid tributaries.
- After the TIPS procedure, the patient is observed in the recovery room for any signs of intraperitoneal hemorrhage, and so on.
- These patients are usually transferred to a "monitored bed".

Conclusion

- The application of TIPS in a patient with chronic Budd–Chiari syndrome provides perhaps the greatest technical challenge.
- In such patients often there is occluded small hepatic vein orifice to attempt placement of the shunt.
- The shunt itself is long, and multiple stents are overlapped. In such patients, extreme care must be taken to avoid placing stents into the right atrium or too far into the portal vein.
- As further experience accumulates, the TIPS procedure plays an increasing role in the management of patients with portal hypertension.
- Although restenosis and shunt thrombosis continue to be problematic.

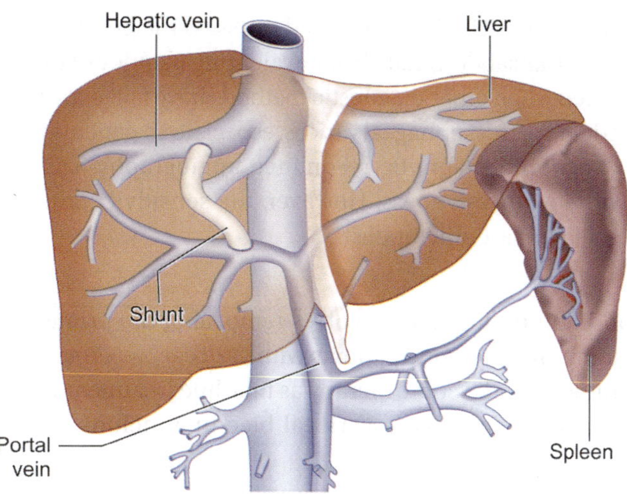

Schematic diagram of TIPS.

15. What do you mean by sectoral portal hypertension? Discuss the etiology, diagnosis, and management of sectoral portal hypertension. ***WBUHS 2021 Supplementary***

Introduction

- Sectoral portal hypertension (SPH), also known as left-sided portal hypertension or Sinistral portal hypertension or segmental portal hypertension, is a rare cause of upper gastrointestinal hemorrhage.
- The main feature of SPH is gastric variceal hemorrhage due to splenic vein thrombosis or occlusion.

Etiology

- Chronic pancreatitis
- Acute severe pancreatitis
- Pancreatic carcinoma
- Pancreatic surgery
- Arteriovenous malformation

Diagnosis

Clinical Features

- Sinistral portal hypertension is most commonly found incidentally in asymptomatic patients.
- In symptomatic patients, the most common presentation (although rare) is gastrointestinal bleeding from esophageal or gastric varices.
- Splenomegaly is common (~70%).
- Cirrhosis and ascites are not common presenting features.

The diagnosis of sinistral portal hypertension should be considered in all those with upper gastrointestinal bleeding associated with splenomegaly and normal liver function tests (LFT).

Investigations

- While diagnosis is mainly clinical and often made by exclusion of systemic portal hypertension, diagnostic imaging plays an important role in confirming the diagnosis in the majority of cases.
- *Angiography of splenic vein* remains the *gold standard* in diagnosing sinistral portal hypertension, although it is less used today by the availability of less invasive methods.
- Transabdominal US with Doppler is often the initial imaging modality utilized, but it is more helpful in excluding presence of systemic portal hypertension and its primary etiologies such as liver cirrhosis.
- The accuracy of transabdominal US is limited in detecting splenic or SMVs thrombosis, which are smaller and more subtle than those of portal veins.

- Recently, endoscopic ultrasound (EUS) has been used to assess the portal vasculature. This method appears to be a more accurate test than transabdominal US for evaluating patency of the splenic vein.
  - EUS should be considered when other diagnostic methods have failed to confirm splenic vein thrombosis as a cause of bleeding gastric or gastroesophageal varices, especially in patients with previous history of pancreatitis.
- Contrast-enhanced CT scan and magnetic resonance angiography are gaining popularity due to faster acquisition of images with low invasiveness. However, the sensitivity and specificity for detection of minor alterations of splenic vasculature are still modest.

Management

- Management of this condition traditionally involves removal of the primary cause if possible, which can be combined with splenectomy. Symptomatic patients with variceal bleeding may be severe and life threatening.
- Current guidelines recommend endoscopic therapy as first-line treatment for bleeding gastric varices.
- Endoscopic therapeutic options for gastric variceal bleeding include band ligation, cyanoacrylate (CYA) injection, and thrombin.
- A patient with active bleeding unresponsive to conservative management should be submitted to an emergent splenectomy, which decreases the venous outflow through the collateral circulation and decompresses the associated varices.
- Embolization of the splenic artery by selective catheterization has been tried with varying success and should be an option in patients who are not medically fit for a splenectomy procedure, depending on local expertise.
- Management of asymptomatic patients is more controversial than the symptomatic ones: splenectomy has been suggested as a prophylactic measure by some while others have not shown any significant benefit of this procedure in survival.
- However, more evidence suggests that watchful waiting as acceptable course of management in asymptomatic individuals.

16. Gastric varices. *WBUHS 2008*

Introduction

Gastric varices are dilated submucosal veins in the stomach, which can be a life-threatening cause of upper gastrointestinal hemorrhage.

Causes

- They are most commonly found in patients with portal hypertension, or elevated pressure in the PV system, which may be a complication of cirrhosis.
- Gastric varices may also be found in patients with thrombosis of the splenic vein, into which the short gastric veins which drain the fundus of the stomach flow.
- The latter may be a complication of acute pancreatitis, pancreatic cancer, or other abdominal tumors.
- In very rare cases, gastric varices are caused by splenic vein occlusion as a result of the mass effect of slow-growing pancreatic neuroendocrine tumors.

Clinical Features

Gastric varices can present in two major ways.

First

- Patients with cirrhosis may be enrolled in screening gastroscopy programs to detect esophageal varices.
- These evaluations may detect gastric varices that are asymptomatic.
- When gastric varices are symptomatic, however, they usually present acutely and dramatically with upper GI hemorrhage.
- The symptoms can include hematemesis, or vomiting blood; melena, passing black, and tarry stools; or passing maroon stools or frank blood in the stools.
- Many patients with bleeding gastric varices present in shock due to the profound loss of blood.

Secondly

- Patients with acute pancreatitis may present with gastric varices as a complication of thrombosis of the splenic vein.
- The splenic vein sits over the pancreas anatomically and inflammation or cancers of the pancreas may result in thrombosis, or clotting of the splenic vein.
- As the short gastric veins of the fundus of the stomach drain into the splenic vein, thrombosis of the splenic vein will result in increased pressure and engorgement of the short veins, leading to varices in the fundus of the stomach.

Investigations

- Laboratory testing usually shows anemia and often thrombocytopenia.
- If cirrhosis is present, there may be coagulopathy manifested by a prolonged INR.
- Both of these may worsen the hemorrhage from gastric varices.
- The *Sarin classification* of gastric varices identifies two types of *gastroesophageal varices*, where esophageal varices are found concurrently, and two types of *isolated gastric varices*, found in the absence of esophageal varices.
- Antral varices, of Sarin classification IGV-2, an unusual class of *gastric varices.*
- Diagnosis of gastric varices is often made at the time of upper endoscopy.

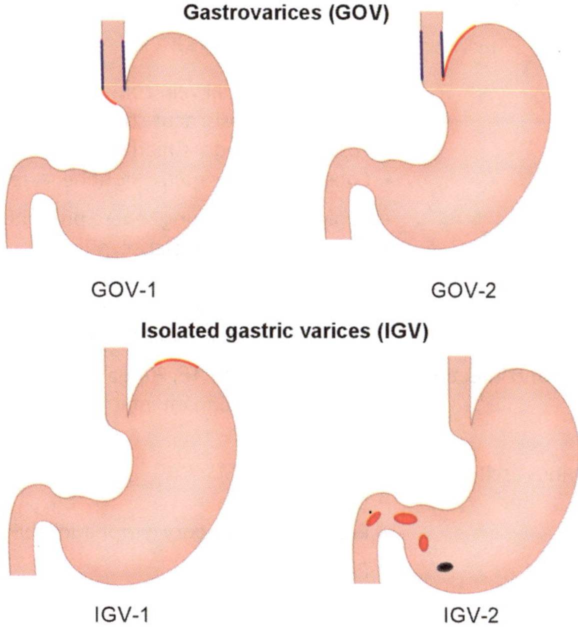

Treatment

- Initial treatment of bleeding from gastric varices focuses on resuscitation, much as with esophageal varices. This includes administration of fluids, blood products, and antibiotics.
- Treatment of gastric varices can include injection of the varices with CYA glue, or a radiological procedure to decrease the pressure in the portal vein, termed transjugular intrahepatic portosystemic shunt or TIPS.
- Treatment with intravenous octreotide is also useful to shunt blood flow away from the stomach's circulation. More aggressive treatment including splenectomy (or surgical removal of the spleen) or liver transplantation may be required in some cases.

Treatment for Refractory Bleeding

- Endoscopic band ligation
- Cyanoacrylate glue

Other techniques for refractory bleeding include:
- Transjugular intrahepatic portosystemic shunts
- Balloon-occluded retrograde transvenous obliteration techniques (BORTO)
- Gastric variceal ligation, although this modality is falling out of favor.
- Intragastric balloon tamponade as a bridge to further therapy: A caveat is that a larger balloon is required to occupy the fundus of the stomach where gastric varices commonly occur.
- Liver transplantation

17. What are the current perspectives in surgical treatment of ascites? ***WBUHS 2019***

Introduction

Ascites is a pathological accumulation of fluid in the peritoneal cavity. Liver cirrhosis (75%) is the most common cause of ascites in adults in the Western World, followed by malignancy (10%), heart failure (3%), tuberculosis (2%), and pancreatitis (1%). An adequate diagnosis is necessary for successful treatment.

Ascites can be classified as:
- *Mild ascites:* Detectable only by US (grade 1)
- *Moderate ascites:* Evident by moderate symmetrical distension of the abdomen (grade 2)
- *Gross or large ascites:* Marked abdominal distension (grade 3)

Pathophysiological mechanism	***Cause of ascites***
Increased portal venous pressure	• *Prehepatic:* Portal vein compression or thrombosis; schistosomiasis • *Hepatic:* Cirrhosis; acute hepatic necrosis; viral hepatitis • *Posthepatic:* Budd–Chiari syndrome; myeloproliferative disorders • *Constrictive pericarditis:* Right heart failure; hypercoagulable state
Hypoproteinemia	• Renal disease causing severe proteinuria • Malnutrition and malabsorption • Protein loosing enteropathy • Acute or chronic liver disease • Severe acute or chronic illness
Chronic peritoneal inflammation and infection	• *Chronic infection:* TB, Fungal infection • Secondary malignant infiltration (carcinomatosis peritonei) • Postirradiation
Leakage of lymphatic fluid (chylous ascites)	• Congenital • Surgical trauma • Primary or secondary lymphatic malignancy
Other fluids	• Pancreatic ascites • Biliary ascites • Urinary ascites

Diagnostic Workup
- *History:* Information about the medical history, medication use, lifestyle, risk factors for liver disease, and infectious disease risk (e.g., migration) are relevant to discover the underlying etiology.
- *Physical examination:*
  - A screening physical examination should be carried out in every patient with awareness of signs of liver disease (erythema palmar, spider naevi, and splenomegaly), heart failure (peripheral edema, jugular venous distension, third heart sound, and pulmonary rales), and malignancy (lymphadenopathy).
  - Flank dullness is found when approximately 1,500 mL of ascites is present.
  - Shifting dullness is determined by a 3-cm flank dullness shift when the patient changes from a supine to a lateral decubitus position.
  - Detection of a fluid wave or puddle sign is less reliable.

- *Blood tests:* Assessment of complete blood cell count, serum creatinine, urea, electrolytes, PT, and LFT is recommended.
- *Abdominal US:* Abdominal US is the first-line imaging method to confirm the presence and quantity of ascites. It can also provide crucial information about the cause of ascites, detect signs of portal hypertension (splenomegaly and portosystemic collaterals) and offer guidance during paracentesis.
- *Abdominal paracentesis and ascitic fluid analysis:* It is the most important step in the diagnostic work-up.
  - *Visual inspection:* It can show a milky, cloudy, bloody, straw colored, or clear appearance. The first impression of the appearance of ascites can steer the direction of diagnosis.
  - *Serum ascites albumin gradient (SAAG):* It is the most sensitive marker to distinguish between ascites due to portal hypertension/hepatic congestion and other causes.
    - A value of ≥1.1 g/dL indicates underlying portal hypertension/hepatic congestion.
    - A value <1.1g/dL indicates etiologies not due to portal hypertension, such as malignancy, pancreatitis, or infection.
  - *Amylase:* The amylase concentration in ascetic fluid should be measured in particular when pancreatic disease is considered. An amylase ascetic fluid/blood serum concentration of 6.0 is indicative for pancreatic disease, considering that a ratio of 0.4 is normal in nonpancreatic ascites.
  - *Triglycerides:* A concentration of triglycerides in the ascitic fluid that exceeds the blood serum level (2.2 mmol/L) indicates chylous ascites; seen mainly in previous abdominal surgery, pancreatitis, trauma, and retroperitoneal lymphoma.
  - *Adenosine deaminase activity (ADA):* It is a reliable marker to differentiate tuberculous ascites from other etiologies. An ADA cut-off value 36–40 IU/L has a high sensitivity (100%) and specificity (97%) for diagnosing abdominal tuberculosis.
  - *Glucose and lactate dehydrogenase:*
    - A lower glucose concentration in ascitic fluid can indicate the presence of bacteria, white blood cells, or cancer cells.
    - A low level of LDH is associated with nonmalignant ascites, high levels suggest a malignant etiology.
  - *Urea and creatinine:* A very uncommon cause of ascites is urinary leakage into the peritoneal cavity. The ascites/plasma creatinine ratio of five is reported in case of urinary ascites.
  - *Polymorphonuclear (PMN) leukocyte count:* A count ≥250 cells/mm^3 confirms the diagnosis of SBP (spontaneous bacterial peritonitis) in the absence of an evident intra-abdominal source of infection. A repeat PMN count 48 hours after antibiotic therapy is recommended to document the efficacy of anti- biotic for SBP; with a decrease suggests SBP and a sustained increase secondary bacterial peritonitis.
  - *Bacterial cultures:* Ascitic fluid should be cultured if SBP is clinically suspected.
  - *Polymerase chain reaction (PCR):* Bacterial DNA of *Mycobacterium tuberculosis* in ascitic fluid can be detected using PCR and can be performed when tuberculous ascites is suspected.
  - *Cytology:* Ascitic fluid cytology should be performed in case of suspicion of malignant ascites or when underlying etiology is in doubt. Positive cytology is highly indicative for peritoneal carcinomatosis (PC).
  - *Diagnostic laparoscopy:*
    - Laparoscopy offers the advantages of visual inspection of the peritoneal cavity in combination with the ability to obtain targeted biopsies for histological and microbiological studies.
    - The procedure may be particularly helpful to diagnose PC, tuberculous peritonitis, and other peritoneal or omental diseases such as mesothelioma and sclerosing peritonitis.

Role of Surgical Therapy in Intractable Ascites

When large-volume paracentesis fails to relieve ascites, patients may be submitted to one of the three following surgical options:

1. Portosystemic shunting
2. Peritoneovenous shunting
3. Liver transplantation

Portosystemic Shunting

- Portosystemic shunting is efficient in clearing ascites, but it is associated with a high rate of encephalopathy or hepatorenal syndrome and liver failure.
- The indications for portosystemic shunting are therefore limited for intractable ascites due to portal hypertension and should be performed only in patient with good liver function in whom all other treatments failed.
- The techniques used are TIPS, Lienorenal shunt (Splenic and renal vein anastomosis) or Portocaval shunt (PV and IVC anastomosis).

Peritoneovenous Shunting

- This is a megalymphatic shunt that returns the ascitic fluid to the central venous system.
- Peritoneovenous shunting is a good procedure and may provide definitive relief of ascites and long-term survival in >50% of the operated patients.
- Commonly used shunts are Denver shunt, LeVeen shunt, both have one way valve situated in the middle.
- Beneficial effects of these shunts include increased cardiac output, renal blood flow, glomerular filtration rate, urinary volume and sodium excretion, and decreased plasma renin activity and plasma aldosterone concentration.
- The AASLD suggests considering peritoneovenous shunting for patients with refractory ascites who are not candidate for paracentesis, transplant or TIPS (class I, level A recommendation).
- Peritoneovenous shunting should not be done when there's history of severe liver failure, SBP, or variceal bleeding.
- Long-term complications include occlusion of the PVS (particularly with bloody or highly proteinaceous or mucoid ascites), SVC thrombosis, bacteremia, and shunt infection, which may lead to subacute bacterial endocarditis (SABE).

Liver Transplantation

The AASLD recommends that patient with cirrhosis and ascites be considered for liver transplantation (class I, level B recommendation).

Special Situations

Malignant Ascites

- It is defined as an accumulation of excess fluid in the peritoneal cavity secondary to a disseminated malignancy.
- It is an ominous sign with an average survival of around 20 weeks from its diagnosis.
- Ovarian malignancy is the most common cause (37%), followed by pancreatobiliary (21%) and gastric malignancy (18%).
- Around 20% patients have unknown primary malignancy.

Pathophysiology

- It is multifactorial, originating from an imbalance between fluid secretion and absorption by peritoneum.
- This is secondary to increased fluid production by tumor cells lining peritoneal cavity in cases of PC
- Alteration in vascular permeability, release of inflammatory cytokines and decreased lymphatic drainage due to tumor involvement and increased portal pressure due to tumor metastasis.
- Obstruction of lymphatics is believed to be the main pathogenic mechanism for malignant ascites.
- Role of matrix metalloproteinase-9 has also been implicated in the pathophysiology of malignant ascites.

Management

- The aim of management is to provide symptomatic relief and specific treatment of the primary pathology.
- Diagnostic laparoscopy and tissue sampling may be utilized to confirm the diagnosis.
- Management options include the conventional methods discussed earlier and newer modalities.
- Newer modalities:

These includes

- Cytoreductive surgery (CRS)
- Hyperthermic intraperitoneal chemotherapy (HIPEC)

- Intraperitoneal instillation of OK-432 (a preparation from *Streptococcus pyogenes*)
- Metalloproteinase inhibitors like Batimastat
- Anti-VEGF therapies such as bevacizumab

These newer modalities of treatment have ongoing trials, without definitive results.

18. Intractable ascites. ***Ayush University, Chhattisgarh 2025***

Intractable ascites (also called *refractory ascites*) refers to *ascites that cannot be mobilized or controlled* adequately with medical therapy (like salt restriction and diuretics). It is a *complication of advanced liver disease*, especially *decompensated cirrhosis*.

Definition (per International Ascites Club)

Refractory ascites is defined as *ascites that cannot be mobilized or that recurs early after therapeutic paracentesis, despite:*

- Sodium restriction
- Maximal diuretic therapy

It's divided into two types:

Type	*Description*
Diuretic-resistant ascites	No response to maximum tolerated diuretic doses
Diuretic-intractable ascites	Diuretics had to be stopped due to complications (e.g., renal failure, electrolyte imbalance)

Causes/Underlying Conditions

- Cirrhosis (most common)
- Portal hypertension
- Hepatorenal syndrome
- Splanchnic vasodilation and RAAS activation

Other less common causes include:

- Malignancy
- Tuberculosis
- Pancreatic disease
- Heart failure

Clinical Features

- Progressive abdominal distension
- Shortness of breath
- Early satiety, nausea
- Weight gain
- Scrotal/labial edema
- Poor response to diuretics

Diagnosis

- *Clinical:*
    - Failure to mobilize ascites despite:
        - Sodium restriction (<2 g/day)
        - Diuretics (Spironolactone up to 400 mg + Furosemide up to 160 mg/day)
- *Imaging:* Abdominal ultrasound (assess fluid, liver size, portal vein flow)
- *Paracentesis:*
    - Diagnostic tap to rule out spontaneous bacterial peritonitis (SBP)
    - Serum-ascites albumin gradient (SAAG) to confirm portal hypertension

Management

- General measures
  - *Salt restriction*
  - *Fluid restriction* (if hyponatremia)
- Serial large-volume paracentesis (LVP)
  - Typically removes ≥5 L
  - *Must give IV albumin* (usually 6–8 g/L of fluid removed) to prevent circulatory dysfunction
- *Midodrine:* An alpha-agonist that improves blood pressure and renal perfusion in cirrhotic patients
- Transjugular intrahepatic portosystemic shunt (TIPS)
  - *Creates a shunt between portal and hepatic veins*
  - Decreases portal pressure
  - *Effective in selected patients* but risk of *hepatic encephalopathy*
- *Liver transplantation:* Definitive treatment if the patient is eligible
- *Avoid nephrotoxic drugs:* NSAIDs, aminoglycosides, etc.

GASTROINTESTINAL HEMORRHAGE

19. Enumerate the causes of upper gastrointestinal tract bleeding. How do you evaluate such a patient coming to the emergency? Outline the management of a case due to portal hypertension. ***WBUHS 2009***

Common causes of upper gastrointestinal hemorrhage.

Nonvariceal bleeding	***(80%)***	***Portal hypertensive bleeding***	***(20%)***
Peptic ulcer disease	30–50%	Gastroesophageal varices	>90%
Mallory–Weiss tears	15–20%	Hypertensive portal gastropathy	<5%
Gastritis or duodenitis	10–15%	Isolated gastric varices	Rare
Esophagitis	5–10%		
Arteriovenous malformations	5%		
Tumors	2%		
Other	5%		

General Approach to the Patient with Acute GI Hemorrhage

Initial Management

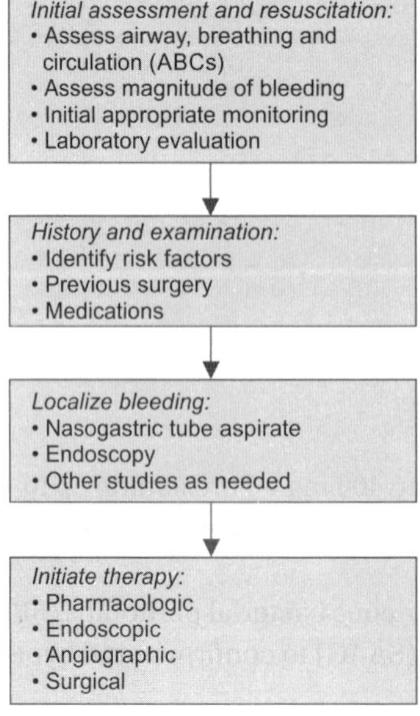

Risk Factors for Morbidity and Mortality in Acute Gastrointestinal Hemorrhage

Age	Comorbid disease	Magnitude of hemorrhage	Transfusion requirement
>60 years	• Renal failure • Liver disease • Respiratory insufficiency • Cardiac disease	• Systolic blood pressure • <100 mm Hg on presentation	• Persistent or recurrent hemorrhage • Onset of hemorrhage during hospitalization • Need for surgery

Algorithm of Management after Initial Resuscitation

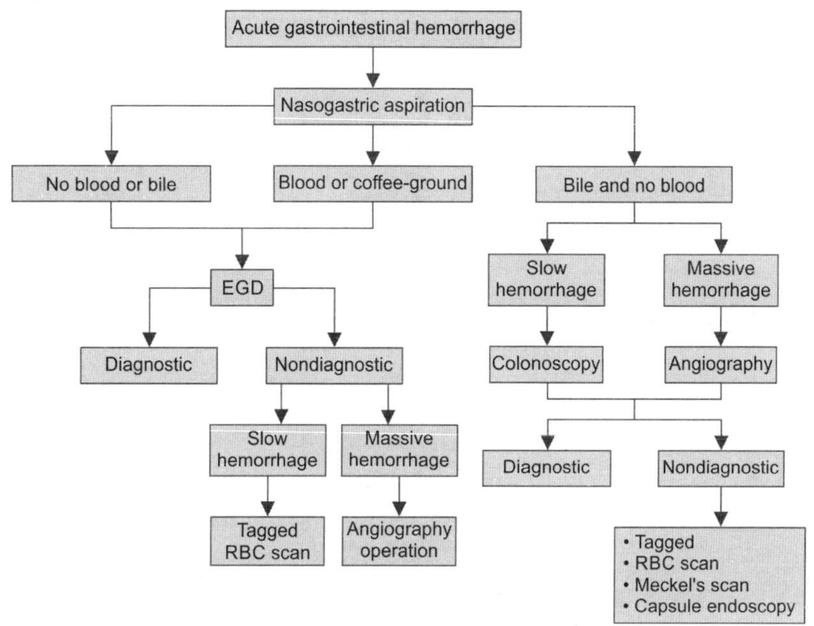

(EGD: esophagogastroduodenoscopy; RBC: red blood cell)

Algorithm for the Diagnosis and Management of Nonvariceal Upper GI Bleeding

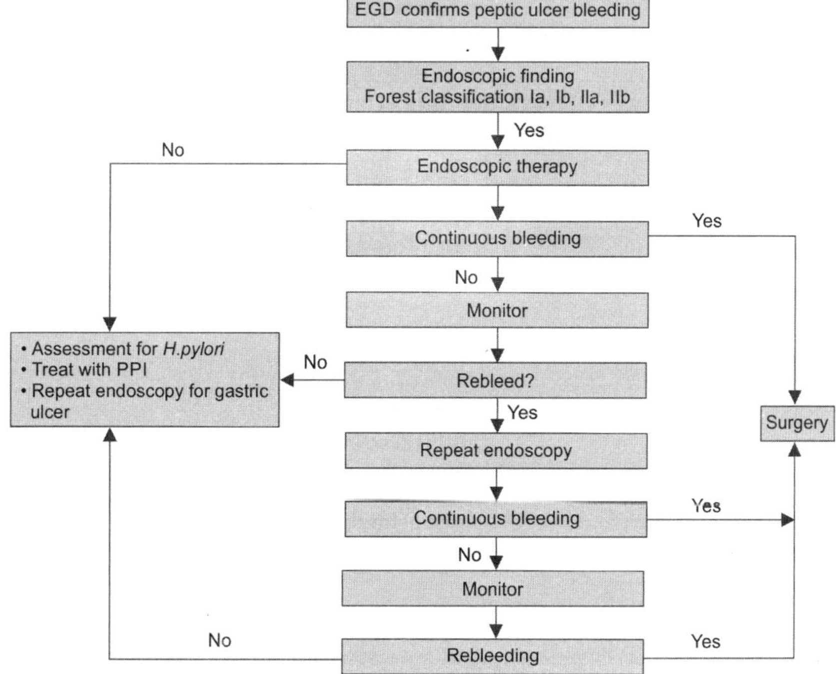

(EGD: esophagogastroduodenoscopy; PPI: proton pump inhibitor)

Indications for Surgery in Gastrointestinal Hemorrhage

- Hemodynamic instability despite vigorous resuscitation (>6 units transfusion)
- Failure of endoscopic techniques to arrest hemorrhage
- Recurrent hemorrhage after initial stabilization (with up to two attempts at obtaining endoscopic hemostasis)
- Shock associated with recurrent hemorrhage
- Continued slow bleeding with a transfusion requirement exceeding 3 units/day.

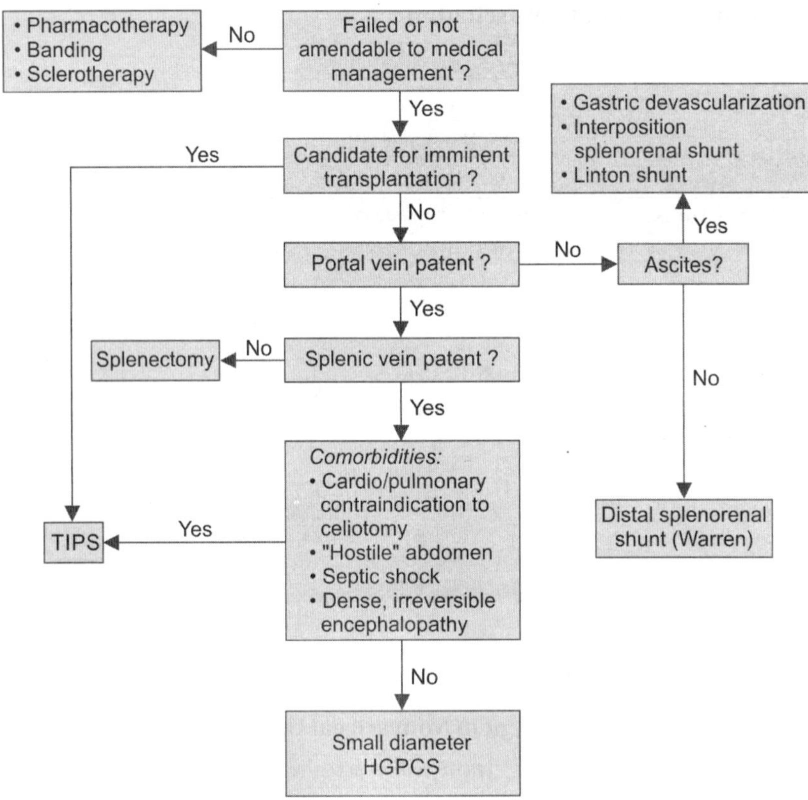

20. What are the common causes of lower GI tract bleeding? Describe in brief how will you investigate and manage a patient with acute lower GI tract bleeding?

Common Causes of lower GI Bleeding

Colonic bleeding (95%)	*Small bowel bleeding (5%)*
Diverticular disease	Angiodysplasias
Ischemia	Erosions or ulcers (potassium, NSAIDs)
Anorectal disease	Crohn's disease
Neoplasia	Radiation
Infectious colitis	Meckel's diverticulum
Postpolypectomy	Neoplasia
Inflammatory bowel disease	Aortoenteric fistula
Angiodysplasia	
Radiation colitis/proctitis	
Other	
Unknown	

Algorithm for Diagnosis and Management of Lower GI Hemorrhage

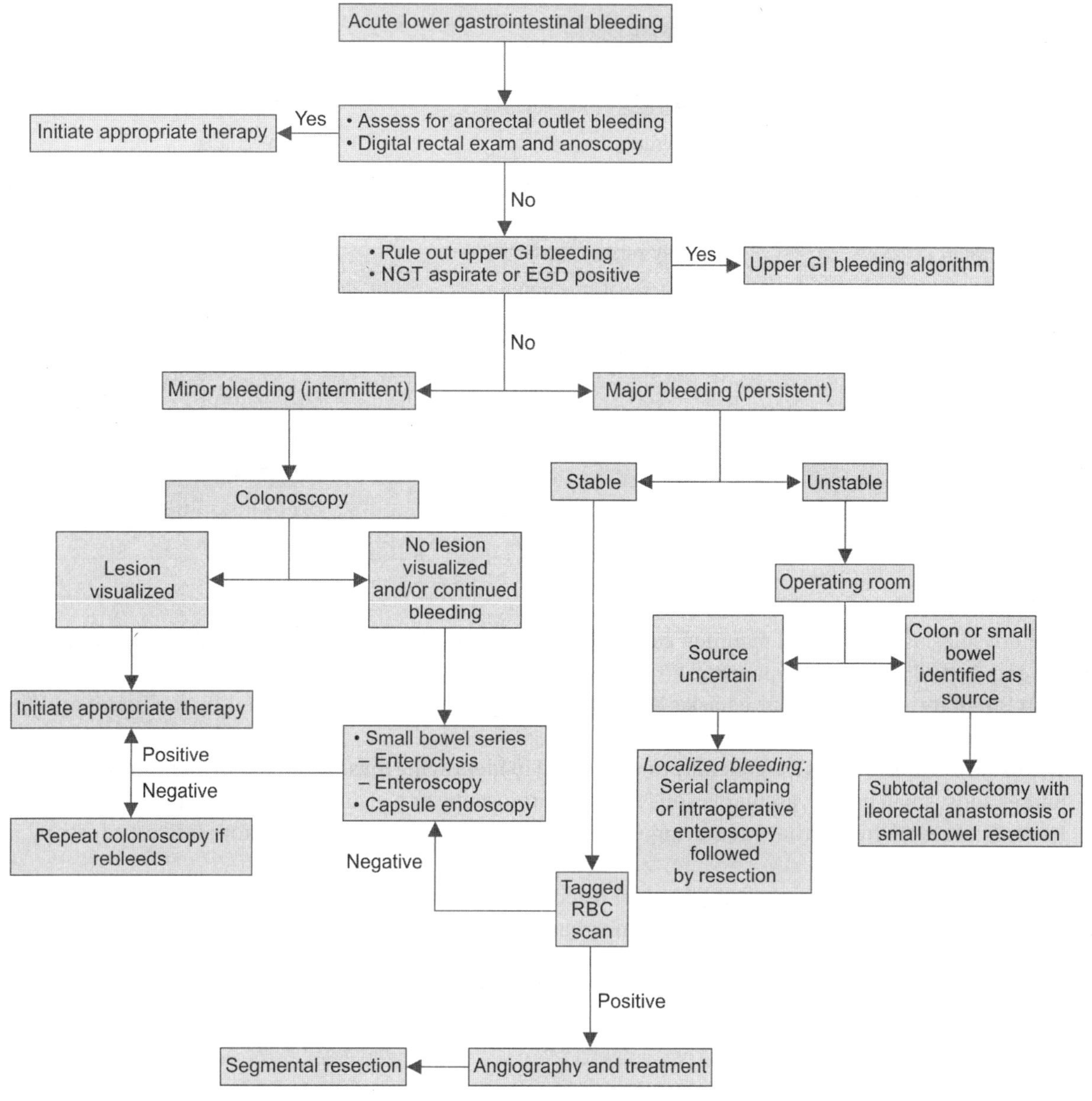

(EGD: esophagogastroduodenoscopy; NGT: nasogastric tube; RBC: red blood cell)

21. Define obscure GI hemorrhage. Discuss briefly the various causes and the investigations required to evaluate obscure GI hemorrhage. ***WBUHS 2022***

22. Presentation and management of obscure GI bleed. ***WBUHS 2021 Supplementary***

23. Describe the management of obscure GI hemorrhage. ***WBUHS 2022***

Introduction

- Obscure gastrointestinal bleeding (OGIB) is defined as recurrent or persistent gastrointestinal bleeding from a source that cannot be identified using upper or lower endoscopy, and is associated with a so-called "gastrointestinal disease of unknown cause.
- Obscure bleeding can be further subdivided into obscure-occult or obscure-overt bleeding.

Differential Diagnosis of Obscure Gastrointestinal Bleeding

Upper GI	Small bowel	Colon
Angiodysplasia	Crohn's disease	Colitis
Peptic ulcer disease	Meckel's diverticulum	Ulcerative colitis
Aortoenteric fistula	Lymphoma	Crohn's colitis
Neoplasia	Radiation enteritis	Ischemic colitis
HIV-related causes	Ischemia	Radiation colitis
Dieulafoy's lesion	HIV-related causes	Infections colitis
Lymphoma	Bacterial infection	Solitary rectal ulcer
Sarcoidosis	Metastatic disease	Amyloidosis
Hemobilia	Angiodysplasia	Lymphoma
Hemosuccus pancreaticus		Endometriosis
GAVE		Angiodysplasia
Metastatic cancer		Neoplasia
		HIV-related causes
		Hemorrhoids

Angiodysplasias

- Angiodysplasias are the most common cause of small intestinal bleeding, accounting for 40% of cases in elderly patients and 10% in younger patients.
- Most small intestinal vascular ectasias appear to occur in the jejunum, followed by the ileum and then the duodenum.
- The usual diagnostic tools are generally unsuccessful in identifying these lesions. Angiography is rarely positive.
- Rather, most small bowel vascular lesions require enteroscopy or capsule endoscopy for identification.
- In cases of severe hemorrhage requiring emergent operative intervention, intraoperative endoscopy may be helpful.
- Endoscope-directed segmental small bowel resection is the treatment of choice. Occasionally, these lesions are diffuse; this may occur in hereditary hemorrhagic telangiectasia (Osler–Weber–Rendu disease), acute renal failure, or von Willebrand's disease.
- In this situation, there has been limited experience with estrogen and progesterone treatment but some studies suggest that these agents may be of benefit.

Neoplasia

- Small bowel tumors are not very common but can be sources of occult or overt GI bleeding. Bleeding typically results from erosion of the mucosa overlying the tumor. GISTs have the greatest propensity for bleeding.
- Small bowel tumors are typically diagnosed by small bowel contrast series or spiral CT scan. Treatment involves surgical resection.

Crohn's Disease

- Patients with Crohn's disease may also present with small bowel bleeding in association with terminal ileitis.
- Bleeding is not generally significant, nor is it usually the only presenting symptom.
- Diagnosis is established by small bowel contrast series, and initial treatment is medical.

Meckel's Diverticulum

- Meckel's diverticulum is a true diverticulum in that it contains all layers of the small bowel wall.
- It is a congenital remnant of the omphalomesenteric duct, occurring in about 2% of the general population.
- Often, heterotopic tissue is present at the base of the diverticulum.

- Bleeding from Meckel's diverticulum is usually from an ulcerative lesion on the ileal wall opposite the diverticulum, caused by acid production by ectopic gastric mucosa.
- If nuclear medicine imaging is negative and bleeding is relatively brisk, angiography may be helpful in the diagnosis.
- Surgical management usually requires a segmental resection incorporating the opposing ileal mucosa, which is typically the site of bleeding.
- *Gastric antral vascular ectasia (GAVE) syndrome,* also known as watermelon stomach, is a significant cause of acute or chronic gastrointestinal blood loss in the elderly. It is characterized endoscopically by "watermelon stripes". Without cirrhosis, patients are 71% female, average age 73, presenting with occult blood loss leading to transfusion-dependent chronic iron-deficiency anemia, severe acute upper gastrointestinal bleeding, and nondescript abdominal pain.

Investigations

Repeat Endoscopy

- The cause of obscure-overt bleeding is often a common lesion that is missed on initial evaluation.
- Repeat upper and lower endoscopy is a valuable tool in identifying missed lesions because up to 35% of patients have the bleeding source identified on second-look endoscopy.
- When repeat endoscopy fails to identify an obscure-overt bleeding source, investigation of the small bowel is warranted.

Conventional Imaging

The next step is probably a tagged RBC scan, although its utility in this setting has not been established, and as discussed previously, it may be misleading.

Tc99-labeled RBC Scan

- It can detect GI bleeding at a rate of >0.1–0.4 mL/min
- Useful in patients with active bleeding
- *Limitations:*
  - Low accuracy in localization
  - Misinterpretation if done after a while bleeding stopped (blood pools down)

Angiography

- It may be more useful but usually requires significant ongoing hemorrhage.
- It can detect both acutely bleeding and nonbleeding lesions, particularly angioectasias.
- Potential to detect bleeding at a rate of >0.5 mL/min
- Successful localization:
  - *With active bleeding:* 50–75%
  - *With cessation of bleeding:* <50%
- Ability to perform therapeutic embolization with use of gelfoam and coils

Small Bowel Enteroscopy

- Small bowel enteroclysis, which uses a tube to infuse barium, methylcellulose, and air directly into the small bowel, provides better imaging than simple small bowel follow-through.
- It is now rarely used. It can identify gross lesions such as small bowel tumors, inflammatory conditions such as Crohn's disease, and small bowel ulcerations.
- The limitation of small bowel radiography is that it cannot visualize angiodysplasias, the main cause of obscure small bowel hemorrhage.
- The hemodynamically stable patient undergoes small bowel enteroscopy. Usually performed with a pediatric colonoscope, this is referred to as *push endoscopy.* It can reach about 50–70 cm past the ligament of Treitz in most cases and permits endoscopic management of some lesions. Overall, push enteroscopy is successful in 40% of patients.

Endoscopic Evaluation

Push Enteroscopy

- Allows limited evaluation of the proximal small bowel, approximately 50–100 cm distal to the ligament of Treitz.
- The diagnostic yield between 3 and 70% with the majority being vascular lesions
- Largely limited to endoscopic therapy in patients with known proximal small bowel lesions

Sonde Enteroscopy

- Dependent on peristaltic propagation of the flexible enteroscope through the small intestine
- Very prolonged in duration
- No longer in practice

Intraoperative Enteroscopy (IOE)

- IOE involves the endoscopic evaluation of the small bowel by surgical assistance via laparotomy or laparoscopy.
- It can be performed orally, rectally, or via surgical enterotomy.
- Surgeon manually telescopes the bowel loops over the tip of the endoscope.

Double Balloon Enteroscopy (DBE)

- High-resolution video endoscope with latex balloons
- Serial inflation and deflation help in negotiation of the enteroscope.
- It can be introduced orally or per rectally.
- Other indications:
  - Unexplained chronic diarrhea
  - HPB pathologies

Single Balloon Enteroscopy

- Most recent balloon-assisted endoscopic technique
- Less procedure time compared with DBE
- Comparable diagnostic yield
- No major complications reported

Spiral Enteroscopy

- New technique of endoscopic evaluation of the small bowel
- Comparable with DBE

Video Capsule Endoscopy

- Capsule endoscopy uses a small capsule with a video camera that is swallowed and acquires video images as it passes through the GI tract.
- This modality permits visualization of the entire GI tract, but offers no interventional capability.
- It is also very time consuming because someone has to watch the video to identify the bleeding source, and then a means to deal with the pathology has to be developed.
- Despite this, capsule endoscopy is an excellent tool in the patient who is hemodynamically stable but continues to bleed.
- This technique has reported success rates as high as 90% in identifying small bowel pathology.
- It is usually well tolerated, although it is contraindicated in patients with obstruction or a motility disorder.

Intraoperative Endoscopy

Intraoperative enteroscopy is reserved for patients who have transfusion-dependent obscure-overt bleeding in whom an exhaustive search has failed to identify a bleeding source.

CT Enterography and CT Enteroclysis

- It can detect both vascular lesions and tumors.
- *Principles:* Ingestion of a large volume of contrastà luminal distensionà visualization of mucosal details and vasculature

- Diagnostic yield of 45%
- *Limitations:*
  - Inadequate bowel distention with oral contrast secondary to bowel obstruction
  - GI dysmotility
  - Patient intolerance
  - Renal insufficiency

CT Angiography (CTA)

- Involves catheterization of the abdominal aorta followed by helical CTA before and after intra-arterial injections of contrast medium.
- Site of hemorrhage→ hyperdense area because of extravasation of contrast medium into the intestinal lumen
- Preferred over CT enteroclysis if the patient is massively bleeding causing intolerance to oral contrast.
- *Sensitivity:* 70%, Specificity: 100%, PPV:100%

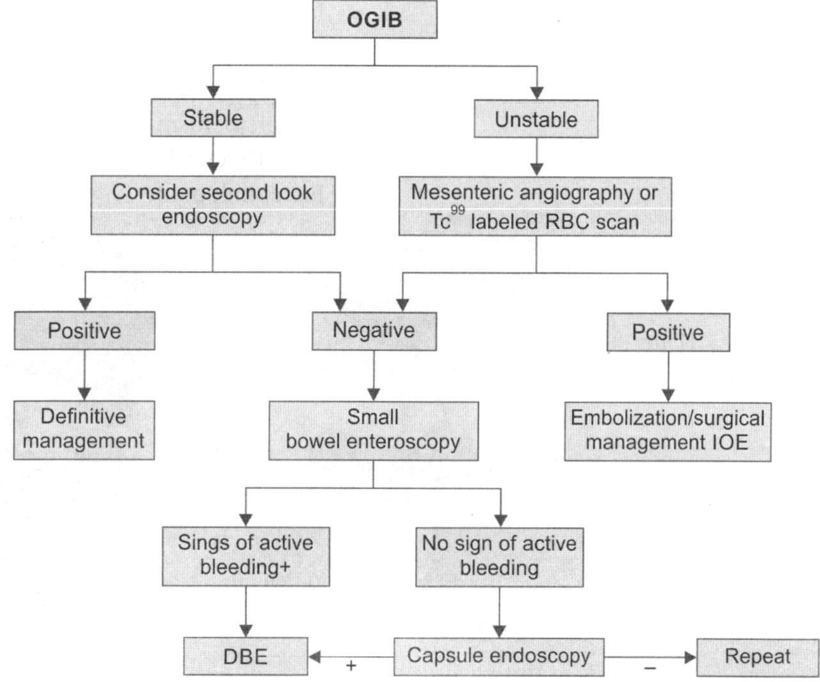

Pharmacotherapy

Indications

- When endoscopic therapy, surgical intervention, or angiographic therapy is not practical or is ineffective, or
- In patients in whom the source of bleeding is unknown or
- The pathology is too diffuse to be amenable to ablative therapy.

Other Options

- Hormonal therapy (estrogen with or without progesterone)—splanchnic vasoconstriction
- Somatostatin analogs-angioectasias and blue rubber bleb nevus syndrome
- Thalidomide-angioectasias and hereditary hemorrhagic telangiectasia
- Erythropoietin-chronic diffuse hemorrhage from GI mucosa by complex effect of erythropoietin on the platelet-subendothelial interactions and also on protein C, protein S, and antithrombin III levels
- von Willebrand factor

EHPVO AND PORTAL BILIOPATHY

24. What is extrahepatic portal venous obstruction (EHPVO)? Describe the clinical features and management of the same. ***WBUHS 2023***

Definition

- Obstruction of the extrahepatic PV with or without involvement of the intrahepatic PVS and does not include isolated thrombosis of SV or SMV
- PV thrombosis or portal hypertension with portal cavernoma formation as a sequel of PV obstruction

Clinical Features

- Variceal bleeding
- Gastroesophageal
- Gastric
- Rectal
- Ectopic
- Mass abdomen
- Pain abdomen
- Ascites
- Jaundice

Sequelae of EHPVO

- Portal biliopathy
- Ectopic varices
- Gastropathy and colopathy
- Hypersplenism
- Growth retardation
- Encephalopathy

Diagnosis

- Ultrasound
- UGI endoscopy
- Complete blood count (CBC) with bone marrow biopsy
- CT scan and MRA
- MRCP
- Liver biopsy

Management

- *Primary and secondary prophylaxis:*
  - Propranolol
  - EST
  - EVL
- *Medical management of variceal bleed:*
  - Vasopressin
  - Terlipressin
  - Somatostatin
- *Other intervention:*
  - Balloon tamponade
  - TIPS

Surgery

- Nonselective
- Selective Shunt
- Devascularization procedure

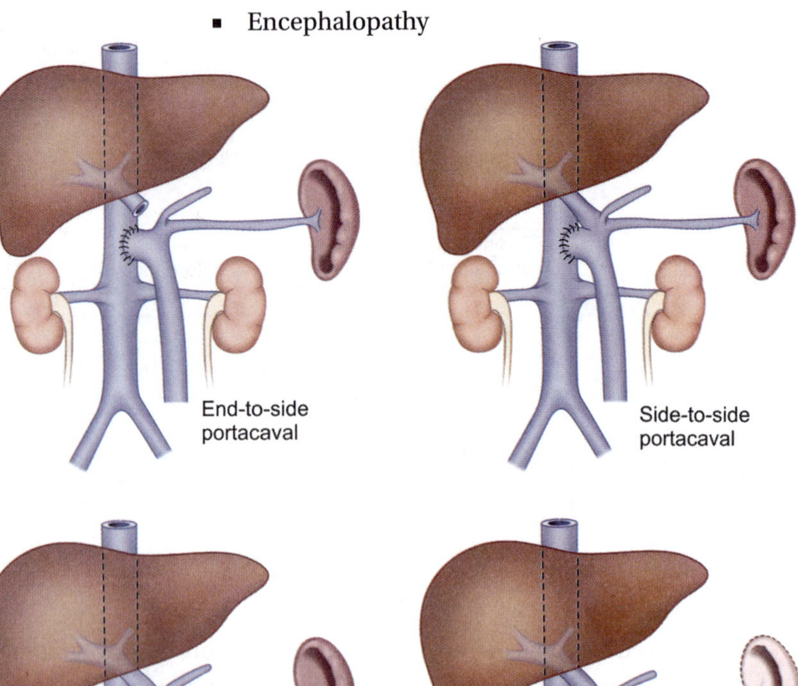

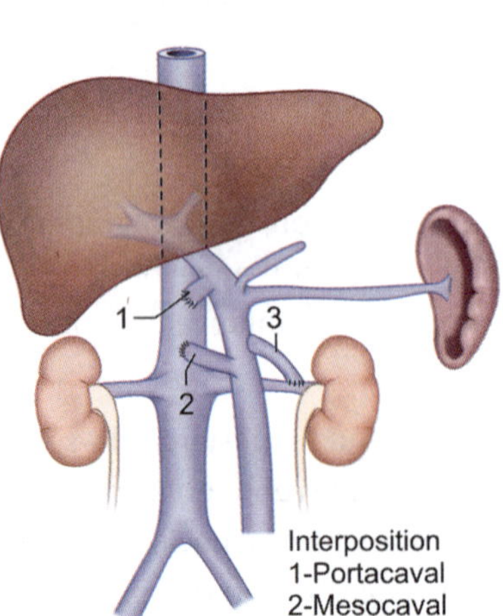

Algorithmic Approach for the Diagnosis of EHPVO and Management of Esophageal and Gastric Varices

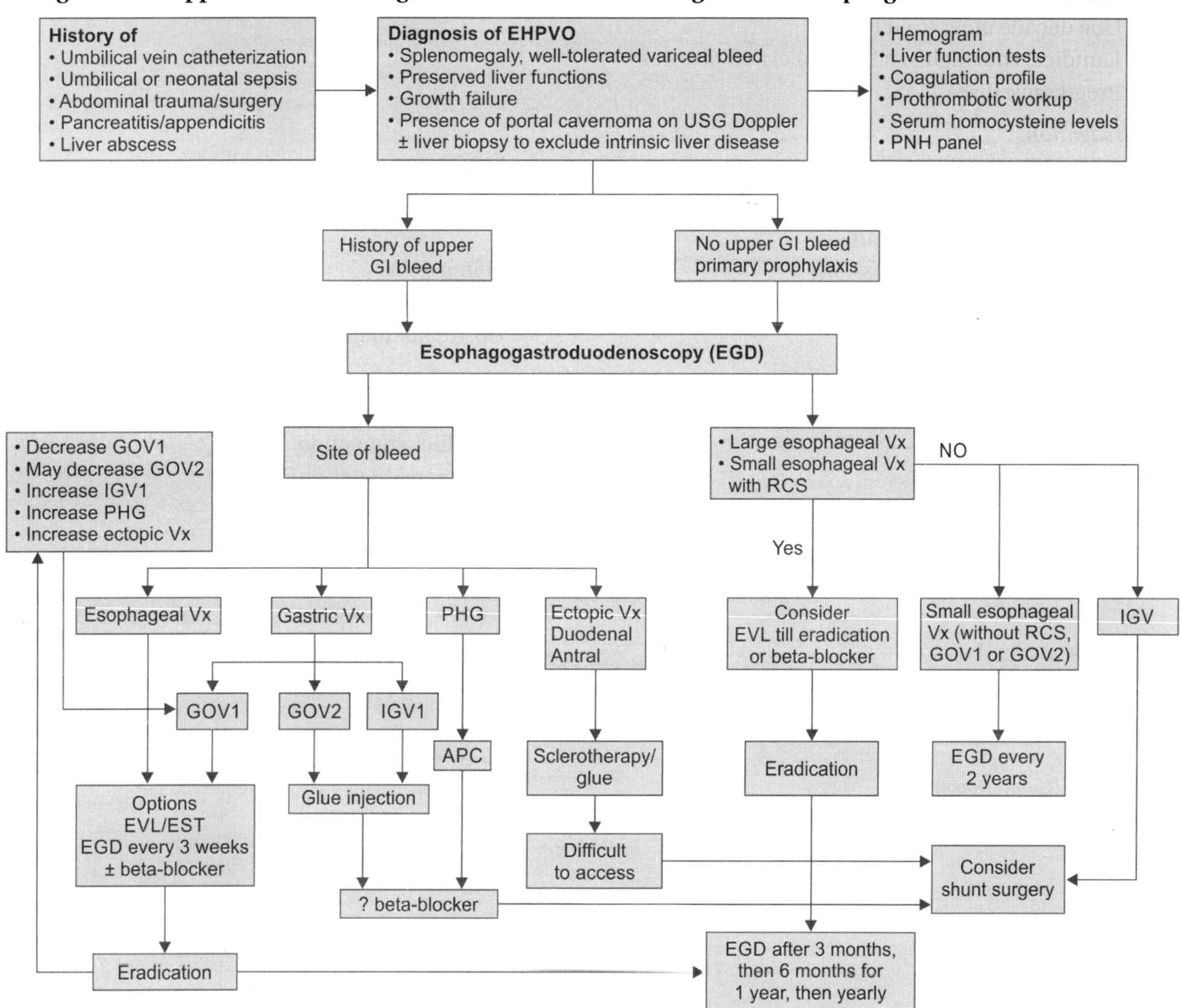

(APC: argon plasma coagulation; EST: endoscopic sclerotherapy; EVL: endoscopic variceal ligation; GOV: gastroesophageal varices; IGV: isolated gastric varices; PHG: portal hypertensive gastropathy; PNH: paroxysmal nocturnal hemoglobinuria; RCS: red color signs; Vx: varix)

25. Portal biliopathy.

Introduction

- Anomalies of intra and extrahepatic bile duct, gallbladder, and cystic duct secondary to portal hypertension
- Occurs in both EHPVO and NCPF (noncirrhotic portal fibrosis)
- *Prevalence:* 80–100%
- *Symptomatic:* 5–30%

Pathogenesis

- Compression theory
- Ischemic theory
- Infective theory
- Left hepatic duct (LHD): 100%, right hepatic duct (RHD): 56%, and common hepatic duct (CHD): 90%
- Secondary biliary cirrhosis

Clinical Features

- One decade older to GI bleed.
- Jaundice, cholangitis, biliary colic, and pruritus
- Progressive disease

Investigations

- CBC/LFT/PT/INR
- USG whole abdomen with color Doppler
- MRCP
- ERC/EUS

Cholangiographic Abnormalities

- Extrinsic/swallow impressions
- Irregular contour
- Stricture
- Filling defect
- Bile duct angulation
- Upstream dilatation

Differential Diagnosis

- Extrinsic/swallow impressions
- Irregular contour
- Stricture
- Filling defect
- Bile duct angulation
- Upstream dilatation

Management

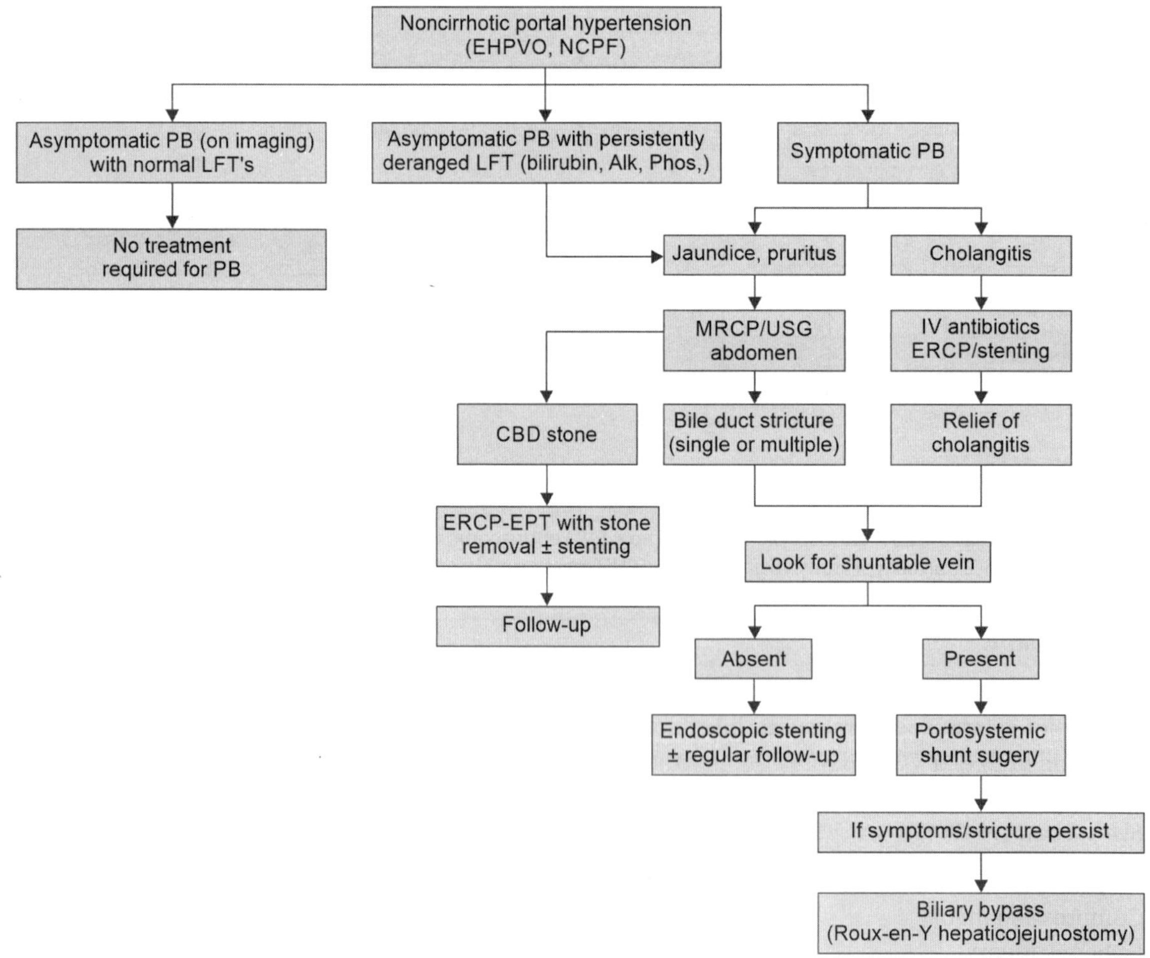

(MRCP: magnetic resonance cholangiopancreatography; NCPF: noncirrhotic portal fibrosis; ERCP: endoscopic retrograde cholangio- and pancreaticography; EPT: endoscopic papillotomy; CBD: common bile duct; EHPVO: extrahepatic portal venous obstruction; PB: portal biliopathy)

26. Left-sided portal hypertension.

Left-sided portal hypertension, also called *sinistral portal hypertension* or *segmental portal hypertension,* is a rare form of portal hypertension that affects *only the splenic vein* and its drainage system, rather than the entire portal venous system.

Definition

Left-sided portal hypertension is *elevated pressure in the splenic venous system* due to *splenic vein obstruction or thrombosis,* leading to increased pressure in the short gastric and gastroepiploic veins.

It does *not* affect the entire portal vein, so:

- *Liver function is typically normal*
- There is *no generalized portal hypertension*

Causes

The most common causes include:

- Pancreatitis (acute or chronic)
- Pancreatic tumors (adenocarcinoma, cystic neoplasms)
- Pancreatic pseudocysts
- Splenic vein thrombosis
- Abdominal trauma or surgery

Clinical Features

- Isolated gastric varices (in the fundus of the stomach)
- Upper GI bleeding (due to variceal rupture)
- Splenomegaly
- Hypersplenism (anemia, leukopenia, thrombocytopenia)

Esophageal varices are typically absent—unlike in generalized portal hypertension.

Diagnosis

- L*maging* is key:
  - *CT angiography or MRI*—shows splenic vein obstruction/thrombosis
  - *Doppler ultrasound*
- *Endoscopy*—reveals isolated gastric varices
- *Liver function tests*—usually normal

Management

- *Splenectomy* is often curative:
  - Removes the source of elevated pressure
  - Prevents further bleeding
- *Endoscopic variceal treatment* (e.g., cyanoacrylate glue for gastric varices) if bleeding
- *Anticoagulation*—in some cases of thrombosis (depending on bleeding risk)
- *Manage underlying cause* (e.g., pancreatitis, tumor resection)

CHAPTER 34

Hernia

LEARNING OBJECTIVES

- **Anterior Abdominal Wall**
- **Myopectineal Orifice of Fruchaud**
- **Newer Classification of Inguinal Hernia**
- **Sliding Hernia**
- **Femoral Hernia**
- **Spigelian Hernia**
- **Stoppa Repair of Abdominal Hernia**
- **Mesh in Hernia Surgery**
- **Biological Mesh and Composite Mesh**
- **Chronic Pain Following Mesh Repair of Inguinal Hernia**
- **Incisional Hernia and Component Separation Technique**

1. Describe the anatomy, blood supply, lymphatic drainage and innervation of abdominal wall.

Gujarat University 2025

Anatomy of the Abdominal Wall

The abdominal wall consists of anterior, lateral, and posterior components and includes muscles, fascia, skin, and peritoneum. It can be divided into:

Layers of the Anterior Abdominal Wall (from superficial to deep):

- Skin
- *Superficial fascia*
  - Camper's fascia (fatty layer)
  - Scarpa's fascia (membranous layer)
- *Muscles and their aponeuroses:*
  - External oblique
  - Internal oblique
  - Transversus abdominis
  - Rectus abdominis (enclosed in rectus sheath)
  - Pyramidalis (small, variable muscle)
- Transversalis fascia
- Extraperitoneal fat
- Parietal peritoneum

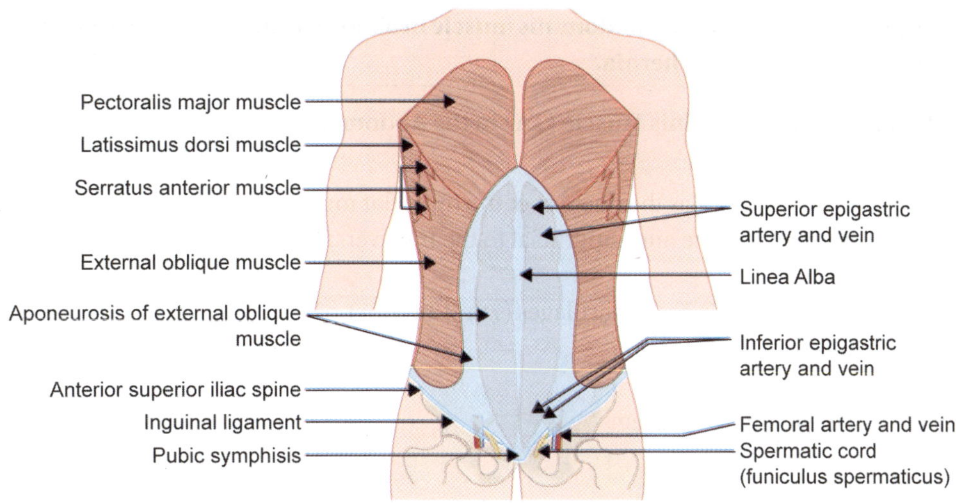

Blood Supply of the Abdominal Wall

Superficial Vessels

- *Superior part:* Branches of musculophrenic artery (from internal thoracic artery)
- *Inferior part:* Branches of superficial epigastric artery and superficial circumflex iliac artery (from femoral artery)

Deep Vessel:

- Superior epigastric artery (from internal thoracic artery)
- Inferior epigastric artery (from external iliac artery)
- Deep circumflex iliac artery (from external iliac artery)
- Intercostal and lumbar arteries

The superior and inferior epigastric arteries anastomose within the rectus sheath, providing collateral circulation.

Lymphatic Drainage of the Abdominal Wall

Superficial Lymphatics

- *Above umbilicus:* Drain to axillary lymph nodes (mainly anterior/pectoral group)
- *Below umbilicus:* Drain to superficial inguinal lymph nodes

Deep Lymphatics:

- Follow deep arteries to drain into:
    - External iliac lymph nodes
    - Common iliac lymph nodes
    - Lumbar (aortic) lymph nodes

Innervation of the Abdominal Wall

The abdominal wall is innervated segmentally by spinal nerves:

Motor and Sensory Innervation:

- Thoracoabdominal nerves (T7–T11) - Continuations of intercostal nerves
- Subcostal nerve (T12)
- Iliohypogastric nerve (L1)
- Ilioinguinal nerve (L1)

These nerves supply the muscles and skin of the anterior and lateral abdominal wall.

2. Describe the disposition of transversus abdominis muscle in abdomen and principle of transversus abdominis release (TAR) for surgery of ventral hernia. ***Gujarat University 2025***

Disposition of Transversus Abdominis Muscle (TA) in the Abdomen

Anatomical Location and Structure

- The Transversus abdominis (TA) is the deepest of the three flat muscles of the anterolateral abdominal wall.
- It lies deep to the internal oblique and superficial to the transversalis fascia.
- *Origin:*
  - Internal surfaces of lower six costal cartilages (7th–12th ribs)
  - Thoracolumbar fascia
  - Iliac crest
  - Lateral third of the inguinal ligament
- *Insertion:*
  - Linea alba (via the aponeurosis)
  - Pubic crest
  - Pectineal line of pubis (via conjoint tendon)

Orientation of Fibers

- Transversely (horizontally) across the abdomen
- Acts like a natural corset providing core stability and increasing intra-abdominal pressure
- *Relations:*
  - *Anteriorly:* Aponeurosis contributes to the rectus sheath
  - *Deep:* Lies above transversalis fascia and peritoneum

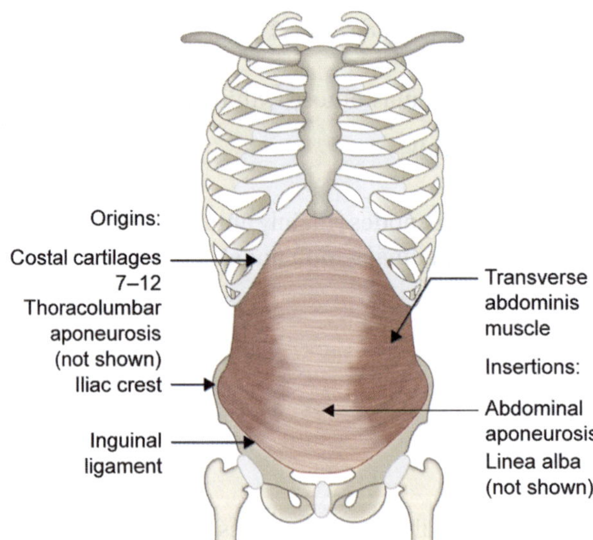

Principle of Transversus Abdominis Release (TAR) in Ventral Hernia Surgery

Background

- Ventral hernias involve a defect in the abdominal wall, often after surgery (incisional hernia).
- Large or complex hernias may not be closed by simple suture or anterior component separation.
- TAR is a posterior component separation technique introduced to allow tension-free closure of large midline abdominal wall defects.

Key Principles of TAR

- Plane Creation
  - In TAR, a retromuscular (sublay) plane is developed between the posterior rectus sheath and the rectus muscle.
  - The posterior rectus sheath is incised, and the transversus abdominis muscle is divided (released) medially.
- Transversus Abdominis Muscle Division
  - Division of the medial portion of the TA muscle exposes the transversalis fascia and preperitoneal space.
  - This creates a large, avascular plane that can be extended laterally to the psoas muscle, cranially to the diaphragm, and caudally into the pelvis.

Mesh Placement

- A large prosthetic mesh is placed in this retromuscular space for a wide, tension-free, posterior reinforcement.
- The posterior layer is closed over the mesh, and then the anterior fascia is approximated.

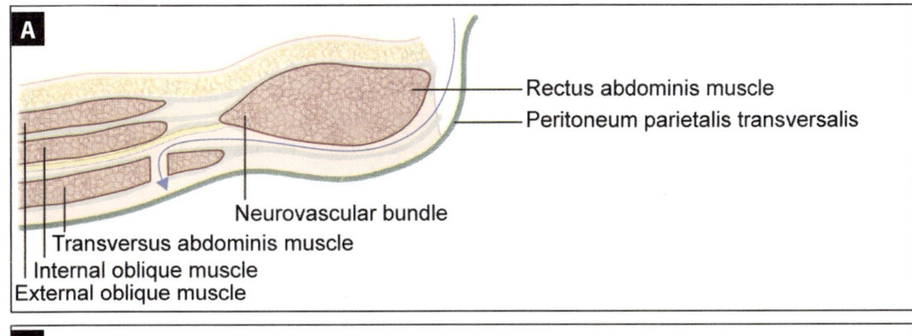

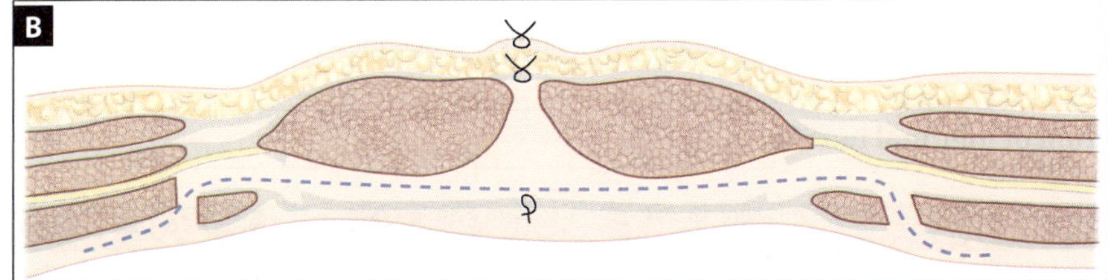

(A) Schematic overview of posterior component technique; (B) final situation after TAR with retro-muscular, preperitoneal mesh in place

Advantages of TAR

- Tension-free closure of large hernia defects
- Avoids skin flaps, reducing wound complications
- Preserves neurovascular supply to abdominal wall muscles
- Allows bilateral release and wide lateral dissection
- Strong and long-lasting repair with lower recurrence

Indications for TAR

- Large midline ventral or incisional hernias
- Loss of domain (abdominal contents outside the abdominal cavity)
- Failed previous hernia repairs
- Need for posterior component separation

3. Myopectineal orifice of Fruchaud. ***WBUHS 2020***

- The term [myopectineal orifice] was coined originally by Dr Henri Fruchaud, and refers to a “distinct area of weakness in the pelvic region”. The term [myopectineal] arises from two root terms which are combined. The root term [-my-] means “muscle” and the term [-pect-] means “comb” or “pectinate”. The word [pectineal] in this case refers to the pelvic bone area of origin of the pectinate muscle of the thigh.

- Fruchaud postulated that the anterior abdominal wall has an area that is inherently weak, and that this area is genetically determined. As such, hernias are part of human nature, or as he stated, "a healthy man is, unknown to himself, a hernia bearer".
- Fruchaud myopectineal orifice is an osseo-myo-aponeurotic tunnel through which all the groin hernia comes out. This orifice is bounded by:
  - Medially by the lateral border of the rectus sheath
  - Laterally by the iliopsoas muscle
  - Below by the pecten pubis and fascia covering it and the Cooper's ligament.
  - Above by the arched fibers of internal oblique, transversus abdominis muscle, and the conjoint tendon

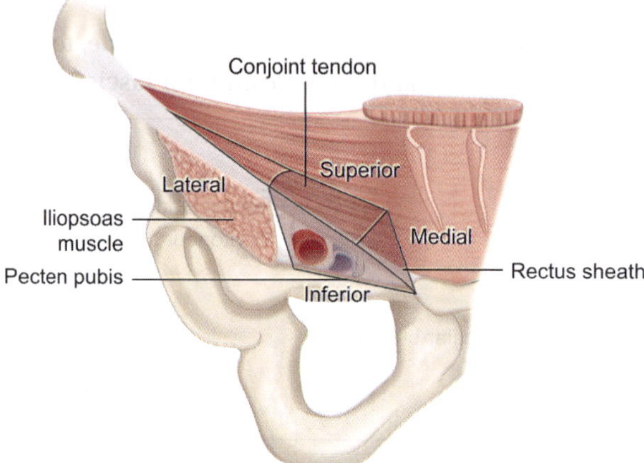

Schematic diagram of Fruchaud's myopectineal orifice.

4. Newer classification of inguinal hernia. ***WBUHS 2006***

Nyhus classification system.	
Type I	Indirect hernia; internal abdominal ring normal; typically in infants, children, and small adults
Type II	Indirect hernia; internal ring enlarged without impingement on the floor of the inguinal canal; does not extend to the scrotum
Type IIIA	Direct hernia; size is not taken into account
Type IIIB	Indirect hernia that has enlarged enough to encroach upon the posterior inguinal wall; indirect sliding or scrotal hernias are usually placed in this category because they are commonly associated with extension to the direct space; also includes pantaloon hernias
Type IIIC	Femoral hernia
Type IV	Recurrent hernia; modifiers A–D are sometimes added, which correspond to indirect, direct, femoral, and mixed, respectively

Gilbert classification system.	
Type 1	Small, indirect
Type 2	Medium, indirect
Type 3	Large, indirect
Type 4	Entire floor, direct
Type 5	Diverticular, direct
Type 6	Combined (pantaloon)
Type 7	Femoral

5. Sliding hernia. ***WBUHS 2010***

Introduction

A sliding hernia results due to slipping of the posterior parietal peritoneum on the underlying structures (usually indirect inguinal in location) and a part of the wall of the hernia sac is formed by an intra-abdominal viscus (usually colon-sigmoid colon and its mesentery on the left, the cecum on the right sometimes, on either side by a portion of the bladder).

Incidence

- Small bowel sliding hernia—1 in 2,000 cases
- Sac less hernia—1 in 8,000 cases

Clinical Features

- It occurs exclusively in male.
- Five out of six are on the left side.
- Bilateral rare
- Age of the patient is nearly always over 40 years. Incidence rises with age.
- It should be suspected in a very large globular inguinal hernia descending well into the scrotum.
- Occasionally, large intestine is strangulated in a sliding hernia; more often, nonstrangulated large intestine is present behind the sac containing strangulated small intestine.

Treatment

- Impossible to control with truss
- Operation is indicated.

Principle of Operation

- It is unnecessary to any of the sliding hernial sac provided, it is freed completely from the cord and the abdominal wall and that it is replaced deep to the repaired fascia transversalis.
- No attempt should be made to dissect the cecum or colon free from the peritoneum.

Complication of Operation

- Peritonitis
- Fecal fistula
- Injury to the vessel of the mesocolon

6. Describe the anatomy of femoral canal. How will you treat a case of strangulated femoral hernia? ***WBUHS 2024***

The femoral canal is the medial compartment of the femoral sheath, an inverted cone-shaped fascial space medial to the common femoral vein within the upper femoral triangle. It is only 1–2 cm long and opens superiorly as the femoral ring.

It serves two purposes:

1. Allows the femoral vein to expand when there is increased venous return from the lower limb
2. A route for efferent lymphatic drainage from the deep inguinal nodes (e.g. Cloquet's node) to the external iliac chain

The femoral ring boundaries are:

- *Medial:* Lacunar ligament
- *Anterior:* Medial part of the inguinal ligament
- *Lateral:* Femoral vein within the intermediate compartment of the femoral sheath
- *Posterior:* Pectineal ligament overlying the pectineus muscle and its fascia covering the superior pubic ramus

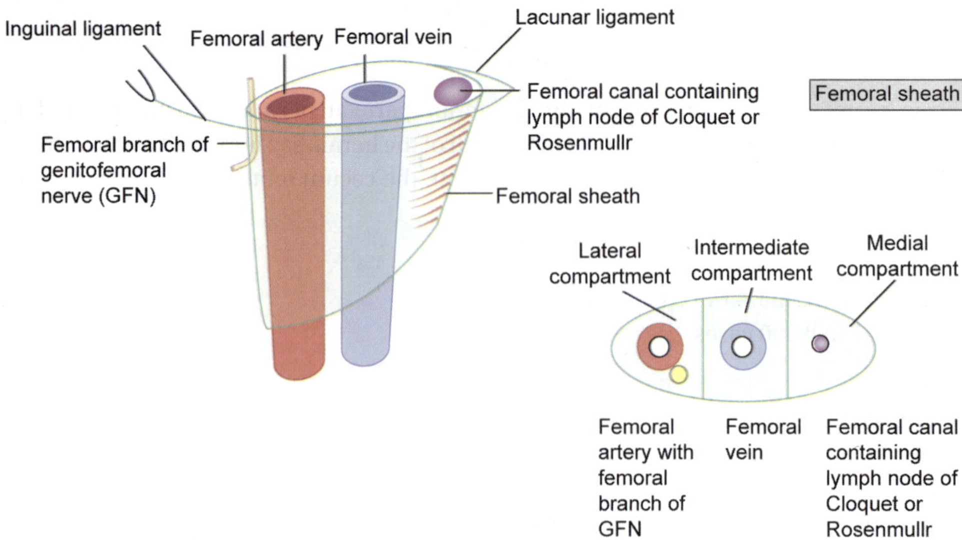

Strangulated femoral hernia is a surgical emergency and requires immediate intervention. A strangulated hernia occurs when the blood supply to the herniated tissue is compromised, leading to ischemia and potential tissue death. This condition can lead to severe complications like bowel necrosis, perforation, or sepsis if not treated promptly.

Treatment of Strangulated Femoral Hernia

Immediate Surgical Intervention:

- *Emergency surgery:* The definitive treatment for a strangulated femoral hernia is surgery. It is typically done under general anesthesia, although local anesthesia may be considered in some cases.
- *Reduction and repair:* The first step is to attempt to reduce the hernia (i.e., push the contents back into the abdominal cavity). However, in the case of strangulation, reduction may not be feasible or safe. If the hernia contents (often a portion of bowel) are viable, they can be reduced, and the hernia defect can be repaired.
- *Resection of necrotic tissue:* If the bowel or other herniated tissue is necrotic, it must be surgically removed. This may involve a bowel resection and anastomosis (joining the remaining healthy bowel).

Hernia Repair:

- *Herniorrhaphy or hernioplasty:* After the reduction or resection of any necrotic tissue, the hernia sac is repaired. This is usually done by closing the defect in the femoral canal with sutures or using a synthetic mesh for reinforcement, depending on the surgeon's preference and the patient's condition.
- *Mesh reinforcement:* A mesh is often used for hernia repair to strengthen the repair and reduce the risk of recurrence, particularly for femoral hernias, which have a high recurrence rate.

Postoperative Care:

- *Monitoring for complications:* After surgery, patients are closely monitored for signs of infection, wound complications, or bowel function. The recovery process may involve gradual reintroduction of oral intake and mobilization.
- *Antibiotics:* Broad-spectrum antibiotics are typically administered to prevent infection, especially when bowel resection is involved.
- *Pain management:* Adequate pain relief is provided to manage postoperative discomfort.

Important Considerations

- *Timing:* The sooner the strangulated hernia is treated, the better the outcomes. Delay in treatment can result in bowel gangrene, septic shock, and increased mortality.

- *Patient factors:* The patient's overall health, comorbidities (e.g., cardiovascular disease, diabetes), and the degree of strangulation may influence surgical options and recovery.

In summary, strangulated femoral hernia is a surgical emergency, and prompt intervention with reduction or resection and hernia repair is essential to prevent severe complications.

7. Spigelian hernia. *WBUHS 2012*

Introduction

- A Spigelian hernia (or lateral ventral hernia) is a hernia through the spigelian fascia, which is the aponeurotic layer between the rectus abdominis muscle medially, and the semilunar line laterally.
- These hernias almost always develop at or below the linea arcuata, probably because of the lack of posterior rectus sheath.
- These are generally interparietal hernias, meaning that they do not lie below the subcutaneous fat but penetrate between the muscles of the abdominal wall; therefore, there is often no notable swelling.

Clinical Features

- Spigelian hernias are usually small and therefore risk of strangulation is high.
- Most occur on the right side.
- *Age:* Fourth to seventh decade of life
- Compared to other types of hernias they are rare.
- Patients typically present with either an intermittent mass, localized pain, or signs of bowel obstruction.

Diagnosis

Ultrasonography or a computed tomography (CT) scan can establish the diagnosis, although CT scan provides the greatest sensitivity and specificity.

Treatment

- These hernias should be repaired because of the high risk of strangulation; fortunately, surgery is straightforward, with only larger defects requiring a mesh prosthesis.
- Laparoscopic repair results in less morbidity and shorter hospitalization compared with open procedures.
- Mesh-free laparoscopic suture repair is feasible and safe. This novel uncomplicated approach to small Spigelian hernias combines the benefits of laparoscopic localization, reduction, and closure without the morbidity and cost associated with foreign material.

8. Stoppa repair of abdominal hernia. *WBUHS 2010*

Introduction

- The Stoppa repair is a tension-free type of hernia repair.
- It is performed by wrapping the lower part of the parietal peritoneum with prosthetic mesh and placing it at a preperitoneal level over Fruchaud's myopectineal orifice.
- It was first described in 1975 by Rene Stoppa.
- This operation is also known as giant prosthetic reinforcement of the visceral sac (GPRVS).
- This technique has met particular success in the repair of bilateral hernias, large scrotal hernias, and recurrent or re-recurrent hernias in which conventional repair is difficult and carries a high morbidity and failure rate.
- The laparoscopic transabdominal preperitoneal (TAPP) repair uses exactly the same principles as the Stoppa repair, however, it is performed laparoscopically.

Retrorectus Mesh Repair

Rives–Stoppa Technique

- This technique utilizes the hernia sac to separate the mesh from the intra-abdominal contents.
- Superior to the umbilicus, dissection is performed above the posterior rectus fascia and under the rectus muscle.
- Below the umbilicus, dissection occurs in the preperitoneal space due to the lack of a posterior rectus sheath.

- A large piece of mesh is placed in the newly formed space, and fixated to the muscle layer above. This repair has decreased recurrences and complications from previous techniques.

Rives–Stoppa repair augmented by laparoscopic components separation is an innovative method for reconstruction of complex abdominal wall defects. Laparoscopic components separation allows fascial closure to be achieved anterior to the mesh in large incisional hernias, which may reduce wound infection rates.

9. Discuss the merits and demerits of different types of mesh used in hernia surgery. ***WBUHS 2018***

10. Prosthesis in hernia surgery.

Properties of an ideal mesh are:

- Strong but pliable and easy to handle.
- Inert, nonallergic, nonbiodegradable, and noncarcinogenic
- Should have an optimum thickness.
- Should stimulate adequate fibroblastic activity and get rapidly incorporated into the tissues.
- Should provide mechanical support through permanent biocompatibility.
- Should achieve early, rapid, and optimum ingrowth of fibrocollagenous tissue to prevent dislocation or migration.
- Macroporous, monofilament, and transparent
- Resistant to infection
- Should provide a barrier to adhesions in intra-abdominal placement.

The mesh materials have been classified based on its biological response and handling characteristics into:

- Nonabsorbable and synthetic
- Nonabsorbable and synthetic with barrier
- Synthetic and partially absorbable
- Combined
- Biological

Nonabsorbable and Synthetic Material

- *Polypropylene (PP)*

Advantages	*Disadvantages*
• High tensile strength • Nonpolar • Highly hydrophobic • Electrostatically neutral • Resistant to biological degradation • Infections can be treated themselves without removal of mesh	• Heavy weight nature • More foreign body reaction • Formation of thick scar • Contraction of mesh/shrinkage • Hernia recurrence • Chronic pain • Intestinal adhesions • Discomfort

- *Polyester*

Special features	*Advantages*	*Disadvantages*
• Composed of polyethylene terephthalate (PET) • Multifilament • Slightly polar • More hydrophilic and hygroscopic	• Coated with collagen • Prevents adhesion • Can be used for intraperitoneal repair • Improves conformability and tissue ingrowth with abdominal wall	• Thick scar formation • Hernia recurrence • Degrades over time • Chronic pain

- Polytetrafluoroethylene (PTFE) and e-PTFE (expanded polytetrafluoroethylene) meshes are smooth, soft, and strong. There are different varieties:
    - Soft tissue patch

- Micromesh
- Micromesh plus
- Dual mesh
- Dual mesh plus
- Dual mesh with holes
- PTFE impregnated with silver and chlorhexidine

These prostheses are suitable for repair of all groin and ventral hernias by open technique as well as by TAPP or totally extraperitoneal (TEP) since they do not come in contact with abdominal viscera.

Advantages	*Disadvantages*
• Less adhesion formation • Inert nature • Smaller pore size • Less tissue ingrowth • Minimal inflammatory reaction • Lower scar density	Weaker hernia repair

- *Nonabsorbable and synthetic with a barrier:*

Advantages	*Barriers used*
• Prevents bowel adhesion when placed intraperitoneally • Minimal biological response • Inhibition of inflammatory cascade • Reduced activation of inflammatory cytokines and cells	• ePTFE • Polyurethane • Oxidized regenerated cellulose • Omega-3-fatty acid • Collagen • Beta-glucan

- *Synthetic and partially absorbable:*
  Example:
  - Polyglactin 910 and poliglecaprone 25
  - Poly(L-lactide-co-glycolide) and PP

Advantages	*Disadvantages*
• Reduces density of biomaterial • Less inflammatory reaction • Less fibrosis • Less structural changes • Larger pores • Less chronic inflammation • Less pain • Less discomfort	• Differences in variety of inflammatory markers • Weaker hernia repair

- *Combined meshes:*
  - Main purpose is to prevent complications by taking advantages of best traits from two different meshes.
  - In case of polyester and PTFE, the former allows abdominal wall tissue ingrowth while the latter prevents occurrence of intestinal adhesions.
  - Synthetic meshes use only a temporary adhesion barrier, hence the use of absorbable polymer coatings.

Advantages	*Disadvantages*
• Absorbable mesh can be used in contaminated fields • Benefit of nonremoval • Formation of collagen upon healing • Can be placed in direct contact with bowel	• Hernia recurrence and catastrophic failure • Weak collagen formation • Nonpromising as a standalone procedure

- *Biological Meshes:*

Advantages	Disadvantages
• Overcome problems of synthetic meshes • Provide mechanical support • Tissue remodeling along mesh scaffold • New vascular access to hernia site • Impeded inflammatory response and immune-mediated rejection • Wound healing response • Potentially resist infection • Good success rate in salvaging contaminated fields • Resistance to adhesion formation	• Connective tissue formed is only 70–80% strong • Greater chance of hernia recurrence • Higher mechanical failure • Disease transmission • High cost

11. Classify various types of meshes used in surgery. Describe the newer meshes for Hernia surgery. ***WBUHS 2023***

- Nonabsorbable and synthetic material
  - Polypropylene (PP)
  - Polyester
  - PTFE—There are different varieties:
    - Soft tissue patch
    - Micromesh
    - Micromesh plus
    - Dual mesh
    - Dual mesh plus
    - Dual mesh with holes
    - PTFE impregnated with silver and chlorhexidine
- Nonabsorbable and synthetic with a barrier
- Synthetic and partially absorbable:
  - *Example:*
    - Polygalactin and poliglecaprone
    - Poly(L-lactide-co-glycolide) and PP
- Combined meshes
- *Biological meshes*

  Chart of biological meshes:

Donor tissues	Product name
Human dermis	Alloderm, Allomax
Porcine dermis	Flex HD, Permacol, Collamend, XenMatrix
Porcine small intestine submucosa	Surgisis
Bovine dermis	Surgi Mend
Bovine pericardium	Veritas

- *Composite mesh:*
  - *Newer meshes—Composite mesh:* Latest technical advances have now made available prosthetic materials, which prevent bowel adhesions.
    - Lightweight composite meshes without adhesion prevention "barrier":
      - VYPRO II
      - ULTRAPRO

- New composite meshes with adhesion prevention "barrier":
  - Repair of ventral and incisional hernia may be undertaken by minimal access surgery rather than the conventional open technique.
  - To achieve this repair, intraperitoneal placement of mesh requires a material which has both high tissue ingrowth towards the abdominal wall and non-adhesiveness on the other side to prevent bowel adhesions.
- Absorbable barrier composite mesh:

- *Sepramesh:*
  - Sepramesh biosurgical composite is a dual-component prosthetic biomaterial composed of macroporous polypropylene on one side, with bioresorbable, nonimmunogenic membrane of sodium hyaluronate and carboxymethyl cellulose on the other side.
  - It was designed to provide protection against intra-abdominal adhesion formation throughout the critical period of remesothelialization during the first postoperative week.
  - The absorbable barrier turns to a gel in 48 hours, remains on the mesh for ~7 days and is cleared from the body in 28 days.
- *Parietex composite mesh and parientene composite mesh:*
  - Parietex composite mesh is composed of multifilament polyester mesh with a purified, oxidized bovine collagen type I coating covered by an absorbable, antiadhesion film of polyethylene glycol and glycerol.
  - Polyethylene glycol is a hydrogel that decreases tissue adherence and glycerol is a hydrophobic lipid. The collagen coating functions to promote collagen ingrowth by increasing the hydrophilicity of the polyester mesh and decreasing the fibrous tissue reaction to the 'foreign' material (mesh).
  - The collagen, polyethylene glycol and glycerol film are resorbed in ~3 weeks.
  - Parientene composite mesh consists of the same antiadhesive barrier but coated to polypropylene.
- *PROCEED surgical mesh:*
  - PROCEED surgical mesh is a sterile multilayered, thin, flexible, laminate mesh comprised of an oxidized regenerated cellulose (ORC) fabric; and prolene soft mesh, a nonabsorbable polypropylene mesh which is encapsulated by a polydioxanne polymer.
  - The polypropylene mesh side of the product allows for tissue ingrowth, while the ORC side provides a bioresorbable layer that physically separates the polypropylene mesh from underlying tissue and organ surfaces during the wound-healing period to minimize tissue attachment to the mesh.
  - The polydioxanone provides a bond to the ORC layer.

It has a lightweight macroporous mesh construction, leaves behind less residual foreign body, allows the fluid to flow through easily and does not harbor bacteria.

- *Nonabsorbable barrier composite mesh:*
  - *Bard composix mesh:*
    - This is a combination of polypropylene that has a thin coat of ePTFE on one side to prevent bowel adhesions.
    - Introduction through a laparoscopic port is difficult because it cannot compress the mesh and hence requires a larger port (12 mm) for its introduction.
  - *GORE-TEX dual mesh:*
    - The Gore-Tex Dual mesh material has two surfaces; one is very smooth (micropores 3 mm) and the other is rough (micropores approximately about 22 mm).
    - It is designed to be implanted with the smooth surface against the visceral organs—tissue to which no or minimal adhesion is desired—and the other surface against which tissue incorporation is desired.

  The use of novel absorbable and nonabsorbable barriers on composite meshes to reduce the incidence of adhesion and adhesion-related complications has been evaluated in animal models and a few clinical studies have been reported. The incidence of adhesions and tenacity of adhesions were reduced for all of the barrier meshes compared with the macroporous polyester mesh.

Selection of mesh: An appropriate mesh should be selected and implanted.

- For inguinal hernia repair by TAPP or TEP, any of the following meshes can be used:
    - Conventional polypropylene mesh
    - PROLENE soft mesh
    - VYPRO II
    - ULTRAPRO
- For intra-abdominal placements, any mesh that will prevent bowel adhesions should be used. It can be either ePTFE, PROCEED surgical mesh or any one of the newly engineered meshes with an absorbable or a nonabsorbable barrier.
- Next important matter to consider is the size of the mesh:
    - It must be at least 15 × 15 cm for an inguinal hernia. For repair of umbilical, ventral and incisional hernia, it should be at least 4 cm wider than the defect.
    - It is better to initially measure the size of the defect with the scale and then select a mesh of appropriate size.
    - It should be wide enough to cover the defect in all directions since a smaller size may lead to protrusion of the mesh into the defect and result in a recurrence.

12. Give an outline of biological mesh and their clinical use. ***WBUHS 2017, 2018***

13. Composite mesh. ***WBUHS 2020***

Introduction

- *Biologic mesh* (or *biomesh*) is a type of surgical mesh made from an organic biomaterial (such as porcine dermis, porcine small intestine submucosa, bovine dermis or pericardium, and the dermis or fascia lata of a cadaveric human).
- *Basic science of biologic meshes:*
    - Most often derived from human or porcine dermis, these materials have been processed to acellular, porous extracellular matrix scaffolds of collagen and elastin.
    - Some source growth factors remain and attract endothelial cells and subsequent fibroblasts into the mesh.
    - These host cells release additional chemoattractants that signal the migration of other structural cells.
    - The three-dimensional nature of the mesh and porosity allows cells to enter the mesh and adhere.
    - What happens from there is a cycle of remodeling consisting of degradation of the biologic mesh and regeneration of the collagen scaffold with host tissue.
    - The balance of this degradation and rebuilding process, and the speed with which it occurs, influences the ultimate strength and structure of the biologic mesh hernia repair.

Biological Mesh

Chart of Biological Meshes

Donor tissues	***Product name***
Human dermis	Alloderm and Allomax
Porcine dermis	Flex HD, Permacol, Collamend, and XenMatrix
Porcine small intestine submucosa	Surgisis
Bovine dermis	Surgi Mend
Bovine pericardium	Veritas

Indications for Use

- *Noncontaminated setting:* The use of biologic mesh in primary or recurrent ventral or inguinal herniorrhaphy in the noncontaminated and previously uninfected field is difficult to justify due to the high-material cost without added benefit.

- *Bridging the gap:* The poor performance of the mesh in terms of laxity in a bridging repair makes this an unacceptable repair in the noncontaminated setting.
- *Reinforcement of the repair:* The use of allograft or xenograft as reinforcement of a primary ventral hernia repair is felt to be a more sound approach.

- *Contaminated setting:* The presence of contamination may limit the applicability of permanent synthetic mesh in some hernia repairs. Biologic mesh may be acceptable for this purpose or for placement in open wounds as a staged closure in complex abdominal wall reconstruction.
- *Prophylaxis during stoma creation:* The role of biologic mesh has been explored in prevention of parastomal hernias.
- *Hiatal hernias:* Biologic mesh has been utilized in the reinforcement of paraesophageal hernia repair.

Composite Mesh

Latest technical advances have now made available prosthetic materials, which prevent bowel adhesions.

- Lightweight composite meshes without adhesion prevention "barrier"
  - VYPRO II.
  - ULTRAPRO.
- *New composite meshes with adhesion prevention "barrier":*
  - Repair of ventral and incisional hernia may be undertaken by minimal access surgery rather than the conventional open technique.
  - To achieve this repair, intraperitoneal placement of mesh requires a material which has both high tissue ingrowth toward the abdominal wall and nonadhesiveness on the other side to prevent bowel adhesions.
- *Absorbable barrier composite mesh:*
  - *Sepramesh:*
    - Sepramesh Biosurgical Composite is a dual-component prosthetic biomaterial composed of macroporous PP on one side, with bioresorbable, nonimmunogenic membrane of sodium hyaluronate and carboxymethyl cellulose on the other side.
    - It was designed to provide protection against intra-abdominal adhesion formation throughout the critical period of remesothelialization during the first postoperative week.
    - The absorbable barrier turns to a gel in 48 hours, remains on the mesh for ~7 days, and is cleared from the body in 28 days.
  - *Parietex composite mesh and parietene composite mesh:*
    - Parietex composite mesh is composed of multifilament polyester mesh with a purified, oxidized bovine collagen type I coating covered by an absorbable, and antiadhesion film of polyethylene glycol and glycerol.
    - Polyethylene glycol is a hydrogel that decreases tissue adherence and glycerol is a hydrophobic lipid. The collagen coating functions to promote collagen ingrowth by increasing the hydrophilicity of the polyester mesh and decreasing the fibrous tissue reaction to the "foreign" material (mesh).
    - The collagen, polyethylene glycol, and glycerol film are resorbed in ~3 weeks.
    - Parientene composite mesh consists of the same antiadhesive barrier but coated to PP.
  - *PROCEED surgical mesh:*
    - PROCEED surgical mesh is a sterile multilayered, thin, flexible, laminate mesh comprised of an oxidized regenerated cellulose (ORC) fabric; and prolene soft mesh, a nonabsorbable PP mesh which is encapsulated by a polydioxanone polymer.
    - The PP mesh side of the product allows for tissue ingrowth, while the ORC side provides a bioresorbable layer that physically separates the PP mesh from underlying tissue and organ surfaces during the wound-healing period to minimize tissue attachment to the mesh.
    - The polydioxanone provides a bond to the ORC layer. It has a lightweight macroporous mesh construction, leaves behind less residual foreign body, allows the fluid to flow through easily, and does not harbor bacteria.

- *Nonabsorbable barrier composite mesh:*
  - *Bard composix mesh:*
    - This is a combination of PP that has a thin coat of ePTFE on one side to prevent bowel adhesions.
    - Introduction through a laparoscopic port is difficult because it cannot compress the mesh and hence requires a larger port (12 mm) for its introduction.
  - *GORE-TEX dual mesh:*
    - The GORE-TEX Dual mesh material has two surfaces; one is very smooth (micropores 3 mm) and the other is rough (micropores approximately about 22 mm).
    - It is designed to be implanted with the smooth surface against the visceral organs—tissue to which no or minimal adhesion is desired—and the other surface against which tissue incorporation is desired. The use of novel absorbable and nonabsorbable barriers on composite meshes to reduce the incidence of adhesion and adhesion-related complications has been evaluated in animal models and a few clinical studies have been reported. The incidence of adhesions and tenacity of adhesions were reduced for all of the barrier meshes compared with the macroporous polyester mesh.

Selection of Mesh

An appropriate mesh should be selected and implanted.

- For inguinal hernia repair by TAPP or TEP, any of the following meshes can be used:
  - Conventional PP mesh
  - PROLENE soft mesh
  - VYPRO II
  - ULTRAPRO
- For intra-abdominal placements, any mesh that will prevent bowel adhesions should be used. It can be either ePTFE, PROCEED surgical mesh or any one of the newly engineered meshes with an absorbable or a nonabsorbable barrier.
- Next important matter to consider is the size of the mesh:
  - It must be at least 15 × 15 cm for an inguinal hernia. For repair of umbilical, ventral, and incisional hernia, it should be at least 4 cm wider than the defect.
  - It is better to initially measure the size of the defect with the scale and then select a mesh of appropriate size.
  - It should be wide enough to cover the defect in all directions since a smaller size may lead to protrusion of the mesh into the defect and result in a recurrence.

14. Causes and management of chronic pain following mesh repair of inguinal hernia. ***WBUHS 2017***

Chronic pain following groin hernia operation:

Classifications of chronic postoperative pain.

- *Somatic (nociceptive) pain:*
  - Most common
  - Pain from preoperative pathological causes
  - Previous ligament/mesh injury
  - New ligament/muscle injury caused by surgery
  - Aggressive scarification reaction
    - Osteitis pubis
  - Reactions to prosthetic material/mesh
- *Neuropathic pain:*
  - Direct nerve damage or injury
  - Incorporation of nerve with staples/sutures/mesh

Contd...

Contd...

Classifications of chronic postoperative pain.

- *Somatic (nociceptive) pain:*
  - Most common
  - Pain from preoperative pathological causes
  - Previous ligament/mesh injury
  - New ligament/muscle injury caused by surgery
  - Aggressive scarification reaction
    - Osteitis pubis
  - Reactions to prosthetic material/mesh
- *Neuropathic pain:*
  - Direct nerve damage or injury
  - Incorporation of nerve with staples/sutures/mesh

- Chronic postoperative groin pain has been defined as pain lasting >30 days and interfering with the patient's activities of daily living or work activities.
- 47% of all patients undergoing all types of inguinal hernia repairs had chronic neuropathic pain.
- The causes for pain included general anesthesia, lengthy surgery, wound infection, and hemorrhage.
- Operations removing the mesh and orchiectomies did not abolish the pain.
- Most complications were related to primary hernia repairs, nonemergency repairs, and the "open" technique.
- Mesh did not increase the rate of chronic pain; however, those factors influencing chronic pain were increased: preoperative pain levels, age fewer than 40 years, pain at other sites (such as back pain), psychosocial issues, and a history of heavy manual labor.
- Technical expertise was also an issue creating variances in postoperative pain.
- Five main factors of causation have been positively identified.
  1. The first factor is that bulky heavyweight mesh material will cause pain.
  2. Secondly, the patient's idiosyncratic reactions with an exaggerated scarification response can generate significant pain.
  3. The third cause of pain is the scenario in which the surgeon exhibits an inattention to the technical details of mesh implantation.
  4. A fourth cause of pain may be allergic reactions to the mesh materials (i.e., PP, polyester, PTFE, and/or the coatings of mesh).
  5. The fifth direct cause of pain emanates from direct or indirect nerve injury or inflammation surrounding the nerves secondary to the mesh affixation process or the mere presence of the mesh.

Recommendations

- Laparoscopic or nonmesh repairs are recommended in patients with recurrent operations or contralateral hernia repair.
- Intraoperative hemorrhage increases postoperative pain and infections.
- Intraoperative contamination is a contraindication for mesh placement.
- Use of biological mesh can be considered in contaminated sites, but not grossly contaminated sites (pus or bowel content).
- Mesh should not be used in patients with allergies to the synthetic material.
- Mesh should not be used in a patient with a history of infection with methicillin resistant *Staphylococcus aureus*.

Nonsurgical Management

- Evaluation and treatment can be very challenging in this patient population.
- Examination and imaging to exclude occult recurrence is important.
- Following that, use of anti-inflammatories, nerve blocks, neuromodulators, and pain clinic referrals should be considered.

- Unless there is evidence of a recurrence, operative intervention should be deferred for at least 1 year since groin pain decreases with time elapsed from surgery.

Surgical Intervention
- *Triple neurectomy and/or mesh removal:* Triple neurectomy of the iliohypogastric, ilioinguinal, and genital femoral nerves.
- Any intervention must be tailored to the individual, with full preoperative disclosure of all potential complications and consideration given to the skills and resources available to the individual surgeon.

15. Classify abdominal wall hernias according to European hernia society. Mention newer terminology in ventral hernia with reference to mesh position. ***WBUHS 2025 Supplementary***

The *European Hernia Society (EHS)* classification system standardizes the description of *abdominal wall hernias,* particularly focusing on *primary and incisional ventral hernias*. It considers the *location* and *size* of the hernia defect.

Classification based on Location
The EHS divides the abdominal wall into *midline* and *lateral* regions:
- *Midline hernias*
  These lie between the *xiphoid process and the pubic bone,* along the linea alba.
  - *M1:* Subxiphoidal (just below the xiphoid process)
  - *M2:* Epigastric (above the umbilicus)
  - *M3:* Umbilical (around the umbilicus)
  - *M4:* Infraumbilical (below the umbilicus)
  - *M5:* Suprapubic (just above the pubic bone)
- *Lateral Hernias*
  These occur lateral to the rectus abdominis muscle.
  - *L1:* Subcostal (below the costal margin)
  - *L2:* Flank (lateral abdominal wall)
  - *L3:* Iliac (above the iliac crest)
  - *L4:* Lumbar (posterior lateral abdominal wall)

  Classification based on size of hernial defect:
  - *W1:* Small (<4 cm)
  - *W2:* Medium (4–10 cm)
  - *W3:* Large (>10 cm)

Putting it Together
A hernia can be described using this classification.
For example:
- *M3W2:* A medium-sized umbilical hernia
- *L2W3:* A large flank hernia

Advantages of EHS classification:
- Standardized terminology
- Aids in surgical planning
- Facilitates research and outcome comparisons

This classification helps in preoperative assessment, choosing surgical approach, and predicting prognosis.

Newer Terminology in Ventral Hernia Surgery: Mesh Position (as per recent consensus and EHS updates)

Modern hernia repair terminology has evolved to standardize the description of *mesh position* in ventral hernia repairs. This helps in surgical planning, reporting, and outcome comparisons.

Here is the *updated terminology for mesh positioning*, largely based on the *European Hernia Society (EHS)* and international consensus guidelines:

Onlay

- *Definition:* Mesh placed *above the anterior rectus sheath,* just beneath the subcutaneous tissue.
- *Advantages:* Easier to perform.
- *Disadvantages:* Higher risk of seroma and infection.

Inlay

- *Definition:* Mesh sutured *edge-to-edge* between the hernia defect margins.
- *Disadvantages:* Weak repair, high recurrence rate; generally not recommended as a standalone technique.

Sublay/Retro-Rectus (Rives–Stoppa technique)

- *Definition:* Mesh placed behind the rectus muscles but in front of the posterior rectus sheath or transversalis fascia.
- *Advantages:* Strong repair with good mesh incorporation; low recurrence and infection rates.
- *Preferred* for open midline hernias.

Preperitoneal

- *Definition:* Mesh placed between the peritoneum and transversalis fascia.
- *Used in:* Some laparoscopic and open repairs, especially in the lower abdomen.

Intraperitoneal (IPOM – Intraperitoneal Onlay Mesh)

- *Definition:* Mesh placed *inside the peritoneal cavity,* directly in contact with abdominal viscera.
- *Used in:* Laparoscopic and robotic ventral hernia repairs.
- *Disadvantages:* Risk of adhesions and erosion; thus, composite or barrier-coated meshes are used.

Extraperitoneal (e.g., eTEP – Extended Totally Extraperitoneal)

- *Definition:* Mesh placed *outside the peritoneal cavity,* often in a retro-rectus or preperitoneal space, *via minimally invasive techniques.*
- *eTEP* is a newer minimally invasive approach for placing mesh in sublay space.

Mesh position	*Location*	*Common technique/approach*
Onlay	Above anterior rectus sheath	Open
Inlay	Bridging the defect edges	Open (less preferred)
Sublay	Retro-rectus space	Rives–Stoppa, Open or eTEP
Preperitoneal	Between peritoneum and transversalis fascia	Open or laparoscopic
Intraperitoneal	Inside peritoneal cavity	Laparoscopic (IPOM), robotic
Extraperitoneal	Outside the peritoneal cavity	eTEP, TAPP-like minimally invasive

INCISIONAL HERNIA AND COMPONENT SEPARATION TECHNIQUE

16. What is abdominal wall reconstruction? Describe the various placement of mesh in abdominal wall surgery for complex ventral hernias. ***Srimanta Sankaradeva University, Assam 2025***

Abdominal wall reconstruction (AWR) is a complex surgical procedure aimed at restoring the integrity, function, and appearance of the abdominal wall, especially after large or complicated hernias, trauma, infection, or prior failed hernia repairs. It often involves extensive dissection, component separation, and the use of prosthetic or biological mesh to provide structural support.

Indications for Abdominal Wall Reconstruction

- Large or complex *ventral hernias*
- *Recurrent hernias* after prior repairs
- *Loss of domain* (where abdominal contents are chronically outside the cavity)
- *Infected or contaminated fields*
- After oncologic resections (e.g., sarcomas)
- *Enterocutaneous fistulas* or open abdomen closure

Mesh Placement in Abdominal Wall Reconstruction

The *placement of mesh* in abdominal wall surgery is crucial for reinforcing the repair and minimizing recurrence. Mesh can be placed in several anatomical planes, each with its own indications, advantages, and disadvantages.

Onlay Mesh

- *Location:* Placed *on top of the anterior rectus sheath*, above the abdominal muscles.
- *Technique:* Requires wide subcutaneous dissection to place the mesh after fascial closure.
- *Advantages:*
  - Technically easier to perform.
  - Useful in contaminated or infected fields (if biological mesh is used).
- *Disadvantages:*
  - Higher risk of *seroma, infection,* and *mesh exposure.*
  - Weaker integration compared to deeper placements.

Inlay Mesh

- *Location:* Mesh is sewn *directly into the defect*, bridging the gap between fascial edges.
- *Technique:* No fascial closure; mesh is used to span the hernia defect.
- *Advantages:*
  - Simple and quick, useful when fascial closure is not possible.
- *Disadvantages:*
  - High tension on the mesh.
  - High *recurrence rate* (due to lack of structural support and tissue ingrowth).
  - Rarely used as a standalone method today.

Sublay Mesh (Retro-Rectus)

- *Location:* Placed *between the posterior rectus sheath and the rectus abdominis muscle.*
- *Technique:* Fascial closure followed by mesh insertion deep to the rectus muscles but above the peritoneum.
- *Advantages:*
  - Excellent *mesh incorporation and low recurrence rates.*
  - Good vascularized bed and coverage.
- *Disadvantages:*
  - Technically more demanding.
  - Not always feasible if posterior sheath is disrupted.

Underlay (Intraperitoneal) Mesh

- *Location:* Placed *inside the peritoneal cavity*, in contact with intra-abdominal organs.
- *Technique:* Often used in laparoscopic or robotic ventral hernia repairs.
- *Advantages:*
  - Minimally invasive approach possible.
  - No need for large subcutaneous dissection.
- *Disadvantages:*
  - Risk of *adhesions, bowel erosion, or fistula formation* (especially with non-coated synthetic meshes).
  - Requires *composite meshes* with anti-adhesive barrier if intraperitoneal.

Preperitoneal Mesh

- *Location:* Placed *between the peritoneum and transversalis fascia.*
- *Technique:* Commonly used in inguinal hernia repair but can be used in ventral hernias.
- *Advantages:*
  - Avoids direct contact with intra-abdominal contents.
- *Disadvantages:*
  - Technically demanding.
  - Peritoneum may be fragile or disrupted in prior surgeries.

Component Separation Technique (CST)

Often combined with mesh placement in complex cases:

- *Anterior CST:* Releases the external oblique to allow medial advancement of rectus muscles.
- *Posterior CST (TAR-Transversus Abdominis Release):* Allows greater medial mobilization and space for sublay mesh placement.

Key Considerations in Mesh Selection and Placement

- *Patient factors:* Comorbidities, infection risk, size of defect.
- *Contamination risk:* Synthetic mesh avoided in grossly contaminated fields; *biologic* or *biosynthetic meshes* preferred.
- *Location of mesh affects:*
  - Recurrence rate
  - Complication profile
  - Integration and tissue remodeling

17. Etiopathogenesis of incisional hernia. Indications and principles of "component separation technique" for incisional hernia repair. ***WBUHS 2025 Supplementary***

18. Describe the pathogenesis of incisional hernia. Discuss the steps of component separation technique of hernia repair. Give a brief comparison of it with preperitoneal mesh repair. ***WBUHS 2015***

19. Indications and techniques of component separation technique. ***KGMU Lucknow 2025***

20. Component separation technique in incisional hernia repair. ***Rajasthan University of Health Sciences 2025***

Introduction

Incisional hernia is one of the common postoperative complication following general surgery. The cumulative incidence has remained constant despite several attempts to improve laparotomy closure. As well as surgical closure technique, individual biological and patient dependent risk factors play a key role.

Incidence

- 11–20% among Indian population
- Seen more in females due to increased incidence of lower uterine cesarean section

Factors Affecting Incisional Hernia Development

- *Surgical technique:*
  - Type of incision
  - Suture material—closure of fascial layer with absorbable sutures
  - Suture technique—faulty abdominal closure technique (ideally length of suture: length of incision should be 4:1) distance between subsequent suture and distance from edge of defect should be 5 mm)
  - Midline incision

- *Other surgical factors:*
  - Postoperative wound infection
  - Incidence is more with emergency surgeries.
- *Patient-related factors:*
  - Wound healing
  - Local wound healing impairment
  - Age—more in elderly people
  - Gender
  - Malnutrition
  - Immunocompromised patients
  - *Concomitant disease:*
    - Obesity
    - Anemia
    - Jaundice
    - Underlying malignancy
    - Diabetes mellitus
    - Abdominal aortic aneurysm
    - COPD, chronic cough
    - Collagen vascular disease
- *Exogenous toxins:*
  - Smoking
  - Certain medicines—steroids, cytotoxic drugs
- *Hereditary connective tissue disorders*

Pathophysiology

- Defective collagen metabolism and synthesis is one of the major factors involved in the development of incisional hernia. Patients with IH have a reduced ratio of collagen I: Collagen III as well as a reduced ratio of matrix metalloproteinase 1 (MMP1) to MMP2. These reductions in the synthesis of different types of collagen and enzymes play a role in the development of IH.
- Biological elements such as copper and zinc are important for the integrity of collagen because they are necessary for the synthesis of the enzyme lysyl oxidase which contribute in the integrity of the collagen molecule.
- The presence of other biological factors (plasminogen activator inhibitor, urokinase plasminogen activator inhibitor) in the scar tissue may contribute in the development of IH.
- Smoking is a well-known risk factor for hernia development. Smokers have fourfold higher risk than non-smokers. Smoking can cause a peripheral tissue hypoxia which hampers collagen deposition and also increases the risk of wound infection by reducing the oxidative killing mechanism of the neutrophils.

Pathogenesis

The development of an incisional hernia is multifactorial. There are two major areas which influence its pathogenesis: surgical technique and patient-related factors.

Surgical Technique

- Most retrospective studies looking at surgical technique as a possible influence of incisional hernia risk has focused on the type of incision, type of suture material, and suture technique.
- Retrospective studies suggest that transverse incisions, Pfannenstiel incisions and other pararectal incisions are associated with reduced incidence of incisional hernia when compared with vertical incisions.
- Regarding type of suture materials, several meta-analyses report the lowest incidences of incisional hernia for monofilamentous, nonresorbable, or long-term resorbable suture materials.

- The theoretical advantage of nonresorbable suture material in hernia prevention must, however, be balanced against a significantly higher incidence of fistula formation and higher rates of postoperative wound pain, due to permanent mechanical tissue irritation.

Patient-related Factors

- A large number of biological factors related to the patient's preexisting disease and its systemic effects have a suspected role in the etiology of incisional hernia.
- *Normal wound healing:*
  - Wound healing is a complex process involving the interaction of several different cell types with the extracellular matrix.
  - The quantity and quality of connective tissue produced is the primary determinant of the degree of normal physiological function and tissue stability achieved during scar formation.
  - The ratio of type I to type III collagen is considered a predictor of connective tissue stability.
  - Of the known collagen variants, type I collagen is, due to its tensile properties, particularly responsible for mechanical tissue resistance.
  - By comparison, type III collagen, expressed primarily during the early wound healing phase, is mechanically less stable and is later replaced by type I collagen.
  - In patients with incisional hernias, a significant decrease in the collagen type I/III ratio relative to normal fascias is observed, suggesting a dysfunction in collagen metabolism. Local disturbances of wound healing—the development of wound infection or seroma significantly increases the risk of incisional hernia.
  - It is established that infections and seromas have an impact on local wound healing via an increase in the production of cytokines and proteases, leading in turn to a reduction in fibroblasts and diminished wound stability.
  - Necrosis resulting from excessive suture tension can also disturb wound healing and stable scar formation.
- *Age and gender:* Age above 45 years emerged as a significant risk factor for incisional hernia.
  - This can be explained by delayed wound healing in older individuals, with changes in fibroblast migration and structural changes with reduced collagen formation as well as the high prevalence of concomitant disease.
  - While many studies suggest that men were at greater risk than women of developing incisional hernia, other studies have not found significant effect of gender.
- *Concomitant disease:* Many studies identify adiposity as a risk factor for incisional hernia development.
  - Poor nutritional status and ill health can also promote incisional hernia formation.
  - Anemia, underlying malignant disorder, and diabetes mellitus were all identified as independent risk factors.
  - The incidence rate of incisional hernia following abdominal aortic aneurysm surgery is at 28–38% significantly higher than the rate observed after laparotomy performed for other indications.
  - It has more recently been shown that these patients suffer in part from genetically determined type III procollagen disorder with concomitant impairment of new collagen synthesis.
- *Environmental influences:* Smoking promotes both hernia recurrence and hernia formation. For example, smokers have been shown to have not only a significantly increased rate of relapse after inguinal hernia repair, but also a fourfold risk of developing incisional hernia.
- In addition, numerous other drugs such as ACE inhibitors, corticosteroids, nonsteroidal anti-inflammatory substances, and chemotherapeutic agents have an impact on the various stages of wound healing.
- *Hereditary connective tissue disorders:* Connective tissue disorders such as Ehlers–Danlos syndrome, osteogenesis imperfecta, and cutis laxa, but also congenital dislocations of the hip are generally associated with an increase in the incidence of hernias or an increase in the relapse rate after primary repair.

Complete prevention of incisional hernia cannot be achieved solely by optimizing the surgical technique for abdominal wall closure. The changes in the extracellular matrix observed in patients with incisional hernia, as well as the observed increased incidence of incisional hernias in patients with additional "endogenous" or "exogenous" risk factors, suggests a multifactorial biological basis for the pathogenesis of incisional hernia.

Component Separation Technique

- Component separation is a reconstructive technique that strategically divides myofascial layers of the abdominal wall in order to achieve tension-free midline fascial approximation. Posterior component separation techniques (CSTs) include the Rives–Stoppa retrorectus dissection and transversus abdominis release (TAR).
- The basic principles of the technique include bilateral midline to lateral dissection in a subcutaneous plane adjacent to the fascia up to a line lateral to the rectus muscles and longitudinal transection of the aponeurosis of the external oblique muscle.
- To manage complex hernias, component separation is one technique that can aid in the repair of these difficult hernias. It is particularly used when there is insufficient muscular wall that can be pulled back together during a conventional hernia repair.
- Component separation is a surgical technique used in hernia repair to facilitate closure of large abdominal wall defects.

Indications for component separation in hernia repair include:

- *Large hernias:* Component separation is typically used in cases where the hernia defect is too large to be closed using primary repair techniques alone.
- *Complex hernias:* Component separation may be used in cases where the hernia repair is complicated by other factors, such as previous failed repairs or infections.
- *Inadequate tissue mobility:* In some cases, the tissues surrounding the hernia defect may be too rigid or inflexible to allow for a tension-free closure. Component separation can help to create additional tissue mobility and facilitate closure.
- *Risk of wound complications:* In some cases, a primary closure of a large hernia defect may put the patient at risk for wound complications, such as dehiscence or infection. Component separation can help to reduce the risk of these complications by allowing for a tension-free closure.
- *Recurrent hernias:* Component separation may be used in cases where a hernia has recurred after previous repair attempts. The technique can help to provide additional tissue for closure and reduce the risk of recurrence.

Overall, the decision to use component separation in hernia repair will depend on the individual patient's specific case and the surgeon's expertise and judgment.

Types of CST

Anterior Component Separation

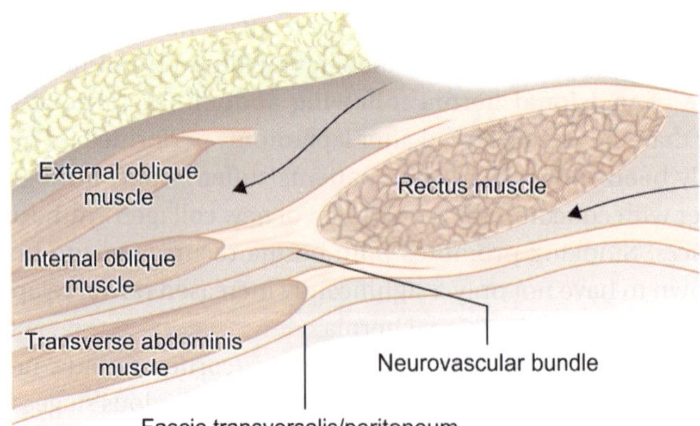

Ramirez developed anterior component separation.

- *Steps:*
  - Wide dissection of subcutaneous space is done
  - Lateral border of rectus muscle and medial border of external oblique muscle is dissected out
  - External oblique muscle is cut 2 cm lateral to rectus border

- Space between external and internal oblique muscle is dissected
- Midline is sutured
- Gain in length is about 8–10 cm in abdominal compartment syndrome (ACS).

Endoscopic Anterior Component Separation

- Incision in upper quadrant made and subcutaneous space is minimally dissected.
- 2 ports (5 mm) are inserted in between the internal and external oblique muscle under vision.
- Dissection is carried out between external and internal oblique muscle.
- About 6 cm advancement on either side can be achieved by this technique.

Benefit: Less surgical site occurrence due to less subcutaneous dissection

Perforator Sparing Anterior Component Separation

- The blood supply of anterior abdominal wall is divided in three zones.
  - *Huger zone 1:* Central abdominal zone, supplied by deep inferior epigastric and superficial epigastric vessels
  - *Huger zone 2:* Lower abdominal zone supplied by superficial inferior epigastric, superficial circumflex iliac, and superficial external pudendal vessels
  - *Huger zone 3:* Lateral abdominal zone supplied by intercostal, subcostal, and lumber vessels.
- In this hernia repair technique, blood supply in and around 3 cm of umbilicus is preserved.

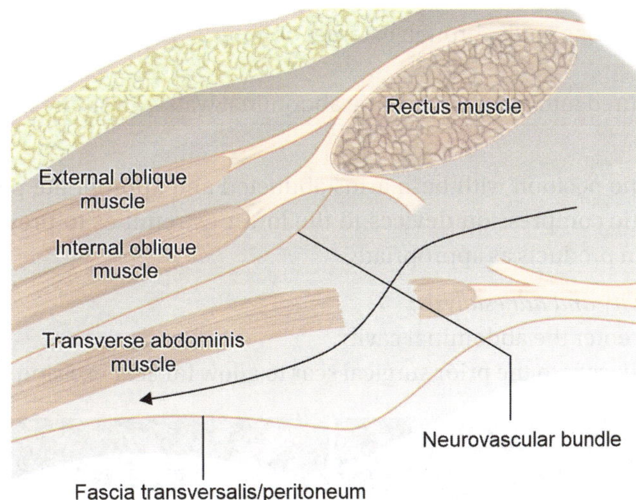

Carbonel introduced posterior component separation technique.

Here retromuscular plane is extended between internal oblique and transversus abdominis.

- *Steps:*
  - Incision is made with in 0.5 cm of medial border of posterior rectus sheath.
  - Incision is extended superiorly and inferiorly along the entire length of external oblique muscle.
  - Dissection carried out medial to lateral preventing injury to epigastric vessel.
  - Lateral limit of the posterior component separation is linea semilunaris.
  - Superiorly it extends up to retroxyphoid or retromuscular space and inferiorly up to space of retzius.
  - Care should be taken to preserve the intercostal neurovasculature.
  - Retrorectus dissection can be extended lateral to linea semilunaris by means of TAR.
  - In this technique, an incision is made 0.5 cm medial to linea semilunaris and transversus abdominis muscle is exposed.
  - With electrocautery transection of transverse abdominis muscle is done
  - Reapproximation of posterior rectus sheath is done in midline using 2-0 polyglactin suture.

Hybrid (Combination of Open and Lap) Release of External Oblique Aponeurosis

Basic Steps to Open CST

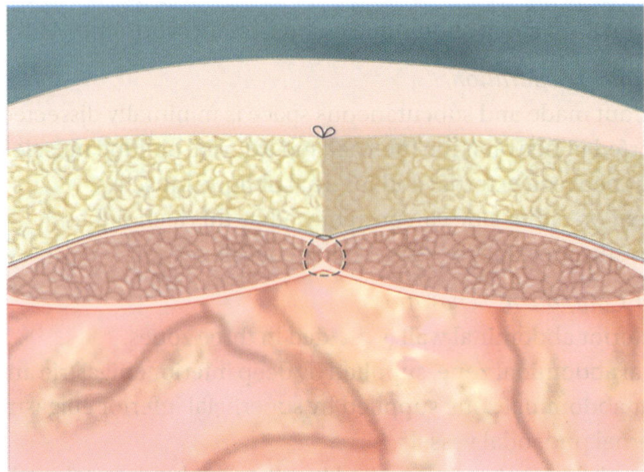

- Enter the abdominal cavity and perform adhesiolysis.
- Bilateral skin flaps raised.
- Bilateral relaxing incisions made through external oblique 2–3 cm lateral to the linea semilunaris.
- Midline closed.
- Surgical Graft is secured into place against the abdominal wall with sutures, followed by skin closure.

Patient Preparation

Place the patient in a supine position with both arms abducted and appropriate padding on all pressure points. Apply sequential pneumatic compression devices to the lower extremities to prevent deep venous thrombosis. Utilize preoperative heparin products as appropriate.

Entering the abdominal cavity and adhesiolysis:

- Use sharp dissection to enter the abdominal cavity.
- The incision is made adjacent to the prior surgical scar to allow for scar excision.

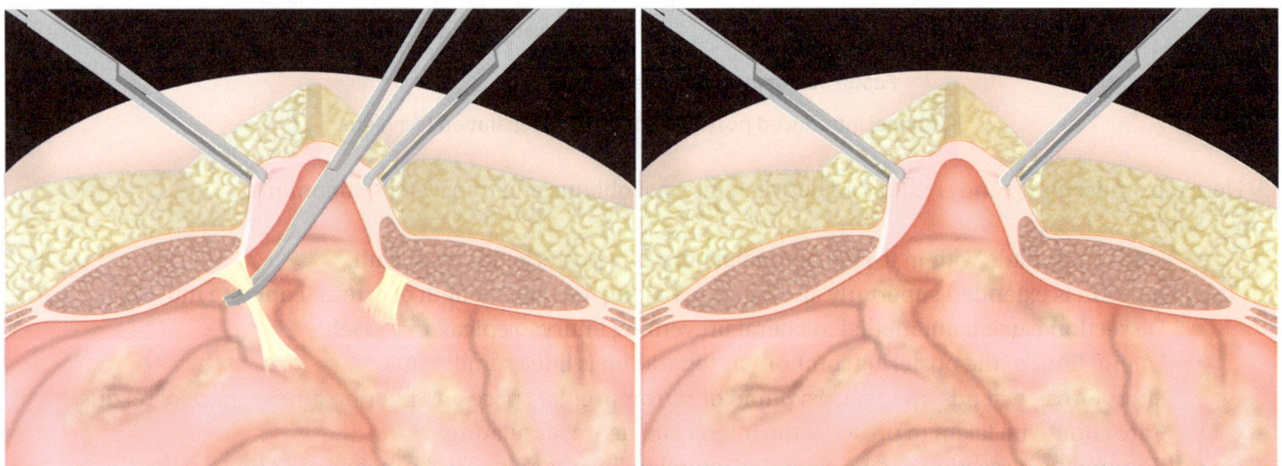

- Enter the abdominal cavity above or below the prior incision to gain access to the peritoneal cavity in an area free of adhesions.
- Open the remainder of the incision.
- Dissect bowel, omentum, and/or other adhered organs from the abdominal wall using direct visualization.

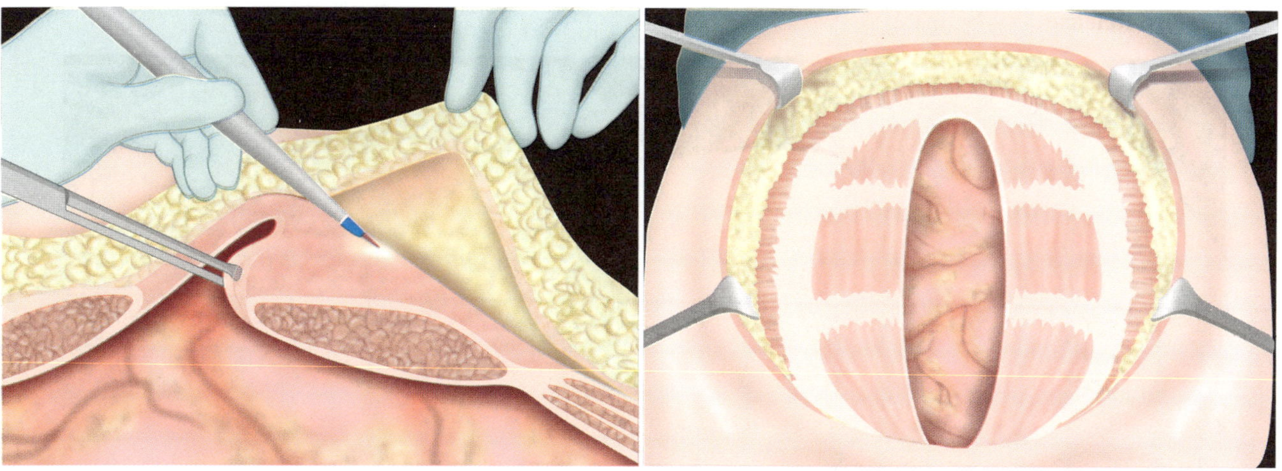

Bilateral Skin Flaps Raised

- Release a flap consisting of skin and subcutaneous tissue from the underlying anterior rectus sheath using cautery.
- Extend laterally beyond the linea semilunaris to the level of anterior axillary line.
- Extend caudally to the inguinal ligament and cephalad to a distance approximately 5 cm above the costal margins.
- In most circumstances, the releases are performed bilaterally.

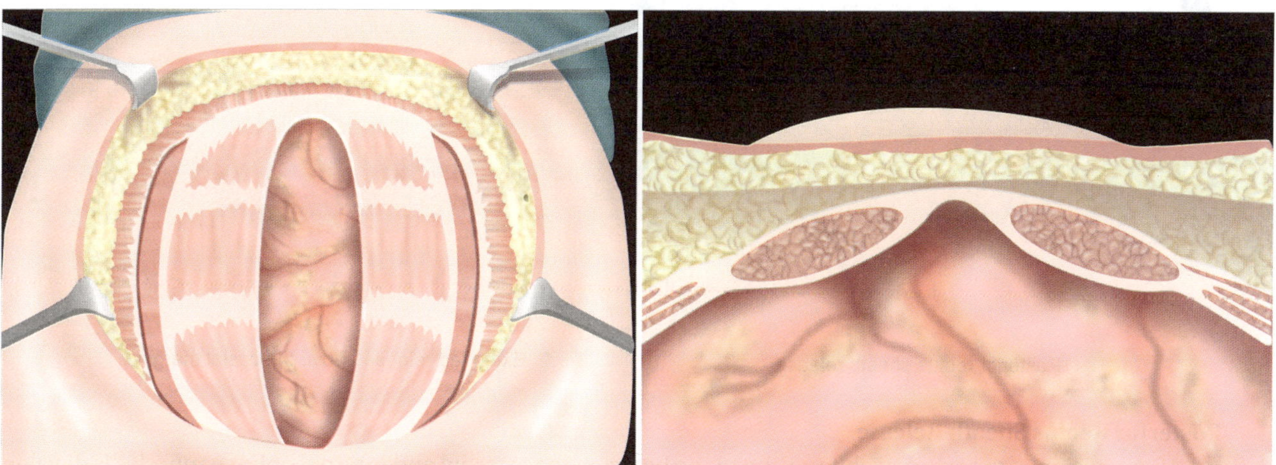

Create Relaxing Incisions

- Create a vertically oriented incision in the external oblique aponeurosis located 2–3 cm lateral to the linea semilunaris.
- The relaxing incision should extend from the inguinal ligament to at least the level of the costal margin.
- In the event of an epigastric defect, the incision should extend several centimeters above the costal margin.

Standard Release

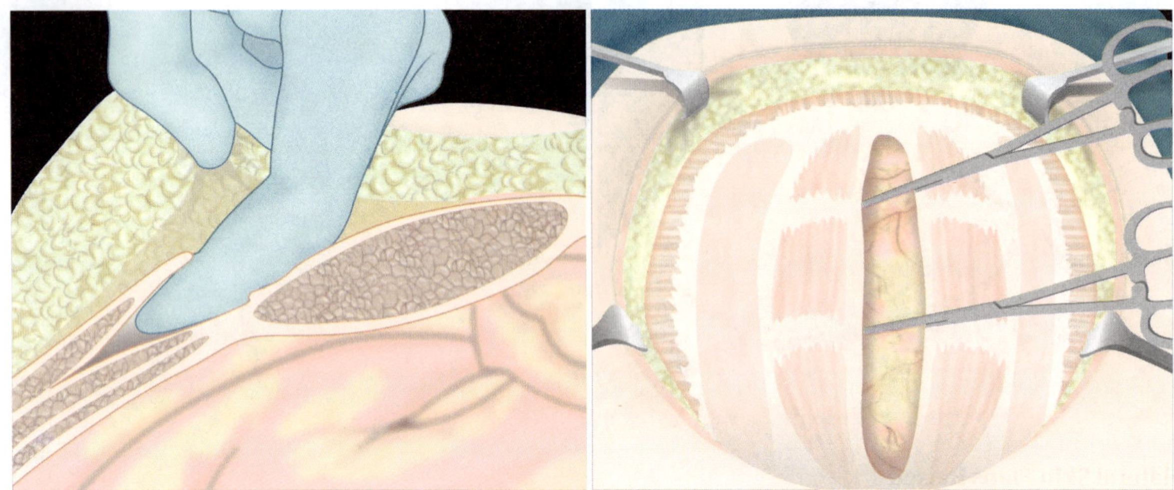

Additional Advancement Options

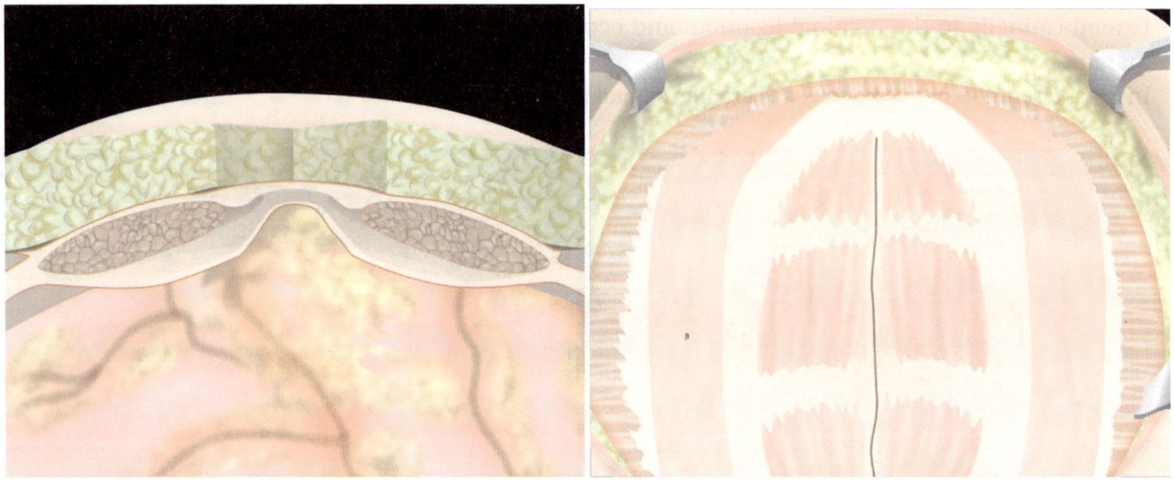

Posterior rectus sheath release

Extended release above the costal margin

Posterior Rectus Sheath Release

- After division of the external oblique, the plane between the external and internal oblique muscles is developed using blunt dissection and extending out to the anterior axillary line.
- Further advancement can be obtained by elevating the rectus from the posterior rectus sheath by incising the posterior rectus sheath 1–2 cm from the midline. The anterior rectus sheath should be left intact for suture placement.
- In most circumstances, the releases are performed bilaterally.

Midline Closure

- The hernia sac and attenuated fascia are debrided from the midline to ensure apposition of healthy well-vascularized tissue as the midline is closed.
- To assess the abdomen for closure, Kocher clamps are applied to the anterior rectus fascia on each side and brought to the midline.

- Monitor peak airway pressures during this maneuver.
- Absent a significant increase in peak airway pressures, plan to close the fascia primarily with interrupted sutures.

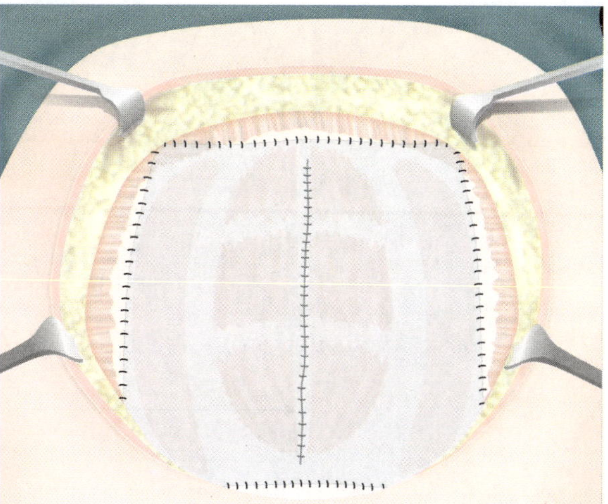

Graft Placement

- Reinforce the hernia repair with a surgical graft in an onlay or underlay position.
- To address larger defects, multiple surgical grafts may be sutured together with a running suture.
- Orient the surgical graft in either a rectangular or diamond configuration to reinforce the entire abdominal wall and secure with a continuous suture.
- For on-lay mesh placement, suture the surgical graft bilaterally to the released lateral edges of the external oblique and sew it to the anterior rectus sheath superiorly and inferiorly.

Retromuscular Placement

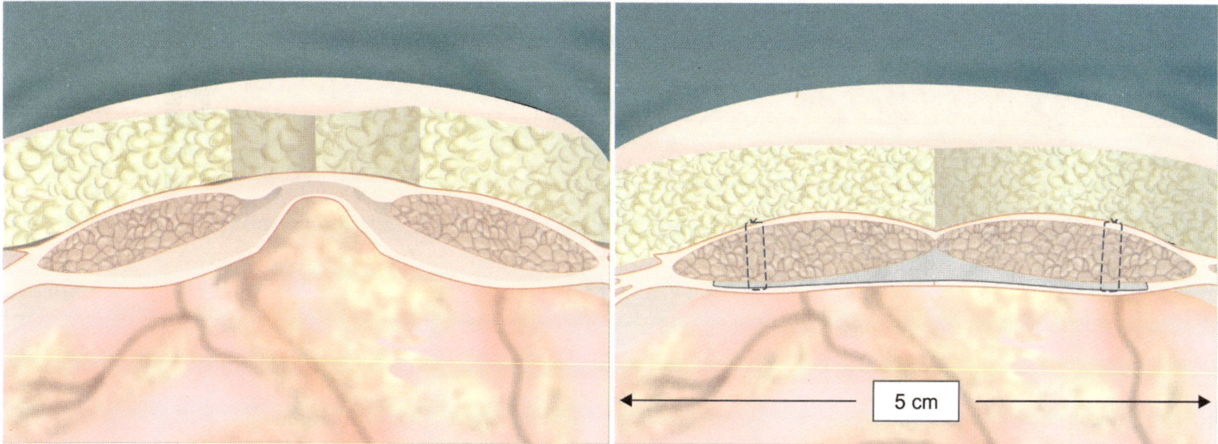

Graft Placement Continued

- For underlay mesh placement, place the surgical graft either as an intraperitoneal graft or in the retrorectus space.
- If placed in the retrorectus space, additional dissection is needed to create a pocket for the graft. Once the retrorectus space has been developed, close the posterior rectus sheath with a running absorbable suture. This will create a space for the surgical graft between the rectus muscle and the posterior rectus sheath.

Intraperitoneal Placement

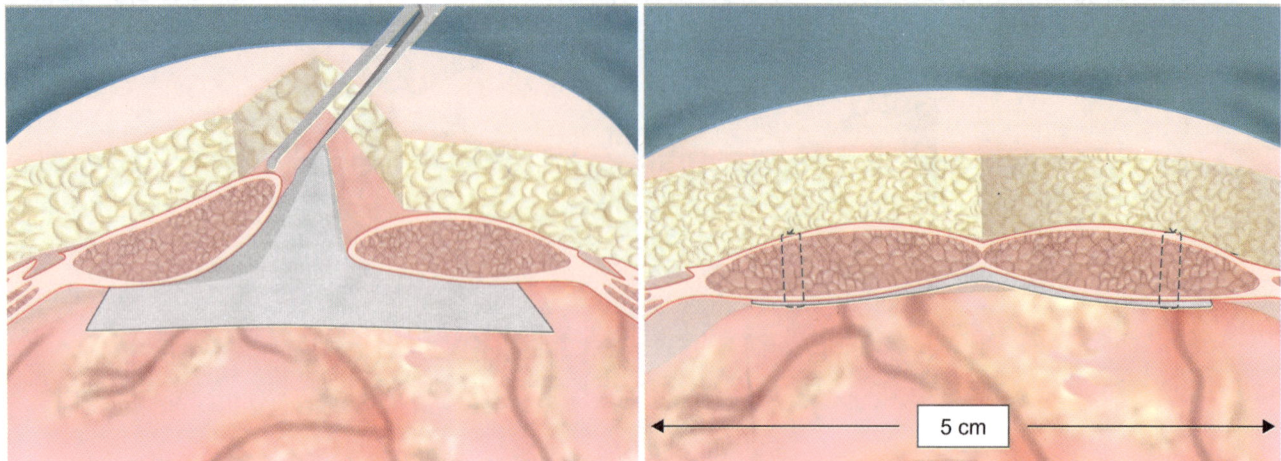

- Reinforce the entire incision by overlapping the surgical graft by approximately 5 cm.
- Suture the graft to the abdominal wall with a series of interrupted horizontal mattress sutures.
- Place the sutures laterally on the abdominal wall to allow for approximation of the midline fascia when the sutures are secured on each side.

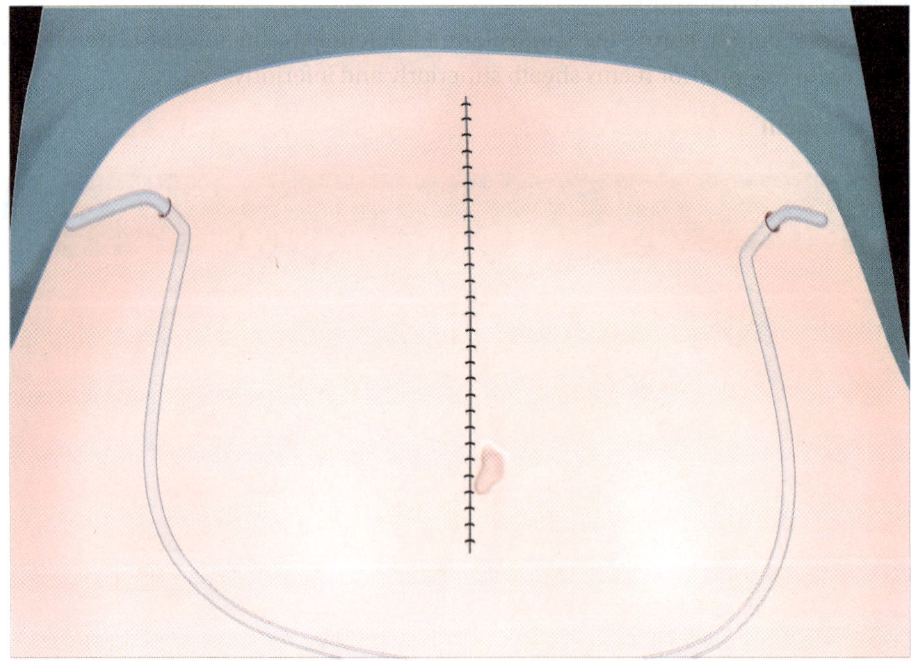

- Irrigate the wound with sterile, normal saline.
- Place closed suction drains beneath the flaps in the subcutaneous plane.
- Maintain the drains until the output decreases to <30 milliliters per day for 2 consecutive days.
- Close the skin in a layered fashion due to the extensive undermining of skin.

Points	Component separation technique	Preperitoneal mesh repair
Indications	• *Size of the defect:* Defects larger than 3 cm and smaller ones in obese patients, recurrent hernias, and special types of hernias such as the spigelian hernia, are best treated laparoscopically. There are no objectively defined selection criteria for the upper limit but some experts have suggested limiting LVHR to cases where transverse separation of the fascial edges is 10 cm. However, there are many reports in the literature of LVHR of far much larger hernias • Obese patients and recurrent hernias • "Swiss-cheese" defects	• Infected abdominal wall with or without mesh • Patients with hernias who are also having a colostomy reversed • Very large ventral hernias. Defects of up to 20 cm at the waistline can be bridged • Multiple defects • Multiple failed attempts at previous repairs • Treatment or prevention of the abdominal compartment syndrome (ACS). May avoid open wound management which usually results in a large ventral hernia and potential skin deficit • In those patients with loss of domain, component separation allows placement of a smaller piece of mesh, thereby minimizing eventration
Contraindications	• Extremely large hernias • End-stage cardiac, liver, and pulmonary disease • Extremely dense adhesions such as in previous multiple laparotomies, peritonitis, or end stage renal disease with peritoneal dialysis, as there may be obliteration of the peritoneal cavity for placement of cannulas and the attendant increased risk of enterotomy • Liver cirrhosis and portal hypertension • General contraindications to laparoscopy, e.g., coagulopathy and ascites • Pediatric age group due to the potential of mesh migration • Strangulated hernias • Lack of abdominal domain. This refers to patients with insufficient space in the abdomen to accommodate the contents of the hernia that are also at great risk for pneumoperitoneum • Hernias in which the fascial edges extend lateral to the midclavicular line may make trocar placement lateral to the defect impossible. Defects in close proximity to the bony margins of the abdomen, especially those near the xiphoid, pose significant challenges for mesh fixation, though this is also true with open incisional herniorrhaphy	• Patients with stoma • Delaying the operation until any risk factors (obesity, smoking, COPD, malnutrition, and steroids) can be eliminated will greatly improve the outcome of the operation
Complications		• Rates of wound sepsis, mesh infection, mesh explantation, and gastrointestinal mesh erosion are low with CST • Recurrence is low
Cost	Low	High

21. Discuss the role of component separation technique for repair of complex or large ventral hernia. ***WBUHS 2018***

22. Discuss the component separation techniques for repair of ventral hernia. ***WBUHS 2025***

Introduction

- A ventral hernia is defined by a protrusion through the anterior abdominal wall fascia.
- These defects can be categorized as spontaneous or acquired or by their location on the abdominal wall.

- Acquired hernias typically occur after surgical incisions and are therefore termed incisional hernias.
- Although not a true hernia, diastasis recti can present as a midline bulge.
- Incisional hernias are twice as common in women as in men.

Principles of Ventral Hernia Repair

- One of the underlying principles of abdominal wall reconstruction is to reestablish the linea alba.
- Restoring the linea alba to the midline provides the advantage of a functional abdominal wall, often protects the mesh from superficial wound issues, and might result in a more durable repair.
- Functions of abdominal wall include protection of the abdominal organs, maintenance of upright posture and support the spine, assist bodily functions requiring generation of Valsalva maneuver like coughing, urination, or defecation and provide aesthetic body image.
- Also, absence of an intact abdominal wall results in loss of the mechanical endpoint of satiety leading to unintentional weight gain.
- There are many different techniques that have been developed for the repair of the incisional hernia.
- The central theme of each repair has become midline reapproximation of the autologous tissue (usually rectus muscles) with physiologic tension and proper mesh reinforcement.
- Suture repair alone is associated with unacceptable recurrence rates and should not be the primary objective.
- Either intraperitoneal or retrorectus placement of the prosthetic mesh is usually advocated by most of the literature, with higher recurrence rates seen with an onlay positioning of the mesh.
- For very large or complex ventral hernia, we adopt the CST. The neurovascular anatomy of the abdominal wall allows for a bilateral myofascial medial advancement of the rectus muscles while maintaining the dynamic functionality of the abdominal wall.

Principle of CST

- Unilateral or bilateral release of one of the three muscles of the abdominal wall through a long relaxing incision leads to weakening of the traction on the remaining wall.
- This firstly helps to slide and advance the remaining vascularized, innervated musculofascial layers of abdomen medially, facilitating midline closure, and secondly increases the total abdominal capacity thereby compensating for the domain loss in very large ventral hernias.

Types of CST based on Approach

- *Open approach:*
  - *Anterior CST:* Release of external oblique aponeurosis
  - *Posterior CST:* Release of transverse abdominis aponeurosis (TAR)
- *Endoscopically assisted anterior component separation:* Release of external oblique aponeurosis
- Hybrid (combination of open and lap) Release of external oblique aponeurosis.

  After CST further procedure: May include augmentation with meshplasty.

Indications for CST

- *Only CST:* Large midline ventral hernias in the presence of infection, patients who are also having a colostomy reversal and prophylaxis/treatment of abdominal compartment syndrome.
- *CST reinforced with mesh:* Large midline ventral hernia, midline hernia with multiple defects, multiple failed repairs of incisional hernias and patients with loss of domain.

Open Component Separation Techniques

Ramirez's Classical Anterior CST (1990)

- The most commonly employed technique involves an anterior or external oblique release described by Ramirez in 1990.
- The procedure is begun with the elevation of subcutaneous flaps from the underlying abdominal musculature to expose the linea semilunaris.

- It is critical to preserve the large periumbilical perforators to prevent ischemia of the skin flaps.
- The external oblique fascia is then incised 1 cm lateral to its insertion into the rectus sheath from above the costal margin to the inguinal ligament.
- This allows for the development of an avascular plane between the external oblique aponeurosis and internal oblique muscle as far as the posterior axillary line.
- The developed myofascial complex allows for an 8- to 10-cm advancement at the waist; 3- to 5-cm advancement in the upper and lower abdomen.
- Additional 2-cm advancement can be achieved if the rectus muscle is elevated off of the posterior sheath. Up to 20 cm defect can be closed.
- However, it is associated with high morbidity including hematoma, seroma, infection, and skin necrosis.
- It is important that patients understand that a lateral bulge can occur after release of the external oblique aponeurosis.

Rives-Stoppa-Wantz

- *Posterior CST (Retro-Rectus Repair) (1989):* This procedure involves opening of the anterior rectus sheath bilaterally to redevelop the posterior facial wall.
- This is followed by reconstruction of the facial wall and insertion of the prosthetics behind the rectus muscle plane in partial contact with the subcutaneous tissue.

Novitsky-Open Posterior CST

- *Transverse abdominis release (TAR) (2012):* This novel technique of transversus abdominis muscle release for posterior component separation during major abdominal wall reconstructions is a modification of the classic retro muscular Stoppa technique to facilitate dissection beyond the lateral border of the rectus sheath.
- Briefly, the retromuscular space is developed laterally to the edge of the rectus sheath.
- The posterior rectus sheath is incised 0.5–1 cm medial to the linea semilunaris to expose the medial edge of the transversus abdominis muscle.
- At this location, the posterior leaflet of the internal oblique and the transversus abdominis muscle are incised to gain access to the space anterior to the transversalis fascia, i.e., the preperitoneum.
- This plane can be extended to the retroperitoneum and eventually to the psoas muscle if necessary.
- Very large sheets of prosthetic mesh can be placed in this location with wide defect coverage.
- The posterior rectus fascia then is advanced medially.
- The mesh is placed as a sublay and the linea alba is restored ventral to the mesh.
- It was associated with low perioperative morbidity and a low recurrence rate.
- The most significant advantage of posterior CST is the avoidance of large subcutaneous skin flaps potentially leading to a reduction in wound morbidity.
- The second advantage is the necessity of creating the retrorectus space for mesh placement, which isolates the prosthetic from the viscera.
- The dissection of the plane between the transverses abdominis and transversalsis fascia allows for a wide piece of mesh to be utilized.
- The disadvantage is the decreased advancement of the rectus muscles compared to the anterior release, which can be problematic in large defects.
- It is important to emphasize that the surgeon cannot perform an anterior release in this situation as the abdominal wall would be severely compromised.

Laparoscopic Component Separation Techniques

- LeBlanc first described a laparoscopic ventral hernia repair (LVHR) in 1993.
- The indications for an LVHR are similar to those for an open procedure. However, not all patients are candidates for the procedure.
- There are two major disadvantages to LVHR. The first is that it requires almost complete lysis of adhesions for trocar placement and wide mesh overlap.

- LVHR is generally avoided in patients with densely incarcerated viscera to prevent iatrogenic bowel injury.
- The second major disadvantage is the inability to close the defect in larger hernia.
- The basic principle of a minimally invasive component separation is to gain direct access to the lateral abdominal wall without creating a lipocutaneous flap.
- Typically, this is performed by a direct cut down through a 1-cm incision off the tip of the 11th rib overlying the external oblique muscle.
- The external oblique is split in the line of its fibers, and a standard bilateral inguinal hernia balloon dissector is placed in between the external and internal oblique muscles, toward the pubis.
- Three laparoscopic trocars are placed in the space created, and the dissection is carried from the pubis to several centimeters above the costal margin.
- The linea semilunaris is carefully identified, and the external oblique is incised from beneath the muscle, at least 2 cm lateral to the linea semilunaris.
- The muscle is released from the pubis to several centimeters above the costal margin. This procedure is performed bilaterally.
- Synthetic or biologic mesh can be used to reinforce the repair of the midline closure.
- These relatively new techniques are feasible, but long-term data demonstrating equivalency to open techniques are lacking.
- It has been shown in several studies that laparoscopic incisional hernia repair results in fewer postoperative complications, lower infection rate, and decreased hernia recurrence.

Endoscopic, Laparoscopic, and Robotic Surgery

LEARNING OBJECTIVES

- Physiological, Pathophysiological and Complications of Pneumoperitoneum
- Safe Laparoscopic Surgery
- Port Site Infection and Port Site Recurrence
- Diagnostic Laparoscopy
- Limitations of Minimal Access Surgery and Access Complications
- Notes and HALS
- Robotic Surgery
- Laparoscopic Hernia Surgery
- Ergonomics in Laparoscopic Surgery
- Endoscopy
- Robotic Surgery
- Artificial Intelligence in Surgery

PNEUMOPERITONEUM

1. What are the gases used for creating pneumoperitoneum? What are the physiological effects of pneumoperitoneum and complications of pneumoperitoneum in laparoscopic surgery?
WBUHS 2022, WBUHS 2025 Supplementary, DY Patil Educational Society Deemed to be University 2020

2. What are the pathophysiologic effect of CO_2 pneumoperitoneum? ***WBUHS 2013***

3. What are the complications of pneumoperitoneum and describe their management?
WBUHS 2016 , DY Patil Educational Society Deemed to be University 2020

Introduction

- Laparoscopic surgery is nowadays a common daily-performed procedure worldwide, replacing many types of open surgeries.
- It has the benefits of small incision, improved cosmetic aspects, less postoperative pain, and quick recovery time to normal activities.
- The most commonly used gas for insufflation is carbon dioxide (CO_2).
- Carbon dioxide pneumoperitoneum and increased intra-abdominal pressure (IAP) can induce many pathophysiologic disturbances, requiring the anesthesiologist to be well alert during the operation for necessary management.
- Moreover, advanced laparoscopic surgeries are being used also on older patients and in critically ill patients, requiring technically demanding anesthesia.

Different Gases Used for Pneumoperitoneum

Most common gas—CO_2

Other gases used are:

Air	Oxygen	N_2O	Helium	Argon	Mixture of these gases

Pathophysiologic Changes

Carbon dioxide pneumoperitoneum and increased IAP can induce many pathophysiologic disturbances, requiring the anesthesiologist to be well alert during the operation for necessary management.

Respiratory Changes

- The physiology of respiratory system is affected by pneumoperitoneum.
- With insufflation, causing an increase in IAP, the diaphragm is pushed upward causing stiffness of the chest wall, causing the total volume of the lungs to be reduced.
- Hence, the pulmonary compliance is decreased to 35–40% and also a non-negligible increase in the maximum respiratory system resistance.
- Hypoxemia may occur from a ventilation-perfusion mismatch and intrapulmonary shunting but is rare in healthy patients.

(CO_2 is usually administered at a rate of 1–2 mL/min being a highly soluble gas, it is readily absorbed into the circulation through the peritoneum, causing hypercapnia and acidosis)

- Several studies have shown the effect of CO_2 pneumoperitoneum on the arterial partial pressure of CO_2 ($PaCO_2$) and end-tidal CO_2 ($ETCO_2$). CO_2 is mainly excreted by the lungs, depending on alveolar and mixed venous CO_2 exchange rates, which are themselves controlled by the cardiac output, alveolar ventilation, and respiratory quotient.
- Normal excretion of CO_2 is 100–200 mL/min and is increased by 14–48 mL/min when CO_2 is administered intraperitoneally.
- After a long laparoscopic operation, achieving a normal CO_2 value can take several hours after desufflation.

Cardiovascular Changes

- Cardiovascular system effects during CO_2 pneumoperitoneum are caused mainly by hypercarbia followed by acidosis and increased IAP.
- Euvolemic status is of great importance prior to surgery to reduce any cardiac depression via reduced preload caused by the pneumoperitoneum.
- Hypercarbia has direct and indirect sympathoadrenal stimulating effects on cardiovascular functions.
- These effects are not pronounced with mild hypercarbia ($PaCO_2$ 45–50 mm Hg).
- Moderate-to-severe hypercarbia affects cardiac function since it is then a myocardial depressant and has direct vasodilatory effect.

Renal Changes

- Oliguria is the most common renal effect of pneumoperitoneum.
- Different mechanisms are involved in the reduction of the urine amount during IAP. IAP also activates of the renin-angiotensin-aldosterone system following decreased renal perfusion, which results in renal cortical vasoconstriction.
- Level of antidiuretic hormone (ADH), renin, and aldosterone significantly increased during laparoscopic gastric bypass (GBP).
- Renal blood flow (RBF) has been measured during increasing IAP, and a gradual decrease in RBF up to 75% was observed upon reaching a pressure of 15 mm Hg.
- Those with maintenance fluid, whereas this change was not noticed in well-hydrated animals with adequate volume loading.

Splanchnic Changes

- The splanchnic circulation is also affected during raised IAP. Depending on IAP, studies in animals have shown to decrease in splanchnic macro and microcirculation.
- Signs of hepatocytic damage were noticed, with increase of glutamic oxaloacetic transaminase and glutamic pyruvic transaminase. Impaired Kupffer cell function and gastric intramucosal pH drop were also noticed.

Complications

Complications due to pneumoperitoneum

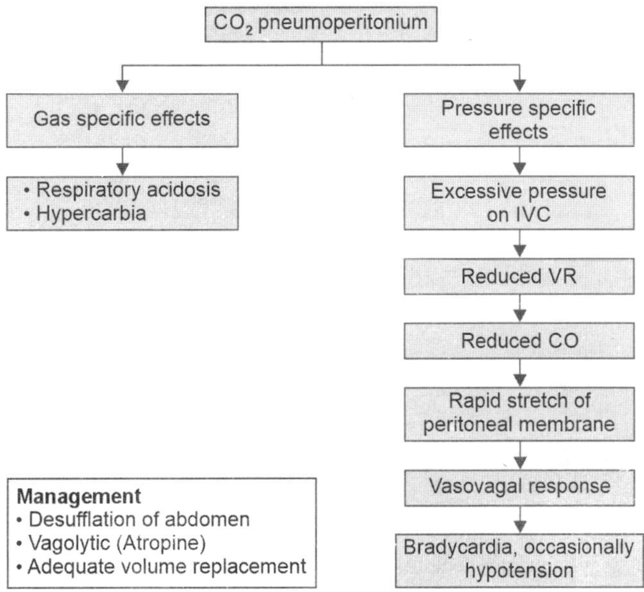

(CO: cardiac output; IVC: inferior vena cava; VR: venous resistance)

Pulmonary Complications of Pneumoperitoneum

- Gas embolism
- Barotraumas, hypoxemia
- Pulmonary edema
- Atelectasis
- Subcutaneous emphysema
- Pneumothorax
- Pneumomediastinum
- Pneumopericardium

Respiratory dysfunction

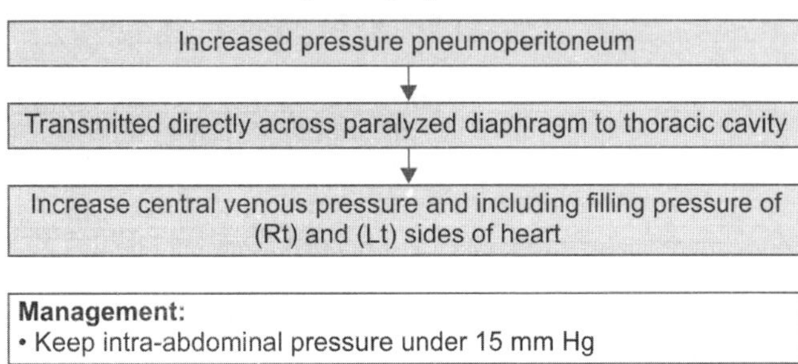

- *Carbon dioxide embolism:*
    - Rare
    - *Incidence:* 0.0014–0.6% of laparoscopic surgeries
    - Mortality rate of about 28%
    - Carbon dioxide enters the circulation through an opening in a damaged vessel under raised IAP.
    - It can also occur if the Veress needle is misplaced into a vessel or parenchymal organ.
    - Transesophageal echocardiography studies have shown bubbling of CO_2 in the right heart chamber in 68% asymptomatic patients during pneumoperitoneum.

- *Clinical manifestations of gas embolism:*
  - Severe drop in blood pressure
  - Cyanosis
  - Cardiac arrhythmias or asystole
  - A mill-wheel murmur may be heard on auscultation of the heart.
  - $ETCO_2$ will increase.

DVT pulmonary embolism

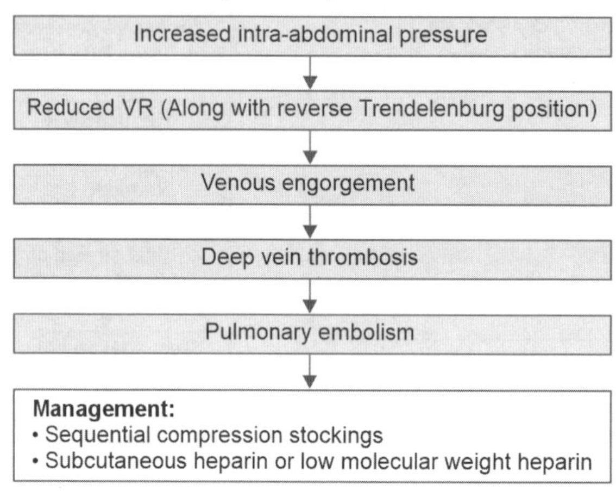

(DVT: deep vein thrombosis; VR: venous resistance)

- *Subcutaneous emphysema:*
  - *Incidence:* 0.3–3.0% laparoscopic surgeries
  - Mild-to-severe subcutaneous emphysema has generally not been shown to have clinical effects, but upper airway obstruction must be considered if there is neck involvement.

Subcutaneous and subfascial emphysema and edema

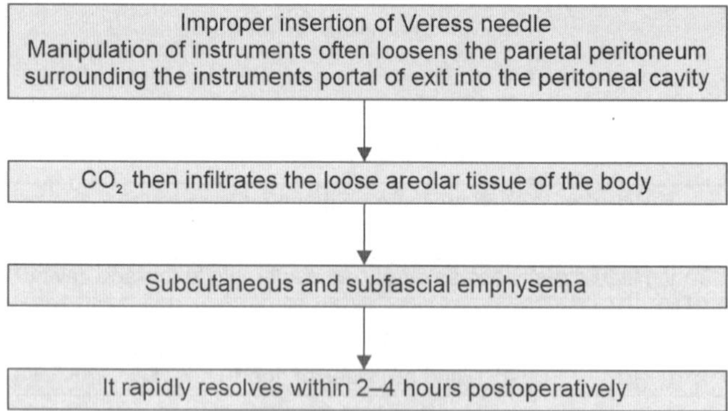

- *Pneumothorax* can occur following peritoneum visceral tear, parietal pleura tear during resection around the esophagus or congenital defect in the diaphragm through which CO_2 gas travels. Pneumothorax should be differentiated with capnothorax following CO_2 diffusion into the intrapleural space.
  - *Diagnosis:* Presence of rapidly falling oxygen saturation or pO_2 together with difficult ventilation and decreased breath sounds.
  - *Management:*
    - Immediate needle thoracostomy
    - Aspiration
    - Chest radiograph
    - Placement of chest tube

- Extension of emphysema can also occur, causing *pneumothorax and pneumomediastinum.*
    - With both pneumothorax and capnothorax, the $ETCO_2$ increases, so capnothorax can be suspected if the mean airway pressure increases with a drop in SpO_2, and confirmation should be made with a chest X-ray.
- *Pneumopericardium* can develop when CO_2 is forced into the mediastinum and pericardium. It can also occur if CO_2 enters the defect in the membranous portion of the diaphragm, resulting in a communication between the pericardial and peritoneal cavities.

Cardiovascular Complications

- Hypertension
- Arrhythmias
- Hypotension and cardiac arrest
    - *Hypertension* seems to have a higher incidence at the beginning of insufflation when the blood volume in the splanchnic vasculature is reduced due to increased IAP, thereby increasing preload and arterial pressure.
    - *Arrhythmias* occur in up to 14–27% of laparoscopies. These must be differentiated from arrhythmias caused by release of catecholamine.
    - *Sinus tachycardia* and *ventricular extrasystoles* are usually more benign, and dangerous ones like bradyarrhythmias (bradycardia, nodal rhythm, atrioventricular dissociation, and asystole) are also seen.
    - *Bradyarrhythmia:*
        - It arises due to the vagal nerve-mediated cardiovascular response following acute stretching of the peritoneum.
    - *Hypotension:*
        - It occurs in up to 13% of laparoscopies, a potentially serious complication. IAP of 20 mm Hg or more results in compression of the inferior vena cava, reducing the venous return. Cardiac output is reduced, leading to hypotension.
        - This complication is aggravated by high intrathoracic pressure.
    - *Vasovagal responses* to quick intraperitoneal CO_2 insufflation and gas embolism have both been related to *cardiac arrest.* The possible development of acute tubular necrosis in response to long-lasting hypoperfusion from pneumoperitoneum is controversial.
    - Free radicals are released by inflation and deflation of the peritoneum. Oxygen and organic free radicals may contribute to ischemia reperfusion phenomena or chemical carcinogenesis. Still, the impact of production of free radicals is smaller than with open surgery injury.

Renal Complications

Effects on renal system

Increased intra-abdominal pressure

Reduced RBF, reduced GFR

Reduced urine output

Including plasma renin activity

Including Na^+ retention

Including ADH activity

Including free water absorption

Management:
• Adequate volume replacement at maintenance rate

(ADH: antidiuretic hormone; GFR: glomerular filtration rate; RBF: renal blood flow)

- The possible development of acute tubular necrosis in response to long-lasting hypoperfusion from pneumoperitoneum is controversial.
  - *Free radicals* are released by inflation and deflation of the peritoneum. Oxygen and organic free radicals may contribute to ischemia reperfusion phenomena or chemical carcinogenesis.

4. Write down the indications, complications, and prevention of complication of carbon dioxide pneumoperitoneum. ***WBUHS 2025***

Carbon Dioxide Pneumoperitoneum

Indications:

- *Laparoscopic surgery:* Used to create a working space in the abdominal cavity for procedures like cholecystectomy, appendectomy, hernia repair, and gynecologic surgeries (e.g., hysterectomy, ovarian cystectomy).
- *Diagnostic laparoscopy:* Facilitates visualization of abdominal organs for diagnostic purposes, such as evaluating chronic abdominal pain or staging malignancies.
- *Minimally invasive procedures:* Employed in robotic surgeries and endoscopic interventions requiring abdominal insufflation.

Complications:

I. *Gas-related complications:*
  - *Hypercarbia:* Excessive CO_2 absorption leading to respiratory acidosis.
  - *Gas Embolism:* Rare but life-threatening; CO_2 bubbles enter the bloodstream, potentially causing cardiovascular collapse.
  - *Subcutaneous emphysema:* CO_2 leaks into subcutaneous tissues, causing swelling and crepitus.
  - *Pneumothorax/pneumomediastinum:* Gas migration into the thoracic cavity or mediastinum.

II. *Pressure-related complications:*
  - *Increased intra-abdominal pressure (IAP):* Can reduce venous return, leading to decreased cardiac output, especially in patients with cardiovascular compromise.
  - *Organ ischemia:* Elevated IAP may impair blood flow to abdominal organs (e.g., kidneys, liver, intestines).
  - *Diaphragmatic splinting:* High pressure restricts diaphragm movement, reducing lung compliance and causing respiratory distress.

III. *Procedure-related complications:*
  - *Visceral or vascular injury:* During trocar insertion or due to excessive pressure.
  - *Postoperative shoulder pain:* Referred pain from diaphragmatic irritation by residual CO_2.
  - *Postoperative nausea/vomiting:* Due to CO_2 absorption or peritoneal irritation.

IV. *Patient-specific complications:*
  - Exacerbation of pre-existing conditions (e.g., chronic obstructive pulmonary disease, heart failure) due to hypercarbia or increased IAP.
  - *Compartment syndrome:* Prolonged high-pressure pneumoperitoneum may lead to abdominal compartment syndrome.

Prevention of Complications

I. *Monitoring and technique:*
  - *Intraoperative monitoring:* Continuous monitoring of end-tidal CO_2, arterial blood gases, and intra-abdominal pressure (typically maintained below 12–15 mm Hg in adults, lower in pediatric patients).
  - *Low-pressure pneumoperitoneum:* Use the lowest effective pressure to minimize cardiovascular and respiratory effects.
  - *Proper trocar placement:* Use open (Hasson) technique or optical trocars to reduce risk of visceral/vascular injury.

- *Gradual insufflation:* Slow initial insufflation to monitor for adverse effects and avoid sudden pressure spikes.

II. *Patient selection and preparation:*
- *Preoperative assessment:* Evaluate cardiopulmonary status to identify patients at risk of complications from hypercarbia or increased IAP.
- *Optimize patient condition:* Correct hypovolemia and stabilize comorbidities before surgery.

III. *Intraoperative strategies:*
- *Ventilation adjustments:* Use adequate positive end-expiratory pressure (PEEP) and adjust tidal volumes to manage hypercarbia and prevent atelectasis.
- *Warming CO_2 gas:* Use warmed, humidified CO_2 to reduce peritoneal irritation and postoperative pain.
- *Limit Procedure Duration:* Minimize duration of pneumoperitoneum to reduce CO_2 absorption and pressure-related effects.

IV. *Postoperative care:*
- *Complete gas evacuation:* Ensure thorough desufflation at the end of surgery to minimize residual CO_2 and reduce shoulder pain.
- *Monitor for complications:* Observe for signs of subcutaneous emphysema, pneumothorax, or gas embolism in the recovery period.
- *Pain management:* Administer analgesics to manage referred shoulder pain or abdominal discomfort.

V. *Special considerations:*
- *Alternative gases:* In high-risk patients, consider helium insufflation (less soluble, lower risk of hypercarbia) if available, though CO_2 remains standard due to safety and availability.
- *Training and expertise:* Ensure surgeons and staffs are trained in laparoscopic techniques to minimize procedural errors.

---

5. Describe peritoneal access in laparoscopic abdominal surgery and principles of VATS.

Srimanta Sankaradeva University, Assam 2025

Peritoneal Access in Laparoscopic Abdominal Surgery

Definition

Peritoneal access is the initial entry into the abdominal cavity to establish pneumoperitoneum (insufflation of CO_2), which allows visualization and working space for laparoscopic instruments.

Methods of Access

- *Closed (Veress Needle Technique)*
  - *Steps:*
    - A small infra- or supra-umbilical incision is made.
    - The *Veress needle* is inserted through the abdominal wall into the peritoneal cavity.
    - Correct placement is confirmed (e.g., saline drop test, low insufflation pressure).
    - CO_2 is insufflated to create pneumoperitoneum (usually 12–15 mm Hg).
    - A trocar is inserted after adequate distension.
  - *Advantages:* Quick, small incision.
  - *Risks:* Blind entry—risk of injury to bowel or major vessels.
- *Open (Hasson Technique)*
  - *Steps:*
    - Small incision at the umbilicus.
    - Layers of abdominal wall dissected under direct vision to enter peritoneum.
    - A blunt-tipped (Hasson) trocar is secured with sutures.
    - CO_2 insufflation is started.
  - *Advantages:* Direct vision reduces injury risk—preferred in patients with prior surgeries or suspected adhesions.

- *Optical trocar/direct entry technique*
  - A trocar with an integrated endoscope is inserted directly through the abdominal wall under visual guidance.
  - *Advantages:* Direct visualization during entry, rapid, less risk of insufflation errors.

Principles of Safe Peritoneal Access

- *Patient positioning:* Usually supine, table level.
- *Empty bladder and stomach* before entry.
- *Choice of site:* Umbilicus is common; alternate sites (Palmer's point) for patients with prior laparotomy or suspected adhesions.
- *Check insufflation pressure:* Should remain low (<10 mm Hg initially).
- *Always confirm intraperitoneal placement* before inserting additional trocars.

Principles of VATS (Video-Assisted Thoracoscopic Surgery)

Definition

VATS is a minimally invasive surgical approach to the thoracic cavity using a thoracoscope and specialized instruments inserted through small intercostal incisions.

Basic Principles

- *Single-lung ventilation:* Achieved with double-lumen endotracheal tube to collapse the operative lung and allow visualization.
- *Port placement:* Typically 2–4 small ports placed strategically depending on the procedure (e.g., lobectomy, pleurodesis).
- *Thoracoscopic visualization:* Camera provides magnified image on video monitor.
- *CO_2 insufflation (optional):* Sometimes used at low pressure to aid collapse and visualization.
- *Instrumentation:* Long, articulated instruments for dissection, stapling, and specimen retrieval.

Advantages

- Smaller incisions, less pain.
- Reduced postoperative complications (less atelectasis, faster recovery).
- Shorter hospital stay and improved cosmetic results.

Limitations/Precautions

- Requires adequate lung isolation and trained anesthetic support.
- Limited tactile feedback.
- Conversion to thoracotomy may be necessary if bleeding or poor visualization occurs.

SAFE LAPAROSCOPIC SURGERY

6. Enumerate the principles of safe laparoscopic surgery. Discuss the technique of primary trocar insertion.

WBUHS 2022

7. Basic principle of port site placement in laparoscopic surgery and technique for primary trocar insertion.

Rajasthan University of Health Sciences 2025

Principles of Safe Laparoscopic Surgery

- Patient positioning and how this aids surgery
- Gaining access into the abdomen
- Methods of establishing pneumoperitoneum
- Maintaining good vision during surgery and how this can be achieved
- Insertion of additional ports
- A description of available laparoscopic instruments

- Limitations of laparoscopy
- Closure of port sites
- Threshold for conversion

Basic Principles of Port Site Placement in Laparoscopic Surgery

Port placement follows *6 core principles* to ensure *safety, efficiency, and ergonomics*:

The 6 Golden Rules

#	*Principle*	*Key rule*	*Purpose*
1	Triangulation	Form a *60°–90° triangle* between camera and two working instruments pointing to the *target organ*	Enables natural manipulation, prevents clashing
2	Target-centric	All ports *converge toward the operative field*	Keeps instruments in view, avoids blind zones
3	Trocar spacing	*≥5–7 cm between ports ≥2–3 cm from bony landmarks*	Prevents external collision, gas leaks, hernia
4	Camera first	Insert *camera port first* (usually *umbilicus*) under direct vision	Establishes safe pneumoperitoneum and overview
5	Tailored to anatomy	Adjust for *BMI, height, prior scars, organ location*	Avoids poor reach, injury, or conversion
6	Ergonomic alignment	Ports at *mid-abdominal level*, surgeon's elbows *90°–110°*	Reduces fatigue and musculoskeletal strain

Standard Camera Port Locations

Procedure Type	*Camera port*
Upper GI/biliary	*Umbilicus or supraumbilical*
Colorectal/pelvic	*Umbilicus or infraumbilical*
Reoperative/adhesions	*Left upper quadrant (Palmer's point)*

Quick Placement Tips

- *Right-hand port*: Slightly *cephalad and lateral* to camera
- *Left-hand port*: *Mirror image* across midline
- *Assistant port*: For *retraction only* (e.g., subxiphoid in cholecystectomy)
- *Avoid midline below umbilicus* for large (>10 mm) ports → ↑ hernia risk
- *Transilluminate* to avoid epigastric vessels

Complications of Poor Placement

Issue	*Cause*	*Fix*
Instrument fighting	Ports too close	Increase spacing
Limited reach	Ports too far	Pre-check with spinal needle
Bleeding	Epigastric injury	Transilluminate
Hernia	Large port in midline	Close fascia, use lateral sites

Technique of Primary Trocar Insertion

- *The open "Hassan" technique* can be likened to the now infrequently used "diagnostic peritoneal lavage" approach.
- Whilst there are minor surgeon-dependent variations in this approach, the technique is standardized.
    - The approach commences with a small vertical skin incision (1 cm) below or above the umbilicus depending on the position of the patient's umbilicus in relation to the territory being operated on.
    - The cicatrix of the umbilicus is then elevated using a clip and dissection is performed to expose the abdominal fascia at the base of the cicatrix.

- The abdominal fascia can then be raised with sutures placed on either side of the midline or with a second clip in order to maximize the distance from the underlying intra-abdominal organs.
- The fascia and peritoneum are then incised in a controlled and progressive manner in order to maintain a truly open technique as opposed to bluntly pushing in instruments, which can easily cause injury.
- A 10-mm trocar and port is generally inserted through this opening, though with the advent of smaller scopes 5-mm ports can now be used instead.
- Inserting the trocar through the fascia has significant potential for iatrogenic injury and reports of aortic or inferior vena cava injury unfortunately occur more frequently than they should.
- Damage to the underlying structures can be minimized by elevating the fascia, ensuring the technique is truly open and by pointing trocars down to the pelvis away from the main vessels on insertion.
- There are several variations to the described method. Some are due to surgeon choice and others are driven by specific surgical indications.

- *Closed method:*
  - A Veress needle can be used to create a pneumoperitoneum prior to port insertion. The Veress needle has a spring-loaded, inner blunt stylet positioned centrally within an outer cannula that has a beveled end.
  - As the Veress needle is pushed through firm tissue, pressure on the tip pushes the blunt stylet into the shaft of the outer cannula, allowing the outer needle to cut through.
  - As the needle passes through the firm layer, the blunt-tipped inner stylet springs out and serves to protect any abdominal viscera from iatrogenic injury by the sharp cannula.
  - Once the Veress needle is in the abdominal cavity, the abdomen is filled with gas before the port is inserted. Patients that have had previous surgery are prone to adhesion formation and carry an increased risk of visceral injury on entry into the abdomen.
  - Special techniques may be required in such circumstances to permit safe entry. One common technique involves an open cut down at a safe site away from scars, such as Palmer's point in the left upper quadrant. An alternative method of entry involves the use of a visual port.
  - The laparoscope is mounted into this port, which is then carefully twisted through the layers of the abdominal wall and into the peritoneal cavity under direct laparoscopic vision. In this instance, it is helpful to have the insufflation gas attached and flowing at the high-flow rate as this aids identifying when the peritoneal cavity has been entered.

PORT SITE INFECTION AND PORT SITE RECURRENCE

8. Discuss the causes of port site infections with particular reference to microbiology. How are they managed?
WBUHS 2018

Introduction

- Mycobacterial infections due to atypical mycobacteria at the laparoscopic port site are a common menace encountered in patients undergoing laparoscopic surgery.
- Atypical mycobacterial colonies often exist in tap water, natural waters, and soil and so can easily contaminate solutions and disinfectants used in hospital settings.
- These infections have been a source of significant morbidity for patients recovering from laparoscopic surgeries.

Port Site Wound Infections in Laparoscopy can be of Two Types

1. The first type occurs immediately within 1 week of laparoscopic surgery due to gram negative or positive bacteria derived from infection acquired during surgery from the infected gall bladder or from the skin or the surgical procedure itself and can be treated by common antibiotics and local wound dressing.
2. The second type is caused by atypical mycobacteria which includes the group of mycobacterial species that is not part of the *Mycobacterium tuberculosis* complex having an incubation period of 3–4 weeks which do not respond to common antibiotics.

Infections with Atypical Mycobacteria

- Infections with atypical mycobacteria have been primarily reported after laparoscopic procedures.
- This is because, unlike open surgery, the instruments used for laparoscopic surgery have a layer of insulation that restricts the use of the autoclave in the sterilization process as the high temperatures involved destroy the insulation on them.
- The standard sterilization procedure has been a 20-minute exposure to 2.0–2.5% glutaraldehyde.
- At the current exposure time, these solutions act only as disinfectants and not as sterilizing agent thus allowing bacterial endospores to survive.
- Also, when proper mechanical cleaning of the instruments is not done, blood and charred tissue deposits are left in the joints of the instruments during laparoscopic surgery.
- These contaminated instruments deposit the endospores on to the subcutaneous tissue during the surgery which then germinate following which clinical symptoms appear after an incubation period of 3–4 weeks.

Prevention

- Disposable laparoscopic instruments are the best solution for prevention of infection and is used in western countries.
- The use of advanced sterilization systems like STERRAD, which utilizes gas plasma technology to kill spores at low temperatures, or using ethylene oxide gas for sterilization of insulated laparoscopic instruments. One can also keep instruments for 24 hours in a formalin gas chamber.

Treatment

- These microorganisms show limited response to first line antituberculosis drugs. The standard treatment consists of combinations of second-line antitubercular drugs including macrolides such as clarithromycin, quinolones like ciprofloxacin, tetracyclines like doxycycline, and aminoglycosides like amikacin.
- The standard treatment starts after manifestation of clinical symptoms which consist of a 28-day regimen of oral clarithromycin and ciprofloxacin or amikacin.
- However, local administration of aminoglycosides has been shown to be highly efficacious in the treatment of particularly stubborn nodules and sinuses that persist after completion of oral therapy.

---

9. Port site recurrences in laparoscopic surgery. ***WBUHS 2006***

Port Site Recurrence

Background

The advent of laparoscopic surgery and the increasing use in intraabdominal and thoracic malignancy has brought forward an uncommon problem of port site recurrence of the primary tumor.

The Diagnosis must Ascertain

- Histologically proven tumor deposit
- A localized circumscribed subcutaneous tumor growth of the abdominal or thoracic wall occurs within the fibrous tissue of the scar as the consequence of a trocar or other sites after laparoscopy, thoracoscopy, or mediastinoscopy.
- Early tumor recurrence (<200 days)
- Port site metastasis is not identical to peritoneal metastasis, serosal invasion, skin metastasis, etc.

Etiology and Pathogenesis

The deposition of metastasis in port site can be attributed due to:

- Increased circulation to parietes in laparoscopic surgery
- *Chimney effect:* At all times, an exodus of the insufflation gas tends to spread the tumor to port site via aerosols.
- Contamination of port by tumor seedling (though not conforming to definition)

Presentation

The revival of the same histologic nature of tumor along the site of extraction of the specimen/unrelated to extraction site may occur in early recurrence. Late recurrence is uncommon.

Diagnosis

As this is diagnosed during follow-up of epithelial cancer the diagnosis is mostly clinical followed by cross-sectional imaging. An excisional biopsy proves the diagnosis.

Treatment

Surgical excision of the port site recurrence with suitable margin (at least 1 cm) along with removal of intra-abdominal recurrence if any.

Prognosis

With a few reports available only port site metastasis does not have a favorable prognosis for epithelial cancers. Though they behave differently from recurrence and thus the longevity is much more than recurrence.

Prevention of Port Site Recurrence

Before resection	*During resection*	*After resection*
• Proper patient selection (exclude patients with very large lesions or lesions invading adjacent organs) • Adequate training and experience of surgeons and assistants • Careful tumor localization • Proper port placement • Anchor all ports	• Avoid gas leaks • Identify tumor bearing segment (intraoperative colonoscopy if needed) • Avoid direct tumor handling or manipulation • Sound surgical techniques (closed resection, en block resection with lymphatic drainage, proximal vessel control, and clearance of resection margin) • Respect oncologic principles • Thorough irrigation and suctioning of abdomen	• Adequate-sized incision for removal of specimen • Wound protector or specimen bag • Microscopic and, if needed microscopic analysis of resected specimen • Thorough irrigation of ports and abdomen with cytotoxic solution or normal saline before closure • Fascial and peritoneal wound closure for ports 10 mm or longer

DIAGNOSTIC LAPAROSCOPY

10. Indications and advantages of diagnostic laparoscopy. *WBUHS 2016*

Diagnostic laparoscopy is often done for the following:

- Find the cause of pain or a growth in the abdomen and pelvic area when X-ray or ultrasound results are not clear.
- After an accident to see if there is injury to the abdomen.
- Before procedures to treat cancer to find out if the cancer has spread. If so, treatment will change.

It is done to examine the following organs:

- Appendix
- Gallbladder
- Liver
- Pancreas
- Small and large bowel
- Spleen
- Stomach
- Pelvic or reproductive organs

It can detect:

- An abdominal mass or tumor
- Fluid in the abdominal cavity
- Liver disease
- The effectiveness of certain treatments
- The degree to which a particular cancer has progressed.

Risks

- Stomach pain that becomes more intense overtime.
- Chills
- Fever
- Redness, swelling, bleeding, or drainage at the incision sites
- Continuous nausea or vomiting
- Persistent cough
- Shortness of breath
- Inability to urinate
- Lightheadedness

Abnormal results may be due to a number of different conditions, including:

- Scar tissue inside the abdomen or pelvis (adhesions)
- Appendicitis
- Cells from inside the uterus grow in other areas (endometriosis)
- Inflammation of the gallbladder (cholecystitis)
- Ovarian cysts or cancer of the ovary
- Infection of the womb, ovaries, or fallopian tubes (pelvic inflammatory disease)
- Signs of injury
- Spread of cancer
- Tumors
- Noncancerous tumors of the womb (uterine fibroids)

11. Diagnostic laparoscopy in staging of gastrointestinal malignancy. *WBUHS 2019*

Introduction

- The staging of gastrointestinal malignancies aims to ensure that each patient receives the most appropriate treatment with minimal morbidity and in a cost-effective manner.
- Thus, the goal of staging is to distinguish patients who have a potentially resectable localized tumor from those with advanced disease and/or distant metastases.
- Accurate staging has become increasingly important in view of the increasing alternatives for neoadjuvant therapy and nonoperative palliative procedures.

Inspection of the Peritoneal Cavity

- The initial step in staging laparoscopy is meticulous inspection of the four quadrants of the peritoneal cavity, which, if done properly, can identify serosal implants as small as 1 mm.
- To facilitate visualization, any ascitic fluid should be aspirated and sent for cytology prior to inspection.
- However, if laparoscopic ultrasonography (USG) is planned during the evaluation, it should be performed before aspiration, as the ascitic fluid is an excellent medium for the transduction of ultrasonic sound waves.

Peritoneal Washings

Peritoneal washings should be obtained, especially if the patient is being evaluated for pancreatic cancer, as the presence of malignant cells has been shown to influence resectability and prognosis.

Biopsy

- When a parenchymal lesion, peritoneal implant, or suspicious lymph node is identified, laparoscopic biopsy can be done with great precision.
- Depending on the size and location, tissue may be obtained by a variety of techniques, including fine-needle, core-needle, forceps, and incisional or excisional biopsy.

Role of Laparoscopic Staging Procedures in Various Regions of them Gastrointestinal Tract

Hepatic Malignancies

- Laparoscopic techniques are well suited to confirm the diagnosis of hepatocellular carcinoma or metastatic liver lesions, in that they can be used to visualize a surface lesion and perform a biopsy.
- Laparoscopy is a reliable method for detecting additional small lesions and peritoneal seeding, which are usually missed by other imaging methods.
  - *Primary liver tumors:*
    - In a recent series of 50 consecutive patients diagnosed with potentially resectable liver tumors, laparoscopy alone demonstrated unresectability in 46%, and nontherapeutic laparotomy was avoided in these patients.
    - Numerous studies have shown that intraoperative ultrasound during open operations is more sensitive for the detection of liver lesions than preoperative imaging modalities, including ultrasound, CT, CT portography, and magnetic resonance imaging (MRI).
    - Based on the results of intraoperative USG, the operative plan was altered in one-third of the study group. Intraoperative USG also may be used to evaluate surrounding structures, including the portal vein and perihilar structures.
    - Laparoscopy and laparoscopic USG averted a nontherapeutic laparotomy.
  - *Liver metastases:* Intraoperative ultrasound may also be used during primary resection of colorectal cancer to identify liver metastases that are not detected by preoperative ultrasound or CT.

Biliary Tract Malignancies

- Malignancies of the biliary tree are relatively rare, and therefore comparisons of staging modalities are difficult to perform. Only a few studies have addressed the usefulness of laparoscopic staging in these diseases
- If, during laparoscopic staging, a gallbladder carcinoma is suspected, conversion to an open surgical approach is recommended.

Pancreatic Cancer

- Pancreatic cancer is notorious for its propensity to metastasize to the liver and peritoneum.
- Most of the patients exhibit local tumor invasion and metastatic spread by the time symptoms occur and therefore have disease that is unresectable for cure.
- Unfortunately, current preoperative imaging methods frequently the disease, and, based on these tests, patients with unsuspected advanced disease undergo laparotomy unnecessarily.
- Studies have demonstrated that over 40% of patients have peritoneal or liver metastasis despite negative preoperative imaging with ultrasound or CT.
- Laparoscopy currently plays a dominant role in the management of pancreatic cancer since it not only has a sensitivity and specificity of 93% and 100%, respectively, for the detection of pancreatic tumors but also enables the biopsy of such lesions.
- Furthermore, peritoneal washings for cytological examination should be obtained during laparoscopic staging of pancreatic malignancies.

Gastric Cancer

- Accurate staging of gastric cancer is increasingly important since more patients are being offered neoadjuvant or palliative therapy without surgical confirmation of disease stage. Endoscopic USG combined with CT is currently the state-of-the-art in staging gastric carcinoma.

- These imaging modalities can miss small metastatic deposits from gastric cancer, resulting in unnecessary laparotomies in patients who already have a poor prognosis.
- Moreover, endoscopic USG has been reported to over stage T-stage in 40% of cases and may result in resectable patients being placed on palliative treatment protocols.
- Several recent reports have addressed the value of laparoscopic staging in gastric cancer.

Esophagogastric Cancer

The use of laparoscopy to stage cancer of the esophagus and gastric cardia remains controversial

Colon and Rectal Cancer

- Currently, there are few absolute indications for staging laparoscopy in the evaluation of a primary colon or rectal malignancy.
- It may be reasonable to perform diagnostic laparoscopy in a patient with an advanced rectal cancer if a suspicious liver lesion is noted on preoperative CT and the patient is being considered for neoadjuvant therapy.
- If the hepatic lesion is proven to be benign by laparoscopy and laparoscopic ultrasound, neoadjuvant therapy could then proceed.
- If malignant, such therapy could be canceled and an immediate palliative procedure performed.

Radioimmunoguided Surgery

- Radioimmunoguided surgery (RIGS) using laparoscopic probes is also on the horizon.
- The RIGS system utilizes a monoclonal antibody CC49-radiolabeled with iodine-125 targeted against a mucin that is highly expressed in human adenocarcinomas, tumor-associated glycoprotein-72 (TAG-72).
- Although the accuracy of RIGS is still being evaluated in open operations, preliminary results of a phase III trial indicate that it accurately determines disease stage and, therefore may influence perioperative therapy and extent of resection.
- Perhaps laparoscopic RIGS will have its greatest impact on improving staging accuracy so that decisions about appropriate neoadjuvant therapy can be made prior to resection, if indicated.

Conclusion

- Although the results of randomized trials comparing laparoscopic and conventional resections for abdominal malignancies will not be available for several years, it is clear that laparoscopic techniques are attaining a prominent role in the diagnosis and staging of many gastrointestinal malignancies.
- The recent addition of laparoscopic USG appears to have achieved an extremely high degree of sensitivity in the evaluation of solid organs without the need for a laparotomy.

---

12. Discuss laparoscopic management of acute abdomen. ***Tripura University 2025; WBUHS 2010***

Introduction

The acute abdomen is characterized by the sudden appearance of abdominal complaints that oblige the surgeon to decide promptly whether to operate immediately to treat conservatively or to observe the patient.

Possibilities for Initial Diagnosis of the Acute Abdomen

Localized peritonitis

- Acute cholecystitis
- Acute appendicitis (right lower abdomen)
- Acute diverticulitis

Generalized Peritonitis of Unknown Origin

- *Peritonitis by perforation:*
  - Perforated gastroduodenal ulcer
  - Perforated acute diverticulitis (colon sigmoid)
  - Small intestinal perforation (typhoid and trauma)
- *Intestinal obstruction*

Role of Laparoscopic Procedure in Different Causes of Acute Abdomen

- Percutaneous transhepatic cholecystostomy is a valuable and effective procedure in a high-risk group of patients with acute cholecystitis.
- Early laparoscopic cholecystectomy is the treatment of choice in patients with acute cholecystitis with acceptable risk.
- Helical CT or an USG will resolve the diagnosis in many patients with right iliac fossa.
- All patients suspected of acute appendicitis should have an USG. Patients will be clinically divided in equivocal and unequivocal appendicitis.
- Unequivocal clinical diagnosis plus positive USG will require diagnostic laparoscopy followed by laparoscopic appendicectomy.
- Unequivocal clinical diagnosis plus negative USG will lead to clinical observation. Helical CT should be done to exclude other diagnoses. If the clinical condition worsens, a diagnostic laparoscopy should be performed.
- An equivocal clinical diagnosis will lead to clinical observation. If local peritonitis develop, a diagnostic laparoscopy should be performed.
- Diagnostic laparoscopy should be performed in all patients with signs of generalized acute abdomen in whom no clear cause is suspected after clinical, radiological, and laboratory investigation. A correct diagnosis will dictate the right surgical approach.
- Laparoscopic closure of perforated duodenal ulcer, in experienced hands, confers superior short-term benefits in terms of postoperative pain and wound morbidity.
- Laparoscopic lavage and drainage in the acute management of perforated acute diverticulitis are a promising alternative to more radical procedures.
- Laparoscopy is an effective procedure for the treatment of acute small bowel obstruction with acceptable risk of morbidity and early recurrence, but conversion rates of 30–40% should be expected.

13. Laparoscopic versus conventional surgery in pregnancy. ***WBUHS 2015***

Introduction

- The advantages of laparoscopic surgery are similar for pregnant and no pregnant women; nevertheless, this procedure had been avoided during pregnancy because of concerns that it may be harmful to the fetus.
- *Potential concerns include:*
  - The rise in IAP during pneumoperitoneum could decrease uteroplacental blood flow and result in fetal hypoxia.
  - Fetal acidosis could develop from absorption of CO_2.
  - The fetus could be injured directly or indirectly if the uterus is perforated by a trocar or Veress needle.
  - Uterine perforation may result in preterm premature rupture of the membranes and preterm delivery.

Advantages of laparoscopy in pregnancy	*Risk of laparoscopy in pregnancy*
Short hospital stay	More chance of uterine injury during port enters as uterus becomes an abdominal organ after first trimester
Early return to normal activities	Problems associated with pneumoperitoneum
Small incision, so rapid postoperative recovery and less incision complications such as hernia, postoperative wound infection, and pain	CO_2 absorption causes increase CO_2 pressure and decrease arterial PH
Less uterine manipulation and hence decrease uterine irritability and fetal loss	Risk of exposure to intra-abdominal smoke including carbon monoxide generated by electro surgery and LASER

Strategies for Safe Laparoscopic Surgery in Pregnancy

- Surgery should be done in second trimester.
- If patient presents in late third trimester, surgery should be postponed if possible until after delivery.

- Nasogastric incubation is a must in all case as there is a high-risk aspiration into the lungs.
- Patient can be placed in dorsal lithotomy position in the first half of pregnancy, but in second half to prevent inferior vena cava compression patient is ideally placed in lateral recumbent position.
- Hypotension should be avoided; proper fluid replacement should be done.
- Ideal method for commencing pneumoperitoneum is open Hasson trocar method. Placement of trocar depends on the size of gravid uterus.
- Tocolysis is indicated if signs of uterine irritability are present.
- Decrease operation time by using adequate number of ports, and using most experienced surgeons.
- Maternal hyperventilation to maintain $ETCO_2$ pressure at 32 mm Hg.
- Lower CO_2 insufflations pressure of <12 mm Hg should be used to avoid fetal acidosis.
- Electrocautery should be used with care; the smokes containing carbon monoxide should be evacuated promptly to avoid toxic effect to fetus.
- Entry of all instruments must be under direct vision; care should be taken to avoid injury to the gravid uterus.
- All specimens should be removed with endobag to avoid spillage.
- Manipulators should never be fixed to vagina or cervix.

Society of American Gastrointestinal Endoscopic Surgery (SAGES) Recommendations

- Obstetrical consultation should be obtained preoperatively.
- When possible, operative intervention should be deferred until the second trimester, when fetal risk is lowest.
- Pneumoperitoneum enhances lower extremity venous stasis already present in the gravid patient and pregnancy induces a hypercoagulable state. Therefore, pneumatic compression devices should be utilized whenever possible.
- Fatal and uterine status, as maternal $ETCO_2$ and/or arterial blood gases, should be monitored.
- The uterus should be protected with a lead shield if intraoperative cholangiography is a possibility.
- Fluoroscopy should be utilized selectively.
- Given the enlarged gravid uterus, abdominal access should be attained using an open technique.
- Dependent positioning should be utilized to shift the uterus away from the inferior vena cava.
- Pneumoperitoneum pressures should be kept at 10 mm Hg.
- Future studies into methods that increase the safety of laparoscopy in pregnant patient should be done.

LIMITATIONS OF MINIMAL ACCESS SURGERY AND ACCESS COMPLICATIONS

14. Limitations of minimal access surgery. ***WBUHS 2022, MAMC 2022***

Surgeons performing laparoscopy should be aware of some special considerations unique to this technique:

- The surgical field is a three-dimensional (3D) space, but most laparoscopes project an image onto a traditional two-dimensional monitor, creating limited depth perception for the surgeon.
- Most laparoscopic instruments can rotate around their long axis, and some may have some degree of articulation at the instrument tip, but they have significantly limited dexterity compared to the human hand and wrist.
- In addition, laparoscopic instruments can transmit some haptic input through the instrument shaft and handle to the operator's hand, but much of the haptic feedback that is central to appropriate tissue handling in open operations is lost during laparoscopy.
- Minimally invasive surgery requires specialized high-end medical equipment.
- Surgeons need specialized training.
- The equipment used with MIS is more expensive.
- There are various procedures, especially the most recent surgeries that may take longer.

15. Access complications. ***WBUHS 2022***

Introduction

- Complications of abdominal access can occur, particularly during blind portions such as Veress needle or blind trocar insertion, including visceral or vascular injuries.
- If bowel contents or blood is aspirated during Veress insertion, the needle should be withdrawn and reinserted and laparoscopic access should proceed.

Complications

- Upon entry into the abdomen, bowel, or other injured organs should be examined and managed per established protocols for traumatic injury to intraperitoneal organs. Veress needle stick to intraperitoneal viscera should prompt close inspection, but in many cases may need only a simple repair or no intervention at all.
- Inadvertent intraluminal insufflation of the bowel with the Veress needle, however, can cause significant injury requiring bowel resection.
- The retroperitoneum should also be closely examined on abdominal exploration, particularly in situations where blood was encountered on initial Veress insertion.
- A stable hematoma in the mesentery or lateral retroperitoneum can usually be observed. However, central or rapidly expanding hematomas require exploration of the retroperitoneum.
- *Trocar insertion can cause injuries far more severe than Veress insertion:*
    - Bowel and visceral injuries should be considered penetrating traumas and managed accordingly, and any central or rapidly expanding retroperitoneal hematoma should be explored.
    - If a rush of blood is encountered on trocar insertion or open cannula placement, the surgeon must assume that a critical vascular injury has occurred and conversion to open must be performed immediately (without yet removing the trocar, which may be partially tamponading the injury).
- Abdominal wall hemorrhage is a common complication of laparoscopic surgery that may be caused by injury to the epigastric arteries, veins, or their tributaries.
    - These are often self-limited and cease with the tamponading effect of the port.
    - If this fails to control the bleeding, control may be attempted using electrosurgical energy or with a transfascial suture.

NOTES AND HALS

16. NOTES. ***WBUHS 2014***

- *Natural orifice transluminal endoscopic surgery (NOTES)* is an experimental surgical technique whereby "scarless" abdominal operations can be performed with an endoscope passed through a natural orifice (mouth, urethra, anus, etc.) then through an internal incision in the stomach, vagina, bladder, or colon, thus avoiding any external incisions or scars.
- Portions of the gastrointestinal tract such as the stomach and colon commonly examined with endoscopy (such as for colon cancer screening) also reside in the peritoneal cavity. Perforation (inadvertent puncture creating a hole) of the gastrointestinal tract has been traditionally considered an undesirable event. Interventions using NOTES, however, intentionally perforate the stomach, bowel, or vagina, thereby allowing the operator to access the peritoneal cavity using a normal body orifice as a conduit. Here, any peritoneal structure is theoretically approachable.
- As an example, in natural orifice surgery the gallbladder might be removed through the mouth. The doctor would insert a tube down the esophagus, make a small incision in the stomach wall to gain access to the abdominal peritoneal cavity and take the gallbladder out by the same route. Potential advantages of the NOTES technique include reduced postoperative pain, shortened recovery times, and improved cosmesis (lack of surgical incision scars).

- A range of procedures might be performed this way, such as GBP, fallopian tube ligation, removal of the ovaries, and diagnostic work. Some operations might be done via the rectum, vagina, urethra, or bladder as well. Because NOTES is so new, research generally has been confined to animals, mainly pigs. Recently, however, human studies have emerged that report the procedures to be feasible. Further studies involving a variety of NOTES procedures, under close supervision by medical experts and Institutional Review Boards, are being performed. The first multicenter human clinical trial in the US is currently underway.
- The last surgical innovation with such radical changes was laparoscopic surgery which was introduced in the late 1980s. Laparoscopic surgery was initially associated with an increased rate of specific complications which threatened to discredit the technique at that time. As a result, extensive research regarding safety measures was conducted in the following years. Laparoscopy is a mature technique today and is the standard procedure for many abdominal operations.

18. HALS (hand-assisted lap surgery). ***WBUHS 2011***

Introduction

- Hand-assisted laparoscopic surgery is an alternative laparoscopic approach in which a mini-laparotomy is planned and performed to enable the surgeon to introduce his or her hand while the pneumoperitoneum is maintained and the dissection maneuvers are performed under video-endoscopic control.
- The insertion of the hand restores the tactile feeling and the sensation of depth, and facilitates the exposure, traction, and retraction maneuvers during the procedure.

HALS Devices

- The simplest way to perform HALS is to insert the hand through a mini-laparotomy performed for that purpose.
- However, it is difficult to keep the seal tight and to avoid loss of gas; in addition, the movements of the arm and the hand are limited.
- Three different devices are available for HALS.
- One type is a glove fixed to a circular platform that adheres to the surface of the skin, around the incision. This device has the drawback of requiring adherence to the skin, which must be well prepared; adhesive substances are needed, and the device itself is easily lifted from the skin by the wound fluid.
- There are also devices with two elements (Hand Port; Smith and Nephew, London, England). The inflatable circular base adapts to the inner contour of the abdominal wall wound and is attached to a sleeve that is fixed to the surgeon's arm, which allows the insertion and withdrawal of the hand. This device is comfortable and easy to install.
- Third, there are single-piece devices that adapt to the inner contour of the wall incision and permit the interchange of hand insertion, either mechanically (LapDisc; Hakko-Medical, Tokyo, Japan) or by inflation (Omniport; Advanced Surgical Concepts, Dublin). Some special surgical instruments have been designed for HALS. These instruments may help some delicate steps of surgical procedures such as those used in splenic or kidney vessel dissection.
- A procedure derived from HALS is finger-assisted LS (fingerscopy). By introducing a finger through a trocar wound the surgeon can free adherences or palpate and identify structures in situations such as appendectomy.

Advantages

- The obvious advantage of HALS is that it recovers the tactile feeling and improves hand-eye coordination despite the fact that the operation is performed under videoscopy.
- The recovery of tactile feeling shortens certain dissection maneuvers, avoids unnecessary movements, favors the smooth traction and exposure of structures, and facilitates the control of unexpected or difficult situations such as hemorrhage or the handling of a voluminous or adherent specimen.
- All of these advantages enhance the efficiency of the endoscopic procedure.

Disadvantages

- The main drawback of HALS is that it requires an additional incision, thus increasing trauma. For this reason, the best indications are those that involve the performance of a mini-laparotomy to extract the specimen.
- The HALS technique requires a new operative strategy to capitalize on the presence of the hand being inside the abdomen, and the scope and the trocars must be correctly placed.
- Furthermore, the hand takes up space inside the abdomen and may hamper certain maneuvers, particularly if the patient is thin or if the surgeon's hand is large.
- Hand-assisted laparoscopic surgery may also induce hand fatigue in long or complicated procedures.

Election of Incision Site for Placement of the HALS Device

- The choice of incision site is likely to depend on whether the intra-abdominal hand is the surgeon's or the assistant's.
- If it is the surgeon's, the nondominant hand is used; if it is the assistant's, the dominant hand is used. If it is the surgeon's hand that is introduced, it should not impair visual field of the scope, so as to permit adequate triangulation over the target organ manipulated by the hand.
- In addition, the hand should not be placed over the structure to be dissected because this may impair the manipulation of the organ.
- When the procedure includes an accessory incision to extract the specimen (e.g., in splenectomy for splenomegaly) or to perform the anastomosis (e.g., in colectomy), the hand may be introduced through the anatomical site at which the incision is performed.
- If it is the assistant who introduces the hand, the accessory incision may be made far away from the introduction points of the operative trocars (Pfannenstiel incision).
- In some situations, the incision should be made in a multifunctional site (for instance, in the periumbilical midline, for a subtotal colectomy).

Indications

- Hand-assisted laparoscopic surgery has been applied in many clinical situations, and its safety and efficacy have been amply demonstrated.
- HALS definitely facilitated the procedure (58% of the surgeons considered that HALS reduced operation time and 88% that the intra-abdominal hand was helpful). Furthermore, immediate postoperative evolution was similar to conventional LS procedures. This suggests that HALS maintains the advantages of LS.
- *Hand-assisted laparoscopic surgery should be considered a priori as an aggressive surgery because:*
  - It requires a mini-laparotomy incision at the beginning of the procedure.
  - This incision is stretched by the HALS device.
  - The area of manipulation and traction is greater than in other procedures that use 5- to 10-mm instruments.

Laparoscopic Procedures Performed with Hand-assisted Laparoscopic Techniques

Stomach and esophagus	***Hepatobiliary and pancreas***	***Colorectal***	***Other operations***
Transhiatal esophagectomy	Hepatectomy	Colorectal cancer	Splenectomy for massive splenomegaly
Preparation of gastric tube	Cryoablation liver metastasis	Colonic polyps	Staging hematological diseases
Nissen fundoplication paraesophageal hernia	Living-donor nephrectomy	Diverticulitis	Adrenalectomy exeresis retroperitoneal tumor
Partial or total gastrectomy	Distal pancreatectomy	Crohn disease	Nephrectomy
Gastric bypass	*Pancreatoduodenectomy*	Rectal prolapse	Vertebral fusion aortobifemoral bypass

Conclusion

- Hand-assisted laparoscopic surgery may be an interesting alternative to conventional laparoscopic splenectomy (LS) or open surgery.
- It simplifies the performance of difficult procedures for experienced surgeons and can initiate less experienced surgeons in advanced LS.
- Comparative trials with well-established laparoscopic techniques are required to define the absolute advantages of HALS.
- However, it may well be a useful resource before conversion to open surgery now that it has been demonstrated that it maintains the advantages of LS.

ROBOTIC SURGERY

19. Enumerate various robotic platforms available for use in surgery. Discuss the components of Da Vinci robotic system. ***AIIMS, Patna 2025***

Various Robotic Platforms Available for Use in Surgery

Here is a non-exhaustive list of major robotic surgical systems currently in clinical use or advanced development (as of 2025). These platforms span general surgery, orthopedics, neurosurgery, and other specialties:

- *da Vinci surgical system* (intuitive surgical)
  - Dominant platform for minimally invasive soft-tissue surgery.
  - *Applications:* Urology (prostatectomy), gynecology (hysterectomy), general surgery (colorectal), cardiothoracic, head and neck.
  - *Generations:* da Vinci Xi (latest multiport), da Vinci SP (single-port), da Vinci 5 (2024 release with enhanced haptics, AI integration, and ion endoluminal system).
- *Senhance surgical system* (Asensus surgical, formerly transenterix)
  - Digital laparoscopy with haptic feedback and eye-tracking camera control.
  - *Applications:* General surgery, gynecology, urology.
  - *Key differentiator:* Reusable instruments and lower cost per procedure.
- *Versius surgical system* (CMR surgical)
  - Modular, portable robotic arms on individual biomimetic trolleys.
  - *Applications:* General surgery, gynecology, urology (especially in Europe and emerging markets).
  - *Advantages:* Small footprint, rapid setup, cost-competitive.
- *Mazor X Stealth edition* (Medtronic)
  - Spine and brain surgery navigation + robotic arm for pedicle screw placement.
  - Integrates with StealthStation navigation.
- *ROSA (Robotic Surgical Assistant)* (Zimmer Biomet)
  - Used in knee arthroplasty (ROSA Knee) and neurosurgery (ROSA Brain).
  - Provides haptic guidance and intraoperative planning.
- *ExcelsiusGPS (Globus Medical):* Spine surgery robot with real-time navigation and rigid robotic arm.
- *MAKO SmartRobotics* (Stryker)
  - Orthopedic surgery (hip, knee, partial knee replacement).
  - Combines 3D planning, AccuStop haptic feedback, and robotic arm.
- *Ion endoluminal system* (Intuitive Surgical)
  - Shape-sensing robotic bronchoscopy for lung biopsy.
  - Catheter-based, reaches peripheral lung nodules.
- *Monarch platform* (Johnson & Johnson/Auris Health)
  - Robotic bronchoscopy and urology (ureteroscopy).
  - Electromagnetic navigation + robotic control.

- *Vicarious surgical system* (Vicarious Surgical)
  - Miniaturized humanoid robots inserted through a single incision.
  - 9-DoF arms, 3D HD vision; in clinical trials (FDA clearance pending).
- *MicroPort MedBot – Toumai* (China): Laparoscopic robot similar to da Vinci; approved in China and expanding globally.
- *Revo-i* (Meere Company, South Korea): Cost-effective da Vinci alternative; used in Asia.
- *Avatera* (Avatera Medical, Germany): Single-use instruments, compact design; CE-marked in Europe.
- *Hugo RAS* (Medtronic): Modular soft-tissue robot; received CE mark and in U.S. clinical trials.
- *Hinotori* (Medicaroid/Kawasaki, Japan): First Japan-made surgical robot; approved in Japan.

Components of the da Vinci Robotic System (Focus on da Vinci Xi/X/5)

The da Vinci system consists of *three primary subsystems*:

I. *Surgeon console (Master Controller)*
  - Ergonomic-seated workstation.
  - *Components*:
    - *Master controllers* (two hand grips with 7-DoF + grip).
    - *Footswitch clutch panel* (camera control, instrument clutch, energy pedals).
    - *3DHD stereoscopic viewer* (dual 1080p displays, 10× magnification, immersive view).
    - *Touchpad* (system settings, telestration, UI).
    - *da Vinci 5 additions*: Integrated TruSense haptics, AI-guided tremor filtration, voice/gesture controls.

II. *Patient cart (Slave Robot)*
  - Four articulated robotic arms mounted on a mobile base.
  - *Components*:
    - *Arm 1–3*: Instrument arms (EndoWrist instruments with 7-DoF, 540° rotation).
    - *Arm 4*: Endoscope arm (0° or 30° 3DHD camera).
    - *Boom system*: Motorized positioning with collision avoidance.
    - *Instrument interface*: Quick-change couplers for sterile adapters.
    - *da Vinci 5*: Force-feedback actuators in arms, dynamic motion scaling.

III. *Vision Cart (Image Processing and Support)*
  - Houses core electronics and peripherals.
  - *Components*:
    - *Vision system*: Image processing unit, light source (xenon/LED), insufflator.
    - *24-inch touchscreen monitor* (for OR team).
    - *Core processor*: Synchronizes motion scaling, tremor filtration, and 3D rendering.
    - *EndoWrist instruments*: Portfolio of >90 reusable instruments (needle drivers, scissors, graspers, staplers, vessel sealers).
    - *Single-port (SP)*: Uses a 25-mm flexible port with four internal channels.

Additional System—Wide Features

- *Motion scaling* (1:1, 3:1, 5:1).
- *Tremor filtration* (6 Hz low-pass filter).
- *Firefly fluorescence imaging* (ICG dye for vascular/perfusion assessment).
- *Integrated OR table compatibility* (Trumpf, Maquet).
- *Skills simulator* (backpack module for training).
- *da Vinci Connect* (remote proctoring/telementoring platform).

19. What are the advantages and limitations of robotic surgery compared to laparoscopic surgery?
WBUHS 2021 Supplementary; Ayush University, Chhattisgarh 2025

Introduction

Robotic surgery was associated with superior ease to laparoscopy in 8 of the 13 factors, including image quality, depth perception, comfort, eye fatigue, dexterity, precision of motion, speed of motion, and range of motion.

- The advantages of robotic surgery over conventional laparoscopic surgery are greater degree of movement, precise dissection, 3D vision, tremor filtration, and a shorter learning curve. The disadvantages are mainly the high cost and lack of haptic feedback.
- Absence of bespoke microsurgical instruments increases in operating time, and high costs associated with robotic-assisted provide a barrier to using such systems effectively for reconstructive microsurgery.

Aspects evaluated	*Robotic surgery*	*Laparoscopy*
Vision	Three dimensional	Two dimensional
Instrument manipulation	360°	Limited
Costs	Extremely high	Lower
Assembly	Extremely long	Faster
Ergonomics	Very good (like human wrist)	Poor
No. of ports	3	3 or more
Port diameter	8 mm	2 mm or more
Diffusion in clinical practice	Rare	In all surgical centers

20. Robotic surgery. ***WBUHS 2008***

Introduction

- Computer-assisted surgery, and robotically assisted surgery are terms for technological developments that use robotic systems to aid in surgical procedures.
- Robotically assisted surgery was developed to overcome the limitations of preexisting minimally-invasive surgical procedures and to enhance the capabilities of surgeons performing open surgery.

Comparison to Traditional Methods

- Major advances aided by surgical robots have been remote surgery, minimally invasive surgery and unmanned surgery.
- Due to robotic use, the surgery is done with precision, miniaturization, and smaller incisions; decreased blood loss, less pain, and quicker healing time.
- Articulation beyond normal manipulation and 3D magnification helps resulting in improved ergonomics.
- Due to these techniques, there is a reduced duration of hospital stays, blood loss, transfusions, and use of pain medication.
- The robot normally costs very high and while it is disposable supply cost is normally also very high per procedure, the cost of the procedure is higher.
- Additional surgical training is needed to operate the system.
- Surgeons report that, although the manufacturers of such systems provide training on this new technology, the learning phase is intensive and surgeons must operate on twelve to eighteen patients before they adapt.
- During the training phase, minimally invasive operations can take up to twice as long as traditional surgery, leading to operating room tie ups and surgical staffs keeping patients under anesthesia for longer periods.
- Patient surveys indicate they chose the procedure based on expectations of decreased morbidity, improved outcomes, reduced blood loss, and less pain.

- Compared with other minimally invasive surgery approaches, robot-assisted surgery gives the surgeon better control over the surgical instruments and a better view of the surgical site.
- In addition, surgeons no longer have to stand throughout the surgery and do not tire as quickly.
- Naturally occurring hand tremors are filtered out by the robot's computer software. Finally, the surgical robot can continuously be used by rotating surgery teams.

Uses

- *General surgery:* In early 2000, the field of general surgical interventions with the da Vinci device was explored by surgeons at Ohio State University.
- *Cardiothoracic surgery:*
    - Robot-assisted MIDCAB and endoscopic coronary artery bypass (TECAB) operations are being performed with the Da Vinci system. Mitral valve repairs and replacements have been performed.
    - The Ohio State University, Columbus has performed CABG, mitral valve, esophagectomy, lung resection, tumor resections, among other robotic assisted procedures and serves as a training site for other surgeons. In 2002, surgeons at the Cleveland Clinic in Florida reported and published their preliminary experience with minimally invasive "hybrid" procedures.
    - These procedures combined robotic revascularization and coronary stenting and further expanded the role of robots in coronary bypass to patients with disease in multiple vessels.
    - Ongoing research on the outcomes of robotic assisted CABG and hybrid CABG is being done.
- *Cardiology and electrophysiology:* The Stereotaxis Magnetic Navigation System (MNS) has been developed to increase precision and safety in ablation procedures for arrhythmias and atrial fibrillation while reducing radiation exposure for the patient and physician, and the system utilizes two magnets to remotely steerable catheters.

  At present, three types of heart surgery are being performed on a routine basis using robotic surgery systems. These three surgery types are:
    1. Atrial septal defect repair—the repair of a hole between the two upper chambers of the heart.
    2. Mitral valve repair—the repair of the valve that prevents blood from regurgitating back into the upper heart chambers during contractions of the heart.
    3. Coronary artery bypass—rerouting of blood supply by bypassing blocked arteries that provide blood to the heart.
- *Colon and rectal surgery:* Results to date indicate that robotic-assisted colorectal procedures outcomes are "no worse" than the results in the now "traditional" laparoscopic colorectal operations. Robotic-assisted colorectal surgery appears to be safe as well.
- *Gastrointestinal surgery:*
    - Multiple types of procedures have been performed with either the "Zeus" or da Vinci robot systems, including bariatric surgery and gastrectomy for cancer. Specific procedures have been more fully evaluated, specifically esophageal fundoplication for the treatment of gastroesophageal reflux and Heller myotomy for the treatment of achalasia.
    - Other gastrointestinal procedures including colon resection, pancreatectomy, esophagectomy, and robotic approaches to pelvic disease have also been reported.
- *Gynecology:* Robotic surgery in gynecology is of uncertain benefit with it being unclear if it affects rates of complications. Using the robotic system, gynecologists can perform hysterectomies, myomectomies, and lymph node biopsies.
- *Neurosurgery:* Several systems for stereotactic intervention are currently on the market. The NeuroMate was the first neurosurgical robot, commercially available in 1997.
- *Orthopedics:* The ROBODOC system was released in 1992 by Integrated Surgical Systems, Inc. which merged into CUREXO Technology Corporation. The Navio System is a navigated, robotics-assisted surgical system that uses a CT free approach to assist in partial knee replacement surgery.

- *Pediatrics:* Surgical robotics has been used in many types of pediatric surgical procedures including: tracheoesophageal fistula repair, cholecystectomy, Nissen Fundoplication, Morgagni's hernia repair, Kasai portoenterostomy, congenital diaphragmatic hernia repair, and others.
- *Radiosurgery:* The Cyber Knife Robotic Radiosurgery System uses image guidance and computer-controlled robotics to treat tumors throughout the body by delivering multiple beams of high-energy radiation to the tumor from virtually any direction.
- *Transplant surgery:* Transplant surgery (organ transplantation) has been considered as highly technically demanding and virtually unobtainable by means of conventional laparoscopy. The development of robotic technology and its associated high-resolution capabilities, 3D visual system, wrist type motion, and fine instruments, gave opportunity for highly complex procedures to be completed in a minimally invasive fashion.
- *Urology:* Robotic surgery in the field of urology has become very popular. It has been most extensively applied for excision of prostate cancer because of difficult anatomical access. It is also utilized for kidney cancer surgeries and to lesser extent surgeries of the bladder.
- *Vascular surgery:* In September 2010, the first robotic operations with Hansen Medical's Magellan Robotic System at the femoral vasculature were performed at the University Medical Centre Ljubljana (UMC Ljubljana), Slovenia.

21. Discuss the advantages and disadvantages of robotic surgery. ***RIMS, 2022***

22. Discuss its present-day role in colorectal surgery. ***WBUHS, 2017***

Advantages

- Major advances aided by surgical robots have been remote surgery, minimally invasive surgery, and unmanned surgery.
- Due to robotic use, the surgery is done with precision, miniaturization, and smaller incisions; decreased blood loss, less pain, and quicker healing time.
- Articulation beyond normal manipulation and 3D magnification helps resulting in improved ergonomics.
- There is a reduced duration of hospital stays, blood loss, transfusions, and use of pain medication.
- The existing open surgery technique has many flaws like limited access to surgical area, long recovery time, long hours of operation, blood loss, surgical scars, and marks.
- Compared with other minimally invasive surgery approaches, robot-assisted surgery gives the surgeon better control over the surgical instruments and a better view of the surgical site. In addition, surgeons no longer have to stand throughout the surgery and do not tire as quickly.
- Naturally occurring hand tremors are filtered out by the robot's computer software. Finally, the surgical robot can be used continuously by rotating surgery teams.
- A Medicare study found that some procedures that have traditionally been performed with large incisions can be converted to "minimally invasive" endoscopic procedures with the use of the *Da Vinci surgical system*, shortening length-of-stay in the hospital and reducing recovery times.

Disadvantages

- Currently, the major limiting factor that is stunting the development of robotic surgery is "latency" which is the time delay between the instructions issued by the surgeon and the movement of the robot which responds to the instructions. With the current level of technology, the surgeon must be in close proximity.
- Robotic technology is extremely expensive both in terms of capital costs, as well as running expenses and will require the training of specialized personnel to properly repair and care for it. Such expenses may far outweigh any savings earned at the present time.

Role of robotic surgery in colorectal surgery: Robotic surgical systems are a step up from both traditional open surgery and minimally invasive laparoscopic procedures because surgeons benefit from:

- *Better visualization:* Robotic surgery provides physicians with a high-resolution 3D screen that provides greater visualization and depth perception of the surgical field.
- *Enhanced dexterity:* The robotic arm can mimic the way a wrist would move. You can rotate it 360° and bend it back or forward. This is an improvement over laparoscopic instruments, which are straight-like chop sticks with no degree of movement.
- *Improved precision:* Physicians can also precisely move the robotic arm and hand, and the movement is scalable. For instance, the physician can move an inch outside the body and program that movement to be one-third of an inch inside the body.

Application of Robotic Surgery in Colon Cancer

- *Hybrid technique:* Hybrid technique is a technique that required two minimums invasive systems in a single patient, thus surgeons have to be adapted and skillful in both laparoscopic and robotic systems. The first part of procedure starts with laparoscopic system to facilitate splenic flexure mobilization as well as mobilization of left colon and inferior mesenteric artery (IMA) ligation branches. Then robotic system comes afterword to pelvic side, as the main advantages maximize during rectal dissection by robotic system utilization.
- *Single port robotic surgery:* Efforts are challenging to further concentrate on the cosmetic outcome of robotic surgery as well as reduce port-related morbidities.
- *Da Vinci Xi system:* Several limitations in robotic Si version in *colorectal surgery*, for instance: inability to perform multi-quadrant operation, fixed heavy arms, need of re-docking and risk of collisions which disrupt working channel and might extent operative time further. Recently, a new innovation of Da Vinci Xi has admitted in the market, which contributed to overcome obstacles and limitations of the previous platform. Rectal cancer surgery is a good example to look at how Da Vinci Xi platform works in multi-quadrant areas smoothly, however potential risk of collision is possible, since totally robotic pelvic procedure has not standardized in Da Vinci Xi yet.

Application of Robotic Surgery in Rectal Cancer

- *Total mesorectal excision (TME):*
  - Caution dissection at IMA root, where superior hypogastric plexus network lied there. If injured, might end with retrograde ejaculation.
  - Mobilization of the rectosigmoid colon from the gonadal vessels and ureters, the hypogastric nerves are at risk at this level. Therefore, the correct surgical plane should be between the rectal proper fascia and prehypogastric nerve fascia.
  - Caution at inferior mesenteric vain (IMV) ligation, as collateral vessel crossing IMV root, if injured, could contribute in blood supply cut down then increase risk of anastomotic leakage.
  - Avoid blunt dissection in the posterior pelvic side, particularly at rectosacral fascia to avoid fascia avulsions and presacral bleeding.
  - Anterior liner incision at the peritoneum reflection with intensive caution to three important structure, which are seminal vesicles in men or vaginal wall in women, watch neurovascular bundles from the pelvic plexus run along the tip of the seminal vesicle (2 o'clock and 10 o'clock directions), and lastly, as deeper you proceed with anterior dissection, as better recognition of Denonvilliers fascia will be, where posterior dissection is recommended to avoid troublesome bleeding and nerves damage, unless if the tumor located anteriorly or threating up front structure, then consider taken down Denonvilliers fascia with the specimen.
  - Final step is to keep circumferential dissection all around the rectum to avoid coning of the mesorectum at the pelvic floor.
- *The intersphincteric resection (ISR):* It is an extended procedure to TME steps with further dissection on the pelvic floor.
- *Abdominoperineal resection (APR)*
- *Hemielevator excision*
- *Robotic-assisted lateral pelvic lymph node dissection (LPLND)*

23. Write in short on concept and functions of surgical robot. ***WBUHS 2024***

Concept of Surgical Robots

Surgical robots are computer-controlled systems comprising two primary components:

Surgeon console: The interface where the surgeon sits and controls the robotic instruments. It provides a high-definition, 3D view of the surgical site and allows the surgeon to manipulate instruments with hand and foot control.

Patient-side robotic arms: These arms hold and maneuver surgical instruments and a camera inside the patient's body. They replicate the surgeon's hand movements with greater precision and range of motion.

The system operates through tiny incisions, offering a minimally invasive approach that can lead to quicker recovery and reduced complications.

Functions of Surgical Robots

- *Enhanced precision and control:* Robotic systems filter out hand tremors and scale down the surgeon's movements, allowing for ultra-precise operations in confined spaces.
- *3D High-definition visualization:* The integrated camera provides a magnified, high-resolution, 3D view of the surgical area, improving depth perception and aiding in delicate procedures.
- *Greater range of motion:* Robotic instruments can rotate and bend in multiple directions, surpassing the human wrist's capabilities, which is particularly beneficial in complex surgeries.
- *Minimally invasive procedures:* By using smaller incisions, robotic surgery reduces trauma to the body, leading to less pain, lower risk of infection, and shorter hospital stays.
- *Remote surgery potential:* Advancements in technology have enabled surgeons to perform procedures remotely. For instance, a Chinese surgeon conducted a prostate surgery between Rome and Beijing, showcasing the potential for global access to specialized car.

Applications in Surgical Fields

Surgical robots are utilized in various specialties, including:

- *Urology:* Prostatectomies and kidney surgeries.
- *Gynecology:* Hysterectomies and fibroid removals.
- *Cardiothoracic surgery:* Heart valve repairs and coronary artery bypass.
- *Orthopedics:* Joint replacements and spinal surgeries.
- *General surgery:* Colorectal procedures and cancer resections.

Benefits

- *Reduced pain and scarring:* Smaller incisions lead to less postoperative discomfort and minimal scarring.
- *Shorter recovery time:* Patients often experience quicker recovery and can return to daily activities sooner.
- *Lower risk of complications:* The precision of robotic systems decreases the likelihood of surgical errors and complications.

Limitations

- *High costs:* The initial investment and maintenance of robotic systems can be expensive.
- *Training requirements:* Surgeons need specialized training to operate robotic systems effectively.
- *Limited availability:* Access to robotic surgery may be restricted in certain regions or healthcare facilities.

24. Robotic surgery—principles, merits and demerits. ***NTRUHS, Vijayawada 2025***

See answers of earlier questions.

25. Discuss the principles of robotic surgery and its application. Compare it to conventional laparoscopic surgery.
Maharashtra University of Health Sciences 2025

See answers of earlier questions.

26. Briefly mention the role of AI in surgery and its limitations. ***WBUHS 2025 Supplementary***

27. Artificial intelligence in surgery. ***The Tamil Nadu Dr MGR Medical University 2025; KGMU 2025***

28. Discuss the role of artificial intelligence in surgery.
AIIMS, Patna 2025; Srimanta Sankaradeva University, Assam 2025

Role of AI in Surgery

- *Preoperative planning:* AI analyzes medical imaging and patient data to help surgeons plan procedures more accurately.
- *Robotic-assisted surgery:* AI-powered surgical robots enhance precision, reduce human error, and allow for minimally invasive techniques.
- *Intraoperative support:* AI provides real-time guidance, monitors vital signs, and assists in decision-making during surgery.
- *Postoperative care:* AI predicts complications, monitors recovery, and personalizes follow-up care based on data analysis.
- *Training and Simulation:* AI-based simulations help train surgeons through realistic virtual environments and feedback systems.

Limitations

- *Data dependency:* AI performance relies on large volumes of high-quality, diverse data, which may not always be available.
- *Lack of human judgment:* AI cannot fully replicate human intuition, adaptability, or ethical reasoning in complex or unexpected surgical situations.
- *Bias and errors:* Algorithms can reflect biases present in training data, leading to inaccurate or unfair outcomes.
- *High costs:* Implementing AI systems and robotic technologies is expensive and may not be accessible in all healthcare settings.
- *Regulatory and legal issues:* There are unresolved legal and ethical concerns regarding responsibility for AI-driven surgical decisions or errors.
- *Limited generalization:* AI models trained for specific tasks may not perform well outside their narrow scope without retraining.

LAPAROSCOPIC HERNIA SURGERY

29. Transabdominal preperitoneal (TAPP) versus totally extraperitoneal (TEP) repair of inguinal hernia.

30. TEP. ***Ayush University, Chhattisgarh 2025***

TEP

- The TEP repair differs from the TAPP in that the abdominal cavity is not entered with the laparoscope.
- All the surgery is performed in the layers outside the peritoneum.
- The risk of bowel injury is therefore less with this technique.
- The TEPP repair is particularly recommended for the repair of bilateral inguinal hernias and recurrent inguinal hernias. The procedure is performed under general anesthesia. Three small incisions are made in the midline between the umbilicus and the pubic bone.

Complications

• Pain • Bleeding	• Wound infection • Mesh infection	• Scar • Difficulty passing urine	• Atrophy of the testicle • Hernia recurrence

Transabdominal preperitoneal repair: It is an alternative keyhole technique for inguinal hernia repair. With this technique, a camera is inserted into the abdominal cavity. Gas is introduced, enabling the surgeon to see the hernia sac. The hernia is repaired using a piece of mesh which is inserted behind the muscle of the abdominal wall.

The principle advantages of this technique over open surgery are:

- Less postoperative pain
- A quicker recovery
- A quicker return to full physical activities
- There is no significant difference in the recovery after TEP or TAPP repair.

Complications

• Pain • Bleeding • Seroma	• Wound infection • Mesh infection	• Scar • Difficulty passing urine	• Atrophy of the testicle (Shrinkage) • Hernia recurrence	• Deep vein thrombosis • Pulmonary embolus • Bowel injury

31. Describe briefly the complications and their anatomical background related to laparoscopic groin hernia repair. ***WBUHS 2021, 2023***

32. Endoscopic anatomy of groin hernia. ***Tripura University 2023***

Introduction

During laparoscopic inguinal hernia repair, it is important to recognize the following important structures in the abdominal cavity: the median umbilical fold, the medial umbilical fold, the lateral umbilical fold, Hesselbach's triangle, the internal inguinal ring, and the femoral ring.

Myopectineal Orifice

- This anatomic region was originally coined by Dr Fruchaud, a French researcher, in 1956. Direct inguinal hernias, oblique inguinal hernias and femoral hernias are all caused by weakness of the abdominal transverse fascia in myopectineal orifice.
- *The inguinal ligament divides the myopectineal orifice into two regions:* The suprainguinal region and the subinguinal region.
- The spermatic cord or the round ligament of the uterus runs through the suprainguinal region, while the femoral nerve, the femoral artery, the femoral vein, and the femoral canal run through the subinguinal region.
- The deep layer of the myopectineal orifice is closed off by the abdominal transverse fascia, which surrounds the spermatic cord, and the femoral sheath, which passes through the myopectineal orifice.
- A single-side repair of the myopectineal orifice can simultaneously and completely repair the site of anatomical weakness for inguinal, direct, and femoral hernias.
- This approach is also the principle of adult laparoscopic inguinal hernia repair.

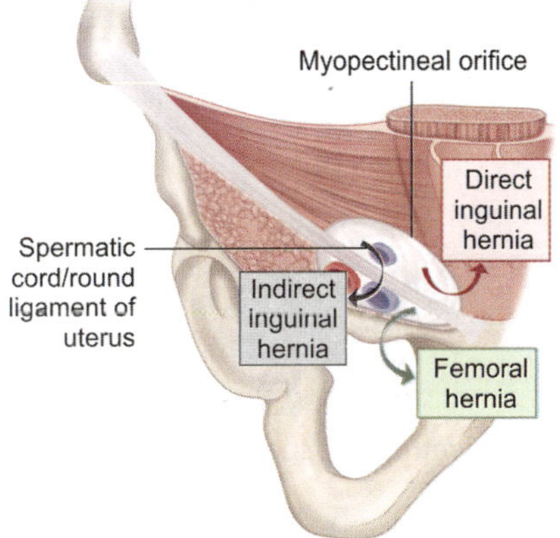

Representation of the myopectineal orifice.

Transverse Fascia

- The transverse fascia is a complicated and contentious anatomical structure.
- It is a thin aponeurotic membrane that lies between the rectus abdominis, the deep layer of the transverse abdominal muscle, and the peritoneum.
- The structure of the transverse fascia is not important in the TAPP approach or the intraperitoneal onlay mesh (IPOM) repair; therefore, the transverse fascia is often neglected.
- However, the transverse fascia has important clinical relevance in the TEP patch repair; a correct understanding of the structure of the transverse fascia can help ensure a smooth operation.

Surgical area	*Important structures*	*Medial*	*Inferior epigastric vessels*	*Lateral*	*Important structures*	*Surgical area*
		Superficial transverse fascia		Superficial transverse fascia	Iliopubic tract Iliac fascia	
	Parietal layer space			Parietal layer space	Spermatic cord	
Preperitoneal retropubic space		Deep transverse fascia		Deep transverse fascia	Internal spermatic fascia	Space of Bogros
		Visceral layer		Visceral layer		
	Space of Retzius	Space		Space		
	Bladder	Peritoneum		Peritoneum	Henna sac	

Lower anterior abdominal wall, transverse fascia, and spaces (the right lower anterior abdominal wall is taken as an example). The surgical area refers to the main surgical field of a laparoscopic inguinal hernia repair.

Preperitoneal Retropubic Space and Extraperitoneal Space Posterior to the Transverse Fascia (Space of Bogros)

- These two spaces are potential non-natural cavities under the lower anterior abdominal wall, and they lie in between the superficial transverse fascia and the peritoneum.
- They are created by blunt separation when performing a laparoscopic inguinal hernia repair.

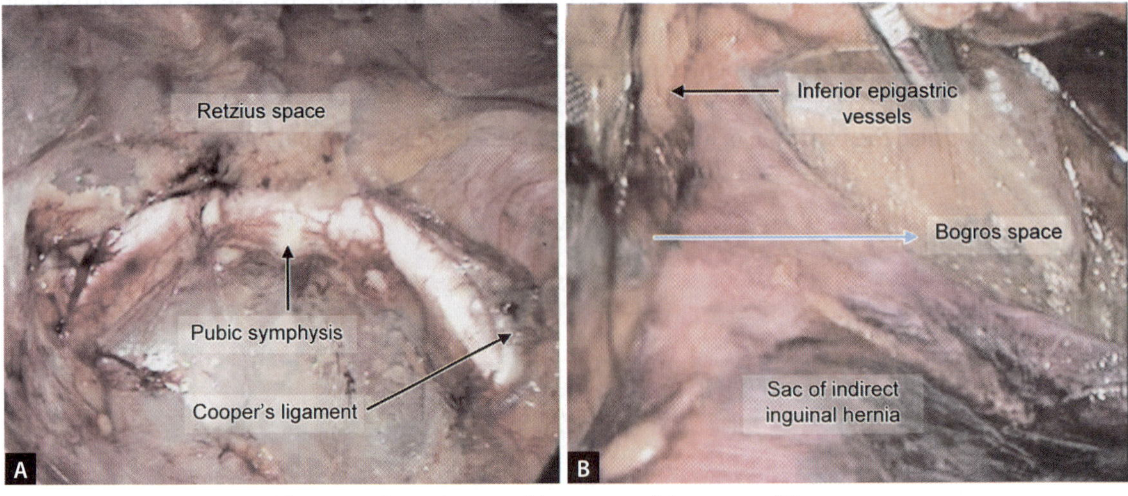

The preperitoneal retropubic space and the space of Bogros

- The preperitoneal retropubic space is located in the midline of the lower abdomen with the superficial transverse fascia and the pubic bone anteriorly, the bladder posteriorly, the umbilicus level superiorly, the pelvic floor muscles inferiorly, and the inferior epigastric arteries laterally.
- It is filled with loose connective tissue and fat, and there are no obvious blood vessels. The space is easily separated; the pubic symphysis and the shiny Cooper's ligament are readily visible after slight blunt separation.
- Usually, the preperitoneal retropubic space is considered to be equivalent to the space of Retzius.
- However, the space of Retzius originally referred to the space formed by the fold of the tight fusion of the deep transverse fascia and the peritoneum between the bladder and the peritoneum, which includes the bladder and is filled with loose connective tissue.
- The preperitoneal retropubic space should include the space of Retzius, a part of the visceral space and a part of the parietal space.
- The space of Bogros is located lateral to the space of Retzius and is bound anteriorly by the superficial transverse fascia, medially by the inferior epigastric blood vessels, laterally by the pelvic wall, and posteriorly by the psoas muscle, the external iliac vessels, and the femoral nerve.
- During laparoscopic inguinal hernia repair, the space of Bogros is explored to access the iliac fossa as well as to make it easier to open the lateral mesh and lay it flat. During surgery, after the preperitoneal retropubic space is separated, care should be taken that the deep transverse abdominal fascia is tightly attached to the anterior abdominal wall at the site lateral to the inferior epigastric blood vessels when separating the space of Bogros.

Important anatomic structures and landmarks: During laparoscopic inguinal hernia repair, it is important to recognize the following important structures in the abdominal cavity:

- The median umbilical fold, the medial umbilical fold, the lateral umbilical fold, Hesselbach's triangle, the internal inguinal ring, and the femoral ring.
- These structures are the landmarks for making a correct diagnosis and performing accurate surgeries.
- Other anatomical structures in the extraperitoneal space that must be recognized include the pubic symphysis, Cooper's ligament, the corona mortis, the inferior epigastric vessels, the vas deferens/the round ligament of the uterus, the testicular vessels, the iliopubic tract, the dangerous triangle (triangle of doom), and the triangle of pain.

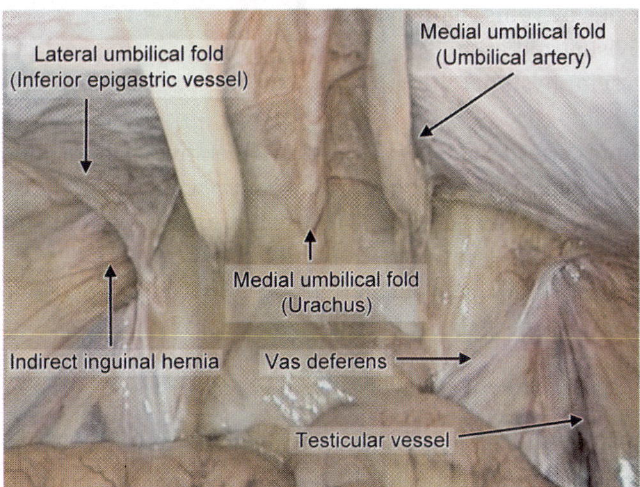

Bilateral inguinal area under laparoscopy.

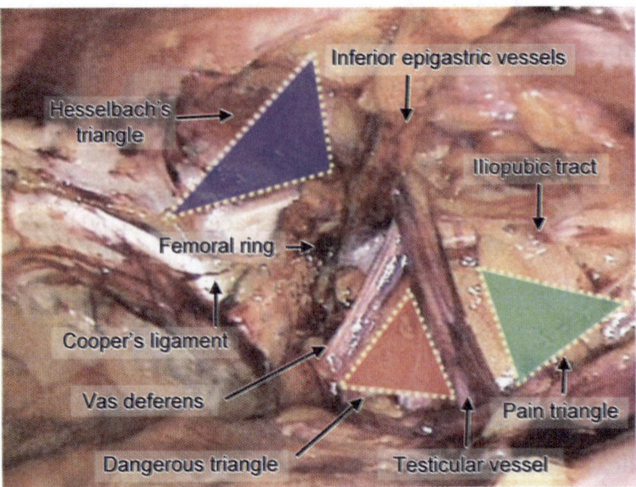

Important Anatomic Landmarks in the Extraperitoneal Space

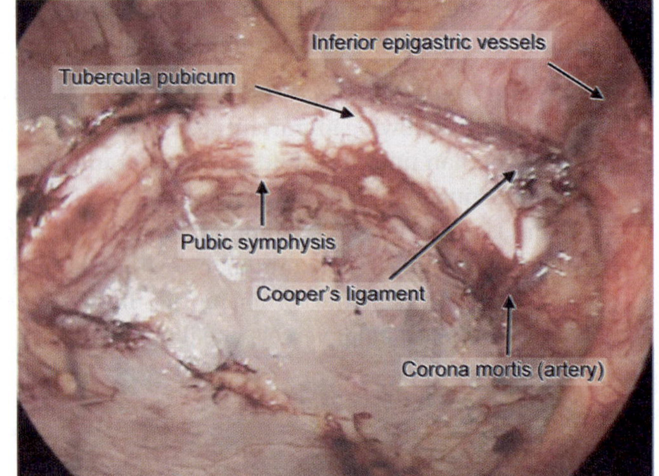

- The pubic symphysis is the first exposed anatomical landmark at separation of the space of Retzius and is the medial reference line when placing mesh.
- Cooper's ligament (also known as the pectineal ligament) is easier to identify because it is white, shiny, and tough tendinous tissue. It is an extension of the lacunar ligament, running inferolaterally along the pectineal line and attaching to the pectineal line. Cooper's ligament is a structure that can hold a mesh and tacks.
- One or a number of anastomotic vessels between the inferior epigastric or the external iliac vessels and the obturator arteries or veins, namely, the corona mortis, can be visualized at the site 5 cm away from the pubic symphysis, arching over Copper's ligament.
- The corona mortis includes arteries and veins, most of which travel alone and leaves the pelvic cavity via the obturator canal. During surgery, significant hemorrhage may occur, and hemostasis may be difficult to achieve if the corona mortis vessels are accidentally cut because they may retract into the obturator canal.
- Therefore, the corona mortis is known as the "crown of death" to remind surgeons to be alert during a procedure such as a separation and fixation on Copper's ligament.

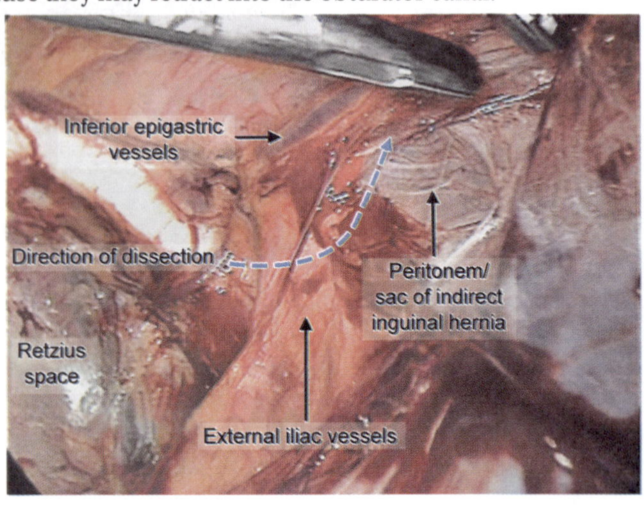

Corona Mortis

- The separation continues laterally along Cooper's ligament and the dark blue external iliac vein; the white, elastic, and pulsating external iliac artery can be seen after passing the corona mortis.
- The slightly thin inferior epigastric arteries and veins can be seen at the top of the external iliac vessels. Most of the inferior epigastric arteries are branches of the external iliac arteries or veins.

- The inferior epigastric artery usually runs with two veins along the back of the rectus abdominis muscle toward the umbilicus.
- The identification of the inferior epigastric vessels is very important before accessing the space of Bogros.
- Separating between the inferior epigastric vessels and the deep transverse abdominal fascia is the only approach to correctly gain access to the space of Bogros.
- Otherwise, it is easy to accidentally damage the inferior epigastric vessels or pierce the peritoneum, which may cause difficulties while performing laparoscopic surgery or even require conversion to open surgery.

Correct Access to the Space of Bogros

- During a laparoscopic inguinal hernia repair, the dangerous triangle (the triangle of doom) refers to a triangular area bound by the vas deferens, the testicular vessels, and the peritoneal fold. Within the boundaries of this area, you can find the external iliac artery and vein. Separation in this area is risky in the setting of an external iliac vascular malformation or aneurysm.
- The triangle of pain is a triangular area located lateral to the dangerous triangle and bound by the iliopubic tract, the testicular vessels, and the peritoneal fold.
- This area from lateral to medial includes the lateral femoral cutaneous nerve, the femoral branch of the genitofemoral nerve and the femoral nerve, which runs on the surface of the psoas muscle and the iliac muscle.
- The femoral nerve is 6 cm above the inguinal ligament and is not easily injured because it is covered by the psoas muscle.
- The lateral femoral cutaneous nerve runs just below the iliac fascia and enters the thigh in the 1- to 4-cm-wide region inferomedial to the anterior superior iliac spine under the iliopubic tract.
- During separation of the space of Bogros, avoiding piercing the iliac fascia and exposing the nerves is one of the most effective methods to reduce the incidence of postoperative chronic neuropathic pain.
- However, these above-mentioned nerves can suffer major damage or entrapment when performing separation or fixation or when controlling bleeding, which may cause abnormal sensation in the nerve-innervated area, especially chronic neuropathic pain, and may even cause motor disorders in the lower extremity.
- It is extremely difficult to manage or improve these symptoms.

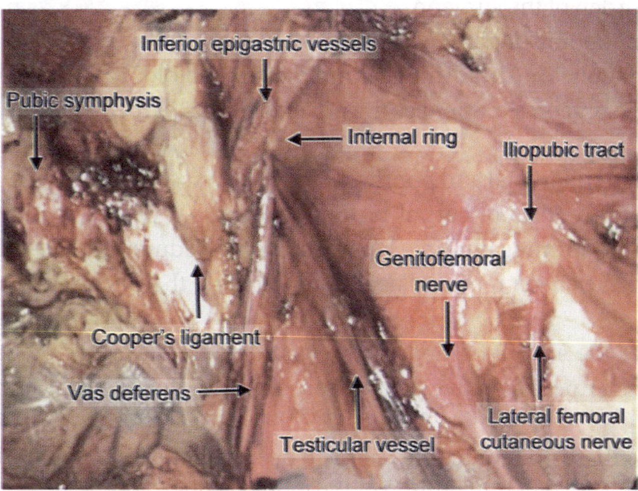

Lateral Femoral Cutaneous Nerve and Genitofemoral Nerve

- The iliopubic tract is a thickened tendinous structure of the transverse abdominal fascia that connects the anterior superior iliac spine and the pubic tubercle and parallels the inguinal ligament.
- It arches medially across the front of the femoral vessels to insert via broad attachment onto the pubic tubercle and Cooper's ligament. The iliopubic tract is the outer boundary of the triangle of pain.

- The lateral part of a mesh should be fixated at a spot just above the level of the iliopubic tract. The white iliopubic tract can be seen at the lower edge of a direct hernia ring or below an internal inguinal ring.
- The simplest method to identify the iliopubic tract is to touch and press the projected spot of the stapler head on the body surface when using a stapler to staple the lateral part of a mesh; the feel of the stapler head indicates that the stapler head is located above the iliopubic tract.
- Otherwise, the stapler head is likely located below the iliopubic tract, and stapling may cause nerve damage.

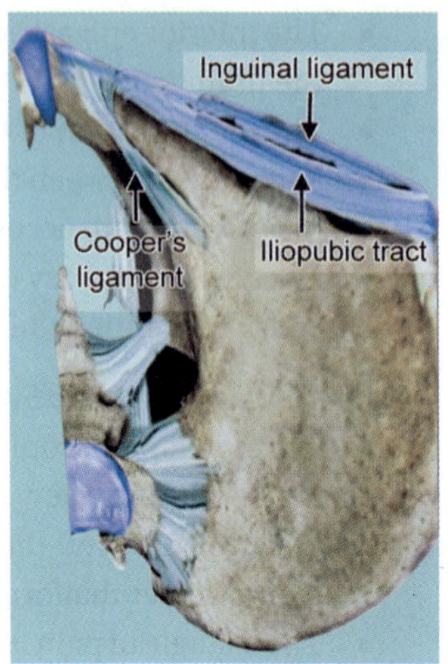

Representation of the right Cooper's ligament, the iliopubic tract, and the inguinal ligament.

The vas deferens/the round ligament of the uterus and testicular blood vessels can be completely exposed only when the internal spermatic fascia is incised and the hernia sac or the peritoneal fold is separated to the cephalad direction.

GO THROUGH ERGONOMICS IN LAPAROSCOPIC SURGERY

33. Describe basic ergonomic concepts in laparoscopic surgery. ***Gujarat Health University 2025***

Introduction

- Laparoscopic surgery provides patients with less painful surgery.
- It is more demanding for the surgeon.
- Increased technological sophistication and sometimes poorly adapted equipment has increased complaints of surgeon fatigue and discomfort during laparoscopic surgery.
- Ergonomic integration and an appropriate laparoscopic operating environment are essential to improve the efficiency, safety, and comfort of the surgical team.
- Understanding ergonomics not only makes the life of the surgeon comfortable in the operating room, but also reduces the physical burden of the surgeon.
- After every progress comes drawback.
- Laparoscopy is no exception. The disadvantages are mainly twofold.
- In the first scenario, the surgeon experiences the adverse effects of the operation, and in the second, the victim is the patient.
- This statement may seem superficial and poorly reflective at first glance, but it answers a much deeper question.
- There have been several reports of carpal tunnel syndrome, eye strain, and cervical spondylosis among unsuspecting surgeons performing multiple laparoscopic procedures in high-volume centers.
- Subsequent neuropathy has been reported as a result of using the uncomfortable thumb grip of laparoscopic pistol grips.
- In the first decade after the advent of laparoscopy, patients too have been found to be experiencing a lot of inconvenience with greater postoperative pain at port sites and due to other complications of the procedure in some cases.
- The mistakes leading to these poor outcomes seem to be completely avoidable with use of simple application of understanding of the physics and functioning of the whole event.

Definition

- The term ergonomics is derived from the Greek words "ergon" meaning work and "nomos" meaning natural laws or arrangement.
- Ergonomics is "the scientific study of people at work, in terms of equipment design, workplace layout, the working environment, safety, productivity, and training." Ergonomics is based on anatomy, physiology, psychology, and engineering, combined in a systems approach.

- In simple words, it is the science of best suiting the worker to his job, or to make the setting and surroundings favorable for the laparoscopic surgeon.
  - The importance of ergonomics in the setting of laparoscopy cannot be overemphasized. Studies have shown that correct ergonomics can reduce suturing time. Pressure-related chronic pain among surgeons has been shown to be relieved by the use of ergonomically designed products.
  - Hence, it is imperative to understand the applications of ergonomics for all surgeons practicing laparoscopy as well as novices yet to be initiated into this field.

The Hawthorne Effect

- It has been a well-observed phenomenon that any individual performs a skill better and with more caution whenever he has the knowledge that he is under observation and assessment. This tends to skew the results toward more positive scores than would otherwise be obtained if the person under study was unaware of the assessment being performed. This constitutes the "Hawthorne effect" which has been found applicable to most scientific assessments of human function and hence an integral knowledge of this aspect is essential for ergonomic purposes.
- Laparoscopy, a surgical skill performed by human skill and coordination, can certainly be judged by ergonomic scales. Although such evaluations must be conducted in secret to avoid biases caused by the Hawthorne effect, this would raise a number of ethical and analytical problems.

Ergonomic Challenges during Laparoscopy

- Initially, it is helpful to identify potential problem areas in the practice of minimal access surgery that present unique ergonomic challenges not encountered by nonlaparoscopic surgeons.
- *The differences between open and laparoscopic surgery are as follows:*
  - In open surgery, there is a lot of freedom and surgeons work along the visual axis.
  - It has 3D live vision and direct tactile feedback.
  - During laparoscopic surgery, two-dimensional vision and some degree of depth perception are monitored. It has a fulcrum, increasing vibrations. There are only 4° of freedom.
  - The biggest limitation is that the sight is not under the control of the surgeon.
  - The biggest nonskill factor affecting the surgeon's efficiency is the decoupling of the visual and motor axis.
  - Tactile reaction also disappears because the surgeon and hands are replaced by instruments.
  - Visual orientation changes when depth perception is impaired due to indirect visual input and also due to loss of peripheral vision due to limited visual spectrum.
  - The laparoscopic surgeon also assumes a relatively static position for most of the procedure, which ergonomically contributes to inefficiency.
- One of the most important cognitive challenges for a general surgeon when he becomes a laparoscopic surgeon is to remove the visual axis and the physical side of the procedure.
- The surgeon cannot look directly at the instruments, his hands, and the operating area at the same time.
- He must learn to adapt to the difficulties of combining these two functions into one channel to skillfully manipulate tissues without direct contact.
- Studies have shown that working in separate coordinate systems degrades efficiency by increasing procedural error rates.
- Performing complex laparoscopic surgeries requires great concentration and skill.
- Therefore, the operating surgeon was observed to adopt a more static position during laparoscopic procedures compared to the earlier open approach.
- These static positions have been shown to be more exhausting and damaging than dynamic positions, as muscles and tendons accumulate lactic acid and toxins when held for long periods of time.
- Sensory ergonomics (manipulation and imaging) increase accuracy, dexterity, and confidence, while physical ergonomics increase surgeon comfort.
- Together, these two elements of ergonomics increased safety, improved performance, and reduced stress.

Ergonomics Concepts in OT

- *OT position:*
  - A surgeon in two different positions can perform laparoscopic cholecystectomy.
  - One is by standing on the left side of patients and other is by standing between the legs.
  - Both the positions are convenient but some find one more ergonomically better.
  - It is usually surgeon's preference or habit of getting adjusted to the position.
  - Though port placement is similar, there is slight change in each position.
- *OT table:* Height of operating table should be adjusted between 64 and 77 cm above floor level since this discomfort and operative difficulty are lowest when instruments are positioned at elbow height.
- *Monitor position:*
  - Ergonomically, the best view for laparoscopy is with the monitor image at or within 25 optimal degrees below the horizontal plane of the eye.
  - This leads to least neck strain according to the available studies.
  - Standard LED monitors placed on a low cart separate from the operating room equipment may be used for best results.
  - It is not advisable to have a "chin-up" arrangement on the part of the surgeon.
  - In operations where surgeons change their ports and positions, the second monitor is essential, e.g., total colectomy. Second monitor for assistants reduces strain on their neck.
- *Trocar placements:*
  - There is no uniform agreement regarding port placement for advanced laparoscopic procedures.
  - Port placement is currently determined by surgeons and based on personal experience.
  - To facilitate smooth manipulation of the instrument and adequate visualization during laparoscopy, trocars are usually placed in a triangular shape.
  - This is called triangulation.

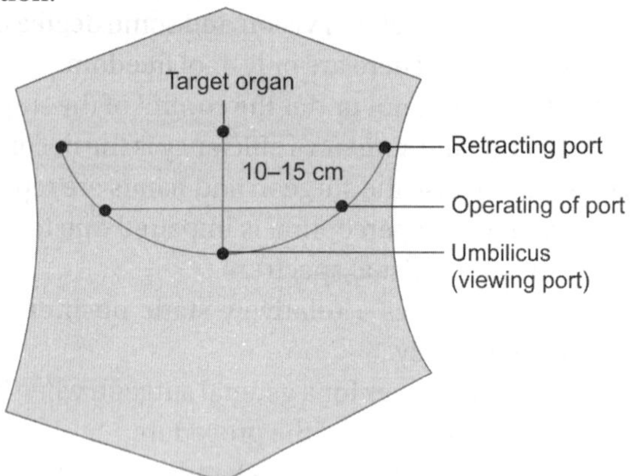

Port placement—triangulation.

- The target organ should be 15–20 cm from the central port used to place the optic trocar.
- Generally, the remaining two trocars are placed in the same 15–20 cm arc 5–7 cm on either side of the optical trocars.
- This allows the instruments to operate at 60–90° angles to the target tissue and avoids the perennial problem of placing ports too far or too close and the problem of abdominal wall interference.
- If necessary, two more withdrawal ports can be placed in the same arc, but on the side so that the instruments do not collide with each other.

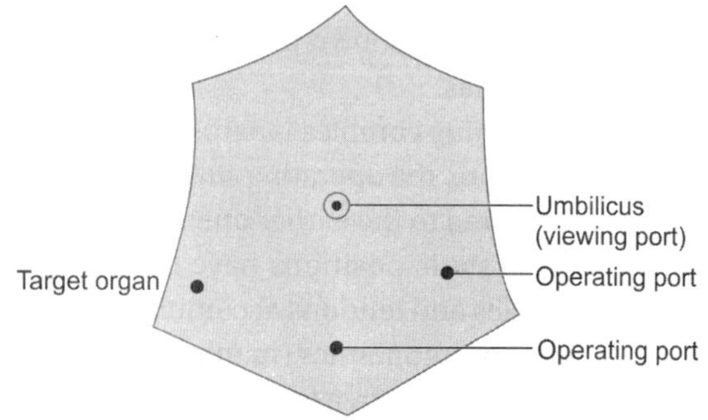

Port placement—sectorization.

- When optical trocar is placed as one of the lateral port trocar, it is called as sectorization.
- This is usually done during appendicectomy when 10-mm trocar is placed in subumbilical region as optical trocar.
- Two other trocars are placed below these trocars laterally. Sectoring of instruments should be avoided by beginners since it requires a greater degree of understanding and experience of the laparoscopic view and significantly different hand-eye coordination.
- Another factor that should be considered when placing trocars is the limited length of the instrument.
- If the trocar is too far from the desired position, the abdominal wall must be elevated a few centimeters toward the target organ.
- This not only makes these movements more imprecise, but also stresses the fingers and hand muscles.
- Similarly, if the angle between the object and the instrument is too wide or obtuse, handling a curved instrument will be very difficult. Most surgeons adjust the position of the trocar.
- If the gate is in the wrong place, you have to push your stomach and your arms start to hurt.

Manipulation Angles for Instrumentation

- Best task efficiency and performance quality are obtained with an ideal manipulation angle between 45° and 60°.
- This can be achieved by correct placement of the ports.
- The 90-manipulation angle had the greatest muscle workload by the deltoid and trapezius of the extracorporeal and intracorporeal limbs and the extracorporeal dominant arm extensor and flexor groups.
- Manipulation angle ranging from 45° to 75° with equal azimuth angles is recommended.
- Manipulation angles below 45° or above 75° are accompanied by increased difficulty and degraded performance.
- Task efficiency was reported be better with equal azimuth angles than with unequal azimuth angles.
- Achieving equal azimuth angles may be difficult in many practical situations, but in principle, azimuth inequality should be avoided because it degrades task efficiency.

There exists a direct correlation between the manipulation and the elevation angles.

- With a manipulation angle of 60°, the corresponding optimal elevation angle which yields the shortest execution time and optimal quality performance is 60°.
- Wide manipulation angles necessitate wide elevation angles for optimal performance and task efficiency.
- When a 30° manipulation angle is imposed by the anatomy or build of the patient, the elevation angle should be also 30° as this combination carries the shortest execution time.
- The best ergonomic layout for endoscopic surgery consists of a manipulation angle ranging from 45° to 75° with equal azimuth angles.

[What's the azimuth? The azimuth is the angle between North, measured clockwise around the observer's horizon, and a celestial body (sun and moon). It determines the direction of the celestial body. For example, a celestial body due North has an azimuth of 0º, one due East 90º, one due South 180º, and one due West 270º].

Equipment-related Challenges

- When performing minimal access surgery, the surgeon usually watches a two-dimensional video image of the surgical field on a television video screen placed at a certain distance of 4–8 meters from the surgeon and the eye.
- Even with the highest quality monitor equipment, the image quality and detail accuracy cannot be compared to direct imaging.
- Another limiting aspect that laparoscopy has to contend with is the loss of peripheral vision, which was one of the cornerstones of his surgical skills in open procedures. He is no longer allowed to see anything other than the immediate surgical area, and he loses the luxury of efficient navigation in the larger surgical workspace.
- A surgeon cannot move his tools endlessly. Currently, the most commonly used laparoscopic instruments offer only 4° of freedom of movement, which are rotation, up/down angles, left/right angles, and in/out movement.
- Laparoscopic instruments reduce efficiency. For example, a laparoscopic gripper transfers force from handle to tip only 1:3, compared to 3:1 for a portable hemostat.

- Therefore, the laparoscope has to work six times harder to achieve similar results.
- Additionally, these laparoscopic instruments are usually available in one standard size, so surgeons of all heights, builds and sizes work with the same instruments, and efficiency suffers somewhere.
- Custom equipment is prohibitively expensive.
- Newer generation 3D imaging cameras significantly improved laparoscopic accuracy in novice and experienced surgeons.
- Skill factors that have a profound effect on outcome are mostly related to intracorporeal suturing techniques.
- These problems arise from the need to suture at odd port sites without triangulation, to suture at an odd angle to the tissue, to suture in the retroperitoneum, and to maintain tension during continuous suturing using less efficient instruments.
- All of the above-mentioned problems associated with this skill area are special challenges of laparoscopy.

Mattern Waller Handles

- Mattern and Waller suggested that improperly designed instrument shapes emphasize the functional areas of the hand.
- They designed the handle based on ergonomic criteria.
- This multi-function grip is designed to fit only one hand and, like a pistol grip, rests continuously on the semiclosed hand, similar to the basic position of the resting hand, between the ring and little fingers, and the thenar performs an encircling grip.
- The longitudinal axis of the instrument is an extension of the rotational axis of the arm.
- This allows pronation and supination to be transmitted directly to the instrument's effector.

Single Port Laparoscopy

- Single port laparoscopy has changed the concept of triangulation used in conventional laparoscopy.
- With single port, the instruments often cross each other, making the procedure "counter-counterintuitive."
- To overcome these difficulties, steerable endoscopes, bent and articulating instrumentation, magnetic anchorage, and guidance systems as well as flexible robotics have been developed.

Robotic Surgery

- Robotic surgery is ergonomically advantageous as it has 7° of freedom as compared to laparoscopic hand surgery.
- This helps one to access deeper areas in abdomen such as esophagus, pancreas, and retroperitoneum.
- It also allows placements of ports in shorter arc without instrument interference.

Physical Constraints to Surgeon due to Inefficient Application of Ergonomics

- Neck pain and spondylosis have been found to be common complaints among surgeons in high-volume centers during the first decade after minimal access surgery.
- The underlying reason was found to be the same height at which the video screen was placed for surgeons of different heights.
- Other physical burdens reported include cervical spondylitis, pain from abduction of the shoulder (chicken wing scapula) during laparoscopy, called "laparoscopic shoulder," back pain, joint pain in the fingers of the hands, tenosynovitis, burning eyes, fatigue, and hand muscle injury.
- The most common reasons why ergonomics cannot be implemented optimally in the field of laparoscopy can be cited as a lack of complete awareness among surgeons, communication between laparoscopy therapists and instrument designers, and insufficient knowledge of potential problems. Users of designer-designed instruments and conflicting expert advice that undermine the credibility of ergonomics as a science.
- The recommended arm position is slight abduction, retroversion, and inward rotation at shoulder level.
- The elbow should be bent approximately 90–120°.
- The surgeon must remember that occasional movement and disengagement of the arms are necessary to prevent lactic acid build-up and fatigue.

- Problems with depth perception, vision, and loss of peripheral visual fields can be reduced by using 10–15x magnification of the optical system and screen output of the recording camera.
- This can make life easier during surgery, especially when dealing with small and complex internal anatomy.
- Laparoscopic surgery offers a less painful operation for patients, but is more demanding for the surgeon.
- Increased technological sophistication and sometimes poorly adapted equipment have increased complaints of surgeon fatigue and discomfort during laparoscopic surgery.
- Better ergonomic integration and understanding of ergonomics will not only make the surgeon's life in the operating room more comfortable, but also reduce the surgeon's physical burden.

34. Microbreaks in surgery. ***AIIMS, Patna 2025***

"Microbreaks in surgery" can refer to two things: *brief, intraoperative pauses for surgeons to stretch and reduce fatigue* or a *surgical procedure called microfracture*, which is used to repair damaged cartilage in joints like the knee. Intraoperative microbreak are short (1–2 minutes) breaks during surgery for staff to stretch, which helps reduce pain, improve focus, and enhance performance without increasing operative time. Microfracture surgery involves creating small holes in a joint to stimulate new cartilage growth to repair damage.

Intraoperative Microbreaks for Surgeons

- *What they are:* Short, periodic breaks (1–2 minutes) taken every 20–40 minutes during long procedures to stretch and relieve strain.
- *What they involve:* Activities like stretching the neck, shoulders, and back, or simply shifting position.
- *Benefits:* They can reduce musculoskeletal pain, improve physical function, enhance mental focus, and increase surgical accuracy and performance.
- *Implementation:* Can be guided by a web-based application and are often designed to be low-disruption, with options to exercise without breaking scrub.

Microfracture (a Surgical Procedure)

- *What it is:* A surgical technique to repair damage to the articular cartilage in a joint, most commonly the knee.
- *How it works:* The surgeon makes tiny holes in the bone to stimulate the growth of new, fibrocartilage tissue to fill the defect.
- *When it's used:* It is most suitable for small areas of damage in younger, active individuals who want to return to sports and have not yet developed widespread arthritis.
- *Limitations:* It is not a suitable treatment for patients with severe or widespread arthritis, or for those unwilling or unable to participate in postsurgery rehabilitation.

THIRD-SPACE ENDOSCOPY

35. Write down the indications and uses of third-space endoscopy. ***WBUHS 2024***

36. Discuss third-space endoscopy. ***SAIMS, Indore 2025; The Tamil Nadu Dr MGR Medical University 2025; Srimanta Sankaradeva University, Assam 2025***

Third-space endoscopy is a minimally invasive procedure used for various therapeutic and diagnostic purposes in the gastrointestinal system, particularly in the submucosal layers. This technique allows for access to areas that are otherwise difficult to reach using conventional endoscopy. Below are the indications and uses of third-space endoscopy:

Background and Concept

The wall of the GI tract consists of several layers:

- Mucosa
- Submucosa (third space)

- Muscularis propria
- Serosa or adventitia

Traditional endoscopic techniques primarily involve working within the *luminal space* (inside the GI tract) or through *full-thickness* incisions (as in NOTES—Natural Orifice Transluminal Endoscopic Surgery).

Third space endoscopy, however, creates and uses a *submucosal tunnel* to access deeper layers without breaching the outer serosal surface. This allows complex interventions while minimizing the risk of perforation.

Principle Steps

1. *Mucosal entry*—A small incision is made in the mucosa.
2. *Submucosal tunnelin* —A saline (or dye)-assisted dissection creates a submucosal tunnel to the target area.
3. *Therapeutic intervention*—The specific procedure (e.g., myotomy, tumor resection) is performed.
4. *Mucosal closure*—The entry point is sealed, typically with endoscopic clips or suturing devices.

This technique is sometimes called *Submucosal Endoscopic Tunnel Technique (SETT).*

Indications of Third-Space Endoscopy

Submucosal tumors: Third-space endoscopy is useful for the resection of submucosal tumors, such as leiomyomas, gastrointestinal stromal tumors (GISTs), or lipomas, that are not amenable to conventional endoscopic removal.

Endoscopic Submucosal dissection (ESD): For the treatment of early cancers or precancerous lesions, especially in the esophagus, stomach, and colon. ESD allows for en bloc resection of large lesions that might otherwise require more invasive surgery.

Esophageal or gastric perforations: Can be used to treat perforations in the esophagus or stomach by creating a working space to apply treatments such as suturing or clipping for closure.

Achalasia treatment: In cases of achalasia, third-space endoscopy can be used for myotomy (cutting of the muscle layers) to treat the condition where the esophagus fails to move food properly into the stomach.

Endoscopic submucosal tunnel (EST): A technique that can be applied to treat conditions like Zenker's diverticulum, where a submucosal tunnel is created to remove the diverticulum.

Peroral endoscopic myotomy (POEM): Used for the treatment of motility disorders like achalasia. It involves creating a submucosal tunnel and performing myotomy to relax the muscle of the esophagus.

Gastrostomy tube placement: Third-space endoscopy can help in placing feeding tubes in patients with difficulty swallowing or when alternative methods are needed.

Surgical treatment of obesity: Used for procedures such as endoscopic sleeve gastroplasty (ESG), where the stomach is sutured or stapled to create a smaller, sleeve-like structure.

Uses of Third-Space Endoscopy

Endoscopic resection of lesions: Removal of benign or early malignant lesions from the gastrointestinal tract.

Diagnostic purposes: To obtain tissue from difficult-to-reach areas, allowing for diagnosis of tumors, ulcers, or other gastrointestinal abnormalities.

Creation of submucosal tunnels: For the treatment of conditions like Zenker's diverticulum and submucosal tumor resection, which can provide significant symptom relief and prevent further complications.

Treatment of motility disorders: Such as POEM for achalasia and other disorders where there is dysfunction in the motility of the esophagus or other parts of the gastrointestinal tract.

Gastrostomy for feeding: Useful in patients who require long-term feeding support, particularly those who have difficulty swallowing due to neurological or muscular conditions.

Management of gastric perforations: Endoscopic techniques can be used to repair or seal perforations in the stomach or esophagus.

In summary, third-space endoscopy is an advanced tool used for minimally invasive treatment of a range of gastrointestinal conditions. It allows for surgical-like interventions, offering both diagnostic and therapeutic benefits without the need for traditional surgery.

CHAPTER 36

Breast

LEARNING OBJECTIVES

- Aberrations of Normal Development and Involution (ANDI)
- Mastalgia and Nipple Discharge
- Gynecomastia
- Phyllodes Tumor
- Percutaneous Management of Benign Breast Lesions
- Granulomatous Mastitis
- Imaging in Breast Diseases
- Fine-needle Aspiration Cytology (FNAC) Scoring of Breast Cancer
- Breast Cancer Prevention
- Lymphatic Manifestation of Breast Carcinoma
- Ductal Carcinoma in Situ (DCIS)
- Sentinel Lymph Node Biopsy (SLNB) and ALND
- Early and Locally Advanced Breast Cancer
- Management of Impalpable Breast Lesions
- Boundaries of Axilla, Diseases Implicating Axilla, and ALND
- Controversies Regarding the Management of Primary Lesion in Presence of Distant Metastasis in Breast Cancer
- Radiotherapy for Breast Cancer
- Breast Conservation Surgery
- Adjuvant Therapy in Carcinoma Breast
- Breast Cancer in Pregnancy
- Breast Reconstruction and Oncoplastic Breast Surgery
- Augmentation and Reduction Mammoplasty

ANDI

1. Aberrations of normal development and involution (ANDI).

WBUHS 2006, DY Patil Educational Society Deemed to be University 2020

The basic principles underlying the aberrations of normal development and involution (ANDI) classification of benign breast conditions are:

- Benign breast disorders and diseases are related to the normal processes of reproductive life and to involution;
- There is a spectrum of breast conditions that ranges from normal to disorder to disease;
- The ANDI classification encompasses all aspects of the breast condition, including pathogenesis and the degree of abnormality.

ANDI Classification of Benign Breast Disorders.

	Normal	*Disorder*	*Disease*
Early reproductive years (age 15–25)	Lobular development	Fibroadenoma	Giant fibroadenoma
	Stromal development	Adolescent hypertrophy	Gigantomastia
	Nipple eversion	Nipple inversion	Subareolar abscess
			Mammary duct fistula

Contd...

Contd...

	Normal	*Disorder*	*Disease*
Later reproductive years (age 25–40)	Cyclical changes of menstruation	Cyclical mastalgia	Incapacitating mastalgia
	Nodularity		
	Epithelial hyperplasia of pregnancy	Bloody nipple discharge	
Involution (age 35–55)	Lobular involution	Macrocysts	
		Sclerosing lesions	
	Duct involution		
	• Dilatation	Duct ectasia	Periductal mastitis
	• Sclerosis	Nipple retraction	
	Epithelial turnover	Epithelial hyperplasia	Epithelial hyperplasia with atypia

2. What is Page—Dupont category of benign breast diseases? Describe the management of breast cyst.

Tripura University 2025

Page-Dupont Classification of Benign Breast Diseases

(Also called the Page and Dupont histopathological classification)

This system classifies benign breast disorders based on *histologic pattern and associated risk of subsequent breast carcinoma.*

Page-Dupont Categories

Category	*Examples/pathology*	*Relative risk of breast cancer*	*Comments*
I. Nonproliferative lesions (simple benign changes)	• Simple cysts • Fibrosis • Mild ductal epithelial hyperplasia • Apocrine metaplasia • Duct ectasia • Fat necrosis	*No increased risk (RR ≈ 1)*	Most common group (~70% of benign breast biopsies)
II. Proliferative disease without atypia	• Moderate/florid ductal or lobular hyperplasia • Sclerosing adenosis • Radial scar/complex sclerosing lesion • Papilloma	*Slightly increased risk (RR 1.5–2)*	Reflects increased epithelial proliferation but normal cytology
III. Proliferative disease with atypia (Atypical hyperplasia)	• Atypical ductal hyperplasia (ADH) • Atypical lobular hyperplasia (ALH)	*Significantly increased risk (RR 4–5)*	Intermediate lesion between benign and carcinoma in situ

Clinical Significance

- The classification helps guide *follow-up and risk reduction strategies.*
  - *Category I:* Routine screening
  - *Category II:* Annual mammography + clinical follow-up
  - *Category III:* Closer surveillance ± chemoprevention (tamoxifen)

Management of Breast Cyst

Definition

A *breast cyst* is a *fluid-filled sac* within the breast, arising from *terminal duct lobular units* due to obstruction and involutional changes.

Common in women aged *35–50 years* (perimenopausal).

Clinical Features

Feature	***Description***
Presentation	Palpable lump—smooth, well-circumscribed, mobile, may fluctuate with cycle
Pain	Often tender, especially premenstrually
Multiple cysts	May be present in both breasts
Nipple discharge	Occasionally present (clear/greenish)

Investigations

Investigation	***Findings/purpose***
Ultrasound breast	Cystic lesion with posterior acoustic enhancement; distinguishes cyst from solid mass
Fine-needle aspiration (FNA)	Diagnostic and therapeutic—confirms cyst (clear or green fluid) and relieves symptoms
Mammography	May show round/oval radiolucent area; used if >40 years or atypical features
Cytology of aspirated fluid	If fluid is blood-stained or cyst recurs, send for cytology (rule out malignancy)

Management Algorithm

- *Simple cyst (benign features)*
  - *Step 1:* Ultrasound confirms simple cyst (thin wall, anechoic, no solid component).
  - *Step 2:*
    - *If asymptomatic:* Reassure; no treatment required.
    - *If symptomatic (painful or tense):* Aspirate the cyst.
  - *Step 3:*
    - *If cyst completely collapses* and fluid is *clear/straw-colored*, discard aspirate.
    - *Follow-up in 4–6 weeks.*
  - *If lump recurs or fluid is blood-stained → Send for cytology + repeat imaging.*
- *Complicated or complex cyst (on ultrasound)*
  - *Features:* Internal echoes, septations, mural nodule, or irregular wall.

Management

  - FNA or *core needle biopsy* to exclude carcinoma.
  - If benign → excision only if recurrent or symptomatic.
  - If suspicious → treat as malignancy.
- *Recurrent or persistent cyst*
  - *Re-aspirate and evaluate cytology.*
  - *Surgical excision (excisional biopsy)* indicated if:
    - Recurrent after 2 aspirations
    - Bloody or suspicious aspirate
    - Residual mass persists after aspiration
    - Associated solid component or atypical imaging features
- *Associated measures*
  - Supportive bra, analgesics (NSAIDs)
  - Avoid caffeine (may help some patients)
  - Reassurance and education about benign nature

3. Enumerate benign breast diseases and its treatment. ***RGHUS Karnataka 2025***

Benign Breast Diseases (BBDs)

Benign breast diseases include a wide range of *noncancerous conditions* of the breast, often related to hormonal influences.

They are much more common than breast cancer, especially in women of reproductive age.

Classification of Benign Breast Diseases

Developmental and Congenital Disorders

- Amastia—absence of breast
- Athelia—absence of nipple
- Polythelia—accessory nipple
- Polymastia— accessory breast tissue
- Juvenile (virginal) hypertrophy

Inflammatory Lesions

Type	***Cause/Features***	***Management***
Acute mastitis (Lactational)	*Staphylococcus aureus* infection during lactation	Antibiotics (e.g., flucloxacillin), analgesics, continued milk drainage, incision and drainage if abscess
Breast abscess	Complication of mastitis	Incision and drainage + antibiotics
Periductal mastitis/Duct ectasia	Chronic inflammation around ducts, may cause nipple discharge and retraction	Antibiotics, duct excision if recurrent
Tuberculous mastitis	Rare, chronic sinus formation	Antituberculous therapy ± surgery

Noninflammatory/Fibrocystic Conditions

Type	***Description***	***Treatment***
Fibrocystic change (Fibroadenosis, ANDI)	Commonest benign breast condition; cyclical pain, nodularity	Reassurance, supportive bra, analgesics; Danazol or evening primrose oil if severe
Simple cysts	Fluid-filled cysts, may be solitary or multiple	Aspiration (both diagnostic and therapeutic)
Galactocele	Milk-filled cyst due to duct obstruction post-lactation	Aspiration or excision if persistent

Benign Tumors

Type	***Features***	***Management***
Fibroadenoma	Common in young women, mobile "breast mouse" lump	Observation if <2 cm; excision if large (>2–3 cm), increasing in size, or patient anxious
Giant (juvenile) fibroadenoma	Rapidly enlarging in adolescents	Excision
Phyllodes tumor (benign/ borderline)	Large, fast-growing, leaf-like tumor; can recur	Wide local excision with margin (≥1 cm); mastectomy if giant/recurrent
Lipoma	Soft, mobile, fatty lump	Excision if symptomatic
Intraductal papilloma	Bloody nipple discharge, usually single duct	Microdochectomy (excision of involved duct)

Nipple and Duct Disorders

Disorder	***Features***	***Treatment***
Nipple discharge (non-bloody)	Often due to duct ectasia or papilloma	Treat underlying cause, microdochectomy if persistent
Nipple eczema (Paget's disease must be excluded)	Eczematous lesion around nipple	Topical steroids, biopsy to rule out malignancy

Traumatic and Miscellaneous

Type	Description	Management
Fat necrosis	Following trauma; may mimic carcinoma	Observation, excision if diagnostic doubt
Breast pain (mastalgia)	Cyclical or non-cyclical	Reassurance, supportive bra, analgesics, hormonal therapy if persistent

General Principles of Management of Benign Breast Disease

- *Triple assessment*
  - Clinical examination
  - Imaging (ultrasound/mammography)
  - FNAC or core needle biopsy
- *Reassurance and education*
  - Most lesions are benign
  - Regular self-examination and follow-up
- *Symptomatic treatment*
  - Analgesics (NSAIDs)
  - Supportive brassiere
  - Hormonal modulation (e.g., danazol, tamoxifen) in severe fibrocystic disease
- *Surgical treatment*
  - Excision biopsy or wide local excision for persistent or suspicious lumps
  - Microdochectomy for single-duct discharge
  - Mastectomy only for giant or recurrent phyllodes tumor

MASTALGIA

4. Discuss the management of mastalgia. ***WBUHS 2020; RIMS, Imphal 2022***

Introduction

- Severe breast pain or mastalgia is a common symptom.
- Affects up to 70% of the female population at some time in their lives.
- It accounts for approximately 50% of referrals to a specialized breast clinic.
- Two-thirds of patients having cyclical and one-third experiencing noncyclical mastalgia, or pain arising from the chest wall deep to the breast.
- After exclusion of breast cancer and proper reassurance, 85% of patients can be discharged from the clinic without specific treatment.
- In only 15% of patients is the pain severe enough to affect their lifestyle and warrant drug therapy.

Diagnosis

- Breast examination
- Imaging by ultrasound is recommended for all ages
- Those over 30 years it is recommended together with mammography

Treatment

- In >75% of people the pain resolves without any specific treatment
- Paracetamol or nonsteroidal anti-inflammatory drugs (NSAIDs)
- A well-fitting bra may also help
- In those with severe pain tamoxifen or danazol may be used
- Bromocriptine may be used as well
- Spironolactone, low-dose oral contraceptives, and low-dose estrogen have helped to relieve pain

- Topical anti-inflammatory medications can be used for localized pain
- Vitamin E is not effective in relieving pain nor is evening primrose oil
- Vitamin B_6 and vitamin A have not been consistently found to be beneficial
- For more severe localized pain, by local anesthetic
- Pain may be relieved by reassurance that it does not signal a serious underlying problem, and an active life style can also effect an improvement
- Counseling
- Women on hormone replacement therapy may benefit from a dose adjustment
- Breasts change during adolescence and menopause and refitting may be beneficial
- Applying heat and/or ice can bring relief
- Dietary changes may also help with the pain. Methylxanthines can be eliminated from the diet to see if a sensitivity is present.
- Patients with severe recurrent or refractory mastalgia may require treatment with tamoxifen, goserelin or testosterone, but the short- and long-term adverse effects of these drugs preclude their use as first-line agents.
- Chest wall pain is usually self-limiting, but symptomatic relief can often be obtained using steroidal and local anesthetic injections or NSAIDs.

NIPPLE DISCHARGE

5. Describe recent advances in management of nipple discharge. ***WBUHS 2019; RIMS, Imphal 2022***

Introduction

- Nipple discharge is a common complaint among women.
- Evaluation and management of nipple discharge can be undertaken with a careful history and examination
- Secretion from nipples can be classified according to its color, cellularity, and biology.
- To be significant a discharge should be true, spontaneous, persistent, and nonlactational.
- Differentiate patients who require surgical intervention from those who do not.
- Surgically significant nipple discharges are watery, serous (yellow), serosanguineous, and bloody.

Discharges from the Nipple

- *Discharge from the surface:*
  - Paget's disease
  - Skin diseases (eczema and psoriasis)
  - Rare causes (e.g., chancre)
- *Discharge from a single duct:*
  - *Blood-stained:*
    - Intraductal papilloma
    - Intraductal carcinoma
    - Duct ectasia
  - *Serous (any color):*
    - Fibrocystic disease
    - Duct ectasia
    - Carcinoma
- *Discharge from more than one duct:*
  - *Blood-stained:*
    - Carcinoma
    - Ectasia
    - Fibrocystic disease
  - *Black or green:* Duct ectasia

- *Purulent:* Infection
- *Serous:*
  - Fibrocystic disease
  - Duct ectasia
  - Carcinoma
- *Milk:* Lactation
- *Rare causes* (hypothyroidism and pituitary tumor)

Nipple Discharge Features based on its Nature

Nature of discharge	*Etiology*	*Localization*	*Ducts involved*
Milky	• Postpartum • Hyperprolactinemia • Medications • Chiari-Frommel syndrome	Bilateral	Multiple
Serous/serosanguinous	Intraductal papilloma or papillomas (papillomatosis) Intraductal cancer	Unilateral	One
Bloody	• Intraductal papilloma or papillomas (papillomatosis) • Intraductal cancer • Inflammation • Trauma*	Unilateral	One or two
Green	Fibrocystic disease	Bilateral	Multiple

*Relatively infrequent causes of nipple discharge.

- Cytology smears of discharge material—classify the cellular material, providing information about normality, atypia, and malignancy, and also about papillary formation of the exfoliated cells.

Cellular arrangement	*Cellular pleomorphism*	*Anisonucleosis nucleoli*		*Chromatin clumping*	*Myoepithelial cells*	*Score*
Monolayer	Absent	Absent	Absent	Absent	Many	1
Nuclear overlapping	Mild	Mild	Micronucleoli	Rare	Moderate	2
Clustering	Moderate	Moderate	Micro and/or rare micronucleoli	Occasional	Few	
Loss of cohesion	Conspicuous	Conspicuous	Predominantly macronucleoli	Frequent	Absent	4

Score 6–10: Nonproliferative breast disease. Score 11–14: Proliferative breast disease without atypia. Score 15–18: Proliferative breast disease with atypia. Score 19–24: Cancer.

- Tests such as Hemoccult help to discover occult blood in the secreted fluid.
- Immunological tests can be performed on cytology smears where occurrence of high lèvels of carcinoembryonic antigen (CEA) could indicate a latent malignancy.
- Galactography investigation is today the state-of-the-art approach to investigate patients with nipple discharge disorders and this examination can demonstrate the size, location, and extent of an intraductal abnormality.
- High-resolution ultrasound techniques are helpful in visualizing intraductal disorders and are becoming a good complementary approach if not an alternative to traditional radiology techniques.

Ultrasonographical Findings in Common Nipple Discharge Etiology

Etiology	*Findings*
Intraductal papilloma	Ovoid hyperechoic mass (image)
Duct ectasia	Single or multiple tubular anechoic subareolar structures
Intraductal carcinoma	Calcifications, irregular shape, and irregular margin contour*, hypoechogenicity and nonuniform internal echotexture#, posterior shadowing and loss of bilateral edge shadowing^

In contrast *to 2 or 3 gentle lobulations, #of the intense, uniform hyperechogenicity and ^of thin, echogenic capsule of benign conditions

- Recently even magnetic resonance (MR) galactography has been shown to be of diagnostic value, but not as informative as regular galactography.
- The most sophisticated investigation method, which can also be used therapeutically, is fiber ductoscopy of the concerned duct in a breast. This technique, although expensive and in its infancy, is a fascinating and promising approach for inspecting the intraductal lumina.

Surgical Diagnosis

- *Biopsy:* Excision of the pathological duct(s) should be performed if nipple discharge persists or when it is bloody.
- *Microdochectomy:* The removal of the duct by a technique that leaves intact the surrounding tissues and the unaffected ducts. The procedure can also be carried out by transnipple pyramidectomy.

Future Perspective

- Endoscopic appearances of ductoscopy should be improved in order to achieve accurate diagnoses in more cases.
- Biopsy tools need further improvements.
- Further evaluation of the potential therapeutic role of guided intraductal biopsy, and of cytology assisted by ductoscopy as a screening tool, is required.
- The mammary pump could be proven to be an essential instrument in nipple discharge screening.

GYNECOMASTIA

6. Gynecomastia. ***WBUHS 2022***

Introduction

- Gynecomastia refers to an enlarged breast in the male.
- Physiologic gynecomastia usually occurs during three phases of life: the neonatal period, adolescence, and senescence.

Key Points

- Common to each of these phases is an excess of circulating estrogens in relation to circulating testosterone.
- Neonatal gynecomastia is caused by the action of placental estrogens on neonatal breast tissues, while in adolescence, there is an excess of estradiol relative to testosterone, and with senescence, the circulating testosterone level falls, resulting in relative hyperestrinism.
- In gynecomastia, the ductal structures of the male breast enlarge, elongate, and branch with a concomitant increase in epithelium.
- During puberty, the condition often is unilateral and typically occurs between ages 12 and 15 years. In contrast, senescent gynecomastia is usually bilateral.
- In the nonobese male, breast tissue measuring at least 2 cm in diameter must be present before a diagnosis of gynecomastia may be made.
- Mammography and ultrasonography are used to differentiate breast tissues.
- Dominant masses or areas of firmness, irregularity, and asymmetry suggest the possibility of a breast cancer, particularly in the older male.
- Gynecomastia generally does not predispose the male breast to cancer.
- However, the hypoandrogenic state of Klinefelter's syndrome (XXY), in which gynecomastia is usually evident, is associated with an increased risk of breast cancer.

Epidemiology

- It can occur at any age
- Tends to have greater prevalence in two groups: adolescent boys and older men

- Prevalence of "asymptomatic" gynecomastia ranges around:
  - *Neonates:* 60–90%
  - *Adolescents:* 50–60%
  - *Men aged 50–69 years:* Up to 70%
- Prevalence of "symptomatic" cases is markedly lower.

Clinical Presentation

Palpation usually demonstrates a palpable, tender, firm, mobile, disk-like mound of tissue.

Pathology

- In gynecomastia, there is enlargement of the male breast due to benign ductal and stromal proliferation.
- A hallmark of gynecomastia is its central symmetric location under the nipple.
- Gynecomastia in most cases tends to be unilateral and/or asymmetrical.
- The imbalance between actions of estrogen relative to actions of androgen at the breast tissue level appears to be a key etiological factor in gynecomastia

Pathophysiologic Mechanisms of Gynecomastia. Estrogen Excess States

- Gonadal origin
  - True hermaphroditism
  - Gonadal stromal (nongerminal) neoplasms of the testis
    - Leydig cell (interstitial)
    - Sertoli cell
    - Granulosa theca
  - Germ cell tumors
    - Choriocarcinoma
    - Seminoma and teratoma
    - Embryonal carcinoma
- Nontesticular tumors
  - Adrenal cortical neoplasms
  - Lung carcinoma
  - Hepatocellular carcinoma
- Endocrine disorders
- Diseases of the liver—nonalcoholic and alcoholic cirrhosis
- Nutrition alteration states

Androgen deficiency states

- Senescence
- Hypoandrogen states (hypogonadism)
  - Primary testicular failure
    - Klinefelter's syndrome (XXY)
    - Reifenstein's syndrome
    - Rosewater, Gwinup, Hamwi familial gynecomastia
    - Kallmann's syndrome
    - Kennedy's disease with associated gynecomastia
    - Eunuchoidal males (congenital anorchia)
    - Hereditary defects of androgen biosynthesis
    - Adrenocorticotropic hormone (ACTH) deficiency
  - Secondary testicular failure
    - Trauma
    - Orchitis
    - Cryptorchidism
    - Irradiation
- Renal failure

Drug-related

Systemic diseases with idiopathic mechanisms

Clinical Classification of Gynecomastia

Grade I	Mild breast enlargement without skin redundancy
Grade IIa	Moderate breast enlargement without skin redundancy
Grade IIb	Moderate breast enlargement with skin redundancy
Grade III	Marked breast enlargement with skin redundancy and ptosis, which simulates a female breast

Diagnostic Approach of Men with Gynecomastia

Medical history collection	*Physical examination*	*First-level laboratory blood tests and instrumental investigations*	*Additional laboratory blood investigations*
Duration of gynecomastia, uni- or bilateral location, tenderness	Uni or bilateral location, size, tenderness	LH, FSH, T, E_2, SHBG	DHEA-S, AA
Previous occurrences of gynecomastia	Height, weight, and body mass index	β-hCG	Karyotype
Previous or current cryptorchidism, fertility status	Thyroid palpation	TSH	DNA for genetic analysis, such as PCR for androgen receptor
Symptoms of testosterone deficiency, hyperthyroidism, or systemic illnesses	General (signs of systemic illnesses) and genital (testicular size, consistency) physical examination	Prolactin	
Complete list of medication, use of recreational drugs and/or supplements		• *Liver function*: SGOT, SGPT, albumin • *Renal function*: creatinine, urea • Testicular ultrasound scan	

(AA: adrenal androgen; β-hCG: β-human chorionic gonadotropin; DHEA-S: dehydroepiandrosterone sulfate; DNA: deoxyribonucleic acid; E_2: estradiol; FSH: follicle-stimulating hormone; LH: luteinizing hormone; PCR: polymerase chain reaction; SGOT: serum glutamic-oxaloacetic transaminase; SGPT: serum glutamate pyruvate transaminase; SHBG: sex hormone binding globulin; T: testosterone; TSH: thyroid-stimulating hormone)

Treatment

- Generally, no treatment is required for physiologic gynecomastia.
- Pubertal gynecomastia resolves spontaneously within several weeks to 3 years in approximately 90% of patients.
- Breasts >4 cm in diameter may not completely regress.
- Identifying and managing an underlying primary disorder often alleviates breast enlargement.
- If hypogonadism (primary or secondary) is the cause of gynecomastia, parenteral or transdermal testosterone replacement therapy is instituted.
- However, testosterone does have the potential to exacerbate gynecomastia through the aromatization of the exogenous hormone into estradiol.
- For patients with idiopathic gynecomastia or with residual gynecomastia after treatment of the primary cause, medical or surgical treatment may be considered.
- A major factor that should influence the initial choice of therapy for gynecomastia is the condition's duration.
- It is unlikely that any medical therapy will result in significant regression in the late fibrotic stage (a duration of 12 months or longer) of gynecomastia. As a result, medical therapies, if used, should be tried early in the condition's course.

Pharmacologic Therapy

Clomiphene	*Tamoxifen*	*Danazol*
An antiestrogen	An estrogen antagonist	Less frequently used
Approximately 50% of patients achieve partial reduction in breast size	It is effective for recent-onset and tender gynecomastia	A synthetic derivative of testosterone

Contd...

Contd...

Clomiphene	Tamoxifen	Danazol
Approximately 20% of patients note complete resolution	Up to 80% of patients report partial to complete resolution	Inhibits pituitary secretion of luteinizing hormone (LH) and follicle-stimulating hormone (FSH), which decreases estrogen synthesis from the testicles
Adverse effects, while rare, include visual problems, rash, and nausea	Nausea and epigastric discomfort are the main adverse effects	

Breast Surgery

- Reduction mammoplasty is considered for patients with macromastia or long-standing gynecomastia or in persons in whom medical therapy has failed. It is also considered for cosmetic reasons (and for accompanying psychosocial reasons).
- More extensive plastic surgery may be required in patients with marked gynecomastia or who have developed excessive sagging of the breast tissue due to weight loss. If surgery is necessary for patients with pseudogynecomastia, liposuction may be warranted.
- Endoscopic subcutaneous mastectomy, without skin excision, could be an effective treatment for gynecomastia.

Complications of Surgery

- Sloughing of tissue due to a compromised blood supply,
- Contour irregularity, hematoma, or seroma formation, and
- Permanent numbness in the nipple-areolar area.

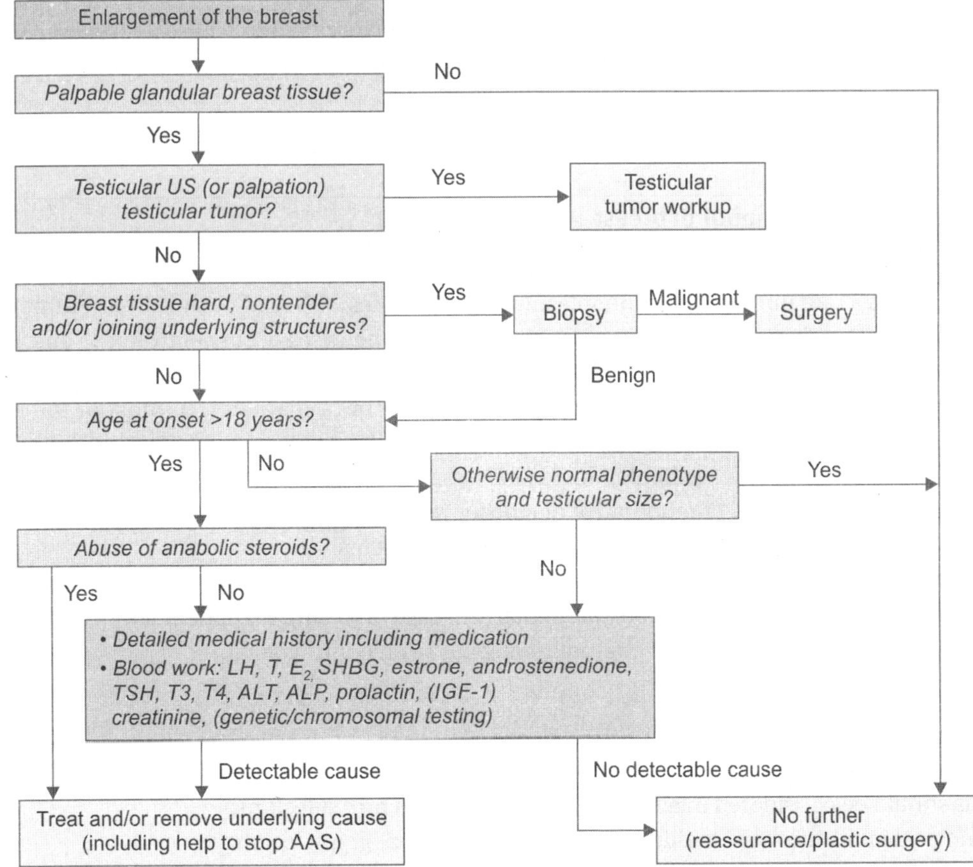

(ALP: alkaline phosphatase; ALT: alanine transaminase; E_2: estradiol; IGF-1: insulin-like growth factor 1; LH: luteinizing hormone; SHBG: sex hormone binding globulin; T: testosterone; TSH: thyroid-stimulating hormone)

PHYLLODES TUMOR

7. How would you determine the criteria for preoperative biopsy (Paddington Clinicopathological Score) and the criteria for the diagnosis of nature (Azzopardi and Salvadori criteria) of phyllodes tumor (PT) of breast? ***WBUHS 2017***

Criteria for preoperative biopsy in PT of breast (Paddington Clinicopathological Suspicious Score)

Clinical Findings
- Sudden increase in size in a long-standing breast lesion.
- Apparent fibroadenoma >3 cm in diameter in a patient >35 years.

Imaging
- Rounded borders with a lobulated appearance at mammography.
- Alteration of cystic areas within a solid mass on high-resolution ultrasound.

Cytopathologic Findings
- Presence of hypercellular stromal fragments.
- Indeterminate features.

Azzopardi and Salvadori Criteria for Diagnosis of Nature of Phyllodes Tumor

Criteria	*Benign*	*Borderline*	*Malignant*
Tumor margins	• Pushing • Well circumscribed	• Unequivocal • Zone of microscopic invasion around tumor margins	Infiltrative
Stromal cellularity	Low	Moderate	High
Mitotic rate (per 10 hpf)	<5	5–9	>10
Pleomorphism	Mild	Moderate	Severe

8. Recent updates of phyllodes tumor of breast. ***WBUHS 2015***

Introduction
- PT of the breast is a rare fibroepithelial neoplasm that constitutes <1% of all female breast tumors.
- It can occur at any age from adolescents to elderly, in most of the cases occurs between 35 and 55 years of age.
- It shows a wide range of clinical and pathological behavior.
- Phyllodes are frequently large in size and may be up to 40 cm in diameter. In most of the patients having unilateral disease, bilateral tumors are rare.
- Clinically, it is very similar to other benign breast masses.
- Uncertain clinical behavior and preoperative diagnoses results in inappropriate management.
- Axillary lymph nodes metastases are found only in <1% of patients.
- Surgery remains the mainstay of management and options vary from wide local excision (WLE) to mastectomy.
- Optimal surgery is still a matter of debate, particularly in case of BL and malignant PT.
- The role of adjuvant radiotherapy and chemotherapy has been controversial.

Diagnosis
- PTs account for <1% of breast neoplasms.
- Median age of presentation is 45 years; 20 years later than that for fibroadenomas.
- Diagnosis should be considered in all rapidly growing benign breast lesions.
- No radiological indicators exist to differentiate benign and malignant lesions.
- Fine-needle aspiration cytology (FNAC) specimens require both epithelial and stromal elements to confirm the diagnosis.

Paddington Clinicopathological Suspicion Score

Clinical findings	*Imaging findings*	*FNAC findings*
Sudden increase in size in a long-standing breast lesion	Rounded borders/lobulated appearance in mammography	Presence of hypercellular stromal fragments
Apparent fibroadenoma >3 cm diameter or in patient >35 years	Attenuation or cystic areas within a solid mass on ultrasonography	Indeterminate features

(FNAC: fine-needle aspiration cytology)

Pathology

- Tumors can grow to over 20 cm in diameter.
- Macroscopically small tumors usually resemble fibroadenomas.
- Large tumors often have a red "meaty" appearance with cystic and necrotic areas.
- Microscopy shows epithelial lined cystic spaces with hypercellular stroma.
- On histological appearance tumors are classified as benign, borderline, or malignant.
- Axillary lymph node metastases occur in approximately 10% of patients.

Prognosis

- Most malignant tumors do not metastasize.
- Some benign tumors may show an unusually aggressive behavior.
- Incomplete excision increases the risk of local recurrence.
- Histological type is the most important predictor for metastatic spread.
- The 5-year survival for benign, borderline, or malignant tumors is 96, 74, and 66%, respectively.

Azzopardi and Salvadori Criteria for Diagnosis of Nature of Phyllodes Tumor

Histological type.			
Criteria	*Benign*	*Borderline*	*Malignant*
Tumor margins	• Pushing • Well circumscribed	• Unequivocal • Zone of microscopic invasion around tumor margins	Infiltrative
Stromal cellularity	Low	Moderate	High
Mitotic rate (per 10 hpf)	<5	5–9	>10
Pleomorphism	Mild	Moderate	Severe

Management

- All rapidly growing benign breast lesions require histological assessment.
- Wide excision or mastectomy should be performed ensuring histological clear margins.
- Mastectomy for malignant tumors offers no survival advantage.
- Axillary nodal dissection is not required.
- The role of adjuvant radiotherapy is unclear.

Recurrent and Metastatic Disease

- 15% of patients develop local recurrence.
- Local recurrence is not associated with distant metastases or reduced survival.
- Local recurrence can often be controlled with further surgery.
- 20% of patients with malignant tumors develop distant metastases.
- The most common sites are lung, bone, and abdominal viscera.
- Good palliation can be obtained with single agent or combination chemotherapy.
- The role of hormonal therapy remains to be defined.

9. Write in brief on Phylloid tumor of breast. ***WBUHS 2024***

Introduction

- Phyllodes tumor (PT) of the breast is a rare fibroepithelial neoplasm that constitutes <1% of all female breast tumors.
- It can occur at any age from adolescents to elderly, in most of the cases occurs between 35 and 55 years of age.
- It shows a wide range of clinical and pathological behavior.
- Phyllodes are frequently large in size and may be up to 40 cm in diameter. In most of the patients having unilateral disease, bilateral tumors are rare.
- Clinically, it is very similar to other benign breast masses.
- Uncertain clinical behavior and preoperative diagnoses results in inappropriate management.
- Axillary lymph nodes metastases are found only in <1% of patients.
- Surgery remains the mainstay of management and options vary from wide local excision (WLE) to mastectomy.
- Optimal surgery is still a matter of debate, particularly in case of BL and malignant PT.
- The role of adjuvant radiotherapy and chemotherapy has been controversial.

Criteria for preoperative biopsy in Phyllodes tumor of breast (Paddington clinicopathological suspicious score)

- *Clinical findings:*
  - Sudden increase in size in a longstanding breast lesion.
  - Apparent fibroadenoma >3 cm in diameter in a patient >35 years.
- *Imaging:*
  - Rounded borders with a lobulated appearance at mammography.
  - Alteration of cystic areas within a solid mass on high-resolution ultrasound.
- *Cytopathologic findings:*
  - Presence of hypercellular stromal fragments.
  - Indeterminate features.

Azzopardi and Salvadori criteria for diagnosis of nature of phyllodes tumor

Histological type.			
Criteria	***Benign***	***Borderline***	***Malignant***
Tumor margins	• Pushing • Well circumscribed	• Unequivocal • Zone of microscopic invasion around tumor margins	Infiltrative
Stromal cellularity	Low	Moderate	High
Mitotic rate (per 10 hpf)	<5	5–9	>10
Pleomorphism	Mild	Moderate	Severe

Diagnosis

- Phyllodes tumors account for less than 1% of breast neoplasms.
- Median age of presentation is 45 years; 20 years later than that for fibroadenomas.
- Diagnosis should be considered in all rapidly growing benign breast lesions.
- No radiological indicators exist to differentiate benign and malignant lesions.
- Fine needle aspiration cytology specimens require both epithelial and stromal elements to confirm the diagnosis.

Paddington Clinicopathological Suspicion Score

Clinical findings	*Imaging findings*	*FNAC findings*
Sudden increase in size in a long standing breast lesion	Rounded borders/lobulated appearance in mammography	Presence of hypercellular stromal fragments
Apparent fibroadenoma >3 cm diameter or in patient >35 years	Attenuation or cystic areas within a solid mass on Ultrasonography	Indeterminate features
Any 2 features mandate core biopsy		

Pathology
- Tumors can grow to over 20 cm in diameter.
- Macroscopically small tumors usually resemble fibroadenomas.
- Large tumors often have a red "meaty" appearance with cystic and necrotic areas.
- Microscopy shows epithelial lined cystic spaces with hypercellular stroma.
- On histological appearance tumors are classified as benign, borderline, or malignant.
- Axillary lymph node metastases occur in approximately 10% of patients.

Prognosis
- Most malignant tumors do not metastasize.
- Some benign tumors may show an unusually aggressive behavior.
- Incomplete excision increases the risk of local recurrence.
- Histological type is the most important predictor for metastatic spread.
- The 5-year survival for benign, borderline, or malignant tumors is 96%, 74%, and 66%. respectively.

Management
- All rapidly growing benign breast lesions require histological assessment.
- Wide excision or mastectomy should be performed ensuring histological clear margins.
- Mastectomy for malignant tumors offers no survival advantage.
- Axillary nodal dissection is not required.
- The role of adjuvant radiotherapy is unclear.

Recurrent and Metastatic Disease
- 15% of patients develop local recurrence.
- Local recurrence is not associated with distant metastases or reduced survival.
- Local recurrence can often be controlled with further surgery.
- 20% of patients with malignant tumors develop distant metastases.
- The commonest sites are lung, bone, and abdominal viscera.
- Good palliation can be obtained with single agent or combination chemotherapy.
- The role of hormonal therapy remains to be defined.

PERCUTANEOUS MANAGEMENT OF BENIGN BREAST LESIONS

10. Percutaneous management of benign breast lesions. ***WBUHS 2014***

Benign Breast Conditions
- *Fibrocystic changes:*
  - Changes in hormone balances during normal, monthly menstrual cycles can create, for some women, symptomatic breast changes that are referred to as fibrocystic changes.
  - Cysts often are described as benign, tiny, fluid-filled sacs that may feel like lumps.

  - Tenderness and lump size commonly increase the week before the menstrual period and lessen a week after.
  - The lumps may be hard or rubbery and can appear as a single breast lump that may be large or small.
  - Fibrocystic changes also can appear as thickening of the breast tissue.
  - Fibrocystic changes can occur in one or both breasts and are the most common cause of benign breast lumps in women age 35–50 years.
  - It is relatively uncommon for postmenopausal women to have symptomatic breast changes because of a lack of hormone stimulation of breast tissue.
- *Simple cysts:*
  - Simple cysts are benign fluid-filled sacs that usually occur in both breasts.
  - They can be single or multiple and can vary in size.
  - Tenderness and lump size often change with the woman's menstrual cycle.
  - Cysts may also be affected by caffeine (coffee, tea, chocolate, energy drinks)
- *Fibroadenomas:*
  - Fibroadenomas are the most common benign solid tumors found in the female breast.
  - They are round, rubbery, slippery lumps that move freely in the breast when pushed.
  - They form as the result of excess formation of lobules (milk-producing glands) and stroma (connective tissue in the breast).
  - Fibroadenomas are usually painless.
  - They occur most often between the ages of 20 and 40 and are more common in African-American women.
- *Intraductal papillomas:*
  - These are small, wart-like growths in the lining of the mammary duct near the nipple.
  - They usually affect women 40–50 years of age and can produce bleeding from the nipple or nipple discharge.
- *Traumatic fat necrosis:*
  - This condition occurs when there is trauma (sudden injury) or surgery to the breast.
  - This causes fat to form in lumps.
  - The lumps are usually round, firm, hard, single, painless, and in the area of a surgical scar.

Diagnostic Tests

- Fine-needle aspiration (FNA)
- *Core biopsy:* The types of core biopsies include ultrasound-guided core biopsy and stereotactic core biopsy.
- *Ultrasound-guided core biopsy:* The exact location of breast tissue is biopsied. The type of echo varies with each type of tissue. Ultrasound can distinguish many benign lesions, such as fluid-filled cysts, from solid lesions. Tissue samples are then taken through the needle.
- *Stereotactic core biopsy:* Computerized mammographic pictures help confirm the needle placement using digital imaging so the exact location of breast tissue is biopsied. Tissue samples are then taken through the needle.
- *Open excisional biopsy:* This is the surgical removal of the entire mass. The tissue is then studied under a microscope. If a rim of normal breast tissue is taken all the way around a lump (lumpectomy), biopsy can also serve as part of breast cancer treatment.

Treatment

- Fibrocystic breast changes do not require treatment.
- Large, painful simple cysts can be treated through FNA, which may take place during or after the evaluation. After fluid is drawn from the cyst, the cyst collapses, and the pain resolves.
- Fibroadenomas of certain size and if painful are recommended to be removed surgically.
- Intraductal papillomas are removed surgically.
- Mastitis can be treated with warm compresses and in some cases, an antibiotic medication may be prescribed.

GRANULOMATOUS MASTITIS

11. Write notes on idiopathic granulomatous mastitis. ***WBUHS 2021 Supplementary***

Introduction

- Idiopathic granulomatous mastitis (IGM) is a rare benign inflammatory breast entity characterized by lobulocentric granulomas.
- IGM has a persistent or recurrent disease course and affects parous premenopausal women with a history of lactation.
- It has also been associated with hyperprolactinemia.
- The most common clinical sign is a palpable tender mass.
- However, the nonspecific manifestations and varied demographic features of this condition, as well as the other similar-appearing and superimposed breast entities, pose substantial diagnostic challenges.

Clinical Manifestations

- The most common clinical manifestation of IGM is a tender palpable unilateral breast mass of variable size (1–20 cm).
- Synchronous bilateral breast findings were estimated to be seen in 1% of cases
- A tender palpable mass with skin erythema and edema and isolated skin induration can be less common clinical manifestations
- Peau d'orange skin changes in some patients and asymmetric breast heaviness or enlargement in fewer patients.
- The nipple is seldom involved; however, nipple retraction, ulceration, and secretions have been documented.
- Axillary lymphadenopathy is only occasionally detected at physical examination
- IGM may manifest with abscess formation, with or without draining skin sinuses, at a variable prevalence
- A cutaneous fistula can develop as a complication of prior percutaneous biopsy or aspiration.
- It is important to note that the presence of an abscess at clinical examination and/or imaging should not preclude tissue biopsy if the clinical course suggests possible malignancy, as inflammatory breast cancer (IBC) also can manifest with fluid collections.

Management

- Ultrasonography (USG) and mammography identified an irregular and ill-defined mass in the majority of patients. The information, obtained from US and mammography is nonspecific and lack of specificity to diagnose IGM or to exclude breast carcinoma.
- Most common US findings were parenchymal heterogeneity, irregular hypoechoic mass, and abscess formation.
- The optimal treatment of IGM remains controversial. Surgical excision still seems to be the best treatment. WLE can be appropriate treatment also provide exact diagnosis and treatment. After WLE, if possible, further therapy is not needed.

12. Idiopathic granulomatous mastitis and tubercular mastitis are they synonymous? Discuss. ***WBUHS 2020***

- IGM, also known as nonpuerperal mastitis or granulomatous lobular mastitis, is a rare benign chronic inflammatory breast disease that was first described by Kessler and Wolloch.
- IGM is characterized by sterile noncaseating lobulocentric granulomatous inflammation. It usually has a recurrent or prolonged natural disease course that eventually leads to lesion burn out.
- IGM usually affects parous premenopausal women with a history of lactation and frequently is clinically associated with hyperprolactinemia.
- The clinical and radiologic findings of IGM are noted to frequently overlap with those of breast cancer and several benign inflammatory breast conditions and thus can often lead to misdiagnosis and delayed treatment.
- IGM is a rare disease of the breast, and its true prevalence is not well established.

- Anecdotal explanations for inflammatory ductal or lobulocentric disease in males include gynecomastia as a predisposing factor and trauma, smoking, and autoimmunity as exacerbating agents.
- There is a strong association between IGM and history of pregnancy and lactation, with most patients reporting having a pregnancy within 5 years before the diagnosis or being diagnosed with IGM within 2 months to 20 years after a pregnancy.
- The manifestation of IGM during pregnancy and lactation is uncommon.
- Hyperprolactinemic states, either drug induced or caused by an intracranial lesion, have been associated with the development of IGM.
- This association lends support for the use of bromocriptine as an optional conservative second-line therapy for patients with IGM.
- The resolution of breast symptoms after the use of antiprolactinemic drugs and the correlation of markedly high prolactin levels with treatment-resistant and highly symptomatic IGM support such an association.
- An association between IGM and Hispanic ancestry in the continental United States was studied in a case control study.
- The most common clinical manifestation of IGM is a tender palpable unilateral breast mass of variable size (1–20 cm).
- Synchronous bilateral breast findings were estimated to be seen in 1% of cases.
- A tender palpable mass with skin erythema and edema (in 11–31% cases) and isolated skin induration (in 20% of cases) as less common clinical manifestations. Investigators in a smaller retrospective study involving 20 cases reported peau d'orange skin changes in 40% of patients and asymmetric breast heaviness or enlargement in approximately 20% of patients. These findings are also seen with IBC.
- IGM may manifest with abscess formation, with or without draining skin sinuses, at a variable prevalence of 6.6–54.0%.
- Ultrasonographically (US)-guided FNA and core-needle biopsy, with or without aspiration of fluid collections, are breast imaging interventions commonly performed in patients with IGM.
- FNA can be used to render a histopathology-based diagnosis; however, its usefulness and reliability have been widely debated
- At imaging, granulomatous mastitis can manifest with a variety of nonspecific appearance, which often mimic the appearances of malignancy.
- Much of the variability in the imaging appearances of IGM might be related to varying histopathologic features, including inflammatory reaction, abscess, and fibrosis.
- Tuberculous mastitis is a rare presentation of tuberculosis that has been called the "great masquerader" due to its multifaceted presentations. Solitary breast mass is the most common clinical presentation of tuberculous mastitis and is associated with inflammatory findings in the majority of cases.
- Tuberculous mastitis typically affects young lactating multiparous women and can present either as an abscess or as a painless breast mass.
- Diagnosis of tuberculous mastitis is usually based on high index of suspicion, finding of granulomatous lesion with Langhans' giant cells and response to anti-tuberculosis treatment (ATT). FNAC and biopsy may also be inconclusive. Acid-fast bacilli (AFB) is not seen in most cases. Prompt diagnosis and adequate treatment can avoid unnecessary operation in these patients.

IMAGING IN BREAST DISEASES

13. Imaging of breast disease.

Imaging Modalities of Breast Diseases

- *Mammography:*
    - Mammography has been the basic imaging method in breast diagnostics, and the only tool suitable for screening breast cancer.

- In screening, its sensitivity and specificity are 90–93% and 93–97%, respectively.
- Mammography has some recognized limitations and disadvantages.
- The sensitivity and specificity are highly dependent on the composition of the breast parenchyma, which for its part is influenced by age, hormonal status, and possible previous interventions.
- In young women, the usefulness of mammography is restricted by high prevalence of dense fibroglandular tissue, which impairs both the detection and the differentiation of the lesion.
- With increasing age, the breast parenchyma usually shows fatty replacement, which makes abnormalities more easily detectable.
- Hormone replacement therapy may decrease the sensitivity of mammography by increasing the breast density and enlarging benign masses, such as cysts and fibroadenomas.
- After breast surgery, mass-like scars and areas of distortion may mimic a tumor or hide subtle signs of malignancy. Radiation after surgical treatment of breast carcinoma leads to skin thickening and increased focal or diffuse density of the breast due to edematous changes. The accuracy of mammography is also impaired in patients with silicon implants.
- Cysts and solid tumors cannot always be definitely differentiated at mammography. Some carcinomas may have a benign appearance, and some fibroadenomas may be irregular and difficult to differentiate from a malignant tumor.
- A palpable mass may be partially or completely obscured by adjacent fibroglandular tissue. Even the spiculations within the fibrous tissue surrounding a cancer may be inconspicuous at mammography, because both the spiculations and the adjacent fibrous tissue are of the same density.
- In addition to standard (craniocaudal, mediolateral oblique, and lateral) views, supplemental mammographic views are often needed to better or more completely visualize the area of special concern.
- The commonly used modified views are spot compression and magnification views.
  - With the spot compression, separation of overlapping structures can be achieved.
  - Coning down with spot compression also reduces scatter radiation and sharpens image details.
  - Magnification provides the ability to define characteristics of microcalcifications and details of masses.
- Also, tangential views, extra lateral craniocaudal views, change-of-angle views, cleavage views and modified compression views (e.g., for patients with breast implants) can be taken.
- Digital mammography has the potential to overcome some of the limitations of conventional mammography.
- Because of the increased contrast and decreased noise of digital systems it is possible to improve image quality, although the spatial resolution is still limited when compared to screen-film mammography.
- *BI-RADS* is an acronym for Breast Imaging-Reporting and Data System, a quality assurance tool originally designed for use with mammography.
- The system is a collaborative effort of many health groups but is published and trademarked by the American College of Radiology (ACR).

BI-RADS assessment categories are:

- 0: Incomplete
- 1: Negative
- 2: Benign
- 3: Probably benign
- 4: Suspicious
- 5: Highly suggestive of malignancy
- 6: Known biopsy—proven malignancy

Other Mammographic Techniques

- In case of spontaneous nipple discharge, galactography has been the method of choice. A mammogram taken after duct cannulation and contrast injection reveals possible intraductal tumors as filling defects, and with the same method, the lesion can also be preoperatively marked with methylene blue dye.

- Galactographic finding helps to localize the origin of nipple discharge but is nonspecific. Sometimes cannulating a secreting duct may be impossible. The latest high resolution US has allowed visualization of the dilated ducts and the intraductal tumors.
- Pneumocystography after an FNA of a cyst may reveal intracystic tumor and help to prevent cyst recurrence.
- Specimen radiography is a sufficient method to confirm removal of a nonpalpable lesion after surgical excision.

Ultrasonography

- *B-mode ultrasonography:*
  - The main indications of breast US have been differentiation between cystic and solid lesions, evaluation of a palpable lesion in a mammographically dense breast (e.g., young, pregnant, or lactating patient), evaluation of a lesion detected at mammography or mammographic asymmetry, detection of an abscess in an infectious breast, evaluation after breast cancer treatment and breast augmentation, evaluation of axillary lymph nodes and guidance for interventional procedures.
  - Ultrasound can detect mammographically occult cancers, but it is generally accepted that US is not suitable for screening.
  - Microcalcifications with no associate mass are not usually reliably detectable at US. The analysis of microcalcifications is, however, only possible with mammographic spot magnification.
  - In the last few years, differentiation between benign and malignant solid breast lesions by means of US has gained increased interest.
  - The individual characteristics for malignant lesions include spiculation, angular margins, marked hypoechogenicity, shadowing, calcification, duct extension, branch pattern, vertical ("taller than wide") orientation and microlobulation. If a single malignant feature is found, the lesion cannot be considered benign. Intense hyperechogenicity, ellipsoid shape, gentle bi- or trilobulations, thin, echogenic pseudocapsule, and lack of malignant findings are considered benign features
  - Currently, most solid breast lesions undergo a diagnostic or preoperative needle biopsy.
- *Doppler techniques:* Doppler enables more accurate detection of the small tumor vessels than conventional color.
  - A considerable problem in tumor diagnostics is that the spatial resolution of Doppler imaging is limited, and only major feeding vessels of the tumors are detectable, not the abnormal complex microvascularity.
  - Color Doppler, or even the more sensitive power Doppler, is not capable of detecting the flow information in small vessels in all directions.
  - The technique is also equipment and operator dependent.
  - Neither examination techniques nor interpretation of the Doppler images are standardized and the results of the studies vary considerably.
- *Contrast-enhanced ultrasonography:*
  - The finding that Doppler signals may be difficult to detect either because of small vessel size or inadequate equipment has led to the development of ultrasound contrast agents.
  - Because US contrast agents do not extravasate from the vessel to the surrounding tissue, any echo received indicates the presence of a vessel.
  - Contrast enhancement improves detection of small vessels with slow and low-volume blood flow.
- *Other ultrasonographic techniques:*
  - Specific imaging techniques for ultrasound contrast agents have been developed to overcome this limitation. In contrast harmonic imaging, the transducer emits at one frequency and receives at the second (or higher) harmonic frequency.
  - Inverted phase imaging, i.e., pulse inversion, is a new variant of second harmonic imaging. The transducer transmits not a single pulse but two pulses that are 180 degrees out of phase. The nonlinear harmonic component from the microbubbles produces a strong signal, while linear signals from the background causing most artifacts are cancelled out. It produces new possibilities for flow detection in both color Doppler

and B-mode. Contrast harmonic imaging together with pulse inversion may overcome the limitations in assessing the microperfusion of tissues.

- In spatial compounding technique, several real-time ultrasound images are acquired using different angles of insonation. These images are combined to provide a single composite image, which has a better signal-to-noise ratio and sharper borders with reduced speckle and clutter compared to a conventional B-mode image.
- Three-dimensional (3D) ultrasound is helpful in determining the exact size and position as well as the surface characteristics of a lesion. With 3D imaging volume measurement is possible, which allows for more accurate follow-up examinations.
- Pathological changes often cause changes in tissue stiffness. In breast diagnostics, breast cancers are firm and less mobile than the surrounding parenchyma. In elasticity imaging, ultrasound is used to monitor the internal tissue displacement responses to externally applied force. This method has many alternative schemes.

Magnetic Resonance Imaging (MRI)

- MR imaging has proved to be the most sensitive method for the detection of invasive breast cancer.
- The detection is based on lesion enhancement after contrast agent administration.
- In various series, the sensitivity for invasive breast cancer has ranged from 88 to 100%, and the specificity from 37 to 97%.
- The value of MR imaging in patients with mammographically detected suspicious microcalcifications and ductal carcinoma in situ (DCIS) has been poor. In cases of nipple discharge, the results have been controversial.

Diagnostic Criteria

- The diagnostic criteria consist of both lesion morphology and enhancement kinetics. The morphologic criteria are comparable to those used at mammography. Well-defined margins indicate benignity, while ill-defined or spiculated lesions are suggestive of malignancy. Internal septations, if seen, are specific for fibroadenomas.
- Enhancement in benign lesions is homogeneous and proceeds centrifugally. Benign lesions also usually enhance less and do so more slowly than malignant lesions. In malignant lesions enhancement is often inhomogeneous or rim-like and tends to proceed centripetally. Diffuse enhancement is a nonspecific finding.
- Relative enhancement >80–90% is a widely used criterion for malignancy, but the quantity of enhancement is highly dependent on the imaging technique (field strength, imaging sequences, dosage of contrast agent, etc.) and thus, it is not generally accepted. Enhancement is not specific for breast pathology, because also normal breast tissue may enhance.
- Due to hormonal changes, transient enhancement has been found in 80% of healthy premenopausal women.
- There is also overlapping between the morphologic and dynamic features of benign and malignant lesions. The most important benign lesions causing false positive findings include fibroadenomas, inflammatory changes, papillomas, proliferative fibrocystic changes and radial scar.
- Post-treatment changes may also be liable to misinterpretations: postoperative scars enhance for 6 months and post radiation therapy (RT) may cause enhancement for 18 months. Hematoma due to core biopsy causes signal increase in some patients, but fine-needle biopsy has not been shown to have influence on MR imaging.

Indications and Contraindications

- Most breast lesions can be diagnosed by using conventional modalities, especially when combined with needle biopsies. It is, however, desirable to be able to reduce the number of biopsies performed for benign causes. In dealing with lesions that remain equivocal after mammographic and sonographic evaluation, MR imaging could be the problem-solving method. A negative MR imaging finding virtually excludes invasive carcinoma.
- The aim of breast imaging is the detection of breast cancer as early as possible, as the prognosis of breast cancer depends on the stage of the disease at the time of diagnosis. MR imaging is not considered suitable for breast screening in a general population, but it might be feasible in imaging the extremely dense breasts of especially young high-risk women (family history, cancer susceptibility genes, and history of contralateral breast cancer).

- It is the best method for detecting an otherwise occult primary breast carcinoma in patients with axillary node metastases. After a cancer diagnosis, MR imaging is the most sensitive tool for preoperative staging and treatment planning.
  - MR imaging can also be an adjunctive method in post-treatment surveillance in conservatively treated breasts with suspected recurrence and evaluation of tumor response to chemotherapy.
  - MR imaging is also the best method for imaging of breasts with silicon prostheses.
  - In addition to general contraindications for MR imaging (e.g., cardiac pacemaker, ferromagnetic incorporated substances) there are some specific limitations concerning breast imaging.
  - It must not be used instead of X-ray mammography, because according to present knowledge, it is not suitable for detecting and evaluating microcalcifications. Due to its variable specificity, MR imaging should not be used for imaging symptomless women without an increased risk of breast cancer.
  - Before breast MR imaging can be a clinically used tool for breast imaging, a proper MR-guided biopsy and localization system must be available for biopsy of suspicious lesions not detected by other modalities.
  - The verification of lesion removal is also a major problem to solve, because MR imaging of the excised specimen is not feasible.

Other MRI Techniques

- In proton MR spectroscopy malignant lesions have been shown as having high levels of choline-containing compounds when compared to benign lesions and normal breast tissue.
- MR elastography is a new imaging modality that produces images with a contrast proportional to the stiffness of the tissue, as in US elasticity imaging. It has been predicted to become a potential adjunctive tool for both lesion detection and characterization.

Other Imaging Modalities

- Computed tomography (CT) has not been recommended for breast imaging, mainly because of high radiation dose. It has been successfully used in regional staging of small breast cancer before breast conserving surgery (BCS).
- Electrical impedance scanning is a new technique, which is based upon the principle that malignant cells exhibit altered local dielectric properties and show measurably higher conductivity values. The method has been presented as a useful tool for further evaluation of equivocal mammographic findings, but its real value remains to be seen.
- The most important task of nuclear medicine with regard to breast cancer is nowadays sentinel node staging using lymphoscintigraphy. In differential diagnostics, nuclear medicine is under investigation as an adjunct to mammography.
- Presented clinical indications for the most commonly used agent Tc 99m sestamibi scintimammography include examining premenopausal dense breasts, palpable lesions with low-suspicion mammographic finding and evaluation of response to neoadjuvant chemotherapy (NACT) for locally advanced breast cancer (LABC).
- Positron emission tomography (PET) scanning might have a role in differential diagnosis and in staging of breast tumors.

FINE-NEEDLE ASPIRATION CYTOLOGY SCORING OF BREAST CANCER

14. FNAC scoring of breast cancer. ***WBUHS 2006***

Introduction

Fine-needle aspiration cytology of the breast is becoming an increasingly popular investigation in the diagnosis of breast malignancies and their further subtyping. The breast lump and cytological specimen were processed and reported routinely.

After FNAC cytology specimens can be graded by the pathologist, without knowledge of the histology result, in accordance with the NHS Breast Screening Programme:

- C1 = insufficient cells for cytological analysis, i.e., fewer than five epithelial cell groups.
- C2 = cells present all benign; no suspicious features.
- C3 = cells suspicious but probably benign.
- C4 = cells suspicious but probably malignant.
- C5 = definitely malignant. Within this unit, this category is used when the degree of diagnostic certainty is such that the pathologist would be happy for the patient to undergo major breast surgery on the basis of the cytology sample alone.

BREAST CANCER PREVENTION

15. Strategies of breast cancer prevention. *WBUHS 2007*

Risk Factors for Breast Cancer

Factors important in populations	*Factors important in individual patients*	*Histologic risk factors*
• Age at menarche and menopause • Parity • Age at first birth • Breastfeeding • Exogenous hormone use or exposure • Alcohol consumption	• Gender (female >> male) • Age (steady increase with age) • Family history (mothers, sisters, and daughters) • History of previous breast cancer (noninvasive or invasive, ipsilateral or contralateral)	• Proliferative breast disease • Atypical ductal hyperplasia (ADH) • Atypical lobular hyperplasia (ALH) • Lobular carcinoma in situ (LCIS)

Management of High-risk Patients

- Prioritize risk factors and consider those that are important to individual patients in making recommendations about screening and intervention. For instance, as discussed earlier, reproductive factors are important for breast cancer incidence in populations but generally insufficient to base a recommendation for medical or surgical intervention.
- *Close surveillance:*
  - Recommendations for women in a family with a breast and ovarian cancer syndrome include monthly breast self-examination beginning at 18–20 years of age, semiannual clinical breast examination beginning at age 25 years, and annual mammography beginning at age 25 years, or 10 years before the earliest age at onset of breast cancer in a family member.
  - Studies of women with known *BRCA1* or *BRCA2* mutations find that half the detected breast cancers were diagnosed as interval cancers; that is, they occurred between screening episodes and not during the course of routine screening. This observation has prompted many groups to add annual screening MRI to mammography, with some doing both simultaneously and others staggering the two examinations.
  - If not done previously, genetic counseling is offered to those with a strong family history of early-onset breast and ovarian cancer, including a discussion of genetic testing for *BRCA1* and *BRCA2* mutations.

Chemoprevention for Breast Cancer

- The only drug currently approved for reducing breast cancer risk is tamoxifen.
- Tamoxifen is an estrogen antagonist with proven benefit for the treatment of estrogen receptor (ER)-positive breast cancer.
- Tamoxifen reduces the incidence of a second primary breast cancer in the contralateral breast of women who received the drug as adjuvant therapy for a first breast cancer
- Data on the efficacy of tamoxifen for reduction of breast cancer risk in *BRCA1* and *BRCA2* mutation carriers are currently too limited to quantify.
- The second prevention trial conducted by the NSABP is the STAR trial, in which tamoxifen was compared with raloxifene.

- In favor of raloxifene, the number of uterine cancers was reduced by 36%, women taking raloxifene had 29% fewer episodes of venous thrombosis, and pulmonary embolism developed in fewer women.

Prophylactic Mastectomy
- Prophylactic mastectomy probably reduces the chance of contracting breast cancer in high-risk women by 90%.
- Women who are screened by mammograms annually have an overall 80% chance of surviving the occurrence of breast cancer.
- Coupled with penetrance figures in the range of 50–60% for mutation carriers, the chance of dying of breast cancer for carriers of *BRCA1* or *BRCA2* mutations is approximately 10% without undergoing preventive mastectomy.

Risk Assessment and Management
- Risk factors for disease provide clues to pathogenesis and identify patients likely to benefit from surveillance and risk reduction interventions.
- Although breast cancer can develop in both sexes, women are at greatly increased risk and breast cancer in males is uncommon.
- Age is a useful risk factor applied every day in clinical practice; breast cancer is rare in women younger than 30 years and very common in women older than 60 years.
- Family history is most significant when breast cancer affects young first-degree relatives (mothers, sisters, and daughters) and when cases of ovarian cancer are found within the same side of the family.
- Histologic risk factors most concerning are atypical ductal hyperplasia (ADH), atypical lobular hyperplasia (ALH), and lobular carcinoma in situ (LCIS).
- A personal history of breast cancer predisposes to contralateral breast cancer in women undergoing mastectomy and to bilateral breast cancer in women undergoing breast conservation with wide excision and radiation.

Significant Risk Factors for Breast Cancer in Women: Assessment and Recommendations

Risk factors	*Mammography screening recommendations*	*Preventive options*
Factors conferring moderate to high risk		
Age >60 years	Annual	Not usually recommended
Atypical hyperplasia (ductal or lobular)	Annual after diagnosis	Tamoxifen, 20 mg/day × 5 years
LCIS	Annual after diagnosis	Tamoxifen, 20 mg/day × 5 years
Personal history of either DCIS or invasive cancer, age>40 years	Annual after diagnosis	No specific preventive recommended
Family history of breast cancer (first-degree relative, age <50 years; two relatives on same side of family)	Annual after age 40 years	Referral for genetic counseling
Factors conferring very high risk		
Therapeutic thoracic radiation (age <30 years)	Annual at 10 years after radiotherapy	No specific preventive recommended
Personal history of DCIS or invasive cancer, age <40 years	Annual after diagnosis	No specific preventive recommended
Family history of breast cancer (two first-degree relatives, age <50 years)	Annual after age 35–40 years	Referral for genetic counseling
Family history of breast and ovarian cancer (first-degree relatives)	Annual after age 35–40 years	Referral for genetic counseling
Known carrier of a mutation in *BRCA1* or *BRCA2* or a first-degree relative with a mutation	Annual after age 25 years; consider annual MRI	Genetic testing for relatives; discuss prophylactic mastectomy or oophorectomy for carriers

(DCIS: ductal carcinoma in situ; LCIS: lobular carcinoma in situ; MRI: magnetic resonance imaging)

16. Describe in brief the molecular biology of breast cancers, particularly in reference to identify a woman at high risk. Describe the presently available medical and surgical options in the risk reduction surgeries.

WBUHS 2014

Molecular subtype	***Luminal (A and B)***		***HER2***	***Basal***
Genetic profile	↑Luminal CKs and ER-related genes (A>B) B ↑in proliferation-related genes		↑HER2-related genes	↑Basal CKs
Histologic correlates	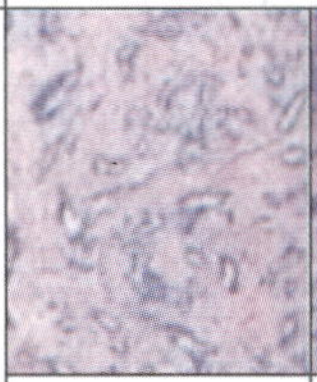	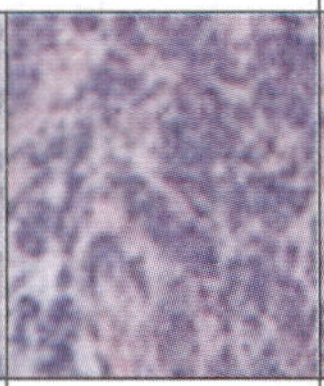	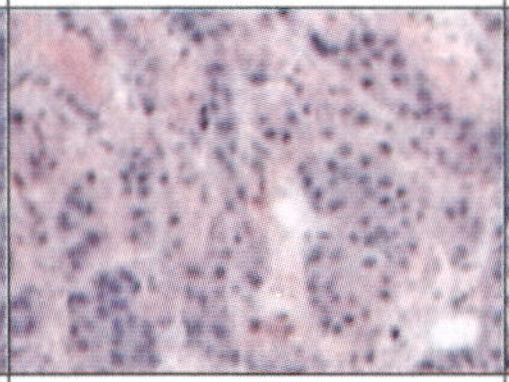	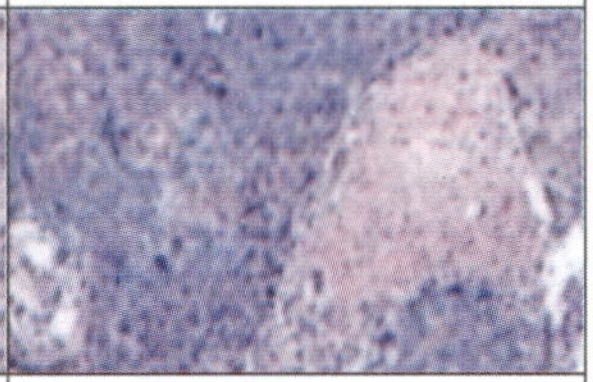
	A Lower-grade ER+	B Higher-grade ER+	High-grade, +/– apocrine features	High-grade, sheet-like necrosis, inflammation *See exceptions
Surrogate markers	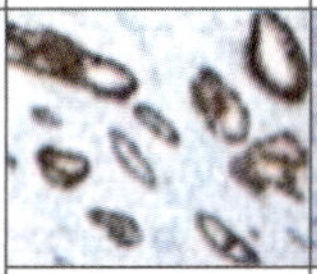	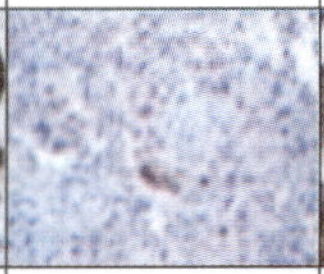	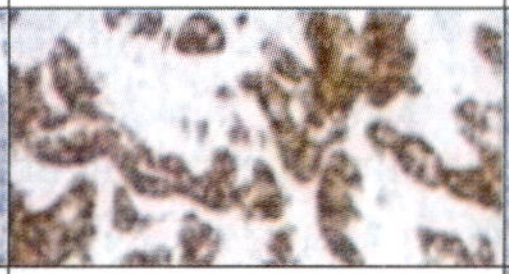	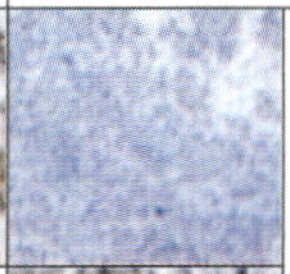 ER/PR- HER2-
	A Strong ER+, PR+/–, HER2-, low Ki67	B Weaker ER+, PR+/–, HER2+/–, 1 K167	HER2+, +/– ER/PR	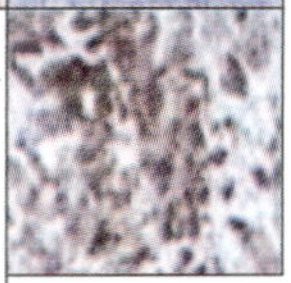 CK5/6+/– EGFR+/–
Prognosis	Good	Intermediate	Worse	Worse
Response to chemotherapy	Lower	Intermediate	Higher	Higher
Targeted therapies	Hormone therapies		HER2-targeted therapies	Currently investigational

Significant Risk Factors for Breast Cancer in Women: Assessment and Recommendations

Risk factors	***Mammography screening recommendations***	***Preventive options***
Factors conferring moderate to high risk		
Age >60 years	Annual	Not usually recommended
Atypical hyperplasia (ductal or lobular)	Annual after diagnosis	Tamoxifen, 20 mg/day × 5 years
LCIS	Annual after diagnosis	Tamoxifen, 20 mg/day × 5 years
Personal history of either DCIS or invasive cancer, age>40 years	Annual after diagnosis	No specific preventive recommended
Family history of breast cancer (first-degree relative, age <50 years; two relatives on same side of family)	Annual after age 40 years	Referral for genetic counseling

Contd...

Contd...

Risk factors	*Mammography screening recommendations*	*Preventive options*
Factors conferring very high risk		
Therapeutic thoracic radiation (age <30 years)	Annual at 10 years after radiotherapy	No specific preventive recommended
Personal history of DCIS or invasive cancer, age <40 years	Annual after diagnosis	No specific preventive recommended
Family history of breast cancer (two first-degree relatives, age <50 years)	Annual after age 35–40 years	Referral for genetic counseling
Family history of breast and ovarian cancer (first- degree relatives)	Annual after age 35–40 years	Referral for genetic counseling
Known carrier of a mutation in *BRCA1* or *BRCA2* or a first-degree relative with a mutation	Annual after age 25 years; consider annual MRI	Genetic testing for relatives; discuss prophylactic mastectomy or oophorectomy for carriers

(DCIS: ductal carcinoma in situ; LCIS: lobular carcinoma in situ; MRI: magnetic resonance imaging)

Risk-reducing Surgery

- For women without a personal history of cancer who have a BRCA mutation, prophylactic (or preventative) surgery reduces the risk of developing cancer.
- Risk-reducing surgery does not completely eliminate the risk of developing cancer as residual risks remain after mastectomy and oophorectomy.
- While prophylactic surgery is effective in cancer risk reduction, women should be counseled preoperatively about the potential morbidity of such procedures, and the possibility that surgery may affect libido, sexual functioning, and body image.
- Oophorectomy in premenopausal women can be associated with increased risks for bone and heart disease, and raises concerns about how to optimally manage surgical menopause and hormone therapy.
- Skin-sparing mastectomy with or without preservation of the nipple-areolar complex followed by immediate breast reconstruction is increasingly being performed as it provides superior cosmetic results.
- There has been considerable debate about whether mutation carriers should undergo hysterectomy at the time of bilateral salpingo-oophorectomy (BSO). Studies have also reported a possible small excess risk of uterine cancers in mutation carriers, the absolute risk is low and it is not clear that the benefits associated with hysterectomy are sufficiently large enough to warrant the risks associated with surgery.

Hormone Replacement Therapy

- Pre- and perimenopausal women who undergo BSO will likely experience side effects of surgically induced menopause.
- The only proven risk-reducing procedure for ovarian cancer in BRCA mutation carriers is BSO. However, there is controversy about whether it is appropriate to perform a salpingectomy alone for BRCA mutation carriers who wish to defer oophorectomy, based upon a possible fallopian tube origin for some ovarian cancers.

Cancer Surveillance

- For patients with a BRCA mutation who do not wish to pursue (or would rather delay) surgical risk reduction, breast cancer surveillance should be offered, and ovarian cancer screening may be performed.
- While breast and ovarian (including fallopian tube and peritoneal) cancers present the greatest risk, individuals with BRCA mutations have elevated risks for other cancers, including prostate cancer and pancreatic cancer.

Breast Examinations

- Beginning at age 18 years, self-breast exams performed periodically may facilitate awareness of changes, and clinical breast examination should be performed every 6–12 months beginning at age 25 years.

- *Annual mammography:* Mammography should begin at age 30 years or be individualized if the earliest age of onset in the family is under age 25 years. However, the sensitivity of mammography for detecting breast cancer in mutation carriers appears to be lower than in other high-risk women, which may be due to:
  - Higher breast density.
  - Differences in morphologic features (e.g., less spiculation due to lack of tumor-surrounding fibrosis).
  - The frequent development of interval malignancies.
- While the risk of radiation-associated breast cancer from breast imaging for the average-risk patient is believed to be small or nonexistent, women at high genetic risk may be more susceptible to radiation-induced carcinogenesis because of the role of BRCA proteins in DNA repair.
- Studies almost exclusively performed in women with a BRCA mutation differ on the effect of diagnostic radiation, but growing evidence suggests the effect depends on the age when exposure occurs and the total dose.
  - A history of having a mammogram before age 30 years in BRCA mutation carriers was associated with a statistically insignificant increased risk of breast cancer.
  - Increased risk of breast cancer among women in this study occurred at radiation dose levels considerably lower than that among women without BRCA.
  - There was no association between breast cancer risk and radiation exposure from ages 30–39 years.

Breast Magnetic Resonance Imaging

- MRI for breast cancer screening is recommended annually beginning at age 25 years and can be scheduled 6 months after annual mammogram.
- The addition of breast MRI to the breast cancer surveillance strategy in high-risk women increases breast cancer detection rates, increases the number of patients diagnosed at an earlier stage of disease, is cost-effective, and is supported in multiple guidelines.
- However, the mortality impact of including breast MRI in the surveillance strategy is not clear.

Breast Ultrasound

Data from large studies evaluating the role of breast ultrasound in addition to other imaging modalities have not demonstrated any additional benefit of this procedure.

Chemoprevention

- Chemopreventive strategies to reduce the risk of breast cancer have focused exclusively on prevention in high-risk women and involve the use of selective estrogen receptor modulators (SERMs) and aromatase inhibitors (AIs) for breast cancer prevention.
- There is also a significant amount of data on the role of oral contraceptives in reducing the risk of hereditary ovarian cancer.
  - Use of *tamoxifen* for risk reduction for women who opt against mastectomies, especially if they are *BRCA2* mutation carriers. However, the option for prophylactic mastectomy should be rediscussed periodically with patients, as medical chemoprevention is less effective than prophylactic mastectomy.
  - Tamoxifen reduced breast cancer risk by 62 percent in *BRCA2* carriers [relative risk [RR] 0.38, 95% confidence interval (CI) 0.06–1.56], but not in *BRCA1* carriers (RR 1.67, 95% CI 0.32–10.07).
  - The use of oral contraceptives in women with a known BRCA mutation is not contraindicated. However, while it may reduce the risk of ovarian cancer, it may increase the risk of breast cancer.
  - Both raloxifene and AIs have been demonstrated to significantly reduce the risk of breast cancer.
  - The main benefit of tamoxifen is in reducing hormone receptor (HR)-positive breast cancer. Whether tamoxifen is effective in reducing recurrence in BRCA mutation carriers with HR-negative breast cancers is unclear.
  - For BRCA mutation carriers with breast cancer who do not opt for contralateral mastectomy, surveillance with clinical breast examination, mammography, and MRI are recommended, as outlined above.

Recommendations

- Women with inherited mutations in breast cancer type 1 and 2 susceptibility genes (*BRCA1* and *BRCA2*) have markedly elevated risks of breast cancer and ovarian cancer. Men with BRCA mutations have increased risk for breast and prostate cancer.
- For women with a known BRCA mutation, risk-reducing mastectomy is a highly effective strategy for breast cancer risk reduction. For BRCA carriers diagnosed with advanced ovarian cancer, we prefer not proceeding with risk-reducing mastectomies until at least 5 years after the ovarian cancer diagnosis, as survival is dominated by the mortality rate of ovarian cancer.
- For women with a BRCA mutation, risk-reducing salpingo-oophorectomy (BSO) is indicated by age 35–40 years and when childbearing is completed. BSO is also indicated for carriers who are diagnosed with early-stage breast cancer.
- Women with a BRCA mutation who do not opt for bilateral mastectomy should undergo breast cancer surveillance with annual mammography and MRI.
- For women with a BRCA mutation who do not opt for risk-reducing mastectomy, chemoprevention with tamoxifen, raloxifene, or an AI is appropriate.
- For women who carry mutations in genes other than BRCA that confer moderate risk for breast cancer (e.g., *PALB2, CHEK2*, and *ATM* gene mutations), the options for breast cancer prevention are similar.
- Oral contraceptive use in BRCA mutation carriers decreases the risk of ovarian cancer and does not appear to increase risk of breast cancer.
- For women with negative or uninformative test results, quantitative models can help identify women with a high lifetime risk of breast cancer of at least 20%. These women are candidates for breast cancer screening with MRI in addition to mammography.
- Women with uninformative negative BRCA results without a family history of ovarian cancer do not appear to be at increased risk of developing ovarian cancer. Thus, BSO is not indicated for ovarian cancer risk reduction.

Other Agents

- A phase III trial randomly assigned 376 patients with metastatic breast cancer with either germline BRCA mutations or triple-negative breast in the first-line setting to treatment with either carboplatin or docetaxel.
- *PARP inhibitors:* PARP inhibitors block the repair of DNA single-strand breaks, and for tumors associated with BRCA mutations, they result in cell death due to inefficiencies in cell repair mechanisms.
- Olaparib is the first of this class to be approved for use in the United States. While specifically approved for the treatment of ovarian cancer in BRCA carriers, it holds great promise in the treatment of breast cancer associated with BRCA mutations.

---

17. A 35-year old lady, G2P2, menarche at age 12 years on oral contraceptive pill (OCP) has a strong family history of breast cancer. She is detected to be carrier of BRCA 1 mutation. How would you proceed for surveillance and undertake prevention strategies for her? ***WBUHS 2017***

Risk management strategies for *BRCA1* mutation carriers include the following:

- Risk-reducing mastectomy and reconstruction
- Risk-reducing salpingo-oophorectomy
- Intensive surveillance for breast and ovarian cancer
- Chemoprevention
- The oral selective ER modulator, tamoxifen, taken daily for 5 years, substantially reduces breast cancer risk for women who are at increased risk owing to their family cancer history, reproductive risk factors, or personal history of atypical hyperplasia or lobular carcinoma *in situ*. Moreover, this benefit is sustained for at least 5 years after ceasing tamoxifen.
- Most breast cancers in *BRCA1* mutation carriers are ER negative at the time of diagnosis.
- Tamoxifen can reduce HR-negative tumors in *BRCA1* mutation carriers, consistent with the prevention properties afforded by BSO.

- In fact, there is strong evidence that female hormones play a critical role in the early ontogeny of *BRCA1*-associated breast cancer. As noted above, BSO in premenopausal *BRCA1* mutation carriers is associated with reduced breast cancer risk.
- For premenopausal women, the main serious side effect of tamoxifen is deep venous thrombosis. The absolute risk, however, is small and similar to the risk associated with the combined OCP. Due to its agonist activity in endometrial tissue, tamoxifen is also associated with endometrial hyperplasia and increased endometrial cancer risk, although the latter appears to be largely confined to women above the age of 50 years.
  - Prophylactic surgery (bilateral mastectomy, BSO, or a combination of both procedures) has proved to be the most effective risk-reducing strategy.
  - Histologically, *BRCA1*-related breast cancers are predominantly of the basal subtype, with predominant lymphocytic infiltration, and are often more aggressive and associated with negative prognostic factors, as characterized by numerous mitoses, pleomorphic pattern, poor differentiation, and higher proliferation rates, as well as a negative estrogen and progesterone receptors (PRs) status. Moreover, a lack of HER-2 expression was observed in breast cancer tumors of *BRCA1* carriers.
  - Most ovarian cancers associated with germ line BRCA mutations are diagnosed at a younger age and are ultimately determined as high-grade and advanced-stage serous carcinomas.
  - Women who have an increased risk of breast and ovarian cancer are advised to consider risk-reducing strategies; however, such methods vary in their effectiveness. These strategies include surveillance [breast self-examination, clinical breast examination, screening using mammography and breast MRI, transvaginal ultrasound scanning and serum (CA125), chemoprevention, and prophylactic surgery (salpingo-oophorectomy and/or mastectomy)].

Surveillance

- The efficacy of surveillance in *BRCA1*/2 mutation carriers is difficult to determine. Importantly, it has been suggested that some *BRCA1*/2 carriers will not develop cancer during their lifetime, although the identification of such individuals is currently impossible.
- The concept of surveillance is based on early detection of cancer rather than cancer prevention.
- It is suggested that women at a high risk of developing breast cancer should perform a monthly breast self-examination, and also undergo bi-annual clinical examination and annual digital mammography.
- Owing to the fact that the sensitivity of mammography is significantly reduced in younger women because of their dense breast tissue and rapid development of breast cancer in *BRCA1*/2 mutations, the use of alternative and more sensitive imaging modalities, such as MRI at shorter intervals, has been recommended.
- Undoubtedly, surveillance is the least invasive option; however, such a method is associated with various negative consequences, such as increased anxiety, false reassurance, and unnecessary biopsies.
- Although MRI is an effective surveillance modality in BRCA mutation carriers—especially in younger women—a significant proportion of women are still found to have node positive breast cancer at the time of diagnosis.
- Furthermore, whilst regular surveillance in women at an increased familial risk of breast cancer is associated with a good clinical outcome if they carry *BRCA2* mutations or no detectable mutation, the outcome in carriers of *BRCA1* mutations is significantly worse, even in the instance that their tumors are diagnosed at an apparently early stage.
- The impact of regular breast screening in this context on overall survival (OS) ultimately remains unclear, and further research is required in order to evaluate the effect of different breast-screening strategies according to the mutation type, type and frequency of screening modality, and age.

Prophylactic Bilateral Mastectomy (PBM)

There are no randomized controlled trials (RCTs) which have previously examined the potential impacts of PBM on survival; therefore, evidence has been derived from retrospective and short follow-up prospective studies in addition to hypothetical mathematical models with variable estimates.

GENE EXPRESSION PROFILING OF BREAST CANCER

18. Gene expression profiling of breast cancer. *WBUHS 2011*

19. Genetic profiling in breast cancer and its role in the management. *MAMC 2022*

- Cancer is a disease characterized by uncontrolled cell growth and proliferation. For cancer to develop, genes regulating cell growth and differentiation must be altered; these mutations are then maintained through subsequent cell divisions and are thus present in all cancerous cells.
- Gene expression profiling is a technique used in molecular biology to query the expression of thousands of genes simultaneously. In the context of cancer, gene expression profiling has been used to more accurately classify tumors.
- The information derived from gene expression profiling often has an impact on predicting the patient's clinical outcome.
- Gene expression profiling is a technique used in molecular biology to query the expression of thousands of genes simultaneously.
- While almost all cells cell in an organism contain the entire genome of the organism, only a small subset of those genes is expressed as messenger RNA (mRNA) at any given time, and their relative expression can be evaluated.
- Techniques include DNA microarray technology or sequenced-based techniques such as serial analysis of gene expression (SAGE).
- DNA labeled with fluorophores (*target*) is prepared from a sample such as a tumor biopsy and is hybridized to the complementary DNA (cDNA) sequences on the gene chip.
- The chip is then scanned for the presence and strength of the fluorescent labels at each spot representing probe-target hybrids.
- The level of fluorescence at a particular spot provides quantitative information about the expression of the particular gene corresponding to the spotted cDNA sequence.
- DNA microarrays evolved from Southern blotting which allows for detection of a specific DNA sequence in a sample of DNA.
- There are a few gene expression profiling tests currently available. Here is a list of those available in the United States or in Europe for breast cancer:
  - *MammaPrint:* This test is designed to help determine how likely early-stage lymph node negative breast cancers are to recur elsewhere in your body.
  - *MapQuant DX:* This test is designed to predict the risk of recurrence of certain types of ER positive breast cancer.
  - *Oncotype DX:* This test is used to help determine whether to use chemotherapy after surgery to treat early-stage ER positive, lymph node negative breast cancers with a low chance of recurrence.
  - *Theros CancerType ID:* This test is designed to help identify women with ER positive breast cancer who are at high risk of recurrence and help predict their response to endocrine adjuvant therapy.
  - *Other tests are in development:*
    - The effectiveness of gene expression profiling is still being studied in a number of clinical trials.
    - While some are using gene expression profiling to plan treatment, others are waiting for the results of these studies.
    - Discuss with specialist the pros and cons of gene expression profiling.
    - These tests are not for people with more advanced breast cancer that has spread to distant parts of the body.

20. Discuss the principle of immunohistochemistry (IHC) and use of molecular markers in diagnosis and prognosis of breast cancer. ***WBUHS 2021***

Introduction

- IHC is a method for detecting antigens or haptens in cells of a tissue section by exploiting the principle of antibodies binding specifically to antigens in biological tissues. The antibody-antigen binding can be visualized in different manners.
- IHC is an important application of monoclonal as well as polyclonal antibodies to determine the tissue distribution of an antigen of interest in health and disease.
- IHC is widely used for diagnosis of cancers; specific tumor antigens are expressed de novo or up-regulated in certain cancers.
- *Major components in a complete IHC experiment:*
  - Primary antibody binds to specific antigen;
  - The antibody-antigen complex is formed by incubation with a secondary, enzyme-conjugated, antibody;
  - With presence of substrate and chromogen, the enzyme catalyzes to generate colored deposits at the sites of antibody-antigen binding.

There are two main steps in IHC:

I. *Sample preparation:* Fixing the sample to preserve the architecture of the collected tissue and prepare it for antibody labeling.

II. *Sample labeling:* Using antibodies to label the protein(s) of interest.

The sample preparation method and antibody selection must be considered carefully to ensure quality results for an IHC experiment.

Antibody type	*Advantages*	*Disadvantages*
Monoclonal antibody	Highly specific to single epitope, therefore less likely to cross react with other proteins and lower background signals	Binds to single epitope therefore more susceptible to changes in antigen conformation (lower signal detection)
Polyclonal antibody	Targets multiple epitopes of same antigen, therefore more resistant to changes in antigen conformation	Multiple epitope targeting increases likelihood for nonspecific signals (increased background)
Fluorophore conjugated	The availability of multiple fluorophores with narrow emission ranges means multiple antigens can be visualized with high spatial specificity	Photobleaching signals
Enzyme conjugated	The chromogenic substrates provide strong signal that is longer lasting	The signal is less spatially specific, and fewer signals can be visualized due to their broad emissions

According to US National Institutes of Health's (NIH) Working Group and Biomarkers Consortium, a molecular marker is a characteristic that is objectively measured as an indicator of pathogenic or normal biological processes, or a pharmacological response to a therapeutic intervention. Although the most of these markers is protein, recently, gene expression patterns and altered DNA identified in tumor tissue have also taken prominence as tumor markers.

Well-established Prognostic and/or Therapeutic Breast Cancer Markers

Hormone Receptors

- The HRs are expressed proteins both in the epithelium and in breast stroma which bind to circulating hormones, mediating their cellular effects.
- The HR best studied in breast cancer are ER and PR.
- Breast cancers classified by positive IHC expression of ER and PR have different clinical, pathological, and molecular characteristics.

- It is postulated that risk factors are closely associated with breast tumors ER+ and PR+ and may involve mechanisms related to exposure to estrogen and progesterone, while etiology of breast cancer ER– and PR– should be independent of hormone exposure.
- The ER and PR are highly associated with patient age at diagnosis, rising continuously with age.
- Tumor cells expressing HRs presented a better response to hormone therapy and patients demonstrated higher survival, both disease free as overall and better prognosis.

Human Epidermal Growth Factor Receptor 2 (HER-2)

- Several names has been given for this gene, such as c-erb-2, cerbB-2, C-erbB-2, HER-2, HER-2/neu, ERBB2, erbB2, erbB2, neu/c-erbB-2/oncogene neu, neu protein, and neu.
- HER-2 amplification is associated with poor prognosis.
- This oncogene is amplified in 20–30% of breast cancers and is considered a marker of poor prognosis.
- The humanized monoclonal antibody trastuzumab, directed against the extracellular domains of HER-2, is indicated for the treatment of HER-2 positive breast cancer cases.
- In addition to Trastuzumab, other therapeutic strategies have been developed to target HER-2 protein, such as tyrosine kinase inhibitor (TKI) lapatinib, which showed improved efficacy after failure of trastuzumab therapy.
- Although HER-2 is associated with aggressive form of cancer, a specific subgroup named triple negative breast cancer (TNBC) arouses special interest, once they are orphan of directed treatment.
- TNBC is a subtype characterized by the lack of ER, PR, and HER-2 expression and it is associated with younger age at diagnosis.
- The clinical behavior of TNBC is classically more aggressive than other types, like luminal A and B molecular subtypes.

Ki-67 Antigen

- Ki-67 score is the most often measured on histological sections by IHC methodology and is defined as the percentage of stained invasive carcinoma cells.
- High expression of Ki-67 in axillary lymph nodes but not in breast tissue is significantly associated with shorter patient survival.
- Patients with higher proliferative activity in lymph nodes metastases might require more aggressive therapy and closer clinical monitoring of their disease.

Tumor Protein p53

- The p53 is involved in several critical pathways including cell cycle arrest, apoptosis, DNA repair, and cellular senescence, which are essential for normal cellular homeostasis and genome integrity maintenance.
- Alteration of *TP53* gene or post-translational modification in p53 protein can alter its response to cellular stress.
- Expression of mutant p53 protein was associated with high tumor proliferation rate, early disease recurrence, and early death in node negative breast cancer.

Carbohydrate 15-3 and Carcinoembryonic Antigens

- Breast cancer is generally no longer curable once metastases are detected by "classical" means: Clinical manifestations of the spread, imaging methods, and serum marker assays, such as those based on carcinoma antigen 15-3 (CA 15-3) or CEA.
- CA 15-3 in combination with CEA is also relevant tumor markers in breast cancer.
- Determination of CEA in breast cancer is indicative of tumor size and nodal involvement.
- Therefore, CEA concentrations >7.5 μg/L are associated with high probability of subclinical metastases.
- Prognosis of patients whose CEA level was within the normal range at the time of diagnosis is significantly better than those with elevated CEA levels.
- Baseline CA 15-3 might be value in the identification of higher risk of relapse, where adjuvant chemotherapy must be introduced.
- Presence of an abnormal CA 15-3 presurgical value is associated with an increased risk of recurrence and death.
- CA 15-3 seems more efficient when compared to CEA.

Breast Cancer Susceptibility Genes (BRCA1 and BRCA2)

- Approximately 80% of the cases related to familial breast cancer are associated with one gene of hereditary susceptibility for breast and ovarian cancer, *BRCA1* and *BRCA2*.
- The *BRCA* genes have been classified as tumor suppressor genes, because the loss of wild-type allele has been observed in tumors of heterozygous carriers.
- BRCA proteins play important roles in different cellular processes, including activation and transcriptional regulation, repair of DNA damage, beyond the control of cell cycle, cellular proliferation, and differentiation.
- *BRCA1* or *BRCA2* are extremely rare in sporadic breast cancer.
- The frequency and spectrum of mutations within *BRCA1* or *BRCA2* genes show considerable variation between ethnic group and geographic region, probably due to interactions between different lifestyle and genetic characteristics.
- Studies have discussed the role of maternal or paternal inheritance of BRCA mutation affecting risk of breast cancer.
- Family history profiles can predict *BRCA1* or *BRCA2* mutation, mainly those characterized by first-degree relatives with ovarian cancer or breast cancer along with young age at diagnosis, bilateral occurrence and increased number of affected relatives.
- If a high-risk status of these women had been recognized, they might have had the opportunity to choose genetic counseling, testing, more effective cancer surveillance, and potentially preventive options, such as prophylactic surgery and/or chemoprevention.
- Among these preventive options, bilateral mastectomy, although invasive, reduces approximately 90% the risk of breast cancer in women with *BRCA1/2* mutations.
- *More susceptible genes have been discovered:*
  - These new findings include rare germline mutations in other high penetrant genes;
  - The most important between them include:
    - TP53 mutations in Li-Fraumeni syndrome,
    - STK11 (serine/threonine kinase 11) mutations in Peutz–Jeghers syndrome, and
    - PTEN (phosphatase and tensin homolog on chromosome ten) mutations in Cowden syndrome.
  - Furthermore, more frequent, but less penetrant, mutations have been identified in families with breast cancer clustering, in moderate or low penetrant genes:
    - CHEK2 (checkpoint kinase 2),
    - ATM (ataxia telangiectasia mutated),
    - PALB2 (partner and localizer of *BRCA2*), and
    - BRIP1 (*BRCA1*-interacting protein C-terminal helicase.

Future Candidate Markers for Prognosis and Therapeutic Responses in Breast Cancer Evolution

- *Proliferating cell nuclear antigen (PCNA):* The PCNA signal transduction has an important impact on growth regulation of breast cancer cells and is associated with poor OS.
- *Caveolin:* Recently, it has been reported a strong association between CAV1 and CAV2 expression and high histological grade, and lack of HRs positivity (ER and PR) in basal-like breast cancer subtype, providing evidence that these proteins can have oncogenic properties.
- *Receptor C-X-C chemokine receptor type 4 (CXCR4):* This receptor is required for migration of breast cancer cells from the primary site to lung, bones, and lymph nodes, which represent organs that secrete high levels of chemokine CXCL12. For this reason, CXCR4 has been found to be a prognostic marker in breast cancer, among other types of cancer.

  Patients who had CXCR4 overexpression had significantly higher incidence of cancer recurrence and cancer-related deaths than those in low CXCR4 expression group.
- *Chemokine (C-C Motif) ligands 2 and 5 (CCL2 and CCL5):* Many studies have addressed the involvement and roles of inflammatory chemokines CCL2 (MCP-1, membrane cofactor protein-1) and CCL5 (RANTES, regulated on activation, normal T-cell expressed and secreted) in breast malignancy. Some studies have shown that CCL2

and CCL5 expressions are higher in breast cancer tissue than in corresponding normal tissue. CCL2 has been correlated with higher tumor grade and has been shown to have significant prognostic value for relapse-free survival.

- *Growth factors: EGF, HGF, IGF, VEGF, and TGF:* The role of growth factors has been extensively analyzed both in cancer risk and tumor progression.
- *V-Myc myelocytomatosis:* Viral Oncogene Homolog (Avian) (MYC). The MYC proto-oncogene family (comprising c-myc, N-myc, and L-muc) ranks among the most exhaustively studied group of genes in biology. Amplification of MYC has been reported in breast cancer as well as in many other cancers.

  The MYC amplification shows strong correlation with ER status, stage of disease (initial), and existence of distant metastasis and tends to be associated with high histologic grade, positive axillary nodal status, and a high S-phase fraction.
- *Forkhead box protein 3 (FOXP3):* Forkhead box protein P3 (FOXP3) plays a critical role in differentiation, development, maintenance, and function of regulatory T-cells. Several studies have examined the distribution of FOXP3 in normal and malignant epithelial breast cells.
- *MicroRNA:* Over the past decades, an increasing amount of evidence has demonstrated applications of microRNAs (miRNAs) as tissue-based markers for classification and prognosis of several human cancers, including breast cancer.

  Genome-wide analyses have identified deregulated miRNA expression in human malignancies and a potential dual role in tumor formation, highlighting that miRNAs can modulate oncogenic or tumor suppressor pathways, including p53, c-MYC, RAS, and BCR-ABL, while expression of miRNAs themselves can be regulated by oncogenes or tumor suppressors.

---

21. Write on importance of cancer genomics in precision of breast cancer. ***WBUHS 2025 Supplementary***

Importance of Cancer Genomics in Precision of Breast Cancer

Cancer genomics plays a pivotal role in the advancement of precision medicine, especially in the diagnosis, prognosis, and treatment of breast cancer. By examining the genetic and molecular profile of breast cancer tumors, researchers and clinicians can tailor therapeutic strategies to the unique characteristics of each patient's cancer. This personalized approach significantly enhances treatment outcomes and minimizes unnecessary side effects.

Understanding Tumor Heterogeneity

Breast cancer is a heterogeneous disease with multiple subtypes, including hormone receptor-positive, HER2-positive, and triple-negative breast cancer (TNBC). Traditional classifications based on histopathology and receptor status provide a basic framework, but cancer genomics offers a deeper understanding by identifying specific mutations, gene expression profiles, and molecular signatures within tumors. This genomic insight enables more accurate classification and risk stratification.

Targeted Therapy Selection

Genomic profiling identifies actionable mutations and alterations, such as BRCA1/2, PIK3CA, ESR1, and HER2 amplifications. These findings guide the use of targeted therapies—for example:

- *HER2 amplification* predicts response to trastuzumab and other HER2-targeted drugs.
- *BRCA1/2 mutations* may indicate suitability for PARP inhibitors.
- *PIK3CA mutations* can inform the use of PI3K inhibitors like alpelisib in HR-positive, HER2-negative breast cancer.

This precision reduces reliance on one-size-fits-all chemotherapy and enhances treatment efficacy.

Minimizing Overtreatment and Side Effects

Genomic tools such as the Oncotype DX, MammaPrint, and PAM50 tests evaluate gene expression patterns to predict the risk of recurrence and the likely benefit of chemotherapy. In early-stage hormone receptor-positive breast cancer, these tests help determine whether chemotherapy can be safely avoided, thus sparing patients from toxic side effects without compromising outcomes.

Monitoring Disease Progression and Resistance

Liquid biopsy technologies, including circulating tumor DNA (ctDNA) analysis, provide a non-invasive method to monitor tumor evolution and detect emerging resistance mutations. This dynamic approach helps adjust treatment strategies in real time and manage metastatic disease more effectively.

Prognostic and Predictive Biomarkers

Cancer genomics enables the identification of biomarkers that predict treatment response or overall prognosis. For example, mutations in TP53 or loss of PTEN are often associated with more aggressive disease and poor outcomes, guiding more intensive monitoring or therapeutic approaches.

Advancing Research and Clinical Trials

Genomic data contribute to the development of novel therapies and inclusion in genotype-matched clinical trials. Patients with rare mutations or resistant tumors may benefit from enrollment in precision oncology trials, accelerating drug development and expanding treatment options.

LYMPHATIC AND CUTANEOUS MANIFESTATIONS OF BREAST CARCINOMA

22. Lymphatic manifestations of breast carcinoma.

Introduction

- Breast cancer cells commonly spread to the lymph nodes, a series of structures that make up part of the immune system.
- Breast cancer spread to the lymph nodes can exhibit a number of symptoms.

Lymphatic manifestations are as follow:

- *Swollen lymph nodes in armpit:*
  - A common symptom initially experienced by patients with breast cancer that has invaded the lymph nodes is lymph node swelling.
  - Patients with invasive breast cancer may notice a swelling in the armpit on the same side as the affected breast, corresponding to swollen lymph nodes.
  - As breast cancer progresses, cancer growth within the lymph nodes leads to node fusion and matting, which also causes a noticeable lump.
- *Lymphedema:*
  - In invasive breast cancer, swelling of the lymph nodes can lead to blockages in the lymphatic system and prevent the circulation and drainage of lymph fluid, called lymphedema.
  - Patients with lymphedema experience swelling of the arm and the hand on the affected side of the body, which often results in pain and difficulty moving the affected limb.
  - Breast cancer patients who have undergone mastectomy to treat cancer may also suffer from lymphedema, since the removal of lymph nodes during surgery disrupts lymph fluid drainage.
- *Chest tenderness and pain:*
  - As the breast cancer progresses, the cancer cells that invaded lymph nodes in the armpit can travel to other lymph nodes throughout the body via the lymphatic system.
  - Breast cancer in the lymph nodes can commonly spread to lymph nodes underneath the breastbone and around the clavicles.
  - When lymph nodes within the chest cavity enlarge, they put pressure on surrounding healthy tissue, which may lead to chest pain.
  - Breast cancer patients experiencing chest pain should seek immediate medical attention to test the extent of cancer metastasis.
- *Lymph nodal metastasis:* Axillary, internal mammary, infraclavicular and supraclavicular nodes can be involved.

23. What are the cutaneous manifestations of carcinoma breast? Enumerate the molecular subtypes of carcinoma breast. How will you manage a case of DCIS? ***WBUHS 2017, 2023***

Cutaneous Manifestations of Breast Carcinoma

- Nodules are the most common clinical manifestations of breast cancer.
- Assessment of cutaneous metastatic disease can be perplexing because the clinical presentation appears similar to other skin maladies such as cellulitis or lymphedema. Patients present with a variety of symptoms ranging from firm, indurated skin to tiny, seed-like solid papules and large egg-sized lesions.
- Lymphedema is a chronic condition characterized by swelling and recurrent skin infections. Characteristic dermatologic findings in cellulitis, a complication of lymphedema, include erythema, edema, tenderness, and warmth. Fibrosis associated with axillary lymph node dissection (ALND) and RT reduces lymphatic flow from the breast and ipsilateral upper extremity, impairing the ability to clear bacteria and, therefore, predisposing patients to infection.
- Cutaneous metastases present similarly to cellulitis and lymphedema. Diagnostic expertise recognizes the manifestation of progressive disease, thus allowing for appropriate treatment interventions.
- Carcinoma erysipeloides is frequently observed in carcinoma breast.

Molecular Subtypes of Breast Carcinoma

Most studies divide breast cancer into four major molecular subtypes:

- Luminal A
- Luminal B
- Triple negative/basal-like
- HER2 type

Luminal A

- Luminal tumor cells look the most like cells of breast cancers that start in the inner (luminal) cells lining the mammary ducts.
- Luminal A tumors tend to be:
  - ER-positive
  - HER2 receptor-negative (HER2-negative)
  - Tumor grade 1 or 2
- About 30–70% of breast cancers are luminal A tumors.
- Of the four subtypes, luminal A tumors tend to have the best prognosis, with fairly high survival rates and fairly low recurrence rates.
- Because luminal A tumors tend to be ER-positive, treatment for these tumors often includes hormone therapy.

Luminal B

- Luminal tumor cells that look like those of breast cancers that start in the inner (luminal) cells lining the mammary ducts.
- Luminal B tumors tend to be ER-positive. They may be HER2-negative or HER2-positive.
- Women with luminal B tumors are often diagnosed at a younger age than those with luminal A tumors.

Compared to luminal A tumors, they also tend to have factors that lead to a poorer prognosis including:

- Poorer tumor grade
- Larger tumor size
- Lymph node-positive
  - About 10–20% of breast cancers are luminal B tumors.
  - Women with luminal B tumors tend to have fairly high survival rates, although not as high as those with luminal A tumors

Triple Negative/basal-like

Triple negative breast cancers are:

- ER-negative
- PR-negative
- HER2-negative
- There are several subsets of TNBC.
- One subset is basal-like. Basal-like tumors have cells that look similar to those of the outer (basal) cells surrounding the mammary ducts.
- Most triple negative tumors are basal-like and most basal-like tumors are triple negative.

HER2 Type

- The molecular subtype HER2 type is not the same as HER2-positive and is not used to guide treatment.
- Although most HER2 type tumors are HER2-positive (and named for this reason), about 30% are HER2-negative.
- HER2 type tumors tend to be:
  - ER-negative
  - PR-negative
  - Lymph node-positive
  - Poorer tumor grade
- About 5–15 percent of breast cancers are HER2 type.
- Women with HER2 type tumors may be diagnosed at a younger age than those with luminal A and luminal B tumors.
- HER2 type breast cancers that are HER2-positive can be treated with anti-HER2 drugs such as trastuzumab (Herceptin)

Molecular subtype	***Biomarker profile***
Luminal A	ER+ and/or PR+, HER2-, and low Ki67 (<14%)
Luminal B	ER+ and/or PR+ and HER2+ (luminal-HER2 group) ER+- and/or PR+, HER2-, and high Ki67 (>14%)
HER2	ER-, PR-and HER2+-
Basal-like	ER—, PR- HER2-, and CK5/6 and/or EGFR+-

	Luminal	***HER2***	***Basel***
Gene expression pattern	High expression of hormone receptors and associated genes (luminal A > luminal B)	• High expression of HER2 and other genes in amplicon • Low expression of ER and associated genes	• High expression of basal epithelial genes, basal cytokeratins • Low expression of ER and associated genes • Low expression of HER2
Clinical features	• ~70% of invasive breast cancers • ER/PR positive • Luminal Â tend to be higher histological grade than luminal A • Some overexpress HER2 (luminal B)	• ~15% of invasive breast cancers • ER/PR negative • More likely to be high grade and node positive	• ~15% of invasive breast cancers • Most ER/PR/HER2 negative (triple negative') • *BRCA1* dysfunction (germline, sporadic) • Particularly common in African-American women
Treatment response and outcome	• Respond to endocrine therapy (but response to tamoxifen and aromatase inhibitors may be different for luminal A and luminal B) • Response to chemotherapy variable (greater in luminal B than in luminal A) • Prognosis better for luminal A than luminal B	• Respond to trastuzumab (Herceptin) • Respond to anthracycline-based chemotherapy • Generally poor prognosis	• No response to endocrine therapy or trastuzumab (Herceptin) • Appear to be sensitive to platinum-based chemotherapy and PARP inhibitors • Generally poor prognosis (but not uniformly poor)

In most cases, treatment options for DCIS include:
- Lumpectomy and RT
- Simple mastectomy

In some cases, treatment options may include:
- Lumpectomy only
- Lumpectomy and the drug tamoxifen

An SN procedure should be considered in the case of:
- Patients with the preoperative diagnosis DCIS, for whom a mastectomy is indicated in relation to size
- Patients with a small DCIS who are eligible for BCT, in which there are risk factors for an invasive component:
  - Younger than 55 years
  - Solid component on the mammogram
  - Suspicion on the basis of histological biopsies
  - Moderate or poorly differentiated DCIS in biopsies

The treatment of DCIS is mastectomy or BCT, consisting of microscopic complete tumor excision and radiotherapy, in which a boost may be considered, particularly for younger patients.

Contraindications for breast conservation therapy (BCT):
- Multicentricity (the presence of DCIS in multiple quadrants of the breast)
- *Residual disease:* mammographic evidence or tumor-positive resection margin
- Axillary staging is not indicated with pure DCIS in the excision sample.
- If postoperative invasive foci are encountered that are larger than 5 mm, lymphogenous staging is recommended.
- Adjuvant (hormonal) treatment after breast-conserving treatment (R0 resection and radiotherapy) is not recommended.

EARLY AND LOCALLY ADVANCED BREAST CANCER

24. Define early breast carcinoma and discuss its management. ***WBUHS 2015***

25. Describe the predisposing factors, clinical features, staging and management of early carcinoma breast in a 32-year-old premenopausal lady. ***KIITS University, Odisha 2025***

Early Breast Cancer

Definition

Early breast cancer refers to *invasive breast carcinoma confined to the breast* (with or without limited axillary lymph node involvement), but *without distant metastasis.*
Includes *Stages I and II* according to TNM classification.

Predisposing (Risk) Factors

Breast cancer is a *multifactorial disease* involving *genetic, hormonal, reproductive, and lifestyle* factors.

Category	*Risk factors*	*Mechanism/explanation*
1. Genetic/Familial	• *BRCA1* and *BRCA2* gene mutations • TP53 (Li-Fraumeni syndrome) • PTEN (Cowden syndrome) • Family history in first-degree relatives	Defective DNA repair mechanisms and inherited oncogenic mutations

Contd...

Contd...

Category	*Risk factors*	*Mechanism/explanation*
2. Hormonal/ reproductive	• Early menarche (<12 years) • Late menopause (>55 years) • Nulliparity or late first pregnancy (>30 years) • Use of combined oral contraceptives or HRT	Prolonged estrogen and progesterone exposure increases mitogenic stimulation of breast epithelium
3. Age	• Risk increases with age, especially >40 years	Accumulation of somatic mutations over time
4. Previous breast disease	• Atypical ductal or lobular hyperplasia • LCIS (lobular carcinoma in situ) • Prior breast cancer	Premalignant or high-risk histologic lesions
5. Radiation exposure	• Chest irradiation (especially before age 30)	DNA damage from ionizing radiation
6. Lifestyle/ environmental	• Obesity (postmenopausal) • High-fat diet • Alcohol consumption • Physical inactivity	Increases estrogen production (via aromatization in adipose tissue)
7. Others	• Diabetes mellitus • Smoking (weak association)	Metabolic and carcinogenic effects

Clinical Features of Early Breast Cancer

In early stages, breast cancer is often *asymptomatic* and detected via *screening (mammography).*

When symptomatic, the findings are usually *localized* to the breast or axilla.

- *Breast lump (most common presentation)*
    - Usually *painless, firm to hard* lump.
    - *Irregular borders,* poorly defined or "gritty" feel.
    - *Non-tender* and *fixed* to surrounding tissue (if invasive).
    - *Common site: Upper outer quadrant* of breast.
- *Changes in breast contour or size*
    - Asymmetry between the two breasts.
    - Localized flattening or distortion of breast contour.
    - May be best seen on *forward leaning* or *arm-raised* position.
- *Skin changes (early local involvement)*
    - *Skin tethering* or *dimpling* (due to involvement of Cooper's ligaments).
    - *Peau d'orange* (orange peel appearance): Due to lymphatic obstruction → skin edema and follicular pitting.
    - *Localized erythema* or thickening (rare in early stage).
- *Nipple and areolar changes*
    - *Nipple retraction or inversion* (recent onset).
    - *Deviation* of nipple position.
    - *Eczematous changes* or *ulceration* of nipple (Paget's disease of the nipple).
    - *Nipple discharge*—may be *bloody,* serous, or clear (though uncommon in early invasive cancer).
- *Axillary findings*
    - *Palpable, firm, discrete lymph node(s)* in axilla (mobile in early stage).
    - May be thc *first sign* detected in some patients.
- *Symptoms due to hormone activity or metastasis*
    - Generally *absent in early stages.*
    - Systemic symptoms (bone pain, weight loss, cough, jaundice) suggest *advanced disease.*

TNM staging system for breast cancer.	
Primary tumor (T): Definitions for classifying the primary tumor (T) are the same for clinical and for pathologic classification. If the measurement is made by physical examination, the examiner will use the major headings (T1, T2, or T3); if other measurements, such as mammographic or pathologic measurements, are used, the subsets of T1 can be used. Tumors should be measured to the nearest 0.1 cm increment	
TX	Primary tumor cannot be assessed
T0	No evidence of primary tumor
Tis	Carcinoma in situ
Tis (DCIS)	Ductal carcinoma in situ
Tis (LCIS)	Lobular carcinoma in situ
Tis (Paget's)	Paget's disease of the nipple with no tumor (*Note:* Paget's disease associated with a tumor is classified according to the size of the tumor)
T1	Tumor 2 cm or less in greatest dimension
T1mic	Microinvasion 0.1 cm or less in greatest dimension
T1a	Tumor >0.1 cm but not >0.5 cm in greatest dimension
T1b	Tumor >0.5 cm but not >1 cm in greatest dimension
T1c	Tumor >1 cm but not >2 cm in greatest dimension
T2	Tumor >2 cm but not >5 cm in greatest dimension
T3	Tumor >5 cm in greatest dimension
T4	Tumor of any size with direct extension to (a) chest wall or (b) skin, only as described below
T4a	Extension to chest wall, not including pectoralis muscle
T4b	Edema (including peau d'orange), or ulceration of the skin of the breast, or satellite skin nodules confined to the same breast
T4c	Both T4a and T4b
T4d	Inflammatory carcinoma
Regional lymph nodes—Clinical (N)	
NX	Regional lymph nodes cannot be assessed (e.g., previously removed)
N0	No regional lymph node metastasis
N1	Metastasis to movable ipsilateral axillary lymph node(s)
N2	Metastases in ipsilateral axillary lymph nodes fixed or matted, or in clinically apparent ipsilateral internal mammary nodes in the absence of clinically evident axillary lymph node metastasis
N2a	Metastasis in ipsilateral axillary lymph nodes fixed to one another (matted) or to other structures
N2b	Metastasis only in clinically apparent ipsilateral internal mammary nodes and in the absence of clinically evident axillary lymph node metastasis
N3	Metastasis in ipsilateral infraclavicular lymph node(s) with or without axillary lymph node involvement, or in clinically apparent ipsilateral internal mammary lymph node(s) and in the presence of clinically evident axillary lymph node metastasis; or metastasis in ipsilateral supraclavicular lymph node(s) with or without axillary or internal mammary lymph node involvement
N3a	Metastasis in ipsilateral infraclavicular lymph node(s)
N3b	Metastasis in ipsilateral internal mammary lymph nodes(s) and axillary lymph node(s)
N3c	Metastasis in ipsilateral supraclavicular lymph node(s)
Distant metastasis (M)	
MX	Distant metastasis cannot be assessed
M0	No distant metastasis
M1	Distant metastasis

TNM stage groupings.

Stage 0	Tis	N0	M0
Stage I	T1[a]	N0	M0
Stage IIA	T0	N1	M0
	T1[a]	N1	M0
	T2	N0	M0
Stage IIB	T2	N1	M0
	T3	N0	M0
Stage IIIA	T0	N2	M0
	T1[a]	N2	M0
	T2	N2	M0
	T3	N1	M0
	T3	N2	M0
Stage IIIB	T4	N0	M0
	T4	N1	M0
	T4	N2	M0
Stage IIIC	Any T	N3	M0
Stage IV	Any T	Any N	M1

[a]T1 includes T1 mic.

Early Invasive Breast Cancer (Stage I, IIa, or IIb)

Management

Confirmation of diagnosis by: Triple assessment—history and clinical examination, digital mammography and core needle biopsy.

Investigations

- Complete blood cell count, complete metabolic panel, and chest X-ray.
- A bone scan if the alkaline phosphatase or calcium level is elevated.
- CT scan of the liver if liver function panel is abnormal.
- CT scan of the thorax to exclude presence of lung secondaries.

Surgical Options

- Mastectomy with or without reconstruction:
    - *Modified radical mastectomy (MRM):* It is indicated for patients with clinically positive lymph nodes or a positive axillary node based on previous sentinel lymph node biopsy (SLNB) or FNAB.
    - Total (simple) mastectomy with SLNB is for patients with a clinically negative axilla. A skin-sparing mastectomy (preserves skin envelope and inframammary ridge) may be performed with immediate reconstruction, resulting in improved cosmesis. The nipple-areolar complex, a rim of periareolar breast skin, and any previous excisional biopsy or partial mastectomy scars are excised.
    - Immediate reconstruction at the time of mastectomy should be offered to eligible patients. Options include latissimus dorsi myocutaneous flaps, transverse rectus abdominis myocutaneous flaps, and inflatable tissue expanders followed by exchange for saline or silicone implants.

Follow-up after mastectomy: Physical examination every 3–6 months for 3 years, then every 6–12 months for the next 2 years, and then annually. Mammography of the contralateral breast should continue yearly. Regular gynecologic follow-up is recommended for all women (tamoxifen increases risk of endometrial cancer)

Breast conservation therapy: Partial mastectomy and SLNB (or ALND) followed by breast irradiation.

Contraindications to BCT

Pregnancy	***Previous radiation therapy (RT)***	***Large breast size***
Multicentric disease	Large tumor/breast ratio	Central tumor
Diffuse indeterminate micro-calcification	Collagen vascular disease	

For patients with large tumors who desire BCT, NACT, or neoadjuvant hormonal therapy may be offered to attempt to reduce the size of the tumor to make BCT attempt possible.

- *Management of the axilla:* Approximately 30% of patients with clinically negative examinations will have positive lymph nodes in an ALND specimen. The presence and number of lymph nodes involved affect staging and thus prognosis.
  - *ALND:* Patients with clinically positive lymph nodes or with positive SLN should undergo ALND for local control.
  - *ALND involves the following:*
    - Removal of level I and level II nodes and, if grossly involved, possibly level III nodes. Motor and sensory nerves are preserved unless there is direct tumor involvement.
    - An ALND should remove 10 or more nodes. The number of nodes identified is often pathologist dependent.
    - Patients with four or more positive lymph nodes should undergo adjuvant radiation to the axilla. Selective patients with 1 to 3 positive nodes may also benefit from RT to the axilla.
    - Intraoperative complications: potential injury to the axillary vessels and neuropathy secondary to injury to the motor nerves of the axilla (the long thoracic, thoracodorsal, and medial pectoral nerves).

Adjuvant chemotherapy is given in appropriate patients after completion of surgery.

- All node-positive patients should receive adjuvant chemotherapy.
  - Regimens are guided by the tumor biomarkers. Typical regimens comprise four to eight cycles of a combination of cyclophosphamide and an anthracycline, followed by a taxane administered every 2–3 weeks.
  - Patients with ER-positive tumors receive adjuvant hormonal therapy for 5 years. Tamoxifen is given to premenopausal women, and AIs are given to postmenopausal women (AIs are not used in premenopausal women).
  - (In postmenopausal women older than 70 years, chemotherapy is performed less frequently. In postmenopausal women with tumors with ER or PR positivity, tamoxifen or an AI is frequently the sole adjuvant medical therapy.)
  - In patients with Her2/neu-positive tumors, polychemotherapy is combined with biological therapy targeting the Her2/neu protein:
    - Trastuzumab is a recombinant monoclonal antibody that binds to Her2/neu receptor to prevent cell proliferation.
    - Adding trastuzumab to a chemotherapy regiment of doxorubicin, cyclophosphamide, and paclitaxel was associated with an increase in the disease-free survival (DFS) by 12% and a 33% reduction in the risk of death at 3 years.
  - Node-negative patients may have increased DFS from adjuvant chemotherapy and/or hormonal therapy.
  - Up to 30% of node-negative women die of breast cancer within 10 years if treated with surgery alone.
  - Node-negative patients who are at high risk and benefit the most from adjuvant chemotherapy include those with tumors >1 cm, higher tumor grade, Her2/neu expression, aneuploidy, Ki-67 expression, increased percentage in S phase, lymphovascular invasion, and ER/PR-negative tumors.
  - Polychemotherapy in combination with tamoxifen was superior to tamoxifen alone in increasing disease-free and OS, especially in ER-negative patients, regardless of tumor size. Adjuvant whole-breast radiation after BCT decreases the breast cancer recurrence rate from 30 to <7% at 5 years.

26. Discuss the principle, indications, method, and significance of sentinel lymph node biopsy in early breast cancer. ***WBUHS 2021 Supplementary, WBUHS 2022***

Principle

- Sentinel nodes are the first lymph nodes where cancer cells might spread from a tumor.
- The concept of sentinel node biopsy is based on two basic principles: the existence of an orderly and predictable pattern of lymphatic drainage to a regional lymph node basin, and the functioning of a first lymph node as an effective filter for tumor cells.

Indications

Role of SLNB in early breast cancer:

- SLNB is primarily used in women with early breast cancers (T1 and T2, N0).
- It also is accurate for T3 N0 cancers, but nearly 75% of these women will have nonpalpable axillary lymph node metastases.
- In women undergoing NACT to permit conservation surgery, SLNB may be used.

Contraindications

- Palpable lymphadenopathy,
- Prior axillary surgery, chemotherapy, or RT, and
- Multifocal breast cancers.

Method

- The combination of intraoperative gamma probe detection of radioactive colloid and intraoperative visualization of isosulfan blue dye (Lymphazurin) is more accurate than the use of either agent alone.
- On the day prior to surgery, or on the morning of surgery, the radioactive colloid is injected. Using a tuberculin syringe and a 25-gauge needle, 0.5 mCi of 0.2-micron technetium-99 sulfur colloid in a volume of 0.2–0.5 mL is injected (three to four separate injections) at the cancer site or subdermally.
- Subdermal injections are given in proximity to the cancer site or subareolar.
- Subsequently, in the operating room, 4 mL of isosulfan blue dye (Lymphazurin) is injected in a similar fashion, but with an additional 1 mL injected between the cancer site and the overlying skin.
- For nonpalpable cancers, the injection is guided by either intraoperative ultrasound or by a localization wire that is placed preoperatively under ultrasound or stereotactic guidance.
- It is helpful for the radiologist to mark the skin overlying the breast cancer at the time of needle localization using an indelible marker.
- In women who have undergone previous excisional biopsy, the injections are made around the biopsy cavity but not into it.
- Women are told preoperatively that the isosulfan blue dye injection will impart a change to the color of their urine and that there is a very small risk of allergic reaction to the dye (1 in 10,000).
- Anaphylactic reactions have been documented. The use of radioactive colloid is safe and radiation exposure is very low.
- A hand-held gamma counter is then employed transcutaneously to identify the location of the sentinel lymph node (SLN).
- The gamma counter is employed to pinpoint the location of the SLN.
- As the dissection continues, the signal from the probe increases in intensity as the SLN is approached.
- The SLN also is identified by visualization of isosulfan blue dye in the afferent lymph vessel and in the lymph node itself.
- The lowest false-negative rates for SLNB have been obtained when all blue lymph nodes and all lymph nodes with radiation counts >10% of the 10-second ex vivo count of the SLN are harvested (10% rule).
- This procedure is repeated until residual radioactivity in the surgical bed is less that 10% of the 10-second ex vivo count of the most radioactive SLN.

Significance

- A SLNB is a procedure in which the SLN is identified, removed, and examined *to determine whether cancer cells are present.* It is used in people who have already been diagnosed with cancer.
- SLNB in breast cancer evolved out of efforts to minimize the morbidity associated with ALND while still providing important staging information.
- The combination of blue dye and isotope has been reported to be better for identification of the SLN; when used in combination, the positive predictive value of the technique approaches 100%, with a negative predictive value close to 95%. The false-negative rate is about 5–10% in most studies.
- The validity of the SLN concept lies in the ability of the SLN to predict the status of the regional lymphatic basin.
- The SLNB procedure is widely used in invasive breast cancer and selectively in DCIS. In certain situations, however, a standard axillary dissection should still be considered, such as when bulky positive axillary nodes are present.
- Previously, the presence of metastases in the SLNB prompted a completion axillary dissection. However, the results of the NSABP-B04 trial, in which some patients did not have their axilla dissected, called into question the value of the axillary dissection as a therapeutic instrument.
- ACOSOG Z0011, a trial designed by the American College of Surgeons Oncology Group, investigated whether foregoing axillary dissection in patients undergoing breast-conserving therapy with 1 or 2 positive SLNs was safe. They reported no difference in local-regional failure, DFS, or OS; the 5-year OS rates were 91.8% (95% CI 89.1–94.5%) with ALND and 92.5% (95% CI 90.0–95.1%) with SLNB alone; the 5-year DFS rates were 82.2% (95% CI 78.3–86.3%) with ALND and 83.9% (95% CI 80.2–87.9%) with SLNB alone.
- In intraductal carcinoma, an SLNB or axillary dissection is generally not indicated. There are special circumstances of intraductal carcinoma, such as high-grade DCIS or extensive DCIS, in which a microinvasive component may be associated with the intraductal carcinoma. In these circumstances, and particularly if a mastectomy is being performed, an SLNB may be considered.

27. Define early and advanced carcinoma breast. How do you manage impalpable lesions of the breast?

WBUHS 2008

TNM staging system for breast cancer.	
Primary tumor (T): Definitions for classifying the primary tumor (T) are the same for clinical and for pathologic classification. If the measurement is made by physical examination, the examiner will use the major headings (T1, T2, or T3); if other measurements, such as mammographic or pathologic measurements, are used, the subsets of T1 can be used. Tumors should be measured to the nearest 0.1-cm increment.	
TX	Primary tumor cannot be assessed
T0	No evidence of primary tumor
Tis	Carcinoma in situ
Tis (DCIS)	Ductal carcinoma in situ
Tis (LCIS)	Lobular carcinoma in situ
Tis (Paget's)	Paget's disease of the nipple with no tumor (*Note:* Paget's disease associated with a tumor is classified according to the size of the tumor)
T1	Tumor 2 cm or less in greatest dimension
T1mic	Microinvasion 0.1 cm or less in greatest dimension
T1a	Tumor >0.1 cm but not >0.5 cm in greatest dimension
T1b	Tumor >0.5 cm but not >1 cm in greatest dimension
T1c	Tumor >1 cm but not >2 cm in greatest dimension

Contd...

Contd...

TNM staging system for breast cancer.	
T2	Tumor >2 cm but not >5 cm in greatest dimension
T3	Tumor >5 cm in greatest dimension
T4	Tumor of any size with direct extension to (a) chest wall or (b) skin, only as described below
T4a	Extension to chest wall, not including pectoralis muscle
T4b	Edema (including peau d'orange), or ulceration of the skin of the breast, or satellite skin nodules confined to the same breast
T4c	Both T4a and T4b
T4d	Inflammatory carcinoma
Regional lymph nodes—Clinical (N)	
NX	Regional lymph nodes cannot be assessed (e.g., previously removed)
N0	No regional lymph node metastasis
N1	Metastasis to movable ipsilateral axillary lymph node(s)
N2	Metastases in ipsilateral axillary lymph nodes fixed or matted, or in clinically apparent ipsilateral internal mammary nodes in the absence of clinically evident axillary lymph node metastasis
N2a	Metastasis in ipsilateral axillary lymph nodes fixed to one another (matted) or to other structures
N2b	Metastasis only in clinically apparent ipsilateral internal mammary nodes and in the absence of clinically evident axillary lymph node metastasis
N3	Metastasis in ipsilateral infraclavicular lymph node(s) with or without axillary lymph node involvement, or in clinically apparent ipsilateral internal mammary lymph node(s) and in the presence of clinically evident axillary lymph node metastasis; or metastasis in ipsilateral supraclavicular lymph node(s) with or without axillary or internal mammary lymph node involvement
N3a	Metastasis in ipsilateral infraclavicular lymph node(s)
N3b	Metastasis in ipsilateral internal mammary lymph nodes(s) and axillary lymph node(s)
N3c	Metastasis in ipsilateral supraclavicular lymph node(s)

TNM stage groupings.			
Stage 0	Tis	N0	M0
Stage I	T1[a]	N0	M0
Stage IIA	T0	N1	M0
	T1[a]	N1	M0
	T2	N0	M0
Stage IIB	T2	N1	M0
	T3	N0	M0
Stage IIIA	T0	N2	M0
	T1[a]	N2	M0
	T2	N2	M0
	T3	N1	M0
	T3	N2	M0
Stage IIIB	T4	N0	M0
	T4	N1	M0
	T4	N2	M0
Stage IIIC	Any T	N3	M0
Stage IV	Any T	Any N	M1

[a]T1 includes T1 mic.

- Early Invasive Breast Cancer is Stage I, IIa, or IIb.
- Advanced Breast Cancer is Stage IIIa or IIIb.

Management of Nonpalpable Lesions

- With the advent of screening mammography breast lesions can be diagnosed early at such a stage where it cannot be palpated. Size <15 mm is considered to be palpable.
- Minimally invasive breast biopsy is the optimal initial tissue acquisition method and procedure of choice for obtaining a pathologic diagnosis of image-detected abnormalities.
- Correlation between pathology results and imaging findings is mandatory.
- Patients with high-risk lesions on image-guided biopsy (ADH, ALH, lobular carcinoma in situ, and radial scar) may have malignancy at the same site and should undergo a surgical biopsy.

Stereotactic Core Biopsy

- It is used for nonpalpable mammographically detected lesions, such as microcalcifications, which cannot be seen with ultrasonography.
- Contraindications include lesions close to the chest wall or in the axillary tail and thin breasts that may allow needle strikethrough.
- Superficial lesions and lesions directly beneath the nipple-areola complex are also often not approachable with stereotactic techniques.
- Nondiagnostic and insufficient specimens should undergo needle-localized excisional biopsy (NLB, see later discussion), as should discordant pathologic findings on core needle stereotactic biopsy.

Vacuum-assisted Biopsy

- It is generally used during stereotactic core biopsies and ultrasound-guided core biopsies.
- Multiple contiguous samples of tissue are collected while the probe remains in the breast.
- Volumes up to 1 mL can be collected during a single insertion.
- This is the preferred approach for lesions presenting with microcalcifications without a visible or palpable mass.

Ultrasound-guided Biopsy

- It is the preferred method if a lesion can be visualized with ultrasound because it is generally easier to perform than a stereotactic core biopsy.
- Lesions with a cystic component are better visualized with ultrasound, and ultrasound-guided biopsy can be used to aspirate the cyst as well as to provide core biopsy specimens.

Needle-localized Excisional Biopsy (NLB)

A needle and hook wire are placed into the breast adjacent to the concerning lesion under mammographic guidance. The patient is then brought to the operating room for an excisional biopsy. Using localization mammograms as a map, the whole hook wire, breast lesion, and a rim of normal breast tissue are removed en bloc. The specimen is oriented, and a radiograph is performed to confirm the presence of the lesion within the specimen.

Magnetic Resonance Imaging

- In the process of evaluating MRI as a means of characterizing mammography abnormalities, additional breast lesions have been detected.
- However, in the circumstance of both a negative mammogram and a negative physical examination, the probability of a breast cancer being diagnosed by MRI is extremely low.
- There is current interest in using MRI to screen the breasts of high-risk women and of women with a newly diagnosed breast cancer.
- In the first case, women with a strong family history of breast cancer or who carry known genetic mutations require screening at an early age, but mammography evaluation is limited because of the increased breast density in younger women.

Wire-guided Localization (WGL)

- WGL is done in impalpable breast lesions.
- Radiologists insert a wire on the day of surgery on the basis of USG guided/mammography guided/stereotactic localization.
- Surgeon operate around 1 cm of the wire localization and takes out the lesion keeping proper 1 cm margin in case of DCIS.
- *Disadvantages:*
  - Wire can cause thermal damage on the skin.
  - Cosmesis can be harmed due to placement of incision based on wire.
  - Wire can cause needle stick injury to surgeon.

ROLL

- Newer technique
- Radio-guided occult lesion localization. Can be done 5 days prior to surgery.
- ^{99}Tc labeled macro albumin is used to detect the lesion.
- Gamma camera can be used by the surgeon.

SNOLL

- Sentinel node with occult lesion localization.
- ^{99}Tc labeled macro albumin is used (injected intratumorally) to detect the lesion and a mobile less dense marker is injected intradermally to detect SLN.
- Nowadays single radiotracer can be used to identify both the lesions and SLN.
- Surgeons can use ROLL and SNOLL better than WGL.
- Lesions can also be detected and taken better with ROLL and SNOLL technique.

RSL

- Radiolabeled seed localization
- ^{125}I labeled titanium seed placed on the basis of USG/mammography/stereotactic localization

USG-guided Cryoprobe

Ice balls can be placed seeing the lesion.

In most cases, treatment options for DCIS include:

- Lumpectomy and RT
- Simple mastectomy

In some cases, treatment options may include:

- Lumpectomy only
- Lumpectomy and the drug tamoxifen

An SN procedure should be considered in the case of:

- Patients with the preoperative diagnosis DCIS, for whom a mastectomy is indicated in relation to size
- Patients with a small DCIS who are eligible for BCT, in which there are risk factors for an invasive component:
  - Younger than 55 years
  - Solid component on the mammogram
  - Suspicion on the basis of histological biopsies
  - Moderate or poorly differentiated DCIS in biopsies

The treatment of DCIS is mastectomy or BCT, consisting of microscopic complete tumor excision and radiotherapy, in which a boost may be considered, particularly for younger patients.

Contraindications for BCT

- Multicentricity (the presence of DCIS in multiple quadrants of the breast)
- *Residual disease:* Mammographic evidence or tumor-positive resection margin

- Axillary staging is not indicated with pure DCIS in the excision sample.
- If postoperative invasive foci are encountered that are larger than 5 mm, lymphogenous staging is recommended.
- Adjuvant (hormonal) treatment after breast-conserving treatment (R0 resection and radiotherapy) is not recommended.
- *Assessment of axillary lymph nodes:*
  - Axillary dissection is not performed for pure DCIS.
  - SNLB (see later discussion) may be considered when there is a reasonable probability of finding invasive cancer on final pathologic examination (e.g., >4 cm, palpable, or high grade).
  - Some surgeons perform SLNB in all patients with DCIS undergoing mastectomy because SLNB cannot be performed postmastectomy if an occult invasive cancer is found. This is an area of ongoing controversy and research.
  - A positive sentinel node indicates invasive breast cancer and changes the stage of the disease; a completion axillary dissection is then indicated.
- *Adjuvant therapy:*
  - For pure DCIS, there is no added benefit from systemic chemotherapy because the disease is confined to the ducts of the breast.
  - However, in those patients with ER-positive DCIS, adjuvant tamoxifen can reduce the risk of breast cancer recurrence by 37% over 5 years and the risk of developing a new contralateral breast cancer (NSABP B-24 trial). However, there is no survival benefit.
  - AIs (e.g., anastrozole, exemestane, and letrozole), which block the peripheral conversion of androgens into estrogens by inhibiting the enzyme aromatase but does not affect estrogen produced by the ovaries, are sometimes used as an alternative in postmenopausal patients.
  - Adjuvant radiation should be given to patients with DCIS treated with partial mastectomy to decrease the local recurrence rate (NSABP B-17 trial).
  - This is especially true for younger women with close margins or large tumors. However, there is no survival benefit.
  - For older patients with smaller, widely excised DCIS of low or intermediate grade, the benefit of RT is so small that adjuvant radiation is not recommended.

Lobular Carcinoma in situ (LCIS)

- LCIS is not considered a preinvasive lesion but rather an indicator for increased breast cancer risk of approximately 1% per year (~20–30% at 15 years) and is not treated as a breast cancer.
- Pleomorphic LCIS is a particularly aggressive subtype of LCIS that is treated more like DCIS; it tends to have less favorable biological markers.
- *Treatment options are:*
  - Lifelong close surveillance
  - Bilateral total mastectomies with immediate reconstruction for selected women with a strong family history after appropriate counseling, or
  - Prophylaxis with tamoxifen

Surgical Options for Stage I and II Breast Cancer

Mastectomy with or without reconstruction.

- *MRM:* It is indicated for patients with clinically positive lymph nodes or a total positive axillary node based on previous SLNB or FNAB.
- Simple mastectomy with SLNB is for patients with a clinically negative axilla. A skin-sparing mastectomy (preserves skin envelope and inframammary ridge) may be performed with immediate reconstruction, resulting in improved cosmesis: The nipple-areolar complex, a rim of periareolar breast skin, and any previous excisional biopsy or partial mastectomy scars are excised.

- Immediate reconstruction at the time of mastectomy should be offered to eligible patients. Options include latissimus dorsi myocutaneous flaps, transverse rectus abdominis myocutaneous flaps, and inflatable tissue expanders followed by exchange for saline or silicone implants. Immediate reconstruction has been shown not to affect patient outcome adversely. The detection of recurrence is not delayed, and the onset of chemotherapy is not changed.

Follow-up after Mastectomy

- Physical examination every 3–6 months for 3 years, then every 6–12 months for the next 2 years, and then annually.
- Mammography of the contralateral breast should continue yearly. Regular gynecologic follow-up is recommended for all women (tamoxifen increases risk of endometrial cancer).

Breast Conservation Therapy

- Partial mastectomy and SLNB (or ALND; see later discussion) followed by breast irradiation.
  - Several trials have demonstrated that BCT with adjuvant RT has similar survival and recurrence rates to those for MRM.
  - *Contraindications for BCT:*
    - A patient who may be unreliable with follow-up or RT (may involve radiation treatment 5 days a week for 5 to 6 weeks)
    - When the extent of disease prevents adequate negative margins;
    - A high tumor-to-breast size ratio, which prevents adequate resection without major deformity
    - Persistently positive margins on reexcision partial mastectomy; and inability to receive adjuvant radiation (e.g., prior radiation to the chest wall; first and second trimester pregnancy in which the delay of radiation to the postpartum state is inappropriate; collagen vascular diseases such as scleroderma).
  - For patients with large tumors who desire BCT, NACT, or neoadjuvant hormonal therapy may be offered to attempt to reduce the size of the tumor to make BCT attempt possible.
  - Partial mastectomy incisions should be planned so that they can be incorporated into a mastectomy incision should that prove necessary. Incisions for partial mastectomy and either SLNB or ALND should be separate.
  - Adjuvant radiotherapy decreases the breast cancer recurrence rate from 30% to <7% at 5 years and is a required component of BCT.
  - *Follow-up after BCT:*
    - Physical examinations are the same as those for mastectomy (*see* earlier discussion).
    - A post-treatment mammogram of the treated breast is performed to establish a new baseline, no earlier than 6 months after completion of RT.
    - Mammograms are then performed every 6–12 months after the new baseline mammogram until the surgical changes stabilize and then annually.
    - Contralateral breast mammography remains on an annual basis.
    - Regular gynecologic follow-up is recommended.
- *Management of the axilla:*
  - Approximately 30% of patients with clinically negative examinations will have positive lymph nodes in an ALND specimen.
  - The presence and number of lymph nodes involved affect staging and thus prognosis.
  - SLNB was developed to provide sampling of the lymph nodes without needing an ALND.
  - SLNB has been established as a standard of care for predicting axillary involvement in most patients with breast cancer.
  - 20–30% of the time more than one SLN is identified.
  - If the SLN is positive for metastasis (micrometastasis 0.2 mm or larger, not isolated tumor cells), a standard ALND is performed. RT can be administered to the axilla if the patient refuses ALND.
    - *ALND:* Patients with clinically positive lymph nodes, with positive SLN, or with positive should undergo ALND for local control. ALND involves the following:

- Removal of level I and level II nodes and, if grossly involved, possibly level III nodes.
- Patients with four or more positive lymph nodes should undergo adjuvant radiation to the axilla.
- Selective patients with one to three positive nodes may also benefit from RT to the axilla.
- *Intraoperative complications:* Potential injury to the axillary vessels and neuropathy secondary to injury to the motor nerves of the axilla (the long thoracic, thoracodorsal, and medial pectoral nerves).
- *Most frequent postoperative complications:* Wound infections and seromas.
- Other complications include pain and numbness in the axilla and upper arm, impaired shoulder mobility, and lymphedema.
  - *Adjuvant chemotherapy* is given in appropriate patients after completion of surgery.
  - All node-positive patients should receive adjuvant chemotherapy.
  - Regimens are guided by the tumor biomarkers. Typical regimens comprise four to eight cycles of a combination of cyclophosphamide and an anthracycline, followed by a taxane administered every 2–3 weeks.
  - Patients with ER-positive tumors receive adjuvant hormonal therapy for 5 years.
  - Tamoxifen is given to premenopausal women, and AIs are given to postmenopausal women (AIs are not used in premenopausal women).
  - In postmenopausal women older than 70 years, chemotherapy is performed less frequently.
  - In postmenopausal women with tumors with ER or PR positivity, tamoxifen or an AI is frequently the sole adjuvant medical therapy.
  - In patients with Her2/neu-positive tumors, polychemotherapy is combined with biological therapy targeting the Her2/neu
  - Adding trastuzumab to a chemotherapy regiment of doxorubicin, cyclophosphamide, and paclitaxel was associated with an increase in the DFS by 12% and a 33% reduction in the risk of death at 3 years. It is usually administered intravenously monthly for 12 months.
  - Node-negative patients may have increased DFS from adjuvant chemotherapy and/or hormonal therapy.
  - Up to 30% of node-negative women die of breast cancer within 10 years if treated with surgery alone.
  - Node-negative patients who are at high risk and benefit the most from adjuvant chemotherapy include those with tumors >1 cm, higher tumor grade, Her2/neu expression, aneuploidy, Ki-67 expression, increased percentage in S phase, lymphovascular invasion, and ER/PR-negative tumors.
  - The NSABP B-20 trial and the International Breast Cancer Study Group trial IX showed that polychemotherapy in combination with tamoxifen was superior to tamoxifen alone in increasing disease-free and OS, especially in ER-negative patients, regardless of tumor size.
  - The St. Gallen Consensus Panel in 1998 suggested that patients who have node-negative disease and whose tumors are 1 cm or less and ER-positive may be spared adjuvant chemotherapy but still may benefit from tamoxifen.

Adjuvant Radiation

Indications

- T3 and T4 tumors
- Attachment to the pectoral fascia
- Positive surgical margins
- Skin involvement
- Involved internal mammary nodes
- Inadequate or no axillary dissection
- Four or more positive lymph nodes
- Residual tumor on the axillary vein.
- Presence of one to three positive axillary nodes is a relative indication.

- Randomized, prospective trials have shown a significantly decreased recurrence and improved survival in premenopausal women with these indications treated with chemotherapy and RT.
- Adjuvant whole-breast radiation after BCT decreases the breast cancer recurrence rate from 30 to <7% at 5 years.

Complications
- Radiation to the chest wall can cause skin changes.
- Infrequent complications include interstitial pneumonitis, spontaneous rib fracture, breast fibrosis, pericarditis, pleural effusion, and chest wall myositis.
- Radiation to the axilla can increase the incidence of lymphedema and axillary fibrosis.
- Angiosarcoma can occur as a late complication.

28. How will you manage a 60-year-old lady with 5 × 5 cm lump in right breast with palpable ipsilateral axillary lymphadenopathy? ***WBUHS 2025 Supplementary***

Managing a *60-year-old woman* with a *5 × 5 cm breast lump* and *palpable ipsilateral axillary lymphadenopathy* raises a high suspicion of *locally advanced breast cancer (LABC).*

29. Discuss the current evidence-based management of locally advanced breast cancer. ***WBUHS 2006***

30. Describe diagnosis and management of locally advanced carcinoma breast [IIIA & IIIB] ***Gujarat Health University 2025***

31. Describe the nonoperative management of carcinoma breast for postmenopausal woman of LABC. ***RGUHS, Karnataka 2025***

Advanced Locoregional Regional Breast Cancer (Stage IIIa or IIIb)

Introduction
- Women with stages IIIa and IIIb breast cancer have advanced locoregional breast cancer.
- Stage IIIa patients are divided into those who have operable disease and those who have inoperable disease.
- Surgical therapy for women with operable stage IIIa disease is usually a MRM, followed by adjuvant chemotherapy, followed by adjuvant RT.
- Adjuvant chemotherapy is used to maximize distant DFS, while RT is used to maximize locoregional DFS.
- In selected stage IIIa patients, initial (neoadjuvant) chemotherapy is used to reduce the size of the primary cancer and permit conservation surgery.
- For inoperable stage IIIa and for stage IIIb breast cancer, NACT is used to decrease the locoregional cancer burden and may permit subsequent surgery to establish locoregional control.
- In this setting, surgery is followed by adjuvant chemotherapy and adjuvant RT.

Treatment for LABC will usually involve a combination of treatments:
- Chemotherapy
- Breast surgery
- Radiotherapy
- Targeted therapies
- Hormonal therapies.

Chemotherapy
- Treatment for LABC often starts with chemotherapy.
- The aim of giving chemotherapy first is to make the breast cancer smaller, and to destroy any cancer cells that may be elsewhere in the body, but cannot be detected using routine tests.

Breast Surgery

- Breast surgery may be recommended for some women with LABC.
- Breast reconstruction may be possible once all initial treatment has been completed but this should be discussed with the treating doctors.

Radiotherapy

Radiotherapy may be used before or after surgery for LABC to destroy cancer cells in the breast, armpit, neck, or surrounding areas.

Targeted Therapies

- Targeted are drugs that stop the growth of particular types of cancer cells.
- Targeted therapies are only suitable for some women.
- They may be used with other breast cancer treatments for LABC.

Hormonal Therapies

- Hormonal therapies used to treat women who have HRs on their breast cancer cells.
- Hormonal therapies may be used alone or with other breast cancer treatments for LABC.

The treatment of LABC must include two major goals:

- Control of locoregional disease and
- Eradication of occult systemic metastases.

The patterns and risk of locoregional recurrence after mastectomy are:

- Functions of the size of the primary tumor
- The degree of regional nodal involvement
- The presence or absence of skin or chest wall involvement, and
- The type of surgical procedure performed.

Patients with LABC have historically had a poor prognosis, and some are initially inoperable. They include:

- Patients with evidence of multiple (≥4) or
- Matted axillary lymph nodes or
- Involvement of the second-echelon nodal basins of the infraclavicular, supraclavicular, and internal mammary lymph nodes (IMLNs).

A clinically distinct but similarly high-risk type of LABC is inflammatory breast cancer.

Breast imaging is important to determine the extent of primary disease and to evaluate for multifocal, multicentric, or contralateral breast cancer.

- *Breast ultrasound:*
  - A bilateral diagnostic mammogram with compression or magnifications views if needed is essential for all breast cancer patients.
  - US may provide additional information regarding breast malignancy and may also be used to evaluate the axilla.
  - US-guided biopsy may be performed for enlarged lymph nodes or lymph nodes demonstrating architectural distortion.
  - The sensitivity of US is low.
- *Magnetic resonance imaging:*
  - It is an important tool in evaluating the extent of disease for LABC.
  - It is useful for detecting abnormal lymph nodes and contralateral disease.
  - It may aid in determining if a mastectomy is feasible without neoadjuvant therapy.
  - MRI can also be used for evaluating response to NACT.
- *CT scan and bone scan:* Because of the high probability of, metastatic disease in patients with LABC, imaging studies including bone scan and CT of the upper abdomen and chest are useful.

- *PET:* PET is sometimes used in lieu of CT of the chest and abdomen, and sometimes bone scan.

Notes:

- For operable patients undergoing mastectomy without irradiation, certain subgroups at higher risk for recurrence were identified.
- The clinical and pathologic status of axillary nodes was found to be an important indicator of preoperative RT was able to convert over 80% of patients to operable status and allow them to undergo mastectomy.
- A randomized trial in stage III breast cancer patients from Helsinki has clearly shown the efficacy of combining all three therapeutic modalities of surgery, chemotherapy, and RT.
  - In this trial, 120 patients with stage IIIA breast cancer were randomized to one of three arms after MRM: Locoregional irradiation alone, systemic VAC (vincristine, adriamycin, and cyclophosphamide) chemotherapy (with or without levamisole), or both VAC and irradiation.
  - At both 3 and 5 years, RT reduced local failures relative to the chemotherapy arm, whereas VAC reduced the number of distant failures.
  - The best DFS and local control rates were seen in the combined-modality arm.

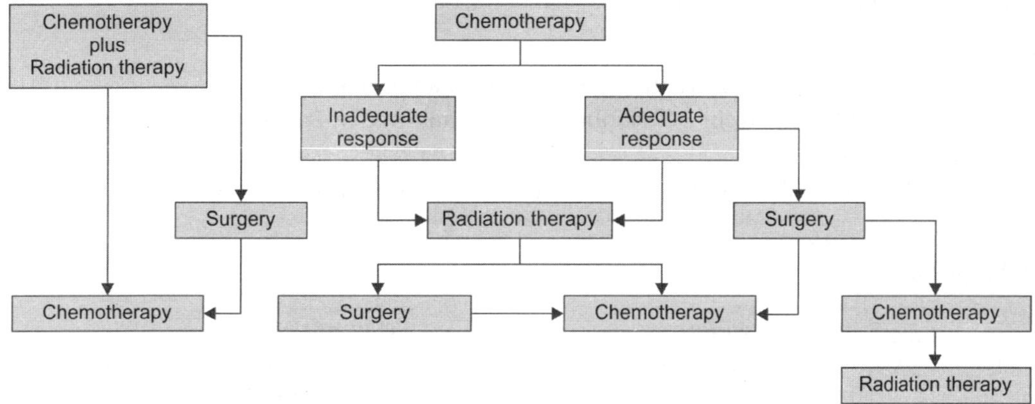

- Although screening mammography has resulted in proportionally fewer cases, LABC remains a difficult clinical problem due to the high rate of relapse and low rate of OS.
- The range of disease encompassed by the term locally advanced is wide and includes patients with large, but operable, primary tumors to patients with rapidly progressing inflammatory carcinomas, who have very different prognoses.
- Thus, treatment decisions must be tailored to the individual patient. Of critical importance in all cases of locally advanced breast tumors is coordination of care among medical oncology, surgical oncology, and radiation oncology, as the vast majority of patients need chemotherapy, surgery, and radiotherapy.
- With continued support of basic and clinical research, further advances in the treatment and prognosis of women with LABC will occur.

Goals of Nonoperative Management

- Downstage the tumor → make it operable (neoadjuvant therapy).
- Control local disease and symptoms (if inoperable).
- Treat systemic micrometastases.
- Improve quality of life and survival.

Components of Nonoperative Management

Neoadjuvant (Primary) Systemic Therapy

- Used before surgery to shrink tumor and control micrometastases.
- Choice depends on receptor status and menopausal state.

A. Endocrine (Hormonal) Therapy

Indicated in postmenopausal, hormone receptor–positive (ER/PR +) tumors.

Drug	Mechanism	Notes
Aromatase inhibitors (Letrozole, Anastrozole, Exemestane)	Block peripheral estrogen synthesis	*Preferred in postmenopausal* women
Tamoxifen	Selective estrogen receptor modulator (SERM)	Alternative if AIs not tolerated
Fulvestrant	ER down-regulator	Used in metastatic/recurrent disease

Duration: Usually 3–6 months before reassessment for operability.

Tumor response monitored clinically and by imaging.

B. Chemotherapy

Used when:

- Tumor is *hormone receptor-negative*
- Rapid response needed (ulceration, bleeding)
- High-grade or inflammatory carcinoma

Common regimens:

- *Anthracycline-based:* FAC (5-FU, Adriamycin, Cyclophosphamide) or FEC
- *Taxane-based:* AC → T (Adriamycin + Cyclophosphamide followed by Paclitaxel or Docetaxel)

Given every 3 weeks × 4–6 cycles.

Response reassessed; if operable → surgery; if not → radiotherapy ± further systemic therapy.

C. Targeted (Biologic) Therapy

Used if HER2-positive.

Drug	Mechanism	Comments
Trastuzumab	Monoclonal antibody against HER2	Combined with chemo (avoid with anthracycline concurrently due to cardiac risk)
Pertuzumab, Lapatinib	Other HER2-targeted agents	Used as per response or resistance

Radiotherapy

Used for:

- *Inoperable LABC* for local control/palliation
- *Postsystemic therapy* when still inoperable
- *Palliative* for ulceration, bleeding, pain, or chest wall recurrence

Dose: 45–50 Gy in 25 fractions over 5 weeks

- Boost to residual lesion if indicated.

Supportive and Palliative Care

- *Analgesics* for pain
- *Wound care* for ulcerated/fungating mass (dressings, odor control with metronidazole)
- *Antibiotics* for secondary infection
- *Psychological support and counseling*
- *Bisphosphonates/Denosumab* if bone metastases present
- *Nutritional and general health optimization*

Assessment of Response

- *Clinical:* Reduction in tumor size, nodal size, and fixation
- *Imaging:* USG/MRI after 3–4 cycles or 3 months of hormonal therapy
- If operable → proceed to *modified radical mastectomy (MRM)* or *breast-conserving surgery* (if suitable).
- If still inoperable → continue *endocrine or radiotherapy palliation.*

Typical Management Plan for Postmenopausal LABC

Step	Treatment
1	Biopsy → confirm diagnosis and ER/PR/HER2 status
2	Start *aromatase inhibitor (Letrozole 2.5 mg daily)*
3	Assess response every 2–3 months
4	If tumor shrinks → proceed to surgery → adjuvant therapy
5	If unresectable → radiotherapy ± continued endocrine therapy
6	Provide symptomatic and palliative care

32. Describe the role of NACT in LABC with relevance to landmark trials. What are the challenges of post-NACT BCS in LABC? ***WBUHS 2022***

33. Discuss the role of NACT in LABC. Discuss the challenges faced in poor responders and how do the challenges can be overcome? ***WBUHS 2024***

Introduction

- Preoperative (neoadjuvant) chemotherapy is used in patients with LABC to reduce tumor volume and allow for definitive surgery.
- It may allow less extensive surgery (e.g., permit breast-conserving surgery in patients who are not candidates for that on initial presentation, or obviate ALND in patients who present with node-positive breast cancer).
- In patients with triple-negative (ER, PR, and HER2) or HER2-positive disease, response to neoadjuvant therapy can guide the selection of adjuvant therapy.

Role of NACT in Breast Cancer

Table of study characteristics as per population, intervention, comparator, and outcome criteria

Study	Information source	Accrual	Accrual period	Population	Intervention	Outcome
Gianni et al., 2009	Full text: Published	902	1996–2002	Operable breast cancer of stage T2-T3, N0-N1, M0	• NACT Arm: 4 × AT + 4 × CMF → (BCS + RT or mast) + TAM for HR + • ACT Arm: BCS + RT or Mast → 4 × AT + 4 × CMF	OS, RFS, LRR, DM, BCS
Taucher et al., 2008	Full text: Published	429	1991–1999	Primary breast cancer patients staged T1-3, N0 or N1 and M0	• NACT Arm: 3 × CMF → BCS/Mast ± RT → 3 × CMF for LN-and 3 × EC for LN + • ACT Arm: BCS/Mast ± RT→ 3 × CMF → 3 × CMF for LN- and 3 × EC for LN +	OS, RFS, LRR, DM, BCS, Toxicity
UK Trial, 2005	Full text: Published	309	1990–1995	Nonmetastatic breast cancer patients of ≤70 years	• NACT Arm: 4 × (3M or 2M) → BCS + RT/ Mast → 4 × (3M or 2M) • ACT Arm: BCS + RT/Mast → 8 × (3M or 2M)	OS, RFS, DM, LRR, BCS
S6 Trial, 1995	Full text: Published	414	1986–1990	Nonmetastatic operable breast tumors of diameter 3–7 cm and with no prior cancer with N0, N1b	• NACT Arm: 4 × CAF → (Mast/BCS)/RT for CR patients • ACT Arm: (Mast/BCS)/RT for CR patients → 4 × CAF	OS, RFS, DM, LRR, BCS, Toxicity
S5, 1991	S5, 1991	196	196	Tb3, N0-1b, M0 breast cancer patients <65 years of age	• NACT Arm: 2 × CAF → RT ± Surgery → 4 × CAF for responders and 4 × AMVT to nonresponders ACT • Arm: RT ± Surgery → 6 × CAF	OS, RFS, LRR, BCS

Contd...

Contd...

Study	Information source	Accrual	Accrual period	Population	Intervention	Outcome
B18, 2008	Full text: Published	1523	1991–1993	Breast cancer patients with operable, palpable breast cancer (T1-3, N0-1, M0)	• NACT Arm: 4 × AC → BCS + RT or MRM • ACT Arm: 4 × AC → BCS + RT or MRM	OS, RFS, DM, LRR, BCS, Toxicity
EORTC, 2009	Full text: Published	698	1991–1999	Primary early breast cancer patients (T1c, T2-3, T4b, N0-1 M0)	• NACT Arm: 4 × FEC → BCS with RT/ • MRM ACT Arm: BCS with RT/MRM → 4 × FEC	OS, RFS, RFS, LRR-, BCS, Toxicity
Forouhi et al., 1995	Full text: Published	79	Not mentioned	Nonmetastatic operable breast cancer larger than 4 cm in maximum diameter	• NACT Arm: ER-: 4 × CAP MRM → 2 × • CAP, ER+: Tamoxifen or Goserelin → • MRM ACT Arm: MRM → 6 × CAP for ER- and Tamoxifen or Goserelin for ER +	Toxicity

(AC: adriamycin and cyclophosphamide; ACT: adjuvant chemotherapy; AMTV: adriamycin, methotrexate, thiotepa, vindesine; AT: adriamycin, taxane; BCS: breast conserving surgery; CAF: cyclophosphamide, adriamycin, and fluorouracil; CAP: cyclophosphamide, adriamycin, and prednisolone; CMF: cyclophosphamide, methotrexate, and 5-fluorouracil; DFS: disease-free survival; DM: distant metastasis; EC: epirubicin and cyclophosphamide; EVM: epirubicin, vincristine, and methotrexate; FEC: fluorouracil, epirubicin, and cyclophosphamide; LN: lymph node; LR: local recurrence; LRR: locoregional recurrence; Mast: mastectomy; MMM/3M: mitoxantrone, methotrexate, and mitomycin; MRM: modified radical mastectomy; MTV: mitomycin, thiotepa, vindesine; NACT: neoadjuvant chemotherapy; OS: overall survival; RFS: relapse-free survival; RM: radical mastectomy; RR: regional recurrence; RT: radiotherapy; TAM: tamoxifen; TMF: thiotepa, methotrexate, 5-fluorouracil; 2M: mitoxantrone and methotrexate; → : followed by)

- RCTs have compared the effectiveness among different patient-related characteristics, varying chemotherapy regimens, and variable end points.
  - A number of RCTs have reported NACT to be beneficial in terms of oncological outcomes as well as functional outcomes NACT may be a preferred choice.
  - NACT is a type of chemotherapy that is administered before surgery in patients with breast cancer.
  - Overall, NACT plays an important role in the management of LABC and is often recommended as part of a multimodal treatment approach.

Role of NACT in LABC

Tumor Downstaging

- NACT reduces the size of the primary tumor and involved lymph nodes, potentially converting inoperable tumors to operable ones.
- Enables breast-conserving surgery (BCS) instead of mastectomy in some patients.

Early Systemic Control

Addresses micrometastatic disease early, which may improve overall survival and disease-free survival.

Biological Response Assessment

- Provides an in vivo assessment of tumor sensitivity to chemotherapy, allowing for prognostication and therapy modification.

Pathological Complete Response (pCR) as a Surrogate Marker

- Achieving pCR is associated with better long-term outcomes, especially in aggressive subtypes like triple-negative and HER2-positive breast cancers.
  - However, this may raise an issue in achieving adequate loco-regional control because of the difficulty of assessing tumor margins after the administration of NACT.
  - Several studies investigated the oncologic safety of BCS after NACT, however data concerning loco-regional recurrence rates are discordant.
  - In particular, there are a few studies evaluating long-term results after NACT with controversial findings.

Challenges in Poor Responders to NACT

Poor responders are patients who show minimal or no reduction in tumor size or progression during NACT. Challenges include:

Limited Surgical Options

Persistent tumor bulk may prevent breast-conserving surgery, necessitating mastectomy or more extensive surgeries.

Worse Prognosis

Poor response is associated with higher recurrence rates and poorer overall survival, especially in triple-negative breast cancer (TNBC).

Treatment Toxicity Without Benefit

Patients endure side effects of chemotherapy without significant clinical gain.

Delay in Definitive Surgery

Continued ineffective treatment may delay surgery, allowing disease progression.

Strategies to Overcome Challenges in Poor Responders

Early Response Monitoring

- Use imaging (MRI, ultrasound, PET-CT) and biomarkers to assess response after 1–2 cycles.
- If poor response is evident early, consider switching chemotherapy regimens or escalating therapy.

Molecular Subtyping and Biomarker-Guided Therapy

- Tailor NACT based on receptor status (ER, PR, HER2) and genomic profiling.
- *For HER2-positive:* Add targeted agents like trastuzumab and pertuzumab.
- *For TNBC:* Consider adding immunotherapy (e.g., checkpoint inhibitors) or platinum-based regimens.

Adaptive Clinical Trials

Enroll poor responders in trials evaluating novel agents (e.g., antibody-drug conjugates, PARP inhibitors).

Multidisciplinary Decision Making

Regular MDT meetings to re-evaluate management strategies, ensuring timely transition to surgery or radiation if response is suboptimal.

Post-NACT Adjuvant Therapy Adjustments

Consider additional adjuvant therapy based on residual disease (e.g., capecitabine for TNBC, T-DM1 for HER2+ residual disease)

Breast conservation surgery (BCS) after neoadjuvant chemotherapy (NACT) is a common treatment approach for locally advanced breast cancer. However, this treatment approach can present several challenges, including:

- *Difficulty in achieving negative surgical margins:*
  - NACT can lead to tumor shrinkage, making it difficult to determine the extent of the tumor and the appropriate margins to remove during surgery.
  - This can increase the risk of positive surgical margins and the need for further surgery.
- *Compromised breast shape and symmetry:*
  - NACT can cause changes in breast volume, shape, and symmetry, which can make it difficult to achieve good cosmetic outcomes.
  - This can lead to dissatisfaction with the appearance of the breast after surgery.
- *Increased risk of complications:*
  - NACT can increase the risk of complications during and after surgery, such as wound healing problems, infections, and bleeding.
  - This can lead to longer hospital stays, delayed recovery, and increased healthcare costs.

- *Difficulty in assessing response to treatment:*
    - NACT can make it difficult to assess the response to treatment and the extent of residual disease before surgery.
    - This can impact the decision-making process for the extent of surgery needed and the need for additional treatment.
- *Need for multidisciplinary approach:*
    - The management of locally advanced breast cancer requires a multidisciplinary approach involving medical oncologists, radiation oncologists, and breast surgeons.
    - Coordination and communication among the different specialties are crucial to ensure optimal treatment outcomes.
        - Overall, BCS after NACT can present several challenges, but with careful planning and management, it remains a viable option for the treatment of locally advanced breast cancer.

IMPALPABLE BREAST LESION

34. How are impalpable breast cancers managed? ***WBUHS 2019***

Breast cancer is the most common cancer diagnosed in the United States, after skin cancer. It is the second leading cause of cancer deaths in women today, after lung cancer. Patients seek medical attention most commonly for an abnormal screening mammogram, a palpable breast mass, breast pain, nipple discharge or skin changes over the breast.

- In most cases, there is a palpable breast lump at presentation, which is discovered by the patient during self breast examination and confirmed by imaging techniques and core needle biopsy as a part of triple assessment.
- There are some early malignant lesions, which are not palpable at presentation, but detected only on imaging. These are known as nonpalpable Ca Breast (NPCB).
- NPCB includes mammographic abnormalities like clustered micro calcifications and areas of abnormal density (architectural distortions and asymmetries) that have not yet produced a palpable finding.
- To avoid unnecessary biopsies for low suspicion nonpalpable mammographic findings, probably benign lesions are designated as BI-RADS 3 and are monitored with short interval mammograms for over a 2 years period during which biopsies are performed for only those lesions which progress during the follow up.
- Almost 75 to 80 % of patients for whom diagnostic biopsy of a nonpalpable mammographic lesion is recommended, have benign findings. Hence, less invasive and less costly image-guided core needle biopsy approach is preferred whenever feasible.

    If the diagnosis is not concordant with imaging findings or there is Atypical Ductal Hyperplasia in a field of microcalcifications that may represent Ductal Carcinoma In Situ (DCIS), most patients should proceed to excisional biopsy for definitive diagnosis.

    - To ensure that the abnormality is completely excised, it should be localized with either a localizing wire or ^{125}I (radioactive Iodine) seed that can be placed adjacent to the lesion under mammographic or ultrasound guidance.
    - Depending on the size of the lesion and the degree of suspicion of malignancy, generally a border of normal tissue around the lesion is also excised to ensure complete removal with a negative margin.
    - After excision, the specimen is sent for specimen radiography to confirm that the targeted lesion has been excised. Patients who have a diagnosis of benign findings on excision should undergo new baseline mammography 4 to 6 months after the surgical procedure.
    - Although wire localization is the most common technique used to localize nonpalpable lesions to facilitate surgical resection, the technique has limitations, including patient discomfort, risk of wire displacement, and a logistic problem because the wire must be placed on the day of surgery.

- Other techniques have been developed to facilitate resection of nonpalpable lesions, including radioactive seed localization, which involves positioning 4.5-mm ^{125}I seeds in the breast tissue, deployed from a preloaded needle under mammographic or ultrasound guidance. Images with the seed in place guide the surgeon.
- In the operating room, a gamma probe, which detects technetium-99m (99mTc), commonly used for sentinel lymph node dissection (SLND), and ^{125}I, can be used to guide the resection. After excision, the specimen is sent for specimen radiography to confirm that the targeted lesion and radioactive seed have been excised.
- In a single-institution report of an initial experience using radioactive seed localization, it was reported that compared with use of localizing wires, use of seeds improved operating room efficiency, and the volume of tissue excised and rates of negative margins were comparable for wire and seed localization.

After biopsy confirmation of the suspicious lesion, we stage the patient appropriately and then can proceed for a definitive surgical plan.

- The selection of surgical procedures takes into account patient characteristics and other clinical and pathologic variables. Patient characteristics, including age, family history, menopausal status, and overall health, are assessed.
- Some patients may undergo genetic testing for *BRCA* gene mutations at the time of diagnosis. Patients with a known mutation are generally counseled toward bilateral mastectomy for treatment of the index breast and reduction of the risk of contralateral breast cancer.
- The location of the tumor within the breast and tumor size relative to breast size are evaluated. Patient preferences for breast preservation versus mastectomy are determined. For patients considering mastectomy, options for immediate reconstruction are discussed.
- Usually in NPCB, the preferred approach is Breast Conservation Surgery (BCS) with SLND ± Axillary clearance followed by Adjuvant Radiotherapy.
- Adjuvant chemotherapy needs to be added if there is axillary lymph node involvement. The breast specimen that is removed is oriented and its edges are inked before sectioning.
- Specimen radiography should be performed for all nonpalpable lesions or if there are microcalcifications associated with the palpable tumor. If a margin appears to be close or is positive histologically on intraoperative assessment (frozen section biopsy), reexcision to remove more tissue frequently achieves a clear margin and allows conservation of the breast.
- Orientation of the surgical specimen allows focal reexcision of involved margins rather than global reexcision and improves the cosmetic result by reducing the amount of normal breast parenchyma that is excised.
- The surgical defect created after lumpectomy is closed in cosmetic fashion, after placing metal clips in the cavity to guide the future radiotherapy.
- There is increasing interest in the use of advancement flap closure and other oncoplastic surgical techniques to maximize the cosmetic result.

AXILLA

35. Describe the surgical anatomy of axilla. Discuss about the diseases that implicate it. ***WBUHS 2006***

Introduction

- The axilla is the area on the human body directly under the joint where the arm connects to the shoulder.
- It contains the axillary vessels, and the brachial plexus of nerves, with their branches, some branches of the intercostal nerves, and a large number of lymph glands, together with a quantity of fat and loose areolar tissue.

Boundaries and Structures in Relation

- The axillary artery and vein, with the brachial plexus of nerves, extend obliquely along the lateral boundary of the axilla, from its apex to its base, and are placed much nearer to the anterior than to the posterior wall, the vein lying to the thoracic side of the artery and partially concealing it.

- At the forepart of the axilla, in contact with the pectorales, are the thoracic branches of the axillary artery, and along the lower margin of the pectoralis minor the lateral thoracic artery extends to the side of the chest.
- At the back part, in contact with the lower margin of the subscapularis, are the subscapular vessels and nerves; winding around the lateral border of this muscle are the scapular circumflex vessels; and, close to the neck of the humerus, the posterior humeral circumflex vessels and the axillary nerve curve backward to the shoulder.
- Along the medial or thoracic side no vessel of any importance exists, the upper part of the space being crossed merely by a few small branches from the highest thoracic artery.
- There are some important nerves, however, in this situation, viz., the long thoracic nerve, descending on the surface of the serratus anterior, to which it is distributed; and the intercostobrachial nerve, perforating the upper and anterior part of this wall, and passing across the axilla to the medial side of the arm.

Boundaries

Superiorly: By the outer border of first rib, superior border of scapula, and posterior border of clavicle	*Anteriorly:* By the pectoral is major, minor, and subclavius posteriorly: by the subscapularis above, and teres major and latissimus dorsi below	*Medially:* By serratus anterior and by the rib cage	*Laterally:* By the intertubercular sulcus (coracobrachialis and the short head of the biceps brachii are in the axilla)	*Floor/base:* By the skin (visible surface of armpit)

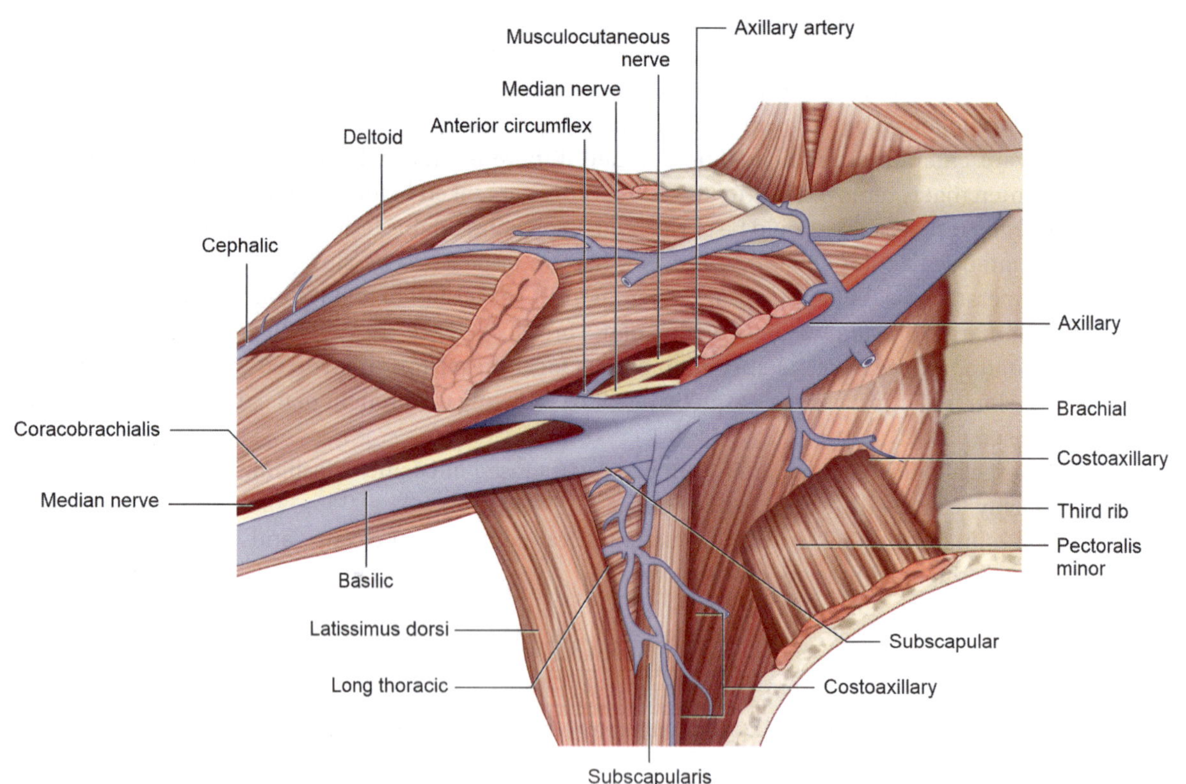

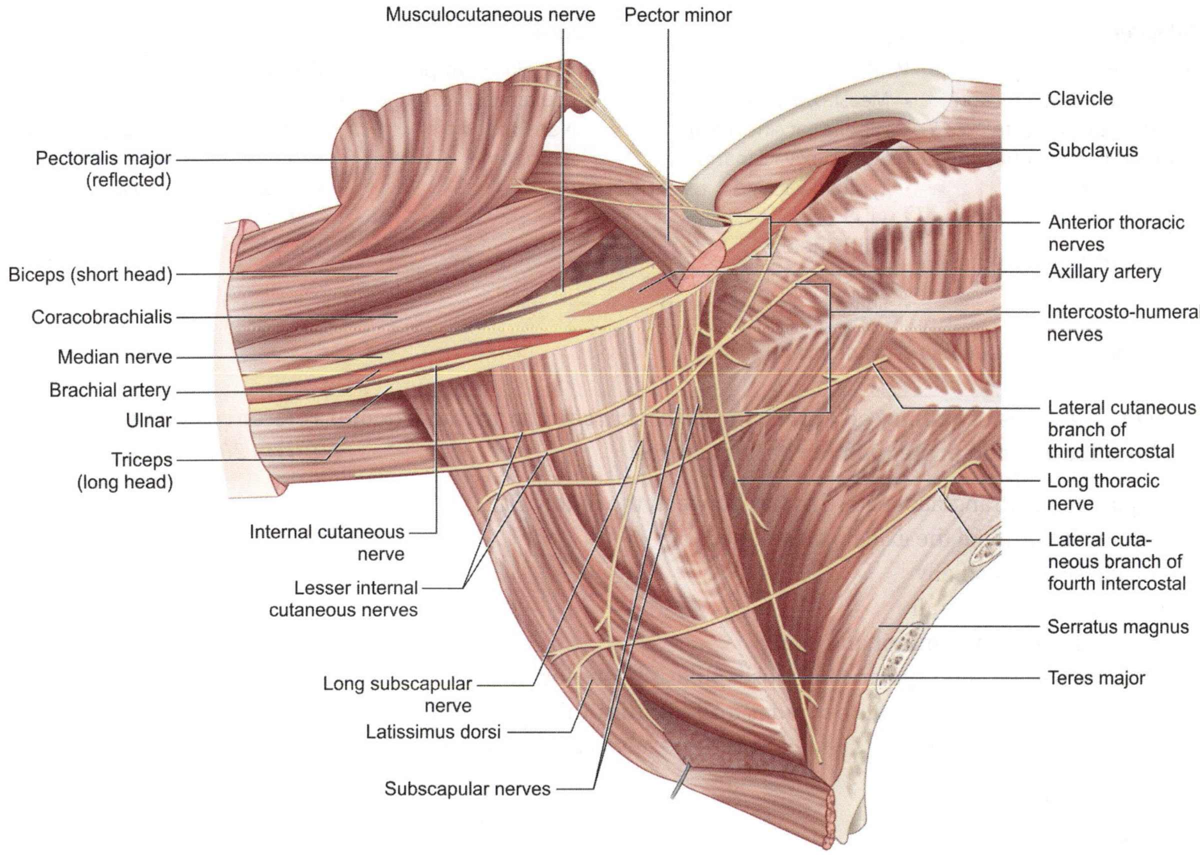

Diseases Implicating Axilla

- Lumps in the axilla have various causes.
- Cysts and infections on the surface of the skin of the armpit may be caused by shaving or use of antiperspirants (as opposed to deodorants). This occurs most frequently in adolescents just beginning to shave. Abscesses under the skin may also produce large, painful lumps in the armpit.
- Lumps may occur when lymph nodes are swollen due to bacterial or viral infections, vaccinations, and cancer.
- Lymph nodes are filters that can catch infectious organisms or cancerous tumor cells. When it happens, lymph nodes increase in size and are easily felt. An armpit lump in a woman should be checked by a healthcare provider immediately, as it may be a sign of breast cancer.

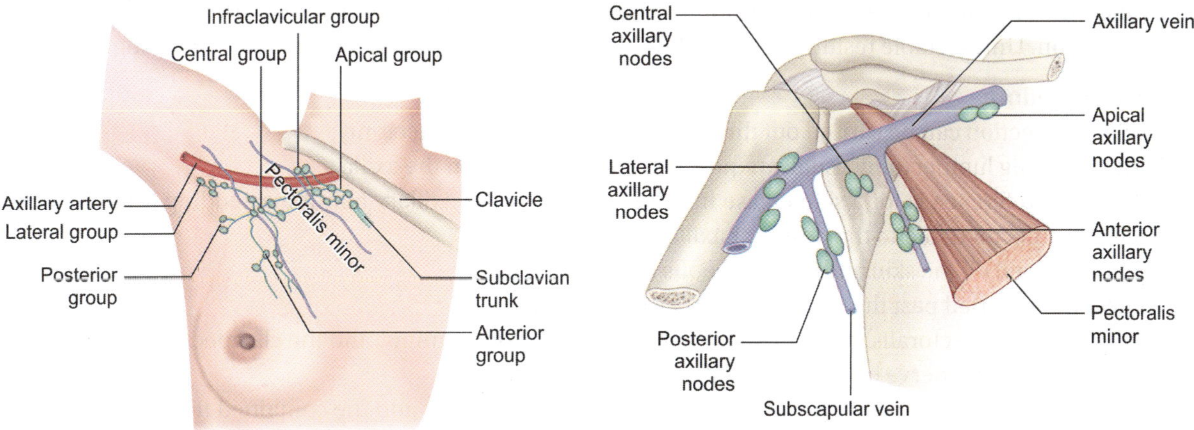

Lymph nodes of the axilla.

Infection		*Cancer*	*Other*
Bacterial: • Arm or breast infection • Cat scratch disease • Ascending lymphangitis • Lymphadenitis *Fungal:* • Sporotrichosis	*Viral:* • Measles, mumps, and rubella vaccine (rare) • Smallpox vaccination • Typhoid vaccine • AIDS • Chickenpox • Infectious mononucleosis • Shingles (herpes zoster)	• Hodgkin's lymphoma • Leukemia • Non-Hodgkin's lymphoma	• Benign cyst • Lipoma • Normal breast tissue (breast tissue extends into the armpit area) • Allergic reaction possibly caused by sulfa drugs, iodine, or penicillin • Vaccinations

(AIDS: acquired immunodeficiency syndrome)

36. Describe the steps of axillary clearance for breast carcinoma with particular reference to anatomical guides for identification and protection of vital structures. ***WBUHS 2016; RIMS, Imphal 2022***

The axilla is a quadrangular space that lies between the following:
- The lower border of the axillary vein superiorly
- The chest wall medially
- The axillary skin laterally
- Pectoralis major and minor anteriorly
- Latissimus dorsi, teres major, and subscapularis posteriorly

Axillary dissection removes all the nodes and fat from this space. Although the nodes are in a continuum, the clearance can be anatomically divided into three levels based on the relationship of the tissue to the pectoralis minor muscle.

Technique
- The extent of ALND within the above boundaries is defined as level I (lateral to the pectoralis minor), level I-II (extending behind the minor), or level I-III (extending to the apex of the axilla, "Halsted's ligament"), and should be based on tumor characteristics, patient anatomy, and intraoperative findings.
- ALND should be sufficient to remove all gross evidence of disease and should in general contain at least 10 nodes.
- Palpably suspicious Rotter's (interpectoral) nodes should be removed if present.
- The pectoralis minor may be divided or excised to facilitate exposure and removal of gross disease at levels II and III.
- The long thoracic, thoracodorsal, and medial pectoral nerves should be identified and, unless grossly involved by tumor, preserved.
- If anatomically suitable, the T2 (intercostobrachial) and T3 sensory nerves may be preserved at the discretion of the surgeon. Unresectable residual disease should be clipped to facilitate RT treatment planning.

Surgical Procedure
- Axillary dissection can be carried out through the incision for a mastectomy.
- Patients having lumpectomy usually require a separate incision in the axilla.
- Often, the preference is for a skin crease incision just below the axillary hairline extending from the posterior edge of the pectoral fold to the posterior axillary line.
- Flaps are raised off the skin and subcutaneous tissue.
- Dissection is carried past the edge of pectoralis major muscle.
- Retraction of the pectoralis major medially exposes the pectoralis minor and the clavipectoral fascia.
- The lateral pectoral nerve bundle is identified and preserved.
- Incision into the clavipectoral fascia allows entry into the axillary fat and the contained nodes.
- These are removed en bloc through the surgery.

- Dissection is carried superiorly along the edge of the pectoralis minor to reach the inferior edge of the axillary vein.
- Once the axillary vein is identified, this is followed medially to reach the axillary apex, where the axillary vein crosses the lateral border of the first rib.
- The axillary contents are then separated from the lateral thoracic wall, which is the medial boundary of the axilla.
- This exposes the long thoracic nerve, which supplies the serratus anterior muscle (injury to which would lead to winging of the scapula).
- During this dissection, branches of the intercostobrachial nerve will be identified as they cross the axilla after emerging from the intercostal spaces.
- The larger trunks should be preserved if possible.
- Ligation and division of the smaller tributaries of the axillary vein as they enter the axilla allows visualization and identification of the subscapular vessels and thoracodorsal nerve as they reach the subscapular and latissimus dorsi muscles posteriorly.
- The axillary fat and nodal tissue between the long thoracic nerve and the subscapular vascular bundle is carefully dissected.
- Often, this is performed en bloc with the specimen, although it sometimes can occur separately if there is extensive nodal involvement.
- The dissection then proceeds toward the apex to include the nodes medial to the pectoralis minor (level III). This is facilitated by flexion of the free draped arm at the shoulder.
- The axillary fat and nodes are finally separated from the axillary tail of the breast to allow the specimen to be excised.
- Careful pathological examination for an axillary dissection will often reveal in excess of 20 lymph nodes.
- The wound is closed in layers over a suction drain.

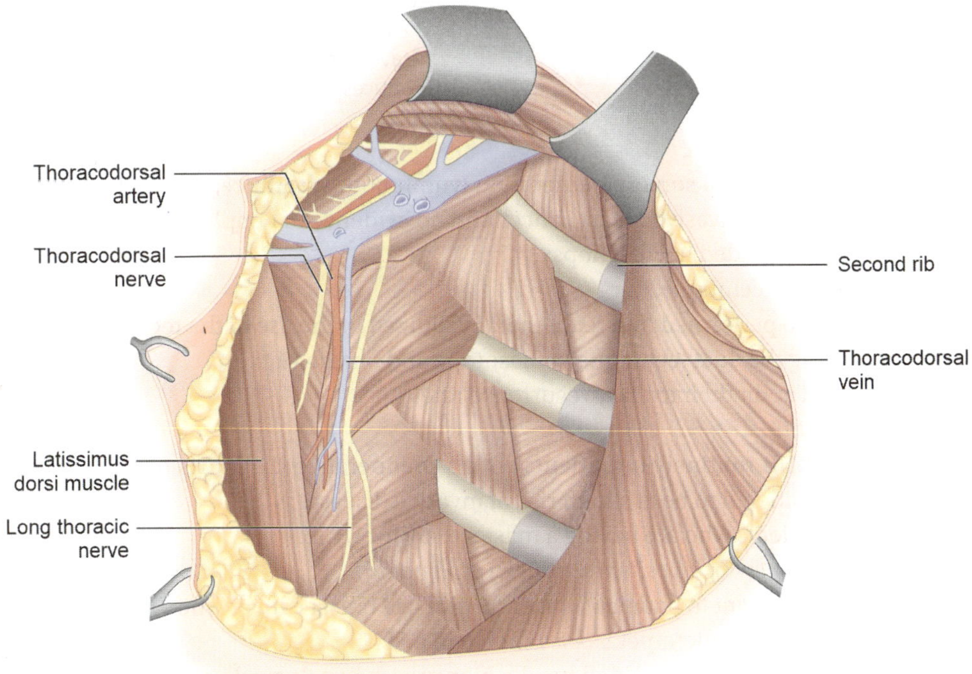

Axillary dissection.

37. Discuss recent trends regarding management of axilla in breast cancer. ***WBUHS 2012***

38. Discuss the current status in management of axilla for breast carcinoma including the landmark trials. ***Tripura University 2025***

Introduction

- The role of axillary surgery in breast cancer is to stage the axilla and in those with lymph node metastases to treat the axilla with axillary clearance.
- Adequate axillary dissection is important in node-positive patients both to ensure removal of all involved nodes to optimize local control and to obtain the maximum prognostic information.
- When staging the axilla, an additional goal, particularly in node-negative patients, is to minimize morbidity.
- Various strategies for doing so have been developed, *the most recent being dual localization SLNB.*
    - SLN mapping has become the standard axillary surgery used for patients who present with Stage I and Stage II breast cancer.
    - This procedure is performed in conjunction with the breast surgery (lumpectomy or mastectomy) or as a stand-alone operation to help determine the patient's need for chemotherapy prior to surgery or eligibility for breast reconstruction procedures.
    - For patients whose SLNs are negative by pathologic review, no additional axillary surgery is recommended.

Arguments for axillary clearance	*Arguments for axillary sampling*
• Axillary clearance both stages and treats the axilla • Sampling potentially misses nodes and understages the axilla • Surgical clearance possibly gains better local control • Avoids complications of axillary radiotherapy • Avoids morbidity of axillary recurrence	• Only stages the axilla • Must be followed by axillary radiotherapy • The 60% of patients with node negative disease have unnecessary surgery • Radical lymphadenectomy in other cancers (e.g., melanoma) produces disappointing results • Avoids morbidity of axillary surgery • The combination of axillary clearance and radiotherapy is to be avoided • Produces unacceptable rate of lymphedema

Surgery to the Axilla

- *Invasive breast cancer:* Minimal surgery, rather than lymph node clearance, should be performed to stage the axilla for patients with early invasive breast cancer and no evidence of lymph node involvement on ultrasound or a negative ultrasound-guided needle biopsy.
    - SLNB is the preferred technique.
    - SLNB should only be performed by a team that is validated in the use of the technique.
    - Perform SLNB using the dual technique with isotope and blue dye.
    - Breast units should audit their axillary recurrence rates.
- *Ductal carcinoma in situ:*
    - Do not perform SLNB routinely in patients with a preoperative diagnosis of DCIS who are having BCS, unless they are considered to be at a high risk of invasive disease.
    - Offer SLNB to all patients who are having a mastectomy for DCIS.
- *Evaluation and management of a positive sentinel lymph node:*
  Offer further axillary treatment to patients with early invasive breast cancer who:
    - Have macrometastases or micrometastases shown in a SLN
    - Have a preoperative ultrasound-guided needle biopsy with histologically proven metastatic cancer.
        - The preferred technique is ALND because it gives additional staging information.
        - Do not offer further axillary treatment to patients found to have only isolated tumor cells in their SLNs. These patients should be regarded as lymph node-negative.

Landmark Trials Shaping Axillary Management

NSABP B-04 (1970s–1980s)

- *Question:* Does radical ALND improve survival in clinically node-negative patients?
- *Findings:*
    - No difference in *overall survival* between radical mastectomy, total mastectomy with ALND, or total mastectomy alone with delayed ALND if nodes became positive.
    - *Conclusion:* Immediate ALND not necessary in all node-negative patients.

NSABP B-32 (2005)

- *Population:* Clinically node-negative, early-stage breast cancer.
- *Comparison:* SLNB vs ALND.
- *Findings:*
    - SLNB accurately staged axilla.
    - *No difference in overall survival or disease-free survival.*
    - Reduced lymphedema, sensory loss, and shoulder morbidity.
- *Conclusion:* SLNB is standard for clinically node-negative patients.

ACOSOG Z0011 (2011)

- *Population:* Women with T1–T2 invasive breast cancer, clinically node-negative, undergoing *breast-conserving surgery and whole breast radiation*, with *1–2 positive sentinel nodes.*
- *Comparison:* SLNB alone vs SLNB + ALND.
- *Findings:*
    - *No difference in overall survival or local recurrence.*
    - ALND did *not provide additional survival benefit.*
- *Impact:* ALND can be *omitted in select patients with limited sentinel node metastasis.*

AMAROS Trial (2014)

- *Population:* Clinically node-negative with positive SLN.
- *Comparison:* ALND vs axillary radiotherapy (ART).
- *Findings:*
    - *Axillary recurrence similar* in both groups.
    - *Less lymphedema* with ART.
- *Conclusion:* Axillary RT is a safe alternative to ALND in selected patients.

IBCSG 23-01 (2013)

- *Population:* SLN micrometastases only.
- *Findings:* ALND did not improve disease-free or overall survival.
- *Conclusion:* ALND can be safely omitted for micrometastases in clinically node-negative patients.

Current Guidelines/Status

- *Clinically node-negative axilla (cN0):*
    - *SLNB* is standard.
    - *ALND* is generally avoided unless:
        - 2 positive SLNs
        - Nonsentinel node disease with extracapsular extension (individualized)
- *Clinically node-positive axilla (cN1) before neoadjuvant therapy:*
    - *ALND* standard.
    - *Neoadjuvant therapy* may *downstage axilla,* allowing SLNB post-treatment in selected patients.
- *SLN positive patients:*
    - *1–2 SLN positive,* breast-conserving surgery + radiation → *ALND can be omitted* (Z0011 criteria).
    - *Micrometastases* → ALND often omitted (IBCSG 23-01).

- *Axillary radiotherapy:* Considered *alternative to ALND* in SLN-positive patients if ALND is omitted (AMAROS trial).

39. Discuss various complications of axillary dissection and their management. ***WBUHS 2020***

- *Various complications of axillary dissection:*
  - The patient may feel discomfort and soreness at the wound site, which is generally managed by taking mild analgesics.
  - A slight risk of wound infection exists after breast surgery, which may result in wound breakdown.
  - Hematoma generally develops within 24 hours after the operation. It is a very rare complication.
  - Patients may notice swelling of the wound site and bruising over the breast or axilla.
  - The observed rates of seroma after axillary surgery range from 2.5 to 51%. It may necessitate needle drainage on one or multiple occasions.
  - Shoulder stiffness is a temporary and self-limited side effect. Physiotherapy can be beneficial.
  - Lymphedema of the arm and breast constitutes a significant long-term sequelae to axillary dissection. This is minimized by limiting the dissection superior to the axillary vein. Studies of reverse axillary mapping may modify the approach to the axilla in the future.
  - A numb patch on the upper arm may be caused by division of intercostobrachial nerve.
- *Precautions during operation:*
  - Care should be taken to ensure the long thoracic nerve is visible and protected as the dissection proceeds to the apex of the axilla.
  - It is often retracted away from chest wall toward the specimen with the traction applied.
  - In cases with excessive nodal involvement, an approach through the interpectoral space is useful.
  - The pectoralis minor is retracted laterally and the pectoralis major medially with the dissection carried out through this space to reach level III.
  - Small vessels at the apex are carefully taken with diathermy.
- *Pre- and postoperative measures:*
  - The patient can be taught a full range of shoulder exercises preoperatively. The range of shoulder movement should be assessed preoperatively.
  - Postoperatively, the same exercises are encouraged to ensure full mobility.
  - Patients are generally advised to avoid any heavy lifting with the arm on the side of the cancer, which will potentially reduce risk of lymphedema and also avoid any unnecessary trauma, including iatrogenic intervention on that arm to reduce risk of infection.

CONTROVERSIES REGARDING THE MANAGEMENT OF PRIMARY LESION IN PRESENCE OF DISTANT METASTASIS IN BREAST CANCER

40. Mention the controversies regarding the management of primary lesion in presence of distant metastasis in breast cancer. ***WBUHS 2020***

Controversies regarding the management of primary lesion in presence of distant metastasis in breast cancer:

- Cure is not possible for these patients, because the cancer cells have spread throughout the body. The aim of treatment is to "prolong survival and palliate symptoms".
- Hormone therapy, chemotherapy and molecular targeted agents are administered, according to their predicted of efficacies, as systemic therapies.
- Recently, appropriate use of new drugs, becoming available annually, has allowed long-term control of symptoms due to metastases and has prolonged the lives of patients. In addition, there have been remarkable advances in diagnostic imaging examinations.

- Extremely small metastases that could not previously be visualized by traditional imaging modalities now can be detected with advanced technology.
- Stage IV breast cancer with small metastases is referred to as minimal Stage IV disease and these patients may have a better prognosis than those with standard Stage IV breast cancer.
- The concept of "oligometastasis" is currently being debated. According to this concept, even distant metastases, depending on their location and number, can potentially be cured with an aggressive treatment strategy that includes surgery.
- Resection of a primary tumor is not actively recommended by guidelines due to lack of high-level evidence indicating prognostic benefit.
- While clinical experience indicates that resection can be useful for alleviating chest symptoms, such as bleeding and ulceration as well as pain due to invasion of the chest wall, no studies or prospective trials have determined whether or not earlier surgery achieves better local control and/or prolongs survival.
- Several recent retrospective studies have demonstrated that resection increases survival time.
- The efficacy of and indications for surgery, as part of an optimal treatment strategy for Stage IV breast cancer tailored to individual situations, require evaluation.
- Defining the role of surgery for Stage IV breast cancer may substantially alter future treatment strategies.
- Distant metastasis is a systemic disease. Cancer cells have already spread throughout the systemic circulation by the time distant metastases are detected. Thus, local therapies do not affect OS.
- Moreover, Fisher et al. raised the possibility that primary tumor resection may promote the progression of distant metastases.
- This might be attributable to resection of the primary tumor triggering surgical dissemination with increased adhesion of circulating tumor cells to the vascular endothelium of target organs, surgery-induced immunosuppression, surgery-induced angiogenic switch or the inflammatory cascade.
- There are several other theories possibly explaining the basic rationale for resection of the primary tumor increasing the survival time of patients with Stage IV breast cancer.
- A reduction in circulating tumor cells according to primary tumor resection reportedly correlates with prognosis.
- Moreover, cancer stem cells, found mainly in the primary tumor, tend to be resistant to systemic drugs.
- Resection of the primary tumor can reduce the tumor volume, including that of cancer stem cells, thereby reactivating autoimmunity and increasing the efficacy of systemic therapies.
- In addition, the concept of "cell seeding" highlights the important features of cancer cells comprising the primary tumor.
- This concept suggests that cancer cells released into the blood from the primary tumor return to be activated in the primary tumor.
- Both of these hypothetical mechanisms are based on the results of basic experiments.
- It is very important to demonstrate similar results clinically by conducting prospective studies.
- At present, whether primary tumor resection for Stage IV breast cancer provides any clinical benefit is unclear.
- According to the results obtained in two trials, routine surgery for all Stage IV breast cancer patients is not warranted, though some do obtain benefits from surgery and it is necessary to establish reliable means of identifying such patients.
- Till date robust and definitive evidence supporting the use of surgery is lacking.
- Breast cancer is not a single disease and there are subtypes which must be considered when devising individual treatment strategies.
- Disease control can be achieved by appropriately using systemic chemotherapeutic agents, based on analyses of cancer biology.
- The treatment goals for Stage IV breast cancer are to prolong the patient's survival time and to control symptoms. Detailed examinations of the results of ongoing clinical trials are anticipated to provide the high-level evidence necessary to optimize the treatments that can be offered to the patients.

- An effective strategy for treating Stage IV breast cancer must incorporate both symptom amelioration and survival prolongation, while remaining mindful of the significance of surgery.
- Recent therapeutic developments, such as the introduction of new cytotoxic agents (taxanes, vinorelbine, capecitabine, gemcitabine, liposomal anthracyclines, etc.), newer hormonal agents, (third-generation AIs and fulvestrant), and biological therapies (trastuzumab, lapatinib, and bevacizumab), have resulted in constant improvements in treatment efficacy and consequently in metastatic breast cancer outcome.

RADIOTHERAPY IN CARCINOMA BREAST

41. Radiotherapy in carcinoma breast. *WBUHS 2019*

Radiation therapy for breast cancer may be delivered in two ways:

- External radiation.
- Internal radiation (brachytherapy)

Radiation after Lumpectomy

After a lumpectomy for breast cancer, RT is typically used.

- *External beam radiation of the whole breast:* The most common types of RT after a lumpectomy is external beam radiation of the whole breast (whole-breast irradiation).
- *Partial-breast irradiation:*
    - For some women with early-stage breast cancer, partial-breast radiation may be an option.
    - The RT is directed to the area around where the tumor was removed, which is at highest risk of having any remaining cancer cells.
    - This radiation can be delivered internally with brachytherapy or externally with X-rays (photons) or protons.
    - Because a smaller area is treated, treatment schedules may be shorter, such as one to two treatments a day over 3–5 days.

Radiation after Mastectomy

- Removal of the entire breast (mastectomy) does not eliminate the risk of recurrence in the remaining tissues of the chest wall or lymph nodes.
- In many situations, the risk of recurrence is high enough that radiation is recommended after mastectomy.
- This type of radiation is called postmastectomy RT and is typically administered 5 days a week for 5–6 weeks.
- Factors that may put you at a high enough risk of breast cancer recurrence in your chest wall or lymph nodes to warrant consideration of radiation after mastectomy include:
    - *Lymph nodes with signs of breast cancer:* Axillary lymph nodes that test positive for cancer cells are an indication that some cancer cells have spread from the primary tumor.
    - *Large tumor size:* A tumor greater than about 2 inches (5 cm) generally carries a higher risk of recurrence than do smaller tumors.
    - *Tissue margins with signs of breast cancer:* After breast tissue is removed, the margins of the tissue are examined for signs of cancer cells. Very narrow margins or margins that test positive for cancer cells are a risk factor for recurrence.

Radiation for LABC

RT can also be used to treat:

- Breast tumors that cannot be surgically removed
- IBC

Radiation for Managing Metastatic Breast Cancer

If breast cancer has spread to other parts of your body (metastasized) and a tumor is causing pain or some other symptom, radiation can be used to shrink the tumor and ease that symptom.

Proton Therapy

- Proton therapy offers more precise radiation dose delivery to the treatment target and protection of nearby healthy tissue.
- This is because proton beams, unlike X-rays, do not travel beyond the target.
- Therefore, researchers hope that proton therapy will decrease the risk of serious long-term complications of RT.
- However, proton therapy still carries risk of side effects because the targeted area may contain skin, muscle, nerves, and other important tissue.
- Proton therapy is being researched in patients with early-stage and LABC.

42. Intraoperative radiotherapy for breast cancer. *WBUHS 2007*

Introduction

- Intraoperative radiotherapy (IORT) is an alternative to conventional postoperative radiotherapy for treatment of early stage invasive breast cancer.
- With IORT, women undergoing BCS (lumpectomy) may receive their radiotherapy at the time of their breast cancer operation while still under anesthesia, completely replacing the need for a 6–7-week course of radiotherapy normally given after surgery.

Good Candidate for Breast IORT

- Patients who participated in trials of breast IORT had low-grade, early-stage breast cancer, with no lymph node involvement and clear surgical margins from a lumpectomy.
- Most participants were women 40 years and older.

Advantages of Intraoperative Radiation Therapy

- Only one radiation treatment needed
- Less patient travel, fewer appointments
- Fewer side effects
- No skin affected by treatment
- Better cosmetic results
- Immediate reconstruction can be done right away
- Adjuvant chemotherapy can be scheduled without conflict
- Faster recovery
- May save cost of treatment

Disadvantages of Intraoperative Radiation Therapy

- Workflow during surgery must be carefully coordinated between surgeons and radiation oncologists
- Small risk of infection
- Difficult to monitor dosage to the radiation site
- Few patients may have access to this technology
- Not yet enough evidence of long-term results

Possible Complications of Breast IORT

- Fat necrosis
- Hematoma
- Mild fibrosis

Outcome

The local cancer recurrence is 1.6%.

BREAST CONSERVATION SURGERY (BCT)

43. Write on newer trends in breast conservation therapy. *RIMS, Imphal 2012*

Introduction

- Carcinoma breast is a local manifestation of a systemic disease. Local radicality does not change survival. Cosmetic considerations and preservation of the nipple, an important sensate focus for younger women.
- Breast-conserving surgery is a less radical cancer surgery than mastectomy. Breast-conserving surgery, as in a lumpectomy removes part of the breast tissue during surgery, as opposed to the entire breast.

Indications

Stage I and II.

Contraindications

Absolute contraindications	*Relative contraindications*
• Pregnancy is an absolute contraindication to the use of breast irradiation. However, in many cases, it may be possible to perform breast-conserving surgery in the third trimester and treat the patient with irradiation after delivery • Women with two or more primary tumors in separate quadrants of the breast or with diffuse malignant-appearing microcalcifications are not considered candidates for breast conservation treatment • A history of prior therapeutic irradiation to the breast region that would require retreatment to an excessively high total-radiation dose to a significant volume is another absolute contraindication • Persistent positive margins after reasonable surgical attempts: the importance of a single focally positive microscopic margin needs further study and may not be an absolute contraindication	• *History of collagen vascular disease:* Most radiation oncologists will not treat patients with scleroderma or active lupus erythematosus, considering it an absolute contraindication. In contrast, rheumatoid arthritis is not a relative or an absolute contraindication • The presence of multiple gross tumors in the same quadrant and indeterminate calcifications must be carefully assessed for suitability • Tumor size is not an absolute contraindication to breast conservation treatment. However, a relative contraindication is the presence of a large tumor in a small breast in which an adequate resection would result in significant cosmetic alteration. In this circumstance, preoperative chemotherapy should be considered • Breast size can be a relative contraindication. Treatment by irradiation of women with large or pendulous breasts is feasible if reproducibility of patient set-up can be assured and the technical capability exists for ≥6 MV photon beam irradiation to obtain adequate dose homogeneity

Special Considerations

- Family history
- Primary tumor histology
- Margin evaluation
- Extensive intraductal component

Methods	*Axillary dissection*	*New investigation modalities*
• Lumpectomy + axillary dissection + RT • Lumpectomy + SLN biopsy + RT • QUART—quadrantectomy + axillary dissection + RT • CTART—chemotherapy + RT	• Better control of locoregional recurrence • Accurate staging of disease • To decide adjuvant therapy • Prognosis	• MRI • Intraoperative ultrasound • Touch preparation cytology • Percutaneous needle biopsy

(RT: radiotherapy)

Role of Neoadjuvant

- Induction chemotherapy
- Drugs
- Selection and monitoring of induction chemotherapy patients

Sequencing of Chemotherapy and RT

• Six cycles of CMF followed by RT • RT followed by six cycles of CMF • Three cycles of CMF followed by RT followed by three cycles of CMF (sandwich therapy)	*BCS:* Procedures • Lumpectomy with 2 cm clearance • Lumpectomy with axillary dissection • Quadrantectomy with axillary dissection

(BCS: breast conserving surgery; CMF: cyclophosphamide, methotrexate, and 5-fluorouracil; RT: radiotherapy)

Indications for BCS	***Contraindications for BCS***
• Small/early tumors in premenopausal women • Lateral than medial tumors • More important to know the contraindications	• Very small breast • Very large breast • Advanced/high grade disease • Lactating breast • Multicentricity • Disease in opposite breast

(BCS: breast conserving surgery)

Newer Frontiers

- Laparoscopic axillary dissection
- Laparoscopic internal mammary clearance
- Technically feasible
- Clearance equal to standard technique
- Acceptability only after it stands the test of time

44. What is triple—negative breast cancer? Describe the various management options used for the diagnosis and treatment of such cancers. ***DY Patil Educational Society Deemed to be University 2020***

Triple-Negative Breast Cancer

Definition

Triple-negative breast cancer (TNBC) is a subtype of breast carcinoma that *lacks expression of the three key receptors* commonly targeted in breast cancer therapy:

1. *Estrogen receptor (ER)*—negative
2. *Progesterone receptor (PR)*—negative
3. *Human epidermal growth factor receptor 2 (HER2/neu)*—negative

Hence the name "Triple-Negative."

Epidemiology and Characteristics

Feature	***Description***
Prevalence	~10–20% of all breast cancers
Demographics	More common in *younger women (<50 years), African or South Asian descent*, and *BRCA1 mutation carriers*
Histology	Mostly *high-grade invasive ductal carcinoma (no special type)*
Behavior	Aggressive—high recurrence rate, early visceral and CNS metastases
Prognosis	Poorer than hormone-positive cancers, especially in first 3–5 years after diagnosis

Pathophysiology and Molecular Features

- *Lack of hormone and HER2 receptors*
  - No ER/PR → insensitive to hormonal therapy (e.g., tamoxifen)
  - No HER2 → cannot use HER2-targeted therapy (e.g., trastuzumab)

- *Molecular subtypes (by Gene Expression)*
  - *Basal-like* (most common): Expresses cytokeratins 5/6, EGFR
  - *Mesenchymal/immunomodulatory* (minor subsets)
  - *BRCA1-related*: Defective DNA repair via homologous recombination
- *Genetic associations*
  - BRCA1 mutation carriers have high incidence of TNBC
  - High genomic instability → chemosensitive but relapse-prone

Clinical Presentation

Similar to other invasive breast cancers, but often:

- Rapidly growing lump
- Firm to hard, irregular mass
- May present with axillary lymphadenopathy
- Higher incidence of *visceral (lung, brain, liver)* and *bone metastasis* at presentation

Diagnosis and Workup

- *Imaging*
  - *Mammography*: Irregular, spiculated mass (often high density, may lack microcalcifications)
  - *Ultrasound / MRI*: For characterization and staging
- *Biopsy: Core needle biopsy* for histopathological confirmation
- *Immunohistochemistry (IHC)*

  Determines receptor status:
  - *ER, PR, HER2—all negative*
  - *Ki-67* often high (indicating proliferation)
  - *Additional markers* (CK5/6, EGFR) may support basal-like phenotype
- *Staging*
  - According to *AJCC TNM system*
  - *CT scan, bone scan, PET-CT* for metastatic workup in advanced disease

Management of Triple-Negative Breast Cancer

Since TNBC lacks targets for endocrine or HER2 therapy, *chemotherapy is the mainstay of treatment.*

- Surgical Management

  Depends on tumor size, nodal status, and patient preference:

Stage/indication	**Surgery**
Early-stage (Stage I–II)	Breast-conserving surgery (BCS) + axillary node sampling or sentinel node biopsy
Locally advanced (Stage III)	Modified radical mastectomy ± reconstruction
Metastatic disease	Palliative surgery (for ulcerated or painful breast lesions)

Adjuvant radiotherapy is indicated after BCS or in high-risk cases post-mastectomy.

- Chemotherapy
  - *Neoadjuvant chemotherapy (before surgery)*
    - Given for large or locally advanced TNBC to downstage the tumor.
    - *Regimens:*
      - Anthracycline + taxane combination (e.g., *Doxorubicin* + *Cyclophosphamide*, followed by *Paclitaxel*)
      - Addition of *Carboplatin* shown to increase pathologic complete response (pCR) in TNBC.

Advantages:

- Shrinks tumor (allows breast conservation)
- Provides early systemic therapy
- Assesses chemosensitivity

- *Adjuvant Chemotherapy (after surgery)*
  - Indicated for all patients with tumor >1 cm or node-positive disease.
  - Same regimens as above.
  - Achieving *pathologic complete response (pCR)* correlates with improved survival.
- *Chemotherapy for metastatic/recurrent TNBC*
  - Single agents preferred for palliation:
    - Taxanes (paclitaxel, docetaxel)
    - Anthracyclines
    - Platinum agents (carboplatin, cisplatin)
    - Capecitabine, eribulin, vinorelbine
    - *PARP inhibitors* in BRCA1/2-mutated cases (see below)

- *Targeted and immunotherapy (Recent advances)*

Class/agent	**Mechanism/indication**	**Comments**
PARP inhibitors (Olaparib, Talazoparib)	Inhibit PARP-mediated DNA repair → effective in *BRCA1/2-mutated TNBC*	Used in metastatic or high-risk early disease
Immune checkpoint inhibitors (Pembrolizumab, Atezolizumab)	PD-1/PD-L1 inhibitors; stimulate immune response against tumor cells	For PD-L1 positive or high tumor mutational burden TNBC
Platinum-based chemotherapy	DNA cross-linking; effective due to defective DNA repair	Often added to standard neoadjuvant regimens
Antibody-drug conjugates (Sacituzumab govitecan)	Trop-2–directed cytotoxic therapy	Used in metastatic TNBC refractory to standard regimens

- *Radiotherapy*
  - Indicated post-BCS or after mastectomy if:
    - Tumor >5 cm
    - Positive margins
    - ≥4 positive axillary lymph nodes
  - Reduces local recurrence and improves survival.

Prognosis

Feature	**Comment**
Aggressive course	High rate of recurrence (especially within 3 years)
Metastatic pattern	Lung, liver, brain more common than bone
5-year survival	60–70% (lower than ER-positive cancers)

ADJUVANT THERAPY IN BREAST CANCER

45. Adjuvant therapy in carcinoma breast.

Adjuvant treatment of breast cancer is designed to treat micrometastatic disease, or breast cancer cells that have escaped the breast and regional lymph nodes but have not yet had an established identifiable metastasis.

Agents used for Adjuvant Therapy

Taxanes (Docetaxel and Paclitaxel)

- Taxanes are among the most active and commonly used chemotherapeutic agents for the treatment of early-stage breast cancer.
- HER2 positivity irrespective of ER status predicted a significant benefit from paclitaxel in terms of reduced disease recurrence.

- Patients with ER-positive, HER2-negative, node-positive breast cancer did not seem to benefit from the addition of a taxane.
- Taxane-based regimens can be used in the treatment of early-stage breast cancer and should be considered in treating women, especially those with HER2-positive disease, using either the weekly paclitaxel or every-3-week docetaxel dosing schedules.

Anthracyclines

- Anthracycline-containing adjuvant chemotherapy regimens have been used in the treatment of early-stage breast cancer.
- Biologically, anthracyclines inhibit topoisomerase IIa, whose gene (*TOP2A*) lies adjacent to the *HER2* gene on chromosome 17. *TOP2A* is coamplified in approximately 35% of HER2-overexpressing breast cancers.
- The original trials demonstrating superiority of anthracycline-based regimens over CMF (cyclophosphamide, methotrexate, 5-fluorouracil) did not include *TOP2A* or *HER2* testing.
- The BCIRG 006 trial, which randomized women with HER2-positive disease to AC followed by T, AC followed by TH (docetaxel/trastuzumab), or TCH (docetaxel and carboplatin plus trastuzumab), did test for*TOP2A* and *HER2* coamplification.
- An anthracycline followed by or concurrent with a taxane is the optimal therapy for "triple-negative" breast cancer patients with no medical contraindications.
- *Adjuvant hormone therapy:* In ER-positive early-stage breast cancer, hormone therapy plays a main role in adjuvant treatment, either alone or in combination with chemotherapy. Hormone treatments function to decrease estrogen's ability to stimulate existing micrometastases or dormant cancer cells.

Adjuvant Hormone Therapy

Adjuvant hormone therapy can reduce the relative risk of distant, ipsilateral, and contralateral breast cancer recurrence by up to 50% in tumors with high ER expression.

- *AIs:*
  - The Food and Drug Administration (FDA) approved endocrine therapies for adjuvant treatment of breast cancer include tamoxifen and the AIs (anastrozole, letrozole, and exemestane).
  - AIs function by inhibiting aromatase, the enzyme (found in body fat, adrenal glands, and breast tissue, as well as tumor cells) responsible for converting other steroid hormones into estrogen.
  - AIs have no effect on ovarian estrogen production.
  - These agents are effective only in postmenopausal women.
  - *Common side effects of AIs include:*
    - Hot flashes
    - Arthralgia/arthritis,
    - Headache,
    - Vaginal dryness, and
    - Mood changes.
- *Tamoxifen:*
  - It is an SERM that binds to and inhibits ER signaling in the breast.
  - It is effective in both premenopausal and postmenopausal women.
  - Tamoxifen has ER-stimulating effects in other tissues, including bone (resulting in preservation of bone density) and endometrium (leading to a two- to fourfold increased risk of endometrial cancer).
  - *Common adverse effects associated with tamoxifen included the following:*
    - Hot flashes (up to 80%)
    - Vaginal bleeding (2–23%)
    - Vaginal discharge (13–55%)
    - Vaginal dryness (<1%)
    - Dyspareunia (3–5%)

  - Urinary frequency or urgency (10%)
  - Mood changes (12–18%)
  - Depression (2–12%)
  - Weight gain (though rare)
- *Advances in targeted therapy:*
  - *Novel antiangiogenic agents:*
    - Small-molecule vascular endothelial cell growth factor receptor (VEGFR) TKIs offer several potential advantages over antibody therapies, including oral administration, a shorter half-life, and multitargeted effects.
    - Sunitinib (Sutent), an oral multitargeted kinase inhibitor of VEGFR and platelet-derived growth factor (PDGF) receptor, as monotherapy showed good result in metastatic breast cancer patients previously treated with an anthracycline and a taxane. Sunitinib has also demonstrated activity in combination with paclitaxel and sequentially with docetaxel as first-line therapy in metastatic breast cancer.
    - Axitinib, another oral TKI of VEGFR, showed promising antitumor activity in combination with docetaxel.
    - Other VEGFR TKIs such as pazopanib, vatalanib, cediranib, and motesanib are under investigation.
  - *Dual blockade by antiangiogenic/HER2 agents:*
    - HER2-targeted therapies have been investigated in combination with angiogenesis inhibitors, with promising results.
    - HER2 overexpression is associated with an increase in VEGF levels in primary breast cancers.
    - Combination therapy targeting HER2, EGFR, and VEGF pathways produces greater inhibition of human breast cancer cell lines than inhibition of any single or dual pathway.
  - *The angiogenesis inhibitor:* Pazopanib, showed promise in a randomized phase II study in combination with lapatinib versus lapatinib alone in chemotherapy-naive, HER2-positive metastatic breast cancer.
  - *Insulin like growth factor–1 receptor inhibitors:*
    - Insulin-like growth factor–1 receptor (IGF-1R) overexpression is associated with the development of breast cancer and correlates with disease-free survival in patients with primary breast cancer.
    - IGF-1R-mediated growth and antiapoptotic signaling occurs through the phosphatidylinositol 3-kinase (PI3K)/Akt and mitogen-activated protein kinase (MAPK) pathways.
    - To date, drug development targeting the IGF pathway has focused on IGF-1R monoclonal antibodies (mAbs).
    - Studies have shown that these compounds yield antitumor activity in several breast cancer models in vitro and in vivo.
    - Breast cancer cell lines with IGF-1R overexpression appear to be more resistant to trastuzumab and ER-targeted therapies; thus, clinical trials are focusing on hormone-refractory and/or HER2-positive disease.
    - This strategy of dual targeting is being employed in an ongoing phase II trial of CP-751,871, a mAb targeting IGF-1R, in combination with the AI exemestane, compared with exemestane alone in postmenopausal patients with HR-positive advanced breast cancer.
  - *PI3K/AKT/mammalian target of rapamycin (mTor) inhibitors:*
    - Among signaling pathways, the PI3K/Akt/mTor pathway is thought to be highly active in human breast cancer development and progression.
    - In breast cancer, this pathway can be activated through PI3K by membrane protein receptors, including the HER family of growth factor receptors, IGF-1R and ER. PI3K activates downstream Akt, leading to mTor phosphorylation and promotion of breast cancer cell survival, as well as resistance to chemotherapy and targeted agents such as trastuzumab and tamoxifen.
    - SF1126 is a chemical conjugate of LY294002, the most studied of the PI3K inhibitors. This compound has a broad spectrum of inhibition via Akt and mTor resulting in antitumor and antiangiogenic activity.

  - *Clinical trials have focused on combination therapy:*
    - Initial randomized trials investigating letrozole alone or in combination with temsirolimus showed no significant clinical benefit in LABC/metastatic breast cancer.
    - A phase I study of letrozole in combination with daily everolimus (RAD001, Afinitor), another selective mTor inhibitor with a good safety profile, proved promising, with 1 complete response and 1 partial response in 18 patients with advanced breast cancer.
- *Heat shock protein 90 (HSP90) inhibitors:*
  - It is a molecular chaperone required for the stability and function of several expressed and/or activated signaling proteins
  - A preclinical study reported that HER2 is particularly susceptible to degradation when exposed to the HSP90 inhibitor tanespimycin (KOS-953).
- *ARP inhibitors:*
  - Poly [adenosine diphosphate (ADP)-ribose] polymerase (PARP) inhibitors were initially developed to investigate the role of PARP-1, a nuclear enzyme involved in DNA repair.
  - These agents have also proven to have antitumor activity in breast cancer cells. *BRCA1*- and *BRCA2*-deficient cell lines are defective in homologous recombination, thus relying on PARP-1 for DNA repair.
  - BRCA-deficient cells treated with PARP inhibitors demonstrate an increase in DNA fragmentation and cell death.
- *Farnesyltransferase inhibitors:*
  - The *Ras* oncogene family is a key component of the MAPK signaling pathway, which promotes mitogenic activity.
  - Aberrant Ras expression resulting in downstream signaling has been reported in breast cancer.
  - Farnesyltransferase inhibitors (FTIs) such as tipifarnib and lonafarnib were developed to block farnesylation and subsequent membrane localization of Ras.
- *Src kinase inhibitors:*
  - Dasatinib (Sprycel) is a novel oral kinase inhibitor that targets the Src family kinases and BCR-abl.
  - Dasatinib is approved by the FDA for the treatment of chronic myelogenous leukemia (CML).
  - A preclinical study revealed a dasatinib-sensitive signature in the basal breast cancer subtype.
  - Additionally, preliminary results from a phase I study of gemcitabine/dasatinib demonstrated antitumor activity in a patient with IBC.

BREAST CANCER IN PREGNANCY

46. Breast cancer in pregnancy. ***WBUHS 2009***

Incidence

Breast cancer occurs in 1 of every 3,000 pregnant women and axillary lymph node metastases are present in up to 75% of these women.

Age

The average age of the pregnant woman with breast cancer is 34 years.

Diagnosis

- Less than 25% of the breast nodules developing during pregnancy and lactation will be cancerous.
- Ultrasonography and needle biopsy are used in the diagnosis of these nodules.
- Open biopsy may be required.
- Mammography is rarely indicated because of its decreased sensitivity during pregnancy and lactation and because of the risk of radiation injury to the fetus.

- Once a breast cancer is diagnosed, complete blood count (CBC), chest X-ray (with shielding of the abdomen), and liver function studies are performed.

Treatment
- Because of the deleterious effects of RT on the fetus, an MRM is the surgical procedure of choice during the first and second trimesters of pregnancy, even though there is an increased risk of spontaneous abortion following first trimester anesthesia.
- During the third trimester, lumpectomy with axillary node dissection is considered if adjuvant RT is deferred until after delivery.
- Lactation is suppressed.
- Chemotherapy administered during the first trimester carries a risk of spontaneous abortion and a 12% risk of birth defects.
- There is no evidence of teratogenicity resulting from administration of chemotherapeutic agents in the second and third trimesters.

Prognosis
- Pregnant women with breast cancer present at a later stage of disease because breast tissue changes that occur in the hormone-rich environment of pregnancy obscure early cancers.
- However, pregnant women with breast cancer have a prognosis, stage by stage, that is similar to that of nonpregnant women with breast cancer.

BREAST RECONSTRUCTION

47. Discuss the principle and surgical options for breast reconstructions.

There are two main techniques for breast reconstruction:
1. *Implant reconstruction:* Inserting an implant that's filled with saline (salt water) or silicone gel.
2. Autologous or "flap" reconstruction.
    - And also reconstruction of nipple areola complex after surgery

Several different types of breast implants can be used to rebuild the breast. Implants are made of a flexible silicone outer shell, and can contain:
- *Saline:* These implants are filled with sterile (germ-free) salt water. These types of implants have been used the longest.
- *Silicone gel:* Gel implants tend to feel a bit more like natural breast tissue. Cohesive gel implants are a newer, thicker type of silicone implant. The thickest ones are sometimes called "gummy bear" implants. They are more accurately called form-stable implants, meaning that they keep their shape even if the shell is cut or broken. They are firmer than regular implants and might be less likely to rupture (break), although this still might happen.

Other types of implants that have different shells and are filled with different materials are being studied, but are only available if you are participating in a clinical trial.
- A tissue flap procedure (also known as autologous tissue reconstruction) is one way to rebuild the shape of your breast after surgery to remove the cancer. As with any surgery, you should learn as much as possible about the benefits and risks, and discuss them with your doctor, before having the surgery.

Tissue flap procedures can also have some potential downsides that need to be considered:
- In general, flaps require more surgery and a longer recovery than breast implant procedures.
- Flap operations leave two surgical sites and scars—one where the tissue was taken from (the donor site) and one on the reconstructed breast. The scars fade over time, but never go away completely.
- Some women can have donor site problems such as abdominal hernias and muscle damage or weakness.

- Because healthy blood vessels are needed for the tissue's blood supply, flap procedures may not be the best option for smokers, and for women who have uncontrolled diabetes, vascular disease (poor circulation), or connective tissue diseases.

Types of Tissue Flap Procedures

- *The most common types of tissue flap procedures are:*
  - Transverse rectus abdominis muscle (TRAM) flap, which uses tissue from the abdomen (tummy)
  - Deep inferior epigastric perforator (DIEP) flap, which uses tissue from the abdomen (tummy)
  - Latissimus dorsi flap, which uses tissue from the upper back
  - Gluteal artery perforator (GAP) flaps (also known as a gluteal free flaps), which uses tissue from the buttocks
  - Transverse upper gracilis (TUG) flaps, which uses tissue from the inner thigh
- *TRAM flap:*
  - The TRAM flap procedure uses tissue and muscle from the tummy. Sometimes an implant is used with this type of flap, but some women have enough tissue in this area to shape the breast so that an implant is not needed.
  - The skin, fat, blood vessels, and at least one abdominal muscle are moved from the belly to the chest.
  - The TRAM flap procedure can tighten the lower belly, resulting in a "tummy tuck," but it can also decrease the strength in your belly muscles.
  - A TRAM flap may not be possible in women who are very thin or who have had abdominal tissue removed before.
  - *There are different types of TRAM flaps:*
    - *A pedicle TRAM flap* leaves the flap attached to its original blood supply and tunnels it under the skin to the chest. It usually requires removing most if not all of the rectus abdominis muscle on that side, which means an increased risk of bulging and/or hernia on one side of the abdomen.
    - *A free TRAM flap* moves tissue (and usually less muscle) from the same part of the lower abdomen, but the flap is completely removed and moved up to the chest. The blood vessels must then be reattached. This requires the use of a microscope (microsurgery) to connect the tiny vessels, and the surgery takes longer than a pedicle TRAM flap. The blood supply to the flap is usually better than with pedicle flaps, there is less risk of losing abdominal muscle strength, and the donor site (abdomen) often looks better. The main risk is that sometimes the blood vessels get clogged and the flap does not work.

Nipple and Areola Reconstruction

- The nipple and areola are usually the final phase of breast reconstruction.
- This is a separate surgery done to make the reconstructed breast look more like the original breast. It can be done as an outpatient procedure.
- It is usually done about 3–4 months after surgery, new breast has had time to heal.
- Ideally, nipple and areola reconstruction tries to match the position, size, shape, texture, color, and projection of the new nipple to the natural one (or to each other, if both nipples are being reconstructed).
- Tissue used to rebuild the nipple and areola comes from the newly created breast or, less often, from skin from another part of your body (such as the inner thigh).
- If a woman wants to match the color of the nipple and areola of the other breast, tattooing may be done a few months after the surgery.
- Nipple prosthetics can also be used.

48. Give a brief account on breast reconstruction.

Patient Selection

- Young healthy patients with early-stage disease are the best candidates for reconstruction.
- Older patients with advanced disease are poorer candidates. However, because of the multitude of different reconstructive options available, all women at least need to be presented with the options before being excluded.

- With the increasing popularity of autogenous breast reconstruction, more stringent guidelines may be needed for the selection of potential reconstructive candidates.
- With regard to mastectomy alone, the greater surgical trauma, increased operative time, increased blood loss, and prolonged recovery mandate that all patients, regardless of their desire for reconstruction, be thoroughly evaluated both physically and psychologically.

Options for Breast Reconstruction

- Autogenous
  - Abdominal-based flaps
    - TRAM
    - Single pedicle
    - Double pedicle
    - Free flap
    - Deep inferior epigastric perforator flap
  - Upper abdominal horizontal flap
  - Vertical abdominal flap
  - Tubed abdominal flap
  - Latissimus dorsi musculocutaneous flap
  - Gluteal flap
    - Superiorly based
    - Inferiorly based
  - Rubens flap
  - Thoracoepigastric flap
  - Lateral thigh flap
  - Breast-splitting procedure
- Alloplastic
  - Silicone gel implant
  - Silicone implant with saline fill
    - Smooth wall
    - Textured wall
    - Round shaped
    - Anatomic shaped
  - Silicone injection
- Combination procedures
  - Latissimus dorsi flap with implant
  - TRAM flap with implant

(TRAM: transverse rectus abdominis myocutaneous)

- The primary part of the procedure can often be carried out immediately following the mastectomy. Patients with significant medical comorbidities (high blood pressure, obesity, and diabetes) and smokers are higher-risk candidates.
- The infection rate may be higher with primary reconstruction (done at the same time as mastectomy), but there are psychological and financial benefits to having a single primary reconstruction.
- Patients expected to receive RT as part of their adjuvant treatment are also commonly considered for delayed autologous reconstruction due to significantly higher complication rates with tissue expander-implant techniques in those patients.
- Waiting for 6 months to a year following may decrease the risk of complications, but this risk will always be higher in patients who have received RT.
- Delayed breast reconstruction is considered more challenging than immediate reconstruction.
- Not just breast volume, but also skin surface area needs to be restored.
- Many patients undergoing delayed breast reconstruction have been previously treated with radiation or have had a reconstruction failure with immediate breast reconstruction.

- In nearly all cases of delayed breast reconstruction tissue must be borrowed from another part of the body to make the new breast.
- Breast reconstruction is a large undertaking that usually takes multiple operations.
- Sometimes these follow-up surgeries are spread out over weeks or months.
- If an implant is used, the individual runs the same risks and complications as those who use them for breast augmentation but has higher rates of capsular contracture and revisional surgeries.

Operative Risk Factors for Breast Reconstruction with the TRAM Flap

- *Moderate:* <25% above ideal body weight
- *Severe:* >25% over ideal body weight
- Light to moderate smoking (1+ pack/day for 2–10 years)
- Chronic heavy smoking (10–20 pack-years)
- Chronic heavy smoking (20–30 pack-years)
- Autoimmune disease (e.g., scleroderma and Raynaud's)
- *Diabetes mellitus:* Noninsulin dependent
- *Diabetes mellitus:* Insulin dependent
- Unstable emotional state (life crisis)
- Personality disorder
- Substance abuse
- If "planned out" of flap design
- *Disruption of vascular perforators:* Transection of superior epigastric vessels (e.g., chevron incision and abdominoplasty)
- Patient unwilling or unable to invest the time required for healing or objects to an abdominal scar
- <10 transverse rectus abdominis muscle (TRAM) flaps
- Chronic lung disease
- Severe cardiovascular disease

Management of the Contralateral Breast

- The challenge of breast reconstruction requires not only creating a natural-appearing breast but also achieving breast symmetry.
- Accordingly, on occasion, breast reconstruction requires an additional procedure on the contralateral breast.
- Occasionally, the mastectomy affords the patient the opportunity to obtain the breast size or shape modification that she had long desired previously.
- In reconstructing postmastectomy breasts, matching preexisting ptosis and larger contralateral breast size is a difficult task.
- In the absence of medical contraindications, a reduction mammoplasty, mastopexy, or insertion of an implant may be required to optimize the breast reconstruction to achieve optimal symmetry.
- Although the risk for development of cancer in the contralateral breast is low (~4%), in reconstructing the contralateral breast, results are best if done with the same reconstructive option.
- BRCA-positive patients require additional counseling to discuss their ultimate risk for a metachronous cancer in the contralateral breast, and such women may opt for simultaneous, bilateral mastectomy with reconstruction.

49. Give a brief account of oncoplastic breast surgery. ***KGMU, Lucknow 2025***

Introduction

- Oncoplastic breast surgery focuses on achieving the best possible aesthetic result in the context of resecting breast tumor with adequate oncologic margins.
- The goal is to retain natural breast size and contour and symmetry with the opposite breast. It is defined as tumor excision with wide margins followed by repair of the defect by local rearrangement/replacement of the breast tissue and the nipple–areola complex to maintain shape and symmetry.
- Volume loss >20–30% or an unfavorable breast-to-tumor ratio requires oncoplastic procedure.

Advantages

- Greater patient satisfaction,
- Less complications, and
- Less local recurrence.

When to Consider Oncoplasty?

- A significant area of skin is to be resected with the tumor
- A large-volume resection is expected
- The tumor is in an area associated with poor cosmetic outcomes (e.g., lower hemisphere below the nipple, for any tumor rescction in the lower breast)
- Resection may lead to nipple malposition
- It is important to correct these deformities before RT because the irradiation may further accentuate any asymmetry and make it more challenging to correct the defect in the future.

Principles of Oncoplasty

Extent of Breast Resection

- The ratio of the anticipated defect to the volume of the remaining breast parenchyma and the type of parenchyma present (fatty replaced vs. dense) is more important than the absolute volume or breast tissue resected.
- In general, oncoplastic surgery should be considered when the size of the surgical defect is likely to be >20–30% of the breast volume.

Breast Size and Body Habitus

- Patients with large breasts could be considered for tumor resection and bilateral reduction mammaplasty to maintain bilateral breast symmetry instead of volume replacement in an already large breast.
- Obese patients should be considered for this approach because they are often poor candidates for autologous tissue reconstruction after mastectomy, and implants are often not large enough to recreate a breast proportional in size to the contralateral breast.
- Breast reduction can also relieve the symptoms of macromastia and also improves outcomes after breast irradiation.

Tumor Location

- Tumors lying directly under the nipple-areolar complex and tumors located between the nipple-areolar complex and inframammary fold require special attention to avoid NAC distortion and contour deformity (which will be exacerbated by radiation).
- In general, the skin and well-vascularized breast parenchyma must be adjusted to correct for the removal of breast tissue in these areas.
- For upper pole lesions techniques such as round block, crescent mastopexy (also provides minor lift), batwing or hemibatwing (more lift).
- Lower pole lesions techniques like a mastopexy based on a superior pedicle flap.
- Lower outer lesions J or V plasty.
- Lower inner quadrant—A Benelli includes a de-epithelization circumferentially around the areola and also provides minor reduction in breast volume.

Timing of Oncoplastic Surgery

- Immediate repair of a partial mastectomy defect is almost always preferred to a delayed approach.
- Oncoplastic techniques done at the time of the initial surgical procedure provide optimal solution as this has not been associated with delay in delivery of adjuvant systemic therapy or radiation.
- In general, oncoplasty cannot be performed on the irradiated breast. Tissue expanders and implants are not recommended because radiation may lead to capsular contracture, distortion, and infection.

- If a cosmetic defect occurs after breast-conserving surgery and RT, reconstruction of the treated breast is generally preferred 1–2 years after RT has been completed. In such cases, use of vascularized tissue from outside the radiation field is favored.
- Mastopexy of the contralateral breast can be considered if the deformity is due to asymmetry with the contralateral breast.

AUGMENTATION AND REDUCTION MAMMOPLASTY

50. Principles of augmentation and reduction mammoplasty.

Reduction Mammoplasty

- Reduction mammoplasty is the resection of excess fat, breast tissue, and skin to achieve a breast size proportional to the body.
- The reduction mammoplasty is to improve the patient's symptoms, decrease the volume of the breast, and to reshape the breast.
- To:
  - Correct ptosis
  - Elevate the breast tissue to an anatomically correct position on the chest wall
  - Reposition the nipple and areola on the reduced and reshaped breast
  - Preserve the nerve supply to the skin and nipple-areola complex
  - Maintain blood supply to the breast tissue, and to minimize scars
- Pedicle is the portion of the breast tissue preserved with its blood and nerve supply while the surrounding breast tissue is removed.
- Vertical reductions are based on the blood supply of the superior and/or medial pedicles.
- In very large breast or gigantomastia, the pedicle is too long, and there is an increased risk of ischemia and necrosis of the nipple-areola complex, thus an amputation style technique or a reduction with subsequent free nipple graft is used.
- Suction-assisted lipectomy is used to remove excess fat laterally, and in patients with mild to moderate hypertrophy, fatty breasts, good skin tone, no ptosis, and good breast shape for whom liposuction alone will reduce volume.
- Before a breast reduction is performed, breast cancer screening is usually done in patient ≥35 years of age.
- In patients younger than 50 years, preoperative mammogram should be performed if there is family history of breast cancer, genetics, and the presence of mass on examination.
- The most frequent complications after reduction mammoplasty are alterations in the nipple-areola sensibility, hematoma, seroma, wound dehiscence, and fat and skin necrosis. The use of drains had led no difference in hematoma rates.

Augmentation Mammoplasty

- Augmentation mammoplasty is the most popular cosmetic procedure performed.
- This procedure is done to resolve the dissatisfaction with small breasts.
- Silicone gel breast implants were developed by Cronin and Gerow in 1963.
- *Newer implants:*
  - New generations of saline implants
  - Highly cohesive form-stable silicone implants
  - Newer gel implants (thicker, more viscous, and cohesive and tend to stay in place, even if the shell of the implant is damaged or ruptured).
  - Saline-filled implants (silicone rubber shells filled in the operating room).

Advantages

- The benign nature of saline
- Some flexibility in adjusting size by varying the amount of fluid put in the implant
- And smaller incisions because the implants are inserted while empty

Disadvantages

- Higher incidence of rippling or wrinkling of the implant under the skin deflation
- Perioperative complications are relatively low
- Bleeding or hematoma
- Wound infections
- Some degree of diminished sensibility of the nipple-areola complex (more frequent when bigger implants are used and in aggressive lateral pocket dissections)
- Capsular contracture
- Implant deflation (due to damage from handling at the time of surgery, pressure from capsular contracture, compression of the implant due to trauma, damage to the implant shell and other reasons that remain unknown)
- Implant rupture
- Implant rotation
- Implant displacement

Incision Options

- The inframammary technique is the most commonly used: provides excellent access without dissection of the mammary parenchyma, although the incision may be noticeable.
- Periareolar incision heals without visible scarring but may alter nipple-areola sensation, and has been associated with an increased risk of capsular contracture due to the less sterile nipple-areola area contents.
- Axillary incision leaves no visible scar on the breast and is ideal for saline implants.

Plane Options

- The implant can be placed in either of the subglandular, subfascial, or submuscular planes.
- Submuscular placement gives better superior upper pole aesthetics and better visualization of the breast by mammography and has less chance for development of capsular contracture, although they have more postoperative discomfort, longer recovery, and potential for breast distortion with pectoralis contraction.
- Silicone gel implants can rupture, but the highly cohesive newer implants may prevent releasing of the gel.
- Thus, it is recommended that gel implants be studied by MRI at intervals of 3 years and every 2 years after to detect silent ruptures.
- A new and more accepted option with use of acellular dermal matrix has been used for secondary breast surgery in the case of capsular contracture, malposition, rippling.

Implant Selection

- Implant selection is important, and comprehensive detailed patient education about the size (volume and diameter) is a critical aspect of the selection.
- The surgeon must determine the size according to the height, weight, chest configuration, and breast anatomy.
- Shape, profile, and surface texture.
- Implant profile (normal, intermediate, and higher) may be used depending on the size of the chest
- Smooth implants are more commonly used and related to more capsular contracture when placed in the subglandular space.
- Surface texture implants have been shown to reduce capsular contracture but are associated with chronic inflammation and recently have been linked to breast

Other Procedures

- Fat grafting to the breast autologous fat injection has become a popular procedure in both cosmetic and reconstructive plastic surgery.

- Autologous fat transfer may compromise the detection of breast cancer and should be administered with caution in patients with high risk of breast cancer.
- The role of fat tissue transfer in cosmetic and reconstructive breast surgery will continue to evolve and today is used for correction lumpectomy after surgical breast reconstruction.

Breast Augmentation
- Breast enhancement with mastopexy
- Correct breast asymmetry due to congenital deformity

Breast Implant-associated Anaplastic Large Cell Lymphoma
- Breast implant-associated anaplastic large cell lymphoma (BIA-ALCL) has been associated with breast implants, and many factors are involved in its pathophysiology, including textured implants, bacterial biofilm formation, immune response, and patient genetics.
- The mean age at onset is in the fifth decade, with implants having been in place for at least 10 years. The most common clinical presentation is a late peri-implant effusion or seroma 1 year after implantation or axillary lymphadenopathy.
- In comparison with patients with silicone implants, patients with textured implants have a higher rate of being diagnosed with BIA-ALCL.

Investigations
- Ultrasound is the first choice of methods to use in cases of breast swelling and can be used to guide FNA.
- MRI is also used.
- Cytologic analysis of the periprosthetic fluid will show large pleomorphic, epithelioid lymphocytes with kidney shape nucleus and prominent nucleolus, CD30 positive, and it is expressed on activated B and T cells.
- PET/CT for staging

Treatment
- Surgical treatment includes removal of the implant, complete removal of any mass with negative margins, and capsulectomy.
- No role for SLNB.

51. India is overdoing mastectomy—criticize. ***WBUHS 2024***

The claim that India is "overdoing" mastectomy, particularly in the context of breast cancer treatment, is a subject of concern and debate within the medical community. While mastectomy has historically been the go-to treatment for breast cancer, especially in cases where the cancer has spread or when other treatments may not be feasible, recent evidence suggests that over-reliance on mastectomy may not always be the most appropriate or effective option. There are several reasons why one might criticize the overuse of mastectomy in India:

Lack of Awareness and Patient Education
- Many women in India are diagnosed with breast cancer at advanced stages due to a lack of early detection and awareness. This leads to unnecessary emphasis on mastectomy as a standard treatment, even when other, less invasive options like breast-conserving surgery (lumpectomy) could be just as effective.
- There is often a lack of information provided to patients about the full range of treatment options available to them. In some cases, mastectomy is recommended because it may be seen as a "one-size-fits-all" solution, without exploring the possibility of breast-conserving surgeries or systemic therapies like chemotherapy or radiation.

Overuse in Early-Stage Cancers
- Mastectomy is sometimes performed even in early-stage breast cancer cases where less invasive options, such as lumpectomy followed by radiation therapy, could provide similar survival rates. Studies have shown that breast-conserving surgery, followed by radiation, can offer the same survival outcomes as mastectomy for

early-stage breast cancer, without the need for the extensive physical and emotional toll associated with the complete removal of the breast.
- Over-reliance on mastectomy can lead to unnecessary physical disfigurement and psychological distress for patients, as well as longer recovery times compared to breast-conserving approaches.

Social and Cultural Pressure
- In some parts of India, societal norms and stigma around breast cancer can contribute to an excessive focus on mastectomy. There is often fear and shame associated with the disease, which may lead both doctors and patients to opt for mastectomy as a "definitive" solution, even when less aggressive treatments would be sufficient.
- Women, particularly in rural or underserved areas, may feel that a mastectomy will "save" their lives, but there is less understanding that treatments like chemotherapy, targeted therapy, or hormone therapy may play just as important a role in managing the disease without requiring a complete removal of the breast.

Surgical Capacity and Resource Constraints
- In some regions of India, the healthcare system faces challenges such as insufficient access to specialized breast cancer treatments, limited availability of radiation therapy, and lack of advanced diagnostic tools. This may lead to an overreliance on mastectomy as a quick, accessible solution, as it can sometimes be seen as the simplest option in settings where more nuanced treatment options are unavailable.
- The overuse of mastectomy may also reflect the shortage of trained oncologists or breast surgeons who are adept at offering breast-conserving surgery or other newer techniques. This contributes to an outdated approach to breast cancer treatment in some parts of the country.

Psychological Impact and Quality of Life
- Mastectomy can have profound psychological consequences for women, including feelings of loss, body image issues, depression, and anxiety. Over-reliance on mastectomy may be harmful in a cultural context where many women face immense pressure to adhere to traditional standards of femininity and beauty.
- The physical scarring and the psychological toll of a mastectomy can significantly affect a woman's quality of life. Alternatives like breast-conserving surgery, followed by appropriate therapies, may offer less trauma while still ensuring effective cancer treatment.

Emerging Evidence Against Over-Surgery
- Recent advances in cancer care have highlighted that many cases of breast cancer can be managed with less invasive techniques. The increasing availability of genomic testing, better screening methods, and the growing understanding of cancer biology have shifted the focus toward personalized treatment plans.
- For example, studies have shown that a significant portion of women with small, localized breast cancers may achieve excellent outcomes with less aggressive treatment (e.g., partial mastectomy, lumpectomy, or even active surveillance), without compromising their survival chances.

Lack of Multidisciplinary Approach

A multidisciplinary approach that includes oncologists, radiologists, psychologists, and reconstructive surgeons can often provide patients with more options and help avoid unnecessary mastectomies. In some parts of India, however, there is still a tendency to make treatment decisions without consulting this broad range of specialists, which can lead to over-surgical approaches.

Economic Factors
- In some cases, mastectomy is perceived as a more cost-effective option for healthcare providers, especially in resource-limited settings. The cost of radiation therapy or the extended treatments needed for breast-conserving surgery can be higher, and there may be limited resources to offer a full range of treatment options.
- However, the long-term costs, including the potential for psychological counseling, reconstructive surgeries, and ongoing care after mastectomy, can outweigh the immediate perceived savings.

Conclusion

While mastectomy remains an essential and life-saving procedure in certain advanced cases of breast cancer, its overuse in India raises concerns. Early-stage breast cancers, in particular, can often be treated effectively with less invasive options that provide comparable survival rates while minimizing the physical and psychological impacts on the patient. There needs to be a concerted effort to educate both healthcare professionals and patients about the full range of treatment options, focusing on personalized, evidence-based care that considers not just survival, but also quality of life. Reducing the over-reliance on mastectomy will help ensure that women receive the most appropriate treatment for their individual cases, leading to better overall outcomes.

52. Describe oncoplastic breast surgery principles. What is role of mammography in the evaluation of breast? Enumerate the genetic markers of carcinoma breast. Mention the molecular classification of breast cancer.
WBUHS 2025

Introduction

- Oncoplastic breast surgery focuses on achieving the best possible aesthetic result in the context of resecting breast tumor with adequate oncologic margins.
- The goal is to retain natural breast size and contour and symmetry with the opposite breast. It is defined as tumor excision with wide margins followed by repair of the defect by local rearrangement/replacement of the breast tissue and the nipple-areola complex to maintain shape and symmetry.
- Volume loss greater than 20%-30% or an unfavorable breast-to-tumor ratio requires oncoplastic procedure.

Principles in of oncoplasty:

- *Extent of breast resection:*
  - The ratio of the anticipated defect to the volume of the remaining breast parenchyma and the type of parenchyma present (fatty replaced vs. dense) is more important than the absolute volume or breast tissue resected.
  - In general, oncoplastic surgery should be considered when the size of the surgical defect is likely to be greater than 20% to 30% of the breast volume.
- *Breast size and body habitus:*
  - Patients with large breasts could be considered for tumor resection and bilateral reduction mammaplasty to maintain bilateral breast symmetry instead of volume replacement in an already large breast.
  - Obese patients should be considered for this approach because they are often poor candidates for autologous tissue reconstruction after mastectomy, and implants are often not large enough to recreate a breast proportional in size to the contralateral breast.
  - Breast reduction can also relieve the symptoms of macromastia and also improves outcomes after breast irradiation.
- *Tumor location:*
  - Tumors lying directly under the nipple-areolar complex and tumors located between the nipple-areolar complex and infra-mammary fold require special attention to avoid NAC distortion and contour deformity (which will be exacerbated by radiation).
  - In general, the skin and well-vascularized breast parenchyma must be adjusted to correct for the removal of breast tissue in these areas.
  - For Upper pole lesions techniques like round block, crescent mastopexy (also provides minor lift), batwing or hemi-batwing (more lift).
  - Lower pole lesions techniques like a mastopexy based on a superior pedicle flap.
  - Lower outer lesions J or V plasty.
  - Lower inner quadrant–A. Benelli includes a de-epithelization circumferentially around the areola and also provides minor reduction in breast volume.

- *Timing of oncoplastic surgery:*
  - Immediate repair of a partial mastectomy defect is almost always preferred to a delayed approach.
  - Oncoplastic techniques done at the time of the initial surgical procedure provide optimal solution as this has not been associated with delay in delivery of adjuvant systemic therapy or radiation.
  - In general oncoplasty cannot be performed on the irradiated breast. Tissue expanders and implants are not recommended because radiation may lead to capsular contracture, distortion, and infection.
  - If a cosmetic defect occurs after breast-conserving surgery and radiation therapy, reconstruction of the treated breast is generally preferred 1 to 2 years after radiation therapy has been completed. In such cases use of vascularized tissue from outside the radiation field is favored.
  - Mastopexy of the contralateral breast can be considered if the deformity is due to asymmetry with the contralateral breast.

Role of Mammography in the Evaluation of Breast

- *Mammography:*
  - Mammography has been the basic imaging method in breast diagnostics, and the only tool suitable for screening breast cancer.
  - In screening, its sensitivity and specificity are 90–93% and 93–97%, respectively.
  - Mammography has some recognized limitations and disadvantages.
  - The sensitivity and specificity are highly dependent on the composition of the breast parenchyma, which for its part is influenced by age, hormonal status, and possible previous interventions.
  - In young women, the usefulness of mammography is restricted by high prevalence of dense fibroglandular tissue, which impairs both the detection and the differentiation of the lesion.
  - With increasing age, the breast parenchyma usually shows fatty replacement, which makes abnormalities more easily detectable.
  - Hormone replacement therapy may decrease the sensitivity of mammography by increasing the breast density and enlarging benign masses, such as cysts and fibroadenomas.
  - After breast surgery, mass-like scars and areas of distortion may mimic a tumor or hide subtle signs of malignancy. Radiation after surgical treatment of breast carcinoma leads to skin thickening and increased focal or diffuse density of the breast due to edematous changes. The accuracy of mammography is also impaired in patients with silicon implants.
  - Cysts and solid tumors cannot always be definitely differentiated at mammography. Some carcinomas may have a benign appearance, and some fibroadenomas may be irregular and difficult to differentiate from a malignant tumor.
  - A palpable mass may be partially or completely obscured by adjacent fibroglandular tissue. Even the spiculations within the fibrous tissue surrounding a cancer may be inconspicuous at mammography, because both the spiculations and the adjacent fibrous tissue are of the same density.
  - In addition to standard (craniocaudal, mediolateral oblique, and lateral) views, supplemental mammographic views are often needed to better or more completely visualize the area of special concern.
  - The commonly used modified views are spot compression and magnification views.
    - With the spot compression, separation of overlapping structures can be achieved.
    - Coning down with spot compression also reduces scatter radiation and sharpens image details.
    - Magnification provides the ability to define characteristics of microcalcifications and details of masses.
  - Also tangential views, extra lateral craniocaudal views, change-of-angle views, cleavage views and modified compression views (e.g., for patients with breast implants) can be taken.
  - Digital mammography has the potential to overcome some of the limitations of conventional mammography.
  - Because of the increased contrast and decreased noise of digital systems it is possible to improve image quality, although the spatial resolution is still limited when compared to screen-film mammography.
  - *BI-RADS* is an acronym for Breast Imaging-Reporting and Data System, a quality assurance tool originally designed for use with mammography.

- The system is a collaborative effort of many health groups but is published and trademarked by the American College of Radiology (ACR).

BI-RADS assessment categories are:

BI-RADS	Description	What it means	Followup
0	Incomplete	More imaging or comparison with prior studies is needed	Additional imaging required
1	Negative	No abnormalities	Routine screening (usually in 1 year)
2	Benign	Non-cancerous finding (like a cyst or fibroadenoma)	Routine screening
3	Probably Benign	<2% chance of cancer	Short-term follow-up (usually 6 months)
4	Suspicious	Abnormality that is not clearly benign	Biopsy recommended
5	Highly Suggestive of Malignancy	>95% chance of cancer	Biopsy and likely treatment
6	Known Biopsy-Proven Malignancy	Cancer already confirmed by biopsy	Used in pre-treatment planning

BI-RADS 4 Subcategories

- *4A:* Low suspicion (2–10%)
- *4B:* Moderate suspicion (10–50%)
- *4C:* High suspicion (50–95%)

Genetic Markers for Breast Cancer

- *BRCA1 and BRCA2 mutations*
  - *Description:* These are the most studied genes linked to breast cancer. Mutations in BRCA1 (chromosome 17) and BRCA2 (chromosome 13) significantly increase the risk of breast and ovarian cancers.
  - *Risk impact:*
    - Women with BRCA1 mutations have a 55–72% lifetime risk of breast cancer.
    - Women with BRCA2 mutations have a 45–69% risk.
    - Men with these mutations also have an elevated risk of breast cancer (about 1–7%).
  - *Prevalence:* About 1 in 400–500 people carry BRCA mutations, with higher prevalence in certain populations (e.g., Ashkenazi Jewish ancestry).
  - *Testing:* Genetic testing for BRCA mutations is recommended for individuals with a strong family history of breast or ovarian cancer.
- *Other high-penetrance genes*
  - *TP53 (Li-Fraumeni syndrome):* Mutations increase breast cancer risk, often at younger ages, and are linked to multiple cancers.
  - *PTEN (Cowden syndrome):* Associated with a 25–50% lifetime risk of breast cancer.
  - *CDH1:* Linked to hereditary diffuse gastric cancer but also increases risk for lobular breast cancer.
  - *STK11 (Peutz-Jeghers syndrome):* Rare mutations associated with a higher breast cancer risk.
  - *PALB2:* Mutations confer a 35–60% lifetime risk of breast cancer, especially when combined with family history.
- *Moderate-penetrance genes*
  - Genes like *CHEK2, ATM, BARD1,* and *RAD51C/D* have a lower risk increase (2–4 times the general population risk) but are significant in combination with other factors.
  - *Example:* CHEK2 mutations (e.g., 1100delC) increase breast cancer risk by about 2–3 times.
- *Low-penetrance genetic variants*
  - Common single nucleotide polymorphisms (SNPs) identified through genome-wide association studies (GWAS) contribute to small increases in risk.
  - Examples include variants in *FGFR2, TOX3,* and *LSP1* genes.
  - These are often population-specific and have a cumulative effect when multiple variants are present.

- *Polygenic risk scores (PRS)*
  - PRS combines multiple low-risk SNPs to estimate an individual's overall genetic predisposition to breast cancer.
  - Used in risk prediction models, especially for women without high-penetrance mutations.

Additional Context

- *Hereditary vs. sporadic:* About 5–10% of breast cancers are hereditary, driven by these genetic markers. The rest are sporadic, influenced by environmental, lifestyle, or unidentified genetic factors.
- *Ethnic variations:* Certain mutations (e.g., BRCA1/2 founder mutations) are more common in specific groups, like Ashkenazi Jews or African Americans.
- *Clinical implications:*
  - Genetic testing (via blood or saliva) can identify these markers, guiding preventive measures like enhanced screening, prophylactic surgeries, or chemoprevention.
  - Guidelines (e.g., NCCN) recommend testing for individuals with a family history, early-onset breast cancer, or specific cancer syndromes.
- *Emerging markers:* Research continues to identify new genes and variants (e.g., *BRIP1*, *RAD50*) through large-scale genomic studies.

Molecular Classification of Breast Cancer

Molecular subtype	*Luminal (A and B)*		*HER2*	*Basal*	
Genetic profile	↑Luminal CKs and ER-related genes (A>B) B ↑in proliferation-related genes		↑HER2-related genes	↑Basal CKs	
Histologic correlates	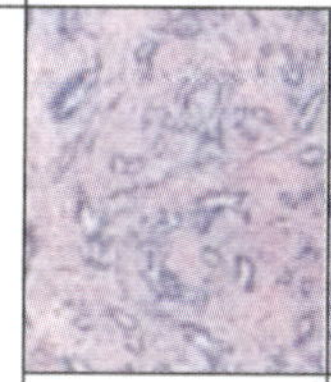	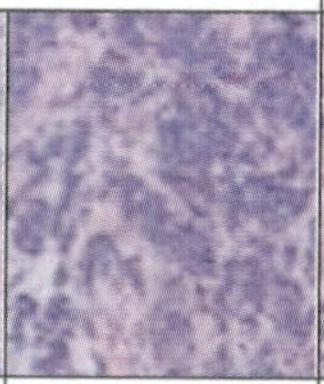	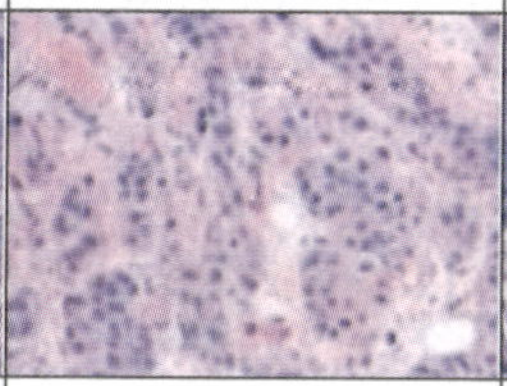	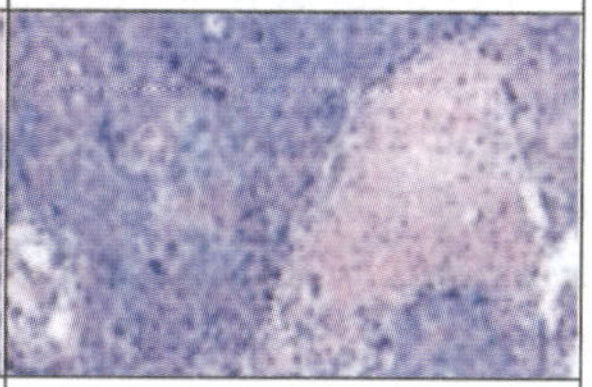	
	A Lower-grade ER+	B Higher-grade ER+	High-grade, +/– apocrine features	High-grade, sheet-like necrosis, inflammation *See exceptions	
Surrogate markers	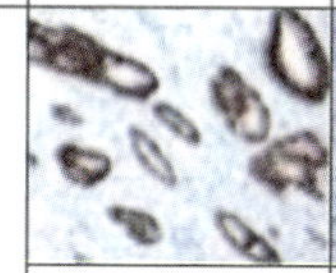	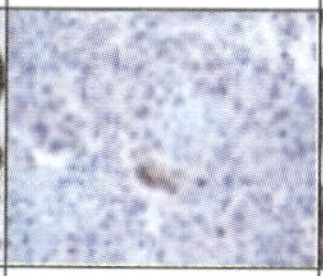	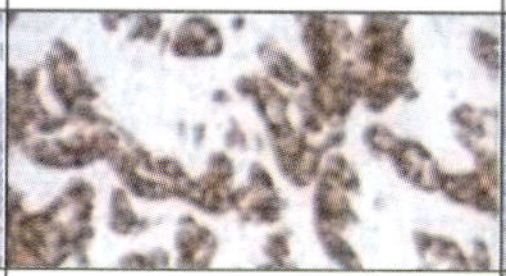	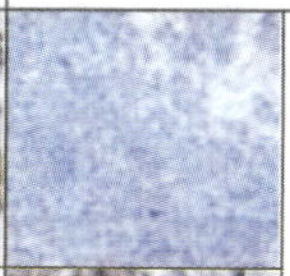	ER/PR- HER2-
	A Strong ER+, PR+/–, HER2-, low Ki67	B Weaker ER+, PR+/–, HER2+/–, 1 K167	HER2+, +/– ER/PR	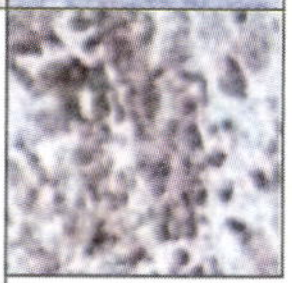	CK5/6+/– EGFR+/–
Prognosis	Good	Intermediate	Worse	Worse	
Response to chemotherapy	Lower	Intermediate	Higher	Higher	
Targeted therapies	Hormone therapies		HER2-targeted therapies	Currently investigational	

53. Discuss genetic counseling and genetic testing in breast cancer. ***Srimanta Sankaradeva University, Assam 2025***

54. Discuss the role of genetic counseling in the management of breast cancer patients. What are the indications for genetic testing in breast cancer patients? Enumerate the types of genetic tests and their pros and cons. ***AIIMS, Patna 2025***

Genetic Counseling and Genetic Testing in Breast Cancer

Introduction

Breast cancer can be caused by both environmental and genetic factors. About *5–10%* of all breast cancers are *hereditary*, resulting from pathogenic variants (mutations) in specific genes that significantly increase cancer risk. Genetic counseling and testing are essential tools in identifying these high-risk individuals, guiding prevention, early detection, and personalized treatment strategies.

Genetic Counseling

Definition: Genetic counseling is a communication process between a healthcare professional (usually a genetic counselor or medical geneticist) and a patient or family to discuss the risk, implications, and management of inherited cancer syndromes.

Goals:

- Assess the individual's and family's risk of hereditary breast cancer.
- Explain the nature of genetic testing, its benefits, limitations, and possible outcomes.
- Support informed decision-making about whether to undergo testing.
- Provide psychological support and discuss implications for family members.

Components of Genetic Counseling

- *Family and medical history assessment*
  - Construction of a detailed *three-generation pedigree.*
  - Identification of patterns suggestive of hereditary breast cancer (e.g., early onset, bilateral breast cancer, multiple related cancers).
- *Risk assessment:* Use of validated models (e.g., Gail, Claus, or BOADICEA models) to estimate risk.
- *Education:* Information about genes associated with hereditary breast cancer, test accuracy, and possible results.
- *Informed consent*: Discussion of test limitations, privacy, and potential discrimination issues.
- *Post-test counseling*: Interpretation of results and guidance on surveillance, preventive measures, or family testing.

Genetic Testing in Breast Cancer

Purpose

To identify pathogenic variants in cancer susceptibility genes that may:

- Explain a patient's cancer predisposition.
- Guide treatment choices.
- Enable predictive testing for relatives.

Commonly Tested Genes

High-penetrance genes	***Associated risks***
BRCA1, BRCA2	60–80% lifetime risk of breast cancer, ↑ ovarian, prostate, pancreatic cancers
TP53 (Li-Fraumeni syndrome)	Early-onset breast cancer, sarcomas, brain tumors
PTEN (Cowden syndrome)	Breast, thyroid, and endometrial cancers
CDH1	Lobular breast cancer, diffuse gastric cancer
STK11 (Peutz-Jeghers syndrome)	Breast, GI, pancreatic cancers

Moderate-Risk Genes

CHEK2, ATM, PALB2, NBN — confer 2–5× increased breast cancer risk.

Types of Genetic Tests

1. *Single-gene testing* (e.g., *BRCA1/2*).
2. *Multi-gene panel testing*—simultaneous analysis of multiple genes.
3. *Whole exome/genome sequencing*—in research or complex cases.

Indications for Genetic Testing

Testing is recommended for individuals with:

- Breast cancer diagnosed *before age 50.*
- *Triple-negative* breast cancer (ER–, PR–, HER2–) diagnosed *before age 60.*
- *Multiple primary breast cancers* (bilateral or recurrent).
- *Strong family history* (≥2 first-degree relatives with breast or ovarian cancer).
- *Male breast cancer.*
- Known familial pathogenic variant.
- *Ashkenazi Jewish ancestry* (higher BRCA1/2 mutation prevalence).

Interpretation of Results

Result	***Meaning***	***Implication***
Pathogenic/Likely Pathogenic Variant	Disease-causing mutation found	Increased surveillance, risk-reducing surgery, family testing
Variant of Uncertain Significance (VUS)	Unclear significance	No change in management; periodic re-evaluation
Negative Result	No mutation detected	Usual population risk (unless strong family history suggests otherwise)

Clinical Implications of Genetic Findings

- *Risk-reducing strategies*
  - *Surveillance:* Annual MRI + mammography starting at earlier age.
  - *Chemoprevention:* Tamoxifen or raloxifene in high-risk women.
  - *Prophylactic surgery:* Bilateral mastectomy or salpingo-oophorectomy in BRCA carriers.
- *Therapeutic implications*
  - *BRCA-mutated cancers:* Increased sensitivity to *PARP inhibitors* (e.g., olaparib).
  - *TP53 mutation:* Avoidance of radiation due to secondary cancer risk.
- *Family cascade testing*: Testing of relatives for the known familial mutation to guide their management.

Ethical, Legal, and Psychosocial Considerations

- *Informed consent* and *confidentiality* are vital.
- Potential for *genetic discrimination* (employment or insurance).
- *Emotional impact*—anxiety, guilt, or relief.
- Importance of *supportive counseling* and multidisciplinary care.

Genetic Testing—Types, Advantages, and Disadvantages

Definition

Genetic testing involves analysis of DNA, RNA, chromosomes, or gene products (proteins or metabolites) to detect *genetic variations* associated with disease, carrier status, or predisposition.

Types of Genetic Tests

Type of test description/principle advantages disadvantages/limitations

- *Karyotyping (conventional cytogenetics)*:
  - Visualization of whole chromosomes under a microscope (e.g., G-banding) to detect large structural or numerical abnormalities.
  - Detects aneuploidies, translocations, deletions, duplications >5–10 Mb.
  - Useful for Down, Turner, Klinefelter syndromes.
  - Low resolution (misses microdeletions).
  - Labor-intensive, needs dividing cells|
- *Luorescence in situ hybridization (FISH)*
  - Uses fluorescent DNA probes to bind specific DNA sequences on chromosomes.
  - Detects microdeletions, duplications, translocations.
  - Works on interphase nuclei (non-dividing cells).
  - Faster than karyotyping.
  - Limited to targeted regions (need to know what you're looking for).
  - Cannot detect unknown or genome-wide changes.
- *Comparative genomic hybridization (CGH)/Array CGH (aCGH)*
  - Compares patient DNA with reference DNA to detect copy number variations (gains/losses).
  - Genome-wide analysis at high resolution.
  - Detects microdeletions and duplications missed by karyotyping.
  - Cannot detect balanced translocations or point mutations.
  - Expensive.
- *Polymerase chain reaction (PCR)-based tests*
  - Amplifies specific DNA sequences to detect small mutations, deletions, or insertions.
  - Sensitive and specific.
  - Rapid, low cost.
  - Small DNA quantity required.
  - Targeted (need to know mutation site).
  - Limited to small regions.
- *Restriction fragment length polymorphism (RFLP)*
  - Detects DNA polymorphisms using restriction enzyme digestion and gel electrophoresis.
  - Simple and inexpensive.
  - Useful for known single nucleotide changes.
  - Low throughput.
  - Largely replaced by newer methods.
- *Sanger sequencing*:
  - Gold standard for detecting small mutations; determines exact nucleotide sequence.
  - High accuracy for small regions.
  - Detects point mutations.
  - Low throughput and expensive for large genes/genomes.
- *Next generation sequencing (NGS)*
  - Massively parallel sequencing of entire genome (WGS), exome (WES), or targeted gene panels.
  - High throughput, detects known and novel mutations.
  - Can sequence multiple genes simultaneously.
  - Expensive data analysis.
  - Variants of uncertain significance common.
  - May reveal incidental findings.
- *Multiplex ligation-dependent probe amplification (MLPA)*
  - Detects deletions or duplications of one or more exons within a gene.
  - Highly sensitive for copy number changes.

  - Faster and cheaper than aCGH for specific genes.
  - Does not detect point mutations.
  - Targeted approach.
- *Southern blot*
  - DNA fragments separated and hybridized with labeled probe.
  - Detects large rearrangements or methylation patterns (e.g., Fragile X).
  - Time-consuming, large DNA required.
  - Largely obsolete.
- *Microarray-based SNP genotyping*
  - Detects single nucleotide polymorphisms (SNPs) across the genome.
  - Detects known polymorphisms, genome-wide association studies (GWAS).
  - Cannot detect novel mutations or structural variants.
- *Biochemical/metabolic genetic testing*
  - Measures enzyme activity or metabolic products in blood/urine.
  - Useful for inborn errors of metabolism.
  - Functional confirmation of genetic defects.
  - Indirect—does not pinpoint exact mutation.
- *Prenatal genetic tests*
  - Includes amniocentesis, chorionic villus sampling, noninvasive prenatal testing (NIPT).
  - Early detection of chromosomal or monogenic disorders.
  - Invasive tests carry fetal risk.
  - Ethical concerns.
- *Epigenetic/methylation studies*
  - Detects DNA methylation abnormalities (e.g., Prader–Willi, Angelman).
  - Identifies imprinting disorders.
  - Complex interpretation.
  - Limited clinical availability.

CHAPTER 37

Endocrine Surgery

LEARNING OBJECTIVES

- Pituitary Tumors
- *Thyroid and Parathyroid:* Development, Surgical Physiology and Surgical Anatomy of Thyroid, Evaluation of Thyroid Function
- Thyrotoxicosis
- Thyroiditis
- Thyroid Nodule, Solitary Thyroid Nodule
- Thyroid Tumor
- The role of USG, CT, MRI, and Radiopharmaceuticals in the Management of Thyroid Malignancies
- Thyroidectomies
- Post-thyroidectomy Phonation Problems
- MEN
- Parathyroid and Calcium Metabolism, Hypercalcemic Crisis, Parathyroid Localization
- Parathyroid Cancer
- Adrenal—Surgical Causes of Hypertension, Pheochromocytoma
- Adrenal Incidentalomas
- Endocrine Pancreas
- Passaro's Triangle

PITUITARY

1. Write short note on pituitary tumors. ***WBUHS 2014***

Introduction

- Almost all tumors of the pituitary gland are noncancerous and do not spread.
- They are sometimes called adenomas.
- Pituitary tumors are either secreting (producing hormones) or nonsecreting tumors (not producing hormones).
- Secreting tumors can release excess amounts of any of the pituitary hormones, and are named after the hormone that is being overproduced, e.g., a prolactin-secreting tumor.

Causes

The cause of pituitary tumors is unknown.

Signs and Symptoms

- Signs and symptoms of pituitary tumors are caused either by direct pressure from the tumor itself or by a change in the normal hormone levels.
- As the tumor grows, it puts pressure on the optic nerve (which leads to the eye) and this often causes headaches and sight problems.
- Symptoms caused by a change in hormone levels usually take a long time to develop.

Prolactin Secreting Tumors

- These are the most common type of secreting tumor.
- Women with this type of tumor may notice that their monthly periods stop and they may also produce small amounts of breast milk.

- Symptoms in men may include impotence (inability to have an erection).
- Infertility (inability to have children) is common in both men and women, and the tumor may be discovered during routine tests for infertility.
- Symptoms of other secreting tumors will relate to the hormones that are released.

Growth Hormone-secreting Tumors

- Excess production of growth hormones can cause a condition called acromegaly.
- This leads to abnormal growth and causes enlargement of the hands, feet, lower jaw, and brows.
- It can also lead to high blood pressure, diabetes, and excess sweating.

Thyroid-stimulating Hormone (TSH)-secreting Tumors

- These tumors may cause symptoms such as weight loss, palpitations, and feeling shaky and anxious.
- These tumors are extremely rare.

Adrenocorticotropic Hormone (ACTH)-secreting Tumors

Overproduction of ACTH can produce a number of symptoms including Cushing's syndrome, which is characterized by a round face (known as moon face), weight gain, increased facial hair in women, and mental changes such as depression.

Other Anterior Pituitary Tumors

Tumors that secrete follicle-stimulating hormone (FSH) or luteinizing hormone (LH) are very rare and are likely to cause infertility.

Posterior Pituitary Tumors

- Tumors in the posterior pituitary are very rare and disturbances in this area are more likely to be caused by pressure being applied to the area from the surrounding tissues.
- The most common symptom of a problem in the posterior pituitary is a condition called diabetes insipidus.

Tests and Investigations

- *Eye tests:* By examining the eyes, pressure on the optic nerve can be detected, which may indicate that a tumor is present. A simple test may also be done to check the visual fields (range of vision).
- Pituitary tumors are often discovered during a blood test. If high levels of pituitary hormones are found in the blood, a CT scan or MRI scan should be done. The scans will normally be able to confirm whether a pituitary tumor is present or not.
- *Imaging:* CT scan and MRI of brain can detect and locate the tumor.

Treatment for Pituitary Tumors

Treatment depends on the type and size of the tumor, and the person's age and general health. Generally, the treatment options include:

- *Surgery:*
  - The tumor is removed using an endoscope or microscope.
  - In rare cases, the tumor may have to be removed through the front of the skull (craniotomy).
  - Surgery is the first-line treatment for all tumors except prolactinomas.
- *Radiation therapy:*
  - Radiosurgery is focused radiotherapy that has improved the accuracy and minimized the risks of treating pituitary tumors.
  - Radiosurgery is used in conjunction with surgery and medications to control the growth of tumors or to stop the activity of hormone-releasing tumors.
- *Medication:*
  - To shrink the tumor and stop it from producing hormones.
  - Medication is the first line of treatment for prolactinoma.
  - Hormone replacement therapy may also be required in cases of pituitary hypofunction or postoperatively.

THYROID AND PARATHYROID

2. Describe the surgical anatomy of the thyroid gland. How do you evaluate its function? ***WBUHS 2009***

3. Describe variations in course of recurrent laryngeal nerve in the neck and its implications in thyroid surgery. ***Gujarat Health University 2025***

4. Describe the anatomy of thyroid gland and write in brief the synthesis of thyroid hormones. ***RIMS, Imphal 2012***

Thyroid Anatomy

- The adult thyroid gland is located posterior to the strap (sternothyroid and sternohyoid) muscles.
- The normal thyroid gland weighs approximately 20 g, but gland weight varies with body weight and iodine intake.
- The thyroid lobes are located adjacent to the thyroid cartilage and connected in the midline by an isthmus which is typically located just inferior to the cricoid cartilage.
- A pyramidal lobe, which represents the most caudal end of the thyroglossal duct, is found in approximately 50% of individuals having thyroid operations.
- The thyroid lobes extend to mid-thyroid cartilage superiorly and lie adjacent to the carotid sheaths and sternocleidomastoid muscles laterally.
- The strap muscles (sternohyoid, sternothyroid, and superior belly of the omohyoid) are located anteriorly and are innervated by the ansa cervicalis (ansa hypoglossi).
- The thyroid gland is enveloped by a loosely connecting fascia that is formed from the partition of the deep cervical fascia into anterior and posterior divisions.
- The true capsule of the thyroid is a thin, densely adherent fibrous layer that sends out septa that invaginate into the gland, forming pseudolobules. The thyroid capsule is condensed into the posterior suspensory or Berry's ligament near the cricoid cartilage and upper tracheal rings.

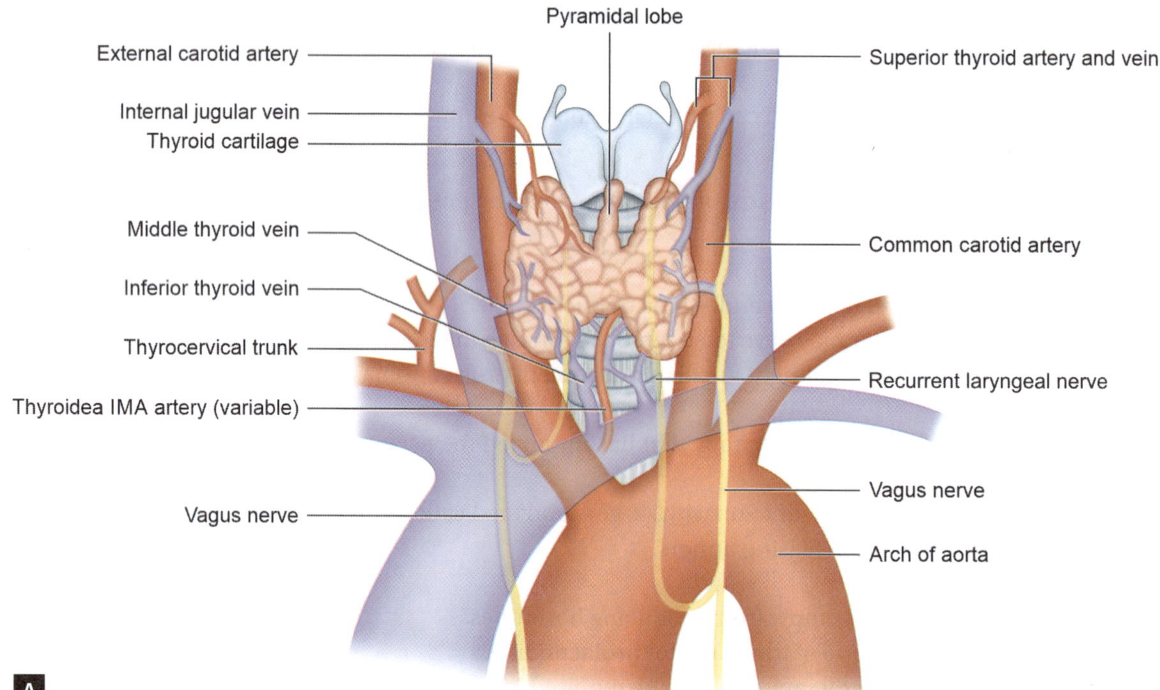

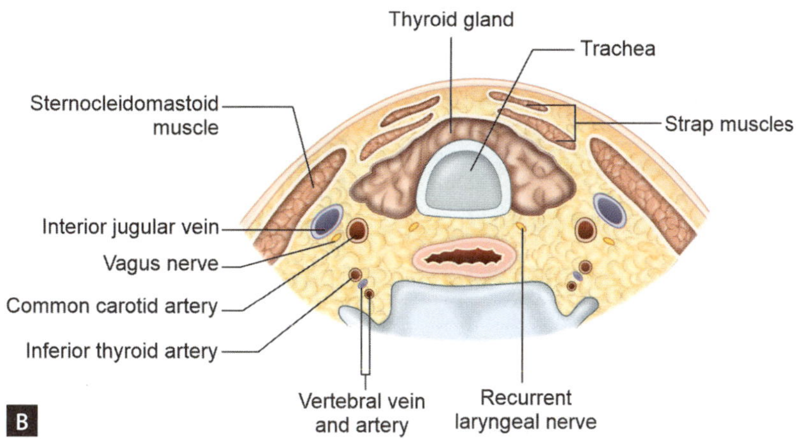

Anatomy of the thyroid gland and surrounding structures, viewed anteriorly (A) and in cross section (B).

Blood Supply

- The superior thyroid arteries arise from the ipsilateral external carotid arteries and divide into anterior and posterior branches at the apices of the thyroid lobes.
- The inferior thyroid arteries are derived from the thyrocervical trunk shortly after their origin from the subclavian arteries. The inferior thyroid arteries travel upward in the neck posterior to the carotid sheath to enter the thyroid lobes at their midpoint.
- A thyroidea IMA artery arises directly from the aorta or innominate in 1–4% of individuals, to enter the isthmus or replace a missing inferior thyroid artery.
- The inferior thyroid artery is intimately associated with the recurrent laryngeal nerve (RLN), necessitating identification of the RLN before the arterial branches can be ligated.
- Venous drainage of the thyroid gland occurs via multiple small surface veins, which coalesce to form three sets of veins—the superior, middle, and inferior thyroid veins. The superior thyroid veins run with the superior thyroid arteries bilaterally.
- The superior and middle veins drain directly into the internal jugular veins, the inferior veins often form a plexus, which drains into the brachiocephalic veins.

Nerves

- The left RLN arises from the vagus nerve where it crosses the aortic arch, loops around the ligamentum arteriosum and ascends medially in the neck within the tracheoesophageal groove.
- The right RLN arises from the vagus at its crossing with the right subclavian artery. The nerve passes posterior to the artery before ascending in the neck, its course being more oblique than the left RLN.
- Along their course in the neck, the RLNs may branch, and pass anterior, posterior or interdigitate with branches of the inferior thyroid artery.
- The right RLN may be nonrecurrent in 0.5–1% of individuals and is often associated with a vascular anomaly in this situation.
- Two nonrecurrent left RLNs are rare, but have been reported in patients with situs inversus and a right-sided aortic arch.
- The RLN may branch in its course in the neck, and identification of a small nerve should alert the surgeon to this possibility. Identification of the nerves or their branches often necessitates mobilization of the most lateral and posterior extent of the thyroid gland, the tubercle of Zuckerkandl, at the level of the cricoid cartilage.
- The last segments of the nerves often course below the tubercle and are closely approximated to the ligament of Berry.
- Branches of the nerve may traverse the ligament in 25% of individuals, and are particularly vulnerable to injury at this junction. The RLNs terminate by entering the larynx posterior to the cricothyroid muscle.

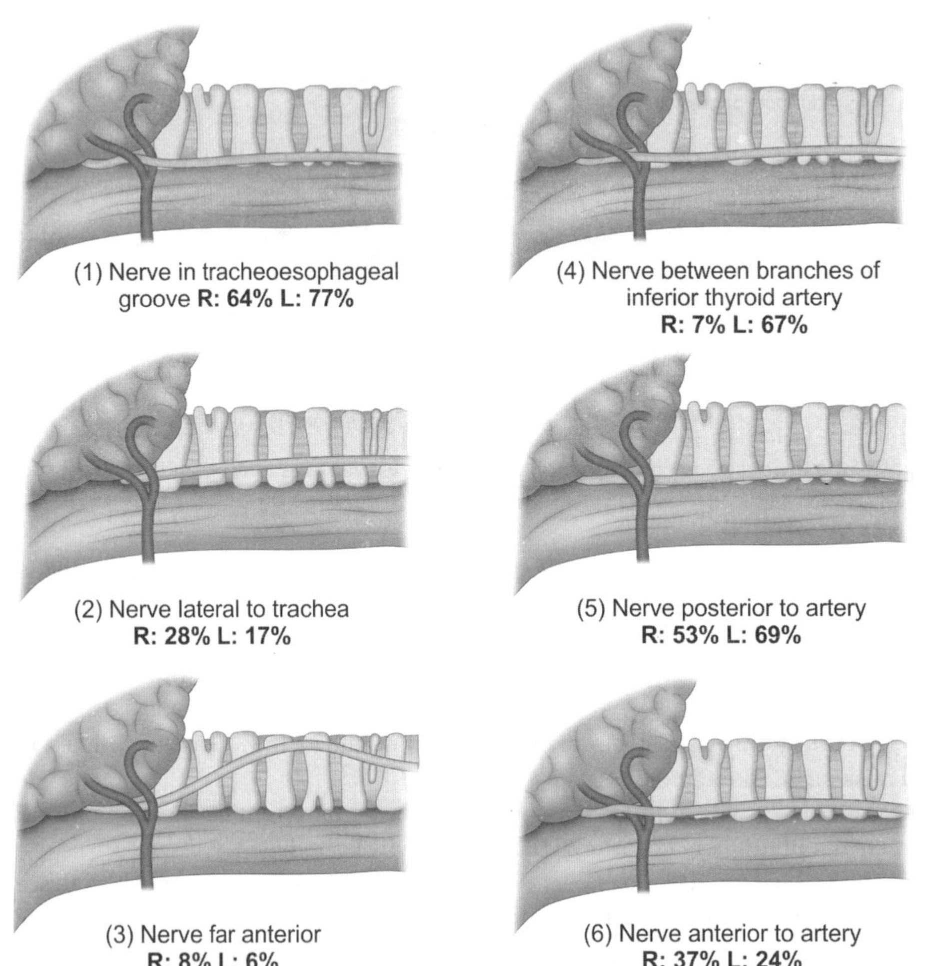

- Relationship of RLN to the inferior thyroid artery. The superior parathyroid is characteristically dorsal to the plane of the nerve, whereas the inferior gland is ventral to the nerve.
- The RLNs innervate all the intrinsic muscles of the larynx, except the cricothyroid muscles, which are innervated by the external laryngeal nerves.
- Injury to one RLN leads to paralysis of the ipsilateral vocal cord, which comes to lie in the paramedian or the abducted position. The paramedian position results in a normal, but weak voice, whereas the abducted position leads to a hoarse voice and an ineffective cough.
- Bilateral RLN injury may lead to airway obstruction, necessitating emergency tracheostomy, or loss of voice.
- The superior laryngeal nerves also arise from the vagus nerves. After their origin at the base of the skull, these nerves travel along the internal carotid artery and divide into two branches at the level of the hyoid bone.
- The internal branch of the superior laryngeal nerve is sensory to the supraglottic larynx. Injury to this nerve is rare in thyroid surgery, but its occurrence may result in aspiration.
- The external branch of the superior laryngeal nerve lies on the inferior pharyngeal constrictor muscle and descends alongside the superior thyroid vessels before innervating the cricothyroid muscle.
  (Cernea and associates proposed a classification system to describe the relationship of this nerve to the superior thyroid vessels. The type 2a variant, in which the nerve crosses below the tip of the thyroid superior pole, occurs in up to 20% of individuals and places the nerve at a greater risk of injury.)
- Therefore, the superior pole vessels should not be ligated en masse, but should be individually divided, low on the thyroid gland, and dissected lateral to the cricothyroid muscle.

- This nerve also has been called the Amelita Galli-Curci or "high note" nerve after the opera singer. Injury to this nerve leads to inability to tense the ipsilateral vocal cord and hence difficulty "hitting high notes," projecting the voice, and voice fatigue during prolonged speech.
- Relationship of the external branch of the superior laryngeal nerve and superior thyroid artery originally described by Cernea and associates.

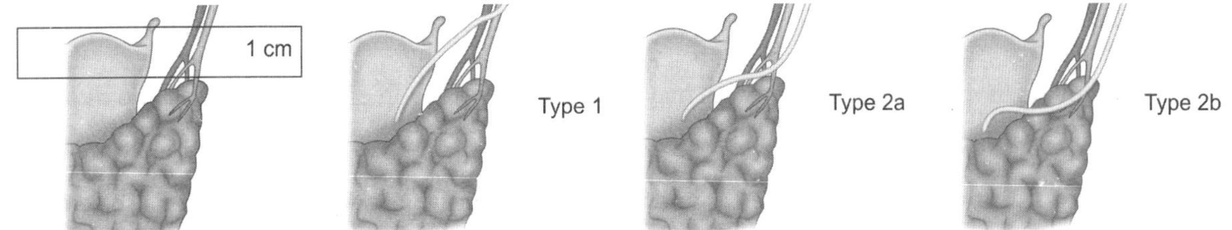

In type 1 anatomy, the nerve crosses the artery 1 cm above the superior aspect of the thyroid lobe. In type 2 anatomy, the nerve crosses the artery <1 cm above the thyroid pole (2a) or below (2b) it.

- Sympathetic innervation of the thyroid gland is provided by fibers from the superior and middle cervical sympathetic ganglia. The fibers enter the gland with the blood vessels and are vasomotor in action. Parasympathetic fibers are derived from the vagus nerve and reach the gland via branches of the laryngeal nerves.

Tests of Thyroid Function

Evaluation of the Pituitary-thyroid Feedback Loop

- *Evaluation of serum TSH:*
  - TSH is measured by an ultrasensitive radioimmunometric assay, which has greatly improved clinical diagnosis.
  - This assay is especially important in the delineation of hypothyroid from euthyroid states. Additionally, clinically euthyroid patients may have suppressed TSH levels (subclinical hyperthyroidism), and the assay can therefore demonstrate hyperthyroidism before it becomes clinically manifested. The sensitivity of the TSH assay is less affected by nonthyroidal disease processes and remains unaffected by changes in thyroid hormone–binding proteins.
- *Serum Triiodothyronine and Thyroxine Levels:*
  - Thyroid production is initially screened by measuring serum free T_4. Total T_4, which measures both free and protein-bound hormone, which can be affected by changes in hormone production or hormone binding to serum proteins; therefore, accurate evaluation of thyroid function requires measurement of free T_4 levels.
- *Calcitonin:*
  - In patients with thyroid masses and in whom multiple endocrine neoplasia type 2 (MEN 2) syndrome or isolated medullary carcinoma is suspected, a baseline calcitonin level can be calculated.
  - If there is doubt about the diagnosis, pentagastrin- or calcium-stimulated calcitonin evaluation, a 4- to 5-hour test, can be performed.
  - Additionally, calcitonin can be used as a screening test in families with MEN 2 syndrome to document clinically in apparent disease.
  - Use of calcitonin screening in patients with a thyroid mass, however, is not cost-efficient or necessary.
- *Radioactive Iodine (RAI) Uptake:*
  - The RAI uptake test is becoming less widely used.
  - A normal result is 15–30% uptake of the radionuclide after about 24 hours.
  - Use of ^{123}I is preferable because of a shorter half-life and lesser radiation exposure than with ^{131}I, which is used to radioablate thyroid neoplasms.

- *Thyroid Autoantibody Levels:*
  - Thyroid antigens are produced in autoimmune thyroid disorders [thyroid-stimulating immunoglobulin (TSI) and antimicrosomal antibodies], including Graves' disease and Hashimoto's thyroiditis.
  - Detection of autoantibodies can be extremely important if either of these autoimmune conditions is suspected. About 95% of patients with Hashimoto's thyroiditis and 80% with Graves' disease have detectable antimicrosomal antibodies.
  - In Graves' disease, circulating antibodies have high affinity for TSH receptor (TSH-R) on thyroid follicular cells.
  - Newer assays have greater sensitivity and may allow earlier detection of Graves' disease and more accurate monitoring of the effects of thyroid medication.

---

5. Describe the surgical anatomy of the thyroid gland. How will you prevent nerve injury during thyroid surgery?
WBUHS 2025

Surgical Anatomy of the Thyroid Gland

The thyroid gland is the largest endocrine gland in the body, weighing approximately 20–25 g in adults, and is located in the anterior neck, overlying the C5 to T1 vertebral levels. It has a butterfly-like shape, consisting of two lateral lobes connected by a central isthmus that crosses the midline at the level of the second and third tracheal rings. Each lobe measures about 5 × 3 × 2 cm and is positioned anterolateral to the larynx and trachea, with the superior pole near the mid-level of the thyroid cartilage and the inferior pole extending toward the fifth tracheal ring. The gland is highly vascular, brownish-red in color, and enveloped by a thin true capsule, which is surrounded by the pretracheal fascia (a layer of the deep cervical fascia). This fascial layer separates the thyroid from adjacent structures, facilitating surgical dissection.

Key Relations

- *Anterior:* Covered by the strap muscles (sternohyoid, sternothyroid, and superior parts of omohyoid).
- *Posterior:* Adheres to the trachea and esophagus via the ligament of Berry (a posterior extension of the true capsule); the recurrent laryngeal nerves (RLNs) course in the tracheoesophageal groove.
- *Lateral:* Adjacent to the carotid sheath (containing the common carotid artery, internal jugular vein, and vagus nerve).
- *Superior:* Near the inferior constrictor muscle and cricoid cartilage.
- *Inferior:* Extends toward the clavicles; may have substernal extensions in cases of goiter.

Blood Supply

The thyroid receives a dual arterial supply:

- *Superior thyroid artery:* Branch of the external carotid artery, entering the superior pole.
- *Inferior thyroid artery:* Branch of the thyrocervical trunk (subclavian artery), supplying the inferior and posterior aspects; it crosses the RLN posteriorly. Venous drainage occurs via superior, middle, and inferior thyroid veins, emptying into the internal jugular and brachiocephalic veins.

Lymphatic Drainage

Primarily follows the arterial supply, draining to prelaryngeal, pretracheal, paratracheal, and deep cervical nodes (levels III–VI). This is clinically relevant for thyroid cancer staging and central neck dissection.

Nerves

- *Recurrent laryngeal nerves (RLNs):* Branches of the vagus nerve (CN X). The right RLN loops under the right subclavian artery and ascends in the right tracheoesophageal groove; the left RLN loops under the aortic arch and ascends similarly on the left. They enter the larynx at the cricothyroid joint (nerve entry point, NEP), innervating all intrinsic laryngeal muscles except the cricothyroid. Surgical injury can cause vocal cord paralysis (transient: 2–11%; permanent: 0.6–1.6%).

- *Superior laryngeal nerve (SLN):* Also from the vagus; its external branch runs near the superior thyroid artery and innervates the cricothyroid muscle (voice pitch control). Vulnerable during superior pole dissection.

Parathyroid Glands

Four small glands (superior pair at the mid-posterior thyroid border; inferior pair near the inferior thyroid artery/RLN crossing) embedded in the false capsule. Supplied mainly by the inferior thyroid artery; injury risks hypocalcemia.

Surgical Landmarks

- *Tubercle of Zuckerkandl:* A posterior-lateral thyroid prominence; reliable for locating the RLN (nerve emerges posterior to it).
- *Ligament of Berry:* Entry point for RLN into larynx; dissection here requires caution.

Variations (e.g., non-recurrent RLN in 0.5–1% of cases, especially right-sided with aberrant subclavian artery) must be anticipated via preoperative imaging.

Preventing Nerve Injury During Thyroid Surgery

Nerve injury, primarily to the RLN (and less commonly the SLN), is a major concern in thyroidectomy, with rates varying by procedure extent and surgeon experience. Prevention relies on meticulous technique, anatomical knowledge, and adjuncts like intraoperative neuromonitoring (IONM). Key strategies include:

Preoperative Measures

- *Vocal Cord Assessment:* Routine flexible laryngoscopy to document baseline function; identifies preexisting paralysis (up to 10% of cases) and informs consent.
- *Imaging:* CT/MRI for anatomical variants (e.g., non-recurrent RLN) or substernal extension; ultrasound for nodule localization.

Intraoperative Techniques

- *Routine nerve identification and dissection:* Visualize the RLN early (e.g., at the ligament of Berry or inferior thyroid artery crossing) using landmarks like the inferior parathyroid or middle thyroid vein. Dissection reduces injury risk (0.5–1% with identification vs. 4–7% without). Avoid skeletonization; gentle handling prevents traction/compression.
- *Capsular dissection:* Stay close to the thyroid capsule to avoid nerves; ligate vessels individually rather than en masse.
- *Minimize traction and thermal injury:* Limit lobe retraction; use energy devices (e.g., harmonic scalpel) judiciously near the NEP (most common injury site, often traction-related). IONM detects loss of signal (LOS) early, allowing staged surgery (e.g., complete one side, assess, then contralateral).
- *High-risk scenarios:* In reoperations (21.7% injury rate vs. 2.8% primary), total thyroidectomy (7.2% vs. 1.9% subtotal), or malignancy (infiltration), proceed cautiously; IONM is particularly beneficial (reduces transient palsy by ~1%).

Intraoperative Neuromonitoring (IONM)

Standardizes RLN/SLN identification; electromyography confirms function. Reduces overall injury risk (5.9% with IONM vs. 6.8% without) and aids in difficult cases (e.g., inflammation). Not a substitute for visualization but complements it.

Postoperative Management

Immediate laryngoscopy for hoarseness; most transient injuries recover within 6 months (speech therapy aids). Permanent cases may require medialization laryngoplasty.

Adhering to these reduces permanent RLN palsy to <1%, emphasizing surgeon experience and a low-threshold for adjuncts.

6. Describe the development and surgical physiology of thyroid gland. How will you manage a case of thyrotoxicosis? ***WBUHS 2022***

Development

- The thyroid gland is the first of the body's endocrine glands to develop, on approximately the 24th day of gestation. This occurs under the influence of fibroblast growth factor signaling pathways.
- The thyroid originates from two main structures: the primitive pharynx and the neural crest.
- The rudimentary lateral thyroid develops from neural crest cells, while the median thyroid, which forms the bulk of the gland, arises from the primitive pharynx.
- The thyroid gland forms as a proliferation of endodermal epithelial cells on the median surface of the developing pharyngeal floor. The site of this development lies between two key structures, the tuberculum impar and the copula, and is known as the foramen cecum. The thyroid initially arises caudal to the tuberculum impar, which is also known as the median tongue bud. This embryonic swelling develops from the first pharyngeal arch and occurs midline on the floor of the developing pharynx, eventually helping form the tongue as the two lateral lingual swellings overgrow it.
- The foramen cecum begins rostral to the copula, also known as the hypobranchial eminence. This median embryologic swelling consists of mesoderm that arises from the second pharyngeal pouch (although the third and fourth pouches are also involved).
- The thyroid gland, therefore, originates from between the first and second pouches. The initial thyroid precursor, the thyroid primordium, starts as a simple midline thickening and develops to form the thyroid diverticulum.
- This structure is initially hollow, although it later solidifies and becomes bilobed. The stem usually has a lumen.
- The thyroglossal duct does not descend into the lateral lobes.
- The two lobes are located on either side of the midline and are connected via an isthmus.

Descent of the Thyroid Gland

- The initial descent of the thyroid gland follows the primitive heart and occurs anterior to the pharyngeal gut.
- At this point, the thyroid is still connected to the tongue via the thyroglossal duct.
- The tubular duct later solidifies into a cord of cells that will form the follicular elements.
- The proximal segment retracts and subsequently obliterates entirely, leaving only the foramen cecum at the posterior aspect of the tongue.
- Nonetheless, in some individuals, remnants of this duct may still persist.
- The foramen cecum represents the opening of the thyroglossal duct into the tongue; its remains may be observed as a small blind pit in the midline between the anterior two thirds and the posterior third of the tongue at the apex of the sulcus terminalis.
- A pyramidal lobe of the thyroid may be observed in as many as 50% of patients. This lobe represents a persistence of the inferior end of the thyroglossal duct that has failed to obliterate.
- The pyramidal lobe itself may be attached to the hyoid bone, similar to a thyroglossal duct cyst, or may be incorporated into a thyroglossal duct cyst. However, the pyramidal lobe can usually be identified along the superior edge of the isthmus, more commonly on the left side.
- The caudal segment of the thyroglossal duct develops as a bilobed, encapsulated gland while reaching its final, orthotopic position.
- Descent of the thyroid gland carries it anterior (or ventral) to the hyoid bone and, subsequently, anterior (or ventral) to the laryngeal cartilages.
- As the thyroid gland descends, it forms its mature shape, with a median isthmus connecting the two lateral lobes. The thyroid completes its descent in the seventh gestational week, coming to rest in its final location immediately anterior to the trachea.
- The caudal segment of the thyroglossal duct undergoes histologic differentiation into follicular elements at gestational weeks 10 and 11.
- The division of these primary follicles results in follicle formation during weeks 11 and 12. Intracellular canaliculi form connections with adjacent cells, and these spaces subsequently fuse, forming a confluent lumen.

- Desmosomes, molecular complexes of adhesion proteins, connect the cells, keeping follicular contents confined within the lumen.
- Colloid then accumulates within the follicles during gestational week 13.
- The connective tissue capsule and the interlobular septa develop from the fourth pharyngeal pouch's neural crest mesenchyme.

Physiology

- *Thyrotropin-releasing hormone (TRH):*
  - TRH secreted by the *hypothalamus* stimulates TSH secretion by the *anterior pituitary gland.*
  - TSH then stimulates thyroid hormone secretion by the thyroid gland. The process of thyroid hormone synthesis begins when dietary iodide is ingested, actively transported into the thyroid, and oxidized by *thyroid peroxidase* (TPO) into iodine.
  - Iodination of tyrosine residues in *thyroglobulin* creates monoiodotyrosine and diiodotyrosine.
  - Coupling reactions of monoiodotyrosine and diiodotyrosine result in the formation of *triiodothyronine (T3) and thyroxine (T4),* both of which are bound to thyroglobulin and stored in thyroid follicles.
  - When released into plasma, >99% of T3 and T4 are bound to carrier proteins, including *thyroxine-binding globulin* (TBG), thyroxine-binding prealbumin, and albumin. Only the unbound or "free" hormones are active (i.e., available to tissues), and T4 is converted to T3 by deiodinases in the peripheral tissues.
  - Compared to T3, T4 has a 20-fold higher circulating concentration but is three to five times less potent. The half-life of T4 (7 days) is significantly longer than the half-life of T3 (1 day).
  - *TSH:* Assessment of thyroid function requires biochemical evaluation and interpretation in the context of clinical findings. Measurement of *TSH* (0.3–4.12 mIU/L) *is the most useful biochemical test in the assessment of thyroid function.*
  - In most patients without hypothalamic or pituitary disease (rare), TSH and free T4 (FT4) vary inversely around a euthyroid state: Increased TSH and low FT4 signify hypothyroidism, while suppressed TSH and high FT4 suggest hyperthyroidism.
- Assessment of FT4 (0.8–1.8 ng/dL) supports identified abnormalities in TSH and provides an index of severity of thyroid dysfunction.

THYROTOXICOSIS

7. Describe in detail the presentation, pathophysiology, management and complications of thyrotoxicosis.

Maharashtra University of Health Sciences 2024

Pathophysiology

Mechanism of Thyrotoxicosis

Excess thyroid hormone leads to:

- *Increased basal metabolic rate (BMR)*
- *Increased oxygen consumption* and *heat production*
- *Enhanced sympathetic activity* (via up-regulation of β-adrenergic receptors)
- *Enhanced protein, carbohydrate, and lipid metabolism*

Causes (for context)

Category	*Examples*	*Mechanism*
Increased hormone synthesis (true hyperthyroidism)	• Graves' disease (autoimmune) • Toxic multinodular goiter • Toxic adenoma	Excessive thyroid hormone production
Destructive thyroiditis (release of preformed hormone)	• Subacute (De Quervain's) thyroiditis • Silent/painless thyroiditis	Leakage of stored hormone due to gland inflammation

Contd...

Contd...

Category	Examples	Mechanism
Exogenous sources	• Factitious thyrotoxicosis • Iodine-induced (Jod-Basedow phenomenon)	Intake of thyroid hormone or iodine
Ectopic sources	• Struma ovarii • Metastatic thyroid carcinoma	Hormone produced outside thyroid gland

Systemic Pathophysiology

- *Cardiovascular:* Increased β_1-receptor sensitivity → tachycardia, palpitations, increased cardiac output, atrial fibrillation, and high-output heart failure.
- *Metabolic:* Enhanced glycolysis, gluconeogenesis, lipolysis → weight loss despite increased appetite.
- *Muscular:* Increased protein catabolism → muscle wasting, weakness.
- *Nervous system:* Increased synaptic activity → tremor, anxiety, hyperreflexia.
- *Thermoregulatory:* Heat intolerance due to increased thermogenesis.
- *Bone metabolism:* Accelerated bone turnover → osteoporosis in chronic cases.

Clinical Presentation

The manifestations reflect the *hypermetabolic* and *adrenergic* effects of thyroid hormone excess.

General/Constitutional

- Weight loss despite increased appetite
- Heat intolerance, excessive sweating
- Fatigue, weakness, hyperactivity
- Menstrual irregularities (oligomenorrhea/amenorrhea)
- Increased bowel movements or diarrhea
- Tremor, irritability, insomnia

Cardiovascular

- Palpitations, tachycardia (resting HR >100/min)
- Bounding pulse
- Systolic hypertension with wide pulse pressure
- Atrial fibrillation (especially in elderly)
- Exertional dyspnea, high-output heart failure (in severe disease)

Neuromuscular

- Fine tremor of hands and tongue
- Proximal muscle weakness and wasting
- Hyperreflexia
- Emotional lability, anxiety, restlessness

Skin and Hair

- Warm, moist, velvety skin
- Increased pigmentation (in Graves')
- Fine, silky hair; alopecia
- Onycholysis (Plummer's nails)

Ocular Manifestations

- *Lid retraction and lag* (from sympathetic overactivity) → "staring" look
- *Exophthalmos/Proptosis* (specific to Graves' disease)
  - Due to autoimmune inflammation of extraocular muscles and orbital tissue
  - Associated with periorbital edema, diplopia, and conjunctival congestion
- *Photophobia, lacrimation, corneal ulceration* in severe cases

Thyroid Gland Findings

- *Diffuse enlargement* (Graves')
- *Nodular goiter* (Toxic multinodular or adenoma)
- *Bruit* over gland (increased vascularity in Graves')

Gastrointestinal

- Increased appetite but weight loss
- Diarrhea, hyperdefecation
- Occasionally mild hepatomegaly

Reproductive

- Oligomenorrhea/amenorrhea
- Infertility due to anovulation
- Gynecomastia and impotence in males

Metabolic and Skeletal

- Negative nitrogen balance
- Osteoporosis and increased fracture risk (long-standing disease)

Complications of Thyrotoxicosis

System/Type	*Complication*	*Explanation*
1. Cardiovascular	• Atrial fibrillation • High-output cardiac failure • Angina or ischemic heart disease	Increased myocardial oxygen demand, tachyarrhythmia, and prolonged workload
2. Skeletal	Osteoporosis	Accelerated bone resorption due to excess thyroid hormone
3. Muscular	Thyrotoxic myopathy	Proximal muscle wasting and weakness
4. Hepatic	Mild hepatic dysfunction, rarely hepatic failure	Hypermetabolism or drug-induced (antithyroid drugs)
5. Reproductive	Infertility, menstrual irregularities	Hormonal imbalance (increased SHBG, altered gonadotropins)
6. Neuropsychiatric	Anxiety, tremor, thyrotoxic periodic paralysis (especially in Asian males)	Hypokalemia due to intracellular K^+ shift
7. Ophthalmic	Severe Graves' orbitopathy → exposure keratitis, optic neuropathy	Autoimmune inflammation of orbit
8. Crisis	Thyroid storm (thyrotoxic crisis)	Life-threatening exaggeration of symptoms: hyperpyrexia, tachyarrhythmia, vomiting, delirium, coma; precipitated by stress, surgery, infection, or trauma

Diagnosis

Thyroid function tests for hyperthyroidism and thyrotoxicosis are as follows:

- TSH
- Free thyroxine (FT4) or free thyroxine index (FTI—total T4 multiplied by the correction for thyroid hormone binding)
- Total triiodothyronine (T3)

Thyroid function study results in hyperthyroidism and thyrotoxicosis are as follows:

- Hyperthyroidism and thyrotoxicosis are marked by suppressed TSH levels and elevated T3 and T4 levels
- Patients with milder hyperthyroidism may have elevation of T3 levels only with a suppressed TSH level
- Subclinical hyperthyroidism features decreased TSH and normal T3 and T4 levels

Autoantibody tests for hyperthyroidism are as follows:

- *Anti-TPO antibody:* Elevation with autoimmune thyroid disease found in 85% of Graves' patients
- *Thyroid-stimulating antibody (TSab):* Also known as TSI, long-acting thyroid stimulator (LATS), or TSH-receptor antibody (TRab); found in 63–81% of Graves' disease; a positive test is diagnostic and specific for Graves' disease

Autoantibody titers in hyperthyroidism and thyrotoxicosis are as follows:

- *Graves' disease:* Significantly elevated anti-TPO, elevated TSI ab
- *Toxic multinodular goiter:* Low or absent anti-TPO and negative TSI ab
- *Toxic adenoma:* Low or absent anti-TPO and negative TSI ab
- Patients without active thyroid disease may have mildly positive anti-TPO and TSI ab
- *Subacute thyroiditis:* Low or absent anti-TPO and negative TSI ab

If the etiology of elevated thyroid hormone levels is not clear after physical examination and other laboratory tests, it can be confirmed by scintigraphy: the degree and pattern of isotope uptake indicate the type of thyroid disorder. Findings are as follows:

- *Graves' disease:* Diffuse enlargement of both thyroid lobes, with uniform uptake of isotope and elevated RAI uptake
- *Toxic multinodular goiter:* Irregular areas of relatively diminished and occasionally increased uptake; overall RAI uptake is mildly to moderately increased
- *Subacute thyroiditis:* Very low RAI uptake, either with a painful thyroid (subacute granulomatous thyroiditis) or occurring within a year of pregnancy (postpartum subacute thyroiditis)

Management

Treatment of hyperthyroidism and thyrotoxicosis includes symptom relief, while hyperthyroidism also requires therapy with antithyroid medications, RAI-131 (^{131}I), or thyroidectomy.

Symptomatic treatment is as follows:

- Oral rehydration for dehydrated patients
- Beta-blockers for relief of neurologic and cardiovascular symptoms
- For mild ophthalmopathy, saline eye drops as needed and tight-fitting sunglasses for outdoors
- For vision-threatening ophthalmopathy, high-dose glucocorticoids, with consideration of orbital decompression surgery, ocular radiation therapy, or a recently approved treatment from the US Food and Drug Administration (FDA), teprotumumab-trbw, a monoclonal antibody that blocks the insulin-like growth factor-1 receptor (IGF-1R) and ameliorates proptosis by reducing inflammation and preventing muscle and fat-tissue remodeling in the orbit

Antithyroid drug treatment is as follows:

- Used for long-term control of hyperthyroidism in children, adolescents, and pregnant women
- In adult men and nonpregnant women, used to control hyperthyroidism before definitive therapy with RAI
- Methimazole is more potent and longer-acting than propylthiouracil
- Propylthiouracil is reserved for use in thyroid storm, first trimester of pregnancy, and methimazole allergy or intolerance
- Antithyroid drug doses are titrated every 4 weeks until thyroid functions normalize
- Patients with Graves' disease may experience remission after treatment for 12–18 months, but recurrences are common within the following year
- Toxic multinodular goiter and toxic adenoma will not go into remission

Radioactive iodine treatment is as follows:

- Preferred therapy for hyperthyroidism
- Administered orally as a single dose in capsule or liquid form
- Causes fibrosis and destruction of the thyroid over weeks to many months
- Hypothyroidism is expected
- Pregnancy, breast feeding, and recent lactation are contraindications
- RAI should be avoided in children younger than 5 years
- RAI is usually not given to patients with severe ophthalmopathy
- RAI is usually not given to patients who cannot comply with physician restrictions for avoidance of radiation exposure to others

Thyroidectomy is reserved for special circumstances, including the following:

- Severe hyperthyroidism in children
- Pregnant women who are noncompliant with or intolerant of antithyroid medication
- Patients with very large goiters or severe ophthalmopathy
- Patients who refuse RAI therapy
- Refractory amiodarone-induced hyperthyroidism
- Patients who require normalization of thyroid functions quickly, such as pregnant women, women who desire pregnancy in the next 6 months, or patients with unstable cardiac conditions.

Ablative Treatment of Graves' Disease with Thyrotoxicosis

Method	*Dose or extent of surgery*	*Onset of responses*	*Complications*	*Remarks*
Surgery	Subtotal excision of gland (leaving about 1–2 g remnant or less)	Immediate	• Mortality: <1% • Permanent hypothyroidism: • 20–30% or greater • Recurrent hyperthyroidism: <15% • Vocal cord paralysis: ~1% • Hypoparathyroidism: ~1%	Applicable in young patients and pregnant women
Radioiodine 5–10 mCi		Several weeks to months	*Permanent hypoparathyroidism:* 50–70% or more, often with delayed onset; multiple treatments sometimes necessary; recurrence possible	Avoid in children or pregnant women

THYROIDITIS

8. Describe autoimmunity. Describe the pathology and management of autoimmune thyroiditis.

WBUHS Supplementary 2025

Autoimmunity is a condition in which the *immune system fails to recognize self-antigens* as "self" and mounts an immune response against the body's own tissues. This can lead to *chronic inflammation, tissue damage, and functional impairment* of the affected organ or system.

Mechanism of Autoimmunity

- *Loss of self-tolerance:* Failure of central (thymic) or peripheral tolerance mechanisms
- *Genetic predisposition:* Certain HLA types (e.g., HLA-DR3, DR5)
- *Environmental triggers:* Infections, drugs, stress, or toxins
- *Molecular mimicry:* Pathogens mimic self-antigens, triggering cross-reactivity
- *Bystander activation:* Inflammation activates autoreactive T-cells nonspecifically

Autoimmune Thyroiditis (Hashimoto's Thyroiditis)

Definition

An *organ-specific autoimmune disease* characterized by chronic inflammation and progressive destruction of the *thyroid gland,* leading to *hypothyroidism.*

Pathology

- *Immune-mediated destruction* of thyroid follicular cells
- Infiltration by *lymphocytes,* formation of *germinal centers*
- Presence of *autoantibodies*:
  - *Antithyroid peroxidase (Anti-TPO)*—most sensitive
  - *Antithyroglobulin (Anti-Tg)*
- May result in *goiter* due to lymphocytic infiltration and fibrosis

Microscopy Features

- Dense lymphocytic infiltrate with germinal centers

- Hurthle cell (oxyphilic) change of follicular epithelial cells
- Fibrosis in late stages

Clinical Features

- *Fatigue, weight gain, cold intolerance*
- *Dry skin, constipation, depression*
- *Bradycardia, menstrual irregularities*
- *Goiter* (firm, nontender, diffuse or nodular thyroid enlargement

Diagnosis

Test	***Findings***
TSH	Elevated (most sensitive marker of hypothyroidism)
Free T4	Low or normal (depending on stage)
Anti-TPO/Anti-Tg Ab	Positive in most patients
Ultrasound of thyroid	Hypoechoic, heterogeneous gland
FNAC (if nodules present)	Lymphocytic infiltrates, Hurthle cells

Management

I. *Thyroid Hormone Replacement*
   - *Levothyroxine* is the treatment of choice
     - Dose individualized based on TSH levels and patient factors
     - Lifelong therapy often required

II. *Monitoring*
   - Regular TSH monitoring (every 6–12 months once stable)
   - Adjust dosage based on TSH response

III. *Management of Goiter*
   - If large, compressive, or cosmetically concerning → may require surgery

IV. *Address Associated Autoimmune Conditions*
   - Often associated with other autoimmune diseases (e.g., Type 1 diabetes, vitiligo, pernicious anemia)
   - Screen as needed

Prognosis

- Generally good with appropriate thyroid hormone replacement
- Risk of developing *other autoimmune disorders*
- Rare risk of *thyroid lymphoma* in long-standing Hashimoto's

THYROID NODULE

9. What are recent guidelines for management of thyroid nodule? ***WBUHS 2020***

10. Discuss the management protocol for solitary thyroid nodule.
KIIT University Odisha 2025; DY Patil Educational Society Deemed to be University 2024

11. Work up and diagnosis of solitary thyroid nodule. ***WBUHS 2016; RIMS, Imphal 2022***

12. Discuss the management of solitary thyroid nodule. ***WBUHS 2024***

13. Investigations of solitary thyroid nodule. ***Gujarat Health University 2025***

14. Evaluation and management of solitary thyroid nodule. ***Maharashtra University of Health Sciences 2024***

Recent guidelines for the management of thyroid nodule:

Modes of detection:

- Incidentalomas on head/neck CTs and MRIs, carotid ultrasound (US), positron emission tomography (PET) scans
- Palpated by primary care physician
- Noticed by patient
- With symptoms of hypo/hyperthyroidism

Solitary Thyroid Nodule

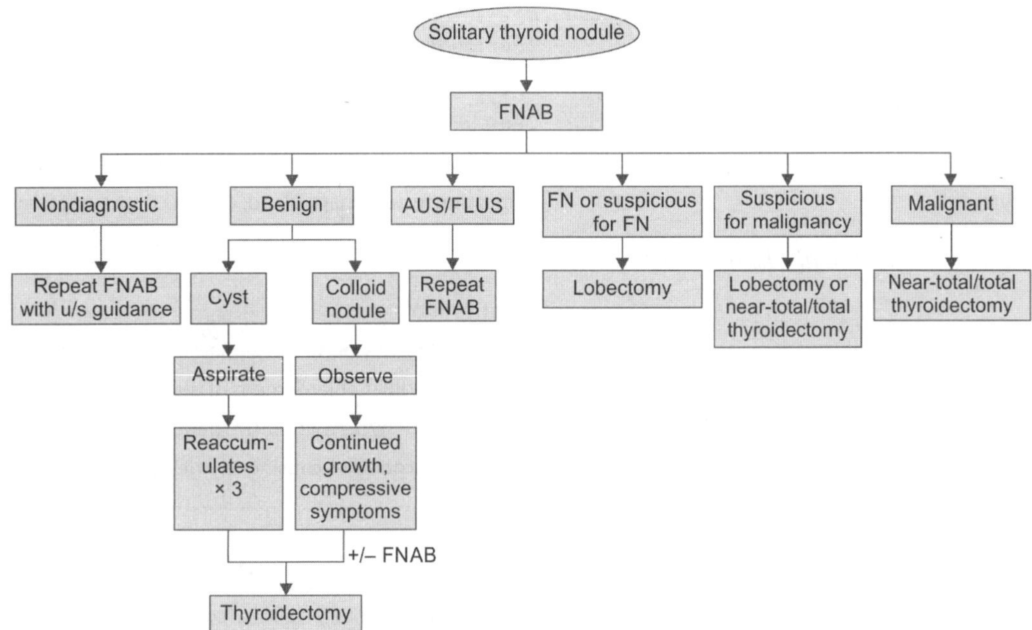

(AUS: atypia of undetermined significance; FLUS: follicular lesions of undetermined significance; FN: follicular neoplasm; FNAB: fine-needle aspiration biopsy)

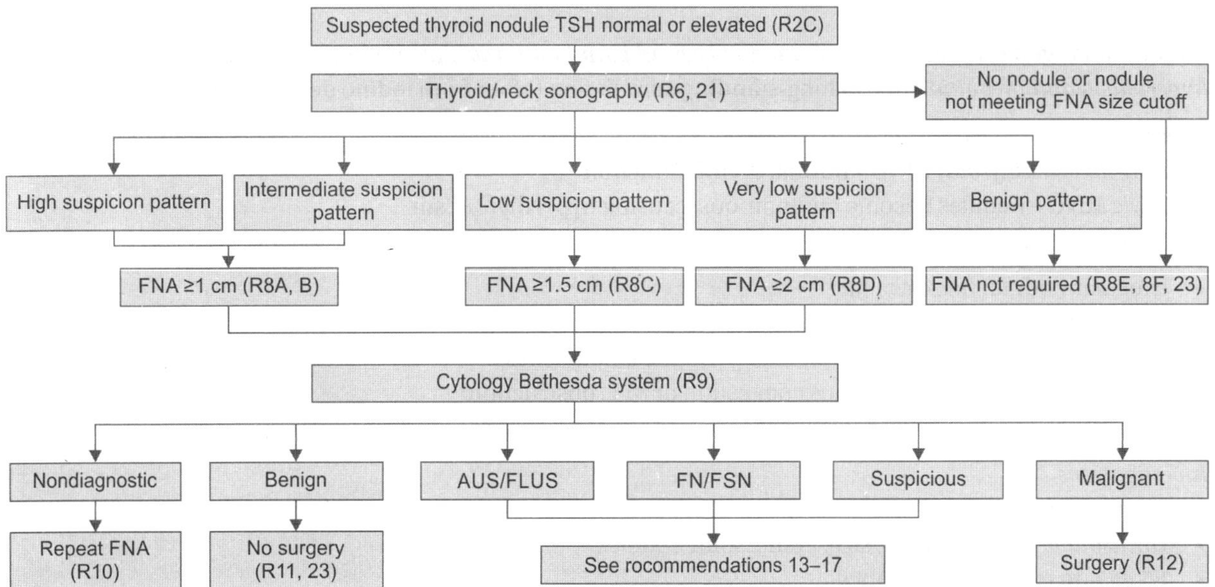

(AUS: atypia of undetermined significance; FLUS: follicular lesions of undetermined significance; FN: follicular neoplasm; FNA: fine-needle aspiration; TSH: thyroid-stimulating hormone)

15. Classify benign conditions of thyroid gland and management of multinodular goiter.

RGUHS 2025; RGUHS Karnataka 2025

Classification of Benign Conditions of the Thyroid Gland

Developmental/Congenital Lesions

I. Ectopic thyroid (e.g., lingual thyroid)
II. Thyroglossal duct cyst
III. Accessory thyroid tissue

Inflammatory Conditions (Thyroiditis)

Type	Key features
Acute suppurative thyroiditis	Bacterial infection, painful swelling, fever
Subacute (De Quervain's) thyroiditis	Post-viral, tender gland, transient thyrotoxicosis
Chronic lymphocytic (Hashimoto's) thyroiditis	Autoimmune, firm goiter, hypothyroidism, anti-TPO antibodies
Riedel's thyroiditis	Fibrosing, woody hard gland, compressive symptoms

Noninflammatory/Functional Disorders

Type	Description
Simple (diffuse) colloid goiter	Iodine deficiency or puberty-related enlargement
Multinodular goiter (MNG)	Irregular nodular enlargement of gland
Graves' disease	Autoimmune hyperthyroidism, diffuse goiter
Toxic nodular (Plummer's) disease	Functioning nodules causing thyrotoxicosis

Benign Neoplasms

Type	Features
Follicular adenoma	Encapsulated, solitary nodule, "cold" on scan
Hurthle cell adenoma	Variant with oncocytic cells

Management of Multinodular Goiter (MNG)

Definition

Multinodular goiter is an *enlargement of the thyroid gland with multiple nodules* resulting from *repeated cycles of hyperplasia and involution* due to long-standing stimulation (often from iodine deficiency).

Types

I. *Non-toxic (euthyroid) MNG* – normal thyroid function
II. *Toxic MNG* – nodules become autonomous, causing hyperthyroidism

Clinical Features

- Irregular nodular neck swelling
- Usually painless, slowly enlarging
- Pressure symptoms (if large): dysphagia, dyspnea, hoarseness
- Retrosternal extension → venous congestion or SVC obstruction
- Features of thyrotoxicosis in toxic MNG

Investigations

- *Thyroid function tests (T3, T4, TSH)*
- *Ultrasound neck* – number, size, cystic/solid nodules
- *FNAC* – to exclude malignancy
- *Thyroid scan (scintigraphy)* – "hot" and "cold" nodules
- *CT/MRI* – if retrosternal or compressive symptoms present

Management

- *General Measures*
  - Ensure adequate iodine intake
  - Maintain euthyroid state before definitive treatment
- *Medical Treatment*
  - *Euthyroid small goiters:* Observation, thyroxine suppression (limited use)
  - *Toxic MNG:*
    - Antithyroid drugs (Carbimazole, Propylthiouracil)
    - Beta-blockers for symptomatic control
    - *Radioiodine (I-131)* in elderly or high-risk surgical patients
- *Surgical Treatment*
  - *Indications:*
    - Large goiter causing compressive symptoms
    - Cosmetic deformity
    - Suspicion or proven malignancy (FNAC)
    - Retrosternal extension
    - Toxic MNG not controlled medically
  - *Surgical Options:*
    - *Near-total thyroidectomy* (preferred)
    - *Total thyroidectomy* – in recurrent or bilateral MNG
    - *Subtotal thyroidectomy* – rarely used now
  - *Complications:*
    - Hemorrhage/hematoma
    - Recurrent laryngeal nerve injury
    - Hypocalcemia (due to parathyroid injury)
    - Hypothyroidism (requiring thyroxine replacement)
- *Postoperative Care*
  - Monitor for airway obstruction and bleeding
  - Check serum calcium levels
  - Lifelong thyroxine replacement (after total thyroidectomy)
- *Follow-up*
  - Regular clinical and thyroid function assessment
  - Ultrasound if residual nodules suspected

16. Solitary thyroid nodule (STN)—management. ***Rajasthan University of Health Sciences 2025***

- The STN is defined as a discrete palpable swelling in an otherwise impalpable gland.
- It is a clinical diagnosis. Many of these cases prove to be multinodular but presenting as a single thyroid nodule.

Diagnostic Tools of Solitary Thyroid Nodule

• Clinical examination • Laboratory studies	• *Radiological studies:* – Neck ultrasonography – Isotope scanning of the thyroid – CT scan	• *Histopathological studies:* – Fine-needle aspiration cytology – Frozen section – Final histopathological examination

Treatment of the Solitary Cold Thyroid Nodule

Nonsurgical	*Surgical*
• No treatment, just follow-up by fine-needle aspiration cytology (FNAC) • Hormone suppressive therapy • Aspiration of a cyst • Ethanol injection • Recently, laser photocoagulation	• Isthmo-lobectomy • Near TT • Total thyroidectomy

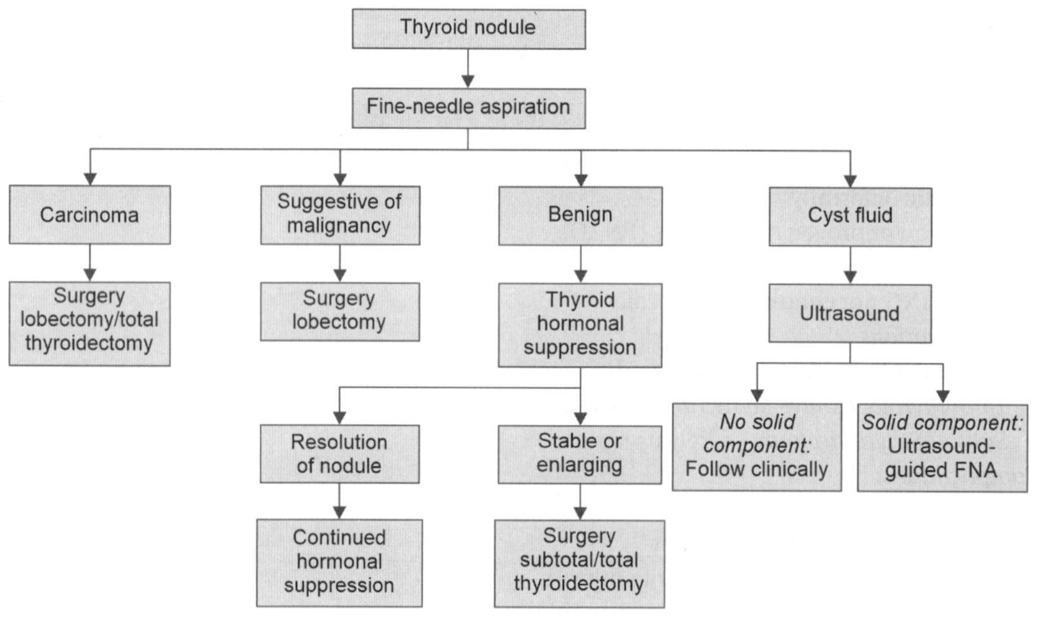

(FNA: fine-needle aspiration)

17. Discuss the modern management of Bethesda 3 and 4 solitary thyroid nodule (STN). ***WBUHS 2023***

The 2023 Bethesda System for Reporting Thyroid Cytopathology: Diagnostic Categories

- *Nondiagnostic*
  - Cyst fluid only
  - Virtually acellular specimen
  - Other (obscuring blood, clotting artifact, drying artifact, etc.)
- *Benign*
  - Consistent with follicular nodular disease (includes adenomatoid nodule, colloid nodule, etc.)
  - Consistent with chronic lymphocytic (Hashimoto) thyroiditis in the proper clinical context
  - Consistent with granulomatous (subacute) thyroiditis
  - Other
- *Atypia of undetermined significance (AUS)*
  - Specify if AUS-nuclear atypia or AUS-other [follicular lesions of undetermined significance (FLUS)]
- *Follicular neoplasm*
  - Specify if oncocytic (formerly Hürthle cell) type
- *Suspicious for malignancy*
  - Suspicious for papillary thyroid carcinoma (PTC)
  - Suspicious for medullary thyroid carcinoma (MTC)
  - Suspicious for metastatic carcinoma

- Suspicious for lymphoma
- Other

- *Malignant*
  - PTC
  - High-grade follicular-derived carcinoma
  - MTC
  - Undifferentiated (anaplastic) carcinoma
  - Squamous cell carcinoma
  - Carcinoma with mixed features (specify)
  - Metastatic malignancy
  - Non-Hodgkin lymphoma
  - Other

The 2023 Bethesda System for Reporting Thyroid Cytopathology: Implied Risk of Malignancy with Expected Ranges Based on Follow-Up of Surgically Resected Nodules with Recommended Clinical Management

Diagnostic category	***Usual management***
Nondiagnostic	Repeat fine-needle aspiration (FNA) with ultrasound guidance
Benign	Clinical and ultrasound follow-up
Atypia of undetermined significance	Repeat FNA, molecular testing, diagnostic lobectomy, or surveillance
Follicular neoplasm	Molecular testing and diagnostic lobectomy
Suspicious for malignancy	Molecular testing, lobectomy, or near-total thyroidectomy
Malignant	Lobectomy or near-total thyroidectomy

The 2023 Bethesda System for Reporting Thyroid Cytopathology in Pediatric Patients with Implied Risk of Malignancy and Possible Management Recommendations

Diagnostic category	***Usual management***
Nondiagnostic	Repeat fine-needle aspiration (FNA) with ultrasound guidance
Benign	Clinical and ultrasound follow-up
Atypia of undetermined significance	Repeat FNA or surgical resection
Follicular neoplasm	Surgical resection
Suspicious for malignancy	Surgical resection
Malignant	Surgical resection

THYROID TUMORS

18. Outline the current trends in management of thyroid malignancies. ***WBUHS 2025 Supplementary***

The management of *thyroid malignancies* has evolved significantly in recent years, with a shift toward more *individualized, risk-adapted, and less aggressive treatment* approaches, particularly for low-risk differentiated thyroid cancers.

Classification of Thyroid Malignancies

1. *Differentiated thyroid carcinomas (DTCs)*—~90% of cases
   - Papillary thyroid carcinoma (PTC)
   - Follicular thyroid carcinoma (FTC)
   - Hürthle cell carcinoma (variant of FTC)

2. *Medullary thyroid carcinoma (MTC)*—3–5%
3. *Anaplastic thyroid carcinoma (ATC)*—<2%
4. *Poorly differentiated thyroid carcinoma (PDTC)*
5. *Thyroid lymphomas and metastases* (rare)

Current Trends in Management

1. *Risk Stratification and Active Surveillance*
    - *Trend:* More conservative management for low-risk DTC
    - *Low-risk microcarcinomas* (<1 cm, confined to thyroid, no nodal disease):
        - Increasing use of *active surveillance* instead of immediate surgery
        - Regular US monitoring every 6–12 months
2. *Minimally Invasive and Conservative Surgery*
    - *Lobectomy* is now preferred over total thyroidectomy in low-risk unilateral DTC
    - *Total thyroidectomy* still reserved for:
        - Bilateral disease
        - Tumor >4 cm
        - Gross extrathyroidal extension
        - Clinically apparent lymph node metastases
    - Use of *nerve monitoring* and *minimally invasive techniques* (e.g., transoral endoscopic thyroidectomy)
3. *Radioactive Iodine (RAI) Therapy*
    - Use of RAI is now *selective*, not routine
    - *Avoided* in:
        - Low-risk PTC (e.g., tumors <2 cm, confined to thyroid, no aggressive histology)
    - *Indicated* for:
        - Intermediate and high-risk DTC
        - Distant metastases or gross residual disease
    - Use of *low-dose RAI* when applicable to reduce side effects
4. *Molecular Testing and Personalized Medicine*
    - *Molecular markers* (e.g., BRAF, RAS, RET/PTC, TERT promoter mutations) increasingly guide:
        - Surgical decisions
        - Prognostication
        - Targeted therapies in advanced disease
    - Genomic profiling standard in *indeterminate nodules* (Bethesda III/IV)
5. *Targeted Therapy and Systemic Treatment*
    - For *RAI-refractory DTC*:
        - *Tyrosine kinase inhibitors (TKIs): Lenvatinib, Sorafenib*
    - For *medullary thyroid cancer*:
        - *RET inhibitors: Selpercatinib, Pralsetinib (selective RET inhibitors)*
    - For *anaplastic thyroid cancer*:
        - *BRAF/MEK inhibitors* (e.g., *Dabrafenib + Trametinib*) in BRAF V600E-positive tumors
        - *Immunotherapy* (e.g., PD-1 inhibitors) in trials or compassionate use
6. *Surveillance and follow-up*
    - *Dynamic risk assessment* model:
        - Follow-up is adapted based on response to initial therapy
    - *Serum thyroglobulin (Tg)* and *neck ultrasound* are key tools
    - Less frequent imaging in low-risk, disease-free patients
7. *Management of Lymph Node Metastases*
    - *Prophylactic central neck dissection* is controversial:
        - *Not recommended* in clinically node-negative (cN0) low-risk PTC
        - *Therapeutic dissection* only if lymph nodes are involved (clinically or radiologically)

8. *Multidisciplinary Care*
   - Management is increasingly handled by *thyroid cancer teams* including:
     - Endocrinologists
     - Endocrine surgeons
     - Nuclear medicine
     - Oncologists
     - Pathologists and genetic counselors
9. *Patient-centered Approach and Shared Decision-Making*
   - Emphasis on *shared decision-making*, especially for:
     - Active surveillance
     - Extent of surgery
     - Use of RAI
   - Attention to *quality of life, cosmetic outcomes*, and *functional preservation*

Emerging and Future Directions

- Development of *AI and radiomics* in ultrasound diagnosis and risk stratification
- Use of *liquid biopsy* (circulating tumor DNA) in surveillance and detection
- New *immune checkpoint inhibitors* and *combination therapies* under clinical trials.

19. Classify thyroid tumors. Discuss the management of well differentiated carcinoma of thyroid.
WBUHS 2007; Maharashtra University of Health Sciences 2024

20. Write the management of well differentiated carcinoma of thyroid. ***RIMS, Imphal 2012***

Classification and Incidence of Thyroid Malignancies

Tumors of follicular cell origin		***Tumors of parafollicular or C-cell origin***	***Other***
Differentiated	*Undifferentiated*	Medullary (5%)	Lymphoma (<1%)
• Papillary (75%) • Follicular (10%) • Hürthle Cell (5%)	Anaplastic (5%)		

Management of Well-differentiated Carcinoma of Thyroid

Investigations

- Thyroid function test
- USG-guided fine-needle aspiration cytology (FNAC)
- CT/USG of neck.
- Indirect laryngoscopy.

Papillary Cancer

- Papillary cancer is the most common malignant thyroid tumor, accounting for 70–80% of all thyroid malignancies.
- Histologically, papillary carcinoma has characteristic features including psammoma bodies, intranuclear grooves, and cytoplasmic inclusions.
- It is multicentric in 30–50% of tumors.
- Papillary cancer tends to spread via the lymphatics with a known propensity for involvement of the mid- and lower-anterior cervical lymph nodes.
- Invasion of adjacent structures and distant metastases at the time of presentation are uncommon.
- Certain subtypes of papillary cancer including tall-cell, columnar cell, and oxyphilic variants tend to be radioiodine resistant, more aggressive, and associated with a poorer prognosis.
- The appropriate extent of surgical therapy for papillary cancer is debated. It is accepted that a lobectomy and isthmusectomy is satisfactory for papillary cancers <1.0 cm in size without lymphatic or systemic metastases. These patients have a recurrence rate of <5% and a death rate of approximately 0.1%.

- Lobectomy with isthmusectomy is also considered acceptable for patients with papillary cancers that are >1.0 cm when patients are categorized as low-risk for recurrence or mortality. Total thyroidectomy (TT) is uniformly accepted for treatment of high-risk papillary carcinoma.
- In addition, patients with a history of head and neck irradiation should undergo TT due to the high incidence of carcinoma at sites other than the nodule and their increased lifetime risk of developing thyroid cancer in the remaining thyroid gland.

Low-versus High-risk Criteria in Papillary Thyroid Cancer

Low-risk	*High-risk*
• Women <50 years • Men <40 years • Well or moderately differentiated tumors • Tumor <4 cm in diameter • Tumor confined to the thyroid gland • No distant metastases	• Women ≥50 years • Men ≥40 years • Poorly differentiated tumors, tall-cell, columnar cell, or oxyphilic variants. • Tumor ≥4 cm in diameter • Local invasion • Distant metastases

Lobectomy and isthmusectomy	*Total thyroidectomy*
• Excellent prognosis for patients with papillary cancer • Lower risk of recurrent laryngeal nerve injury and permanent hypoparathyroidism • >5% of recurrences occur in the thyroid bed, and that half of local recurrences can be cured surgically • Tumor multicentricity has little clinical significance	• Associated with the lowest incidence of local and regional recurrence and that when combined with postoperative ^{131}I ablation there is improved survival • Performing a total thyroidectomy also allows for the use of serum thyroglobulin (Tg) and radioiodine for early detection and treatment of metastatic disease • It eliminates the 1% risk of anaplastic transformation of cancer that remains in the residual lobe and avoids future reoperative surgery, which is associated with an increased risk of complications

- Furthermore, the role of lymph node dissection is also debated. Most series in the United States and Europe report a 30–40% incidence of cervical lymph node metastases. Prophylactic lymph node dissection is not warranted.
- Enlarged lymph nodes in the central and lateral neck should be removed and submitted for frozen section exam. If positive in the central neck, a central neck dissection should be performed.
- If positive in the lateral neck, a modified radical neck dissection should be undertaken. Modified radical neck dissection, also known as a functional neck dissection, refers to removal of lymph nodes anterior and posterolateral to the internal jugular vein from the mastoid process superiorly to the subclavian vessels inferiorly and laterally to the spinal accessory nerve, levels two through five.
- The internal jugular vein, spinal accessory nerve, and sternocleidomastoid muscle are preserved. Formal lymph node dissection is preferable.

Follicular Cancer

- Follicular cancer accounts for approximately 10% of all thyroid cancer.
- The female/male ratio is 3:1 and the mean age at presentation is 50 years. It usually presents as a painless solitary nodule or as a rapidly growing nodule within a multinodular goiter.
- Follicular cancers spread hematogenously with a predilection for the lungs and bones.
- Multicentricity and lymph node metastases are less common in patients with follicular carcinoma compared with papillary carcinoma.
- Approximately 10% will have spread to cervical lymph nodes.
- A follicular carcinoma is distinguished from a follicular adenoma based on the presence of capsular or vascular invasion determined by microscopic examination of a tissue sample.
- Fine-needle aspiration biopsy (FNAB), which evaluates cellular features alone, is unable to distinguish a benign from a malignant follicular neoplasm.
- Patients with a FNAB that is interpreted as a follicular neoplasm should undergo a lobectomy and isthmusectomy.
- Frozen section is also unreliable in distinguishing an adenoma from a malignant carcinoma.

- A completion thyroidectomy is recommended when the permanent section shows a clinically significant follicular cancer.
- A lobectomy and isthmusectomy are adequate for minimally invasive follicular cancer because it has an indolent course and patients have a near-normal life expectancy.
- A minimally invasive tumor is almost indistinguishable from a benign follicular adenoma except for the presence of limited capsular invasion.
- Invasive follicular carcinoma, defined by major capsular invasion and angioinvasion, is more aggressive, and affected patients are treated with either a near-total or TT.
- TT facilitates radioiodine ablation, the use of radioiodine for detection and treatment of metastatic disease,
- The use of serum Tg as a marker for persistent or recurrent disease.
- Lymph node dissection is performed only for gross metastatic disease.

Hürthle Cell Cancer

- Hürthle cell cancer accounts for approximately 5% of all thyroid cancers.
- Hürthle cell cancers have many clinicopathologic features that are similar to follicular cancers including difficulty in distinguishing a Hürthle cell carcinoma from a Hürthle cell adenoma and a propensity for vascular invasion.
- Hürthle cell carcinomas have many features that are distinct from follicular carcinomas including a greater tendency to spread to cervical lymph nodes, a higher incidence of distant metastases, and a failure to concentrate radioiodine.
- Less than 10% of Hürthle cell cancers take up radioiodine. Hürthle cell cancers have a higher tumor recurrence rate and a higher mortality rate.
- The mortality for patients with Hürthle cell carcinoma has been reported to be 30% at 10 years.

21. How will you prognosticate differential thyroid carcinoma? Describe management of a FNAC proved follicular neoplasm of right lobe of thyroid in a 45 years old female. ***WBUHS 2014***

Prognostication of Differentiated Thyroid Carcinoma

Low-versus High-risk Criteria in Papillary Thyroid Cancer

Low-risk	High-risk
• Women <50 years • Men <40 years • Well or moderately differentiated tumors • Tumor <4 cm in diameter • Tumor confined to the thyroid gland • No distant metastases	• Women ≥50 years • Men ≥40 years • Poorly differentiated tumors, tall-cell, columnar cell, or oxyphilic variants • Tumor ≥4 cm in diameter • Local invasion • Distant metastases

Prognostic risk Classification for Patients with Well-differentiated Thyroid Cancer (AMES or AGES)

	Risk	
Parameter	**Low**	**High**
Age (year)	<40	>40
Gender	Female	Male
Extent	No local extension, intrathyroidal, no capsular invasion	Capsular invasion, extrathyroidal extension
Metastasis	None	Regional or distant
Size	<2 cm	>4 cm
Grade	Well differentiated	Poorly differentiated

(AGES: age, pathologic grade of tumor, extent, and size of the primary tumor; AMES: age distant metastasis, extent of primary tumor size of primary tumor)

MACIS is an Abbreviation for the Factors Taken into Account to Predict Survival

- Metastasis (distant) or spread of the cancer to areas outside the neck,
- Age of the patient at the time the tumor was discovered,
- Invasion into surrounding areas of the neck as seen by the naked eye,
- Completeness of surgical resection (or removal) of the tumor, and
- Size of the tumor.

Prognostic Scoring Systems for AGES, AMES, and MACIS

AGES	*Prognostic score = 0.05 × age (if age ≥40)* • + 1 (if grade 2) • + 3 (if grade 3 or 4) • + 1 (if extrathyroid) • + 3 (if distant spread) • + 0.2 × tumor size (cm maximum diameter) *Survival by AGES score (20 years):* • ≤3.99 = 99% • 4–4.99 = 80% • 5–5.99 = 67% • ≥6 = 13%
AMES	*Low-risk: Younger patients (men ≤40, women ≤50)* • With no metastases • Older patients (intrathyroid papillary, minor capsular invasion for follicular lesions) • Primary cancers <5 cm • No distant metastasis (men >40, women >50) *Survival by AMES risk-groups (20 years):* • Low-risk = 99% • High-risk = 61%
MACIS	*Score = 3.1 (if age <40 years) or 0.08 ×* age *(if age <40 years)* • + 0.3 × tumor size (cm maximum diameter) • + 1 (if incompletely resected) • + 1 (if locally invasive) • + 3 (if distant spread) *Survival by MACIS score (20 years):* • <6 = 99% • 6–6.99 = 89% • 7–7.99 = 56% • ≥8 = 24%

(AGES: age, pathologic grade of tumor, extent, and size of the primary tumor; AMES: age distant metastasis, extent of primary tumor size of primary tumor; MACIS: metastasis, age at presentation, completeness of excision, invasion, size)

Treatment of follicular carcinoma is primarily surgical: Current National Comprehensive Cancer Network (NCCN) guidelines recommend lobectomy plus isthmusectomy as the initial surgery for patients with follicular neoplasms, with prompt completion of thyroidectomy if invasive follicular thyroid carcinoma (FTC) is found on the final histologic section. Therapeutic neck dissection of involved compartments is recommended for clinically apparent/biopsy-proven disease.

- The diagnosis of the carcinoma cannot be determined by preoperative FNA or intraoperative frozen section diagnosis of a follicular lesion.
- If the lesion is 2 cm or smaller and well contained within one thyroid lobe, thyroid lobectomy and isthmusectomy can be done.
- If the lesion is larger than 2 cm, then TT should be done.
- If the follicular lesion is larger than 4 cm, the risk for cancer is higher than 50%, and TT is an obvious choice.
- Current recommendations support performing completion thyroidectomy if TT would have been offered if the diagnosis had been secured preoperatively.

- The prognosis after treatment of follicular cancer depends on age.
  - Patients younger than 40 years have the best prognosis, with survival rates approaching 95% at 5 and 10 years.
  - Series comparing follicular cancer with PTC have shown a poorer prognosis for follicular cancer, although this disparity is more prominent after 10–15 years.
  - Poorly differentiated follicular cancer and well-differentiated follicular cancer have 60% and 80% 10-year survival rates, respectively.

Postoperative Treatment

- Accepted postsurgical management of well-differentiated follicular thyroid cancers involves the use of radioiodine ablation and long-term monitoring of Tg.
- ^{131}I contains high energy (gamma rays) and medium-energy (beta particles), which enhances the therapeutic effect.
- Patients are usually withheld from thyroid replacement therapy so that TSH levels may become elevated, rendering the thyroid iodine avid and thus maximizing the effect of ^{131}I.
- Several studies have suggested that ^{131}I ablation reduces disease-specific mortality in patients with primary tumors measuring at least 1 cm.
- If a patient has undergone complete thyroid ablation, Tg levels should be undetectable.
- The recent development of human recombinant TSH has redefined the efficacy of monitoring stimulated Tg levels as evidence of recurrence.

22. Discuss the role of USG, CT, MRI, and radiopharmaceuticals in the management of thyroid malignancies. ***WBUHS 2018***

Role of USG in the Management of Thyroid Malignancy

- Ultrasonography can detect multiple nodules in patients with clinically STN. A dominant palpable nodule should be managed as STN even if USG reveals additional non palpable nodular disease. Even a 1 mm size nodule could be detected with high resolution USG.
- Nonpalpable nodule >1.0–1.5 cm represents an absolute indication to perform an US-guided fine-needle biopsy.
- It can also help in differentiating malignant from benign nodules by detecting hypoechogenicity in solid nodules (up to 55% of benign nodules are hypoechoic compared to thyroid parenchyma, making nodule hypoechogenicity less specific), presence of microcalcifications, irregularity in shape, intranodular vascular spots, and absence of halo and cystic elements, which suggested high chance of malignancy. Features with the highest specificities for thyroid cancer are microcalcification, irregular margins, and tall shape.
- Thyroid nodules diagnostic FNA is recommended for:
  - Nodules >1 cm in greatest dimension with high suspicion pattern.
  - Nodules >1 cm in greatest dimension with intermediate suspicion sonographic pattern.
  - Nodules >1.5 cm in greatest dimension with low suspicious sonographic pattern.

  The FNAB is recommended for nodules smaller than 10 mm if clinical information or US features are suspicious.
- US-guided FNA of thyroid nodules has a distinct role in the primary diagnostic process of thyroid carcinoma.
- Also during the follow-up US has a clear added value: US imaging is presently the most sensitive imaging modality for the early detection of locoregional recurrence and/or metastases, especially cervical lymph node metastases. Size and location of cervical lymph nodes are the most important predictors of metastatic disease.
- The US procedure may be easily combined with FNA biopsies from suspected lesions. US of the neck has been recommended as a standard procedure during follow-up of thyroid carcinoma.

Computed Tomography and Magnetic Resonance Imaging

- CT and MRI do not add significantly to the workup of uncomplicated thyroid nodules that are otherwise well characterized by US.
- However, either modality may be helpful in evaluating local extension in more advanced stages of thyroid cancer.

- CT or MRI is particularly appropriate for a suspicious mass (or biopsy-proven cancer) with bulky cervical lymph nodes. Additionally, either modality can be used for postoperative follow-up, particularly for suspicion of recurrent disease.
- CT is advisable in preoperative planning for larger thyroid masses that are believed to have a substernal component based on physical examination, US, or chest radiograph.
- CT scan has role in detecting local neck or upper thoracic spread and compression of neighboring structures.
- There is no standard role for computed tomography (CT) scans in the follow-up of patients with thyroid carcinoma; the use of this modality is at the discretion of the attending physician.
- CT scans can be done to visualize the anatomic substrate of a focus of I-131 uptake or 18-FDG uptake, or possibly to demonstrate metastases in Tg-positive, I-131 negative patients.
- *Magnetic resonance imaging (MRI):* There is no defined role for MRI in the treatment and follow-up of thyroid carcinoma.
- MRI can serve as an imaging modality for detection of metastases. As a result of the high protein (Tg) content of PTC and FTC, cervical lymph node metastases are sometimes identified by MRI. However, the low specificity will not allow its use as a screening technique in this area.

Radiopharmaceuticals used in Thyroid Cancer

Radiopharmaceutical	*Radiation emission*	*Clinical utility*
^{131}I	Gamma, beta	• Imaging thyroid nodules[a] • Whole body imaging to stage DTC • Postoperative ablation of thyroid remnant • Treating metastatic DTC
^{123}I	Gamma	• Imaging thyroid nodules • Whole body imaging to stage DTC
[^{99}mTc]pertechnetate	Gamma	• Imaging thyroid nodules • Imaging local metastases[b]
[^{99}mTc]MDP	Gamma	Identify bone metastases
^{124}I	Positron	Whole body imaging to stage DTC[b]
[^{111}In]pentetreotide	Gamma	Somatostatin receptor imaging in DTC and MCT
[^{123}I]MIBG	Gamma	Amine uptake imaging in MCT
[^{99}mTc]DMSA(V)	Gamma	Staging of MCT
[^{18}F]FDG	Positron	Staging of DTC and MCI[b]
^{201}T1	Gamma	Characterization of thyroid nodule[a]
[^{99}mTc]sestamibi	Gamma	• Characterization of thyroid nodule[a] • Staging of DTC
[^{131}I] MIBG	Gamma, beta	• Staging of MCT[a] • Treating MIBG positive metastatic MCT
[99Y] octreotide/tate	Beta	• Treating [^{111}In]penteterotide positive MCT[b] • Treating [^{111}In]pentetreotide positive, ^{131}I negative DTC

(DMSA: dimercaptosuccinic acid; DTC: differentiated thyroid cancer; FDG: fluorodeoxyglucose; MCT: medullary cell cancer of the thyroid; MDP: methyl diphosphosphate; MIBG: meta-iodobenzylguanidine)
[a]No longer used routinely.
[b]Experimental.

- Following (near) TT, patients with differentiated thyroid cancer are usually treated with I-131 ablation of residual normal and neoplastic thyroid tissue. This serves multiple purposes: firstly, it destroys remaining (normal or neoplastic) thyroid tissue, thereby increasing the specificity of thyroglobulin measurements during the follow-ups.

- Secondly, I-131 may destroy occult microcarcinoma, thereby minimizing the incidence of recurrence. Thirdly, a high I-131 dose permits postablation I-131 whole body scintigraphy (WBS) which can detect occult metastases.
- I-131 ablation in addition to (near) TT significantly reduces the risk of recurrence and cancer-specific mortality in patients with differentiated thyroid cancer.
- Diagnostic scintigraphy with I-131 preceding ablation is controversial; it may or may not cause "stunning" of the remaining thyroid tissue (i.e., diminished I-131uptake) and thus reduce the efficacy of the I-131 ablative dosage.
- Thallium-201 SPECT and Planar Scintigraphy Thallium-201 thallous chloride (Tl-201) scanning has no specific advantages in the follow-up of thyroid carcinoma.
- This specific tumor-seeking agent can be employed for the detection of I-131-negative lesions if 18-FDG PET is unavailable.

23. Current concept in the management of different types of thyroid carcinoma. *WBUHS 2016*

Investigations

- *TSH and FT3, FT4.*
- *High-resolution US:* Halo sign, comet tail sign, and type 3 intranodular vascularity of malignancy are helpful. Involvement of trachea, vessels, and strap muscles can be made out.
- *Fine-needle aspiration cytology:* Cellular diagnosis of DTC is now feasible; ultrastructural study, and histocytochemistry are of great help.
- *Tru-cut Biopsy:* Selected indication is in inoperable cases to plan out management. Also to differentiate lymphoma from anaplastic carcinoma.
- *Monoclonal antibodies for lymphoma:* This can differentiate anaplastic carcinoma from lymphoma.
- *Imprint smear:* Better interpretation than FNAC/frozen section.
- *CT/MRI:* Specific indication is to know extent of tumor spread and local tissue plane infiltration.
- *Scintiscan:* Presently limited use. Cold nodule classically in malignancy. Still helpful in solitary nodule thyroid.
- *Tumor markers:* Very significant is TGB which if done before and after management helps in follow-up and can indicate recurrence/metastasis. Carcinoembryonic antigen (CEA), CD-34, MVD, and p53 protein have also correlation.
- *X-ray chest and X-ray of bone met site:* Demonstrates local secondary deposit.
- *US liver:* Done to detect liver metastases wherever suspected.
- *Skeletal survey:* Done by radionuclide scan (gamma camera) wherever indicated can alter the clinical staging of the disease.

MACIS Score

MACIS Score = 3.1 (if age <40 years) or 0.8 × age (if age ≥40 years)

- + 0.3 × tumor size (cm maximum diameter)
- + 1 (if incompletely resected)
- + 1 (if locally invasive)
- + 3 (if distant spread)

AGES Score

AGES	Prognostic score = 0.5 × age (if age ≥40 years) • + 1 (if grade 2) • + 3 (if grade 3 or 4) • + 1 (extrathyroid) • + 3 (if distant spread) • + 0.2 × tumor size (cm maximum diameter)	*Survival by AGES score (20 years):* • ≤3.99 = 99% • 4–4.99 = 80% • 5–5.99 = 67% • ≥6 = 13%

AMES Score

Low-risk

- Younger patients (men ≤40, women ≤50)
- With no metastasis
- Older patients (intrathyroid papillary, minor capsular invasion for follicular lesions)
- Primary cancers <5 cm
- No distant metastases

High-risk

- All patients with distant metastasis
- Extrathyroid papillary, major capsular invasion for follicular lesions
- Primary cancers ≥5 cm in older patients (Men >40, women >50)

Survival by AMES Risk Groups (20 years)

- Low-risk = 90%
- High-risk = 61%

Treatment

Low- versus High-risk Criteria in Papillary Thyroid Cancer

Low-risk	*High-risk*
• Women <50 years • Men <40 years • Well or moderately differentiated tumors • Tumor <4 cm in diameter • Tumor confined to the thyroid gland • No distant metastases	• Women ≥50 years • Men ≥40 years • Poorly differentiated tumors, tall-cell, columnar cell, or oxyphilic variants • Tumor ≥4 cm in diameter • Local invasion • Distant metastases

Surgical Treatment

- A lobectomy and isthmusectomy is satisfactory for papillary cancers <1.0 cm in size without lymphatic or systemic metastases.
- Lobectomy with isthmusectomy—for patients with papillary cancers that are >1.0 cm when patients are categorized as low-risk for recurrence or mortality.
- TT is uniformly accepted for treatment of high-risk papillary carcinoma.
- In addition, patients with a history of head and neck irradiation should undergo TT due to the high incidence of carcinoma at sites other than the nodule and their increased lifetime risk of developing thyroid cancer in the remaining thyroid gland.

Role of Postoperative Remnant Ablation

Indications

- Stage III and IV disease
- All patients with stage II disease younger than age 45 years
- Most patients with stage II disease 45 years or older
- Selected patients with stage I disease, especially those with multifocal disease, nodal metastases, extrathyroidal or vascular invasion, and/or more aggressive histologies.

Protocol of Thyroid Hormone Withdrawal for Remnant Ablation

Aim: Achieve TSH of >30 mU/L

- Single-dose exogenous rTSH results in TSH levels between 51 and 82 mU/L
- Endogenous TSH elevation can be achieved by
    - Stopping levothyroxine (LT4) and switching to levotriiodothyronine (LT3) for 2–4 weeks followed by withdrawal of triiodothyronine (T3) for 2 weeks

- Discontinuation of LT4 for 3 weeks without use of T3
- rTSH stimulation can be used for remnant ablation.

Role of Postoperative Diagnostic RAIU Scan

Indication

- When the extent of thyroid remnant cannot be assessed from the surgical report/USG
- If the result is likely to alter the subsequent management
- If the result is likely to alter the dose of RAI treatment
- If used, low dose I-131 (1-3 mCi)/I-123 scan recommended
    - Low iodine diet (50 μg/day for 1–2 weeks) is recommended prior to scan
- *Post-therapy scan:*
    - Detects additional foci in 10–26% cases, alters the stage in 10%
    - Done 1 week post radioiodine therapy.

Role of TSH Suppression Therapy

Mechanism of action:

- Decreases the expression of thyroid specific proteins
- Decreases the rate of cell growth
- *High-risk patients:*
    - Keep TSH <0.1 mIU/L
    - After remission continue suppressive therapy × 3–5 years
- *Low-risk patients:*
    - TSH = 0.1–0.5 mIU/L
    - After remission keep it between 0.5 and 1 mIU/mL

  There is no role for routine adjunctive chemotherapy.

Surgery for Follicular Carcinoma

- From clinicopathological stand point these carcinomas are divided into low-risk and high-risk.
- Three important risk factors, viz., vascular invasion, metastases, and age >45 years.
- The result of cytological and frozen section histology in this tumor is high in accuracy of both in interpretation.
    - In low-risk patient with intrathyroidal (noninvasive) lesion <2.5 cm in size (determined on scan) a hemithyroidectomy with isthmusectomy suffices.
    - Completion thyroidectomy is indicated if histology reveals a more invasive form of carcinoma postoperatively.
    - In all other follicular carcinoma, a total or near TT is indicated.

      This is recommended in presence of even metastases (the incidence of which is fairly high with this carcinoma) as it facilitates adjuvant treatment with I-131.

      If nodes are involved, ipsilateral functional block dissection with central compartment clearance is to be undertaken.

Hürthle Cell Tumors

- Hürthle cell, though modified follicular cell is now considered a separate tumor altogether, contrary to earlier belief, majority of Hürthle cell tumor (HCN) are benign.
- Capsular and vascular invasion on histology and metastases clinically characterize malignant HCN.
- There is an indeterminate form also. The potential incidence of indeterminate forms creates controversy regarding extent of surgery.
- The undisputed benign forms are best treated by hemithyroidectomy.
- For aggressive benign type, indeterminate type and frankly malignant HCN, a total or near thyroidectomy is the standard.

- If malignancy is found on postoperative histology in a preoperative diagnosed benign lesion, a completion thyroidectomy is then indicated.
- The approach to lymph nodes is same as in follicular carcinoma; if nodes are involved, ipsilateral functional block dissection with central compartment clearance is to be undertaken.

Medullary Carcinoma Thyroid

- All patients should receive TT, a complete central neck dissection (removal of all lymph nodes and fatty tissues in the central area of the neck), and removal of all lymph nodes and surrounding fatty tissues within the side of the neck which harbored the tumor.
- RAI therapy is not useful.
- Prophylactic thyroidectomy recommended before the age of 5 years in patients with familial medullary carcinoma, MENIIa, and IIB.

Anaplastic Carcinoma Thyroid

Patients tend to present late. Compressive symptoms of neighboring structures can be common.

- *CT:* Useful for assessment of tumor invasion as well as metastatic burden. Lymph node ± metastatic involvement is generally common at time of CT assessment. Typically seen as a highly infiltrative lesion about the thyroid gland
- Nuclear imaging—radioiodine: Usually has no uptake

External irradiation or chemotherapy may provide limited palliation.

THYROIDECTOMIES

24. Completion thyroidectomy.

Completion thyroidectomy plays an important role in the treatment of patients with thyroid cancer. Recently, not all patients have undergone TT, which is the preferred operation for cancer treatment.

One of the reasons is the difficulty of perioperative diagnosis of cancer which can lead to inappropriate procedures.

Completion thyroidectomy is still believed to have increased complication rates, but other authors in the literature describe no higher incidence of complications. Several studies that are designed to decrease the complication risk have focused on the timing of completion surgery and the care for, or attention to, the surgical technique.

Completion Thyroidectomy

- When a lobectomy is performed and the pathology comes back that the lobe had cancer, the remaining lobe is surgically removed as well.
- It involves removing the remaining thyroid tissue after a patient has had a previous partial thyroid resection (i.e., lobectomy).
- It may be done years later or it may be done soon after a lobectomy (as early as the next week).
- The reasons for completion thyroidectomy are the same as for a lobectomy or TT.
- TT—removal of the whole thyroid. All patients who undergo a completion thyroidectomy will need to be on life-long thyroid hormone replacement after surgery.

25. Describe the recent advances of thyroid surgery and enumerate ten complications of thyroidectomy.

RGUHS Karnataka 2025

Recent Advances in Thyroid Surgery

Thyroid surgery has evolved considerably over the past two decades — from conventional open thyroidectomy to minimally invasive and image-guided, function-preserving procedures. The goals of these advances are to *reduce morbidity, improve cosmesis, preserve function,* and *enhance oncological safety.*

I. *Minimally Invasive and Remote Access Techniques*

- *Minimally Invasive Video-assisted Thyroidectomy (MIVAT)*
  - Developed by *Miccoli et al.*
  - Uses a small (2–3 cm) central incision.
  - Performed under endoscopic vision.
  - *Advantages:*
    - Smaller scar and better cosmesis
    - Less pain and shorter hospital stay
    - Comparable oncological safety in selected patients (small nodules, early cancers)
  - *Limitations:* Not suitable for large goiters or advanced cancers.
- *Endoscopic Thyroidectomy (Remote Access)*

  These techniques avoid a neck scar by using remote incisions:

Approach	*Access incision*	*Remarks*
Transaxillary approach	Axilla	Common in East Asia; good cosmetic results; unilateral access only
Bilateral axillo-breast approach (BABA)	Axilla + periareolar	Allows bilateral access
Retroauricular/Facelift approach	Behind ear	Excellent cosmesis; technically demanding
Transoral vestibular approach (TOETVA)	Oral vestibule	Truly scarless; increasingly popular worldwide

  - *Advantages:*
    - No visible neck scar ("scarless thyroidectomy")
    - Good visualization of recurrent laryngeal nerve and parathyroids
  - *Limitations:*
    - Longer operative time, learning curve
    - Risk of mental nerve injury (in TOETVA)
    - Not suitable for large or invasive cancers

II. *Robotic Thyroid Surgery*

- Uses *da Vinci robotic system* with 3D magnified vision and articulated instruments.
- Approaches: *Transaxillary, BABA, Retroauricular, Transoral*
  - *Advantages:*
    - Precise dissection with tremor filtration
    - Better visualization of critical structures
    - Excellent cosmetic results
  - *Disadvantages:*
    - High cost
    - Longer operative time
    - Limited availability

III. *Intraoperative Neuromonitoring (IONM)*

- Used to identify and preserve *recurrent laryngeal nerve (RLN)* function.
- *Two main types:*
  - *Intermittent IONM:* Nerve stimulated intermittently with a handheld probe
  - *Continuous IONM:* Ongoing real-time feedback using an electrode on the endotracheal tube
- *Advantages:*
  - Reduces risk of RLN injury
  - Helps decide on staging bilateral thyroidectomy if loss of signal occurs

IV. *Parathyroid Preservation and Autotransplantation*

- *Intraoperative parathyroid identification* improved by:
  - *Near-infrared autofluorescence imaging* (detects natural parathyroid fluorescence)
  - *Indocyanine green (ICG) angiography* (assesses vascularity)
- *Parathyroid autotransplantation* (into sternocleidomastoid) helps prevent permanent hypocalcemia.

V. *Energy-based Devices*

- *Used for hemostasis and dissection:*
  - *Harmonic scalpel (ultrasonic coagulator)*
  - *LigaSure (bipolar vessel sealing system)*
- *Advantages:*
  - Reduces operative time
  - Minimizes blood loss
  - Less lateral thermal damage than conventional electrocautery

VI. Enhanced Recovery after Surgery (ERAS) Protocols

- Shorter hospital stay and faster recovery.
- *Elements include:*
  - Preoperative counseling and optimization
  - Early mobilization and feeding
  - Minimal drains and dressings

VII. *Image-guided and Adjunctive Technologies*

- Intraoperative Ultrasound
  - For localization of nodules and lymph nodes.
- Nearinfrared Fluorescence (NIR)
  - Enhances visualization of parathyroid glands and vascularity.
- Navigation and Augmented Reality
  - 3D imaging helps in orientation during complex or reoperative thyroid surgery (emerging technology).

VIII. *Molecular and Oncologic Advances (Adjuncts to Surgery)*

- *Molecular testing* (e.g. BRAF, RAS, RET mutations) improves diagnosis and guides surgical extent.
- *Active surveillance* for low-risk papillary microcarcinomas — reducing unnecessary surgery.

Answer of 2nd part of the question is in the next answer.

---

26. Discuss the preventive measure, diagnosis, and complications of total thyroidectomy.

The Tamil Nadu Dr MGR Medical University 2025; WBUHS 2008

Postoperative Complications

- *Hemorrhage:*
  - A tension hematoma deep to the cervical fascia is usually due to reactionary hemorrhage from one of the thyroid arteries.
  - Occasionally, hemorrhage from a thyroid remnant or a thyroid vein may be responsible.
  - This is a rare but desperate emergency.
  - Urgent exploration of wound followed by securing the bleeding site should be done.
  - If releasing the tension hematoma does not immediately relieve airway obstruction, the trachea should be intubated at once.
  - An endotracheal tube can be left in place for several days; steroids are given to reduce edema and a tracheostomy is rarely necessary.

- Intubation in the presence of laryngeal edema may be very difficult and should be carried out by an experienced anesthetist.
- Repeated unsuccessful attempts may aggravate the problem and, in a crisis, it is safer to perform a needle tracheostomy as a temporary measure; a large bore 12 G intravenous (IV) cannula (diameter 2.3 mm) is satisfactory.

▪ *Recurrent laryngeal nerve paralysis and voice change:*
  - RLN injury may be unilateral or bilateral, transient, or permanent.
  - Early routine postoperative laryngoscopy reveals a much higher incidence of transient cord paralysis than is detectable by simple assessment of the integrity of the voice and cough.
  - Such temporary dysfunction is not clinically important, however, but voice and cord function should be assessed at the first follow-up 4 weeks postoperatively.
  - Permanent paralysis is rare if the nerve has been identified at operation.
  - Injury to the external branch of the superior laryngeal nerve is more common because of its proximity to the superior thyroid artery.
  - This leads to loss of tension in the vocal cord with diminished power and range in the voice.
  - Patients, particularly those who use their voices professionally, must be advised that any thyroid operation will result in change to the voice even in the absence of nerve trauma.
  - Fortunately, for most patients the changes are subtle and only demonstrable on formal voice assessment.

▪ *Thyroid insufficiency:*
  - Following subtotal thyroidectomy this usually occurs within 2 years;
  - The incidence is considerably higher than was previously thought and rates of 20–45% at 10 years have been reported.
  - This results from a change in the autoimmune response, from stimulation to destruction of the thyroid cells.
  - There is a definite relationship between the estimated weight of the thyroid remnant and the development of thyroid failure after subtotal thyroidectomy for Graves' disease.
  - Thyroid insufficiency is rare after surgery for a toxic adenoma because there is no autoimmune disease present.

▪ *Parathyroid insufficiency:*
  - This is due to removal of the parathyroid glands or to infarction through damage to the parathyroid end artery; often, both factors occur together.
  - Vascular injury is probably far more important than inadvertent removal.
  - The incidence of permanent hypoparathyroidism should be <1% and most cases present dramatically 2–5 days after operation; however, very rarely the onset is delayed for 2–3 weeks or a patient with marked hypocalcemia is asymptomatic.

▪ *Thyrotoxic crisis (storm):*
  - This is an acute exacerbation of hyperthyroidism.
  - It occurs if a thyrotoxic patient has been inadequately prepared for thyroidectomy and is now extremely rare.
  - Very rarely, a thyrotoxic patient presents in a crisis and this may follow an unrelated operation.
  - Symptomatic and supportive treatment is for dehydration, hyperpyrexia, and restlessness.
  - This requires administration of IV fluids, cooling the requiring urgent decompression by opening the layers of the wound, not simply the skin closure, to relieve tension before urgent transfer to theatre to secure the bleeding vessel.
  - A subcutaneous hematoma or collection of serum may form under the skin flaps and require evacuation in the following 48 hours.
  - This should not be confused with the potentially life-threatening deep tension hematoma.

- *Respiratory obstruction:*
  - This is very rarely due to collapse or kinking of the trachea (tracheomalacia).
  - Most cases are caused by laryngeal edema.
  - The most important cause of laryngeal edema is a tension hematoma.
  - However, trauma to the larynx by anesthetic intubation and surgical manipulation are important contributory factors, particularly if the goiter is very vascular, and may cause laryngeal edema without a tension hematoma.
  - Unilateral or bilateral recurrent nerve paralysis will not cause immediate postoperative respiratory obstruction unless laryngeal edema is also present but it will aggravate the obstruction.
  - Patient with ice packs, the administration of oxygen, diuretics for cardiac failure, digoxin for uncontrolled atrial fibrillation, sedation, and IV hydrocortisone.
  - Specific treatment is with carbimazole 10–20 mg 6-hourly,
  - Lugol's iodine 10 drops 8-hourly by mouth or sodium iodide 1 g intravenously.
  - Propranolol intravenously (1–2 mg) or orally (40 mg 6-hourly) will block β-adrenergic effects.
- *Wound infection:*
  - Cellulitis requiring prescription of antibiotics.
  - A significant subcutaneous or deep cervical abscess is exceptionally rare and should be drained.
- *Hypertrophic or keloid scar:*
  - This is more likely to form if the incision overlies the sternum and in dark-skinned individuals. Intradermal injections of corticosteroid should be given at once and repeated monthly if necessary.
  - Scar revision rarely results in significant long-term improvement.
- *Stitch granuloma:*
  - This may occur with or without sinus formation and is seen after the use of non-absorbable, particularly silk, suture material.
  - Absorbable ligatures and sutures must be used throughout thyroid surgery.
  - Some surgeons use a subcuticular absorbable skin suture rather than the traditional skin clips or staples.
  - Skin staples, if used, can be removed safely in <48 hours because the skin closure is supported by the platysma stitch.

Postoperative Care

- If the voice is normal and the cough occlusive it is not essential to carry out laryngoscopy before leaving hospital.
- Transient cord palsies are probably more common than generally appreciated.
- Even if routine cord visualization is not part of the normal postoperative review, persisting voice change requires visualization of the cords.
- Hypocalcemia depends not only on the identification but also on the preservation of the parathyroid glands with an intact blood supply. In addition, metabolic bone disease, "hungry bones syndrome," results in the rapid influx of serum calcium into bones, particularly if preoperative preparation has been with β-blockade rather than normalization of the serum T4.
- Hypocalcemia is more common after total than subtotal thyroidectomy and reflects the increased trauma to the parathyroids.
- About 25% of patients develop transient hypocalcemia and oral calcium may be necessary (1 g three or four times daily).
- If associated symptoms are severe and the serum calcium less, 10 mL of 10% calcium gluconate (equivalent to 8.4 mg or 2.3 mmol calcium) should be given.
- To screen for parathyroid insufficiency the serum calcium should be measured at the first review attendance 4–6 weeks after operation.
- After subtotal resection, stability in terms of thyroid function takes time.

- It is important that biochemical (subclinical) thyroid failure should not be an indication for treatment during the first year, as the majority of patients with early subclinical failure, which is common, ultimately regain normality.
- Even when there are clinical features of failure, thyroxine should be withheld if possible during the first 6 months.
- Most patients who develop thyroid failure do so within the first 2 years but there is a continuing incidence thereafter.
- Recurrent thyrotoxicosis may occur at any time after operation and follow-up should therefore be for life.
- Once a stable situation has been achieved, follow-up after thyroid surgery should be carried out by an automated computerized system, which dramatically reduces the number of patient attendances at the thyroid clinic.

POST-THYROIDECTOMY PHONATION PROBLEMS

27. What are the types of phonation problems encountered after thyroid surgery? How are they prevented or treated? ***WBUHS 2018***

The voice problems after thyroid surgery include breathiness with loss of air during vocalization, change in pitch, inability to project the voice, and early vocal fatigue, any and all of which can impair communication.

- Voice change is a known complication after thyroid surgery. There are two sets of nerves near the thyroid gland that help control the voice. These are the RLN and the external branch of the superior laryngeal nerve. Damage to a RLN can cause patient "to lose his/her voice." The chance that one of the RLNs will be permanently damaged is about 1%. A more subtle change in vocal function may be noticeable if the patient is a professional voice singer or public speaker.
- Temporary voice changes, such as mild hoarseness, voice tiring, and weakness are more common and can happen in 5–10% of patients. The temporary problem usually occurs because one or more of the nerves are irritated either by moving them out of the way during the operation or because of the inflammation that happens after the surgery. Although the voice usually improves in the first few weeks after surgery, it can last up to 6 months.
- If both RLNs are damaged, the vocal cords may close and not allow air to pass from the mouth and nose into the lungs. In this case, a tracheostomy tube may need to be placed to allow passage of air into the lungs. This is extremely rare.
- If the external branch of the superior laryngeal nerve is injured and not functioning properly, the vocal cord may move normally. However, it may cause a problem in making high-pitched noises or yelling. These changes are slightly more common, but may be so subtle that they are difficult to notice.
- If any of these voice changes last for >6 months after the operation, they are likely to be permanent. An otolaryngologist/ear, nose, and throat (ENT) doctor or vocal specialist can be very helpful in determining the specific problem and can perform different procedures to reposition the vocal cord to improve voice quality (vocal cord medialization).

Signs and symptoms of vocal cord paralysis may include:

- A breathy quality to the voice
- Hoarseness
- Noisy breathing
- Loss of vocal pitch
- Choking or coughing while swallowing food, drink, or saliva
- The need to take frequent breaths while speaking
- Inability to speak loudly
- Loss of your gag reflex

Algorithm for management of unilateral recurrent laryngeal nerve paralysis (URLNP) after thyroid surgery.

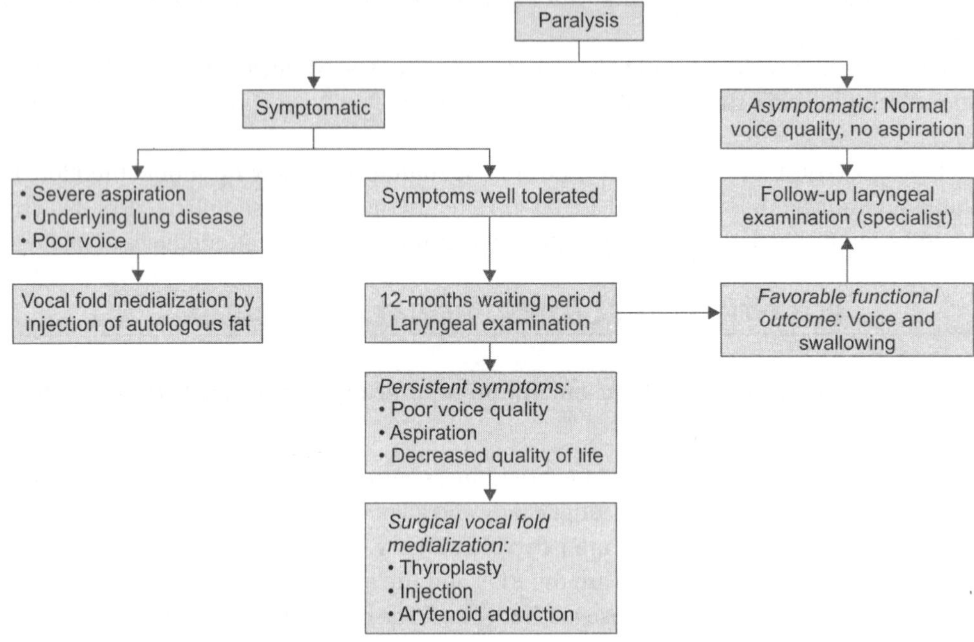

MULTIPLE ENDOCRINE NEOPLASIA

28. Classify MEN syndrome. Discuss the management of MEN 2. ***WBUHS 2022, 2024***

Endocrine features	***Nonendocrine features***
Primary hyperparathyroidism (PHPT)—Parathyroid hyperplasia (90%)	Lipomas (30%)
Enteropancreatic tumor	Facial angiofibromas (85%)
1. Gastrinoma (40%)	
2. Insulinoma (10%)	Collagenomas (70%)
3. Nonfunctioning (NF) including pancreatic polypeptide (20%)	Ependymoma (1%)
4. *Other rare types:* (2%) • Glucagonoma • VIPoma • Somatostatinoma, etc. • Foregut carcinoid • Thymic carcinoid NF (2%) • Bronchial carcinoid NF (2%) • Gastric enterochromaffin-like tumor NF (10%) • Anterior pituitary tumor • Prolactinoma (20%) • *Other:* Growth hormone (GH) + PRL1 GH1 NF (each 5%) • Adrenocorticotropic hormone (ACTH) (2%), thyroid-stimulating hormone (TSH) (rare) • Adrenal cortex NF (25%) • Pheochromocytoma (<1%)	

MEN 2

Clinical Features of Sporadic MTC, MEN 2A, MEN 2B, and FMTC

Clinical setting	*Features of MTC*	*Inheritance pattern*	*Associated abnormalities*	*Genetic defect*
Sporadic MTC	Unifocal	None	None	Somatic RET mutations in >20% of tumors
MEN 2A	Multifocal, bilateral	Autosomal dominant	Pheochromocytomas, hyperparathyroidism	Germline missense mutations in extracellular cysteine codons of RET
MEN 2B	Multifocal, bilateral	Autosomal dominant	Pheochromocytomas, mucosal neuromas, megacolon, skeletal abnormalities	Germline missense mutation in tyrosine kinase domain of RET
FMTC	Multifocal, bilateral	Autosomal dominant	None	Germline missense mutations in extracellular or intracellular cysteine codons of RET

(FMTC: familial medullary thyroid carcinoma; MEN: multiple endocrine neoplasia; MTC: medullary thyroid cancer)

Management of MEN 2

- Genetic testing is the mainstay in the diagnosis of MEN 2 syndromes. Perform genetic screening for RET mutations in all index patients. If a mutation is identified, also screen family members who are at risk.
- For individuals identified with a mutation or for persons who are at risk, biochemical screening consists of baseline calcitonin levels, serum calcium and parathyroid hormone (PTH) levels, along with urine collection for catecholamines and metanephrines concentrations. However, a plasma metanephrine level can be used for screening. Note that one-fourth of patients with apparently sporadic pheochromocytoma may be carriers of mutations characteristic of syndromes associated with pheochromocytomas.
- If a patient's calcitonin level is within reference ranges, a pentagastrin and/or Ca^{++} stimulation test may be used as a guide to assess the necessity of a central compartment or modified neck dissection.
- Patients who have been diagnosed with MTC require serial calcitonin (with or without provocative testing) and CEA testing after neck surgery to assess for persistent or recurrent disease.

Genetic Testing

Germline RET proto-oncogene mutations (on chromosome arm 10q) discovered in MEN 2-related syndromes include the following:

- *MEN 2A:* The majority of cases show substitutions of conserved cysteine residues in exons 10 and 11.
- *MEN 2B:* 95% of cases show threonine-for-methionine substitution in codon 918 of exon 16.
- *Familial medullary thyroid carcinoma (FMTC):* Most commonly seen with mutations in exons 10, 13, and 14.
- Initial testing for MEN 2A is either a single or multi-tiered analysis to detect RET mutations in the following:
  - Exon 10 (codons 609, 611, 618, and 620)
  - Exon 11 (codons 630 and 634)
  - Exons 8, 13, 14, 15, and 16.

  Sequencing of the entire coding region should be reserved for situations in which no RET mutation is identified or the identified genotype is inconsistent with the MEN 2 phenotype.

Initial testing for MEN 2B should be to detect the RET codon M918T mutation (exon 16), and if negative, then testing for the RET codon A883F mutation (exon 15) should be completed. If no mutations are identified in these two exons the entire RET coding region should be sequenced.

Screening for Cancer and Hyperparathyroidism

- Calcitonin is the principal biochemical marker in MTC; measurement of calcitonin is used for detection, staging, postoperative management, and determining prognosis.
- The higher the calcitonin levels are above normal, the greater the likelihood of MTC; basal levels of >100 pg/mL have been found to have 100% positive predictive value for MTC. Very rarely, patients with clinically apparent MTC may not have elevated calcitonin levels.
- Traditionally, a pentagastrin-induced rise in calcitonin secretion has been used to diagnose MTC; however, pentagastrin is not available in the United States, and deoxyribonucleic acid (DNA) testing for RET has replaced this diagnostic method in familial cases

- Calcitonin and CEA determinations remain useful serologic tests to identify recurrent disease.
- Serum calcium and PTH levels screen for hyperparathyroidism. An inappropriately normal or elevated PTH level in relation to the elevated serum calcium is consistent with primary hyperparathyroidism (PHPT). If the 24-hour urine calcium level is low, the presence of familial hypocalciuric hypercalcemic syndrome should be considered.

Urinary catecholamine and metanephrine levels screen for pheochromocytomas. If these are elevated, imaging studies of the adrenals are recommended.

Imaging Studies

- CT scanning or MRI of the adrenals.
- A meta-iodobenzylguanidine (MIBG) or DOTATATE scan is useful for localizing pheochromocytomas in case of nonvisualization of pheochromocytomas by traditional radiologic studies.
- If calcitonin levels are elevated at either baseline or with provocative testing, evaluate the chest and abdomen for metastatic disease. Available modalities include CT scanning, MRI, octreotide scanning, and, in some instances, laparoscopy.
- Radionuclide scanning may reveal the extent of metastasis. OctreoScan provides a whole-body examination and is used to examine the spread of MTC.
- For this procedure the somatostatin analog octreotide, which is used for the treatment of hormone-related symptoms, is labeled with the isotope indium-111 (^{111}In) and injected intravenously.
- The next day, the patient is examined with a gamma camera, which can detect the accumulation of radioactivity.

Other Tests

Fine-needle Aspiration

Avoid the removal of cells from thyroid masses for cytology in patients with MEN 2 who have had their diagnosis previously confirmed by either genetic analysis or elevated calcitonin levels. These patients have an established diagnosis, and a biopsy increases the possibility of tumor spread. A fine-needle aspiration biopsy is primarily used in an index patient who presents with a thyroid nodule when the clinician considers the presence of MTC to be unlikely.

Treatment

- TT indicated in patients identified by genetic screening. Symptomatic patients need TT and cervical nodal dissection for the lymph nodes on the involved side.
- Laparoscopic adrenalectomy for pheochromocytoma.
- Parathyroidectomy for MTC in patients belonging to families in which hyperparathyroidism is frequently associated.

29. MEN Syndrome. ***KGMU Lucknow 2025***

30. Describe MEN syndrome and management of medullary carcinoma of thyroid. ***WBUHS 2019***

Introduction

- MEN syndromes are familial conditions characterized by the occurrence of tumors involving two or more endocrine glands in a patient and family members.
- There are two major forms of MEN, namely MEN-type 1 (MEN 1 → Werner's syndrome) and MEN-type 2 (MEN 2, Sipple's syndrome); each form is characterized by the development of tumors of specific endocrine glands.
- The MEN syndromes are uncommon, but because they are inherited as autosomal dominant disorders, the finding of MEN in a patient has important implications for other family members. First degree relatives of a patient with known MEN have about a 50% risk of developing the disease.
- Occasionally, the MEN syndromes may arise sporadically (i.e., without a family history).

MEN 1

- Autosomal dominant.
- The *MEN 1* gene was originally mapped to chromosome 11q13 by a combination of genetic linkage studies and tumor deletion mapping. It encodes a protein merlin.
- The *MEN 1* gene consists of 10 exons spanning 9 kb of genomic DNA and encodes a 610-amino acid protein product termed menin.

Features of MEN 1

Major disease components	***Associated tumors***
• Primary hyperparathyroidism • Pancreatic endocrine tumors (PET) • Anterior pituitary tumor	• Facial angiofibroma • Collagenoma • Adrenal cortical tumor • Lipoma • Foregut carcinoid

Components of MEN-1 with estimated penetrance (in parentheses) at age 40 year:

Endocrine features	***Nonendocrine features***
Primary hyperparathyroidism (PHPT)—Parathyroid hyperplasia (90%)	Lipomas (30%)
Enteropancreatic tumor	Facial angiofibromas (85%)
1. Gastrinoma (40%)	
2. Insulinoma (10%)	Collagenomas (70%)
3. Nonfunctioning (NF) including pancreatic polypeptide (20%)	Ependymoma (1%)
4. *Other rare types:* (2%) • Glucagonoma • VIPoma • Somatostatinoma, *etc.* • Foregut carcinoid • Thymic carcinoid NF (2%) • Bronchial carcinoid NF (2%) • Gastric enterochromaffin-like tumor NF (10%) • Anterior pituitary tumor • Prolactinoma (20%) • *Other:* Growth hormone (GH) + PRL1 GH1 NF (each 5%) • Adrenocorticotropic hormone (ACTH) (2%), thyroid-stimulating hormone (TSH) (rare) • Adrenal cortex NF (25%) • Pheochromocytoma (<1%)	

- Parathyroid gland tumors. By age 40, 95% of patients have hypercalcemia which is the most common manifestation.
- Pancreatic islet cell tumors.
  - Prevalence of 30–75%.
  - Usually multicentric, slow-growing.
  - Secrete multiple polypeptides (insulin and gastrin are most common).
  - Gastrinoma leads to Zollinger–Ellison syndrome (ZES) (recurrent and multiple peptic ulcers, severe reflux esophagitis, and diarrhea).
  - Rarer tumors are VIPoma, glucagonoma, and somatostatinoma.
- Anterior pituitary tumors.
  - Detected in 15–40%.
  - Most common is prolactinoma.
  - Rarer are GH (causes acromegaly) or ACTH (causes Cushing's disease) secreting tumors.

Carcinoid tumors (thymus, lungs, and foregut), adrenal tumors, lipomas, and pinealomas have also been reported to appear in MEN-1 patients.

MEN 2A	*MEN 2B*
Medullary thyroid carcinoma	Medullary thyroid carcinoma
Pheochromocytoma	Pheochromocytoma
Hyperparathyroidism	Marfanoid body habitus
Lichen planus amyloidosis	Mucosal neuromas
Hirschsprung's disease	Ganglioneuromatosis of the gastrointestinal tract

MEN 2

Clinical Features of Sporadic MTC, MEN 2A, MEN 2B, and FMTC

Clinical setting	*Features of MTC*	*Inheritance pattern*	*Associated abnormalities*	*Genetic defect*
Sporadic MTC	Unifocal	None	None	Somatic RET mutations in >20% of tumors
MEN 2A	Multifocal, bilateral	Autosomal dominant	Pheochromocytomas, hyperparathyroidism	Germline missense mutations in extracellular cysteine codons of RET
MEN 2B	Multifocal, bilateral	Autosomal dominant	Pheochromocytomas, mucosal neuromas, megacolon, skeletal abnormalities	Germline missense mutation in tyrosine kinase domain of RET
FMTC	Multifocal, bilateral	Autosomal dominant	None	Germline missense mutations in extracellular or intracellular cysteine codons of RET

(FMTC: familial medullary thyroid carcinoma; MEN: multiple endocrine neoplasia; MTC: medullary thyroid cancer)

Treatment

Surgical Treatment

MEN-1

- Parathyroidectomy.
- *Pancreatic tumors:* Enucleation of individual tumors in the head of the pancreas and distal pancreatectomy for tumors in the tail/body.
- Hypophysectomy and external beam irradiation are considered for pituitary tumors.

MEN-2

- TT indicated in patients identified by genetic screening. Symptomatic patients need TT and cervical nodal dissection for the lymph nodes on the involved side.
- Laparoscopic adrenalectomy for pheochromocytoma.
- Parathyroidectomy for MTC in patients belonging to families in which hyperparathyroidism is frequently associated.

Medical Treatment:

MEN-1: Prolactinomas can be treated with dopamine agonists (bromocriptine/cabergoline).

Management of Medullary Carcinoma Thyroid

Treatment

- Surgery is the primary modality of treatment of MTC whether sporadic or inherited.
- Pheochromocytoma must be carefully excluded and if present treated surgically before embarking on the surgical management of MTC to avoid intraoperative catecholamine crisis.
- All patients with palpable disease localized to thyroid must undergo TT with central node dissection from the hyoid bone to the innominate veins and ipsilateral mid jugular node sampling and if found positive, then

functional ipsilateral lymph node dissection preserving jugular vein, sternocleidomastoid muscle and accessory nerve is recommended.

- A prophylactic contralateral neck dissection should be done when the primary tumor is bilateral and when there is extensive lymphadenopathy on the side of the primary tumor.
- Parathyroids needs to be identified and preserved in absence of clinical hyperparathyroidism or frank parathyroid enlargement. In patient with hereditary MTC presenting with palpable disease, TT must be combined with bilateral functional neck dissection.
- Clinically detectable cervical node metastasis calls for radical neck dissection of the affected site.
- Patients with biochemical evidence of PHPT must undergo bilateral neck exploration and total parathyroidectomy and autotransplantation of 30–60 mg. of most normal parathyroid tissue to the nondominant forearm if asymmetric parathyroid hyperplasia is present.
- Patients with FMTC should have a continued follow-up for pheochromocytoma and PHPT.

Prophylactic Thyroidectomy

- Prophylactic thyroidectomy has been recommended in hereditary MTC.
- *MEN 2A:* In most centers, thyroidectomy is performed in patients by the age of 5 years or when a mutation is identified.
- *FMTC:* Some centers recommend management similar to that of MEN 2A
- *MEN 2B:* In most centers, surgery is performed with in first 6 months of life, preferably within first month, because of early age of MTC onset and particularly aggressive behavior.

Treatment of Residual Disease

- By definition the surgical cure of MTC means normal postoperative serum calcitonin levels. Elevation of postoperative calcitonin levels or rising levels indicate persistent or recurrent disease.
- The other sites of persistent or recurrent disease are mediastinal lymph nodes, lungs, and liver. Liver metastasis are difficult to pick up with available imaging and nuclear medicine techniques.
- Reoperation for minimal residual disease with curative intent is controversial.
- Palliative debulking surgery in patients with advanced MTC does have a role in controlling compression on vital structures in the mediastinum and in large liver metastasis for poorly controlled diarrhea and flushing.
- Cytoreductive procedures such as radiofrequency ablation or cryoablation for liver metastases should be considered in symptomatic patients to reduce tumor burden.
- External beam radiotherapy may give some relief.
- Combination chemotherapy using dacarbazine, cyclophosphamide, and vincristine has been shown to exhibit some response in pheochromocytoma.
- Chemotherapy or radioactive immunotherapy (iodine-131 labeled CEA monoclonal antibody) protocols have been advocated in patients with nonoperable widely metastatic progressing MTC.
- Biological response modifiers such as somatostatin analogs and interferon have been shown to be of some benefit in reliving the symptoms of paraneoplastic syndrome.
- Monoclonal antibodies to CEA have been found to be unsuccessful.

Prognostic Factors

- Screening for MTC and early treatment (total thyroidectomy with central node clearance) gives nearly 100% cure rate.
- A high proportion of patients continue to receive less than optimal initial surgical treatment.
- Patients with postoperative hypercalcitonemia without clinical or radiological evidence of residual tumor after apparently curative surgery enjoy a long-term survival but have occult metastasis.
- Age at presentation and clinical staging have been found to independent predictors of survival.
- Patients without capsular invasion have been shown to have 92% survival at 10 years compared to only 67% in those with capsular invasion.
- Calcitonin immunostaining is another important prognostic indicator. Calcitonin immunostaining if positive in>50% of cells is attended with 87% survival as compared to only <60% in those with <10% staining. Calcitonin levels per se are not of much predictive value.

31. Classify thyroid malignancies. Explain surgical management of a patient with proven medullary carcinoma thyroid. *DY Patil Educational Society Deemed to be University 2020*

Already discussed in earlier answers

PARATHYROID AND CALCIUM METABOLISM

32. Describe MEN I and MEN II. Describe diagnosis and management of parathyroid adenoma. *Gujarat Health University 2024*

First part of the question already discussed

Parathyroid Adenoma

Definition

A *parathyroid adenoma* is a *benign neoplasm* of a single parathyroid gland that causes *autonomous overproduction of parathyroid hormone (PTH)*, leading to *primary hyperparathyroidism* and *hypercalcemia.*

Pathophysiology

- Normally, PTH secretion is regulated by serum calcium via negative feedback.
- In adenoma, the tumor cells *lose feedback control*, secreting *excess PTH* →
  - ↑ Bone resorption (osteoclast activation)
  - ↑ Renal tubular calcium reabsorption
  - ↑ Conversion of 25(OH)D to 1,25$(OH)_2$D → ↑ intestinal calcium absorption
    → *Result: Hypercalcemia + Hypophosphatemia*

Clinical Features

- General Features of Hyperparathyroidism
  "Stones, bones, groans, and psychic moans"

System	*Manifestations*
Renal (Stones)	Nephrolithiasis, nephrocalcinosis, polyuria, polydipsia
Skeletal (Bones)	Bone pain, osteitis fibrosa cystica ("brown tumors"), fractures
Gastrointestinal (Groans)	Peptic ulcers, pancreatitis, constipation, nausea
Neuropsychiatric (Moans)	Fatigue, depression, confusion
Cardiovascular	Hypertension, arrhythmias
Muscular	Weakness, myalgia

- *Asymptomatic cases*
  - Many patients today are detected incidentally during *routine calcium testing.*

Diagnosis

- *Biochemical findings*

Test	*Typical finding*	*Comment*
Serum calcium	↑ Elevated	Hallmark feature
Serum phosphate	↓ Low	PTH inhibits renal phosphate reabsorption
PTH level	↑ Inappropriately high	Confirms PTH-mediated hypercalcemia
24-hour urinary calcium	↑ High	To differentiate from familial hypocalciuric hypercalcemia
Alkaline phosphatase	↑ High	Reflects increased bone turnover
Vitamin D (25-hydroxy)	May be low/normal	Secondary to increased metabolism

- *Localization studies*
  Performed *after biochemical confirmation* of primary hyperparathyroidism to identify the adenoma for surgical planning.

Modality	Purpose/Findings
Neck ultrasound	Detects enlarged parathyroid gland (sensitivity ~70–80%)
Tc-99m sestamibi scan	Most widely used; localizes hyperfunctioning parathyroid tissue
4D-CT/MRI	For ectopic adenomas (mediastinal, retroesophageal)
Intraoperative PTH monitoring	Confirms complete removal during surgery (PTH falls >50% within 10–15 min)

Management

Definitive Treatment—Surgical Removal

- *Indications for Parathyroidectomy*
  - *Symptomatic* hyperparathyroidism (renal stones, bone pain, etc.)
  - *Asymptomatic* but meets *NIH criteria*:
    - Serum calcium >1 mg/dL above normal
    - Age <50 years
    - Reduced bone mineral density (T-score ≤ –2.5 or fragility fracture)
    - Creatinine clearance <60 mL/min
    - Nephrolithiasis or nephrocalcinosis
    - 24-hour urinary calcium >400 mg/day
- *Types of surgery*

Approach	Description	Indication
Focused (Minimally Invasive) Parathyroidectomy	Removal of localized adenoma through small incision under image guidance	Single localized adenoma
Bilateral Neck Exploration	Exploration of all 4 glands; abnormal one excised	If localization unclear or multigland disease suspected
Intraoperative PTH monitoring	Confirms adequacy of excision (rapid fall in PTH after adenoma removal)	Common adjunct

Postoperative Management

Aspect	Notes
Monitor serum calcium	Transient hypocalcemia (due to "hungry bone syndrome") may occur; treat with calcium + vitamin D
Monitor PTH	Should normalize or fall significantly
Symptom resolution	Fatigue, bone pain, and mental symptoms usually improve
Recurrence surveillance	Annual calcium checks

Medical/Conservative Management

For *patients unfit for surgery* or with *mild, asymptomatic disease.*

Therapy	Purpose
Hydration and mobility	Prevent stones, reduce calcium
Avoid thiazides, lithium	These elevate calcium
Cinacalcet (calcimimetic)	Increases calcium receptor sensitivity → ↓ PTH, ↓ serum calcium
Bisphosphonates/Denosumab	Improve bone mineral density
Monitor	Calcium, renal function, and bone density periodically

Complications

Intraoperative/Early	*Late*
Recurrent laryngeal nerve injury	Recurrent or persistent hypercalcemia
Hemorrhage/hematoma	Hypocalcemia (hungry bone syndrome)
Hypocalcemia/tetany	Hypoparathyroidism (if multiple glands removed)

Prognosis

- *Cure rate >95%* with successful adenoma removal.
- *Recurrence* rare but possible (especially in multiple gland disease).
- *Long-term follow-up* with annual calcium monitoring.

33. Write in brief physiology of parathyroid and calcium homeostasis. *WBUHS 2025 Supplementary*

Physiology of Parathyroid and Calcium Homeostasis (Brief):

- *Parathyroid glands:*
  - Small glands located behind the thyroid.
  - Secrete *parathyroid hormone (PTH)*, the primary regulator of calcium balance.
- *Parathyroid hormone (PTH)* functions:
  - *Bone:* Stimulates osteoclast activity → increases bone resorption → releases calcium and phosphate into blood.
  - *Kidneys:*
    - Increases calcium reabsorption in the distal tubules.
    - Decreases phosphate reabsorption (phosphaturia).
    - Stimulates conversion of vitamin D to its active form (*calcitriol*).
  - *Intestines:* Indirectly increases calcium absorption via activated vitamin D (calcitriol).
- *Calcium homeostasis:*
  - Normal serum calcium: ~8.5–10.5 mg/dL.
  - *Low calcium* → stimulates PTH release.
  - *High calcium* → inhibits PTH release (via negative feedback).
  - *Calcitonin* (from thyroid C-cells): Opposes PTH by inhibiting bone resorption, minor role in humans.
  - *Vitamin D (Calcitriol):* Enhances calcium and phosphate absorption from the gut, aids in bone mineralization.

Together, PTH, vitamin D, and calcitonin regulate calcium levels in the blood, ensuring proper function of muscles, nerves, and bone metabolism.

Distribution (mmol/L) of calcium in normal human plasma.		
Total diffusible		1.34
Ionized (Ca^{2+})	1.18	
Complexed to HCO_3^-, citrate, etc.	0.16	
Total nondiffusible (protein-bound)		1.16
Bound to albumin	0.92	
Bound to globulin	0.24	
Total plasma calcium		2.50

- The normal plasma level of intact PTH is 10–55 pg/mL. The half-life of PTH is approximately 10 minutes, and the secreted polypeptide is rapidly cleaved by the Kupffer cells in the liver into mid region and carboxyl terminal fragments that are probably biologically inactive. PTH and these fragments are then cleared by the kidneys.

- PTH acts directly on bone to increase bone resorption and mobilize Ca^{2+}. In addition to increasing the plasma Ca^{2+} and depressing the plasma phosphate, PTH increases phosphate excretion in the urine.
- This *phosphaturic action* is due to a decrease in reabsorption of phosphate in the proximal tubules. PTH also increases reabsorption of Ca^{2+} in the distal tubules, although Ca^{2+} excretion is often increased in hyperparathyroidism because the increase in the amount filtered overwhelms the effect on reabsorption. PTH also increases the formation of 1, 25-dihydroxycholecalciferol, and this increases Ca^{2+} absorption from the intestine.

On a longer time scale, PTH stimulates both osteoblasts and osteoclasts. The net effect varies, but with mildly elevated plasma PTH levels it is usually anabolic.

Actions of Major Calcium-regulating Hormones

	Bone	*Kidney*	*Intestine*
Parathyroid hormone	Stimulates resorption of calcium and phosphate	Stimulates resorption of calcium and conversion of $25(OH)D_3$; inhibits resorption of phosphate and bicarbonate	No direct effects
Vitamin D	Stimulates transport of calcium	Inhibits resorption of calcium	Stimulates calcium and phosphate absorption
Calcitonin	Inhibits resorption of calcium and phosphate	Inhibits resorption of calcium and phosphate	No direct effects

34. Discuss calcium metabolism in health and surgical disease. ***WBUHS 2010***

35. Write in short the calcium metabolism in human body. ***RIMS, Imphal 2012***

Distribution (mmol/L) of calcium in normal human plasma.		
Total diffusible		*1.34*
Ionized (Ca^{2+})	1.18	
Complexed to HCO_3^-, citrate, etc.	0.16	
Total nondiffusible (protein bound)		*1.16*
Bound to albumin	0.92	
Bound to globulin	0.24	
Total plasma calcium		*2.50*

- The normal plasma level of intact PTH is 10–55 pg/mL. The half-life of PTH is approximately 10 minutes, and the secreted polypeptide is rapidly cleaved by the Kupffer cells in the liver into mid region and carboxyl terminal fragments that are probably biologically inactive. PTH and these fragments are then cleared by the kidneys.

- PTH acts directly on bone to increase bone resorption and mobilize Ca^{2+}. In addition to increasing the plasma Ca^{2+} and depressing the plasma phosphate, PTH increases phosphate excretion in the urine.
- This *phosphaturic action* is due to a decrease in reabsorption of phosphate in the proximal tubules. PTH also increases reabsorption of Ca^{2+} in the distal tubules, although Ca^{2+} excretion is often increased in hyperparathyroidism because the increase in the amount filtered overwhelms the effect on reabsorption. PTH also increases the formation of 1, 25-dihydroxycholecalciferol, and this increases Ca^{2+} absorption from the intestine.

On a longer time scale, PTH stimulates both osteoblasts and osteoclasts. The net effect varies, but with mildly elevated plasma PTH levels it is usually anabolic.

Actions of Major Calcium-regulating Hormones

	Bone	*Kidney*	*Intestine*
Parathyroid hormone	Stimulates resorption of calcium and phosphate	Stimulates resorption of calcium and conversion of 25(OH)D_3; inhibits resorption of phosphate and bicarbonate	No direct effects
Vitamin D	Stimulates transport of calcium	Inhibits resorption of calcium	Stimulates calcium and phosphate absorption
Calcitonin	Inhibits resorption of calcium and phosphate	Inhibits resorption of calcium and phosphate	No direct effects

Hypoparathyroidism

Hypoparathyroidism is an endocrine disorder in which hypocalcemia and hyperphosphatemia are the result of a deficiency in PTH secretion or action.

Causes of hypoparathyroidism are:

- *Iatrogenic:* Damage to the parathyroid glands during thyroidectomy (most common), but it also can occur after parathyroid exploration.
- It can occur as part of a multiglandular endocrine deficiency syndrome (type 1) characterized most commonly by hypoparathyroidism, adrenal insufficiency, and mucocutaneous candidiasis.
- Disorders in which there is abnormal or absent formation of the parathyroid glands are associated with hypocalcemia, e.g., DiGeorge syndrome occurs when the third and fourth branchial pouches develop abnormally.
- Parathyroid gland function can be impaired by infiltrative involvement of the glands in diseases such as hemochromatosis, Wilson's disease, sarcoidosis, tuberculosis, or amyloidosis.
- Exposure to external radiation or very large doses of ^{131}I for Graves' disease or well-differentiated thyroid cancer has rarely been associated with hypocalcemia.
- Abnormalities in magnesium levels are associated with a reversible abnormality of PTH secretion.
- Parathyroid gland function can be impaired by infiltrative involvement of the glands in diseases such as hemochromatosis, Wilson's disease, sarcoidosis, tuberculosis, or amyloidosis. Exposure to external radiation or very large doses of ^{131}I for Graves' disease or well-differentiated thyroid cancer has rarely been associated with hypocalcemia. Finally, abnormalities in magnesium levels are associated with a reversible abnormality of PTH secretion.

Signs and Symptoms of Hypocalcemia

- The signs and symptoms of hypocalcemia are caused by neuromuscular excitability from reduced plasma ionized calcium.
- Early manifestations include perioral numbness and tingling in the fingers.
- Anxiety or confusion can follow, anxiety often results in hyperventilation, which can then lead to respiratory alkalosis and a further reduction in the serum calcium level.
- Tetany, marked by carpopedal spasm, convulsions, or laryngospasm (or any combination of the three), may follow and can be fatal.
- Physical examination includes testing for a Chvostek sign, which is contraction of the facial muscles after tapping on the facial nerve anterior to the ear.
- Approximately 15% of normal individuals have a positive Chvostek sign.

Causes of Hypercalcemia

Disease	*Confirmatory test*
Primary hyperparathyroidism	
Sporadic	Intact parathyroid hormone
Familial	
Malignancy	
Humoral/multiple myeloma	Parathyroid hormone-related protein
Osteolytic	
Endocrinopathy	
Hyperthyroidism	Thyroid-stimulating hormone
Addison's disease	Adrenocorticotropic hormone stimulation test
Drug-related	
Vitamin D intoxication	25-hydroxyvitamin D_3
Thiazide diuretics	
Granulomatous disease	
Sarcoidosis	Angiotensin-converting enzyme 1,25-dihydroxyvitamin D_3
Familial hypocalciuric hypercalcemia	*Urine calcium:* Creatinine ratio

Hyperparathyroidism

- *PHPT* is a syndrome of inappropriate secretion of PTH by one or more abnormal parathyroid glands.
- Most cases of PHPT occur sporadically, with a female preponderance of nearly 4 to 1. Familial syndromes of PHPT account for relatively few cases.
- These syndromes include MEN, types 1 and 2; familial isolated hyperparathyroidism; and hereditary hyperparathyroidism jaw tumor syndrome.
- A single parathyroid adenoma accounts for between 85 and 90% of cases of PHPT.
- Multiple gland disease, in the form of either multiple adenomas or hyperplasia of all parathyroid glands, occurs in the remaining 10–15%.
- Parathyroid carcinoma is a rare (<1%) cause of PHPT.
- The molecular mechanisms underlying most sporadic cases of PHPT remain poorly understood.

Clinical Presentation

- The parathyroid glands function to preserve serum calcium in a tightly controlled range (8.5–10.2 mg/dL).
- Most patients present with hypercalcemia and few, if any, symptoms.
- Most patients come to clinical attention by identification of hypercalcemia on routine chemistry panels.
- Increasingly, otherwise asymptomatic patients are being identified during evaluation of osteoporosis.
- Classic manifestations of moderate PHPT include nephrolithiasis, osteoporosis, arthralgia, and myopathy.
- Subtle manifestations of PHPT may include hypertension, neuropsychiatric disorders, dyspepsia, and constipation.
- Severe manifestations of PHPT occur uncommonly and include osteitis fibrosa cystica, osteoclastomas (Brown tumors), and nephrocalcinosis.
- Severe PHPT may still be seen today in populations not routinely screened with the multichannel serum chemistries.
- Familial cases of PHPT are uncommon but must be discerned through careful determination of family history, in order to either exclude the possibility of familial hypocalciuric hypercalcemia (FHH) or alert the surgeon to the possibility of multiple gland disease.

- *Secondary hyperparathyroidism (2HPT)* is the result of chronic overstimulation leading to hypersecretion and hyperplasia of intrinsically normal parathyroid glands in response to derangements in mineral metabolism.
  This phenomenon occurs to some degree in nearly all patients with chronic renal failure (CRF) but can also be seen in patients with celiac disease, malabsorption, and vitamin D resistance.
- *Tertiary hyperparathyroidism (3HPT)* occurs in the setting of longstanding 2HPT in which long-standing parathyroid hyperplasia leads to autonomous function despite correction of the underlying cause, usually by means of a kidney transplant. It manifests as either failure of resolution of hyperparathyroidism after renal transplantation or refractory hypercalcemia despite aggressive medical management in a patient with previously medically controlled 2HPT.

36. Write down the differential diagnosis of hypercalcemia. Mention the radiologic features of primary hyperparathyroidism. ***WBUHS 2021***

Causes of Hypercalcemia

Disease	***Confirmatory test***
Primary hyperparathyroidism	
Sporadic	Intact parathyroid hormone
Familial	
Malignancy	
Humoral/multiple myeloma	Parathyroid hormone-related protein
Osteolytic	
Endocrinopathy	
Hyperthyroidism	Thyroid-stimulating hormone
Addison's disease	Adrenocorticotropic hormone stimulation test
Drug-related	
Vitamin D intoxication	25-hydroxyvitamin D_3
Thiazide diuretics	
Granulomatous disease	
Sarcoidosis	Angiotensin-converting enzyme 1,25-dihydroxyvitamin D_3
Familial hypocalciuric hypercalcemia	*Urine calcium:* Creatinine ratio

[*Note: Causes of hypercalcemia covers the differential diagnosis. I have also provided the confirmatory tests for the benefit of the students*]

Radiologic Features of Primary Hyperparathyroidism

- Subperiosteal bone resorption
  - Classically affects the radial aspects of the proximal and middle phalanges of the second and third fingers
  - Medial aspect of tibia, femur, and humerus
  - *Lamina dura:* Floating teeth (not specific)
- Subchondral resorption
  - Lateral end of the clavicles
  - Symphysis pubis
  - Sacroiliac joints
- Subligamentous resorption
  - Ischial tuberosity
  - Trochanters
  - Inferior surface of calcaneus and clavicle

- *Intracortical resorption:* Cigar/oval-shaped or tunnel-shaped radiolucency in the cortex
- Terminal tuft erosion (acro-osteolysis)
- Rugger jersey spine
- Osteopenia
- Brown tumors
- Salt and pepper sign in the skull (pepper pot skull)
- Chondrocalcinosis

37. Describe the clinical features and biochemical abnormalities associated with primary hyperparathyroidism. Outline the work up protocol and indications of parathyroidectomy in a patient with primary hyperparathyroidism. ***AIIMS, Patna 2025***

38. Primary hyperparathyroidism - diagnostic work up. ***AIIMS, Raipur 2025***

Primary Hyperparathyroidism (PHPT)

Definition

Primary hyperparathyroidism is an endocrine disorder characterized by autonomous overproduction of parathyroid hormone (PTH) from one or more parathyroid glands, leading to hypercalcemia and associated metabolic disturbances.

- *Clinical features*

  Classically summarized by the mnemonic: "Bones, Stones, Groans, and Psychic Overtones."
  - *Skeletal (Bones)*
    - Bone pain and tenderness
    - Pathological fractures
    - Osteitis fibrosa cystica (rare, advanced form)
    - Subperiosteal bone resorption (especially in phalanges and skull)
    - Reduced bone mineral density (mainly cortical bone loss)
  - *Renal (Stones)*
    - Nephrolithiasis (calcium oxalate or phosphate stones)
    - Nephrocalcinosis
    - Polyuria, polydipsia (due to nephrogenic diabetes insipidus from hypercalcemia)
    - Chronic kidney disease (late)
  - *Gastrointestinal (Groans)*
    - Anorexia, nausea, vomiting
    - Constipation
    - Abdominal pain, peptic ulcers (from increased gastrin secretion)
    - Pancreatitis (rare association)
  - *Neuropsychiatric (Psychic Overtones)*
    - Fatigue, weakness
    - Depression, irritability
    - Cognitive dysfunction, confusion
    - In severe cases: stupor or coma (hypercalcemic crisis)
  - *Cardiovascular*
    - Hypertension
    - Shortened QT interval on ECG
    - Arrhythmias (in severe hypercalcemia)
  - *Others*
    - Proximal myopathy
    - Corneal calcifications (band keratopathy)

- *Biochemical abnormalities*

Parameter	Finding	Mechanism
Serum calcium	↑ (usually mild–moderate)	Excess PTH increases bone resorption and renal calcium reabsorption
Serum phosphate	↓	PTH increases renal phosphate excretion
Serum PTH	↑ (inappropriately elevated for calcium level)	Autonomous secretion
Alkaline phosphatase (ALP)	↑ (variable)	Increased bone turnover
Urinary calcium	↑ or normal	High filtered calcium load
Vitamin D (1,25(OH)$_2$D)	↑	PTH stimulates renal 1α-hydroxylase
Chloride:phosphate ratio	>33 (suggestive of PHPT)	Due to hypophosphatemia

- *Work-up/diagnostic protocol*
  - *Confirm Diagnosis*
    - *Serum calcium:* Corrected for albumin or measure ionized calcium
    - *PTH assay:* Intact PTH elevated or inappropriately normal
    - *Exclude secondary causes:* Check vitamin D, renal function
  - *Assess Target Organ Damage*
    - *Renal:*
      - Serum creatinine and eGFR
      - 24-hour urinary calcium and creatinine
      - Renal ultrasound (stones or nephrocalcinosis)
    - *Skeletal:*
      - Dual-energy X-ray absorptiometry (DEXA) at lumbar spine, hip, and distal radius
      - X-rays if symptomatic (subperiosteal resorption, cysts)
  - *Localizing Studies (for surgical planning only; not diagnostic)*
    - Neck ultrasound
    - Sestamibi scan (99mTc-sestamibi scintigraphy)
    - 4D-CT or MRI (for ectopic or difficult cases)
- *Indications for parathyroidectomy*
  According to the Fourth International Workshop Guidelines (2014):
  - *Symptomatic PHPT*
    - *Any of the following:*
      - *Nephrolithiasis or nephrocalcinosis*
      - *Fractures or osteitis fibrosa cystica*
      - *Hypercalcemic symptoms (neuropsychiatric, GI, etc.)*
  - *Asymptomatic PHPT – Surgery indicated if any of the following present:*

Category	Indication
Serum calcium	>1.0 mg/dL (0.25 mmol/L) above upper limit of normal
Skeletal	T-score ≤ −2.5 at any site (spine, hip, or distal radius) OR vertebral fracture
Renal	Creatinine clearance <60 mL/min OR nephrolithiasis/nephrocalcinosis OR 24-hr urinary calcium >400 mg/day with stone risk
Age	<50 years

  - *Patient Preference*
    - In patients who prefer definitive surgical cure, provided there are no contraindications.

- Alternatives/Nonsurgical Management
  For patients not meeting surgical criteria or unfit for surgery:
  - Maintain hydration
  - Avoid thiazide diuretics and lithium
  - Moderate calcium and vitamin D intake
  - Bisphosphonates or denosumab (for bone protection)
  - Cinacalcet (calcimimetic) to reduce calcium levels

39. Describe the management of primary hyperparathyroidism. ***Srimanta Sankaradeva University, Assam 2025***

Primary Hyperparathyroidism (PHPT) – Overview

Definition:

A disorder characterized by *autonomous overproduction of parathyroid hormone (PTH),* leading to *hypercalcemia* and *hypophosphatemia.*

Common Causes:

- *Single parathyroid adenoma* (~85%)
- *Parathyroid hyperplasia* (10–15%)
- *Parathyroid carcinoma* (<1%)

Initial Evaluation and Diagnosis

- Biochemical Tests
  - ↑ *Serum calcium*
  - ↑ *PTH (inappropriately elevated or non-suppressed)*
  - ↓ *Serum phosphate*
  - ↑ *24-hour urinary calcium excretion*
  - *Bone mineral density* (DEXA scan) for osteopenia/osteoporosis
- Localization Studies (for surgical planning)
  - *Neck ultrasound*
  - *Sestamibi (Tc-99m) scan*
  - *4D-CT* or *MRI* if localization unclear

Management Overview

- *Definitive Treatment—Parathyroidectomy*
  - Indications (NIH Guidelines/International Workshop Criteria):
    Surgery is recommended for *symptomatic* patients and for *asymptomatic* patients meeting any of the following:

Category	***Criteria***
Serum calcium	>1.0 mg/dL (0.25 mmol/L) above upper normal limit
Skeletal	T-score ≤ –2.5 at lumbar spine, hip, or distal radius, or fragility fracture
Renal	Creatinine clearance <60 mL/min, nephrolithiasis or nephrocalcinosis, or 24-hour urine calcium >400 mg/day
Age	<50 years

  - *Surgical options:*
    - *Focused (minimally invasive) parathyroidectomy:* if single adenoma localized.
    - *Bilateral neck exploration:* if localization negative or multigland disease suspected.
    - *Subtotal or total parathyroidectomy with autotransplantation:* for hyperplasia.

  - *Postoperative care:*
    - Monitor *serum calcium* for *transient hypocalcemia* (may need calcium and vitamin D supplementation).
    - Watch for *"hungry bone syndrome"* after surgery.
- *Nonsurgical (Conservative) Management*
  For *asymptomatic patients not meeting surgical criteria* or those *unfit for surgery*.
  - *Lifestyle and Monitoring:*
    - Maintain *adequate hydration* to prevent nephrolithiasis.
    - *Avoid thiazide diuretics and lithium,* which increase calcium.
    - *Moderate calcium intake* (do not restrict severely).
    - Regular *exercise* to maintain bone density.
    - *Monitor:*
      - Serum calcium and creatinine annually.
      - DEXA scan every 1–2 years.
  - *Medical Therapy:*
    - *Calcimimetics (e.g., cinacalcet):*
      - Increases sensitivity of calcium-sensing receptor, lowering serum calcium.
      - Especially useful in patients with *severe hypercalcemia* who cannot undergo surgery.
    - *Bisphosphonates or Denosumab:*
      - Improve *bone mineral density*; used when osteoporosis is present.
    - *Vitamin D supplementation:*
      - If deficiency present; may modestly lower PTH levels.
- *Management of Acute Severe Hypercalcemia ("Hypercalcemic Crisis")*
  - *Aggressive IV hydration* (normal saline)
  - *Loop diuretics (e.g., furosemide)* after rehydration to enhance calciuresis
  - *IV bisphosphonates* (e.g., zoledronic acid) to inhibit bone resorption
  - *Calcitonin* for rapid, temporary calcium reduction
  - *Dialysis* if refractory or renal failure

Follow-Up and Prognosis

- *Post-surgical cure rate:* >95% in experienced hands.
- *Recurrence:* Possible if multigland disease or incomplete removal.
- *Long-term monitoring:* Periodic calcium and PTH measurements.

40. Hypercalcemic crisis. *WBUHS 2015*

Introduction

- Hypercalcemic crisis or severe hypercalcemia represents a life-threatening emergency. The most common cause is hypercalcemia of malignancy, although granulomatous diseases, previously undetected PHPT, medication-induced hypercalcemia, and a few rarer causes may result in this endocrine emergency as well.
- The clinical presentation and prognosis depend on the acuity of the development of hypercalcemia, the degree of hypercalcemia, and the underlying cause.

Clinical Presentation

- The clinical presentation of patients with hypercalcemic crisis varies depending once again on the underlying cause and degree and rapidity of the hypercalcemia.
- Most patients experience some constitutional symptoms, neurologic symptoms, gastrointestinal symptoms, and renal manifestations of hypercalcemia.

Treatment

Medical Treatment

- Hypercalcemic crisis needs aggressive rehydration.
- Establish large caliber IV access. Give 1 L in first hour, further 4–6 L in first 24 hours.
- Monitor urine output and central venous pressure until normalized.
- Frusemide can be added to increase urinary excretion of calcium once rehydration is adequate.
- Bisphosphonates (e.g., IV pamidronate) should be avoided in PHPT when parathyroidectomy is anticipated, since they impair the ability to maintain normocalcemia after the excision of an overactive parathyroid adenoma.

Group	*Drug*	*Side effect*
Diuretic	Normal saline	
	Furosemide	Hypokalemia
Anti resorptive	Bisphosphonates	Osteonecrosis of jaw
	Calcitonin	Diarrhea
	Plicamycin	• Hepatotoxic • Nephrotoxic • Thrombocytopenia
Decrease calcium absorption	Glucocorticoids	Systemic
	Intravenous (IV) phosphate	Extraskeletal calcium deposition
Extractive	Hemodialysis	

41. Discuss the causes of hypercalcemia in surgical practice and how to correct it. *WBUHS 2017*

Causes of Hypercalcemia

Disease	*Confirmatory test*
Primary hyperparathyroidism	
Sporadic	Intact parathyroid hormone
Familial	
Malignancy	
Humoral/multiple myeloma	Parathyroid hormone-related protein
Osteolytic—breast cancer, lung cancer, renal cell carcinoma (RCC) and gastrointestinal tract (GIT) cancer	
Endocrinopathy	
Hyperthyroidism	Thyroid-stimulating hormone
Addison's disease	Adrenocorticotropic hormone stimulation test
Drug-related	
Vitamin D intoxication	25-hydroxyvitamin D_3
Thiazide diuretics	
Granulomatous disease	
Sarcoidosis	Angiotensin-converting enzyme 1,25-dihydroxyvitamin D_3
Familial hypocalciuric hypercalcemia	*Urine calcium:* Creatinine ratio

Management

- *Calcimimetics:* This type of drug mimics calcium circulating in the blood, so it can help control overactive parathyroid glands.
- *Bisphosphonates:* IV osteoporosis drugs can help rebuild bone weakened by hypercalcemia.
  Risks associated with this treatment include osteonecrosis of the jaw and certain types of thigh fractures.
  - Risedronate
  - Ibandronate
  - Alendronate
  - Zoledronic acid
  - Pamidronate
- *Other drugs stopping breakdown of bones:*
  - Calcitonin
  - Plicamycin
  - Gallium nitrate
- *Prednisone:* If hypercalcemia is caused by high levels of vitamin D, short-term use of steroid pills such as prednisone might be helpful.
- *IV fluids and diuretics:* Extremely high calcium levels can be a medical emergency. Hospitalization for treatment with IV fluids and diuretics to promptly lower the calcium level may be needed to prevent heart rhythm problems or damage to the nervous system.
- *Surgical and other procedures:* Problems associated with overactive parathyroid glands often can be cured by surgery to remove the malfunctioning tissue. In many cases, only one of a person's four parathyroid glands is affected. A special scanning test uses an injection of a small dose of radioactive material to locate the gland or glands that aren't working properly.

---

42. Parathyroid localization. ***WBUHS 2014; RGUHS Karnataka 2025***

- No consensus on whether preoperative localization necessary
- Preoperative localization can allow for unilateral focused parathyroidectomy.
  - *The combination often used is:*
    - Sestamibi for localization
    - US for information on size and relationship of the abnormal glands to surrounding tissue
    - Sestamibi scanning limited in identifying multiple adenomas and four-gland hyperplasia
    - Preoperative localization essential in reoperation cases.

Preoperative Evaluation

- Neck US
- MRI
- Thallium-technetium dual isotope scintigraphy
- Technetium-99m sestamibi scan
- Single-photon emission computed tomography (SPECT) sestamibi scan: allows for 3-D localization but is expensive
- Angiography with or without selective venous sampling (angioablation)

Intraoperative Localization

- Intraoperative US
- Intraoperative rapid PTH (50 and 80%)
- Hand-held gamma probe

PARATHYROID CANCER

43. What are the clinical features, laboratory parameters and molecular markers that set parathyroid carcinoma apart from other pathologies of the parathyroid gland? Discuss the treatment policy of parathyroid carcinoma.
WBUHS 2023

Parathyroid Cancer

Clinical Manifestations

- Parathyroid cancer is a rare disease, accounting for <1% of patients with PHPT
- Most (>90%) of parathyroid carcinomas are biochemically functional
- Nausea and vomiting
- Anorexia and constipation
- Frequent urination
- Feeling of thirst
- Tiredness and depression
- Memory loss
- Muscle aches, cramps weakness
- Approximately 50% of patients have a palpable neck mass
  - They are typically hard, firm, and adherent to surrounding tissues.
  - Their average size at presentation is around 3 cm, as they are often otherwise asymptomatic.
  - They tend to present with local invasion into adjacent structures, especially the ipsilateral thyroid.
  - Invasion of the trachea, strap muscles, and RLN are possible in more advanced disease, but are rare presenting findings.
- Regional metastases are rare and distant metastases even more so, but if present can occur in the lungs, bone, mediastinal nodes, liver, and kidney.

Laboratory Parameters

- Serum calcium levels may exceed 15 mg/dL.
- PTH levels are often five times the upper limit of normal (≥300 pg/mL).
- Patients with parathyroid carcinoma tend to have extremely high PTH levels compared to patients with benign PHPT, and almost always have a refractory, elevated, serum calcium also.
- A PTH three times the upper limit of normal is suspicious for malignancy, while a PTH of 10 times the upper limit of normal has a positive predictive value of 84% for parathyroid carcinoma.

Localization and Diagnosis

- USG and 99mTc sestamibi imaging can help localize disease, but diagnosis depends on histologic findings of vascular or capsular invasion, metastases, or gross invasion of local structures.
- CT scan is the imaging study of choice for a newly discovered neck mass and may reveal a perithyroid mass and potential thyroid invasion. This has the advantage of concurrently evaluating the remaining neck compartments for invasion or lymphadenopathy suspicious for metastasis.
- PET scans may be helpful in determining metastasis and staging, though the reliability of PET in parathyroid carcinoma is unknown.
- X-rays of the hand a skull may be performed to evaluate for osteoporosis, but are extremely nonspecific and are not recommended as a screening examination.
- US-guided fine-needle aspiration has been reported, but the ability to distinguish benign hyperplastic parathyroid from malignant parathyroid remains in question.

Etiology and Molecular Markers

- Most parathyroid carcinomas are idiopathic and sporadic, though there are well-documented syndromic associations with MEN syndrome types I and IIa, as well as with hyperparathyroidism-jaw tumor syndrome (HPT-JT).
- It is reported that parathyroid carcinoma is the cause of PHPT in 0.1–5% of cases.
- It is uncertain whether parathyroid carcinoma begins as benign parathyroid lesions, but it has been hypothesized by some that parathyroid carcinoma may arise in the presence of primary parathyroid hyperplasia, though the potential for malignant transformation remains theoretical.
- *HRPT2* gene:
  - Mutation of HRPT2 (CDC73), a tumor suppressor gene, has been described in the molecular pathogenesis of parathyroid carcinoma.
  - This gene is located on chromosome 1 and encodes for the protein parafibromin, which is involved in the inhibition of cell proliferation.
  - The HRPT2 mutation is found in hyperparathyroidism-jaw tumor syndrome and sporadic parathyroid carcinoma.
  - Patients with hyperparathyroidism-jaw tumor syndrome develop ossifying fibromas of the jaw, cysts, and neoplasms of the kidneys.
  - They are at an increased risk for parathyroid carcinoma.
  - Studies show 15% of patients with hyperparathyroidism-jaw tumor syndrome develop parathyroid carcinoma.
  - A profile including serum calcium and PTH levels and tissue expression of APC, parafibromin, PGP9.5, galectin 3 and Ki67 is proposed.
  - *Telomerase repeat amplification protocol (TRAP):* A new molecular marker for parathyroid carcinoma.

Medical Management of Hypercalcemic Crisis

- Patients with parathyroid cancer and some patients with benign HPT may develop hypercalcemic crisis with serum calcium levels of 16–20 mg/dL and azotemia.
- Symptoms of this acute, sometimes fatal illness, include profound muscular weakness, nausea and vomiting, drowsiness, and confusion.
- Ultimate treatment is surgery, but volume and electrolyte abnormalities should be addressed first.
- First-line therapy involves IV infusion of 0.9% sodium chloride at 300–500 mL/hour to restore intravascular volume and to promote renal excretion of calcium.
- After urinary output exceeds 100 mL/hour, furosemide (80–100 mg intravenously every 2–6 hours) may be given to promote further renal sodium and calcium excretion, though consequent hypokalemia and hypomagnesemia should be corrected.
- Thiazide diuretics impair calcium excretion and should be avoided.
- If diuresis alone is unsuccessful in lowering the serum calcium, other agents may be used, including the bisphosphonates pamidronate and etidronate, mithramycin, and salmon calcitonin.
- Orthophosphate, gallium nitrate, and glucocorticoids also have calcium-lowering effects.
- Both cinacalcet, an activator of calcium sensing receptor, and denosumab, a monoclonal antibody to RANKL, may be used to manage hypercalcemia associated with unresectable disease.

Operative Strategy

- Surgical treatment of parathyroid cancer can be curative, and entails radical local excision of the tumor en bloc with surrounding soft tissue, lymph nodes, and ipsilateral thyroid lobe.
- Reoperation should be considered for local and distant recurrences to control malignant hypercalcemia.
- Tumor debulking.
- Metastasectomy.
  - Chemotherapy and radiation therapy are not commonly used to treat parathyroid cancer.

ADRENAL

44. List out the surgical causes of hypertension. How would you approach a case of hypertension associated with an adrenal mass? ***WBUHS 2022***

Frequencies of the Most Common Causes of Surgical Hypertension

Endocrine	*Vascular*
Primary hyperaldosteronism (<1%)	Renal artery stenosis (<3%)
Cushing's syndrome (<1%)	Coarctation of aorta (<0.1%)
Pheochromocytoma (<0.1%)	

Prevalence of Diagnosis in Patients with an Incidentally Discovered Adrenal Mass

Condition	*Prevalence per 10,000 patients*
Pheochromocytoma	650
Aldosterone producing adenoma	700
Glucocorticoid producing adenoma	3.5
Adrenal carcinoma	5.8

All four classes of adrenal hormones can cause high blood pressure.

These four classes of adrenal hormones are:

1. Aldosterone,
2. Cortisol,
3. Catecholamines, and
4. Sex-steroid hormones.

- Overproduction of all of these hormones can cause secondary hypertension.
- That means primary hyperaldosteronism (Conn's syndrome), Cushing's syndrome, pheochromocytomas, and sex-steroid hormone-producing tumors are all associated with hypertension.
- Of patients with adrenal incidentalomas (AIs), 5.1% have been proven to have pheochromocytoma, but the prevalence of pheochromocytoma would be expected to be higher in patients with a hypertensive crisis with adrenal masses. Surveys of AI generally exclude patients with severe hypertension.
- Approximately 10% of AIs are either hyperfunctional or significantly autonomous.

Screening Tests to Assess Hormonal Function of an Adrenal Mass

Pheochromocytoma	*Primary hyperaldosteronism*	*Cushing's syndrome*
• 24-hour urine fractionated metanephrines + catecholamines or • Plasma free metanephrine	• Morning aldosterone/plasma renin activity ratio ≥20 when absolute aldosterone ≥15 ng/dL with potassium ≥3.5 µg/L • Studies can be performed on all drugs except spironolactone, eplerenone or amiloride	• *Dexamethasone suppression test:* 1 mg dexamethasone between 11 PM and midnight: 8.00 AM cortisol level should be <2.5 µg/dL • 24-hour urine free cortisol level, 4-50 µg/24 hours

- More extensive hormonal testing of incidentally discovered adrenal masses may reveal evidence of subclinical hypercortisolism.
- Adrenocortical carcinoma is associated with hypertension, and extra-adrenal carcinoma metastatic to the adrenal glands is also a consideration when an adrenal mass is discovered.
- Size and imaging phenotype are the important considerations when assessing the malignant potential of an incidentally noted adrenal mass.

- A diameter >4 cm was shown to have a 90% sensitivity and a 24% specificity for the detection of adrenocortical carcinoma.
- The characteristics of the mass on computerized imaging, or imaging phenotype, provides an important assessment of intracytoplasmic fat content, which is high in adrenal adenomas and low in malignancy.
- High adrenal intracytoplasmic fat content is associated with low attenuation on unenhanced CT. The Hounsfield scale is a semiquantitative assessment of X-ray attenuation on the CT imaging spectrum which ranges from air (black) to bone (white).
- MRI characteristics have likewise been employed to decide the malignant potential of adrenal lesions, but many adrenal masses are indeterminate with conventional spin-echo MRI.
- As with CT, mild enhancement with rapid washout of gadolinium-DPTA-enhanced MRI favors adenoma, whereas greater enhancement and a slower washout of contrast favor malignancy. Imaging phenotype features used to distinguish AIs are summarized here.

Characteristics of adrenal incidentalomas on imaging (imaging phenotype).

Variable	*Adrenocortical adenoma*	*Adrenocortical carcinoma*	*Pheochromocytoma*	*Metastasis*
Size	Small, usually ≤3 cm in diameter	Large, usually >4 cm in diameter	Large, usually >3 cm in diameter	Variable, frequently <3 cm
Shape	Round or oval, with smooth margins	Irregular, with unclear margins	Round or oval, with clear margins	Heterogeneous, with mixed densities
Texture	Homogeneous	Heterogeneous, with mixed densities	Heterogeneous, with cystic areas	Heterogeneous, with mixed densities
Laterality	Usually solitary, unilateral	Usually solitary, unilateral	Usually solitary, unilateral	Often bilateral
Attenuation (density) on unenhanced CT	≤10 HU	>10 HU (usually >25)	>10 HU (usually >25)	>10 HU (usually >25)
Vascularity on contrast-enhanced CT rapidity of washout of contrast medium	Not highly vascular ≥50% at 10 minutes	Usually vascular <50% at 10 minutes	Usually vascular <50% at 10 minutes	Usually vascular <50% at 10 minutes
Appearance on MRI	Isointense in relation to liver on T2-weighted image	Hyperintense in relation to liver on T2-weighted image	Markedly hyperintense in relation to liver on T2-weighted image	Hyperintense in relation to liver on T2- weighted image
Necrosis, hemorrhage, or calcifications	Rare	Common	Hemorrhage and cystic areas common	Occasional hemorrhage and cystic areas
Growth rate	Usually stable over time or very slow (<1 cm/year)	Usually rapid (>2 cm/year)	Usually slow (0.5–1.0 cm/year)	Variable, slow to rapid

45. Briefly discuss the embryology and blood supply of adrenal gland. ***AIIMS, Bhopal 2021***

Embryology of Adrenal Glands

The *adrenal glands* (also called *suprarenal glands*) are *paired endocrine organs* located above the kidneys. They have two distinct parts with different embryological origins:

- *Cortex (Outer Layer)*
  - *Origin:* Mesoderm, specifically from the intermediate mesoderm (coelomic epithelium near the developing gonads).

- *Development:*
  - Begins in the *5th–6th week* of gestation.
  - The *fetal cortex* forms first and later involutes.
  - The *definitive cortex* (zona glomerulosa, fasciculata, and reticularis) develops later and becomes functional after birth.
- *Medulla (Inner Layer)*
  - *Origin: Ectoderm,* specifically from *neural crest cells.*
  - *Development:*
    - Neural crest cells migrate into the developing adrenal gland.
    - They differentiate into *chromaffin cells,* which produce *catecholamines* (epinephrine and norepinephrine).

Blood Supply of Adrenal Glands

Each adrenal gland has a *rich blood supply* due to its endocrine function.

Arterial Supply (Three main sources):

1. *Superior suprarenal arteries*
   - From *inferior phrenic artery* (branch of the abdominal aorta)
2. *Middle suprarenal artery*
   - Directly from the *abdominal aorta*
3. *Inferior suprarenal artery*
   - From the *renal artery*

These arteries form a *subcapsular plexus* and supply both the cortex and medulla.

Venous Drainage

- Blood drains from a *single central suprarenal vein* on each side:
  - *Right suprarenal vein* → drains into the *inferior vena cava*
  - *Left suprarenal vein* → drains into the *left renal vein*

---

46. Pheochromocytoma. (Describe the etiology, pathology, clinical features and management of pheochromocytoma.) ***AIIMS, Bhopal 2021***

---

47. Outline the perioperative pharmacological management in a patient of pheochromocytoma. ***WBUHS 2018, 2020, 2024***

---

48. Investigations and treatment in pheochromocytoma. ***Rajasthan University of Health Sciences 2025***

Introduction

- Pheochromocytoma affects approximately 0.2% of hypertensive individuals.
- Males and females are affected equally.
- The peak incidence in sporadic cases lies between the ages of 40 and 50 years, whereas familial cases tend to be manifested earlier.
- A subset of patients have the classic triad of headache, diaphoresis, and palpitations, although almost all patients will display at least one of these symptoms.
- Hypertension is present in 90% of cases and may be episodic or sustained.
- The principal challenge in making the diagnosis of pheochromocytoma arises from the fact that essential hypertension is common and the clinical features suggestive of pheochromocytoma are nonspecific.
- Previously, pheochromocytoma was dubbed the "10% tumor" for the reason that 10% are bilateral, 10% malignant, 10% extra-adrenal, and 10% familial.

Molecular Genetics of Pheochromocytoma

Pheochromocytoma was known to be associated with:

- MEN type 2 syndromes (40–50% penetrant),
- Von Hippel–Lindau syndrome (10–20% penetrant), and
- Neurofibromatosis type 1 (1–5% penetrant).
- Germline mutations in the B and D subunits, which are inherited in an autosomal dominant fashion, have been identified in approximately 10% of apparently sporadic pheochromocytoma cases.
- 21–30% of pheochromocytomas are familial. Familial cases occur at an earlier age and are more likely to be multifocal.
- Succinate dehydrogenase B mutation carriers have high rates of extra-adrenal (abdominal or thoracic) pheochromocytomas and malignant disease, whereas succinate dehydrogenase D carriers tend to have multiple tumors and hormonally inactive paragangliomas of the head and neck.
- Genetic counseling and testing is encouraged for patients in whom pheochromocytoma is diagnosed before the age of 50.

Symptoms and Signs

- Headache, palpitations, and diaphoresis constitute the "classic triad" of pheochromocytomas.
- Symptoms such as anxiety, tremulousness, paresthesias, flushing, chest pain, shortness of breath, abdominal pain, nausea, vomiting, and others are nonspecific and may be episodic in nature.
- Cardiovascular complications, such as myocardial infarction and cerebrovascular accidents, may ensue.
- These symptoms can be incited by a range of stimuli including exercise, micturition, and defecation. The most common clinical sign is hypertension.
- The hypertension related to this tumor may be paroxysmal with intervening normotension, sustained with paroxysms, or sustained hypertension alone.
- Sudden death may occur in patients with undiagnosed tumors who undergo other operations or biopsy.

Algorithm for the Diagnosis, Localization, and Management of Pheochromocytoma

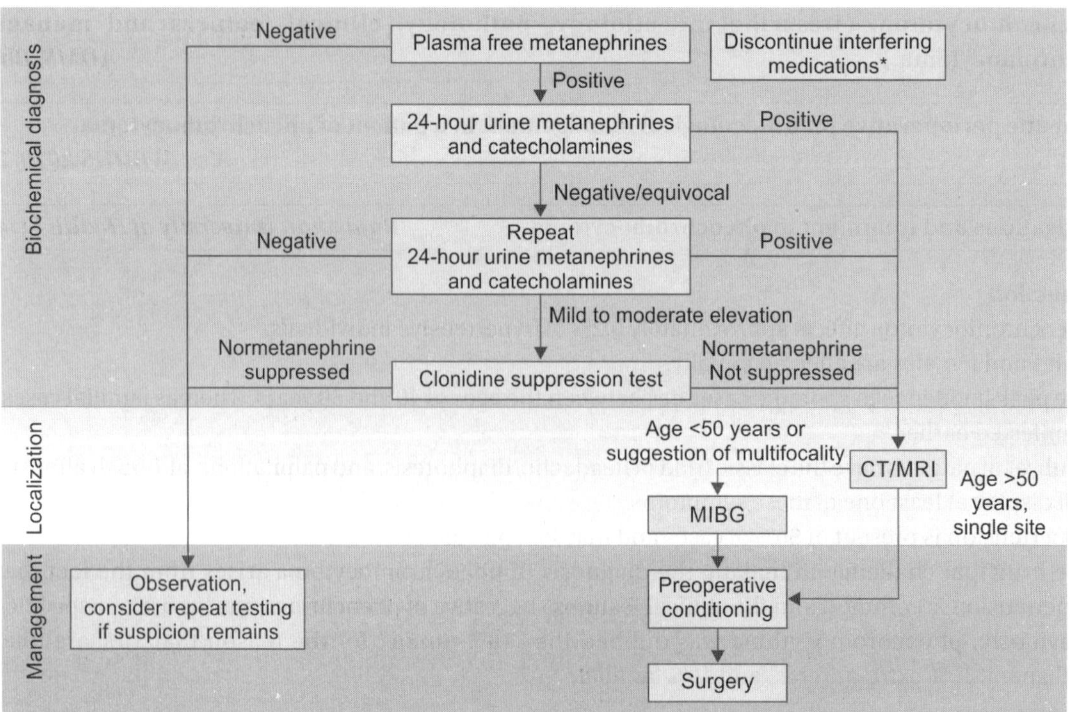

*Including sympathomimetics, phenoxybenzamine, acetaminophen, many psychotropic drugs.
(MIBG: meta-iodobenzylguanidine)

Perioperative Care

- The adverse perioperative hemodynamic changes that are most commonly observed with pheochromocytoma are intraoperative hypertension and postoperative hypotension.
- Intraoperative hypertension may be caused by stimulation of catecholamine release by anesthetic induction agents, as well as direct manipulation of the tumor.
- Postoperative hypotension may be profound. It results from a state of hypovolemia created by the presence of excess circulating catecholamines.
- Sudden withdrawal of this stimulus after tumor removal leads to peripheral arteriolar vasodilation, in addition to a dramatic increase in venous capacitance, which together may precipitate cardiovascular collapse.
    - As soon as the biochemical diagnosis of pheochromocytoma has been confirmed, α-adrenergic blockade is initiated to protect against hemodynamic lability. Start with phenoxybenzamine, 10 mg twice daily. The dosage can be titrated upward every 2–3 days to a maximum of 40 mg three times daily to achieve normalization of heart rate and blood pressure. The period of preoperative conditioning lasts at least 2 weeks to allow adequate reversal of α-adrenergic receptor downregulation. Phenoxybenzamine is a nonspecific, noncompetitive (irreversible), long-acting (half-life of 24 hours) α-adrenergic antagonist.
    - β-blockers may be administered after adequate α-blockade has been achieved in the subset of patients with persistent tachycardia. β-blockers are never the first agent administered because a decrease in peripheral vasodilatory β-receptor stimulation results in unopposed α-adrenergic tone, which may exacerbate hypertension.
    - Clinical suspicion of hypovolemia needs to remain high in the postoperative period, and patients need to be aggressively resuscitated if they become hypotensive or oliguric.
    - Some patients may require vasopressors after tumor removal, especially if preoperative α-blockade is incomplete.

Surgical Management and Outcomes

- Successful operative treatment of pheochromocytoma is dependent on close communication between the surgeon and anesthesiologist.
- Invasive hemodynamic monitoring is required, and fluid management must be meticulous. Manipulation of the tumor needs to be minimized, and the anesthetic team must be prepared to administer supplemental IV α- and β-blockers, as well as vasopressors, when necessary.
- Surgery is curative in >90% of pheochromocytoma cases.
- Although these tumors are highly vascular and tend to adhere to adjacent structures, the great majority of them can be removed successfully via a laparoscopic approach.
- Laparoscopic resection is contraindicated when preoperative imaging demonstrates local invasion.
- Functional image-guided focused exploration has replaced bilateral adrenal and retroperitoneal exploration and has led to diminished rates of solid organ injury.

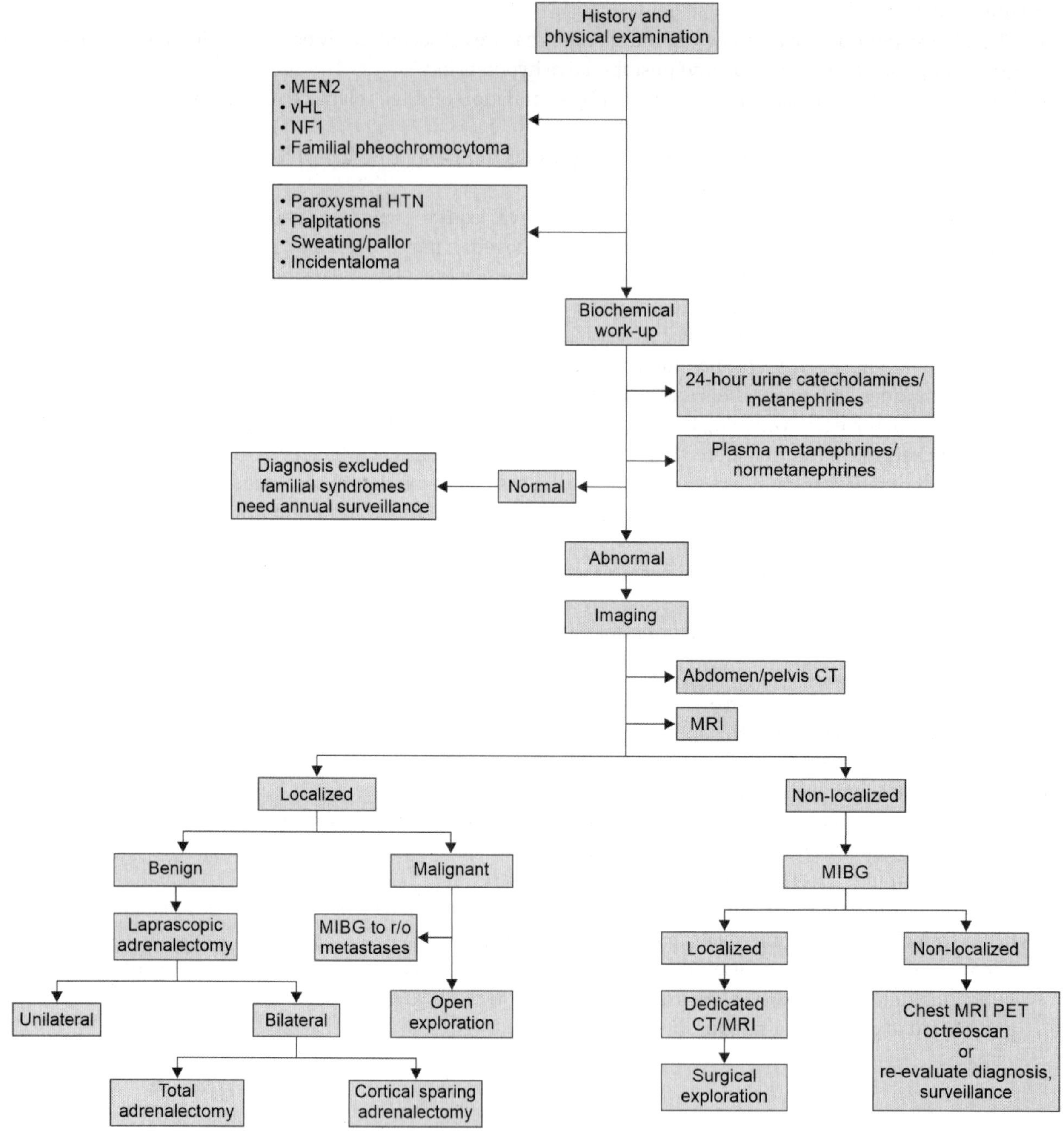

(HTN: hypertension; MIBG: meta-iodobenzylguanidine; PET: positron emission tomography)

49. What are the extra-adrenal sites of pheochromocytoma? Name the genetic factors predispose to pheochromocytoma. How will you investigate a case of pheochromocytoma and differentiate between benign and malignant tumor? ***WBUHS 2017***

A classification system for extra-adrenal pheochromocytomas (EAPs) proposed by Glenner and Grimley in 1974 divided the tumors into four groups based on location:

- Branchiomeric
- Intravagal
- Aorticosympathetic
- Visceroautonomic
- The branchiomeric and intravagal tumors occur in the head and neck, are rarely functional, and generally stain negative for chromaffin.
- The aorticosympathetic group is found along the length of the aorta, between the renal arteries, around the iliac bifurcation, and includes the organ of Zuckerkandl.
- The visceroautonomic division occurs in association with blood vessels or visceral organs like the bladder.
- The latter two groups tend to be functional and usually are chromaffin positive.

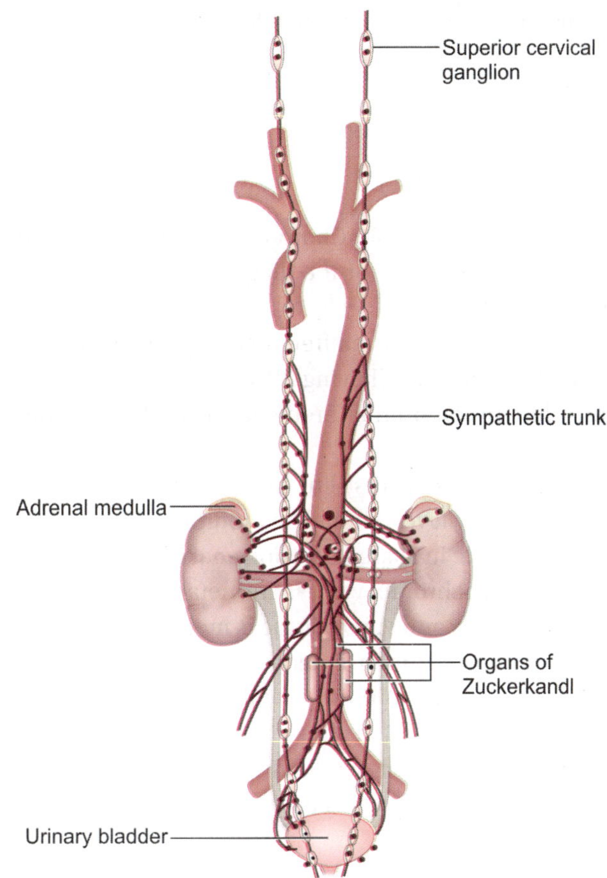

Extra-adrenal Paraganglioma

- Carotid body
- Jugulotympanic
- Vagal
- Laryngeal

- Aorticopulmonary
- Gangliocytic
- Cauda equine
- Orbital nasopharyngeal

Extra-adrenal Sympathetic Paraganglioma

- Superior and inferior para-aortic paraganglioma
- Urinary bladder
- Intrathoracic and cervical paravertebral

Gene(s)	*Associated finding(s)*	*Syndrome name*
SDHA, SDHAF2, SDHB, SDHC, and SDHD	Paraganglioma, pheochromocytoma, kidney cancer, thyroid cancer, and gastrointestinal stromal tumors (GISTs)	Hereditary paraganglioma and pheochromocytoma syndrome
VHL	Pheochromocytoma, kidney cancer, kidney and pancreatic cysts, retinal angiomas, and hemangioblastomas	Von Hippel-Lindau syndrome
RET	Pheochromocytoma, medullary thyroid cancer, mucosal, and gastrointestinal neuromas	Multiple endocrine neoplasia syndrome type II (MEN 2)
NF1	Pheochromocytoma, breast cancer, neurofibromas, and other noncancerous findings	Neurofibromatosis type 1
MAX	Pheochromocytoma	
TMEM127	Paraganglioma and pheochromocytoma	

Investigations

The Endocrine Society, the American Association for Clinical Chemistry, and the European Society of Endocrinology (ESE) have released clinical practice guidelines for the diagnosis and management of pheochromocytoma and paraganglioma (jointly referred to as PPGL).

- Biochemical testing via measurement of plasma free metanephrines or urinary fractionated metanephrines should be performed in patients suspected of having PPGL.
- Patients with a known germ-line mutation that predisposes to PPGL should undergo periodic biochemical testing.
- CT, rather than MRI, is recommended as the first-line imaging technique.
- Blood pressure, heart rate, and glucose levels should be monitored immediately after surgery.
- Patients with PPGLs should participate in shared decision-making for genetic testing.
    - Catecholamines produced by pheochromocytomas are metabolized within chromaffin cells. Norepinephrine is metabolized to normetanephrine and epinephrine is metabolized to metanephrine.
    - Because this process occurs within the tumor, independently of catecholamine release, pheochromocytomas are best diagnosed by measurement of these metabolites rather than by measurement of the parent catecholamines.
    - Guidelines from the North American Neuroendocrine Tumor Society (NANETS) recommend biochemical testing for pheochromocytoma in the following cases:
        - Symptomatic patients
        - Patients with an AI
        - Patients who have a hereditary risk for developing a pheochromocytoma or paraganglioma (EAP)
    - The choice of diagnostic test should be based on the clinical suspicion of a pheochromocytoma.
    - General laboratory features of pheochromocytoma include the following:
        - Hyperglycemia
        - Hypercalcemia
        - Erythrocytosis

Imaging

- Imaging studies should be performed only after biochemical studies have confirmed the diagnosis of pheochromocytoma.
- CT scanning or MRI can be used for detection of the disorder.
- Scintigraphy may be used when these techniques fail to localize the tumor.
- PET scanning has shown promising results as an imaging modality for pheochromocytoma.

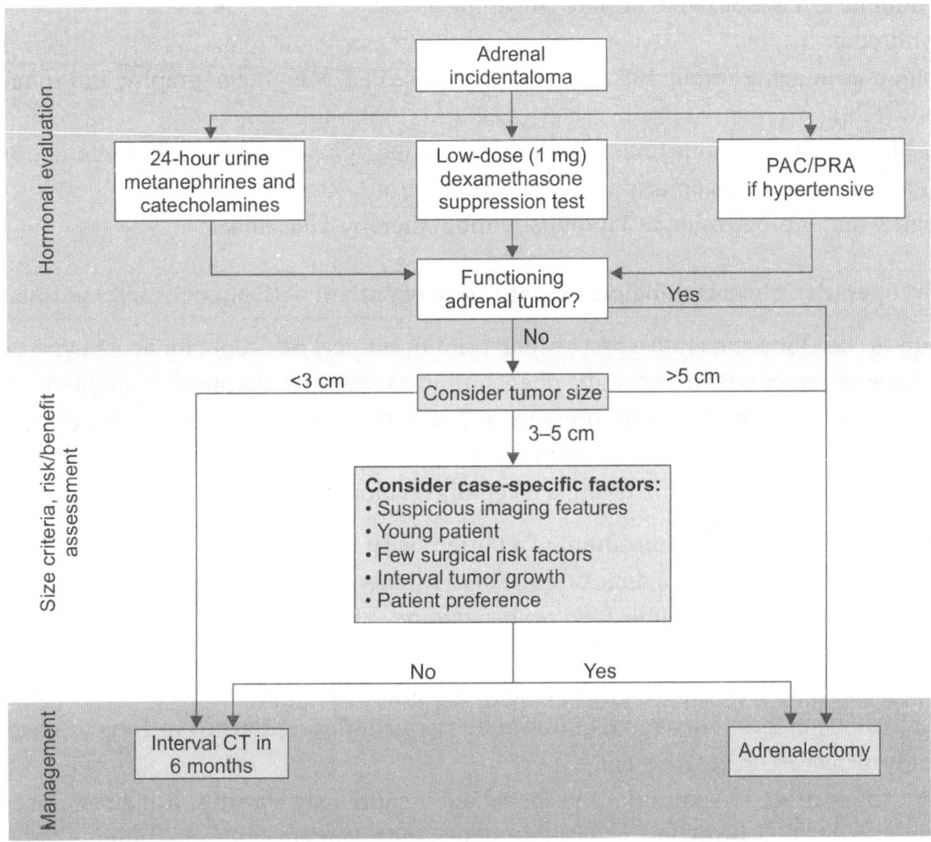

Algorithm for the Management of an Adrenal Incidentaloma

- Adrenalectomy is recommended for all patients with functional tumors.
- For nonfunctioning tumors, the risk for malignancy is assessed according to size.
- Tumors >5 cm on CT carry a >25% risk for malignancy and need to be removed. Those <3 cm can be safely observed.
- Case-specific factors must be considered for intermediate sized tumors. PAC, plasma aldosterone concentration, PRA, plasma renin activity.

Differentiating features malignant from benign pheochromocytoma:

- Vascular invasion, cellular atypia, and even local recurrence do not definitively identify a pheochromocytoma as malignant. Currently, a malignant pheochromocytoma is defined only by the presence of metastasis.
- A younger age at diagnosis has been suggested to be a clinical risk factor for malignant.
- Pheochromocytoma of the Adrenal gland Scaled Score (PASS) was proposed as a scoring system for malignancy risk. However, there have been conflicting reports regarding its reliability in predicting malignancy. Thompson et al. found that tumors with a PASS >4 exhibited increased metastatic potential.
- Norepinephrine- or dopamine-producing tumors have a higher risk of malignancy.
- Extra-adrenal paragangliomas are more commonly malignant than intra-adrenal paragangliomas.

Things to be noted:

- Age and gender.
- Primary tumor location (if multiple tumors are present, the tumor that is >5 cm and/or associated with local spread or regional positive lymph nodes is considered the primary tumor).
- Hormone- and tumor-related symptoms, including hypertension, constipation, and pain.
- Serum chromogranin A levels and urinary and/or plasma metanephrine, normetanephrine, and methoxytyramine levels indexed to urinary creatinine levels.
- Genetic syndrome.
- Best scintigraphic imaging among 18F-fluorodeoxyglucose PET, MIBG scintigraphy, and somatostatin receptor scintigraphy (SRS).
- Bone, lung, liver, and lymph node tumor burden determined by head and neck, thoracic, abdominal, and pelvic CT and/or MRI in early arterial phase and guided CT and/or MRI.
- Morphological tumor progression at 3 months, without therapy if feasible.

50. Outline the preoperative pharmacological management of patient with pheochromocytoma.

Medical therapy is used for preoperative preparation prior to surgical resection, for acute hypertensive crises, and as primary therapy for patients with metastatic pheochromocytomas. Preoperative preparation requires combined alpha and beta blockade to control blood pressure and to prevent an intraoperative hypertensive crisis. Alpha-adrenergic blockade, in particular, is required to control blood pressure and prevent a hypertensive crisis. High circulating catecholamine levels stimulate alpha receptors on blood vessels and cause vasoconstriction.

Perioperative Pharmacological Management of a Patient with Pheochromocytoma

- Preoperative preparation includes administration of α-adrenergic blocker to control hypertension and to permit re-expansion of intravascular volume. Phenoxybenzamine, 10 mg orally twice a day, is initiated and increased to 20–40 mg orally twice a day until the desired effect or prohibitive side effects are encountered.
- Other selective competitive alpha 1 adrenergic antagonist like prazosin can also be used. It has a short elimination half-life of 2–3 hours and requires more frequent dosing starting at 1 mg three to four times daily and gradually increased up to 12 mg daily.
- Whichever drug is used, it is important to introduce it cautiously starting with small doses and increasing gradually until orthostatic hypotension develops indicating adequate alpha blockade.
- Postural hypertension is expected and is the desired endpoint. β-adrenergic blockade (e.g., propranolol) may be added if tachycardia or arrhythmias develop but only after complete α-adrenergic blockade.
- Beta adrenergic blockade should be avoided in patients with catecholamine induced cardiomyopathy as it can lead to development of intractable hypotension, bradycardia and asystolic arrest. Selective beta I adrenoceptor antagonists such as atenolol (100 mg day-1) or bisoprolol (10–20 mg day-1) should be used in order to minimize undesirable side effects in the bronchi or peripheral vasculature.
- Calcium channel blockers have also been employed in the preoperative and intraoperative hemodynamic control, such as nifedipine 30–90 mg/day and nicardipine infusion starting at 5 mg/hour, increasing by 2.5 mg/hour every 5 minutes to a maximum of 15 mg/hour.
- High-sodium diet with fluid intake to prevent severe hypotension after removal of the tumor.
- Preoperative sedation and anxiolysis, preferably with a benzodiazepine, and assurance by the anesthesiologist will decrease anxiety and prevent marked hemodynamic fluctuation in the immediate preoperative period.
- Medication for alpha and beta blockade should be continued until the day of the operation except phenoxybenzamine which may be stopped the day before surgery as it has a long half-life and can cause postoperative hypotension.
- Blood pressure, heart rate, and glucose levels should be monitored.

51. Describe multiple endocrine neoplasia syndromes. describe the clinical presentation of pheochromocytoma and how will you prepare your patient preoperatively.

DY Patil Educational Society Deemed to be University 2024

Discussed in earlier questions

52. Incidentalomas. *WBUHS 2011*

53. Adrenal incidentalomas. *AIIMS, Raipur 2025*

54. How will you evaluate a patient of Adrenal incidentaloma? *WBUHS 2024*

Introduction

An AI is a mass lesion >1 cm in diameter, serendipitously discovered by radiologic examination. This entity is the result of technological advances in imaging such as CT and MRI. Discovery of an adrenal mass raises two questions that determine the degree of evaluation and the need for therapy.

Definition

It is an asymptomatic adrenal tumor that is discovered on an imaging test (CAT scan, MRI, etc.) which was ordered to evaluate a problem that is unrelated to adrenal disease.

Differential Diagnosis of Adrenal Incidentalomas

Primary adrenal neoplasm		***Metastasis***
Nonfunctioning	***Functioning***	• Lung • Kidney • Breast • Gastrointestinal • Melanoma
• Cortical adenoma/carcinoma • Cyst • Myelolipoma • Ganglioneuroma • Hemorrhage/hematoma	*Cortical adenoma/carcinoma:* • Hypercortisolism and hyperaldosteronism • Pheochromocytoma	

Algorithmic approach for the evaluation of adrenal incidentaloma.

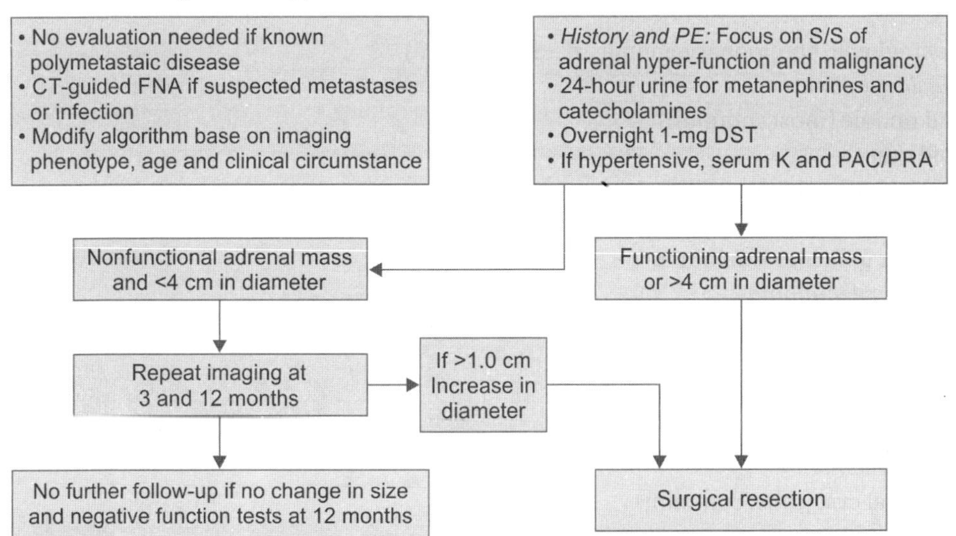

(FNA: fine-needle aspiration; PAC: plasma aldosterone concentration; PRA: plasma renin activity)

55. Enumerate the likely etiologies of incidentalomas. Outline the preoperative work up and treatment options of a patient having symptomatic pheochromocytoma of 5 cm size in the left adrenal gland.

AIIMS, Patna 2025

Incidentalomas

Definition

An incidentaloma is an incidentally discovered, usually asymptomatic mass or lesion found during imaging or investigations done for unrelated reasons.

Such lesions may arise in any organ, but are most commonly found in adrenal glands, pituitary, thyroid, parathyroid, lung, kidney, and liver.

Common Sites and Likely Etiologies

- Adrenal Incidentaloma *(Most common site for incidentalomas)*
  - *Benign causes:*
    - Nonfunctioning adrenal adenoma (most common)
    - Adrenal cyst
    - Adrenal myelolipoma
    - Adrenal hemorrhage (old resolving hematoma)
    - Adrenal hyperplasia (nodular)
  - *Malignant or functional causes:*
    - Adrenocortical carcinoma
    - Metastasis (e.g., lung, breast, kidney)
    - Pheochromocytoma
    - Functioning adenoma (Cushing's, Conn's)
- Pituitary Incidentaloma
  - *Benign:*
    - Nonfunctioning pituitary microadenoma
    - Cystic lesions (Rathke's cleft cyst, arachnoid cyst)
  - *Functional:*
    - Prolactinoma
    - GH or ACTH secreting adenoma
  - *Others:*
    - Meningioma, craniopharyngioma, metastasis (rare)
- *Thyroid Incidentaloma*
  - Colloid nodule (most common)
  - Thyroid cyst
  - Hashimoto's thyroiditis nodule
  - Follicular adenoma
  - Papillary or follicular carcinoma
- *Parathyroid Incidentaloma*
  - Parathyroid adenoma
  - Parathyroid hyperplasia
  - Parathyroid cyst
  - Parathyroid carcinoma (rare)
- *Renal Incidentaloma*
  - Simple renal cyst (most common)
  - Angiomyolipoma
  - Oncocytoma

- Renal cell carcinoma (RCC)
- Metastasis (less common)

- *Hepatic Incidentaloma*
  - Hemangioma (most common benign)
  - Focal nodular hyperplasia (FNH)
  - Hepatic adenoma
  - Simple cyst
  - Hepatocellular carcinoma (HCC)
  - Metastases
- *Pulmonary Incidentaloma (Solitary Pulmonary Nodule)*
  - Granuloma (TB, fungal infections)
  - Hamartoma
  - Primary bronchogenic carcinoma
  - Metastatic nodule
- *Other Less Common Sites*

Site	***Common etiologies***
Pancreas	Cystic neoplasms, neuroendocrine tumors, pseudocyst
Ovary	Simple cyst, endometrioma, dermoid cyst, cystadenoma/carcinoma
Prostate	Benign prostatic hyperplasia nodule, carcinoma
Spleen	Cyst, hemangioma, lymphoma

Rest part of the question has already been answered previously.

56. Describe the modern investigation tools for localizing and diagnosing functioning adrenal tumors with special reference to bifunctional chelate-based nuclear scans. ***WBUHS 2021 Supplementary***

Introduction

Adrenal masses are often discovered incidentally and are then termed AIs. They are often discovered after an imaging procedure is performed that is unrelated to the adrenal gland. Usually, the patient has no signs of hormonal excess or obvious underlying malignancy.

The following tests may be used to diagnose an adrenal gland tumor:
Biochemical tests used in the assessment of AIs include evaluation of the following:

- *Pheochromocytoma:* Urine-free and plasma-free metanephrines
- *Primary aldosteronism:* Plasma aldosterone-to-renin ratio
- *Adrenocortical carcinoma:* Urine 17-ketosteroids
- *Cushing or "silent" Cushing syndrome:* Overnight 1-mg dexamethasone test

Diagnosis

Guidelines issued in 2009 by the American Association of Clinical Endocrinologists (AACE) and American Association of Endocrine Surgeons (AAES) for the management of AIs recommend that evaluation of patients with an AI include clinical, biochemical, and radiographic testing for the following:

- Hypercortisolism
- Aldosteronism (if hypertensive)
- Pheochromocytoma or a malignant tumor
  - The simplest screening test for autonomous cortisol secretion from an incidentaloma is a 1-mg overnight dexamethasone suppression test.

- Salivary cortisol, dexamethasone suppression, and urine free cortisol testing can be used if clinical suspicion is high (e.g., in patients with hypertension, obesity, diabetes mellitus, or osteoporosis).
- Primary aldosteronism is confirmed by lack of aldosterone suppression on a 24-hour urine study with salt loading.
- To determine the incidentaloma subtype, high-resolution CT scanning should be performed in all patients. In addition, adrenal venous sampling should be performed in most patients older than 40 years.

Clinical practice guidelines for AI management issued in 2016 by the ESE, in collaboration with the European Network for the Study of Adrenal Tumors (ENSAT), include the following diagnostic recommendations:

- That clinicians aim to establish if an adrenal mass is benign or malignant at the time of initial detection
- That all AIs undergo an imaging procedure to determine if the mass is homogeneous and lipid-rich and therefore benign; for this purpose, the use of noncontrast CT scanning is recommended
- That every patient with an AI undergo careful assessment, including clinical examination, for symptoms and signs of adrenal hormone excess
- That all patients with AIs undergo a 1-mg overnight dexamethasone suppression test to exclude cortisol excess
- That post-dexamethasone serum cortisol levels between 51 and 138 nmol/L (1.9-5.0 μg/dL) be considered evidence of possible autonomous cortisol secretion and that post-dexamethasone cortisol levels of over 138 nmol/L (over 5.0 μg/dL) be taken as evidence of autonomous cortisol secretion
- That pheochromocytoma be excluded by measurement of plasma-free metanephrines or urinary fractionated metanephrines
- That in patients with concomitant hypertension or unexplained hypokalemia, the aldosterone/renin ratio be used to exclude primary aldosteronism
- That sex hormones and steroid precursors be measured in patients with clinical or imaging features suggestive of adrenocortical carcinoma
- That if the adrenal mass is indeterminate on noncontrast CT scan and the results of the hormonal workup do not indicate significant hormone excess, three options be considered by a multidisciplinary team acknowledging the patient's clinical context: immediate additional imaging with another modality, interval imaging in 6–12 months (noncontrast CT or MRI scan), or surgery without further delay.

For evaluation of possible adrenocortical carcinomas, the 2012 European Society for Medical Oncology (ESMO) guidelines utilize the 2005 proposed diagnostic workup of ENSAT. The recommended workup includes the following tests.

Hormonal Work-up

These studies include the following:

- Glucocorticoid excess (minimum three of four tests)
- Dexamethasone suppression test (1 mg, 23:00 hours)
- Excretion of free urinary cortisol (24-hour urine)
- Basal cortisol (serum)
- Basal ACTH (plasma)

Sexual Steroids and Steroid Precursors

These studies include the following:

- Dehydroepiandrosterone-S (serum)
- 17-OH-progesterone (serum)
- Androstenedione (serum)
- Testosterone (serum)
- 17-beta-estradiol (serum, only in men and postmenopausal women)
- 24-hour urine steroid metabolite examination

Mineralocorticoid Excess

These studies include the following:

- Potassium (serum)
- Aldosterone/renin ratio (only in patients with arterial hypertension and/or hypokalemia)

Catecholamine Excess

These studies include the following:

- Normetanephrine, metanephrine, and methoxytyramine (plasma)
- *Alternatively:* Fractionated metanephrine excretion (24-hour urine)

Imaging

- CT or MRI scan of abdomen and CT thorax scan
- Bone scintigraphy (when suspecting skeletal metastases)
- Fluorodeoxyglucose-PET (FDG-PET) scan (optional)
- MIBG scintigraphy, DOTATATE-PET scan, or dopa/dopamine PET scan if pheochromocytoma is proved

Imaging Characteristics of Adrenal Masses

Adrenal mass	*Imaging characteristics*
Adrenocortical adenoma	• Unilateral, <4–5 cm in diameter • Round, homogeneous density with smooth border • Low attenuation on CT scan (<10 HU) • Rapid, intense contrast enhancement followed by early contrast washout (absolute percent washout >60%, relative percent washout >40%) • Intracellular fat with signal loss on opposed-phase MRI images
Myelolipoma	• Macroscopic fat on CT • Calcification • Hyperintense signal on Tl MRI
Pheochromocytoma	• Hypervascularity with cystic areas in larger lesions • Rapid, intense contrast enhancement with variable delayed washout • High 12 MRI signal intensity (light-bulb sign)
Adrenocortical carcinoma	• Unilateral, >4–5 cm • Irregular shape, heterogeneous, central tumor • Necrosis, local invasion • Calcification • Increased attenuation on CT (>10 HU) • Delay in contrast washout • No loss of signal on opposed-phase MRI • Elevated standardized uptake value (SUV) on positron emission tomography (PET)
Adrenal metastasis	• Irregular shape, heterogeneous • Maybe bilateral or with other metastatic disease • Increased attenuation on CT (>10 HU) • Delay in contrast washout • No loss of signal on MRI • Elevated SUV on PET

In patients with biochemical evidence pheochromocytoma and negative CT and MRI, further imaging with scintigraphic or PET scanning can help identify occult tumors.

- Scintigraphic scanning after the administration of 123I-MIBG provides a functional and anatomic test of hyperfunctioning chromaffin tissue. *MIBG scanning* is very specific for both intra-adrenal pheochromocytomas and EAPs but is expensive and somewhat difficult to use.
- *68-Ga DOTATATE PET* scanning has the highest sensitivity and can be helpful in identifying occult tumors or metastatic disease in patients with high-risk of metastatic disease (paraganglioma or large tumor).

[Go Through-Gallium-68 Bifunctional Chelators (BFC) in the Neuroendocrine Tumor Imaging]

- The bifunctional chelators are compounds acting as a conjugate between the radioisotope and a vector. The BFC's key features are the ability to quickly and steadily incorporate the isotope and create covalent bonds with biomolecules, responsible for targeting.
- The macrocyclic chelators with three or four nitrogen atoms in a ring have been established as frequently considered routes for the introduction of gallium-68. Between them, the molecules with tri- and tetraaza-ring have become the most prevalent since irreversible complexation of the gallium atom, thermodynamic stability, and superior kinetic even at room temperature. External substituents, usually in the form of carboxyl groups allow convenient conjugation to various targeting molecules.
- DOTA (1,4,7,10-tetraazacyclododecane-1,4,7,10-tetraacetic acid) remains the most frequently used chelator because of its availability and well-recognized coordination chemistry.
- A significant number of compounds, similar to DOTA and NOTA have been used for specific applications: bifunctional derivatives of NOTA–NODAGA (1,4,7-triazacyclononane,1-glutaric acid-4,7-acetic acid) and NODASA (1,4,7-triazacyclononane-1-succinic acid-4,7-diacetic acid) are limited to coupling peptides through an amide bond, NODAPA (1,4,7-triazacyclononane-1,4-diacetic acid-7-p-phenyl-acetic acid) with hydroxyl group (NODAPA-OH) or thiocyanate groups [NODAPA-(NCS)n] have been successfully applied as versatile bifunctional chelators.
- ^{68}Ga-DOTA-peptides are a group of PET tracers that specifically bind to somatostatin (SST) receptors that are overexpressed on the neuroendocrine tumor (NET) cells. Targeting agents are coupled via the BFC leveraging standard intermediates that enable covalent attachment of peptides, including active octapeptides (octreotide, OC) and related peptide analogs, TOC (Tyr^3-OC), TATE (Tyr^3-Thr^8-OC), and NOC (NaI^3-OC).
- Despite the variations in SST receptors affinity, all described compounds (^{68}Ga-DOTA-TOC, -NOC, -TATE) have been reported to be accurate for the localization of well-differentiated NET lesions, performing better than CT.
- Comparing to other modalities, studies have shown the superiority of PET over ^{111}In-pentetreotide-SPECT in the detection of metastases and unknown primary neuroendocrine tumors.
- PET imaging using ^{68}Ga-SSTR has also been found to be more accurate than ^{18}F-FDOPA-PET in noncarcinoid tumors. [^{68}Ga]-DOTA-TATE detected more tumor sites than [^{123}I]-MIBG in patients with the neural crest tumors (including paragangliomas).
- Only one bone lesion in one patient with adrenal paraganglioma was detected on [^{123}I]-MIBG scan but not in [^{68}Ga]-DOTA TATE.23, 24, 25, 26, 27, 28, 29
- Radionuclide-labeled DOTA-SSTR analogs are used for diagnostics and therapy of the neuroendocrine tumors.
- Typically, ^{68}Ga-DOTA-TOC is used for diagnosis, while the same compound labeled with high- or medium-energy β-emitters such as yttrium-90 or lutetium-177 is used for therapy.
- The use of coupled diagnostic and therapeutic isotopes with ligand for treatment of NET allows better planning of therapy and to evaluate the therapeutic outcome as in personalized medicine where the diagnosis is tailored to the subsequent therapy.
- It influenced radiopharmaceutical sciences with the "theranostics" concept, which combines gallium-68 diagnostics with trivalent therapeutic radiometals (yttrium-90, lutetium-177, bismuth-213) with improved personal dosimetry.

---

57. Compare the different imaging modalities for adrenal masses with special reference to Linos formula. How will manage a patient with bilateral adrenal incidentalomas? ***WBUHS 2023***

The "Linos formula" is a mathematical formula applied for the correct measurements of the adrenal gland tumor in CT.

Linos formula (Histologic size (cm) = 0.85 + [(1.09) (CT major size in cm)]

- Based on the results of various clinical series, adrenal tumors are discovered incidentally on 0.35–5.00% of abdominal CT scans obtained for different reasons.

- Once an adrenal tumor is found and hormone hypersecretion is ruled out, decision has to be taken between surgical excision and close observation.
- Imaging phenotype and mass size are the two major predictors of malignancy.
- Some radiologic characteristics may help in the differential diagnosis between benign and malignant adrenal tumors.
- Considering that most AIs have a nonspecific appearance using imaging techniques, decisions are based mainly on the diagnostic likelihood of each specific tumor.
- Moreover, the imaging phenotype is not accurate in many cases, often varying with the visual interpretation
- In the absence of imaging characteristics suggestive of malignancy, tumor size has shown the closest correlation to malignancy.
- The number of asymptomatic nonfunctioning tumors <3 cm that are malignant is low compared to the high prevalence of malignancy in tumors >6 cm.
- CT scanning is the method most commonly used to evaluate AIs.
- Discrepancies in the measurement may arise from two aspects: The accuracy of the procedure itself and the way measurements are performed.
- For most CT scans the anteroposterior and lateral axes are measured, and the cephalocaudal axis is taken into account less frequently.
- To improve these discrepancies, measurements must be taken considering all three axes.
- Mantero and Arnaldi found good correlation between radiologic size (CT or MRI) and the size measured at pathologic examination ($r = 0.92$, $p < 0.0001$), with higher accuracy of MRI for lesions <3 cm.
- In contrast, Linos and Jossart found that the adrenal mass size determined by radiology using CT scans was usually inferior to the size reported by pathology.
- To avoid underestimating any of the axes, all three axes were routinely measured on all CT scans; moreover, considering that decisions are usually based on the largest diameter, the largest diameter was chosen for our evaluations.
- On the bivariate analysis, the direct measurement and the corrected value using the Linos formula were similar.
- However, when the overestimation and underestimation of real dimensions were taken into account, the Linos correction resulted in fewer underestimated values.
- Overestimation would lead to an increase in the number of patients selected for surgical treatment; and underestimation would deprive patients with adrenal cortical carcinomas proper medical attention.
- Therefore, for the purpose of this particular pathology and considering that the risk of laparoscopic adrenalectomy is negligible in most patients,
- CT scanning tends to underestimate the real dimension of adrenal tumors. However, for predicting the real pathologic size of the tumor the two methods—direct and corrected measurements using the Linos formula—provided similar results in 83.1% of the patients.

Differential Diagnosis of Imaging Phenotypes by CT Scanning: Benign Versus Malignant Masses

Management of Bilateral Adrenal Incidentaloma

Radiologic morphology	*Benign*	*Malignant*
Size	Small (<4 cm)	Large (>5 cm)
Shape	Round to oval	Irregular
Margins	Smooth	Unclear or blurred
Texture	Homogeneous	Heterogeneous
Density (without contrast)	<10 Hounsfield units	>10 Hounsfield units
MR imaging (compared with liver)	Isointense	Hyperintense
Necrosis/hemorrhage	Rare	Common
Growth	Very slow	Usually rapid

Key Points

- Diagnosis for bilateral AIs is based on the same principles as for patients diagnosed with solitary AI.
- The first step is to determine, based on a patient's clinical history and imaging phenotype, whether these adrenal lesions could be malignant and if they are indicative of hormonal excess. However, there are issues unique to bilateral AIs including the differential diagnosis, the evaluation and the management depending on the underlying cause.
- Patients with bilateral AIs are more likely to demonstrate hormone excess, although rarely adrenal insufficiency may occur if there is marked bilateral infiltration of the adrenal glands as in cases of lymphoma, amyloidosis, or infection.
- In some clinical settings, congenital adrenal hyperplasia (CAH) and adrenal hemorrhage may also be present. Familial syndromes may also be present in bilateral AIs.
- In cases where bilateral pheochromocytomas occur, familial syndromes must be considered.

Evaluation

- Approximately 15% of AIs occur bilaterally.
- Whereas most unilateral masses are benign or nonfunctional, the bilateral adrenal mass is more likely metastatic disease, hemorrhage, infiltrative disease, CAH, macronodular Cushing's syndrome, or bilateral cortical adenomas/Bilateral pheochromocytomas are also possible, especially as part of a familial syndrome.
- In evaluating the hormone function of any AI, testing for subclinical Cushing's, pheochromocytoma, and hyperaldosteronism (in patients with hypertension) should be performed.
- In the case of the bilateral AI, patients who present with symptoms such as hypotension, dizziness, weight loss, or abdominal pain in the setting of bilateral adrenal masses should be evaluated for adrenal insufficiency using an ACTH stimulation test.
- CAH infrequently manifests as bilateral adrenal disease. CAH is unlikely to present as an adult, since most patients are diagnosed in childhood or have symptoms of adrenal insufficiency, virilization, or salt-wasting. If CAH is suspected, screening for adrenal insufficiency as well as mutation analysis for CYP21B is recommended.
- Specific attention should be paid to the unique clinical situation of the bilateral pheochromocytoma, which account for approximately 10% of pheochromocytomas.

Recommended screening tests in AIs. Additional analyses in bilateral incidentalomas listed below will depend on the clinical presentation and family history.

Recommended screening for all incidentalomas	***Test***
Cushing's syndrome	1 mg overnight dexamethasone suppression test
Pheochromocytoma	24-hour urine collection for fractionated metanephrines and catecholamines
Primary aldosteronism (screen only in hypertensive patients)	Plasma aldosterone to plasma renin activity ratio
Additional screening recommended for bilateral incidentalomas	***Test***
Adrenal insufficiency	Morning cortisol and ACTH (or corticotrophin stimulation test)
MEN2	*RET* gene mutation analysis, evaluation for hyperparathyroidism, medullary thyroid cancer, or mucosal neuromas
Von Hippel-Lindau syndrome	*VHL* gene mutation analysis and evaluation for additional tumors (such as renal, retinal, or nervous system)
Neurofibromatosis type 1	*NF1* gene mutation analysis
Pheochromocytoma-paraganglioma syndrome	*SDHB/SDHD* gene mutation analysis

All guidelines recommend that bilateral AIs should undergo the same clinical, radiological, and hormonal evaluations as unilateral AIs.

This new approach to bilateral diseases is suggested in the 2023 ESE guideline in cases with the following radiological and hormonal results:

- Bilateral (macronodular) hyperplasia;
- Bilateral adrenal adenomas;
- Two morphologically similar but nonadenoma-like adrenal masses;
- Two morphologically different adrenal masses. In particular, the assessment of comorbidities attributable to cortisol excess is recommended in patients with bilateral macronodular hyperplasia.

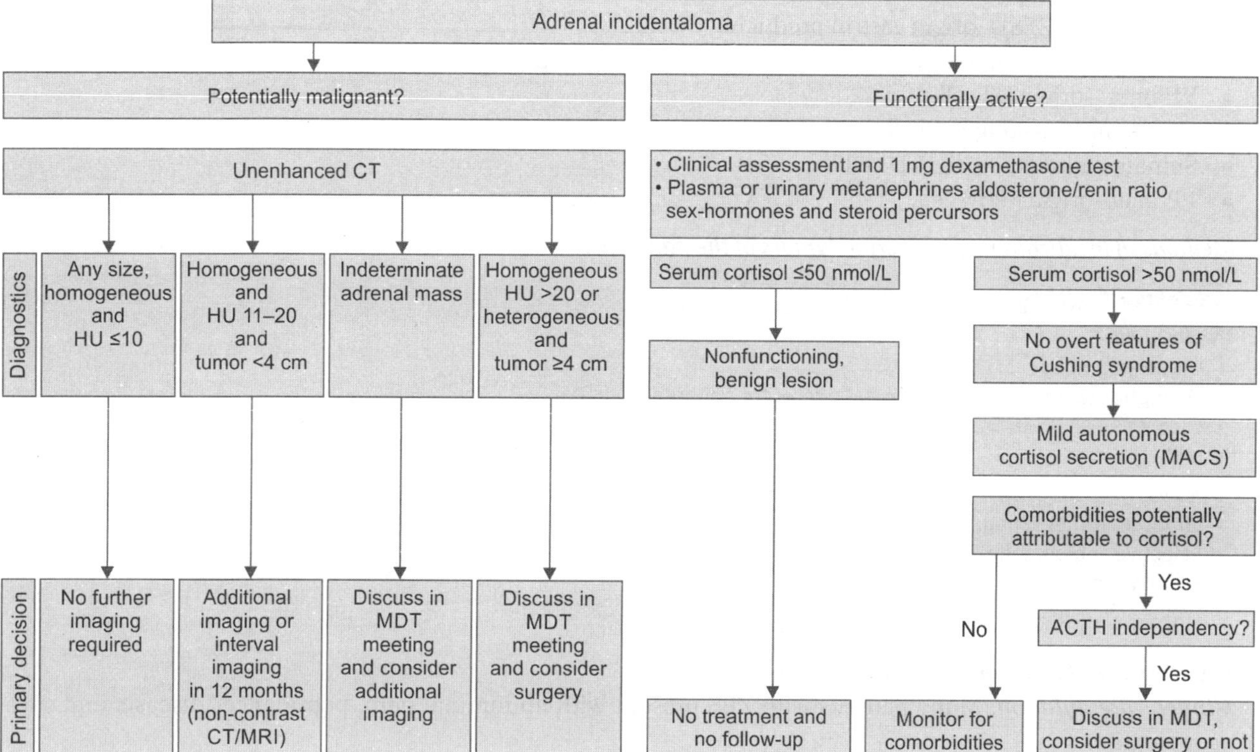

Definite Treatment

- Definitive treatment for bilateral adrenal masses is surgical resection of both adrenal glands in most cases, except in the case of aldosterone secreting tumors, in which case medical options may be the preferred approach.
- Special care is needed in the case of the bilateral pheochromocytoma given the added morbidity of adrenal insufficiency after bilateral adrenalectomy.
- No specific guidelines exist addressing the optimal surgical approach to the bilateral pheochromocytoma; alpha-blockade followed by beta-blockade (with or without metyrosine) along with IV volume expansion remains the mainstay of preoperative management.
- Following bilateral adrenalectomy, care must be taken to ensure proper glucocorticoid, and mineralocorticoid replacement.

ENDOCRINE PANCREAS

58. Tumors of endocrine pancreas. ***WBUHS 2010***

59. Describe in brief on neuroendocrine tumor of pancreas. ***WBUHS 2024***

60. Glucagonoma. ***WBUHS 2010***

61. Zollinger Ellison Syndrome. ***Gujarat Health University 2025***

62. Write on gastrinoma. ***RIMS, Imphal 2012***

Tumors of Endocrine Pancreas

Tumors of endocrine pancreas are:

- Gastrinoma (ZES)—origin gastrin producing G cell.
- Insulinoma—origin B cell.
- VIPoma—origin D2 cell.
- Glucagonoma—origin A cell.
- Somatostatinoma—origin D cell.
- PPoma—origin PP(F) cell.

Methods of localization of endocrine tumors of the pancreas:

Modality
Noninvasive: • Ultrasonography • Octreotide radioimaging [somatostatin receptor scintigraphy (SRS)] • CT • MRI
Invasive: • Endoscopic ultrasonography • Selective angiography • Portal venous sampling • *Provocative angiography:* Calcium for insulinoma; secretin for gastrinoma

Gastrinoma (Zollinger-Ellison Syndrome)

Clinical presentation: Many patients with ZES present with abdominal pain, peptic ulcer disease, and severe esophagitis.

Aspects of peptic ulcer disease that raise suspicion for ZES:

- Ulcers in atypical locations
- Multiple ulcers
- Ulcers that fail to respond to conventional treatment
- Ulcers that recur after conventional treatment
- Peptic ulcer disease in association with diarrhea
- Ulcers in association with hyperparathyroidism

- *Serologic testing:* The diagnosis of ZES is made by measuring the serum gastrin level. It is important that patients stop taking proton pump inhibitors for this test. In most patients with gastrinomas, the level is >1,000 pg/mL, but it can be in the 150-1,000 pg/mL range or even normal.
- *Tumor localization:* The next step is to localize the gastrinoma(s) and to determine if metastases are present. This is best accomplished preoperatively if possible. In 70-90% of patients, the primary gastrinoma is found in Passaro's triangle; an area defined by a triangle with points located at the junction of the cystic duct and common bile duct, the second and third portion of the duodenum, and the neck and body of the pancreas.
- The test of choice is SRS in combination with CT.
- *Endoscopic ultrasound (EUS)* is another new modality that assists in the preoperative localization of gastrinomas. It is particularly helpful in localizing tumors in the pancreatic head or duodenal wall where gastrinomas are usually <1 cm. A combination of OctreoScan and EUS detects >90% of gastrinomas.

Surgery

Pharmacologic control of acid secretion has rendered total gastrectomy unnecessary. Omeprazole therapy is so effective that every patient with ZES is a candidate for a tumor removal operation until proved otherwise because of systemic illness or widespread metastases.

Although gastrinomas have a high rate of malignancy, efforts at surgical cure are clearly justified.

- Every attempt is made to localize the tumor before surgery, and CT and MRI are effective with larger tumors and especially with hepatic metastases. Gastric secretion is controlled during the perioperative period with either oral or parenteral proton pump inhibitors.
- Intraoperative USG plus palpation is effective in localizing 90–98% of pancreatic gastrinomas.
    - Tumors within the pancreas are enucleated if at all possible. If they are adjacent to a duct, care must be taken to not injure the duct, but if the duct is injured, it is fine-sutured and a drain placed. Large tumors located distally can be excised by distal pancreatectomy. Tumors within the head are enucleated if at all possible.
    - Treatment of metastatic disease has undergone serial changes but is still unsatisfactory. Radiation therapy and chemotherapy are largely ineffective.
    - The combination of doxorubicin, streptozotocin, and 5-fluorouracil has a low, temporary response rate, but it is highly toxic and has no impact on survival.
    - Surgical treatment of distant metastases by cytoreduction procedures (debulking) appears to be useful, and some patients with solitary localized metastatic disease have prolonged postoperative disease-free survival.

Insulinoma: Insulinoma is the most common functioning tumor of the pancreas.

Clinical Features and Diagnosis

The diagnostic hallmark of the syndrome is the so-called Whipple triad, namely, symptoms of hypoglycemia (catecholamine release) and low blood glucose (40–50 mg/dL) and relief of symptoms after the IV administration of glucose.

- The symptom complex may be due to autonomic nervous overactivity, as expressed by fatigue, weakness, fearfulness, hunger, tremor, sweating, and tachycardia, or alternatively, a central nervous system disturbance with apathy (or irritability or anxiety), confusion, excitement, loss of orientation, blurring of vision, delirium, stupor, coma, or convulsions.
- The pathognomonic finding is an inappropriately high (>5 mU/mL) level of serum insulin during symptomatic hypoglycemia.
- A possible mechanism for this high level of insulin in the face of hypoglycemia may be overexpression of the insulin splice variant.
- A diagnostic ratio of blood insulin (in microunits per milliliter) to glucose (in milligrams per deciliter) of >0.4 or C peptide levels higher than 2 nmol/L have proved valuable in diagnosis.
- *The best way to induce hypoglycemia is with fasting:* Two-thirds of patients will experience hypoglycemic symptoms in 24 hours, and nearly all other patients experience symptoms by 72 hours of fasting.

Localization

- Insulinomas are small (usually <1.5 cm), usually single (only 10% are multiple and those are usually associated with MEN 1 syndrome), usually benign (only 5–10% are malignant), and generally hard to find.
- Plain abdominal radiographic and US studies are rarely helpful, but contrast-augmented CT and MRI locate 50–60% of tumors.
- Because few insulinomas have many somatostatin receptors, SRS is not highly successful. Success in localization by selective arteriography varies with the size of the tumor; 90% accuracy rates have been reported with insulinomas.
- Selective portovenous sampling is also helpful for measurement of insulin levels in pancreatic venous tributaries, a method that does not absolutely localize the site of the tumor but, in about 75% of cases, does provide accurate information on the region of the pancreas from which high levels of insulin are released.

- Highly promising test has been developed for localizing insulinomas by means of selective intra-arterial injection of calcium (into the gastroduodenal, superior mesentery, right hepatic, or splenic arteries) and obtaining samples for radioimmunoassay of insulin from the right hepatic vein.
- Localization study is useful in identifying the tumor by intraoperative US.

Surgery

Treatment of insulinoma is surgical and performed by either open or laparoscopic approaches:

- Most insulinomas are benign and can be enucleated.
- Care needs to be taken during enucleation to avoid injury to ductal structures, and if a duct is injured, it is sutured and drained.
- If malignant, the tumor is resected in a cancer-type operation, and if metastatic, it is worthwhile to try to remove all primary and metastatic tumor tissue in an effort to minimize persistent hyperinsulinism.
- Persistent hyperinsulinemia after surgery for metastatic islet cell tumors may be managed by hepatic artery tumor embolization, by diazoxide, or by streptozotocin plus fluorouracil.

Verner–Morrison Syndrome (VIPoma)

- VIPomas are endocrine tumors usually arising from pancreatic islets that secrete VIP and cause a syndrome of profound watery diarrhea, hypokalemia, and achlorhydria.
- The diarrhea persists despite fasting (which qualifies it as a secretory diarrhea) and despite nasogastric aspiration (which differentiates it from the diarrhea of ZES).
- Verner–Morrison syndrome is highly variable. Constant features are diarrhea, hypovolemia, hypokalemia, and acidosis; variable features are achlorhydria or hypochlorhydria, hypercalcemia, hyperglycemia, and flushing with rash.

Diagnosis

- The diagnostic triad in Verner–Morrison syndrome is a secretory diarrhea, high levels of circulating vasoactive intestinal peptide (VIP), and a pancreatic tumor.
- Diarrhea volumes are often massive, 3 to 5 L/day, and the diagnosis of VIPoma is unlikely if stool volume is <700 mL/day. VIPomas alone show elevated levels of VIP; normal levels are lower than 200 pg/mL, and VIPoma patients have levels ranging from 225 to 2,000 pg/mL.
- The best localization is achieved either by SRS or by endoscopic US. Most tumors are large, and localization is often achieved with enhanced CT or MRI or with arteriography.
- About 50% of patients have metastatic spread by the time of diagnosis. If abdominal studies fail to locate the tumor, thoracic CT is performed because as many as 10% of the tumors are intrathoracic.

Treatment

- As soon as the diagnosis is established, treatment with the long-acting somatostatin analog octreotide is used to control fluid loss.
- Surgical removal of VIPoma is attempted in all patients.
- Most VIPomas can be excised by distal pancreatectomy.
- The adrenals and retroperitoneal tissue are carefully examined if no pancreatic tumor is found.
- In the 50% of patients with metastatic disease, local excision of as much tumor as can be safely removed (debulking) is indicated.
- Partial pancreatectomy plus resection of liver metastases has been reported to bring about resolution of recurrent Verner–Morrison syndrome.
- In patients with nonresectable tumors, chemotherapy is rarely effective, but octreotide is helpful in the control of diarrhea.

Glucagonoma

- It is a tumor of islet alpha cells.

- Glucagonoma causes a syndrome of a characteristic rash, diabetes mellitus, anemia, weight loss, and elevated circulating levels of glucagon.
- The characteristic skin lesion is a necrolytic migrating erythema.
- The syndrome is rare, and most patients are initially recognized by their skin lesions and referred to surgeons by dermatologists.
- Glucagonoma was found to be associated with anemia, glossitis, and most importantly, a low level of amino acids; parenteral administration of amino acids was found to bring about disappearance of the skin lesions.
- Diabetes is usually mild.
- A pseudoglucagonoma syndrome has been described in patients who have necrolytic migratory erythema without a pancreatic tumor; the cause is unknown, but the condition is associated with several chronic illnesses, and only a few patients show elevated levels of glucagon.

Diagnosis

- The diagnosis of glucagonoma is made from the characteristic skin lesion, elevated levels of glucagon (whose release can be provoked by secretin, if necessary), and a pancreatic tumor. The upper limit of normal for glucagon is 150–190 pg/mL; glucagonoma patients have levels of 200–2,000 pg/mL.
- The islet tumor may be demonstrated by enhanced CT or MRI or by selective angiography.

Localization and Treatment

- Once the diagnosis is made, the patient is prepared by the administration of total parenteral nutrition containing amino acids, along with simultaneous octreotide for symptomatic relief.
- Tumors are best localized by CT, MRI, and intraoperative USG.
- Because a third of these patients have been reported to have thrombotic complications after surgery, perioperative heparin is indicated.
- Treatment is surgical excision of the tumor, which usually lies in the body or tail of the pancreas. Nearly all glucagonomas are malignant, but an aggressive approach to removal of the primary and metastatic tumor is warranted.
- Even so, the cure rate appears to be only 30%, and long-term chemotherapy has proved disappointing for metastatic disease.
- Symptomatic relief can be achieved with octreotide.

Somatostatinoma

- All endocrine tumors of the pancreas are rare; somatostatinomas are exceedingly rare.
- Full syndrome (steatorrhea, diabetes mellitus, hypochlorhydria, and gallstones).
- The features of the syndrome are variable and do not always coincide with the predictable effects of high circulating levels of somatostatin.
- Most patients have mild diabetes, but 10% have symptoms of hypoglycemia.
- This illustrates the unpredictability of hormone-hormone interactions: in the case of diabetes, the suppressive effect of somatostatin on insulin release predominates; in hypoglycemic patients, the predominant inhibition affects glucagon.
- The clinical findings are unpredictable; obstructive jaundice caused by pressure on the common bile duct by tumor has developed in some patients, whereas initial findings in other patients have been diarrhea and gallstones.
- Some duodenal somatostatinomas have been associated with von Recklinghausen's neurofibromatosis.
- Tumors can be localized by CT, MRI, arteriography, and even SRS because somatostatinomas do possess functioning somatostatin receptors.
- Treatment is surgical. 70–90% of tumors have been reported to be malignant. Most tumors are located in the tail of the pancreas, and caudal pancreatectomy is indicated.

- Localization is rarely a problem because the tumors are generally large. Hepatic metastases are common and debulking of metastatic tumor tissue is indicated.
- The large size and frequency of malignancy dictate resection rather than enucleation of the pancreatic tumor.
- Metastases are, of course, excluded before consideration is given to a Whipple resection of the head of the pancreas. Small duodenal tumors can be treated by local excision.
- At surgery, cholecystectomy is performed regardless of whether the patient has gallstones because if they are not present, they will probably occur.

Still-Rarer Tumors

- Various functional tumors of the endocrine pancreas have been reported, with some secreting growth hormone-releasing factor (GRF), neurotensin, PTHrP, PP, or ACTH, with the appropriate resultant endocrine syndrome.
- GRFomas are invariably associated with MEN 1 syndrome; 30% of GRF tumors originate in the pancreas, 50% in the lung, and 10% in the small bowel.
- Forty percent of patients with GRFoma have ZES, and 40% have Cushing's syndrome.
- Patients with ACTH-secreting tumors usually have other endocrine syndromes, most frequently ZES. They have classic symptoms of Cushing's syndrome (which occurs in 5% of all ZES patients and in 20% of patients with both ZES and MEN 1).
- Neurotensinomas cause hypokalemia, weight loss, hypotension, cyanosis, flushing, and diabetes. They are usually malignant.
- PPomas are associated with high circulating PP levels and no characteristic symptoms, although patients with PPomas have been reported with watery diarrhea and rash. PPomas are almost always large and, except when associated with MEN 1 syndrome, are usually solitary and in the head of the pancreas. Elevated levels of PP are often seen with other islet cell tumor syndromes.

---

63. Passaro's triangle. ***WBUHS 2006***

Passaro's Triangle

In 70–90% of patients, the primary gastrinoma is found in Passaro's triangle, an area defined by a triangle with points located at the junction of the cystic duct and common bile duct, the second and third portion of the duodenum, and the neck and body of the pancreas.

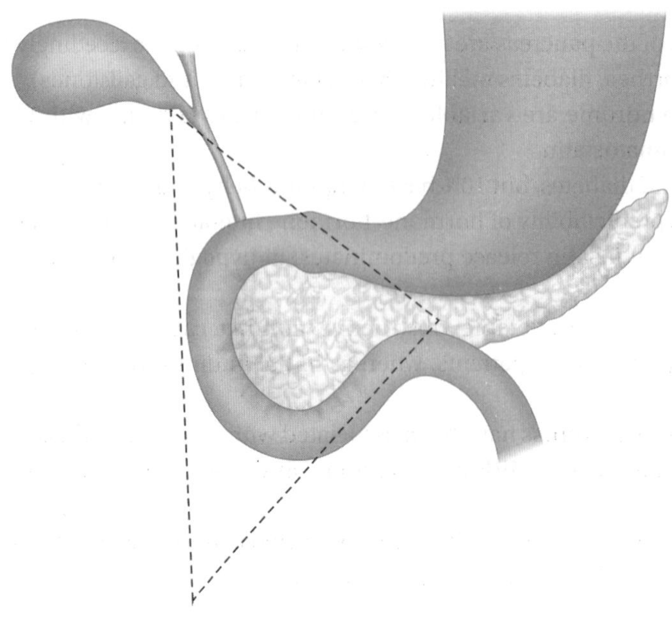

64. Discuss about diagnosis and localization of insulinomas. ***WBUHS 2007***

65. What are the latest biochemical diagnostic criteria and imaging done for diagnosis and localization of insulinoma? ***WBUHS 2021 Supplementary***

Diagnosis

The diagnostic hallmark of insulinoma is the so-called Whipple triad:

- Symptoms of hypoglycemia (catecholamine release) and
- Low blood glucose (40–50 mg/dL) and
- Relief of symptoms after the IV administration of glucose.
- The triad is not entirely diagnostic.

The clinical syndrome of hyperinsulinism may follow one of two patterns or sometimes a combination of both.

- The symptom complex may be due to autonomic nervous overactivity, as expressed by fatigue, weakness, fearfulness, hunger, tremor, sweating, and tachycardia, or alternatively, a central nervous system disturbance with apathy (or irritability or anxiety), confusion, excitement, loss of orientation, blurring of vision, delirium, stupor, coma, or convulsions.
- The pathognomonic finding is an inappropriately high (>5 mU/mL) level of serum insulin during symptomatic hypoglycemia.
- A diagnostic ratio of blood insulin (in microunits per milliliter) to glucose (in milligrams per deciliter) of >0.4 or C peptide levels higher than 2 nmol/L have proved valuable in diagnosis.

The biochemical diagnosis is established in 95% of patients during prolonged fasting when the following parameters are found:

- Serum insulin levels of 10 μU/mL or more (normal <6 μU/mL)
- Glucose levels of <40 mg/dL
- C-peptide levels exceeding 2.5 ng/mL (normal <2 ng/mL)
- Proinsulin levels ≥22 pmol/L, or >25% (or up to 90%) that of immunoreactive insulin

As Soon as a Patient with Insulinoma is Identified

- Care must be taken to prevent severe hypoglycemia with possible loss of cerebrocytes.
- The diet is modified to include frequent meals, even awakening at night to eat.
- The standard drug is diazoxide, which is helpful in about two thirds of patients but discontinued at least a week before surgery because it may cause intraoperative hypotension.
- The long-acting somatostatin analog octreotide, though helpful in children with nesidioblastosis, has been effective only rarely in adults.

Localization

- Insulinomas are small (usually <1.5 cm), usually single (only 10% are multiple and those are usually associated with MEN 1 syndrome), usually benign (only 5–10% are malignant), and generally hard to find.
- *Plain abdominal radiographic* and *US* studies are rarely helpful, but *contrast-augmented CT* and *MRI* locate 50–60% of tumors.
- Because few insulinomas have many somatostatin receptors, *SRS* is not highly successful.
- Success in localization by *selective arteriography* varies with the size of the tumor.
- Demonstration of islet tumors by enhanced CT, enhanced MRI, or arteriography depends, of course, on the relatively rich blood supply to islet tumors as compared with the rest of the pancreatic parenchyma.
- *Selective portovenous sampling* is also helpful for measurement of insulin levels in pancreatic venous tributaries, a method that does not absolutely localize the site of the tumor but, in about 75% of cases, does provide accurate information on the region of the pancreas from which high levels of insulin are released. The method has a relatively high incidence of problems with bleeding into the peritoneal cavity or biliary tree. It is expensive and requires skill.

- Calcium is known to release insulin. *Selective intra-arterial injection of calcium* (into the gastroduodenal, superior mesentery, right hepatic, or splenic arteries) and obtaining samples for radioimmunoassay of insulin from the right hepatic vein is useful to localize insulinomas.

The presence of MEN 1 must be evaluated by excluding the following:

- Hyperprolactinemia due to a pituitary adenoma
- Hyperparathyroidism due to parathyroid hyperplasia
- Hypergastrinemia due to a gastrinoma.

Imaging studies should be started only after the diagnosis has been confirmed biochemically, because 80% of insulinomas are <2 cm in size and may not be visible by CT scanning or transabdominal USG.

Successful preoperative tumor localization is achieved in about 60% of patients.

Computed Tomography and Magnetic Resonance Imaging

- Helical or multislice CT has 82–94% sensitivity. In one study, dual-phase helical CT proved more sensitive than single-phase for detection of insulinoma.
- Volume perfusion CT (VPCT) is significantly more accurate than CECT for insulinoma detection, and 3 Tesla magnetic resonance imaging (3T MRI) with diffusion-weighted imaging (DWI) is better. Lesions were more conspicuous on MRI than on VPCT, and conspicuity with both was better than with CECT.
- Tumor-to-pancreatic duct distance was better appreciated on MRI than on VPCT and CECT.

Arteriography

- The accuracy of selective arteriography varies but is around 60% in the best hands.
- Arteriography with catheterization of small arterial branches of the celiac system combined with calcium injections (which stimulate insulin release from neoplastic tissue but not from normal islets), and simultaneous measurements of hepatic vein insulin during each selective calcium injection localizes tumors in 90% of patients.

Nuclear Medicine

- Insulinomas have been shown to have a very high density of glucagon-like peptide–1 (GLP-1) receptors, and radiolabeling GLP-1 analogs (e.g., exendin-4) with appropriate radioisotopes can provide noninvasive localization of benign insulinomas. For example, indium-111 (^{111}In)–labeled exendin-4 (^{111}In-DOTA-exendin-4) has successfully been used to localize small insulinomas both preoperatively and, with the use of a gamma probe, intraoperatively.
- Malignant insulinomas can be missed by GLP-1 target imaging because these tumors often lack GLP-1 receptors. However, these tumors often express somatostatin receptor subtype 2 (SSTR2), which can be detected with indium-111 (^{111}In)-pentetreotide single-photon CT (SPECT).

Ultrasonography

- EUS detects 77% of insulinomas in the pancreas.
- Combining EUS with CT can increase the yield, resulting in the detection and localization of the majority of sporadic insulinomas.

CHAPTER 38

Diabetes

LEARNING OBJECTIVES

- Surgical Complications of Diabetes Mellitus
- Clinical Importance of HbA1c
- Perioperative Management of a Patient having Diabetes Mellitus

1. Describe surgical complications of diabetes mellitus (DM). Clinical importance of glycated hemoglobin A1c (HbA1c) test in monitoring the treatment. ***WBUHS 2021 Supplementary***

Surgical complications of DM are due to the following reasons:

- Microvascular changes involving the capillaries of the retina, kidneys, and peripheral nerves
- Macrovascular changes characterized by atherosclerotic lesions of the coronary and peripheral arterial circulation
- Diabetic neuropathy
- Infection in glucose-loaded tissue

The following are the prominent surgical complications:

- Bacterial infections, such as abscesses, carbuncles, chronic balanitis, and diabetic foot. Fungal infections, such as candidiasis and mucormycosis
- Emphysematous cholecystitis, emphysematous pyelonephritis, necrotizing fasciitis, and Fournier's gangrene
- Sexual dysfunctions

The diabetic foot:

- Most feared and devastating complication of diabetes
- Most common cause for leg amputations
- The classic pathological triad of the diabetic foot is vascular disease, neuropathy, and infection

Surgery in diabetic patients:

- Diabetic patients are prone to develop sudden hyperglycemia or hypoglycemia during surgery; so, frequent monitoring of blood glucose is necessary.
- Short-acting insulin is given as intravenous (IV) during surgery and in the immediate postoperative period
- They are admitted a few days ahead of surgery.
- Oral hypoglycemic drugs are stopped a few days before major surgery and insulin is started, to bring about better control of blood sugar. Insulin is continued for a few days in the postoperative period also.
- They are prone to cardiac arrest, thromboembolism, and cerebrovascular accidents.
- Wound healing is likely to be poor and prolonged
- HbA1c is an *important indicator of long-term glycemic control* with the ability to reflect the cumulative glycemic history of the preceding 2–3 months. HbA1c not only provides a reliable measure of chronic hyper- glycemia but also correlates well with the risk of long-term diabetes complications.

- *The higher the percentage is, indicates higher blood sugar levels over the last few months.* For <5.7% means one does not have diabetes. About 5.7–6.4% signals prediabetes. For about 6.5% or higher means a diabetes diagnosis.
- HbA1c is not only a useful biomarker of long-term glycemic control but also a good predictor of lipid profile; thus, monitoring of glycemic control using HbA1c could have additional benefits of identifying diabetes patients who are at a greater risk of cardiovascular complications.
- Thus, a single HbA1c test provides valuable information that can be used for the management of chronic diseases.
- HbA1c exhibited direct correlations with cholesterol, triglycerides, and low-density lipoprotein cholesterol and an inverse correlation with high-density lipoprotein cholesterol.
- There was a linear relationship between HbA1c and dyslipidemia as the levels of serum cholesterol and triglycerides were significantly higher and that of high-density lipoprotein cholesterol was significantly lower in patients with worse glycemic control as compared to patients with good glycemic control.
- Elevated level of HbA1c has been identified as a significant risk factor for cardiovascular diseases and stroke in subjects who may have diabetes.
- High levels of HbA1c were associated with an increased risk of recurrence of atrial tachyarrhythmia in patients with type II DM and paroxysmal atrial fibrillation undergoing catheter ablation.
- HbA1c is a useful tool for the diagnosis of a previously undiagnosed DM in critically ill patients, and HbA1c at admission is significantly associated with intensive care unit mortality.

2. Discuss the perioperative management of a patient having DM as a comorbidity.

WBUHS 2018; RIMS, Imphal 2022

General Preoperative Assessment

History

- Suggestive symptoms (e.g., polyuria/polydipsia and blurred vision)
- Eating patterns, nutritional status, exercise history, and weight history
- Current treatment of diabetes, including medication regimen, diet, exercise, and glucose monitoring results
- Frequency, severity, and etiology of acute complications (e.g., ketoacidosis and hypoglycemia)
- Previous or current infections (e.g., skin, foot, dental, and genitourinary)
- Symptoms and treatment of chronic microvascular or macrovascular complications (e.g., eye; kidney; nerve; genitourinary, bladder, and gastrointestinal function; heart; peripheral vascular; foot; and cerebrovascular complications)
- Nondiabetic medications that may affect blood glucose levels (e.g., corticosteroids)
- Risk factors for atherosclerosis (e.g., smoking, hypertension, obesity, dyslipidemia, and family history)
- History and treatment of other conditions (e.g., endocrine and eating disorders)
- Family history of DM and endocrine disorders
- Lifestyle, cultural, psychosocial, and economic factors that might influence DM management.
- Tobacco, alcohol, and controlled substance use

Physical Examination

- The physical examination includes assessment for orthostatic hypotension, a potential sign of autonomic neuropathy.
- A funduscopic examination may provide insight into the patient's risk of developing postoperative blindness, especially following prolonged spinal surgery in the prone position and cardiac surgery requiring cardiopulmonary bypass.
- Type I DM is associated with a "stiff joint" syndrome, which poses a significant risk during airway management at the time of general anesthesia. The temporomandibular, atlantooccipital, and other cervical spine joints may be affected.

- Further airway evaluation should include assessment of thyroid gland size, as patients with type I DM have a 15% association with other autoimmune diseases, such as Hashimoto's thyroiditis and Graves' disease.
- Finally, the degree of preoperative neurologic dysfunction is important to document, especially before the administration of regional anesthesia or peripheral nerve blocks, to assess the degree of subsequent nerve injury.

The physical examination should include the following:

- Blood pressure (including orthostatic measurements)
- Funduscopic examination
- Airway examination
- Thyroid palpation
- Cardiac examination
- Abdominal examination (hepatomegaly)
- Evaluation of pulses by palpation and with auscultation
- Feet examination
- Skin examination (insulin-injection sites)
- Neurologic examination

General Preoperative Management

- Given that patients with DM are treated with a variety of regimens and are scheduled for surgery at varying times of the day, there is no established consensus for optimal perioperative management. However, using general management principles to minimize the likelihood of hypoglycemia and to limit the incidence of excessive hyperglycemia should guide decision-making.
- In general, on the day of surgery, patients on oral regimens should be advised to discontinue these medications:
  - Secretagogues (e.g., sulfonylureas and meglitinides) have the potential to cause hypoglycemia
  - In addition, sulfonylureas may interfere with ischemic myocardial preconditioning and may theoretically increase the risk of perioperative myocardial ischemia and infarction.
  - Patients taking metformin should be advised to discontinue this drug preoperatively because of the risk of developing lactic acidosis.
- Insulin-dependent patients are typically advised to reduce their bedtime dose of insulin the night before surgery to prevent hypoglycemia while nil per os (NPO). Maintenance insulin may be continued, based on the history of glucose concentrations and the discretion of the advising clinician.
- Patients may be advised to consult with their anesthesiologist and diabetes-managing practitioner for individualized recommendations regarding their diabetes plan.
- Additionally, patients should be monitored preoperatively to assess for hyperglycemia and hypoglycemia.

Metabolic Response to Anesthesia and Surgery

- Surgery induces a considerable stress response mediated by the neuroendocrine system through the release of catecholamines, glucagon, and cortisol.
- The principal mechanism lies with the elevation of sympathetic tone, with a subsequent release of cortisol and catecholamines during surgery.
- This compensatory mechanism is impaired in diabetic patients through a relative insulin deficiency (type II) or an absolute insulin deficiency (type I), necessitating supplemental insulin in the perioperative period.
- Thus, patients with type 1 DM usually require intravenous insulin therapy, depending on the nature of the surgery, and are more predisposed to end-organ complications than patients with type II DM.
  - Patients with type II DM need to have their oral hypoglycemic drugs discontinued preoperatively, with intravenous insulin administered if dictated by the extent of the procedure.
  - Multiple randomized controlled studies have shown that controlling serum glucose levels in all patients, not merely those with DM, impacts the outcome of surgical patients who are critically ill. This effect does not appear to be related to the dose of insulin but rather to the absolute level of serum glucose achieved.

- Anesthetic agents can affect glucose metabolism through the modulation of sympathetic tone; in vitro, data suggest that inhalational agents suppress insulin secretion.
- The resulting relative insulin deficiency often leads to glucose dysregulation and hyperglycemia.
- This deficiency is compounded in diabetic patients, particularly those with insulin resistance, raising the risk of ketoacidosis.
- The use of regional anesthesia or peripheral nerve blocks may mitigate these concerns, but no data suggest that these forms of anesthesia improve postoperative survival in patients with DM.

Consensus Recommendations for Target Inpatient Blood Glucose Concentrations

Patient population	*Blood glucose target*	*Rationale*
General medical/surgical*	• *Fasting:* 90–126 mg/dL • *Random:* <200 mg/dL	Decreased mortality, shorter length of stay, and lower infection rates
Cardiac surgery*	<150 mg/dL	Reduced mortality and reduced risk of sternal wound infections
Critically ill†	<150 mg/dL	Beneficial effect on short-term mortality and morbidity; length of stay
Acute neurologic disorders‡	80–140 mg/dL	Lack of data and consensus on specific target; consensus for controlling hyperglycemia

*American Diabetes Association
†Society Critical Care Medicine
‡American Heart Association/American Stroke Association

Methods of Achieving Glycemic Control

Class of oral agent	*Example*	*Considerations*
Alpha-glucosidase inhibitors	Acarbose	Inhibit enzymes that metabolize carbohydrates; no benefit if NPO
Secretagogues (e.g., sulfonylureas and meglitinides)	Glyburide and glimepiride	Hypoglycemia, prolonged action, may be unpredictable, and difficult to titrate
Biguanides	Metformin	Risk of lactic acidosis; use cautiously in the presence of renal or hepatic insufficiency chronic heart failure (CHF); may be found in combination medications
Thiazolidinediones	Rosiglitazone	Increased intravascular volume (CHF), slow onset of effect, and difficult to titrate
Dipeptidyl peptidase-4 (DPP-4) inhibitor	Sitagliptin	Slows inactivation of incretin hormones to enhance physiologic glucose control; dosage reduction required for renal insufficiency

Perioperative Methods for Achieving Glycemic Control

- Establish separate intravenous access for a "piggyback" infusion of regular insulin (100 U per 100 mL 0.9% saline).
- The infusion rate can be determined by using the following formula: Insulin (U/hour) = serum glucose (mg/day)/150.
- Intra-arterial catheter placement is recommended to facilitate checking blood glucose concentrations every 1–2 hours intraoperatively and postoperatively
- A second intravenous catheter may be used for intravascular volume replacement with a normal saline solution.

Numerous insulin protocols are available, with varying reliability and validation. In addition, computer-based systems are available that calculate the continued dosing based on glucose concentration and rate of change.

Diabetic Complications and Perioperative Management Considerations

Diabetic complication	*Potential complication*	*Therapeutic considerations/strategies*
Atherosclerotic vascular disease	Myocardial infarction	• Low threshold to evaluate for myocardial ischemia • Perioperative β-blockers • Glycemic control • Lipid-lowering therapy • Aspirin (antiplatelet therapy) • Maintain BP <130/80 mm Hg*
	Stroke	• Perioperative beta-blocker • ACE inhibitor/ARB • Glycemic control • Antiplatelet agents as appropriate • Lipid-lowering therapy
Peripheral neuropathy	Lower extremity ulceration	• Foot and heel protection • Close evaluation for pressure ulcers
	Increased infection rates	• Glycemic control • Vaccinations (e.g., influenza and pneumococcal)
	Inhibited wound healing	• Glycemic control • Close evaluation of wound status
Autonomic neuropathy	Decreased bladder tone	Avoid aggravating medications (e.g., anticholinergics)
	Gastroparesis	• Minimize opiate analgesics • Gradual dietary progression • Prokinetic agents (e.g., metoclopramide)
Nephropathy	Renal insufficiency	• Avoid hypotension/optimize BP control • Glycemic control • Pretreat for contrast-induced nephropathy • ACE inhibitor/ARB • Judicious use of nephrotoxic agents (e.g., aminoglycosides, NSAIDs) • Limit protein intake to 0.8 g/kg/day • Optimal room lighting • Assistance with ambulation
Retinopathy	Limited visual acuity for ambulation	• Glycemic control • Optimal BP control • Proper intraoperative eye protection
	Disorientation/greater risk for delirium	• Temporal and spatial orientation • Minimize medications that may cause delirium

*If no contraindication with agent shown to be effective in lowering cardiovascular events. Other disease states (critical illness) may necessitate higher amounts of protein.

(ACE: angiotensin-converting enzyme; ARB: angiotensin receptor blocker; BP: blood pressure; NSAIDs: nonsteroidal anti-inflammatory drugs)

CHAPTER 39

Oncology

LEARNING OBJECTIVES

- Oncogene
- Tumor Markers
- Biomarkers and Biologically Targeted Therapy
- Immunotherapy in Cancer
- Gene Therapy for Cancer
- Paraneoplastic Syndrome
- Micro- and Macroanatomy of Lymph Node
- Sentinel Lymph Node Biopsy
- Radiofrequency Thermal Ablation for Malignant Lesions
- Targeted Therapy
- Stereotactic Surgery
- Drug Delivery System

1. Oncogene.

Introduction

- An oncogene is a gene that has the potential to cause cancer.
- In tumor cells, they are often mutated or expressed at high levels.
- Many abnormal cells normally undergo a programed form of death (apoptosis). Activated oncogenes can cause those cells to survive and proliferate instead.
- Most oncogenes require an additional step, such as mutations in another gene or environmental factors, such as viral infection to cause cancer.
- A proto-oncogene is a normal gene that can become an oncogene due to mutations or increased expression.

Activation

The proto-oncogene can become an oncogene by a relatively small modification of its original function.

There are three basic activation types:

1. A mutation within a proto-oncogene can cause a change in the protein structure, causing:
   - An increase in protein (enzyme) activity
   - A loss of regulation
2. An increase in protein concentration, caused by:
   - An increase of protein expression (through misregulation)
   - An increase of protein [messenger ribonucleic acid (mRNA)] stability, prolonging its existence and its activity in the cell
   - A gene duplication (one type of chromosome abnormality), resulting in an increased amount of protein in the cell
3. A chromosomal translocation (another type of chromosome abnormality), causing:
   - An increased gene expression in the wrong cell type or at wrong times

- The expression of a constitutively active *hybrid protein*. This type of aberration in a dividing stem cell in the bone marrow leads to adult leukemia

The expression of oncogenes can be regulated by *micro-RNAs* (miRNAs), small *RNAs* 21–25 nucleotides in length that control gene expression by *downregulating* them.

Mutations in such *micro-RNAs* (known as *oncomiRs*) can lead to activation of oncogenes. *Antisense* messenger RNAs could theoretically be used to block the effects of oncogenes.

Classification

Category	*Examples*	*Description*
Growth factors or mitogens	c-Sis	Usually secreted by specialized cells to induce cell proliferation in themselves, nearby cells, or distant cells. An oncogene may cause a cell to secrete growth factors even though it does not normally do so. It will thereby induce its own uncontrolled proliferation *(autocrine loop)* and proliferation of neighboring cells. It may also cause production of growth hormones in other parts of the body
Receptor tyrosine kinases	EGFR, PDGFR, VEGFR, and HER2/neu	Kinases add phosphate groups to other proteins to turn them on or off. Receptor kinases add phosphate groups to receptor proteins at the surface of the cell (which receive protein signals from outside the cell and transmit them to the inside of the cell). Tyrosine kinases add phosphate groups to the amino acid tyrosine in the target protein. They can cause cancer by turning the receptor permanently on (constitutively), even without signals from outside the cell
Cytoplasmic-tyrosine kinases	Src-family, Syk-ZAP-70 family, and BTK family of tyrosine kinases, and the Abi gene in CML—Philadelphia chromosome	—
Cytoplasmic serine/threonine kinases and their regulatory subunits	RAF kinase and cyclin-dependent kinases (through overexpression)	—
Regulatory GTPases	Ras protein	Ras is a small GTPase which hydrolyses GTP into GDP and phosphate. Ras is activated by growth factor signaling (i.e., EGF, TGF-alpha) and acting like a binary switch (on/off) in growth signaling pathways. Downstream effectors of Ras include RAF, MEK, MEKK, MAPK, and ERK, most of which in turn regulate genes that mediate cell proliferation
Transcription factors	Myc gene	They regulate transcription of genes that induce cell proliferation

(BTK: Bruton's tyrosine kinase; CML: chronic myeloid leukemia; EGF: epidermal growth factor; EGFR: EGF receptor; ERK: extracellular signal-regulated kinases; GDP: guanosine diphosphate; GTP: guanosine triphosphate; HER2: human EGF receptor 2; MAPK: microtubule-associated protein kinase; MEK: mitogen-activated protein kinase; MEKK: mitogen-activated protein kinase kinase; PDGFR: platelet-derived growth factor receptor; RAF: rapidly accelerated fibrosarcoma; TGF: transforming growth factor; VEGFR: vascular endothelial growth factor receptor)

There are two mechanisms by which proto-oncogenes can be converted to cellular oncogenes:

1. *Quantitative:* Tumor formation is induced by an increase in the absolute number of proto-oncogene products or by its production in inappropriate cell types.
2. *Qualitative:* Conversion from proto-oncogene to transforming gene (c-onc) with changes in the nucleotide

2. Tumor markers and their role in surgery.

Introduction

- Tumor markers are indicators of cellular, biochemical, molecular, or genetic alterations by which neoplasia can be recognized.
- These surrogate measures of the biology of the cancer provide insight into the clinical behavior of the tumor.
- This is particularly useful when the cancer is not clinically detectable.
- The information provided may:
  - Be diagnostic and distinguish benign from malignant disease
  - Correlate with the amount of tumor present (so-called tumor burden)
  - Allow subtype classification to more accurately stage patients
  - Be prognostic, either by the presence or absence of the marker or by its concentration
  - Guide choice of therapy and predict response to therapy

The ideal tumor marker has three defining characteristics:

1. The marker is expressed exclusively by the particular tumor
2. Collection of the specimen for the tumor marker assay is easy.
3. The assay itself is reproducible, rapid, and inexpensive.
   - Tumor markers fall into three broad categories—proteins, genetic mutations, and epigenetic changes.
   - All three may be found in the tumor tissue itself.
   - Tumor markers found in body fluids, particularly blood and urine, have the greatest potential for clinical application because of the ease of access to these fluids for analysis and because repeated sampling allows in vivo monitoring of the malignancy for such features as disease progression or recurrence, metastasis, and response to therapy.

Potential nonprotein tumor markers
RNA-based markers: • Overexpressed/underexpressed transcripts • Regulatory RNA (e.g., micro-RNA)
DNA-based markers: • Single-nucleotide polymorphisms (SNPs) • Chromosomal translocations—BCR-ABL (Philadelphia) • Changes in DNA copy number • Microsatellite instability • Epigenetic changes (e.g., differential promoter region methylation)

(DNA: deoxyribonucleic acid; RNA: ribonucleic acid)

Protein Tumor Markers

- *Carcinoembryonic antigen (CEA):*
  - Predominantly used clinically in patients with cancer of the colon and rectum
  - It is an oncofetal protein that is normally present during fetal life but can be seen in low concentration in healthy adults
  - *Testing:*
    - Normal serum levels are <2.5 ng/mL, borderline if 2.5–5.0 ng/mL, and elevated if >5.0 ng/mL.
    - Borderline levels occur with benign disorders such as inflammatory bowel disease, pancreatitis, cirrhosis, chronic obstructive pulmonary disease, and smoking can also increase CEA—the upper limit of normal in smokers is considered 5 ng/mL.
  - *Screening:* CEA is not useful as a screening test because of its low sensitivity in early-stage disease—elevated CEA levels occur in only 5–40% of patients with localized disease.

- *Prognosis:*
  - Elevated CEA levels reflect the burden of tumor present.
  - The degree of CEA elevation correlates with increasing stage of disease, and therefore CEA levels have prognostic value.
  - Preoperative serum CEA is an independent predictor of survival—the higher the preoperative serum level, the poorer the prognosis.
  - This effect persists even after patients are stratified for resectability and extent of local tumor invasion.
  - 5-year survival is significantly worse in patients with elevated preoperative CEA levels than in those with a normal preoperative CEA level.
- *Monitoring:*
  - The most common application of CEA is to monitor patients for recurrent disease.
  - CEA is most sensitive for hepatic or retroperitoneal metastasis and relatively insensitive for local, pulmonary, or peritoneal involvement.
  - About 75% of patients with recurrent colorectal cancer (CRC) have an elevated serum CEA level before the development of symptoms.
  - A confirmed rising trend in CEA prompts evaluation for recurrent disease.

■ *α-fetoprotein (AFP):*
- AFP is used for the detection and management of hepatocellular carcinoma (HCC).
- It is an oncofetal antigen that consists of a single-chain polypeptide with a molecular weight of 700 kD.
- Levels are elevated in the fetus, decrease sharply after birth, and are increased during pregnancy.
- *Testing:*
  - AFP is measured with immunoassay kits, either enzyme-linked immunoassays or radioimmunoassays.
  - The upper limit of normal for a healthy, nonpregnant adult is <25 ng/mL.
  - 10–20% of HCCs do not have detectable levels of AFP. Levels are also raised in nonseminomatous testicular cancer, for which it is a valuable tumor marker.
  - 20% of patients with gastric or pancreatic cancer and 5% of patients with colorectal or lung cancer have significant elevations (>5 ng/mL) in serum AFP levels.
  - Elevated levels are also seen in hepatitis, inflammatory bowel disease, and cirrhosis.
- *Screening:* AFP has an estimated sensitivity of 25–75%, a specificity of 76–94%, and a positive predictive value of 9–50%.
- *Prognosis:*
  - The AFP concentration reflects tumor size, with levels higher than 400 ng/mL being associated with larger tumors.
  - As a result, it has been shown that AFP correlates with stage and prognosis.
  - The rate of increase, expressed as AFP doubling time, has also been associated with poorer prognosis.
- *Monitoring:*
  - AFP has been shown to decline after resection or ablation.
  - After complete resection, AFP levels should drop and remain at <10 ng/mL.
  - Tumor regrowth after chemoembolization does not correlate with rate of increase in AFP or tumor burden.
  - AFP levels usually decline in response to effective chemotherapy.
  - Monitoring of AFP therefore avoids prolonged use of ineffective and potentially toxic chemotherapy.

■ *Carbohydrate antigen 19-9 (CA 19-9):*
- CA 19-9 is widely used as a serum marker for pancreas cancer, but its use is limited to monitoring response to therapy not as a diagnostic marker.
- The CA 19-9 epitope is normally present within the biliary tree.
- Biliary tract disease, both acute and chronic, can elevate serum CA 19-9 levels.

- *Testing:*
  - CA 19-9 is detected with an immunoassay and the upper limit of normal for a healthy adult is 37 U/mL.
  - Patients with benign biliary tract disease can have levels up to 400 U/mL, with 87% having concentrations higher than 70 U/mL.
  - Significant numbers of patients with pancreatitis, either acute or chronic, also have elevated levels.
  - Besides pancreatic cancer, CA 19-9 levels are also elevated in patients with other cancers, including those of the biliary tree (95%), stomach (5%), colon (15%), liver (HCC, 7%), and lung (13%).
  - For CRC, CA 19-9 levels add little clinically useful information to determination of CEA levels.
- *Screening:*
  - CA 19-9 is not useful as a screening modality because of its low sensitivity in early-stage disease.
  - With increasing levels of CA 19-9, the diagnosis of pancreatic cancer becomes more accurate.
  - Because of its frequent elevation in benign biliary tract disease, CA 19-9 is not useful in distinguishing benign from malignant distal common bile duct strictures.
- *Prognosis:*
  - In patients with pancreatic cancer who have CA 19-9 detectable in their serum, the level has been shown to correlate with tumor burden.
  - For example, higher CA 19-9 levels typically correlate with higher tumor stage and >95% of patients with unresectable disease have levels >1,000 U/mL
- *Monitoring:*
  - Serial measurement of CA 19-9 is used to monitor response to therapy.
  - A rise in CA 19-9 after curative resection has been shown to precede clinical or computed tomographic evidence of recurrence by 2–9 months.
  - In patients with unresectable/metastatic disease, failure of CA 19-9 levels to fall with chemotherapy reflects poor tumor response.

- *Prostate-specific antigen (PSA):*
  - PSA is a serine protease that is formed in the prostatic epithelium and secreted into the prostatic ducts.
  - PSA is considered a tissue-specific rather than a prostate cancer-specific marker—patients who have undergone curative radical prostatectomy, as well as females, have no detectable PSA.
  - *Testing:*
    - PSA is detected with an immunoassay.
    - Besides BPH, other instances in which serum PSA levels may be elevated include prostatitis, prostatic massage, prostatic biopsy, and digital rectal examination.
    - Upper limit of normal for PSA at 4 ng/mL, with levels >10 ng/mL being suspicious for malignancy and levels of 4–10 ng/mL being indeterminate.
  - *Screening:*
    - PSA is widely used as a screening tool for prostate cancer because it enables early detection and diagnosis of this disease.
    - Screening detects prostate cancer earlier.
  - *Monitoring response to therapy:*
    - After operative resection, the PSA level is expected to normalize after 2–3 weeks.
    - In patients whose PSA level remained elevated 6 months after radical prostatectomy, recurrent disease eventually developed.
    - In contrast, it takes 3–5 months for PSA to normalize after radiotherapy.
    - However, failure of the PSA level to normalize after radiotherapy also predicts relapse.
    - A rise in serum PSA is usually the first sign of either local recurrence or metastatic progression.
    - In patients with advanced disease, PSA levels are also used to monitor response to systemic therapy.

- *Carbohydrate antigen 125 (CA 125):*
  - CA 125 is a carbohydrate epitope on a glycoprotein carcinoma antigen.
  - It is present in the fetus and in derivatives of the celomic epithelium, including the peritoneum, pleura, pericardium, and amnion.
  - In healthy adults, CA 125 has been detected by immunohistochemistry in the epithelium of the fallopian tubes, endometrium, and endocervix.
  - *Testing:*
    - CA 125 levels are measured with an immunoassay, with the upper limit of normal set at 35 U/mL.
    - Elevated levels are detected in 80% of patients with ovarian cancer.
    - In patients with ovarian masses, an elevated CA 125 level has a sensitivity of 75% and a specificity of approximately 90% for malignancy.
    - It is also detectable in a high percentage of patients with cancer of the fallopian tube, endometrium, and cervix, as well as in nongynecological malignancies of the pancreas, colon, lung, and liver.
    - Benign conditions in which CA 125 is elevated include endometriosis, adenomyosis, uterine fibroids, pelvic inflammatory disease, cirrhosis, and ascites.
    - As for CA 19-9 in patients with pancreatic cancer, CA 125 is an adjunct to diagnosis rather than being diagnostic by itself.
  - *Screening:* Alone, CA 125 is not useful as a screening tool for ovarian cancer because of its poor specificity.
  - *Prognosis:*
    - Patients with elevated CA 125 levels at the time of diagnosis have a worse prognosis than patients with normal levels do.
    - Absolute levels of CA 125 do not clearly correlate with tumor stage, although with increasing stage, greater percentages of patients have elevated CA 125 levels.
  - *Monitoring response to therapy:*
    - CA 125 is of value in monitoring the disease course.
    - Partial or complete response to therapy is associated with a decrease in CA 125 levels in >95% of patients.
    - Increasing levels of CA 125 correlate with disease recurrence and precede clinical or imaging evidence of recurrence by a median of 3 months.
    - When rising CA 125 levels are used as an indication for second-look laparotomy, recurrent disease is found approximately 90% of the time.
    - CA 125 levels in peritoneal fluid may be more sensitive than serum levels.
    - The upper limit of normal for peritoneal fluid CA 125 is 200 U/mL.
- *AFP and human chorionic gonadotropin (hCG) in testicular germ cell tumors:*
  - Nonseminomatous testicular cancers comprise several different histologic types, including embryonal carcinoma, syncytiotrophoblasts (choriocarcinoma), yolk sac tumors, and teratomas.
  - Marker expression can be predicted on the basis of the predominant histologic type—hCG is detected in >90% of choriocarcinomas, whereas AFP is expressed by 90–95% of yolk sac tumors, 20% of teratomas, and 10% of embryonal carcinomas.
  - *Diagnosis:*
    - Of patients with proven nonseminomatous testicular germ cell tumors, about 50% will have elevated serum levels of hCG and 60% will have elevated AFP, with either marker being elevated in 90% of cases.
    - In addition to the high rate of marker positivity, there have been very few cases of spuriously elevated serum levels of hCG or AFP in patients without testicular cancer.
    - The presence of a testicular tumor in combination with an elevated level of AFP or hCG is suggestive of testicular cancer, without being diagnostic.
    - Elevated levels of these markers in a man younger than 40 years without signs of a testicular tumor may indicate extratesticular germ cell cancer.

- *Prognosis:*
  - An absolute AFP concentration >500 ng/mL or an hCG level >1,000 ng/mL is predictive of a poor prognosis.
  - These tumor markers are useful in identifying biologically distinct categories of morphologically similar tumors.
- *Monitoring:*
  - In the majority of patients with nonseminomatous germ cell tumors, tumor marker levels correlate with response to chemotherapy.
  - The rate of marker decline (half-life), calculated from weekly determinations after initiation of chemotherapy, can be used for early identification of patients who will respond poorly to chemotherapy.

Deoxyribonucleic Acid (DNA)-based Markers

- Specific mutations in oncogenes, tumor-suppressor genes, and mismatch repair genes can serve as biomarkers.
- These mutations may be germline, such as the RET proto-oncogene of MEN 2 and the APC gene of familial adenomatous polyposis (FAP), or somatic mutations, such as the occurrence of *p53* mutations in a wide variety of tumors.
- Chromosomal abnormalities such as the 9:22 translocation that creates the BCR-ABL oncogene are also useful biomarkers.
- Specific single-nucleotide polymorphisms have been identified that are associated with increased risk for specific cancers and haplotype assessment has been shown to predict susceptibility to several cancers, including prostate, breast, lung, and colon cancer.

Epigenetic Changes

- Testing for epigenetic changes is still at an early discovery stage and has not yet reached the clinic.
- First, DNA assays for aberrant methylation are easier and more sensitive than those for point mutations.
- Second, cancer-specific DNA methylation patterns can be detected in tumor-derived free DNA in the bloodstream and in epithelial tumor cells shed into the lumen.
- This ease of access to sample medium may facilitate efforts at detection and monitoring of cancer.
- Third, DNA-methylation profiles are more chemically and biologically stable than RNA or most proteins. As a result, they may be more reliably detected in diverse biologic fluids.
  - Methylation biomarker studies have been performed in a variety of cancers, including breast, esophageal, gastric, colorectal, and prostate cancer. Sources of the DNA have included plasma/serum, urine, sputum, and saliva.
  - Combining DNA methylation assays may complement existing screening methods with high sensitivity but low specificity, such as PSA in prostate cancer. The use of panels of methylation targets in these studies improved the clinical sensitivity of the assay.

Potential Applications

- *Early detection:*
  - Although abnormal epigenetic silencing of genes can occur at any time during carcinogenesis, it appears to occur most frequently early in the transformation process.
  - Aberrant crypt foci that contain preneoplastic hyperplastic colonic epithelial cells have been found to demonstrate abnormal methylation in promoter regions of genes involved in abnormal activation of the Wnt signaling pathway.
  - Detection of abnormal methylation patterns in histologically normal cells may emerge as a useful marker for assessment of cancer risk.
- *Predict response to therapy:* Methylation of specific genes can be linked to the biologic behavior of the tumor.
- *Prognostication:* Abnormal methylation of combinations of genes has been associated with a poor outcome.

RNA-based Markers

- RNA-based markers have been identified in the context of global mRNA expression by high-throughput technologies.
- These microarrays (gene chips) allow us to measure the expression of 30,000–40,000 human genes in a single experiment.

Proteomic Profiling

- Proteomics is the study of all the proteins expressed by the genome.
- Proteomic profiling using mass spectrometry technologies generates complex fingerprints of ion peaks corresponding to protein concentrations, which can be correlated with disease states.
- Numerous studies using samples of blood (plasma or serum), urine, and pancreatic juice have demonstrated the feasibility of this technology for discovery of biomarkers and early detection of ovarian, breast, prostate, and pancreatic cancer.
- Identification of reproducible protein signatures of specific diseases has the potential to achieve much higher diagnostic sensitivity and specificity than possible with currently available biomarkers.
- Proteomic profiling lacks a standardized methodology and remains time and labor intensive.

---

3. Write down the criteria for ideal tumor biomarkers and advantages of uses of tumor markers. Enlist the three broad categories of tumor marker with examples. ***WBUHS 2025***

The ideal tumor marker has three defining characteristics:

1. The marker is expressed exclusively by the particular tumor
2. Collection of the specimen for the tumor marker assay is easy.
3. The assay itself is reproducible, rapid, and inexpensive.

- Tumor markers fall into three broad categories—proteins, genetic mutations, and epigenetic changes.
- All three may be found in the tumor tissue itself.
- Tumor markers found in body fluids, particularly blood and urine, have the greatest potential for clinical application because of the ease of access to these fluids for analysis and because repeated sampling allows in vivo monitoring of the malignancy for such features as disease progression or recurrence, metastasis, and response to therapy.

Advantages of Tumor Biomarkers

- *Early detection and diagnosis:*
    - Tumor biomarkers enable the identification of cancer at an early stage, often before symptoms appear, improving the chances of successful treatment.
    - *Example:* Elevated PSA (prostate-specific antigen) levels can indicate prostate cancer, prompting further diagnostic tests.
- *Personalized treatment:*
    - Biomarkers help tailor treatments to individual patients by identifying specific molecular characteristics of the tumor.
    - *Example:* HER2 overexpression in breast cancer guides the use of targeted therapies like trastuzumab (Herceptin).
- *Monitoring disease progression:*
    - Biomarkers allow clinicians to track the progression or recurrence of cancer during and after treatment.
    - *Example:* Rising CEA (carcinoembryonic antigen) levels may indicate colorectal cancer recurrence.
- *Predicting treatment response:*
    - Biomarkers can predict how a patient will respond to specific therapies, enabling the selection of the most effective treatment while avoiding unnecessary toxicity.

- *Example:* KRAS mutation status in colorectal cancer predicts response to anti-EGFR therapies like cetuximab.
- *Prognostic information:*
  - Biomarkers provide insights into the likely course of the disease, helping clinicians estimate patient outcomes and survival rates.
  - *Example:* High levels of CA-125 in ovarian cancer are associated with poorer prognosis.
- *Non-invasive monitoring:*
  - Many biomarkers can be detected through blood, urine, or other bodily fluids, offering a non-invasive way to monitor cancer compared to biopsies or imaging.
  - *Example:* Circulating tumor DNA (ctDNA) in liquid biopsies can detect mutations without invasive procedures.
- *Screening high-risk populations:*
  - Biomarkers facilitate targeted screening for individuals at high risk of developing cancer, improving early intervention.
  - *Example:* BRCA1/BRCA2 mutations identify individuals at risk for breast and ovarian cancer, guiding preventive measures.
- *Guiding drug development:*
  - Biomarkers are critical in clinical trials to identify suitable patient populations, assess drug efficacy, and monitor safety.
  - *Example:* PD-L1 expression levels help select patients for immunotherapy trials with checkpoint inhibitors.
- *Improved Disease Management:*
  - Biomarkers enable real-time assessment of treatment effectiveness, allowing timely adjustments to therapy plans.
  - *Example:* Monitoring AFP (alpha-fetoprotein) levels in hepatocellular carcinoma helps evaluate response to chemotherapy.
- *Cost-effectiveness:* By enabling early detection, personalized treatment, and efficient monitoring, biomarkers can reduce healthcare costs associated with advanced-stage cancer treatment or ineffective therapies.

Three Broad Categories

I. *Tumor-specific antigens:*
  - These are molecules uniquely or predominantly expressed by cancer cells, often associated with specific tumor types.
  - *Examples:*
    - *PSA (Prostate-specific antigen):* Used for prostate cancer screening and monitoring.
    - *CA-125 (Cancer antigen 125):* Associated with ovarian cancer.

II. *Oncofetal antigens:*
  - These are proteins expressed during fetal development but typically absent or at low levels in healthy adults, re-expressed in certain cancers.
  - *Examples:*
    - *AFP (Alpha-fetoprotein):* Elevated in hepatocellular carcinoma and germ cell tumors.
    - *CEA (Carcinoembryonic antigen):* Associated with colorectal cancer and other adenocarcinomas.

III. *Tumor-associated markers:*
  - These include enzymes, hormones, or other molecules produced in higher quantities by cancer cells or in response to cancer, not necessarily specific to tumors.
  - *Examples:*
    - *LDH (Lactate dehydrogenase):* Elevated in various cancers, including lymphoma and leukemia.
    - *β-hCG (Beta-human chorionic gonadotropin):* Associated with testicular cancer and trophoblastic tumors.

4. Biomarkers and biologically targeted therapies.

5. What are the different molecular markers for cancer? Give an outline of targeted therapy for cancer.
WBUHS 2017

Cancer	*Biomarker*	*Therapy*
Breast	Estrogen and progesterone receptor	Tamoxifen/aromatase inhibitors
Lymphoma	CD20	Rituximab
CML	BCR-ABL	Imatinib
GIST	c-kit	Imatinib
Non-small cell lung cancer	EGFR mutation	Gefitinib
Breast	HER2/neu	Trastuzumab

(CML: chronic myelogenous leukemia; EGFR: epidermal growth factor receptor; GIST: gastrointestinal stromal tumor; HER2: human epidermal growth factor receptor 2)

Molecular Cancer Biomarkers

Tumor type	*Biomarker*
Breast	• ER/PR (estrogen receptor/progesterone receptor) • HER2/neu • EGF
Colorectal	• KRAS • UGT1A1
Gastric	HER-2/neu
GIST	• c-KIT • CD20 • CD30 • FIP1L1-PDGFR-alpha • PDGFR
Leukemia/ Lymphoma	• Philadelphia Chromosome (BCR/ABL) • PML/RAR-alpha • TPMT • UGT1A1 • EML4/ALK
Lung	• EGFR • KRAS
Melanoma	BRAF
Pancreas	Elevated levels of leucine, isoleucine, and valine

Other Examples of Biomarkers

- *Tumor suppressors lost in cancer:* For example, *BRCA1* and *BRCA2*
- *RNA:* For example, mRNA and microRNA
- *Proteins found in body fluids or tissue:* For example, PSA and CA 125

Types of Targeted Therapy

- Most targeted therapies are either small-molecule drugs or monoclonal antibodies.
- Small-molecule drugs are small enough to enter cells easily, so they are used for targets that are inside cells.
- Monoclonal antibodies are drugs that are not able to enter cells easily. Instead, they attach to specific targets on the outer surface of cancer cells.

Mechanisms of Action

- Help the immune system destroy cancer cells
- Stop cancer cells from growing
- Stop signals that help form blood vessels
- Deliver cell-killing substances to cancer cells
- Cause cancer cell death
- Starve cancer of the hormones it needs to grow

Types of Target Therapies

- Hormone therapies slow or stop the growth of hormone-sensitive tumors. Hormone therapies act by preventing the body from producing the hormones or by interfering with the action of the hormones. Hormone therapies have been approved for both breast cancer and prostate cancer.
- Signal transduction inhibitors block the activities of molecules that participate in signal transduction, the process by which a cell responds to signals from its environment. During this process, once a cell has received a specific signal, the signal is relayed within the cell through a series of biochemical reactions that ultimately produce the appropriate response(s). In some cancers, the malignant cells are stimulated to divide continuously without being prompted to do so by external growth factors. Signal transduction inhibitors interfere with this inappropriate signaling.
- Gene expression modulators modify the function of proteins that play a role in controlling gene expression.
- Apoptosis inducers cause cancer cells to undergo a process of controlled cell death called apoptosis.
- Angiogenesis inhibitors block the growth of new blood vessels to tumors (a process called tumor angiogenesis). Some targeted therapies that inhibit angiogenesis interfere with the action of vascular endothelial growth factor (VEGF), a substance that stimulates new blood vessel formation. Other angiogenesis inhibitors target other molecules that stimulate new blood vessel growth.
- Immunotherapies trigger the immune system to destroy cancer cells. Some immunotherapies are monoclonal antibodies that recognize specific molecules on the surface of cancer cells.
- Monoclonal antibodies that deliver toxic molecules can cause the death of cancer cells specifically. Once the antibody has bound to its target cell, the toxic molecule that is linked to the antibody—such as a radioactive substance or a poisonous chemical—is taken up by the cell, ultimately killing that cell. The toxin will not affect cells that lack the target for the antibody, i.e., the vast majority of cells in the body.
- Cancer vaccines and gene therapy

Targeted Therapies Approved for Specific Types of Cancer

- *Adenocarcinoma of the stomach or gastroesophageal junction (GEJ):* Trastuzumab and ramucirumab
- *Bladder cancer:* Atezolizumab
- *Brain cancer:* Bevacizumab and everolimus
- *Breast cancer:* Everolimus, tamoxifen, toremifene, trastuzumab, fulvestrant, anastrozole, exemestane, lapatinib, letrozole, and pertuzumab
- *CRC:* Cetuximab, panitumumab, and bevacizumab
- *Dermatofibrosarcoma protuberans:* Imatinib mesylate
- *Head and neck cancer:* Cetuximab
- *Gastrointestinal (GI) stromal tumor:* Imatinib mesylate and sunitinib
- *Giant cell tumor of the bone:* Denosumab
- *Kidney cancer:* Bevacizumab, sorafenib, sunitinib, temsirolimus, and everolimus
- *Liver cancer:* Sorafenib
- *Lung cancer:* Bevacizumab and erlotinib
- *Neuroblastoma:* Dinutuximab
- *Pancreatic cancer:* Erlotinib, everolimus and sunitinib
- *Prostate cancer:* Cabazitaxel

- *Soft tissue sarcoma:* Pazopanib
- *Systemic mastocytosis:* Imatinib mesylate
- *Thyroid cancer:* Cabozantinib

6. Current status of immunotherapy in cancer patients.

7. Discuss the role of immunotherapy in malignancies. ***Srimanta Sankaradeva University, Assam 2025***

Name of the drug	*Mechanism of action*	*Others*
Sorafenib	Sorafenib is a small inhibitor of several tyrosine protein kinases, such as VEGFR, PDGFR, and RAF family kinases (more avidly C-RAF than B-RAF)	Used in renal cell carcinoma
Sunitinib	Sunitinib is an oral, small-molecule, multitargeted RTK	Also used in imatinib-resistant GIST
Temsirolimus	Temsirolimus works by blocking a cell protein known as *mTOR,* which normally helps cells grow and divide	Used in renal cell carcinoma
Everolimus		It is used to treat advanced kidney cancers after other drugs such as sorafenib or sunitinib have been tried
Bevacizumab	• Targets VEGF-A • Bevacizumab is in the angiogenesis inhibitor and monoclonal antibody families of medication. It works by slowing the growth of new blood vessels	• It may help some people with kidney cancer when used with interferon-alpha • Used for colon cancer, lung cancer, and glioblastoma • For age-related macular degeneration, it is given by injection into the eye
Pazopanib	Pazopanib is a potent and selective multitargeted receptor tyrosine kinase inhibitor that blocks tumor growth and inhibits angiogenesis	Also given in soft tissue sarcoma
Cabozantinib	Cabozantinib, is a small molecule inhibitor of the tyrosine kinases c-Met and VEGFR2, and has been shown to reduce tumor growth, metastasis, and angiogenesis	Used in renal cell carcinoma
Lenvatinib	It acts as a multiple kinase inhibitor against the VEGFR1, VEGFR2, and VEGFR3 kinases	Also used in thyroid cancer

(GIST: gastrointestinal stromal tumor; *mTOR*: mammalian target of rapamycin; PDGFR: platelet-derived growth factor receptor; RAF: rapidly accelerated fibrosarcoma; RTK: receptor tyrosine kinase; VEGFR: vascular endothelial growth factor receptor; VEGF-A: vascular endothelial growth factor A)

- Patients with moderate-to-high-grade disease often receive intravesical immunotherapy with a weakened, live bacterium, bacillus Calmette–Guérin (BCG). BCG was the first Food and Drug Administration (FDA)-approved immunotherapy and helps reduce the risk of bladder cancer.
- *Brain tumor:*
  - *Bevacizumab:* A monoclonal antibody that targets the VEGF/VEGFR pathway and inhibits tumor blood vessel growth; approved for advanced glioblastoma
  - *Dinutuximab:* A monoclonal antibody that targets the GD2 pathway; approved for first-line treatment of high-risk pediatric neuroblastoma
- *Esophageal cancer (EC):*
  - Targeted antibodies
    - *Ramucirumab:* A monoclonal antibody that targets the VEGF/VEGFR2 pathway and inhibits tumor blood vessel growth; approved for subsets of patients with advanced GE cancer

- *Trastuzumab:* A monoclonal antibody that targets the HER2 pathway; approved for subsets of patients with advanced, HER2-positive GE cancer, including as a first-line therapy
- Immunomodulators
  - *Pembrolizumab:* A checkpoint inhibitor that targets the PD-1/PD-L1 pathway; approved for subsets of patients with advanced, PD-L1-positive GE cancer
- *Malignant melanoma:*
  - Immunomodulators
    - *Ipilimumab:* A checkpoint inhibitor that targets the CTLA-4 pathway; approved for subsets of patients with advanced melanoma, including as a first-line therapy
    - *Nivolumab:* A checkpoint inhibitor that targets the PD-1/PD-L1 pathway; approved for subsets of patients with advanced melanoma
    - *Pembrolizumab:* A checkpoint inhibitor that targets the PD-1/PD-L1 pathway; approved for subsets of patients with advanced melanoma, including in the adjuvant (presurgical) setting
    - The combination of nivolumab and ipilimumab, which target the PD-1/PD-L1 and the CTLA-4 pathways, respectively; approved for subsets of patients with advanced melanoma
    - *Aldesleukin:* A cytokine that targets the interleukin 2 (IL-2)/IL-2R pathway; approved for patients with advanced melanoma
    - *Interferon-alpha-2b (IFNAR-2b):* A cytokine that targets the IFNAR1/2 pathway; approved for subsets of patients with melanoma
    - *Peginterferon alfa-2b:* A cytokine that targets the IFNAR1 pathway; approved for subsets of patients with melanoma
- Oncolytic virus therapy
  - *Talimogene laherparepvec (T-VEC):* A modified herpes simplex virus (HSV) that infects tumor cells and promotes their destruction; approved for subsets of patients with advanced melanoma.

8. Outline the current understanding of cancer immunology. Discuss the role of check-point inhibitors in modem oncology. ***WBUHS 2025***

Introduction to Cancer Immunology

Cancer immunology is the study of the interaction between the immune system and cancer cells. It underpins the development of immunotherapies, which aim to harness or modify the immune system to recognize and eliminate tumor cells.

- *Immune surveillance and tumor escape*
  - *Immune surveillance:* The immune system continuously monitors tissues to detect and destroy emerging tumor cells.
  - *Tumor immune escape:* Despite surveillance, some tumors develop mechanisms to evade immune detection or suppress immune responses.
- *Cancer-immunity cycle*

  The process by which the immune system identifies and attacks cancer cells includes:
  - *Release of cancer cell antigens.*
  - *Antigen presentation* by dendritic cells.
  - *Priming and activation* of T cells in lymph nodes.
  - *Trafficking of T cells* to tumors.
  - *Infiltration of T cells* into tumors.
  - *Recognition of cancer cells* by T cells.
  - *Killing of cancer cells,* leading to further antigen release.

Tumors can interrupt this cycle at multiple points to avoid immune destruction.

Key Players in Tumor-Immune Interactions

- *Innate immune cells*
  - *Macrophages:* Can be tumor-promoting (M2) or tumor-suppressing (M1).
  - *Natural killer (NK) cells:* Recognize and kill tumor cells lacking MHC I.
  - *Dendritic cells:* Present tumor antigens to T cells.
- *Adaptive immune cells*
  - *CD8+ Cytotoxic T lymphocytes (CTLs):* Directly kill tumor cells.
  - *CD4+ Helper T cells:* Support cytotoxic responses and coordinate immune activity.
  - *Regulatory T cells (Tregs):* Suppress immune responses and are often co-opted by tumors to inhibit antitumor immunity.
- *Tumor Microenvironment (TME):* Often immunosuppressive, containing cytokines (e.g., IL-10, TGF-â), immune checkpoint ligands (e.g., PD-L1), and metabolic by-products (e.g., adenosine) that inhibit immune cell function.

Immune Checkpoints and Tumor Immune Evasion

- *Immune checkpoints*

  These are regulatory pathways that prevent autoimmunity and limit immune responses.

  Key checkpoints:
  - *CTLA-4 (Cytotoxic T-Lymphocyte Antigen 4):* Inhibits early T cell activation.
  - *PD-1 (Programmed Death-1):* Inhibits T cell activity in peripheral tissues during inflammation.
  - *PD-L1 (Programmed Death Ligand-1):* Often expressed on tumor cells to deactivate T cells.
- *Tumor use of immune checkpoints*
  - Tumors exploit checkpoint pathways to avoid immune destruction.
  - Upregulation of PD-L1 on tumor cells binds to PD-1 on T cells, leading to T cell exhaustion and reduced cytotoxicity.

Checkpoint Inhibitors in Modern Oncology

Checkpoint inhibitors are monoclonal antibodies that block immune checkpoints, thereby restoring T-cell activity against cancer.

- *Approved checkpoint Inhibitors*
  - *Anti-CTLA-4: Ipilimumab*
  - *Anti-PD-1: Nivolumab, Pembrolizumab*
  - *Anti-PD-L1: Atezolizumab, Durvalumab, Avelumab*
- *Clinical applications*

  Checkpoint inhibitors are now standard-of-care for multiple cancers:
  - *Melanoma:* Dramatic survival improvements.
  - *Non-small cell lung cancer (NSCLC)*
  - *Renal cell carcinoma*
  - *Head and neck squamous cell carcinoma*
  - *Triple-negative breast cancer*
  - *Microsatellite instability-high (MSI-H) cancers:* Regardless of tissue origin.
- *Combination therapies*
  - Dual checkpoint blockade (e.g., CTLA-4 + PD-1) offers enhanced efficacy in some cancers.
  - Combination with chemotherapy, targeted therapy, or radiation is under active investigation.

Challenges and Limitations

- *Primary and acquired resistance*

  Not all patients respond; resistance mechanisms include:
  - Lack of tumor-infiltrating lymphocytes.
  - Defective antigen presentation.
  - Mutations in interferon signaling pathways.

- *Immune-related adverse events (irAEs)*
  - Checkpoint inhibition can lead to inflammation in normal tissues (e.g., colitis, dermatitis, pneumonitis).
  - Management often requires immunosuppressants like corticosteroids.
- *Biomarkers for response*
  - *PD-L1 expression:* Imperfect predictor.
  - *Tumor mutational burden (TMB):* High TMB may predict response.
  - *MSI status:* Strong predictor of benefit.
  - *T cell inflamed gene expression profiles*
- *Future directions*
  - Development of *novel checkpoint targets* (e.g., LAG-3, TIGIT, TIM-3).
  - Use of *personalized cancer vaccines* to enhance T cell priming.
  - *Adoptive cell therapies* (e.g., CAR T-cells, TIL therapy).
  - Improved *biomarker discovery* for patient stratification.
  - Strategies to *modulate the tumor microenvironment* to favor immune activity.

9. Write short note of genetic testing in cancer diagnosis. ***WBUHS 2024***

Genetic testing plays a crucial role in the *diagnosis, prognosis, and treatment planning* of cancer. It involves analyzing DNA to identify inherited or acquired (somatic) mutations that may increase the risk of cancer or affect tumor behavior.

Types of Genetic Testing in Cancer

- *Germline testing*
  - Detects inherited mutations (e.g., BRCA1/2, TP53, APC).
  - Used for risk assessment in families with strong cancer histories.
  - Helps in early detection and preventive strategies.
- *Somatic (Tumor) testing*
  - Identifies mutations in the tumor cells (e.g., EGFR, KRAS, HER2).
  - Guides targeted therapy decisions and predicts response to treatment.

Applications in Cancer Diagnosis

- *Risk stratification:* Identifies individuals at high genetic risk (e.g., BRCA in breast/ovarian cancer).
- *Early detection:* Enables surveillance and preventive measures.
- *Therapy selection:* Facilitates precision medicine (e.g., EGFR inhibitors in lung cancer).
- *Prognosis:* Some mutations indicate aggressive disease or higher recurrence risk.

10. Gene therapy for cancer. ***WBUHS 2006***

Introduction

- Advances in understanding and manipulating genes have set the stage for scientists to alter a person's genetic material to fight or prevent disease.
- Gene therapy is an experimental treatment that involves introducing genetic material (DNA or RNA) into a person's cells to fight disease.
- Gene therapy is being studied in clinical trials (research studies with people) for many different types of cancer and for other diseases.
- It is not currently available outside a clinical trial.

Strategies of Gene Therapy for Cancer

- Enhancing the immunogenicity of the tumor, for example, by introducing genes that encode foreign antigens
- Enhancing immune cells to increase antitumor activity, for example, by introducing genes that encode cytokines
- Inserting a "sensitivity" or suicide gene into the tumor, for example, by introducing the gene that encodes *HSVtk*.

- Blocking the expression of oncogenes, for example, by introducing the gene that encodes antisense K-RAS message.
- Inserting a wild-type tumor-suppressor gene, for example, *p53* or the gene involved in Wilms tumor
- Protecting stem cells from the toxic effects of chemotherapy, for example, by introducing the gene that confers multiple drug resistance type 1 (MDR-1).
- Blocking the mechanisms by which tumors evade immunological destruction, for example, by introducing the gene that encodes antisense insulin-like growth factor 1 (IGF-1) message
- Killing tumor cells by inserting toxin genes under the control of a tumor-specific promoter, for example, the gene that encodes diphtheria A chain

Approaches to Ex Vivo Gene Transfer

- *Genetically engineered tumor cells:*
  - Various groups are investigating the production of autologous cellular vaccines for the treatment and prevention of cancer.
  - This is most commonly attempted by surgically removing tumor cells from the patient, growing them in tissue culture and inserting immunostimulatory genes in vitro.
  - These cells are then reinjected into the patient in an effort to induce a significant systemic immune response that will both destroy tumor cells and protect the patient against a recurrence of the tumor.
  - Treating cells that produce cytokines has been shown to result in systemic immunity in mice.
  - Alteration of syngeneic tumors with the genes that encode IL-1 b, IL-2, IL-4, IL-6, tumor necrosis factor alpha (TNF-α), granulocyte-macrophage colony-stimulating factor (GM-CSF), or r-interferon results in immunological destruction of the tumor cells in vivo.
  - In human gene therapy trials, patients are injected with either autologous or allogeneic genetically modified tumor cells.
  - These trials involved the insertion of retroviral vectors carrying the gene that encodes either IL-2, TNF-α, or GM-CSF into melanoma, colorectal renal cell carcinoma, neuroblastoma, or breast cancer cells in vitro.
  - One modification of this technique is the insertion of the gene for either IL-2 or IL-4 into autologous fibroblasts, which are then mixed with irradiated tumor cells from the patient and reinjected.
  - This approach has the advantage that growing fibroblasts in vitro is much easier than culturing tumor cells from a large number of individuals.
  - Besides modifying tumor cells to produce immune activating cytokines; another strategy is to block the production of IGF-1.
  - Many tumors such as breast cancer produce high levels of IGF-1. Insertion of an antisense gene that stops production of IGF-1 in the tumor allows immunological rejection of the genetically altered tumor after reimplantation.
  - Destruction of the tumor is mediated by cytotoxic T lymphocytes.
  - The precise mechanism by which IGF-1 mediates tumor protection in vivo remains unclear.
- *Genetically engineered T lymphocytes:*
  - T lymphocytes have the capacity to hone in on tumor tissue.
  - This property has been used to deliver cytokines directly to tumor masses for human gene therapy.
  - The secretion of cytokines locally at the tumor site by the effector T lymphocytes will enhance their anti-tumor activity and avoid the side effects that result from the systemic administration of cytokines.
  - For the trial of TNF-modified tumor-infiltrating T lymphocytes
  - T lymphocytes are difficult to transduce with retroviral vectors and tend to downregulate expression of the cytokine gene carried by the vector.
  - These two problems of poor gene transfer efficiency and poor cytokine expression have so far limited the application of this approach and have shifted the emphasis from modification of T lymphocytes toward the genetic alteration of tumor cells, which are much easier to grow in culture and more readily engineered.

- *Insertion of a sensitivity gene:*
  - Gene therapy uses the genes to activate a relatively nontoxic prodrug to form a highly toxic agent.
  - The most widely studied system uses the thymidine kinase gene of the HSV (*HSVtk*).
  - The *HSVtk* gene confers sensitivity to the antiherpes drug, ganciclovir (GCV), by phosphorylating GCV to a monophosphate form (GCV-MP). Phosphorylation to the triphosphate form (GCV-TP) by cellular kinases results in inhibition of DNA polymerase, and leads to cell death.
  - In this procedure, GCV kills tumor cells which express KSVtk and the adjacent cells that lack the gene are also destroyed.
  - This is termed the bystander effect phenomenon.
  - To use the bystander effect to kill human cancer in vivo, the irradiated ovarian tumor cells that contain the *HSVtk* gene will be injected into the peritoneal cavity of patients who will be given GCV.
  - These *HSVtk*-expressing cells will destroy bystander tumor cells in vivo.
- *Protection of hematopoietic stem cells (HSCs):*
  - Protection of HSCs from the toxic effects of chemotherapy by using the gene that confers MDR-1 is another possible strategy for human cancer therapy.
  - The MDR-1 gene will be isolated from tumor cells, where it functions to pump chemotherapy drugs (including daunorubicin, doxorubicin, vincristine, vinblastine, VP-16, VM-26, taxol, and actinomycin-D) from within the cell.
  - Transfer of a retroviral vector carrying the MDR-1 gene into bone marrow stem cells and their subsequent reintroduction will protect stem cells in vivo from the effects of large doses of taxol.
- *Genetic alteration of cancer cells in situ:*
  - *Liposome-mediated gene transfer:*
    - The genetical modification of tumors in situ involves the direct injection of liposomes containing an allogene that encoded *HLA-B7*, a foreign antigen that is transiently expressed on the cell surface and includes an immune reaction against the altered tumor cells.
    - Antitumor immune response is significantly increased when some of the tumor cells express foreign antigens on their cell surface.
    - The transient expression of immunostimulatory genes in tumors might have potential as a treatment and as a vaccination against certain malignancies.
  - *Retrovirus-mediated gene transfer:*
    - In vivo gene transfer using murine retroviral vectors has been applied to the treatment of brain tumors.
    - In this process, murine fibroblasts that are actively producing retroviral vectors, so-called retroviral vector producer cells (VPCs), are implanted directly into growing tumors.
    - The gene transferred by the retroviral vectors into the surrounding tumor cells is the *HSVtk* gene.
    - The *HSVtk* gene should integrate only into the proliferating tumor cells because retrovirus-mediated gene transfer is limited to mitotically active cells.

Some Uses

- Gene therapy alters immune cells for treatment of advanced melanoma.
- Gene therapy is also used for human breast cancer.
- Can also be used to treat prostate cancer
- Used in oral cancers
- HLA-B7 is the most common gene used in bladder cancer.
- Novel suicide gene therapy used to treat malignant brain tumors
- Gene therapy-based soluble fms-like tyrosine kinase 1 (sFLT-1) approach for carcinoma of the ovary
- It is also used in liver cancer.
- Mesothelioma may be particularly well suited for gene therapy treatment owing to its accessibility, allowing both intrapleural and intratumoral gene delivery.
- It is also used in blood cancers.

11. Paraneoplastic syndrome.

Introduction

A *paraneoplastic syndrome* is a syndrome (a set of signs and symptoms) that is the consequence of cancer in the body but that, unlike mass effect, is not due to the local presence of cancer cells. These phenomena are mediated by humoral factors (by hormones or cytokines) excreted by tumor cells or by an immune response against the tumor.

- Paraneoplastic syndromes are typical among middle-aged to older patients and they most commonly present with cancers of the lung, breast, ovaries, or lymphatic system (a lymphoma).
- Sometimes, the symptoms of paraneoplastic syndromes show before the diagnosis of a malignancy, which has been hypothesized to relate to the disease pathogenesis.
- In this paradigm, tumor cells express tissue-restricted antigens (e.g., neuronal proteins), triggering an anti-tumor immune response which may be partially or, rarely, completely effective in suppressing tumor growth and symptoms.
- Patients then come to clinical attention when this tumor immune response breaks immune tolerance and begins to attack the normal tissue expressing that (e.g., neuronal) protein.
- Paraneoplastic syndromes can be divided into four main categories—(1) endocrine, (2) neurological, (3) mucocutaneous, and (4) hematological paraneoplastic syndromes, as well as others that may not fit into any of the above categories:

Syndrome class	*Syndrome*	*Main causal cancers*	*Causal mechanism*
Endocrine	Gushing syndrome	• Small-cell lung cancer • Pancreatic carcinoma • Neural tumors • Thymoma	Ectopic ACTH and ACTH-like substance
	SIADH	• Small-cell lung cancer • CNS malignancies	Antidiuretic hormone
	Hypercalcemia	• Lung cancer (typically squamous cell) • Breast carcinoma • Renal carcinoma • Multiple myeloma (may occur independent of osteolytic lesions) • Adult T cell leukemia/lymphoma • Ovarian carcinoma	PTHrP, TGF-β, TNF, IL-1
	Hypoglycemia	• Fibrosarcoma • Other mesenchymal sarcomas • Insulinoma • Hepatocellular carcinoma	Insulin or insulin-like substance or "big" IGF-2
	Carcinoid syndrome	• Bronchial adenoma (carcinoid type) • Pancreatic carcinoma	Serotonin, bradykinin
	Anti-NMDA receptor encephalitis	Teratoma	Autoimmune reaction against NMDA receptor subunits
	Polymyositis	• Non-Hodgkin lymphoma • Lung cancer • Bladder cancer	
	Acanthosis nigricans	• Gastric carcinoma • Lung carcinoma • Uterine carcinoma	• Immunologic • Secretion of EGF

Contd...

Contd...

Mucocutaneous	Dermatomyositis	• Bronchogenic carcinoma • Breast carcinoma • Ovarian cancer • Pancreatic cancer • Stomach cancer • Colorectal cancer • Non-Hodgkin lymphoma	Immunologic
	• Leser–Trélat sign • Necrolytic migratory erythema • Sweets syndrome • Florid cutaneous papillomatosis • Pyoderma gangrenosum • Acquired generalized hypertrichosis	Glucagonoma	
	Granulocytosis	Bladder cancer	G-CSF
	Polycythemia		See hematological paraneoplastic syndromes
	Hyperaldosteronism	• Adrenal adenoma/Conn's syndrome • Non-Hodgkin's lymphoma • Ovarian carcinoma • Pulmonary	Aldosterone
Neurological	LEMS	Small-cell lung cancer	Immunologic
	Paraneoplastic cerebellar degeneration	• Lung cancer • Ovarian cancer • Breast carcinoma • Hodgkin's lymphoma	
	Encephalomyelitis		Inflammation of the brain and spinal cord
	Limbic encephalitis	Small-cell lung carcinoma	
	Brainstem encephalitis		
	Opsoclonus myoclonus ataxia syndrome	• Breast carcinoma • Ovarian carcinoma • Small-cell lung carcinoma • Neuroblastoma (in children)	Autoimmune reaction against the RNA-binding protein Nova-1
	Anti-NMDA receptor encephalitis	Teratoma	Autoimmune reaction against NMDA receptor subunits
	Polymyositis	• Non-Hodgkin lymphoma • Lung cancer • Bladder cancer	
Mucocutaneous	Acanthosis nigricans	• Gastric carcinoma • Lung carcinoma • Uterine carcinoma	Immunologic Secretion of EGF
	Dermatomyositis	• Bronchogenic carcinoma • Breast carcinoma • Ovarian cancer • Pancreatic cancer • Stomach cancer • Colorectal cancer • Non-Hodgkin lymphoma	Immunologic

Contd...

Contd...

	Leser–Trélat sign		
	Necrolytic migratory erythema	Glucagonoma	
	Sweet's syndrome		
	Fiord cutaneous papillomatosis		
	Pyoderma gangrenosum		
	Acquired generalized hypertrichosis		
	Granulocytosis		G-CSF
Hematological	Polycythemia	• Bladder cancer • Renal carcinoma • Cerebellar hemangioma • Hepatocellular carcinoma	Erythropoietin
	Trousseau sign	• Pancreatic carcinoma • Bronchogenic carcinoma	Mucins that activate clotting, others
	Nonbacterial thrombotic endocarditis	Advanced cancers	Hypercoagulability
	Anemia	Thymic neoplasms	Unknown
Others	Membranous glomerulonephritis	Various	• Tumor antigens • Immune complexes
	Tumor-induced osteomalacia	• Hemangiopericytoma • Phosphaturic mesenchymal tumor	FGF-23
	Stauffer syndrome	Renal cell carcinoma	
	Neoplastic fever		

(ACTH: adrenocorticotropic hormone; CNS: central nervous system; EGF: epidermal growth factor; FGF-23: fibroblast growth factor-23; G-CSF: granulocyte colony-stimulating factor; IGF-2: insulin-like growth factor 2; IL-1: interleukin 1; LEMS: Lambert–Eaton myasthenic syndrome; NMDA: N-methyl-D-aspartate; PTHrP: parathyroid hormone-related protein; SIADH: syndrome of inappropriate antidiuretic hormone secretion; TGF: transforming growth factor; TNF: tumor necrosis factor)

Neurological

- A particularly devastating form of paraneoplastic syndromes is a group of disorders classified as paraneoplastic neurological disorders (PNDs).
- These paraneoplastic disorders affect the central or peripheral nervous system; some are degenerative, though others [such as Lambert–Eaton myasthenic syndrome (LEMS)] may improve with treatment of the condition or the tumor.
- Symptoms of PNDs may include ataxia (difficulty with walking and balance), dizziness, nystagmus (rapid, uncontrolled eye movements), difficulty swallowing, loss of muscle tone, loss of fine motor coordination, slurred speech, memory loss, vision problems, sleep disturbances, dementia, seizures, and sensory loss in the limbs.

The most common cancers associated with PNDs are breast, ovarian and lung cancer, but many other cancers can produce paraneoplastic symptoms as well.

Treatment Options Include

- Therapies to eliminate the underlying cancer such as chemotherapy, radiation, and surgery.
- Rapid diagnosis and treatment are critical for the patient to have the best chance of recovery. Since these disorders are relatively rare, few doctors have seen or treated PNDs.
- Therefore, it is important that PND patients consult with a specialist with experience in diagnosing and treating PNDs.

12. Discuss the micro- and macroanatomy of lymph nodes. Mention the imaging criteria for metastatic lymph nodes. Discuss the role of sentinel node biopsy in common malignancies.

Lymph Nodes

- The lymph nodes are small, round, or ovoid bodies placed along the course of lymphatic vessels.
- They are surrounded by a fibrous capsule from which trabeculae penetrate into the nodes.
- The node can be differentiated into an *outer cortex* and *an inner medulla.*
- In the cortex are accumulations of lymphocyte primary lymphoid follicles, within which germinal centers (secondary follicles) develop during antigenic stimulation.

  The follicles contain:
  - Proliferating lymphocytes
  - Dendritic macrophages which capture and process the antigen
- In the medulla, the lymphocytes are arranged as elongated branching bands (medullary cords). The cortical follicles and medullary cords contain B lymphocytes and constitute the bursa-dependent areas.
- Between the cortical follicles and medullary cords, there is a broad, ill-defined, intermediate zone (paracortical area) which contains T lymphocytes and constitutes the thymus-dependent area.

Functions of Lymph Node

- Lymph nodes act as a filter for the lymph, each group of nodes draining a specific part of the body.
- They phagocytose foreign materials including microorganisms.
- They help the proliferation and circulation of T and B cells.
- They enlarge following local antigen stimulation.

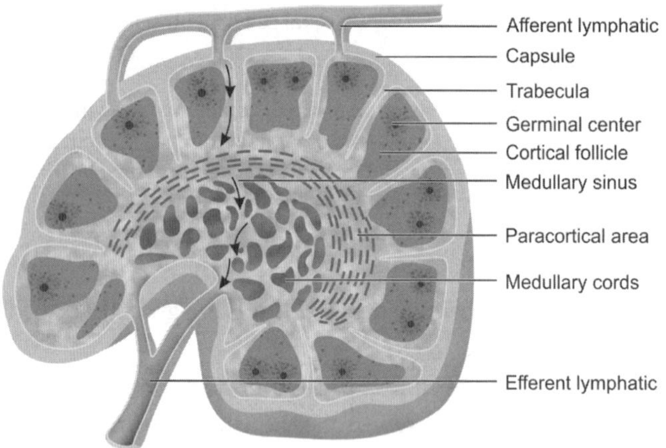

Diagrammatic section of a lymph node.

Imaging Criteria for Metastatic Lymph Nodes

- *Ultrasonography (USG) criteria:*
  - Size of the lymph node greater than 1.0 cm
  - Necrosis
  - Shape of a lymph node is determined by measurements taken vertically (maximum longitudinal or minimal axial diameter) L/T ratio >1
  - Eccentric enlargement of nodal cortex

- *Computed tomography (CT) and magnetic resonance imaging (MRI) criteria:*

• A discrete mass greater than 1.0 cm • An ill-defined mass in a lymph node area • Multiple nodes of 6–15 mm • Obliteration of tissue planes around vessels in a nonirradiated neck • A nodal mass with central low density is specifically indicative of tumor necrosis	• A nodal mass with central low density is specifically indicative of tumor necrosis • If neoplastic process progresses, lymph node gains a spheric appearance due to an increase in node size • Original node structure shows defeats due to tumor infiltration, desmoplastic reaction, and necrosis • In this stage, either a decrease or an increase can be seen in vascularization under influence of angiogenic factors

- The assessment of lymph nodes using these modalities relies on lymph node anatomy rather than function and physiology.
- On cross-sectional imaging, a normal lymph node usually measures <1 cm in size, has a smooth and well-defined border, and shows uniform, homogeneous density or signal intensity.
- Most benign nodes have a central fatty hilum, which has a distinctive feature on CT and MRI.

Role of Sentinel Lymph Node (SLN) Biopsy in Different Malignancies

- *Carcinoma breast:*
  - SLN biopsy is primarily used in women with early breast cancers (T1 and T2, N0).
  - It also is accurate for T3 N0 cancers, but nearly 75% of these women will have nonpalpable axillary lymph node metastases.
  - In women undergoing neoadjuvant chemotherapy to permit conservation surgery, SLN biopsy may be used.

Contraindications to the Procedure

- Palpable lymphadenopathy
- Prior axillary surgery, chemotherapy, or radiation therapy
- Multifocal breast cancers
- The combination of intraoperative gamma probe detection of radioactive colloid and intraoperative visualization of isosulfan blue dye (Lymphazurin) is more accurate than the use of either agent alone.
- On the day prior to surgery, or on the morning of surgery, the radioactive colloid is injected. Using a tuberculin syringe and a 25-gauge needle, 0.5 mCi of 0.2-micron technetium-99 sulfur colloid in a volume of 0.2–0.5 mL is injected (three to four separate injections) at the cancer site or subdermally.
- Subdermal injections are given in proximity to the cancer site or subareolar.
- Subsequently, in the operating room, 4 mL of isosulfan blue dye (Lymphazurin) is injected in a similar fashion, but with an additional 1 mL injected between the cancer site and the overlying skin.
- For nonpalpable cancers, the injection is guided by either intraoperative ultrasound or by a localization wire that is placed preoperatively under ultrasound or stereotactic guidance.
- It is helpful for the radiologist to mark the skin overlying the breast cancer at the time of needle localization using an indelible marker.
- In women who have undergone previous excisional biopsy, the injections are made around the biopsy cavity but not into it.
- Women are told preoperatively that the isosulfan blue dye injection will impart a change to the color of their urine and that there is a very small risk of allergic reaction to the dye (1 in 10,000).
- Anaphylactic reactions have been documented. The use of radioactive colloid is safe and radiation exposure is very low.
  - A handheld gamma counter is then employed transcutaneously to identify the location of the SLN.
  - The gamma counter is employed to pinpoint the location of the SLN.
    - By using a combination of isotope lymphatic mapping, an intraoperative handheld gamma probe, and intraoperative injection of blue dye, the SLN could be identified in >95% of cases in the groin and axilla, with identification in the head/neck region being slightly lower (85%).

  - There was great anatomic variation, resulting in drainage to multiple or uncommon sites.
  - Detailed pathologic analysis of the sentinel nodes via step sections enabled detection of micro- metastases that could be missed by standard techniques.
  - The probability of finding a positive sentinel node can be predicted by using a nomogram derived from multifactorial analysis.
  - In most cases, a positive sentinel node was the only positive node.
  - No prognostic factors were found that accurately identified a subpopulation of SLN-positive patients at zero risk of harboring other positive nodes.
- As the dissection continues, the signal from the probe increases in intensity as the SLN is approached.
- The SLN also is identified by visualization of isosulfan blue dye in the afferent lymph vessel and in the lymph node itself.
- The lowest false-negative rates for SLN biopsy have been obtained when all blue lymph nodes and all lymph nodes with radiation counts >10% of the 10-second ex vivo count of the SLN are harvested (10% rule).
- This procedure is repeated until residual radioactivity in the surgical bed is <10% of the 10-second ex vivo count of the most radioactive SLN.

Malignant melanoma: Management of regional lymph nodes:

- After wide local excision (WLE) of the primary tumor, the most common sites of first recurrence are regional (lymph nodes, in-transit metastases, and local recurrences).
- Nodal metastases generally appear in the basin or basins draining from the primary site. This is a predictable pattern for extremity melanomas; however, truncal and head and neck melanomas may drain to more than one site.
- Lines of drainage for truncal melanomas are divided by the midline and the line of Sappey, which extends from the umbilicus across the iliac crest and around to the spine at the level of L2.
- This sequence of recurrences led surgeons to conclude that resection of nodal basins containing occult metastases could provide an increase in survival. This procedure, termed elective lymph node dissection (ELND), was commonly practiced.
- As prognostic factors became better understood, it was postulated that patients with thin tumors (<1 mm in thickness) would have a low risk of metastases at any site and patients with thick tumors (>4 mm in thickness) would have a high risk of distant as well as regional metastases. In contrast, patients with intermediate-thickness melanoma (1–4 mm) would have an elevated risk for nodal metastases without a high risk for distant disease.

Development of the SLN concept ended one debate over ELND, changed clinical management, and opened a new series of questions about the tumor biology of melanoma.

Carcinoma penis: Not used nowadays. Biopsy of the lesion is taken to confirm the diagnosis.

13. Radiofrequency thermal ablation of malignant tumors. *WBUHS 2007*

Introduction

- In 1868, the French scientist Jaques-Arsène D'Arsonval described the basic principle of radiofrequency ablation (RFA), demonstrating that an alternating electric current greater than 10 kHz could pass through living tissue without neuromuscular effect.
- Since then, more studies have proved the utility and essential efficacy of RFA in treating discrete tumors in humans.
- Many different ablation systems have been explored, including monopolar, bipolar, and multipolar electrodes, cooled tip electrodes, and expandable electrodes with multiple times, with the aim of improving local thermal efficacy and thereby, oncological results.
- In the last decade, this technique has been increasingly used as an alternative, or as an adjunct or bridge, to surgery and/or transplant in the treatment of liver tumors. More recently, RFA has confirmed its usefulness in the treatment of renal, adrenal, lung, and other focal cancers.

Principle

Radiofrequency ablation works by converting electromagnetic energy into heat but its effectiveness is influenced by thermal conductivity and perfusion of the target tissue.

RFA can be performed via a percutaneous approach, laparoscopically or during open laparotomy. For liver and renal tumors, RFA is usually performed under ultrasound guidance. For lung tumors, the procedure is necessarily performed under CT guidance.

Use

- *In liver:* The ideal lesion for RFA using current technology is around 3 cm in diameter, not superficial, and distant from large bowel and large vascular structures. Caution should be taken when treating lesions near the proximal bile ducts, large vessels, diaphragm, and gut to avoid possible complications such as bleeding, infection, bilomas, biliary strictures, hemothorax, and colonic perforation due to heat transmission.

  Radical surgical resection is the best treatment for discrete, nontransplantable HCC in favorable patients. RFA plays an important role as an alternative treatment for primary lesion when surgery is not possible and has been shown to be more effective than other local therapies such as percutaneous ethanol injection and cryotherapy.
- *In colorectal liver metastases:* RFA plays an important role in the treatment of nonresectable liver colorectal metastases and as a complement to surgical resection.

  The fibrotic nature of the colorectal liver metastases, surrounded by normal parenchyma may compromise the efficacy of RFA. Lesions >3 cm in diameter are considered at significantly higher risk of recurrence.
- *In metastatic neuroendocrine tumors:* RFA alone or in combination with surgery appears to be a useful "cytoreductive" tool which can improve neuroendocrine symptomatology from metastatic neuroendocrine tumors.
- *In renal tumors:* Minimally invasive therapy can be employed for the treatment of small volume (<4 cm), T1a disease renal malignancy. RFA under imaging guidance appears well suited to this task.
- *In lung malignancies:* RFA has shown to be feasible, effective, and safe in the treatment of poorly resectable primary and secondary lung malignancies.

14. Classify anticancer drugs. What is the role of chemotherapy in the management of carcinoma breast?
WBUHS 2016

Anticancer Drugs

According to drug acting directly on cells:

- Alkalyting agent
  - Nitrogen mustard

For example, mechlorethamine (mustine HCL), cyclophosphamide, and ifosfamide

- Ethylenimine

For example, thiotepa

- Alkyl Sulfonate

For example, busulfan

- Nitrosourea

For example, carmustine and lomustine

- Triazine

For example, dacarbazine

- Antimetabolites
  - Folate antagonist

For example, methotrexate

- Purine antagonist

For example, 6-mercaptopurine, 6-thiogunine, and azathioprine

- Pyrimidine antagonist

For example, 5-fluorouracil (5-FU) and cytarabine

- Vinka alkaloids

For example, vincristine and vinblastine

- Taxanes

For example, paclitaxel

- Epipodophyllotoxin

For example, etoposide

- Antibiotics

For example, actinomycin, doxorubicin, daunorubicin, mitoxantrone, bleomycins, and mithramycin

- Miscellaneous

For example, hydroxyurea and procarbazine L-asparaginase, cisplatin, and carboplatin Drug-altering hormonal milieu

- Glucocorticoids

For example, prednisolone and its derivatives

- Estrogen

For example, fosfestrol and ethinylestradiol

- Antiestrogen

For example, tamoxifen

- Antiandrogen

For example, flutamide

- 5-α-reductase inhibitor

For example, finasteride

- Gonadotropin-releasing hormone (GnRH) analogs

For example, nafarelin and goserelin

According to mechanism of action:

- Drugs affecting biosynthesis of nucleic acid
- Drugs destroying DNA structure and function
- Drugs interfering with transcription and blocking

RNA synthesis:

- Drugs affecting protein synthesis
- Hormonal agents

Drug affecting nucleic acid synthesis: Hydroxyurea

Drugs destroying DNA structure and its function: Alkylating agent, camptothecins, antitumor antibiotics, cisplatin, and carboplatin

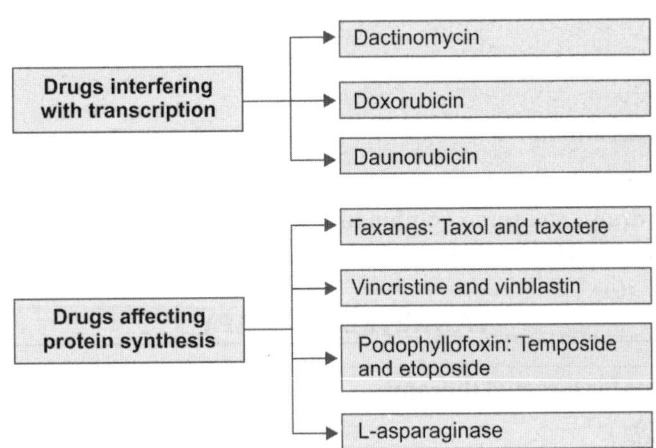

Chemotherapy in Carcinoma Breast

Not all women with breast cancer will need chemo, but there are several situations in which chemo may be recommended:

- *After surgery (adjuvant chemotherapy):* Adjuvant chemo is used after surgery to try to kill any cancer cells that may have been left behind or spread but cannot be seen, even on imaging tests. If these cells were allowed to grow, they could form new tumors in other places in the body. Adjuvant chemo can reduce the risk of breast cancer coming back.
- *Before surgery (neoadjuvant chemotherapy):* Neoadjuvant chemo is given before surgery. It can be used to try to shrink the tumor so that it can be removed with less extensive surgery. Because of this, neoadjuvant chemo is often used to treat cancers that are too big to be removed at the time of diagnosis (called *locally advanced* cancers). Also, by giving chemo before the tumor is removed, doctors can better see how the cancer responds to it. If the first set of chemo drugs does not shrink the tumor, your doctor will know that other drugs are needed.
- *For advanced breast cancer:* Chemo can be used as the main treatment for women whose cancer has spread outside the breast and underarm area, either when it is diagnosed or after initial treatments. The length of treatment depends on how well the chemo is working and how well you tolerate it.

Chemotherapeutic Drugs are used for Breast Cancer

In most cases (especially as adjuvant or neoadjuvant treatment), chemo is most effective when combinations of more than one drug are used. Today, doctors use many different combinations, and it is not clear that any single combination is clearly the best.

The most common drugs used for adjuvant and neoadjuvant chemotherapy include:

- Anthracyclines, such as doxorubicin (adriamycin) and epirubicin (Ellence)
- Taxanes, such as paclitaxel (taxol) and docetaxel (taxotere)
- 5-fluorouracil
- Cyclophosphamide (cytoxan)
- Carboplatin (paraplatin)

Most often, combinations of 2 or 3 of these drugs are used.

Chemotherapy for Advanced Breast Cancer

Chemo drugs useful in treating women with breast cancer that has spread include:

- Docetaxel
- Paclitaxel
- Platinum agents (cisplatin and carboplatin)
- Vinorelbine
- Capecitabine
- Liposomal doxorubicin

- Gemcitabine
- Mitoxantrone
- Ixabepilone
- Albumin-bound paclitaxel eribulin

Although drug combinations are often used to treat early breast cancer, advanced breast cancer is more often treated with single chemo drugs. Still some combinations, such as carboplatin or cisplatin plus gemcitabine, are commonly used to treat advanced breast cancer.

TARGETED THERAPY

15. Discuss the different agents for targeted therapy. ***WBUHS 2023***

Targeted Therapy

Targeted therapy is a type of cancer treatment that targets proteins that control how cancer cells grow, divide, and spread.

Types

- Monoclonal antibodies
- Small-molecule inhibitors

Monoclonal Antibodies

Monoclonal antibodies can be classified as targeted therapy or immunotherapy, depending on the type of monoclonal antibody.

Types of targeted therapy monoclonal antibodies include:

Type	*Mechanism of action*	*Examples*
Angiogenesis inhibitors	These drugs reduce the blood supply to a tumor to slow or stop it growing. They target various proteins linked with the growth of new blood vessels and stop them from working	Bevacizumab
Human epidermal growth factor receptor 2- (HER2)-targeted agents	High levels of the protein HER2 cause cancer cells to grow uncontrollably. Some targeted therapy drugs destroy the HER2 positive cancer cells or reduce their ability to divide and grow	• Trastuzumab • Pertuzumab
Anti-CD20 monoclonal antibodies	These drugs target a protein called CD20 found on some B-cell leukemia and non-Hodgkin lymphomas	• Rituximab • Obinutuzumab

Small Molecule Inhibitors

These drugs are small enough to get inside cancer cells and block certain proteins that tell cancer cells to grow.

Types of small molecule inhibitors include:

Type	*Mechanism of action*	*Examples*
Tyrosine kinase inhibitors (TKIs)	TKIs block proteins called tyrosine kinases from sending signals that tell cancer cells to grow, multiply, and spread. Without this signal, the cancer cells may die	• Erlotinib • Sunitinib • Imatinib • Dasatinib
Mammalian target of rapamycin (mTOR) inhibitors	These drugs block mTOR, a protein that tells cancer cells to grow and spread	Everolimus
Poly (ADP-ribose) polymerase (PARP) inhibitors	These drugs block PARP, a protein that repairs damaged DNA in cancer cells	Olaparib
Cyclin-dependent kinase (CDK) inhibitors	These drugs block cyclin-dependent kinase (CDK) from sending signals that tell cancer cells to grow, multiply, and spread. Without this signal, the cancer cells may die	• Palbociclib • Ribociclib • Abemaciclib

16. Write short notes on targeted therapy in GI malignancy.

Introduction

- GI cancers are among the top 10 most prevalent and deadliest tumors worldwide.
- It accounts for 26% of global cancer incidence and 35% of all cancer-related deaths.
- Surgical resection remains the primary treatment option for patients with CRC, gastric cancer (GC), and EC.
- Despite advances in adjuvant and neoadjuvant chemoradiotherapy (CRT), a fair number of patients still develop distant metastases and therapy resistance.
- To improve the prognosis of GI cancers, new therapeutic strategies are urgently needed. Over the last few decades, immune-targeted therapy has emerged as a revolutionary option for cancer treatment.
- However, the regulatory role of the immune system underlying GI cancers remains to be clarified.
- With the development of immunotherapy, cancer immunotherapy mainly based on checkpoint inhibitors has shown great prospects in clinical research, which shows the importance of immunotherapy in cancer treatment.

Molecular targets and signaling pathways of various targeted therapies used in the treatment of GI cancers.

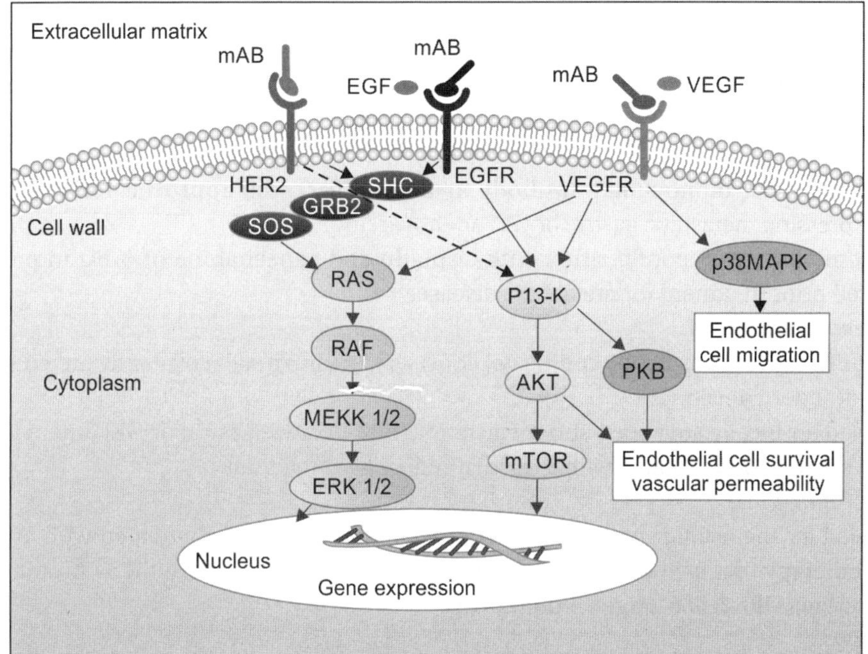

Agents	*Antibodies*	*TKIs*	*Blocks intracellular pathways*
Mechanism of action	Blocks membrane receptors	Prevents phosphorylation	Affects various pathways in the cell
Examples			
Targeting EGFR (HER-1)	• Cetuximab • Panitumunab	• Erlotinib • Gefitinib	Rapamycin and everolimus—blocks mTOR pathway
Targeting EGFR (HER-2)	Trastuzumab	Lapatinib	Sorafenib—inhibits RAF pathway
Targeting VEGFR	• Bevacizumab (binds VEGFR) • Ramucirumab (binds VEGFR)	• Sunitinib • Sorafenib • Apatinib	
Targeting PDGFR		Sorafenib	
Targeting HGFR	Onartuzumab	• Foretinib • Crizotinib	

(EGFR: epidermal growth factor receptor; HER: human epidermal growth factor receptor; HGFR: hepatocyte growth factor receptor; mTOR: mammalian target of rapamycin; PDGFR: platelet-derived growth factor receptor; RAF: rapidly accelerated fibrosarcoma; TKIs: tyrosine kinase inhibitors; VEGFR: vascular endothelial growth factor receptor)

Immunotherapeutic Strategies in GI Cancer

- Activating the immune response—cytokines
- Immune checkpoint inhibitors
- Chimeric antigen receptor (CAR) T cell therapy
- Targeted therapy-mediating immune cells
- Tumor vaccines

Clinical Applications

- *GE cancer:*
  - *Ramucirumab:*
    - The angiogenesis inhibitor ramucirumab (cyramza) is for the treatment of advanced stomach cancer or GEJ adenocarcinoma in patients with unresectable or metastatic disease following therapy with a fluoropyrimidine- or platinum-containing regimen.
  - *Pembrolizumab:*
    - Pembrolizumab is approved, in combination with trastuzumab, fluoropyrimidine- and platinum-containing chemotherapy, for the first-line treatment of locally advanced unresectable or metastatic gastric or GEJ adenocarcinoma that is positive for human epidermal growth factor receptor 2 (HER2).
    - Pembrolizumab received approval for gastric or GEJ carcinoma in patients expressing PD-L1 with disease progression on or after 2 or more prior lines of therapy.
  - *Trastuzumab:*
    - Trastuzumab, a monoclonal antibody against HER2, was approved for the treatment of HER2-overexpressing metastatic gastric or GEJ adenocarcinoma.
    - It is administered in combination with cisplatin and capecitabine or 5-FU in patients who have not received prior treatment for metastatic disease.
  - *Trastuzumab deruxtecan:*
    - First HER2-directed antibody conjugate, consists of trastuzumab covalently linked to the topoisomerase I inhibitor deruxtecan.
    - It is used for locally advanced and metastatic HER2-positive gastric or GEJ adenocarcinoma in patients who were previously treated with a trastuzumab-based regimen.
  - *Tipiracil/trifluridine:*
    - It is used for metastatic gastric or GEJ adenocarcinoma previously treated with at least 2 prior lines of chemotherapy that included a fluoropyrimidine; a platinum agent; either a taxane or irinotecan; and if appropriate, HER2/neu-targeted therapy.
  - *Nivolumab:*
    - It is used for first-line immunotherapy in combination with fluoropyrimidine- and platinum-containing chemotherapy for advanced or metastatic GC, GEJ cancer, and esophageal adenocarcinoma.
  - *Bevacizumab:*
    - Bevacizumab, a monoclonal antibody against VEGF has been evaluated for use in advanced GC.
- *Colorectal cancer:*

VEGFR inhibitors	*EGFR inhibitors*	*BRAF inhibitor*	*HER2 inhibitors*	*Target cells with NTRK gene*	*Multi kinase inhibitor*
• Bevacizumab • Ramucirumab • Zivaflibercept	• Cetuximab • Panitumumab	Encorafenib	• Trastuzumab • Pertuzumab • Tucatinib • Lapatinib • Famtrastuzumab deruxtecan	• Larotrectinib • Entrectinib	Regorafenib

(EGFR: epidermal growth factor receptor; HER2: human EGF receptor 2; NTRK: neurotrophic tyrosine receptor kinase; VEGFR: vascular endothelial growth factor receptor)

- *Pancreatic neuroendocrine tumors (PNETS):*
  - Two targeted therapy drugs are approved for the treatment of advanced PNETs:
    - Sunitinib
    - Everolimus
- *Bile duct cancer:*
  - Fibroblast growth factor receptor 2 (FGFR2) inhibitors:
    - Pemigatinib
    - Infigratinib
    - Futibatinib
- *Gallbladder cancer:*
  - Two types of immunotherapy are approved to treat gallbladder tumors with a certain genetic marker called microsatellite instability.
    - Pembrolizumab
    - Nivolumab
- *HCC:*

Kinase inhibitors		***VEGFR inhibitors***
• Sorafenib • Lenvatinib	• Regorafenib • Cabozantinib	• Bevacizumab • Ramucirumab

- *Small bowel cancers:*
  - Insulin-like growth factor receptor (IGFR) inhibitors:
    - Cetuximab
    - Panitumumab
- *GI stromal tumors:* The targeted drugs used to treat GISTs are called tyrosine kinase inhibitors (TKIs), because they target proteins that are tyrosine kinases, such as KIT and platelet-derived growth factor receptor alpha (PDGFRA).
- *Imatinib:*
  - This drug is used to treat most people with GISTs at some point
  - Tumors can be tested for certain mutations in the *KIT* and *PDGFRA* genes before treatment, which can help tell how likely it is that imatinib will be helpful
  - This drug targets both the KIT and PDGFRA proteins, blocking their ability to help tumor cells grow and divide. In most GISTs, the cells have too much of one of these proteins
  - Imatinib can be helpful in different situations.
- *Sunitinib:*
  - This drug can be useful in treating GISTs if imatinib is no longer working or if a person cannot take imatinib for some reason.
  - Sunitinib targets the KIT and PDGFRA proteins, as well as several other proteins that imatinib does not target.
- *Regorafenib:*
  - Regorafenib can be used to treat advanced GISTs if imatinib and sunitinib stop working, or if a person cannot take these drugs for some reason.
  - This drug targets many proteins, including KIT and PDGFRA.
- *Ripretinib:*
  - Ripretinib is typically used to treat advanced GISTs if other TKIs such as imatinib, sunitinib, and regorafenib are no longer helpful, or if a person cannot take these drugs for some reason.
  - This drug targets many kinase proteins, including KIT and PDGFRA.

- *Avapritinib:*
  - This is another TKI that targets PDGFRA and KIT, as well as several other proteins.
  - Avapritinib is used mainly to treat advanced GISTs whose cells have a change in the PDGFRA gene known as an exon 18 mutation.
  - These cancers typically do not respond well to treatment with the TKIs mentioned above.
- *Other TKIs:*
  - Sorafenib
  - Nilotinib
  - Dasatinib
  - Pazopanib

STEREOTACTIC SURGERY AND DRUG DELIVERY SYSTEM

17. Explain the principles of "stereotactic surgery" and its applications. ***WBUHS 2023***

18. What are the recent advances in drug delivery systems (DDS) for enhancing drug penetration into tumors? ***WBUHS 2023***

Introduction

Stereotactic radiosurgery utilizes externally generated ionizing radiation to inactivate or eradicate defined targets in the head or spine without the need to make an incision. This concept requires steep-dose gradients to reduce injury to adjacent normal tissue while maintaining treatment efficacy in the target.

Main Principles

- Basic principles of radiation biology have been traditionally referred to as the four Rs: Repair, repopulation, reoxygenation, and reassortment.
- Stereotactic radiosurgery allows precise delivery of a single high-radiation dose to a defined target volume and rapid dose falloff outside this volume.
- Stereotactic surgery aims at introducing cannula or electrodes with high precision into the deeply located small brain structures along a straight path.
- The required target point is determined by consulting CT/MR images of the patient and is achieved by means of a mechanically precise apparatus.

Mechanical Components of the Stereotactic System

The system consists of the following main components:

- *Basic ring:* This is rigidly fixed (under anesthesia) on the patient's skull. It provides a fixed reference system in all three directions of the room.
- *Localization disks:* These are attached to the ring and used to calculate the coordinates of the destination from CT/MR images. The stereotactic frame in CT with laser must be aligned exactly parallel to the gantry.

Uses

- To treat various brain cancers, benign, and functional disorders of the brain
- This is sometimes combined with whole brain radiotherapy can be used for single brain metastasis.
  - *Amongst the malignant brain disorders are:* Brain metastasis and glioblastoma.
  - *The benign brain disorders:* Meningioma, cerebral arteriovenous malformation, vestibular schwannoma, and pituitary adenoma
  - *Functional disorders:* Trigeminal neuralgia, Parkinson's disease, and epilepsy.

Recent DDS are formulated with improved properties such as smaller particle size, increased permeability, increased solubility, efficacy, specific site targeting, stability, toxicity, and sustained delivery.

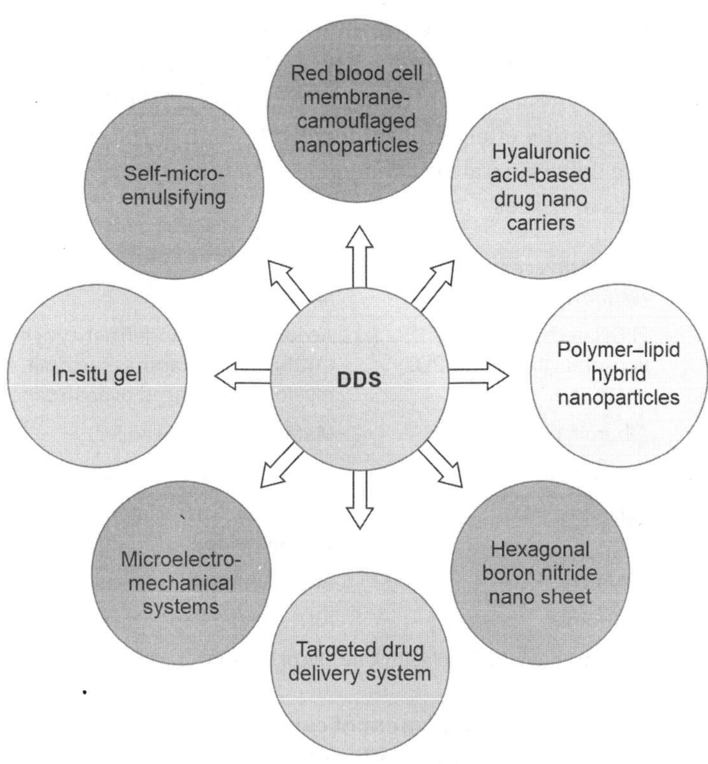

(DDS: drug delivery system)

Recent drug delivery system	***Advantages***	***Disadvantages***	***Therapeutic use***
Red blood cell membrane-camouflaged nanoparticles drug delivery system	• Avoids triggering the immune system and achieves long- term circulation • Inherent biocompatibility and biodegradability which avoid accumulation-related toxicity	Being camouflaged as part of the biological system, complex issues of regulation may arise; also, protein identification, purification, and conjugation may be bypassed	• Erythrocyte membrane-coated • Nanoformulations have been applied in antitumor and anticancer research to substantial accomplishment
Hyaluronic acid-based drug nanocarriers drug delivery systems	Good biocompatibility, biodegradable, and nonimmunogenicity; it has the ability to recognize overexpressed cells and kill them	They may increase cell proliferation when they interact with certain protein receptors, potentially hazardous to cancer patients	Cancer chemotherapy
Hexagonal boron nitride nanosheet drug delivery system	Biocompatibility, very little to no level of toxicity, high drugloading ability	Hydrophobicity makes it challenging to function in a biological system	Used in tumor labeling and sensing
Polymer–lipid hybrid nanoparticles drug delivery system	Physical stability in encapsulation and biocompatibility, in vivo cell delivery efficacy	Poor drug entrapment and loading capacity inflammation and tissue damage can affect or inactivate lipids in serum	Targeted anticancer therapy
Self-micro-emulsifying drug delivery system	Bioavailability of poor solubility drugs, long duration stability, protection of drug sensitive materials, availability of the liquid and solid forms of	Interaction of drugs could potentially accelerate physical aging in patients due to interactions of glyceride and oxidation of vegetable oil	Used In the treatment of pulmonary infections

The advanced drug delivery systems such as liposomes, nanoparticles, and dendrimer have enhanced pharmacokinetic properties for anticancer therapeutics. For earlier detection of cancer biomarkers in the blood circulation, new, advanced drug delivery systems were designed with increased selectivity and sensitivity.

Nanocarriers can enhance the targeting effect on tumor cells through surface modifications to precisely deliver drugs to tumor tissue. Such a precise delivery strategy can increase the tumor accumulation of drugs, thereby reducing their toxic side effects on normal cells or tissues.

Therapeutic agent	*Drug delivery system technology*	*Indication*	*Administration route*
Doxil (doxorubicin)	PEGylated or stealth liposomal (liposome-PEG)	Acquired immunodeficiency syndrome (AIDS)-related Kaposi's sarcoma, multiple myeloma, advanced ovarian cancer	IV
Abraxane (paclitaxel)	Albumin bound	Metastatic breast cancer	IV
DepoCyt (cytarabine)	Liposomal	Malignant lymphomatous meningitis	IT
Neulasta (pegfilgrastim)	Polymeric (PEG)	Neutropenia associated with cancer chemotherapy	SC
Oncaspar (L-asparaginase)	Polymeric (PEG)	Acute lymphoblastic leukemia	IV, IM
DaunoXome (daunorubicin)	Liposomal	AIDS-related Kaposi's sarcoma	IV

(IM: intramuscular; IT: intrathecal; IV: intravenous; PEG: polyethylene glycol; SC: subcutaneous)

19. Discuss multidisciplinary approach in management of cancer.

Srimanta Sankaradeva University, Assam 2025; KIIT University, Odisha 2025

A *multidisciplinary approach* in the management of cancer is a coordinated, team-based strategy that brings together *specialists from different medical and allied health disciplines* to provide *comprehensive, patient-centered care.*

This approach ensures that *all aspects of the disease—medical, surgical, psychological, and social—are addressed,* improving outcomes, quality of life, and patient satisfaction.

Concept and Rationale

Cancer is a *complex, multisystem disease* involving:

- Variable biology and behavior,
- Multiple treatment modalities (surgery, chemotherapy, radiotherapy, targeted therapy, etc.),
- Significant psychosocial and economic impact.

No single specialist can manage all these dimensions effectively. Hence, *a multidisciplinary team (MDT)* is essential.

Goals of a Multidisciplinary Approach

- *Comprehensive evaluation* of each patient's disease and overall health.
- *Individualized treatment planning* based on tumor type, stage, comorbidities, and patient preference.
- *Optimal sequencing and integration* of therapies (e.g., neoadjuvant vs. adjuvant).
- *Improved communication* among professionals and with patients.
- *Enhanced psychosocial, nutritional, and palliative support.*

Members of the Multidisciplinary Cancer Team

Specialist	*Primary Role in Care*
Medical Oncologist	*Systemic therapy:* Chemotherapy, targeted therapy, immunotherapy
Surgical Oncologist/Surgeon	Tumor resection, biopsy, staging surgery
Radiation Oncologist	Radiation planning and delivery

Contd...

Contd...

Specialist	*Primary Role in Care*
Pathologist	Diagnosis, grading, staging, molecular profiling
Radiologist/Nuclear Medicine Specialist	Imaging for diagnosis, staging, treatment response
Palliative Care Specialist	Symptom control, end-of-life care, quality of life
Oncology Nurse/Nurse Navigator	Patient education, coordination, monitoring side effects
Pharmacist	Chemotherapy safety, drug interactions, dose adjustment
Nutritionist/Dietitian	Nutritional optimization during and after therapy
Physiotherapist/Occupational Therapist	Rehabilitation and functional recovery
Psychologist/Psychiatrist / Social Worker	Mental health, counseling, social and financial support
Genetic Counselor	Risk assessment, familial cancer syndromes
Primary Care Physician	Continuity of care, management of comorbidities

MDT Workflow

- *Case presentation*: The patient's history, imaging, pathology, and current condition are presented at an *MDT meeting.*
- *Discussion*: Each specialist gives input based on their expertise.
- *Consensus plan*: The team agrees on a treatment plan that balances efficacy, safety, and patient preference.
- *Implementation*: The plan is communicated to the patient and executed in a coordinated manner.
- *Follow-up and review*: Outcomes and side effects are reviewed regularly; plan is modified if needed.

Advantages of the Multidisciplinary Approach

Clinical Benefits

- More accurate diagnosis and staging.
- Evidence-based, individualized treatment.
- Improved survival and functional outcomes.
- Reduced risk of over- or under-treatment.

Patient-centered Benefits

- Better understanding of treatment options.
- Shared decision-making.
- Improved psychosocial support and quality of life.

Systemic Benefits

- Efficient use of resources.
- Enhanced communication among healthcare professionals.
- Improved adherence to clinical guidelines.

Challenges in Multidisciplinary Cancer Care

- *Coordination difficulties* (scheduling, communication).
- *Resource constraints* in low- and middle-income settings.
- *Variation in expertise* among institutions.
- *Data management and documentation* challenges.
- *Maintaining patient-centered focus* amidst complex decision-making.

Examples of Multidisciplinary Management

- *Breast cancer*
  - *Team:* Surgeon, radiologist, pathologist, medical and radiation oncologists, reconstructive surgeon, psychologist, nurse.

- *Plan:* Neoadjuvant chemo → surgery → radiation → hormonal or targeted therapy → follow-up and psychosocial care.
- *Colorectal cancer*
  - *Team:* Gastroenterologist, surgeon, oncologist, radiologist, pathologist, stoma therapist, nutritionist.
  - *Plan:* Preoperative staging → neoadjuvant chemoradiation (if rectal) → surgery → adjuvant therapy → surveillance.
- *Head and neck cancer*
  - *Team:* ENT surgeon, radiation oncologist, medical oncologist, speech therapist, dietitian, psychologist.
  - *Plan:* Combined chemoradiation or surgery + reconstruction → speech/swallowing rehabilitation → psychosocial support.

Role of MDT in Palliative and Survivorship Care

- Early integration of *palliative care* improves quality of life, symptom control, and sometimes survival.
- *Survivorship programs* address long-term issues: rehabilitation, fertility, secondary prevention, and mental health.

Conclusion

The *multidisciplinary approach* is the cornerstone of modern oncology practice.
It ensures that:

- Every patient benefits from the collective expertise of specialists
- Management is evidence-based yet individualized
- Physical, emotional, and social needs are addressed holistically.

20. What do you understand by personalized care in oncology? Describe its key components. ***AIIMS, Patna 2025***

Personalized care in oncology, often referred to as precision or personalized medicine, refers to an approach that tailors cancer prevention, diagnosis, treatment, and management to the unique characteristics of each patient. This includes factors such as their genetic profile, tumor biology, lifestyle, environment, and personal preferences, moving away from a one-size-fits-all model to optimize outcomes, minimize side effects, and improve quality of life.

Key Components

The main elements of personalized care in oncology typically include:

- *Genomic and molecular profiling:* Analyzing the patient's DNA, RNA, proteins, and tumor biomarkers to identify specific genetic mutations or alterations that drive the cancer. This informs targeted interventions and helps predict treatment responses.
- *Targeted therapies and precision treatments:* Using drugs or therapies designed to attack specific molecular targets in the cancer cells, such as tyrosine kinase inhibitors for certain mutations, while sparing healthy cells to reduce toxicity.
- *Immunotherapy customization:* Tailoring immune-based treatments, like checkpoint inhibitors or CAR-T cell therapy, based on the patient's immune system profile and tumor microenvironment to enhance the body's natural defenses against cancer.
- *Patient-centered assessment and planning:* Conducting holistic needs assessments to create individualized care plans that incorporate the patient's values, preferences, and overall health status, including supportive care for symptoms, mental health, and lifestyle factors.
- *Multidisciplinary collaboration:* Involving a team of specialists (e.g., oncologists, geneticists, pathologists, and nutritionists) to integrate diverse expertise and ensure comprehensive decision-making.
- *Informed consent and ethical considerations:* Ensuring patients are fully educated about potential benefits, risks, and alternatives, with ongoing monitoring to adjust plans as needed based on response and new data.

CHAPTER 40

Head and Neck

LEARNING OBJECTIVES

- Deep Cervical Fascia
- Jaw Tumors
- Neck Dissection
- Pathogenesis of Oral Cancer, Carcinoma Tongue
- Salivary Glands

1. Describe different layers of deep cervical fascia. Write down its significance and surgical importance.

WBUHS 2025 Supplementary

The *deep cervical fascia* is a complex and multilayered structure that surrounds the neck and supports the muscles, blood vessels, nerves, and organs within the neck. It acts as both a structural and functional framework for the cervical region. There are three primary layers of the deep cervical fascia, each with distinct anatomical and clinical significance:

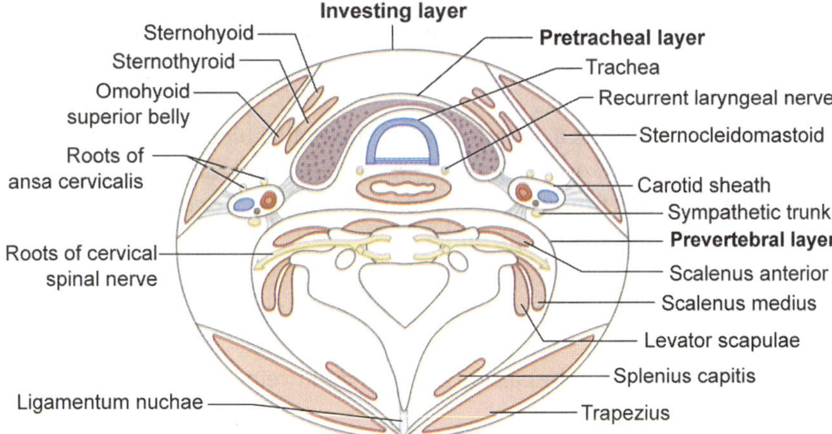

- **Superficial Layer (Investing Layer):**
  - *Anatomy:*
    - The superficial layer of the deep cervical fascia is the outermost layer. It completely surrounds the neck, enclosing structures like the sternocleidomastoid (SCM) and trapezius muscles.
    - It extends from the base of the skull to the upper thoracic region, forming a dense connective tissue sheath around the neck.
    - This layer divides into two parts around the sternocleidomastoid and trapezius muscles, creating a space known as the "prevertebral space."

- *Significance:*
  - Provides protection and structural support to the muscles and organs in the neck.
  - Limits the spread of infection or abscesses within the neck, acting as a barrier between different fascial compartments.
- *Surgical importance:*
  - Surgeons encounter the superficial layer during neck dissections, for example, when removing tumors in the neck or performing lymph node dissections. It may also be involved in procedures like tracheostomy.
  - If infected, it can limit the spread of a deep neck abscess, but in cases of severe infection, it may become involved, requiring careful dissection.

- **Middle Layer (Pretracheal and Prevertebral Fascia):**
  - *Anatomy:*
    - The *pretracheal fascia* surrounds the trachea, thyroid gland, and esophagus. It is a thin, delicate layer of fascia that encloses these structures and extends to the mediastinum.
    - The *prevertebral fascia* surrounds the vertebral column, cervical muscles, and the brachial plexus. It forms a sheath for the muscles of the cervical spine and helps anchor them in place.
  - *Significance:*
    - The *pretracheal fascia* is essential in maintaining the position of the thyroid gland, trachea, and esophagus within the neck and preventing displacement.
    - The *prevertebral fascia* provides structural support to the cervical spine and protects the deep cervical muscles and nerves.
  - *Surgical importance:*
    - The middle layer is vital during surgery for neck masses, particularly when dealing with the thyroid gland or trachea. It forms an important reference point for procedures like thyroidectomy and carotid endarterectomy.
    - Infections or abscesses in the middle layer can spread along the fascial planes to other regions, particularly into the chest, which can lead to life-threatening conditions.
    - The *prevertebral fascia* can become a key area to address in spinal surgery or cervical nerve surgery.
- **Deep Layer (Carotid Sheath):**
  - *Anatomy:*
    - The deep layer of fascia forms a sheath around the major blood vessels and nerves of the neck. This includes the *common carotid artery, internal jugular vein,* and the *vagus nerve.*
    - The carotid sheath extends from the base of the skull to the root of the neck and is in close association with the sympathetic trunk and lymph nodes.
  - *Significance:*
    - The carotid sheath contains critical neurovascular structures, and its integrity is essential for the proper function of these structures.
    - It acts as a protective barrier for the carotid artery, jugular vein, and vagus nerve from external mechanical forces or infections.
  - *Surgical importance:*
    - During carotid surgery, such as in carotid endarterectomy or carotid artery repair, the carotid sheath is often encountered and must be carefully dissected to avoid damaging the neurovascular structures it contains.
    - In neck trauma or surgeries, knowledge of the carotid sheath is essential for avoiding inadvertent injury to the carotid artery or jugular vein.
    - The carotid sheath is also important when addressing tumors or infections in the neck, as it helps surgeons understand the relationship between these structures and adjacent organs.

Clinical Significance of the Deep Cervical Fascia

The deep cervical fascia plays several crucial roles in clinical medicine, particularly in preventing the spread of infection and providing anatomical guidance for surgical procedures. It is of particular importance in:

- *Infections:*
  - Infections in the neck often spread along fascial planes. The deep cervical fascia can compartmentalize and limit the spread of infections, but when these fascial planes become involved (e.g., in a deep neck abscess), it can lead to significant morbidity.
  - An understanding of the fascial layers is crucial for effective drainage and treatment of deep neck infections.
- *Trauma:* In the case of blunt or penetrating trauma to the neck, understanding the fascial layers is essential to prevent damage to critical neurovascular structures. Surgical intervention may involve the release of the deep cervical fascia to access and repair injured structures.
- *Surgical Procedures:*
  - In procedures like thyroidectomy, lymph node dissection, or carotid endarterectomy, knowledge of the deep cervical fascia is important for identifying and preserving critical anatomical structures.
  - In some cases, the fascia is incised to expose deeper structures, but care must be taken to avoid damaging important nerves and vessels.
- *Cancer:* For cancers of the head and neck, the deep cervical fascia plays a role in the staging and prognosis, as the spread of malignancies may be limited by fascial boundaries. The fascia also serves as a guide in the planning of resection or radiation therapy.

---

2. Jaw tumors. ***WBUHS 2010***

Malignant Jaw Tumors

Malignancies are usually encountered in the upper jaw. Those in the mandible are rare. The malignant tumors of upper jaw are:

- Columnar cell cancer—carcinoma maxillary antrum
- Osteogenic sarcoma
- Squamous cell carcinoma (SCC)—from epithelium overlying hard palate, tooth socket, and gums
- Invasion of maxilla by sarcoma of ethmoid
- Lymphoma—Burkitt tumor

Osteogenic Sarcoma

- Seen in women over 40 years usually, men are infrequently involved
- It is usually of periosteal variety and the anterior part of the bone is usually involved.
- Later, the palatal and nasal walls get affected. Pain, nasal obstruction, and epiphora usually occur late in the disease.
- Histologically, it is of round cell variety, but rarely, it is highly differentiated fibromyxochondroma.
- Treatment is radiotherapy and outcome is fatal.

Carcinoma Maxillary Antrum

- This is the most common jaw malignancy and is seen beyond the age of 40 years, almost equal in both the sexes.
- Most of the patients have associated secondary infection of nasal sinuses.
- Clinical features—a line diagonal drawn from the inner canthus of the eye to the angle of the mandible divides the maxilla into two parts, a lower antro-alveolar and an upper antro-ethmoidal.
- Tumors in the antro-alveolar segment present with:
  - Bulge in lateral nasal wall
  - Bulge on the palate
  - Pain in teeth, not relieved by regular dental checkup

- Foul purulent blood-stained discharge from nose
- Free bleeding associated with antral puncture
- Tumors originating in the antro-ethmoidal segment present with
  - Bulge on the anterior face
  - Frog face
  - Proptosis and diplopia
  - Epiphora
  - Intracranial extension medially and infratemporal extension laterally
  - Trismus—involvement of pterygoid muscles
  - Palatal anesthesia—involvement of greater palatine nerve

Metastasis occurs late in the disease:

- The jugulodigastric lymph node is first to be involved.
- In one third of the cases, metastasis is seen as the first presenting symptom.
- Lymph nodes are only involved when the antrum is breached and lymphatic-rich hard palate and cheek get involved.

Biopsy

- This is best done by a diagnostic Caldwell-Luc operation.
- Antral lavage for exfoliative cytology is a poor second choice.

Treatment

- A judicious combination of radiotherapy and surgery is employed.
  - *Step 1:* A course of high voltage radiation 6,000 rads in 6 weeks or gamma ray from teleradium unit.
  - *Step 2:* Once the inflammation of radiotherapy subsides in 6–8 weeks, surgery is performed.
  - *Step 3:* This depends on the presence or absence of residual disease in the antrum
- Recurrences are treated by total maxillectomy or by radical maxillectomy, which include the eye and cribriform plate by adding a Dieffenbach extension and/or bicoronal incision with frontal craniotomy.
- Presence of lymph nodes in the neck—radical neck dissection
- Cytotoxic drugs are also used for recurrences with limited success.

Malignancies of the Mandible

- This is rarely a site for primary or even secondary tumor
- It often gets directly involved in carcinomas originating from the tongue, floor of mouth, or gingivolabial/gingivobuccal sulcus.
- Another method of neoplastic involvement is from the involved facial lymph node lying in juxtaposition to the mandible near the facial artery groove.
- The node once involved may invade the mandible.
- The treatment is hemimandibulectomy followed by mandibular reconstruction by free iliac bone graft or vascularized fibula.
- Radiation routinely causes osteoradionecrosis of the mandible.

Benign Jaw Tumors

Fibro-osseous Group

- Fibrous dysplasia
  - Monostotic—leontiasis ossea
  - Polyostotic
- Cherubism
- Paget's disease of jaw

Giant Cell Tumors

- Giant cell reparative granuloma

- Aneurysmal bone cyst
- Osteoclastoma
- Brown tumor of hyperparathyroidism

Fibrous Dysplasia

- It is a lesion of unknown etiology, uncertain pathology, and diverse histology.
- It is not strictly a neoplasm but behaves like one.
- It is a developmental derangement of bones caused by an aberrant activity of bone-forming mesenchymal tissue, resulting in abnormal proliferation of undifferentiated mesenchymal bone-forming cells.
- The bony lesion exhibits general histological features of fibrosis with varying degrees of simultaneous resorption and repair.
- The disease is either monostotic or polyostotic.
- Polyostotic variety is further classified into:
  - Fibrous dysplasia involving variable number of bones although most of the skeleton is normal and accompanied by pigmented lesions or café-au-lait spots—Jaffe type
  - A more severe disease involving nearly all the bones of the skeleton, accompanied by pigmented skin lesions and endocrine disturbances of various types—Albright's syndrome

Monostotic fibrous dysplasia is a totally different disease altogether and will not march on to become polyostotic type. It also does not manifest extra-skeletal lesions as seen in the polyostotic variety.

Treatment of polyostotic fibrous dysplasia is aimed at achieving facial symmetry. Total extirpation of tumor may not be the ultimate goal.

Monostotic lesions in the mandible are excised en-bloc and the mandible is reconstructed by vascularized bone graft.

Paget's Disease of the Jaws

- This may be a part of generalized Paget's disease or confined mainly to the jaws.
- A differential diagnosis of polyostotic fibrous dysplasia
- It occurs in older people.
- It is painful and radiological appearance of teeth, if they are any, show apical club-shaped swellings—cementosis.
- Treatment is aimed at achieving facial symmetry by bone contouring.
- Sarcomas develop more often in the jawbones affected by Paget's disease.

Giant-cell Reparative Granuloma

- Females are more prone to develop this type of lesion than males.
- Nearly, always between the age of 10 and 25 years
- Usually, a history of trivial trauma and a painless swelling in the jaw, usually the mandible
- X-ray reveals expansion of both tables with a unilocular or multilocular cystic appearance. Other giant cell tumors are always in the differential diagnosis along with ameloblastoma.
- The lesion is not locally malignant, so if the inner table is thick, it can be treated by curettage and bone chip filling.
- If the condition recurs, hyperparathyroidism should be suspected, as even histologically it is very difficult to distinguish it from Brown tumor of hyperparathyroidism.

NECK DISSECTION

3. Discuss the different lymph node levels in the neck. ***WBUHS 2020***

4. What are the indications, types, and basic steps of radical neck dissection?
WBUHS 2007, 2023; RIMS, Imphal 2022

5. Discuss the role of radical neck dissection for the management of head and neck cancer. ***WBUHS 2016***

6. Types of neck node dissection and their indications. ***WBUHS 2025 Supplementary***

7. List the different types of neck dissections. Describe the operative steps of one of the types.
RGUHS Karnataka 2025

The cervical lymphatic nodal basins contain between 50 and 70 lymph nodes per side and are divided into seven levels:

- *Level I is subdivided into IA and IB:*
  - Level IA is bounded by the anterior belly of the digastric muscle, the hyoid bone, and the midline.
  - Level IB is bounded by the anterior and posterior bellies of the digastric muscle and the inferior border of the mandible. Level IB contains the submandibular gland.
- *Level II:* It is bounded superiorly by the skull base, anteriorly by the stylohyoid muscle, inferiorly by a horizontal plane extending posteriorly from the hyoid bone, and posteriorly by the posterior edge of the sternocleidomastoid muscle (SCM). Level II is further subdivided into IIA and IIB.
  - Level IIA is anterior to the spinal accessory nerve.
  - Level IIB, or the so-called submuscular triangle, is posterior to the nerve.
- *Level III:* It begins at the inferior edge of level II and is bounded by the laryngeal strap muscles anteriorly, by the posterior border of the SCM posteriorly, and by a horizontal plane extending posteriorly from the inferior border of the cricoid cartilage.
- *Level IV:* It begins at the inferior border of level III and is bounded anteriorly by the strap muscles, posteriorly by the posterior edge of the SCM, and inferiorly by the clavicle.
- *Level V:* It is posterior to the posterior edge of the SCM, anterior to the trapezius muscle, superior to the clavicle, and inferior to the base of skull.
- *Level VI:* It is bounded by the hyoid bone superiorly, the common carotid arteries laterally, and the sternum inferiorly. Although level VI is large in area, the few lymph nodes that it contains are mostly in the para- tracheal regions near the thyroid gland.
- *Level VII (superior mediastinum):* It lies between the common carotid arteries and is superior to the aortic arch and inferior to the upper border of the sternum.

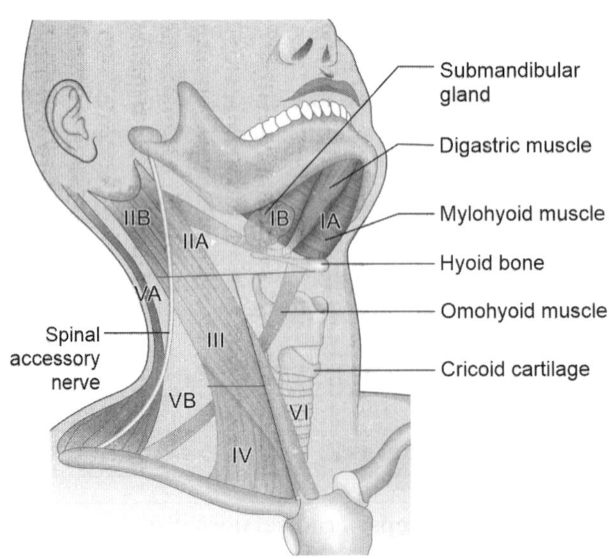

Classification of Different Types of Neck Dissection with Clinical Indications

Comprehensive	*Nodal levels removed*	*Structures preserved*	*Indications*
Radical neck dissection	Levels I–V	None	N+ neck for SCC where SAN involved
Modified radical neck dissection type I	Levels I–V	SAN	N+ neck for SCC where SAN free of disease
Modified radical neck dissection type II	Levels I–V	SAN, SCM	N+ neck for SCC where IJV involved but SAN free of disease
Modified radical neck dissection type III	Levels I–V	SAN, SCM, IJV	Metastatic differentiated thyroid carcinoma
Selective			
Supraomohyoid neck dissection	Levels I–III	SAN, SCM, IJV	N0 neck for SCC of oral cavity and oropharynx (include level 4). N0 neck malignant melanoma where primary site is anterior to ear (includes parotidectomy for face and scalp)
Extended supraomohyoid neck dissection	Levels I–IV	SAN, SCM, IJV	N0 neck for SCC of lateral tongue
Lateral neck dissection	Levels II–IV	SAN, SCM, IJV	N0 neck for SCC of larynx and hypopharynx
Posterolateral neck dissection	Levels II–V, suboccipital, retroauricular nodes	SAN, SCM, IJV	N0 neck malignant melanoma where primary site is posterior to ear
Lateral neck dissection	Levels II–IV	SAN, SCM, IJV	N0 neck for SCC of larynx and hypopharynx
Posterolateral neck dissection	Levels II–V, suboccipital, retroauricular nodes	SAN, SCM, IJV	N0 neck malignant melanoma where primary site is posterior to ear

(SAN: spinal accessory nerve; SCC: squamous cell carcinoma; SCM: sternocleidomastoid muscle; IJV: internal jugular vein)

Basic Steps of Radical Neck Dissection

The surgical incision is made starting at the lateral neck from beneath the jaw to the supraclavicular area.

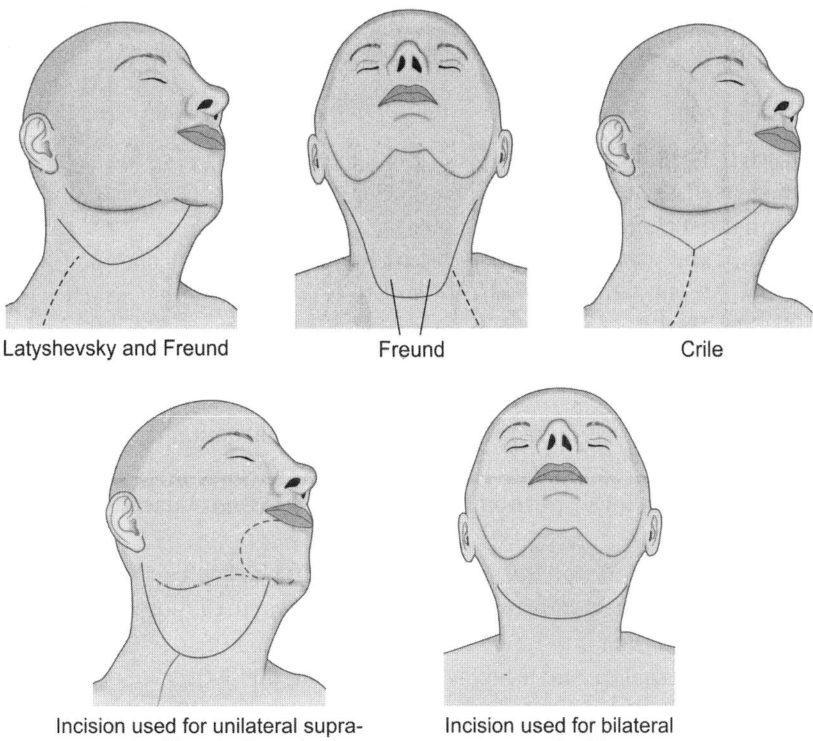

- Skin flaps are mobilized, while hemostasis is achieved using fine hemostats as well as ligatures on bleeding vessels.
- Once the skin flaps are freed, traction sutures are placed in different areas of the skin flap, and then a hemostat on the end.
- This is done to retract the skin flap for better exposure. Using curved scissors, the anterior trapezius muscle is exposed as well as the external jugular vein.
- The trapezius muscle and the external jugular vein are clamped, ligated, and divided.
- The internal jugular vein (IJV) is dissected out, isolated, and divided.
- The omohyoid muscle is identified and transected.
- The fatty tissue in the neck contains lymph nodes.
- These lymph nodes are dissected away from other structures, and the common carotid artery and vagus nerve are identified.

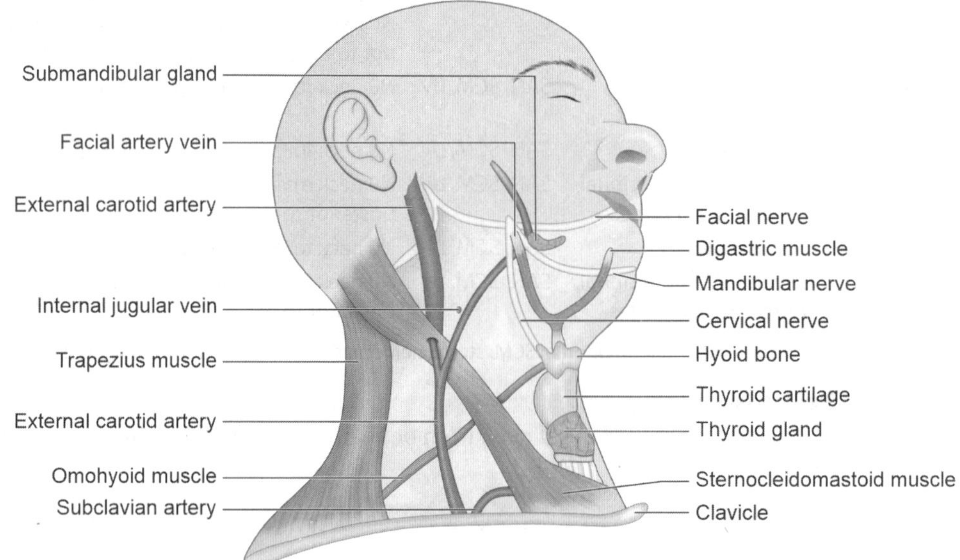

- The thyrocervical artery is then clamped, divided, and ligated.
- The posterior triangle is dissected starting at the anterior of the trapezius muscle up to the brachial plexus, the levator scapulae, and the scalene muscles.
- Branches of the cervical and suprascapular arteries are identified and then clamped, ligated, and divided. Once the anterior dissection is complete, the omohyoid muscle is severed where it attaches to the hyoid bone.
- Hemostasis is controlled and all hemostats are removed.
- The surgical field is then covered with warm, moist, sterile packs. After that, the SCM is cut and retracted out of the way.
- At this point, the submental space is dissected from fatty tissue that contains lymph nodes, starting upward and working down.
- The fascia lying deep into the lower portion of the mandible is then incised and the facial vessels are then divided and ligated.
- Submandibular triangle is entered, and the submandibular duct is divided and ligated.
- The submandibular glands that have fatty tissue and lymph nodes surrounding them are dissected going toward the digastric muscle.
- The facial branch of the external carotid artery is identified and divided.
- Parts of the digastric, as well as the stylohyoid muscles are then cut, where they attach to the hyoid bone and mastoid.

- The top end of the IJV is elevated and divided and the mass is removed.
- The entire surgical site is checked for any bleeding and irrigated with warm saline solution.
- If a skin graft is needed, it is placed over the bifurcation of the carotid artery downward about 4 inches, then sutured using 4-0 absorbable suture on a small, cutting needle.
- Hemovac drain, as per preference of the surgeon, is placed in the wound.
- The skin flaps are then approximated and closed with interrupted, fine nonabsorbable sutures or skin staples.
- A pressure dressing is applied to the neck, which also depends on the surgeon's preference.

Surgical Procedure

Radical Neck Dissection

- Procedure is done under general anesthesia.
- *Position:* Reverse Trendelenburg's position with neck extended at atlantoaxial joint and head elevated 10° above the table. Face should be turned to the opposite side of the dissection.
- Neck skin should be cleaned.
- Draping of the operating site is done.
- Preferred incision for radial neck dissection (RND) is Lahey's lateral utility incision in post-irradiated patients. Modified Schobinger's incision has been found to be useful in patients undergoing commando operation. MacFee's double horizontal incision can be used in some selected post-irradiated cases.
- Incision is marked with surgical marker pen, infiltrate with 10–15 mL of 1% xylocaine with 1:4 lacs adrenaline solution.
- After waiting for 5 minutes, skin incision is made with 10 number surgical blade, subplatysmal flap is raised superiorly till lower border of mandible, mastoid tip posteriorly, midline of neck anteriorly, anterior border of trapezius posteriorly, and till clavicle inferiorly.
- Then the lower part of SCM is cut with electrocautery, 2 cm above clavicle after dissecting it carefully from IJV.
- Dissect the IJV from its fascial attachments with common carotid artery and vagus nerve.
- The lower end of IJV is ligated at the level of common tendinous attachment of 2 bellies of omohyoid muscle crossing over IJV.
- Transfixation of the IJV is done after ligating with double ligatures. IJV is put up gradually with SCM after holding with Babcock forceps.
- Lymph nodes are dissected. Lymphatics, fat, and fascia from the supraclavicular fossa including level-5 nodes are cleared.
- Care has to be taken to avoid injuring brachial plexus, phrenic nerve, and transverse cervical vessels. At the junction of upper one third and lower two thirds of SCM muscle, greater auricular nerve (GAN) can be seen exiting from cervical plexus crossing over external jugular vein along posterior border.
- GAN winds around the posterior border of SCM and crosses obliquely upward to enter into the tail of parotid gland. Spinal accessory nerve also exits at this point, known as Erb's point and runs in the posterior triangle to enter into trapezius muscle.
- These nerves have to be dissected from cutaneous branches supplying the fascia and skin. Middle thyroid vein is ligated at the level of thyroid cartilage and all lymph nodes along the middle one third of IJV are removed, thus clearing level 3 and 4.
- After reaching the upper end of IJV, dissect at the level of posterior belly of digastric muscle, which is the landmark for ligating the upper end. Bony landmark is the transverse process of atlas.
- Ligate with double ligatures, transfix with 3-0 silk suture, and cut the IJV after ligating the venae comitantes for hypoglossal nerve.
- This will clear level 2a and 2b lymph nodes. Last step is removal of level 1a and 1b nodes along with submandibular gland. Remove the complete specimen en bloc.
- The field is irrigated with normal saline and dilute povidone iodine solution.
- After securing hemostasis, negative suction 14–16 FG size drain is placed.

- After repositioning the skin flap, first layer is sutured with 3-0 absorbable suture and skin with staples/3-0 monofilament sutures.
- Apply pressure dressing and check the drain function before extubating the patient.
- Postoperatively, patient is kept in Fowler's position and given intravenous (IV) antibiotics for 5 days.
- Drain is removed when collection is <10 mL.
- Sutures can be removed on 7th postoperative day.

Points to Remember

- Lymph node metastasis reduces the survival of patients with SCC by half.
- The survival rate is <5% in patients who previously underwent surgery and have a recurrent metastasis in the neck.
- Therefore, the control of cancer that has spread to the neck is one of the most important aspects in the successful management of these particular cancers.
- The neck dissection is a standardized procedure that was developed to ensure the complete removal of cancer that has spread to the lymph nodes of the neck.

8. Discuss the N1 cervical lymph nodes at level 2 with unknown primary. *WBUHS 2023*

- *N1:* The cancer has spread to a single lymph node on the same side as the primary tumor and the cancer found in the node is 3 cm or smaller.
- Level II nodes are internal jugular nodes above the level of the hyoid bone.
- In early stages (N1), neck dissection and radiotherapy seem to have similar efficacy.

First-echelon Lymph Nodes for Various Primary Sites

Level 1: Oral cavity, oropharynx
Level 2: Oral cavity, oropharynx, larynx, nose, hypopharynx, parotid, nasopharynx
Level 3: Oral cavity, oropharynx, larynx, hypopharynx, thyroid, nasopharynx
Level 4: Larynx, thyroid, hypopharynx, esophagus
Level 5: Nasopharynx, hypopharynx, thyroid, oropharynx
Level 6: Thyroid, larynx, hypopharynx, cervical esophagus

Diagnostic Workup

- *Clinical evaluation:*
  - Personal history, focusing on tumor history
  - Performance status, respiratory system, and cardiovascular evaluation with electrocardiography (ECG); complete ear, nose, and throat (ENT) clinical and fiberscopic evaluation, careful examination of surgical scars
- *Imaging:* Chest X-ray, thyroid, and neck ultrasound (US)
- *Fine needle aspiration (FNA) biopsy (slides review if biopsied elsewhere):*
  - Examinations following cyto/histopathological diagnosis:
    - *SCC or undifferentiated carcinoma:*
      - Magnetic resonance imaging (MRI)/computed tomography (CT)
      - Positron emission tomography (PET)-CT
      - Anti-Epstein–Barr virus (EBV) antibodies evaluation (in case of undifferentiated carcinoma)
      - Physical examination under general anesthesia, including inspection and palpation of the oral cavity, base of tongue, oropharynx, and nasopharynx.
      - Direct laryngoscopy and pharyngoscopy.
      - Biopsy of any abnormal mucosa. If there are no visible or palpable abnormalities and the FNA suggests SCC or poorly differentiated malignancy, biopsy of sites of suspected primary, depending on the position of the involved nodes.

This usually includes biopsies of the nasopharynx, base of the tongue, and pyriform sinus.

- *Adenocarcinoma:*
  - MRI/CT
  - PET-CT
  - Prostate-specific antigen (PSA), cancer antigen 125 (CA-125), and carcinoembryonic antigen (CEA) assay.
  - Liver enzymes and function tests (since nodal disease in the neck may be manifestation of meta- static disease from a primary site below the clavicle, in which case, metastatic liver disease may also be present)
  - Salivary glands, thyroid, lungs physical and imaging evaluation, mammography
  - CT scan of the abdomen and pelvis, and gastrointestinal (GI) imaging or endoscopy/colonoscopy according to the location of the neck node, the patient's age, individual risk factors, and the results of pelvic/rectal examinations.
- Lymphomas
- Lymph node biopsy

Management

Various therapeutic approaches are being employed for carcinoma with unknown primary (CUP) including surgery and radiotherapy alone or combined treatment (surgery, radiotherapy, and chemotherapy). The choice of the treatment depends on the histology and the stage of the disease.

- *SCC:*
  - Biopsy and neck dissection and radiotherapy
  - N1 disease without extracapsular extension and with no history of incisional or excisional biopsy—surgery followed by radiotherapy
  - N1 disease with previous biopsy—postoperative irradiation
  - In the head and neck cancer management, hyperfractionated radiotherapy was used in CUP patients, although its superiority over conventional irradiation remains to be established.
  - Another innovative strategy tested in CUP patients was the combination of radiotherapy and hyperthermia.
- *Adenocarcinoma:*
  - Excisional biopsy
  - If clinical and pathological evaluation cannot identify the source of the primary, then neck dissection (levels I–V) can be done, including parotidectomy if indicated, generally followed by radiotherapy.

9. Give an account of "secondaries neck" and its management. ***Tripura University, 2024***

Definition

- *"Secondaries in the neck"* refer to *metastatic deposits of malignant cells in the cervical lymph nodes* originating from a *primary malignancy located elsewhere*—most commonly in the *upper aerodigestive tract (UADT)* (oral cavity, oropharynx, larynx, nasopharynx, etc.).
- These metastatic nodes are of *squamous cell carcinoma (SCC)* origin in most cases, as SCC is the commonest cancer type in the head and neck region.

Pathophysiology

Malignant cells from the primary tumor spread via *lymphatic channels* to the *regional cervical lymph nodes.*

- Lymphatic drainage of the *oral cavity and pharynx* determines which group of cervical nodes are affected.
- Once tumor cells lodge in the lymph node, they proliferate and may:
  - Replace nodal tissue
  - Break through the capsule (→ *extracapsular spread*)
  - Invade surrounding soft tissues (→ *fixed node*).

Common Primary Sites for Neck Secondaries

Neck level involved	*Common primary site*
Level I (Submental, Submandibular)	Oral cavity (lip, anterior tongue, floor of mouth)
Level II (Upper jugular)	Oral cavity, oropharynx, parotid, nasopharynx
Level III (Mid-jugular)	Oropharynx, hypopharynx, larynx
Level IV (Lower jugular)	Hypopharynx, thyroid, cervical esophagus
Level V (Posterior triangle)	Nasopharynx, scalp, thyroid, lymphoma
Level VI (Central compartment)	Thyroid, larynx, trachea, esophagus

Clinical Features

- *Neck mass:* Firm, non-tender, usually unilateral (may be bilateral in nasopharyngeal carcinoma).
- *Mobility:* Mobile in early stage → fixed in advanced stage (due to extracapsular spread).
- *Associated features:*
  - Dysphagia, odynophagia, voice change.
  - Non-healing ulcer or lesion in oral cavity/pharynx.
  - Sometimes *no obvious primary*—termed *"Carcinoma of Unknown Primary (CUP)"*.

Diagnosis

- *Clinical Examination*
  - Full head and neck examination to locate possible primary site.
  - Palpation of all neck levels.
- *Imaging*
  - *Ultrasound neck + FNAC* (Fine Needle Aspiration Cytology)—confirms metastatic SCC.
  - *CT/MRI neck:* Extent and relation to surrounding structures.
  - *PET-CT scan:* Especially useful in identifying occult primary.
- *Biopsy*
  - FNAC preferred over excision biopsy (to avoid disturbing lymphatic drainage).
  - If FNAC inconclusive → *core needle biopsy.*
- *Endoscopic Examination:* Panendoscopy (examination of nasopharynx, oropharynx, hypopharynx, larynx, esophagus) under anesthesia to detect primary lesion.

Staging (Nodal Stage – AJCC 8th Edition)

Stage	*Description*
N1	Single ipsilateral node ≤3 cm, no extracapsular spread
N2a	Single ipsilateral node 3–6 cm, no extracapsular spread
N2b	Multiple ipsilateral nodes ≤6 cm
N2c	Bilateral or contralateral nodes ≤6 cm
N3	Node >6 cm or any node with extracapsular spread

Management

- *Identify and Treat the Primary Tumor*
  - Essential step
  - Management tailored according to the *primary site, stage,* and *general condition* of the patient
- *Neck Management*

  Surgical Treatment

  Neck dissection is the mainstay for resectable metastatic nodes.

Types of Neck Dissection

Type	Description	Indication
Radical Neck Dissection (RND)	Removal of all lymph nodes (levels I–V) along with sternocleidomastoid (SCM), internal jugular vein (IJV), and spinal accessory nerve (SAN)	Grossly involved, fixed nodes; extracapsular spread
Modified Radical Neck Dissection (MRND)	Same as RND, but one or more non-lymphatic structures (SCM, IJV, SAN) are preserved	Most common type; for clinically positive but mobile nodes
Selective Neck Dissection (SND)	Removes selected nodal levels only (e.g., I–III, II–IV)	Elective or limited nodal involvement
Extended Neck Dissection	Includes additional structures or nodal groups beyond standard RND	Advanced cases with spread beyond typical levels

Radiotherapy (RT)

- *Used:*
  - As *adjuvant* after surgery (positive margins, extracapsular spread)
  - As *definitive treatment* in inoperable or medically unfit patients
  - As *postoperative adjuvant* RT for high-risk features

Chemoradiotherapy

- Combined *cisplatin-based chemoradiation* for:
  - Unresectable disease
  - Extracapsular nodal spread
  - Advanced nodal disease (N2/N3)
  - Carcinoma of unknown primary (CUP)
- Management of "Neck Secondaries with Unknown Primary"
- When no primary site is found despite thorough work-up:
  - *Ipsilateral (or bilateral) modified radical neck dissection,* followed by: *Radiotherapy* to likely mucosal sites (nasopharynx, oropharynx, base of tongue) and neck
  - If histology suggests SCC, upper aerodigestive tract is presumed primary

Prognosis

- *Depends on:*
  - Size and number of involved nodes
  - Presence of extracapsular spread
  - Primary site and histologic grade
- *Single small mobile node:* 5-year survival ~70–80%
- *Multiple/fixed nodes:* 5-year survival drops to <40%

10. Pathogenesis of oral cancer. *WBUHS 2006*

Risk Factors for Oral Cancer

- *Tobacco:*
  - In India and other Asian countries, oral neoplasia has been associated with chewing tobacco with betel quid (BQ), while in Western countries, smoking and heavy alcohol consumption are the main risk factors.
  - Consumption of chewing tobacco-containing BQ increases exposure to carcinogenic tobacco-specific nitrosamines (TSNA) and nitrosamines derived from areca nut alkaloids.
  - In addition, significant amounts of reactive oxygen species (ROS) are formed in the oral cavity during chewing, which are involved in multistep carcinogenesis.
- *Betel quid and areca nut:*
  - Betel chewing is found to be the most important factor for the development of oral submucosal fibrosis.

  - Use of betel and tobacco-containing areca nuts is associated with a much higher relative risk of oral cancer of 8–15 times compared to 1–4 times the risk associated with no tobacco use.
- *Alcohol:* Alcohol can act both independently as well as synergistically with smoking in oral carcinogenesis
- *Viruses:*
  - Human papillomavirus (HPV) is closely associated with benign and malignant oral lesions.
  - This virus can be isolated from condylomas, focal epithelial hyperplasia, squamous cell papilloma, and malignant oral lesions.
- *Diet:*
  - Fruits and vegetables high in vitamins A and C are protective in oral neoplasia.
  - Meat and red chili powder are risk factors.
  - Vegetables and fruits rich in beta-carotene and vitamins C and E are protective due to their antioxidant property.
  - Iron deficiency, resulting in oral epithelial atrophy and the Plummer–Vinson (Patterson Brown Kelly) syndrome, is associated with cancer of upper air and food passages and dietary iron may play a protective role in maintaining the thickness of the epithelium.
- *Family history of head and neck SCC (HNSCC):* Epidemiological evidence from case-control studies of HNSCC indicates that a family history of head and neck cancer is a risk factor.
- *Immune deficiency:*
  - In a person infected with the human immunodeficiency virus (HIV), a defective immune response can promote cancer.
  - The most common oral malignancy in HIV-infected patients is Kaposi's sarcoma, which is caused by human herpes virus type 8 (HHV-8).
  - Lymphoma, mostly non-Hodgkin B-cell lymphoma in HIV-infected individuals, or other immunosuppressed states, is commonly associated with EBV and may occur in the head and neck.
  - Oral SCC of the lip is more likely to occur in transplant patients who receive immunosuppressive treatment, but HIV infection is not a risk factor for intraoral carcinogenesis.
- *Candida:*
  - *Candida albicans* can induce epithelial proliferation and can produce carcinogens from procarcinogens in vitro.
  - Chronic hyperplastic candidosis presents as nodular or speckled, white mucosal plaques.
  - They are potentially malignant oral epithelial lesions.

Molecular Changes in Oral Cancer

- Cancer occurs through multiple steps, each characterized by the sequential stimulation of additional genetic defects, followed by clonal expansion.
- The genetic alterations observed in head and neck cancer are mainly due to oncogene activation and tumor suppressor gene inactivation, leading to deregulation of cell proliferation and death.
- These genetic alterations include gene amplification and overexpression of oncogenes such as c-myc, c-erbB-2, epidermal growth factor receptor (EGFR), cyclin D1 and mutations, deletions, and hypermethylation, leading to *p16* and *p53* tumor suppressor gene (TSG) inactivation.

TSGs and Growth Regulators

- Growth regulators and TSGs act as transducers of negative growth signals.
- Genetic alterations involving the tumor suppressor genes *p16* and *p53,* are frequently observed in head and neck tumors.
- Genetic abnormalities inactivating the *p16* gene might confer cell growth defects, contributing to the tumorigenic process.
- These genes are involved in cell cycle regulation, including cell cycle arrest and apoptosis.
- Alteration in both alleles of a gene is required for the loss of function.

Genomic Instability

- The evaluation of the genomic stability can be done using techniques such as loss of heterozygosity (LOH) screening and comparative genomic hybridization (CGH).
- LOH of the *p53* allele has been reported in 20% of oral SCC (OSCCs), as well as in 22% of premalignant oral lesions.
- The risk of progression from premalignancy to cancer is low—when no genetic changes were seen, intermediate—if there is genetic loss on the short arms of chromosomes 3 and 9 (3p and 9p), and high—if there is 3p and 9p loss accompanied by genetic loss on additional chromosome arms, including 4q, 8p, 11q, 13q, and 17p.
- The LOH of the *H-ras* allele may encompass a tumor suppressor gene in the vicinity of the oncogene. Loss of chromosome 11 alleles has been reported in a number of tumors.

Role of Deregulated Apoptosis in the Pathogenesis of Oral Cancer

- The deregulation of apoptosis-related genes aids in successful carcinogenesis.
- The relative contribution of apoptosis and proliferation to disease progression in the oral mucosa was examined using terminal deoxynucleotidyl transferase nick end-labeling (TUNEL) assay and Ki-67 staining.
- Further apoptosis-related cell cycle regulators, namely retinoblastoma (Rb), cyclin D1, and fragile histidine triad gene (FHIT) were analyzed for LOH, gene amplification, and aberrant transcripts, respectively, in oral cancer samples.
- Status of *p53*, bcl-2, and Bax members of the *p53*-dependent apoptotic pathway were evaluated in oral cancers/oral lesions by immunohistochemistry.
- Frequent overexpression of apoptosis regulators *p53*, bcl-2, and Bax was observed in oral cancers and a subset of oral lesions.
- It was further revealed that there is overexpression of antiapoptotic members of the bcl-2 family namely, bclxL and Mcl-1 in oral cancer cell lines.
- These studies thus indicate that evasion of apoptosis via abnormal expression of bcl-2, bclxL, mcl-1, and *p53* may contribute to oral cancer pathogenesis.

Enhanced Telomerase Activity

The ribonucleoprotein enzyme telomerase extends the telomeric repeat sequences at the chromosomal ends and it is active in a majority (90%) of human neoplasia but inactive in most normal cells.

Neovascularization

- The steps critical to successful angiogenesis include the degradation of the extracellular matrix, endothelial cell proliferation, migration, and assembly of endothelial cells into higher-order structures.
- In the majority of cancers, highly vascularized tumors showed a poor prognosis and the influence of tumor angiogenesis proved to be independent of conventional prognostic indicators.

Cytokine Profile

- Suppression of *Th1* cytokine genes was reported due to increase in tumor load and lymph node invasion, which skewed it toward a *Th2*-like cytokine response.
- HNSCCs express interleukin-4 receptors in situ and interleukin-13 was secreted by HNSCCs but does not modulate their growth in vitro.
- It has been postulated that these cytokines, in addition to others, were responsible for the growth pattern of these tumors and could be responsible for their active spread.

---

11. What are the predisposing factors for carcinoma tongue? What are the premalignant conditions for carcinoma tongue? Discuss about role of neck dissection in carcinoma tongue.

Predisposing Factors for Carcinoma Tongue

- Tobacco smoking and alcohol ingestion are major risk factors.
- Riboflavin and iron deficiencies are known to produce dysplastic changes to the oral mucosa. This may partly explain its relationship to alcoholism, which may result in riboflavin deficiency and oral cancer.

- HPV is an etiological factor for SCC.
- Sharp teeth and spicy food
- Hematopoietic stem cell transplantation
- Vitamins A and C, along with the carotenoids, may be protective against epithelial cancers.

Premalignant Conditions for Carcinoma Tongue

- White patches (leukoplakia)
- Red patches (erythroplakia) or mixed red and white patches (erythroleukoplakia or "speckled leukoplakia")
- Oral lichen planus (particularly the erosive type)
- Oral submucous fibrosis
- Actinic cheilitis
- Plummer–Vinson syndrome

Lymphatic Drainage of Tongue

- *Anterior tongue:* Level Ia nodes (submental nodes)
- *Lateral tongue:*
    - *Level Ib nodes:* Submandibular
    - *Level Ii nodes:* Upper jugulodigastric nodes
    - Potentially drain directly to level IV nodes
- *Posterior tongue:* Level II nodes (upper jugulodigastric nodes)

Role of Neck Dissection

- *Neck dissection is warranted for T3/T4 oral cavity carcinoma,* but there has been an ongoing controversy in the treatment of clinically negative neck in T1/T2.
- The risk of occult metastases in N0 SCC of the oral cavity is 20–30% and was found highest for tongue carcinoma.
- Elective supraomohyoid neck dissection (SOHND) detects occult metastases in early node-negative oral tongue SCC and is sufficient to remove the majority of lymph node metastases.
- Patients with early oral SCC, exhibiting occult metastases should be considered as high-risk patients.
- Elective neck dissection (END) significantly reduced mortality by lymph nodal metastasis and increased the 5-year free survival especially in patients with stage T2 OSCC and suggested END as a preferred treatment strategy for tongue carcinoma in stage T2.

---

12. Discuss the pre-malignant condition of oral cancer. Describe the management of early cancer tongue.

KIIT University, Odisha 2025

Definition

Pre-malignant (potentially malignant) condition refers to a generalized state of the oral mucosa associated with a significantly increased risk of cancer development *anywhere* in the oral cavity.

- The World Health Organization (WHO) now uses the term "Oral Potentially Malignant Disorders" (OPMDs) instead of "pre-cancerous conditions and lesions."

Classification

OPMDs can be divided into two groups:

I. *Pre-malignant Lesions:*
   Localized alterations in oral mucosa with a higher risk of malignant transformation.

- *Leukoplakia:*
    - *Definition:* A *white patch or plaque* that cannot be characterized clinically or pathologically as any other disease.
    - *Risk:* 5–25% may show dysplasia or carcinoma on biopsy.

- *Common sites:* Buccal mucosa, tongue, floor of mouth.
- *Types:* Homogeneous (flat, thin, uniform) and non-homogeneous (nodular, speckled, verrucous).

- *Erythroplakia*
  - *Definition:* A *bright red, velvety patch* that cannot be classified as another condition.
  - High-risk lesion — over 90% show severe dysplasia, carcinoma in situ, or invasive carcinoma.
- *Speckled Leukoplakia (Erythroleukoplakia)*
  - Mixed red and white lesion, higher malignant potential than homogeneous leukoplakia.

II. *Pre-malignant Conditions*

Generalized disorders associated with an increased risk of oral cancer development.

- *Oral Submucous Fibrosis (OSMF)*
  - Chronic, progressive condition caused mainly by areca nut (betel nut) chewing.
  - *Features:* Stiffness of oral mucosa, trismus, burning sensation, blanching.
  - Malignant transformation rate: 7–13%.
- *Lichen Planus (Oral Lichen Planus - OLP)*
  - Immune-mediated mucocutaneous disorder.
  - *Common forms:* Reticular (lace-like), erosive, atrophic.
  - Erosive and atrophic forms carry higher malignant potential (~1–3%).
- *Discoid Lupus Erythematosus (DLE)*
  - Chronic autoimmune condition affecting skin and oral mucosa.
  - Malignant transformation: 1–2%.
- *Syphilitic Glossitis*
  - Seen in tertiary syphilis; causes epithelial atrophy and scarring.
  - Predisposes to carcinoma of the tongue.
- *Xeroderma Pigmentosum*
  - Genetic disorder with defective DNA repair mechanism.
  - Increased risk of skin and mucosal malignancies.

Management of Early Cancer Tongue

Definition

Early cancer of the tongue refers to *carcinoma of the oral tongue (anterior two-thirds)* that is confined to the tongue and has *not yet metastasized extensively* to lymph nodes or distant sites.

According to the *TNM staging (AJCC 8th edition)*, early cancer of the tongue usually corresponds to:

- *Stage I:* T1 N0 M0 → Tumor ≤2 cm in greatest dimension, depth of invasion (DOI) ≤5 mm, no nodal or distant metastasis.
- *Stage II:* T2 N0 M0 → Tumor 2–4 cm or DOI 5–10 mm, no nodal/distant metastasis.

Objectives of Management

- Achieve *complete local tumor control.*
- Prevent *regional lymph node metastasis.*
- Preserve *speech, swallowing, and appearance* (functionally and cosmetically acceptable outcome).
- Provide *close surveillance* for recurrence.

Evaluation and Staging

Before treatment, the patient undergoes:

- *Clinical examination* of the oral cavity and neck.
- *Imaging:*
  - MRI/CT scan—to assess local invasion and depth of infiltration.
  - Ultrasound neck ± FNAC - for lymph node evaluation.
- *Biopsy*—to confirm squamous cell carcinoma (SCC) and grade it histologically.

Treatment Modalities

A. *Primary Tumor Management*

Choice depends on tumor size, site, depth of invasion, and patient's condition.

- Surgery (Preferred for Most Cases)
  - Wide local excision (WLE) with adequate margins (1 cm clinically/5 mm histologically).
  - For small T1/T2 lesions:
    - *Partial glossectomy* (for lateral lesions).
    - *Hemiglossectomy* if lesion involves midline.
  - *Reconstruction* may be done with local flaps (e.g., primary closure, skin grafts, or myocutaneous flaps) to preserve tongue mobility and function.
- *Radiotherapy (RT)*
  - Alternative to surgery for small T1 lesions (especially in medically unfit or non-surgical candidates).
  - *Modalities:*
    - *External beam radiotherapy (EBRT)* or
    - *Interstitial brachytherapy* (Iridium-192).
  - *Radiation dose:* Typically 60–70 Gy.
- *Combined modality*
  - Surgery followed by adjuvant RT if:
    - Close/positive margins,
    - Perineural or lymphovascular invasion,
    - DOI >10 mm,
    - Poor differentiation.

B. *Management of the Neck*

Even in early tongue cancers, *occult metastasis* to lymph nodes occurs in ~20–30% cases.

- *N0 Neck (Clinically Negative Nodes)*
  - *Elective neck dissection (END)* is recommended if:
    - Depth of invasion (DOI) >3–4 mm.
    - Poorly differentiated tumor.
  - *Types of END:*
    - *Supraomohyoid neck dissection (SOHND)* – levels I, II, III.
    - *Selective neck dissection (levels I–III).*
  - Alternatively, *watchful waiting* with close follow-up if DOI ≤3 mm.
- *N+ Neck (Clinically Positive Nodes)*
  - *Therapeutic neck dissection* (modified radical or selective) + adjuvant RT/chemoradiation depending on histopathology.

C. *Adjuvant Therapy*

- *Postoperative radiotherapy (PORT)* indicated for:
  - Positive/close margins,
  - Lymphovascular or perineural invasion,
  - DOI >10 mm,
  - Node-positive disease.
- *Chemoradiotherapy* is reserved for:
  - Positive margins not amenable to re-excision,
  - Extracapsular spread in lymph nodes.

Rehabilitation

- *Speech and swallowing therapy* after surgery.

- *Nutritional support* – nasogastric feeding initially, then oral rehabilitation.
- Physiotherapy to maintain tongue mobility.

Follow-Up

- Regular follow-up is critical for early detection of recurrence.
    - Every 1–3 months for the first 2 years.
    - Every 3–6 months for the next 3 years.
    - Annual check-ups thereafter.
- Inspection and palpation of tongue and neck at each visit.
- Imaging if recurrence is suspected.

Prognosis

- *Stage I:* 5-year survival ~80–90%.
- *Stage II:* 5-year survival ~70–80%.
- Prognosis worsens with nodal involvement, poor differentiation, or deeper invasion.

13. Treatment plan for carcinoma tongue anterior two-thirds and management of secondary in neck from with occult primary. ***WBUHS 2017***

Treatment

- Surgery
- Radiotherapy
- Chemotherapy

Surgery

- *Tumor <1 cm in size/carcinoma in situ:*
    - Wide excision with 1 cm clearance in margin and depth
    - Laser (CO_2/diode) can be used.
- *Tumor between 1 and 2 cm in size:* Partial glossectomy with 2 cm clearance from the margin with removal of one third of anterior two-thirds of the tongue.
- *Tumor >2 cm:*
    - Hemiglossectomy is done with removal of anterior one third of tongue on one side up to sulcus terminalis.
    - Raw area can be left alone when area is wide, allowing it to granulate and heal by epithelialization.
    - If area is small, like in wide excision, it can be closed by primary suturing.
    - Wide raw area can also be covered with pectoralis major myocutaneous flap (PMMF) or quilted split-skin graft.
- *Larger primary tumor:*
    - Preoperative radiotherapy can be given, followed by hemiglossectomy.
    - Ipsilateral palpable, mobile lymph nodes are removed by radical neck block dissection.
    - Bilateral mobile lymph nodes are dealt with one side radical block and other side functional block dissection with essentially retaining IJV (on opposite side) to maintain the cerebral venous blood flow.
    - Another option is doing same-side radical neck dissection and on opposite side supraomohyoid block dissection.

Treatment and Prognosis

- For small tumors, excision is possible with a hemiglossectomy or partial hemiglossectomy. Reconstruction of the tongue depends on the size of the defect.
- When less than a third of the tongue has been resected, primary closure is possible. Larger defects require pedicle or free-flap reconstruction.

- Larger lesions which cross the midline, although sometimes technically resectable with a total glossectomy, are usually not resected due to the operation being poorly tolerated.
- In tumors that extend laterally across the floor of mouth and into the mandible, resection is challenging, often requiring segmental mandibulectomy and reconstruction.
- *Radiotherapy* is often used either in conjunction with surgery or alone in advanced cases.
  - Patients treated with local or regionally advanced disease are treated most successfully with a combined modality therapy of surgery, radiation therapy, and chemotherapy.
  - Concomitant chemotherapy [with 5-fluorouracil (5-FU) and cisplatin] and radiation therapy appear to be the most effective sequencing of treatment.
- Patients with recurrent and/or metastatic disease are with few intentions treated with palliative intent. Chemotherapy can be used for transient symptomatic benefit.
- Drugs with single-agent activity in this setting include methotrexate, 5-FU, cisplatin, paclitaxel, and docetaxel. Combinations of cisplatin and 5-FU, carboplatin and 5-FU, and cisplatin and paclitaxel are also used.

PAROTID GLANDS

14. Sjögren syndrome. ***WBUHS 2010***

Essentials of Diagnosis

- 90% of patients are female; the average age is 50 years.
- Dryness of eyes and dry mouth (sicca components) are the most common features; they occur alone or in association with rheumatoid arthritis or other connective tissue disease.
- Rheumatoid factor and other autoantibodies common
- Increased incidence of lymphoma

General Considerations

- Sjögren syndrome is a systemic autoimmune disorder whose clinical presentation is usually dominated by dryness of the eyes and mouth due to immune-mediated dysfunction of the lacrimal and salivary glands.
- The disorder is predominantly seen in women, with a ratio of 9:1; most cases develop between the ages of 40 and 60 years.
- Sjögren syndrome can occur in isolation ("primary" Sjögren syndrome) or in association with another rheumatic disease.
- Sjögren syndrome is most frequently associated with rheumatoid arthritis.
- It can also occur with systemic lupus erythematosus (SLE), primary biliary cirrhosis, scleroderma, poly- myositis, Hashimoto thyroiditis, polyarteritis, and interstitial pulmonary fibrosis.

Symptoms and Signs

- Keratoconjunctivitis sicca results from inadequate tear production caused by lymphocyte and plasma cell infiltration of the lacrimal glands.
- Ocular symptoms are usually mild burning, itching, and the sensation of having a foreign body or a grain of sand in the eye occur commonly.
- For some patients, the initial manifestation is the inability to tolerate wearing contact lenses. Many patients with more severe ocular dryness notice ropy secretions across their eyes, especially in the morning. Photophobia may signal corneal ulceration resulting from severe dryness.
- Most of the patients experience dryness of the mouth (xerostomia). The persistent oral dryness causes most patients to carry water bottles or other liquid dispensers from which they sip constantly.
- A few patients have such severe xerostomia that they have difficulty speaking.

- Persistent xerostomia results often in rampant dental carries; carries at the gum line strongly suggest Sjögren syndrome.
- Some patients experience loss of taste and smell.
- Parotid enlargement, which may be chronic or relapsing, develops in one third of patients. Desiccation may involve the nose, throat, larynx, bronchi, vagina, and skin.
- Systemic manifestations are dysphagia, vasculitis, pleuritis, obstructive lung disease (in the absence of smoking), neuropsychiatric dysfunction (most commonly peripheral neuropathies), and pancreatitis; they may be related to the associated diseases noted earlier.
- Renal tubular acidosis (type I, distal) occurs in 20% of patients.
- Chronic interstitial nephritis, which may result in impaired renal function, may be seen.
- A glomerular lesion is rarely observed but may occur secondary to associated cryoglobulinemia.

Laboratory Findings

- Laboratory findings include mild anemia, leukopenia, and eosinophilia.
- Polyclonal hypergammaglobulinemia, rheumatoid factor positivity (70%), and antinuclear antibodies (95%) are all common findings.
- Antibodies against the cytoplasmic antigens SS-A and SS-B (also called Ro and La, respectively) are often present in primary
- Sjögren syndrome tends to correlate with the presence of extraglandular manifestations.
- Thyroid-associated autoimmunity is a common finding among patients with Sjögren syndrome.
- Useful ocular diagnostic tests include the Schirmer test, which measures the quantity of tears secreted.
- Lip biopsy reveals characteristic lymphoid foci in accessory salivary glands.
- Biopsy of the parotid gland should be reserved for patients with atypical presentations such as unilateral gland enlargement that suggest a neoplastic process.

Differential Diagnosis

- Chronic hepatic C can cause sicca symptoms.
- Minor salivary gland biopsies reveal lymphocytic infiltrates but not to the extent of Sjögren syndrome and tests for anti-SS-A and anti-SS-B are negative.
- Diffuse infiltration of CD8 T cells producing parotid gland enlargement can develop in HIV-infected individuals.
- Involvement of the lacrimal or salivary glands, or both in sarcoidosis can mimic Sjögren syndrome; biopsies reveal noncaseating granulomas.
- Rarely, amyloid deposits in the lacrimal and salivary glands produce sicca symptoms.

Treatment and Prognosis

- Treatment is symptomatic and supportive.
- Artificial tears applied frequently will relieve ocular symptoms and avert further desiccation.
- The mouth should be kept well lubricated. Sipping water frequently or using sugar-free gums and hard candies usually relieve dry mouth symptoms.
- Pilocarpine (5 mg orally four times daily) and the acetylcholine-derivative cevimeline (30 mg orally three times daily) may improve xerostomia symptoms.
- Atropinic drugs and decongestants decrease salivary secretions and should be avoided. A program of oral hygiene, including fluoride treatment, is essential in order to preserve dentition.
- If there is an associated rheumatic disease, its systemic treatment is not altered by the presence of Sjögren syndrome.

Prognosis

- Sjögren syndrome may compromise patients' quality of life significantly.
- The disease is usually consistent with a normal life span.

- Poor prognosis are influenced mainly by the presence of systemic features associated with underlying disorders, the development in some patients of:
  - Lymphocytic vasculitis
  - Painful peripheral neuropathy
  - Complication (in a minority of patients) of lymphoma
- The patients (3–10% of the total Sjögren population) at greatest risk for developing lymphoma are those with severe exocrine dysfunction, marked parotid gland enlargement, splenomegaly, vasculitis, peripheral neuropathy, anemia, and mixed monoclonal cryoglobulinemia.

---

15. Describe the anatomy of submandibular triangle with its clinical importance.

WBUHS 2025 Supplementary

Anatomy of the Submandibular Triangle:

The *submandibular triangle* is one of the subdivisions of the anterior triangle of the neck. It is located beneath the mandible and contains important anatomical structures.

Boundaries:

- *Superior:* Inferior border of the mandible
- *Anterior:* Anterior belly of the digastric muscle
- *Posterior:* Posterior belly of the digastric muscle
- *Floor:* Mylohyoid, hyoglossus, and part of the middle pharyngeal constrictor muscles
- *Roof:* Skin, superficial fascia, platysma, and deep cervical fascia

Contents:

I. *Submandibular gland* (major salivary gland)
II. *Facial artery and vein*
III. *Submental artery (branch of facial artery)*
IV. *Hypoglossal nerve (CN XII)*
V. *Mylohyoid nerve* (branch of mandibular nerve - CN V3)
VI. *Lymph nodes:* Submandibular lymph nodes

Clinical Importance:

- *Submandibular gland pathologies:*
  - Common site for *sialolithiasis* (salivary stones), especially in Wharton's duct.
  - *Submandibular gland infections* or tumors can cause swelling in the triangle.
- *Surgical access:*
  - Important area for *submandibular gland excision* or *lymph node biopsy.*
  - Risk of injury to the *marginal mandibular branch of the facial nerve, hypoglossal nerve,* or *lingual nerve* during surgery.
- *Lymphadenopathy:*
  - *Submandibular lymph nodes* can become enlarged in infections of the oral cavity, face, or upper respiratory tract.
  - Metastasis from cancers of the *tongue, floor of the mouth,* or *salivary glands* may present here.
- *Vascular considerations:* Injury to the *facial artery or vein* can cause significant bleeding during procedures.

16. Management of stones of submandibular salivary gland and duct. ***WBUHS 2015***

Diagnosis and Investigations:

- Radiographs of the submandibular gland and duct are helpful, although many calculi are not radio-opaque.
  - Lower occlusal X-ray of the teeth will show a stone in the submandibular duct.
  - A lateral oblique X-ray of the mandible will show a calculus in the submandibular gland.
- Submandibular duct radiography (sialography) is technically difficult and rarely gives more information than plain radiographs, although the flushing effect of the radio-opaque dye may give a therapeutic benefit.

Treatment

The traditional approach to obstructive salivary diseases recommends duct dilatation, incision, and dissection (sometimes followed by marsupialization with the risk of postoperative stricture) for distal stones and sialadenectomy for proximal, hilar, or intraparenchymal sialoliths.

Although sialolithiasis has been associated with a high incidence of chronic inflammation, suggesting that salivary gland obstruction has caused irreversible parenchymal damage, recent scintigraphic and histopathological studies have shown that recovery of secretory function after lithotomy is ensured in most cases. If general anesthesia is administered, the stones in the inner part of the ducts may be excised.

- Babcock forceps is used to steady the stone and incise is given directly over it. The stone is removed, and the duct is marsupialized.
- If stone/stones within the submandibular gland, removal of the submandibular gland is needed.
- Sialolithotripsy [extracorporeal shock wave lithotripsy (ESWL)] is a noninvasive method of fragmenting salivary stones into smaller portions in order to flush them out from the salivary duct system spontaneously or after salivation induced by citric acid or other sialogogues.

The Exclusion Criteria for ESWL

- Stones with a diameter of <2 mm
- Which cannot be identified using a US probe
- The presence of complete distal duct stenosis

Contraindications

- Patients with acute sialadenitis
- Acute inflammation in the head and neck region
- Patients with cardiac pacemakers.
- The main limitation of ESWL is that it does not always completely clear the calculus but leaves stone fragments inside the duct system that may subsequently become the nidus of recurrent sialolithiasis.

Other Treatment Modalities

- *Intracorporeal lithotripsy:* The shock waves reach the stone surface through a lithotripsy probe placed inside the salivary duct system under endoscopic guidance.
- Endoscopically guided intracorporeal laser lithotripsy
- Endoscopically controlled intracorporeal electrohydraulic lithotripsy
- Endoscopically controlled intracorporeal pneumatic lithotripsy
- Initially used for diagnostic purposes, sialoendoscopy is now scheduled interventionally in the case of obstructive salivary gland disease.
- Fluoroscopically guided stone retrieval is currently the best therapeutic option. It is indicated for mobile stones located in the middle and proximal portion of the submandibular ductal system.
- Endoscopically assisted removal of submandibular stones
- Botulinum toxin therapy

17. Surgical pathology of salivary gland tumors. *WBUHS 2007*

Tumors of the Major and Minor Salivary Glands

Benign	*Malignant*
• Pleomorphic adenoma • Warthin's tumor • Capillary hemangioma • Oncocytoma • Basal cell adenoma • Canalicular adenoma • Myoepithelioma • Sialadenoma papilliferum • Intraductal papilloma • Inverted ductal papilloma	• Acinic cell carcinoma • Mucoepidermoid carcinoma • Adenoid cystic carcinoma • Polymorphous low-grade adenocarcinoma • Epithelial–myoepithelial carcinoma • Basal cell adenocarcinoma • Sebaceous carcinoma • Papillary cystadenocarcinoma • Mucinous adenocarcinoma • Oncocytic carcinoma • Salivary duct carcinoma • Adenocarcinoma • Myoepithelial carcinoma • Malignant mixed tumor • Squamous cell carcinoma • Small cell carcinoma • Lymphoma • Metastatic carcinoma • Carcinoma ex pleomorphic adenoma

Pleomorphic Adenoma

- Remarkable histologic diversity
- Also been called mixed tumors
- They represent about 60% of tumors in the parotid, are less common in the submandibular glands, and are relatively rare in the minor salivary glands.
- They are benign tumors.
- They are derived from a mixture of ductal (epithelial) and myoepithelial cells and therefore show both epithelial and mesenchymal differentiation.
- They also have epithelial elements dispersed throughout a matrix along with varying degrees of myxoid, hyaline, chondroid (cartilaginous), and even osseous tissue.
- In some tumors, the epithelial elements predominate; in others, they are present only in widely dispersed foci.
- Equally uncertain is the histogenesis of the various components.
- A currently popular view is that all neoplastic elements, including those that appear mesenchymal, are of either myoepithelial or ductal reserve cell origin (hence the designation pleomorphic adenoma).
- *Morphology:* Most pleomorphic adenomas present as rounded, well-demarcated masses, rarely exceeding 6 cm in greatest dimension. Although they are encapsulated in some locations (particularly the palate), the capsule is not fully developed and expansile growth produces tongue-like protrusions.

Gross pathology	*Histology*
• Smooth • Well demarcated • Solid • Cystic changes	• Mixture of epithelial, myoepithelial, and stromal components • *Epithelial cells:* Nests, sheets, ducts, and trabeculae • *Stroma:* Myxoid, chondroid, fibroid, and osteoid • No true capsule • Tumor pseudopods

Warthin's Tumor

Gross pathology	Histology
• Encapsulated • Smooth/lobulated surface • Cystic spaces of variable size, with viscous fluid, and shaggy epithelium • Solid areas with white nodules, representing lymphoid follicles	• Papillary projections into cystic spaces surrounded by lymphoid stroma • *Epithelium:* Double cell layer • Luminal cells • Basal cells • *Stroma:* Mature lymphoid follicles with germinal centers

Oncocytoma

Gross pathology	Histology
• Encapsulated • Homogeneous, smooth • Orange/rust color	• Cords of uniform cells and thin fibrous stroma • Large polyhedral cells • Distinct cell membrane • Granular, eosinophilic cytoplasm • Central, round, vesicular nucleus

Mucoepidermoid Carcinoma

Gross pathology	Histology
• Well circumscribed to partially encapsulated to unencapsulated • Solid tumor with cystic spaces	• Low grade • Mucus cell > epidermoid cells • Prominent cysts • Mature cellular elements

18. Discuss etiology, presentation, and management of pleomorphic adenoma. *AIIMS, Bhopal 2023*

Etiology

Pleomorphic adenoma, also known as *benign mixed tumor,* is the *most common benign salivary gland tumor,* particularly affecting the *parotid gland* (~80% of cases).

Origin

- Arises from *epithelial and myoepithelial cells* of the salivary glands.
- Called "pleomorphic" due to its *histological diversity* – contains *epithelial, myoepithelial,* and *mesenchymal-like (stromal)* elements (e.g., cartilage, myxoid tissue).

Risk Factors/Associations

- Radiation exposure
- Female gender (more common in females, M:F = ~1:2)
- *Age:* Most common in *30–60 years*
- No strong genetic link, but certain chromosomal abnormalities (e.g., *PLAG1, HMGA2* gene rearrangements) have been noted.

Clinical Presentation

Symptoms:

- *Painless, slow-growing mass* (most commonly in the parotid region)
- Firm and mobile on palpation (unless deep-lobe or fixed)
- Usually *unilateral*
- No facial nerve involvement (unless malignant transformation)
- May be present for *months to years* before diagnosis

Common sites:

- *Parotid gland* (most common)
- Submandibular gland
- Minor salivary glands (e.g., palate, upper lip)

Management

Diagnosis:

Clinical examination: Mobile, firm, painless swelling in salivary gland region

Imaging:

- *Ultrasound:* Useful for initial assessment of superficial lesions
- *MRI* or *CT scan:* For deep lobe involvement or large tumors
  - Well-defined, lobulated mass
  - May show mixed solid and cystic components

Fine-needle aspiration cytology (FNAC):

- Common preoperative diagnostic tool
- Confirms benign nature but cannot definitively rule out malignancy

Treatment

Surgical Excision – Mainstay of Treatment

- *Superficial parotidectomy* (for tumors in superficial lobe of parotid)
- *Total conservative parotidectomy* (if deep lobe involved)
- *Wide local excision* (for minor salivary gland tumors)

Enucleation is contraindicated – high risk of recurrence due to incomplete removal or spillage of tumor cells.

Prognosis and Follow-up:

- Excellent prognosis if *completely excised*
- *Recurrence rate:* ~2–5% after proper surgery
- *Risk of malignant transformation:* ~2–10% over long duration (especially in long-standing or recurrent tumors)
  - Converts to *carcinoma ex pleomorphic adenoma* (aggressive)

---

19. Mention the anatomical landmarks for preoperative facial nerve identification during parotid surgery.

WBUHS 2021 Supplementary

---

20. Mention the different landmarks used in identifying facial nerve during superficial parotidectomy. Complications of superficial parotidectomy and how to prevent them?

WBUHS 2021 Supplementary, 2023; Tripura University 2023

---

21. Classify Parotid tumors. Enumerate the landmarks for intraoperative identification of facial nerve. What is pathophysiology of Frey's syndrome? Mention the causes of parotid fistula.

Classification of Parotid Tumor

I. Based on Nature

Benign tumors	***Malignant tumors***
• Pleomorphic adenoma *(most common overall)* • Warthin tumor *(second most common, almost always in parotid)* • Basal cell adenoma • Oncocytoma • Canalicular adenoma • Sebaceous adenoma • Myoepithelioma	• Mucoepidermoid carcinoma *(most common malignant parotid tumor)* • Adenoid cystic carcinoma • Acinic cell carcinoma • Carcinoma ex pleomorphic adenoma • Salivary duct carcinoma • Polymorphous low-grade adenocarcinoma • Adenocarcinoma NOS • Squamous cell carcinoma (primary or metastatic)

II. Based on Histological Origin

Epithelial Tumors (majority)	*Nonepithelial Tumors*
Include all of the above benign and malignant tumors	• Lymphoma • Sarcomas (rare) • Lipoma

III. WHO Classification (2022 Update)

The *World Health Organization (WHO)* classifies *salivary gland tumors* under the following categories:

Benign epithelial tumors	*Malignant epithelial tumors*
• Pleomorphic adenoma • Warthin tumor • Basal cell adenoma • Canalicular adenoma • Oncocytoma • Myoepithelioma • Sebaceous adenoma • Others	• Mucoepidermoid carcinoma • Adenoid cystic carcinoma • Acinic cell carcinoma • Salivary duct carcinoma • Secretory carcinoma • Epithelial-myoepithelial carcinoma • Carcinoma ex pleomorphic adenoma • Polymorphous adenocarcinoma • Basal cell adenocarcinoma • Others

During parotidectomy, after incising the deep cervical fascia, the lower pole of the parotid gland is dissected and lifted up. The digastric muscle is dissected up to its origin. The junction of the bony and cartilaginous part of the external auditory canal is delineated. The styloid process is palpated. The facial nerve emerges at this point through the stylomastoid foramen.

Landmarks

- Surgical landmarks to the facial nerve include the tympanomastoid suture line, the tragal pointer, and the posterior belly of the digastric muscle. The posterior belly of digastric muscle is inserted into the mastoid process just behind the stylomastoid foramen. By dissection at the medial border of the posterior belly of digastric near its insertion, facial nerve may be identified. The tympanomastoid suture line lies between the mastoid and tympanic segments of the temporal bone and is approximately 6–8 mm lateral to the stylomastoid foramen.
- The styloid process itself can be palpated superficial to the stylomastoid foramen and nerve is identified just lateral to the styloid process.
- There is a palpable groove between the bony external auditory meatus and the mastoid process which is filled with fibrofatty tissue. The facial nerve lies deep in this groove. The nerve lies at the junction of cartilaginous and bony part of external auditory canal.
- The main trunk of the nerve can also be found midway between (10 mm posteroinferior to) the cartilaginous tragal pointer of the external auditory canal and the posterior belly of the digastric muscle.
- The nerve is usually located inferior and medial to the pointer.

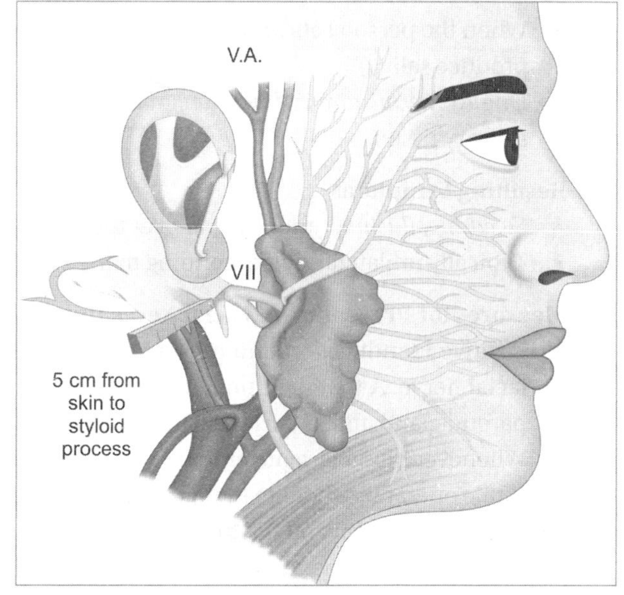

Potential complications of parotidectomy include facial nerve injury, Frey's syndrome, salivary leakage, ear numbness, facial asymmetry, flap necrosis, and tumor recurrence.

Complications of Superficial Parotidectomy

- Hematoma formation
- Infection
- Temporary facial nerve weakness
- Transection of the facial nerve and permanent facial weakness
- Sialocele
- Facial numbness
- Permanent numbness of the ear lobe associated with great auricular nerve transection
- Frey's syndrome

Pathophysiology of Frey's Syndrome

Frey's syndrome, also known as *gustatory sweating,* is a condition where a person sweats on the cheek or temporal region during eating or thinking about food. It most commonly occurs *after parotid gland surgery,* especially *parotidectomy.*

Normal Anatomy and Physiology

- The *parotid gland* receives *parasympathetic innervation* from the *auriculotemporal nerve,* a branch of the *mandibular division of the trigeminal nerve (CN V3).*
- This nerve carries *preganglionic parasympathetic fibers* from the *glossopharyngeal nerve (CN IX),* via the *otic ganglion,* to stimulate *saliva secretion.*
- The *sympathetic fibers* innervate *sweat glands* of the overlying skin via *postganglionic fibers* from the *superior cervical ganglion.*

Pathophysiology of Frey's Syndrome

Injury to Auriculotemporal Nerve

During *parotid surgery,* the *auriculotemporal nerve* (carrying parasympathetic fibers) is often *damaged* or *severed.*

Aberrant Regeneration (Miswiring)

- During healing, *parasympathetic fibers regenerate abnormally.*
- Instead of reconnecting to the *parotid gland,* they *grow into the sweat glands and blood vessels of the overlying skin* (usually preauricular or temporal region).

Stimulus Mismatch

- When the person eats or thinks about food, the *parasympathetic system is activated* (as it normally would be to produce saliva).
- Due to the *misdirected nerve regrowth,* these signals now stimulate *sweat glands and vasculature* instead of salivary tissue.

Resulting Symptoms

- *Sweating, flushing,* and *warmth* over the cheek during meals or salivation.
- Typically unilateral, corresponding to the side of surgery or trauma.

Measures for Prevention of Facial Nerve Injury

- Positive identification and preservation of the facial nerve are essential for preventing inadvertent injury to facial nerve. A thorough understanding of the anatomy of the stylomastoid foramen, the facial nerve, and the parotid gland and its surrounding structures is essential for the identification and preservation of the nerve.
- Whenever possible, a normal cuff of parotid tissue should be resected around a tumor to prevent recurrence.
- While operating a benign tumor, if a facial nerve branch is found directly on the tumor capsule, the nerve should be gently dissected off the tumor.
- In case of a malignancy, consideration should be given to sacrificing as opposed to preserving the nerve.

- Raw gland surface contributes to postoperative salivary leakage (sialocele or salivary fistula). In addition, raw gland in vicinity to skin provides a ready pathway for postganglionic parasympathetic fibers to migrate from the salivary tissue and cross-innervate facial sweat glands, resulting in gustatory sweating (Frey's syndrome).
- The parotid capsule should be closed after removal of a parotid tumor or a portion of the gland. If closure of the capsule is not possible, consideration should be given to interposing tissue (e.g., dermal fat graft) or implantable biologic material (e.g., acellular dermis) between the raw gland and the skin.
- Injury to the posterior branch of the GAN, which supplies sensation to the ear, is often avoidable. If the nerve has to be cut, it can be marked with a stitch to facilitate re-approximation at the conclusion of the case.
- Patients should be warned to expect at least temporary earlobe numbness and should take precautions to prevent heat or cold injury to the insensate area (e.g., frostbite or curling iron burns).
- Closed suction drainage is used in most cases to prevent postoperative hematoma or seroma.

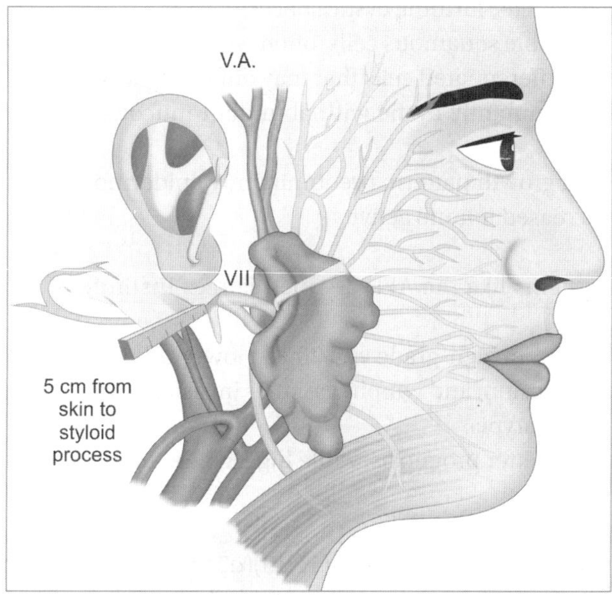

22. Discuss the clinical features, pathology and management of Mucoepidermoid carcinoma of the Parotid gland.
KGMU, Lucknow 2025

Mucoepidermoid carcinoma (MEC) is the most common malignant tumor of the parotid gland, accounting for approximately 30–35% of salivary gland malignancies. It arises from the salivary gland epithelium and is characterized by a mix of mucous, epidermoid (squamous), and intermediate cells. Below is a detailed discussion of its clinical features, pathology, and management.

Clinical Features

- **Presentation:**
  - *Mass:* Typically presents as a slowly growing, painless mass in the parotid gland region (preauricular area). It may be firm or fluctuant, depending on the cystic component.
  - *Pain:* Pain is uncommon but may occur in high-grade tumors due to local invasion or perineural spread.
  - *Facial nerve involvement:* Facial weakness or paralysis is rare but suggests a high-grade tumor with nerve invasion.
  - *Lymphadenopathy:* Regional lymph node involvement is uncommon in low-grade tumors but may be present in high-grade cases.
  - *Other symptoms:* High-grade tumors may cause symptoms like rapid growth, fixation to surrounding tissues, or skin ulceration.

- *Demographics:*
  - Occurs across a wide age range, with a peak incidence in the 3rd to 6th decades.
  - Slight female predominance.
  - More common in the parotid gland than in minor salivary glands.
- *Behavior:*
  - MEC is classified into low-grade, intermediate-grade, and high-grade tumors based on histological features.
  - Low-grade tumors are often indolent with a good prognosis, while high-grade tumors are aggressive, with a higher risk of metastasis (lungs, bones, lymph nodes).

Pathology

- *Histological Features:*
  - MEC is composed of three cell types:
    1. *Mucous cells:* Secrete mucus, forming cystic spaces.
    2. *Epidermoid cells:* Resemble squamous cells, often with keratinization in high-grade tumors.
    3. *Intermediate cells:* Undifferentiated cells that may differentiate into mucous or epidermoid cells.
  - *Low-grade tumors:* Predominantly cystic with abundant mucous cells, minimal atypia, and low mitotic activity.
  - *High-grade tumors:* Solid growth pattern, predominantly epidermoid and intermediate cells, with marked atypia, necrosis, and increased mitotic activity.
- **Grading Systems:**
  - Grading is based on systems like the AFIP (Armed Forces Institute of Pathology) or Brandwein criteria, which consider:
    - Cystic component (<20% in high-grade vs. >20% in low-grade).
    - Necrosis, perineural invasion, and lymphovascular invasion (more common in high-grade).
    - Mitotic rate and cellular atypia.
  - Low-grade tumors have a better prognosis, while high-grade tumors are associated with higher recurrence and metastasis rates.
- *Molecular Features:*
  - A characteristic chromosomal translocation, t(11;19)(q21;p13), results in the CRTC1-MAML2 fusion gene, present in ~50–70% of MECs. This is more common in low-grade tumors and is associated with a better prognosis.
  - High-grade tumors may show additional genetic alterations, such as p53 mutations or EGFR amplification.
- *Spread:*
  - Local invasion into surrounding tissues (skin, muscle, bone) is more common in high-grade tumors.
  - Lymphatic spread to cervical lymph nodes occurs in 10–15% of cases, primarily in high-grade tumors.
  - Distant metastasis (lungs, bones, liver) is rare but occurs in advanced high-grade cases.

Management

- *Diagnosis:*
  - *Imaging:*
    - *Ultrasound:* First-line imaging to assess the mass and guide fine-needle aspiration cytology (FNAC).
    - *CT/MRI:* MRI is preferred for assessing tumor extent, soft tissue involvement, and perineural spread. High-grade tumors may show irregular margins, necrosis, or invasion.
  - *Fine-needle aspiration cytology (FNAC):* Helps confirm malignancy and grade the tumor, though core biopsy may be needed for definitive histology.
  - *Biopsy:* Excisional biopsy is avoided due to the risk of tumor seeding; incisional or core biopsy is preferred for preoperative planning.
- *Staging:*
  - Based on the TNM system (AJCC 8th edition):

    - *T (tumor size and extent):* T1 (<2 cm) to T4 (invasion of skin, bone, or nerves).
    - *N (nodal involvement):* N0 (no nodes) to N3 (extensive nodal spread).
    - *M (metastasis):* M0 (no distant metastasis) to M1 (distant metastasis).
  - Stage I-II (early, localized) vs. Stage III-IV (advanced, with nodal or distant spread).
- *Treatment:*
  - *Surgery:*
    - *Primary Treatment:* Superficial or total parotidectomy with preservation of the facial nerve (if not involved). Total parotidectomy is preferred for high-grade or large tumors.
    - *Neck Dissection:* Elective neck dissection is considered for high-grade tumors or clinically positive nodes (N+).
    - *Reconstruction:* Required in cases of extensive resection (e.g., skin or nerve involvement).
  - *Radiotherapy:*
    - *Adjuvant:* Indicated for high-grade tumors, positive margins, perineural invasion, lymph node involvement, or advanced-stage disease.
    - *Primary:* Rarely used as a primary modality in inoperable cases or patients unfit for surgery.
    - Intensity-modulated radiotherapy (IMRT) is preferred to minimize damage to surrounding structures (e.g., facial nerve, oral cavity).
  - Chemotherapy:
    - Limited role in MEC; reserved for palliative treatment in metastatic or unresectable high-grade tumors.
    - Agents like cisplatin, 5-fluorouracil, or taxanes may be used, but evidence of efficacy is limited.
  - *Targeted Therapy:*
    - Emerging therapies targeting CRTC1-MAML2 or EGFR pathways are under investigation but not yet standard.
    - Clinical trials may be considered for advanced cases.
- *Follow-Up:*
  - Regular follow-up with clinical examination and imaging (MRI/CT) to monitor for recurrence or metastasis.
  - *Low-grade tumors:* Follow-up every 6–12 months for 5–10 years.
  - *High-grade tumors:* More frequent follow-up (every 3–6 months initially) due to higher recurrence risk.
- *Prognosis:*
  - *Low-grade:* Excellent prognosis, with 5-year survival rates of ~90–95%.
  - *High-grade:* Poorer prognosis, with 5-year survival rates of ~50–60%.
  - *Factors affecting prognosis*: Tumor grade, stage, margin status, perineural invasion, and CRTC1-MAML2 fusion status.

23. Parotid fistula. ***WBUHS 2013***

Introduction

A parotid fistula is a communication between the skin and a salivary duct or gland through which saliva is discharged.

Causes

- Parotid gland and duct injuries are rare complications following surgery of parotid gland and temporomandibular joint.
- Various other causes of parotid injury are rupture of parotid abscess, inadvertent incision of parotid abscess, complication of superficial parotidectomy, gunshot wounds, and trauma.

Clinical Features

- Clinical features include salivary extravasations into the tissues causing swelling over or adjacent to parotid gland (sialocele), expanding neck mass and cutaneous fistula formation.
- In glandular fistulas, discharge is less and tends to heal spontaneously with conservative treatment, whereas ductal fistulas continuously discharge saliva and spontaneous healing is very rare.

- *Classification of parotid injuries:*
  - An injury classification system has been devised by Van Sickels.
  - This system divides the parotid injuries into three regions:
    - Posterior to the masseter or intraglandular (site A)
    - Overlying the masseter (site B)
    - Anterior to the masseter (site C)

Diagnosis

- Injury to the parotid duct may be difficult to diagnose; therefore, the initial examining physician must have a high index of suspicion for injuries occurring in the parotid region. If not recognized, it will lead to salivary fistula and sialocele formation, which will not heal spontaneously because of continuous flow of saliva. Successful treatment depends on early recognition and appropriate early intervention.
- Examination of parotid injuries should include assessment of location, size, shape, type (e.g., puncture, laceration, avulsion, crush, and abrasion), asymmetry, drainage (i.e., quality, character, and odor) tenderness, surrounding erythema, edema, cellulitis, or crepitation and facial nerve status.
- The most straightforward way to diagnose a parotid duct injury is to cannulate the intraoral parotid duct papilla with a small silastic tube and observe if the tube is visible in the wound. This test does require patient cooperation; therefore, it may be difficult or impossible in children, individuals with intoxication, or individuals with mental disabilities. If any question regarding the diagnosis remains, a small amount of saline may be injected through the tube and observed for flow through the wound.
- Methylene blue probably should not be injected through the tube because it terribly discolors tissues and makes subsequent operation even more challenging.
- Sialography may be performed but is usually not necessary to establish the diagnosis of parotid duct injury. If performed, water-soluble contrast material should be employed because it is more easily drained and absorbed and it does not remain as an irritant to the gland.
- In doubtful cases, fluid can be sent for laboratory analysis; raised salivary amylase levels confirm the diagnosis.
- CT fistulography can be performed to look for the extent of the fistula.

Treatment Options

- Aspiration and pressure dressings
- Anti-sialogogues
- Radiation therapy
- Parasympathetic denervation (tympanic denervation)
- Cauterization of the fistulous
- Reconstruction of the duct
- Superficial or total parotidectomy tract

24. Percutaneous tracheostomy (PT). ***WBUHS 2008; NTRUHS Vijayawada 2025***

Background

PT has gained an increasing acceptance as an alternative to the conventional surgical tracheostomy (ST). In experienced hands and with proper patient selection, it is safe, easy, and quick. The advantages of PT are that it is a simple, fast, and minimally invasive bedside procedure, leading to less stress to the patient compared with ST.

Advantages of PT over ST

- It is a relatively simpler technique suitable for trained staff in the critical care setting.
- It does not require an operating theater, and the procedure is usually performed under local anesthetic, sedation, and neuromuscular blockade as appropriate.
- It forms a stoma between tracheal rings, resulting in reduced blood loss as there is usually no disruption of blood vessels. Moreover, the tracheostomy tube is fitted snugly in the stoma thereby minimizing any tendency to bleeding after the procedure.

- Infection rates for PT range from 0 to 3.3%, whereas those for open tracheostomy have been reported to be as high as 36%.
- Stenosis rates for PT range from 0 to 9%. The reported incidence of late complications resulting from open tracheostomy such as tracheal stenosis, tracheomalacia, fistula, and scarring varies widely.
- Small and neat stoma of dilatational tracheostomy generally results in a more cosmetic scar.

Indications

- Facilitate weaning from positive pressure ventilation and sedation
- Bypass an obstruction of the upper respiratory tract
- Prevent aspiration from the pharynx or GI tract
- Facilitate removal of secretion by aspiration
- Facilitate long-term airway management

Techniques

Ciaglia's method is the most commonly applied, but no study has shown superiority of any of the percutaneous techniques described. A variant of the original Ciaglia technique using a single tapered dilator known as a "blue rhino" is the most commonly used of these newer techniques and has largely taken over from the early multiple dilator technique.

Complications

Perioperative complications are comparable with those of ST and these are mostly minor. An important advantage of PT over ST is that there is no need to move a critically ill patient to the operating room and the rate of stomal infection is very low.

- *Complications of insertion:*
  - *Early:*
    - During the procedure:
      - Hypoxia due to failure of ventilation.
      - Ventilation of the patient may also be difficult if the cuff of the endotracheal tube is inadvertently punctured.
    - Pneumothorax, pneumomediastinum, or creation of a false passage and subcutaneous emphysema due to the placement of the tracheostomy tube in the paratracheal space.
    - Tracheoesophageal fistula due to damage or injury to the posterior tracheal wall
    - Bleeding:
      - Major bleeding is unusual.
      - Minor bleeding can usually be controlled by pressure or occasionally a suture.
      - Hemorrhage into the airway is potentially dangerous as it may result in a blood clot obstructing the airway.
    - Needle puncture on the lateral wall of trachea may subsequently lead to stenosis.
    - Dislodgement of the tracheostomy tube soon after the procedure may be hazardous as the entry to the trachea is small and deep; hence, replacement of the tube may be impossible.
    - The PT tube should not be pushed blindly back in but replaced after proper dilation of the track following orotracheal reintubation.
    - Secondary hemorrhage:
      - Infection
      - Erosion of vessels
- *Late:*
  - The incidence of clinically significant subglottic stenosis is low in PT.
  - Causes of subglottic stenosis:
    - Laryngeal edema

- Damage to the tracheal mucosa
- High pressure exerted by the endotracheal cuff
- Prolonged translaryngeal intubation

Go Through

The House-Brackmann Facial Nerve Grading System is widely used to characterize the degree of facial paralysis (this has come as question in one of the papers of AIIMS, Bhopal).

Grade	*Appearance*	*Forehead*	*Eye*	*Mouth*
1	Normal	Normal	Normal	Normal
2	Mild weakness, normal resting tone	Medium-good movement	Full closure with minimum effort	Slightly asymmetrical
3	Nondeforming weakness, normal resting tone	Weak-medium movement	Full closure with maximum effort	Mild weakness with maximum effort
4	Deforming weakness, normal resting tone	N/A	Incomplete closure	Asymmetrical with maximum effort
5	Minimum movement, asymmetric resting tone	N/A	Incomplete closure	Slight movement
6	Asymmetric	N/A	N/A	N/A

Benign Skin Lesions and Soft Tissue Tumor

LEARNING OBJECTIVES

- Scalp Tumors
- Skin and Soft Tissue Infections: Erysipelas, Fournier's Gangrene, Necrotizing Fasciitis
- Pressure Sore
- Neurofibromatosis, Desmoid Tumors
- Skin Malignancy—Premalignant Skin Lesions, Marjolin's Ulcer, Basal Cell Carcinoma
- Malignant Melanoma
- Soft Tissue Sarcoma
- Retroperitoneal Tumor, Retroperitoneal Sarcoma, Retroperitoneal Liposarcoma

SKIN AND SOFT TISSUE INFECTIONS

1. Scalp tumors. ***WBUHS 2021***

Scalp tumors can refer to a wide range of growths that appear on the scalp. They may be *benign (non-cancerous)* or *malignant (cancerous)*. Here is a general breakdown to help you understand the types, features, and management:

Types of Scalp Tumors

Benign Tumors

- *Epidermoid (Sebaceous) cyst*
  - Slow-growing, firm lump under the skin
  - Often contains keratin; may get infected
- *Lipoma*
  - Soft, movable lump of fatty tissue
  - Usually painless
- *Pilar (Trichilemmal) cyst*
  - Common on the scalp
  - Originates from hair follicles
- *Seborrheic keratosis*
  - Warty, pigmented lesion
  - Often mistaken for melanoma
- *Hemangioma*
  - Vascular tumor; more common in children
  - Red to purple in color
- *Neurofibroma*
  - Associated with neurofibromatosis
  - Soft, sometimes painful

Malignant Tumors

- *Basal cell carcinoma (BCC)*
  - Most common skin cancer
  - Pearly appearance, may ulcerate
  - Rarely spreads but can be locally destructive
- *Squamous cell carcinoma (SCC)*
  - More aggressive than BCC
  - Scaly, crusted surface; may ulcerate or bleed
- *Melanoma*
  - Dangerous and aggressive skin cancer
  - Asymmetrical, irregular borders, multicolored
  - Can metastasize early
- *Cutaneous metastases*
  - Secondary deposits from internal cancers (e.g., breast, lung)
  - Firm, nodular, often multiple
- *Angiosarcoma*
  - Rare but aggressive vascular tumor
  - Common in elderly; bruised or purplish appearance

Diagnosis:

- Clinical examination
- Dermatoscopy
- Biopsy (excisional or incisional)
- Imaging (CT/MRI if deep or large lesion suspected)

Treatment:

- *Benign tumors:*
  - Observation if asymptomatic
  - Surgical excision if large, painful, or cosmetically concerning
- *Malignant tumors:*
  - Surgical excision with clear margins
  - Mohs micrographic surgery (especially for BCC/SCC)
  - Radiation therapy
  - Chemotherapy or immunotherapy (e.g., for melanoma)

Consider Biopsy if:

- Rapid growth
- Bleeding or ulceration
- Irregular pigmentation or borders
- Pain or tenderness
- Non-healing lesion

SKIN AND SOFT TISSUE INFECTIONS

2. Erysipelas. ***WBUHS 2011***

Erysipelas is an acute *Streptococcus* bacterial infection of the deep epidermis with lymphatic spread.

Risk Factors

This disease is most common among the elderly, infants, and children. People with immune deficiency, diabetes, alcoholism, skin ulceration, fungal infections, and impaired lymphatic drainage (e.g., after mastectomy, pelvic surgery, and bypass grafting) are also at increased risk.

Signs and Symptoms

- Patients typically develop symptoms including high fevers, shaking, chills, fatigue, headaches, vomiting, and general illness within 48 hours of the initial infection.
- The erythematous skin lesion enlarges rapidly and has a sharply demarcated raised edge. It appears as a red, swollen, warm, hardened, and painful rash.
- More severe infections can result in vesicles, bullae, and petechiae, with possible skin necrosis. Lymph nodes may be swollen, and lymphedema may occur.
- Occasionally, a red streak extending to the lymph node can be seen.
- The infection may occur on any part of the skin including the face, arms, fingers, legs, and toes, but it tends to favor the extremities.
- Fat tissue is most susceptible to infection, and facial areas typically around the eyes, ears, and cheeks.
- Repeated infection of the extremities can lead to chronic swelling (lymphadenitis).

Etiology

- Most cases of erysipelas are due to *Streptococcus pyogenes* (also known as beta-hemolytic group A streptococci), although non-group A streptococci can also be the causative agent.
- Historically, the face was most affected; today the legs are affected most often.
- The rash is due to an exotoxin.
- Erysipelas infections can enter the skin through minor trauma, eczema, surgical incisions, and ulcers, and often originate from strep bacteria in the subject's own nasal passages.
- Infection sets in after a small scratch or abrasion spreads resulting in toxemia.
- Erysipelas does not affect subcutaneous tissue. It does not release pus, only serum or serous fluid.
- Subcutaneous edema may lead the physician to misdiagnose it as cellulitis, but the style of the rash is much more well circumscribed and sharply marginated than the rash of cellulitis.

Diagnosis

- This disease is diagnosed mainly by the appearance of well-demarcated rash and inflammation. Blood cultures are unreliable for diagnosis of the disease, but may be used to test for sepsis.
- Erysipelas must be differentiated from herpes zoster, angioedema, contact dermatitis, and diffuse inflammatory carcinoma of the breast.
- Erysipelas can be distinguished from cellulitis by its raised advancing edges and sharp borders. Elevation of the antistreptolysin O (ASO) titer occurs after around 10 days of illness.

Treatment

- Depending on the severity, treatment involves either oral or intravenous antibiotics, using penicillins, clindamycin, or erythromycin. While illness symptoms resolve in a day or two, the skin may take weeks to return to normal.
- Because of the risk of reinfection, prophylactic antibiotics are sometimes used after resolution of the initial condition. However, this approach does not always stop reinfection.

Complications

- Spread of infection to other areas of body through the bloodstream (bacteremia), including septic arthritis and infective endocarditis (heart valves)
- Septic shock
- *Recurrence of infection:* Erysipelas can recur in 18–30% of cases even after antibiotic treatment.
- Lymphatic damage
- *Necrotizing fasciitis:* Commonly known as "the flesh-eating bug." A potentially deadly exacerbation of the infection if it spreads to deeper tissue.

3. Fournier's gangrene. *WBUHS 2009, 2022*

Definition

Fournier gangrene is defined as a polymicrobial necrotizing fasciitis of the perineal, perianal, or genital areas. Necrotizing process commonly originates from infection in anorectum, urogenital tract, or skin of genitalia.

Etiology and Risk Factors

Etiology

Anorectal causes	*Urogenital causes*	*Dermatologic causes*	*Other less common causes*
• Infection in the perineal glands • Manifestation of colorectal injury, malignancy or diverticulitis	• Infection in the bulbourethral glands • Urethral injury • Iatrogenic injury • Lower urinary tract infections	• Hidradenitis suppurativa • Ulceration from scrotal pressure • Trauma to scrotum or perineum	• Consequence of bone marrow malignancy • Systemic lupus erythematosus • Crohn's diseases

Diabetes mellitus	Malignancies	Chronic steroid use	Malnutrition
Alcoholism	Cirrhosis liver	HIV infection	Morbid obesity

Causative Bacteria

- Polymicrobial infection
- Minimum of four isolates per case
- Most common aerobe—*E. coli*
- Most common anaerobes—bacteroides
- *Others: Streptococcus*, *Staphylococcus*, MRSA (methicillin-resistant *Staphylococcus aureus*), *Klebsiella, Pseudomonas, Proteus*, and *Clostridium*

Pathogenesis

Bacteria act synergistically causing obliterative endarteritis and production of various enzymes causing destruction. There is imbalance between host immunity and virulence of organism.

Pathology

Pathognomonic findings on pathological evaluation of tissue are:

- Necrosis of superficial and deep fascial planes
- Fibrinoid coagulation of the nutrient arterioles
- Polymorphonuclear cell infiltration
- Presence of microorganisms within the involved tissues
- Air in the perineal tissue

Incidence

- *Age:* 30–60 years
- *Sex:* 10 times more common in males
- *Social habits:* More common in males homosexuals (more prone for rectal injury)

Clinical Features

- Begins with insidious onset of pruritus and discomfort of external genitalia
- Prodromal symptoms of fever and lethargy, which may be present for 2–7 days before gangrene.
- The hallmark of Fournier gangrene is out of proportion pain and tenderness in the genitalia.
- Increasing genital pain and tenderness with progressive erythema of the overlying skin
- Dusky appearance of the overlying skin; subcutaneous crepitation; feculent odor
- Obvious gangrene of a portion of the genitalia; purulent discharge from wounds
- As gangrene develops, pain subsides (nerve necrosis)

Investigations

- Complete blood count (CBC)
- Electrolytes
- Blood urea nitrogen (BUN)/serum creatinine
- Blood sugar
- Arterial blood gas (ABG)
- Blood and urine culture with sensitivity
- Coagulation profile for disseminated intravascular coagulopathy (DIC)

Imaging

- *Conventional radiography:* Presence of gas in soft tissue
- *Ultrasonography:*
  - Presence of gas in scrotal tissue
  - Excludes other conditions
  - Testicular blood flow—normal
  - Limitations—direct pressure on involved tissue causes inconvenience
- *Computed tomography (CT) scanning:*
  - Can detect smaller amount of soft tissue gas
  - Defines extent more specifically
  - Identifies underlying causes, e.g., small perineal abscess
- *Magnetic resonance imaging (MRI):*
  - Yields greater soft tissue details
  - Creates logistic challenges, especially in critically ill patients

Medical Treatment

- Restoration of normal organ perfusion
- Reduction of systemic toxicity
- Broad-spectrum antibiotics to cover anaerobes as well (ciprofloxacin + clindamycin + metronidazole)
- Vancomycin for MRSA
- Tetanus prophylaxis
- Irrigation with super oxidized water
- Hyperbaric oxygen therapy
- Intravenous (IV) immunoglobulins to neutralize super antigen as streptotoxin A and B (as adjuvant)
- Antifungal—if required
- Nonconventional—dressing with gauge soaked with zinc per oxide

Surgical Treatment

- Repeated aggressive debridement
- Preservation of testes (subcutaneous pocket from desiccation)
- Reconstruction after infection is over
- Fecal diversion
- Urinary diversion
- Vacuum-assisted closure (VAC)

Complications

Acute renal failure (ARF)	Septicemia and gram-negative shock	Tetanus
Acute respiratory distress syndrome (ARDS)	Multiple systems organ failure (MSOF)	Death

4. Discuss the etiology, clinical features, and management of different types of synergistic gangrene. What is necrotizing fasciitis? ***WBUHS 2018***

Type	*Etiology*	*Clinical presentation*	*Management*
Fournier gangrene is necrotizing fasciitis of the perineum. It is a true urological emergency due to the high mortality rate but fortunately, the condition is rare	• Fournier gangrene is typically seen in diabetic men aged 50–70 years, rarely in women. • Other predisposing factors include: – Diabetes mellitus – Immunosuppression – Alcoholism – Debility	• Perineal/scrotal pain, swelling, redness • Crepitus from soft tissue gas (up to 65%) • Systemically unwell • Fever and leukocytosis	Management options include: • Immediate radical surgical debridement of necrotic tissue • Intravenous antibiotics • Hyperbaric oxygen therapy • Testes replaced into the remaining scrotum or covered by skin graft (once infection settled)
Meleney's gangrene is a rare, rapidly spreading destructive subcutaneous tissue infection	• Most commonly occurs at post-surgical sites—caused by *Staphylococcus aureus* and *Streptococcus* organisms • Most patients with postoperative synergistic: Gangrene have pre-existing immunosuppressive conditions such as chronic renal failure, HIV, diabetes mellitus, or are elderly	• Initial signs are not specific • One of the identifying symptoms is the presence of extremely painful lesions, which usually form in the 2nd week after surgery or minor trauma • The ulcers that form at the center of the lesion are usually covered by a black eschar and encircled by a gangrenous margin	• With introduction of newer antimicrobials, zinc oxide was replaced with modern day antibiotics as the choice of treatment • Surgical debridement is most important. Serial debridements are usually necessary to completely remove the dead, devitalized tissue • Additional treatment measures such as hyperbaric oxygen therapy can be used as an adjunct to this
Synergistic gangrene of breast	• History of trauma • Diabetes mellitus	• Cellulitis of breast • Growing necrotic ulceration	• Resuscitation and supportive treatment • Broad-spectrum antibiotics • Surgical debridement

Necrotizing fasciitis (rare plural: necrotizing fasciitides) refers to a rapidly progressive and often fatal necrotizing soft tissue infection primarily involving and spreading along the fascia.

The most common risk factor is diabetes mellitus, especially in combination with peripheral arterial disease. Other predisposing factors include immunocompromise due to HIV infection, cancer, alcoholism, and organ transplants. However, infections can occur in otherwise healthy individuals following surgery, penetrating trauma, minor wounds such as insect bites or abrasions, or even blunt trauma with no clear portal of entry.

Microbiologically, there are two major recognized forms:

1. *Polymicrobial (Type I):* Most common; involves both anaerobic and aerobic organisms, such as *Clostridium*, *Bacteroides*, and *Peptostreptococcus* in the former group, and *Enterobacteriaceae* family members and *Staphylococcus aureus* in the latter group.
2. *Monomicrobial (Type II):* Less common (10–15%); most commonly involves group a streptococci, the "flesh-eating bacteria" and may be complicated by toxic shock syndrome. Less commonly due to *Staphylococcus aureus*.

Necrotizing Fasciitis

- It is a rapidly progressive and often fatal necrotizing soft tissue infection primarily involving and spreading along the fascia.
- The most common risk factor is diabetes mellitus, especially in combination with peripheral arterial disease.
- Other predisposing factors include immunocompromise due to HIV infection, cancer, alcoholism, and organ transplants.

- However, infections can occur in otherwise healthy individuals following surgery, penetrating trauma, minor wounds such as insect bites or abrasions, or even blunt trauma with no clear portal of entry.

---

5. Describe necrotizing soft tissue infection. ***WBUHS 2012***

Definition

Necrotizing soft tissue infection is a rare but very severe type of bacterial infection that can destroy the muscles, skin, and underlying tissue. Necrotizing refers to something that causes tissue death.

Causes, Incidence, and Risk Factors

- Many different types of bacteria can cause this type of infection. A very severe and usually deadly form of necrotizing soft tissue infection is due to *Streptococcus pyogenes*, which is sometimes called "flesh-eating bacteria",
- Necrotizing soft tissue infection develops when the bacteria enter the body, usually through a minor cut or scrape. The bacteria begin to grow and release harmful substances (toxins) that:
  - Directly kill tissue
  - Interfere with the blood flow to the tissue
  - Breakdown materials in the tissue, which rapidly spread the bacteria, leading to widespread effects such as shock.

Signs and Symptoms

- The first sign of infection may be a small, reddish, painful spot or bump on the skin. This quickly changes to a very painful bronze- or purple-colored patch that grows rapidly.
- The center may become black and die off. The skin may break open and ooze fluid. The wound may quickly grow in less than an hour.
- Symptoms may include general ill feeling, fever, sweating, chills, nausea, dizziness, profound weakness, and finally shock. Without treatment, death can occur rapidly.

Tests

- Often a patient will be diagnosed in the operating room by a surgeon. Imaging tests, such as CT scans, are sometimes helpful.
- Tests performed on blood, fluids, or tissue from the area may determine the bacteria that are causing the infection.

Treatment

- Powerful, broad-spectrum antibiotics must be given immediately through a vein (IV). Surgery is required to open and drain infected areas and remove dead tissue. Sometimes donor immunoglobulins (antibodies) are given by vein to help fight the infection.
- Skin grafts may be needed after the infection goes away. If an arm or leg infection cannot be controlled, amputation of the limb may be considered.
- If the bacteria are determined to be an oxygen-avoiding organism (anaerobe), the patient may receive hyperbaric oxygen therapy. This involves placing the patient in a chamber that delivers 100% oxygen at high pressure.

Complications

- Local spread of infection, progressive tissue damage
- Systemic spread of infection, sepsis, shock
- Scarring and disfigurement
- Functional loss of an arm or leg
- Death

Prevention

Always clean the skin thoroughly after a cut, scrape, or other skin injury.

6. Necrotizing fasciitis. ***WBUHS 2007***

7. Clinical features and recent concept of management of necrotizing fasciitis. ***WBUHS 2019***

Introduction

Necrotizing fasciitis (NF) is a severe life-threatening, rapidly advancing soft tissue infection that progresses along fascia and subcutaneous tissue, characterized by a fulminant course and a high mortality.

Clinical Features

- Necrotizing fasciitis is difficult to diagnose in early stages and a high index of suspicion with low threshold to prompt surgical intervention should be the dictum.
- Patient may present with early features of localized evidence of skin inflammation (pain, erythema, and edema) or with later systemic symptoms of sepsis (pyrexia, tachycardia, hypotension, tachypnea, and altered mental state).

Clinical Stages of Necrotizing Fasciitis

Stage 1	*Stage 2*	*Stage 3*
Tenderness	Blister and bullae formation	Tissue necrosis
Erythema		Hyposensitivity
Edema		Anesthesia
Warm skin		Tissue crepitation
Fever		Hemorrhagic bullae

Pathophysiology

- NF is a deep-seated infection with deep fascia as the primary site of pathology that results in progressive destruction of fascia and fat with sparing of the skin initially.
- The cutaneous manifestations are secondary changes as a consequence of progressive ischemia.
- Muscles usually are not affected.
- Organisms spread rapidly along superficial and deep fascial tissue planes facilitated by the production and release of bacterial enzymes (hyaluronidase), toxins, and endogenous cytokines.

The major pathological events include:

- Extensive destructions of tissues and spread of bacteria along fascial planes
- Thrombosis of blood vessels
- Ischemia and tissue necrosis
- Damage to superficial nerves producing localized anesthesia.

Microbiology

- Necrotizing soft tissue infection (NSTI) can be classified into bacteriological classes.
- While it can affect any part of the body, 50% of cases involve the lower extremities. Other common areas include the upper extremities, the perineum (Fournier gangrene), and head and neck region. In neonates, the most common area involved is the trunk.

Type I (polymicrobial)	*Type II (monomicrobial)*	*Type III (salt water NF)*	*Type IV (fungal)*
• Most common (80%) • Synergism among bacteria lead to fulminant infection • *Gram-positive cocci*: *Staphylococcus aureus, Streptococcus pyogenes,* enterococci • *Gram negative*: *E. coli, Pseudomonas* • *Anaerobes*: *Clostridium perfringens, C. septicum, C. sordellii*	• Around 20% cases • Group A *Streptococcus* (GAS) alone or with *Staphylococcus aureus* • Can lead to shock (toxic shock syndrome) and multiorgan failure	• Marine contamination of an open wound • *Gram-negative marine organisms:* Vibrio species (*V. vulnificus*) • High mortality (25%) despite aggressive therapy	• Fungal infections following traumatic wounds or burns • Rapidly progressive • Zygomycetes, aspergilla, *Candida*

Investigations

- Necrotizing fasciitis is a clinical diagnosis and a surgical emergency.
- The Laboratory Risk Indicators for Necrotizing Fasciitis (LRINEC) described by Wong et al. is an effective tool to help distinguish NF from other soft tissue infections or abscesses.
- LRINEC score of ≥6 is highly suspicious of NF and >8 is diagnostic, with positive predictive value of 92% and negative predictive value of 96%.

Variables	*Value*	*Score*
CRP (mg/dL)	<150	0
	>150	4
TLC (/mm^3)	<15k	0
	15–25k	1
	>25k	2
Hemoglobin (g/dL)	>13.5	0
	11.0–13.5	1
	<13.5	2
Serum sodium level (mmol/L)	<135	0
	>135	2
Serum creatinine level (μmol/L)	<141	0
	>141	2
Serum glucose (mmol/L)	<10	0
	>10	1

(CRP: C-reactive protein; TLC: total leukocyte count)

Imaging

- Plain film radiography can show gas within the soft tissues in presence of polymicrobial infection. This is a nonspecific sign.
- Ultrasound can have a role in determining the presence or absence of an abscess and can reveal subcutaneous gas and edema along the fascial planes.
- Magnetic resonance imaging (MRI) scans are highly sensitive, if no fascial thickening is found, NF can be excluded.

Surgical Diagnosis

- The gold standard for detection of NF is tissue biopsy.
- An incision over the site of maximal skin change is needed to assess the underlying tissue. Healthy subcutaneous fat and fascia indicates that further resection is not needed.
- If the exploration reveals the presence of dusky gray necrotic subcutaneous fat and fascia, lack of bleeding, thrombosed vessels, noncontracting muscle, dish water-colored fluid (dish water pus) seeping from the wound, and a positive finger test result; the diagnosis of NF is confirmed.
- A positive finger test is characterized by lack of resistance to finger dissection in tissue.

Treatment

Necrotizing fasciitis is a surgical emergency needing a high index of suspicion, early diagnosis, and aggressive surgical debridement. The treatment for NF follows the same principles for any kind of surgical infection:

- Source control
- Antimicrobial therapy
- Support
- Monitoring

Resuscitation, Antibiotic, and Critical Care

- The degree of respiratory, hemodynamic, renal, and metabolic compromise must be quickly assessed.
- Early resuscitation with intravenous fluids or colloids should be initiated and inotrope should be added if required.
- All patients should be started with broad-spectrum antibiotics to cover *Staphylococcus, Streptococcus, gram-negative rods and anaerobes.*
- Recommended regimens include single agents such as Meropenem, Imipenem, Ertapenem, Piperacillin-Tazobactum, but may be changed according to sensitivity.
- The commonly used multidrug regime includes a high dose of Penicillin, Clindamycin and a fluoroquinolone or an aminoglycoside for Gram-negative coverage.

Surgical Treatment

- NF is one of the excellent examples highlighting a very important role played by source control in management of surgical infection.
- Radical surgical debridement is the mainstay of treatment.
- Patients should be consented regarding the seriousness of the infection and informed that the risk of mortality is increased without wide surgical excision.
- A generous incision is made and the macroscopic features of the lesion are used to decide the extent of debridement, with excision of all nonviable tissue including the fascia, drainage of all abscesses, and extensive fasciotomy.
- Healthy, viable, bleeding tissue at the edge of excision site should be the end point of debridement.
- To ensure that infectious process has not extended, a repeat surgical exploration 24–48 hours later become essential.
- After the initial debridement, patient should be preferably managed in an intensive care unit which allows to provide a good physiological support along with close monitoring of the patient.
- Reconstructive surgery should be planned once the patient is stabilized and infection is fully eradicated.
- Sterile dressings with alginate or hydrogel are used for wound coverage during the interim. Skin cover can be provided either with secondary skin suturing, split skin grafting, or tissue transfer.
    - *Negative pressure wound therapy (NPWT)* is the vacuum-assisted closure of wound. It improves healing and helps in reducing the size of larger defects that would have been difficult to manage with simply on their own.
    - *Other forms of surgery* which may be necessary include amputations for necrotizing infections of the extremities and a defunctioning colostomy for perineal wounds to prevent continuous fecal contamination.

Adjunct Measures

- *Hyperbaric oxygen therapy:*
    - It has been used with controversial status in literature.
    - It involves intermittent inhalation of 100% O_2 under pressure exceeding the atmospheric pressure, which leads to enhanced oxygenation in blood and tissues.
    - This prevents further necrosis.
- *Intravenous immunoglobulin (IVIG)* is reasonable and desirable option to neutralize Streptococcal toxins.

Complications of NF

- Septic shock
- Cardiovascular collapse
- Renal failure
- Scarring with cosmetic deformity
- Limb loss
- Toxic shock syndrome

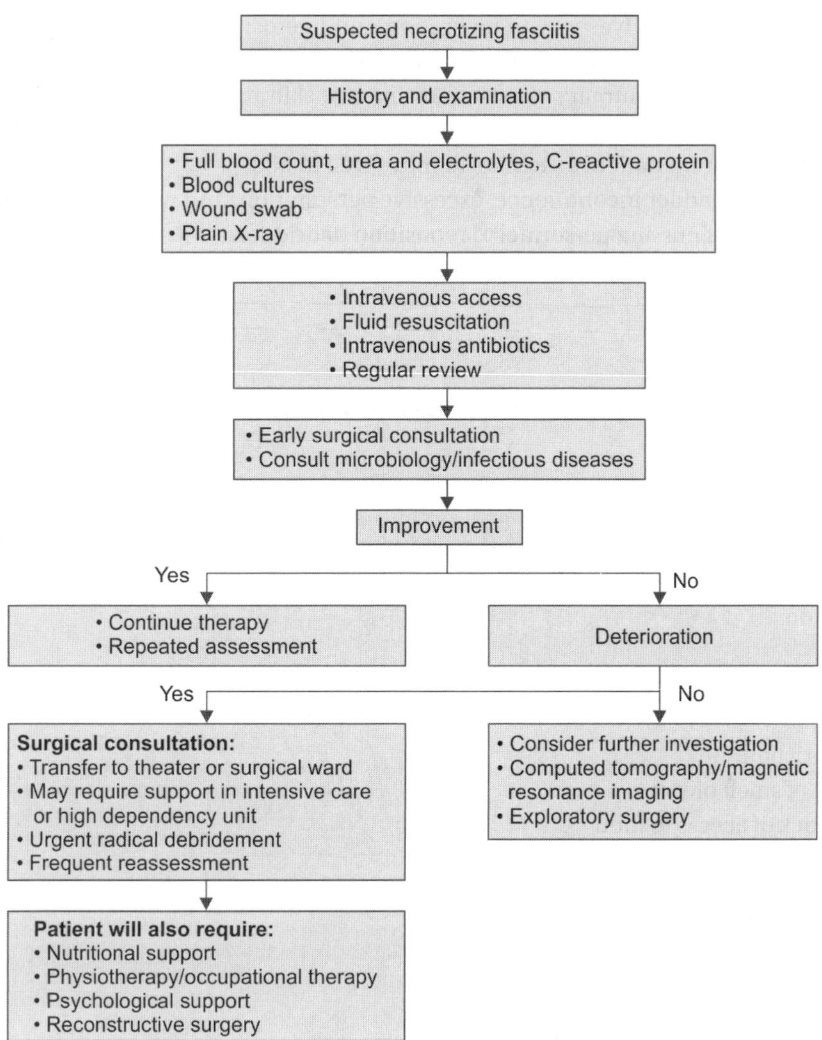

8. Enumerate causes and prevention and management of pressure sore. ***WBUHS 2019***

9. Write short note on pressure sores. ***RIMS, Imphal 2012***

- Prolonged weight bearing, as in an immobilized or paralyzed patient, can elevate tissue pressure above arterial capillary perfusion pressure (32 mm Hg) and result in compromised oxygenation, ischemia, and eventual tissue necrosis.
- In models of ischemia, external pressure >60 mm Hg for 2 hours leads to irreversible tissue damage, and clinical studies have confirmed this.
- The clinical sequelae of this damage are pressure sores with ulceration, infection, and exposure of bone.
- In order of occurrence, the surfaces most commonly involved are those over the sacrum, calcaneus, ischium, and greater trochanter.

Etiopathogenesis of Pressure Ulcer

- *Extrinsic factors:*
  - *Pressure from any hard surface (e.g., bed, wheelchair, stretcher):* The intensity and duration of such pressure govern the severity of the ulcer, pressure over an area for a moderate period (1–2 hours), produces tissue ischemia and increased capillary pressure leading to edema and multiple small vessel thrombosis.

- An inflammatory reaction gives way to ulceration and necrosis of ischemic cells. In turn, necrotic tissue predisposes to bacterial invasion and subsequent infection.
- Shearing forces—from involuntary muscle movements, skin moves one way and the bone underneath it moves another way.
- *Friction:* Abrasion—from patient's inability to move well in bed
- *Moisture:* Bowel or bladder incontinence, excessive perspiration, and wound drainage
- *Immobility:* Failure of nursing personnel to reposition bedridden

- *Intrinsic factors*
  - Limited mobility
  - Spinal cord injury
  - Cerebrovascular accident
  - Progressive neurologic disorders (Parkinson disease, Alzheimer disease, and multiple sclerosis)
  - Pain
  - Fractures
  - Postsurgical procedures
  - Coma or sedation
  - Arthropathies
  - Poor nutrition
  - Anorexia
  - Dehydration
  - Poor dentition
  - Dietary restriction
  - Weak sense of smell or taste
  - Poverty or lack of access to food
  - *Comorbidities:*
    - Diabetes mellitus
    - Depression or psychosis
    - Vasculitis or other collagen vascular disorders
    - Peripheral vascular disease
    - Decreased pain sensation
    - Immunodeficiency or use of corticosteroid therapy
    - Congestive heart failure
    - Malignancies
    - End-stage renal disease
    - Chronic obstructive pulmonary disease
    - Dementia
  - *Aging skin:*
    - Loss of elasticity
    - Decreased cutaneous blood flow
    - Changes in dermal pH
    - Flattening of rete ridges
    - Loss of subcutaneous fat
    - Decreased dermal–epidermal blood flow

Braden scale has reasonable predictive capacity, with high reliability. This scale accounts for several extrinsic and intrinsic causative factors by scoring six subscales—sensory perception, moisture, activity, mobility, nutrition, and friction and shear.

Stages of Pressure Ulcers

National pressure ulcer advisory panel staging system—

Classification Description

Stage I: Intact skin with nonblanchable redness
Stage II: Partial-thickness loss of dermis; may present as blister
Stage III: Full-thickness loss of dermis with visible subcutaneous fat (no deeper structures exposed)
Stage IV: Full-thickness loss of dermis with exposed bone, tendon, or muscle
Unstageable: Full-thickness loss of dermis with ulcer base obscured by eschar

Prevention of Pressure Sore

It is first and foremost.

- Movement and exercise improve circulation and prevent sores.
- A healthy diet keeps skin healthy and better able to resist breakdown.
- Protective skin care—once a pressure sore is developed it needs proper cleansing, treatment, and dressing procedure.
- *Mattresses and cushions:* Protection is the best way to prevent ulcers. Patients who are at risk of developing pressure ulcers should have the skin carefully inspected for any damage or redness (particularly over bony areas) twice daily.
- The skin should be kept clean and dry.
- Any pressure causing damage to skin or tissue should be immediately eliminated.
    - Use of special mattresses, cushions, and by many protective devices
    - Two or three times per day, check the skin of bedridden for possible changes in color, turgor, temperature, and sensation. Examine an existing ulcer for any change in size or degree of damage.
    - Turning and repositioning—every 2 hours, around the clock as much as possible, should be turned in bed, or repositioned in a wheelchair. Allow to change his own position as long as he can by himself.
    - Range of motion (ROM) exercises—again allow to do as much by himself as he can, but when it becomes evident that he no longer can do it, passively exercise the arms, legs and move the head as well.
    - Provide meticulous skin care.
    - Change bed linens frequently who are diaphoretic or incontinent
    - Diet good nutrition is essential to healing ulcers and preventing new ones. Encourage foods rich in protein and certain vitamins and mineral
    - *Topical agents:* Gentle soap, Dakins solution, zinc oxide cream, absorbable gelatin sponge, granulated sugar (mechanical irritation to enhance granulation), dextranomer (inert, absorbing beads), karaya gum powder, topical antibiotics (only when infection is confirmed by culture and sensitivity testing of wound exudate), silver sulfadiazine cream (antimicrobial agent) for necrotic areas, water vapor permeable dressings, duoderm, and tegaderm dressings.

Treatment of Pressure Sore

- Where possible, treatment of ulcers is planned with an aim to reverse the factors that have originally caused the ulcer.
- Careful assessment is needed before planning for treatment. In general, the possible causative factor should be removed (pressure, shear, and friction) and the associated general condition should be taken into the control (like treatment of associated comorbid illness and improvement in the nutrition).
- Wound healing requires adequate protein, iron, vitamin-C, and zinc. Supplements may be prescribed if they are deficient in the diet.

Cleaning and Debridement

- *Conventional surgical debridement:* Cleaning of the wound and meticulous skin care are the most essential part of the treatment. The process involves removal of surface contamination and meticulous excision of all dead tissue.
- *Mechanical debridement*—which includes use of repeated wet to dry dressings to remove slough
- Some mechanical debridement techniques include:

- *Cleansing and pressure irrigation:* Where dead tissue is removed using high-pressure water jets. There is no evidence available to support any specific and effective cleansing techniques or solution, in particular.
- *Ultrasound:* Dead tissue is removed using low-frequency energy waves.
- *Laser:* Dead tissue is removed using focused beams of light.

- *Enzymatic debridement:* Using enzymes to liquefy dead tissue in the wound and remove them with the dressings and biological debridement or maggots and larval therapy—in which the larvae eat all the dead tissue and make the wound clean without harming the living tissues.

Wound Dressings

- The dressing used for various stages of wound healing is specialized for every stage.
- Dressings are usually occlusive, so the ulcers heal better in a moist environment.
- If the ulcer is clean and dry, occlusive dressings are usually changed weekly, and more frequent changes are avoided as dressing changes remove healthy cells along with debris.
- Contaminated or weeping wounds may require more frequent dressing changes, sometimes every few hours.
- Heavily contaminated ulcers are treated with negative pressure wound therapy (NPWT).
- Specialized dressings and bandages are used to protect and speed up the healing process of the pressure ulcers.

These dressings include:

- *Hydrocolloid dressings:* These contain a special gel that encourages the growth of new skin cells in the ulcer and keeps the nearby healthy area of skin dry.
- *Alginate dressings:* These are made from seaweed that contains sodium and calcium known to speed up the healing process.
- *Nano silver dressings:* These use the antibacterial property of silver to clean the ulcer.
- *Creams and ointments:* To prevent further tissue damage and help speed up the healing process, topical preparations, such as cream and ointments are frequently used.

Antibiotics

- All pressure sores do not require antibiotics.
- Antibiotics are usually only prescribed to treat an infected pressure ulcer and prevent the infection from spreading.
- If tissue infection exists, antibiotics are necessary to treat the infection, but effort must be made to debride the ulcer thoroughly and leave all viable tissues only, otherwise antibiotics alone will not clean up the ulcer.
- Antibiotics are adjunct to surgical debridement and not an alternative to it.
- Topical antibiotics should be avoided because their use may increase antibiotic resistance and allergy.
- Antiseptic cream may also be applied topically to pressure ulcers to clear out any bacteria that may be present.

Biofilm

- It has been noticed that the long-standing pressure ulcers are frequently colonized by microorganisms in a biofilm.
- The biofilm may be composed of bacteria, fungi, or other organisms, which are embedded in and adherent to the underlying wound.
- The organisms are protected from the effect of conventional antibiotics; unnecessary prescription of antibiotics may, in fact, select more resistant organisms.

Negative Pressure Wound Therapy (NPWT)

- This is an invaluable tool in the management of pressure sores and involves the application of subatmospheric pressure to a wound using a computerized unit to intermittently or continuously convey negative pressure to promote wound healing.
- NPWT is effective for deep, cavitating, infected and copiously discharging pressure ulcers, particularly with exposed bone.

Newer Research

There are many supportive therapies to promote healing of pressure ulcers. While some are in clinical use, others are in the realm of research. Many products are available to aid wound healing but should be prescribed only under strict medical advice, as they still require further research to determine their effectiveness.

These include:

- Growth factors and cytokines
- Hyperbaric oxygen (HBO) to increase tissue oxygen tension
- Skin graft substitutes (bioengineered skin)
- Connective tissue matrix
- Expanded epidermis
- Epidermal stem cells
- Bone marrow (BM) or adipose tissue derived stem cell (ASC) therapy

Reconstructive Surgery

- Sometimes the severe pressure ulcer (Grade III or IV) fails to heal, in such cases, surgery is required to fill the wound and prevent any further tissue damage.
- This is usually done by cleaning the wound and closing it by bringing together the edges of the wound (direct closure), application of various type skin grafts or using local and regional flaps and free tissue transfer.
  - *The available reconstructive options are:*
    - *Split thickness skin grafting:* When the ulcer is superficial and vital tissues such as bone, vessels, nerves, or tendons are not exposed, and the ulcer is not copiously discharging.
    - *Local flaps:* Local transposition, rotation, and Limberg flap are the available options.
    - *Regional flaps:* For sacral pressure sores gluteus maximus myocutaneous flap, superior gluteal artery-based rotation fasciocutaneous flap, superior gluteal artery perforator flaps, perforator based V-Y advancement flap, lateral or medial calcaneal flaps, reverse sural flap, varieties of fasciocutaneous flaps may provide a huge reconstructive option.
    - *Microvascular free flaps:* Microvascular free flaps are usually reserved for some selected cases where the local and regional flap options are either not available or have failed.

---

10. Neurofibromatosis. ***WBUHS 2021***

Introduction

Neurofibromatoses (NF) comprise a number of clinically and genetically distinct inherited conditions that carry a high risk of tumor formation. They fall under the wider classification of phakomatoses. The tumors particularly involve the central and peripheral nervous systems:

- Neurofibromatosis type 1
- Neurofibromatosis type 2
- Schwannomatosis

Neurofibromatosis Type 1

Neurofibromatosis type 1 (NF1), also known as *von Recklinghausen disease*, is a multisystem neurocutaneous disorder, the most common phakomatosis, and a RASopathy. Additionally, it is also one of the most common inherited central nervous system (CNS) disorders, autosomal dominant disorders, and inherited tumor syndromes.

Epidemiology

- Neurofibromatosis affects 1:2,500–3,000 individuals
- In half of the cases, the disease is inherited as an autosomal dominant condition. In the other half, the disease is due to a de novo mutation.
- There is a variable expression but 100% penetrance by 5 years of age.

Clinical Presentation

As is the case with many phakomatoses, NF1 results in a variety of abnormalities of variable severity. To make the clinical diagnosis, two or more of the following are required:

- Cafe-au-lait spots evident during 1 year (prepubertal >0.5 cm, postpubertal >1.5 cm in size)
- Two or more neurofibromas or one plexiform neurofibroma
- Optic nerve glioma
- Distinctive osseous lesion (such as sphenoid wing dysplasia or thinning of long bone cortex with or without pseudoarthrosis)
- Two or more iris hamartomas (Lisch nodules)
- Axillary or inguinal freckling
- A primary relative with NF1 with above criteria

In addition, ~45% (range 30–60%) of patients have learning disabilities, and approximately 1% have hypertension due to renal artery stenosis.

It is important to consider that NF1 has a much earlier age of onset than schwannomatosis and NF2, with approximately 50% of patients meeting the diagnostic criteria for NF1 by the age of 1 year.

Neoplasms

It should come as no surprise that a disease due to inactivation of a tumor suppressor gene (see below) is also associated with an increased incidence of numerous tumors:

- Pheochromocytoma
- Malignant peripheral nerve sheath tumor (MPNST) (~10% of patients)
- Wilms tumor
- Rhabdomyosarcoma
- Renal angiomyolipoma
- *Glioma:*
    - Juvenile pilocytic astrocytoma (~20% of patients)
    - Optic nerve glioma
    - Diffuse brainstem glioma
    - Spinal astrocytoma and spinal pilocytic astrocytoma
- Carcinoid tumor
- Leiomyoma
- Leiomyosarcoma
- Ganglioglioma
- Leukemia

Pathology

The *NF1* gene locus is on chromosome 17q11.2 and the gene product is neurofibromin, which acts as a tumor suppressor of the Ras/MAPK pathway; inactivation of the gene thus predisposes to tumor development.

The disease primarily is a hamartomatous disorder that involves the ectoderm and mesoderm. Usually, three types of neurofibromas occur in this disorder and are distinguished on the basis of their gross and microscopic appearances.

i. *Localized neurofibroma (cutaneous neurofibroma):* The most common type
ii. Diffuse neurofibroma (subcutaneous neurofibroma)
iii. Plexiform neurofibroma

Radiographic Features

Breast—neurofibromatosis of the breast.

Central Nervous System

- *FASI (focal areas of signal intensity):* Occur in deep white matter and basal ganglia or corpus callosum, areas of T2/FLAIR hyperintensity with no contrast enhancement

- Optic nerve glioma or optic pathway glioma (may manifest as enlarged optic foramen)
- Progressive sphenoid wing dysplasia
- Lambdoid suture defects
- Dural calcification at the vertex
- Moyamoya phenomenon (rare)
- Buphthalmos

Cutaneous—cutaneous and subcutaneous neurofibromas: Benign peripheral nerve sheath tumors

Skeletal

- Kyphoscoliosis
- Posterior vertebral scalloping
- Hypoplastic posterior elements
- Enlarged neural foramina
- Ribbon rib deformity, rib notching, and dysplasia
- Dural ectasia
- Tibial pseudoarthrosis or, less commonly, ulnar pseudoarthrosis
- Bony dysplasias—especially affecting tibia
- Severe bowing, gracile bones
- Multiple nonossifying fibromas
- Limb hemihypertrophy

Thoracic

- *Mediastinal masses:*
    - Neurofibroma
    - *Lateral thoracic meningocele:* Typically, on the convex side of scoliosis (through widened neural foramina)
    - Extra-adrenal pheochromocytoma
- *Lung parenchymal disease:* ~20%
    - *Diffuse interstitial fibrosis:* Lower zone
    - *Bullae formation:* Upper zone
    - Secondary pulmonary arterial hypertension and cor pulmonale

Vascular

- Aneurysms/arteriovenous malformations
- Renal artery stenosis
- Coarctation of aorta

Treatment and Prognosis

No single treatment exists, and a combination of supportive and surgical therapies is employed depending on the specific tumors and anomalies present.

Although prognosis is very variable, overall life-expectancy is approximately half that of nonaffected individuals. Tumors or cardiovascular complications are the most common causes of mortality.

Neurofibromatosis Type 2

Neurofibromatosis type 2 (NF2) is a rare autosomal-dominant neurocutaneous disorder (phakomatosis) manifesting as a development of multiple CNS tumors. Unlike neurofibromatosis type 1 (NF1), it is not associated with neurofibromas. Instead, patients with this disease have:

- *Intracranial schwannomas:* Mostly vestibular schwannomas sometimes patients may have spinal schwannomas
- Intracranial and spinal meningiomas
- Intraspinal-intramedullary ependymomas

These features give rise to the acronym MISME, which describes *Multiple Inherited Schwannomas Meningiomas and Ependymomas*. In fact, labeling this disorder *neurofibromatosis type 2* is a misnomer, because neurofibromas are not a part of its constellation of abnormalities.

Epidemiology
- The disease is rare with an estimated prevalence of 1:50,000.
- NF2 usually presents in young adults (age 18–24 years).
- Of patients with NF2, 50% have an affected parent (autosomal dominant inheritance) and 50% having a de novo mutation.

Pathology
- The *NF2* gene is located on the long arm of chromosome 22 (22q12) and encodes the merlin protein (also known as "schwannomin").
- Mutations in NF2 cause loss of protein function, resulting in a predisposition to tumor formation throughout the nervous system

Associations: There can also be associated syringohydromyelia with lesions in the spine as well as cataracts.

Radiographic Features
- Meningioma
- *Schwannoma:*
- Usually arise from the inferior vestibular division of the vestibulocochlear nerve
- Can also be from the facial nerve
- *Ependymoma:* Usually spinal intramedullary (not intracranial/intraventricular)

Bilateral vestibular schwannomas are diagnostic of NF2, but care should be taken because bilateral internal acoustic meatus masses are not specific for vestibular schwannoma and can represent, for example, sarcoidosis or metastases.

11. Give an account of abdominal desmoid tumors. ***WBUHS 2021***

12. Discuss the etiology, diagnosis, and treatment of desmoid tumor. ***WBUHS 2014, 2024***

Introduction
- Desmoid tumors are benign, noninflammatory fibroblastic tumors with a tendency for local invasion and recurrence but without metastasis.
- The terms desmoid tumor and aggressive fibromatosis are occasionally used synonymously.

Epidemiology
- They are rare tumors, thought to account for only ~0.03% of all neoplasms.
- Desmoid tumors are found in all age groups but are most frequently encountered between 20 and 40 years of age.
- They are seen more in women (2:1).
- They are rare lesions with an estimated incidence of 3.7 new cases per million population per year.

Associations
- Some cases have been associated with pregnancy and estrogen therapy.
- Gardner syndrome
- In the case of mesenteric desmoid, they are seen either sporadically or in association with familial polyposis coli syndrome (FAP): 9–18% of FAP cases may have a desmoid tumor.

Clinical Presentation

Desmoid tumors present as masses, and as such presentation depends on location.

Pathology
- Their exact etiology remains uncertain, although they are frequently associated with previous trauma or surgical incision.

- On the molecular level, desmoids are characterized by mutations in the β-catenin gene, *CTNNB1*, or the adenomatous polyposis coli (*APC*) gene.

Location

Frequent locations in the abdomen are the abdominal wall, the root of the mesentery, and the retroperitoneum.

Classification

Desmoid-type fibromatosis is listed in the WHO classification of soft tissue tumors under the category "fibroblastic/myofibroblastic tumors."

Radiographic Features

- *Ultrasound:*
  - Desmoid tumors are the most common neoplasms of the abdominal wall and typically appear as homogeneously hypoechoic masses.
  - They may have a similar appearance to muscle, may be lobulated, and may show vascularity on color Doppler interrogation.
- *CT:*
  - Most desmoid tumors are well-circumscribed masses, although in some cases, they may appear more aggressive with ill-defined margins.
  - Most are relatively homogeneously or focally hyperattenuating when compared to soft tissue on the noncontrast scan.
  - Most will demonstrate enhancement following administration of intravenous contrast.
- *MRI:*
  - MRI, as is the case with other soft tissue tumors, is more sensitive to local tumor extension.
  - Their appearance is accounted for by their dense cellularity. Typical signal characteristics include:
    - *T1:* Low-signal intensity
    - *T2:* Low-signal intensity
    - *T1 C+ (Gd):* May show homogeneous, inhomogeneous, or no significant enhancement

Treatment and Prognosis

- Watchful waiting is now considered a reasonable option in selected asymptomatic patients.
- Other management options include:
  - Surgical resection (traditionally used, although recurrence rate is high)
  - NSAIDs and antiestrogens can be used to reduce the rate of recurrence
  - Radiotherapy
- *Differential diagnosis:*
  - Carcinoid tumor
  - Sclerosing mesenteritis—tends to be more central at the "root" of the mesentery

SKIN MALIGNANCY

13. Describe premalignant conditions of skin. ***WBUHS 2014, WBUHS 2025 Supplementary***

- Actinic keratosis
- Arsenical keratosis
- Chronic radiation keratosis
- Bowen's disease
- Erythroplasia of Queyrat
- Erythroplakia
- Leukoplakia

Actinic Keratosis

Etiology	*Pathogenesis*	*Clinical features*
• Age >60–80% chances of development • M>F • Phenotype of fair skin which burn and freckles easily and rarely tan • Blue or light-colored eyes and blond hair • Immunosuppression • Genetic syndromes—xeroderma pigmentosum and albinism	• Sunlight exposure • UV-induced mutation in • Tumor-suppressor gene p53	• In elderly patient, 80% of lesions found on chronically sun-exposed sites—head, neck, forearms, and dorsum of hand • Erythematous, flat, scaly, yellow-colored papules • Hypertrophic—cutaneous horn • Actinic cheilitis

Bowen's Disease

Etiology	*Clinical features*	*Treatment*
• Squamous cell carcinoma in situ • Affects both skin and mucous membranes—having potential to progress into invasive carcinoma • Age >60 rarely before 30 years of age • Can occur at any body parts—sun or nonsun-exposed areas of body • Sun exposure • Arsenic exposure • Ionizing radiation • Immunosuppression • Infection with HPV-16 especially anogenital Bowen's disease	• Discrete • Slowly enlarging • Pink to erythematous • Thin plaque with well demarcated, irregular borders • Overlining scales or crust • Hyperkeratotic verrucous lesions • 5% of BD progress to invasive SCC	• Surgical excision • Cryosurgery • Curettage • 5 fu topical chemotherapy • Imiquimod 5% cream • Laser • Photodynamic therapy

(SCC: squamous cell carcinoma)

Erythroplasia of Queyrat

Etiology	*Clinical features*
• EQ—is carcinoma in situ affecting the mucosal surfaces of penis in uncircumcised males • Age 20–80 years • Uncircumcised • Poor hygiene • Smegma • HSV infection • HPV-16 and -18 infection	• Glistening • Red • Velvety plaque on glans penis, prepuce, or urethra • Usually solitary plaque • Localized pain or pruritus • Difficulty in retracting fore • Bleeding or crusting may be there at the lesion • Enlarge slowly and persist for several years • 33% of cases progress to invasive SCC

Leukoplakia

- It is fixed predominantly white lesion of mucosa
- Oral and anogenital mucosal surfaces
- Alcohol and tobacco use
- Age >50–70 years
- 5–25% risk of becoming invasive
- Clinically
- Asymptomatic
- Asymmetric
- White plaque
- At floor of mouth
- Lateral and ventral tongue

- Soft palate
- Diagnosis by biopsy
- Surgical excision of the lesion

14. Describe staging of squamous cell carcinoma. ***WBUHS 2006***

American Joint Committee on Cancer System for Classification and Staging of Squamous Cell Carcinoma

Primary tumor (T)			
TX	Primary tumor cannot be assessed		
T0	No evidence of primary tumor		
Tis	Carcinoma in situ		
T1	Tumor ≤2 cm in greatest dimension		
T2	Tumor >2 cm, but not >5 cm, in greatest dimension		
T3	Tumor >5 cm in greatest dimension		
T4	Tumor invades deep extradermal structures (i.e., cartilage, skeletal muscle, or bone)		
Regional lymph nodes (N)			
NX	Regional lymph nodes cannot be assessed		
N0	No regional lymph node metastasis		
N1	Regional lymph node metastasis		
Distant metastasis (M)			
MX	Distant metastasis cannot be assessed		
M0	No distant metastasis		
M1	Distant metastasis		
Stage grouping			
Stage 0	Tis	N0	M0
Stage I	T1	N0	M0
Stage II	T2	N0	M0
	T3	N0	M0
Stage III	T4	N0	M0
	Any T	N1	M0
Stage IV	Any T	Any N	M1

15. Marjolin's ulcer. ***RGUHS, Karnataka 2025***

Introduction

- Marjolin's ulcer refers to an aggressive ulcerating squamous cell carcinoma presenting in an area of previously traumatized, chronically inflamed, or scarred skin.
- They are commonly present in the context of chronic wounds including burn injuries, venous ulcers, ulcers from osteomyelitis, and postradiotherapy scars.

Appearance: Slow growth, painlessness (as the ulcer is usually not associated with nerve tissue), and absence of lymphatic spread due to local destruction of lymphatic channels

Characteristics

- Histologically, the tumor is a well-differentiated squamous cell carcinoma.

- This carcinoma is aggressive in nature, spreads locally, and is associated with a poor prognosis. 40% occur on the lower limb and the malignant change is usually painless.
- This malignant change of the wound happens a long time after initial trauma, usually 10–25 years later. Its edge is everted and not always raised.

Diagnosis

Wedge biopsy is the favored method of diagnosis. Tissue specimens obtained should be taken from both the center and margin of lesion, as the central ulcerated deposits may be necrotic.

Treatment

Treatment is usually surgical, with a wide excision of the lesion; typically a 1 cm margin all around is required. Radiation therapy is also a good alternative in most cases.

16. Write in brief about basal cell carcinoma.

Epidemiology and Etiology

- >400,000 new patients annually
- Age usually over 40 years
- Sex males > females
- Race rare in brown- and black-skinned patient

Clinical Features

Pearly papules or nodules	Rolled border	Telangiectasias	Central ulcer
Crusting	Bleed easily	Rodent ulcer	Locally malignant

Sites: Teardrop cancer—

Head, neck	Cheeks	Ears
Forehead	Nose	Upper trunk

Biopsy

Shave Punch Excision	Specimen to reliable dermatopathologist or pathologist

Treatment

- Electrodesiccation and curettage
- Excision
- Cryosurgery
- Moh's surgery
- Radiation
- 5-fluorouracil
- Aldara (imiquimod)

MALIGNANT MELANOMA

17. What are the different layers of epidermis and dermis? Describe the clinical types, clinical features, and management of melanoma. ***Tripura University 2023***

Epidermis

- *Type:* Stratified squamous keratinized epithelium

- *Thickness:* 0.05–1.5 mm (thin/thick skin variation)
- *Avascular:* Gets nutrients via diffusion from dermis
- *Cells:* Keratinocytes (~90%), melanocytes, Langerhans cells, Merkel cells

The epidermis has *5 layers (strata)* from *deep to superficial*:

Layer	*Other name*	*Characteristics/function*
Stratum basale	Basal layer, stratum germinativum	• Single layer of cuboidal/columnar cells • Mitotically active (stem cells) • Contains melanocytes and Merkel cells • Hemidesmosomes attach to basement membrane
Stratum spinosum	Prickle cell layer	• Several layers of polygonal keratinocytes • Cells connected by desmosomes (appear "spiny" under microscope) • Langerhans cells present
Stratum granulosum	Granular layer	• 3–5 layers of flattened keratinocytes • Keratohyalin granules (precursor of keratin) • Lamellar bodies → barrier function
Stratum lucidum	Clear layer (only in thick skin: palms/soles)	• Thin, translucent layer of dead keratinocytes • Homogenous, eosinophilic cytoplasm
Stratum corneum	Horny layer	• Many layers of dead, keratinized, enucleated cells (corneocytes) • Provides barrier against water loss, pathogens, and mechanical stress

Dermis

- *Type:* Dense irregular connective tissue
- *Thickness:* 0.6–3 mm (thin/thick skin)
- *Vascularized:* Supplies nutrients to epidermis, regulates temperature
- *Cells:* Fibroblasts, mast cells, macrophages, adipocytes (in reticular layer)

The dermis has two layers:

Layer	*Characteristics/features*
Papillary dermis	• Superficial layer, loose connective tissue • Dermal papillae interdigitate with epidermal ridges • Rich in capillaries, lymphatics, and sensory receptors (Meissner corpuscles) • Provides nutrients to epidermis
Reticular dermis	• Deeper layer, dense irregular connective tissue • Collagen bundles (types I and III) provide strength • Contains sweat glands, sebaceous glands, hair follicles, Pacinian corpuscles (pressure), blood vessels

Notes

- *Basement membrane* separates epidermis from dermis:
  - Composed of lamina lucida, lamina densa, and sublamina densa (anchoring fibrils)
  - *Role:* Structural support and selective permeability
- *Skin appendages* (hair, nails, glands) originate from *epidermis but extend into dermis.*

Answer of the next part of the question is written below.

18. Enumerate the pigmented lesions of the skin. ***WBUHS 2017***

19. Variants of melanoma.

20. Describe the clinical types of cutaneous melanoma. Write down clinical staging and management of malignant melanoma. ***WBUHS 2025 Supplementary***

21. Discuss the etiology, diagnosis, and management of melanoma. ***WBUHS 2012***

22. Discuss the pathology and management of malignant melanoma. ***WBUHS 2016***

23. Briefly discuss the roll of immunotherapy/biological therapy in malignant melanoma. ***WBUHS 2017***

Classification of Pigmented Lesions of Skin

Nonmelanocytic Lesions

- *Inflammatory:*
  - Postinflammatory hyperpigmentation
  - Dermatofibroma
- *Hamartomas:*
  - Collagenous nevus, papillary dermal type
  - Nevoid hyperkeratosis of the nipple
- *Benign neoplasms:*
  - Solar lentigo, including lichen planus-like keratosis
  - Seborrheic keratosis
- *Malignant neoplasms:*
  - Basal cell carcinoma, pigmented
  - Solar keratosis, pigmented

Melanocytic Lesions

- *Benign:*
  - Melanosis
  - Simple lentigo
  - Nevus of Ota, nevus of Ito
  - *Nevi:*
    - *Congenital:*
      - Classic acral
      - Superficial
      - Superficial and "deep"
      - Masson's blue neuronevus
      - Common blue (Jadassohn-Tieche)
      - Combined
      - Miescher's
      - Unna's
      - Nevus spilus
      - Persistent
      - Special site
      - Yet to be classified
  - *Superficial congenital nevus, probable:*
    - *Acquired:*
      - Clark's
      - Spitz's
      - Reed's

- *Yet to be classified:*
  - Clark-like
  - Spitz-like
  - Reed-like
- *Malignant:*
  - *Melanoma:*
    - In situ
    - No longer in situ ("invasive")
    - Persistent
    - In association with a nevus
    - Metastatic

Malignant Melanoma

Introduction

The incidence and outcome of melanoma are related to multiple factors.

- Melanoma is prevalent in whites.
- This disease is less common in Asian and Black populations.
- Melanoma develops 20 times more frequently in Whites than in Blacks.
- The disease occurs slightly more often in men than women, and the prognosis is slightly better for women.
- The anatomic distribution of melanoma varies between the two genders. Melanomas arise more commonly on the lower extremity in women and more often on the trunk and head and neck in men.
- Melanoma can occur at any age from birth to advanced age. The median age at diagnosis is in the range of
- 45–55 years. Tumors rarely develop before the age of puberty; however, there is a significant incidence in the third and fourth decades of life.

Risk Factors

- *Skin type:* People with white racial background have ten times melanoma incidence of African Americans and seven times the melanoma incidence of American Hispanics.
- *Age:* The incidence of melanoma increases with age.
- *Gender:* Incidence of melanoma is higher in men than in women.
- *Tanning bed use:* The use of a tanning bed more than ten times per year is associated with a doubling in the risk of melanoma for patients age 30 years or older.
- Previous melanoma
- *Sunlight exposure:* Occasional or recreational exposure to sunlight, especially a history of severe blistering sunburn, has been associated with increased risk of melanoma. Sunburns after the age of 20 years may be associated with an increased risk of melanoma. The effects of sunlight have been attributed to UV-B radiation.
- *Benign nevi:* The presence of large numbers of nevi has been consistently associated with an increased risk of melanoma. Persons with more than 50 nevi, all of which are greater than 2 mm in diameter, have 5–17 times the melanoma risk of persons with fewer nevi.
- *Family history:* A family history of melanoma increases a person's risk of melanoma by 3–8 times. Persons who have two or more family members with melanoma are at a particularly high risk for developing melanoma.
- *Genetic predisposition:*
  - Specific genetic alterations have been implicated in the pathogenesis of melanoma.
  - At least 4 distinct genes—located on chromosomes 1p, 6q, 7 and 9—may play a role in melanoma.
  - A tumor suppressor gene located on chromosome 9p21 is probably involved in familial and sporadic cutaneous melanoma.

  - Deletions or rearrangements of chromosome 10 and 11 are also well documented in cutaneous melanoma.
  - Another tumor suppression gene *p16* also plays a role in the development of melanoma.
  - Another genetic alteration that may play role is mutation in the *BRAF* gene.
- Atypical mole and melanoma syndrome
- Additional factors that increase the risk for development of melanoma include:
  - Dysplastic nevus (DN) syndrome
  - Xeroderma pigmentosum
  - A history of nonmelanoma skin cancer (NMSC)
  - A family history of melanoma

Diagnosis Choice of Biopsy

- Clinical management of melanoma begins with an accurate diagnosis.
- The classic signs of melanoma include a skin lesion with changing characteristics such as *irregular borders, varying degrees of pigmentation, an irregular surface, bleeding, itching, and ulceration.*
- The decision to perform a biopsy is frequently based on clinical experience. The specific method of biopsy depends on the size of the lesion and its anatomic location.
- Regardless of the method, biopsy specimens are full thickness into subcutaneous tissue. For small lesions, an excisional biopsy is commonly performed that includes a narrow (1–2 mm) margin of surrounding skin.
- *Shave biopsies are* commonly performed for benign-appearing lesions, this technique must not be used when melanoma is suspected. A shave biopsy may lead to a pathology report showing extension of tumor to the deep margins of excision.
- In these circumstances, the most important prognostic factor, tumor thickness, will not be accurate and could lead to incorrect decisions regarding *wide local excision (WLE), SLN biopsy,* and *adjuvant therapy.*
- The clinical appearance of melanoma may be deceptively benign, which is why the use of cautery or cryoablation may lead to a delay in the diagnosis of melanoma.
- If a skin lesion reappears at the site of a previously cauterized or frozen skin lesion, excisional biopsy and histopathologic analysis are required.
- The biopsy removes the full thickness of skin, including a layer of the underlying fatty tissue and the entire visible tumor.
- Care must be taken to not crush or otherwise traumatize the specimen so that histologic interpretation is not compromised.
- The biopsy is a full-thickness specimen and includes a margin of adjacent normal skin if possible.
- When biopsy of a large lesion is performed, at least one punch is placed through the most elevated portion to accurately classify its thickness.

Pathology

Histologically, melanoma is divided into four major types based on growth pattern and location: lentigo maligna melanoma (LMM), superficial spreading melanoma (SSM), acral lentiginous melanoma (ALM), and nodular melanoma (NM).

Melanomas arise as proliferations of melanocytes in the basal layer of the skin. As they multiply, these cells expand radially in the epidermis and superficial dermal layer. With time, growth begins in a vertical direction and the skin lesion may become palpable. NMs are an exception to this pattern in that the vertical growth phase is present from an early point in tumor development. It is the vertical growth phase more than any other histologic parameter of the primary tumor that determines prognosis.

Variant of Melanoma

Superficial spreading melanoma (SSM)	***Nodular melanoma***	***Lentigo maligna melanoma***	***Acral lentiginous melanoma***
Most common form of melanoma (80%)	Most aggressive form	Usually found in older patients as a large melanotic freckle on the temple or malar region known as Hutchinson freckle	Occurs on the palms, soles, and nailbeds
Approximately one-half arising from a pre-existing mole	Rapidly becoming a palpable, elevated, firm nodule that may be dense black or reddish blue–blackish	It is usually slow growing but becomes large, often reaching 5–6 cm in diameter	Occurs primarily in darker skinned people
The lesions usually are slow growing and brown, with small discrete nodules of differing colors	A distinct convex nodular development indicates deep dermal invasion	Initially, it is flat, but it becomes raised and thicker, with discrete brown to black nodules and irregular edges	Metastasizes more frequently than do other melanomas possibly related to later stage at presentation
SSM tends to spread laterally but can be slightly elevated	Nodular melanomas arise from the epidermal–dermal junction and invade deeply into the dermis and subcutaneous tissue		
SSM is found most commonly on the back in men and women and on the lower extremities of women	Approximately 5% are amelanotic		

Familial Melanoma

- Approximately 5–10% of melanoma patients have a family history of the disease. When compared with patients who have sporadic melanoma, the age of onset is earlier, the incidence of DNs is higher, and multiple primary melanomas are more common.
- Chromosome mapping studies have shown evidence of linkage and heterogeneity to chromosomes 1p and 9p. Chromosome 1p contributes to both sporadic and familial melanoma, whereas 9p contributes more to sporadic melanoma alone. All reported kindreds are white.

In-transit metastases and satellites both signify a poor prognosis with a high risk of local recurrence and distant metastasis. In-transit metastases are lesions in the skin >2 cm from the primary lesion; they arise from tumor cells in intradermal lymphatics. Satellites are metastatic lesions in the skin within 2 cm of the primary tumor.

Early Signs of Malignant Melanoma

- *A:* Asymmetry
- *B:* Border irregularity
- *C:* Color variegation
- *D:* Diameter >6 mm
- *E:* Evolving or enlarging lesion

Prognostic Factors

Clark and associates described a classification of melanoma based on the extent of tumor invasion relative to the anatomic layers of the skin and showed that the level of invasion was related to survival.

Clark's Classification (Level of Invasion) of Melanoma

Level I: Lesions involving only the epidermis (*in situ* melanoma); not an invasive lesion

Level II: Invasion of the papillary dermis but does not reach the papillary–reticular dermal interface *Level III:* Invasion fills and expands the papillary dermis but does not penetrate the reticular dermis *Level IV:* Invasion into the reticular dermis but not into the subcutaneous tissue

Level V: Invasion through the reticular dermis into the subcutaneous tissue

In some cases, determining the Clark level was found to be difficult, and readings of the same slides could differ between pathologists (especially in the level 3 to 4 range).

Breslow described a more straightforward system based on measuring the vertical thickness of the tumor in millimeters. This method was found to be accurately reproducible between pathologists, and there was excellent correlation with 5-year survival. The prognosis worsens with increasing thickness as a continuous logarithmic function without stair-step areas or natural breakpoints.

Breslow's Staging
Stage I: <0.75 mm
Stage II: 0.76–1.5 mm
Stage III: 1.51–4.0 mm
Stage IV: >4.0 mm

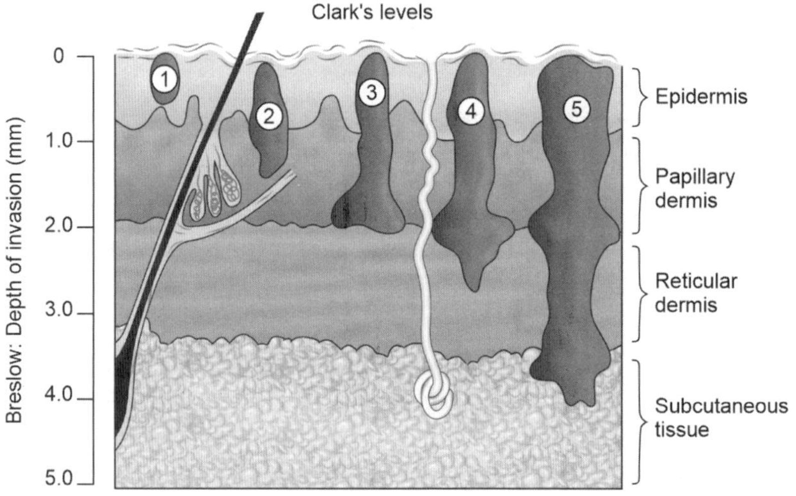

American Joint Committee on Cancer TNM Melanoma Classification—2002

Primary tumor (T)	
TX	Primary tumor cannot be assessed (e.g., shave biopsy or regressed melanoma)
T0	No evidence of primary tumor
Tis	Melanoma in situ
T1	Melanoma ≤1.0 mm in thickness, with or without ulceration
T1a	Melanoma ≤1.0 mm in thickness and level II or III, no ulceration
T1b	Melanoma ≤1.0 mm in thickness and level IV or V or with ulceration
T2	Melanoma 1.01–2.0 mm in thickness, with or without ulceration
T2a	Melanoma 1.01–2.0 mm in thickness, no ulceration
T2b	Melanoma 1.01–2.0 mm in thickness, with ulceration
T3	Melanoma 2.01–4.0 mm in thickness, with or without ulceration

Contd...

Contd...

T3a	Melanoma 2.01–4.0 mm in thickness, no ulceration
T3b	Melanoma 2.01–4.0 mm in thickness, with ulceration
T4	Melanoma >4.0 mm in thickness, with or without ulceration
T4a	Melanoma >4.0 mm in thickness, no ulceration
T4b	Melanoma >4.0 mm in thickness, with ulceration
Regional lymph Nodes (N)	
NX	Regional lymph nodes cannot be assessed
N0	No regional lymph node metastasis
N1	Metastasis in one lymph node
N1a	Clinically occult (microscopic) metastasis
N1b	Clinically apparent (macroscopic) metastasis
N2	Metastasis in two or three regional nodes or intralymphatic regional metastasis without nodal metastases
N2a	Clinically occult (microscopic) metastasis
N2b	Clinically apparent (macroscopic) metastasis
N2c	Satellite or in-transit metastasis without nodal metastasis
N3	Metastasis in four or more regional nodes, matted metastatic nodes, in-transit metastasis, or satellites with metastasis in regional node(s)
Distant metastasis (M)	
MX	Distant metastasis cannot be assessed
M0	No distant metastasis
M1	Distant metastasis
M1a	Metastasis to skin, subcutaneous tissue, or distant lymph nodes
M1b	Metastasis to lung
M1c	Metastasis to all other visceral sites or distant metastasis at any site associated with elevated serum lactate dehydrogenase

Treatment Surgery:

- *Wide local excision* is the primary treatment for most melanomas and premalignant lesions.
- Melanoma in situ (MIS) should be excised to clean margins.
- For all other malignant melanomas, the width of the surgical margin depends on the Breslow tumor thickness.
- Thin melanomas (Breslow <1 mm) should have a margin of 1 cm; lesions thicker than 1 mm and all scalp lesions should have a margin of at least 2 cm.

Recommended margins for surgical resection of primary melanoma:

Tumor thickness (mm)	***Margin radius (cm)***
In situ	0.5
<1.0	1.0
1-2	1.0-2.0
>2.0	≥2.0

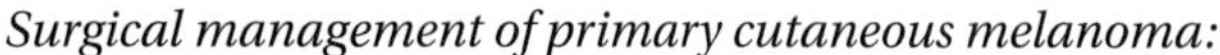

Surgical management of primary cutaneous melanoma:

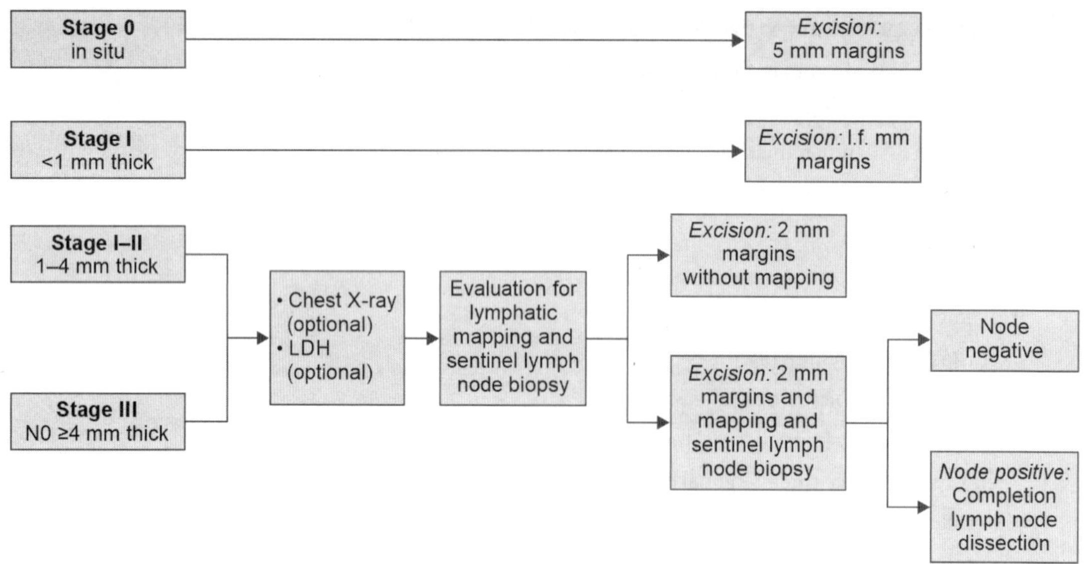

(LDH: lactate dehydrogenase)

- *Moh's micrographic surgery* has been advocated for areas where wide and deep excisions are difficult.
- *Elective lymph node dissection (ELND):* The term "elective" refers here to lymph node dissection done in the absence of clinically evident, palpable nodes. ELND provided an element of local control and reasonably accurate staging for patients with occult lymph node metastases.
- *Sentinel lymph node biopsy (SLNB):*
  - SLNB has greatly enhanced accurate staging of melanoma patients.
  - This technique is based on the documented pattern of lymphatic drainage of melanomas to a specific, initial lymph node, termed the sentinel lymph node, before further spread.
  - The histology of the SLN is highly (although not perfectly) reflective of the rest of the nodal basin.
  - *If the SLN is negative for metastases, a more radical and morbid lymph node dissection can be avoided.*
  - SLNB appears to be most beneficial for intermediate-thickness melanomas (Breslow 1–4 mm). SLNB appears to be a better diagnostic procedure than clinical staging or ELND in terms of sensitivity and morbidity, but some controversy remains over its absolute benefit.
- *Therapeutic lymph node dissection:*
  - It should be performed for involved axillary and superficial inguinal lymph nodes unless unresectable distant metastases are present.
  - Ideally, therapeutic lymph node dissection (LND) provides optimal locoregional control of disease and a chance of cure, with 5-year survival rates of 20–40.
  - Deep inguinal node dissection should be reserved for patients whose survival is thought to justify the potential morbidity of the procedure. In some cases, nodal dissection will not benefit patients with advanced disease and should, therefore, be carefully considered.
- *Resection of metastases:*
  - The surgical options for patients with metastatic melanoma can be divided into two categories: curative or palliative.
  - Curative interventions for metastatic melanoma should carefully weigh the risks of the surgery against the potential benefits.
  - Recent data on the surgical management of metastatic melanoma note that certain factors are associated with an improved overall survival:

- Ability to achieve a complete resection with negative margins
- The initial site of metastasis
- Extent of metastatic disease (single or multiple sites)
- Disease-free interval after surgical removal of the primary melanoma
- Stage of initial disease
- Favorable sites for resection include the skin, subcutaneous tissue, lymph nodes, lung, and gastrointestinal tract. Skin and subcutaneous metastases demonstrated the best long-term results after resection.
- *Unfavorable sites include metastases to the brain, adrenal, and liver.*

Isolated limb perfusion:

- Isolated limb perfusion (ILP) is used for recurrent limb melanoma that is locally advanced and cannot be resected by simple surgical means.
- ILP delivers high-dose regional chemotherapy and establishes a hyperthermic environment to an extremity while its circulation has been isolated from the rest of the body.
- Melphalan is commonly used. Adding tumor necrosis factor-α (TNF-α) to melphalan has been suggested to increase the complete response rate to 60–85%.
- Patients who are elderly or who have medical comorbidities or systemic metastases are generally not suitable for this therapy.

Immunotherapy:

- Complete and durable regression of stage IV melanoma has been reported using interleukin-2 (IL-2)-based immunotherapy alone.
- Interleukin-2 plays a central role in the activation and stimulation of T-lymphocytes and natural killer (NK) cells. In response to IL-2 stimulation, these cells acquire cytolytic properties which are believed to enhance their anti-tumoral properties.
- It can be used in:
  - Metastatic malignant melanoma
  - Advanced melanoma
  - Intralesional IL-2 for in-transit lesions
- Although patients can be cured of metastatic melanoma solely using high-dose IL-2, the response rate is low. This has led to the use of IL-2 in conjunction with other treatments, including vaccines, monoclonal antibodies, and adoptive transfer of T lymphocytes.
- Recently, a 50% response rate according to *Response Evaluation Criteria in Solid Tumors (RECIST)* criteria was reported in patients with metastatic melanoma treated with in vitro expanded tumor-infiltrating lymphocytes and IL-2.
- *Interferon α:* The immunotherapeutics approved by the FDA for the adjuvant treatment of melanoma are interferon α-2b and peginterferon α-2b.
- *Adoptive immunotherapy:*
  - The adoptive cell therapy (ACT) approach utilizes ex vivo cultured autologous lymphocytes.
  - These lymphocytes can be derived from resected metastasis or from peripheral blood.
  - The optimization of the host environment prior to cell transfer appears to be very important for the success of this procedure: high-dose chemotherapy is needed to induce lymphodepletion to eliminate immune regulatory elements (both cellular and humoral) that could affect homing and activity of transferred cells.
  - Recent advances in ACT involve the use of autologous engineered T-cells that express T-cell receptors specific for various tumor-associated antigens (such as *MART-1-TCG* genes), or that secrete specific cytokines.

Biological therapy:

- *Anti-CTLA-4:* The cytotoxic T-lymphocyte antigen 4 (CTLA-4) is a receptor that interacts with CD80 (B7-1) and CD86 (B7-2) and downregulates T-cell response.

- *Ipilimumab and tremelimumab (CP-675206)* are monoclonal antibodies that block CTLA-4 and allow CD28 to bind to B7-1 receptors, which leads to IL-2 secretion, cytotoxic T-cell activation, and proliferation.
- *Anti-CTLA-4 antibodies in metastatic melanoma:* Clinical studies confirm that the CTLA-4 inhibitor ipilimumab can induce durable responses and improve overall survival in patients with advanced melanoma. Also used in adjuvant therapies.
- *Anti-PD-1 and PDL-1:* Programmed death-1 (PD-1) receptor, also known as CD279, is a protein receptor that is inducibly expressed on $CD4^+$ T-cells, $CD8^+$ T-cells, natural killer T-cells, and B-cells. PD-1, interacting with programmed death ligand 1 (PDL-1) and PDL-2 negatively regulates immune responses.
  - *Nivolumab* is a human monoclonal antibody targeting PD-1.
  - *Pembrolizumab is also* PD-1 inhibitor.
- *CD40 agonist:* CD40 is a costimulatory molecule expressed on dendritic cells, B-cells, and monocytes. Its ligand, CD40L, is expressed on $CD4^+$ T-cells. It can be used in metastatic melanoma.
- *CD137 agonist:* CD137 is an inducible T-lymphocyte surface molecule of the tumor necrosis factor (TNF) receptor superfamily. Its ligand, CD137L, can be expressed by most immune and many nonimmune cells as a transmembrane protein. CD137 signaling enhances T-lymphocyte proliferation and T-helper-1 cytokine production, protecting $CD8^+$ T-lymphocytes from apoptosis. It can be used in metastatic melanoma.
- *Agonistic antibodies targeting OX40:* OX40 and its ligand, OX40L, are key TNF members that augment T-cell expansion, cytokine production, and cell survival. OX40 is a co-stimulatory molecule expressed transiently on the surface of T-cells. Agonistic antibodies targeting OX40 have been shown to have antitumor activity.
- *Anti-TIM-3 antibody:* T-cell immunoglobulin mucin-3 (TIM-3) is another inhibitory receptor expressed on a subset of tumor reactive T-cells. Blockage of TIM-3 has been shown to improve the function. It can be used in malignant melanoma.

Systemic Treatment of Melanoma

- Most of the increase in the incidence of melanoma is attributable to thin melanomas with an excellent prognosis. Unfortunately, the number of deaths from melanoma is also rising.
- The most common areas of metastasis are the lung, liver, bone, and brain.
- The most frequently used drug for systemic therapy is dacarbazine.
- A doubling of the response rate has been observed with CVD (cisplatin, vinblastine, dacarbazine) combined with interferon-α, interleukin-2, or a combination of these two biological.
- The combination of CVD, interferon, and interleukin-2 (frequently called biochemotherapy) has a response rate of 50% and a complete response rate of 15%.
- Temozolomide is also being used in combination with other drugs.
- Current recommendations for chemotherapy are summarized in the National Comprehensive Cancer Network guidelines stage IV patients are also candidates for investigational protocols involving the use of immunotherapy.
- An extensive history of immunotherapy for melanoma, this modality remains investigational. It is postulated that stage IV patients who can undergo resection of all detectable disease will be a group of patients who will benefit from systemic therapies such as immunotherapy.

Adjuvant Systemic Therapy

Clinical investigators have been attempting to identify an effective adjuvant therapy for melanoma for >40 years, but no treatment regimen has shown a conclusive benefit.

Monitoring of Patients after Surgical Therapy

- After primary treatment of melanoma, prediction of the pattern of recurrence can be based on the same factors used to estimate survival (tumor thickness, ulceration, and lymph node status).
- The risk of the first metastasis being at a distant site increases with thick primary tumors and resected regional positive nodes.
- Follow-up examinations focus on detection of treatable metastases.

- The most common sites of initial recurrence are local and regional.
- Patients are informed about the common symptoms and signs of recurrence so that they can report important changes arising between scheduled examinations.
- Such changes include local swelling, itching, new lesions in and beneath the skin, enlargement of lymph nodes, central nervous system changes, and pulmonary and gastrointestinal symptoms.
- The physical examination is the most important aspect of the return visit.
- A complete skin examination is performed with inspection and palpation of the primary site and skin surfaces leading to regional nodal basins. In-transit metastases may be palpable but not visible.
- *The follow-up examination* schedule reflects the risk for recurrence. Initially, patients are seen at 3–6-month intervals until they have reached the 3-year anniversary.
- By this time, 75% of patients in whom a metastasis would ever develop would have had that event occur. Annual examinations are scheduled thereafter.
- Patients with early melanoma, stage IA, are monitored without radiologic or laboratory studies. For asymptomatic patients, a chest radiograph and serum lactate dehydrogenase assay may be performed at 6- to 12-month intervals, although there is no evidence that the routine use of these follow-up tests results in a survival benefit.
- The routine use of screening computed tomography (CT), magnetic resonance imaging, or positron emission tomography (PET) has not been shown to be cost-effective and remains a subject of investigation for stage III patients
- PET scan results change treatment decisions in up to 20% of cases; however, the rate is very low in patients with a single microscopic nodal metastasis. Scans and other tests may be required for patients participating in clinical protocols.

Surgical Considerations for Metastases

Approximately 80% of patients who are treated for melanoma are cured of their disease. Recurrent disease appears locally, regionally, systemically, or in a combination of these sites.

Regional Nodal Recurrence

- Regional nodal metastases are the most common site of first recurrence in patients who undergo WLE alone. When palpable lymph nodes develop, the diagnosis is most rapidly made by fine-needle aspiration (FNA) performed during the office visit.
- If positive, complete resection of the nodal basin will control regional disease in a large proportion of patients.
- If FNA is negative or insufficient, excisional biopsy is performed to verify the diagnosis. If nodes are positive, long-term survival is unfortunately low.
- Even with a single palpable nodal metastasis, the 5-year survival rate is 40–50%.
- Before complete regional lymphadenectomy, a full metastatic workup is performed, including CT scans of the head, chest, abdomen, and pelvis, although these scans are normal in the majority of patients who are otherwise asymptomatic.
- The risk for further loco-regional recurrence after complete lymph node basin dissection is increased in the presence of multiple positive nodes, especially those containing extracapsular extension.
- Postoperative irradiation of the involved areas has been advocated in some centers as a way to further reduce recurrences; however, such radiotherapy has not been tested in a prospective, randomized trial.

Local and Regional Recurrences

- True local recurrence (N2c, stage III) is defined as tumor appearing in skin or subcutaneous tissue within a 5-cm radius of the primary wide excision site. Factors that predict local recurrence are the same as those predicting overall survival.
- Local recurrence is treated by surgical resection to attain histologically clear margins. WLE guidelines for primary tumors do not apply to local recurrences.
- Amputation for extensive local-regional recurrence is seldom indicated.

- Occasionally, patients have indolent locoregional disease for which amputation is indicated only after other attempts at locoregional tumor control have been unsuccessful.
- Patients with multiple recurrences on the limbs may be candidates for isolated hyperthermic limb perfusion (IHLP). Interleukin-2, tumor necrosis factor, and multiple other chemotherapeutic agents have also been used. Response rates exceed 80%, and complete responses are seen in 10–15% of patients.
- Reperfusion of extremities can be performed in patients who have an excellent initial response. Based on encouraging results with therapeutic IHLP, a randomized trial was designed to test the value of prophylactic perfusion in patients with high-risk melanoma (>1.5 mm in thickness). After >6 years' median follow-up, there was no improvement in overall survival. Therefore, IHLP is recommended only for patients with established multiple in-transit metastases.

Distant Metastases

- The most common sites of initial distant metastases are the brain, lung, and liver and less commonly the skin, bone, and other gastrointestinal tract sites.
- The prognosis varies significantly with the site of first metastases. In the majority of cases, metastases appear at multiple sites simultaneously.
- In such circumstances, systemic therapy is indicated for palliation. Occasionally, metastases develop that are apparently isolated to a single site.
- These patients are evaluated for surgical resection because the long-term disease-free survival rate after metastasectomy is reported to range from 10 to 20%.
- Patients being considered for resection of visceral metastases undergo complete staging, including CT and PET scans.
- In general, the prognosis for metastases to distant sites is related to the number of metastases and the disease-free interval between primary therapy and recurrent disease.
- Highly selected patients may undergo excision of multiple intra-abdominal metastases with a favorable outcome.

One-year Survival Rates for Patients with Distant Metastases

Stage	*Metastatic site(s)*	*Approximate 1-year survival (%)*
M1a	Skin, subcutaneous tissues, lymph nodes	60
M1b	Lung	55
M1c	Other visceral sites	40

24. Enumerate the risk factors and prognostic factors of malignant melanoma. Principles of management of malignant melanoma. ***WBUHS 2021 Supplementary***

Primary risk factors and clinical warning signs for melanoma include the following:

- Changing mole (most important clinical warning sign)
- *Presence of xeroderma pigmentosum or familial atypical mole melanoma syndrome:* These genodermatoses confer a 500- to 1,000-fold greater relative risk of developing melanoma.
- Clinical atypical/dysplastic nevi in familial melanoma
- Sporadic (nonfamilial) clinical atypical/dysplastic nevi (particularly >5–10)
- Melanoma in first-degree relative(s) (especially multiple)
- Large numbers of common nevi (>100)
- Previous melanoma
- Male sex
- Age >50 years
- Sun sensitivity/history of excessive sun exposure or sunburns

- Large (giant) congenital nevi (>20 cm diameter in an adult)
- Prior nonmelanoma skin cancer (basal cell and squamous cell carcinoma)
- Immunosuppression

The most important prognostic factors include the following:

- Thickness and/or level of invasion
- Mitotic index (mitoses per millimeter)
- Ulceration or bleeding at the primary site
- Number of regional lymph nodes involved, with distinction of macrometastasis and micrometastasis
- Systemic metastasis, including the site (nonvisceral versus lung versus all other visceral sites) and serum lactate dehydrogenase (LDH) level elevation

Positive prognostic factors include the following:

- Younger age
- Female sex
- Melanoma located on the extremities

Principles of Management of Malignant Melanoma

- Surgery is the definitive treatment for early-stage melanoma. In patients with solitary or acutely symptomatic brain metastases, surgical management or treatments such as gamma knife radiation may alleviate symptoms and provide local control of disease.
- Because the definitive treatment of cutaneous melanoma is surgery, medical management is reserved for adjuvant therapy of patients with advanced melanoma. Less than one-half of patients with deep primaries
- (>4 mm) or regional lymph node involvement have long-term disease-free survival; consequently, these patients are classified as high risk and should be considered for adjuvant therapy.

By stage, standard treatment options for melanoma are as follows:

- *Stage 0:* Excision
- *Stage I:* Excision, with or without lymph node management
- *Stage II:* Excision, with or without lymph node management
- *Resectable stage III:* Excision, with or without lymph node management; adjuvant therapy and immunotherapy
- *Unresectable stage III, stage IV, and recurrent melanoma:* Intralesional therapy, immunotherapy, signal transduction inhibitors, chemotherapy, palliative local therapy

Multiple options for adjuvant treatment of node-positive melanoma have become available:

- BRAF and BRAF/MEK inhibitor combinations are useful in some patients to slow the progression of disease.
- In patients with no BRAF mutation (i.e., wild-type BRAF), current guidelines from the National Comprehensive Cancer Network (NCCN) recommend single-agent immunotherapy with the programmed cell death-1 (PD-1) inhibitor pembrolizumab or nivolumab or combination therapy with nivolumab plus ipilimumab.
- For patients with a BRAF mutation, the NCCN recommends targeted combination therapy with dabrafenib/trametinib or vemurafenib/cobimetinib.
- Targeted therapy is preferred if clinically needed for early response. Current targeted therapies can slow tumor growth (e.g., BRAF inhibition) or release the brakes on the immune response, resulting in tumor lysis (e.g., PD-1 inhibition).
- Interferon α-2b was approved in 1995 for adjuvant treatment after excision in patients who are free of disease but are at high risk for recurrence.
- Regional therapy with isolated limb perfusion (ILP) or isolated limb infusion (ILI) of chemotherapy can be used for recurrent or in-transit extremity melanoma that is locally advanced and/or unresectable.
- Intralesional therapy is indicated for unresectable satellite or in-transit metastasis.

25. Describe the Clerk level and Breslow depth classification of malignant melanoma. Outline management of a malignant melanoma of forearm 3 cm diameter. ***WBUHS 2022, Tripura University 2025***

26. Describe the Clerk level and Breslow depth classification of malignant melanoma. Outline treatment of malignant melanoma of cheek 2 cm diameter. ***WBUHS 2025 Supplementary***

Clark's Classification (Level of Invasion) of Melanoma

Level I	Lesions involving only the epidermis (*in situ* melanoma); not an invasive lesion
Level II	Invasion of the papillary dermis but does not reach the papillary-reticular dermal interface
Level III	Invasion fills and expands the papillary dermis but does not penetrate the reticular dermis
Level IV	Invasion into the reticular dermis but not into the subcutaneous tissue
Level V	• Invasion through the reticular dermis into the subcutaneous tissue • In some cases, determining the clark level was found to be difficult, and readings of the same slides could differ between pathologists (especially in the level 3 to 4 range)

Breslow described a more straightforward system based on measuring the vertical thickness of the tumor in millimeters. This method was found to be accurately reproducible between pathologists, and there was excellent correlation with 5-year survival. The prognosis worsens with increasing thickness as a continuous logarithmic function without stair-step areas or natural breakpoints.

Breslow's staging:
Stage I: <0.75 mm
Stage II: 0.76–1.5 mm
Stage III: 1.51–4.0 mm
Stage IV: >4.0 mm

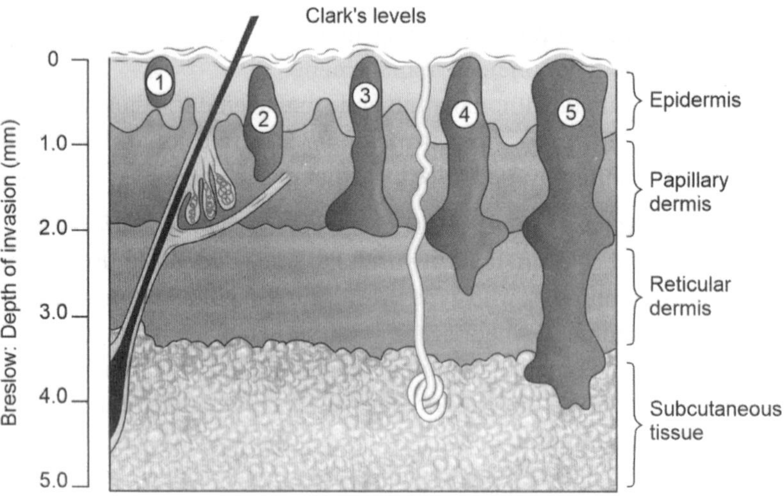

Treatment

Staging Workup

- Any lesion that is clinically suspicious for melanoma should ideally undergo a complete elliptical excisional biopsy with narrow margins.
- Examination of the entire pigmented lesion allows for the greatest chance of accurate diagnosis and also for the measurement of *Breslow* thickness and the assessment of other prognostic factors.

- If the lesion is large or located on certain anatomical sites, a full-thickness incisional biopsy can be performed, reaching to the adipose tissue. This biopsy should be obtained from the most elevated or darkest area of the lesion, although there is not always a correlation between clinical appearance and the thickest part of the lesion.
- If initial biopsy confirms melanoma with subtotal excision and if there is significant amount of residual lesion, a narrow margined re-excision should be immediately made, to evaluate if the patient is a candidate for sentinel lymph node biopsy.

Evaluation for Regional Metastasis

Macroscopic Metastases

- First step should always be history taking and physical examination.
- A careful lymph node examination of the whole body should be made, particularly the regions close to the site of the primary lesion.
- Also because of the aberrant lymphatic drainage pathways to unexpected nodal basins and to interval nodes between the primary site and expected regional nodal basin, a search for clinically detectable nodal disease in unexpected locations is crucial.
- If there is a palpable lymph node during physical examination, first a fine-needle aspiration biopsy should be performed to make a histological confirmation. If the result of the fine-needle aspiration is inconclusive, an excisional biopsy can be made.
- For the detection of small nodal metastases, best noninvasive methods seem to be ultrasound imaging and positron emission tomography, with sensitivity and specificity being lower than tissue diagnosis.

Microscopic Metastases

- Sentinel lymph node biopsy (SLNB)
- The node is removed and subjected to pathological examination using immunohistochemistry (S100 and HMB-45)
- The value of SLNB in patients with tumors of *Breslow* thickness 4 mm or thicker is questionable (if the intent is therapeutic as well as being a staging tool) because the risk of hematogenous spread is so high.

Evaluation for Distant Metastasis

- For the evaluation of distant metastases, a thorough examination of the neurologic, psychiatric, musculoskeletal, skin, lymphatic, endocrine, cardiovascular, and respiratory systems is necessary.
- Patients with newly diagnosed melanoma require a complete cutaneous and physical examination with particular attention to lymphadenopathy and hepatomegaly, and a baseline chest radiograph.
- Current imaging techniques such as computed tomography, magnetic resonance imaging, PET, chest X-ray, and laboratory tests like LDH are not routinely indicated as their sensitivity and specificity are low.

Treatment of Primary Melanoma

- The standard treatment for primary cutaneous melanoma is wide local excision.
- The aim of wide excision is to reach histopathologically confirmed tumor-free margins, as well as preventing local recurrence.

Treatment of Regional Metastasis

- *Macrometastatic nodal disease:*
  - One of the main causes of melanoma-related morbidity with an important negative effect on quality of life is the poor control of the nodal disease. Therefore, current standard of therapy for microscopic or macroscopic melanoma in lymph nodes is complete dissection of the node in the involved regional basin.
  - According to the current guidelines, adequate lymphadenectomy is described as at least 10 nodes in the groin region, 15 lymph nodes in the axillary region, and 15 lymph nodes in the neck area.
- *Micrometastatic nodal disease:*
  - Thus, there is no role for elective lymph node dissection today, especially considering its significant morbidity and the availability of sentinel lymph node biopsy.

- For the identification of micrometastatic nodal disease, sentinel node biopsy is the tool of choice. According to current trials of investigations, immediate complete lymph node dissection has a higher survival rate than delayed dissection.

Adjuvant Therapy

- Adjuvant therapy is usually given after surgical resection of the primary lesion. It is preferred in patients with increased relapse risk. When thickness of the primary lesion is higher than 4 mm or when there is nodal involvement, adjuvant therapy is necessary.
- Up to now, interferon-a2b (IFN-a2b) is the only form of adjuvant therapy, which is approved by US Food and Drug Administration.
- *Melanoma vaccines:* Vaccines stimulate specific immune response against melanoma-associated antigens.

Satellite Metastases

- For localized disease, limited to one extremity only, first choice of treatment should ideally be surgical excision with clear margins if possible.
- But in case of multiple lesions, chance of performing an ideal excision may be low, so in that case, isolated limb perfusion can be considered.
- Main idea about isolated limb perfusion is giving high doses of chemotherapeutic agents locally, to avoid systemic toxicity, and obtain more therapeutic effect. The technique of this method involves perfusing an isolated arm or leg in a hyperthermic environment, with cytotoxic agents. Conventionally chemotherapeutic agent used in this procedure is melphalan. Approximately in half of the patients, complete disappearance of the lesion is observed.

Treatment of Distant or Disseminated Metastasis

In case of stage 4 melanoma, with distant metastasis, mean survival is 6–8 months and there is currently no effective systemic treatment, to increase survival rate. For this reason, main treatment goal is the palliation of symptoms.

Radiation Therapy

Radiation therapy plays a role in the management of primary cutaneous melanoma in definitive, adjuvant, and palliative settings. The role for radiation therapy in early stage primary melanoma is limited as the treatment is adequate excision.

Systemic Therapies

Chemotherapy

- For systemic chemotherapy, first-line chemotherapeutic agent is dacarbazine, an alkylating agent.
- Temozolomide is also an alkylating agent. This chemotherapeutic agent can also be used orally.
- For metastatic melanoma to brain, a combination of temozolomide and thalidomide, along with radiation, can be beneficial. For dacarbazine, increased response rates are reported, when combined with other cytotoxic agents like cisplatin, vinblastine, carmustine, or tamoxifen.

Immunotherapy

Among immunotherapeutic agents, interleukin-2 (IL-2) is the only agent, which has an approval from FDA.

Biochemotherapy

Biochemotherapy alone has not shown any increase in overall survival rate, but when compared to other systemic chemotherapeutic agents like dacarbazine or interferon, vaccines, IL-2, it can show better results.

Novel Therapies

- About the etiopathology of intrinsic resistance of malignant melanoma to chemotherapy, the antiapoptotic protein B-cell lymphoma 2 (Bcl-2) is found to play an important role. A new antisense Bcl-2 oligonucleotide, Oblimersen, is targeting Bcl-2 messenger RNA selectively and this leads to the degradation of the Bcl-1, thus decreasing the levels of Bcl-2 in the body. Oblimersen can also be used in combination with conventional systemic chemotherapeutic agents, like dacarbazine.

- Also in two-thirds of melanomas, there is a mutation in *B-RAF* gene. An RAF inhibitor, Sorafenib, inhibits both B-RAF and C-RAF, and also used orally.
- Currently under preclinical investigation includes SB590885, dabrafenib (GSK2118436), AZ628, XL281, GDC-0879, and vemurafenib (RG704, PLX4032/4720)

Vaccines

- Melanoma is considered as a rather "immunogenic" tumor.
- A variety of strategies, including peptide and protein vaccines, recombinant DNA and viral vectors, and the use of autologous and allogeneic whole cell vaccines, have been tested in patients.

The treatment of a *2-cm malignant melanoma on the cheek* depends on several factors including depth (Breslow thickness), ulceration status, mitotic rate, and staging (based on sentinel lymph node involvement and possible metastasis).

Initial Evaluation

- *Clinical Examination:* Full skin exam, check for lymphadenopathy.
- *Dermatoscopy & Biopsy:* Excisional biopsy with 1–2 mm margins preferred to determine Breslow thickness and histologic subtype.
- *Staging Workup* (if indicated):
  - Sentinel lymph node biopsy (SLNB) usually considered if Breslow thickness ≥ 0.8 mm or ulcerated.
  - Imaging (CT/PET/MRI) if nodal or distant disease suspected.

Definitive Surgical Treatment

Wide Local Excision

- *Margins based on Breslow thickness:*
  - *<1 mm:* 1 cm margin
  - *1–2 mm:* 1–2 cm margin
  - *>2 mm:* 2 cm margin
- *Reconstruction of defect* (especially on face/cheek):
  - Local flaps (e.g., rotation, advancement, or transposition flaps)
  - Full-thickness skin graft if needed, considering cosmetic outcome

Sentinel Lymph Node Biopsy

- Typically offered for:
  - Tumors ≥ 0.8 mm in thickness
  - Ulcerated melanomas regardless of thickness
  - High mitotic rate or regression

Adjuvant Therapy (if node-positive or high-risk features)

- *Immunotherapy:* Anti-PD-1 agents (e.g., nivolumab, pembrolizumab)
- *Targeted therapy:* If BRAF mutation-positive (e.g., dabrafenib + trametinib)
- *Clinical trials:* Consider for eligible patients

Follow-up and Surveillance

- Regular dermatologic exams every 3–12 months depending on stage
- Education on self-examination and sun protection
- Imaging if high-risk or advanced-stage

Multidisciplinary management: Involvement of dermatology, surgical oncology, medical oncology, plastic surgery, and possibly radiation oncology (rarely used).

SOFT TISSUE SARCOMA

27. Discuss the etiopathology, diagnosis and treatment of soft tissue sarcomas. ***WBUHS 2010***

28. Discuss in brief the pathology, staging, and management of soft tissue sarcoma. ***WBUHS 2018***

Introduction

- Soft tissue sarcomas (STS) are a heterogeneous group of solid neoplasm's arising from cells of mesenchymal origin.
- There are >50 subtypes, but pleomorphic sarcoma, liposarcoma, leiomyosarcoma, synovial sarcoma, and malignant peripheral nerve sheath tumor account for 75%.
- Approximately 50% arise in the extremities, but the trunk wall, retroperitoneum, and head and neck are also fairly common locations.

Etiopathology

Predisposing Factors for Sarcomas

- *Genetic predisposition:*
  - Neurofibromatosis (von Recklinghausen's disease)
  - Li-Fraumeni syndrome
  - Retinoblastoma
  - Gardner's syndrome (familial adenomatous polyposis)
- *Lymphedema:*
  - Postsurgical
  - Postirradiation status
  - Parasitic infection (filariasis)
- *Radiation exposure:* Therapeutic radiation in the orthovoltage and megavoltage range
- *Chemical:*
  - 2,3,7,8-tetrachlorodibenzodioxin (TCDD)
  - Polyvinyl chloride
  - Hemochromatosis
  - Arsenic
- *Trauma:*
  - Postpartum status
  - Extremity

Histologic type		
• Synovial sarcoma • Myxoid/round cell liposarcoma • Ewing's sarcoma • Alveolar rhabdomyosarcoma • Extraskeletal myxoid chondrosarcoma	• Dermatofibrosarcoma protuberans • Desmoplastic small round cell tumor • Clear cell sarcoma • Infantile fibrosarcoma • Alveolar soft part sarcoma	• Atypical lipomatous tumor/well-differentiated liposarcoma • Leiomyosarcoma • Malignant fibrous histiocytoma • Malignant peripheral nerve sheath tumor

Age is a factor in histopathology: Embryonal rhabdomyosarcoma is most common in childhood, synovial sarcoma is more likely to be seen in young adults (<35 years), and there is an even distribution of liposarcoma and MFH as the predominant types in the older population.

- Many MFH is currently being reclassified as myofibrosarcoma, pleomorphic sarcoma, or dedifferentiated liposarcoma. Sarcoma histiotype and liposarcoma subtype are generally important determinants of prognosis and a predictor of distinctive patterns of behavior. Biologic behavior is currently best predicted on the basis of histologic type, histologic grade, tumor size, and depth.

- Genetic alterations that play a role in the development of soft tissue sarcoma segregate into two major types:
  I. Sarcomas with specific genetic alterations that result in simple karyotypes, including fusion genes secondary to reciprocal translocations and specific point mutations such as *KIT* mutations in gastrointestinal stromal tumors (GISTs) and *APC*/b-catenin mutations in desmoid tumors.
  II. Sarcomas with nonspecific genetic alterations and typically complex unbalanced karyotypes representing numerous genetic losses and gains

Staging

G, Histologic grade	*T, Primary tumor size*	*N, Regional nodes*	*M, Distant metastasis*
GX: Grade cannot be assessed	*TX:* Primary size cannot be assessed	*NX:* Regional nodes cannot be assessed	*MX:* Presence of distant metastasis cannot be assessed
G1: Well differentiated	*T0:* No evidence of primary tumor	*N0:* No regional lymph node metastasis	*M0:* No distant metastasis
G2: Moderately differentiated	*T1:* Tumor <5 cm	*N1:* Regional lymph node metastasis	*M1:* Distant metastasis present
G3: Poorly differentiated	*T1a:* Superficial tumor		
G4: Undifferentiated	• *T1b:* Deep tumor • *T2:* Tumor 5 cm or greater • *T2a:* Superficial tumor • *T2b:* Deep tumor		

Diagnosis

- Preoperative biopsy is required to determine the grade and histological subtype of sarcoma.
- Generally, it is recommended that—any soft tissue mass that is symptomatic or enlarging, any superficial mass that is >5 cm (unless an obvious subcutaneous lipoma), and all deep-seated masses irrespective of size should be sampled.
- Inappropriate biopsy scar can turn a limb salvage surgery into amputation so outmost care should be given when performing the biopsy.
- Biopsy incision or core track should be placed in a way that it can be removed en bloc during surgery without sacrificing extra skin or any vital structure.
- *Role of core needle/tru-cut biopsy:*
  - For most soft tissue masses, core needle/tru-cut biopsy (USG or CT guided) is usually preferred.
  - Core-needle biopsy has a diagnostic accuracy of 93% and now is the preferred modality for taking biopsy, and can be then advocated as the first step in the diagnostic armamentarium.
- *Role of incisional biopsy:*
  - Guidelines recommend incisional biopsy when core needle biopsy cannot produce adequate tissue for diagnosis or when findings on core needle biopsy are nondiagnostic.
  - The disadvantages of incisional biopsy include the need to schedule the procedure, the need for general anesthesia, and high costs.
  - In addition, inappropriately placed incisions can necessitate more extensive definitive resection to encompass the biopsy site.
- *Role of excisional biopsy:* Excision biopsy recommended only for small cutaneous or subcutaneous tumors, usually <3 cm, in which a wide re-excision (if required) is usually straightforward.

Imaging

Imaging should be done before any biopsy attempt as it helps in better targeting from representative area and sometimes helps pathologist in difficult situations.

- *MRI* is usually the preferred procedure for imaging extremity soft tissue masses. MRI enhances the contrast between tumor and adjacent structures and provides excellent three-dimensional definition of fascial planes.
- *CT* is a predominantly anatomic imaging modality.
- Therefore, CT plays mainly a complementary role to MRI in evaluation of the extent of tumor.
- MRI, with its superior soft tissue contrast resolution, is the dominant imaging modality for the evaluation of extremity sarcomas.
- CT is useful for evaluation of the tumor matrix, especially for small calcifications and the evaluation of subtle cortical involvement.
- MRI is limited in the detection of small calcifications within a mass because calcium distorts the magnetic field.
- CT may also be useful in patients for whom MRI is contraindicated or cannot be tolerated. Once the diagnosis and grade are known, evaluation for sites of potential metastasis can be performed.
- Chest X-ray (CXR) and chest computed tomography (CT) scans are important to survey the lungs for hematogenous spread of soft tissue sarcomas.
- Additionally, for sarcomas of the abdomen and pelvis, the liver and peritoneal contents are at risk for metastatic disease and should be surveyed either by MRI or CT.

Lymph Node Metastases

- It occurs in <3% of adult soft tissue sarcomas.
- Lymph node metastasis is present in certain histological types of childhood sarcoma.
- For extremity lesions, the lung is the principal site for metastasis; for visceral lesions and some histologic types of retroperitoneal sarcoma, the liver is the principal site.
- Thus, CT is the most commonly and minimally used modality to evaluate pulmonary metastases.
- Patients with visceral and retroperitoneal lesions should have their liver imaged as part of the initial abdominal CT.

Fluorodeoxyglucose-positron Emission Tomography (FDG-PET)

- It is used to evaluate distant metastases and, when combined with CT and conventional imaging, may improve the diagnostic accuracy of preoperative staging.
- The current role of PET seems to be primarily in the identification of unsuspected sites of metastasis in patients with recurrent high-grade tumors, given the high rate of metastatic disease in this setting.
- PET may also become useful for determining early responses to systemic therapy for soft tissue sarcoma.

Prognostic Factors in Extremity Sarcoma

- Factors that increased risk of local recurrence were age, recurrent presentation, positive margin, and fibrosarcoma, malignant peripheral nerve sheath tumor (mPNST), or leiomyosarcoma histology.
- Factors that increased distant recurrence rates were large tumor size, high histologic grade, deep location, recurrent disease at presentation, and histologic subtype of leiomyosarcoma.
- Liposarcoma was associated with decreased distant recurrence compared with other histologic types.
- Factors that increased the risk of disease-specific death were recurrent presentation, size >5 cm, tumor depth and grade, positive margin, and mPNST or leiomyosarcoma histology.
- Prognosis is related to the site of origin, resectability, presence of metastasis, number of metastatic sites, and histopathological features.
- Grade is a dominant factor in early metastasis, but in late recurrence initial size becomes equally important. Best prognosis is seen in extremity STS and best prognostic factor of extremity STS is grading.
- Death from local recurrence is uncommon in those with extremity lesions but occurs frequently in patients with retroperitoneal liposarcoma. Most common cause of death in extremity STS is metastasis.

Management

Recommendations for the management of soft tissue masses:

- Soft tissue tumors that are enlarging or >3 cm should be evaluated with radiologic imaging [ultrasonography or computed tomography (CT)], and a tissue diagnosis should be made using core needle biopsy.

- Once a sarcoma diagnosis is established, obtain imaging (magnetic resonance imaging for extremity lesions and CT for other anatomic locations) and evaluate for metastatic disease with chest CT for intermediate- or high-grade (grade 2 or 3) or large (T2) tumors.
- A wide local excision with 1- to 2-cm margins is adequate therapy for low-grade lesions and T1 tumors.
- Radiation therapy plays a critical role in the management of large (T2), intermediate- or high-grade tumors.
- Patients with locally advanced high-grade sarcomas or distant metastases should be evaluated for chemotherapy.
- An aggressive surgical approach should be taken in the treatment of patients with an isolated local recurrence or resectable distant metastases.

Surgery

- Surgery remains the principal therapeutic modality in STS, the extent of surgery required, along with the optimum combination of radiotherapy and chemotherapy, remains controversial.
- Wide en bloc resection is used most often. Historical attempts to resect all muscle bundles from origin to exertion have been supplanted by an encompassing resection, aiming to obtain a 1- to 2-cm margin of uninvolved tissue in all directions.
- The limiting factor is usually neurovascular or, occasionally bony juxtaposition. Because very few soft tissue sarcomas invade bone directly, only rarely does bone need to be resected.
- Similarly, few soft tissue sarcomas involve the skin, and so major skin resection should be limited.
- If a primary or recurrent tumor does involve the skin or if the tumor is so extensive that skin is involved, then one should consider free flap or rotational flap closure, particularly in those patients who are candidates for subsequent adjuvant radiation therapy.
- Primary tumors with no evidence of distant metastasis are managed with surgery alone or, when wide pathologic margins cannot be achieved because of anatomic constraints and/or the grade is high, surgery plus radiation therapy.
- The type of surgical resection is determined by several factors, including tumor location, tumor size, depth of invasion, involvement of nearby structures need for skin grafting or autogenous tissue reconstruction, and the patient's performance status.

Wide Local Excision

- The preferred treatment for extremity sarcomas is wide local excision that includes resection of the biopsy site.
- The goal of wide local excision is to remove the tumor with approximately 1–2 cm of surrounding normal soft tissue, but narrower margins may be necessary to preserve uninvolved critical neurovascular structures.
- If the tumor is adjacent to or displacing major neurovascular structures, these do not need to be resected, but the adventitia or perineurium should be removed.
- Surgical clips should be placed to delineate the extent of the resection bed for patients likely to require postoperative radiation therapy.
- Recent reports demonstrate encouraging results following radical en bloc resection with vascular reconstruction in the lower extremities.
- While en bloc resection with vascular reconstruction has been associated with increased rates of postoperative complications.
- In cases of bone invasion, bone resection is required to obtain an adequate surgical margin and to achieve local control.
- Soft tissue sarcomas abutting bone and in the absence of frank cortical bone penetration, periosteum was an adequate surgical margin in patients treated with wide local excision and radiation.
- Soft tissue sarcomas arising in the distal extremities, particularly the hands and feet, present unique technical challenges.

Amputation remains a reasonable option for patients with soft tissue sarcomas of the distal extremities when acceptable oncologic or functional outcomes cannot be achieved using available limb salvage techniques. All patients undergoing resection of extremity sarcomas should undergo physical therapy beginning immediately after surgery and continuing until maximum function is achieved.

Locoregional Lymphadenectomy

- Patients with clinically or radiologically suspicious regional nodes should have metastases confirmed before radical lymphadenectomy.
- Ultrasound-guided fine-needle aspiration of lymph nodes in selected patients with suspicious clinical or radiologic findings can be done.

Radiation Therapy

- The addition of radiation therapy to less radical surgical resection has made limb salvage possible in most cases.
- Radiation therapy is part of the standard treatment for intermediate or high-grade extremity and trunk wall STS either in the pre or postoperative setting.
- Patients with low-grade tumors or small, superficial high-grade tumors that have been resected with adequate margins may safely avoid radiation therapy.
- The standard treatment guidelines required radiation therapy after surgery for all patients with intermediate- or high-grade tumors of any size.
- However, small tumors (≤5 cm) have not generally been associated with local recurrence, and radiation therapy for such tumors may not be necessary.
- The optimal mode of radiation therapy [external-beam radiation therapy (EBRT), brachytherapy, or intensity-modulated radiation therapy (IMRT)], and timing of radiation therapy (preoperative, intraoperative, or postoperative) have yet to be defined.

External-beam Radiation Therapy (EBRT)

- It can be delivered using photons or particle beams (electrons, protons, pions, or neutrons).
- Conventional fractionation is usually 1.8–2 Gy per day.
- The optimal radiation margin is not well defined: a margin of 5–7 cm is standard, but some centers advocate wider margins for tumors >15 cm.
- At most institutions, the typical preoperative dose is 50 Gy given in 25 fractions, and resection is performed
- 4–8 weeks after completion of radiation therapy to allow acute radiation changes to subside.
- Postoperative radiation therapy planning is based on tumor site, tumor grade, and surgical margins. The entire surgical scar and drain sites should be included in the field, so that a near-full dose can be administered to the superficial skin.
- Doses of 60–70 Gy are usually necessary for postoperative treatment.
- For some radiosensitive histologic subtypes, such as myxoid liposarcoma, preoperative radiation therapy may shrink the tumor, facilitating resection with negative margins.
- Reconstructive surgical techniques with advanced tissue transfer procedures are being used more often in these high-risk wounds and reportedly result in better outcomes.
- The higher doses generally required for postoperative radiation therapy have also been shown to be associated with greater long-term functional impairment.
- *Late radiation toxic effects* (e.g., fibrosis, joint stiffness, and edema) were more common with postoperative than preoperative radiation therapy because of higher postoperative radiation doses and larger treatment field sizes.

Brachytherapy

Brachytherapy involves the placement of multiple radioactive seeds through catheters inserted in the tumor resection bed. The primary benefit of brachytherapy is the shorter overall treatment time of 4–6 days, compared to the 4–6 weeks generally required for preoperative or postoperative radiation therapy regimens.

Chemotherapy

- The chemosensitivity of STS varies by histological subtype.

- Synovial sarcoma, myxoid/round cell liposarcoma, and uterine leiomyosarcoma are sensitive to chemotherapy, whereas pleomorphic liposarcoma, myxofibrosarcoma, epithelioid sarcoma, leiomyosarcoma, mPNSTs, angiosarcomas, and desmoplastic round cell tumors have intermediate sensitivity to chemotherapy.
- Relatively chemoresistant histological subtypes include clear cell sarcoma, endometrial stromal sarcoma, alveolar soft part sarcoma, and extra skeletal myxoid chondrosarcoma.
- Doxorubicin and ifosfamide are the two most active agents against soft tissue sarcoma.
- The European guidelines recommend doxorubicin 75 mg/m^2 every 3 weeks as first-line treatment for advanced disease.
- Ifosfamide is the recommended second-line treatment and is recommended for first-line treatment in patients with cardiac morbidity. Other Systemic Therapies:

Novel Chemotherapeutic Agents

- *Trabectedin*, a marine-derived alkaloid that binds DNA, affecting transcription and inducing the formation of DNA double-strand breaks has shown benefit in the treatment of advanced soft tissue sarcomas, particularly leiomyosarcoma, myxoid liposarcoma, and other translocation-related sarcomas.
- *Palifosfamide* is a stabilized formulation of the active metabolite of ifosfamide that has been reported to be better tolerated than ifosfamide.
- *Pazopanib* is an oral angiogenesis inhibitor that targets vascular endothelial growth factor receptors, platelet-derived growth factor receptor (PDGFR), and c-kit.
- Inhibitors of the mammalian target of rapamycin pathway, including temsirolimus, *everolimus* and *ridaforolimus* have also shown activity against some soft tissue sarcomas.

Management of Recurrent Sarcoma

- For patients with extremity sarcomas, achieving negative margins on resection of recurrent disease frequently requires amputation.
- However, in some patients with recurrent extremity sarcoma, function-preserving resection combined with additional radiation therapy, with or without chemotherapy, can produce acceptable rates of local.

Management of Recurrent and Distant Metastatic Sarcoma

- In selected individuals with distant metastatic disease, surgical resection of a primary soft tissue sarcoma may be appropriate as a palliative procedure.
- The decision should be based on the patient's symptoms, which often include pain, ability to achieve local tumor control, comorbidities, anticipated morbidity of the surgical procedure, and the extent of metastases.
- The most common initial site of distant metastasis of soft tissue sarcomas is the lung.
- Selected patients with a limited number of pulmonary nodules (less than four nodules), long disease-free intervals, and no endobronchial invasion may become long-term survivors after pulmonary resection
- Favorable prognostic factors included:
  - Microscopically tumor-free margins
  - Age <40 years
  - Grade 1 or 2 tumor
- For patients who are surgical candidates, pulmonary resection alone can be more effective than watchful waiting, chemotherapy, or chemotherapy plus surgery.

Chemotherapy for Distant Metastatic Sarcoma

- Doxorubicin, either alone or combined with other agents, has been the primary treatment modality for patients with advanced or distant metastatic sarcomas for several decades.
- Although most patients with metastatic disease are not curable, some patients with limited disease experience stabilization of disease with multidisciplinary treatment, which often includes surgery and radiation therapy in addition to chemotherapy.

- *Isolated liver metastases:* If stable over several months, may be amenable to resection, radiofrequency ablation, or chemoembolization.

Palliative Surgery

In cases of metastatic settings, a palliative resection or amputation is required in cases of bleeding, fungation, infection, or intractable pain.

Palliative Radiation Therapy

- Definitive radiation therapy can be considered when no acceptable surgical option is available (e.g., in patients with significant medical co-morbidities).
- In this setting, radiation doses greater than 63 Gy yielded superior tumor control, but doses greater than 68 Gy resulted in increased rates of major complications.

Algorithm for the Management of Extremity and Superficial Trunk Sarcoma

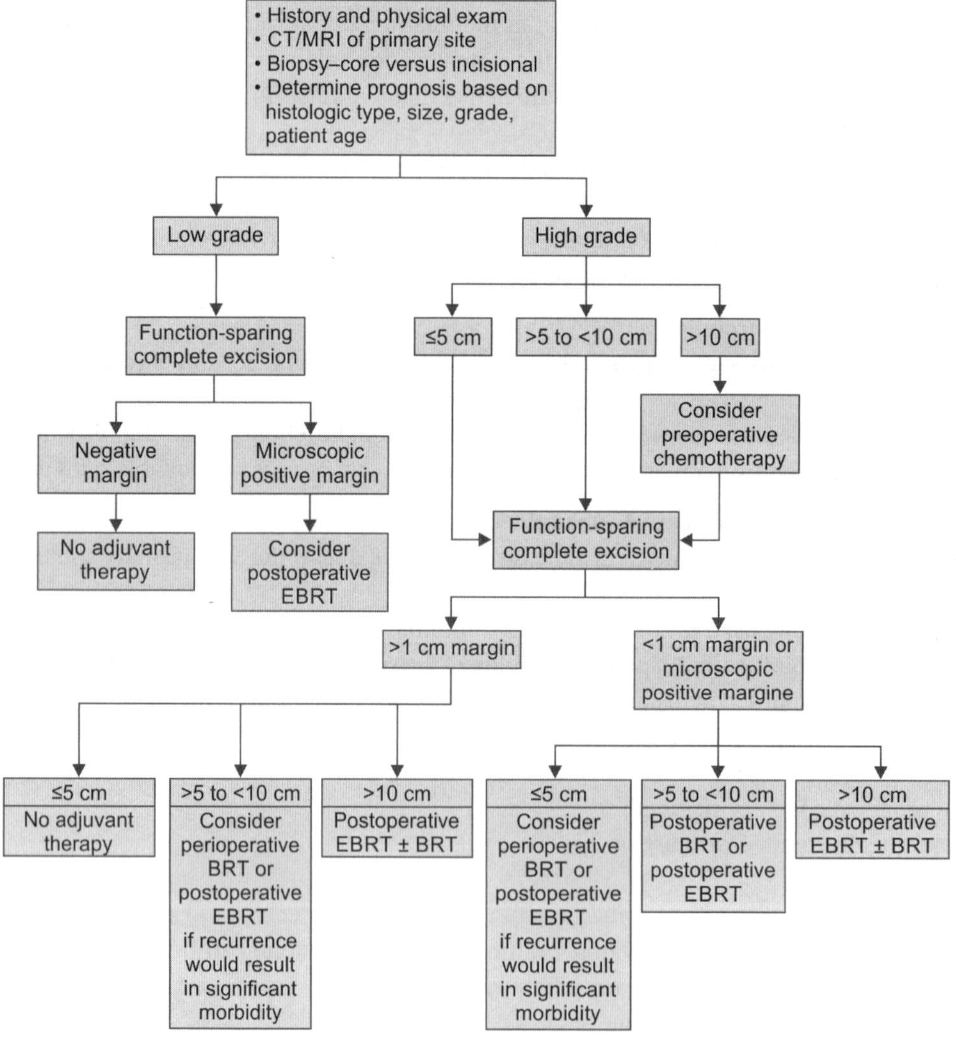

29. Describe retroperitoneal sarcoma.

Introduction

- Retroperitoneal sarcomas occur in the retroperitoneum.
- This is an area behind the peritoneum, the lining of the abdominal space that covers the abdominal organs.

- The retroperitoneum is deep in the abdomen and pelvis, behind the abdominal lining, where organs such as the major blood vessels, kidneys, pancreas, and bladder are located.

The main types of sarcoma that occur in the retroperitoneum are:
- Liposarcoma—cancer of the fatty tissue
- Leiomyosarcoma—cancer of the involuntary muscle

Other less common types in the retroperitoneum include:
- Solitary fibrous tumor
- Pleomorphic sarcoma
- Malignant nerve sheath tumor
- Synovial sarcoma
- Ewing's sarcoma

Signs and Symptoms
Symptoms of retroperitoneal sarcoma can vary depending on the size and location of your tumor.

They may include:
- A noticeable lump in the abdomen
- Increase in abdominal girt
- Dull pain in the abdomen or back
- Intense abdominal pain with bleeding
- Other rare symptoms include early satiety (meaning feeling full after eating a small amount of food), weight loss, hernia, or anemia.

Following tests to be done:
- Physical examination—looking at and feeling any lump
- A scan—taking pictures of the inside of the body using ultrasound, X-ray, CT, EUS, PET, or MRI
- A biopsy—taking and testing a tissue sample

Types of Diagnostic Scans and Tests
- *Ultrasound:* A scan that uses sound waves to create images from within the body.
- *CT:* The computed tomography (CT) scan takes a number of X-rays to make a 3D image of an affected area.
- *MRI:* Magnetic resonance imaging (MRI) uses magnets to create an image of the tissues of the body.
- *Histopathology:* Examination of a tissue sample by a pathologist under a microscope to identify disease
- Blood test

Grading
- Low-grade means the cancer cells are slow-growing, look quite similar to normal cells, are less aggressive, and are less likely to spread.
- Intermediate-grade means the cancer cells are growing slightly faster and look more abnormal.
- High-grade means cancer cells are fast growing, look very abnormal, are more aggressive and are more likely to spread.

Staging
Most sarcomas are staged by looking at:
- The size and grade of the tumor
- Whether the tumor is deep in the body or superficial. This means closer to the surface.
- Whether it has spread to another part of the body

Most retroperitoneal sarcomas are >5 cm in size and deep in the body. This makes the grade of the cancer a more important factor when finding out the stage of your cancer.
- Stage 1 means the cancer is low grade, small (<5 cm), and has not spread to other parts of the body.

- Stage 2 means the cancer is of any grade, usually larger than stage one but has not spread to other parts of the body.
- Stage 3 means a high-grade cancer that has not spread to other parts of the body.
- Stage 4 means a cancer of any grade or size that has spread to any other part of the body.

Surgery

Surgery is the main treatment for this type of sarcoma.

As retroperitoneal sarcomas can sometimes touch or press on surrounding organs, the surgeon will aim to remove the tumor along with any organs next to it "en bloc" meaning, as a whole. This is to ensure they remove all cancer cells including those that are not clearly visible.

30. What are the different types of retroperitoneal sarcomas? How do you diagnose, stage, and treat a case of retroperitoneal liposarcoma? When is a biopsy indicated? ***WBUHS 2021, 2022***

Retroperitoneal Sarcoma

Retroperitoneal sarcoma represents approximately 15% of all soft tissue sarcomas (STS).

The most frequent retroperitoneal sarcoma subtypes are:

- Liposarcoma
- Leiomyosarcoma
- MFH (malignant fibrous histiocytoma)
- Undifferentiated pleomorphic sarcoma

The predominant intraperitoneal STS subtypes are:

- GIST
- Leiomyosarcoma

Histological Types

- *Common:*
    - Liposarcoma
    - Leiomyosarcoma
    - Undifferentiated
- *Rare:*
    - MPNST
    - Solitary fibrous tumor
    - RMS
    - Extra-skeletal OGS
    - Synovial sarcoma
    - Desmoplastic SRCT
    - Malignant PEComa

Investigations

- CT and MRI are widely used for the evaluation of retroperitoneal sarcoma, because of their excellent spatial resolution and reproducible axial image acquisition.
- The advantages of CT scan include rapid image acquisition, nearly universal availability, and a concise image.
- The advantages of MRI include a wider range of soft tissue differentiation, but the disadvantages include an increased susceptibility to claustrophobia and motion artifact, the more limited availability, and a greater number of implant-related contraindications compared with CT scan.
- The patient must be carefully evaluated along with the imaging studies to verify that the retroperitoneal mass does not represent an unappreciated lymphoma, germ cell tumor, or metastasis from another primary tumor.
- The preoperative CT scan often contains enough information to proceed with treatment without a preoperative biopsy as long as the other basic considerations in the differential diagnosis are considered excluded.

- Biopsy for retroperitoneal sarcoma is not mandatory and has drawbacks in certain situations.
  - By definition, a surgical biopsy ruptures the tumor, seeding the operative field and potentially reducing the possibility of a margin-negative resection.
  - Preoperative biopsy can be particularly misleading in patients with large tumors as the biopsy are susceptible to a significant degree of sampling bias. This sampling bias can provide inappropriately reassuring information.
  - If preoperative biopsy is obtained from a heterogeneous mass, the specimen should be obtained from the most concerning region under image guidance.

American Joint Committee on Cancer Staging for Soft Tissue Sarcoma

Tumor (T)

- *T0:* No evidence of primary tumor
- *T1:* 5 cm or less in greatest dimension
- *T2:* >5 cm and ≤10 cm in greatest dimension
- *T3:* >10 cm and ≤15 cm in greatest dimension
- *T4:* >15 cm in greatest dimension

Definition of Regional Lymph Node (N)

- *N0:* No regional lymph node metastasis or unknown lymph node status
- *N1:* Regional lymph node metastasis

Definition of Distant Metastasis (M)

- *M0:* No distant metastasis
- *M1:* Distant metastasis

Grading

- Most important indicator of recurrence (after gross total excision), metastases, and overall survival
- Decides adjuvant chemotherapy

FNCLCC Grading is based on three Parameters

- Differentiation (1–3)
- Mitotic activity (1–3)
- Necrosis (0–2)

Definition of Grade (G)—FNCLCC Histologic Grade

- *GX:* Grade cannot be assessed
- *G1:* Total differentiation, mitotic count and necrosis score of 2 or 3
- *G2:* Total differentiation, mitotic count and necrosis score of 4 or 5
- *G3:* Total differentiation, mitotic count and necrosis score of 6, 7, or 8

Treatment

- When possible, treatment should proceed with a complete gross resection.
- Given the much larger tumor dimensions of most retroperitoneal sarcomas, it is not practical and often impossible to microscopically evaluate 100% of the surgical specimen margin surface area.
- Consequently, most of the retroperitoneal sarcoma literature refers to complete gross resection.
- In 75% of patients, achieving complete gross resection may mean resecting contiguous or inseparable adjacent organs, such as the kidney, bowel, or pancreas and vascular structures.
- Resection requiring pancreaticoduodenectomy, major vascular resection, or splenectomy was more likely to result in a major postoperative complication, but a major postoperative complication does not appear to adversely affect long-term survival or recurrence.
- Predictors of poor prognosis include gross residual disease after resection, unresectable disease (either metastatic or locally advanced), and high-tumor grade.

- Even with optimal chemotherapy and radiation therapy, the median survival of patients with unresectable disease is 10 months.
- The role of multimodality therapy is more controversial in retroperitoneal sarcoma.
- Given the success of adjuvant radiation in extremity STS, this approach has been applied to retroperitoneal sarcoma, but with fewer randomized data to support its efficacy.
- An advantage of neoadjuvant radiation is that the in situ tumor displaces the bowel anteriorly, thus facilitating the delivery of a higher radiation dose posteriorly, which is the most likely site of a positive histologic margin.
- For patients with metastatic retroperitoneal sarcoma, there are few effective chemotherapeutic options.
- Single or combination therapy with anthracyclines can be used as first-line therapy.
- A second-line regimen is gemcitabine and docetaxel.
- The experience with immunotherapy agents in STS patients has been disappointing.
- One encouraging finding is that patients with undifferentiated pleomorphic sarcoma or dedifferentiated liposarcoma have a somewhat more promising objective response rate than those with other STS subtypes when treated with pembrolizumab.

Retroperitoneal Liposarcomas

- Retroperitoneal liposarcomas can be difficult to treat.
- Patients with retroperitoneal liposarcomas have higher rates of local recurrence and disease-specific death than patients with liposarcomas of the extremities.
- The primary treatment is surgical resection with a negative margin, which improves local control; however, the role for resection of contiguous organs remains controversial.
- Reports have described the efficacy of chemotherapy and/or radiation therapy in treating retroperitoneal sarcomas, although recommendations regarding neoadjuvant and adjuvant therapy differ greatly even among major sarcoma treatment centers.
- For retroperitoneal liposarcomas, the clinical objective is to remove all macroscopic disease. Although there are some published reports that support en bloc resection of uninvolved adjacent organs to improve local control
- No randomized controlled trial supports extended resection beyond R0 resection.
- Therefore, unless the tumor is inseparable from adjacent organs and is likely to cause impending morbidity such as bowel obstruction, we do not advocate liberal en bloc organ resection.
- However, owing to the high recurrence rate and aggressive nature of retroperitoneal dedifferentiated liposarcoma, neoadjuvant chemotherapy with/without radiation therapy is often considered.
- Therefore, an accurate subtype-specific diagnosis is critical for the appropriate consideration of neoadjuvant therapy.

Role of Biopsy

- In addition, pathological confirmation of dedifferentiation is routinely required as part of eligibility for novel therapeutic clinical trials in patients who are not appropriate candidates for surgery.
- The preoperative tissue diagnosis of retroperitoneal liposarcoma often employs image-guided core needle biopsy (CNB) or fine-needle aspiration (FNA).
- Previously, investigators have reported on the efficacy of image-guided FNA and CNB for diagnosing retroperitoneal soft tissue tumors; however, only one study has assessed the accuracy of FNA and CNB in the subtype-specific diagnosis of liposarcoma.
- There has not been a study that has compared preoperative pathologic biopsy findings with final operative pathologic reports to assess the subtype-specific accuracy of preoperative percutaneous biopsy.
- There is need to analyze the accuracy of preoperative percutaneous biopsy in the subtype-specific diagnosis of retroperitoneal liposarcoma and the reliability of percutaneous biopsy in guiding clinical decisions regarding neoadjuvant treatment.

CHAPTER 42

Radiotherapy

LEARNING OBJECTIVES

- Brachytherapy
- Intraoperative Radiotherapy

1. Brachytherapy.

Introduction

- Also known as *internal radiotherapy, sealed source radiotherapy, curietherapy,* or *endocurietherapy*, is a form of radiotherapy where a sealed radiation source is placed inside or next to the area requiring treatment.
- Brachytherapy can be used alone or in combination with other therapies, such as surgery, external beam radiotherapy (EBRT), and chemotherapy.
- Brachytherapy represents an effective treatment option for many types of cancer. Treatment results have demonstrated that the cancer cure rates of brachytherapy are either comparable to surgery and EBRT or are improved when used in combination with these techniques.
- In addition, brachytherapy is associated with a low risk of serious adverse side effects.

Types

Different types of brachytherapy can be defined according to:

1. The placement of the radiation sources in the target treatment area
2. The rate or "intensity" of the irradiation dose delivered to the tumor
3. The duration of dose delivery.

Source Placement

The two main types of brachytherapy treatment in terms of the placement of the radioactive source are: (1) *Interstitial* and (2) *contact.*

- In the case of interstitial brachytherapy, the sources are placed directly in the target tissue of the affected site, such as the prostate and breast.
- Contact brachytherapy involves the placement of the radiation source in a space next to the target tissue. This space may be a body cavity (*intracavitary* brachytherapy), such as the cervix, uterus, and vagina; a body lumen (*intraluminal* brachytherapy), such as the trachea and esophagus; and externally (*surface* brachytherapy), such as the skin. A radiation source can also be placed in blood vessels (*intravascular* brachytherapy) for the treatment of coronary in-stent restenosis.

Dose Rate

The dose rate of brachytherapy refers to the level or "intensity" with which the radiation is delivered to the surrounding medium and is expressed in Grays per hour (Gy/h).

- *Low-dose rate (LDR)* brachytherapy involves implanting radiation sources that emit radiation at a rate of up to 2 Gy/h. LDR brachytherapy is commonly used for cancers of the oral cavity, oropharynx, sarcomas, and prostate cancer.

- *Medium-dose rate (MDR)* brachytherapy is characterized by a medium rate of dose delivery, ranging between 2 and 12 Gy/h.
- *High-dose rate (HDR)* brachytherapy is when the rate of dose delivery exceeds 12 Gy/h. The most common applications of HDR brachytherapy are in tumors of the cervix, esophagus, lungs, breasts, and prostate. Most HDR treatments are performed on an outpatient basis, but this is dependent on the treatment site.
- *Pulsed-dose rate (PDR)* brachytherapy involves short pulses of radiation, typically once an hour, to simulate the overall rate and effectiveness of LDR treatment. Typical tumor sites treated by PDR brachytherapy are gynecological and head and neck cancers.

Duration of Dose Delivery

Permanent brachytherapy is often performed for prostate cancer using "seeds"—small radioactive rods implanted directly into the tumor.

Clinical Applications

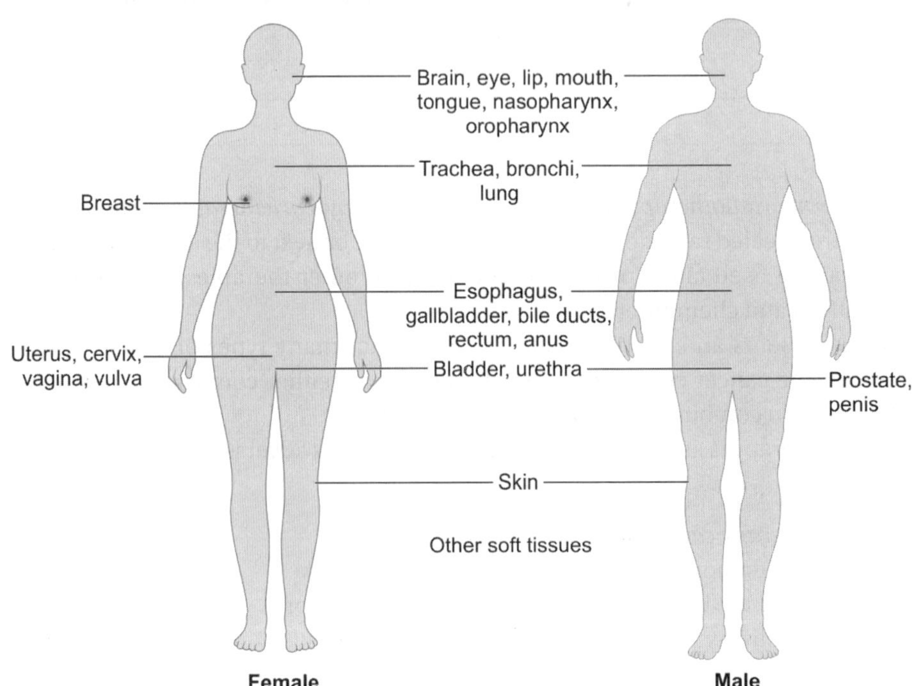

Uses

- Cervical cancer
- Prostate cancer
- Breast cancer
- Skin cancer
- *Coronary/vascular:* Brachytherapy can be used in the treatment of coronary in-stent restenosis, in which a catheter is placed inside blood vessels, through which sources are inserted and removed.

There are two methods that can be used to deliver breast brachytherapy:

1. *Interstitial breast brachytherapy* using multiple catheters
2. *Intracavitary breast brachytherapy* using a balloon catheter

Side Effects

- *Acute:*
    - Acute side effects associated with brachytherapy include localized bruising, swelling, bleeding, discharge, or discomfort within the implanted region.

- Brachytherapy treatment for cervical or prostate cancer can cause acute and transient urinary symptoms, such as urinary retention, urinary incontinence, and painful urination (dysuria).
- Transient increased in bowel frequency, diarrhea, constipation, or minor rectal bleeding may also occur.
- Acute and subacute side effects usually resolve over a matter of days or a few weeks. In the case of permanent (seed) brachytherapy for prostate cancer, there is a small chance that some seeds may migrate out of the treatment region into the bladder or urethra and be passed through the urine.
- Brachytherapy for skin cancer may result in a shedding of the outer layers of skin (desquamation) around the area of treatment in the weeks following therapy, which typically heals in 5–8 weeks. If the cancer is located on the lip, ulceration may occur as a result of brachytherapy but usually resolves after 4–6 weeks.
- Most of the acute side effects associated with brachytherapy can be treated with medication or through dietary changes, and usually disappear over time (typically a matter of weeks), once the treatment is completed.
- The acute side effects of HDR brachytherapy are broadly similar to EBRT.

- *Long-term:*
  - In a small number of people, brachytherapy may cause long-term side effects due to damage or disruption of the adjacent tissues or organs.
  - Long-term side effects are usually mild or moderate in nature, e.g., urinary and digestive problems may persist as a result of brachytherapy for cervical or prostate cancer and may require ongoing management.
  - Brachytherapy for prostate cancer may cause erectile dysfunction in approximately 15–30% of patients. However, the risk of erectile dysfunction is related to age (older men are at a greater risk than younger men) and also the level of erectile function prior to receiving brachytherapy.
  - Brachytherapy for breast or skin cancer may cause scar tissue to form around the treatment area. In the case of breast brachytherapy, fat necrosis may occur as a result of fatty acids entering the breast tissues. This can cause the breast tissue to become swollen and tender. Fat necrosis is a benign condition and typically occurs 4–12 months after treatment and affects about 2% of the patients.

Safety Around Others

- If temporary brachytherapy is used, no radioactive sources remain in the body after treatment; therefore, there is no radiation risk to friends or family from being in close proximity with them.
- If permanent brachytherapy is used, low-dose radioactive sources (seeds) are left in the body after treatment—the radiation levels are very low and decrease over time. In addition, the irradiation only affects tissues within a few millimeters of the radioactive sources (i.e., the tumor being treated).
- As a precaution, some people receiving permanent brachytherapy may be advised to not hold any small children or be too close to pregnant women for a short time after treatment.

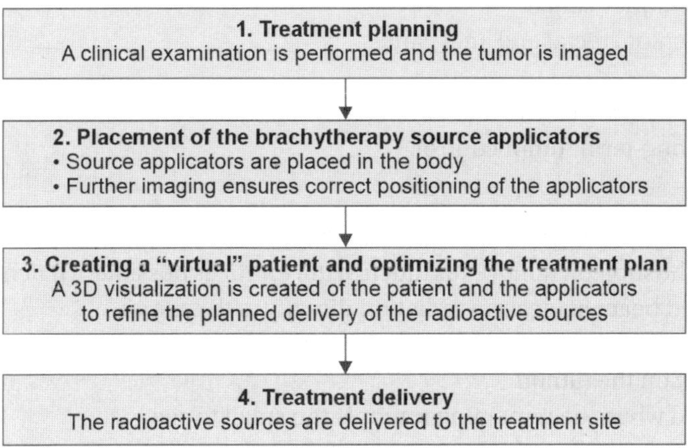

Typical Stages of a Brachytherapy Procedure

Radiation Sources

Commonly used radiation sources (radionuclides) for brachytherapy.

Radionuclide	*Type*	*Half-life*	*Energy*
Cesium-131 (^{131}Cs)	Electron capture, ε	9.7 days	30.4 keV (mean)
Cesium-137 (^{137}Cs)	Beta particles	30.17 years	0.662 MeV
Cobalt-60 (^{60}Co)	Beta particles	5.26 years	1.17, 1.33 MeV
Iridium-192 (^{192}Ir)	γ-rays	73.8 days	0.38 MeV (mean)
Iodine-125 (^{125}I)	Electron capture, ε	59.6 days	27.4, 31.4, and 35.5 keV
Palladium-103 (^{103}Pd)	Electron capture, ε	17.0 days	21 keV (mean)
Ruthenium-106 (^{106}Ru)	Beta particles	1.02 years	3.54 MeV
Radium-226 (^{226}Ra)	Beta particles	1599 years	

Electronic Brachytherapy

Electronic brachytherapy involves the placement of miniature low-energy X-ray tube sources into a prepositioned applicator within body/tumor cavities to rapidly deliver high doses to target tissues while maintaining low doses to distant nontarget tissues.

2. Intraoperative radiotherapy. *WBUHS 2008*

Introduction

Intraoperative radiation therapy (IORT) is an intensive radiation treatment that delivers a concentrated beam of radiation to tumors as they are located during surgery. IORT allows direct radiation to the tumor while sparing normal surrounding tissue.

Conditions Treated with IORT

Intraoperative radiation therapy is used for cancer that cannot be cured with surgery alone and for tumors that are either attached or close to vital tissues.

Intraoperative Radiation Therapy is Used to Treat

- Recurrent rectal cancer
- Cervical, uterine, and ovarian cancers
- Breast cancer
- Prostate, bladder, and kidney cancer
- Stomach, pancreatic, colon, rectal and anal cancer
- Soft-tissue sarcoma
- For people who have recurring cancer and people who have locally advanced cancers, IORT can be an effective therapy in achieving long-term tumor control.

Working Principle

- IORT is almost always used along with external radiation prior to surgery.
- During surgery, after the surgeon removes as much of the tumor as possible, a machine called a linear accelerator delivers a concentrated beam of electron radiation directly to the tumors.
- The surgeon moves healthy organs out of the radiation field to prevent damage, and special tubes are used to focus the beams safely on the tumor.
- IORT also may be used when the remaining tumor is too small to see.

Advantages of IORT

- IORT allows to administer of high doses of radiation to tumors without exposing nearby healthy organs to radiation.
- A single dose of intraoperative radiation may have as much effect on the tumor as 10–20 daily radiation treatments.
- *IORT offers the following benefits:*
  - Higher radiation dosage to cancer cells
  - Faster radiation delivery during surgery
  - Decreased radiation exposure to normal surrounding tissue
  - Safer application compared with traditional radiation treatments.

CHAPTER 43

National Health Programme for Cancer

LEARNING OBJECTIVES

- Algorithm of Screening of Common Malignancies in India
- Cervical Cancer Screening
- Oral Cancer Screening
- Breast Cancer Screening

1. Algorithm of screening of common malignancies in India from the perspective of the National Health Mission. *WBUHS 2017, 2025*

Prevention of Cancers

- Create awareness about the ills of tobacco and advocate avoidance
- Encourage and assist habitual tobacco users to quit the habit
- Promote healthy dietary practices and physical activity

Early Detection of Cancers

- Create awareness about the early warning signs of cancer
- Encourage breast awareness
- Encourage oral self-examination
- Create awareness about the symptoms of cervical cancer
- Examine the oral cavity of patients with a history of tobacco use as a routine
- Offer clinical breast examination to any woman over 30 years presenting to the health center
- Offer screening for cervical cancer to any woman over 30 years presenting to the health facility
- Promptly refer any person with a suspicious lesion for diagnosis and appropriate treatment

C	Change in bowel or bladder habits
A	A wound that does not heal
U	Unusual bleeding or discharge
T	Thickening or lump in the breast or elsewhere
I	Indigestion or difficulty in swallowing
O	Obvious change in wart or mole
N	Nagging cough or hoarseness of voice

Treatment of Cancers

- Ensure that every patient complies with therapy advised
- If follow-up care is required at the health center level, make sure that detailed instructions are provided by the treating institutions

Palliative Care

- Ensure that the patient is free from pain as far as possible. Learn and provide the step-ladder approach of the World Health Organization (WHO) of pain management, refer to the appropriate center for oral morphine
- Achieve control of unwanted symptoms to the extent possible
- Provide psychological support to the patient to accept the diagnosis and treatment
- Involve the family in diagnosis, treatment, and care as far as possible

Screening for Cervical Cancer

Cervical Cancer Screening

Visual inspection with acetic acid (VIA): Visual inspection of the uterine cervix, after application of 3–5% acetic acid (VIA) is a simple test for the early detection of cervical precancerous lesions and early invasive cancer. The results of VIA are immediately available and do not require any laboratory or specialist support. The categorization of the result of VIA depends upon the color changes observed on the cervix. This test can be performed by any trained paramedical health worker and not necessarily only by a doctor. Only minimal duration training is all that is required for performing this test.

Exclusion Criteria

- Menstruation
- Pregnancy
- Within 12 weeks of delivery/abortion
- Previous history of treatment for cancer cervix

If any woman who does not fall under inclusion criteria but has any symptoms should also be immediately referred to the Medical Officer of Primary Health Care (PHC) for further evaluation.

Criteria for categorizing visual inspection with acetic acid (VIA) test results as negative or positive or invasive cancer.

VIA category	*Description*
Negative	• No acetowhite lesions • Transparent lesions or faint patchy lesions without definite margins • Nabothian cysts becoming acetowhite • Faint line-like acetowhitening at the junction of columnar and squamous epithelium
Positive	• Acetowhite lesions far away from the transformation zone • Distinct, opaque acetowhite area • Margin should be well defined, and may or may not be raised • Abnormality close to the squamocolumnar junction in the transformation zone and not far away from the os
Invasive cancer	Obvious growth or ulcer in the cervix. The acetowhite area may not be visible because of the bleeding

Algorithm for Screening and Management of Cervical Cancer

Visual examination using acetic acid (VIA)

- VIA negative → Repeat VIA after 5 years
- VIA positive → Refer to gynecologist/Lady Medical Officer wherever available PHC/CHC/DH
  - Lesions eligible for cryotherapy → Cryotherapy → Follow-up after 1 year with VIA
  - Lesions not eligible for cryotherapy → Biopsy (naked eye or colposcopic guided)
    - Low grade (CIN 1) → Cryotherapy → Follow-up after 1 year with VIA
    - High grade (CIN 2 and 3) → LEEP → Follow-up after 1 year with VIA
    - Cancer → Refer to TCC

Please note: The accuracy of VIA decreases in postmenopausal women. However, in facilities where there are no resources for Pap, women may be screened using VIA till 65 years of age

(CHC: Community Health Center; CIN: cervical intraepithelial neoplasia; DH: District Hospitals; LEEP: loop electrosurgical excision procedure; PHC: Primary Health Centers)

Eligibility for Cryotherapy

- The lesion should not be spread over more than two quadrants of the cervix
- The entire lesion is located in the ectocervix without extension to the vagina and/or endocervix
- The lesion is visible to an entire extent
- The lesion can be adequately covered by the largest available cryotherapy probe.
- There is no suspicion of invasive cancer.

Cryotherapy is not recommended if:

- *Symptoms:*
  - Postcoital bleeding
  - Postmenopausal bleeding
- *On examination:*
  - Overt cervical growth
  - Irregular surface
  - Bleeds on touch

Screening for Oral Cancer

- *Risk factors:*
  - Tobacco chewing is the single most important risk factor for oral cancer.
  - Other risk factors include alcohol use, betel nut chewing, and chronic trauma to oral mucosa by sharp tooth or ill-fitting dentures. Chronic exposure to these risk factors causes changes in the oral mucosa and

these changes are visible as precancerous lesions. Over a period of time, malignancy may develop in these lesions.

- *Precancerous lesions:* Precancerous lesions or conditions are local/generalized disturbances that predispose to malignancy in a particular site. Leukoplakia, erythroplakia, palatal changes associated with reverse smoking or beedi smoking, and submucous fibrosis are local precancerous lesions. Plummer-Vinson syndrome, syphilis, and erosive lichen planus are generalized precancerous conditions. All these conditions are amenable to early diagnosis, and treatment is possible in many cases.

Leukoplakia: This is defined as a white patch that cannot be characterized as any other disease clinically or pathologically.

They can be of four types:

I. *Homogeneous leukoplakia:* Low risk of cancer
II. *Ulcerated or erosive leucoplakia:* High risk of cancer
III. *Speckled or nodular leucoplakia:* High risk of cancer
IV. *Verrucous leukoplakia:* Very high risk of cancer

Two or more types of leucoplakia may be present in the oral cavity at the same time. Confirmatory diagnosis is by biopsy.

Erythroplakia:

- This is a bright, velvety area sometimes surrounded by faint plaques which cannot be characterized as any other lesion clinically or pathologically
- About 90% of these lesions show cellular dysplasia or malignancy.
- The risk of malignancy in erythroplakia is higher than in leukoplakia.

Basic considerations:

- The most common cancer seen in the oral cavity is squamous cell carcinoma.
- It presents as a painless ulcer, mass, or fissure.
- As the disease advances, the patient may have excessive salivation, trismus, and difficulty in chewing, swallowing, or cervical lymphadenopathy.
- Distant metastasis is uncommon in oral cancers

Inclusion criteria:

- Any individual aged 30 years old and above should be screened at all screening centers.
- Any abnormal finding on oral visual examination should be considered positive and the patient should be managed according to the screening and management algorithm for oral cancer.

Screening for Breast Cancer

Breast cancer is the most common cancer among women all over the world.

Risk Factors

- *Reproductive and hormonal factors:*
  - The older a woman is when she has her first child, the greater the chance of having breast cancer.
  - Early menarche (before the age of 12 years), late menopause (after the age of 55 years) or never had children are also at greater risk.
  - Women who take menopausal hormone therapy (estrogen and progesterone) for 5 years or more after menopause also appear to have an increased risk.
- *Family history:* Risk of breast cancer increases in women with a first-degree relative with breast cancer.
- *Other factors:*
  - Being obese after menopause
  - Physical inactivity
  - Alcohol intake: Some studies suggest that the risk of breast cancer increases with increased intake of alcoholic beverages.

High-risk Group for the Occurrence of Breast Cancer

- Personal history of breast cancer
- Family history of breast, ovarian, and colon cancer
- Chronic benign breast disease

Prompt diagnosis of breast cancer in the early stage is very important. This is possible by increasing the level of awareness among women and healthcare professionals. The following methods may be used for early detection.

Breast Awareness

The first person to detect any lump in the breast is the woman herself which is by teaching the woman to be aware of any of the following signs at the earliest possible:

- A change in size.
- A nipple that is pulled in or changes in position or shape.
- A rash on or around the nipple.
- Discharge from one or both nipples
- Puckering or dimpling of skin
- Lump or thickening in the breast
- Constant pain in the breast or armpit
- In case a woman notices any such change, she should promptly visit the health center or health professional.
- All women >30 years of age will be received by the staff nurse/auxiliary nurse midwife (ANM) at the screening center, will be provided a preprocedure counseling, and then screened using clinical breast examination (CBE). Clinical breast examination is to be performed by a trained physician, nurse, or health worker.

Algorithm for Screening and Management of Breast Cancer

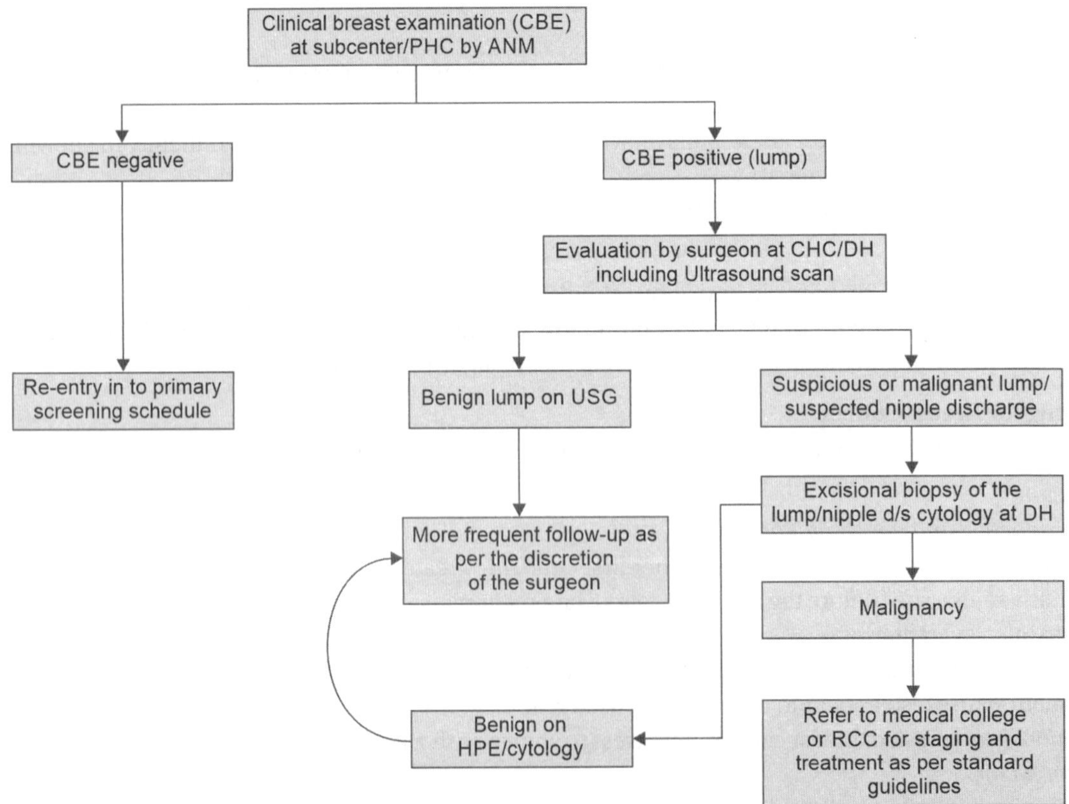

(CHC: Community Health Center; DH: District Hospitals; HPE: histopathological examination; RCC: renal cell carcinoma; USG: ultrasonography)

Organ Transplantation

LEARNING OBJECTIVES

- Allograft Rejection
- Brain Death and Organ Procurement
- MHC
- Liver Transplantation
- Child's Criteria
- Orthotopic Liver Transplantation
- Bowel Transplantation
- Renal Transplantation
- TOLL-Like Receptors

ALLOGRAFT REJECTION

1. Types of rejection following transplant. *WBUHS 2016*

2. Management of acute rejection. *WBUHS 2016*

3. Allograft rejection. *WBUHS 2010*

4. What are the different types of allograft rejection? Discuss the management policy. *WBUHS 2017*

Allograft

It is an organ or tissue transplanted from one individual to another.

Allografts trigger a graft rejection response because of allelic differences at polymorphic genes that give rise to histocompatibility antigens (transplant antigens), of which ABO blood group antigens and human leucocyte antigens (HLA) are the most important.

	Class I	*Class II*
HLA loci	HLA-A, -B, and -C	HLA-DR, -DP, and -DQ
Structure	Heavy chain and β2 microglobulin	α- and β-chain
Distribution	All nucleated cells	B-cells, dendritic cells, and macrophages

Types of rejection following transplant:

Hyperacute rejection (HAR):

- It is mediated by preformed antibodies that bind to antigens of ABO blood groups, nonself HLA, and xenografts that are similar to antigens found on bacteria and viruses.
- It results in immediate tissue edema, hemorrhage, and thrombosis.

Acute rejection:

It is a function of both the innate and the adaptive immune system, triggered by the recognition of foreign major histocompatibility complex (MHC) and foreign peptides presented by self MHC, by T-cells, and results in tissue destruction over days to many months after transplant.

Chronic Rejection

- It is a poorly understood vasculopathy that occurs over years. It is probably a function of the adaptive immune system mediated predominantly through indirect recognition.
- Chronic rejection occurs after the first 6 months.
- Nonimmune factors may contribute to pathogenesis. It is the most common cause of graft rejection and is characterized by myointimal proliferation in great arteries leading to ischemia and fibrosis.
- Chronic rejection manifests as allograft coronary artery disease, detectable in over half of cardiac transplant patients within 5 years of transplantation, and within months in a few patients.
- Other processes that have been associated with allograft coronary disease include increased donorage, hyperlipidemia, and *Cytomegalovirus* (CMV) infection. Ischemia is frequently silent as the heart is denervated.
- The clinical picture includes ventricular arrhythmias, congestive cardiac failure, and sudden death.
- Coronary angiography is the gold standard investigation but may underestimate the extent of the disease as the morphology is diffuse, smooth, and intimal proliferation.
- There is no effective treatment apart from retransplantation.
- Prophylaxis centers on the same risk reduction strategies used in native ischemic heart disease.

Types of Graft Rejection

- *Hyperacute rejection:*
    - Immediate graft destruction due to ABO or preformed anti-HLA antibodies
    - Characterized by intravascular thrombosis and interstitial hemorrhage
- *Acute rejection:*
    - Usually occurs during the first 6 months
    - T cell-dependent
- Maybe cell-mediated, antibody-mediated, or both
    - Usually, reversible
- *Chronic rejection:*
    - Occurs after first 6 months
    - Most common cause of graft failure
    - Antibodies play an important role
    - Nonimmune factors contribute to pathogenesis characterized by myointimal proliferation in graft arteries leading to ischemia and fibrosis

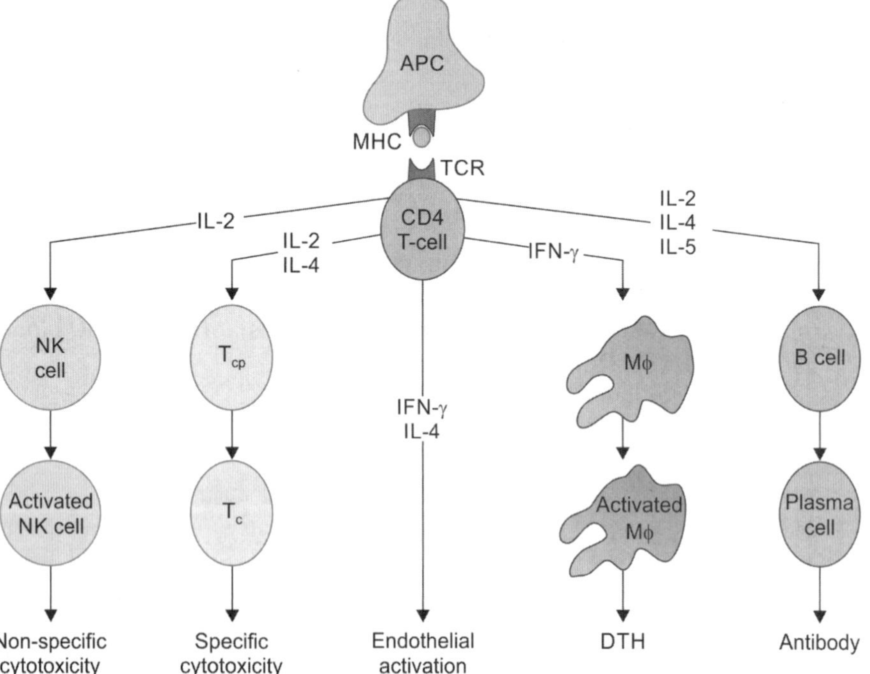

The central role of the CD4 T-cell in orchestrating the various effector mechanisms responsible for allograft rejection. (APC: antigen-presenting cell; DTH: delayed-type hypersensitivity; IFN-γ: interferon-gamma; IL: interleukin; Mϕ: macrophage; MHC: major histocompatibility complex; NK: natural killer; Tc: T cytotoxic cell; Tcp: T cyto-toxic precursor cell; TCR: T-cell receptor).

Diagnosis and Treatment

- *Hyperacute rejection* manifests severely and within minutes, so the treatment is immediate—removal of the tissue.

Acute rejection: Definitions (Adapted from Banff '07 Update)	
Antibody-mediated	***T cell-mediated***
"Rule of three" PMNs >> monocytes C4d$^+$ Presence of anti-donor antibodies (anti-DSA) *Acute tissue injury:* ATN-like (minimal inflammation) Capillary and/or glomerular inflammation and/or thromboses Arterial inflammation	"Is it in the tubules/interstitium, or in the vessels?" • Monocytes >> PMNs • *IA:* >25% interstitial infiltration, *4–10* mononuclear cells/tubular cross-section • *IB:* >25% interstitial infiltration, >*10* mononuclear cells/tubular cross-section • *IIA:* Intimal arteritis—mild-to-moderate (*0–25%* of the lumenal area) • *IIB:* Intimal arteritis—severe (>*25%* of the lumenal area) • *III: Transmural* arteritis and/or fibrinoid change and necrosis of the medial smooth muscle cells with accompanying lymphocyte inflammation
"Suspicious" 2 of 3 above (C4d, DSA, or injury)	*Borderline* For about 10–25% interstitial infiltration, <4 mononuclear cells/tubular cross-section

(ATN: acute tubular necrosis; anti-DSA: anti-donor-specific antibodies; PMNs: polymorphonuclear neutrophils)

- Biopsy is recommended before treating acute rejection unless the biopsy will substantially delay treatment
- Subclinical and borderline acute rejection should be treated
- Administer corticosteroids for the initial treatment of acute cellular rejection
- Recommendation is to add or restore maintenance prednisone in patients, not on steroids who have a rejection episode
- It has been suggested to use lymphocyte-depleting antibodies or OKT3 for acute cellular rejections that do not respond to corticosteroids, and for recurrent acute cellular rejections.
- It is better to treat antibody-mediated acute rejection with one or more of the following alternatives, with or without corticosteroids:
  - Plasma exchange
  - Intravenous immunoglobulin (IVIg)
  - Anti-CD20 antibody
  - Lymphocyte-depleting antibody
  - For patients who have a rejection episode, it is better to add mycophenolate if the patient is not receiving mycophenolate or azathioprine, or switching azathioprine to mycophenolate, OKT3, and muromonab (anti–T-cell antibody)

Acute rejection—treatment	
Antibody-mediated	***T cell-mediated***
• IVIg • Plasmapheresis • Rituximab • Novel therapies	• High dose corticosteroids • Depleting T cell therapy (rATG and ATGAM) • Novel therapies
Steroids versus depleting Ab for acute rejection?	
• Meta-analysis of 14 trials (965 patients) compared therapies for first AR episodes • Ab was better than steroid in reversing rejection (RR: 0.57) and preventing graft loss (death-censored RR 0.74) • No difference in preventing subsequent rejection or death at 1 year	

(ATGAM: antithymocyte globulin equine; IVIg: intravenous immunoglobulin; rATG: rabbit antithymocyte globulin; RR: relative risk)

Diagnosis of Chronic Rejection

- Clinical features include low-grade fever, malaise, reduced exercise tolerance, pericardial rub, supraventricular arrhythmias, low cardiac output, and signs of congestive cardiac failure.
- Blood tests reveal a lymphocytosis
- As all patients are on immunosuppression, symptoms may be minimal until rejection is quite advanced, so routine surveillance is undertaken.
- Hemodynamic measurements with a pulmonary artery (PA) catheter may be helpful, but the gold standard diagnostic tool is right ventricle (RV) endomyocardial biopsy: usually via a right internal jugular percutaneous approach.
- This is carried out every 7–10 days for a month, tapering to 2–6 months intervals.
- Lymphocyte infiltration and myocyte necrosis is used to grade the severity of cellular rejection.
- Biopsy-negative cardiac dysfunction raises the possibility of accelerated coronary artery disease or vascular rejection.

Management

- Asymptomatic mild rejection is monitored but not routinely treated
- Myocyte necrosis is a definite indication for increased immunosuppression, but intermediate grades are treated according to the clinical context.
- Up to 3 days IV methylprednisolone 1,000 mg/day for acute rejection within 3 months of transplant, or for severe episodes.
- 100 mg/day PO methylprednisolone on a reducing dose over several weeks for all other episodes.
- *Repeat endomyocardial biopsy after 7–10 days:* Repeat steroid course if no improvement, or give rescue therapy if hemodynamically unstable.
- Rescue protocols include methylprednisolone + OKT3, or methotrexate.
- Total lymphoid irradiation and photophoresis have been used in refractory rejection.
- Retransplantation is no longer performed in many centers for refractory rejection as results are extremely poor
- Take care of risk factors
- Proper and adequate immunosuppression

Agent	*Principal mode of action*
Corticosteroids	Widespread anti-inflammatory effects
Azathioprine	Prevents lymphocyte proliferation
Mycophenolic acid preparations	Prevents lymphocyte proliferation
Calcineurin inhibitors (ciclosporin/tacrolimus)	Blocks IL-2 gene transcription
mTOR inhibitors	Blocks IL-2 receptor signal transduction
ALG	Depletion and blockade of lymphocytes
Anti-CD25 mAb	Targets activated T cells
Anti-CD52 mAb	Depletion of lymphocytes
Anti-CD2O	Depletion of B lymphocytes
CTLA-41g	Blocks T-cell costimulation

(ALG: antilymphocyte globulin; CTLA-41g: cytotoxic T-lymphocyte associated protein 4; mTOR: mammalian target of rapamycin)

Immunosuppressive agents

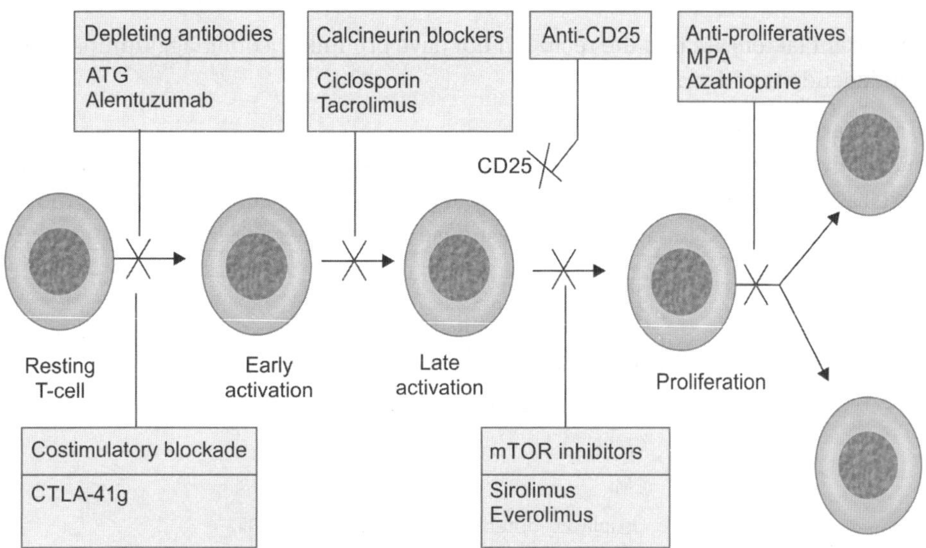

Site of action of immunosuppressive agents on T-cell. (ATG: antithymocyte globulin; CTLA-41g: cytotoxic T-lymphocyte associated protein 4; MPA: mycophenolic acid; mTOR: mammalian target of rapamycin)

- *Corticosteroids:* Corticosteroids inhibit the immune response at many levels. They decrease the production of interferon and interleukins that would normally cause upregulation of the lymphocyte response and reduce macrophage function
- *Cyclosporin (CYA):* Cyclosporin is a calcineurin inhibitor—it inhibits the production of interleukin-2 (IL-2) by T helper cells, selectively reducing the cytotoxic T-cell response.
- *Tacrolimus (FK506):* Tacrolimus is also a calcineurin inhibitor with a similar profile
- *Mycophenolate mofetil (MMF):* MMF inhibits purine synthesis in lymphocytes, reducing clonal expansion and lymphocyte count.
- *Azathioprine (AZA):* Azathioprine causes dose-related bone marrow suppression by suppression of purine synthesis.
- *Sirolimus (rapamycin):* Sirolimus stops IL-2 triggering the clonal expansion of T-lymphocytes.
- *Daclizumab and basiliximab: IL-2 receptor blockers* that prevent clonal expansion of T-cells.
- *OKT3:* OKT3 is a monoclonal antibody produced in mice that binds the cluster of differentiation 3 (CD3) receptor site on cytotoxic T-cells, preventing antigen recognition and clonal expansion
- *Polyclonal antibodies, e.g., antithymocyte globulin (ATG):* These are produced by animals after immunization with HLA: they attach to most circulating lymphocytes effecting a reduction in cell counts to <10% of normal.
- *Simvastatin:* Simvastatin has a moderate protective effect against chronic rejection—it suppresses T-cell function.

5. Graft rejection in transplants. ***WBUHS 2015***

Transplant rejection occurs when transplanted tissue is rejected by the recipient's immune system, which destroys the transplanted tissue. Transplant rejection can be lessened by determining the molecular similitude between donor and recipient and by the use of immunosuppressant drugs after transplant.

ABO-incompatible Transplants

- Because very young children (generally under 12 months, but often as old as 24 months) do not have a well-developed immune system, it is possible for them to receive organs from otherwise incompatible donors.
- This is known as ABO-incompatible (ABOi) transplantation.

- Graft survival and patient mortality is approximately the same between ABOi and ABO-compatible (ABOc) recipients.

  The most important factors are that the recipient not have produced isohemagglutinins and that they have low levels of T cell-independent antigens.

Immunologic Mechanisms of Rejection

Rejection is an adaptive immune response via cellular immunity (mediated by killer T-cells inducing apoptosis of target cells) as well as humoral immunity (mediated by activated B cells secreting antibody molecules), though the action is joined by components of innate immune response (phagocytes and soluble immune proteins).

Tissue	*Mechanism*
Blood	Antibodies (isohemagglutinins)
Kidney	Antibodies and cell-mediated immunity (CMI)
Heart	Antibodies, CMI
Skin	CMI
Bone marrow	CMI
Cornea	Usually accepted unless vascularized: CMI

- *Medical categories of rejection:*
  Types of graft rejection
  - *Hyperacute rejection:*
    - Immediate graft destruction due to ABO or preformed anti-HLA antibodies
    - Characterized by intravascular thrombosis and interstitial hemorrhage
  - *Acute rejection:*
    - Usually occurs during the first 6 months
    - T-cell dependent
    - Maybe cell-mediated, antibody-mediated, or both
    - Usually, reversible
  - *Chronic rejection:*
    - Occurs after first 6 months
    - Most common cause of graft failure
    - Antibodies play an important role
    - Nonimmune factors contribute to pathogenesis characterized by myointimal proliferation in graft arteries leading to ischemia and fibrosis
    - Types of graft rejection
- *Rejection due to nonadherence:* One principal reason for transplant rejection is non-adherence to prescribed immunosuppressant regimens. This is particularly the case with adolescent recipients, with nonadherence rates near 50% in some instances.

Rejection Detection

- Diagnosis of acute rejection relies on clinical data—patient signs and symptoms but also calls on laboratory data, such as tissue biopsy.
- The laboratory pathologist generally seeks three main histological signs:
  1. Infiltrating T-cells, perhaps accompanied by infiltrating eosinophils, plasma cells, and neutrophils, particularly in telltale ratios
  2. Structural compromise of tissue anatomy, varying by tissue type transplanted
  3. Injury to blood vessels
- Tissue biopsy is restricted, however, by sampling limitations and risks/complications of the invasive procedure.
- Cellular magnetic resonance imaging (MRI) of immune cells radiolabeled *in vivo* might offer noninvasive testing.

Rejection Treatment

- *Hyperacute rejection* manifests severely and within minutes, so treatment is immediate—removal of the tissue.
- *Acute rejection* is treated with one or multiple of a few strategies.
  - Administer corticosteroids for the initial treatment of acute cellular rejection.
  - Recommendation is to add or restore maintenance prednisone in patients, not on steroids who have a rejection episode.
  - It has been suggested to use lymphocyte-depleting antibodies or OKT3 for acute cellular rejections that do not respond to corticosteroids, and for recurrent acute cellular rejections.
  - It is better treating antibody mediated acute rejection with one or more of the following alternatives, with or without corticosteroids:
    - Plasma exchange
    - IVIg
    - Anti-CD20 antibody
    - Lymphocyte depleting antibody
  - For patients who have a rejection episode, it is better to add mycophenolate if the patient is not receiving mycophenolate or azathioprine, or switching azathioprine to mycophenolate, OKT3, and muromonab (anti-T-cell antibody)
    - Chronic rejection is generally considered irreversible and poorly amenable to treatment—only retransplant is generally indicated if feasible—though inhaled cyclosporine is being investigated to delay or prevent chronic rejection of lung transplants.

Immunosuppressive Therapy

- A short course of high-dose corticosteroids can be applied and repeated.
- Triple therapy adds a calcineurin inhibitor and an anti-proliferative agent.
- Where calcineurin inhibitors or steroids are contraindicated, mTOR inhibitors are used.

Immunosuppressive Drugs

Corticosteroids	*Calcineurin inhibitors*	*Antiproliferatives*	*mTOR inhibitors*
Prednisolone	Cyclosporin	Azathioprine	Sirolimus
Hydrocortisone	Tacrolimus	Mycophenolic acid	Everolimus

Antibody-based Treatments

- Antibody specific to select immune components can be added to immunosuppressive therapy.
- The monoclonal anti-T-cell antibody OKT3, once used to prevent rejection, and still occasionally used to treat severe acute rejection, has fallen into disfavor, as it commonly brings severe cytokine release syndrome and late post-transplant lymphoproliferative disorder (OKT3 is available in the United Kingdom for named-patient use only.)

Antibody Drugs

- *Monoclonal anti-interleukin-2 receptor α (anti-IL-2Rα) receptor antibodies*
  - Basiliximab
  - Daclizumab
- *Polyclonal anti-T-cell antibodies*
  - ATG
  - Antilymphocyte globulin (ALG)
- *Monoclonal anti-CD20 antibodies:* Rituximab

Blood Transfer

Cases refractory to immunosuppressive or antibody therapy are sometimes given blood transfusions—removing antibody molecules specific to the transplanted tissue

Marrow Transplant

- Bone marrow transplant can replace the transplant recipient's immune system with the donor's one, and the recipient accepts the new organ without rejection.
- The marrow's hematopoietic stem cells—the reservoir of stem cells replenishing exhausted blood cells including white blood cells forming the immune system—must be of the individual who donated the organ or of an identical twin or a clone.
- There is a risk of graft-versus-host disease (GVHD); however, whereby mature lymphocytes entering with marrow recognize the new host tissues as foreign and destroy them.

6. Describe the tissue response to solid organ transplantations and methods of immune suppression. ***WBUHS 2025***

7. Describe the tissue response to solid organ transplantations. ***Srimanta Sankaradeva University, Assam 2025***

Tissue Response to Solid Organ Transplantation

When a *solid organ transplant* (e.g., kidney, liver, heart) is performed, the recipient's body responds in two major ways:

I. *Nonimmune (innate) responses* – immediate tissue injury and inflammation.
   Nonimmune (Injury-related) tissue response:
   - Ischemia–Reperfusion Injury (IRI)
     - Occurs during the period between organ harvest and revascularization.
     - Causes oxidative stress, endothelial injury, and release of inflammatory cytokines (IL-1, TNF-α).
     - Activates innate immunity and predisposes to rejection.
   - Wound Healing and Fibrosis
     - Surgical trauma induces healing response.
     - Chronic inflammation can lead to fibrosis and scarring, which may impair graft function.

II. *Immune (adaptive) responses* – directed against donor antigens, especially *HLA (human* leukocyte antigen) molecules.
   Immune (adaptive) tissue responses:
   - *Antigen Recognition*
     - Recipient *T-lymphocytes* recognize donor *HLA antigens via:*
       - *Direct pathway* – Recipient T-cells recognize intact donor MHC on donor antigen-presenting cells (APCs).
       - *Indirect pathway* – Recipient APCs process donor antigens and present them to recipient T-cells.
       - *Semi-direct pathway* – Recipient APCs acquire donor MHC via exosomes and present them.

This recognition triggers activation of *$CD4^+$ helper T cells, $CD8^+$ cytotoxic T-cells,* and *B-cells,* leading to rejection.

- *Hyperacute Rejection*
  - *Timing*: Occurs within minutes to hours post-transplant.
  - *Mechanism*: Pre-existing antibodies in the recipient (e.g., anti-ABO or anti-HLA antibodies) react with antigens on the donor organ's vascular endothelium, activating the complement system and causing rapid thrombosis, ischemia, and graft failure.
  - *Histology*: Characterized by vascular thrombosis, hemorrhage, and neutrophil infiltration.
  - *Clinical Features*: Immediate graft dysfunction, often irreversible.
  - *Prevention*: Prevented by ABO blood group matching and crossmatching to detect preformed antibodies.
- *Acute Rejection*:
  - *Timing*: Occurs days to months post-transplant (most common within the first 6 months).
  - *Mechanism*: Primarily T-cell-mediated (cellular rejection) or antibody-mediated (humoral rejection).
    - *Cellular Rejection*: $CD4^+$ and $CD8^+$ T-cells recognize donor HLA via direct (donor antigen-presenting cells) or indirect (recipient antigen-presenting cells) pathways, leading to cytotoxic damage to the graft.

  - *Antibody-Mediated Rejection (AMR)*: Donor-specific antibodies (DSAs) bind to graft endothelium, activating complement and causing inflammation.
- *Histology*: Lymphocytic infiltration, endothelialitis, and parenchymal damage (cellular); C4d deposition, vasculitis, and microcirculatory injury (AMR).
- *Clinical Features*: Graft dysfunction (e.g., rising creatinine in kidney transplants), fever, or tenderness.
- *Management*: Treated with high-dose corticosteroids, anti-thymocyte globulin (ATG), or plasmapheresis for AMR.

- *Chronic Rejection*:
  - *Timing*: Develops months to years post-transplant.
  - *Mechanism*: Complex interplay of immune and non-immune factors, including repeated episodes of acute rejection, chronic low-grade inflammation, and non-immunological factors (e.g., ischemia-reperfusion injury, hypertension). Primarily antibody-mediated, leading to progressive fibrosis and vascular occlusion.
  - *Histology*: Fibrosis, intimal thickening of arteries (transplant vasculopathy), and organ-specific changes (e.g., glomerulopathy in kidneys, bronchiolitis obliterans in lungs).
  - *Clinical Features*: Gradual decline in graft function, often irreversible.
  - *Management*: Limited options; focus on optimizing immunosuppression and managing comorbidities.

Cellular Mechanisms in Immune Response

- T-cell–mediated
  - $CD8^+$ cytotoxic T-cells destroy graft parenchyma directly.
  - $CD4^+$ helper T-cells recruit macrophages and other inflammatory cells.
  - Cytokines (IL-2, IFN-α) amplify inflammation.
- B-cell- and Antibody-mediated
  - B-cells produce anti-donor antibodies.
  - Complement activation → endothelial injury → thrombosis and graft dysfunction.
  - *C4d deposition* (on biopsy) is a hallmark of antibody-mediated rejection.

Long-term (Chronic) Changes

- Progressive *fibrosis* and *vascular narrowing (arteriosclerosis).*
- Loss of functional tissue → organ failure.
- Driven by repeated subclinical rejection, chronic inflammation, and non-immune factors (e.g., hypertension, calcineurin inhibitor toxicity).
- The goal of immunosuppression in transplantation is to control the immune response so that the graft survives and functions.

Modulating the Response

- *Immunosuppressive therapy* (e.g., calcineurin inhibitors, corticosteroids, antimetabolites, mTOR inhibitors).
- *Tissue matching* (HLA typing, crossmatching).

Tolerance induction (experimental): Aiming to reprogram the immune system to accept the graft without lifelong immunosuppression.

Methods of Immune Suppression

To prevent or manage rejection, immunosuppressive therapies are used to dampen the recipient's immune response while minimizing side effects like infection or malignancy. These are typically divided into induction, maintenance, and rescue therapies.

I. *Induction therapy:*
  - *Purpose:* Provides intense immunosuppression immediately post-transplant to prevent early acute rejection.
  - *Agents:*
    - *Anti-Thymocyte Globulin (ATG):* Polyclonal antibodies targeting T-cells, depleting them via apoptosis or complement-mediated lysis. Used in high-risk patients.

    - *Basiliximab:* Monoclonal antibody targeting the IL-2 receptor (CD25) on activated T-cells, preventing T-cell proliferation. Used in low-to-moderate risk patients.
    - *Alemtuzumab:* Anti-CD52 monoclonal antibody, depletes T- and B-cells. Less commonly used due to prolonged lymphopenia.
  - *Administration:* Administered perioperatively (IV) during or shortly after transplant.
  - *Side effects:* Cytokine release syndrome (ATG), increased infection risk.

II. *Maintenance therapy:*
  - *Purpose:* Long-term immunosuppression to prevent acute and chronic rejection while balancing side effects.
  - *Common regimens:* Typically involve a combination of drugs targeting different immune pathways:
    - *Calcineurin inhibitors (CNIs):*
      - *Tacrolimus* (preferred) or *Cyclosporine*: Inhibit T-cell activation by blocking calcineurin, preventing IL-2 production.
      - *Side effects:* Nephrotoxicity, hypertension, neurotoxicity, diabetes.
    - *Antiproliferative agents:*
      - *Mycophenolate mofetil (MMF)* or *azathioprine:* Inhibit purine synthesis, reducing T- and B-cell proliferation.
      - *Side effects:* Gastrointestinal upset (MMF), bone marrow suppression.
    - *mTOR inhibitors:*
      - *Sirolimus* or *Everolimus*: Inhibit mTOR, blocking T-cell proliferation and angiogenesis.
      - *Side effects:* Delayed wound healing, hyperlipidemia, pneumonitis.
    - *Corticosteroids:*
      - *Prednisone:* Broadly suppress inflammation by inhibiting cytokine production and immune cell activity.
      - *Side effects:* Osteoporosis, diabetes, weight gain, infection risk.
  - *Administration:* Oral, lifelong unless tolerance is achieved (rare).
  - *Monitoring:* Drug levels (e.g., tacrolimus trough levels) to optimize dosing and minimize toxicity.

III. *Rescue therapy:*
  - *Purpose:* Treat acute rejection episodes.
  - *Agents:*
    - *High-dose corticosteroids:* First-line for cellular rejection (e.g., IV methylprednisolone).
    - *ATG:* Used for steroid-resistant cellular rejection.
    - *Plasmapheresis/IVIG:* Removes DSAs in AMR, often combined with rituximab (anti-CD20) to deplete B-cells.
    - *Bortezomib:* Proteasome inhibitor targeting plasma cells in severe AMR.
  - *Side effects:* Similar to induction agents, with higher infection risk due to intense immunosuppression.

IV. *Emerging and adjunctive therapies:*
  - *Costimulation blockade:*
    - *Belatacept:* Inhibits CD28-B7 interaction, preventing T-cell activation. Used as a CNI alternative in kidney transplants.
    - *Advantage:* Less nephrotoxicity; Disadvantage: Higher acute rejection risk.
  - *Tolerance Induction:* Experimental approaches (e.g., mixed chimerism, regulatory T-cell therapy) aim to induce immune tolerance, reducing the need for lifelong immunosuppression.
  - *Desensitization:* For sensitized patients with preformed antibodies, protocols include plasmapheresis, IVIG, and rituximab to reduce antibody levels pre-transplant.

Additional Considerations

- *Infection risk:* Immunosuppression increases susceptibility to opportunistic infections (e.g., cytomegalovirus, Pneumocystis jirovecii). Prophylactic antimicrobials (e.g., valganciclovir, trimethoprim-sulfamethoxazole) are standard.

- *Malignancy risk:* Long-term immunosuppression increases risk of cancers (e.g., post-transplant lymphoproliferative disorder, skin cancer). Regular screening is essential.
- *Individualization:* Immunosuppression is tailored based on patient risk (e.g., HLA mismatch, sensitization status, organ type) and comorbidities.

Monitoring: Regular biopsies, blood tests (e.g., creatinine for kidney function), and DSA monitoring guide therapy adjustments.

BRAIN DEATH AND ORGAN PROCUREMENT

8. Define brain death. ***WBUHS 2010, 2021***

9. Describe surgical technique of procurement of multiple organs. (Lung, Kidney, Liver, Pancreas). ***WBUHS 2021***

10. Discuss the principles and technique of organ procurement. ***Tripura University 2025***

11. Brain death. ***WBUHS 2010***

Brain Death

A brain-dead individual has no clinical evidence of brain function upon physical examination.

This includes no response to pain and no cranial nerve reflexes.

- *Reflexes include:*
    - Pupillary reaction to light (fixed pupils)
    - Vestibulo-ocular reflex
    - Corneal reflex
    - Gag reflex
    - Motor response to central pain,
    - Apnea test—apnea despite a carbon dioxide increase to >6.65 kPa.

All reflexes must be absent and are tested twice by two doctors.

Organ Procurement

- Organ procurement is an essential step for organ transplantation, from which a quality organ is received for subsequent transplantation.
- As the demand for organ transplantation continues to grow, multiorgan donation including the heart, lung, liver, pancreas, kidneys, and small intestine from one potential donor is always a priority to meet the demand.
- The donor is generally rigorously assessed for suitability of organ donation prior to proceeding to organ procurement.
- The quality of the organ from multiorgan procurement is usually satisfactory without jeopardizing its transplantation.

Procurement of Lungs

- Donation after cardiac death (DCD) is an evolving method for lung transplantation with the potential for increasing the limited donor pool.
- Satisfactory outcomes have been reported from early experience with this technique. DCD lung procurement requires a systematic approach for efficient utilization of resources.
- It is important to minimize the ischemic time during lung procurement.
- The lung procurement operation is usually performed through a median sternotomy.
- In sequence, the pulmonary arteries are dissected free from the ascending aorta, and the superior vena cava is dissected free up to the innominate bifurcation.

Procurement of the Liver

- Following the procurement of the heart and lung by the cardiothoracic team, the liver is taken first for the abdominal organs if the small intestine is not for procurement.
- The gastroduodenal artery is tied and divided.
- The portal vein is divided at the level of 1 cm proximal to the junction of the splenic vein and superior mesentery vein if the pancreas is retrieved for transplantation.
- Otherwise, the division can be at the level of the confluence of the splenic vein and superior mesenteric vein (SMV).
- The splenic artery is divided 0.5 cm from its origin arising from the celiac trunk and left gastric artery.
- However, if the left accessory hepatic artery is present arising from the left gastric artery, then the left gastric artery is preserved on the celiac trunk for its continuity to the left hepatic accessory artery.
- Along the celiac trunk, the celiac complex and lymphatic tissues are divided at the left side of the aorta, and the aorta is exposed. An aortic patch is excised around the ostium of the celiac trunk.
- If the right accessory or replacement hepatic artery is present, then the superior mesenteric artery (SMA) is better included in the aortic patch with celiac trunk.
- If the pancreas is also harvested for transplant, then the SMA is divided just above the level where the accessory hepatic artery arises. So, both liver and pancreas are suitable for transplant without jeopardizing its vasculature.
- After that the attention is directed to the inferior vena cava (IVC). The anterior wall of the IVC is incised transversely above the level of the renal vein.
- Both entrances of the left and right renal vein are checked, and the IVC is transected.
- The IVC is lifted anteriorly by the insertion of a finger from the suprahepatic end, and its posterior side is dissected to reach the suprahepatic end.
- The posterior side of the IVC is dissected superiorly to the level of division just below the atrium.
- Care is taken during IVC dissection without jeopardizing the quality of renal vein for kidney transplantation. The right hepatic triangle ligament is dissected, and part of the diaphragm is taken with the liver during the procurement.
- The liver is now removed freely from the abdomen and immersed in the ice-slush-filled basin.
- One technical point is that liver laceration is easy to occur at the location where the adhesion band is present; therefore, gentle handling of the liver is always emphasized during the dissection and procurement of the liver to avoid potential injury.

Procurement of the Pancreas

- The pancreas can be retrieved in favor with the liver as an en bloc as described in a separate paragraph.
- We should consider a technique for pancreas retrieval as a subsequent procedure following the liver procurement.
- A 6/0 polypropylene suture is placed at the transection of the port vein and splenic artery, respectively, as a mark during the liver procurement if known the pancreas is also procured.
- A segment of the duodenum is routinely procured with the pancreas as exocrine drainage.
- A gastrointestinal anastomosis (GIA) stapler is used to divide the duodenum from the stomach distal to the pylorus.
- Care is taken to ensure that the nasogastric tube (NGT) tube is positioned proximal to the pylorus without being caught in the GIA stapler.
- A reload GIA is needed to divide the distal part of the duodenum at the level of the fourth part of the duodenum or at the beginning of the jejunum.
- The distal part of the SMA and SMV is tied, respectively, by preplaced 2/0 Vicryl tie and divided. The transverse mesocolon is divided to free the inferior edge of the pancreas.
- On the left the dissection is continued to the splenic flexure and on the right to the duodenocolic ligament, which are divided together with the root of mesentery. So, the pancreas with attached duodenum is now free from its attachment.

- Then, the pancreas is lifted anteriorly by holding the spleen, and the dissection to its posterior attachment is performed from the tail toward the body of the pancreas.
- At this point, the SMA is excised with a small aortic patch, and the pancreas is removed from the abdomen and placed in the ice-slush-filled basin.
- Care must be taken during excision of the SMA without jeopardizing the renal artery.

Procurement of the Liver and Pancreas as an En Bloc

- The liver and pancreas are preferred to have en bloc procurement to minimize warm ischemic injury to these organs.
- Following cold perfusion, the proximal and distal part of the duodenum is transected by using a GIA stapler at the level distal to the pylorus and the fourth part of the duodenum, respectively.
- The distal part of the SMA and SMV is tied by a preplaced 2/0 Vicryl tie and divided.
- The transverse mesocolon is divided, and the division is continued on the left to the splenic flexure and on the right to the duodenocolic ligament, which are also divided and the colon retracted inferiorly.
- The spleen is lifted anteriorly as a handle of the pancreas for dissection posterior to the pancreas.
- SMA is excised at the inferior edge with a small aortic patch that is extended superiorly to include the celiac trunk on the same aortic patch.
- The left gastric artery is divided. The attention is directed to the IVC. The IVC is divided just proximal to the level of the entrance by the renal veins, and the dissection to its posterior is continued superiorly to reach the suprahepatic end of the IVC.
- At this stage, the liver and pancreas are free to be removed from the abdominal cavity and immersed in an ice basin for separation from each other on the back table.

Procurement of the Kidneys

- The kidneys are the last procured abdominal organs.
- Therefore, care must be taken during the cooling and procurement phase to ensure that the kidneys are properly cooled by placing enough ice slush at its surroundings, in particular at its posterior and lateral sides.
- The right kidney is retrieved first.
- The bowel is placed superiorly, and the kidneys, the vena cava, and the aorta are left in situ.
- The perfusion cannula is removed, and the aorta is transected at this level.
- The superior end of the aorta is also transected at the level where the SMA aortic patch is excised.
- The left renal vein is excised with a small patch from the vena cava and dissected away from the aorta.
- The anterior part of the aorta is split open as well as the posterior part of the aorta.
- Care is taken to keep an equal aortic patch with each side of the renal artery.
- The renal arteries are inspected at this point and are remained on its patch.
- The IVC is transected at the level of the confluence of common iliac veins.
- The right ureter is divided at the level of iliac vessels.
- The ureter is lifted anteriorly, and its posterior is dissected toward the kidney along the plane anterior to the major psoas muscle.
- Care is taken to retain plenty of surrounding tissues with the ureter. Then, the kidney is lifted anteriorly within Gerota's fascia together with the ureter, and its posterior side is dissected from the psoas muscle.
- The dissection is continued posteriorly to the IVC, and the right half of the aortic patch until the kidney is free from the attachment.
- The right kidney is then removed as a pack from the abdomen and placed in the basin filled with ice slush.
- Care is taken to ensure that the dissection is along the surface of the psoas muscle and spine. So, the injury to the renal artery and renal vein is prevented.
- The left kidney is procured in the same method as the right kidney.

12. Brain death. *WBUHS 2010*

The concept of brain death emerged in the 1960s, as the ability to resuscitate individuals and mechanically keep the heart and lungs functioning became prevalent.

Brainstem death is defined by the irreversible loss of consciousness, loss of brainstem reflexes, and apnea and these patients are therefore mechanically ventilated in the intensive care setting.

Diagnosis of Brainstem Death in three Stages

1. Identification of the cause of irreversible coma.
2. Exclusion of irreversible causes of coma.
3. Clinical demonstration of the absence of brainstem reflexes.

Medical Criteria

- A brain-dead individual has no clinical evidence of brain function upon physical examination.
- This includes no response to pain and no cranial nerve reflexes.
- *Reflexes include:*
  - Pupillary reaction to light (fixed pupils)
  - Vestibulo-ocular reflex
  - Corneal reflex
  - Gag reflex
  - Motor response to central pain
  - *Apnea test:* Apnea despite a carbon dioxide increase to >6.65 kPa

All reflexes must be absent and are tested for twice by two doctors.

It is important to distinguish between brain death and states that may mimic brain death (e.g., barbiturate overdose, alcohol intoxication, sedative overdose, hypothermia, hypoglycemia, coma, or chronic vegetative state.

Some comatose patients can recover, and some patients with severe irreversible neurological dysfunction will nonetheless retain some lower brain functions, such as spontaneous respiration, despite the losses of both cortex and brainstem functionality.

Thus, anencephaly, in which there is no higher brain present, is generally not considered brain death, though it is certainly an irreversible condition in which it may be appropriate to withdraw life support.

One has been declared dead, and would not have met UK test conditions in any case. This is clearly a case of negligent misdiagnosis.

Organ Donation

- Brain death may result in legal death, but still with the heart beating, and with mechanical ventilation all other vital organs may be kept completely alive and functional, providing optimal opportunities for organ transplantation.
- Most organ donation for organ transplantation is done in the setting of brain death. In some nations (for instance, Belgium, Poland, Portugal, and France) everyone is automatically an organ donor, although some jurisdictions (such as Singapore, France, and New Zealand) allow opting out of the system.
- Elsewhere, consent from family members or next of kin is required for organ donation.
- The nonliving donor is kept on ventilator support until the organs have been surgically removed. If a brain-dead individual is not an organ donor, ventilator, and drug support is discontinued and cardiac death is allowed to occur.

13. Preparing a patient for organ transplant. *RGUHS Karnataka 2025*

Preparing a patient for *organ transplantation* is a *comprehensive, multidisciplinary process* aimed at ensuring the patient is *medically, surgically, psychologically, and socially fit* to undergo the procedure and the lifelong post-transplant care that follows.

Preparation involves *evaluation, optimization, counseling, and education*—all coordinated by a *transplant team.*

Goals of Pretransplant Preparation

- *Confirm indication* for transplantation.
- *Assess suitability*—medical, surgical, and psychosocial.
- *Identify and optimize comorbid conditions.*
- *Prevent transmissible infections* and immunological incompatibility.
- *Educate and prepare* the patient and family for post-transplant responsibilities.
- *Ensure ethical and legal compliance.*

Steps in Preparing a Patient for Organ Transplant

Referral and Initial Assessment

- Referred to a *transplant center* when end-stage organ failure is diagnosed (kidney, liver, heart, lung, pancreas, etc.).
- *Initial evaluation includes:*
  - Confirmation of *end-stage disease.*
  - Review of *previous treatments* and prognosis without transplantation.
  - Assessment of *urgency* and eligibility.

Comprehensive Medical Evaluation

- *General medical workup*
  - Detailed history and physical examination.
  - *Review of comorbidities:* Hypertension, diabetes, cardiovascular disease, malignancy, infection.
  - *Baseline investigations:*
    - CBC, renal and liver function, electrolytes.
    - Coagulation profile.
    - ECG, echocardiography, chest X-ray.
    - Blood glucose and lipid profile.
    - Nutritional assessment (BMI, albumin).
- *Organ-specific evaluation*

Each organ transplant has its own set of investigations:

Type of transplant	***Key evaluations***
Kidney	GFR, renal imaging, cardiovascular screening
Liver	MELD/Child-Pugh score, imaging, endoscopy for varices
Heart	Echocardiogram, coronary angiography, pulmonary pressures
Lung	Pulmonary function tests, CT thorax, ABG, right heart cath
Pancreas	C-peptide levels, glucose control, vascular studies

Immunological Evaluation

- Blood typing (ABO compatibility)
- HLA typing (human leukocyte antigen profile)
- *Crossmatching: Complement-dependent cytotoxicity (CDC)* or *Flow cytometry crossmatch* to detect preformed antibodies.
- *Panel Reactive Antibody (PRA)* test to measure sensitization.
- Helps determine *donor-recipient compatibility* and risk of rejection.

Infectious Disease Screening and Vaccination

Tests/Vaccinations	***Purpose***
HIV, Hepatitis B & C, CMV, EBV, Syphilis, Tuberculosis	Identify latent or active infections
COVID-19, Influenza, Pneumococcal, Hepatitis B vaccines	Immunization before immunosuppression
Dental, ENT, skin, and urine cultures	Identify potential infection foci

All infections must be treated or controlled before transplantation.

Psychosocial and Psychiatric Evaluation

- Assess *mental health, adherence potential, social support, and substance use.*
- Evaluate for *depression, anxiety, cognitive impairment*, and *coping ability*.
- Identify a *support network* (family or caregivers).
- Counseling about *lifestyle modification* and *post-transplant compliance.*

Nutritional and Functional Assessment

- Evaluate for *malnutrition or obesity*.
- Dietary advice for optimizing health before surgery.
- Encourage *physical conditioning* and rehabilitation to improve recovery.

Financial, Ethical, and Legal Preparation

- *Financial counseling* for transplant and post-transplant costs.
- *Legal verification of organ source:*
  - For *living donors*: Ensure voluntary, non-commercial donation, and obtain authorization as per local transplant laws (e.g., Human Organ Transplant Act).
  - For *deceased donors*: Ensure consent and documentation.
- *Ethics committee approval* where required.

Patient Education and Counseling

- *Explain:*
  - The *transplant procedure* and possible complications.
  - The need for *lifelong immunosuppression*.
  - *Infection prevention* and regular follow-up.
  - *Lifestyle changes* (diet, exercise, avoiding alcohol/tobacco).
- Involve family or caregivers in counseling sessions.

Listing and Waiting Period

- *Once medically and psychosocially cleared:*
  - The patient is *listed on the transplant registry.*
  - For *deceased donor transplants*, the patient waits for a matched organ.
  - For *living donor transplants*, synchronization of donor and recipient workup follows.
- Regular re-evaluation is required during the waiting period.

Preoperative Preparation (Once Organ is Available)

- *Confirm compatibility* (ABO, crossmatch).
- *Final infection screen* (to rule out new infection).
- *Dialysis (if renal transplant)* within 24 hrs before surgery.
- *Optimize medical condition:* BP, blood sugar, electrolytes.
- *Informed consent* for surgery and immunosuppression.
- *Premedication:* antibiotics, immunosuppressive induction (e.g., basiliximab, ATG).
- *Anesthetic and surgical planning.*

14. Discuss principles of organ transplantation. ***RIMS-IMPHAL 2022***

Immunological Principles

A. *Histocompatibility*
- Matching *human leukocyte antigens (HLA)* between donor and recipient reduces the risk of rejection.
- The more similar the HLA profile, the better the transplant outcome.

B. *Graft Types*

Graft type	*Description*
Autograft	Same person (e.g., skin graft)
Isograft	Between genetically identical individuals
Allograft	Between genetically different individuals
Xenograft	Between different species (e.g., pig to human)

C. *Rejection Types*

Type of rejection	*Timing*	*Mechanism*
Hyperacute	Minutes–hours	Preformed antibodies
Acute	Days–weeks	T-cell mediated
Chronic	Months–years	Immune and nonimmune fibrosis

D. *Immune Suppression*
- Use of *immunosuppressive drugs* (e.g., cyclosporine, tacrolimus, steroids) to prevent rejection.
- Balance is needed to avoid *infections or malignancy* due to over-suppression.

Donor and Recipient Selection

- *Donor evaluation:* Brain death confirmation, organ function assessment, infectious disease screening.
- *Recipient evaluation:* Disease severity, likelihood of benefit, immunological match, psychosocial suitability.

Ethical and Legal Principles

- *Informed consent* from donor or family.
- *Noncommercialization:* Organ trade is illegal.
- *Equity:* Fair allocation based on urgency, compatibility, and waiting time.
- *Brain death criteria:* Legally accepted definition for deceased organ donation.

Indications for Organ Transplantation

Organ	*Indication*
Kidney	End-stage renal disease
Liver	Cirrhosis, hepatic failure
Heart	Heart failure, cardiomyopathy
Lungs	COPD, pulmonary fibrosis
Pancreas	Type 1 diabetes (selected cases)
Intestine	Short bowel syndrome

Outcomes and Follow-up

- *Survival rates* vary by organ type and match quality.
- *Lifelong follow-up required for:*
  - Rejection monitoring
  - Infection surveillance

- Immunosuppressant side effects
- Graft function

Summary Mnemonic: "MATCHED"

- **M** – Matching HLA
- **A** – Avoid rejection
- **T** – Type of graft
- **C** – Consent and ethics
- **H** – Host immune suppression
- **E** – Evaluation of donor/recipient
- **D** – Disease-specific indications

15. Give an account on the procedures of organ donation and organ procurement for transplantation.

WBUHS 2023

Steps of Organ Donation

- Registering a donor
- Medical care of potential donors
- Brain death testing
- Role of organ procurement organizations (OPOs)
- Authorizing donation
- The matching process
- Recovering and transporting organs
- Transplanting the organs

Organ Donation Step by Step

- The organ recovery process involves a complex series of events coordinated by medical professionals in OPOs and hospitals.
- The National Organ Transplant Act of 1984 (NOTA) was enacted to help ensure the process is carried out in a fair and efficient way, leading to equitable distribution of donated organs.
- The act established the National Organ Procurement and Transplantation Network (OPTN) for matching donor organs to waiting recipients.
- The OPTN is managed through the United Network for Organ Sharing (UNOS) located in Richmond, Virginia. United Network for Organ Sharing works with 58 federally designated OPOs across the country to place organs locally, regionally, and nationally.

Steps in the process are as follows:

- *Identification of the potential donor by the hospital:*
  - Medical professionals at a hospital identify a potential candidate for donation.
  - The nature of the injury leads a physician to determine whether the patient is brain dead or a potential DCD candidate.
- *Evaluation of donor eligibility:*
  - OneLegacy is called on all patient deaths and imminent patient deaths.
  - Information is provided on the patient's medical status
  - OneLegacy recovery coordinator evaluates the patient.
  - The evaluation includes a medical and social history and physical examination of the patient.
  - This determines whether or not the patient is a suitable candidate for donation.
- *Authorization for organ recovery:*
  - If the patient is a candidate for organ and/or tissue donation, at an appropriate time the legal next-of-kin is approached with the opportunity of donation.

- If a donor designation or individual authorization by the decedent cannot be identified, the family must give their consent in order for the donation process to proceed.
- If the family consents, the legal next-of-kin signs a donor consent form.

- *Medical maintenance of the patient:*
  - Once family consent or donor designation has been provided, the OneLegacy clinical coordinator, in concert with the hospital staff, maintains the patient medically.
  - In some cases, physician support is requested on a consultation basis.
- *Matching organs to potential recipients:*
  - Information on the organs available for donation, the donor's blood type, and body size is provided to UNOS by the OneLegacy clinical coordinator.
  - The UNOS computer then matches the donated organs to potential recipients.
  - Recipient selection is based on blood type, body size, medical urgency, and length of time on the waiting list.
  - The heart, liver, and lungs are matched by blood type and body size.
  - In matching the pancreas and kidneys, genetic tissue type is also considered.
- *Offering organs regionally, then nationally:* A computerized list of waiting patients in the matching blood group is provided to the OneLegacy coordinator who seeks to match organs with recipients in the OneLegacy's donation service area. If a match cannot be made for a specific organ within this area, the organ is offered on a regional basis, then nationally, if necessary.
- *Placing organs and coordinating recovery:*
  - When a recipient match has been found, the OneLegacy coordinator calls the transplant center for the patient who matches the donated organ(s).
  - The patient's transplant surgeon is responsible for making the decision whether to accept the organ.
  - If the surgeon declines the organ for that patient, the OneLegacy coordinator contacts the transplant surgeon of the next patient on the list.
  - This process continues for each organ until all of the organs have been appropriately matched with recipients.
  - The OneLegacy coordinator then arranges for the operating room (for the recovery of the organs) and the arrival and departure times of the transplant surgery teams.
- *Surgical recovery of organs:*
  - When the surgical team arrives, the donor is taken to the operating room where the organs and tissues are recovered through a dignified surgical procedure.
  - In accordance with law, physicians recovering the organs do not participate in the donor's care prior to the determination of brain death.
- *Preparing recipients for surgery:*
  - Once the recipients have been identified, they are called by their transplant surgeons for the final preoperative preparations while the organ recovery process is occurring at the donor hospital.
  - Upon the organ's arrival at the transplant hospital, the recipients are taken to surgery and the transplants are performed.
- *Distribution of organs:*
  - The OneLegacy coordinator takes a sample of the lymph node tissue to a laboratory for tissue typing and subsequent matching with recipients.
  - Other organs are taken directly to the recipients by the surgical recovery teams.
- *Funeral and burial plans:*
  - After the recovery process has occurred, the donor family can proceed with funeral or burial plans, which are not affected by organ donation.
  - Organ and tissue donation is a dignified and respectful process.
- *Follow-up with family and hospital:* OneLegacy follows up each donation by sending letters to the donor family, hospital staff, physicians, and nurses regarding the organs and tissues that have been recovered.

Organ Procurement for Transplantation

- *Regulation:*
  - Organ procurement is tightly regulated by UNOS. In the United States, there are a total of 58 organ procurement organizations that are responsible for evaluating the candidacy of deceased donors for organ donation and coordinating the procurement of the organs. Each OPO is responsible for a particular geographic region and is under the regulation of the OPTN.
  - *In India:* The Transplantation of Human Organs Act (THOA) 1994 was enacted to provide a system of removal, storage, and transplantation of human organs for therapeutic purposes and for the prevention of commercial dealings in human organs. THOA is now adopted by all the states except Andhra and Jammu and Kashmir, who have their own similar laws.

    Section 11 of the THO Amendment Act of 2011 forbids any donor or person empowered to give authority for the removal of any human organ or tissue from doing so for any reason other than therapeutic purposes.

Laws and Rules Governing Organ Transplantation in India

The primary legislation related to organ donation and transplantation in India, the Transplantation of Human Organs Act, was passed in 1994 and is aimed at regulation of removal, storage, and transplantation of human organs for therapeutic purposes and for prevention of commercial dealings in human organs.

In India, matters related to health are governed by each state. The Act was initiated at the request of Maharashtra, Himachal Pradesh, and Goa (who therefore adopted it by default) and was subsequently adopted by all states except Andhra Pradesh and Jammu and Kashmir. Despite a regulatory framework, cases of commercial dealings in human organs were reported in the media. An amendment to the act was proposed by the states of Goa, Himachal Pradesh, and West Bengal in 2009 to address inadequacies in the efficacy, relevance, and impact of the Act. The amendment to the Act was passed by the parliament in 2011, and the rules were notified in 2014. The same is adopted by the proposing states and union territories by default and may be adopted by other states by passing a resolution.

The main provisions of the Act (including the amendments and rules of 2014) are as follows:

A. Brain death is identified as a form of death. Process and criteria for brain death certification defined (Form 10)

B. Allows transplantation of human organs and tissues from living donors and cadavers (after cardiac or brain death)

C. Regulatory and advisory bodies for monitoring transplantation activity and their constitution defined.
   i. *Appropriate Authority (AA):* Inspects and grants registration to hospitals for transplantation enforces required standards for hospitals, and conducts regular inspections to examine the quality of transplantations. It may conduct investigations into complaints regarding breach of provisions of the Act and has the powers of a civil court to summon any person, request documents, and issue search warrants.
   ii. *Advisory Committee:* Consisting of experts in the domain who shall advise the appropriate authority.
   iii. *Authorization Committee (AC):* It regulates living donor transplantation by reviewing each case to ensure that the living donor is not exploited for monetary considerations and to prevent commercial dealings in transplantation. Proceedings are to be video recorded and decisions are notified within 24 hours. Appeals against their decision may be made to the state or central government.
   iv. *Medical board (Brain Death Committee):* Panel of doctors responsible for brain death certification. In case of the nonavailability of a neurologist or neurosurgeon, any surgeon, physician, anesthetist, or intensivist, nominated by the medical administrator in-charge of the hospital may certify brain death.

D. Living donors are classified as either near relatives or nonrelated donors.
   i. A near-relative (spouse, children, grandchildren, siblings, parents, and grandparents) needs permission of the doctor in-charge of the transplant center to donate his organ.
   ii. A nonrelated donor needs the permission of an Authorization Committee established by the state to donate his organs.

E. *Swap transplantation:* When a near relative living donor is medically incompatible with the recipient, the pair is permitted to do a swap transplant with another related unmatched donor/recipient pair.

F. Authorization for organ donation after brain death:
   i. May be given before death by the person himself/herself Or
   ii. By the person in legal possession of the body. A doctor shall ask the patient or relative of every person admitted to the ICU whether any prior authorization has been made. If not, the patient or his near relative should be made aware of the option to authorize such donation.
   iii. Authorization process for organ or tissue donation from unclaimed bodies outlined.

G. Organ retrieval is permitted from any hospital with an intensive care unit (ICU) facility once registered with the appropriate authority. Any hospital having ICU facilities along with manpower, infrastructure, and equipment as required to diagnose and maintain the brainstem dead person and to retrieve and transport organs and tissues including the facility for their temporary storage, can register as a retrieval center.

H. Cost of donor management, retrieval, transportation, and preservation to be borne by the recipient, institution, government, nongovernmental organization (NGO), or society, and not by the donor family.

I. Procedure for organ donation in medicolegal cases defined to avoid jeopardizing determination of the cause of death and delay in retrieval of organs.

J. Manpower and facilities required for registration of a hospital as a transplant center are outlined.

K. Infrastructure, equipment requirements, guidelines, and standard operating procedures for tissue banks are outlined.

L. Qualifications of transplant surgeons, cornea, and tissue retrieval technicians defined.

M. Appointment of transplant coordinators (with defined qualifications) made mandatory in all transplant centers.

N. NGO, registered societies, and trusts working in the field of organ or tissue removal, storage or transplantation will require registration.

O. The central government to establish a National Human Organs and Tissues Removal and Storage Network, i.e., National Organ and Tissue Transplant Organization (NOTTO), Regional Organ and Tissue Transplant Organization (ROTTO), and State Organ and Tissue Transplant Organization (SOTTO). Manner of establishing National or Regional State Human Organs and Tissues Removal and Storage Networks and their functions clearly stated.

P. The central government shall maintain a registry of the donors and recipients of human organs and tissues.

Q. Penalties for removal of organs without authority, making or receiving payment for supplying human organs, or contravening any other provisions of the Act have been made very stringent in order to serve as a deterrent for such activities.

The various forms outlined in the rules are as follows:

- *Form 1:* Near-relative consent
- *Form 2:* Spouse consent
- *Form 3:* Other than near-relative donor consent
- *Form 4:* Psychiatrist evaluation of the donor
- *Form 5:* HLA deoxyribonucleic acid (DNA) profiling report
- *Form 7:* Self-consent for deceased donation
- *Form 8:* Consent for organ donation from family (also applicable for minors)
- *Form 9:* Consent for organ donation from unclaimed bodies
- *Form 10:* Brain death declaration form
- *Form 11:* Joint transplant application by donor/recipient
- *Form 12:* Registration of hospital for organ transplantation
- *Form 13:* Registration of hospital for organ retrieval
- *Form 16:* Grant of registration
- *Form 17:* Renewal of registration
- *Form 18:* Decision by hospital authorization committee
- *Form 19:* Decision by district authorization committee

- *Form 20:* Verification of domicile for non-near relative
- *Form 21:* Letter from embassy

Procedure

- If the organ donor is human, most countries require that the donor be legally dead for consideration of organ transplantation (e.g., cardiac or brain dead).
- For some organs, a living donor can be the source of the organ, for example, living donors can donate one kidney or part of their liver to a well-matched recipient.
- Organs cannot be procured after the heart has stopped beating for a long time. Thus, donation after brain death is generally preferred because the organs are still receiving blood from the donor's heart until minutes before being removed from the body and placed on ice. In order to better standardize the evaluation of brain death.
- The American Academy of Neurology (AAN) published a new set of guidelines in 2010. These guidelines require that three clinical criteria be met in order to establish brain death: (1) coma with a known cause, (2) absence of brain stem reflexes, and (3) apnea.
- DCD involves surgeons taking organs within minutes of the cessation of respirators and other forms of life support for patients who still have at least some brain activity.
- Once life support has been withdrawn, there is a 2–5 minutes waiting period to ensure that the potential donor's heart does not start beating again spontaneously.
- After this waiting period, organ procurement surgery begins as quickly as possible to minimize the time that the organs are not being perfused with blood.
- If consent is obtained from the potential donor or the potential donor's survivors, the next step is to perform a match between the source (donor) and the target (recipient) to reduce rejection of the organ by the recipient's immune system.
- Coordination between teams working on different organs is often necessary in case of multiple-organ procurement. Multiple-organ procurement models are also developed from slaughtered pigs to reduce the use of laboratory animals.

Preservation and Transport

- After organ procurement the organs are often rushed to the site of the recipient for transplantation or preserved for later study.
- The faster the organ is transplanted into the recipient, the better the outcome.
- While the organ is being transported, it is either stored in an icy cold solution to help preserve it or it is connected to a miniature organ perfusion system which pumps an icy solution (sometimes enriched with potassium) through the organ.
- This time during transport is called the "cold ischemia time." Heart and lungs should have <6 hours between organ procurement and transplantation.
- For liver transplants, the cold ischemia time can be up to 24 hours, although typically surgeons aim for a much shorter period of time.
- For kidney transplants, as the cold ischemia time increases, the risk of delayed function of the kidney increases.
- Sometimes, the kidney function is delayed enough that the recipient requires temporary dialysis until the transplanted kidney begins to function.
- In recent years novel methods of organ preservation have emerged that may be able to improve the quality of donated organs or assess their viability.
- The most widely used technique involves machine perfusion of the organ at either hypothermic (4–10°C) or normothermic (37°C) temperatures.
- Hypothermic perfusion of kidneys is a relatively widespread practice. For the heart normothermic preservation has been used in which the heart is provided with warm oxygenated blood and so continues to beat ex vivo during its preservation.

- For the liver, hypothermic and normothermic techniques are being used with evidence to suggest that both may be beneficial.

Human Immunodeficiency Virus Organ Policy Equity (HOPE) Act

The HOPE Act allows for clinical research on organ transplantation from human immunodeficiency virus (HIV)+ donors to HIV+ recipients.

Ethics of Organ Transplantation

- Although the procedure of organ transplantation has become widely accepted, there are still a number of ethical debates around related issues.
- The debates center around illegal, forced, or compensated transplantation such as organ theft or organ trade, fair organ distribution, and to a lesser degree, animal rights, and religious prohibition on consuming some animals, such as pork.

Because of the significant need for organs for transplantation, there is an ethical debate about where the organs can be obtained from and whether some organs are obtained illegally or through coercion.

MAJOR HISTOCOMPATIBILITY COMPLEX AND PRINCIPLES OF LIVER TRANSPLANTATION

16. What is MHC and its function? Principles of liver transplantation. ***WBUHS 2021***

Major Histocompatibility Complex

- The MHC is a group of genes that encode proteins on the cell surface that have an important role in immune response. Their main role is in antigen presentation where MHC molecules display peptide fragments for recognition by appropriate T-cells.
- MHC class I and class II proteins play a pivotal role in the adaptive branch of the immune system. Both classes of proteins share the task of presenting peptides on the cell surface for recognition by T-cells.

Function of MHC

- MHC is the tissue antigen that allows the immune system (more specifically T-cells) to bind to, recognize, and tolerate itself (autorecognition). Major histocompatibility complex is also the chaperone for intra- cellular peptides that are complexed with MHCs and presented to T-cell receptors (TCRs) as potential foreign antigens. MHC interacts with TCR and its coreceptors to optimize binding conditions for the TCR-antigen interaction, in terms of antigen binding affinity and specificity, and signal transduction effectiveness.
- Essentially, the MHC-peptide complex is a complex of autoantigen/alloantigen. Upon binding, T-cells should in principle tolerate the auto-antigen, but activate when exposed to the alloantigen. Disease states occur when this principle is disrupted.
- *Antigen presentation:* MHC molecules bind to both T-cell receptor and CD4/CD8 coreceptors on T lymphocytes, and the antigen epitope held in the peptide-binding groove of the MHC molecule interacts with the variable Ig-like domain of the TCR to trigger T-cell activation.
- *Autoimmune reaction:* Having some MHC molecules increases the risk of autoimmune diseases more than having others, for example, HLA-B27. It is unclear how exactly having the HLA-B27 tissue type increases the risk of ankylosing spondylitis and other associated inflammatory diseases, but mechanisms involving aberrant antigen presentation or T-cell activation have been hypothesized.
- *Tissue allorecognition:* MHC molecules in complex with peptide epitopes are essential ligands for TCRs. T-cells become activated by binding to the peptide-binding grooves of any MHC molecule that they were not trained to recognize during positive selection in the thymus.

Principles of Liver Transplantation

- A liver transplant involves the removal of and preparation of the donor's liver, removal of the diseased liver, and implantation of the new organ.

- The liver has several key connections that must be reestablished for the new organ to receive blood flow and to drain bile from the liver.
- The structures that must be reconnected are the inferior vena cava, the portal vein, the hepatic artery, and the bile duct.
- The exact method of connecting these structures varies depending on the specific donor and anatomy or recipient anatomic issues and, in some cases, the recipient's disease.

Organ Allocation

- Child–Pugh classification and model of end-stage liver disease (MELD) score
- Pediatric end-stage liver disease (PELD) score, similar to the adult MELD score used to determine priority
- PELD calculator
- PELD consists of bilirubin, international normalized ratio (INR), serum albumin, age <1 year, and growth failure. Additional PELD points for hepatopulmonary syndrome, urea cycle defects, and neoplasms
- PELD is not a predictor of 30 days or long-term outcome following transplantation

Graft Options

- Whole organ transplantation is ideal
- Split liver transplantation where a single liver can be used with two recipients

Living Donor Transplantation

- Graft to recipient body weight ratio (GRWR) used to determine optimal graft volume with a GRWR of 1–3%
- Grafts from pediatric donors have improved outcomes in the pediatric population than grafts from adult donors

Computed tomography (CT) of liver volumetry is an essential imaging study in preoperative assessment for living donor liver transplantation (LDLT).

Major General Principles

- Maintain patency of the graft vascular anastomoses (particularly the hepatic artery but also the portal and hepatic veins)
- Provide normal to slightly supraphysiologic blood pressure to ensure adequate perfusion of the graft while avoiding significant hypertension that may predispose to bleeding
- Communication with the transplant team is key

For someone undergoing liver transplantation, the sequence of events in the operating room is as follows:

- *Incision:* Evaluation of the abdomen for abnormalities that would preclude liver transplantation (for example, undiagnosed infection or malignancy). Mobilization of the native liver (dissection of the liver attachments to the abdominal cavity)
- Isolation of important structures (the inferior vena cava above, behind, and below the liver; the portal vein; the common bile duct; the hepatic artery)
- Transection of the aforementioned structures and removal of the native, diseased liver.
- *Sewing in the new liver*: First, venous blood flow is reestablished by connecting the donor's and the recipient's inferior vena cava and portal veins. Next, arterial flow is reestablished by sewing the donor's and recipient's hepatic arteries. Finally, biliary drainage is achieved by sewing the donor's and recipient's common bile ducts.
- Ensuring adequate control of bleeding
- Closure of the incision

---

17. Live-related liver transplant. ***WBUHS 2008, 2015***

Introduction

- *Liver transplantation* or *hepatic transplantation* is the replacement of a diseased liver with a healthy liver allograft.
- The most commonly used technique is orthotopic transplantation, in which the native liver is removed and replaced by the donor organ in the same anatomic location as the original liver.

- Liver transplantation nowadays is a well-accepted treatment option for end-stage liver disease and acute liver failure.
- It is also one of the most expensive treatments in modern medicine.
- Typically, three surgeons and one anesthesiologist is involved, with up to four supporting nurses.
- The first human liver transplant was performed in 1963 by a surgical team led by Dr Thomas Starzl of Denver, Colorado, United States.

Living Donor Liver Transplantation

- It has emerged in recent decades as a critical surgical option for patients with end-stage liver disease such as cirrhosis and/or hepatocellular carcinoma often attributable to one or more of the following:
  Long-term alcohol abuse, long-term untreated hepatitis C infection, and long-term untreated hepatitis B infection.
- *The concept of LDLT is based on the following:*
  - The remarkable regenerative capacities of the human liver
  - The widespread shortage of cadaveric livers for patients awaiting transplants. In LDLT, a piece of healthy liver is surgically removed from a living person and transplanted into a recipient, immediately after the recipient's diseased liver has been entirely removed.
- Historically, LDLT began as a means for parents of children with severe liver disease to donate a portion of their healthy liver to replace their child's entire damaged liver.
- The first report of successful LDLT was by Dr Christoph Broelsch at the University of Chicago Medical Center in November 1989.
- The risk of complications in the donor is around 10%, and very occasionally a second operation is needed.
- Common problems are biliary fistula, gastric stasis, and infections; they are more common after removal of the right lobe of the liver.
- In a typical adult recipient LDLT, 55–70% of the liver (the right lobe) is removed from a healthy living donor.
- The donor's liver will regenerate approaching 100% function within 4–6 weeks, and will almost reach full volumetric size with recapitulation of the normal structure soon thereafter.
- It may be possible to remove up to 70% of the liver from a healthy living donor without harm in most cases. The transplanted portion will reach full function and the appropriate size in the recipient as well, although it will take longer than for the donor.
- Living donors are faced with risks and/or complications after the surgery.
- Blood clots and biliary problems have the possibility of arising in the donor postoperative, but these issues are remedied fairly easily.
- Although death is a risk that a living donor must be willing to accept prior to the surgery, the mortality rate of living donors in the United States is low.
- The LDLT donor's immune system does diminish as a result of the liver regenerating, so certain foods that would normally cause an upset stomach could cause serious illness.

Indications

- Liver transplantation is potentially applicable to any acute or chronic condition resulting in irreversible liver dysfunction, provided that the recipient does not have other conditions that will preclude a successful transplant.
- Uncontrolled metastatic cancer outside the liver, active drug or alcohol abuse, and active septic infections are absolute contraindications.
- While infection with HIV was once considered an absolute contraindication, this has been changing recently.
- Advanced age and serious heart, pulmonary, or other disease may also prevent transplantation (relative contraindications).
- Most liver transplants are performed for chronic liver diseases that lead to irreversible scarring of the liver, or cirrhosis of the liver. Another cause is cryptogenic liver disease.

Liver Donor Requirements

Any member of the family, parent, sibling, child, spouse, or volunteer can donate their liver. The criteria for a liver donation include:

- Being in good health
- Having a blood type that matches or is compatible with the recipient's
- Having a charitable desire of donation without financial motivation
- Being between 18 and 60 years old
- Being of similar or bigger size than the recipient
- Before one becomes a living donor, the donor must undergo testing to ensure that the individual is physically fit. Sometimes CT scans or MRIs are done to image the liver. In most cases, the workup is done in 2–3 weeks

Screening for Donors

- Living donor transplantation is a multidisciplinary approach
- All living liver donors undergo a medical evaluation
- Every hospital that performs transplant have dedicated nurses who provide specific information about the procedure and answer questions that families may have
- During the evaluation process, confidentially is assured on the potential donor
- Every effort is made to ensure that organ donation is not made by coercion from other family members
- The transplant team provides both the donor and family thorough counseling and support which continues until full recovery is made.
- All donors are assessed medically to ensure that they can undergo the surgery.
- Blood type of the donor and recipient must be compatible but not always identical
- Other things assessed prior to surgery include the anatomy of the donor's liver.
- However, even with mild variations in blood vessels and bile duct, surgeons today are able to perform transplantation without problems.
- The most important criterion for a living liver donor is to be in excellent health.

Complications

- Living donor surgery is done at a major center.
- Very few individuals require any blood transfusions during or after surgery.
- Even though the procedure is very safe, all potential donors should know there is a 0.5–1.0% chance of death.
- Other risks of donating a liver include bleeding, infection, painful incision, the possibility of blood clots, and a prolonged recovery.
- The vast majority of donors enjoy complete and full recovery within 2–3 months.

Pediatric Transplantation

In children, living liver donor transplantations have become very accepted. The accessibility of adult parents who want to donate a piece of the liver for their children/infants has reduced the number of children who would have otherwise died waiting for a transplant. Having a parent as a donor also has made it a lot easier for children—because both patients are in the same hospital and can help boost each other's morale.

Benefits

There are several advantages of living liver donor transplantation over cadaveric donor transplantation, including:

- Transplant can be done on an elective basis because the donor is readily available.
- There are fewer possibilities for complications and death while waiting for a cadaveric organ donor.
- Because of donor shortages, UNOS has limited the cadaveric organ allocation to foreigners who seek medical help in the USA. However, with the availability of living donor transplantation, this will now allow foreigners a new opportunity to seek medical care in the USA.

18. Child's criteria for assessment of hepatic function. ***WBUHS 2008***

Introduction

Determination of functional liver reserve is necessary for patients who are going to have hepatic surgery.

Pugh's modification of Child's grading of cirrhosis.			
Measurements	***One point***	***Two points***	***Three points***
Bilirubin (mg/dL)	1–1.9	2–2.9	>2.9
Prothrombin time prolongation (secs)	1–3	4–6	>6
Albumin (g/dL)	>3.5	2.8–3.4	<2.8
Ascites	None	Mild	moderate to severe
Encephalopathy	None	Grade 1 or 2	Grade 3 or 4

Interpretation

Child's A: For about 5–6 points; B: 7–9 points; and C: 10–15 points.

- Functionally well-compensated cirrhosis is classified as Pugh–Child's classification grade A; decompensating cirrhosis is grade B; and decompensated cirrhosis is grade C.
- *Usefulness:* Generally, partial hepatectomy is only offered to patients who are Pugh–Child's A and the most favorable class B patients.
- In general, Child's class C patients are only offered supportive care, since even nonsurgical ablative methods such as embolization is associated with a procedure-related mortality in one-third of the patients.

19. Enumerate indications and contraindications of liver transplant and write a note on extended donor criteria for liver transplant. ***DNB 2024 October***

20. Discuss about indications, selection criteria, techniques and complications of orthotopic liver transplant (OLT).

Indications for Liver Transplantation

Adults	***Children***
• Noncholestatic cirrhosis • Viral hepatitis B and C • Alcoholic • Cryptogenic • Cholestatic • Primary biliary cirrhosis • Primary sclerosing cholangitis • Autoimmune • Malignant neoplasm • Miscellaneous	• Biliary atresia • Inborn errors of metabolism • Cholestatic • Primary sclerosing cholangitis • Alagille syndrome • Autoimmune • Viral hepatitis • Miscellaneous

The selection of donors for adult-to-adult right hepatic lobe LDLT is one of the most important aspects of this procedure. Criteria for donor selection are evolving as experience with the procedure increases. However, the two fundamental purposes of the donor evaluation are to ensure that (1) the donor operation may be performed safely and (2) the donor is able to yield a suitable graft for the recipient.

Phases of Living Donor Evaluation

Phase I

- Age ≥18 and ≤55 years
- Identical or compatible blood type with the recipient

- Absence of previous significant abdominal surgery and/or medical problems
- Significant long-term relationship with the recipient
- Normal liver function test results, serum electrolyte levels, complete blood count with differential cell count, and negative hepatitis B surface antigen, and hepatitis C antibody results

Phase II

- Complete medical history and physical examination laboratory tests—serum ferritin, iron, transferrin, ceruloplasmin, α1-antitrypsin level and phenotype, rapid plasma reagin, CMV antibody (immunoglobulin G), Epstein–Barr virus antibody (immunoglobulin G), antinuclear antibody, human immunodeficiency antibody, toxicology/substance abuse screen, urinalysis, and blood oxygen saturation
- Chest radiograph
- Electrocardiogram
- Formal surgical evaluation *of* donor
- Anesthesia preoperative evaluation
- Magnetic resonance imaging of the liver, biliary system, and hepatic vasculature

Phase III

- Other tests or consultations to clarify any potential problems uncovered during evaluation, e.g., endoscopic retrograde cholangiopancreatography, hepatic angiogram, liver biopsy, echocardiogram, and stress echocardiogram (some centers routinely perform these tests as part of the donor evaluation)
- Body size compatibility between the donor and recipient is an important preliminary consideration in the donor evaluation. The donor and recipient should be within approximately 30% body weight of each other.
- Two formulas are used to assess graft size adequacy: (1) Graft-recipient body weight ratio and (2) graft weight as a percentage of standard liver mass.

Special Considerations and/or Issues in Donor Evaluation

- *Obesity:* Obesity [body mass index (*BMI*)—28 kg/m^2) in potential donors is an increasingly common problem.
- *Liver biopsy:* The role of liver biopsy in the donor evaluation process varies greatly from center to center.
- *Cost of donor evaluation:* Financial considerations of the donor evaluation and hepatectomy are important to consider because the process is complex and expensive.
- *Donor advocate:* An important recent development in the donor evaluation process is the recommendation for a donor advocate.
- *Hepatitis B core antibody-positive donor:* Donors who are hepatitis B virus (*HBV*) surface antigen positive are excluded from donation. However, donors who have HBV core antibody and HBV surface antigen negative have been successfully used as living liver transplant donors.

Patient Selection Criteria for Liver Transplantation

In both categories of liver diseases, factors that are listed below are often the precipitating reason for proceeding with liver transplantation:

- Severe fatigue
- Unacceptable quality of life
- Recurrent variceal bleeding
- Intractable ascites
- Recurrent or severe hepatic encephalopathy
- Spontaneous bacterial peritonitis
- Hepatorenal syndrome
- Development of small hepatocellular carcinoma on hepatic imaging

Techniques

- Before transplantation, liver-support therapy might be indicated (bridging-to-transplantation). Artificial liver support like liver dialysis or bio-artificial liver support concepts are currently under preclinical and clinical evaluation.

- Virtually all liver transplants are done in an orthotopic fashion, that is, the native liver is removed and the new liver is placed in the same anatomic location.
- The transplant operation can be conceptualized as consisting of the hepatectomy (liver removal) phase, the anhepatic (no liver) phase, and the postimplantation phase.
- The operation is done through a large incision in the upper abdomen. The hepatectomy involves the division of all ligamentous attachments to the liver as well as the common bile duct, hepatic artery, hepatic vein, and portal vein.
- Usually, the retrohepatic portion of the inferior vena cava is removed along with the liver, although an alternative technique preserves the recipient's vena cava ("piggyback" technique).
- The donor's blood in the liver will be replaced by an ice-cold organ storage solution, such as the University of Wisconsin (UW) and histidine tryptophan ketoglutarate (HTK) until the allograft liver is implanted.
- Implantation involves anastomoses (connections) of the inferior vena cava, portal vein, and hepatic artery.
- After blood flow is restored to the new liver, the biliary (bile duct) anastomosis is constructed, either to the recipient's own bile duct or to the small intestine.
- The surgery usually takes between 5 and 6 hours but may be longer or shorter due to the difficulty of the operation and the experience of the surgeon.
- The large majority of liver transplants use the entire liver from a nonliving donor for the transplant, particularly for adult recipients.
- A major advance in pediatric liver transplantation was the development of reduced-size liver transplantation, in which a portion of an adult liver is used for an infant or small child.
- Further developments in this area included split liver transplantation, in which one liver is used for trans- plants for two recipients, and LDLT, in which a portion of a healthy person's liver is removed and used as the allograft.
- LDLT for pediatric recipients involves the removal of approximately 20% of the liver (Couinaud segments two and three).
- Further advance in liver transplant involves only resection of the lobe of the liver involved in tumors and the tumor-free lobe remains within the recipient. This speeds up the recovery and the patient's stay in the hospital quickly shortens to within 5–7 days.
- Many major medical centers are now using radiofrequency ablation of the liver tumor as a bridge while awaiting for liver transplantation. This technique has not been used universally and further investigation is warranted.

Complications

- Surgical complications requiring reoperation are common, and they relate to any of the five anastomoses between the donor and the recipient
- Hepatic artery thrombosis is especially common in children (5–10%) and often requires retransplantation
- Biliary complications are also fairly common
- Anastomotic strictures are more common than leaks, and these usually happen early. Late strictures can be related to rejection.
- Post-transplant death is usually related to multiple organ failure. It is usually brought on by a combination of infection or rejection plus nephrotoxicity from cyclosporine or tacrolimus.
- Recurrence of hepatitis. Hepatitis B recurrence can be treated with lamivudine.
- Recurrence of hepatitis C is universal and usually takes an insidious course.
- The long-term outcome of recurrent hepatitis C is mild or no hepatitis in 40%, moderate hepatitis in 45%, and recurrent cirrhosis.
- *Rejection:* Rejection is the most common complication following transplant surgery. It happens when the immune system, which defends the body against foreign agents, such as viruses and bacteria, treats a transplanted organ as foreign and will try to attack it.
    - Acute rejection usually manifests as increased liver function tests and occurs in about 40% of the recipients. Fever or jaundice can occur with rejection. Diagnosis is made by liver biopsy. Rejection is almost always reversible.

- Chronic rejection, also called *vanishing bile duct syndrome*, represents an immunologic attack on the bile ducts and the small arteries that nourish them. This is uncommon but may require retransplantation because it is generally untreatable.

- *Infection:* As a liver transplant recipient, the recipient will be more susceptible to infection because of intake of immunosuppressant medications to help prevent rejection. The risk of infection from bacteria and viruses is greatest in the early period after transplant when immunosuppressant dosages are at their highest.
- *Hypertension:* Many transplant recipients take medications to control hypertension or high blood pressure, since prednisone and cyclosporine, two of the medications used to prevent rejection, can raise blood pressure.
- *Renal dysfunction:* Some of the medications that patients are required to take after transplant to prevent rejection can have an adverse effect on the kidney's filtering function. The transplant team will use caution when considering the use of other drugs that can also be toxic to the kidneys in light of the potential adverse effects of the transplant medications.
- *Hyperlipidemia:* Hyperlipidemia can occur early post-transplant due to the effects of cyclosporine and Prograf. Patients may be placed on a cholesterol-lowering medication immediately following transplant for lipid control.
- *Post-transplant diabetes:* Some of the immunosuppressant medications may increase the risk of developing diabetes.
- *CMV:* It is a very common virus. About 70% of the adults have been exposed to CMV at some time. It usually causes a flu-like illness with fever, general body aches, and decreased appetite which lasts two or three days. Because of the immunosuppressant medications, one will be at risk for infection with CMV after transplant. During the first few months, while the immunosuppressant doses are highest and the immune system is especially weak, the CMV virus can reactivate or "wake up." A CMV infection can range from flu-like symptoms to more serious infections involving your stomach and lungs (pneumonia).

Liver Donor Requirements

Any member of the family, parent, sibling, child, spouse, or volunteer can donate their liver. The criteria for a liver donation include:

- Being in good health
- Having a blood type that matches or is compatible with the recipient's
- Having a charitable desire of donation without financial motivation
- Being between 18 and 60 years old
- Being of similar or bigger size than the recipient
- Before one becomes a living donor, the donor must undergo testing to ensure that the individual is physically fit. Sometimes CT scans or MRIs are done to image the liver. In most cases, the workup is done in 2–3 weeks.

Complications

- Very few individuals require any blood transfusions during or after surgery.
- Even though the procedure is very safe, all potential donors should know there is a 0.5–1.0% chance of death.
- Other risks of donating a liver include bleeding, infection, painful incision, the possibility of blood clots, and a prolonged recovery.
- The vast majority of donors enjoy complete and full recovery within 2–3 months.

BOWEL TRANSPLANTATION

21. Bowel transplantation. ***Ayush University Chhattisgarh 2025***

Bowel Transplantation (Intestinal Transplantation)

Bowel transplantation, also known as *intestinal transplantation (ITx)*, is a *life-saving procedure* for patients with *intestinal failure (IF)* who can no longer be sustained on *total parenteral nutrition (TPN)* due to life-threatening complications. It involves replacing the diseased small intestine (and often other organs) with a donor graft. First attempted in the 1960s, modern success stems from *advances in immunosuppression, surgical techniques, and postoperative care* (e.g., tacrolimus-based regimens, vigilant rejection monitoring via endoscopy/biopsies).

Indications

- *Primary: Short bowel syndrome (SBS)* (73% of cases) from trauma, volvulus, Crohn's disease, mesenteric ischemia, tumors (e.g., desmoids), or congenital defects (pediatrics).
- *TPN failures:* Recurrent catheter infections, loss of vascular access, *TPN-associated liver disease (IFALD)* leading to cirrhosis.
- *Other:* Motility disorders (e.g., intestinal pseudo-obstruction), *high-output fistulas,* or *multivisceral tumors* (e.g., Gardner syndrome).
- *Absolute:* Impending death from TPN complications; *relative:* Poor quality of life on TPN.

Contraindications: Active malignancy (except GI stromal tumors), uncontrolled sepsis, poor psychosocial support.

Types of Transplants

Type	*Components*	*Indications*	*Advantages*
Isolated small bowel	Small intestine ± colon	No liver disease	Simpler, better short-term survival
Liver + small bowel	Liver + intestine	IFALD/cirrhosis	Liver protects against rejection
Modified multivisceral (MMVT)	Stomach/duodenum/pancreas + intestine	Extensive disease, no liver fail	Tailored "cherry-picking"
Full multivisceral (MVT)	Stomach + pancreas + intestine + liver ± kidney	Catastrophic abdominal pathology	Comprehensive rescue

Donor Sources

- *Deceased Donor (DD):* 98% of cases; full/segmental bowel.
- *Living Donor (LD):* <2%; 150–220 cm distal ileum (sparing ileocecal valve for donor). Advantages: HLA-matching, short ischemia time, elective timing. Outcomes comparable to DD; no donor mortality reported (minor complications ~15%).

Surgical Procedure (Key Steps)

- *Recipient*: Excision of native organs; vascular reconstruction (superior mesenteric artery/vein to aorta/portal vein or cava).
- *Graft implantation*: Orthotopic placement; enteric anastomosis; *protective ostomy* (e.g., Bishop-Koop) for surveillance.
- *Duration*: 8–12 hours; *multidisciplinary OR team.*
- *Innovations*: *Robotic-assisted LD ileal segmentectomy* (less pain, faster recovery).

Postoperative Management

- *Immunosuppression:* Induction (thymoglobulin/alemtuzumab); maintenance (tacrolimus + steroids); *rapamycin* for long-term.
- *Monitoring: Protocol endoscopy/biopsies* (q7–10 days initially); DSA testing for antibody-mediated rejection.
- *Infections:* Prophylaxis (CMV, EBV, fungi); gut decontamination.
- *Nutrition:* TPN → enteral feeds; >75% off TPN long-term.

Outcomes and Survival (2025 Data)

Era/graft type	*1-year patient*	*5-year patient*	*1-year graft*
Overall	80–90%	50–75%	70–80%
Pediatric Isolated	89%	76%	–
Adult MVT	65–80%	35–55%	–
LD-ITx	Comparable to DD	Comparable	Comparable

Complications

Category	Incidence	Management
Rejection	50–80% (acute/chronic)	Steroids/OKT3; retransplant (10%)
Infections	High (CMV, fungi)	Prophylaxis; monitor viral loads
PTLD	15–30%	Rituximab; reduce immunosuppression
GVHD	5–15%	Steroids
Vascular	10%	Thrombectomy/stenting
Other	Leaks, strictures	Endoscopy/surgery

Recent Advances (2024–2025)

- *Liver inclusion:* Reduces rejection/DSA.
- *Tolerance protocols:* Bone marrow co-transplant, spleen inclusion.
- *Rehab alternatives:* Teduglutide (GLP-2 analog), STEP – *reduced transplant need by 50%.*
- *Tissue engineering:* Stem cell "organoids" (preclinical).
- *Outcomes rival home TPN* in isolated ITx.

Future: *AI monitoring, xenotransplants, full tolerance* to eliminate lifelong immunosuppression. *Referral early* to rehab/transplant centers saves lives.

RENAL TRANSPLANTATION

22. Dual cadaver renal transplant. ***Gujarat Health University 2024***

Dual Cadaveric (Deceased Donor) Renal Transplantation

Definition

A *dual cadaver renal transplant (DKT)* involves transplanting *both kidneys from a single deceased donor into one recipient.* It is done when each kidney *individually may not provide sufficient function*, but *together they can achieve adequate renal performance.*

Rationale and Background

In kidney transplantation, the quality of the donor organ strongly influences graft survival. Sometimes, kidneys from *"marginal" or "expanded criteria" donors* (ECD) — such as elderly donors or those with comorbidities — may have *reduced nephron mass* or *impaired function.*

Implanting both kidneys into one recipient helps *compensate for this reduced function.*

Indications for Dual Kidney Transplantation

Donor-Related Factors

- Older donor age (commonly >60 years; or 50–59 years with comorbidities).
- High terminal serum creatinine (suggesting impaired function).
- *Histological findings:*
  - Moderate to severe glomerulosclerosis (>20%).
  - Arteriolar hyalinosis or interstitial fibrosis.
- *Small kidney size or low nephron mass.*

Recipient-related Factors

- Typically older recipients or those with low metabolic demand.
- Recipients who may not tolerate re-transplantation if single kidney fails.

Donor Kidney Assessment

Before deciding on dual transplantation, *biopsy and functional assessment* are usually performed:

- *Pre-implantation biopsy:* Evaluates glomerulosclerosis, interstitial fibrosis, tubular atrophy, and vascular changes.
- *Split renal function (DTPA or MAG3 scan)* may help assess differential function (if available).

If both kidneys are structurally intact but marginal in function, *dual implantation* is planned.

Surgical Techniques

There are *two main approaches*:

1. *Ipsilateral (Same Side) Placement*
   - Both kidneys are placed in the same iliac fossa (usually right).
   - The *renal veins and arteries* of both kidneys are *anastomosed separately or together* to the *iliac vessels.*
   - *Ureters* may be:
     - Implanted *separately* into the bladder, or
     - *Joined together (ureteroureterostomy)* and implanted as one.

   Advantages:
   - Single surgical field, shorter operative time, less morbidity.
   - Useful when the other iliac fossa is not suitable (due to previous surgery or scarring).
2. *Bilateral (One Kidney Each Side) Placement*
   - One kidney implanted in each iliac fossa.
   - Each anastomosed to the ipsilateral iliac vessels.

   Advantages:
   - Better space accommodation.
   - Easier vascular anastomosis if vessels are short or multiple.

   Disadvantages:
   - Longer surgery, two incisions.

Postoperative Management

- *Similar to standard renal transplant,* with standard immunosuppression (calcineurin inhibitor, antimetabolite, corticosteroid).
- *Close monitoring of renal function,* urine output, and Doppler ultrasonography for vascular patency.
- *Complications* (e.g., vascular thrombosis, ureteric leak, lymphocele) may be slightly higher due to the complex anatomy.

Outcomes

- *Graft survival and function* are comparable to single standard-criteria kidney transplants.
- *Better utilization* of marginal donor organs that might otherwise be discarded.
- *Reduced waiting list mortality,* especially in older or high-risk recipients.

Several studies and registry data (e.g., UNOS, Eurotransplant) have shown:

- *1- and 5-year graft survival rates* are excellent when dual transplantation criteria are well-selected.
- *Creatinine levels* and *glomerular filtration rates (GFR)* typically approach those of standard single transplants within months.

Advantages

Benefits	***Explanation***
Better function from marginal kidneys	Two kidneys provide adequate nephron mass
Efficient organ utilization	Prevents discarding suboptimal donor kidneys
Similar long-term outcomes	Comparable to standard single kidney transplants
Flexible surgical options	Can use ipsilateral or bilateral techniques

Disadvantages/Challenges

Limitations	***Details***
Longer operative time	Especially in bilateral implantation
Technical complexity	More vascular and ureteric anastomoses
Higher surgical risk	Thrombosis, leak, or lymphocele
Space constraints	Especially in smaller recipients
Donor variability	Quality assessment is critical

Recent Advances

- *Machine perfusion and functional assessment* have improved marginal kidney selection.
- *Histology-based scoring systems* (e.g., Remuzzi score) guide whether to use kidneys singly or in pairs.
- *Minimally invasive approaches* (laparoscopic recipient surgery) are emerging.

23. Renal transplant—steps. *WBUHS 2011*

Introduction

- Kidney transplantation or renal transplantation is the organ transplant of a kidney into a patient with end-stage renal disease (ESRD).
- Kidney transplantation is typically classified as deceased-donor (formerly known as cadaveric) or living- donor transplantation depending on the source of the donor organ.
- Living-donor renal transplants are further characterized as genetically related (living-related) or nonrelated (living-unrelated) transplants, depending on whether a biological relationship exists between the donor and recipient.

Indications of Renal Transplantation

- *ESRD, regardless of the primary cause:*
  - This is defined as a glomerular filtration rate <15 mL/min/1.73 m^2.
  - Common diseases leading to ESRD include:
    Malignant hypertension, infections, diabetes mellitus, and focal segmental glomerulosclerosis; genetic causes include polycystic kidney disease, a number of inborn errors of metabolism, and autoimmune conditions, such as lupus and Goodpasture's syndrome.
    - Diabetes is the most common cause of kidney transplantation, accounting for approximately 25%.
    - The majority of renal transplant recipients are on some form of peritoneal dialysis, or a similar process of hemofiltration—at the time of transplantation. However, individuals with chronic renal failure who have a living donor available may undergo preemptive transplantation before dialysis is needed.

Procedure for a Living Kidney Donor

If you are donating a kidney, you will be placed under general anesthesia before surgery. This means you will be asleep and pain-free. Usually, surgeons today can use small surgical cuts with laparoscopic techniques.

Procedure for the Person Receiving the Kidney (Recipient)

People receiving a kidney transplant are given general anesthesia before surgery. The surgeon makes a cut in the lower belly area.

- Surgeon places the new kidney inside the lower belly. The artery and vein of the new kidney are connected to the artery and vein in your pelvis. The tube that carries urine (ureter) is then attached to the bladder.
- Patient's kidneys are left in place, unless they are causing high blood pressure, infections, or are too large for your body. The wound is then closed.

Kidney transplant surgery takes about 3 hours. People with diabetes may also have a pancreas transplant done at the same time. This will usually add another 3 hours to the surgery.

Procedure

In most of the cases, the barely functioning existing kidneys are not removed, as this has been shown to increase the rates of surgical morbidities. Therefore, the kidney is usually placed in a location different from the original kidney, often in the iliac fossa, so it is often necessary to use a different blood supply:

- The renal artery of the kidney, previously branching from the abdominal aorta in the donor, is often connected to the external iliac artery in the recipient.
- The renal vein of the new kidney, previously draining to the inferior vena cava in the donor, is often connected to the external iliac vein in the recipient.

24. Cadaveric renal transplantation. *WBUHS 2015*

Introduction

Kidney transplantation or *renal transplantation* is the organ transplant of a kidney into a patient with ESRD. Kidney transplantation is typically classified as deceased-donor (formerly known as cadaveric) or living-donor transplantation depending on the source of the donor organ.

Deceased Donors can be Divided into Two Groups

1. Brain-dead (BD) donors
2. Donation after cardiac death donors
    - Although brain-dead (or "beating heart") donors are considered dead, the donor's heart continues to pump and maintain circulation. This makes it possible for surgeons to start operating while the organs are still being perfused (supplied blood).
    - "DCD" donors are patients who do not meet the brain-dead criteria but, due to the unlikely chance of recovery, have elected via a living will or through the family to have support withdrawn. In this procedure, treatment is discontinued (mechanical ventilation is shut off).
    - Several ethical and procedural guidelines must be followed; most importantly, the organ recovery team should not participate in the patient's care in any manner until after death has been declared.

Compatibility

- In general, the donor and recipient should be ABO blood group and crossmatch (HLA antigen) compatible.
- If a potential living donor is incompatible with their recipient, the donor could be exchanged for a compatible kidney. Kidney exchange, also known as "kidney paired donation" or "chains" has recently gained popularity over the past few years.
- In an effort to reduce the risk of rejection during incompatible transplantation, ABO-incompatible, and desensitization protocols utilizing IVIg have been developed, with the aim to reduce ABO and HLA antibodies that the recipient may have to the donor.

Procedure

In most cases, the barely functioning existing kidneys are not removed, as this has been shown to increase the rates of surgical morbidities; therefore, the kidney is usually placed in a location different from the original kidney, often in the iliac fossa, so it is often necessary to use a different blood supply:

- The renal artery of the kidney, previously branching from the abdominal aorta in the donor, is often connected to the external iliac artery in the recipient.
- The renal vein of the new kidney, previously draining to the inferior vena cava in the donor, is often connected to the external iliac vein in the recipient.

Urological Complications

- Urine leakage
- Obstruction of the upper urinary tract

- *Other urological complications:*
  - Urethral strictures
  - Urinary stone

25. What are the ethical issues of consent and organ trade? Mention strategies to increase donor numbers.

Tripura University 2024

Ethical Issues of Consent and Organ Trade, and Strategies to Increase Donor Numbers

Introduction

Organ transplantation saves countless lives but raises serious *ethical, legal, and social challenges*—especially concerning *consent, organ procurement*, and *organ trade.*

Ethical practice requires balancing *respect for autonomy, justice, beneficence*, and *nonmaleficence* while ensuring equitable access and preventing exploitation.

Ethical Issues Related to Consent in Organ Donation

Consent is the *cornerstone* of ethical organ donation. It ensures that organs are procured *voluntarily*, with *informed understanding* and *respect for autonomy.*

Types of Consent

- *Explicit (Opt-in) consent:*
  - Individuals voluntarily register as donors during their lifetime.
  - *Example:* India, USA, UK.
  - *Ethical advantage:* Respects individual autonomy.
  - *Limitation:* Donor rates often low due to inaction or lack of awareness.
- *Presumed (Opt-out) consent:*
  - All individuals are considered donors unless they have explicitly refused.
  - *Example:* Spain, Austria, Belgium.
  - Ethically controversial: May compromise autonomy if people are unaware of the law, but generally increases donation rates.
- *Mandated choice:*
  - Individuals are required to make a choice (yes/no) about organ donation during official procedures (e.g., driver's license renewal).
  - Encourages active participation and respects autonomy.

Ethical Issues in Consent

Issue	*Description /Concern*
Informed Consent	Donor or family must fully understand the process, risks, and implications
Coercion or Pressure	Consent must be free from family, social, or economic coercion—especially in living donors
Consent after Death	Family override of deceased person's consent raises conflict between *autonomy* and *family wishes*
Vulnerable Populations	Poor, illiterate, or mentally impaired individuals may not give valid consent
Children and Mentally Incapacitated Donors	Ethical and legal restrictions; require proxy consent and strict oversight
Transparency and Trust	Lack of public confidence in the organ retrieval system undermines willingness to consent

Ethical principle

Consent must be *informed, voluntary, and based on adequate understanding.*

Ethical Issues Related to Organ Trade

Organ trade refers to the *buying and selling of human organs* for transplantation—a practice condemned worldwide as *unethical and illegal.*

Key Ethical Concerns

Issue	***Ethical violation***
Exploitation of the poor	Wealthy recipients exploit economically disadvantaged donors
Commodification of the human body	Treats organs as market commodities, violating human dignity
Coercion and trafficking	Many donors are forced, deceived, or trafficked
Inequity and injustice	Only the rich can afford to buy organs, worsening healthcare inequality
Loss of altruism	Undermines the spirit of voluntary donation
Health risks to donors	Poor medical follow-up, increased morbidity, and psychological harm

Legal and Ethical Prohibitions

- *WHO* and *Declaration of Istanbul (2008)* condemn organ trafficking and transplant tourism.
- *Indian Law: Transplantation of Human Organs and Tissues Act (THOTA), 1994* (amended 2011)
    - Prohibits organ sale.
    - Allows living donation only from near relatives or for altruistic reasons with authorization.
    - Enforces legal penalties for commercial transactions.

Ethical Principle

Organs should be donated *freely and altruistically*, never sold.

Strategies to Increase Donor Numbers (Ethical & Practical Approaches)

To meet growing transplant needs while maintaining ethical standards, several strategies can be adopted:

- *Public awareness and education*
    - Campaigns to improve understanding of brain death and the importance of donation.
    - School and community programs to promote altruism and dispel myths.
- *Improving consent systems*
    - *Opt-out (presumed consent)* systems (as in Spain)—shown to increase donation rates significantly.
    - *Mandated choice* during official documentation (license, voter ID).
    - *Donor registries* and *national databases* to simplify registration.
- *Enhancing hospital infrastructure*
    - Establish *transplant coordination* units in hospitals.
    - Train healthcare professionals in *approaching families for consent* sensitively.
    - Ensure timely identification and maintenance of potential brain-dead donors.
- *Legislative and policy measures*
    - Strengthen laws to ensure transparency and prevent organ trafficking.
    - Streamline procedures for cadaveric donation and interstate organ sharing.
    - Incentivize hospitals for successful organ retrieval programs (non-monetary).
- *Living donor support*
    - *Provide medical, psychological, and financial support* (reimbursement of expenses, leave benefits).
    - Ensure long-term health monitoring of living donors.
- *Building public trust*
    - Transparency in organ allocation (via systems like NOTTO in India).
    - Media coverage of success stories and gratitude ceremonies to promote altruistic culture.
- *Use of expanded donor criteria*
    - Use of *marginal or extended-criteria donors* (older or less-than-perfect organs) after proper evaluation.
    - Encourage *dual kidney* or *split liver transplants* to optimize organ use.

- *International collaboration*
  - Data sharing and mutual assistance through international registries.
  - Strict adherence to ethical frameworks such as the Declaration of Istanbul and WHO guidelines.

TOLL–LIKE RECEPTORS

26. Discuss TOLL-like receptors. ***KIIT University Odisha 2025***

TOLL-Like Receptors (TLRs)

Introduction

Toll-like receptors (TLRs) are a family of *pattern recognition receptors (PRRs)* that play a *crucial role in innate immunity*, the body's first line of defense against infection.

They recognize *pathogen-associated molecular patterns (PAMPs)* and *damage-associated molecular patterns (DAMPs)*—conserved molecular structures found in microbes or released from damaged cells—and activate immune responses.

Discovered first in *Drosophila* (fruit flies) for their role in embryonic development ("Toll" meaning *amazing* in German), TLRs were later found to have a vital immune function in mammals.

Distribution and Structure

Location

- Expressed on a variety of immune and non-immune cells, including:
  - *Macrophages*
  - *Dendritic cells*
  - *Neutrophils*
  - *B cells*
  - *Epithelial cells*
- Found on:
  - *Cell surface* → detect extracellular microbes (e.g., bacteria, fungi)
  - *Endosomal membranes* → detect intracellular microbes (e.g., viruses)

Structure

Each TLR is a *type I transmembrane protein* with:

- *Extracellular domain:* Contains *leucine-rich repeats (LRRs)* → recognizes PAMPs.
- *Transmembrane domain*
- *Cytoplasmic tail:* Contains *Toll/IL-1 receptor (TIR) domain* → initiates intracellular signaling.

Classification of TLRs (in Humans)

Humans have *10 functional TLRs (TLR1–TLR10)*, each recognizing specific microbial or host-derived molecules.

TLR	*Location*	*Ligand Recognized (PAMP/DAMP)*	*Typical Microorganism Targeted*
TLR1/2 (heterodimer)	Cell surface	Bacterial lipoproteins, lipopeptides	Gram-positive bacteria
TLR2/6 (heterodimer)	Cell surface	Peptidoglycan, lipoteichoic acid	Gram-positive bacteria, fungi
TLR3	Endosome	Double-stranded RNA	Viruses
TLR4	Cell surface	Lipopolysaccharide (LPS)	Gram-negative bacteria
TLR5	Cell surface	Flagellin	Motile bacteria
TLR7 & TLR8	Endosome	Single-stranded RNA	RNA viruses
TLR9	Endosome	Unmethylated CpG DNA	Bacteria, DNA viruses
TLR10	Cell surface	Not fully defined (may regulate other TLRs)	Possibly viruses, bacteria

Signaling Pathways of TLRs

Upon ligand binding, TLRs recruit *adaptor proteins* via their *TIR domains*, triggering intracellular signaling cascades that activate transcription factors.

Major Adaptor Proteins

- *MyD88 (Myeloid differentiation primary response 88)*—used by most TLRs.
- *TRIF (TIR-domain-containing adapter-inducing interferon-α)*—mainly used by TLR3 and TLR4.

Downstream Effects

- Activation of transcription factors:
  - *NF-κB* → induces pro-inflammatory cytokines (TNF-α, IL-1, IL-6).
  - *IRF3 and IRF7 (Interferon regulatory factors)* → induce type I interferons (IFN-α, IFN-β).
- Upregulation of:
  - *Costimulatory molecules* (CD80, CD86)
  - *MHC molecules*
  - *Cytokines and chemokines*

Result

- Activation of *innate immunity*
- Initiation and shaping of *adaptive immune responses*

Biological Functions of TLRs

Function	Description
Pathogen recognition	Detect PAMPs from bacteria, viruses, fungi, parasites
Activation of innate immunity	Induce cytokine production, complement activation, and inflammation
Bridge to adaptive immunity	Activate dendritic cells → stimulate T-cell responses
Tissue repair and homeostasis	Recognize DAMPs released from injured tissues → promote repair
Role in vaccines	Synthetic TLR ligands used as *vaccine adjuvants* (e.g., CpG motifs for TLR9)

Clinical and Pathological Significance

Protective Role

- Essential in defense against infections:
  - *TLR4 deficiency* → ↑ susceptibility to Gram-negative infections.
  - *TLR3 deficiency* → ↑ susceptibility to viral encephalitis.

Pathological Role (Overactivation or Dysregulation)

- *Sepsis:* Excessive TLR4 activation by LPS → cytokine storm, shock.
- *Autoimmune diseases:* TLR7 and TLR9 recognize self-nucleic acids → implicated in SLE.
- *Chronic inflammation:* TLR activation contributes to atherosclerosis, IBD, and asthma.
- *Cancer:* Chronic TLR signaling may promote tumor growth and immune evasion.

Therapeutic Potential

- *TLR agonists:* Used as vaccine adjuvants or cancer immunotherapy (e.g., Imiquimod - TLR7 agonist for skin cancers).
- *TLR antagonists:* Potential therapy for sepsis, autoimmune and inflammatory diseases.

CHAPTER 45

Stem Cell Therapy

LEARNING OBJECTIVE

➢ Stem Cell Research and its Uses in Surgery

STEM CELL RESEARCH IN SURGERY

1. Stem cell research in surgery. ***WBUHS 2015, RIMS, IMPHAL 2022***

2. Write an essay on applications of stem cell (SC) therapy in surgical practice. ***WBUHS 2021***

Introduction

- Stem cells are the body's raw materials—cells from which all other cells with specialized functions are generated. Under the right conditions in the body or a laboratory, SCs divide to form more cells called daughter cells.
- These daughter cells become either new SCs or specialized cells (differentiation) with a more specific function, such as blood cells, brain cells, heart muscle cells, or bone cells. No other cell in the body has the natural ability to generate new cell types.
- Early SC research has traditionally been associated with the controversial use of embryonic SCs. The new focus is on nonembryonic adult mesenchymal stem cells (MSCs) which are found in a person's own blood, bone marrow, and fat.

Research and Uses

- *Urology:*
  - Interstitial cystitis
  - Peyronie's disease
  - Erectile dysfunction
  - Male incontinence
- *Orthopedics:*
  - Neck arthritis and spine disease
  - Back arthritis and spine disease
  - Knee problems
  - Hip problems
  - Elbow and hand problems
  - Shoulder problems

Applications

- Plastic surgeons perform procedures in the fields of skin and adipose tissue grafting, reconstruction of compound tissue loss and congenital malformations, treatment of acute and chronic wounds and burns, and cosmetic surgery.

- SCs are increasingly frequently employed in in vitro experiments, animal models, and clinical trials.
- The most commonly utilized SCs for these purposes are adult stem cells (ASCs), which are present in small amounts in every tissue; among these are two types of cells: (1) Bone marrow (BM)-MSCs and (2) adipose-derived stem cells (ADSCs).
- Many studies have described the progress of trials using ADSCs and BM-MSCs mainly in the treatment of compound tissue loss and chronic wounds. The use of their paracrine, proangiogenic, and osteogenic functions is emphasized. However, because of the very high harvesting and culturing expenses and the limited availability of data on their safety for human use, SCs are not a first-choice therapy.
- The use of MSCs derived from ASCs is under preliminary research for potential orthopedic applications in bone and muscle trauma, cartilage repair, osteoarthritis, intervertebral disc surgery, rotator cuff surgery, and musculoskeletal disorders.
- SCs can also be used to stimulate the growth of human tissues.

Cell-based Approach in Neurosurgery

Cell types	*Donor source*	*Advantages*	*Disadvantages*
Embryonic stem cell (ESC)	Embryo	• Unlimited expansion in undifferentiated state • Enormous differentiation potential	• Difficulty in directing in vitro differentiation • Potential of teratoma formation
Neural Stem/progenitor cells	Fetal brain	• Long-term in vitro expansion • Large differentiation potential • Safe	Lack of ability to differentiate into projection neurons
• Neuronal • Restricted progenitor cells	Embryo or fetal brain	• Predictable differentiation to neuronal phenotype • Safe	• Restricted neuronal differentiation potential • Very limited expandability
Primary neural cells	Fetal brain	• Predictable phenotypic differentiation • Safe	• Lack of expandability and restricted differentiation potential • Require stage-specific embryonic source • Mixed/inconsistent cell types
Adult stem cells	Adult "self" neural or non-neural	• Avoid ethical and immunological constraints • Expandable in culture • Possible autologous transplant • Safe	• Greatly restricted potential in neural differentiation • Questionable functional differentiation and integration
• Xenotransplant cells • Induced pluripotent stem cells (iPSCs)	Nonhuman adult somatic cells with nuclear transfer	• Readily available • Possible genetic modification • Immunosuppression avoided • Large differentiation potential • Expandable	• Tendency to immune rejection • Possible zoonoses • Difficulty in directing in vitro differentiation • Potential of teratoma formation

Uses

Harvest progenitors	*Resolve immune response*	*Transplant in utero*	*Organ generation/ tissue engineering*	*Gene discovery/drug screen*
• Replace damaged and lost cells • Deliver molecules and growth factors	• Recombined strategies • Bank of matched cells • Somatic cell nuclear transfer (SCNT)	• Observe developmental strategies • Target genetic disorder and childhood disease	• Mold to guide regeneration • Creation of biohybrid • Synthetic biological interface	• Normal/mutated cells of defined phenotype • Scale up of cells for testing of drugs • Preliminary test before human trials

CHAPTER 46

Hair Transplantation

LEARNING OBJECTIVE

➢ Steps and Complications of Hair Transplantation

STEPS AND COMPLICATIONS OF HAIR TRANSPLANTATION

1. The steps and complications of hair transplantation. ***WBUHS 2021 Supplementary***

Introduction

- Hair transplantation is a surgical procedure that involves removing hair follicles from any part of the body, such as the face or legs, and transplanting them into hairless areas.
- This procedure is also used to transfer hair to eyelashes and eyebrows.
- The newest method is permanent and removes hair follicular clusters.
- This process is called follicular hair transplantation (FUT) and it is of two types, strip harvesting and follicular unit extraction (FUE)
- In strip harvesting, with good hair growth, the skin strips are removed manually and transplanted into the hairless area where the hair follicles are rooted.

Steps of Hair Transplantation

- *Prepare for hair transplant:* In the first step of hair transplant, hair follicles from the back of the head are removed and transplanted to the scalp.
- *Donor area is cut:* Before the operation, the hair in the donor area is cut.
- *The donor area is prepared for surgery:* After cutting the hair in the donor area, local anesthesia is given.
- *Tissue in the donor area is removed and the donor area is sutured:* The tissue containing hair follicles in the donor area is surgically removed and the donor area is sutured.
- *Thin hair in the stitched donor area:* The stitches in the donor area are hidden by the patient's hair.
- These stitches are removed 10 days after the hair transplant surgery.
- *Donor tissue is cut into follicular unit grafts:* A microscope is then used by the surgical technician to dissect and prepare the hair transplant from the donor tissue follicular unit.
- *Scalp preparation:* After the patient is given local anesthesia, the scalp is prepared for the surgical procedure.
- *Parts made in the constricted area:* Follicular unit grafts are placed in small parts made in a regular pattern in the recipient area.
- *Graphics are placed according to density:* The smallest graphics (one and two) are placed in front of the hairline, and three and four (closer than one and two) are placed in the back.
- *After hair transplant surgery:* After hair transplant surgery, patients will see small patches of short hair at the surgery site.

- *Closure of hair transplant surgery:* The incision scar heals naturally and the redness at the recipient site disappears within a week.

Complications

- Bleeding
- Infection
- Swelling of the head
- Bluishness around the eyes
- A crust that forms on the scalp where the hair has been removed or transplanted.
- Swelling or numbness in the treated area of the scalp.
- Confusion
- Inflammation or infection of hair follicles, known as folliculitis.
- Sudden loss or sudden but usually temporary loss of transplanted hair
- Unnatural hair texture

CHAPTER 47

Research in Surgery: Levels of Evidence

LEARNING OBJECTIVES

- Ethics
- Levels of Evidence
- Sample Size Estimation
- Clinical Audit, Surgical Audit
- Informed Consent
- Different Types of Scientific Studies
- Simulation in Surgical Training

1. Ethics and law in surgical practice. ***WBUHS 2015, RIMS, Imphal 2022***

Introduction

The fundamental contract in surgery is an undertaking by one individual to cure another by operation in the expectation of reward.

- Ethics is an essential discipline in the practice of surgery
- Represents your best understanding of moral responsibility
- Requires an ability to distinguish degrees of value or lack thereof
- Evolves as reasoned reflection on clinical experience
- Ethical study that investigates what our character and conduct should be.
- Morality is subject to reexamination and improvement
- Ideas of justice and fairness require critical assessment and improvement
- Ethical argument should maintain relevance and integrity

Autonomy	*Beneficence*	*Nonmaleficence*	*Justice*
• Respect for informed consent for surgery • Truth-telling • Consent for involvement of trainees in surgical procedures • Confidentiality • Respecting patient's requests (for procedures/ particular surgeons) • Good communication skills	• Surgical competence • Ability to exercise sound judgment • Continuous professional development • Research and innovation in surgery • Responsible conduct • Functioning equipment and optimal operating conditions • Minimizing harm (including pain control) • Good communication skills	• Surgical competence • Continuous professional development • Ability to exercise sound judgment • Recognizing the limits of one's professional competence • Research and auditing • Disclosure and discussion of surgical complications including medical errors • Good communication skills	• Allocation of scarce resources • Competing needs • Rights and obligations • Legal issues

Role of the Surgeon is to Act as the Patient's Fiduciary

Expectations

- Patient will get better.
- Patient's interests are paramount
- Resolution of the presenting problem

Surgical Obligations

Knowledge, technical ability, and ethical integrity

Informed consent and disclosure

- *Physician responsibilities:*
  - Explanation of the patient's disease
  - Explanation of untreated natural history
  - Recommendation of the most appropriate treatment
  - Discussion of risks and benefits
  - Anticipated outcome
  - Treatment alternatives
- Only adult patients are competent to decide which treatments to accept or reject.
- Information provided to the patient should be accurate and reasonably complete.
- Reasonable person standard "identify clinically salient information about the patient's condition and its management."
- Patients do not have the right to dictate treatment.

2. Discuss "Doctrine of Double Effect: Law, Ethics and Intent". ***Tripura University 2023***

Doctrine of Double Effect (DDE): Law, Ethics and Intent

Introduction

The *Doctrine of Double Effect (DDE)* is an important principle in *moral philosophy, medical ethics, and law* that helps determine when it is morally or legally permissible to perform an action that has *two effects*—one *intended and good*, and the other *unintended but potentially harmful or bad.*

This doctrine is especially relevant in *medical practice*, particularly in *end-of-life care, pain management*, and *palliative sedation,* where treatments intended to relieve suffering may also hasten death.

Origin and Background

- The doctrine originates from *Thomas Aquinas (13th century)* in his *Summa Theologica.*
- Aquinas discussed it in the context of *self-defense*—that killing an aggressor might be permissible if the *intention* was to save one's own life, not to kill the aggressor.
- Over time, the doctrine was extended to medical and legal ethics to justify actions that have both beneficial and harmful outcomes.

The Core Principle

The *Doctrine of Double Effect* holds that an action producing both a good and a bad outcome may be morally permissible *if certain conditions are met*—specifically concerning *intention, means, and proportionality.*

Conditions for Applying the Doctrine

Traditionally, four conditions must be satisfied:

Condition	***Explanation***
The act itself must be morally good or at least neutral	The action (e.g., giving analgesics) must not be intrinsically wrong
The good effect must be intended; the bad effect only foreseen, not intended	The physician's intention must be to relieve pain, not to hasten death
The bad effect must not be the means of achieving the good effect	The relief of pain should not occur because the patient dies
There must be proportionality between the good and bad effects	The anticipated good (relief of suffering) must outweigh the potential harm (possible life-shortening)

When all four criteria are satisfied, the action may be ethically and legally acceptable, even if it results in a foreseeable negative outcome.

Ethical Perspective

In Medical Ethics:

- The DDE is often invoked in *palliative care*:
  - *Example:* Administering high-dose opioids or sedatives to relieve severe pain or dyspnea in a terminally ill patient, knowing that it may suppress respiration and hasten death.
- The physician's *intent* is key:
  - If the intent is *pain relief*, the act is ethically permissible.
  - If the intent is *to cause death*, it becomes euthanasia, which is ethically and legally prohibited in most jurisdictions.

Ethical Justification:

- Based on *respect for patient dignity, beneficence* (doing good), and *nonmaleficence* (avoiding harm).
- The doctrine allows clinicians to relieve suffering without moral guilt, provided they act with *right intent* and *proportionate means.*

Legal Perspective

In Law:

- The DDE has influenced *medical jurisprudence* in end-of-life care.
- Courts in several countries (e.g., UK, US, India) have recognized the distinction between:
  - *Intentionally causing death* (unlawful euthanasia), and
  - *Foreseeably hastening death* as a *side effect of lawful symptom relief.*

Example:

- The UK's *House of Lords in the Bland Case (1993)* accepted that doctors may give treatment to relieve pain even if it may incidentally shorten life, provided the *primary intention* is to relieve suffering.

In Indian Context:

- Active euthanasia is illegal, but *palliative sedation and pain control* under the DDE principle are ethically and legally defensible if the intent is not to cause death.

The Role of Intent

Intent is the *moral and legal cornerstone* of the doctrine.

Intent	***Ethical/legal status***
Relief of pain (good effect)	Morally and legally acceptable
Causing death (bad effect)	Morally and legally impermissible
Foreseeing death (without intending it)	Acceptable under DDE, if proportionate and unavoidable

Hence, *the moral quality of an action depends on the agent's intent,* not solely on the consequences.

Applications in Medicine

Clinical situation	***Good effect (intended)***	***Bad effect (foreseen)***
High-dose opioid in terminal illness	Relief of pain, comfort	Respiratory depression, hastened death
Palliative sedation	Relief of intractable suffering	Loss of consciousness, potential shortening of life
Withdrawal of life-sustaining treatment	Respect for patient autonomy, allowing natural death	Death due to disease progression

Criticisms of the Doctrine

- *Difficult to assess true intent*—clinicians' motives may be ambiguous.
- *Consequences matter too,* not just intentions—utilitarian critics argue that foreseeable harm cannot be ignored.
- *Potential for misuse*—may be used to justify morally questionable acts.
- *Cultural and legal variability*—interpretation differs among societies and legal systems.

Despite these critiques, DDE remains an important moral framework guiding complex medical decisions.

3. Informed consent. ***RGUHS, Karnataka 2025; AIIMS, Bhopal 2023***

4. Disclosures prior to consent. ***Rajasthan University of Health Sciences 2025***

Definition

Informed consent is a legal and ethical process by which a patient voluntarily agrees to undergo a medical treatment, procedure, or participation in research after being fully informed about the relevant details, including the risks, benefits, and alternatives.

It reflects the patient's autonomy and right to make decisions about their own body and medical care.

Key Elements of Informed Consent

i. *Disclosure:*
   - The healthcare provider must explain:
     - Nature and purpose of the procedure/treatment
     - Risks and complications
     - Benefits
     - Alternatives (including doing nothing)
     - Expected outcomes and prognosis

ii. *Comprehension:*
   - The patient must understand the information.
   - Language should be clear, non-technical, and appropriate for the patient's level of understanding.

iii. *Voluntariness:* The decision must be made freely, without coercion, pressure, or manipulation.

iv. *Competence/Capacity:*
   - The patient must have the mental capacity to make the decision (i.e., be conscious, oriented, and of sound mind).
   - If not, a legal guardian or next of kin must provide consent.

v. *Consent:* The patient gives permission, typically in written form (signed consent form), though verbal consent may be valid in some situations.

Types of Informed Consent

- *Written consent:* For major procedures, surgeries, and research
- *Verbal consent:* For minor or routine procedures
- *Implied consent:* Assumed through patient's actions (e.g., extending arm for blood draw)

Exceptions to Informed Consent

- Medical emergency where patient is unconscious or unable to consent, and delay could be life-threatening.
- *Waiver:* Patient waives the right to be informed.
- *Therapeutic privilege:* Rare cases where full disclosure may cause harm (controversial and used cautiously).

Importance of Informed Consent

- Protects patient autonomy
- Builds trust between patient and provider

- Legally protects the healthcare provider
- Ethically required in medical and research settings

5. Discuss the moral and legal boundaries and practical difficulties of informed consent. ***WBUHS 2024***

Moral and Legal Boundaries and Practical Difficulties of Informed Consent

Informed consent is a fundamental principle in ethics and law, particularly in healthcare, research, and legal agreements. It ensures that individuals have the necessary information to make autonomous decisions. However, there are moral and legal boundaries, as well as practical difficulties, that complicate its implementation.

Moral Boundaries of Informed Consent

Autonomy vs. Paternalism

- A core ethical dilemma in informed consent is balancing an individual's right to make decisions (autonomy) with the duty of professionals to act in the person's best interest (paternalism).
- For example, in medical settings, a doctor may withhold certain distressing information to prevent emotional harm, potentially compromising full transparency.

Competency and Understanding

- Some individuals, such as minors, people with cognitive impairments, or those under extreme stress, may lack the capacity to fully comprehend information.
- Determining the threshold for competence is ethically complex, as it requires weighing individual rights against their ability to make an informed decision.

Coercion and Manipulation

- True-informed consent must be given voluntarily, without pressure or undue influence.
- Subtle coercion, such as financial incentives for research participation or a doctor's authority over a patient, can undermine genuine consent.

Legal Boundaries of Informed Consent

Standard of Disclosure

- Different legal systems have different standards regarding what information must be disclosed.
- The reasonable person standard requires that all information a typical patient would need to know is provided.
- The professional practice standard relies on what medical experts consider appropriate, potentially limiting the scope of disclosure.

Exceptions to Consent

- *Emergency Situations:* When immediate action is required to save a life, consent may be bypassed.
- *Legal Incompetency:* When individuals are deemed legally incompetent, guardians or courts may provide consent on their behalf.
- *Public health justifications:* In cases like infectious disease outbreaks, individual consent may be overridden for the greater public good.

Documentation and Legal Liability

- Written consent forms are often required to provide legal protection, but they may not fully ensure that true understanding has been achieved.
- Lawsuits can arise if patients claim they were not adequately informed, making legal documentation a crucial yet imperfect safeguard.

Practical Difficulties of Informed Consent

- *Complexity of information:*
  - Many medical, legal, or research-related decisions involve complex terminology that laypeople struggle to understand.
  - Professionals must balance thoroughness with simplicity to ensure comprehension.
- *Language and cultural barriers:*
  - Language differences can lead to miscommunication, making it necessary to provide interpreters or translated documents.
  - Cultural beliefs may also impact the decision-making process, affecting how consent is understood and given.
- *Time constraints:*
  - In fast-paced environments like emergency rooms or high-pressure legal negotiations, obtaining fully informed consent may not be feasible.
  - Patients or participants may feel rushed, leading to incomplete understanding.
- *Emotional state of the individual:*
  - People facing life-altering decisions, such as terminal illness treatment, may be in a distressed or vulnerable state, affecting their ability to process information rationally.

---

6. Discuss the level of evidences in scientific research. How will you calculate sample size for a research project? ***WBUHS 2023***

---

7. What is evidence-based medicine? Enumerate the different levels of evidence. ***AIIMS, Raipur 2024***

---

8. Sample size calculation. ***AIIMS, Raipur 2024***

---

9. Discuss about levels of evidence. ***WBUHS 2008***

---

10. What is understood by a 'blinded' trial? Why is it necessary to calculate a sample size? What is meant by lead time bias? Explain with an example. What is meant by a 'systematic review' and 'meta-analysis'? What are the 'levels of evidence'? ***DNB, June 2018***

---

11. What are the levels of evidence? Describe the role of meta-analysis in rational therapy.
KIIT University, Odisha 2025

Evidence-based medicine (EBM) is a systematic approach to healthcare that uses the best available scientific evidence, combined with clinical expertise and patient values, to make informed decisions about patient care.
Definition: EBM is defined as "the conscientious, explicit, and judicious use of current best evidence in making decisions about the care of individual patients".

Key Components

- *Best research evidence:* This includes high-quality clinical trials, systematic reviews, and other relevant research findings.
- *Clinical expertise:* The knowledge, skills, and experience of healthcare professionals in diagnosing and treating patients.
- *Patient values and preferences:* The individual's unique circumstances, beliefs, and preferences regarding their health and treatment options.

LEVELS OF EVIDENCE

Levels of Evidence

Level	Description
1a	Systematic review (or meta-analysis) (with homogeneity) of randomized controlled trials (RCTs)
1b	Individual RCT (with narrow confidence Interval)
1c	All or none
2a	Systematic review (with homogeneity) of cohort studies
2b	Individual cohort study (Including low-quality RCT, e.g., <80% follow-up)
2c	"Outcomes" research; ecological studies
3a	SR (with homogeneity) of case-control studies
3b	Individual case-control study
4	Case-series (and poor-quality cohort and case-control studies)
5	Expert opinion without explicit critical appraisal or based on physiology, bench research, or "first principles"

Homogeneity/heterogeneity—in a systematic review of results from different studies, when there are worrisome variations in the direction and degree of results between individual studies, it is called heterogeneity. Studies without significant variations are "homogeneous."

When there is either a single result with a wide confidence interval or a systematic review with troublesome heterogeneity add a minus "–" sign. The grade of recommendation then becomes D.

All or none studies: When all patients died before the Rx became available, but some now survive on it; or when some patients died before the Rx became available, but none now die on it.

Grades of Recommendations

Grade	Description
A	Consistent level 1 studies
B	Consistent level 2 or 3 studies or extrapolations from level 1 studies
C	Level 4 studies or extrapolations from level 2 or 3 studies
D	Level 5 evidence or troublingly inconsistent or inconclusive studies of any level

It is important to remember, however, that evidence-based practice is not just blindly following published evidence—it has to be combined with two other important elements—clinical expertise and patient wishes and expectations.

Calculating sample size is crucial in research and data analysis to ensure that the study is statistically sound, reliable, and provides meaningful results. A sample that is too small may not accurately represent the population, leading to inaccurate conclusions. Conversely, a sample that is too large can be a waste of resources and potentially unethical.

The four ways to determine sample size are:

1. Power analysis
2. Convenience sampling
3. Random sampling
4. Stratified sampling

Assuming RCT has two comparison groups and both groups have the same size of subjects; sample size calculation depends on the type of primary outcome measures.

- *Parameter definitions:*
  - N = size per group; p = the response rate of standard treatment group; p_0= the response rate of new drug treatment group; z_x = the standard normal deviate for a one or two sided x; d= the real difference between two treatment effect; δ_0= a clinically acceptable margin; S^2= Polled standard deviation of both comparison groups.
  - *Dichotomous variable:*
    - For non-inferiority design, the formula is:

$$N = 2 \times \left(\frac{z_{1-\alpha} + z_{1-\beta}}{\delta_0} \right)^2 \times p \times (1-p)$$

    - For equivalence design, the formula is:

$$N = 2 \times \left(\frac{z_{1-\frac{\alpha}{2}} + z_{1-\beta}}{\delta_0} \right)^2 \times p \times (1-p)$$

    - For statistical superiority design, the formula is:

$$N = \frac{1}{2} \times \left(\frac{z_{\frac{\alpha}{2}} + z_{\beta}}{\arcsin\sqrt{p} - \arcsin\sqrt{p_0}} \right)^2$$

    - For clinical superiority design, the formula is:

$$N = 2 \times \left(\frac{z_{1-\alpha} + z_{1-\beta}}{d - \delta_0} \right)^2 \times p \times (1-p)$$

  - *Continuous variable:*
    - For non-inferiority design, the formula is:

$$N = 2 \times \left(\frac{z_{1-\alpha} + z_{1-\beta}}{\delta_0} \right)^2 \times s^2$$

    - For equivalence design, the formula is:

$$N = 2 \times \left(\frac{z_{1-\frac{\alpha}{2}} + z_{1-\beta}}{\delta_0} \right)^2 \times s^2$$

    - For statistical superiority design, the formula is:

$$N = 2 \times \left(\frac{z_{1-\frac{\alpha}{2}} + z_{1-\beta}}{\delta} \right)^2 \times s^2$$

    - For clinical superiority design, the formula is:

$$N = 2 \times \left(\frac{z_{1-\alpha} + z_{1-\beta}}{\delta - \delta_0} \right)^2 \times s^2$$

- *Calculating proportion:*

$$N=4PQ/D^2$$

  P = Prevalence (from previous studies)
  Q = 100 – P
  D = Allowable error (5–20% of *P*)
- Calculating difference in proportions:

$$N=\frac{15.7\times\rho\times Q}{(P_1-P_2)^2}$$

Where,
  - P_1 and P_2 are the proportions of the 2 groups
  - ρ is the average of P_1 and P_2
  - Q is 100 – ρ
- *Calculating the mean:*

$$N=4\sigma^2/d^2$$

Where,
  - σ (Sigma) is the standard deviation as in similar studies done previously
  - d = Allowable error (5–20% of σ)
- *Calculating difference in means:*

$$N = 15.7\,(\sigma_1 \times \sigma_2)/d^2$$

Where,
  - σ_1 and σ_2 are the standard deviations of the 2 study groups.
  - d is the smallest meaningful difference that can be measured.

Lead time bias occurs when a diagnostic approach merely identifies the disease earlier and gives the impression that survival is prolonged, thus increasing perceived survival without significant modification of the disease course.

For example, the genetic disorder Huntington's disease is diagnosed when symptoms appear at around 50, and the person dies at around 65. The typical patient, therefore, lives about 15 years after diagnosis. A genetic test at birth makes it possible to diagnose this disorder earlier.

A systematic review identifies, selects, appraises, and summarizes all relevant studies addressing a specific research question. A meta-analysis, which may or may not follow a systematic review, is a statistical method to combine and analyze data from multiple studies to produce a quantitative summary of the evidence.

Systematic Review
- Aims to comprehensively identify and synthesize all relevant empirical research on a specific question.
- Uses explicit and reproducible methods to minimize bias.
- Includes a thorough search strategy across multiple databases.
- Appraises the quality and validity of included studies.
- May be qualitative (summarizing findings) or quantitative (including meta-analysis).

Meta-analysis
- A statistical method used to combine and analyze data from multiple studies.
- Requires studies to be sufficiently similar in terms of research question and methodology.
- Provides a quantitative estimate of the overall effect.
- May be used within a systematic review or on its own (though systematic review is preferred to minimize bias).

Feature	Systematic review	Meta-analysis
Method	Comprehensive literature search, study selection, and synthesis	Statistical analysis of pooled data
Output	Qualitative summary or quantitative synthesis (if meta-analysis is included)	Quantitative summary of effect
Relationship	A meta-analysis is often, but not always, a component of a systematic review	Can be done without a systematic review, but this is not recommended

Role of Meta-analysis in Rational Therapy

Introduction

Rational therapy means using medications or interventions based on the *best available scientific evidence*, ensuring *maximum efficacy, safety, and cost-effectiveness* for patients.

A *meta-analysis* is a *statistical technique* that combines and analyzes data from multiple independent studies addressing the same clinical question. It sits at the *top of the hierarchy of evidence* and plays a key role in *evidence-based medicine (EBM)*—the foundation of rational therapy.

What is Meta-analysis?

- It is a *quantitative, systematic review* method that pools results from several studies to obtain a *more precise and reliable estimate* of treatment effect.
- It increases statistical power and resolves uncertainty when individual studies give conflicting results.

Steps in Conducting a Meta-analysis

i. *Define the clinical question* (using PICO—Patient, Intervention, Comparison, Outcome).
ii. *Systematic literature search* for all relevant studies.
iii. *Selection and critical appraisal* of high-quality studies (often RCTs).
iv. *Data extraction and pooling* using statistical models (fixed- or random-effects).
v. *Assessment of heterogeneity*, publication bias, and sensitivity analysis.
vi. *Interpretation* of pooled results to guide clinical decisions.

Role in Rational (Evidence-based) Therapy

Role/contribution	Explanation
Establishes efficacy of therapy	By combining results from multiple RCTs, meta-analysis determines whether a drug or intervention truly works better than placebo or standard therapy
Improves precision of estimates	Larger pooled sample size gives more reliable estimates of treatment effects and adverse outcomes
Resolves conflicting evidence	When individual trials show differing results, meta-analysis provides an overall conclusion
Detects small but clinically important effects	May identify benefits or risks too small to be detected in single studies
Guides clinical practice guidelines	Meta-analyses form the core evidence for recommendations by WHO, NICE, and other health authorities
Supports cost-effective therapy	By clarifying comparative efficacy, meta-analysis helps choose treatments that give best outcomes for least cost
Identifies gaps in knowledge	Highlights areas needing further research or better trial design
Assists in risk–benefit assessment	Summarizes both efficacy and adverse effects across trials for balanced therapeutic decisions

Examples

- *Antihypertensive therapy:* Meta-analyses of major RCTs established that thiazide diuretics reduce stroke and mortality, guiding their use as first-line drugs.
- *Statins:* Pooled data confirmed their role in primary and secondary prevention of cardiovascular events.
- *Antimicrobial therapy:* Meta-analyses guide antibiotic choice by comparing cure rates and resistance patterns.
- *Cancer therapy:* Combined trial data determine effectiveness of new chemotherapy regimens or targeted agents.

Advantages

- High level of evidence (Level I).
- Reduces random error and bias (if well-designed).
- Supports development of *clinical practice guidelines* and *standard treatment protocols*.
- Enhances rational prescribing by summarizing global evidence.

Limitations

- *Quality dependent:* Poor-quality or heterogeneous studies can give misleading results ("garbage in, garbage out").
- *Publication bias:* Positive studies are more likely to be published and included.
- *Heterogeneity:* Differences in study design, populations, or interventions may complicate interpretation.
- *Statistical complexity:* Requires expertise to perform and interpret correctly.

Despite these, when carefully conducted, meta-analysis remains the most powerful tool for evidence synthesis.

12. Gompertzian growth. *DNB 2021 June; AIIMS, Bhopal 2023*

Gompertzian growth refers to a type of mathematical model used to describe growth that starts exponentially but then slows down as it approaches a maximum limit (asymptote). It is widely used in biology, particularly for modeling tumor growth, population dynamics, and aging.

The general form of the Gompertz function is:

$$N(t)=K\cdot \exp\left(-e^{-b(t-t0)}\right)$$

Where

- N(t) is the size at time.
- K is the upper asymptote (maximum size or carrying capacity).
- b is the growth rate constant.
- t_0 is the inflection point (where growth rate starts slowing).
- exp is the exponential function.

Key Characteristics

- *Initially exponential:* At the beginning, the growth resembles an exponential curve.
- *Decelerating growth:* As time goes on, the growth rate decreases.
- *Asymptotic behavior:* Eventually, the function approaches a maximum value (carrying capacity), but never quite reaches it.

Applications

- *Tumor growth modeling:* Reflects how cancer cells grow quickly early on and then slow down due to resource limitations.
- *Population ecology:* Models animal or microbial populations with resource constraints.
- *Actuarial science:* Describes mortality rates and aging processes.

AUDIT

13. What is a clinical audit (AIIMS, Bhopal 2023)? How many types of audit exist and what role do they serve? How does it differ from research? ***WBUHS 2021 Supplementary***

14. Audit cycle. ***DNB 2021 June***

Clinical audit is a process that has been defined as a quality improvement process that seeks to improve patient care and outcomes through systematic review of care against explicit criteria and the implementation of change.

Types of Audit

- *Random audit:*
  - A random audit is one of the most efficient and commonly used audit types, designed to get a glimpse of the medical organization and the way it functions. The examination is done on an ad-hoc basis and does not have a known scheduled date. The purpose of a random audit is to sample a variety of different claims and compare them to relevant data and regulations.
  - This focuses more on the amount of money spent or received on different claims. So that will tell the healthcare auditors a glimpse about the whole thing if the organization is fine or needs to be reviewed in a closer way rather than the random way.
  - The benefit of a random medical audit is that it can quickly identify whether a more systematic and detailed review is necessary to improve the way a particular provider is functioning. It offers a quick snapshot of whether there is an underlying problem that needs further investigation.
- *Comprehensive audit:*
  - This approach of auditing does not take samples randomly, but it focuses on claims that are audited before but in a closer way; samples of the comprehensive audit are chosen in two different ways, electronic and manual. However, if the organization looking for a refund of its spent money, they usually trust this way compared to the random auditing-approach because a complete inspection goes into more detail than the random audit.
  - Due to this, it is one of the most common types of medical audits used when specific claims are in dispute, or a particular institution is asking for a refund for a specific claim.
- *Hybrid audit:*
  - It is a mix of the previous two types of healthcare auditing which are random and comprehensive. During a hybrid review, the auditors select samples for both random and thorough inspections at the same time. This kind of auditing provides a better insight into different types of claims. It avoids errors missed during a random or just comprehensive audit.
  - This kind of audit is usually more accurate when it comes to auditing different cases and claims and eventually results in inaccurate statistics to be used in the future to compensate for the money spent for no reason.
- *Quality improvement audit:*
  - Quality improvement medical audits focus on both providers and patients at the same time. This type goes all over the year to get results that will improve the patient's treatment and decrease the financial costs and the health providers to give more quality and decrease the money spent on treatments. This type chooses different patients before the progress of curing to be enrolled in the auditing process till they get back to their normal condition.

- During a quality improvement audit, an independent auditor will track and measure the quality of services performed, patient satisfaction, and the financial cost to both the patient and the provider in achieving the desired result. Quality improvement audits provide a roadmap for providers on how to improve their services and provide the best possible health care in a cost-efficient way.

The clinical audit process seeks to identify areas for service improvement, develop, and carry out action plans to rectify or improve service provision and then to reaudit to ensure that these changes have an effect.

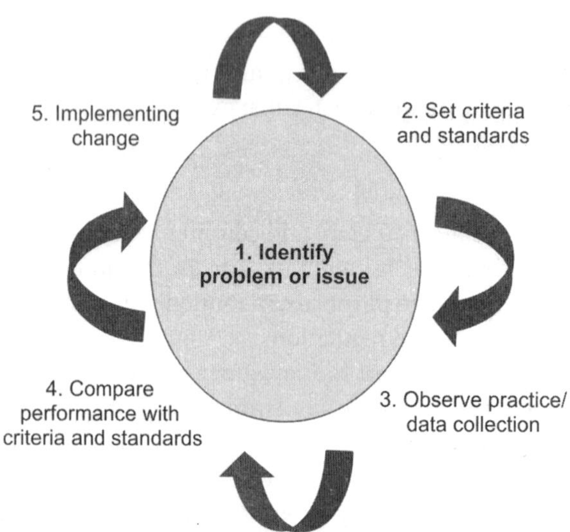

Audit	*Research*
Never involves experiments, whether on healthy volunteers or patients as volunteers	May involve experiments on human subjects whether patients, patients as volunteers, or healthy volunteers
Is a systematic approach to the peer review of medical care in order to identify opportunities for improvement and to provide a mechanism for bringing them about	Is a systematic investigation which aims to increase the sum of knowledge
Never involves allocating patients randomly to different treatment groups	May involve allocating patients randomly to different treatment groups
Never involves a completely new treatment	May involve a completely new treatment
Never involves a disturbance to the patients beyond that required for normal clinical management	May involve extra disturbance or work beyond that required for normal clinical management
May involve patients with the same problem being given different treatments but only after full discussion of the known advantages and disadvantages of each treatment. The patients are allowed to choose freely which treatment they get	May involve the application of strict selection criteria to patients with the same problem before they are entered Into the research study
Measures against a standard	Usually involves an attempt to test a hypothesis

15. Surgical audit. ***WBUHS 2008; Ayush University, Chhattisgarh 2025; KIIT University, Odisha 2025***

16. Discuss the role of surgical audit. ***RIMS, Imphal 2022***

17. Surgical audit—Definition, methods and advantages. ***NTRUHS, Vijayawada 2025***

18. Write down the purpose of surgical audit. How does it affect the quality of surgical care? ***WBUHS 2024***

Surgical audit is an unbiased, systematic, and critical analysis of the quality of surgical care, reviewed by peer(s) against explicit criteria or recognized standards. The purpose of an audit is to examine whether what you think is happening really is, and whether audited outcomes meet existing standards.

Possible reasons for conducting clinical audit:

- As a result of local clinical interests
- As a result of clinical incident reporting
- To comply with regional or national initiatives
- To inform patients about surgical results
- To drive continuous quality improvement
- For healthcare regulation

A surgical audit aims to: Identify ways of improving and maintaining the quality of care for patients—assist in the continuing education of surgeons, and—help make the most of resources available for the provision of surgical services.

Surgical audit is typically based on a five-step cycle

Step 1: Determine scope

Step 2: Define standards

Step 3: Collect data

Step 4: Present and interpret results (with peer review)

Step 5: Make changes and monitor progress

Data to be Used for Audit

- *Routine hospital data:*
  - Ideally, hospitals should have clearly defined systems in place to use the data.
  - The data may be incorrect or there may be issues about classification or attribution that explain away an apparent alert, but structured investigation should improve the organization's and the clinician's knowledge about their data systems and may lead to impressions that necessitate improvements in patient care.
- *Specialty-specific multicenter data:* These are usually clinically driven and have benefits above routine hospital data in that a more useful dataset can be designed for specific purposes and in particular can look in more detail at subtleties of case mix and specific clinical outcomes in a way that is more robust and sensitive than that derived from routine hospital administration systems.
- *Locally derived data:* Individual hospital departments will often decide to audit a specific theme that may be chosen because of clinical risk management issues, subspecialist interest, or other concerns.

To maximize the chances of improving care as a result of audit, the following should be considered:

- Will the sample size be big enough to be useful? What dataset is needed? Will that data be accessible from existing hospital case notes or will prospective data collection be necessary?
- Is there an existing robust benchmark to which the results of the audit can be compared? How will the "significance" of the results be analyzed?
- Does conducting the audit have financial implications?
- Will the potential results of the audit have financial implications?
- Are all stakeholders who may need to change their behavior as a result of the audit involved in the process?

Good Practice in Audit

- A clinical department should benefit from a clear forward plan about its audit activity that should be developed by the multidisciplinary team in conjunction with patients and their caregivers.

- The audit activity should include an appropriate mix of national, local, and risk management driven issues and the specifics should depend on the configuration of services and local preferences.
- The plan should include thoughts about dissemination of results to users and potential users of the services.
- The multidisciplinary team should include doctors, professionals allied to medicine, and administration staff.
- Adherence to the audit plan should be monitored through the departmental operational management structures.
- For the department to be successful in improving care as a result of audit, there should be clear understanding of effective techniques of change management.

Arguments against Audit

- In the United Kingdom, audit has been an essential part of all doctors' job plans for a number of years, but audit activity remains sporadic.
- In some high-profile specialties such as cardiac surgery, comprehensive audit has been led by clinicians and driven by politicians and the media. In other areas, there has been little or no coordinated national audit activity.
- This may be due to a perceived lack of benefits from audit from clinicians along with failure to meet challenges in gaining consensus or difficulties in securing adequate resource.
- The experience from cardiac surgery is that structured national audit improves the quality of mortality outcomes.
- It is likely that other issues such as complication rates are also reduced with associated costs savings, and as such effective audit may well pay for itself.

Research	*Clinical audit*	*Service evaluation*
The attempt to derive generalizable new knowledge including studies that aim to generate hypotheses as well as studies that aim to test them	Designed and conducted to produce best care information to inform the delivery of best care	Designed and conducted solely to define or judge current care
• Quantitative research—designed to test a hypothesis • Qualitative research—identifies/explores themes following established methodology	*Designed to answer the question:* "Does this service reach a predetermined standard?"	*Designed to answer the question:* "What standard does this service achieve?"
Addresses clearly defined questions, aims, and objectives	Measures against a standard	Measures current service without reference to a standard
Quantitative research—may involve evaluating or comparing interventions, particularly new ones Qualitative research—usually involves studying how interventions and relationships are experienced	Involves an intervention in use only (The choice of treatment is that of the clinician and patient according to guidance, professional standards, and/or patient preference)	Involves an intervention in use only. (The choice of treatment is that of the clinician and patient according to guidance, professional standards, and/or patient preference)
• Usually involves collecting data that are additional to those for routine care but may include data collected routinely • May involve treatments, samples, or investigations additional to routine care	Usually involves analysis of existing data but may include administration of simple interviews or questionnaires	Usually involves analysis of existing data but may include administration of simple interviews or questionnaires
• Quantitative research—study design may involve allocating patients to intervention groups • Qualitative research uses a clearly defined sampling framework underpinned by conceptual or theoretical justifications	No allocation to intervention groups—the healthcare professional and patient have chosen intervention before clinical audit	No allocation to intervention groups—the healthcare professional and patient have chosen intervention before clinical service evaluation
May involve randomization	No randomization	No randomization

SCIENTIFIC STUDIES

19. Give an overview of the types of scientific studies. ***DNB 2021 June***

Scientific studies are broadly categorized based on their purpose, design, and methodology. Here is an overview of the main types:

I. By Purpose:

1. *Descriptive studies:*
    - *Aim:* Describe characteristics of a population or phenomenon.
    - *Example:* A study that reports the average age of patients with a disease.
    - *Types:*
        - Case reports
        - Case series
        - Cross-sectional studies
2. *Analytical studies:*
    - *Aim:* Investigate associations, causes, or effects.
    - Compare groups to test hypotheses.
    - *Types:*
        - Observational studies
        - Experimental studies

II. By Design:

A. Observational Studies:

Researchers observe without intervening.

1. *Cross-sectional:*
    - Snapshot at a single point in time.
    - Used to assess prevalence.
    - *Example:* Survey of smoking rates among teenagers.
2. *Case-control:*
    - *Retrospective:* Compares people with a condition (cases) to those without (controls).
    - Good for rare diseases.
    - *Example:* Comparing past exposure to asbestos in lung cancer patients vs. healthy controls.
3. *Cohort studies:*
    - Follow groups over time based on exposure.
    - Can be prospective or retrospective.
    - *Example:* Tracking smokers and non-smokers to compare lung cancer incidence.

B. Experimental (Interventional) Studies:

Researchers actively intervene to study effects:

1. *Randomized controlled trials (RCTs)*
    - Participants randomly assigned to treatment or control groups.
    - Gold standard for testing efficacy of interventions.
    - *Example:* New drug vs. placebo for treating hypertension.
2. *Field trials:* Conducted in the general population, often for preventive measures (e.g., vaccines).
3. *Community trials:*
    - Interventions applied to entire communities.
    - *Example:* Fluoridation of water in one city vs. another.

III. Other Specialized Types

1. *Systematic reviews:*
   - Synthesizes results from multiple studies using a predefined methodology.
   - May or may not include meta-analysis.
2. *Meta-analyses:* Statistical analysis that combines results of several studies to increase power and resolve uncertainty.
3. *Qualitative studies:*
   - Focus on understanding human behavior, experiences, and meaning.
   - *Methods:* Interviews, focus groups, thematic analysis.
4. *In vitro and in vivo studies:*
   - *In vitro:* Laboratory experiments on cells or biological molecules outside living organisms.
   - *In vivo:* Experiments conducted in living organisms (e.g., animal models).

20. Presenting and publishing an article. ***Rajasthan University of Health Sciences 2025***

Presenting and Publishing a Surgical Article: Step-by-Step Guide (2025 Edition)

Phase 1: Preparation (Before Submission)

Step	***Action***	***Tips***
1. Choose target	Select *journal* (impact factor, scope, audience)	Use *SCImago, PubMed, Journal Citation Reports*
2. Study guidelines	Download *Author Instructions*	Follow *word count, structure, references, CONSORT/ STROBE/PRISMA*
3. Confirm authorship	Apply *ICMJE criteria*	*All listed:* Substantial contribution, drafting, approval, accountability
4. Register trial	*ClinicalTrials.gov* or *WHO ICTRP*	Required for RCTs, prospective studies
5. Ethics and consent	IRB approval, *COI disclosure*, patient consent for images	Include in manuscript

Phase 2: Manuscript Writing (IMRAD + Extras)

Section	***Key content***	***Pro tips***
Title	≤15 words, specific, *no abbreviations*	"Robotic vs Laparoscopic Colectomy: A Propensity-Matched Analysis"
Abstract	*Structured (250–300 words):* Background, Methods, Results, Conclusion	Use *PICO* framework
Introduction	3 paragraphs: Problem → Knowledge gap → Study aim	End with *clear objective*
Methods	*STROBE* checklist; detail stats (software, α=0.05, power)	Include *STROBE flowchart*
Results	*Tables/Figures first*, then text	*Max 6* (no data duplication)
Discussion	4–5: Summary → Context → Strengths → Limitations → Future	First line = answer to aim
References	Vancouver style, ≤40 (reviews ≤100)	Use *EndNote/Zotero/Mendeley*
Supplementary	Raw data, protocols, videos	*MP4 <50MB*, annotated

Phase 3: Submission

Platform	***Examples***
Editorial Manager	Annals of Surgery, JACS
ScholarOne	JAMA Surgery, Surgical Endoscopy
Evise/Editorial System	World J Surgery

Submission Checklist:

- Cover letter (novelty, no prior submission)
- Title page (authors, affiliations, corresponding)
- Blinded manuscript
- Figures (300 dpi, TIFF/JPEG)
- *ORCID iD* for all authors
- *Data availability statement*

Phase 4: Peer Review Response

Reviewer comment	***Response strategy***
Major revision	Point-by-point *table*, highlight changes in *yellow*
Stats critique	Consult *biostatistician*, re-run analysis
"Add more cases"	Politely justify sample size (power calculation)
Reject	Revise → submit elsewhere (never resubmit same data)

Timeline:

- *Initial decision: 2–8 weeks*
- *Revision: 2–4 weeks* to resubmit
- *Final acceptance: 1–3 months*

Phase 5: Presentation (Abstract → Podium/Poster)

Abstract Submission
Structure: Background → Methods → Results (with *p-value*) → Conclusion

Podium Presentation (8–10 minutes)

Time	***Slide***	***Content***
0–1 minutes	1	Title + Disclosure
1–2 minutes	2–3	Background + Gap
2–3 minutes	4	Aim + Study Design
3–5 minutes	5–7	Methods (flowchart)
5–7 minutes	8–10	Results (graphs, tables)
7–8 minutes	11	Conclusion + Take-home
8–10 minutes	—	Q&A

Design Tips:

- *Font ≥24 pt, ≤6 lines/slide*
- *High-contrast* (dark blue background, white text)
- *One graph/table per slide*
- *No paragraphs*—bullet points

Poster Presentation

Section	***Size***
Standard	*4 ft* × *6 ft* (ACS) or *A0* (Europe)

Layout (Left → Right):

Title → Intro → Methods → Results → Conclusion → QR code (full paper)

Pro Move

- Include *3-minute audio summary* via QR code (Record in PowerPoint → export MP3)

Phase 6: Post-publication

Action	***Tool***
Share	Twitter/X, ResearchGate, institutional repo
Altmetrics	PlumX, Altmetric.com
Press Release	EurekAlert (for high-impact)
Video Abstract	YouTube (≤2 minutes), embed in journal

SIMULATION IN SURGICAL TRAINING

21. Discuss the role of simulation in surgical training. Enumerate the types of simulation platforms available for surgical training. ***AIIMS, Patna 2025***

22. Simulation-based learning in surgery. ***RGUHS, Karnataka 2025***

23. Opine about role of simulation in surgery. ***KIIT University, Odisha 2025***

Role of Simulation in Surgical Training

Simulation has transformed surgical education from the traditional Halstedian "see one, do one, teach one" model into a *proficiency-based, patient-safe paradigm*. Its core roles are:

Skill Acquisition in Zero-risk Environment

- Trainees practice motor, cognitive, and decision-making skills without endangering patients.
- Enables deliberate practice with immediate feedback and repeatable scenarios.

Proficiency-based Progression

- Objective metrics (time, economy of motion, error rates) define competency (e.g., FLS, MISTELS, OSATS).
- Trainees must achieve benchmarks before OR privileges.

Crisis Management and Team Training

- Simulates rare events (anastomotic leak, massive hemorrhage, malignant hyperthermia).
- Integrates CRM (Crew Resource Management) for multidisciplinary teams.

Credentialing and Re-credentialing

- Mandatory for FLS (fundamentals of laparoscopic surgery), FES (flexible endoscopy), and robotic certification (da Vinci).
- Used for maintenance of certification (MOC) and hospital privileging.

Curriculum Integration

- ACS/AEISim Consortium, SAGES, AORN guidelines mandate simulation hours in residency.
- Boot camps (e.g., ACS Transition to Residency) use simulation for PGY-1 orientation.

Technological Familiarity

Pre-trains surgeons on robotic consoles, energy devices, and VR anatomy before first case.

Research and Innovation

Validates new instruments, techniques (e.g., NOTES, SP surgery), and AI-guided training.

Types of Simulation Platforms for Surgical Training

Type	*Description*	*Examples*	*Validation level*
1. Benchtop/Box Trainers	Physical models with real instruments under laparoscopic camera	FLS Trainer Box, EO Sim, Lap Mentor physical module	High (FLS validated)
2. VR (Virtual Reality) Simulators	Computer-based 3D environments with haptic feedback.	LapSim (Surgical Science), MIST-VR, Simbionix LAP Mentor	High (transfer studies)
3. AR (Augmented Reality)	Overlays digital data on real-world view (e.g., HoloLens).	Microsoft HoloLens for anatomy, Proximie AR telementoring	Emerging
4. Full-Physics Robotic Simulators	Console-based training for robotic systems.	da Vinci Skills Simulator, RoSS, dV-Trainer, RobotiX Mentor	High (Intuitive certification)
5. Cadaveric Simulation	Fresh or Thiel-preserved human cadavers	Fresh Tissue Labs, IRCAD cadaver courses	Gold standard (anatomy)
6. Live Animal Models	Porcine, canine models for physiologic response	Swine laparoscopy labs (IRCAD, EITS)	Limited (ethical)
7. 3D-Printed Task-Specific Models	Patient-specific or generic anatomy via additive manufacturing	3D-printed kidney tumors, vascular aneurysms, pediatric hearts	Growing
8. Hybrid Simulation	Combines part-task trainers with human actors (standardized patients)	TraumaMan + actor for ATLS, laparoscopic inguinal hernia with SP	High (team training)
9. Synthetic Organ Models	Silicone/rubber organs with realistic haptics	Chamberlain Group hearts, Syndaver livers, Limbs and Things bowel	Moderate
10. Screen-based Simulation	2D serious games or branching scenario software	Touch Surgery, Incision Academy, Level EX	Low–Moderate
11. Full-scale OR Mockups	High-fidelity operating room with mannequins	Laerdal SimMan 3G in mock OR, ORCAMP (Japan)	High (crisis management)
12. Perfusion-based Models	Pulsatile, blood-perfused cadaveric or synthetic systems	Strategic Operations "Cut Suit", Pulsatile Organ Perfusion (POP) Trainer	High (hemodynamics)
13 AI-Driven Adaptive Simulators	Machine learning adjusts difficulty in real-time	Osso VR (adaptive modules), Fundamental Surgery (AI analytics)	Emerging

Hierarchy of Simulation Fidelity

Fidelity level	*Type*	*Use case*
Low	Screen-based, 2D apps	Cognitive priming, anatomy review
Medium	VR, box trainers	Psychomotor skill acquisition
High	Robotic consoles, hybrid	Procedure-specific rehearsal
Ultra-High	Perfused cadavers, live OR	Crisis management, team coordination

Key Validated Curricula Using Simulation

Program	*Simulator type*	*Certification*
FLS	Box trainer + VR	SAGES/ACS
FES	GI Mentor (VR)	SAGES
da Vinci Training	Skills Simulator + RoSS	Intuitive Surgical
Fundamentals of Robotic Surgery (FRS)	Multi-platform (VR, dry lab)	Multisociety
ATLS/ACS BEST	Hybrid (mannequin + SP)	ACS

Future Directions

- *Patient-specific rehearsal:* 3D-printed models from CT/MRI for complex cases (e.g., conjoined twin separation).
- *AI-proctored training:* Real-time error detection and coaching (e.g., Intuitive's Iris analytics).
- *Remote VR mentorship:* 5G-enabled telementoring with haptic overlay.
- *Metaverse ORs:* Fully immersive multiuser training environments.

CHAPTER 48

Fast-track Surgery

LEARNING OBJECTIVE

- Fast-track surgery

FAST-TRACK SURGERY

1. Write a short note on fast-track surgery. ***WBUHS 2009***

- Fast-track surgery is a multimodal, evidence-based comprehensive program aimed at enhancing postoperative recovery and outcome by attenuating stress-related organ dysfunction.
- It is important to understand that the discharge criteria (mobile patient, pain-free on oral analgesia, and complete recovery of gut and bladder functions) in fast-track surgery remain unaltered but achieved sooner.
- The modern concepts of patient education, preoptimization, improved analgesia and surgical techniques, and better understanding of perioperative care principles with enforced early oral feeding and ambulation have led to the success of fast-track surgery.
- Published evidence confirms the benefits of fast-track surgery including reduced hospitalization, low morbidity, cost-effectiveness, patient satisfaction, and safety, with very low readmission rates.
- Organization and team delivery with strict attention to the protocols are vital to the success of a fast-track surgery program.
- An analysis of outcome is essential to success and a database should be maintained to aid this assessment.

Mediators and Modulators of Catabolic Pathways after Surgery

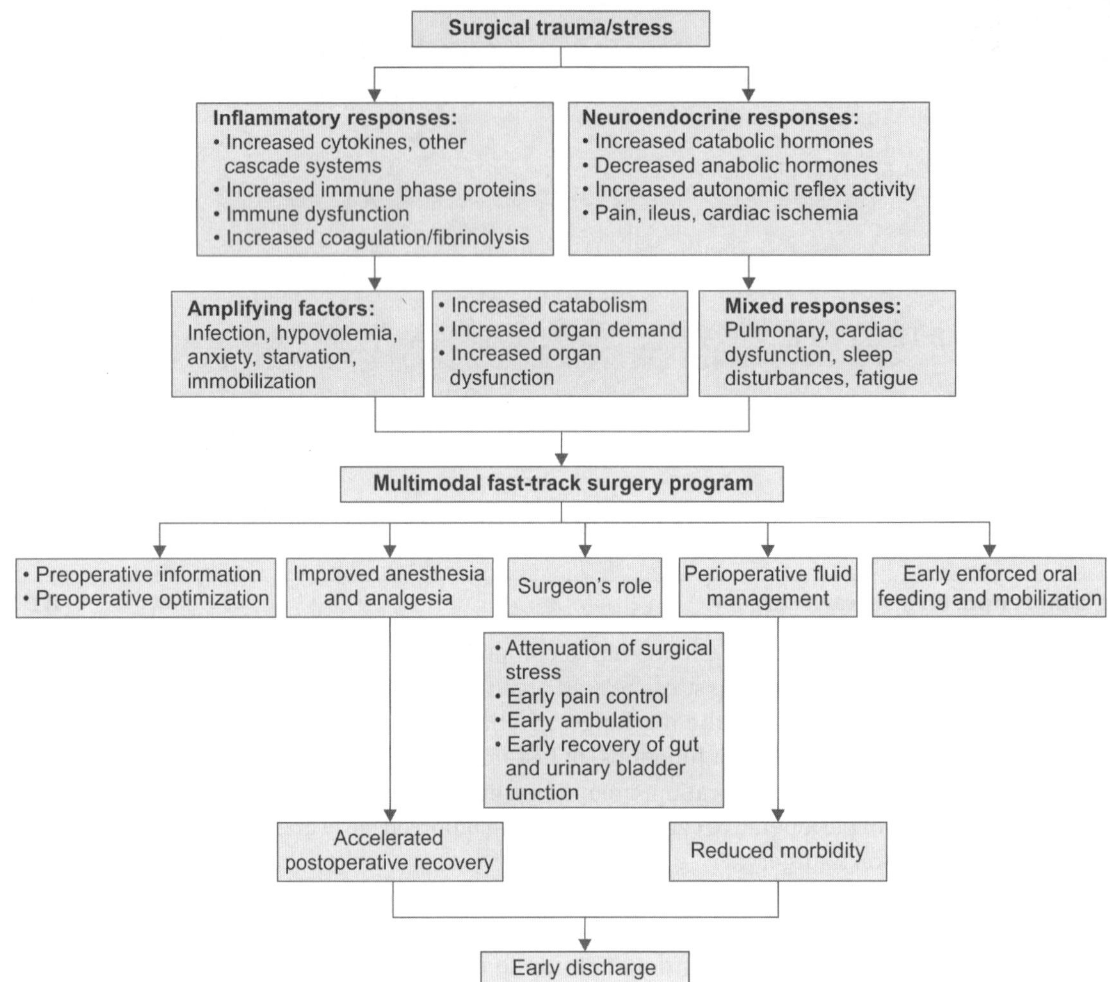

Vein, Artery, Nerve, and Lymphatics

LEARNING OBJECTIVES

- CEAP Classification, Clinical Features, and Investigations of Varicose Veins
- Treatment of Varicose Veins
- Recurrent Varicose Veins
- Venous Ulcer
- Deep Vein Thrombosis (DVT) and Pulmonary Embolism (PE)
- Thromboprophylaxis in Coronary Artery Bypass Graft (CABG)
- Lymphedema
- Chronic Limb Ischemia and Raynaud's Phenomenon
- Pharmacotherapy of Peripheral Arterial Disease
- Extra-anatomic Leg Bypass and Femoropopliteal Bypass
- Endovascular Approaches to Arteriovenous Fistula (AVF)
- Chronic Foot Ulcer and Diabetic Foot
- Median Nerve Injury
- Limb Edema

Vein

VARICOSE VEINS

1. Write notes on: CEAP classification, clinical features, and investigations of a case of varicose veins.
WBUHS 2021, 2023

2. Give an outline of endovenous intervention techniques for varicose veins. ***WBUHS 2021***

CEAP: Classification of chronic lower extremity venous disease.

Classification	*Definition*
C	*Clinical classification*
	C0: No visible or palpable signs of venous disease *C1:* Telangiectasias or reticular veins *C2:* Varicose veins; distinguished from reticular veins by a diameter of 3 mm or more *C3:* Edema *C4:* Changes in skin and subcutaneous tissue secondary to CVD • *C4a:* Pigmentation or eczema • *C4b:* Lipodermatosclerosis or atrophie blanche *C5:* Healed venous ulcer *C6:* Active venous ulcer
	S: Symptomatic (includes aching, pain, tightness, skin irritation, heaviness, muscle cramps, and other complaints attributable to venous dysfunction) *A:* Asymptomatic

Contd...

Contd...

Classification	*Definition*
E	*Etiologic classification*
	Ec: Congenital *Ep:* Primary *Es:* Secondary (i.e., post-thrombotic) *En:* No venous cause identified
A	*Anatomic distribution*
	As: Superficial veins involved *Ap:* Perforator veins involved *Ad:* Deep veins involved *An:* No venous location identified
P	*Pathophysiologic dysfunction*
	Pr: Reflux *Po:* Obstruction *Pr, o:* Reflux and obstruction *Pn:* No venous pathophysiology identified

(CVD: chronic venous disease)

Clinical Features

- *Signs and symptoms:*
  - Aching and heavy legs
  - Appearance of spider veins (telangiectasia) in the affected leg
  - Ankle swelling
  - A brownish-yellow shiny skin discoloration near the affected vein
  - Redness, dryness, and itchiness of areas of skin, termed stasis dermatitis, or venous eczema
  - Muscle cramps when making sudden movements, such as standing
  - Abnormal bleeding or healing time for injuries in the affected area
  - Lipodermatosclerosis or shrinking skin near the ankles
  - Restless legs syndrome appears to be a common overlapping clinical syndrome in people with varicose veins and other chronic venous insufficiency (CVI)
  - Atrophie blanche, or white, scar-like formations
  - Burning or throbbing sensation in the legs
- *Complications:*
  - Most varicose veins are reasonably benign, but severe varicosities can lead to major complications due to the poor circulation through the affected limb
  - Pain, tenderness, heaviness, and inability to walk or stand for long hours
  - Skin conditions/dermatitis which could predispose skin loss.
  - Skin ulcers especially near the ankle, usually referred to as venous ulcers
  - Development of carcinoma or sarcoma in longstanding venous ulcers
  - Severe bleeding from minor trauma, of particular concern in the elderly
  - Blood clotting within affected veins, termed superficial thrombophlebitis
  - Acute fat necrosis can occur, especially at the ankle of overweight people with varicose veins. Females have a higher tendency of being affected than males

Investigations

- *Noninvasive studies:*
  - *Duplex scanning—B-mode ultrasound (US)* imaging combined with Doppler frequency shift display is used to assess venous valvular competence, obstruction, and presence of acute or chronic deep vein thrombosis (DVT).

Duplex US is considered to be the "gold standard" for the assessment of venous hemodynamics and anatomy (duplex anatomy) to determine the appropriate treatment for each patient.

- There is no evidence to recommend multidetector computed tomography or other diagnostic tests for the diagnosis and treatment planning of varicose veins.
- *Plethysmography* is a noninvasive venous test that measures each potential component of the pathophysiologic mechanisms of CVI, including reflux, obstruction, and muscle pump dysfunction. Venous volume, venous refilling times, maximum venous outflow, segmental venous capacitance, and ejection fraction can be determined Because of its complexity of use, the use of this technique is limited to academic or hospital settings when Doppler ultrasound (DUS) does not provide definitive information on the pathophysiology of CVI.
- *Computed tomography and magnetic resonance venography:* Although advancements in computed tomography (CT) and magnetic resonance (MR) images have allowed for better evaluation of venous disease, these techniques are rarely required to determine the cause and plan treatment for CVI.

Endovascular Therapy

- *Radiofrequency (RF) ablation:*
  - The intervention employs RF energy-mediated heating of the vein wall to destroy the intima and denature collagen in the media with resulting fibrous occlusion of the vein.
  - The procedure is usually performed under conscious sedation and local anesthesia (LA) in an outpatient setting.
  - The catheter is preferably introduced into the saphenous vein at the knee percutaneously under US guidance or through a small incision and direct exposure of the vein.
  - The position of the catheter at the saphenofemoral junction (SFJ) is confirmed by US.
  - Local tumescent anesthetic is instilled in the subcutaneous tissues superficial to the vein under US guidance.
  - The vein wall temperature is allowed to equilibrate at 85°C after turning on the circuit and graduated withdrawal of the catheter is performed at a rate of 3 cm/min.
  - The heating is controlled by monitoring temperature and impedance of the vein wall via a feedback system.
  - Veins up to 12 mm in diameter are treated.
  - The treated vein should be relatively straight, free of severe tortuosity, or thrombus and without aneurysm.
  - Contraindications include a postphlebitic vein that cannot be accessed, a mega saphenous vein (>12 mm), and significant dilation of the proximal saphenous vein with an aneurysmal SFJ.
- *Endovenous laser therapy:*
  - Endovenous laser therapy (EVLT) is similar to RF ablation, but laser energy is used for ablation of the saphenous vein.
  - The procedure is faster and easier to perform than RF ablation and there is no size limitation of the saphenous vein that can be treated.
  - Both the 810-nm and the 940-nm diode lasers are effective in inducing thrombotic vessel occlusion.
  - Laser-induced indirect local heat injury of the inner vein wall by steam bubbles originating from boiling blood is proposed as the pathophysiological mechanism of action of EVLT.
  - This causes collagen contraction and endothelial damage.
  - The result is thickening of the vein wall and contraction or thrombosis of the lumen.
  - The use of diode laser energy to ablate the saphenous vein is a method that obviates the need for general anesthesia and is associated with less pain than traditional surgical stripping of the great saphenous vein (GSV).

---

3. Modified Brodie-Trendelenburg test. ***Gujarat Health University 2025***

Modified Brodie-Trendelenburg Test

Purpose: To *differentiate between saphenofemoral junction (SFJ) incompetence* and *perforator vein incompetence* in patients with *varicose veins.*

Principle: The test assesses how quickly superficial veins refill when the patient stands, and whether this refilling comes from *above (SFJ reflux)* or *below (incompetent perforators).*

Procedure

- *Position:*
  - Patient lies *supine.*
  - *Elevate the affected leg* (≈45°) to *empty the superficial veins.*
- *Apply a tourniquet:*
  - Place a *tourniquet just below the saphenofemoral junction* (i.e., at the upper thigh).
  - The tourniquet should *compress only the superficial veins,* not the deep veins.
- *Ask the patient to stand:* Observe the veins for filling.
- *Observe for venous filling:*
  - If *veins remain collapsed* → SFJ valves are competent (no reflux from above).
  - If *veins fill rapidly despite tourniquet* → reflux through *incompetent perforator veins* (from deep → superficial).
- *Release the tourniquet:* If there is *sudden rapid filling* from above after release → indicates *SFJ incompetence.*

Interpretation

Observation	***Inference***
No filling while standing, then rapid filling after releasing tourniquet	Incompetent saphenofemoral junction (SFJ reflux)
Gradual filling while tourniquet still on	Incompetent perforator veins
No filling before or after release	Competent valves (normal)

Diagrammatic Summary (Text Description)

Step 1: Leg raised → veins empty

Step 2: Tourniquet at SFJ level

Step 3: Patient stands

- Veins fill slowly → perforator incompetence
- Veins fill rapidly after release → SFJ incompetence

Clinical Significance

- Helps to *localize the site of valvular incompetence.*
- Guides *surgical planning*:
  - *SFJ incompetence* → high saphenous ligation.
  - *Perforator incompetence* → subfascial ligation or perforator surgery.

Modified vs. Original Test

Aspect	***Original Brodie–Trendelenburg test***	***Modified version***
Tourniquet	Applied and released in two steps	Single tourniquet, observed in one step
Purpose	Distinguish between superficial and perforator incompetence	Simplified approach, more practical clinically
Current use	Historical value	Modified test more commonly demonstrated

4. Recent trends in management of varicose veins. ***WBUHS 2013***

5. Describe the different surgical options for the management of varicose vein. ***WBUHS 2020***

6. Surgery of varicose veins. ***WBUHS 2012***

Physical Examination

The physical examination should include inspection of the limb in a standing position. Notation should be made of:

- Ankle venous flare
- Telangiectasias (dilated intradermal venules <1 mm)
- Reticular veins (nonpalpable subdermal veins 1–3 mm)
- Varicose veins (>3 mm)
- Edema
- Skin pigmentation
- Venous ulcers–chart on a diagram and note size, depth, and character of the ulcer base.

Photo documentation is increasingly being used to:

- Evaluate the response to therapy
- Track the natural progression of the disease
- Decide when to refer
- Keep a medicolegal record (remember to get consent from the patient to take and store a photograph as part of the medical record).

It is also important to document arterial pulses in all patients. In unusually sited or appearing varicosities, consider arteriovenous malformation. Traditional noninvasive office-based testing (e.g., Trendelenburg) has largely been replaced by duplex US.

Diagnostic Testing

Venous duplex US has become the standard of care for the investigation of varicose veins. Duplex US should document the:

- Patency and competency of the deep system
- Patency and competency of the superficial system, including site of incompetent segments, site of junctions, and perforators
- Location and relationships of the saphenopopliteal junction
- Diameter of the affected vein—this may be important in some endoluminal applications

Magnetic Resonance Venography

- MR venography is safe, does not involve ionizing radiation as phlebography and is not operator-dependent like duplex US.
- At present MR venography is in its infancy but its role will undoubtedly increase in future.
- The efficacy of MR venography in DVT have been assessed against duplex US, contrast phlebography or both using a variety of MR techniques and it has been shown that in many cases MR can be as effective as or, on occasion, superior to other imaging studies. But, it is expensive and not available at all places.

Treatment

- Conservative treatment with stockings and external compression is an acceptable alternative to surgery, but worsening cutaneous findings or symptoms despite these measure usually warrant intervention. Nonetheless, a patient's desire for surgical management over conservative treatment or for cosmetic purposes alone are both reasonable relative indications for surgery.
- Patients with venous outflow obstruction should not have their varicosities ablated, because they are important bypass pathways that allow blood to flow around the obstruction.
- Those patients who cannot remain active enough to reduce the risk of postoperative DVT should not undergo surgery.
- Surgery during pregnancy is contraindicated because many varicose veins of pregnancy spontaneously regress after delivery.

- Choice of treatment depends on many factors, including local expertise. Taking into account age, general health and symptomatology, patients with varicose veins may be offered one or more of the following management options:
  - Reassurance only
  - Conservative management with compression therapy
  - Endovenous therapy
  - Sclerotherapy—using liquid or foam [can be ultrasound-guided foam sclerotherapy (UGFS)]
  - EVLT
  - Radiofrequency ablation (RFA)
  - Mechanical—using steam or rotating catheter
  - Surgical treatment

A recent review of the literature revealed the following:

- No significant difference in short-term outcomes between the modalities
- Complications were few and mostly minor
- New varices may develop in 10% of patients within the first year after any treatment.
- The technical failure rate was highest with UGFS.
- Both RFA and UGFS were associated with a faster recovery and less postoperative pain than EVLT and stripping
- The shortest time to return to work was seen in the UGFS and RFA groups.
- There were significantly more cases of superficial phlebitis in the UGFS and RFA groups.
- The mean cost per treatment was lowest in the UGFS group and highest in the RFA and EVLT groups.
- Recent guidelines recommend against UGFS alone for the treatment of GSV incompetence.
- Overly large (>2 cm diameter)—thermal treatment may fail, and there is a high risk of DVT.
- Overly tortuous—endoluminal catheters may not pass up the vein.
- Very close to the skin—skin burns are more likely, and in cases of thrombophlebitis—endoluminal catheters may not pass up the vein.

Open Surgery

Surgical treatment of varicose veins:

Indications for Treatment

- When recognizable changes appear in the skin of the lower leg, i.e., presence of ankle flare, lipodermatosclerosis, or venous ulcer.
- If there are problems with hemorrhage or recurrent superficial thrombophlebitis
- If the patient wishes to be treated for symptomatic or cosmetic reasons
- Those who are medically unfit because of presence of varicose veins.

Options available for surgical treatment of varicose veins are as follows:

- Ablation of saphenous vein reflux: greater or smaller
- Incompetent perforators interruptions
- Elimination of residual varicosities
- Surgical interventions should be individualized according to the patient's preoperative evaluation. An important principle is to "treat the patient and not the duplex scan". A combination of ligation, axial stripping, and stab phlebectomy may be applied as needed to the GSV, short saphenous vein (SSV), tributary veins, and perforating veins.

Alternatives to Stripping

New venous surgical techniques have been developed in an effort to reduce the number and size of lower-extremity incisions and hematomas, to eliminate postoperative discoloration, and to reduce the recuperation time.

- *RFA:* The intervention employs RF energy-mediated heating of the vein wall to destroy the intima and denature collagen in the media with resulting fibrous occlusion of the vein.

- *EVLT:* EVLT is similar to RF ablation, but laser energy is used for ablation of the saphenous vein. The procedure is faster and easier to perform than RF ablation and there is no size limitation of the saphenous vein that can be treated.
- *Foam sclerotherapy:* An increasing number of authors have recently reported successful injection of incompetent GSV with 3% polidocanol in the form of foam.

Open Surgeries

- *Saphenopopliteal ligation:* Some surgeons advocate routine stripping of the SSV should be disconnected and never stripped. The SSV operation should be carried out first, if a long saphenous vein operation is to be performed under the same anesthetic.
- *Ligation of the lower leg perforating veins:* Surgery for these veins is usually required in patients with lipodermatosclerosis or ulceration. The presence of incompetent perforators in patients with advanced CVI (clinical classes 4 to 6) is an indication for surgical treatment in a fit patient. Whereas open perforator ligation is done only in those with healed ulceration, a clean, granulating open ulcer is not a contraindication for subfascial endoscopic perforator surgery (SEPS).

Endoscopic Surgery

Not preferred now.

- *SEPS:*
  - The major drawback of open procedure was a high incidence of wound complications. Edwards in 1976 designed a device called the phlebotome to ablate the incompetent perforators from sites remote from the diseased skin.
  - SEPS is a minimally invasive surgical technique used to treat chronic venous ulcers caused by perforating veins that may have been damaged due to DVT or CVI.
  - The goal of treatment is to heal the ulcer to prevent serious complications or to prevent ulcer recurrence.
  - Patients with chronic venous ulcers may have developed CVI as a result of damage to their perforating veins, which are veins located above the ankle that carry blood from the superficial veins into the deep veins.
  - If not corrected, patients may experience prolonged symptoms of severe CVI and recurrent venous stasis ulcer formation.

---

7. Recurrent varicose vein. ***WBUHS 2007, 2015***

Introduction

Recurrence of varicose veins after conventional surgery is common. Recurrence rates of 25–50% are found following SSV surgery after a follow-up period of 3–5 years. Incomplete dissection, filling by tributaries or residual veins, neovascularization to a network of superficial veins, and reflux from another origin may all contribute to varicose vein recurrence.

Definition

Recurrent varicose veins occur when you have previously had treatment for varicose veins. Treatment can include injections such as sclerotherapy, avulsions, cuts in the groin, or cuts behind the knee.

Causes

There are several reasons for veins coming back after treatment:

- Normal veins become varicose. If the person had varicose veins in the past then the patient is more likely to develop more varicose veins
- *Neovascularization:*
  - When a cut has been made in the skin, the wound heals because living tissue has the ability to regenerate.
  - When this happens, new blood vessels grow to provide a means for blood to get to the new skin.
  - The same process is thought to happen in the area where varicose veins have been treated by surgery.
  - The new veins appear to grow from the site of the vein ligation, most commonly the SFJ.

- The new veins are like weeds growing in the garden.
- If they connect up to an original main vein, then blood flows through them, runs into the area of varicose veins in the leg.
- This will cause recurrence of your varicose veins.
- If the long saphenous vein in your leg was not removed at the original operation, then the new veins can connect with it and cause recurrence.
- People who have this type of recurrence may be suitable for VNUS treatment to remove their veins.

- Inadequate initial treatment
- *Pudendal and pelvic varicose veins:* Some recurrent varicose veins are caused by connections to veins inside the pelvis. In some people the problem can arise in the veins that run from the testicles or ovaries (gonadal veins). If the blood runs in the wrong direction in these veins (gonadal reflux) then there can be a long column of blood pushing blood out of the pelvis and down the leg.

Treatment

In much the same way as primary varicose veins (those that have not been operated upon). It is important to know exactly where and how the recurrent veins are formed.

- Surgery on the type of recurrence one has.
- If one needs another cut in the groin, he/she may be suitable for VNUS (minimally invasive treatment for superficial venous reflux)
- New techniques such as VNUS, EVLT, and Varicofoam can avoid these complications.
- If the patient needs another cut behind the knee, then he/she has recurrent short saphenous disease. He/she may need a much larger cut than before so that the surgeon can carefully identify the blood vessels and nerves behind the knee.
- With this operation, patient may be at increased risks of wound infection and damage to nerves.
- It might be worth considering Varicofoam therapy if patient have recurrent SSV disease.
- In 20% of the cases, inadequate surgery was considered to be the cause of recurrence and as soon as 2 weeks after surgery up to 23% of patients showed reflux on duplex scanning.
- In the last decade, endovenous techniques, including endovenous laser ablation (EVLA) and RFA, have been successfully introduced. Recurrence of varicose veins after conventional surgery is common. Recurrence rates of 25–50% are found following SSV surgery after a follow-up period of 3–5 years. Incomplete dissection, filling by tributaries or residual veins, neovascularization to a network of superficial veins, and reflux from another origin may all contribute to varicose vein recurrence.

VENOUS ULCER

8. Discuss pathophysiology of varicose veins and management of venous ulcer.

Srimanta Sankaradeva University, Assam 2025

Normal Venous Physiology

- Venous blood in the lower limbs is returned to the heart against gravity through:
    - *Superficial veins:* Great and small saphenous veins.
    - *Deep veins:* Femoral, popliteal, tibial veins.
    - *Perforator veins:* Connect superficial to deep systems.
- One-way valves in both superficial and perforating veins direct flow from superficial → deep → central veins.
- Muscle pump (especially calf muscles) and respiratory changes in intrathoracic pressure assist venous return.

Pathophysiological Basis of Varicosity

Varicose veins develop due to a failure of this normal mechanism, leading to sustained venous hypertension.

Venous Valve Incompetence (Primary Factor)

- *Primary varicose veins:* Congenital or idiopathic incompetence of venous valves (especially at saphenofemoral or saphenopopliteal junctions).
- *Secondary varicose veins:* Due to damage to valves from—
  - Deep vein thrombosis (DVT)
  - Trauma
  - Pregnancy or pelvic tumors causing obstruction

Result: Retrograde (reverse) flow of blood during standing → increased venous pressure in distal veins.

Venous Hypertension

- Normally, standing venous pressure ≈ 80–90 mm Hg, but muscle contraction reduces it to ~30 mm Hg.
- When valves are incompetent, pressure remains elevated even during exercise, causing chronic venous hypertension.

Venous Wall Changes

- *Chronic high pressure and turbulent flow cause:*
  - Dilatation and elongation of vein segments.
  - Degeneration of vein wall connective tissue (loss of elastin and smooth muscle atrophy).
  - Progressive valve cusp separation, worsening reflux → a vicious cycle of further dilation and valve failure.

Microcirculatory Effects

Persistent venous hypertension leads to:

- Capillary distension and increased permeability → leakage of plasma proteins and RBCs into interstitium.
- Pericapillary fibrin cuff formation → impairs oxygen and nutrient diffusion.
- Inflammation and tissue hypoxia → skin changes (eczema, lipodermatosclerosis, pigmentation).
- Ulcer formation in severe cases (venous ulcers, typically near the medial malleolus).

Contributing Factors

Factor	***Mechanism***
Genetic predisposition	Weakness of venous wall or valves
Prolonged standing/sedentary lifestyle	Increases hydrostatic pressure
Pregnancy	Hormonal relaxation of vessel wall + increased venous pressure
Obesity	Raised intra-abdominal pressure impedes venous return
Deep vein obstruction	Increases pressure in superficial system via perforators

Summary of Pathophysiological Sequence

- Valve incompetence (superficial, deep, or perforator).
- Retrograde flow of blood → venous reflux.
- Sustained venous hypertension during standing and walking.
- Vein wall dilation and remodeling → varicosity.
- Microcirculatory changes → edema, skin pigmentation, eczema, ulceration.

Diagram Summary

Valve incompetence → Reflux → ↑ Venous pressure

↓

Venous distension → Further valve separation

↓

Chronic venous hypertension → Capillary leakage, inflammation

↓

Skin changes and ulceration

Answer of the 2nd part of the question – see the answers of next questions

9. Venous ulcer.

WBUHS 2010, 2015; RIMS, Imphal 2012

Introduction

- Chronic venous disease, including CVI and chronic venous ulceration, is a common and important medical problem that causes significant morbidity. Venous ulcers are expensive to treat and adversely impact patient's quality of life.
- Venous ulcers occur more commonly in the elderly, the peak prevalence occurring between ages 60 and 80 years.
- A venous leg ulcer can develop after a minor injury if there is a problem with the circulation of blood in your leg veins. If this happens, the pressure inside the veins increases.

Risk Factors

- Obesity—this increases the risk of high pressure in the leg veins.
- Not being able to move for a long period of time—this can weaken the calf muscles, which can affect circulation in the leg veins.
- Having previously had DVT—blood clots that develop in the leg, which can damage valves.
- Varicose veins—swollen and enlarged veins caused by malfunctioning valves.
- Previous injury to the leg, such as a broken or fractured bone, which may cause DVT.
- Previous surgery to the leg, such as a hip replacement or knee replacement, which can prevent you from moving about.
- Increasing age—as people generally find it harder to move about as they get older.

Pathophysiology

- *Venous hypertension:* DVT, perforator insufficiency, superficial and deep vein insufficiencies, arteriovenous fistulas (AVFs), and calf muscle pump insufficiencies lead to increased pressure in the distal veins of the leg and finally DVT.
- *Fibrin cuff theory:* Fibrin gets excessively deposited around capillary beds leading to elevated intravascular pressure. This causes enlargement of endothelial pores resulting in further increased fibrinogen deposition in the interstitium. The "fibrin cuff" which surrounds the capillaries in the dermis decreases oxygen permeability 20-fold. This permeability barrier inhibits diffusion of oxygen and other nutrients, leading to tissue hypoxia causing impaired wound healing.
- *Inflammatory trap theory:* Various growth factors and inflammatory cells, which get trapped in the fibrin cuff promote severe uncontrolled inflammation in surrounding tissue preventing proper regeneration of wounds. Leukocytes get trapped in capillaries, releasing proteolytic enzymes and reactive oxygen metabolites, which cause endothelial damage. These injured capillaries become increasingly permeable to various macromolecules, accentuating fibrin deposition. Occlusion by leukocytes also causes local ischemia thereby increasing tissue hypoxia and reperfusion damage.
- *Dysregulation* of various cytokines.
- *Dysregulation* of various proinflammatory cytokines and growth factors such as tumor necrosis factor-α (TNF-α), transforming growth factor-β (TGF-β), and matrix metalloproteinases lead to chronicity of the ulcers.
- *Miscellaneous:* Thrombophilic conditions such as factor V Leiden mutation, prothrombin mutations, deficiency of antithrombin, presence of antiphospholipid antibodies, protein C and S deficiencies, and hyperhomocysteinemia are also implicated.

Clinical Features

Venous leg ulcers are open, often painful, sores in the skin that take more than 4 to 6 weeks to heal. They most often develop on the inside of the leg, just above the ankle.

Symptoms

- Swollen ankles (edema)
- Discoloration and darkening of the skin around the ulcer.

- Hardened skin around the ulcer, which may make your leg feel hard and resemble the shape of an upside-down champagne bottle.
- A heavy feeling in your legs
- Aching or swelling in your legs
- Red, flaky, scaly, and itchy skin on your legs (varicose eczema)
- Swollen and enlarged veins on your legs (varicose veins)
- An unpleasant and foul-smelling discharge from the ulcer

Signs of an Infection

A venous leg ulcer can be susceptible to bacterial infection. Symptoms of an infected leg ulcer can include:

- Worsening pain
- A green or unpleasant discharge coming from the ulcer.
- Redness and swelling of the skin around the ulcer.
- A high temperature (fever)

Nonsurgical Treatment

A. Infected Ulcers

- Necessitate treatment of the infection first.
- *Staphylococcus aureus*, *Streptococcus pyogenes*, and *Pseudomonas* species are responsible for most infections.
- Usually treated with local wound care, wet-to-dry dressings, and oral antibiotics.
- Topical antiseptics should be avoided.
- Severe infections require intravenous antibiotics.

B. Leg Elevation

- Leg elevation can temporarily decrease edema and should be instituted when swelling occurs.
- This should be done before a patient is fitted for stockings or boots.

C. Compression Therapy: Compression therapy is the primary treatment for CVI.

- *Elastic compression stockings:*
  - Fitted to provide a compression gradient from 30 to 40 mm Hg, with the greatest compression at the ankle.
  - Donned on arising from bed and removed at bedtime.
  - Effective in healing ulcers but can take months to obtain good results.
  - Stockings do not correct the abnormal venous hemodynamics and must be worn after the ulcer has healed to prevent recurrence.
  - Principal drawback is patient compliance.
- *Unna boots:*
  - Paste gauze compression dressings that contain zinc oxide, calamine, and glycerin.
  - Used to help prevent further skin breakdown.
  - Provide nonelastic compression therapy.
  - Changed once or twice a week.
  - Healing time for ulcers is less than that of elastic compression alone.
- *Pneumatic compression devices:*
  - Provide dynamic sequential compression.
  - Used primarily in the prevention of deep vein thrombi in hospitalized patients.
  - Also used successfully to treat venous insufficiency.

D. Topical Medications

- Largely ineffective as a stand-alone therapy for venous stasis ulcers.
- Topical therapy is directed at absorbing wound drainage and avoiding desiccation of the wound.
  - Antiseptics can be counterproductive. Hydrogen peroxide, povidone-iodine, acetic acid, and sodium hypochlorite are toxic to cultured fibroblasts and should be used for the shortest duration necessary to control ulcer infection.

E. Surgical Therapy

- Skin grafting
  - Occasionally used to speed healing of large ulcers.
  - Ulcer bed should be dry and free of infection.
  - Fenestrated split-thickness skin graft is preferred to allow for serous drainage.
  - Bed rest is recommended until the ulcer has healed completely.
  - Recurrence is common unless the underlying venous pathology is corrected or conservative support (elastic compression) is initiated and maintained after skin grafting. Cultured skin substitutes are now commonly used to minimize patient discomfort and avoid possible donor-site complications.
  - Stripping the greater saphenous vein.

---

10. Outline the current approach in the investigation and management of venous ulcer.

WBUHS 2025 Supplementary

The current approach to *investigation and management of venous ulcers* is comprehensive, aiming to address both the underlying *venous insufficiency* and the *local wound* environment.

Investigation of Venous Ulcers

Clinical Assessment

- *History:*
  - Chronicity of ulcer, previous episodes, trauma
  - *Risk factors:* age, varicose veins, DVT, obesity, immobility
  - *Symptoms:* leg heaviness, aching relieved by elevation
  - *Physical examination:*
    - *Ulcer features:* Typically above medial malleolus, irregular edges, shallow base
    - *Associated signs:* Varicosities, edema, lipodermatosclerosis, hemosiderin deposition

Ankle-Brachial Pressure Index (ABPI)

- Performed using Doppler ultrasound
- *Purpose:* Exclude arterial disease before compression therapy
- *Interpretation:*
  - *>0.8:* safe for compression
  - *0.5–0.8:* mild-to-moderate arterial disease—cautious compression
  - *<0.5:* severe arterial disease—avoid compression, refer to vascular specialist

Duplex Doppler Ultrasound

- Gold standard to assess venous *reflux* and *obstruction*
- Identifies sites of valvular incompetence or DVT

Other Investigations

- *Blood tests:* FBC, HbA1c, CRP, albumin (to assess anemia, diabetes, inflammation, nutrition)
- *Wound swab:* Only if signs of infection present (e.g., cellulitis, increasing pain, exudate)

Management of venous ulcers

Compression Therapy (cornerstone of treatment)

- *Goal:* Improve venous return and reduce edema
- *Types:*
  - Multilayer compression bandaging (e.g., four-layer or two-layer systems)
  - Compression stockings (for maintenance post-healing)
- Must confirm ABPI > 0.8 before starting

Wound Care

- *Cleansing:* Use of normal saline or wound cleansers
- *Dressings:* Aim to maintain moist wound environment and manage exudate
    - Hydrocolloids, alginates, foams depending on exudate levels
    - Antimicrobial dressings (e.g., silver) if signs of local infection
- *Debridement:* Sharp, autolytic, or enzymatic if necrotic/sloughy tissue present

Treatment of Infection

- *Topical or systemic antibiotics:* Only if clinical signs of infection
- *Biofilm management:* Debridement and antimicrobial dressings may be used

Adjunctive Therapies

- *Pentoxifylline:* Improves microcirculation and shown to enhance healing
- Aspirin (some studies support its anti-inflammatory effect)
- *Skin grafts or bioengineered tissue:* In refractory or large ulcers
- *Negative Pressure Wound Therapy (NPWT):* May help in selected cases

Surgical/Interventional Approaches

- Endovenous ablation (laser or radiofrequency)
- Sclerotherapy or ligation/stripping for superficial venous incompetence
- Indicated in recurrent or large ulcers where reflux persists

Lifestyle and Risk Factor Modification

- Leg elevation
- Exercise to activate calf muscle pump
- Weight reduction, smoking cessation, diabetes control

Patient Education and Follow-up

- Adherence to compression therapy
- Skin care to prevent recurrence
- Long-term follow-up to monitor recurrence

Prevention of Recurrence

- Continued use of compression stockings (Class II or III)
- Treat underlying venous insufficiency (e.g., surgery or ablation)
- Regular skin moisturization to prevent breakdown

---

11. How will you diagnose and manage a case of chronic leg ulcer? ***WBUHS 2023***

Symptoms

- Swollen ankles (oedema)
- Discoloration and darkening of the skin around the ulcer
- Hardened skin around the ulcer, which may make your leg feel hard and resemble the shape of an upside-down champagne bottle
- A heavy feeling in your legs
- Aching or swelling in your legs
- Red, flaky, scaly and itchy skin on your legs (varicose eczema)
- Swollen and enlarged veins on your legs (varicose veins)
- An unpleasant and foul-smelling discharge from the ulcer

Signs of an infection

A venous leg ulcer can be susceptible to bacterial infection. Symptoms of an infected leg ulcer can include:

- Worsening pain

- A green or unpleasant discharge coming from the ulcer
- Redness and swelling of the skin around the ulcer
- A high temperature (fever)

Physical examination: The physical examination should include inspection of the limb in a standing position. Notation should be made of—Venous ulcers - chart on a diagram and note size, depth, character of the ulcer base.

Photo documentation is increasingly being used to:

- Evaluate the response to therapy
- Track the natural progression of the disease
- Decide when to refer
- Keep a medicolegal record (remember to get consent from the patient to take and store a photograph as part of the medical record).

It is also important to document arterial pulses in all patients. In unusually sited or appearing varicosities, consider arteriovenous malformation. Traditional non-invasive office based testing (e.g., Trendelenburg) has largely been replaced by duplex ultrasound.

Diagnostic Testing

Venous duplex ultrasound has become the standard of care for the investigation of varicose veins. Duplex ultrasound should document the:

- Patency and competency of the deep system
- Patency and competency of the superficial system, including site of incompetent segments, site of junctions and perforators
- Location and relationships of the saphenopopliteal junction
- Diameter of the affected vein—this may be important in some endoluminal applications.

Magnetic Resonance Venography

- Magnetic resonance venography is safe, does not involve ionizing radiation as phlebography and is not operator dependent like duplex ultrasound.
- At present Magnetic resonance venography is in its infancy but its role will undoubtedly increase in future.
- The efficacy of Magnetic resonance venography in deep vein thrombosis have been assessed against duplex ultrasound, contrast phlebography or both using a variety of MR techniques and it has been shown that in many cases MR can be as effective as or, on occasion, superior to other imaging studies. But, it is expensive and not available at all places.

Nonsurgical Treatment

Infected Ulcers

- Necessitate treatment of the infection first.
- Staphylococcus aureus, *Streptococcus* pyogenes, and *Pseudomonas* species are responsible for most infections.
- Usually treated with local wound care, wet-to-dry dressings, and oral antibiotics.
- Topical antiseptics should be avoided.
- Severe infections require intravenous antibiotics.

Leg Elevation

- Leg elevation can temporarily decrease edema and should be instituted when swelling occurs.
- This should be done before a patient is fitted for stockings or boots.

Compression Therapy

Compression therapy is the primary treatment for CVI.

- *Elastic compression stockings:*
  - Fitted to provide a compression gradient from 30 to 40 mm Hg, with the greatest compression at the ankle.
  - Donned on arising from bed and removed at bedtime.

- Effective in healing ulcers but can take months to obtain good results.
- Stockings do not correct the abnormal venous hemodynamics and must be worn after the ulcer has healed to prevent recurrence.
- Principal drawback is patient compliance.

- *Unna boots:*
  - Paste gauze compression dressings that contain zinc oxide, calamine, and glycerin.
  - Used to help prevent further skin breakdown.
  - Provide non-elastic compression therapy.
  - Changed once or twice a week.
  - Healing time for ulcers is less than that of elastic compression alone.
- *Pneumatic compression devices:*
- Provide dynamic sequential compression.
- Used primarily in the prevention of deep vein thrombi in hospitalized patients.
- Also used successfully to treat venous insufficiency.

Topical Medications

- Largely ineffective as a stand-alone therapy for venous stasis ulcers.
- Topical therapy is directed at absorbing wound drainage and avoiding desiccation of the wound.
- Antiseptics can be counterproductive. Hydrogen peroxide, povidone-iodine, acetic acid, and sodium hypochlorite are toxic to cultured fibroblasts and should be used for the shortest duration necessary to control ulcer infection.

Surgical Therapy

- *Skin grafting*
  - Occasionally used to speed healing of large ulcers.
  - Ulcer bed should be dry and free of infection.
  - Fenestrated split-thickness skin graft is preferred to allow for serous drainage.
  - Bed rest is recommended until the ulcer has healed completely.
  - Recurrence is common unless the underlying venous pathology is corrected or conservative support (elastic compression) is initiated and maintained after skin grafting. Cultured skin substitutes are now commonly used to minimize patient discomfort and avoid possible donor-site complications.
  - Stripping the greater saphenous vein.

12. Discuss the principles of different modalities of surgery for chronic venous stasis of inferior extremities.
WBUHS 2018

Venoablation

Venoablation is reserved for those with discomfort or ulcers refractory to medical management. The primary goal of surgical and endovenous approaches is to correct venous insufficiency by removing the major reflux pathways.

Techniques for venoablation include the following:

- Ligation with stripping
- Simple ligation and division
- Sclerotherapy (with or without ligation)
- Stab evulsion (with or without ligation)
- RFA
- EVLT
  - All methods of venoablation are effective (although there is some disagreement between the medical and the surgical literature as to the prevalence and timing of varicose recurrences). Once the overall volume of

venous reflux is reduced below a critical threshold by any mechanism, venous ulcerations heal, and patient symptoms are resolved.

- In general, vein ligation is reserved for cases of CVI involving reflux in the saphenous system that causes severe symptoms.
- Thus, a diagnosis of reflux must be established preoperatively, usually with photoplethysmography or duplex imaging.
- In patients with symptomatic varicosities of the GSV, deep occlusion must be ruled out; it is an absolute contraindication to vein ligation. Venography of the deep venous system before superficial vein ligation is imperative.
- Sclerotherapy is performed by injecting or infusing a sclerosing substance into the refluxing vessel to produce endothelial destruction and fibrosis of the treated vessel. Injection of a sclerosing agent directly into veins usually is reserved for telangiectatic lesions rather than CVI.
- Phlebotonics have not been proven to be beneficial for CVI.
- EVLT is performed by passing a laser fiber from the knee to the groin and then delivering laser energy along the entire course of the vein. Destruction of the vascular wall is followed by fibrosis of the treated vessel. It has been shown to yield excellent long-term (>5 years) results and a low rate of complications, which vary with the laser wavelength used.
- RFA is performed by passing a special RF catheter from the knee to the groin and then carrying out controlled and preset heating of the targeted vessel until thermal injury causes shrinkage. The process is repeated every 7 cm along the course of the vein. Initial thermal injury is followed by fibrosis of the treated vessel. RFA has been shown to be effective, with a low rate of complications. It has produced excellent results that have been confirmed with up to 10 years of follow-up.
- SEPS has also been employed to treat CVI. Endoscopic techniques are used to find and ligate perforating veins. Preliminary reports showed that after SEPS, the average healing time for ulcers was 42 days, with a recurrence rate of 3%, and that ulcers treated with SEPS healed 4 times faster than ulcers treated conventionally. In addition, the morbidity of SEPS was significantly lower than that of traditional operations.

DEEP VEIN THROMBOSIS (DVT) AND PULMONARY EMBOLISM (PE)

13. Deep vein thrombosis. ***SAIMS, Indore 2025; WBUHS 2014***

14. Diagnosis and management of DVT. ***WBUHS 2013***

15. Discuss the prophylaxis and management of deep vein thrombosis. ***WBUHS 2023, DNB 2024 October***

16. Risk factors for venous thromboembolism and recommended thromboprophylaxis in surgical patients. ***Maharashtra University of Health Sciences 2024***

Causes

- May develop in association with abnormalities of the vein wall, blood flow, or constituents of blood (Virchow's triad).
- May be due to vein compression or stasis (immobility, trauma, mass, bed rest, surgery, paralysis, and long-distance travel including airline travel).
- May be due to inherited hypercoagulability (factor V Leiden, protein C, protein S, or antithrombin insufficiency).
- May be due to acquired hypercoagulability [surgery, malignancy, polycythemia, smoking, hormone replacement therapy (HRT), oral contraceptive pill (OCP), and dehydration].

- Severity may vary from isolated asymptomatic tibial/calf thrombosis to severe iliofemoral segment thrombosis with phlegmasia cerulea dolens (venous gangrene).

Documented risk factors for deep vein thrombosis (DVT)

- Increasing age
- Obesity
- Prolonged immobility
- Varicose veins
- Stroke
- Cardiac dysfunction
- Paralysis
- Indwelling central venous catheters
- Previous venous thromboembolism
- Inflammatory bowel disease
- Cancer and its treatment
- Nephrotic syndrome
- Major surgery
- Pregnancy or estrogen use
- Trauma

Clinical Features

- Clinical manifestations may be absent.
- Local features of venous engorgement and stasis
- Limb swelling
- Pain
- Erythema and warmth to the touch
- Mild fever and tachycardia resulting from release of inflammatory mediators.
- Homan's sign calf pain on dorsiflexion of the foot is very unreliable and should not be performed.
- *Complications:*
    - PE
    - Venous gangrene (phlegmasia dolens)

Diagnosis and Investigations

- Aim to confirm presence and extent of thrombosis (to decide on necessity and type of treatment, risk of embolization).
- *Fibrin and fibrinogen assays:* The basis of fibrin or fibrinogen can be assayed by measuring the degradation of intravascular fibrin. The D-dimer test measures cross-linked degradation products, which is a surrogate of plasmin's activity on fibrin. It is shown that in combination with clinical evaluation and assessment, the sensitivity exceeds 90–95%. The negative predictive value is 99.3% for proximal evaluation and 98.6% for distal evaluation. In the postoperative patient, D-dimer is causally elevated due to surgery, and, as such, a positive D-dimer assay for evaluating for DVT is of no use. However, a negative D-dimer test in patients with suspected DVT has a high negative predictive value, ranging from 97 to 99%.
- *Ascending venography:* Rarely used now.
- *Duplex scan:* Investigation of choice. Visualizes anatomy and gives extent of thrombosis. Relies on flow of blood and compressibility of vein. Is operator-dependent and has lower sensitivity for calf DVT.
- *VQ scan:* If suspicion or evidence of PE.
- *CT pulmonary angiography (CTPA):* Safest, most sensitive, and most specific investigation for suspected PE.

Risk stratification for thromboembolism after surgery.

Level of risk	*Age (years)*	*Type of surgery*	*Additional risk factors*	*Incidence of proximal DVT (%)*	*Incidence of PE (%)*
Low	<40	Minor	None	0.4	<0.5
Moderate					
A B C	Any <40 40–60	Minor Major Nonmajor	Present None None		
High				4–8	2–4
A B C	>60 >40 <40	Nonmajor Major Major	± Other None Present		
Highest risk				10–20	4–10
B	>40	Major	Prior VTE Cancer Hypercoagulable state		

(DVT: deep vein thrombosis; PE: pulmonary embolism; VTE: venous thromboembolism)

Recommendations

- *Low-risk patients:* No prophylaxis is needed other than early ambulation
- *Moderate risk:* Low dose unfractionated heparin (LDUH) (5,000 U) BID or low-molecular-weight heparin (LMWH) (<3,400 U) QD or intermittent pneumatic compression stocking (IPCS). There is some data suggesting multiple modalities may be synergistic.
- *High risk:* LDUH (5,000 U) BID or TID or LMWH (<3,400 U) QD or IPCS
- *Highest risk:* LDUH (5,000 U) BID or TID or LMWH (<3,400 U) QD and IPCS

Arguments Against of Heparin Prophylaxis

- *Bleeding:* 2–3% increase risk compared with placebo
- *Heparin-induced thrombocytopenia:* Occurs in 1–5% of people and usually resolves with d/c of heparin. LMWHs have even a lower incidence.
- *Cost:* Cost-based analysis has shown heparin prophylaxis is far more cost effective when considering the decreased incidence of DVT and PE.

Treatment

Prophylaxis

- *Conservative measures:* Bed rest, elevation, and good hydration.
- *Uncomplicated DVT:* LMWH, initially in hospital; may be given on an outpatient basis via a dedicated DVT clinic. Subsequent treatment is with oral anticoagulation with warfarin for 3–6 months.
- *Complicated DVT:* Initially with IV unfractionated heparin (UFH) whilst converting to oral anticoagulation with warfarin.
  - Thrombolysis or surgical thrombectomy are reserved for severe thrombosis with venous gangrene.
  - Vena cava filter percutaneously inserted via jugular vein into infrarenal inferior vena cava (IVC) to catch thromboembolism and prevent PE.
    - *Used for patients:* With recurrent PEs despite treatment; at risk of major central PE; requiring urgent surgery despite high risk that DVT is present.
    - Risks include IVC obstruction, renal vein thrombosis, complications of insertion.

Thromboprophylaxis

The prevention of clots forming in the veins can be achieved in three ways: chemical thromboprophylaxis; mechanical thromboprophylaxis; or, a combination of chemical and mechanical.

Risks which Increase the Risk of Venous Thromboembolism (VTE)

- *Age:* There is an exponential increase in risk with age. In the general population:
  - <40 years—annual risk 1/10,000
  - 60–69 years—annual risk 1/1,000
  - 80 years—annual risk 1/100
  - This may reflect immobility and coagulation activation
    - *Obesity:* The risk of VTE is increased by three times if body mass index (BMI) ≥ 30 kg/m^2, again this may reflect immobility and coagulation activation.
    - *Varicose veins:* The risk is increased by 1.5 times when a patient with varicose veins undergoes major orthopedic or general surgery. However, the risk of VTE is low after varicose vein surgery.
    - *Immobility:* Bed rest >3 days. Lower limb immobility with plaster cast.
    - *Dehydration:* Increases the viscosity of the blood.
    - *Previous VTE:* Recurrence rate is 5%/year and this is increased by surgery.
    - Family history of VTE
    - Unidentified inherited thrombophilias will be risk factors which may be undiagnosed at time of admission.
    - *Surgery:* Without prophylaxis the rates of VTE after major orthopedic surgery are 40–60%. Major surgery includes >90 minutes duration.
    - *Pregnancy/postpartum:* There is a 10-fold increase in thrombotic risk throughout pregnancy and the puerperium. The same factors that increase thrombotic risk in nonpregnant patients also increase the risk of thrombosis associated with pregnancy. During pregnancy additional risk factors such as preeclampsia and delivery, particularly operative delivery, must be considered. If a patient is admitted to a general ward and is pregnant, the obstetric team must be informed and the appropriate risk assessment carried out.
    - *Thrombophilias:*
      - Low coagulation inhibitors (antithrombin, protein C or S)
      - Activated protein C resistance (e.g., factor V Leiden)
      - High coagulation factors (I, II, VIII, IX, and XI)
      - Antiphospholipid syndrome
      - High homocysteine

All patients with thrombophilias having major surgery should have their care discussed with a consultant hematologist. There may be a need for extended thromboprophylaxis.

- *Other thrombotic states:*
  - Malignancy 7X risk compared to the general population
  - Heart failure
  - Recent myocardial infarction/stroke
  - Acute infection
  - Inflammatory bowel disease and nephrotic syndrome
  - Polycythemia and paraproteinemia
  - Behçet's disease and paroxysmal nocturnal hemoglobinuria
- *Travel:* >3 hours within 4 weeks (pre and post) of surgery
- *Lower limb cast or similar appliance:* These inhibit venous return and increase the risk of pooling in the calf veins.
- *Medicines which increase the risk of VTE:*
  - Oral contraceptives/HRT and hormone therapy.
  - The use of oral contraceptives (estrogen and estrogen/progestogen) or HRT confers an increased risk of thromboembolism on all patients regardless of whether they are undergoing a surgical procedure.
  - *Progestogen:* Progestogen-only contraception—no increased risk is conferred on the patient. Therefore, advise patient to continue the contraceptive and risk assess the patient according to procedure and other thromboembolic or clinical risk factors.

  - *High-dose progestogens:* There is evidence of an association of VTE with higher doses of progestogen used for other therapeutic indications (e.g., menstrual disorders) therefore the patient will need at least 20 mg enoxaparin (dose dependent on other risk factors)
  - Combined oral contraceptives (COCPs) and HRT
  - Estrogen receptor antagonists—tamoxifen
  - Aromatase inhibitors
  - Thalidomide

The options available for thromboprophylaxis are:

- Mechanical thromboprophylaxis
  - Antiembolism stockings
  - Intermittent-pneumatic compression devices or foot impulse devices (may be used in theater)
  - IVC filter
- Pharmacological thromboprophylaxis
  - LMWH—enoxaparin
  - Oral anticoagulant—rivaroxaban for use in elective total hip replacement (THR) and total knee replacement (TKR) only
  - Unfractionated heparin (UFH)

---

17. Pulmonary embolism. ***WBUHS 2008***

Introduction

Pulmonary thromboembolism (PE) constitutes a problem of immense clinical importance. Diagnosis is often difficult because PE may mimic a variety of cardiopulmonary conditions.

Etiology

- Respiratory difficulty in the setting of elevated risk for thrombosis indicates a likelihood of PE.
- The highest rates of PE are documented in patients older than 60 years and those in the highest quintile of weight.
- Heavy tobacco use and hypertension were also risk factors for PE.
- Women taking hormone replacements have a two to three times increased risk of PE depending on the formulation.
- Patients with cancer and those undergoing surgery are also at increased risk for PE.

Clinical Features

- Dyspnea is the most common presenting symptom, and tachypnea is the most common sign.
- Pleuritic chest pain, cough, and/or hemoptysis can also occur.
- Helpful findings on physical examination include those that indicate right ventricular dysfunction, namely, bulging neck veins with V waves, a left parasternal lift, an accentuated pulmonic component of S_2, and a systolic murmur at the lower left sternal border that increases in inspiration.
- The differential diagnosis includes pneumonia, bronchitis, myocardial infarction, pulmonary edema, aortic dissection, pneumothorax, worsening chronic obstructive pulmonary disease, carcinoma of the lung, and primary pulmonary hypertension.

Investigations

- The diagnostic workup should include at the outset an electrocardiogram (ECG) and a chest radiograph. The most common ECG abnormality is T-wave inversion in the anterior precordial leads. Prominence of the S wave in lead I and a Q-wave and T-wave inversion in lead III may occur when right ventricular strain is present (S1Q3T3 pattern).
- Abnormalities seen on chest X-ray film include focal oligemia (Westermark's sign), a peripheral wedged-shaped density above the diaphragm (Hampton's hump), and an enlarged right descending pulmonary artery (Palla's sign).

- Arterial blood gases may be helpful in the differential diagnosis and should be analyzed when PE is suspected. Hypoxemia and/or hypocapnia are suggestive of but not specific for the diagnosis, and PE can occur in the setting of normal blood gas analyses.

Three more specific tests are helpful in the diagnosis of PE:

1. Perfusion lung scanning is the most useful screening test to rule out clinically significant PE. Normal results or results indicating a high probability of PE are useful. When the degree of clinical suspicion is high, low probability results should be considered non-diagnostic and further studies carried out.
2. Spiral CT with contrast is most accurate for PE involving the proximal pulmonary arteries.
3. Pulmonary arteriography should be used in the setting of high clinical suspicion with inconclusive scan results.

Ancillary tests include:

- *D-dimer ELISA:* The D-dimer lacks specificity and may be elevated in patients with myocardial infarction, pneumonia, heart failure, or cancer.
- *Lower extremity venous US:* Venous ultrasonography is accurate for the diagnosis of DVT, but a normal examination does not rule out a PE.
- *Transthoracic echocardiography:* Transthoracic echocardiography is useful in critically ill patients suspected of having a PE.
- Venous ultrasonography is accurate for the diagnosis of DVT, but a normal examination does not rule out a PE.
- The combination of right ventricular pressure overload, right ventricular hypokinesis, and positive findings on venous US of the leg veins is pathognomonic of PE.

Treatment

- Anticoagulation with heparin is the treatment of choice in all patients with PE unless contraindications such as active bleeding exist. Heparin should be given to all patients with a moderate or high clinical suspicion of PE during the definitive diagnostic workup. UFH should be given as an initial bolus of 5,000–10,000 units followed by a continuous infusion of 18 U/kg of body weight per hour (not to exceed 1,600 units per hour) with a target of a partial thromboplastin time of 60–80 seconds.
- LMWH may be given to hemodynamically stable patients with PE with comparable safety and efficacy. Heparin therapy is directed to the source of the embolus rather than the offending thrombus in the pulmonary artery.
- Thrombolysis is an established therapy for patients with PE and hemodynamic instability. These agents have been shown to dissolve thrombi and improve both pulmonary perfusion and right ventricular function.
- The patients with PE undergo echocardiography to assess the degree of right ventricular dysfunction and if moderate or severe receive intravenous alteplase in addition to heparin. Catheter-directed therapy allows the infusion of thrombolytic agents directly into the pulmonary artery thrombus. Wedging the catheter into the thrombus also allows for some thrombofragmentation with the potential for more rapid thrombolysis.
- Transvenous catheter embolectomy, percutaneous thrombofragmentation, or surgical embolectomy should be considered in patients with hemodynamic instability and contraindications to thrombolysis. Pulmonary embolectomy has been advocated as the procedure of last resort in patients with circulatory collapse and PE.
- In situations of hemodynamic collapse, percutaneous cardiopulmonary support systems can be used at the bedside as a bridge to emergent surgical embolectomy. These systems are compact, battery-operated portable units that employ femoral arterial and venous cannulas, a centrifugal pump, and a membrane oxygenator.
- Indications for aggressive intervention in a patient with a pulmonary embolism (at least one of the following should be present)

1. Arterial hypotension
2. Cardiogenic shock
3. Echocardiographic evidence of right ventricular failure
4. Precapillary pulmonary hypertension
5. Arterial-alveolar O_2 gradient >50 mm Hg
6. Contraindication to anticoagulation

Role of Caval Interruption

- Interruption of the IVC by either ligation, plication, or insertion of an intravascular device has been used for the prevention of PE. In some centers, filters have been used as an alternative to heparin therapy for primary prevention of PE in patients with DVT of the lower extremity thought to have contraindications to anticoagulation.
- Filters should be reserved for secondary prevention or in those patients with contraindications for anticoagulation.
- *Indications for inferior vena cava filter (IVCF) placement:*
  - *Contraindication to anticoagulation.*

Absolute indications	***Relative indications***
• Failure of anticoagulation—pulmonary embolism (PE) or recurrent deep vein thrombosis (DVT) while anticoagulated • Complications of anticoagulation • DVT/PE with contraindication to anticoagulation • Failure of previously placed filter • After pulmonary embolectomy	• Large free-floating thrombus • DVT in patients with poor cardiopulmonary reserve • Protection during thrombolytic therapy • High-risk trauma patients • High-risk surgical patients • Cancer patients with DVT/PE • High-risk patients with prolonged bed rest • Pregnant patients

  - Complication with anticoagulation.
  - Recurrent PE despite anticoagulation or presence of another device.
  - Prophylaxis in the presence of DVT/PE.
  - Following pulmonary embolectomy.

Prevention

Recommendations for venous prophylaxis

Surgical risk	***Recommendation***
Low: <40 years, minor procedure	Early ambulation
Moderate: Minor procedures with thrombosis risk factors, age 40-60 years, major surgery in patients <40 years	Elastic stockings or IPC or low-dose UFH (5,000 IU SC q 12h)
High: >60 years, >40 years with major procedures and risk factors for thrombosis	LMWH or IPC
Very high: >60 years with associated risk factors for thrombosis	LMWH and IPC
Total Joint replacement	LMWH or warfarin started preoperatively or Immediately postoperatively and continued
Very high with additional high risk for bleeding	IPC

(IPC: intermittent pneumatic compression; LMWH: low-molecular-weight heparin; SC: subcutaneously; UFH: unfractionated heparin)

18. Inferior vena caval (IVC) filter. ***Gujarat Health University 2024***

Definition

An *IVC filter* is a *metallic device* implanted in the *inferior vena cava* to *trap emboli* (usually thrombi from the lower limbs or pelvis) and *prevent pulmonary embolism (PE)*, while still allowing blood flow.

Indications

Absolute Indications (Classical)

Used in patients with *documented venous thromboembolism (VTE)* who *cannot receive anticoagulation.*

Absolute indication	***Example***
Contraindication to anticoagulation	Active bleeding (e.g., GI bleed, intracranial hemorrhage)
Complication of anticoagulation	Heparin-induced thrombocytopenia
Failure of anticoagulation	Recurrent PE despite adequate anticoagulation
High risk of PE with DVT	Extensive iliofemoral thrombosis, free-floating thrombus

Relative/Extended Indications

(Controversial, individualized)

- Prophylaxis in major trauma or spinal cord injury (high PE risk)
- Perioperative protection in high-risk orthopedic or neurosurgical patients
- Following pulmonary embolectomy (to prevent recurrence)
- Massive PE with residual DVT when anticoagulation is temporarily contraindicated

Types of IVC Filters

Type	*Description*	*Example*
Permanent filters	Designed for lifelong implantation	Greenfield filter
Retrievable (optional) filters	Can be removed once PE risk subsides	Günther Tulip, Celect, Option Elite
Temporary filters	Short-term use (attached via catheter)	Less commonly used

Site of Placement

- Usually placed *below the renal veins* (infrarenal IVC) to preserve renal venous drainage.
- *Suprarenal placement* indicated if:
  - Thrombus extends above renal veins
  - Pregnancy
  - IVC duplication or anomalies

Insertion Technique

- *Access:* Via *right internal jugular* or *femoral vein* (under fluoroscopic or ultrasound guidance).
- *IVC venography:* Performed to confirm anatomy and select site.
- *Filter deployment:* Expanded to engage the IVC walls.
- *Postprocedure imaging:* To confirm correct position and patency.

Mechanism of Action

- Filter acts as a *mechanical barrier*, trapping large emboli from deep venous thrombi before they reach the lungs.
- Blood continues to flow around and through the filter's struts.

Complications

Early/procedural	*Late/long-term*
Venous injury or perforation	IVC thrombosis or occlusion
Malposition or migration	Recurrent DVT (due to stasis)
Filter tilt or fracture	Penetration into adjacent structures (aorta, duodenum)
Access site hematoma	Difficulty removing retrievable filter

Retrievable filters should be *removed once PE risk has passed* (usually within weeks to months) to reduce long-term complications.

Follow-up

- Periodic *imaging (Doppler/CT/fluoroscopy)* to check position and patency.
- Resume *anticoagulation* as soon as it is safe, even with a filter in place.
- *Filter retrieval* if indication resolved and device is retrievable.

19. Discuss the perioperative management of a patient on thromboprophylaxis [postcoronary artery bypass graft (CABG) status] requiring emergency exploratory laparotomy. ***WBUHS 2018***

Introduction

- Perioperative management of anticoagulant therapy is constantly evolving, with the primary aim being a balance between reducing the risk of systemic arterial and venous embolism and reducing perioperative bleeding risk.

- The traditional strategy to "bridge" interrupted warfarin therapy for atrial fibrillation with the administration of LMWH is under review, following the results of large and influential studies such as the BRIDGE trial.
- The use of novel oral anticoagulants (NOACs) is also increasing and so it is crucial to understand both the pharmacokinetics of these drugs and their use in the perioperative period. Recommendations related to drugs used to modify coagulation:

Drug	*Time to peak effect*	*Elimination half-life*	*Acceptable time after drug for block performance*	*Administration of drug while spinal or epidural catheter in place*	*Acceptable time after block performance or catheter removal for next drug dose*
Warfarin	3–5 days	4–5 days	INR 1–4 or below	Not recommended	After catheter removal
Rivaroxaban prophylaxis (creatinine clearance >30 mL min^{-1})	3 hours	7–9 hours	18 hours	Not recommended	6 hours
Rivaroxaban treatment (creatinine clearance >30 mL min^{-1})	3 hours	7–11 hours	48 hours	Not recommended	6 hours
Apixaban prophylaxis	3–4 hours	12 hours	24–48 hours	Not recommended	6 hours
Dabigatran prophylaxis or treatment					
Creatinine clearance >80 mL min^{-1}	0.5–2 hours	12–17 hours	48 hours	Not recommended	6 hours
Creatinine clearance 50–80 mL min^{-1}	0.5–1 hours	15 hours	72 hours	Not recommended	6 hours
Creatinine clearance 30–50 mL min^{-1}	0.5–2 hours	18 hours	96 hours	Not recommended	6 hours

Management of patients undergoing emergency surgery while taking dabigatran.

Dabigatran	
<30 ng/mL	Operate
APTT <1.2	
Dabigatran >30 ng/mL 200 ng/mL APTT >1.2 <1.5	• Wait 12 hours and obtain new test • If emergent, operate and antagonize anticoagulant effect as needed
Dabigatran >200 ng/mL APTT >1.5	• Wait 12 hours and obtain new lest delay surgery as much as possible • Discuss hemodialysis, especially if creatinine clearance <50 mL/min • If emergent, operate and antagonize anticoagulant effect as needed
Dabigatran >400 ng/mL	• Major hemorrhagic risk • Hemodialysis

(APTT: activated partial thromboplastin time)

Management of patients undergoing emergency surgery while taking rivaroxaban.

Rivaroxaban	
<30 ng/mL	Operate
APTT <1.2 and PT <1.2	
Rivaroxaban >30 ng/mL <200 ng/mL APTT >1.2 <1.5 and PT >1.2	• Wait 12 hours and obtain new test • If emergent, operate and antagonize anticoagulant effect as needed
Rivaroxaban >200 ng/mL APTT >1.5	• Wait 12 hours and obtain new test • Delay surgery as much as possible • If emergent, operate and antagonize anticoagulant effect as needed
Rivaroxaban >400 ng/mL	Major hemorrhagic risk

(APTT: activated partial thromboplastin time; PT: prothrombin time)

If no specific reversal agent is available, nonspecific hemostatic agents can be used for reversal of excessive bleeding.

- Recombinant factor 7a initiates thrombin generation by activating factor 10.
- Four-factor prothrombin complex concentrates contain large amounts of nonactivated vitamin K-dependent factors 2, 7, 9, and 10.
- Three-factor prothrombin complexes contain small amounts of nonactive factor 7 relating to 2, 9, and 10.
- Activated prothrombin complex concentrate contains activated factor 7 and factors 2, 9, and 10.

One of the specific characteristics of emergency surgery is its limitation in patient preparation.

- Elimination of certain patient-related factors to lower the operative risk is difficult and often impossible.
- Effects of some drugs being used by the patients in the emergency setting, such as anticoagulant drugs, may therefore raise important issues.
- The introduction of anticoagulant drugs represented a major breakthrough in the treatment and prophylaxis of some cardiovascular diseases.
- Similarly, the possibility of safe oral administration allowed the patients to treat themselves in the comfort of their homes.
- Therefore, the introduction of oral anticoagulant drugs was welcomed by both patients and clinicians.

The reversal agent used for warfarin is a synthetic preparation of phytomenadione (vitamin K_1). The presence of vitamin K is essential for formation of prothrombin, factor 7, factor 9, and factor 10.

- Major bleeding—stop warfarin sodium; give 5 mg phytomenadione (vitamin K_1) by intravenous injection; give four-factor prothrombin complex (factors 2, 7, 9, and 10); if prothrombin complex unavailable. Fresh-frozen plasma can be given but is less effective.
- International normalized ratio (INR) > 8.0, minor bleeding—stop warfarin sodium; give 1–3 mg phytomenadione (vitamin K_1) by slow IV injection; repeat dose of phytomenadione if INR still too high after 24 hours; restart warfarin sodium when INR < 5.0.
- INR > 8.0, no bleeding—stop warfarin sodium; give 2.5 mg phytomenadione (vitamin K_1) by mouth using the IV preparation orally; repeat dose of phytomenadione if INR still too high after 24 hours; restart warfarin when INR <5.0.
- INR 5.0–8.0, minor bleeding—stop warfarin sodium; give 1–3 mg phytomenadione (vitamin K_1) by IV injection; restart warfarin sodium when INR <5.0.
- INR 5.0–8.0, no bleeding—withhold one or two doses of warfarin sodium and reduce subsequent maintenance dose.

Unexpected bleeding at therapeutic levels—always investigate the possibility of underlying cause, e.g., unsuspected renal or gastrointestinal (GI) tract pathology.

20. Prevention and management of Deep Venous Thrombosis in COVID-19 patient. Add note on newer oral anticoagulants. ***DY Patil Educational Society, Deemed to be University 2025***

Deep Venous Thrombosis (DVT) in COVID-19 Patients

Definition

Deep venous thrombosis (DVT) refers to *formation of a thrombus in the deep veins,* usually of the lower limbs, which may lead to *pulmonary embolism (PE)* and *venous thromboembolism (VTE).* In COVID-19, the risk of DVT and VTE is significantly increased due to the *prothrombotic (hypercoagulable) state* associated with the infection.

A. Pathophysiology of DVT in COVID-19

COVID-19–associated coagulopathy results from a combination of *Virchow's triad*:

Factor	Mechanism in COVID-19
Endothelial injury	SARS-CoV-2 infects endothelial cells via ACE2 receptors → endotheliitis → release of von Willebrand factor and tissue factor
Hypercoagulability	Cytokine storm (IL-6, TNF-α) → increased fibrinogen, factor VIII, D-dimer → excessive thrombin generation
Venous stasis	Prolonged immobilization, hypoxia, sedation, mechanical ventilation

Additional contributors:
- Platelet activation
- Complement activation
- Hypoxia-induced vasoconstriction and erythrocytosis
- Disseminated intravascular coagulation (DIC)-like state in severe cases

B. Prevention of DVT in COVID-19 patients
- *General preventive measures*

Measure	Details
Early mobilization	Encourage movement, physiotherapy, and limb exercises in stable patients
Hydration	Maintain adequate fluid intake to prevent hemoconcentration
Compression devices	Graduated compression stockings or intermittent pneumatic compression if not contraindicated
Avoid risk factors	Discontinue estrogen therapy, avoid dehydration, correct sepsis and hypoxia promptly

- *Pharmacologic prophylaxis*

All hospitalized COVID-19 patients (unless contraindicated) should receive *thromboprophylaxis.*

Clinical setting	Recommended prophylaxis
Non-ICU (moderate disease)	Low molecular weight Heparin (LMWH), e.g. *Enoxaparin 40 mg SC once daily*
ICU/severe disease	Intermediate or full-dose LMWH (e.g. *Enoxaparin 40 mg SC twice daily* or 1 mg/kg SC BID)—based on institutional protocols and D-dimer levels
Renal impairment (CrCl <30 mL/min)	*Unfractionated heparin (UFH)* 5000 units SC every 8–12 hours
Contraindicated to anticoagulation (active bleeding)	Mechanical prophylaxis (compression stockings) only

Duration:
- Continue until patient is ambulatory.
- *Postdischarge prophylaxis* (2–6 weeks) may be considered in high-risk cases (elevated D-dimer, cancer, prolonged immobility).

C. Diagnosis of DVT

Investigation	Findings
D-dimer	Elevated (nonspecific but sensitive)
Compression venous ultrasonography	Gold standard for limb DVT
CT pulmonary angiography	If pulmonary embolism suspected
Coagulation profile	May show high fibrinogen and mildly prolonged PT/aPTT

D. Management of established DVT in COVID-19
- *Anticoagulation therapy*

Drug	Regimen	Remarks
LMWH (Enoxaparin)	1 mg/kg SC every 12 hours (therapeutic dose)	Preferred; predictable effect, less monitoring
UFH (Heparin infusion)	Continuous IV, titrated to aPTT	For patients with renal impairment or high bleeding risk
Transition to oral anticoagulant	After stabilization (usually 5–10 days)	Can switch to warfarin or NOACs (DOACs)

- *Monitoring*
- Platelet count (for HIT)
- aPTT (for UFH)
- D-dimer and fibrinogen trends
- Clinical signs of bleeding
- *Supportive and adjunctive measures*
- Adequate oxygenation (hypoxia worsens thrombosis)
- Manage comorbidities (diabetes, obesity)
- Compression stockings after acute phase to prevent post-thrombotic syndrome

E. Complications of DVT
- *Pulmonary embolism (PE)* → sudden dyspnea, chest pain, hemoptysis, shock
- *Post-thrombotic syndrome* → chronic leg pain, swelling, ulceration
- *Recurrent venous thromboembolism (VTE)*
- *Heparin-induced thrombocytopenia (HIT)*

Newer Oral Anticoagulants (NOACs/DOACs)

Types

Class	Drugs	Mechanism of action
Direct factor Xa inhibitors	*Rivaroxaban, Apixaban, Edoxaban*	Inhibit factor Xa → prevent thrombin generation
Direct thrombin inhibitor	*Dabigatran etexilate*	Inhibits thrombin (Factor IIa) directly

Advantages
- Oral administration, fixed dosing
- No need for routine INR monitoring
- Rapid onset and offset of action
- Fewer food and drug interactions than warfarin
- Predictable pharmacokinetics

Disadvantages
- High cost
- Contraindicated in severe renal or hepatic impairment
- Limited availability of specific reversal agents (though now available: *Idarucizumab* for *dabigatran, andexanet* alfa for Xa inhibitors)
- Short half-life—missing doses increases thrombotic risk
- Not suitable for mechanical heart valves or pregnancy

Typical Regimens (for DVT/VTE)

Drug	Dosage	Remarks
Rivaroxaban	15 mg twice daily × 21 days, then 20 mg once daily	Take with food
Apixaban	10 mg twice daily × 7 days, then 5 mg twice daily	Dose adjust in renal dysfunction
Dabigatran	150 mg twice daily (after 5–10 days parenteral anticoagulation)	Avoid in CrCl <30 mL/min

Lymphatics

21. Primary lymphedema. *WBUHS 2010*

Primary lymphedema.

	Congenital hyperplasia (10%)	*Distal obliteration (80%)*	*Proximal obliteration (10%)*
Age of onset	Congenital	Puberty (praecox)	Any age
Sex distribution	Male > female	female > male	Male = female
Extent	Whole leg	Ankle and calf	Whole leg and thigh only
Laterality	Unilateral = bilateral	Often bilateral	Usually unilateral
Family history	Often positive	Often positive	No
Progression	Progressive	Slow	Rapid
Response to compression therapy	Variable	Good	Poor
Comments	Lymphatics are Increased In number; although functionally defective, there Is usually an Increased number of lymph nodes. May have chylous ascites, chylothorax and protein-losing enteropathy	Absent or reduced distal superficial lymphatics. Also termed aplasia or hypoplasia	There Is obstruction at the level of the aortoiliac or Inguinal nodes. If associated with distal dilatation, the patient may benefit from lymphatic bypass operation. Other patients have distal obliteration as well

ARTERY

22. Write in brief on investigations and management of peripheral occlusive arterial disease. *WBUHS 2024*

Peripheral Occlusive Arterial Disease (POAD): Investigations and Management

Investigations

Clinical Assessment

- *History:* Intermittent claudication, rest pain, non-healing ulcers.
- *Examination:* Pulse examination, capillary refill time, skin changes.

Noninvasive Tests

- *Ankle-Brachial Index (ABI):* ABI < 0.9 suggests POAD.
- *Duplex ultrasonography:* Assesses blood flow and location of occlusion.

Imaging

- *CT angiography or MR angiography:* Detailed vascular mapping.
  - CTA is another modality used to image arterial disease. It does have some pitfalls, such as the requirement for large amounts of contrast media, the necessity of synchronizing the image acquisition with the media administration, and the need for an upgraded CT scanner with postprocessing techniques to reconstruct helpful images. However, advances in technology now allow three-dimensional (3D) and four-dimensional (4D) reconstructions providing temporal information.
  - MRA is useful for imaging large and small vessels. Although it was initially considered to provide inadequate images, this is no longer the case. With improved imaging capabilities, MRA can be used not only to diagnose but also to help plan the type of indicated intervention.
  - A study that compared MRA with conventional angiography in regard to quality of life and cost-effectiveness found that although MRA was nearly 20% cheaper, there was no difference in quality of life.

- *Digital Subtraction Angiography (DSA):* Gold standard for diagnosis and pre-intervention planning.

Laboratory Tests

- Lipid profile, blood glucose, renal function, coagulation profile.

In July 2014, the Society for Cardiac Angiography and Interventions (SCAI) issued a consensus statement on the treatment of infrapopliteal arterial disease.

The statement indicated the following:

- Endovascular intervention is not appropriate for most single-vessel, mildly symptomatic, or asymptomatic blockages of infrapopliteal vessels.
- It is not appropriate to treat most cases of moderate-to-severe claudication or major tissue loss in one-vessel disease and mild claudication in one-, two-, or three-vessel disease.
- Primary amputation should be the preferred intervention in non-ambulatory patients with a limited life expectancy and extensive necrosis or gangrene.
- Consider surgical bypass and evaluate its associated risks for ambulatory patients with a patent infrapopliteal artery that has direct flow to the foot and an adequate autologous venous conduit.
- Use balloon angioplasty for clinically significant infrapopliteal arterial disease; consider bailout bare-metal and drug-eluting stents for tibial arterial disease that is refractory to treatment with balloon angioplasty.

Moreover, the SCAI indicated that intervention for infrapopliteal disease is appropriate in patients with two- or three-vessel disease and (1) moderate-to-severe claudication with a focal arterial lesion; (2) ischemic foot pain during rest (Rutherford classification 4); or (3) minor and major (skin necrosis, gangrene) tissue loss.

Management

- *Lifestyle modifications:*
  - Smoking cessation
  - Regular supervised exercise programs
  - Diet control for dyslipidemia and diabetes
- *Medical management:*
  - *Antiplatelets:* Aspirin or clopidogrel
  - *Statins:* For lipid control and plaque stabilization
  - Antihypertensives & Diabetes control
- *Endovascular treatment:*
  - Angioplasty with or without stenting
- *Surgical management:*
  - *Bypass surgery:* For long-segment occlusion or failed endovascular therapy
  - *Endarterectomy:* In selected cases
  - Advanced Therapies (in critical limb ischemia):
  - Amputation (if limb is non-viable)
  - Stem cell or gene therapy (experimental)

---

23. Acute limb ischemia. ***Ayush University, Chhattisgarh 2025***

---

24. Describe acute lower limb ischemia and its management. ***Gujarat Health University 2025.***

---

25. Mention the causes of acute limb ischemia. Discuss briefly the clinical features and management of acute limb ischemia. ***WBUHS 2025***

Definition

Acute limb ischemia is a *sudden decrease in limb perfusion* that threatens the *viability of the limb* and occurs *within 14 days* of symptom onset.

It is a *vascular emergency* requiring prompt recognition and management to prevent limb loss or death.

Etiology (Causes)

- *Embolism (≈ 40–50%)*
  - Common source: *Heart*
    - Atrial fibrillation (most common)
    - Mural thrombus after MI
    - Valvular heart disease (mitral stenosis)
    - Prosthetic valves, infective endocarditis
  - Usually *sudden onset, previously normal limb, no collaterals*
- *Thrombosis (≈ 40%)*
  - Occurs on *pre-existing atherosclerotic artery*
  - May be precipitated by:
    - Plaque rupture
    - Low flow (e.g. hypotension)
    - Trauma or dissection
  - *History of claudication, presence of collaterals*
- *Trauma:*
  - Arterial injury (penetrating or blunt trauma)
  - Iatrogenic (e.g., during catheterization)
- *Dissection:* Aortic dissection extending into limb vessels
- *Hypercoagulable states:*
  - Malignancy
  - Antiphospholipid syndrome
  - Protein C/S or antithrombin III deficiency

Pathophysiology

↓ Arterial perfusion → ↓ Oxygen delivery →
→ Ischemia → Cellular hypoxia → Tissue necrosis

Time is Muscle

Irreversible changes start within *6 hours* of complete ischemia.

Clinical Features

Classic "6 P's" of Acute Limb Ischemia

Feature	***Explanation***
Pain	Sudden, severe distal limb pain
Pallor	Pale, cold limb
Pulselessness	Absence of distal pulses
Paresthesia	Tingling, sensory loss (ischemic neuropathy)
Paralysis	Late sign—muscle infarction
Poikilothermia	Limb cold to touch

Additional Signs

- Demarcation line between viable and ischemic skin
- Mottling or cyanosis (indicates severe ischemia)

Classification (Rutherford Classification of ALI)

Grade	*Findings*	*Limb viability*
I—Viable	No sensory/motor deficit, audible Doppler signals	Not immediately threatened
IIa—Marginally threatened	Minimal sensory loss (toes), no motor loss	Salvageable if treated promptly
IIb—Immediately threatened	Sensory loss > toes, mild–moderate weakness	Requires *immediate revascularization*
III—Irreversible	Profound anesthesia, paralysis, rigor	*Major tissue loss inevitable, amputation indicated*

Investigations

- *Bedside*
  - *Doppler ultrasound*: Absence of arterial flow
  - *Ankle-brachial index (ABI)* <0.3 indicates severe ischemia
- *Laboratory*
  - CBC, coagulation profile
  - Renal function, electrolytes
  - Serum CK (muscle necrosis indicator)
- *Imaging*
  - *CT angiography (CTA)*: Gold standard for defining level of occlusion
  - *Duplex Doppler ultrasound*: Quick, bedside
  - *Catheter-based angiography*: Diagnostic and therapeutic (for thrombolysis)

Management

Goal: Restore perfusion as early as possible to prevent irreversible damage. Treatment depends on *cause, site,* and *limb viability.*

Immediate (Initial) Management

- *Hospital admission*
- *Anticoagulation:* IV unfractionated *heparin bolus (5000 U)* then infusion → Prevents propagation of thrombus
- *Analgesia:* Opioids
- *Limb care:*
  - Keep limb *dependent (not elevated)*
  - Avoid heat or cold
- Protect from trauma
- *IV fluids* (prevent myoglobinuria-induced renal failure)

Definitive Management

Depends on severity (viability of the limb) and cause:

- *Embolectomy or thrombectomy:*
  - Open surgical or catheter-directed
  - Especially for embolic occlusion
- *Thrombolysis:*
  - Catheter-directed intra-arterial thrombolysis with agents like alteplase
  - Used for select patients with viable limbs
- *Bypass surgery:* In cases of thrombosed chronic occlusion
- *Percutaneous transluminal angioplasty (PTA) and stenting:* Minimally invasive option for selected cases
- *Amputation:* If limb is nonviable and revascularization is not possible

Cause/Grade	Treatment
Embolism (Grade IIb)	*Urgent surgical embolectomy* (Fogarty catheter) ± intraoperative angiography
Thrombosis (Grade IIa–IIb)	*Catheter-directed thrombolysis* (tPA, urokinase) or *angioplasty/stenting*
Viable limb (Grade I)	Medical management + observation ± delayed revascularization
Irreversible (Grade III)	*Primary amputation* to prevent sepsis, myoglobinuria
Adjuncts	Fasciotomy if reperfusion injury or compartment syndrome develops

Postrevascularization Care

- Monitor for *reperfusion injury* (hyperkalemia, myoglobinuria, renal failure)
- Continue anticoagulation (heparin → warfarin or DOAC)
- Treat *underlying cause* (e.g., control AF, diabetes, atherosclerosis)

Complications

- Reperfusion injury
- Compartment syndrome
- Myonephropathic metabolic syndrome (myoglobinuria → renal failure)
- Infection and gangrene
- Amputation
- Death (from sepsis or renal failure)

Prognosis

- *Limb salvage rate:* 70–80% (if treated promptly)
- *Amputation rate:* Up to 30% in delayed cases
- *Mortality:* 15–25% (often due to cardiac comorbidities)

26. Chronic limb ischemia. *WBUHS 2009*

Upper limb ischemia occurs less frequently than lower limb ischemia.

Causes

- Previous trauma or axillary irradiation leading to arterial stenosis.
- Buerger's disease. Affects small vessels of the hands and feet, principally in smokers, associated with Raynaud's phenomenon. Mostly young men but women may be affected. Presents with digital gangrene/ischemia and may present with acute limb ischemia in young people.
- Subclavian steal syndrome. Reversed flow in the vertebral artery/diminished hindbrain perfusion (dizziness/syncope), arm claudication.
- Takayasu's arteritis. Uncommon in Europe; major arch/upper limb vessels affected.
- Thoracic outlet syndrome
    - Term used to cover a spectrum of symptoms resulting from the compression of the neurovascular bundle as it leaves the chest to enter the upper limb, in an area enclosed by the first rib, clavicle, and scalenus anterior.
    - Presents as a variable combination of neural, arterial, and venous symptoms exacerbated by elevation of the limb, with pain, paresthesias, weakness, or arm claudication. 95% are neurogenic and 5% are arterial or venous manifestations.

Clinical Features

- Weakness, cramp, or exercise-related pain and digital ischemia/gangrene.
- Examine bilateral upper limb pulses, BP in both arms (elevated/at sides), wrist Doppler pressures.
- *Roos test:* Arm abducted to 90 Â°, hands up with elbows braced backward, chin elevated, hands serially clenched/opened for 1–2 minutes. Test positive if pain or weakness in hand or forearm.

- *Adson's test:* Pulse diminishes or absent on elevation/abduction of arm with head turned to contralateral side. Reliability improved by using in conjunction with arterial duplex.
- *Allen's test:* Assesses integrity of the palmar arch and dominant vessel (radial or ulnar).
- *Tinel's test:* To exclude carpal tunnel syndrome.

Diagnosis and Investigations

- Cervical spine and thoracic outlet X-rays; wrist Doppler pressures.
- CT/MRI to exclude fibrous bands/ribs.
- Arterial duplex or angiography to exclude proximal arterial lesions.

Treatment

- *Thoracic outlet syndrome:*
  - *Mild neurogenic problem:* Simple analgesia and advice on risk factors
  - Surgery has good results for those with arterial or venous symptoms/complications
  - Excision of the first rib/band will improve symptoms in over 90%.
  - Careful evaluation is needed prior to surgery for pure neurological symptoms, e.g., nerve conduction studies.
- Cervical sympathectomy in upper limb disease

Indications

- Palmar hyperhidrosis (not axillary)
- Buerger's disease/small vessel disease with digital gangrene

Complications

- Horner's syndrome
- Pneumothorax
- Hemorrhage
- Compensatory truncal hyperhidrosis
- Frey's syndrome (gustatory sweating)
  - *Axillary hyperhidrosis:* Treatment of choice is now subcutaneous (SC) botulinum toxin injections to the axillary sweat glands, repeated as necessary.

Chronic Lower Limb Ischemia

Introduction

- Atherosclerosis is a generalized disease and has a predilection for the coronary, cerebral, and peripheral circulations.
- In the lower limb it may affect the aortoiliac, femoral or popliteal, and calf vessel levels singly or in combinations.
- Single-level disease usually results in intermittent claudication (IC) and two-level disease in critical limb ischemia (CLI).
  - *La Fontaine classification of lower limb ischemia:*
    - Asymptomatic
    - C
    - Rest pain
    - Ulcers/gangrene

  Grades III and IV = CLI
  - *Intermittent claudication*

Key Facts

- Affects 7% of men over 50 years of age.
- M:F ratio is 2:1.
- One-third of patients improve, one-third remain stable, and one-third deteriorate.
- 4% require an intervention and 1% result in amputation.

Intermittent claudication: Risk factors and associations.	
Risk factors	***Associations***
• Hypertension • Hyperlipidemia • Diabetes mellitus • Tobacco smoking • Positive family history	• Obesity • Diet • Sedentary lifestyle • Gender • Occupation

Clinical Features

- *Pain on exercise of the affected limb:* Worsened with increasing level of exercise; relieved by rest.
- *Differential diagnosis.*
  - *Spinal stenosis:* Symptoms caused by drop in distal corda equina blood flow due to exercise leading to neurogenic pain.
  - Osteoarthritis, especially hip joint.
  - Nerve root entrapment.
  - Popliteal artery entrapment due to compression of popliteal artery over medial head of gastrocnemius during exercise. Distal pulses reduced/absent on plantar flexion alone. Treated by surgical release after MRI defines anatomy.

Diagnosis and Investigation

- Diagnosis is clinical and not based on imaging.
- Serum fasting glucose, serum cholesterol, blood pressure (BP) checked on initial presentation.
- Imaging is only conducted for worsening symptoms, failure to respond to conservative management, and consideration of surgery.
  - Angiography [usually digital subtraction angiography (DSA), perhaps CT angiogram, or magnetic resonance angiography (MRA)].
- Abdominal US if aneurysm disease suspected.

Treatment

- *Risk factor modification:*
  - 40% of patients with peripheral vascular disease have coronary or cerebral arterial disease. The mainstay of treatment is aggressive risk factor modification.
  - Stop smoking, oral statin treatment, increased exercise, control of BP, and serum glucose.
- *Endovascular treatment:*
  - Angioplasty ± stent. Excellent results in the aortoiliac segment (over 90% success) and good results in the superficial femoral segment (90% success and 60–80% patency at 2 years).
  - Usually performed under LA, percutaneously as a day case.
  - Rarely performed for claudication in the popliteal and tibial segments due to high risk of occlusion.
- *Surgery:*
  - *Indications for surgery are as follows:*
  - *Failure/unsuitability for endovascular treatment (EVT) in the aortoiliac segments. Procedures available are:*
    - *Aortobifemoral graft:* 5-year patency of over 90% but carries a 5–8% mortality and a risk of impotence; used for younger patients;
    - *Femorofemoral crossover bypass graft:* Used for isolated unilateral iliac disease. 90% 1-year patency
    - *Common femoral endarterectomy:* Used for isolated common femoral disease; good results; and a low complication rate.
  - Short distance claudication, severe lifestyle limitation, or failed medical therapy in infrainguinal (superficial femoral, popliteal, and distal) disease. Risks are significant. Procedures available are:
    - *Femoro-above knee popliteal bypass:* 80% 2-year patency with vein or prosthetic graft
    - *Femoro-below knee popliteal bypass:* 70% 2-year patency with vein graft
    - *Femoro-distal (below knee) bypass:* 5-year patency <35%. Usually reserved only for critical ischemia.

27. Raynaud's phenomenon. ***WBUHS 2007, 2015***

Introduction

- In 1862, Maurice Raynaud was the first to document that some individuals developed discoloration of their digits upon cold exposure, which was presumed to be an abnormal response of the CNS.
- It is now recognized that this phenomenon is secondary to vasoconstriction of the digital arteries, precapillary arterioles, and cutaneous arteriovenous shunts.
- Although the exact mechanism of this vasospastic abnormality remains elusive and in most patients the etiology ill defined, recent investigations suggest that elevated levels of homocysteine or recent viral infection may play a role in at least a subset of patients.
- In addition, Raynaud's syndrome may occur in response to interferon treatment, as a paraneoplastic syndrome from non-small-cell lung cancer, or as a generalized vasospastic disorder associated with Prinzmetal's angina, migraines, or scleroderma.

Presentation

- In its classic form, Raynaud's syndrome presents with digital ischemia in response to a cold exposure.
- It typically commences in one or several fingers and then spreads to both hands.
- The duration of the attack is variable and culminates in an erythematous recovery known as reactive hyperemia.
- Before recovery, the digits can turn white, blue, and red.
- The lack of a clinical history of tricolor changes excludes the diagnosis of Raynaud's syndrome.
- Women are more commonly affected than men, and although this gender discrepancy occurs in both pediatric and adult populations, the syndrome most commonly arises in the second and third decades of life.
- The syndrome is more common in geographic regions with cooler daily temperatures and in winter months.
  - *Primary versus secondary Raynaud's syndrome:* Raynaud's syndrome is classically divided into primary and secondary and each is defined by certain clinical criteria.
  - *Primary Raynaud's syndrome* occurs in patients with symmetric attacks; absence of tissue necrosis, ulceration, or gangrene; the absence of a secondary cause on the basis of history and physical examination; normal nail-fold capillaries; a negative test for antinuclear antibody; and a normal erythrocyte sedimentation rate.
  - *Secondary Raynaud's syndrome* is suggested by an age at onset of older than 30 years; episodes that are intense, painful, asymmetric, or associated with ischemic skin lesions; clinical features suggestive of an underlying connective tissue disorder; specific autoantibodies; and evidence of microvascular disease on microscopy of nailfold capillaries.
    - Recent work has suggested that duplex determination of carotid elasticity and stiffness may also assist in differentiating between the two forms.
    - A clear distinction between primary and secondary Raynaud's syndrome may be difficult.

Management

- The initial therapy for Raynaud's syndrome is avoidance of a cold stimulus and use of appropriate attire that minimizes cold exposure such as gloves and stockings. Because Raynaud's syndrome is a sympathetic-mediated response, anxiety can provoke vasospasm. Thus, reduction of anxiety or avoidance of stressful situations can assist in reducing symptom occurrence.
- Although smoking has never been implicated as a causative factor in the development of Raynaud's syndrome, it adversely effects digital blood flow and should be avoided. In addition to these recommendations, a variety of pharmacologic and surgical approaches are available for managing this disorder.

Medication

- *Nifedipine* is a calcium channel blocker—a type of medication that encourages the blood vessels to dilate.
- Angiotensin-converting enzyme (ACE) inhibitors
- Fluoxetine—which was widely used in the treatment of depression

- Sildenafil—which is used to treat erectile dysfunction (inability to get or maintain an erection)—5 phosphodiesterase inhibitors.

Surgery

Surgery for Raynaud's is rare. It is usually only recommended if the symptoms are so severe that there is a risk the affected body part, such as your fingers, could lose their blood supply and begin to die.

- Sympathectomy is sometimes used. It involves cutting the nerves causing the affected blood vessels to spasm.
- The results of a sympathectomy are often only temporary and further treatment and possibly more surgery may be required after a few years.

---

28. Discuss Buerger's disease of lower limb.

Ayush University Chhattisgarh 2025, Maharashtra University of Health Sciences 2025

---

29. Thromboangiitis obliterans. ***NTRUHS, Vijayawada 2024***

Definition

Buerger's disease, or *thromboangiitis obliterans (TAO)*, is a *non-atherosclerotic, segmental, inflammatory occlusive disease* of *small- and medium-sized arteries and veins* of the limbs, leading to *ischemia and gangrene.*

It almost exclusively affects *young male smokers.*

Epidemiology

- *Age:* 20–40 years
- *Sex:* Male >> Female (though rising in female smokers)
- *Common in:* Middle East, India, Southeast Asia
- *Strong association with: Tobacco use (smoking or chewing)*

Etiopathogenesis

- *Smoking (Tobacco)*
  - Nicotine and other toxins cause *endothelial injury* → *inflammation* and *thrombosis.*
  - Disease improves only after *complete cessation* of tobacco.
- *Immune mechanisms*
  - Hypersensitivity to tobacco extracts.
  - Circulating antiendothelial antibodies.
- *Genetic Predisposition:* Association with *HLA-A9, HLA-B5.*

Pathology

- *Segmental, inflammatory, thrombotic* process involving *small- and medium-sized arteries and veins* (tibial, peroneal, radial, ulnar).
- *Thrombosis with microabscesses* in vessel lumen.
- *Preserved internal elastic lamina* (distinguishes from atherosclerosis).
- Adjacent *veins and nerves* often involved ("vascular triad").

Sites Commonly Affected

- *Lower limb:* Tibial, peroneal, dorsalis pedis arteries.
- *Upper limb:* Radial and ulnar arteries (often bilateral).

Clinical Features

- *Limb ischemia*
  - *Intermittent claudication:* Calf or foot pain on walking.
  - *Rest pain:* Especially at night, relieved by hanging foot over bed.
  - *Coldness, numbness, and paresthesia.*

- *Trophic changes*
  - Thin, shiny, hairless skin.
  - Brittle nails.
  - *Ulcers and gangrene* at tips of toes or fingers.
- *Raynaud's phenomenon:* Episodic digital pallor and cyanosis due to vasospasm.
- *Superficial thrombophlebitis:* Migratory thrombophlebitis (painful, cord-like veins)—characteristic feature.
- *Absent peripheral pulses:* Dorsalis pedis and posterior tibial pulses absent; femoral usually palpable.

Clinical Staging (Shionoya Criteria)

- Smoking history
- Onset before age 50
- Infrapopliteal arterial occlusion
- Upper limb involvement or migratory thrombophlebitis
- No other atherosclerotic risk factors

Diagnosis is confirmed when *all 5 criteria* are met.

Investigations

- *Noninvasive*
  - *Doppler study/Duplex scan:* Diminished distal flow.
  - *Ankle-brachial index (ABI):* Reduced (<0.5).
  - *Allen's test:* Positive (delayed filling indicates radial/ulnar involvement).
- *Imaging*
  - *Conventional or CT angiography:*
    - *Segmental occlusions* with *"corkscrew collaterals"* (vasa vasorum proliferation).
    - Distal arteries affected; proximal arteries spared.
- *Laboratory:* Usually *normal* (used to rule out diabetes, autoimmune, hypercoagulable states).

Management

- *Absolute smoking cessation*
  - *Most important and only curative measure.*
  - Even minimal tobacco use causes relapse or progression.
- *Medical therapy*
  - *Vasodilators:* e.g. nifedipine, cilostazol, pentoxifylline (symptomatic relief).
  - *Antiplatelets/anticoagulants:* Limited benefit.
  - *IV prostaglandin analogues (Iloprost):* May improve distal perfusion.
  - *Analgesics* for pain.
  - *Wound care* for ulcers and gangrene.
- *Surgical treatment*
  - *Lumbar sympathectomy:*
    - Causes arteriolar dilatation → relieves rest pain, promotes healing.
    - Indicated in *rest pain without gangrene.*
  - *Arterial bypass:* Rarely feasible (distal disease, lack of target vessel).
  - *Amputation:*
    - For *irreversible gangrene* or *infection.*
    - Aim: *Minor amputation* if possible (toe or transmetatarsal).
- *Newer/adjunctive therapies*
  - *Stem cell therapy/therapeutic angiogenesis* (experimental).
  - *Spinal cord stimulation*—pain relief, improves microcirculation.

Prognosis

- Progression depends entirely on *smoking cessation.*
- With continued smoking → recurrent episodes → *progressive gangrene* and *amputation.*
- Complete abstinence → stabilization and sometimes improvement.

30. Thoracoscopic sympathectomy. *WBUHS 2008*

Thoracoscopic sympathectomy resolves primary hyperhidrosis, Raynaud's phenomenon and excessive facial blushing.

- During the procedure, a surgeon partially disables the nerve that controls the sweat glands as well as the dilation of blood vessels near the surface of the skin of the face and fingers.
- Performed as a minimally invasive procedure, thoracoscopic sympathectomy has few risks, but people who undergo the surgery often experience later sweating problems in other parts of their bodies.
- *Procedure:* During a thoracoscopic sympathectomy, a surgeon severs and seals the right-hand side of the sympathetic nerve, which runs along the inside of the spinal column. The nerve gets cut at a point parallel to the space between the second and third ribs. Most thoracoscopic sympathectomies are now performed as endoscopic procedures, in which the surgeon makes a small incision below the right armpit to access the sympathetic nerve and uses a flexible camera cable to guide the application of surgical instruments. Patients undergoing endoscopic thoracoscopic sympathectomy receive general anesthesia and must have their right lung deflated during the surgery, but patients generally do not need to stay in the hospital overnight. Full recovery occurs within a few days.

Risks and complications:

- Patients can expect some pain following a thoracoscopic sympathectomy.
- Also, an initial thoracoscopic sympathectomy does not always resolve a patient's problem, so a second procedure may be necessary.
- Rarer risks from the procedure include a collapsed lung caused by the collection of air in the chest cavity during surgery and inadvertent damage to other nerves near the sympathetic nerve.
- Some patients have developed Homer's syndrome following thoracoscopic sympathectomy, experiencing drooping eyelids, constricted pupils and reduced facial sweating.

31. Pharmacotherapy of Peripheral Arterial Disease. *WBUHS 2014*

- Lifestyle changes may be enough treatment for some people with peripheral artery disease (PAD), others may require medication.
- Examples of medications used to treat PAD include *antiplatelet or anticlotting agents,* cholesterol-lowering drugs such as statins, medications that increase blood supply to the extremities such as cilostazol and pentoxifylline and medications that control high BP.
  - *Antiplatelet medications* (such as aspirin and clopidogrel):
  - They make the blood platelets less likely to stick to one another to form blood clots.
  - Low dose aspirin (81–325 mg/day) is usually prescribed indefinitely because it is also helpful in preventing strokes and heart attacks in patients with PAD.
  - Clopidogrel (Plavix) is an alternative to aspirin for those who are allergic or cannot tolerate aspirin.
  - Antiplatelet medications also help prevent occlusion of blood vessels after angioplasty or bypass surgery.
- *Anticoagulant medications:*
  - They act to prevent blood clotting. Both heparin and warfarin (Coumadin) are anticoagulant medications.
  - Anticoagulants are sometimes prescribed for people with PAD if they are at increased risk for formation of blood clots; these agents are used much less frequently than antiplatelet agents in patients with PAD.

- *Cholesterol-lowering drugs* of the statin family:
  - They have been shown in numerous large clinical trials to help prevent heart attacks and strokes and prolong survival among patients with atherosclerosis.
  - Statins have also been shown to slow the progression of PAD, decrease arthrosclerosis in the arteries, and improve claudication symptoms.
- *Cilostazol:*
  - It is a medication that can help increase physical activity (enabling one to walk a greater distance without the pain of claudication).
  - Cilostazol works by causing dilation of the arteries and an increased supply of oxygenated blood to be delivered to the arms and legs.
  - Cilostazol is recommended for some patients with claudication when lifestyle modifications and exercise are ineffective.
  - Cilostazol should be taken on an empty stomach either a half an hour before or two hours after meals.
  - High fat meals, grapefruit juice, and certain medications such as omeprazole and diltiazem can increase the absorption, and hence, the blood levels of cilostazol.
  - Side effects are generally mild that include headache, diarrhea, and dizziness.
  - Cilostazol should not be used in patients with heart failure because of concern over increased mortality in heart failure patients using medications similar to cilostazol.
- *Pentoxifylline:*
  - It improves blood flow to the extremities by decreasing the viscosity ("stickiness") of blood, enabling more efficient blood flow.
  - Side effects are fewer than with cilostazol, but its benefits are weaker and have not been conclusively proven by all studies.
- Drugs to control hypertension may also be prescribed.
- Current recommendations are to treat hypertension in patients with PAD to prevent strokes and heart attacks.

32. Femoropopliteal bypass. *WBUHS 2011*

- Femoropopliteal bypass surgery is a procedure in which surgeons reroute femoral and popliteal blood flow either through a blood vessel transplanted from a healthier part of the leg or through a prosthetic vessel. It is a sort of detour around blocked or damaged blood vessels near the knee. The transplanted vessel then serves as a conduit between the femoral and popliteal arteries.
- Femoropopliteal bypass surgery begins with a consultation where the surgeon determines whether to redirect the flow through an existing vein, or to use a graft material. Most prefer to use an alternate vein. Studies suggest that using alternate veins produce better results.
- Patients can expect to remain in the hospital for 2–4 days after the procedure, although initial recovery (sitting up and walking around) may begin as early as 24 hours later. Although femoropopliteal bypass surgery is typically successful in alleviating blockage symptoms, it is usually viewed as a last resort when more conservative treatments have not worked.
- The surgery is reserved for patients whose symptoms are so severe that amputation is a potential consideration.
- Like most procedures, fem-pop bypass surgery carries a number of risks. Patients should discuss potential side effects such as infection, failed or blocked grafts, excessive bleeding, heart attack, and swelling.
- During the operation, the blocked native artery is bypassed using either a section of the patient's own vein (autologous vein), human umbilical vein (HUV), or an artificial graft, e.g., Dacron or polytetrafluoroethylene (PTFE).

Reasons a femoral popliteal bypass surgery or percutaneous transluminal angioplasty (PTA) of the femoral artery may be performed include, but are not limited to, the following:

- Medical management that has not improved symptoms, or worsening of symptoms despite medical management

- Severe disability (IC that causes interference with lifestyle and/or ability to work)
- Nonhealing wounds
- Infection or gangrene
- Ischemic rest pain (lack of oxygen and nutrients to the leg resulting in pain at rest)
- Danger of losing the limb due to decreased blood flow
    - Not all peripheral arterial disease can be treated with PTA. Your doctor will decide the best treatment of your PAD based on your individual circumstances.
    - There may be other reasons for your doctor to recommend femoral popliteal bypass surgery or PTA.

Risks of the Procedure

As with any surgical procedure, complications can occur. Some possible complications may include, but are not limited to, the following:

Myocardial infarction (heart attack)	Wound infection	Pulmonary edema (fluid in the lungs)	Restenosis (blockage in the blood vessels after PTA procedure)
Cardiac arrhythmias (irregular heartbeats)	Leg edema (swelling of the leg)	Bleeding at the catheter insertion site (usually the groin) after percutaneous transluminal angioplasty (PTA) procedure	Nerve injury
Hemorrhage (bleeding)	Thrombosis (clot in the leg)	Blood clot or damage to the blood vessel at the insertion site (PTA)	Graft occlusion (blockage in the graft used in bypass surgery)

- Patients who are allergic to or sensitive to medications, contrast dyes, iodine, shellfish, or latex should notify their doctor.
- There may be other risks depending on your specific medical condition. Be sure to discuss any concerns with your doctor prior to the procedure.

33. Extra-anatomic bypass for leg ischemia. ***WBUHS 2007***

Key Points

- Chronic CLI is manifested by pain at rest, nonhealing wounds, and gangrene.
- Ischemic rest pain is typically described as a burning pain in the arch or distal foot that occurs while the patient is recumbent but is relieved when the patient returns to a position in which the feet are dependent.
- Objective hemodynamic parameters that support the diagnosis of CLI include an ankle-brachial index of 0.4 or less, an ankle systolic pressure of 50 mm Hg or less, or a toe systolic pressure of 30 mm Hg or less.
- Intervention may include conservative therapy, revascularization, or amputation.
- Progressive gangrene, rapidly enlarging wounds or continuous ischemic rest pain can signify a threat to the limb and suggest the need for revascularization in patients without prohibitive operative risks.
- Bypass grafts are usually required because of the multilevel and distal nature of the arterial narrowing in CLI.
- Patients with diabetes are more likely than other patients to have distal disease that is less amenable to bypass grafting.
- Compared with amputation, revascularization is more cost-effective and is associated with better perioperative morbidity and mortality.
- Limb preservation should be the goal in most patients with CLI.
- As with all occlusive arterial diseases it is important to identify and treat any risk factors that may be accelerating or aggravating the condition.
- In CLI the collateral arteries have reached the limit of their ability to compensate and spontaneous improvement is unlikely.

- CLI is strongly associated with arterial disease elsewhere, particularly in the heart, and this increases the risk of serious complications.
- In general, unless some action is taken, a patient with CLI has a significant chance of developing gangrene in the affected leg and requiring an amputation.
- The most effective treatment is an operation to bypass the blocked arteries and to restore a good blood flow to the leg and foot.
- This is a major operation and can only be offered if the patient is well enough to undergo an anesthetic.
- Occasionally it is possible to do a lesser operation which does not completely relieve all the occlusions but improves the blood supply sufficiently to relieve the worst symptoms and avoid an amputation.
- In some cases it is possible to improve the blood supply by angioplasty.
- In order to decide which form of treatment is possible an angiogram is necessary.

Bypass Operation–Working Formulation

- The essential problem in all patients undergoing bypass surgery to the lower legs is that insufficient blood and hence oxygen is able to reach the tissues of the leg and foot.
- The tissues are starved of oxygen and this is what leads to pain, gangrene, and ulceration.
- Bypass operations work by improving the blood supply and hence the oxygen supply to the tissues that have been starved of oxygen.
- To do this the surgeon must take blood from a good artery above the area where the artery is blocked, and take the blood along a tube (the conduit) to a good artery below the blocked segments.
- There are variations on this principle when blood can be taken from one side of the body to the other (femorofemoral crossover) or blood is diverted from arteries to the arms down to the legs (axillobifemoral grafting).

Extra-anatomic bypass are as follows:

- *Infrainguinal bypass:* Above knee and below knee femoropopliteal bypass grafting has been used using saphenous vein and PTFE as the graft material. Comparative studies have shown that while saphenous is superior to PTFE in graft patency at 2 years for below knee level, the results are equivocal for above knee level but favor the use of vein.
- *Suprainguinal bypass:* Aortobifemoral bypass has >90% patency at 1 year but higher mortality.

Specific risks for aortobifemoral bypass surgery include:

- Leg swelling
- Failed or blocked grafts
- Sexual dysfunction caused by nerve damage in the pelvis
  - Cross femoral or iliofemoral by pass have similar success rates for unilateral disease with lower mortality rates
  - Axillobifemoral grafts have a lower patency rate and are not justifiable for claudication

They can also be classified as follows:

- *Inflow operations:*
  - Inflow operations are performed to restore blood flow to the top of the leg.
  - When the blood flow is normal to the legs, femoral pulses can be felt around the groin area.
  - If major blood vessels (aorta or iliac arteries) are blocked then the blood flowing into the leg is severely reduced. An inflow operation is required to restore this flow to normal.

There are many operations to restore inflow to the legs, but the most common are:

Aortobifemoral grafting	***Axillobifemoral grafting***	***Femorofemoral cross-over grafting***	***Iliofemoral bypass grafting***
• These grafts originate on the aorta and take blood to the femoral arteries at the groins • These are major operations with an approximately 5% (1 in 20) risk of dying • Aortobifemoral grafting Is the most successful type of Inflow operation, but is also the most traumatic • A Dacron graft (usually) is stitched to the aorta in the abdomen, just below the level of the kidneys • The graft has two legs which are then tunneled under the abdominal muscles into the groins to be attached to the femoral arteries	• These grafts originate from the axillary arteries and take blood to the femoral arteries • This Is sometimes the best option in very elderly or very unfit patients as It Is a less traumatic alternative to aortobifemoral grafting	• These grafts originate from a normal femoral artery in the groin on one leg and take blood to the femoral artery in the groin on the opposite leg • At least one of the arteries running to the legs must be flowing normally in order to perform this operation	• These grafts originate from the iliac arteries in the pelvis and take blood to the femoral arteries in the groins • These can be useful If there Is enough normal Iliac artery in the pelvis

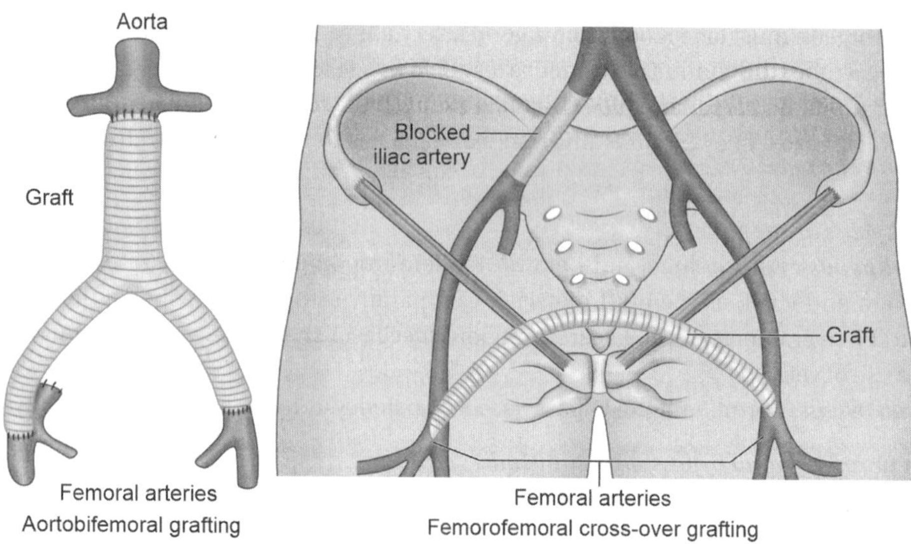

Aortobifemoral grafting

Femorofemoral cross-over grafting

- The common theme with these operations is that they restore good blood flow to the femoral artery at the top of the leg in the groin region.
- Restoring the inflow to normal levels is often all that is required in many patients, even if there is disease in the arteries further down the leg.
- The improvement in inflow alone can be enough to permit healing or reduce symptoms to a more bearable level.

- *Outflow operations:*
  - If the arterial flow to the femoral artery is good and there are good femoral pulses in the groin, an inflow operation is not required.
  - If the patient has a shortage of blood to the leg and good femoral pulses, then the arterial problem must lie at a lower level in the thigh and/or the calf arteries.
  - These operations are frequently prolonged and complex procedures.
  - There are many operations to restore blood flow to the legs, but the most common are:

Femoropopliteal bypass	*Femorodistal or femorocrural bypass*	*Pedal bypasses*
These grafts originate from the femoral artery in the groin and take blood to the popliteal artery either just above or below the knee	These grafts originate from the femoral artery at the groin and take blood to one of the three calf blood vessels (anterior and posterior tibial arteries and peroneal artery)	These grafts can originate from any artery in the leg (femoral, popliteal and rarely tibial) and take blood to arteries below the level of the ankle Joint (dorsalis pedis artery and posterior tibial artery or their branches)

- For pedal and distal bypasses the arteries are small and difficult to stitch with the naked eye so magnifying glasses are required to perform these operations reliably.
- Femoral endarterectomy is a similar operation to carotid endarterectomy in which the diseased lining of the artery can be removed and blood flow restored.

General Graft Principles

- For inflow operations it is better to use artificial grafts. They perform well when the arterial flow is high and have been shown over years to provide durable results. The most common material used for inflow operations is Dacron.
- For outflow operations it is generally better not to use artificial materials. Sometimes artificial materials have to be used as no vein is available and in these circumstances. PTFE is the most common material in use, although there is some reasonable evidence that for femoropopliteal bypasses that Dacron impregnated with heparin can perform better.

In general with any graft, it is better to make the grafts as short as possible and to avoid crossing joints, but quite frequently, grafts have to be long and cross joints to salvage the leg and foot.

Complications

- *Local complications:*
  - Graft failure
  - Wound infection
  - Graft infection
  - Leg swelling
- *General complications:*
  - Chest infections
  - Heart attacks
  - Strokes

Maintenance and follow-up:

- A small dose of aspirin every day.
- Clopidogrel is being used more frequently. It has little advantage over aspirin alone.
- There is increasing evidence that the combination of aspirin and clopidogrel may be more beneficial than either alone.
- In some patients aspirin alone is not considered a strong enough treatment to prevent blood clotting. In these patients warfarin can be used either alone or with aspirin to reduce the chances of clots.
- There is good evidence that use of warfarin prolongs the patency of bypass grafts in the legs but for various reasons it is not used as frequently as it probably should.
- In addition to aspirin the vascular risk factors should be treated.
  - *Duplex surveillance:*
    - In about one-third of grafts performed with veins a narrowing develops after the operation.
    - To identify patients who develop narrowing.
    - Duplex scanning of the graft is usually recommended at frequent intervals over the first 2 years.
    - This enables problems to be identified at an early stage when they can be corrected before the graft blocks.

- Once a graft blocks it is usually more difficult to rescue the situation and restore normal blood flow.
- This sort of scanning is most useful in patients with vein grafts.

- Only a few patients are unsuitable for a bypass operation or angioplasty, and in for these unfortunate cases the treatment options are limited. There are no drugs or other treatments that have been shown to be very effective.
- Often strong pain killers are the only option to control the symptoms.
- If the pain is uncontrollable or gangrene and infection become established then an amputation may be necessary as a life protecting operation because without it there is a risk of the infection spreading and causing blood poisoning.

34. Mention the endovascular approaches of arteriovenous fistula. ***WBUHS 2021***

Endovascular Approaches of Arteriovenous Fistula

Introduction

An *AVF* is an abnormal connection between an adjacent artery and vein.

Locations

These can occur in multiple locations with the more common ones having separate articles as follows:

- Cerebral AVF
  - Dural AVF
  - Pial AVF
- Scalp AVF (also called cirsoid aneurysm)
- Spinal AVF
  - Spinal dural AVF
- Coronary AVF
- Renal AVF

Endovascular Treatment

- EVT can be performed for size and grade reduction, presurgical devascularization, size reduction before radiosurgery, targeted embolization, and as stand-alone treatment for cure. Targeted embolization can address intranidal or flow-related aneurysms and high flow arteriovenous shunts.
- EVT of arteriovenous malformations (AVMs) is most often performed with liquid embolic material such as Onyx or N-butyl cyanoacrylate (NBCA) to occlude the nidus while avoiding migration or extravasation into the draining veins.
- Total EVT is achieved in approximately 20% of cases.
- Embolization complication rates range from 9 to 30% and the natural history needs to be considered during decision making.
- Traditional EVT uses embolic material via a transarterial route; however, recently transvenous and combined approaches have been described.
- Endovascular embolization uses liquid embolics such as NBCA and ethylene vinyl alcohol.
- Stereotactic radiosurgery is used for the treatment of cerebral AVMs. The ideal AVM for treatment with SRS is small, <3 cm in diameter or <10 cm^3, in noneloquent regions where the margin can receive a dose of 16–25 Gy. Larger AVMs should be staged and thoughtful consideration should be given to multimodal therapy.
- Renal AVMs are rare vascular malformations that cause hematuria. Treatment for renal AVMs has evolved from open nephrectomy to transcatheter arterial embolization (TAE).
- Embolization of congenital renal AVMs using ethanol and coil.
- Most intracranial dural arteriovenous fistulae (DAVFs) involve the transverse-sigmoid sinus (TSS), and various types of EVT have been involved in managing TSS DAVFs.

35. Discuss the etiology, diagnosis, and outline the management of chronic ulcer foot. ***WBUHS 2013***

Introduction

- A foot ulcer is an open sore on the foot.
- A foot ulcer can be a shallow red crater that involves only the surface skin. A foot ulcer also can be very deep. A deep foot ulcer may be a crater that extends through the full thickness of the skin. It may involve tendons, bones, and other deep structures.
- People with diabetes and people with poor circulation are more likely to develop foot ulcers. It can be difficult to heal a foot ulcer. In people with these conditions, even a small foot ulcer can become infected if it does not heal quickly.
- If an infection occurs in an ulcer and is not treated right away, it can develop into:
  - An abscess (a pocket of pus)
  - A spreading infection of the skin and underlying fat (cellulitis)
  - A bone infection (osteomyelitis)
  - Gangrene is an area of dead, darkened body tissue caused by poor blood flow
- Among people with diabetes, most severe foot infections that ultimately require some part of the toe, foot, or lower leg to be amputated start as a foot ulcer.

Etiology

Causes of leg ulcers.

Vascular	***Infection***	***Neuropathic***	***Panniculitis***	***Tumors***
• Venous • Arterial • Mixed	• Bacterial • Fungal • Protozoal	• Diabetes • Tabes • Syringomyelia	• Necrobiosis lipoidica • Fat necrosis	• Basal cell carcinoma • Squamous cell carcinoma
Hematological	***Infection***	***Trauma***	***Metabolic***	***Pyoderma gangrenosum***
• Sickle cell disease • Cryoglobulinemia	• Bacterial • Fungal • Protozoal	• Pressure • Injury • Burns	• Diabetes • Gout • Prolidase deficiency	Special-hypertensive ulcer

Foot ulcers are especially common in people who have one or more of the following health problems:

- *Peripheral neuropathy:*
  - People with peripheral neuropathy may not be able to feel when they have stepped on something sharp or when they have an irritating pebble in their shoes.
  - They can injure their feet significantly and never know it, unless they examine their feet routinely for injury.
  - Many elderly people and diabetics with vision problems also cannot see their feet well enough to examine them for problems.
- *Circulatory problems:*
  - Any illness that decreases circulation to the feet can cause foot ulcers.
  - Poor circulation in the leg arteries is called PAD.
  - It also causes pain in the leg or buttock during walking.
  - It is caused by atherosclerosis.
  - This is a disease in which fatty deposits of cholesterol build up inside arteries.
- *Abnormalities in the bones or muscles of the feet:*
  - Any condition that distorts the normal anatomy of the foot can lead to foot ulcers.
  - Examples are claw feet, feet with fractures, and cases of severe arthritis.

More than any other group, people with diabetes have a particularly high risk of developing foot ulcers.

In addition to diabetes, other medical conditions that increase the risk of foot ulcers include:

- *Atherosclerosis:* This condition involves poor circulation to the legs.

- *Raynaud's phenomenon:* This condition causes sudden episodes of decreased blood flow to the fingers and toes. During these episodes, the fingers and toes turn white as the blood supply diminishes. They turn blue, and red again as the circulation returns to normal.

Assessment of foot ulcer	
Patient	• History of ulcer development • Past and current medical problems • General health status, nutrition • Social, occupation • Mobility problem, limitations to self-care • Obesity
Skin changes	• Arterial, malignant, autoimmune
Vascular assessment	• Pedal pulse • Ankle brachial pressure index
Limb factors	• Edema • Circumferences • Lymphedema • Orthopedic problems • Sensation and pain
Ulcer	• Site—venous, arterial, and pressure • Size—measure • Appearance • Wound base and exudate level • Surrounding skin

Investigations

- The Ankle Brachial Pressure Index (ABPI) using a handheld DUS and sphygmomanometer can be carried out for more accurate assessment of arterial perfusion.
- The results are used to determine the likelihood of arterial insufficiency and can be used to guide the management plan.
- When Doppler tests indicate arterial insufficiency, arterial duplex ultrasonography will (noninvasively) provide accurate anatomic and hemodynamic information on the site and extent of the arterial disease.
- When indicated, further detailed anatomic information for treatment planning can be obtained from MRA, computer tomographic angiography, or DSA.

Ankle brachial pressure index (ABPI) symptoms: Management correlation guide.

Index	*Symptoms*	*Severity of disease*	*Management*
>0.8–0.95	None/mild intermittent claudication	Mild arterial disease	• Modify risk factors • Stop smoking • Regular exercise • Consider antiplatelet therapy
>0.5–0.8	Intermittent claudication	Moderate arterial disease	• As for patients with ABPI between 0.8 and 0.95 together with routine referral to a vascular surgeon • Possible arterial Doppler scan/angiogram
>0.3–0.5	Severe intermittent claudication and rest pain	Severe arterial disease	• As for patients with ABPI between 0.8 and 0.95 together with routine referral to a vascular surgeon • Possible arterial Doppler scan/angiogram

Contd...

Contd...

Index	*Symptoms*	*Severity of disease*	*Management*
0.3 or below or ankle systolic pressure <50 mm Hg	Critical ischemia (rest pain for >2 weeks duration) with or without tissue loss (ulcer, gangrene)	Severe arterial disease and risk of losing limb	Urgent referral to the vascular emergency surgical or radiological intervention team and possible on-call
Abnormally high ABPI (>1.3)	Variable	Vessel calcification	As for patients with ABPI between 0.8 and 0.95 together with routine referral to a vascular surgeon

- Accurate and regular measurement of the wound is important to give an objective assessment of the effectiveness of the current management plan.
- The Leg Ulcer Measurement Tool (LUMT) is a validated tool that has been developed to quantify leg ulcer assessment and can be used to track change in wound status over time.
- Blood investigations such as complete blood count, erythrocyte sedimentation rate, blood sugar, lipid profile, renal function tests, and liver function tests are essential in patients with chronic leg ulcers.
- The plain radiography of the foot along with CT and MRI should be done to rule out osteomyelitis and malignancy.
- *Laboratory screening tests for vasculitis:* Urine analysis for proteinuria, hematuria, cylindruria, routine and immunohistopathology of skin biopsies, antinuclear antibodies, rheumatoid factor, complement C4, circulating immune complexes, paraproteins, immunoglobulin fractions, antineutrophil cytoplasmic antibodies, serological tests, and cultures for underlying infections.
- *Laboratory screening tests for clotting disorders:* Activated partial thromboplastin time, prothrombin time, thrombin time, factor V (Leiden) mutation, factor II (prothrombin) mutation, antithrombin III, protein C and protein S, and lupus anticoagulant anticardiolipin.
- Venography may be performed as an investigational procedure prior to valvular surgery. Lower extremities arteriography is indicated in patients with ischemic rest pain, intolerable claudication, impending gangrene, or the presence of nonhealing ulcers of suspected arterial origin.
- Color duplex US scanning which is becoming the de facto standard for evaluation of venous obstruction is also used to assess the location and extent of reflux in venous ulcers.
- Plethysmography and venous pressure data are important in determining the need for surgical bypass or valve replacement. Quantitative data on venous obstruction, calf muscle pump ejection fraction, and reflux are provided by air plethysmography, whereas venous pressure studies assess the physiological importance of anatomic obstruction because the collaterals may or may not provide adequate compensation for an obstructed pathway.
- A quantitative bacterial culture is more specific and should be performed once wound infection is suspected.
- The quantitative biopsy is the current gold standard for assessing the quality and quantity of microbial pathogens within wound. Quantitative biopsies containing $>10^5$ organisms per gram of tissue are considered significant, and systemic antibiotic therapy should be considered. If osteomyelitis is suspected, representative cultures need to be obtained from the bone or deepest tissue layers.
- Ulcer biopsy is important in making a correct diagnosis and to rule out malignancy as these ulcers are prone to malignant transformation.
- Chronic ulcers are sometimes biopsied for experimental protocols:
  - To obtain information regarding the wound bed or the wound edge.
  - To grow cells in vitro from nonhealing wound.
- The clinical application of gene variant analysis and evaluation in patients with venous leg ulcers implies that the high-risk minority of patients could be identified in advance by means of a simple blood test that would act as a genetic screening device.

Treatment options for common foot ulcers.	
Ulcer type	***Management***
Venous	• Leg elevation • Compression therapy • Aspirin • Pentoxifylline • Surgical management
Arterial	• Revascularization • Antiplatelet medication • Management of risk factors
Neuropathic	• Off-loading of pressure • Topical growth factors • Tissue engineered skin
Pressure	• Off-loading of pressure • Reduction of excessive moisture, sheer, and friction • Adequate nutrition

Recent Advances in Management

Several researchers are still discovering other modalities of treatment.

- The knowledge of microribonucleic acid (miRNA) function in the regulation of wound healing and developing improved miRNA modulation techniques in the skin will help in translating this knowledge into more effective therapies.
- The clinical practices could be strongly influenced by the results of the HFE genetic test. The presence of *C282Y* mutation would strengthen the indications and priorities for surgical correction of superficial venous insufficiency.
- Chronic wounds are characterized by changes in cell receptors (integrins). The activation or inhibition of integrin receptors by various agents may provide an excellent means of influencing wound healing.
- Venous leg ulcers can be healed with a spray formulation of allogeneic neonatal keratinocytes and fibroblasts without the need for tissue engineering, at an optimum dose of cells per mL every 14 days.
- The regenerative medicine is utilizing therapeutic potential of the stem cells to promote skin regeneration.
  - Stem cell-based therapies offer tremendous potential for skin regeneration following injury and disease.
  - Functional stem cell units have been described throughout all layers of human skin, and the collective physical and chemical microenvironmental cues that enable this regenerative potential are known as the stem cell niche.
  - Stem cells in the hair follicle bulge, interfollicular epidermis, dermal papillae, and perivascular space have been closely investigated as model systems for niche-driven regeneration.
  - These studies suggest that stem cell strategies for skin engineering must consider the intricate molecular and biologic features of these niches.
  - Innovative biomaterial systems that successfully recapitulate these microenvironments will facilitate progenitor-cell-mediated skin repair and regeneration.
- According to Frade et al., the natural biomembrane of latex extracted from *Hevea brasiliensis* proved to be safe as a dressing.
- The vegetal biomembrane was important for the induction of the healing, especially on the inflammatory stage, confirmed by the abundant exudation and debridement of the ulcers in relation of the control treatment of chronic venous ulcers, which seems to be directly related to the intense vascular formation followed by reepithelialization.
- Topical application of F-5 peptide promoted acute and diabetic wound closure in mice far more effectively than did platelet-derived growth factor-BB (PDGF-BB).

36. Diabetic foot. ***WBUHS 2009***

37. Write a note on diabetic foot. ***WBUHS 2024***

38. Diabetic foot—recent trend in management. ***WBUHS 2011; Srimanta Sankaradeva University, Assam 2025***

Surgeons are frequently called upon to evaluate and treat the complications of diabetic foot disease. In the diabetic population, foot disease is the leading cause of hospitalization.

- *Pathophysiology:*
  - Diabetic foot disease involves a complex sequence of changes that lead to the destruction of the foot's function and structure.
  - Peripheral neuropathy, arthropathy, arterial insufficiency, and infection are the major derangements underlying diabetic foot disease.
  - The final common pathway is often one of ulceration, gangrene, and limb loss.
- *Peripheral neuropathy:*
  - Peripheral neuropathy is common among diabetics and is the most difficult component of diabetic foot disease to treat.
  - Its severity ranges from minimal somatosensory changes to total anesthesia with the complete absence of sweating.
  - Diabetic neuropathy affects the motor, sensory, and autonomic nervous systems, which leads to multiple pathologic conditions.
  - Destruction of myelinated motor fibers produces a *motor polyneuropathy* that tends to be bilateral and symmetric.
  - Attenuation of the Achilles reflex is an early sign of motor neuropathy.
  - Progression leads to loss of function and atrophy of the lumbricals and intrinsic muscles of the foot.
  - Unopposed, the extrinsic muscles distort the foot, leading to depression of the metatarsal heads, digital contractures, "clawing" of the toes, and a varus malformation.
  - These alterations allow pressure points and ulcers to develop over the proximal interphalangeal joints and beneath the metatarsal heads.
  - *Sensory neuropathy* involving type A myelinated fibers leads to loss of proprioception, light tough, pressure, and vibration and is noted to develop early.
  - Compromise of these nerves leads to an ataxic gate and pressure ulceration.
  - Loss of type C sensory fibers limits a patient's ability to detect painful or noxious stimuli, which contributes to neuroarthropathy, injuries, and the formation of ulcers.
  - C fibers also participate in nociceptive or neuroinflammatory responses that blunt the signs of trauma and infection in diabetic feet.
  - *Sensory neuropathy* can also paradoxically produce pain and paresthesias.
  - Neuropathic pain can be severe and quite difficult to differentiate from other foot problems.
  - Diabetic paresthesias are characterized by hyperesthesia, burning, or tingling sensations and tend to resolve over time.
  - *Autonomic neuropathy* produces abnormal vasomotor responses.
  - Autosympathectomy increases arteriovenous shunting, which leads to osteopenia.
  - Hypohidrosis results in dry, cracked skin, which compromises the skin barrier and increases the susceptibility to infections.
- *Neuroarthropathy:*
  - Neuroarthropathy or Charcot's foot is a condition in which extensive destruction of the joints occurs within the foot consequent to a loss in muscular stability, osteopenia, and insensitivity to pain.
  - It is present in many disorders of peripheral nerves but is most common in diabetics.

  - Sensory neuropathy permits mechanical insults to go unrecognized by the patient, which produce severe stresses on osteopenic bone.
  - Bony dissolution and loss of structural integrity follow, leading to collapse of the midfoot arch.
  - Minor foot trauma (e.g., minor fracture, sprain, and contusion) often catalyzes neuropathic skeletal changes.
  - Localized warmth and swelling at the site occur initially; this is usually nontender and out of proportion to the injury.
  - The warmth and swelling of this inflammatory stage of neuropathic osteoarthropathy can be difficult to distinguish from infection.
  - Chronically, skeletal encroachment occurs in the tarsometatarsal and metatarsophalangeal joints followed by collapse of the arch.
  - Subluxation or even lateral dislocation of the forefoot occurs, producing a bowed, "rocker-bottom" foot, which is extremely susceptible to ulceration.
- *Arterial insufficiency:*
  - Altered glucose metabolism in diabetics leads to changes in response to endothelial injury, dyslipidemia, enhanced platelet activity, and increased blood viscosity.
  - These factors contribute to an increased incidence of atherosclerotic occlusive disease and hypercoagulability in diabetic patients.
  - Arterial insufficiency contributes to the development of neuropathy, limits a patient's ability to heal ulcers and traumatic injuries, and in the worst case, produces ischemic ulcers.
  - The distribution of atherosclerotic disease in diabetics typically involves the femoropopliteal and tibial vessels with relative sparing of aortoiliac and pedal vessels.
  - Consequently, femoral to distal tibial or pedal bypasses are feasible for limb salvage in many diabetics with critical ischemia.
- *Infections:*
  - Diabetic foot infections range from superficial cellulitis to wet gangrene and abscess formation.
  - Peripheral neuropathy and neglected skin lesions or ulcers often initiate deep-space infections.
  - Fungal infections contribute to ulceration and secondary bacterial infection either by direct microscopic breaks in the skin or through toenail loss.
  - Loss of proprioception facilitates traumatic injury.
  - Arterial insufficiency and the diminished inflammatory response allow for rapid progression of an infection.
  - The hallmark of diabetic foot infections is a polymicrobial infection.
  - Gram-positive species, including streptococci, staphylococci, enterococci, and gram-negative anaerobes are present.

Assessment

- History with attention given to the presence of cardiac disease, renal disease, peripheral vascular disease, smoking history, and habits of foot care.
- A thorough laboratory studies include a basic chemistry, a complete blood cell count, a hemoglobin A1cconcentration, and a urinalysis.
- A comprehensive physical examination with emphasis on the neurologic and vascular function of the lower extremities is essential.
- The feet should be carefully examined for capillary refill, nail thickening, ulcers or ischemic lesions, signs of infection, intrinsic muscle wasting, bony prominences, and evidence of tenderness.
- Ischemic ulcers tend to occur in the toes, whereas neuropathic ulcers present over bony prominences and the heel in patients who are bed bound.
- Gentle probing of ulcers to determine whether there is palpable bone at the base is encouraged as a highly specific and accurate test for the detection of osteomyelitis.
- Superficial wound cultures are of little utility.

- Pulse assessment of the femoral, popliteal, dorsalis pedis, and posterior tibial arteries should be performed.
- In the absence of palpable pulses, a continuous-wave Doppler probe should be used to assess for the presence of signals.
- Neurologic examination begins with examination of vibratory sense in the toes and ankle and proceeds to the deep-tendon reflexes of the Achilles and patellar tendons.
- Finally, sensation of pain, light touch, and temperature in the feet should be evaluated.
- Inability to feel the pressure from a Semmes-Weinstein 5.07 nylon monofilament applied to multiple points on the plantar surface is a sensitive screening test for the detection of neuropathy.
- Noninvasive laboratory studies are often helpful in assessing the degree of vascular insufficiency and predicting healing potential.
- Studies may include segmental limb pressures with Doppler waveforms, calculation of ankle-brachial indices, and toe pressures.
- Any gradient >30 mm Hg between any level indicates the presence of a high-grade stenosis or occlusion.
- Calcification within the arterial wall often renders diabetic vessels incompressible and waveform interpretation must be used to identify disease.
- In diabetics, toe or partial foot amputations require ankle pressures of at least 55 mm Hg and toe pressures of at least 30 mm Hg to heal.
- Transcutaneous oxygen measurements may also predict healing if there is at least a pressure of 30 mm Hg.

Imaging

- Plain radiographs are useful in the assessment of the diabetic foot. They can identify soft tissue calcifications, gas from bacterial infections, the presence of foreign bodies, and fractures. Plain radiographs can detect osteomyelitis but are most sensitive in the later stages when bony destruction has occurred.
- Three-phase bone scans are highly sensitive for osteomyelitis except in the presence of severe vascular disease.
- Arteriography:
  - It is required when foot perfusion appears inadequate and arterial reconstruction is planned.
  - The location and degree of occlusive disease are readily assessed with arteriography.
  - Assessment of the outflow vessels and, in particular, communication of the pedal vessels with the pedal arch is also important.
  - MRA is highly accurate in the detection of large-vessel disease and is useful in patients who are intolerant of contrast dyes.
- Magnetic resonance imaging (MRI) of the diabetic foot provides unparalleled imaging of the soft tissues.
  - Contrast-enhanced sequences can be used to determine the extent of osseous and soft tissue infection and can delineate areas of ischemia or necrosis
  - MRI is increasingly becoming the preferred imaging test for osteomyelitis. Osteomyelitis is characterized by an altered bone marrow signal. Sensitivity of MRI for osteomyelitis ranges from 77 to 100%, with a specificity from 79 to 100%.

Management

- Optimal treatment of diabetic patients requires a comprehensive program involving control of hyperglycemia, foot protection, and the timely treatment of ulcers, osteoarthropathy, and infections.
- Diabetics with high-risk foot conditions benefit from education regarding risk factors and their appropriate management.
- Successful treatment of diabetic foot ulcers consists of addressing these three basic issues: debridement, offloading, and infection control.
- *Prevention:*
  - Prevention of ulceration is imperative to prevent limb loss.
  - Every diabetic patient should have an annual foot examination by a physician and, if the patient has neuropathy, at every visit with a healthcare professional.

- Self-examinations should occur daily.
- Hyperglycemia should be controlled to slow the development of neuropathy.
- The risk of ulceration is increased in diabetic patients with longstanding diabetes, male gender, poor glucose control, neuropathy, or the presence of vascular, renal, or cardiac disease complications of diabetes.
- Patients with signs of increased plantar pressure such as erythema, warmth, or callus formation should use protective footwear that cushions and redistributes weight appropriately.
- Nonambulatory or bed-bound patients should also have their feet protected; the Rooke boot is a sheepskin and foam boot that is ideal for this purpose.
- Calluses should be debrided by a specialist.
- Dryness and fungal infections should be treated appropriately with petroleum-based products (e.g., Aquaphor ointment) and topical antifungals, respectively.

▪ *Neuropathic ulcers:*
- Diabetic foot ulcerations fall into two main categories, ischemic and neuropathic, with some overlap between.
- In about 30% of patients with plantar neuropathic ulcerations, ischemia will prolong healing times.
- Vascular assessment is always required to ascertain the presence of coexisting occlusive disease.
- However, even with adequate arterial inflow, neuropathic ulcers may remain unchanged for months secondary to impaired inflammatory and healing responses.
- These ulcers are subject to the constant risk of infection, and prolonged ulcer healing lengthens the exposure to this risk. Infection requires prompt management when it arises.
- The extent and anatomic site of neuropathic ulcers direct their management.
- They are most commonly located beneath one of the metatarsal heads or the interphalangeal joint of the hallux.
- Aggressive *debridement* is essential in establishing the depth of the ulcer.
- This requires removal of excessive callus and all necrotic debris.
- Daily wound care minimizes the risk of infection.
- Protecting the weight bearing surface of the foot and *offloading* mechanical stress is paramount in the treatment of neuropathic ulcers not associated with ischemia.
- Non-weight bearing for 6 to 12 weeks is an ideal, though poorly tolerated, method to promote healing.
- An alternative treatment is total contact casting (TCC), which uses a protective short leg cast to mechanically offload the foot at the ulcer site and control edema while allowing some degree of ambulation.
- Neuropathic ulcers 3 cm or less in diameter can be treated with TCC unless severe ischemia, deep ulceration, infection, or significant edema is present.
- When casting or specialized footwear alone is inadequate, surgical correction of architectural deformities may be necessary.
- Correction of clawed toes at the metatarsophalangeal or proximal interphalangeal joints, arthrodesis of the interphalangeal joint of the hallux, resection of the head of one or more metatarsals, or even lengthening of the calcaneus tendon may be needed to maintain closure of an ulcer.
- Adequate perfusion must be confirmed before any surgical procedure is performed.
- Once the ulcer is healed, the foot must be continually protected in appropriate footwear.
- In the diabetic foot, all calluses should be considered preulcerative
- Calluses should be reduced, bony prominences padded or relieved, and skin lotion used after bathing the feet once or twice daily, drying well between the toes.
- Antibiotics are used in neuropathic and ischemic foot ulcers only in the presence of cellulitis, abscess, osteomyelitis, or pyarthrosis.

▪ *Ischemic ulcers and gangrene:*
- Patients with dry gangrene without signs of infection should undergo a careful vascular evaluation to determine healing potential.

- If the healing potential is inadequate, evaluation for revascularization should be undertaken with amputations delayed until this can be safely performed.
- Dry gangrene in this setting is almost never the cause of systemic infection.
- Aggressive arterial reconstruction has been paramount in reducing amputation rates over the past several decades.
- With current techniques, 90% of diabetics presenting with ischemic ulceration or gangrene are found to have surgically correctable occlusive disease.
- Vascular reconstruction in diabetic patients typically involves bypass from the femoral or popliteal arteries to tibial, peroneal, or pedal vessels.
- In the absence of continuous tibial vessels, a bypass to a patent pedal vessel or a peroneal artery with good ankle collaterals is a reasonable option.
- A vein should be used whenever possible because synthetic grafting to infrageniculate vessels has poor long-term patency.
- Although EVT of flow-limiting arterial stenosis and occlusions has not achieved the long-term patency of distal bypass with autologous vein grafts, this modality is effective in short-term improvements in circulation.
- Endovascular therapy may be preferable in patients unable or unwilling to undergo traditional bypass.

▪ *Invasive foot infections:*
  - Infection often originates in areas of recent trauma or chronic ulceration and may progress rapidly to acute foot sepsis.
  - Pain and tenderness, for instance, may be absent depending on the degree of sensory neuropathy.
  - Infection alters glucose metabolism further in the diabetic, and extreme hyperglycemia or even keto-acidosis may occur.
  - The initial management is directed at resuscitation and control of the foot infection.
  - Drainage and debridement of necrotic tissues are the primary goals in invasive diabetic foot infections with revascularization delayed until the infection has been controlled.
  - Diabetic foot infections are often much more extensive than assumed given the propensity of infection to track along the tendon and fascial sheaths.
  - Wound and sinus tracts should be opened to permit free drainage; involved bone or joints should be resected.
  - Subsequent procedures may be necessary to ensure adequate drainage.
  - Deep cultures of the wound should be obtained.
  - Initial broad-spectrum antibiotics should be administered and refined based on culture and sensitivity data.
  - Mild to moderate infections with localized cellulitis can be treated on an outpatient basis with oral antibiotics such as cephalexin, amoxicillin with clavulanate potassium, moxifloxacin, or clindamycin. The antibiotics should be started after initial cultures are taken and changed as necessary.
  - Partial foot amputations may be warranted to control sepsis.
  - These amputations are left open, and are designed to remove large areas of devitalized tissue, destroyed bones, and septic joints.
  - Careful consideration must be given to preserve as much functional tissue as possible.
  - Guillotine amputation at or above the ankle is required when infection extends proximal to the midfoot and is associated with hindfoot ischemia.
  - Definitive amputation follows when infection has been controlled and metabolic derangements improve.

▪ *Amputation:*
  - Amputations are indicated for removal of gangrenous or necrotic tissue.
  - The level of amputation depends on the proximal extent of the disease and the degree of vascular insufficiency.
  - With normal circulation, amputation can usually be performed just proximal to the extent of the necrotic tissue.

  - Distal toe ulcers will often slough once revascularization has occurred and should be followed for several months before amputation is offered.
  - Although some allow dry gangrenous digits to autoamputate, button, or ray amputations are preferable to spare the discomfort and distress autoamputations can cause patients.
  - Resection of the distal metatarsal head and removal of all cartilage and sesamoid bones are essential maneuvers in the performance of ray amputations.
  - A transmetatarsal amputation is considered if multiple toes or the distal forefoot is involved. A transmetatarsal amputation is inadequate in the presence of the midplantar foot ischemia, especially if the medial two or lateral three rays must be sacrificed. In this scenario, midfoot or hindfoot amputations (e.g., Chopart's) along with the appropriate tenotomies may be considered.
  - Even if successful, however, hindfoot amputations leave patients with a "peg leg", which may not be as functional as a below-knee amputation. If ischemic disease or infection involves the proximal foot, a below-knee amputation is indicated in the ambulatory patient.
  - Furthermore, in the presence of extensive neuropathic osteoarthropathy involving the tarsal bones with total collapse of the midfoot, a below-knee amputation may be preferable to extensive attempts at reconstruction.
  - Above-knee amputations may be appropriate in chronically non-ambulatory patients, patients with fixed knee contractures, or patients with marginal, unreconstructible, and distal circulation.
- *Adjunctive therapies:*
  - Despite good wound care, adequate offloading, and treatment of infection, diabetic foot ulcers will occasionally be recalcitrant to standard care.
  - Several therapies exist to improve wound healing, including hyperbaric oxygen therapy, platelet-derived growth factors, bioengineered skin and dermal substitutes, granulocyte colony-stimulating factor, and vacuum-assisted dressings.
  - Vacuum-assisted compression dressings have been particularly useful in stimulating reepithelialization and granulation tissue formation and are well tolerated by patients.

Nerve

39. Classify nerve injuries. ***Gujarat Health University 2025***

Classification of nerve injuries: There are *two main systems* commonly used:

1. *Seddon's classification (1943)*—simpler, 3 types.
2. *Sunderland's classification (1951)*—more detailed, 5 degrees (expands on Seddon's).

Seddon's Classification (1943)

Type	*Pathology*	*Key features*	*Recovery*
Neuropraxia	Conduction block without axonal disruption	• Myelin sheath affected, axon intact • No Wallerian degeneration • Usually due to mild compression or ischemia	Complete recovery within days to weeks
Axonotmesis	Axonal disruption with intact endoneurium and supporting connective tissue	• Axon and myelin destroyed • Wallerian degeneration distal to lesion • Endoneurial tubes guide regeneration	Recovery possible but slow (1–3 mm/day)
Neurotmesis	Complete transection of nerve (axon + connective tissue)	• Wallerian degeneration occurs • No pathway for regeneration	No spontaneous recovery — needs surgical repair

Sunderland's Classification (1951)

(Expands Seddon's three into five degrees based on the extent of structural damage.)

Degree	*Structures damaged*	*Pathology*	*Recovery/prognosis*
1st degree	Local myelin injury only	Equivalent to *Neuropraxia*	Full recovery in days–weeks
2nd degree	Axon and myelin	Equivalent to *Axonotmesis*	Axon regenerates within intact endoneurium → good recovery
3rd degree	Axon + endoneurium	Perineurium intact; fibrosis possible	Incomplete recovery—some misdirected fibers
4th degree	Axon + endoneurium + perineurium	Only epineurium intact; internal scarring blocks regeneration	Poor recovery → needs surgical repair
5th degree	Complete transection of nerve	Equivalent to *Neurotmesis*	No recovery without surgery

Clinical Correlation

Finding	*Neuropraxia*	*Axonotmesis*	*Neurotmesis*
Cause	Compression, ischemia	Crush, stretch	Laceration, severe trauma
Tinel's sign	Negative	Positive (advancing)	Absent (no regeneration)
Muscle wasting	None	Yes (transient)	Severe (permanent without repair)
Electrophysiology	Conduction block only	Denervation potentials	No response

40. Discuss median nerve injury at different levels. Outline the management. ***WBUHS 2025***

41. Clinical features of median nerve injury at various levels and its management. ***WBUHS 2016***

42. Median nerve injury. ***WBUHS 2013***

Anatomy

- Mixed nerve (contain motor and sensory fibers).
- *Root value:* C5,6,7,8, and T1
- Runs in the median plane of the forearm, so it is called median nerve.
- *Arises in the axilla by joining:*
  - Lateral cord of the brachial plexus
  - Medial cord of the brachial plexus.
- *Axilla:* After being from lateral cord and medial cord of brachial plexus runs on the lateral aspect of axillary artery.
- *Arm:* Continues to run lateral to the brachial artery till the mid-arm—crosses the artery anteriorly and passes anterior to the elbow joint into forearm.
- *Forearm:* Enters to the forearm between two heads of pronator teres—runs deep to the fibrous arch of flexor digitorum superficialis (FDS), in proximal one-third—in mid forearm it descends between FDS and flexor digitorum profundus (FDP)—about 5 cm above wrist, it comes to lie on the lateral side of the FDS, becomes superficial just above wrist.
- *Hand:* Passes deep to the flexor retinaculum and enters the hand—muscular branches supply muscles of Thenar eminence:
  - Abductor pollicis brevis
  - Opponens pollicis
  - Flexor pollicis brevis
- *Hand:* Divides into four to five palmar digital branches supplying lateral three and half digit and their nail beds—motor branches to the first and second lumbrical muscles

- *Other branches:*
    - *Articular branches:* Supply the proximal radioulnar joint
    - *Palmar cutaneous branch:* Supplies skin over thenar eminence

Injury can occur:

- Occasionally in the elbow region in supracondylar fractures of the humerus
- Commonly injured by stab wounds or broken glass just proximal to the flexor retinaculum
    - *High median nerve injuries*—injury proximal to the elbow—due to forearm fractures or elbow dislocation—stab injuries and GSW's—paralysis of all the muscles supplied by the median nerve in the forearm and hand.
    - *Low median nerve injuries*—injury in the distal third of the forearm—sparing of the forearm muscles—muscles of the hand paralyzed—anesthesia over the median nerve distribution in the hand—thenar eminence is wasted and thumb abduction and opposition are weak—sensation lost over the radial three and half digits and trophic changes may seen
- *Injury at elbow (motor):*
    - Here it lies between the tendons of flexor carpi radialis and FDS.
    - Rarely injured due to its protected position beneath the biceps brachii muscle
    - If injured high up in the arm, the biceps, and coracobrachialis are paralyzed, and brachialis is weakened.
    - Sensory loss along the lateral side of the forearm occurs.
    - When the patient tries to make a fist, the index, and middle fingers tend to remain straight.
    - Only ring and little fingers flex
    - Flexion in these fingers is weakened by the loss of the FDS.
    - Flexion of terminal phalanx of thumb is lost because of paralysis of flexor pollicis longus.
    - The thumb is laterally rotated and adducted.
    - Muscles of thenar eminence are paralyzed.
    - The hand looks flattened and ape-like.
- *Injury at elbow (sensory):*
    - Skin sensation is lost on the palmar aspect of the lateral three and half fingers.
    - Sensory loss occurs on the skin of the distal part of the dorsal surfaces of the lateral three and half fingers.
    - Total area of anesthesia is less.
- *Injury at elbow (vasomotor changes):*
    - The skin areas involved in sensory loss are warmer and drier than normal.
    - Arteriolar dilatation and absence of sweating resulting from loss of sympathetic control.
- *Injury at elbow (Trophic changes)*

In long standing cases:

- Skin is dry and scaly.
- Nails crack easily.
- Atrophy of the pulp of the fingers
- *Injury at wrist:*
    - Almost all the clinical findings are same as injury of the median nerve at elbow.
    - In addition, a delicate pincer-like movement is not possible.
- *Carpal tunnel syndrome:*
    - The carpal tunnel is formed by the concave anterior surface of carpal bones and closed by flexor retinaculum.
    - Clinically, the syndrome consists of a burning pain or pins and needles along the distribution of the median nerve.
    - Lateral three and half fingers are involved.
    - The exact cause is difficult to determine.
    - Condition is relieved by decompressing the tunnel by making a longitudinal incision through the flexor retinaculum.

Examination

- *Flexor pollicis longus:* Tested by holding thumb at its base and patient asked to flex the terminal phalanx.
- *FDS and profundus (Ochsner's clasping test):* Patient is asked to clasp the hands, the index finger of affected side fails to flex.
- *Flexor carpi radialis:* Hand deviates to the ulnar side when flexed against resistance.
- *Muscles of thenar eminence:* Abductor pollicis brevis (Pen test)—hand laid flat on the table—pen held above the palm and the patient is asked to touch the pen with his thumb.
- *Opponens pollicis:* Brings the tip of the thumb toward the tips of other fingers.
- *Opponens polices:* Benedict sign, Klein Nioh/OK Sign, Ape thumb.

Principles of Surgical Management

- *Direct injury:* Nerve repair
- *Compression neuropathies:* Decompression
- *Long standing cases:*
    - *Tendon transfers:*
    - *Low median nerve:* Re-routing of ring/middle finger superficial flexor around FCU to APB to aid thumb opposition.
    - *High median nerve:* Suturing of profundus tendons to ring and small finger tendons for restoration of IP joint movements—ECU re-routing and attachment to dorsal radius/transfer of biceps insertion from medial to lateral part of radius for weak forearm pronation
- Median nerve compression syndromes
    - Carpal tunnel
    - Pronator
    - Interosseous
- *Carpal tunnel syndrome:* Compressive neuropathy as the nerve passes through the carpal tunnel.
    - *Causes:*
        - Idiopathic
        - Rheumatoid arthritis
        - Wrist osteoarthritis
        - Post-traumatic
        - *Bone thickening-endocrine:* Myxedema and acromegaly
        - Pregnancy
        - Gout
        - *Repetitive wrist movements:* Typists and computer users
    - *Symptoms:*
        - Hand and wrist pain
        - Paresthesia
        - Hypoesthesia
        - Sparing of palmar cutaneous branch supply
        - Patient wakes at night with burning or aching pain and shakes the hand to obtain relief and restore sensation.
        - Aggravated by elevation of hand.
        - Thenar atrophy and weakness of thumb opposition and abduction may develop late.
    - *Diagnosis:*
        - History
        - *Clinical examination:*
            - Thenar wasting
            - Phalen's sign
            - Tinel's sign
            - Carpal compression test/Durkan's test
        - *Electrodiagnostic studies:* Very reliable for evaluation—atypical cases may be present.

- *Management:*
  - *Splinting:* Prevents wrist flexion
  - Corticosteroid/anesthetic injection
  - *Surgical decompression:* Division of the transverse carpal ligament (open/endoscopic)
- *Complications:*
  - Injury to palmar cutaneous/recurrent motor branch of the median nerve
  - Hypertrophic scarring
  - Hematoma/arterial injury
  - Pillar pain

- *Pronator teres syndrome:*
  - High compression neuropathy
  - It is rare compared to CTS and AIS
  - Proximal forearm median nerve involved
  - Misnomer compression
- *Symptoms and signs:*
  - Symptoms are similar to those of carpal tunnel syndrome.
  - Sensory disturbances—Thumb and index > Middle finger
  - Night pain is unusual and forearm pain is more common.
  - Hand numbness on gripping
  - Phalen's test negative
  - Double crush phenomena
  - Symptoms provoked by resisted elbow flexion with forearm supinated (tightening of bicipital aponeurosis)
  - By resisted forearm pronation with the elbow extended (pronator tension)
- *Management:*
  - No relief with steroids
  - Surgical decompression
- *Anterior interosseous syndrome (AIS):* Damage to the anterior interosseous nerve
  - *Causes:* Injury to elbow—injury during open/closed reduction
  - *Signs/symptoms:*
    - Pain in the forearm
    - Weakness of the gripping movement of the thumb and index finger (unable to make ok sign)
  - *Management:*
    - Corticosteroids
    - *Surgery:* Resection/detachment of deep head of pronator teres

43. Write in brief the different modalities of management of lower limb edema. ***WBUHS 2024***

Management of lower limb edema involves identifying and treating the underlying cause, along with symptomatic relief. The main modalities include:

- *Lifestyle modifications:*
  - Elevation of legs above heart level
  - Regular physical activity and leg exercises
  - Weight loss if overweight
  - Avoiding prolonged standing or sitting
- *Compression therapy:*
  - Compression stockings or bandages to promote venous return
  - Pneumatic compression devices in severe cases
- *Pharmacological treatment:*
  - Diuretics for fluid overload (e.g., in heart failure or renal disease)
  - Medications for underlying conditions (e.g., antihypertensives, anticoagulants)

- *Treatment of underlying conditions:*
  - *Venous insufficiency:* Compression, venous surgery
  - *Lymphedema:* Manual lymphatic drainage, specialized massage
  - *Cardiac, renal, hepatic causes:* Specific organ-based treatments
  - *Infections (e.g., cellulitis):* Antibiotics
- *Surgical and interventional procedures:*
  - Varicose vein surgery (e.g., sclerotherapy, vein stripping)
  - Lymphatic bypass or debulking procedures in severe lymphedema
- *Skin and wound care:*
  - Prevention and treatment of ulcers
  - Moisturizers to prevent dryness and cracking
- Accurate diagnosis of the cause is crucial for effective management.

---

44. Surgical management of filarial lymphedema of lower limb. ***Gujarat Health University 2025***

Filarial Lymphedema of Lower Limb

Definition

A *chronic lymphatic obstruction* caused by *Wuchereria bancrofti* (rarely Brugia malayi), leading to *progressive swelling, fibrosis, and deformity* of the limb.

Pathophysiology (Brief Overview)

- Adult filarial worms live in *lymphatic channels*, causing: *Inflammation, fibrosis*, and *obliteration* of lymphatic vessels.
- This leads to: *Lymphatic stasis → tissue edema → fibrosis → elephantiasis* (irreversible stage).
- *Chronic changes:* Thickened skin, papillomatosis, fibrosis, and secondary infections.

Goals of Surgical Management

- Reduce limb volume.
- Restore or improve lymphatic drainage.
- Prevent recurrent infections and ulceration.
- Improve function and cosmesis.

Staging (for Surgical Planning)

Stage	***Features***	***Surgical indication***
Grade I (pitting, reversible)	Edema subsides with elevation	*Conservative* only
Grade II (non-pitting, fibrotic)	Chronic swelling, skin thickening	*Physiologic procedures*
Grade III (elephantiasis)	Massive deformity, papillomatosis	*Excisional/reductive procedures*

Types of Surgical Procedures

Physiologic (Reconstructive/Drainage) Procedures

Aim: Restore lymph flow by creating new drainage pathways between lymphatic vessels and veins or by bypassing obstructed lymphatics.

- *Lymphatic–venous anastomosis (LVA)*
  - *Principle:* Connect functional lymphatics to nearby venules → lymph drained directly into venous system.
  - *Technique:* Microsurgical; end-to-end or end-to-side anastomosis under microscope (8×–25× magnification).
  - *Indications:* Early to moderate stages (before gross fibrosis).
  - *Advantages:* Physiologic, less invasive.
  - *Limitations:* Requires patent lymphatics; technically demanding.
- *Vascularized lymph node transfer (VLNT)*
  - *Principle:* Transfer lymph node flaps (e.g., from supraclavicular or groin region) with their blood supply to the affected limb.

- *Mechanism:* Lymphangiogenesis and establishment of new lymphatic drainage.
- *Indications:* Chronic lymphedema (Stage II–III).
- *Limitations:* Microsurgical expertise required.

- *Omental transposition/Omentoplasty*
  - *Principle:* Mobilized omentum (rich in lymphatics) is tunneled subcutaneously into the limb to facilitate lymph drainage.
  - *Indications:* Moderate-to-severe cases when local lymphatics destroyed.

Excisional (Reductive/Ablative) Procedures

Aim: Remove fibrotic, hypertrophied, nonfunctional tissue in late-stage elephantiasis.

- *Charles' procedure (1901)*
  - *Principle:* Radical excision of affected skin and subcutaneous tissue down to deep fascia → cover with *split-thickness skin grafts.*
  - *Indications:* Gross, irreversible elephantiasis with papillomatosis.
  - *Advantages:* Effective in volume reduction.
  - *Disadvantages:* Poor cosmetic result, prolonged healing, graft breakdown risk.
- *Modified Charles/Kondoleon/Homan procedures*

Procedure	***Principle***	***Key feature***
Kondoleon's (1912)	Subfascial excision to create lymphatic communication with deep system	Partly physiologic
Homan's (1936)	Excision of subcutaneous tissue while preserving skin flaps	Better cosmesis
Thompson's operation (1962)	Buried dermal flaps (deepithelialized skin) create lymphatic drainage channels	Combines excision + physiologic mechanism
Modified Charles	Limited excision + preservation of dermal flaps	Improved healing, less morbidity

- *Liposuction/debulking:* Useful adjunct for residual fibrofatty hypertrophy after physiologic surgery.
- *Supportive measures (pre- and postoperative)*
  - *Preoperative limb care:*
    - Treat infection (antibiotics, antifilarial drugs—DEC).
    - Skin hygiene and antifungal treatment.
  - *Compression therapy* after healing to maintain reduction.
  - *Physiotherapy* to preserve mobility and prevent contractures.
  - *Regular follow-up* for recurrence or ulceration.
- *Choice of procedure*

Stage	***Procedure type***	***Example***
Early (pitting edema)	Conservative	Limb elevation, compression, DEC therapy
Moderate (nonpitting, fibrosis)	Physiologic	LVA, VLNT, omentoplasty
Late (elephantiasis)	Excisional/debulking	Charles, Homan, Thompson procedures

- *Complications*
  - Infection and wound breakdown
  - Graft loss (in excisional procedures)
  - Recurrence of swelling
  - Persistent lymphorrhea
  - Disfigurement (especially after radical excision)

CHAPTER 50

Abdominal Aortic Aneurysms

LEARNING OBJECTIVES

- Classification of Abdominal Aortic Aneurysm
- Clinical Features
- Management

CLASSIFICATION OF ABDOMINAL AORTIC ANEURYSM

1. Define aneurysm. Classify aneurysm. Discuss recent advances in the management of aneurysm. (Abdominal Aortic Aneurysm) ***WBUHS 2025***

Definition of Aneurysm

An aneurysm is a permanent, localized dilation of a blood vessel, usually defined as an enlargement of at least 50% beyond the vessel's normal diameter. In the context of the abdominal aorta, this enlargement is referred to as an Abdominal Aortic Aneurysm (AAA) when the abdominal aortic diameter is ≥3 cm.

Classification of Aneurysms

- *By pathology/wall involvement*
  - *True aneurysm:* Involves all three arterial wall layers (intima, media, and adventitia). Examples include atherosclerotic, syphilitic, and congenital aneurysms *Wikipedia PMC*
  - *False aneurysm (Pseudoaneurysm):* A contained rupture where blood leaks outside the vessel but is confined by surrounding tissue *Wikipedia*
  - *Dissecting aneurysm:* Occurs when blood infiltrates a tear in the intima, splitting the vessel wall. These are typically classified via Stanford and DeBakey systems in the thoracic aorta context and less commonly in aneurysms PMC
- *By morphology*
  - *Fusiform aneurysm:* Uniform, circumferential dilation. Most AAAs fall into this category Saccular aneurysm: Localized outpouching on one side of the vessel with a distinct neck *Wikipedia*
- *By location*
  - *Abdominal aortic aneurysm (AAA):* Most common; infrarenal segment of the aorta
  - *Thoracic aortic aneurysm (TAA):* Occurs within the chest; less common
  - *Thoracoabdominal aortic aneurysm (TAAA):* Spans both thoracic and abdominal segments; notably complex and often classified using the Crawford classification
- *By size*
  - *Small:* <3 cm
  - *Medium:* 3–5.5 cm

  - *Large:* ≥5.5 cm (AAA), ≥6 cm (TAAA)
  - *Giant:* ≥10 cm
- *Inflammatory AAA (IAA):* A subtype characterized by thickened, inflamed aneurysm walls with peri-aneurysmal fibrosis. Represents about 5–10% of AAAs. Symptoms may include back pain, elevated ESR, and systemic signs; corticosteroids and immunosuppressive therapy may reduce inflammation and fibrosis.

Recent Advances in Management of AAA

- *Personalized biomechanical and imaging-based risk assessment*
  - Traditional risk stratification relies on diameter thresholds (≥ 5.5 cm in men, ≥ 5 cm in women) and growth rates, but these have limitations—smaller AAAs can rupture and large ones may remain stable.
  - Emerging approaches incorporate wall stress, wall strength, hemodynamic factors, and advanced imaging modalities:
    - Ultrasound elastography, CT/MR-based biomechanical modeling, and finite element analysis (FEA) enhance predictions of rupture risk by assessing mechanical forces and tissue integrity
    - A novel Relative Structural Integrity Index (RSII) derived from 4D-CTA imaging combined with wall strain and tension measurements allows noninvasive, patient-specific mapping of wall integrity
    - Geometric deep learning models utilizing SE (3)-transformers can predict localized AAA growth and accurately forecast when a patient may become eligible for elective repair.
- *Precision/personalized medicine and ai integration*
  - Reviews emphasize the future of AAA management lying in precision medicine: integrating biomechanical assessments with AI-driven imaging, biomarkers, and genotypic data for individualized risk profiling and timing of intervention.
  - Advanced imaging combined with AI models improves diagnostic accuracy and enables early detection without relying solely on contrast agents (e.g., U-net models for CT image segmentation).
- *Pharmacological and novel therapies (experimental stage)*
  - *Experimental strategies include:* Nanoparticle-based drug delivery, stem cell therapies, and gene editing (e.g., CRISPR-Cas9) targeting aneurysm wall strengthening and progression slowdown.
  - *Additional emerging therapeutic targets:*
    - Inhibition of BMP4 showed promise in reducing inflammation and endothelial-mesenchymal transition in experimental AAA models.
    - Other approaches like mesoporous silica nanoplatforms, ferroptosis modulation, or anti-inflammatory compounds (e.g., Atractylenolide-I) are under investigation.
- *Surgical and endovascular repair*
  - *Elective repair thresholds remain:* ≥ 5.5 cm in men, ≥ 5.0 cm in women, or rapid growth/symptoms.
  - Endovascular aneurysm repair (EVAR) is associated with lower perioperative morbidity and mortality than open repair, though long-term survival differences become comparable after ~2 years; requires lifelong imaging surveillance due to complications like endoleaks.
  - Endoleak classification (post-EVAR) includes Types I–V, guiding ongoing monitoring and reintervention.

---

2. Classify Abdominal Aortic Aneurysm and discuss its management. ***WBUHS 2017***

---

3. Classify aortic aneurysm. What are the clinical features and management of aortic aneurysm? ***WBUHS 2023***

- Infrarenal
- Juxtarenal
- Pararenal
- Suprarenal

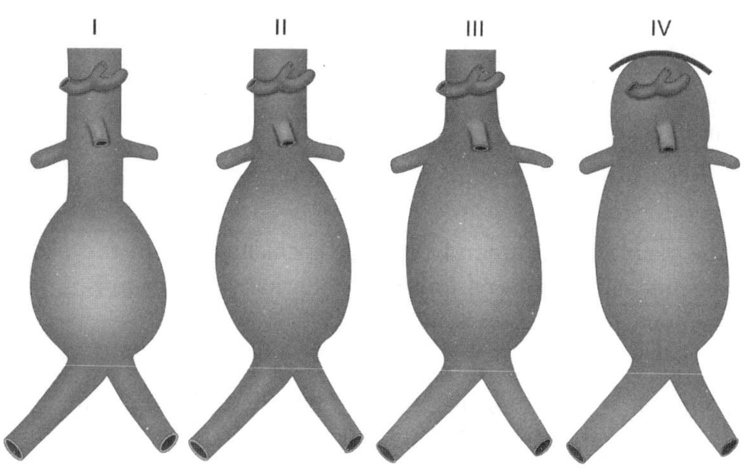

Risk Factors for Rupture of AAA

Risk factor	*Low risk*	*Average risk*	*High risk*
Diameter	<5 cm	5–6 cm	>6 cm
Expansion	<0.3 cm/year	0.3–0.6 cm/year	>0.6 cm/year
Smoking and COPD	None, mild	Moderate	Severe/steroids
Family history	No relatives	One relative	Numerous relatives
Hypertension	Normal blood pressure	Controlled	Poorly controlled
Shape	Fusiform	Saccular	Very eccentric
Gender		Male	Female

(COPD: chronic obstructive pulmonary disease)

CLINICAL FEATURES

- *Clinical presentation:*
  - Most AAAs are asymptomatic.
  - Diagnosed incidentally
  - Presents with severe symptoms when it leaks or ruptures.
  - Unruptured aneurysms may present with abdominal or back pain—though uncommon
  - Large aneurysms may present as a pulsatile abdominal mass.
- *Complications:*
  - The most significant complication is abdominal aortic rupture, which presents with severe abdominal or back pain, hypotension, and shock. The mortality rate from a ruptured AAA is very high.
  - *Other complications include:*
    - Pseudoaneurysm from chronic contained leak/rupture
    - Aortic fistulas
    - Aortocaval fistula
    - Aortoenteric fistula
    - Aorto-left renal vein fistula (very rare)
    - Distal thromboembolism
    - Thrombotic occlusion of a branch vessel
    - Infection/mycotic aneurysm (actually a pseudoaneurysm)
    - Compression of adjacent structures from large aneurysms (rare)
    - Anterior vertebral scalloping

Role of Imaging

- Detection of AAA
- Monitoring of growth rate
- Preoperative planning
- Postoperative follow-up

Plain Radiograph

- An aneurysm may be visible as an area of curvilinear calcification in the paravertebral region on either abdominal or lumbar spine radiographs performed for alternative indications.
- Radiographs are not optimal for detection or follow-up.

Ultrasound

- Ultrasound assessment is simple, safe, and inexpensive. It has a reported sensitivity of 95% and specificity close to 100%.
- It is usually the preferred choice for the monitoring of small aneurysms.
- The measurement error for ultrasound evaluation of AAA is 4 mm.

Computed Tomography (CT)

- CT angiography (CTA) is considered the imaging gold standard but exposes the patients to high-radiation doses.
- It is excellent for preoperative planning as it accurately delineates the size and shape of the AAA and its relationship to branch arteries and the aortic bifurcation. Oblique reformations enable accurate measurements in nonorthogonal planes.
- CTA is superior to ultrasound in detecting and measuring common iliac artery aneurysms.

Signs of frank rupture include:

- Retroperitoneal hematoma
- Para-aortic fat stranding
- Contrast extravasation from the aorta into the retroperitoneum

Signs of impending rupture or contained leakage:

- Draped aorta sign (contained rupture)
- High-attenuation crescent sign
- Thrombus fissuration
- Focal discontinuity of intimal calcification
- Tangential calcium sign

An increasing diameter of the aneurysmal sac of 10 mm over a 12-month interval or a diameter of 7 cm is also considered to be at high risk for rupture and warrants urgent repair.

Magnetic Resonance (MR) Angiography

Offers lack of ionizing radiation, but is more costly, less widely available, and the examination is substantially lengthier.

Angiography

- Digital subtraction angiography (DSA) does not show the true aneurysm size if there is a mural thrombus but is superb at delineating branch vessels.
- Barring certain contraindications, endovascular repair of AAA is usually the first treatment choice.

Treatment and Prognosis

- The natural history of AAAs is that of slow expansion, with possible eventual rupture having devastating consequences.
- The risk of rupture is proportional to the size of the aneurysm and the rate of growth. Differing rates of rupture for a given aneurysm size have been reported in the literature, but the general consensus is that aneurysms

>5.0 cm in diameter in women and 5.5 cm in men carry a significantly increased risk of rupture and should be treated.

- Furthermore, aneurysms that expand at a rate of >10 mm per annum are also at a significant risk of rupture and are considered for treatment even when <5.0 cm.
- In patients with a connective tissue disorder, especially those with a bicuspid aortic valve, surgical treatment may be considered even with a diameter smaller than 5.0 cm.
- Follow-up intervals for imaging an enlarged infrarenal abdominal aorta from initial detection
  - *<2.5 cm:* Follow-up is not needed.
  - *2.5–2.9 cm:* 5-year interval
  - *3.0–3.4 cm:* 3-year interval
  - *3.5–3.9 cm:* 2-year interval
  - *4.0–4.4 cm:* 1-year interval
  - *4.5–4.9 cm:* 6-month interval
  - *5.0–5.5 cm:* 3–6-month interval
  - *>5.5 cm:* Treatment

MANAGEMENT

Management options include:

- Endovascular aneurysm repair (EVAR)
- *Open surgical repair:*
  - Open repair is indicated in young patients as an elective procedure, or in growing or large, symptomatic or ruptured aneurysms.
  - The aorta must be clamped off during the repair, denying blood to the abdominal organs and sections of the spinal cord; this can cause a range of complications.
  - It is essential to make the critical part of the operation fast, so the incision is typically made large enough to facilitate the fastest repair.
  - Recovery after open AAA surgery takes significant time.
  - The minimums are a few days in intensive care, a week total in the hospital, and a few months before full recovery.

CHAPTER 51

Stents in Surgical Practice

LEARNING OBJECTIVE

- Stents in Surgical Practice

STENTS IN SURGICAL PRACTICE

1. Stents in surgical practice. ***WBUHS 2015***

Definition

A stent is a small, expandable tube inserted into a vessel or duct to keep it open, often used to treat narrowed or blocked passages.

- Coronary stents are placed during a percutaneous coronary intervention, also known as angioplasty. The most common use for coronary stents is in the coronary arteries, into which a bare-metal stent, a drug- eluting stent, a bioabsorbable stent, a dual-therapy stent (combination of both drug and bioengineered stents), or occasionally a covered stent is inserted.
- Vascular stents are commonly placed as part of peripheral artery angioplasty. Common sites treated with peripheral artery stents include the carotid, iliac, and femoral arteries. Because of the external compression and mechanical forces subjected to these locations, flexible stent materials such as nitinol are used in a majority of peripheral stent placements.
- A stent graft or covered stent is a type of vascular stent with a fabric coating that creates a contained tube but is expandable like a bare-metal stent. Covered stents are used in endovascular surgical procedures such as endovascular aneurysm repair. Stent grafts are also used to treat stenoses in vascular grafts and fistulas used for hemodialysis.
- Ureteral stents are used to ensure the patency of a ureter, which may be compromised, e.g., by a kidney stone. This method is sometimes used as a temporary measure to prevent damage to a blocked kidney until a procedure to remove the stone can be performed.
- Prostatic stents are placed from the bladder through the prostatic and penile urethra to allow drainage of the bladder through the penis. This is sometimes required in benign prostatic hypertrophy.
- Esophageal stents are a palliative treatment for advanced esophageal cancer.
- Biliary stents provide bile drainage from the gallbladder, pancreas, and bile ducts to the duodenum in conditions such as ascending cholangitis due to obstructing gallstones.
- Other types are duodenal stents, colonic stents, and pancreatic stents, the name referring to the location of their placement.

Specialty	***Use of stents***
Cardiothoracic surgery	*Coronary artery stents* – used during percutaneous coronary intervention (PCI) to open narrowed arteries
Vascular surgery	*Peripheral vascular stents* – used in peripheral artery disease to maintain blood flow
Urology	*Ureteral stents* – placed to relieve or prevent obstruction of the ureter (e.g., after stone removal or due to malignancy)
Gastrointestinal surgery	*Esophageal, biliary, and colonic stents* – used for obstruction due to malignancy or strictures
Neurosurgery/Interventional radiology	*Intracranial stents* – for aneurysms or stenosed cerebral vessels
Plastic/Reconstructive surgery	Used to maintain patency of reconstructed ducts or passages, e.g., lacrimal stents

CHAPTER 52

Cardiothoracic and Vascular Surgery

LEARNING OBJECTIVES

- Arterial System of Heart
- Myocardial Revascularization Procedures
- Central Venous Catheterization and Vascular Access for Dialysis
- Portal Vein Embolization
- Complications of Endovascular Stents
- Empyema Thoracis and ARDS
- Complications of Chest Injury, Flail Chest, and Tension Pneumothorax
- Thoracic Outlet Syndrome and Thoracic Inlet Syndrome
- Minimally Invasive Thoracic Procedures
- VATS and CABG
- Pulmonary Hydatid Disease
- Mediastinal Tumors
- Pancoast Tumor

1. Draw the diagram of arterial system of heart. What are the methods of myocardial revascularization procedures and the materials used? ***RGUHS Karnataka 2025***

Arterial System of Heart

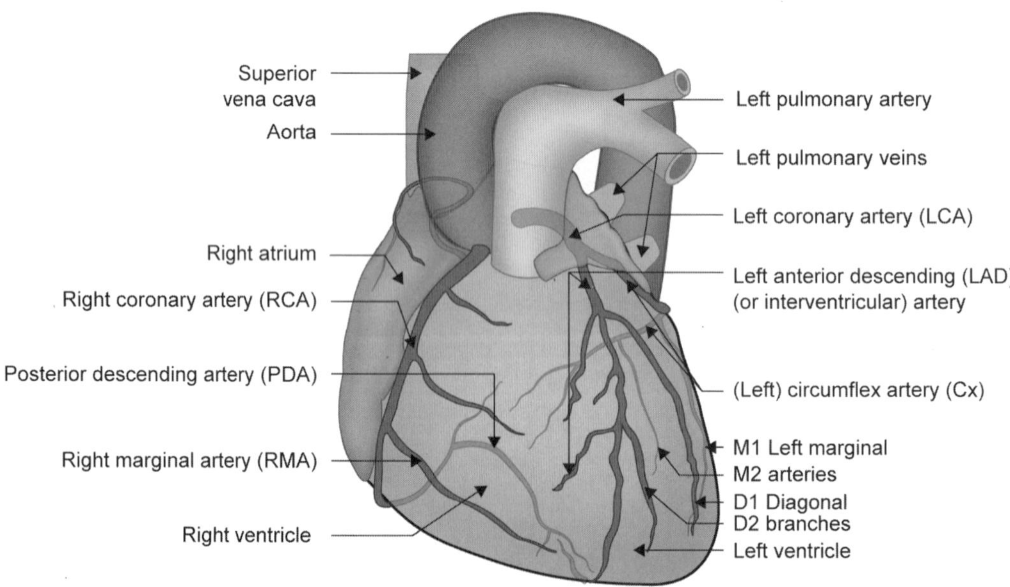

Myocardial Revascularization

Introduction

Myocardial revascularization refers to any procedure that restores blood flow to ischemic (underperfused) areas of the heart caused by *coronary artery disease (CAD).*

There are two main categories:

I. *Percutaneous (catheter-based) methods:* Non-surgical
II. *Surgical methods:* Coronary artery bypass grafting (CABG)

Percutaneous Coronary Revascularization (PCI)

Also known as *percutaneous coronary intervention (PCI),* these are catheter-based procedures performed through the femoral or radial artery.

Techniques

- *Balloon angioplasty (PTCA - Percutaneous transluminal coronary angioplasty)*
  - A balloon-tipped catheter is inserted into the coronary artery and inflated to dilate the stenotic segment.
  - Often followed by stent placement.
- *Coronary stenting*
  - After angioplasty, a *stent* (a small mesh tube) is inserted to keep the artery open.
  - *Types of stents:*
    - *Bare-metal stents (BMS):* Simple metallic framework.
    - *Drug-eluting stents (DES):* Coated with antiproliferative drugs (e.g., sirolimus, everolimus) to reduce restenosis.
    - *Bioresorbable vascular scaffolds:* Dissolvable materials (e.g., polylactic acid).
- *Atherectomy techniques*
  - Used for heavily calcified or complex lesions.
  - *Types:*
    - *Rotational atherectomy:* Diamond-tipped burr ablates plaque.
    - *Directional atherectomy:* Cuts plaque mechanically.
    - *Laser atherectomy:* Vaporizes plaque with laser energy.
- *Intravascular lithotripsy (IVL)*
  - Uses sonic pressure waves to fracture calcium in the vessel wall, facilitating stent deployment.

Surgical Myocardial Revascularization (CABG)

Coronary Artery Bypass Grafting (CABG) creates alternate routes (bypasses) for blood to reach the myocardium beyond blocked arteries.

Techniques

- *Conventional (on-pump) CABG*
  - Heart-lung machine (cardiopulmonary bypass) is used.
  - The heart is stopped (cardioplegia), and grafts are attached.
- *Off-pump CABG (OPCAB)*
  - Surgery performed on a *beating heart* using stabilization devices.
  - Avoids cardiopulmonary bypass—useful in high-risk patients.
- *Minimally Invasive Direct Coronary Artery Bypass (MIDCAB)*
  - Small thoracotomy incision without sternotomy.
  - Typically used for left anterior descending (LAD) artery lesions.
- *Robot-Assisted or Totally Endoscopic CABG (TECAB)*
  - Robotic instruments and cameras used through small ports.
  - Least invasive surgical option.

Graft Materials Used in CABG

Type of graft	*Common vessel used*	*Features/advantages*	*Typical use*
Arterial grafts			
Internal mammary (thoracic) artery (usually LIMA – left internal mammary artery)	Excellent long-term patency (>90% at 10 years)	Gold standard for LAD artery	
Right internal mammary artery (RIMA)	Often used in bilateral grafting	LAD or RCA territory	
Radial artery (from forearm)	Good patency, muscular wall—spasm risk (needs vasodilators)	Second conduit for obtuse marginal or diagonal branches	
Gastroepiploic artery	Used in selected patients	Posterior descending artery	
Venous grafts			
Great saphenous vein	Easy to harvest, flexible	Shorter patency (~50% at 10 years), prone to atherosclerosis	
Small saphenous or arm veins	Alternative if great saphenous not available	Less common	
Synthetic/Prosthetic Grafts	PTFE (polytetrafluoroethylene) or Dacron	Rarely used—poor patency in coronary circulation	Used in experimental or hybrid cases

Hybrid Revascularization

- *Combines* surgical and percutaneous methods.
- *Example:*
  - *LIMA–LAD* graft surgically (for main vessel), and
  - *PCI with stent* for other lesions.
- Minimizes invasiveness and maximizes long-term graft survival.

Summary

Method	*Approach*	*Anesthesia*	*Materials used*	*Advantages*	*Limitations*
PCI	Catheter-based	Local	Balloons, stents (metal, drug-eluting, bioresorbable)	Minimally invasive, rapid recovery	Restenosis, stent thrombosis
CABG (on-pump)	Surgical (open)	General	Arterial and venous grafts	Long-term patency, complete revascularization	Invasive, longer recovery
OPCAB	Surgical (off-pump)	General	Same as CABG	Avoids CPB complications	Technically demanding
MIDCAB/TECAB	Minimally invasive	General	LIMA or radial grafts	Less trauma, faster recovery	Limited to certain vessels
Hybrid	Combined	General + local	LIMA + stent	Best of both approaches	Requires specialized setup

2. Write short note on central venous catheterization. ***WBUHS 2012***

Introduction

- A central venous catheter ("central line", "CVC", "central venous line" or "central venous access catheter") is a catheter placed into a large vein in the neck (internal jugular vein) chest (subclavian vein or axillary vein) or groin (femoral vein).

- It is used to administer medication or fluids, obtain blood tests (specifically the "mixed venous oxygen saturation"), and directly obtain cardiovascular measurements such as the central venous pressure.

Indications for the use of central lines include:

Therapeutic	Delivery of drugs that are prone to cause phlebitis in peripheral veins (caustic)	Procedures	Need for intravenous therapy when peripheral venous access is impossible
• Monitoring of the central venous pressure (CVP) in acutely ill patients to quantify fluid balance • Long-term intravenous antibiotics • Long-term parenteral nutrition especially in chronically ill patients • Long-term pain medications • Chemotherapy	• Calcium chloride • Chemotherapy • Hypertonic saline • Potassium chloride • Amiodarone • Vasopressors (e.g., epinephrine and dopamine)	• Plasmapheresis • Peripheral blood stem cell collections • Dialysis • Frequent blood draws • Frequent or persistent requirement for intravenous access	• Blood • Medication • Rehydration

Central venous catheters usually remain in place for a longer period of time than other venous access devices, especially when the reason for their use is longstanding (such as total parenteral nutrition in a chronically ill patient).

Insertion

- The skin is cleaned, and local anesthetic applied if required.
- The location of the vein is then identified by landmarks or with the use of a small ultrasound device.
- A hollow needle is advanced through the skin until blood is aspirated; the color of the blood and the rate of its flow help distinguish it from arterial blood (suggesting that an artery has been accidentally punctured), although this method is inaccurate. Ultrasound probably now represents the gold standard for central venous access and skills, within North American and Europe, with landmark techniques are diminishing.

The Line is then Inserted Using the Seldinger Technique

- A blunt guidewire is passed through the needle, then the needle is removed.
- A dilating device may be passed over the guidewire to slightly enlarge the tract.
- Finally, the central line itself is then passed over the guidewire, which is then removed.
- All the lumens of the line are aspirated (to ensure that they are all positioned inside the vein) and flushed.
- A chest X-ray is typically performed afterward to confirm that the line is positioned inside the superior vena cava and, in the case of insertion through the subclavian vein, no pneumothorax was caused as a side effect.
- Vascular positioning systems can also be used to verify tip placement during insertion without the need to a chest X-ray, but this technique is not yet a standard of practice.

Complications

Mechanical Complications

- Arterial puncture, hematoma, and pneumothorax are the most common mechanical complications during the insertion.
- *Frequency of mechanical complications, according to the route of catheterization:*
    - Overall, internal jugular catheterization and subclavian venous catheterization carry similar risks of mechanical complications.
    - Subclavian catheterization is more likely than internal jugular catheterization to be complicated by pneumothorax and hemothorax.
    - Internal jugular catheterization is more likely to be associated with arterial puncture.
- Hematoma and arterial puncture are common during femoral venous catheterization.

Infectious Complications

Catheter-related infections are thought to arise by several different mechanisms: Infection of the exit site, followed by migration of the pathogen along the external catheter surface; contamination of the catheter hub, leading to intraluminal catheter colonization; and hematogenous seeding of the catheter.

Thrombotic Complications

- Patients who require central venous catheterization are at high risk for catheter-related thrombosis.
- The risk of catheter-related thrombosis varies according to the site of insertion:
- Subclavian venous catheterization carries the lowest risk of catheter-related thrombosis.

Scope of Therapeutic Embolism of Surgical Diseases

- Embolization involves the selective occlusion of blood vessels by purposely introducing emboli, in other words deliberately blocking a blood vessel.
- Embolization is used to treat a wide variety of conditions affecting different organs of the human body.

The treatment is used to occlude:

- Recurrent coughing up of blood
- Cerebral aneurysm
- Gastrointestinal bleeding
- Nosebleed
- Varicocele
- Primary postpartum bleeding
- Surgical bleeding
- Traumatic bleeding such as splenic rupture or pelvic fracture
- *Growths:* The treatment is used to slow or stop blood supply thus reducing the size of the tumors—
  - Kidney lesions
  - Liver lesions, typically hepatocellular carcinoma (HCC). Treated either by particle infarction or trans-catheter arterial chemoembolization (TACE).
  - Uterine fibroids
  - Arteriovenous malformations (AVMs)
  - Juvenile nasopharyngeal angiofibroma
- *Malignant hypertension:* It could be useful for managing malignant hypertension due to end-stage kidney failure.
- *Other:* Portal vein embolization (PVE) prior to liver resection.

Agents

- *Liquid embolic agents*—used for AVM, these agents can flow through complex vascular structures so the surgeon does not need to target his catheter to every single vessel. Onyx is an example for a liquid embolic agent.
- N-butyl cyanoacrylate (NBCA)
  - Ethiodol
- *Sclerosing agents*—these will harden the endothelial lining of vessels. They require more time to react than the liquid embolic agents. Therefore, they cannot be used for large or high-flow vessels.
  - *Ethanol:* This permanent agent is very good for treating AVM.
  - *Ethanolamine oleate:* This permanent agent is used for sclerosing esophageal varices.
  - *Sotradecol:* This agent is used for superficial lower extremity varicose veins. It can cause hyperpigmentation of the region in 30% of patients.
- *Particulate embolic agents*—these are only used for precapillary arterioles or small arteries. These are also very good for AVM deep within the body. The disadvantage is that they are not easily targeted in the vessel.
  - Gelfoam hemostasis—temporarily occludes vessels for 5 weeks.
  - Polyvinyl alcohol (PVA)—these are permanent agents.

- Embolization microspheres—these are superior permanent or resorbable particulate embolic agents available in different well-calibrated size ranges for precise occlusion. Embolization microspheres may comprise additional functionality such as drug loading and elution capability, specific mechanical properties, imageability, or radioactivity.
- *Mechanical occlusion devices*—these fit in all vessels. They also have the advantage of accuracy of location; they are deployed exactly where the catheter ends.
  - Coils—these are used for AVF, aneurysms, or trauma.
  - Detachable balloon treats AVF and aneurysms.

3. Vascular access for dialysis. *WBUHS 2011*

Preparing a vascular access is an important step before starting regular hemodialysis sessions, which is the site on the body where blood is removed and returned during dialysis. To maximize the amount of blood cleansed during hemodialysis treatments, the vascular access should allow continuous high volumes of blood flow.

- A vascular access should be prepared weeks or months before the starting of dialysis. The early preparation of the vascular access will allow easier and more efficient removal and replacement of blood with fewer complications.
- The three basic kinds of vascular access for hemodialysis are an arteriovenous (AV) fistula, an AV graft, and a venous catheter.

AV Fistula

- A fistula is an opening or connection between any two parts of the body that are usually separate.
- The AV fistula is considered the best long-term vascular access for hemodialysis because it provides adequate blood flow, lasts a long time, and has a lower complication rate than other types of access.
- If an AV fistula cannot be created, an AV graft or venous catheter may be needed.
- An AV fistula requires advance planning because a fistula takes a while after surgery to develop—in rare cases, as long as 24 months. Properly formed fistulas tend to last many years—longer than any other kind of vascular access.
- A surgeon creates an AV fistula by connecting an artery directly to a vein, frequently in the forearm. Connecting the artery to the vein causes more blood to flow into the vein. As a result, the vein grows larger and stronger, making repeated needle insertions for hemodialysis treatments easier.

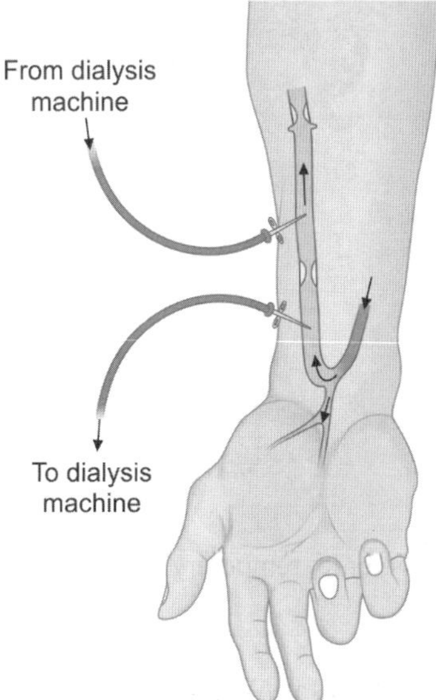

Forearm arteriovenous fistula

Arteriovenous Graft

- It can be used when vein for dialysis is small or short.
- A graft does not need to develop as a fistula does, so it can be used sooner after placement, often within 2 or 3 weeks.
- Compared with properly formed fistulas, grafts tend to have more problems with clotting and infection and need replacement sooner. However, a well-cared-for graft can last several years.

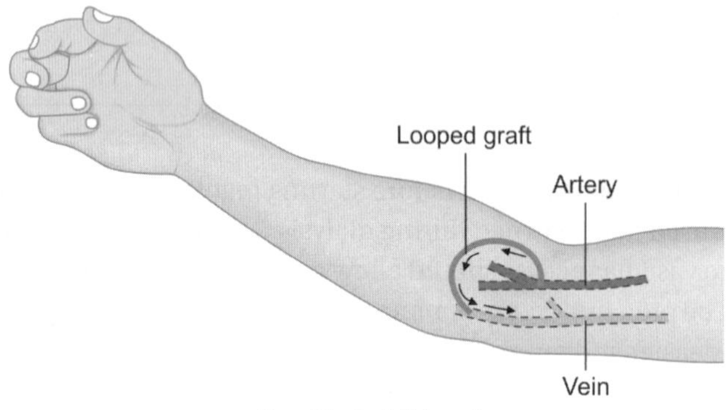

One kind of AV graft

Venous Catheter for Temporary Access

- If kidney disease has progressed quickly, one may not have time to get a permanent vascular access before you start hemodialysis treatments. It is wise to use a venous catheter as a temporary access.
- A catheter is a tube inserted into a vein in the neck, chest, or leg near the groin. It has two chambers to allow a two-way flow of blood. Once a catheter is placed, needle insertion is not necessary.
  - Catheters are not ideal for permanent access. They can clog, become infected, and cause narrowing of the veins in which they are placed. It is useful to start hemodialysis immediately; a catheter will work for several weeks or months while permanent access develops.

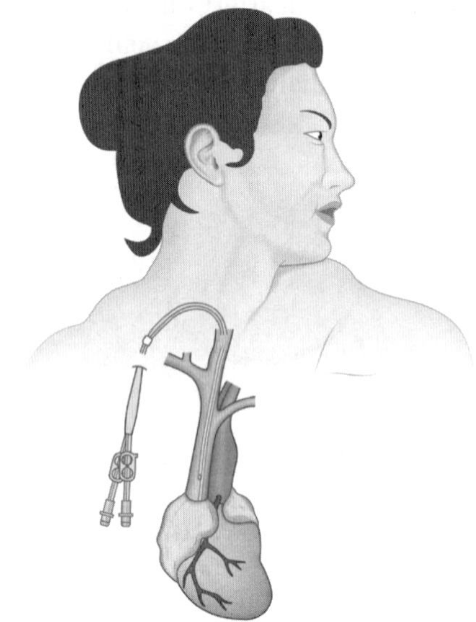

Venous catheter for temporary hemodialysis access

Complications of Vascular Access

- All three types of vascular access—AV fistula, AV graft, and venous catheter—can have complications that require further treatment or surgery. The most common complications are access infection and low blood flow due to blood clotting in the access.

- Venous catheters are most likely to develop infection and clotting problems that may require medication and catheter removal or replacement.
- AV grafts can also develop low blood flow, an indication of clotting or narrowing of the access. In this situation, the AV graft may require angioplasty, a procedure to widen the small segment that is narrowed. Another option is to perform surgery on the AV graft and replace the narrow segment.
- Infection and low blood flow are much less common in properly formed AV fistulas than in AV grafts and venous catheters. Still, having an AV fistula is not a guarantee against complications.

Care of Vascular Access

- Make sure that nurse or technician checks your access before each treatment.
- Keep the access clean at all times.
- Use the access site only for dialysis.
- Be careful not to bump or cut the access.
- Do not let anyone put a blood pressure cuff on the access arm.
- Do not wear jewelry or tight clothes over the access site.
- Do not sleep with the access arm under the head or body.
- Do not lift heavy objects or put pressure on the access arm.
- Check the pulse in the access every day.

---

4. Portal vein embolization. *WBUHS, 2012*

Introduction

- Portal vein embolization is a procedure carried out radiologically (using X-rays), in order to help toward treating cancer of the liver.
- It is not a treatment for cancer but it may enable potentially curative/beneficial surgery to take place.
- It is achieved by blocking off the portal venous flow to part of the affected liver, enabling the nonaffected part to grow bigger.

Indications

- PVE is performed in patients who have liver cancer that is suitable for surgical resection but where the potential remaining liver is of inadequate size in order to work properly.
  - This could lead to hepatic (liver) failure after the operation.
  - Therefore, PVE is carried out before surgery.
  - The aim is to shrink the part of liver affected with cancer and enlarge the healthy/normal part of liver.
  - PVE therefore blocks blood flow into the cancerous part of the liver that will be removed later during surgery.
  - Blocking off this part of liver causes shrinkage of this segment and in turn causes extra growth of the remaining healthy part of the liver.
  - Therefore by the time surgery is done, the remaining liver is already enlarged, reducing the risk of liver failure.

Procedure

- The procedure itself involves a puncture of the liver to inject glue like material into the relevant branch of the portal vein.
- This is done in the X-ray department by a radiologist, using ultrasound and angiography techniques to direct the needle into the correct position.
- It is usually done as a day case or involves an overnight stay in hospital.
- Alternatively, the branch of the portal vein may be tied off during a surgical operation.

Complications

- There are some risks involved, including bleeding or bile leak from the puncture into the liver.
- Spillage of the glue into parts of the circulation is another small risk. It is difficult to predict exactly how much liver growth this procedure will cause in a particular patient, and one has to wait and see.

5. Complications in endovascular stents. ***WBUHS 2012***

Introduction

- An endovascular stent graft is a tube composed of fabric supported by a metal mesh called a stent.
- It can be used for a variety of conditions involving the blood vessels, but most commonly is used to reinforce a weak spot in an artery called an aneurysm.
- Over time, blood pressure and other factors can cause this weak area to bulge like a balloon and it can eventually enlarge and rupture.
- The stent graft is designed to seal tightly with your artery above and below the aneurysm.
- The graft is stronger than the weakened artery and it allows your blood to pass through it without pushing on the bulge.
- Endovascular stent grafting is commonly used to treat abdominal aortic aneurysms (AAAs), but they also use it to treat thoracic aortic aneurysms (TAAs) and less commonly, aneurysms in other locations.

The potential complications of endovascular stent grafting include:

- Leaking of blood around the graft ("endoleaks")—endovascular stent grafts can sometimes leak blood through the areas where the graft components join together, or they can allow blood to leak back into the aneurysm sac through small arteries feeding the aneurysm sac. These leaks are called "endoleaks". Lifelong CT scans are advocated.
- Infection
- Movement of the graft away from the desired location ("migration")
- Graft fracturing
- Blockage of the blood flow through the graft
- Sometimes fever and an increase in white blood cell count can happen shortly after endovascular stent grafting. These symptoms usually last 2–10 days and are treated with medications such as aspirin and ibuprofen.
- Other complications that are rare but serious include a burst artery, injury to kidney, paralysis, blocked blood flow to abdomen or lower body, and delayed rupture of AAA.

6. Empyema thoracis. ***RGUHS, Karnataka 2025; WBUHS 2006; Ayush University Chhattisgarh 2025***

7. Discuss the etiology, diagnosis and management of empyema thoracis. ***KGMU Lucknow 2025***

8. Write down the investigations and management of empyema thoracis. ***WBUHS 2023***

9. Discuss the surgical options in the management of empyema thoracis. ***WBUHS 2020***

Introduction

Empyema thoracis is the condition of pus formation in the pleural space.

Etiology

- The pleural effusion which accompanies infective conditions of the lung may itself become infected and form pus.
- A lung abscess may burst into the pleural space.
- Hemothorax may become infected.

Clinical Features

- The symptoms which the condition produces depend on the amount of pus present, and the degree of compression of, or disease in, the underlying lungs.
- There is some embarrassment of respiration, and "swinging" fever, typically present whenever pus has accumulated in the body.

- Fever may sometimes be absent, especially if the patient is being treated with antibiotics.
- The patient with an empyema is severely toxic, looks ill, loses weight rapidly, and becomes severely anemic.
- If the pus is sufficiently thin to be removed through a needle, then the treatment is entirely by aspiration.

Investigations

Laboratory Studies

Relevant laboratory studies include the following:

- A CBC with differential may reveal a leukocytosis and a left shift.
- Collect sputum for Gram staining, culturing, and sensitivity testing.
- If tuberculosis is suspected, acid-fast bacilli testing should be obtained.
- In the presence of fever, obtaining a blood culture may be appropriate.

Additional potentially useful tests include the following:

- Pulse oximetry to assess oxygenation
- Arterial blood gas (ABG) or venous blood gas (VBG) analysis to assess respiratory adequacy
- Transtracheal aspiration for culturing (if sputum findings are nondiagnostic)

Imaging Studies

- *Chest radiography:*
  - It can diagnose and differentiate pneumonia, pulmonary abscess, and empyema.
  - On the chest radiograph, a lung abscess appears as a solitary cavitary area with an air-fluid level, which typically is present in a dependent portion of the lung. A surrounding patchy area of infiltrate aids in differentiating a pulmonary abscess from a cavitary lung cancer.
  - On the chest radiograph, findings that suggest empyema, as opposed to lung abscess, include extension of the air-fluid level to the chest wall, extension of the air-fluid level across fissure lines, and a tapering border of the air-fluid collection.
  - The costophrenic angle should be closely inspected on the chest radiograph to assess the presence of fluid that suggests effusion or empyema.
  - A lateral chest decubitus radiograph, obtained with the patient on his or her side, reveals whether the pleural fluid is mobile and forms layers or whether it is loculated.

Ultrasonography

- It is useful for needle-guided aspiration and drainage of a potential pleural effusion or empyema.
- *Some empyema characteristics found with ultrasound are:*
  - Homogeneous echogenicity
  - Anechoic effusion with hyperechoic septation
  - Pleural thickening and split pleural
  - Separation of the parietal, and visceral pleural by the fluid
- Color Doppler ultrasonography can also assist in differentiating empyema from peripheral air-fluid pulmonary abscess.

CT of the Chest

- It can assess for pneumonia, lung abscess, tumor, pleural effusions and septations, other pleural diseases, or pleural thickening.
- CT of the chest has shown increased sensitivity for detection of pulmonary infections compared to chest radiograph, especially for immunocompromised individuals.
- Chest CT may be considered when the index of suspicion for significant pulmonary infection is high despite a negative radiograph findings.
- *Thoracocentesis:* Both diagnostic and therapeutic

Treatment

- Penicillin or other antibiotic solution may be injected into the pleural space after the withdrawal of the pus.
- Aspiration needs to be repeated daily until lung expansion is adequate.
- If the pus becomes too thick for aspiration, the empyema is treated by one of two surgical methods:
    1. A small intercostal incision is made and a large self-retaining catheter placed into the pleural space to allow the escape of pus. The catheter is connected to an underwater seal. This method of intercostal drainage is rarely used but it is sometimes suitable for children.
    2. Rib resection and drainage by a wide-bore tube. Part of one rib is removed and the pleural space opened through its periosteum. This tube may be left open at its outer end or may be attached to an underwater seal. One type of tube is the 'Tudor-Edward' empyema tube which has an additional small rubber side tube through which the empyema cavity can be irrigated.

Operations for empyema thoracis are conventionally performed by open thoracotomy, whereas the video-assisted thoracic surgery (VATS) approach remains controversial.

Thoracoscopy

- Thoracoscopy is an alternate therapy for multiloculated empyema thoracis.
- In patients with multiloculated parapneumonic pleural effusions, the loculations in the pleural space can be disrupted with a thoracoscope, and the pleural space can be drained completely.
- If extensive adhesions are present or thick pleural peel entraps the lung, the procedure may be converted to open thoracostomy and decortication.

VATS

- It is safe and effective for treatment
- Earlier intervention with VATS can produce better clinical results.
- Compared with thoracotomy. Morbidity and mortality rates were similar among all groups.
- VATS debridement had a lower postoperative hospital stay and shorter duration of chest drainage and greater improvement in a subjective dyspnea score.

Wang and colleagues proposed a new technique using an electronic endoscope (bronchoscope or gastroscope): Inserted through the chest tube to directly visualize, irrigate, and break down the loculation effectively in various pleural diseases, including 13 cases of empyema thoracis.

Thoracocentesis (Tapping)

- *Drainage:*
    - *Simple:*
        - Empyema tube (von Petzer's drain)
        - Negative passive drain (underwater drain/von Bülau's system/Heimlich's valve)
    - *Active:*
        - Intermittent suction
        - Continuous suction
    - *Irrigation:*
        - Cystic (tidal) one tube or more
        - Continuous suction—irrigation (two or more tubes)
    - Chemical decortication (fibrinolysis)
- *Debridement:*
    - Open
    - VATS
- *Decortication (Fowler-Delorme procedure)*
- *Thoracoplasty*
    - Without plomb
    - With plomb

  - Muscle
  - Omentum
  - Other
- *Open window thoracostomy:*
  - Eloesser and modifications
  - Without flap (fenestration)
- *Combined procedures:*
  - Clagett procedure
  - Welder procedure

10. Surgical management of pyothorax. ***Ayush University Chhattisgarh 2025***

Surgical management of pyothorax, a condition characterized by pus in the pleural cavity, is typically reserved for cases where medical management (e.g., antibiotics, pleural drainage) fails or complications arise. The approach depends on the severity, chronicity, and underlying cause of the pyothorax.

Indications for Surgical Management

- Failure of medical management (persistent infection despite antibiotics and drainage).
- Organized empyema (thickened pleural peel trapping the lung).
- Chronic or loculated pleural collections.
- Complications like bronchopleural fistula or lung abscess.
- Significant pleural thickening causing lung restriction.

Surgical Approaches

I. *Thoracentesis and Chest Tube Drainage (Minimally Invasive)*
  - *Procedure:* Ultrasound- or CT-guided needle aspiration or chest tube insertion to drain pus.
  - *Use:* Early-stage empyema (exudative phase) or small, accessible collections.
  - *Limitations:* Ineffective for loculated or organized empyema.

II. *Video-Assisted Thoracoscopic Surgery (VATS)*
  - *Procedure:* Minimally invasive surgery using a thoracoscope to visualize and debride pleural cavity, break down loculations, and remove pus and fibrinous material.
  - *Indications:* Multiloculated empyema or early organization not responsive to drainage.
  - *Advantages:* Less invasive, faster recovery, reduced morbidity compared to open surgery.
  - *Considerations:* Requires general anesthesia; may not be suitable for advanced cases with thick pleural peel.

III. *Open Thoracotomy with Decortication*
  - *Procedure:* Open chest surgery to remove the thickened pleural peel, evacuate pus, and free the trapped lung to restore expansion.
  - *Indications:* Chronic empyema with organized pleural peel, lung entrapment, or failure of VATS.
  - *Types:*
    - *Limited decortication:* Removal of localized peel.
    - *Complete decortication:* Extensive removal of pleural rind and debris.
  - *Risks:* Higher morbidity, longer recovery, and risks of bleeding or infection.

IV. *Pleurodesis*
  - *Procedure:* Chemical or mechanical irritation of pleural surfaces to promote adhesion, typically after drainage.
  - *Use:* Recurrent effusions or persistent pleural space issues.
  - *Agents:* Talc, doxycycline, or bleomycin (chemical pleurodesis).
  - *Note:* Less common in pyothorax unless malignancy or chronic effusion is present.

V. *Open Window Thoracostomy (Eloesser Flap)*
- *Procedure:* Creation of a permanent opening in the chest wall to allow continuous drainage of pus, often packed and cleaned regularly.
- *Indications:* Severe, chronic empyema in patients unfit for major surgery (e.g., elderly, comorbidities) or with persistent bronchopleural fistula.
- *Considerations:* Used as a last resort; requires long-term wound care.

VI. *Rib Resection or Drainage Procedures*
- *Procedure:* Resection of a portion of the rib to facilitate drainage in chronic empyema.
- *Use:* Rare, typically in complex cases with persistent infection or poor response to other treatments.

Adjuncts to Surgery
- *Antibiotics:* Broad-spectrum initially, tailored based on culture and sensitivity results, continued post-surgery (4–6 weeks for empyema).
- *Imaging:* CT chest to assess loculations, pleural thickening, or lung involvement before surgery.
- *Nutritional Support:* Optimizes healing, especially in debilitated patients.
- *Pulmonary Rehabilitation:* Post-operative physiotherapy to improve lung expansion and function.

Complications of Surgical Management
- Bleeding, infection, or injury to lung/diaphragm.
- Persistent air leak or bronchopleural fistula.
- Incomplete lung re-expansion.
- Chronic pain or wound complications.

Considerations
- *Timing:* Early intervention (VATS or drainage) improves outcomes in acute cases; delayed surgery may require decortication.
- *Patient Factors:* Comorbidities, nutritional status, and overall fitness influence the choice of procedure.
- *Multidisciplinary Approach:* Involves thoracic surgeons, pulmonologists, and infectious disease specialists.

---

11. ARDS. *WBUHS 2013*

Introduction
- *Acute respiratory distress syndrome (ARDS),* previously known as *respiratory distress syndrome (RDS), acute lung injury (ALI), adult RDS, or shock lung,* is a severe, life-threatening medical condition characterized by widespread inflammation in the lungs. While ARDS may be triggered by a trauma or lung infection, it is usually the result of sepsis.
- The syndrome has a high mortality.
- The mortality rate with ARDS varies widely based on disease severity, a person's age, and the presence of other medical conditions.

Pathology
- ARDS is a disease of the microscopic air sacs of the lungs (alveoli) that leads to decreased exchange of oxygen and carbon dioxide (gas exchange).
- ARDS is associated with several pathologic changes: the release of inflammatory chemicals, breakdown of the cells lining the lung's blood vessels, surfactant loss leading to increased surface tension in the lung, fluid accumulation in the lung, and excessive fibrous connective tissue formation.

Signs and Symptoms
- The signs and symptoms of ARDS often begin with 2 hours of an inciting event, but can occur after 1–3 days.
- Signs and symptoms may include shortness of breath, fast breathing, and a low oxygen level in the blood. A chest X-ray frequently demonstrates generalized infiltrates or opacities in both lungs, which represent fluid accumulation in the lungs.

- Other signs and symptoms that occur in people with ARDS may be associated with the underlying disease process. For example, those with ARDS from sepsis may have low blood pressure and fever, while a person with pneumonia may have a cough.

Cause

- The predisposing factors of ARDS are numerous and varied.
- Common causes of ARDS include sepsis, pneumonia, trauma, multiple blood transfusions, babesiosis, lung contusion, aspiration of stomach contents, and drug abuse or overdose.
- Other causes of ARDS include burns, pancreatitis, near drowning, or the inhalation of chemical irritants such as smoke, phosgene, or chlorine gas.
- Some cases of ARDS are linked to large volumes of fluid used during post-trauma resuscitation.

Diagnosis

Acute respiratory distress syndrome is characterized by the following criteria:

- Lung injury of acute onset, within 1 week of an apparent clinical insult and with progression of respiratory symptoms
- Bilateral opacities on chest imaging not explained by other lung pathology (e.g., pleural effusion, pneumothorax, or nodules)
- Respiratory failure not explained by heart failure or volume overload
- *Decreased arterial PaO_2/FiO_2 ratio:*
    - *Mild ARDS:* Ratio is 201–300 mm Hg (≤39.9 kPa)
    - *Moderate ARDS:* 101–200 mm Hg (≤26.6 kPa)
    - *Severe ARDS:* ≤100 mm Hg (≤13.3 kPa)

[A minimum positive end-expiratory pressure (PEEP) of 5 cmH_2O is required; it may be delivered noninvasively with CPAP to diagnose mild ARDS]. A decreased PaO_2/FiO_2 ratio indicates reduced arterial oxygen content relative to that of the inhaled gas, indicating a failure of the lung to transport oxygen into the blood.

The above characteristics are the "Berlin criteria" of 2012 by the European Society of Intensive Care Medicine, endorsed by the American Thoracic Society and the Society of Critical Care Medicine. They are a modification of the previously used criteria:

- Acute onset
- Bilateral infiltrates on chest radiograph sparing costophrenic angles
- Pulmonary artery wedge pressure <18 mm Hg (obtained by pulmonary artery catheterization), if this information is available; if unavailable, then lack of clinical evidence of left atrial hypertension if PaO_2:FiO_2 <300 mm Hg (40 kPa) ALI is considered to be present if PaO_2:FiO_2 <200 mm Hg (26.7 kPa) ARDS is considered to be present.

An arterial blood gas analysis and chest X-ray allow formal diagnosis. Although severe hypoxemia is generally included, the appropriate threshold defining abnormal PaO_2 has never been systematically studied.

A severe oxygenation defect is not synonymous with ventilatory support. Any PaO_2 below 100 (generally saturation <100%) on a supplemental oxygen fraction of 50% meets criteria for ARDS. This can easily be achieved by high-flow oxygen supplementation without ventilatory support.

While CT scanning leads to more accurate images of the lung tissue in ARDS, it has little use in the clinical management of patients with ARDS and remains largely a research tool.

Treatment

- Acute respiratory distress syndrome is usually treated with mechanical ventilation in the intensive care unit (ICU).
- Ventilation is usually delivered through orotracheal intubation, or by tracheostomy whenever prolonged ventilation (≥2 weeks) is deemed inevitable.

- The possibilities of noninvasive ventilation are limited to the very early period of the disease or to prevention in individuals with atypical pneumonias, lung contusion, or major surgery patients, who are at risk of developing ARDS.
- Treatment of the underlying cause is imperative.
- Appropriate antibiotic therapy must be administered as soon as microbiological culture results are available.
- Empirical therapy may be appropriate if local microbiological surveillance is efficient.
- The origin of infection, when surgically treatable, must be operated on.
- When sepsis is diagnosed, appropriate local protocols should be enacted.
- Commonly used supportive therapy includes particular techniques of mechanical ventilation and pharmacological agents whose effectiveness with respect to the outcome has not yet been proven.

Mechanical Ventilation

- The overall goal is to maintain acceptable gas exchange and to minimize adverse effects in its application.
- The parameters PEEP (to maintain maximal recruitment of alveolar units), mean airway pressure (to promote recruitment and predictor of hemodynamic effects), and plateau pressure (best predictor of alveolar overdistention) are used.

Airway pressure release ventilation (APRV): No particular ventilator mode is known to improve mortality in APRV.

Well-documented advantages to APRV ventilation include:

- Decreased airway pressures
- Decreased minute ventilation
- Decreased dead-space ventilation
- Promotion of spontaneous breathing, almost 24-hour-a-day alveolar recruitment
- Decreased use of sedation
- Near elimination of neuromuscular blockade
- Optimized arterial blood gas results
- Mechanical restoration of FRC (functional residual capacity)
- A positive effect on cardiac output (due to the negative inflection from the elevated baseline with each spontaneous breath)
- Increased organ and tissue perfusion and potential for increased urine output secondary to increased kidney perfusion.

Positive End-expiratory Pressure

- PEEP is used in mechanically ventilated patients with ARDS to improve oxygenation.
- PEEP can be harmful; high PEEP necessarily increases mean airway pressure and alveolar pressure, which can damage normal alveoli by overdistension resulting in diffuse alveolar disease.

Prone Position

- Distribution of lung infiltrates in ARDS is nonuniform.
- Repositioning into the prone position (face down) might improve oxygenation by relieving atelectasis and improving perfusion.
- If this is done early in the treatment of severe ARDS, it confers a mortality benefit of 26% compared to supine ventilation.

Fluid Management

Several studies have shown that pulmonary function and outcome are better in patients that lost weight or pulmonary wedge pressure was lowered by diuresis or fluid restriction.

Corticosteroids

A study found improvement in ARDS using modest doses of corticosteroids. The initial regimen consists of methylprednisolone. After 3–5 days a response must be apparent. In 1–2 weeks, the dose can be tapered. But high-dose steroid therapy has no effect on ARDS when given within 24 hours of the onset of illness. This study involved a small number of patients in one center.

Nitric Oxide (NO)

- Inhaled NO potentially acts as selective pulmonary vasodilator.
- Rapid binding to hemoglobin prevents systemic effects. It should increase perfusion of better ventilated areas.
- Almitrine bismesylate stimulates chemoreceptors in carotid and aortic bodies.
- It has been used to potentiate the effect of NO, presumably by potentiating hypoxia-induced pulmonary vasoconstriction.
- In case of ARDS, it is not known whether this combination is useful.

Surfactant Therapy

To date, no prospective-controlled clinical trial has shown a significant mortality benefit of exogenous surfactant in adult ARDS.

ECMO (Extracorporeal Membrane Oxygenation)

12. Complications of chest injury. *WBUHS 2010, 2020*

Early after primary survey

Open pneumothorax	*Flail chest*	*Massive hemothorax*	*Cardiac tamponade*
• Occlude with a three-sided dressing • Follow by immediate insertion of an intercostal drain through a separate incision	• Results in paradoxical motion of the chest wall. Hypoxia is caused by restricted chest wall movement and underlying lung contusion • If the segment is small and respiration is not compromised, nurse patient in HDU with adequate analgesia. Encourage early ambulation and vigorous physiotherapy. Regular blood gas analysis to be done • In more severe cases, endotracheal intubation with positive-pressure ventilation is required	• Accumulation of >1,500 mL of blood in pleural cavity • Suspect when shock is associated with dull percussion note and absent breath sounds on one side of chest • Simultaneously restore blood volume and carry out decompression by inserting a wide bore chest drain • Consider need for urgent thoracotomy to control bleeding if there is continued brisk bleeding and need for persistent blood transfusion. Consult with a regional thoracic center	• Most commonly results from penetrating injuries but blood can also accumulate in pericardial sac after blunt trauma • *Recognize by hemodynamic instability:* Hypotension, tachycardia, raised jugular venous pressure, pulsus paradoxus, and faint heart sounds • If critically ill with suspected tamponade perform blind pericardiocentesis and call cardiothoracic or general surgeons to consider emergency thoracotomy • If unwell but responding to treatment arrange urgent transthoracic echo or focused abdominal ultrasound

After Secondary Survey

- *Simple pneumohemothorax:* Treat with a chest drain if large or symptomatic or in any patient likely to undergo a general anesthetic.
- *Pulmonary contusion:* Most common potentially lethal chest injury. Risk of worsening-associated consolidation and local pulmonary edema. Treat with analgesia, physiotherapy, and oxygenation. Consider respiratory support for a patient with significant hypoxia.
- *Tracheobronchial rupture:*
  - Suspect when there is persistent large air leak after chest drain insertion. Seek immediate (cardiothoracic) surgical consultation.
  - Thoracic CT scan usually diagnostic.

- *Blunt cardiac injury (myocardial contusion/traumatic infarction):* Suspect when there are significant abnormalities on ECG or echocardiography. Seek cardiological/cardiothoracic surgical advice.
- *Aortic disruption:*
  - Patients survive immediate death because the hematoma is contained.
  - Suspect when history of decelerating force and where there is widened mediastinum on chest X-ray.
  - Thoracic CT scan is diagnostic.
  - Consider cardiothoracic surgical referral.
- *Diaphragmatic rupture:*
  - Usually, secondary to blunt trauma in restrained car passengers (seat belt compression causes burst injury commonly on the left side).
  - Suspect in patient with a suitable history and a raised left hemidiaphragm on CXR.
  - Penetrating trauma below the fifth intercostal space can produce a perforation.
  - Thoracoabdominal CT scan usually diagnostic.

13. Flail chest. ***SAIMS, Indore 2025; WBUHS 2009, 2013, 2015, 2019***

14. Discuss the pathophysiology and management of flail chest and tension pneumothorax. ***WBUHS 2018***

15. What is flail chest? Mention physiological changes that develop after flail chest. Outline its management. ***WBUHS 2021 Supplementary***

- Multiple injuries to multiple ribs can result in an island of chest wall that is not fixed to the surrounding thoracic cage.
- Results in paradoxical motion of the chest wall. Hypoxia is caused by restricted chest wall movement and underlying lung contusion.
- If the segment is small and respiration is not compromised, nurse patient in HDU with adequate analgesia. Encourage early ambulation and vigorous physiotherapy. Regular blood gas analysis is needed.
- In more severe cases, endotracheal intubation with positive-pressure ventilation is required.
- The management of flail chest should focus on the size and degree of anticipated pulmonary contusion. The contusion is often underestimated initially because it does not appear on X-ray film until 24 hours later.
- Small flail segments can usually be managed conservatively with pain control. Larger flail segments hinge on pain control and management of underlying pulmonary contusion. As the pulmonary contusion improves, the respiratory mechanics related to the area of flail will improve.
- Surgical stabilization of severe flail injuries remains controversial. Surgical devices such as wires, compression plates, absorbable surgical ties, straps, and fixators have been described and proponents claim shorter time on the ventilator with less pain. These procedures are often performed via an extrapleural approach. Thoracotomy solely to perform open reduction and internal fixation of flail segments has generally not been recommended. Operative fixation of the flail chest remains an extremely uncommon procedure. Some authors have adapted the approach that they may attempt fixation of ribs in a patient who is undergoing thoracotomy for another reason.

Physiological changes in flail chest:

- During normal inspiration, the diaphragm contracts and intercostal muscles pull the rib cage out. Pressure in the thorax decreases below atmospheric pressure, and air rushes in through the trachea. The flail segment will be pulled in with the decrease in pressure while the rest of the rib cage expands.
- During normal expiration, the diaphragm and intercostal muscles relax increasing internal pressure, allowing the abdominal organs to push air upwards and out of the thorax. However, a flail segment will also be pushed out while the rest of the rib cage contracts

- A flail segment of the chest wall will negatively affect respiration in three ways: ineffective ventilation, pulmonary contusion, and hypoventilation with atelectasis. There is ineffective ventilation because of increased dead space, decreased intrathoracic pressure, and increased oxygen

	Pathophysiology	***Management***
Flail chest	• Flail chest results from deceleration injury and can be associated with life-threatening aortic disruption, tracheo-bronchial disruption, and sternal fracture. The anatomical basis of the flail chest is the presence of multiple rib fractures. When a series of adjacent ribs is fractured in two places (anteriorly and posteriorly) because of a blunt trauma that segment of the chest wall (the flail) may lose its mechanical continuity with the rest of the thorax. The flail section of the chest wall becomes unstable and moves inward during inspiration. A flail segment of the chest wall can lead to inefficient ventilation, pulmonary contusion, and atelectasis resulting in derangement of ventilation function and gas exchange • The excessive mobility of the flail segment not only causes significant pain but also leads to inefficient ventilation, inability to cough leading to accumulation of tracheobronchial secretions with its sequel. The associated pulmonary contusion can produce arteriovenous shunting and alters the alveolar ventilation-perfusion ratio resulting in hypoxemia and respiratory distress	Patients with flail chest and multiple injuries present with shock will require control of the airway preferably by endotracheal intubation. Traditional management focuses on treatment of the flail segment to ameliorate the flail respiration or on treating the underlying pulmonary contusion to improve gas exchange. Treatment of the flail chest depends on the severity of the ventilation dysfunction and physiologic impairment (attributable to the flail segment). Methods available for stabilizing a flail chest include surgical stabilization, treatment in a respirator (physiologic stabilization), or a combination of both. Surgical fixation may decrease morbidity, but conservative treatment with positive pressure ventilation is recommended when there are multiple injuries to other intrathoracic organs
Tension pneumothorax	• Intrapleural pressure is normally negative (less than atmospheric pressure) because of inward lung and outward chest wall recoil. In pneumothorax, air enters the pleural space from outside the chest or from the lung itself via mediastinal tissue planes or direct pleural perforation. Intrapleural pressure increases, and lung volume decreases • Tension pneumothorax is a pneumothorax causing a progressive rise in intrapleural pressure to levels that become positive throughout the respiratory cycle and collapses the lung, shifts the mediastinum, and impairs venous return to the heart. Air continues to get into the pleural space but cannot exit. Without appropriate treatment, the impaired venous return can cause systemic hypotension and respiratory and cardiac arrest (pulseless electrical activity) within minutes. Tension pneumothorax most commonly occurs in patients receiving positive-pressure ventilation (with mechanical ventilation or particularly during resuscitation). Rarely, it is a complication of traumatic pneumothorax, when a chest wound acts as a one-way valve that traps increasing volumes of air in the pleural space during inspiration	• Immediate needle decompression for tension pneumothoraces • Observation and follow-up X-ray for small, asymptomatic, primary spontaneous pneumothoraces • Catheter aspiration for large or symptomatic primary spontaneous pneumothoraces • Tube thoracostomy for secondary and traumatic pneumothoraces • Patients should receive supplemental oxygen until chest X-ray results are available because oxygen accelerates pleural reabsorption of air. Treatment then depends on the type, size, and effects of the pneumothorax. Primary spontaneous pneumothorax that is <20% and that does not cause respiratory or cardiac symptoms can be safely observed without treatment if follow-up chest X-rays done at about 6 and 48 hours show no progression. Larger or symptomatic primary spontaneous pneumothoraces should be evacuated by catheter aspiration. Tube thoracostomy is an alternative

16. How will you approach a case of acute hemopneumothorax following chest injury?
WBUHS 2025 Supplementary

Approaching a case of acute hemopneumothorax following chest injury involves rapid assessment and intervention, prioritizing airway, breathing, and circulation (ABCs), and addressing life-threatening thoracic injuries.

Initial Assessment and Stabilization (Primary Survey)

Airway

- Ensure the airway is patent.
- If compromised or patient is unconscious: secure with endotracheal intubation.

Breathing

- Assess respiratory rate, effort, symmetry of chest movements.
- *Look for:*
  - Dyspnea
  - Decreased breath sounds
  - Hyperresonance (pneumothorax) or dullness (hemothorax)
  - Tracheal deviation (suggests tension pneumothorax)
- Administer high-flow oxygen.

Circulation

- Check for signs of shock: hypotension, tachycardia, cold extremities.
- Establish 2 large-bore IV lines.
- Begin fluid resuscitation (crystalloids ± blood products).
- Monitor vital signs and urine output.

Diagnostic Evaluation

Focused Imaging

- *Chest X-ray (CXR):* Confirms presence of both air (pneumothorax) and fluid (hemothorax) in pleural space.
- *Ultrasound (eFAST):* Quickly identifies fluid in pleural cavity and lung sliding (or absence in pneumothorax).
- *CT chest (after stabilization):* More detailed assessment of extent of lung injury, rib fractures, vascular involvement.

Emergency Management

Tube Thoracostomy (Chest Tube Insertion)

- *Indication:* All cases of significant hemopneumothorax.
- Insert large-bore chest tube (28–36 Fr) in the 5th intercostal space, mid-axillary line.
- Attach to an underwater seal drainage system.
- *Monitor:*
  - Air leak
  - Blood drainage (amount and rate)

Assess Output:

- Immediate drainage >1,500 mL → indication for thoracotomy.
- Ongoing bleeding >200 mL/hr for 3 consecutive hours → also consider thoracotomy.

Definitive Management Based on Findings

Findings	*Management*
Stable after chest tube insertion	Continue drainage and observation
Massive initial output	Emergency thoracotomy
Persistent air leak (bronchopleural fistula)	Surgical consultation
Hemodynamic instability	Consider resuscitative thoracotomy

- **Additional Supportive Care**
  - *Pain control:* IV opioids or intercostal nerve blocks.
  - *Antibiotics:* May be given to prevent empyema in some protocols.
  - Tetanus prophylaxis if penetrating injury.
  - Blood transfusion if hemothorax is large.
  - Monitor serial CXR and hemoglobin levels.
- **Monitor for Complications**
  - Tension pneumothorax
  - Retained hemothorax
  - Empyema
  - Fibrothorax
  - Respiratory failure

17. Discuss the surgical anatomy of thoracic outlet syndrome. How is such a patient surgically treated? ***WBUHS 2018***

18. Discuss about Thoracic outlet syndrome. ***WBUHS 2007; KGMU Lucknow 2025***

Introduction

- The term thoracic outlet syndrome (TOS) describes a complex of signs and symptoms caused by compression of the neurovascular structures of the arm as they exit the thoracic outlet.
- The neurovascular bundle has three components: nerve, artery, and vein, each of which can be individually compressed, producing a distinct symptom complex different from the others.
- Specifically, TOS is categorized as neurogenic, arterial, or venous in origin, with the neurogenic form constituting the most common form (greater than 95%) followed by the venous (2 to 3%) and the arterial forms (1%).

Anatomy

- Thoracic outlet is bounded by manubrium sternae anteriorly, the spine posteriorly, and the first rib laterally. The interscalene space is bounded by the anterior scalene muscle anteriorly and the middle scalene muscle posteriorly and the first rib inferiorly.
- The costoclavicular space is bounded by the clavicle and the subclavius muscle anteriorly, the anterolateral border of the first rib medially and the scapula posteriorly. The subclavian artery, vein and the branchial plexus pass from neck into the upper extremity through these spaces, where they are liable to get compressed.
- The first rib is strategically located. It is the only bony structure to border the three anatomic spaces through which the neurovascular bundle passes.
- It also serves as the osseous framework to which muscle and ligaments are attached. It is hypothesized that the first rib is the common denominator against which the various structures compress the neurovascular bundle and the removal of the first rib will ameliorate all the symptoms

Etiology

Neurogenic Thoracic Outlet Syndrome

- Compression of elements of the brachial plexus most often results from variations in scalene muscle anatomy as they insert on the first rib.

- A history of neck trauma can be identified in approximately 80% of neurogenic TOS cases.
- The most common type is hyperextension trauma (e.g., a whiplash injury from an auto accident) that stretches the scalene muscles causing hemorrhage and edema.
- These swollen and scarred muscle fibers can compress the adjacent brachial plexus leading to irritation and resultant neurologic symptoms.
- Scalene trauma can also result from repetitive stress injury such as is seen in jobs requiring repeated, frequent movements of the neck and upper extremity (e.g., assembly line worker or shelf stocker), or prolonged neck hyperextension (e.g., keyboard operator).
- Other predisposing factors include osseous abnormalities (e.g., cervical ribs) and congenital bands and ligaments narrowing the thoracic outlet, and less commonly, sagging shoulders from poor posture and significant macromastia.

Arterial Thoracic Outlet Syndrome

- Arterial compression is almost universally associated with a bony abnormality of the thoracic outlet.
- Cervical ribs, which occur in 0.5–1.5% of the normal population, are present in >95% of patients with arterial TOS.
- Other abnormalities include elongated transverse processes of C7, anomalies of the first rib (anterior agenesis, exostoses), and scarring associated with clavicular fractures.
- These osseous structures are usually associated with anomalous myofascial bands that elevate and "pinch" the subclavian artery with abduction of the arm.
- Repetitive compression and trauma to the subclavian artery lead to intimal injury/ulceration at the site of compression or poststenotic dilation/aneurysmal degeneration of the artery just distal to the point of compression.
- Mural thrombus forming at the site of the damaged intima or within an aneurysm can then embolize down the arm, leading to ischemic symptomatology.

Venous Thoracic Outlet Syndrome

- Compression of the subclavian vein usually occurs at the junction of the clavicle and first rib. During strenuous hyperabduction of the arm, the vein can be crushed between the overlying clavicle (and subclavius muscle/tendon) and the first rib.
- Repetitive trauma at this location produces intimal injury and perivenous scarring eventually followed by clot formation.
- The result is primary subclavian-axillary vein thrombosis, also known as Paget–Schroetter syndrome or effort thrombosis because it often occurs after exertion of the affected extremity.
- Secondary subclavian-axillary vein thrombosis is usually the result of direct subclavian trauma (e.g., from an indwelling CVC) and is much more common and better tolerated than primary thrombosis.

Diagnosis

Neurogenic Thoracic Outlet Syndrome

- The major symptoms of neurogenic TOS are upper extremity pain and paresthesias. The most common pattern is irritation of all the nerve roots, followed by the lower plexus (ulnar nerve distribution), and lastly the upper plexus (median nerve distribution).
- Pain can also occur in the neck (from scalene muscle spasm), shoulder, parascapular area, and anterior chest wall; it usually radiates down the arm into the hand with paresthesias and numbness in the fingertips.
- Occipital headache is a common complaint and probably represents referred pain from scalene muscle spasm.
- Women typically outnumber men, and most patients are in their thirties or forties.
- In patients with a history of neck trauma, symptoms typically begin within a few days of the injury; in patients with work-related overactivity, the onset of symptoms is more gradual.
- Symptoms can be precipitated (or aggravated) by activities that stretch the plexus (e.g., hair combing, reaching up to a shelf, or even grasping a steering wheel).

- *Physical examination:*
  - Often reveals tenderness over the scalene muscles or supraclavicular fossa on the involved side.
  - Radiating pain or paresthesias in the affected arm can often be elicited by pressing on the scalene muscles, tapping over the brachial plexus, or by tilting the head to the opposite side.
  - Abducting the arms to 90° in external rotation (the so-called "stick-em-up" position) can also elicit symptoms.
  - Decreased grip strength and loss of light touch in the affected hand is common.
  - Atrophy of the ulnar innervated intrinsic musculature of the hand is an uncommon and late finding.
  - Much has been made of the loss of radial pulse with provocative positioning. Adson's sign (loss of radial pulse produced by head rotation to the affected side with deep inspiration) and other tests, however, are positive in up to 50% of normal individuals and hence have no diagnostic utility in neurogenic TOS.
- *Investigations:*
  - Nerve compression is usually not severe enough to cause neurophysiologic abnormalities.
  - Electromyography and nerve conduction studies are therefore of little help in patients with neurogenic TOS.
  - Cervical spine films should be obtained to determine the presence of osseous abnormalities.
  - Cross-sectional imaging with CT or MRI (magnetic resonance imaging) can be helpful to rule out cervical spine disease.
  - Other conditions that can mimic the neurogenic TOS include carpal tunnel syndrome and shoulder tendonitis.

Arterial Thoracic Outlet Syndrome

- Patients with symptomatic arterial TOS most commonly present with symptoms of digital ischemia related to microembolization of platelet aggregates formed on intimal lesions or mural thrombus from poststenotic aneurysms.
- Early symptoms may include unilateral Raynaud's syndrome, or complaints of digital cyanosis, pallor, coldness, pain, and paresthesias. Findings are most common in the thumb and index finger because of the direct pathway of the radial artery.
- If the arterial lesion is not diagnosed and corrected, repeated embolization will lead to obliteration of the distal arterial bed, with worsening ischemia leading to digital ulceration and gangrene.
- Macroembolization to the larger arteries of the arm presents as acute limb ischemia, the severity of symptoms depending on the patency of the distal arterial tree.
- Thrombotic occlusion of the subclavian artery can also occur.
- *Physical examination:*
  - May be normal or reveal signs of ischemia of varying degrees and extents.
  - A supraclavicular bruit or pulsatile mass may occasionally be detected.
  - Concomitant symptoms of neurogenic TOS may be present but are often overshadowed by ischemic symptomatology.
- *Investigations:*
  - Because the most common etiologic agent is a cervical rib, cervical spine films are extremely helpful.
  - Recognition of arterial TOS usually requires a high index of suspicion.
  - Patients with Raynaud's symptoms or subtle signs of digital ischemia should always undergo segmental pressure testing including the digital waveforms to rule out an occlusive process.
  - In the absence of a documented collagen vascular disorder or severe arteriosclerosis, the presence of small artery (palmar/digital) occlusive disease should always lead to arteriography.
  - Patients with macroemboli and no obvious cardiac source should also undergo arteriography to exclude a proximal arterial source. Arteriography should include complete views from the aortic arch to the fingertips.
  - If the subclavian artery appears normal in the neutral position, repeat view should be obtained with the arm abducted.
  - Magnified views of the hand following vasodilator injection are helpful in distinguishing embolic occlusions from intrinsic disease.

- Arteriographic findings can be subtle, ranging from minor wall irregularities and minimal poststenotic dilation to frank aneurysms.
- Duplex scanning may be useful in patients who present with pulsatile supraclavicular masses or questionable findings on arteriography.

Venous Thoracic Outlet Syndrome

- Primary axillosubclavian venous thrombosis is characterized by the sudden development of swelling and pain in the affected extremity.
- Edema is typically nonpitting and involves the entire arm. Additional signs can include prominence of superficial veins over the shoulder and anterior chest wall and varying degrees of cyanosis.
- Symptoms are worsened by use of the affected extremity.
- Patients are typically young, healthy adults (males outnumber females 2:1) with a history of strenuous or repetitive activity (e.g., weightlifting) before symptom onset.
- *Investigations:*
  - Patients with suspected axillosubclavian venous thrombosis should undergo duplex ultrasonography to confirm the diagnosis.
  - Phlebography remains the "gold standard" testing modality and should be used whenever intervention is contemplated or the diagnosis is in doubt following duplex scanning.
  - In the absence of thrombus, additional views should be obtained with the arm fully abducted or held behind the head to exclude extrinsic compression.
  - Special attention should be focused on the subclavian vein at the costoclavicular junction where intrinsic lesions are most often found.

Treatment

Neurogenic Thoracic Outlet Syndrome

- Initial treatment for neurogenic TOS should almost always be conservative, except in rare cases when patients present with longstanding symptoms and evidence of distal muscle atrophy.
- Start patients on an aggressive home physical therapy regimen consisting of neck stretching exercises, posture improvement, and avoidance of aggravating activities.
- Patients are given modest doses of analgesics and muscle relaxants.
- Majority of patients improve significantly on this regimen.
- Operative intervention is offered only to stable patients whose symptoms remain significantly disabling after a minimum of 6–12 months of this conservative therapy.
- The goal of surgery is to decompress the brachial plexus.
- The traditional operative approach calls for resection of all of the rigid scalene triangle structures that may be compressing the plexus—the first rib and any other osseous abnormalities (e.g., cervical ribs) inferiorly, the anterior scalene muscle anteriorly, and the middle scalene posteriorly.
- Thoracic outlet decompression with first rib resection is associated with greater morbidity and greater length of stay than when the first rib is spared, with no difference in neurologic outcome.
- Which approach (supraclavicular versus transaxillary) to use for surgical decompression of the brachial plexus remains controversial.
- A supraclavicular approach for neurogenic TOS provides the best exposure of the brachial plexus and associated myofascial/bony pathology.
- A transaxillary approach does provide good exposure for first rib resection, but identification of offending soft tissue pathology and complete brachial plexus neurolysis is difficult if not impossible through this approach.

Arterial Thoracic Outlet Syndrome

- Therapy for arterial TOS must address not only the pathologic lesion in the involved subclavian artery but also any clot that may have embolized into the distal arterial tree.

- The timing and sequence of intervention depend on the severity and acuteness of the patient's ischemic symptoms.
- Patients with arterial TOS most commonly present with symptoms of chronic ischemia in which limb viability is not immediately threatened. In this situation, treat the subclavian artery pathology first; postponing any attempt at distal vascular reconstruction (i.e., bypass surgery) until after the proximal emboligenic site has been eliminated.
- In situations of acute upper extremity ischemia, however, distal thromboemboli should be cleared by standard techniques before treating the subclavian artery.
- Although in some situations both lesions can be treated at the same operation, postponing surgery on the thoracic outlet at least several days may be safer.
- Arterial vasospasm at the site of distal thromboembolectomy and residual surgically inaccessible clot can compromise the outcome of the subclavian repair. Treatment with heparin anticoagulation allows time for resolution of distal arterial vasospasm and maximizes the chances for endogenous lysis of remaining thrombus.
- Catheter-directed thrombolysis has been a useful modality for treating some patients with acute limb ischemia.
- Thoracic outlet decompression for arterial TOS requires elimination of the causative compressive pathology as well as correction of the resulting arterial pathology.
- As discussed earlier, the overwhelming majority of patients have a bony anomaly, most commonly a cervical rib. Isolated myofascial bands and scalene anomalies have been described with arterial TOS but are exceedingly rare. Identification of the causative pathology is usually straightforward during exposure of the subclavian artery. Resection of these compressive elements proceeds before arterial reconstruction, taking care to avoid undue manipulation of the artery with the potential for further distal embolism. In rare situations with clavicular pathology (e.g., hypertrophic callus from a previous fracture), medial claviculectomy may be required.
- If there is any concern about significant ulceration or residual mural thrombus, the involved arterial segment must be opened and the culprit lesion removed.
- A limited superficial thromboendarterectomy (intimectomy) of a focal lesion can usually be performed through a longitudinal arteriotomy.
- The approach to patients with poststenotic dilation or aneurysmal changes without intraluminal thrombus/ulceration must be tailored to the specific lesion.
- In cases of minimal poststenotic dilation (only 1 or 2 mm larger than the adjacent normal artery), treatment is decompression alone without arterial reconstruction. With more significant degrees of dilation, arterial placation can be performed; When the dilated segment approaches twice the normal arterial diameter, arterial resection may be the only choice. In these situations, it necessary to place an interposition graft; saphenous vein graft is preferred.
- If concomitant first rib resection is required, there is often enough arterial redundancy to allow a primary end-to-end anastomosis.
- In patients with severely compromised distal circulation, we always consider concomitant cervicodorsal sympathectomy at the time of thoracic outlet decompression.

Venous Thoracic Outlet Syndrome

- Traditional management of primary axillosubclavian vein thrombosis has been conservative—systemic anticoagulation with rest and elevation of the affected limb.
- Current management of primary subclavian vein thrombosis has evolved in an attempt to avoid this outcome. Modern therapy is designed to restore venous patency, relieve extrinsic compression on the vein, and eliminate any venous scarring/stenosis that may be impeding flow.
- When thrombosis is confirmed, catheter-directed thrombolysis is initiated using recombinant tissue plasminogen activator or urokinase according to institutional preference/protocol. It is rarely necessary to continue thrombolysis beyond 36–48 hours.
- Following successful thrombolysis, careful phlebographic assessment of the subclavian vein is performed (using arm elevation if necessary) to demonstrate extrinsic compression or intrinsic stenosis.

- Narrowing of the vein at the costoclavicular junction is almost universally present. Relief of this narrowing is necessary to prevent recurrent thrombosis or, in the absence of thrombosis, and activity-induced upper extremity venous congestion.
- Angioplasty with or without stenting has been advocated as a good technique for treating this lesion, although recent experience suggests a high failure rate for this approach without concomitant first rib resection.
- Optimal timing of operative intervention remains controversial, with opinions ranging from treating patients urgently following successful thrombolysis to placing them on anticoagulation for several weeks to allow time for the venous endothelium to heal and the surrounding inflammatory response to subside.
- Prolonged waiting, however, risks recurrent thrombosis and delays return to normal activity for these young, healthy patients. In our practice, patients are anticoagulated following thrombolysis and undergo operation electively during the same hospitalization.

19. Discuss about thoracic inlet syndrome. ***WBUHS 2014***

Thoracic Inlet Syndrome

The thoracic inlet allows unobstructed passage of the neurovascular bundle (nerves, arteries, and veins) from the root of the neck to the axilla (from the neck to the arm pit).

Causes

- Signs and symptoms of thoracic inlet syndrome occur if there is some restriction of the passage of the neurovascular bundle between the shoulder and the neck.
- There are many factors that may be involved, including tight neck muscles or abnormal muscular attachment onto the ribs, cervical ribs (either calcific or fibrous), or postural causes.

Presentation

- The patient will normally present with numbness and pins and needles through one or both arms. Neurological symptoms (pins and needles and pain) predominate in 90% of people and vascular in 10%.
- They may also complain of incoordination, muscle weakness and pain particularly in the hands and fingers.
- The symptoms are generally worse with sustained overhead activity and positions. It is quite common in weightlifters and carpenters, or in people who are overweight or with very poor posture.

Observation

- What is observed depends on whether there is a predominance of vascular or neurological causes.
- Typically, one will observe some form of numbness, muscle weakness and in the later stages, wasting especially of the intrinsic finger muscles and thumb muscles.
- If the cause is primarily vascular a decrease of the radial pulse may be felt in sustained shoulder abduction, a blush discoloration in the hand when down by the side and venous symptoms may also be present such as edema (swelling).

Treatment

- Physiotherapy treatment will address faulty neck/back postures and joint mobility with mobilizing of joints and posture correction exercises.
- Tightness of neck musculature, in particular the scalenes, can be decreased through stretching and retraining of shoulder girdle muscles.
- The stabilizing muscles of the neck and thoracic spine (such as longus colli, lower trapezius, and serratus anterior) are also retrained and strengthened.
- Modifying household activities and exercise routines is important for positive long-term outcomes. Initial manual physiotherapy can speed recovery and is best combined with a prescribed home exercise program.
- Results from conservative treatment can be very successful with 70–90% resolution of symptoms.
- *Thoracoscopic sympathectomy:*

- Thoracoscopic sympathectomy resolves primary hyperhidrosis, Raynaud's phenomenon, and excessive facial blushing.
- During the procedure, a surgeon partially disables the nerve that controls the sweat glands as well as the dilation of blood vessels near the surface of the skin of the face and fingers.
- Performed as a minimally invasive procedure, thoracoscopic sympathectomy has few risks, but people who undergo the surgery often experience later sweating problems in other parts of their bodies.

- *Risks and complications:*
  - Patients can expect some pain following a thoracoscopic sympathectomy.
  - Also, an initial thoracoscopic sympathectomy does not always resolve a patient's problem, so a second procedure may be necessary.
  - Rarer risks from the procedure include a collapsed lung caused by the collection of air in the chest cavity during surgery and inadvertent damage to other nerves near the sympathetic nerve.
  - Some patients have developed Homer's syndrome following thoracoscopic sympathectomy, experiencing drooping eyelids, constricted pupils, and reduced facial sweating.

20. Describe the anatomy of scalenus anterior muscles and describe its importance in thoracic outlet syndrome.

RGUHS Karnataka 2025

Scalenus Anterior Muscle (Anterior Scalene): Anatomy and Clinical Significance

Anatomy

- *Location*
  - The *scalenus anterior* (anterior scalene) is one of the *three scalene muscles* in the lateral neck: *Scalenus anterior, scalenus medius,* and *scalenus posterior.*
  - It lies in the *posterior triangle of the neck,* forming an important landmark for major neurovascular structures.
- *Origin and Insertion*

Feature	***Description***
Origin	From the *anterior tubercles* of the *transverse processes of the 3rd to 6th cervical vertebrae (C3–C6)*
Insertion	Into the *scalene tubercle* and upper surface of the *first rib,* between the grooves for the *subclavian vein (anteriorly)* and *subclavian artery (posteriorly)*

- *Nerve Supply*
  - *Ventral rami of C4, C5, and C6* spinal nerves.
- *Actions*
  - *Unilateral contraction:* Flexes neck laterally to the same side.
  - *Bilateral contraction:* Flexes the neck forward.
  - *Accessory muscle of inspiration:* Elevates the *first rib* during deep inspiration
- *Relations*

  Anterior (in front of scalenus anterior):
  - *Phrenic nerve* (descends obliquely on its surface)
  - *Transverse cervical* and *suprascapular arteries*
  - *Subclavian vein* (runs anterior to the muscle)
  - *Prevertebral fascia*

  Posterior (behind scalenus anterior):
  - *Brachial plexus roots and trunks*
  - *Subclavian artery*

  Medial
  - *Longus colli* muscle

Lateral
- *Scalenus medius* muscle
- *Brachial plexus* passes between scalenus anterior and medius

- *Anatomical Triangle:* Scalene (Interscalene) Triangle

  Formed by
  - *Anteriorly:* Scalenus anterior
  - *Posteriorly:* Scalenus medius
  - *Inferiorly:* First rib

  Contents
  - *Subclavian artery (3rd part)*
  - *Roots/trunks of the brachial plexus*

Note: The *subclavian vein* does *not* pass through this triangle — it lies anterior to scalenus anterior.

Importance in Thoracic Outlet Syndrome (TOS)

Definition

Thoracic Outlet Syndrome (TOS) refers to a group of disorders caused by *compression of neurovascular structures* as they pass from the neck into the upper limb through the *thoracic outlet.*

The thoracic outlet is bordered by:
- *First rib,*
- *Clavicle,* and
- *Scalene muscles (mainly scalenus anterior and medius).*

Role of Scalenus Anterior in TOS

Compression Site
- The *interscalene triangle* (between scalenus anterior and medius) is a *common site* of compression of:
  - *Brachial plexus trunks* → neurological TOS
  - *Subclavian artery* → vascular TOS

Causes
- *Hypertrophy or spasm* of the *scalenus anterior* (often due to repetitive use or trauma).
- *Presence of a cervical rib* or *fibrous band* arising from C7 vertebra that tethers the muscle and compresses underlying structures.
- *Postural abnormalities* causing narrowing of the scalene triangle.
- *Anomalous insertion* of scalenus anterior onto the first rib.

Types of TOS Related to Scalenus Anterior

Type	*Structures compressed*	*Symptoms*
Neurogenic TOS (≈90%)	Brachial plexus (lower trunk, C8–T1)	Pain, paresthesia, weakness, numbness in ulnar distribution
Arterial TOS	Subclavian artery	Ischemia, coldness, pallor, diminished radial pulse
Venous TOS (less related to scalenus anterior)	Subclavian vein (anterior to scalenus anterior)	Arm swelling, cyanosis, venous distension

Clinical Implications
- *Scalene Anticus Syndrome:* An older term for *TOS caused by hypertrophy or spasm of the scalenus anterior* compressing the neurovascular bundle.
- *Adson's Test:*
  - Used to diagnose TOS due to scalenus anterior compression.

- The patient extends the neck and turns the head toward the affected side while taking a deep breath.
- A *diminished or absent radial pulse* suggests compression of the subclavian artery in the scalene triangle.

- *Surgical Importance:*
  - *Scalenectomy* (removal or release of scalenus anterior) or *first rib resection* may be performed to decompress the thoracic outlet.
  - Care must be taken to protect the *phrenic nerve* lying on its surface.

Summary

Feature	*Scalenus anterior*
Origin	Transverse processes of C3–C6
Insertion	Scalene tubercle on 1st rib
Nerve supply	Ventral rami of C4–C6
Action	Flexes neck laterally; elevates 1st rib
Relations	Phrenic nerve on surface; subclavian artery and brachial plexus posterior; subclavian vein anterior
Clinical relevance	Compression of neurovascular bundle in Thoracic Outlet Syndrome (Scalene Anticus Syndrome)

21. Discuss in brief about the minimally invasive thoracic procedures.

Minimally invasive thoracic procedures are surgical techniques performed in the chest (thoracic cavity) using small incisions, specialized instruments, and often a camera (thoracoscope), aiming to reduce trauma, pain, and recovery time compared to traditional open surgery (thoracotomy).

Key Techniques:

- **Video-Assisted Thoracoscopic Surgery (VATS)**
  - A small camera (thoracoscope) and instruments are inserted through 2–4 small incisions.
  - Performed under general anesthesia.
  - Commonly used for:
    - Lung biopsy or lobectomy (lung cancer)
    - Pleural effusion drainage
    - Decortication for empyema
    - Wedge resection of lung lesions
- **Robot-Assisted Thoracic Surgery (RATS)**
  - Surgeon operates robotic arms with enhanced precision via a console.
  - Offers 3D visualization and improved dexterity.
  - Used for complex lung resections, mediastinal tumor removal, etc.

Advantages of Minimally Invasive Thoracic Surgery:

- Smaller incisions
- Less postoperative pain
- Shorter hospital stay
- Faster recovery and return to normal activities
- Lower complication rates (e.g., infection, bleeding)

Common Indications

- Lung cancer
- Pneumothorax
- Empyema
- Mediastinal masses
- Esophageal diseases (e.g., achalasia, cancer)

22. Write in brief about VATS. ***WBUHS 201***

23. VATS. ***Rajiv Gandhi Institute of Health Sciences 2019; KIIT University, Odisha 2025***

24. What is VATS? Briefly point out the indications and complications of VATS. ***NTRUHS Vijayawada 2025***

Video-assisted thoracoscopic surgery (VATS) is a minimally invasive surgical technique used to diagnose and treat problems in your chest. During this surgery, a tiny camera (thoracoscope) and surgical instruments are inserted in the chest through small incisions. The thoracoscope transmits images of the inside of your chest onto a video monitor, guiding the surgeon in performing the procedure.

Video-assisted thoracoscopic surgery can be used for many purposes, ranging from a biopsy to removal of tumors or entire lobes from the lung. Its advantages include:

- Less pain and need for pain medication
- Smaller scar
- Shorter hospital stay
- Faster recovery time

Uses for VATS

- *Pleural diseases:* The pleura is a two-layer membrane that lines the chest cavity and surrounds both lungs. VATS is used to remove air or fluid which can collect in the pleural cavity following a chest injury or disorder and lung surgery. Surgeons may also use VATS to perform pleurodesis, a procedure where medicine is injected into your chest to fuse the space between the lung and chest wall and prevent fluid from returning to the chest.
- *Mesothelioma:* A rare cancer of the membranes lining the chest, abdominal cavity, or heart, mesothelioma can be diagnosed with a VATS biopsy.
- *Lung cancer:* VATS is used to remove pieces (wedge resection), lobes (lobectomy), fluid-filled lumps (nodules), and any suspicious spots on the lung along with a surrounding margin of healthy tissue. These tissue samples are then analyzed by an experienced pathologist to determine the stage of cancer.
- *Interstitial lung disease:* VATS is used to gather pieces of lung to make the proper diagnosis and guide treatment decisions.
- *Empyema:* An empyema is a collection of pus and fluid that develops from a lung infection such as pneumonia. VATS is used to drain the excess fluid and allow the lung to re-expand.
- *Granulomas:* VATS can be used to diagnose and remove swollen (inflamed) tissue called a granuloma which can develop in the lungs.
- *Lymphomas:* Surgeons can remove tissue samples of abnormal lymph nodes from the chest cavity with a VATS biopsy to determine the type of lymphoma present.
- *Hyperhidrosis (excessive sweating):* Chest surgeons use VATS to remove or cut the nerves that cause sweating (sympathectomy).
- *Pericardial effusion:* VATS can be used to drain fluid from the sac surrounding the heart (pericardium), caused by a range of diseases and conditions.

The best candidates for VATS procedures are:

- Individuals who have never had chest surgery. Scar tissue from previous procedures can impede access to the chest cavity.
- People who are at high risk for complications if they undergo traditional, open chest surgery.

Complications of VATS

- Air leak
- Partially collapsed lung (atelectasis)
- Abnormal heart rhythms
- Excess bleeding

- Pneumonia
- Empyema
- Wound infection
- Blood clot—this can lead to pulmonary embolism or stroke.

25. What do you understand by nonintubated video assisted thoracoscopic surgery (NIVATS)? What are indications and advantages and disadvantages of NIVATS? ***AIIMS, Patna 2025***

Nonintubated video-assisted thoracoscopic surgery (NIVATS) refers to performing thoracic (chest) surgery using *video-assisted thoracoscopic techniques (VATS) without endotracheal intubation or general anesthesia with mechanical ventilation.*

Instead of traditional intubation and muscle relaxation, the patient breathes *spontaneously* under *regional anesthesia* (e.g., thoracic epidural, paravertebral block, intercostal block, or local infiltration) combined with *sedation.* Oxygen is provided via face mask, nasal cannula, laryngeal mask airway (LMA), or high-flow nasal oxygen.

Concept and Rationale

Traditional VATS requires *general anesthesia, intubation, and one-lung ventilation* using a double-lumen tube.

However, mechanical one-lung ventilation can cause:

- Barotrauma
- Volutrauma
- Inflammatory lung injury
- Airway trauma from intubation

NIVATS avoids these by allowing *spontaneous breathing* throughout the procedure.

Anesthetic Techniques

- *Sedation:* Propofol, dexmedetomidine, or remifentanil infusions.
- *Regional anesthesia:* Thoracic epidural, paravertebral block, or intercostal nerve blocks.
- *Airway management:* Facemask, nasal cannula, LMA, or high-flow oxygen.
- CO_2 rebreathing and coughing are managed with mild sedation or local lidocaine.

Indications

- *Appropriate/Feasible for*
- *Diagnostic procedures*
  - Pleural biopsy
  - Lung biopsy
  - Mediastinal biopsy
- *Pleural conditions*
  - Pleural effusion (decortication, pleurodesis)
  - Pneumothorax (bullectomy, bleb resection)
- *Selected therapeutic lung surgeries*
  - Wedge resection for peripheral nodules
  - Lung volume reduction (selected cases)
- *Patients with high risk for general anesthesia*
  - Severe COPD or poor pulmonary reserve
  - Cardiovascular comorbidities
  - Difficult airway anatomy

Contraindications

- Uncooperative or anxious patient
- Obesity (difficult spontaneous ventilation)
- Significant hypoxemia or hypercapnia

- Central lesions needing extensive dissection
- Expected major bleeding or prolonged operation
- Dense pleural adhesions
- Need for airway control (e.g., massive hemoptysis)

Advantages

Physiological/Clinical

- Avoids intubation and mechanical ventilation injury
- Preserves natural breathing mechanics
- Less airway trauma and postoperative sore throat
- Reduced postoperative pulmonary complications
- Faster recovery and earlier mobilization
- Shorter hospital stay
- Lower postoperative pain (due to less anesthetic and muscle relaxant use)
- Avoidance of residual neuromuscular blockade

Economic/Logistical

- Shorter anesthesia and operating time
- Potentially reduced costs

Disadvantages/Challenges

Anesthetic

- Airway control is limited—risk if conversion needed
- Patient movement or coughing during surgery
- CO_2 accumulation due to hypoventilation
- Inadequate analgesia or sedation

Surgical

- Lung movement may obscure operative field
- More challenging in obese or anxious patients
- Possible need to convert to general anesthesia with intubation intraoperatively (reported rates 2–10%)

Team factors

- Requires experienced anesthesiology and surgical team
- Not suitable for emergency or complex resections

26. Pulmonary hydatid disease.

Diagnosis

- In the majority of cases, a combination of imaging and serological methods usually yields the diagnosis of cystic echinococcosis.
- A patient who has lung cysts should be investigated for associated liver cysts.

Treatment

- Surgery remains the treatment of choice for hydatid cysts of the lung, and a parenchyma-saving operation is usually possible.
- *Medical treatment:* Medical therapy with benzimidazoles is valuable in disseminated disease, including secondary lung or pleural hydatidosis, poor surgical risk patients and when there is intraoperative spillage of hydatid fluid.
- *PAIR therapy for hydatid cyst.*
  - *PAIR*—percutaneous therapy by puncture, aspiration, injection, and reaspiration combined with albendazole is a good method for the treatment of hydatid cyst.

- *Scolicidal agents used in PAIR:*
  - 95% sterile ethanol
  - Absolute alcohol
  - Mebendazole 2.4 ug/mL

27. CABG. ***WBUHS 2011***

Coronary artery bypass grafting or CABG is an open-heart procedure to relieve the blockages of the arteries of the heart.

Indications for CABG depend on various factors, mainly on the individual's symptoms and severity of disease.

Some of these include:

- Left main artery disease or equivalent
- Triple vessel disease
- Abnormal left ventricular function
- Failed percutaneous transluminal coronary angioplasty (PTCA)
- Immediately after myocardial Infarction (to help perfusion of the viable myocardium)
- Life-threatening arrhythmias caused by a previous myocardial infarction
- Occlusion of grafts from previous CABGs

Bypass grafting may be contraindicated in patients, e.g., absent viable myocardium or the artery that needs grafting is too small.

Choice of Grafts for Coronary Artery Bypass Grafting

There are three types of grafts—venous grafts, arterial grafts, and synthetic grafts.

- *Venous grafts:*
  - The most commonly used vein is the long saphenous vein.
  - If the long saphenous vein is diseased with varicosities, then short saphenous vein can be used.
  - The saphenous vein graft is usually harvested by the assistant and can be taken through a long skin incision or recently by the endoscope (EVH).
  - Benefits of endoscopic vein harvesting include more cosmetic incision and lower incidence of infection.

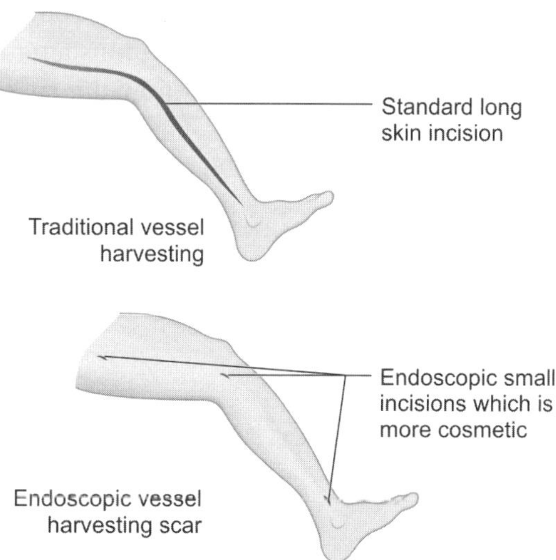

Arterial grafts: Certain arteries in the body can be harvested without doing much problems to the areas they were taken from. Here are examples of some of the arteries which can be harvested:

- *The left internal mammary artery:*

    - Very commonly used vessel which is also called the left internal thoracic artery.
    - It is usually freed in its lower part and its upper part is kept attached to its branch of origin from the aorta where it gets the blood from.
    - After freeing its lower part, it is sutured to the left anterior descending coronary, which generally is the most important coronary artery for bypass.
    - The very good thing about the left internal mammary artery is its excellent patency rate in which there is about a 95% chance it will remain open for 20 or more years later.
    - Sometimes its size is a disadvantage. It may only be a millimeter or less in diameter which is smaller than the coronary artery being bypassed, and sometimes the blood flow through it is inadequate.
    - Occasionally, the internal mammary artery will not reach the point on the coronary that it needs to be grafted.
    - That obstacle can frequently be overcome by disconnecting the upper end and sewing one end to the coronary and one to the aorta or another artery.
- *The right internal mammary:*
    - It is frequently used to bypass blockages in the coronary arteries.
    - This artery usually reaches the right coronary, the left anterior descending, and some branches of the circumflex. If it does not, the approach is generally the same.
    - The upstream end of the artery is disconnected, and one end is sewn on the coronary artery and the other is attached to the aorta or to another bypass graft.
    - One of the disadvantages of harvesting the internal mammary arteries is that they are the arteries which give blood supply to the breastbone. In some patients, the healing of the breastbone, which is opened during surgery, is delayed, and can be infected as well.
- *Radial artery:*
    - Before harvesting the radial artery, surgeons will do special tests and sometimes
    - Doppler ultrasound to make sure that the ulnar artery can take over and supply the hands when the radial artery is removed.
    - The patency rates with radial arteries so far indicate that it has a greater chance of staying open longer than saphenous vein grafts but not quite as long as the left internal mammary artery.
    - One of the disadvantages of the radial artery is that it can develop some spasm and narrowing after harvesting.
    - This can be overcome by bathing the artery in some solutions after harvesting and by giving you special intravenous drugs in the ICU that will protect the artery from this spasm.

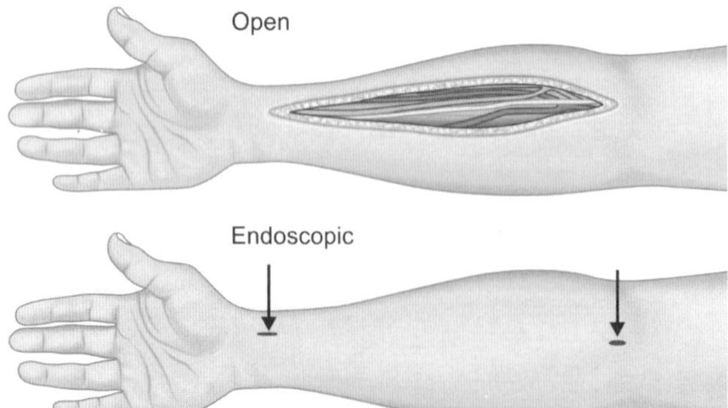

- *Gastroepiploic artery*
    - It can sometimes be used as the bypass graft.
    - The gastroepiploic artery can also be used as a free graft when both ends are disconnected. In this case, the other end is sewn to the aorta or another coronary bypass graft.

- The gastroepiploic artery graft seems to have a better patency rate than the saphenous vein graft but a somewhat poorer patency rate than the left internal mammary artery.
- The disadvantage of using this artery is that the surgeon has to make a second major incision to open the abdomen and take part of the blood supply of a portion of the stomach.

- *Synthetic grafts* made of Dacron or other material have also been used. These grafts generally work quite well in other areas of the body, particularly in the larger arteries and the aorta, but the patency rates for coronary artery grafting have not been very good, and these synthetic arteries are not routinely used.
- A new concept, called *total arterial revascularization,* is now emerging in which arterial grafts are only used because of their patency rates.

On Pump CABG

- The surgeon or an assistant surgeon removes the graft from legs or hands, ensuring the other ends are ligated properly.
- Meanwhile, the chest layers are cut open right in the middle almost on top of the sternum.
- When the sternum is reached, the bone is sawed and the ribcage is retracted to expose the heart.
- The patient is connected to a heart lung machine by diverting blood from the systemic circulation through sterile plastic tubes.
- The blood is oxygenized and filtered in the machine and sent back to the aorta thereby maintaining oxygen and nutrient supply to other vital organs.
- When the heart stops working, the surgeon identifies the block, makes incision (small cut) below the block.
- Surgeon then sutures the graft to that incision.
- Then the top end of the graft is sutured to the aorta.
- The left internal mammary artery that comes as a branch from aorta is left connected to its origin, however, the distal or far end of the artery is divided for connection to the diseased coronary artery.
- When all the grafts are in place and sutured, the heart is allowed to fill with blood and the heart lung machine is slowly weaned off.
- The surgeons make sure that there are no leaks in the connection between the graft and the aorta.
- Once the heart regains its function the pacing wires and drainage tubes are placed in the chest cavity to drain any fluid that normally collects after the procedure.
- The ribs are usually brought together and closed together with sternal wires and the rest of the muscles are closed in layers. The graft-harvested area is also sutured or closed in layers.
- Following the surgery, the chest wound is cleaned of the blood marks and dressed. The leg wound is dressed and bandaged with pressure to prevent swelling or limb edema.
- Throughout the procedure an anesthesiologist will monitor the blood pressure, oxygen saturation, and body temperature.
- Few blood tests may be repeated in intervals, especially when the patient is connected to the bypass machine.

Off-Pump Coronary Artery Bypass (OPCAB) Surgery

- The same procedure can be performed without the use of the heart lung machine. It is often called as OPCAB or off-pump coronary artery bypass.
- This procedure can be performed when the heart is still beating.
- Exposure of the heart is done by cutting the sternum open.
- Then a stabilizing device is used to hold and stabilize pertinent regions of the myocardium or heart muscle.
- Beating heart has to be handled very carefully, hence the lesions present on the front or anterior side is easier to graft as opposed to the ones on the lateral or posterior sides.
- Similar restrictions can be found in minimally invasive procedure, where the incision is made on the left side of the chest.
- A part of the ribcage is removed making the anterior part of the heart accessible.
- Patients with single vessel disease, who need one or two grafts, can be opted for OPCAB procedures.

Complications

- Coronary artery bypass surgery is a major surgical procedure, and it carries some risks and complications.
- These complications are higher in patients who are heavy smokers or if they have a major problem with this other vital organs such as kidneys or lungs or have reduced blood supply to the brain.
- Infection and bleeding are examples of risks and complications any surgery may present.
- Some of these complications may be uncommon.

Complications after surgery include:

- Ankle swelling
- Heart attack
- *Stroke:* Incidence of stroke is about 1–2%
- Emboli
- Arrhythmias
- Vein graft occlusion
- Kidney failure or temporary shutdown
- Death
- Stress and depression could be long-term problem.
- Some patients may lose some of their cognitive ability, especially older women, however, most will regain it within 6–12 months.
- The risk of death from CABG is approximately 1%. The main reason of death is heart attacks occurring during or immediately after surgery. Heart attacks occur in about 5% of the patients.
- Neurological complications are minimal and occur more in women than men, especially elder. Long-term studies show that exercise reduces mortality rate by 20%.

28. Classify mediastinal tumors. How do you investigate such a tumor? Discuss the clinical features and management of such a patient. ***WBUHS 2009***

Classification of Primary Mediastinal Tumors and Cysts

- *Neurogenic tumors*
  - Neurofibroma
  - Neurilemoma
  - Paraganglioma
  - Ganglioneuroma
  - Neuroblastoma
  - Chemodectoma
  - Neurosarcoma
- *Thymoma*
  - Benign
  - Malignant
- *Lymphoma*
  - Hodgkin's disease
  - Lymphoblastic lymphoma
  - Large cell lymphoma
- *Germ cell tumors*
  - Teratodermoid
    - Benign
    - Malignant
  - Seminoma
  - Nonseminoma

  - Embryonal
  - Choriocarcinoma
  - Endodermal
- *Primary carcinomas*
  - *Mesenchymal tumors*
    - Fibroma/fibrosarcoma
    - Lipoma/liposarcoma
    - Leiomyoma/leiomyosarcoma
    - Rhabdosarcoma
    - Xanthogranuloma
    - Myxoma
    - Mesothelioma
    - Hemangioma
    - Hemangioendothelioma
    - Hemangiopericytoma
    - Lymphangioma
    - Lymphangiomyoma
    - Lymphangiopericytoma
  - *Endocrine tumors*
    - Intrathoracic thyroid
    - Parathyroid adenoma/carcinoma
    - Carcinoid
  - *Cysts*
    - Bronchogenic
    - Pericardial
    - Enteric
    - Thymic
    - Thoracic duct
    - Nonspecific
  - *Giant lymph node hyperplasia*
    - Castleman's disease
  - Chondroma
  - Extramedullary hematopoiesis

Tumors of Anterior Mediastinum

- *Thymic tumors:* Thymomas represent the most common mediastinal neoplasm, as well as the most common anterior compartment neoplasm, constituting approximately 40–50% of the anterior compartment masses and 15% of all mediastinal masses.
- *Lymphoma:* Lymphomas constitute the second most common anterior compartment neoplasm in adults and the most common neoplasm in the pediatric population.
- *Germ cell tumor:* Benign teratomas, seminomas, and nonseminomatous germ cell tumors are a heterogeneous group of benign and malignant neoplasms thought to originate from primordial germ cells that fail to complete migration from the urogenital ridge during embryogenesis.
- *Thyroid and parathyroid tumors and cysts*

Tumors of Middle Mediastinum

- Lymphomas
- *Cystic masses:* Bronchogenic cysts, neurenteric cysts, and pericardial cysts
- Mesenchymal tumors

Tumors of Posterior Mediastinum

- *Neurogenic tumors:*
  - *Originating from peripheral nerves:*
    - Schwannoma (or neurilemoma)
    - Neurofibroma
    - Malignant nerve sheath tumors
  - *Originating from sympathetic ganglia:*
    - Ganglioneuroma
    - Ganglioneuroblastoma
    - Neuroblastoma
  - *Originating from the paraganglionic cell:*
    - Pheochromocytomas
    - Chemodectomas
- Cystic masses
- Mesenchymal tumors

Tumors of Superior Mediastinum

- Lymphomas.
- *Thyroid and parathyroid tumors and cysts*

Investigations

- *Anterior mediastinal tumors:*
  - *CT scan of the chest:*
    - An anterior compartment mass in a patient with a history of myasthenia gravis can almost be assumed to represent a thymoma.
    - On CT scan mediastinal goiters are well-encapsulated, lobulated, and heterogeneous tumors.
    - Coarse or punctate calcifications are common and goiters often demonstrate intense and sustained contrast enhancement.
    - The continuity between the cervical and mediastinal components of the thyroid gland on CT scan is usually diagnostic without the need for biopsy.
    - Parathyroid tumors are usually located on the posterior capsule of the thyroid but may be in ectopic positions.
    - Parathyroid hormone (PTH) levels can localize metabolically active parathyroid adenomas to the anterior mediastinal compartment.
  - *Tumor markers:*
    - For any young adult male presenting with a mass in the anterior compartment, simply obtaining serum tumor marker (STM) levels, which include beta-human chorionic gonadotropin (beta-hCG) and alpha-fetoprotein (AFP) is essential.
    - A significant elevation of STM is virtually diagnostic of a nonseminomatous germ cell tumor primarily arising in the mediastinum (PMNSGCT).
  - Following initial clinical and CT evaluation, biopsy of the anterior compartment mass may be indicated.
  - Video-assisted thoracic surgery:
    - It provides excellent exposure to the anterior compartment for biopsy purposes; however, the pleural space is traversed and selective lung ventilation with a double-lumen endobronchial tube is required.
    - Moreover, if thymoma is a diagnostic possibility, pleural space seeding can potentially occur during VATS biopsy efforts.
- *Middle mediastinal tumors:*
  - Chest X-ray and CT chest should be done first.
    - Because a wide variety of conditions may cause lymphadenopathy in this compartment, a thorough history and physical examination, in addition to a complete chest and upper abdominal CT scan, are essential for the initial evaluation.

- Occasionally, elevated serum levels of angiotensin-converting enzyme (ACE) can be indicative of sarcoidosis.
- Elevated serum histoplasmosis or coccidioidomycosis antigen or antibody titers can be suggestive of the etiology of mediastinal lymphadenopathy but should not be totally relied on for a definitive diagnosis.
- Extensive paratracheal and bilateral hilar lymphadenopathy in an otherwise asymptomatic patient is often a result of sarcoidosis.
- In contrast, extensive paratracheal lymphadenopathy in a patient who presents with a new onset of a cough, weight loss, shortness of breath, and a smoking history would be suspicious for metastases from either small-cell or inoperable nonsmall-cell lung cancer.
- As CT-guided FNA biopsy cannot safely be performed on most masses in the middle mediastinum, other diagnostic procedures are required. Biopsy of upper and lower paratracheal masses is best performed with transcervical mediastinoscopy.
- If a diagnosis cannot be established by cytology, biopsy either by a VATS, or a limited right thoracotomy approach would be recommended.

- *Posterior mediastinal tumors:*
  - Typically, benign nerve sheath tumors present in adult patients with symptoms such as minor back discomfort or asymptomatic masses found on incidental chest radiograph.
  - *CT scan:* Chest CT or MRI should be used to initially define the characteristics and location. A well-circumscribed, smooth-walled mass in the paravertebral sulcus is a typical finding for a benign nerve sheath tumor.
  - CT scan or MRI will also assess the relationship between the mass and potentially adjacent structures such as the esophagus, aorta, and spinal cord. If the CT scan demonstrates the tumor to abut the costovertebral angle.
  - MRI is indicated to rule out extension into the neural foramen.
  - CT-guided FNA biopsy can be confirmatory, although surgical extirpation is usually recommended for both diagnostic and therapeutic purposes.
  - Transesophageal ultrasound can also differentiate between solid and cystic intraluminal esophageal masses, which are often not discernible by CT scan.
  - Typically, pericardial cysts are observed radiologically, reserving surgical intervention if a foregut cyst or cystic neoplasm cannot be ruled out.

Mediastinal tumor	*Clinical features*	*Treatment*
Thymoma	Thymomas usually present in the fourth and fifth decades of life, although cases have been reported from childhood well into the ninth decade of life. There is no clear sex predisposition. One-third to one-half of patients present with an asymptomatic anterior mediastinal mass on chest radiograph or CT, one-third present with local symptoms (e.g., cough, chest pain, phrenic nerve palsy, superior vena cava syndrome, and dysphagia), and one-third are detected during the evaluation of myasthenia gravis. Distant metastases are uncommon at initial presentation. However, when present, the most common metastatic site is the pleura. Metastasis to the kidney, bone, liver, and brain is rarely seen *Paraneoplastic syndromes associated with thymoma:* • *Cardiac disorders* – Acute pericarditis – Myocarditis	*Surgical resection:* The basic principles underlying successful surgical therapy are: (1) median sternotomy; (2) complete wide resection of the tumor; (3) resection of all normal thymic tissue; (4) extended en bloc resection of invasive tumors (Masaoka stage III), including, if necessary, pericardium, lung, brachiocephalic vein, or superior vena cava; and (5) excision of all pleural implants or lung metastases. For tumors confined to the thymus gland, wide excision should still be performed, extending from phrenic nerve to phrenic nerve and from the superior thymic poles to the diaphragm. Lesser resection even for small and seemingly encapsulated tumors is not appropriate

Contd...

Mediastinal tumor	Clinical features	Treatment
	• *Collagen disorders* – Polymyositis – Rheumatoid arthritis – Scleroderma – Systemic lupus erythematosus • *Dermatologic disorders* – Alopecia areata – Pemphigus (vulgaris, erythematosus) • *Endocrine disorders* – Addison's disease – Cushing's syndrome – Panhypopituitarism – Thyroiditis • *Gastrointestinal disorders* – Ulcerative colitis • *Hematologic disorders* – Agranulocytosis – Erythrocytosis – Hemolytic anemia – Pancytopenia – Pernicious anemia – Red cell aplasia • *Immune deficiency syndromes* – Hypogammaglobulinemia – DiGeorge syndrome • *Neuromuscular syndromes* – Myasthenia gravis – Myositis – Limbic encephalopathy – Myotonic dystrophia – Stiff-person syndrome • *Renal disorders* – Minimal change nephropathy – Nephrotic syndrome	*Induction (neoadjuvant) therapy:* With cisplatin, epirubicin, and etoposide before and after resection has resulted in complete or partial responses in most patients, with dramatic improvements in survival for higher stage. Patient selection for induction therapy is generally based on the size of the tumor, because tumors >10 cm appear to be invasive in most cases and associated with poorer outcome
Lymphoma	Cough, chest pain, fever, and weight loss	Combination chemotherapy
Germ cell tumors	Chest pain, cough, and hoarseness	Seminoma - surgical resection+ postoperative radiotherapy
Neurogenic tumors	Located in the paravertebral gutter. About 10-20% are malignant. Chest pain is the most common symptom. May cause spinal cord compression	Surgical excision. In malignant tumors, postoperative radiotherapy is helpful
Pericardial cyst	Usually asymptomatic	Surgery is usually done as a diagnostic procedure to identify the lesion

PANCOAST TUMOR

29. Write in brief on Pancoast tumor. ***WBUHS 2025 Supplementary***

A *Pancoast tumor* (also known as a *superior sulcus tumor*) is a type of *lung cancer* that occurs at the *apex (top) of the lung,* typically involving the *superior pulmonary sulcus.* It is a *non-small cell lung carcinoma (NSCLC)* in most cases, especially *squamous cell carcinoma* or *adenocarcinoma.*

Anatomical Location

- Apical region of the lung
- Involves structures of the *thoracic inlet*, including:
  - *Brachial plexus*
  - *Subclavian vessels*
  - *Ribs (1st and 2nd)*
  - *Vertebrae*
  - *Stellate ganglion*

Clinical Features (Pancoast Syndrome)

Due to involvement of adjacent structures:

- *Shoulder and Arm Pain*
  - Most common symptom
  - Radiates along the *ulnar nerve distribution* (C8–T1)
- *Horner's Syndrome*
  - Due to involvement of the *stellate ganglion* (sympathetic chain)
    - *Ptosis* (drooping eyelid)
    - *Miosis* (constricted pupil)
    - *Anhidrosis* (loss of sweating on the affected side)
    - *Enophthalmos* (sunken eyeball)
- *Weakness/Atrophy of Hand Muscles*
  - Due to *brachial plexus* involvement
- *Supraclavicular Mass*
  - May be palpable

Diagnosis

- *Imaging:*
  - *Chest X-ray:* Apical mass
  - *CT/MRI:* Defines extent, chest wall/brachial plexus involvement
  - *PET-CT:* For staging
- *Biopsy:*
  - CT-guided, bronchoscopy, or surgical

Histology

Most commonly *non-small cell lung cancer* (NSCLC):

- *Squamous cell carcinoma*
- *Adenocarcinoma*

Treatment

Multimodal approach (due to complex anatomy):

- *Neoadjuvant chemoradiotherapy*
  - Shrinks tumor and improves resectability
- *Surgical Resection*
  - Lobectomy or extended resection of involved structures
- *Postoperative Radiotherapy/Chemotherapy* (as indicated)

Prognosis

- Depends on stage and resectability
- *Better outcomes* with multimodal therapy and complete resection

CHAPTER 53

Neurosurgery

LEARNING OBJECTIVES

- Spinal Cord Injury
- Extradural and Subdural Hematoma
- Brain Tumors
- Hydrocephalus
- Spina Bifida
- Carotid Endarterectomy

SPINAL CORD INJURY

1. Describe clinical features, diagnosis and management of spinal cord injury. ***WBUHS 2019***

2. Classify spinal cord injury. Describe clinical features, diagnosis, and principles of management in spinal cord injury. ***WBUHS 2025***

Introduction

Spinal cord injury can manifest as a wide variety of clinical syndromes resulting from damage to the spinal cord or its surrounding structures. It can result from minor injury if the spine is weakened from disease such as ankylosing spondylitis or if there is pre-existing spinal stenosis. It is an emergency which may require urgent surgical intervention to prevent long-term neurological complications of spinal cord injury.

Clinical Presentation

- Clinical presentation is very variable ranging from minor neurological dysfunction to complete paralysis (e.g., in spinal cord transection).
- Damage to the cord not only can vary in severity but also only affect certain tracts and result in incomplete cord syndromes.
- In addition to neurological signs (e.g., altered sensation, limb weakness, autonomic dysfunction, and sphincter disruption) there is usually pain due to related injury to the musculoskeletal components of the spine.
- A complete SCI produces total loss of all motor and sensory function below the level of injury.
- Nearly
- 50% of all SCIs are complete. Both sides of the body are equally affected.
- In an incomplete SCI, some function remains below the primary level of the injury. A person with an incomplete injury may be able to move one arm or leg more than the other or may have more functioning on one side of the body than the other.

Treatment Depends on Severity

Rehabilitation and assistive devices allow many people with spinal cord injuries to lead productive, independent lives. Treatments include drugs to reduce symptoms and surgery to stabilize the spine.

SCIs are graded according to the American Spinal Injury Association (ASIA) grading scale, which describes the severity of the injury. The scale is graded with letters:

- *ASIA A:* Injury is complete spinal cord injury with no sensory or motor function preserved.
- *ASIA B:* A sensory incomplete injury with complete motor function loss.
- *ASIA C:* A motor incomplete injury, where there is some movement, but less than half the muscle groups are anti-gravity (can lift up against the force of gravity with a full range of motion).
- *ASIA D:* A motor incomplete injury with more than half of the muscle groups are anti-gravity.
- *ASIA E:* Normal

Pathology

There are several types of traumatic spinal cord injury:

- Spinal cord swelling
- Spinal cord contusion/edema
    - *Cord edema only:* Most favorable prognosis
    - *Cord edema and contusion:* Intermediate prognosis
    - *Cord contusion only:* Worse prognosis
- Intramedullary hemorrhage
- Extrinsic compression, e.g., from fracture fragment or disc herniation
- Spinal cord transection

Principles of Management in Spinal Cord Injury

Management of SCI involves early recognition, stabilization, prevention of secondary injury, rehabilitation, and long-term care. The goal is to preserve neurological function, minimize complications, and optimize recovery and quality of life.

Initial Assessment and Stabilization (Pre-hospital and Emergency Care)

- ABCDE Approach (Trauma Protocol)
    - *A—Airway:* Ensure a patent airway with cervical spine protection (use cervical collar).
    - *B—Breathing:* Monitor for respiratory compromise, especially in cervical injuries (C3–C5).
    - *C—Circulation:* Manage hypotension (neurogenic shock); maintain MAP ≥ 85 mm Hg.
    - *D—Disability:* Quick neuro assessment using GCS and ASIA scale.
    - *E—Exposure:* Remove clothing to inspect for associated injuries.

Spinal precautions must be maintained during all transfers.

Neurological Assessment

- Use the ASIA Impairment Scale (AIS) to grade severity.
- Determine level of injury (motor, sensory, reflexes).
- Perform serial exams to monitor progression or improvement.

Imaging

- *X-ray (Trauma series):* Cervical spine, thoracolumbar spine.
- *CT scan:* For bony injuries, instability.
- *MRI:* Essential for soft tissue, cord compression, hemorrhage, edema.

Prevention of Secondary Injury

- *Hemodynamic support:* Maintain MAP ≥ 85–90 mm Hg for the first 7 days.
- *Oxygenation:* Prevent hypoxia.
- *Immobilization:* Hard cervical collar or spine board.

- *High-dose steroids:* Controversial (e.g., methylprednisolone within 8 hours)—not routinely recommended now due to side effects.

Surgical Management
- *Indications*
  - Spinal instability
  - Cord compression (e.g., fracture-dislocation, hematoma)
  - Progressive neurological deficit
- *Procedures*
  - Decompression (laminectomy, corpectomy)
  - Stabilization (instrumentation, fusion)

Timing: Early surgery (<24 hours) is associated with better outcomes in selected patients.

Medical Management and Complication Prevention
- *DVT prophylaxis:* LMWH or compression stockings
- *Bladder care:* Intermittent catheterization, prevent UTIs
- *Bowel care:* Bowel regimen to avoid constipation
- *Pressure sore prevention:* Frequent turning, special mattresses
- *Respiratory support:* Chest physiotherapy, ventilatory support if high cervical injury
- *Infection prevention:* Aseptic techniques, early mobilization
- *Pain management:* Neuropathic and musculoskeletal pain

Rehabilitation
- Begins as early as possible, ideally in specialized centers.
- Multidisciplinary approach
- *Physiotherapy:* Mobility, muscle strengthening
- *Occupational therapy:* Daily activities, assistive devices
- *Psychological support:* Coping, adjustment
- *Vocational therapy:* Return to work or education

Long-term Follow-up and Psychosocial Support
- Regular neurological reassessment
- *Monitor for late complications:* Spasticity, syringomyelia, osteoporosis
- *Mental health care:* Anxiety, depression, PTSD
- Family education and caregiver support

---

3. Discuss overall management of a case of traumatic quadriplegia. ***WBUHS 2017***

Active Physiological Conservative Management
- Active simultaneous, nonsurgical management, from the early hours of injury, of the injured spine
- The multisystem neurogenic effects of SCI on respiratory, cardiovascular, urinary, gastrointestinal, dermatological, sexual, reproductive functions
- The associated psychological effects
- Rehabilitation
- Environmental modifications

SCI Terminology and Classification
- The International Standards for Neurological and Functional Classification of Spinal Cord Injury (ISNCSCI) is a widely accepted system describing the level and extent of injury based on a systematic motor and sensory examination of neurologic function.

- The following terminology has developed around the classification of spinal cord injuries:
  - *Tetraplegia (replaces the term quadriplegia):* Injury to the spinal cord in the cervical region, with associated loss of muscle strength in all four extremities
  - *Paraplegia:* Injury in the spinal cord in the thoracic, lumbar, or sacral segments, including the cauda equina and conus medullaris.
    - The percentage of spinal cord injuries as classified by the ASIA is as follows:
      - *Incomplete tetraplegia:* 29.5%
      - *Complete paraplegia:* 27.9%
      - *Incomplete paraplegia:* 21.3%
      - *Complete tetraplegia:* 18.5%
      - The most common neurologic level of injury is C5. In paraplegia, T12 and L1 are the most common levels.

Quadriplegia

C1–4 Quadriplegia

- *C1 and C2:* May have functional phrenic nerves
- *C3:* Impaired breathing, ventilator dependent
- *C4:* May be free from advanced respiratory support but require functional equipment need as C3 (C1–4: Quadriplegics require assistance for all personal care, turning, and transfer functions.)

C5 Quadriplegia

- Have functional deltoid and/or biceps musculature
- Can feed themselves, perform oral facial hygienic and bladder care, and for transfers

C6 Quadriplegia

- Has musculature that permits more shoulder motion, elbow bending but not strengthening and active wrist extension
- Can perform upper and lower body dressing without assistance
- Can perform some transfers independently with a transfer board

C7–8 Quadriplegia

- Have functional triceps, they can bend and strengthen their elbows
- May also have enhanced finger extension and wrist flexion
- They can turn and perform most transfers independently

Management

- An early and accurate diagnosis of lesions of the spine and cervical spinal cord in tetraplegic patients is important.
- CT scan and MRI are important tools for early diagnosis.
- The initial assessment of individuals with acute SCI should include a complete history and physical and neurologic examination to determine the level of injury as accurately as possible.
- Physical assessment should include an evaluation of breathing pattern and effectiveness of cough. The most common abnormal breathing pattern is an isolated diaphragmatic breathing with chest wall retraction during inspiration.
- The neurologic examination, more specific the motor and sensory examinations, of tetraplegia includes:
  - The International Standards for Neurological Classification of Spinal Cord Injury (ISCSCI)
  - *Electrophysiological measures:* Stimulated muscle testing, strength-duration (SD) testing, evoked potential testing, nerve conduction velocity (NCV) testing, and needle and dynamic electromyography (EMG) testing.
- These motor and sensory examinations could be used for the assessment of muscles strength and sensation.

- For the assessment of upper limb in tetraplegia, the Sollerman hand function test, capabilities of the upper extremity (CUE) instrument, the motor capacity scale, and the tetraplegia hand activity questionnaire are useful instruments. At least one or a battery of several of these tools should be used for the assessment of the hand function and to collect evidence for interventions.

Treatment

- The medical management of tetraplegia could be the treatment of the cause, an invasive technique might be used to release pressure or attempts can be made to repair damage. Most of these techniques are still in an experimental stage (e.g., use of stem cells).
- *Medications:*
  - Methylprednisolone is a treatment option for an acute SCI.
    - If given within 8 hours of injury, some people experience mild improvement.
      - Reducing damage to nerve cells and decreasing inflammation near the site of injury
    - Not a cure for SCI
- More often the treatment is aimed on the functional recovery. The ability to use the upper limb(s) has an important influence on the independency of the patient (use of a wheelchair, pressure relief maneuvers, independent transfers, etc. Therefore, procedures such as the transfer of the teres minor motor branch for triceps reinnervation and biceps-to-triceps transfer for elbow extension could give the patient an improvement in function.
- Patients who lost their ability to breathe autonomously are ventilated through a tracheotomy and are more likely to get a respiratory infection and/or decease. A better technique is the use of a diaphragm-pacing system which electrically stimulates the phrenic nerve to pace the diaphragm. This technique has promising results.

Physical Therapy Management

- The ability to use the upper limbs is considered crucial to regain independence.
- There is some evidence that suggests that task-specific training is ideal to improve the hand function. Almost all studies showed an improvement in arm and hand function and/or activity level.
- If the surgeon and physician decide to use a procedure as mentioned earlier, the physiotherapist's task will be to reinforce the muscle and teach the patient to control his muscle individually.
- Furthermore, the lack of physical activity which is often paired with chronic SCI should be one of the key points a physical therapist should address. Innovative techniques such as the use of functional electrical stimulation (FES) lowers extremities; cycling, treadmill gait; and electrical stimulation during gait are used to regain/maintain muscle mass in the legs, strengthen the bones, and to gain many other benefits from physical activity (cardiovascular).
- Hypotension and orthostatic hypotension is often seen is these patients; a patient should be instructed to get up (form a lying or seated position) gradually and slowly. Circulatory exercises before standing up might be helpful to stimulate the blood flow. Furthermore, medication, a special diet (with enough water and salt), and regular exercise therapy should be given to prevent hypotension.
- For the respiratory problems that can come with tetraplegia secretion removal techniques, use of expiratory flow devices are recommended and the improvement of various components of cough (vital capacity, flow rate, and maximum respiratory pressures) are recommended.
- Intermittent positive pressure breathing (IPPB) can be used as a treatment for or to prevent atelectasis. The efficacy for quadriplegics has not been proven, but it is suggested that this will help the respiration as it does for chronic obstructive pulmonary disease (COPD) patients.

Surgery

- Remove fragments of bones, foreign objects, herniated disks, or fractured vertebrae
- Needed to stabilize the spine to prevent future pain or deformity

FES

- Functional electrical stimulation has been applied to various nerves in the lower limb (LL) to facilitate a more normal gait.
- Theory is that FES applies the appropriate sensory input necessary to normalize reflex output of the spinal cord
- Therefore, the disruption caused by the SCI is removed.

EXTRADURAL AND SUBDURAL HEMATOMA

4. Epidural hematoma of the head. ***WBUHS 2009***

5. Discuss the clinical presentation and management of extradural hematoma. ***KIIT University, Odisha 2025***

Introduction

Epidural or extradural hematoma (haematoma) is a type of traumatic brain injury (TBI) in which a buildup of blood that occurs between the dura mater and the skull. The dura mater also covers the spine, so epidural bleeds may also occur in the spinal column. Often due to trauma, the condition is potentially deadly because the buildup of blood may increase pressure in the intracranial space and compress delicate brain tissue. The condition is present in 1–3% of head injuries. Between 15 and 20% of patients with epidural hematomas die of the injury.

Signs and Symptoms

- Epidural bleeds are extra-axial bleeds, occurring outside of the brain tissue, while intra-axial hemorrhages, including intraparenchymal and intraventricular hemorrhages occur within it.
- Epidural bleeding is rapid because it is usually from arteries, which are high pressure. Epidural bleeds from arteries can grow until they reach their peak size at 6–8 hours post-injury, spilling from 25–75 cm^3 of blood into the intracranial space. As the hematoma expands, it strips the dura from the inside of the skull, causing an intense headache.
- Epidural bleeds can become large and raise intracranial pressure (ICP), causing the brain to shift, lose blood supply, or be crushed against the skull. Larger hematomas cause more damage.
- Epidural bleeds can quickly expand and compress the brainstem, causing unconsciousness, abnormal posturing, and abnormal pupil responses to light.
- Epidural hematomas may occur in combination with subdural hematomas, or either may occur alone. CT scans reveal subdural or epidural hematomas in 20% of unconscious patients.

Causes

- There are sharp ridges inside the skull from which the moving brain can be damaged.
- The main cause of epidural hematoma is usually traumatic, although spontaneous bleeding can occur.
- Bleeding is usually caused by trauma and transverse forces caused by acceleration and deceleration. 10% of epidural hemorrhages may be venous injuries caused by surgical damage caused by rotational forces.
- An epidural hematoma is usually caused by a blow to the side of the head. The region of the pterion above the middle meningeal artery is relatively weak and prone to damage. Thus, only 20–30% of epidural hematomas occur outside the temporal bone region.
- The brain can be damaged by bumps on the inside of the skull if it scrapes past them.
    - An epidural hematoma is usually found on the same side of the brain that was affected by the stroke, but in very rare cases, it can be caused by contrecoup injury.
- In the hallmark of epidural hematoma, patients may regain consciousness during what is called a lucid interval, only to descend suddenly and rapidly into unconsciousness later. The lucid interval, which depends on the extent of the injury, is a key to diagnosing epidural hemorrhage. If the patient is not treated with prompt surgical intervention, death is likely to follow.

Imaging

- On CT scans and MRIs, epidural hematomas usually appear convex in shape.
- The lens-like shape of the hematoma leads the appearance of these bleeds to be called "lentiform."

Treatment

- Surgical aspiration of blood can be done to remove the mass, thus reducing the ICP.
- The hematoma is evacuated through a burr hole or craniotomy.
- Trephination may be performed in the emergency department.

Prognosis

- TBI patients with epidural hematomas have a better prognosis if the patient has a clear interval than if the patient was comatose from the time of injury.
- Unlike most forms of TBI, people with an epidural hematoma and a Glasgow Coma Score of 3 (the lowest score) have a good outcome if they get surgery quickly.

---

6. Discuss the diagnosis and management of extradural hematoma. ***WBUHS 2024***

Diagnosis and Management of Extradural Hematoma

Extradural hematoma (EDH), also known as epidural hematoma, is a type of traumatic brain injury characterized by the accumulation of blood between the dura mater (the outermost membrane covering the brain) and the skull. This condition typically results from a traumatic head injury, often caused by a blow to the head, leading to the rupture of the middle meningeal artery or venous sinuses. EDH is considered a neurosurgical emergency due to the potential for rapid neurological deterioration if not treated promptly.

Diagnosis of Extradural Hematoma

- *Clinical presentation:* The symptoms of EDH can vary depending on the size and location of the hematoma, as well as the speed of its expansion. Common signs and symptoms include:
  - *Loss of consciousness:* Often, patients experience an initial loss of consciousness after the traumatic injury (which may last briefly) followed by a lucid interval, during which the patient appears relatively normal. This period may last from minutes to hours before a rapid decline in consciousness occurs.
  - *Headache:* A common symptom due to the pressure exerted by the blood on the brain.
  - *Nausea and vomiting:* Associated with increased intracranial pressure.
  - *Focal neurological deficits:* These can include weakness, numbness, difficulty speaking, or changes in vision, depending on the location of the hematoma.
  - *Seizures:* Less common but may occur due to pressure on the brain tissue.
  - *Cushing's reflex:* A combination of hypertension, bradycardia, and irregular breathing patterns seen in severe cases of intracranial pressure increase.
- *Imaging studies*
  - *CT (computed tomography) scan:* The gold standard for diagnosing EDH. A *CT scan without contrast* is typically the first-line imaging modality. It typically shows a *biconvex, lens-shaped* hyperdense (bright) area between the dura and the skull. This shape reflects the fact that the hematoma is confined by the rigid skull and does not cross suture lines (distinct from subdural hematomas, which can cross suture lines).
  - *MRI (Magnetic Resonance Imaging):* MRI can also be used, though it is less commonly the first choice for acute trauma. It provides better contrast for soft tissue structures but is often reserved for cases with atypical presentations or when further evaluation is needed.
- *Neurological examination*
  - Neurological examination involves assessing the patient's level of consciousness using the *Glasgow Coma Scale (GCS)*, as well as testing cranial nerve function, motor function, and reflexes. Any deterioration in neurological function suggests increasing intracranial pressure or hematoma expansion.

Management of Extradural Hematoma

Management of EDH depends on the size of the hematoma, the patient's clinical condition, and the timing of intervention. Prompt and effective management is crucial to prevent irreversible brain damage or death.

- *Initial stabilization*
  - *Airway, breathing, circulation (ABC):* The primary concern in any head injury is ensuring that the patient's airway is secure, they are breathing adequately, and their circulation is stable. If the patient has a reduced level of consciousness or is intubated, ensuring proper oxygenation and ventilation is vital.
  - *Intravenous access:* IV fluids and medications are given as needed to stabilize the patient.
  - *Monitoring:* Continuous monitoring of vital signs, including intracranial pressure (if available), and neurological status.
- *Surgical management*
  - *Emergency craniotomy:* The definitive treatment for EDH is surgical intervention. A *craniotomy* is performed to evacuate the hematoma and relieve the pressure on the brain. This involves making a small opening in the skull to access the hematoma and remove the accumulated blood. This is typically performed as an emergency procedure.
    - *Indications for surgery* include:
      - A large hematoma causing significant midline shift or compression of brain structures.
      - Neurological deterioration or deterioration in the GCS score.
      - Rapidly increasing size of the hematoma.
  - *Burr hole:* In some cases, a smaller incision may be made using a burr hole to drain the hematoma. This is less invasive than a craniotomy and can be used if the hematoma is not very large and there is no significant shift or brain compression.
- *Medical management*
  - *Management of increased intracranial pressure (ICP):* If the hematoma is small or if surgery cannot be performed immediately, measures to control increased ICP may include:
    - *Mannitol* or *hypertonic saline* to decrease cerebral edema and reduce ICP.
    - Sedation to reduce metabolic demand and agitation.
    - Elevating the head of the bed to 30 degrees to facilitate venous drainage.
    - Hyperventilation to lower CO_2 levels, causing vasoconstriction and reducing cerebral blood flow (though this is used cautiously due to potential complications).
  - *Anticonvulsants:* Seizures can occur in some patients after EDH, and anticonvulsants (such as phenytoin or levetiracetam) may be prescribed prophylactically in certain cases.
- *Postoperative care*
  - *Neuro-monitoring:* After surgery, patients should be closely monitored in an intensive care unit (ICU) for signs of recurrent bleeding, increasing ICP, or other neurological deterioration.
  - *Repeat imaging:* CT scans or MRI may be repeated after surgery to assess the success of hematoma evacuation and detect any residual bleeding or complications.
  - *Rehabilitation:* Depending on the extent of neurological damage, rehabilitation in the form of physical therapy, occupational therapy, and speech therapy may be required.
- *Conservative management:* In some cases, if the EDH is small, stable, and not causing significant neurological deficits or elevated intracranial pressure, conservative management may be considered. This may involve:
  - Close observation in a hospital setting with repeat CT scans to monitor for progression.
  - Regular neurological assessments.
- *Prognosis:* The prognosis of EDH largely depends on the size of the hematoma, the rapidity of intervention, and the degree of neurological damage at the time of presentation.
  - *Good prognosis:* Most patients with a small EDH who receive prompt treatment have a good recovery rate, especially if there is no significant brain damage or long-term neurological deficits.
  - *Poor prognosis:* Delayed diagnosis or intervention, large hematomas, or those that cause significant shifts in brain structures, are associated with poorer outcomes, including permanent neurological deficits or death.

7. Decompressive hemicraniectomy. ***WBUHS 2014***

Introduction

Decompressive hemicraniectomy and durotomy is a surgical technique used to relieve the increased ICP and brain tissue shifts that occur in the setting of large cerebral hemisphere mass or space-occupying lesions. In general, the technique involves removal of bone tissue (skull) and incision of the restrictive dura mater covering the brain, allowing swollen brain tissue to herniate upward through the surgical defect rather than downward to compress the brainstem.

Indications

Hemicraniectomy has been used to treat brain swelling and mass effect secondary to a middle cerebral artery (MCA) territory infarction, hemispheric encephalitis, and large parenchymal intracerebral hemorrhage in subarachnoid hemorrhage.

Procedure

- Hemicraniectomy involves removal of a substantial portion of the skull on one side of the head over the area of cerebral infarction.
- The landmarks for the portion of bone removed are anterior—frontal to the midpupillary line; posterior—posterior to the external auditory meatus; superior—to the lateral edge of the superior sagittal sinus; and inferior—to the floor of the middle cranial fossa at the origin of the zygomatic arch.
- Surgeons avoid the sigmoid and superior sagittal sinuses to prevent the possibility of sinus thrombosis or hemorrhage.

Complications

Complications associated with hemicraniectomy include infection, cerebrospinal fluid (CSF) leak, shunt-dependent hydrocephalus, subdural fluid collection, and seizure.

8. Subdural hematoma. ***WBUHS 2007***

9. What are the pathogenesis, clinical presentation, and treatment of acute subdural hematoma? ***RGUHS, Karnataka 2025***

A subdural hematoma or subdural haematoma (British spelling), also known as a subdural hemorrhage (SDH), is a type of hematoma and a form of TBI. Blood gathers within the outermost meningeal layer, between the dura mater, which adheres to the skull and the arachnoid mater, which envelops the brain. Usually resulting from tears in bridging veins which cross the subdural space, SDHs may cause an increase in ICP, which can cause compression of and damage to delicate brain tissue. Subdural hematomas are often life-threatening when acute. Chronic subdural hematomas, however, have better prognosis if properly managed.

Classification

Subdural hematomas are divided into acute, subacute, and chronic, depending on their speed of onset.

Acute subdural hematomas that are due to trauma are the most lethal of all head injuries and have a high mortality rate if they are not rapidly treated with surgical decompression.

- Though much faster than chronic subdural bleeds, acute subdural bleeding is usually venous and therefore slower than the usually arterial bleeding of an epidural hemorrhage.
- The mortality rate associated with acute subdural hematoma is around 60–80%.

Chronic subdural bleeds develop over the period of days to weeks, often after minor head trauma, though such a cause is not identifiable in 50% of patients.

- They may not be discovered until they present clinically months or years after a head injury. The bleeding from a chronic bleed is slow, probably from repeated minor bleeds, and usually stops by itself. Since these bleeds progress slowly, they present the chance of being stopped before they cause significant damage.

Signs and Symptoms

Hematoma type	*Epidural*	*Subdural*
Location	Between the skull and the dura	Between the dura and the arachnoid
Involved vessel	• Temporoparietal locus (most likely)—middle meningeal artery • Frontal locus—anterior ethmoidal artery • Occipital locus—transverse or sigmoid sinuses • Vertex locus—superior sagittal sinus	Bridging veins
Symptoms	Lucid interval followed by unconsciousness	Gradually increasing headache and confusion
Appearance on CT	Biconvex lens	Crescent shaped

- Chronic subdural hematomas are common in the elderly.
  Other signs and symptoms of subdural hematoma can include any combination of the following:

A history of recent head injury	*Numbness*	*Loss of appetite*	*Disorientation*
Loss of consciousness or fluctuating levels of consciousness	Nausea or vomiting	Personality changes	Amnesia
Irritability	Hearing loss or hearing ringing (tinnitus)	Inability to speak or slurred speech	Weakness or lethargy
Seizures	Headache (either constant or fluctuating)	Ataxia or difficulty walking	Blurred vision
Pain	Dizziness	Altered breathing patterns	Deviated gaze or abnormal movement of the eyes

Causes

- Subdural hematomas are most often caused by head injury, when rapidly changing velocities within the skull may stretch and tear small bridging veins. Subdural hematomas due to head injury are described as traumatic.
- Much more common than epidural hemorrhages, SDHs generally result from shearing injuries due to various rotational or linear forces.
- SDH is a classic finding in shaken baby syndrome, in which similar shearing forces classically cause intra- and preretinal hemorrhages.
- Subdural hematoma is also commonly seen in the elderly and in alcoholics who have evidence of cerebral atrophy.
- It is also more common in patients on anticoagulants, especially aspirin and warfarin.

Risk Factors

- Factors increasing the risk of a subdural hematoma include very young or very old age. In juveniles, an arachnoid cyst is a risk factor for a subdural hematoma.
- Other risk factors for subdural bleeds include taking blood thinners (anticoagulants), long-term alcohol abuse, and dementia.

Pathophysiology

- Collected blood from the subdural bleed may draw in water due to osmosis, causing it to expand, which may compress brain tissue and cause new bleeds by tearing other blood vessels. The collected blood may even develop its own membrane.
- In some subdural bleeds, the arachnoid layer of the meninges is torn and CSF and blood both expand in the intracranial space, increasing pressure.
- Substances that cause vasoconstriction may be released from the collected material in a subdural hematoma, causing further ischemia under the site by restricting blood flow to the brain. When the brain is denied adequate blood flow, a biochemical cascade known as the ischemic cascade is unleashed and may ultimately lead to brain cell death.
- The body gradually reabsorbs the clot and replaces it with granulation tissue.

Diagnosis

- On a CT scan, subdural hematomas are classically crescent shaped, with a concave surface away from the skull. However, they can have a convex appearance, especially in the early stage of bleeding.
- A more reliable indicator of SDH is its involvement of a larger portion of the cerebral hemisphere since it can cross suture lines, unlike an epidural hemorrhage.
- Subdural blood can also be seen as a layering density along the tentorium cerebelli.
- A chronic bleed can be the same density as brain tissue (called isodense to brain), meaning that it will show up on CT scan as the same shade as brain tissue, potentially obscuring the finding.

Treatment

- Assessment including a complete neurological examination
- CT or MRI scans will usually detect significant subdural hematomas.
- Treatment of a subdural hematoma depends on its size and rate of growth. Some small subdural hematomas can be managed by careful monitoring until the body heals itself.
- Other small subdural hematomas can be managed by inserting a temporary small catheter through a hole drilled through the skull and sucking out the hematoma; this procedure can be done at the bedside.
- Large or symptomatic hematomas require a craniotomy, the surgical opening of the skull.
- Postoperative complications include increased ICP, brain edema, new or recurrent bleeding, infection, and seizure. The injured vessels must be repaired.
- It is also worth noting that dependent on the size and deterioration, age of the patient and anesthetic risk posed, some subdurals will be inoperable and palliative management is the suitable treatment option.

10. Craniotomy. ***Rajasthan University of Health Sciences 2025***

A *craniotomy is a surgical procedure* in which a section of the skull (called a *bone flap*) is temporarily removed to access the brain.

Craniotomies are performed for various reasons, including:

- Removing brain tumors
- Clipping or repairing aneurysms
- Evacuating blood clots (hematomas)
- Relieving pressure after brain injury or swelling
- Performing biopsies
- Treating epilepsy or other neurological disorders

Procedure Overview

- *Anesthesia:* The patient is placed under general anesthesia.
- *Incision:* A scalp incision is made, and the skin and muscles are carefully moved aside.
- *Bone flap removal:* A piece of skull bone is removed using specialized surgical tools.
- *Brain access:* The surgeon performs the necessary operation on the brain tissue or vessels.
- *Closure:* The bone flap is replaced and secured (usually with plates or screws), and the scalp is sutured.

Recovery

- *Hospital stay:* Typically several days to weeks, depending on the condition.
- *Full recovery:* May take weeks to months, often involving physical or cognitive rehabilitation.

Risks

- Infection or bleeding
- Brain swelling
- Neurological deficits (e.g., weakness, speech issues)
- Seizures
- Reactions to anesthesia

BRAIN TUMORS

11. Enumerate the commonly encountered intra-axial brain tumors and give the common clinical presentation of an intracranial tumor. Discuss the role of CT and contrast-enhanced MRI in its diagnosis. ***WBUHS 2022***

Intra-axial Brain Tumors

Primary

- Glioblastoma (GBM)
- Astrocytoma
- Primary central nervous system (CNS) lymphoma
- Ganglioglioma
- Oligodendroglioma

Cerebral Metastases

Symptoms caused by primary tumors and metastatic tumors are the same. Many symptoms are caused by increased ICP:

- Headache
- Deterioration of mental state
- Focal brain dysfunction

Headache is the most common symptom. Headaches may be most severe when patients awaken from deep non-rapid eye movement (non-REM) sleep (usually several hours after falling asleep) because of hypoventilation, which increases cerebral blood flow and therefore, ICP is usually maximal during non-REM sleep.

Papilledema develops in approximately 25% of brain tumor patients but may be absent even when ICP is high.

- In infants and very young children, increased ICP can cause the head to enlarge.
- If the ICP rises high enough, a brain herniation occurs.

Deterioration of mental status is the second most common symptom.

- Obvious symptoms include drowsiness, lethargy, personality changes, disturbed behavior, and cognitive impairment, especially in malignant brain tumors.
- Airway reflexes may be impaired.

Focal dysfunction of the brain causes certain symptoms.

- Depending on the location of the tumor, focal neurological deficits, endocrine dysfunction or focal seizures (sometimes secondarily generalized) may occur.
- Focal defects often indicate the location of the tumor.
- However sometimes, the focal defects do not correspond to the location of the tumor.
- Such errors, known as *false localizing signs*, include:
    - Unilateral or bilateral lateral rectus palsy (abductor palsy) due to increased ICP compressing the sixth cranial nerve.
    - Ipsilateral hemiplegia due to compression of the contralateral brainstem against the tentorium (Kernohan's notch).
    - Ipsilateral visual field defect due to ischemia in the contralateral occipital lobe
- Generalized seizures may occur, more often in primary than metastatic brain tumors.
- Loss of consciousness can result from herniation, brainstem dysfunction, or bilateral cortical dysfunction.
- Some tumors cause inflammation of the meninges, leading to subacute or chronic meningitis.

Diagnosis

- The diagnosis of a suspected brain tumor depends on appropriate brain imaging and histopathology.
- Gadolinium-enhanced MRI is the preferred modality because of its resolution and contrast enhancement.

- If MRI cannot be performed (e.g., patients with metal implants, embedded devices, or claustrophobia), CT of the head and spine is acceptable, although the resolution is not as high as MRI and it cannot adequately assess lesions in the MR posterior fossa and spine.
- Disadvantages of MR include incompatibility with certain medical devices, longer imaging time (increased risk of motion artifact), and poor visualization of the subarachnoid space.
- Neither CT nor MR can be used to distinguish between tumor recurrence and radionecrosis.

Imaging

- T1-weighted MRI with gadolinium or CT with contrast
  Early-stage brain tumors are often misdiagnosed.

  A brain tumor should be considered in patients with any of the following:
  - Progressive focal or global deficits of brain function
  - New seizures
  - Persistent, unexplained, recent-onset headaches, particularly if worsened by sleep
  - Evidence of increased ICP (e.g., papilledema and unexplained vomiting)
  - Pituitary or hypothalamic endocrinopathy

Similar findings may result from other intracranial masses (e.g., abscess, aneurysm, arteriovenous malformation, intracerebral hemorrhage, subdural hematoma, granuloma, and parasitic cysts such as neurocysticercosis) or ischemic stroke.

- A complete neurologic examination, neuroimaging, and chest X-rays (for a source of metastases) should be done. T1-weighted MRI with gadolinium is the study of choice.
- CT with contrast agent is an alternative.
- MRI usually detects low-grade astrocytomas and oligodendrogliomas earlier than CT and shows brain structures near bone (e.g., the posterior fossa) more clearly.
- If whole-brain imaging does not show sufficient detail in the target area (e.g., sella turcica, cerebellopontine angle, and optic nerve), closely spaced images or other special views of the area are obtained.
- If neuroimaging is normal but increased ICP is suspected, idiopathic intracranial hypertension should be considered and lumbar puncture to be done.
- Sometimes brain biopsy is required.

HYDROCEPHALUS

12. Hydrocephalus. ***WBUHS 2006, 2016***

13. Classify hydrocephalus. Discuss clinical features, diagnosis and management of hydrocephalus. ***DNB, June 2019***

Introduction

Hydrocephalus is a medical condition in which there is an abnormal accumulation of CSF in the ventricles or cavities of the brain. This may cause increased ICP inside the skull and progressive enlargement of the head, convulsion, and mental disability. Hydrocephalus can also cause death.

Signs and Symptoms

- *Symptoms of increased ICP:*
  - Headaches, vomiting, nausea, papilledema, sleepiness, or coma
  - Elevated ICP may result in uncal and/or cerebellar tonsil herniation, with resulting life-threatening brainstem compression.
  - The triad (Hakim triad) of gait instability, urinary incontinence, and dementia is a relatively typical manifestation of the distinct entity normal pressure hydrocephalus (NPH).

- Focal neurological deficits may also occur, such as abducens nerve palsy and vertical gaze palsy (Parinaud syndrome due to compression of the quadrigeminal plate, where the neural centers coordinating the conjugated vertical eye movement are located).

NPH

The symptoms depend on the cause of the blockage, the person's age, and how much brain tissue has been damaged by the swelling.

In infants with hydrocephalus, CSF fluid builds up in the CNS, causing the fontanelle (soft spot) to bulge and the head to be larger than expected.

Early symptoms may also include	*Symptoms that may occur in older children can include*	
• Eyes that appear to gaze downward • Irritability • Seizures • Separated sutures • Sleepiness • Vomiting	• Brief, shrill, high-pitched cry • Changes in personality, memory or the ability to reason or think • Changes in facial appearance and eye spacing • Crossed eyes or uncontrolled eye movements • Difficulty feeding • Excessive sleepiness • Headache • Irritability, poor temper control	• Loss of bladder control (urinary incontinence) • Loss of coordination and trouble walking • Muscle spasticity (spasm) • Slow growth (child 0–5 years) • Slow or restricted movement • Vomiting

Epidemiology

- Hydrocephalus affects both pediatric and adult patients. Pediatric hydrocephalus affects one in every 500 live births, making it one of the most common developmental disabilities.
- It is the leading cause of brain surgery for children in the United States.
- Pediatric hydrocephalus may also be a heritable condition and mainly affects males.
- Hydrocephalus may be detectable during prenatal ultrasound examinations.
- Hydrocephalus also causes infection in the CSF. It can also result from maternal infection during birth.

Pathology

- Hydrocephalus is usually due to blockage of CSF outflow in the ventricles or in the subarachnoid space over the brain.
- In a person without hydrocephalus, CSF continuously circulates through the brain, its ventricles, and the spinal cord and is continuously drained away into the circulatory system.
- Alternatively, the condition may result from an overproduction of the CSF fluid, from a congenital malformation blocking normal drainage of the fluid, or from complications of head injuries or infections.
- Compression of the brain by the accumulating fluid eventually may cause convulsions and mental retardation.
- These signs occur sooner in adults whose skulls no longer are able to expand to accommodate the increasing fluid volume within.
- Fetuses, infants, and young children with hydrocephalus typically have an abnormally large head, excluding the face because the pressure of the fluid causes the individual skull bones—which have yet to fuse—to bulge outward at their juncture points.
- Another medical sign, in infants, is a characteristic fixed, downward gaze with whites of the eyes showing above the iris, as though the infant were trying to examine its own lower eyelids.
- The elevated ICP may cause compression of the brain, leading to brain damage and other complications.
- Conditions among affected individuals vary widely. Children who have had hydrocephalus may have very small ventricles and presented as the "normal case."
- If the foramina of the fourth ventricle or the cerebral aqueduct are blocked, CSF can accumulate within the ventricles. This condition is called *internal hydrocephalus* and it results in increased CSF pressure.
  - The production of CSF continues even when the passages that normally allow it to exit the brain are blocked.

- Consequently, fluid builds inside the brain, causing pressure that compresses the nervous tissue and dilates the ventricles.
- Compression of the nervous tissue usually results in irreversible brain damage. If the skull bones are not completely ossified when the hydrocephalus occurs, the pressure may also severely enlarge the head.
- The cerebral aqueduct may be blocked at the time of birth or may become blocked later in life because of a tumor growing in the brainstem.

- Internal hydrocephalus can be successfully treated by placing a drainage tube (shunt) between the brain ventricles and abdominal cavity to eliminate the high internal pressures. There is some risk of infection being introduced into the brain through these shunts; however, and the shunts must be replaced as the person grows. A subarachnoid hemorrhage may block the return of CSF to the circulation.
- If CSF accumulates in the subarachnoid space, the condition is called *external hydrocephalus*. In this condition, pressure is applied to the brain externally, compressing neural tissues and causing brain damage.

Classification

- Hydrocephalus can be caused by impaired CSF flow, reabsorption, or excessive CSF production.
- The most common cause of hydrocephalus is CSF flow obstruction, hindering the free passage of CSF through the ventricular system and subarachnoid space—stenosis of the cerebral aqueduct or obstruction of the interventricular foramina—*foramina of Monro* secondary to tumors, hemorrhages, infections, or congenital malformations.
- Hydrocephalus can also be caused by overproduction of CSF (relative obstruction) (e.g., papilloma of choroid plexus).
- Based on its underlying mechanisms, hydrocephalus can be classified into *communicating* and *noncommunicating* (obstructive). Both forms can be either *congenital* or *acquired.*
  - *Communicating:* Communicating hydrocephalus, also known as nonobstructive hydrocephalus, is caused by impaired CSF resorption in the absence of any CSF flow obstruction between the ventricles and subarachnoid space. Various neurologic conditions may result in communicating hydrocephalus, including subarachnoid/intraventricular hemorrhage, meningitis, Chiari malformation, and congenital absence of arachnoidal granulations (Pacchioni's granulations). Scarring and fibrosis of the subarachnoid space following infectious, inflammatory, or hemorrhagic events can also prevent resorption of CSF, causing diffuse ventricular dilatation.
    - *NPH:* It is a particular form of communicating hydrocephalus, characterized by enlarged cerebral ventricles, with only intermittently elevated CSF pressure. The diagnosis of NPH can be established only with the help of continuous intraventricular pressure recordings (over 24 hours or even longer), since more often than not, instant measurements yield normal pressure values. Dynamic compliance studies may be also helpful. Altered compliance (elasticity) of the ventricular walls, as well as increased viscosity of the CSF may play a role in the pathogenesis of NPH.
    - *Hydrocephalus ex vacuo* also refers to an enlargement of cerebral ventricles and subarachnoid spaces and is usually due to brain atrophy (as it occurs in dementias), post-traumatic brain injuries, and even in some psychiatric disorders, such as schizophrenia. As opposed to hydrocephalus, this is a compensatory enlargement of the CSF spaces in response to brain parenchyma loss—it is not the result of increased CSF pressure.
  - *Noncommunicating:* Noncommunicating hydrocephalus, or obstructive hydrocephalus, is caused by a CSF flow obstruction, ultimately preventing CSF from flowing into the subarachnoid space (either due to external compression or intraventricular mass lesions).
    - *Foramen of Monro obstruction* may lead to dilation of one or if large enough (e.g., in colloid cyst), both lateral ventricles.

- *The aqueduct of Sylvius*, normally narrow to begin with, may be obstructed by a number of genetically or acquired lesions (e.g., atresia, ependymitis, hemorrhage, and tumor) and lead to dilation of both lateral ventricles as well as the third ventricle.
- *Fourth ventricle obstruction will lead to dilatation of the aqueduct as well as the lateral and third ventricles.*
- *The foramina of Luschka and foramen of Magendie may be obstructed due to congenital failure of opening (e.g., Dandy-Walker malformation).*

- *Congenital:* The cranial bones fuse by the end of the third year of life. For head enlargement to occur, hydrocephalus must occur before then. The causes are usually genetic but can also be acquired and usually occur within the first few months of life, which include (1) intraventricular matrix hemorrhages in premature infants, (2) infections, (3) type II Arnold-Chiari malformation, (4) aqueduct atresia and stenosis, and (5) Dandy-Walker malformation.
- *Acquired:* This condition is acquired as a consequence of CNS infections, meningitis, brain tumors, head trauma, or intracranial hemorrhage (subarachnoid or intraparenchymal) and is usually extremely painful.

Effects

Because hydrocephalus can injure the brain, thought and behavior may be adversely affected. Learning disabilities including short-term memory loss are common among those with hydrocephalus, who tend to score better on verbal intelligence quotient (IQ) than on performance IQ, which is thought to reflect the distribution of nerve damage to the brain. However, the severity of hydrocephalus can differ considerably between individuals and some are of average or above-average intelligence. Someone with hydrocephalus may have motion and visual problems, problems with coordination, or may be clumsy. They may reach puberty earlier than the average child. About one in four develops epilepsy.

Treatment

- Hydrocephalus treatment is surgical. It involves the placement of a ventricular catheter (a tube made of silastic) into the cerebral ventricles to bypass the flow obstruction/malfunction in arachnoidal granulations and drain the excess fluid into other body cavities, from where it can be resorbed.
- Most shunts drain the fluid into the peritoneal cavity (ventriculoperitoneal shunt), but alternative sites include the right atrium (ventriculoatrial shunt), pleural cavity (ventriculopleural shunt), and gallbladder.
- A shunt system can also be placed in the lumbar space of the spine and have the CSF redirected to the peritoneal cavity (lumbar-peritoneal shunt).
- An alternative treatment for obstructive hydrocephalus in selected patients is the endoscopic third ventriculostomy (ETV), whereby a surgically created opening in the floor of the third ventricle allows the CSF to flow directly to the basal cisterns, thereby shortcutting any obstruction as in aqueductal stenosis.

SPINA BIFIDA

14. Meningocele. ***WBUHS 2009, 2014***

Introduction

Meningocele: The least common form of spina bifida is a posterior meningocele (or meningeal cyst). In a posterior meningocele, the vertebrae develop normally; however, the meninges are forced into the gaps between the vertebrae. As the nervous system remains undamaged, individuals with meningocele are unlikely to suffer long-term health problems, although there are reports of tethered cord.

Causes

- Teratoma and other tumors of the sacrococcyx and of the presacral space
- Currarino syndrome, bony defect with outpouching of meninges.

Symptoms

- Asymptomatic
- Bowel dysfunction
- Hydrocephalus
- Bladder dysfunction
- Spinal defect
- Paralyzed legs
- Spinal mass
- Pain

Investigations

- Second-trimester maternal serum alpha-fetoprotein screening
- Fetal ultrasound
- Multiple-marker screens
- Amniocentesis

Diagnosis

In most cases, a meningocele diagnosis is made before birth.

Meningocele Repair

Meningocele repair (also known as myelomeningocele repair) is surgery to repair birth defects of the spine and spinal membranes.

Description

- A meningocele repair is a surgical procedure performed to repair an abnormal opening in the spinal column (called spina bifida) by draining excess fluid and closing the opening.
- For both meningoceles and myelomeningoceles, the surgeon will close the opening in the back.
- After birth, the defect is covered by a sterile dressing. The child may then be transferred to a neonatal intensive care unit (NICU) and cared for by a medical team experienced in caring for children with spina bifida.
- Baby will likely have an MRI or ultrasound of the back. An MRI or ultrasound of the brain may be done to look for hydrocephalus
- If the myelomeningocele is not covered by skin or a membrane when your child is born, surgery will happen within 24–48 hours after birth to prevent infection. If the child has hydrocephalus, the doctor may put a shunt (plastic tube) in their brain to drain the extra fluid to the stomach. This prevents pressure that could damage the baby's brain.
- The child should not be exposed to latex before, during, and after surgery. Many of these children have very bad allergies to latex.

Risks

- *Anesthesia-related risks:*
  - Breathing problem
  - Reactions to medications
- *Surgery-related risks:*
  - Infection
  - Bleeding
  - Hydrocephalus
  - Increased chance of urinary tract infection (UTI) and bowel-related problems
  - Paralysis, weakness, or sensation changes due to loss of nerve function

15. Meningomyelocele (MMC). ***WBUHS 2016***

16. Describe the pathology, clinical features, and management of myelomeningocele. ***WBUHS 2025***

Introduction

It is a type of spina bifida, a kind of birth defect in which the spinal canal and the backbone do not close before birth. This type of birth defect is also called a neural tube defect. The spinal cord and the meninges (the tissue that covers the spinal cord) may actually protrude through the child's back.

- Failure of closure of the neural tube during the third week of gestation leads to the constellation of defects observed in patients with MMC.
- The open neural tube is continuous with the surface of the skin. For this reason, infants with MMC are at risk for bacterial meningitis due to the spinal defect.
- Leak of CSF leak is commonly observed.
- The major indication for early-operative repair (within 48 hours of delivery) is prevention of infection.
- Although protection of the exposed neural tissue from trauma and drying is essential, the neurological deficit caused by MMC is fixed and rarely improves following repair.
- Deterioration, however, can occur.

Diagnosis and Preoperative Management

- Currently, MMC is usually diagnosed prenatally by ultrasound during the second trimester.
- Positive screening for maternal serum alpha-fetoprotein—fetal ultrasound
- Although all MMC patients have a Chiari II malformation (hindbrain herniation) visualized, on MRI, only a minority will be symptomatic at birth.
- This may consist of stridor and upper airway obstruction.
- *If infant did not undergo prenatal repair of MMC:*
  - Careful examination to be done to estimate the anatomic level of lesion and whether sac is intact.
  - A small amount of CSF usually "weeps" from the translucent edges of the neural placode. If the sac ruptures, it usually decompresses and drops to the level of the back.
  - Using sterile technique, cover lesion with sterile Telfa dressing soaked in bacitracin (50,000 units/1,000 mL of 0.9% NaCl) and apply transparent dressing
  - Once the dressing is in place and if repair is planned within 24–48 hours, do not change dressing unless it is soiled. If closure is delayed greater than 48 hours, change the dressing bid and keep it moist with bacitracin solution.
  - Avoid contamination of site and dressing from stool and urine.
- *If infant did have prenatal repair of MMC:*
  - Examine operative site for evidence of breakdown, leakage of CSF, or inflammation.
  - If operative site is well healed, no special wound care is needed.
  - If there is leakage of CSF, breakdown of site, or evidence of inflammation, cover lesion with sterile Telfa dressing soaked in bacitracin (50,000 units/1,000 mL of 0.9% NaCl) and apply transparent dressing.
  - Consult with neurosurgery and pediatric surgery units regarding possible need for further surgery and/or special treatment.
  - Perform a careful neurological examination to determine the levels of the sensory and motor defects. Note the presence of any orthopedic deformities such as clubfeet.
  - Measure the head circumference and look carefully for clinical findings of hydrocephalus. Obtain a baseline head ultrasound.
  - The decision to place a ventriculoperitoneal shunt is individualized for each patient. In general, symptomatic hydrocephalus, progressive increase in head size, or leakage of CSF from the repaired defect site are indications for shunt placement. Usually a shunt is placed several days after the initial repair, although infrequently, this may need to be done at the same time as the repair.
  - Keep infant flat and either prone or on side.

- Monitor infant closely for signs of meningitis.
- Check with neurosurgery regarding further investigation (e.g., cranial and abdominal ultrasound and radiograph of spine), timing of surgical repair, and whether feedings can be started.

Postoperative Management

- After surgical repair, a dry Tela dressing should be applied to the incision daily or PRN if soiled. Gently clean the incision with sterile normal saline and apply a layer of bacitracin ointment. Place diderm around the incision and use paper tape to prevent skin breakdown.
- Postoperative cranial ultrasounds
- Abdominal and hip ultrasound
- Urology and orthopedic consults for evaluation of urinary function and associated orthopedic abnormalities

17. Repair of meningomyelocele. ***WBUHS 2008***

Introduction

- Spina bifida can be associated with a wide variety of meningeal and neural herniations, from a small meningeal protrusion to a complete rachis.
- Meningoceles and myelomeningoceles **(Figs. 1A and B)** are presented in various locations, shapes, sizes, and coatings.
- Neurological function varies from complete paralysis below the level of the lesion to neurologically intact in patients.
- The most common location for these birth defects is the lumbosacral region.
- These children may also have many other congenital anomalies.
- In most cases, myelodysplasia should be treated surgically as soon as possible after birth, regardless of whether there is a rupture of the meninges.
- The goal of surgery is to protect the neural elements, remove excess skin tissue, and obtain a watertight hard closure to prevent infection without exacerbating neurological deficits.

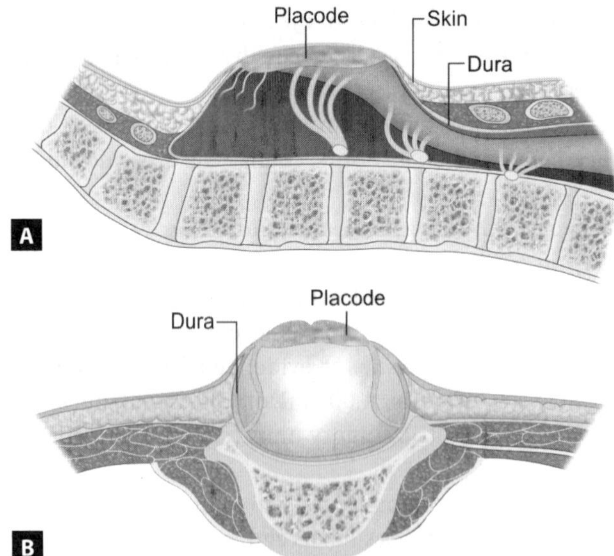

Figs. 1A and B: (A) Midsagittal section; (B) Cross-section of a lumbar myelomeningocele.

Procedure

- For both meningeal and myelomeningoceles, the surgeon closes the opening in the back.
- After delivery, the defect is covered with a sterile bandage.
- The baby can then be transferred to the NICU and cared for by a team of doctors experienced in treating children with spina bifida.

- Appointment of MRI and ultrasonography (USG) of the back
- A brain MRI or ultrasound may be done to look for hydrocephalus.
- If the myelomeningocele is not covered by skin or membrane at birth, surgery is performed within 24–48 hours after birth to prevent infection.
- If the child has hydrocephalus—ventriculoperitoneal shunt
- Children should not be exposed to latex before, during, or after surgery. Many of these children are highly allergic to latex.

Rationale
- Repair of a meningocele or myelomeningocele is needed to prevent infection and further injury to the child's spinal cord and nerves.
- Surgery cannot correct the defects in the spinal cord or nerves.

Risks

Risks for any anesthesia are:
- Breathing problems
- Reactions to medications

Risks for surgery are:
- Bleeding
- Infection
- Hydrocephalus
- Increased chance of UTI and bowel problems
- Infection or inflammation of the spinal cord
- Paralysis, weakness, or sensation changes due to loss of nerve function

Before the procedure:
- A healthcare provider often will find these defects before birth using fetal ultrasound.
- Close monitoring of the fetus till birth
- Full-term baby with cesarean section (C-section) is better. This will prevent further damage to the sac or exposed spinal tissue.

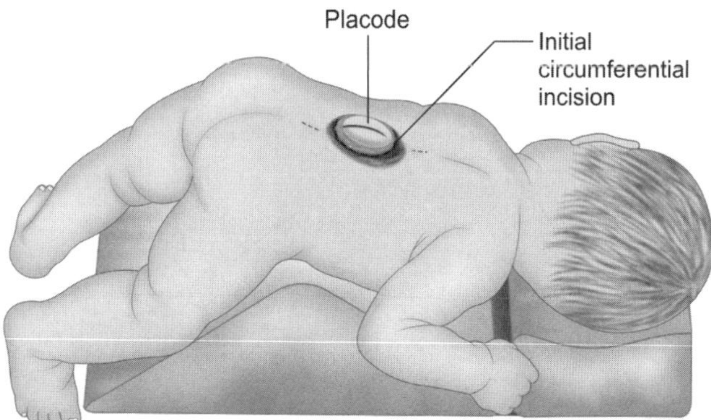

Fig. 2: Surgical position of the patient. The lumbar region is elevated relative to the head, which reduces the loss of cerebrospinal fluid. Circumcision preserves as much healthy skin as possible.

Technique
- After general anesthesia, the child is placed lying on the operating table with the head slightly under the back, so that the CSF is not replaced by air **(Fig. 2)**.
- The surgical site is properly cleaned.
- The myelomeningocele is irrigated with very warm sterile saline and the surrounding skin is cleaned with betadine.

- The anus is closed from the operative area with a suitable drape.
- A skin incision is drawn on the child's back.
- Vertical extensions are designed to weaken the skin and close the midline if possible.
- A skin incision is made immediately adjacent to the exposed meninges **(Fig. 3)**.
- Even if the skin extends well to the dome of the lesion, it must be preserved.
- Excess skin is cut off later.
- The cut is made downward and often into the brainstem, initially in an area without nerve elements.
- The edges of the skin are pulled in laterally. Nerve roots returning to the spinal canal are mobilized in the sac wall.
- Some neural elements are atretic and terminate in the sac itself and can be sacrificed.
- To revive (restore) spinal configuration, the edges of the neural plate are folded and sutured with interrupted 6-0 monofilament nylon **(Figs. 4A and B)**.
- The filum terminale can often be identified in the spinal canal.
- It must be cut sharply to release the associated spinal cord attachment.

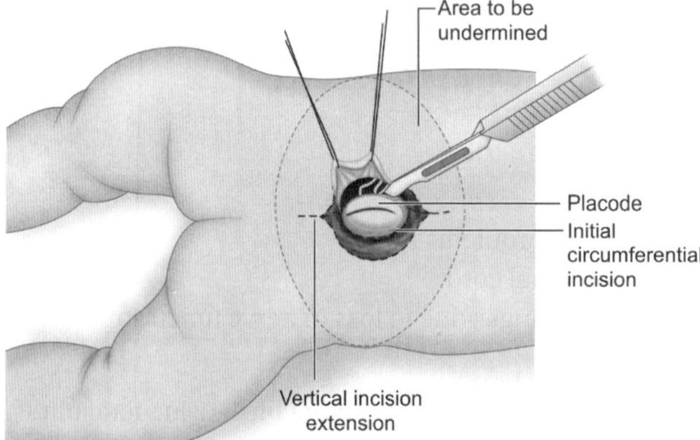

Fig. 3: Operative field as viewed by the surgeon. Dashed lines indicate circumferential incision at the edge of the placode and its rostral and caudal extensions. Dotted lines indicate the extent of the undermined skin needed to accomplish closure.

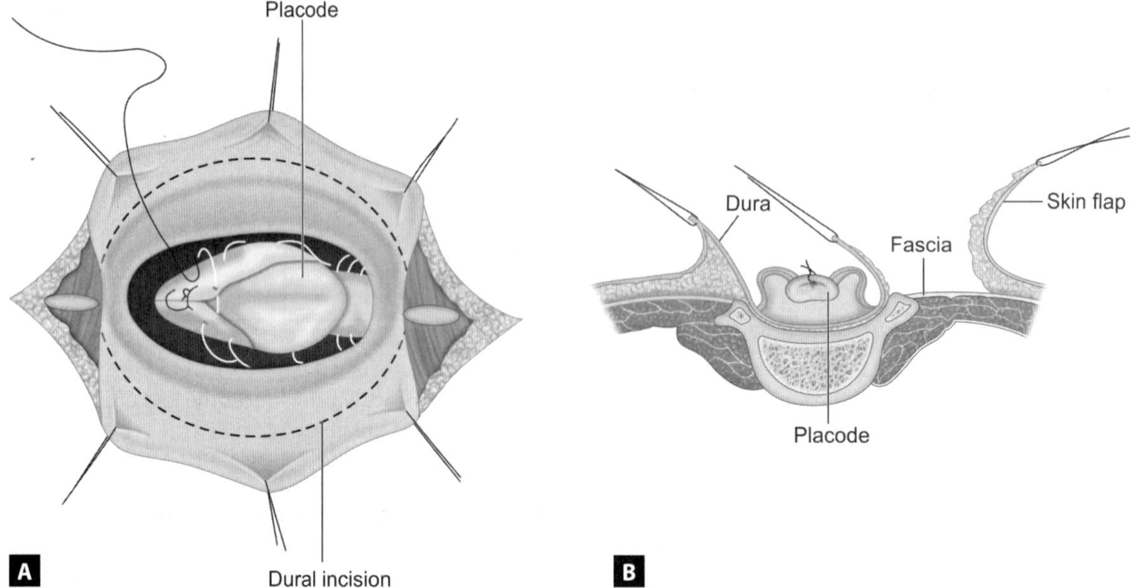

Figs. 4A and B: (A) Surgeon's view of the neuron during closure. Dashed lines indicate dural incision; (B) Cross-section of closed squares. The dura is incised and mobilized. A skin flap is cut from the fascia subcutaneously, starting from the edge of the bony defect.

- The dura is then excised from the subcutaneous tissue and lumbosacral fascia **(Figs. 4A and B)**.
- A water seal is essential and can be ensured by the anesthetist performing the Valsalva maneuver on the patient.
- To strengthen the dural suture line, the paravertebral muscles and fascia are mobilized to, if possible, close in the midline and restore the correct position of the spine in relation to the elements of the spine **(Figs. 5A and B)**.
- Alternatively, semilunar flaps of lumbosacral fascia can be swung across the midline and sutured to the base of the opposite side **(Figs. 6A and B)**.
- The skin margins are undermined to the extent that the wound can be reapproximated without tension, often far out to the lateral flank areas bilaterally.
- Placement of small subcutaneous drains bilaterally along the flank is optional and helps prevent seromas that might be confused with CSF leakage from the spinal column (1–2 days of drainage is adequate) **(Figs. 7A and B)**.
- A layer of absorbable, undyed suture is used to close the subcutaneous dissection.

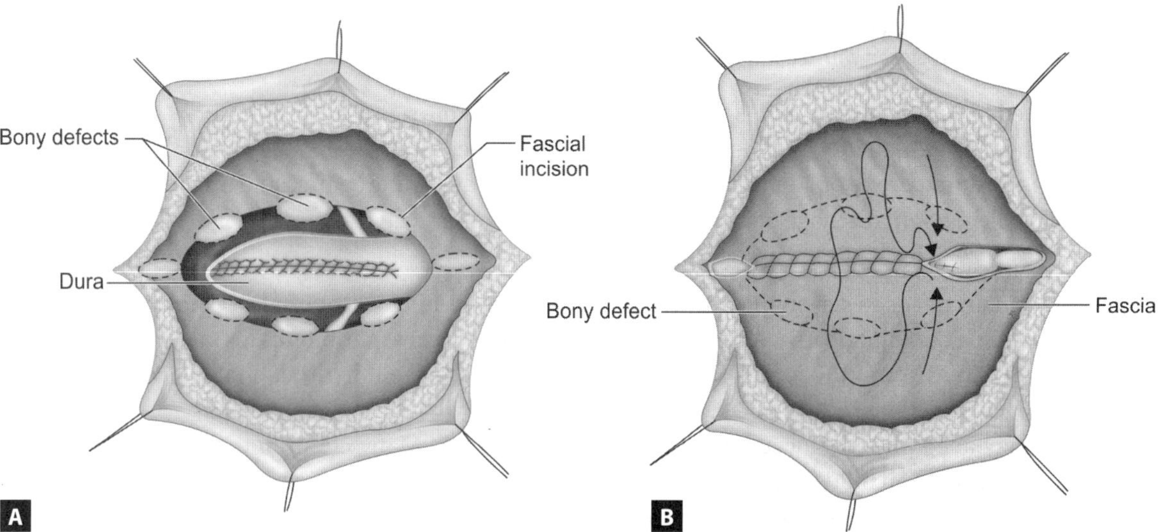

Figs. 5A and B: (A) Dural closure and fascial incision (dashed lines); (B) Closure of the fascia and paravertebral muscles along the midline. The bony defect is ghosted below the closure.

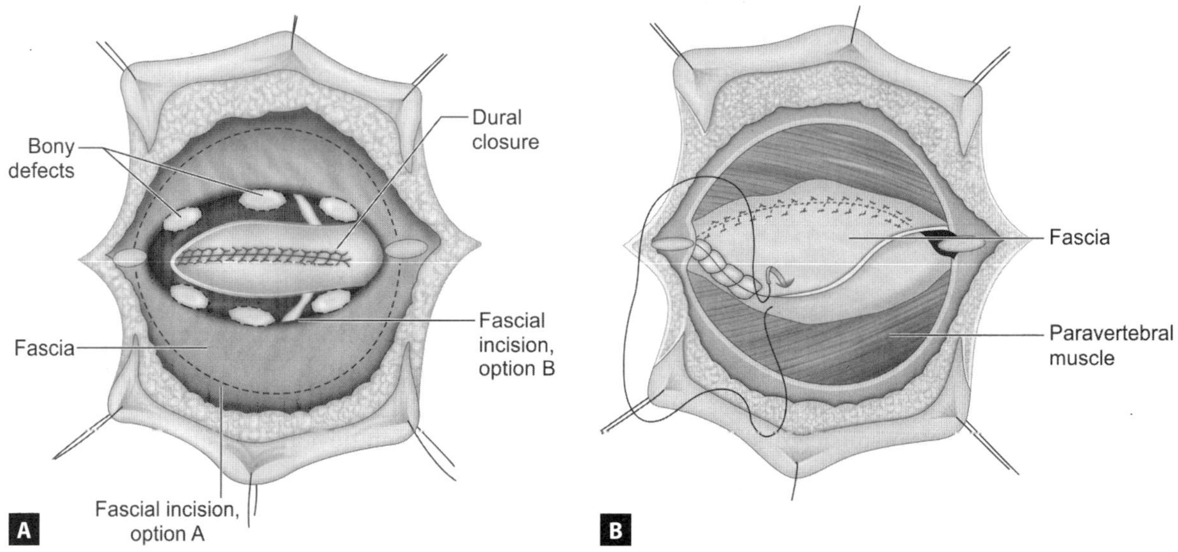

Figs. 6A and B: (A) Alternate fascial closure using semilunar flaps. The dashed lines indicate the fascial incision; (B) Each semilunar flap is sutured across the midline to the other fascial flap.

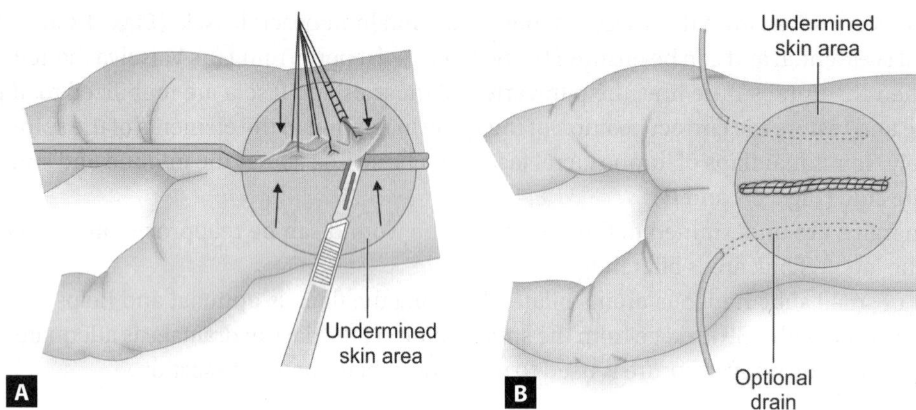

Figs. 7A and B: (A) The skin is approximated and trimmed. The subcutaneous undermining is indicated by the circled area; (B) The skin is closed with a continuous suture. Optional subcutaneous epifascial drains are shown.

- Nylon is used to suture the skin and is left in place for about 10 days.
- The dressing must remain dry and the wound isolated from feces.
- The child is nurtured prone or lateral 3–4 days after surgery to avoid undue pressure on the fresh surgical wound and to allow dependent drainage of urine and feces.

After the procedure

- The child usually needs to stay in the hospital for about 2 weeks after the operation. The child should lie down without touching the injured area. After surgery, the child will receive antibiotics to prevent infections.
- After surgery, an MRI or ultrasound of the brain is repeated to see if hydrocephalus occurs after the SCI is repaired.
- The child may need physical, occupational and speech therapy. Many children with these problems already have severe (major) and mild (minor) motor and swallowing disorders at an early age.
- A child can often see a team of spina bifida specialists after leaving hospital.

Prognosis

- How well a child does depend on the initial state of his spinal cord and nerves. After the meningocele heals, children often do well and have no other brain, nerve, or muscle problems.
- Children with myelomeningocele usually have paralysis or weakness of the muscles in the lower spine where the defect is located. They may also not be able to control their bladder or bowels. They are likely to need medical and educational support for many years.
- The ability to walk and control bowel and bladder function depends on where the fetal lesion was in the spine. Defects below the spinal cord may give a better result.

18. Carotid endarterectomy. *WBUHS 2022*

Introduction

- *Carotid endarterectomy (CEA)* is a surgical procedure that involves removing atherosclerotic plaque, causing internal carotid artery stenosis in order to prevent ischemic stroke. It can be used in both in the setting of symptomatic and asymptomatic carotid stenosis.
- More recently, percutaneous carotid arterial stenting (CAS) has been developed as an alternative to CEA, particularly in patients at high risk for postsurgical complications.

Indications

According to the National Institute for Health and Care Excellence (NICE) [United Kingdom (UK)] guidelines patients with suspected transient ischemic attack (TIA) or nondisabling stroke should be considered for endarterectomy if:

- Symptomatic carotid stenosis of 50–99% according to the NASCET (North American Symptomatic Carotid Endarterectomy Trial) criteria
- Symptomatic stenosis of 70–99% according to the ECST (European Carotid Surgery Trial) criteria

The European Society for Vascular Surgery guidelines advice CEA if:

- >50% carotid stenosis in patient with one or more TIA in the last 6 months

There is less consensus on prophylactic CEA in patients who are found to have significant carotid artery stenosis without neurological symptoms.

However, the ASCT-1 (Autologous Stem-Cell Transplantation) trial evaluated the prophylactic endarterectomy for asymptomatic stenosis and found a significant reduction in 10-year mortality. Unfortunately, they did not use a uniform minimum value for luminal stenosis and this is being further evaluated by ASCT-2.

Contraindications

Absolute contraindications include:

- Significantly disabling stroke, precluding benefits of further surgical prophylaxis
- Acute carotid occlusion

Relative Contraindications

High risk of surgical complications with no benefit in overall risk when compared to medical therapy

Preprocedural Planning

- Carotid artery disease may be either symptomatic or asymptomatic.
- Symptoms include TIA, stroke, stroke in evolution, or crescendo TIA.
- In symptomatic patients, imaging should begin with carotid duplex USG.
- Carotid duplex imaging uses qualitative and quantitative information to determine the severity of carotid artery stenosis with an overall accuracy of 80–97%.
- If duplex imaging demonstrates severe stenosis or ulcerative plaque that correlates with clinical symptoms, no further carotid imaging is required in most cases.
- In patients with mild-to-moderate disease (<50%) on duplex imaging and hemispheric TIAs, alternative causes may be sought with magnetic resonance angiography (MRA), CT angiography (CTA), or catheter-based angiography of the chest, neck, and brain.

Monitoring and follow-up:

- As a rule, if no complication occurs, patients are discharged home on postoperative day 1. They continue their antiplatelet and secondary preventative therapy.
- At 2–6 weeks after CEA, carotid duplex US should be performed. If the findings from duplex imaging are satisfactory, another duplex study should be done 6 months to 1 year later, then every year thereafter. If there is evidence of moderate contralateral disease or recurrent carotid artery stenosis, scanning may be performed at intervals of 6–12 months.

Complications

- Stroke (3% incidence at 30 days)
- Myocardial infarction
- Nerve injury (commonly hypoglossal, accessory, laryngeal, or mandibular nerves)
- *Hyperperfusion syndrome after CEA (1–2%):* Headache, seizures, and intracranial hemorrhage

19. Enumerate the indications and techniques of endarterectomy. ***KIIT University, Odisha 2025***

Definition

An *endarterectomy* is a *surgical procedure* in which *atheromatous plaque* and the inner lining of an artery are *removed* to restore normal blood flow.

Indications

Endarterectomy is indicated when *arterial narrowing (stenosis)* or *occlusion* due to *atherosclerosis* causes significant compromise of blood flow, leading to ischemic symptoms or high risk of stroke.

- *General indications:*
  - Symptomatic arterial occlusive disease with significant stenosis.
  - Asymptomatic but hemodynamically significant stenosis with high risk of future ischemic events.
  - Failure of medical management (e.g., antiplatelets, statins).
  - Lesions accessible surgically and not suitable for endovascular procedures.
- *Common specific indications:*
  - *Carotid endarterectomy (CEA)*
    - Symptomatic carotid stenosis of:
      - ≥70% (by NASCET criteria)
      - 50–69% with recurrent symptoms or plaque ulceration
    - Asymptomatic stenosis ≥60% in selected patients (low surgical risk, high stroke risk on imaging).
  - *Femoral endarterectomy*
    - Common femoral artery occlusive disease, causing:
      - Claudication
      - Rest pain
      - Nonhealing ulcers
  - Often performed as part of *hybrid procedures* with angioplasty.
- *Aortic, iliac, or popliteal endarterectomy:* Selected cases of *segmental atherosclerosis* where bypass is not indicated or feasible.

Techniques

- *Conventional (open) endarterectomy*
  - *Exposure* of the affected artery.
  - *Arteriotomy* (longitudinal incision along the artery).
  - *Plaque dissection and removal* from the intimal plane.
  - *Flushing* to clear debris and check distal runoff.
  - *Arteriotomy closure:*
    - *Primary closure* (direct suturing) or
    - *Patch angioplasty* (using vein or synthetic patch to widen lumen and prevent restenosis).
- *Eversion endarterectomy (specific for carotid arteries)*
  - The internal carotid artery (ICA) is transected at its origin.
  - The artery is everted (turned inside out), and the plaque is peeled off circumferentially.
  - The ICA is then reattached to the common carotid artery.

  Advantages: Lower restenosis rate, shorter clamp time, no patch needed.
- *Semi-closed or Closed Endarterectomy:* Plaque is removed through limited arteriotomies using special ring strippers (less common today).

Postoperative Care

- Antiplatelet therapy (e.g., aspirin, clopidogrel)
- Blood pressure control
- Monitoring for restenosis or complications (e.g., stroke, thrombosis)

Complications

- Stroke or embolization (carotid)
- Arterial thrombosis or restenosis
- Cranial nerve injury (especially in CEA)
- Hemorrhage or hematoma
- Infection

CHAPTER 54

Plastic and Reconstructive Surgery

LEARNING OBJECTIVES

- Functions of Skin
- Survival of Skin Graft
- Management of Skin Loss
- Flaps in Surgery
- Skin Grafting
- Tissue Engineering and Regenerative Surgery
- Tissue Expansion
- Skin Substitutes
- Development of Face
- Cleft Lip and Cleft Palate
- Hand Injury

FUNCTIONS OF SKIN

1. Functions of skin. How does a skin graft survive?

Functions of Skin

- *Protection:* An anatomical barrier from pathogens and damage between the internal and external environment in bodily defense. Langerhans cells in the skin are part of the adaptive immune system.
- *Sensation:* Contains a variety of nerve endings that jump to heat and cold, touch, pressure, vibration, and tissue injury
- *Thermoregulation:* Eccrine (sweat) glands and dilated blood vessels (increased superficial perfusion) aid heat loss, while constricted vessels greatly reduce cutaneous blood flow and conserve heat. Erector pili muscles in mammals adjust the angle of hair shafts to change the degree of the insulation provided by hair or fur.
- *Control of evaporation:* The skin provides a relatively dry and semi-impermeable barrier to reduce fluid loss.
- *Storage and synthesis:* It acts as a storage center for lipids and water.
- *Absorption through the skin:* Oxygen, nitrogen, and carbon dioxide can diffuse into the epidermis in small amounts. Some medications are absorbed through the skin.
- *Water resistance:* The skin acts as a water-resistant barrier, so essential nutrients are not washed out of the body. The nutrients and oils that help hydrate the skin are covered by the most outer skin layer, the epidermis. This is helped in part by the sebaceous glands that release sebum, an oily liquid. Water itself will not cause the elimination of oils on the skin, because the oils residing in our dermis flow and would be affected by water without the epidermis.
- *Camouflage:* Whether the skin is naked or covered in fur, scales, or feathers, and skin structures provide protective coloration and patterns that help to conceal animals from predators or prey.

Graft Survival

- After graft placement, an initial adherence to the wound bed via a thin fibrin network temporarily anchors the graft until definitive circulation and connective-tissue connections are established. This adherence begins immediately and is probably maximized by 8 hours postgrafting.

- The period of time between grafting and revascularization of the graft is referred to as the phase of plasmatic imbibition. The graft imbibes wound exudate by capillary action through the sponge-like structure of the graft dermis and through the dermal blood vessels. This prevents graft desiccation, maintains graft vessel patency, and provides nourishment for the graft.
- This process is entirely responsible for graft survival for 2–3 days until circulation is reestablished. During this time, the graft typically becomes edematous and increases in weight by 30–50%.
- Revascularization of the graft begins at 2–3 days postgrafting by a mechanism that is not completely understood. Inosculation is the establishment of direct anastomoses between graft and recipient blood vessels.
- Alternatively, some investigators have demonstrated vascular ingrowth of recipient bed vessels into the graft along the channels of previous graft vessels.
- Several important aspects of skin graft healing deserve further discussion. Wound contraction may present serious functional and cosmetic concerns, depending on the location and severity. Contraction probably begins shortly after initial wounding, progressing slowly over 6–18 months following grafting. Myofibroblasts are believed to cause contraction.
    - The spectrum of wound contraction from least to most is as follows:
    - *Full-thickness skin grafts (FTSG):* Least contraction
    - Thick split-thickness skin graft (STSG)
    - Thin STSG
    - Open wounds—most contraction
- Epithelial appendages must be regenerated following grafting. Hair rarely grows from STSG as the follicles are not transferred with the graft. Sweat glands and sebaceous glands initially degenerate the following grafting because only a portion of the gland is transferred, the remaining portion may not regenerate. Sweat gland regeneration is dependent on the reinnervation of the skin graft with recipient bed sympathetic nerve fibers. Once this ingrowth has occurred, the skin graft assumes the sweating characteristics of the recipient site. Sebaceous gland regeneration is independent of graft reinnervation and retains the characteristics of the donor site.
- Reinnervation of the graft occurs from the recipient bed and from the periphery along the empty neurolemma sheaths of the graft. Sensation returns to the periphery of the graft and proceeds centrally. Usually, this process begins during the first month but is not complete for several years following grafting.
- A general recommendation is to keep the graft be protected from direct sunlight for at least 12 months postgrafting.

2. Management of skin loss. ***WBUHS 2010***

The reconstructive ladder: The reconstructive ladder of soft-tissue coverage begins with consideration of the simplest approach (healing by secondary intention) and culminates with the most complex (free tissue transfer), maximizing opportunities for success.

- Healing by secondary intention is the simplest approach but is not always feasible. Absolute contraindications include exposed vessels, nerves, tendons, viscera, or bone. Relative contraindications include a large or poorly vascularized wound with a prolonged (>3 weeks) anticipated period of healing and undesirable aesthetic consequences.
- Primary closure may provide the most aesthetically pleasing result, but excessive tension on the skin may cause displacement of neighboring structures (e.g., lower eyelid) or necrosis of the skin flaps.
- Skin grafting is the most common method of large-wound closure. Skin grafts require a healthy, uninfected bed, protected from shear forces, to survive. Wound surfaces such as bare tendon, desiccated bone or cartilage, or infected tissue beds will not support skin graft survival. In addition, exposed vessels, nerves, or viscera are relative contraindications for skin grafting.
- Local tissue transfers of skin, fascia, and muscle may be used in regions with healthy adjacent tissue. If the adjacent tissue cannot be adequately mobilized or the wound requires more bulk than is locally available, the sole use of local flaps may not be adequate.

- Distant tissue transfers were the mainstay of difficult wound closure until the advent of free tissue transfer. This involves transferring healthy tissue into the wound bed while leaving it attached to its native blood supply. The pedicle is divided in a subsequent procedure. Inherent disadvantages of this technique include multiple operations, prolonged wound healing, immobilization for at least 3 weeks, and a limited choice of donor sites.
- Free tissue transfer is the most technically demanding approach to wound closure but has several potential advantages, including single-stage wound closure, a relatively wide variety of flaps to ensure closure specifically tailored to coverage needs, and in many cases, an aesthetically pleasing outcome.
- Vacuum-assisted closure has altered wound management by decreasing bacterial load and accelerating granulation. Wounds may be treated adequately with vacuum-assisted closure that would not traditionally be candidates for healing by secondary intention. Furthermore, it may convert a wound that would otherwise need an adjacent or free tissue transfer into a wound that needs only STSG.

3. Write down the basic concept of flaps and graft. ***WBUHS 2024***

Flaps and grafts are two fundamental techniques in reconstructive surgery used to repair tissue defects.

Flaps

A *flap* is a section of living tissue that is transferred from one part of the body to another along with its own blood supply. Flaps can be classified based on their blood supply, composition, or method of transfer.

Types of Flaps:

- *Local flaps:* Tissue is moved from an adjacent area without severing its blood supply.
- *Regional flaps:* Tissue is moved from a nearby region while maintaining its vascular connection.
- *Free flaps:* Tissue is completely detached and reattached at a new site using microsurgery.

Grafts

A *graft* is a piece of tissue that is transplanted from one site to another without its own blood supply. The graft relies on the recipient site to develop new blood vessels for survival.

Types of Grafts:

- *Skin grafts:* Used for wound coverage and burn treatment.
    - *Split-thickness grafts* (epidermis and part of the dermis).
    - *Full-thickness grafts* (epidermis and entire dermis).
- *Bone, cartilage, and fat grafts:* Used for reconstructive procedures.

Key difference: Flaps retain their original blood supply, while grafts depend on the recipient site for vascularization

FLAPS IN SURGERY

4. Give an account of flaps used in reconstructive surgery.
WBUHS 2021, DY Patil Educational Society, Deemed to be University 2024

5. Flaps in Surgery. ***WBUHS 2007, 2009***

6. Define skin flap. Name commonly used skin flaps for reconstruction. Principles of flap used in surgery.
***WBUHS 2021 Supplementary, 2025 Supplementary,* RIMS-IMPHAL 2022**

A flap is any tissue that is transferred to another site with an intact blood supply.

Definition

A flap is a unit of tissue that is transferred from one site (donor site) to another (recipient site) while maintaining its own blood supply.

Classification based on Blood Supply

- *Random cutaneous flaps* are used to cover adjacent defects.

    - Blood supply from the dermal and subdermal plexus without a single dominant artery.
    - Length-to-width ratio (usually 3:1), varies by anatomic region (e.g., the face has a ratio of up to 5:1).
    - Flaps that rotate about a pivot point include rotation flaps and transposition flaps.
        - The effective length shortens through the arc of rotation
        - The further from the base of the flap, the greater the risk of necrosis.
        - *More complex rotation flaps:* Bilobed flaps and rhomboid flaps.
- Advancement of skin directly into a defect without rotation.
    - Simple advancement
    - V-Y advancement
    - Bipedicle advancement flap

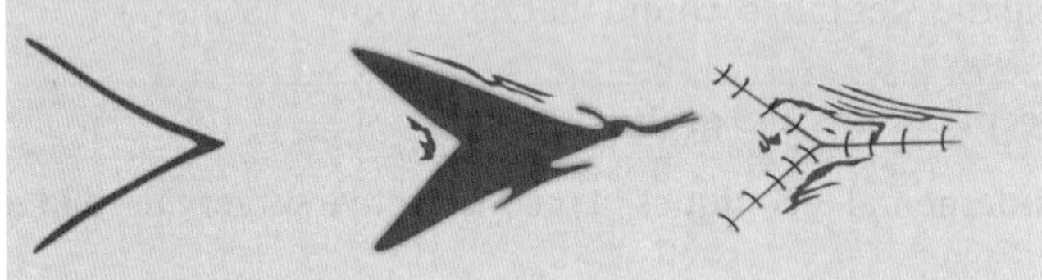

V-Y advancement. The skin to the sides of the V is advanced.

- *Axial cutaneous flaps* contain a single dominant arteriovenous system, allowing for a potentially greater length-to-width ratio.
    - *Peninsular flap:* Skin and vessels are moved together as a unit.
    - *Island flaps:* Skin is divided from surrounding tissue and maintained on an isolated, intact vascular pedicle.
    - *Free flaps:* Vascular pedicle is isolated and divided, then re-anastomosed at a new anatomic site.
        - *Axial (named blood vessel) Mathes and Nahai classification:*
            - One vascular pedicle (e.g., tensor fascia lata)
            - Dominant pedicle(s) and minor pedicle(s) (e.g., gracilis)
            - Two dominant pedicles (e.g., gluteus maximus)
            - Segmental vascular pedicles (e.g., sartorius)
            - One dominant pedicle and secondary segmental pedicles (e.g., latissimus dorsi)

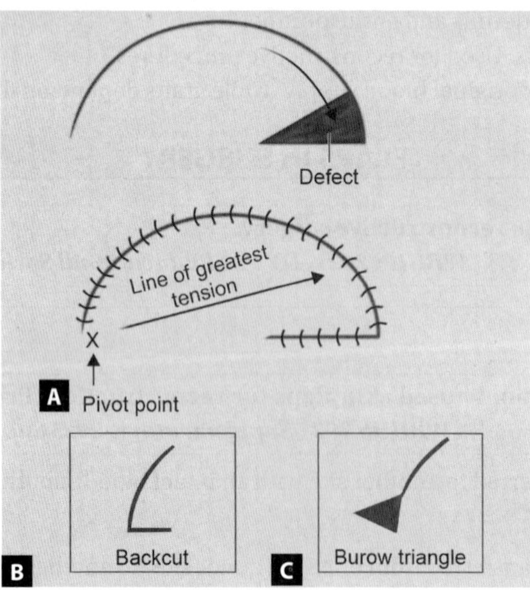

- *Rotation flap:*
    - *A:* The edge of the flap is four to five times the length of the base of the defect triangle.
    - *B, C:* A back cut or Burow's triangle can be useful if the flap is under tension.

- Flaps that rotate around a pivot point include rotation flaps and transposition flaps. Planning for shortening of the effective length through the arc of rotation is important when designing these flaps. More complex rotation flaps include bilobed flaps and rhomboid flaps.
- Advancement of skin directly into a defect without rotation can be accomplished with a simple advancement, a V-Y advancement, or a bipedicle advancement flap.

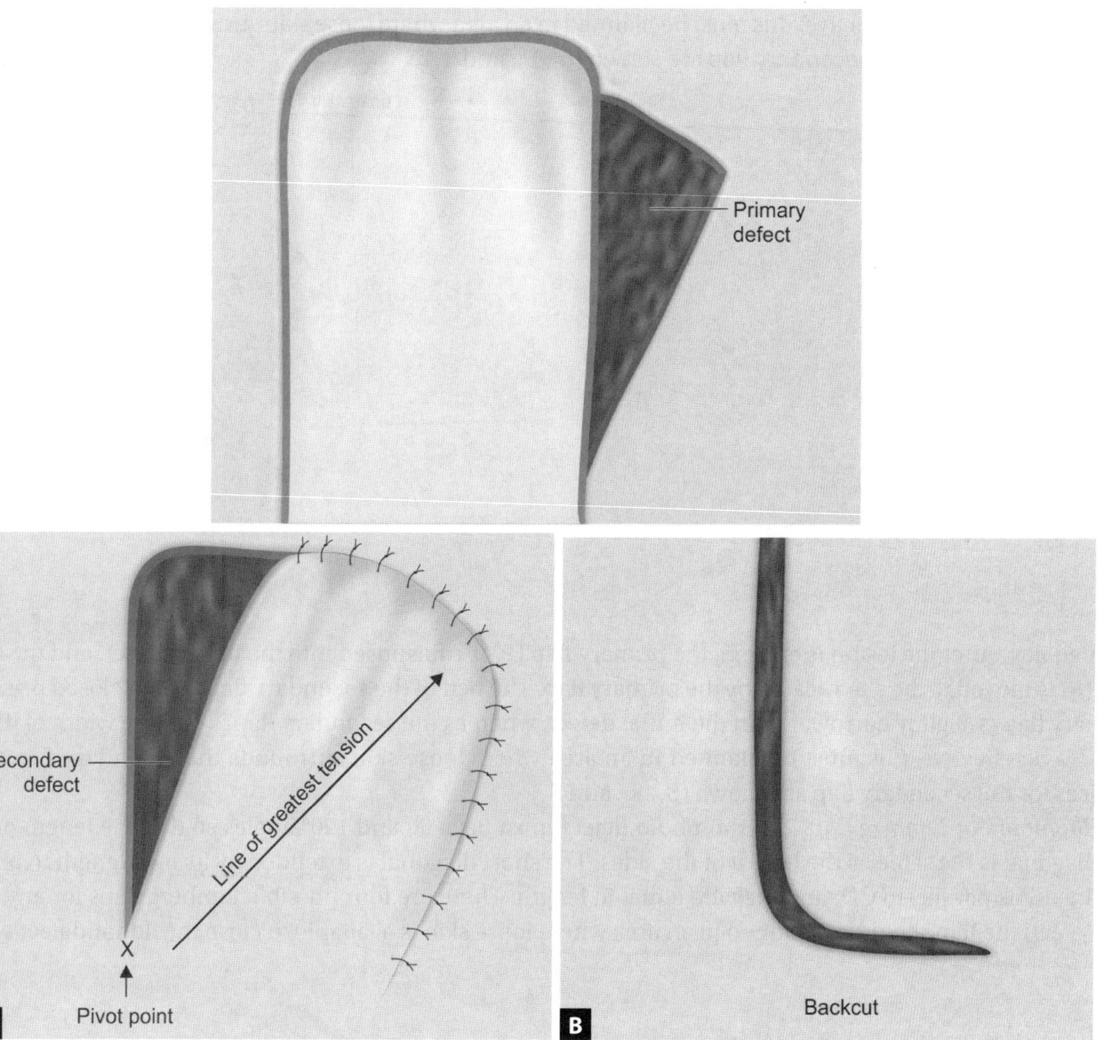

- *Transposition flap:* The secondary defect is typically covered with a skin graft. B: A back cut may be added to reduce tension at the pivot point.

Classification Based on the Tissue Type

- *Fascial/fasciocutaneous flaps* are used when thin, well-vascularized coverage is needed (e.g., dorsum of the hand or foot).
  - *Fascia:* Temporoparietal fascia.
  - *Fasciocutaneous flaps:* Radial forearm, anterolateral thigh, lateral arm, and groin flaps.
  - *Muscle or musculocutaneous flaps* are used when the muscle is needed for bulk, to obliterate dead space, or when robust well-vascularized coverage is needed.
  - *Muscle:* Sartorius, rectus femoris, and gracilis muscle for groin coverage.
  - *Musculocutaneous:* Latissimus dorsi or pectoralis major for chest, or rectus abdominis or gracilis for perineal coverage.

- *Vascularized bone flaps* are used for critical bony defects >8 cm

Specialized Flaps

- *Bilobed flap:* After the lesion is excised, the primary flap (P) is transposed into the initial defect, and the secondary flap (S) is moved to the site vacated by the primary flap. The bed of the secondary flap is then closed primarily. The primary flap is slightly narrower than the initial defect, whereas the secondary flap is half the width of the primary flap. To be effective, this must be planned in an area where loose skin surrounds the secondary flap site. Three choices for the secondary flap are shown (S_1, S_2, and S_3).

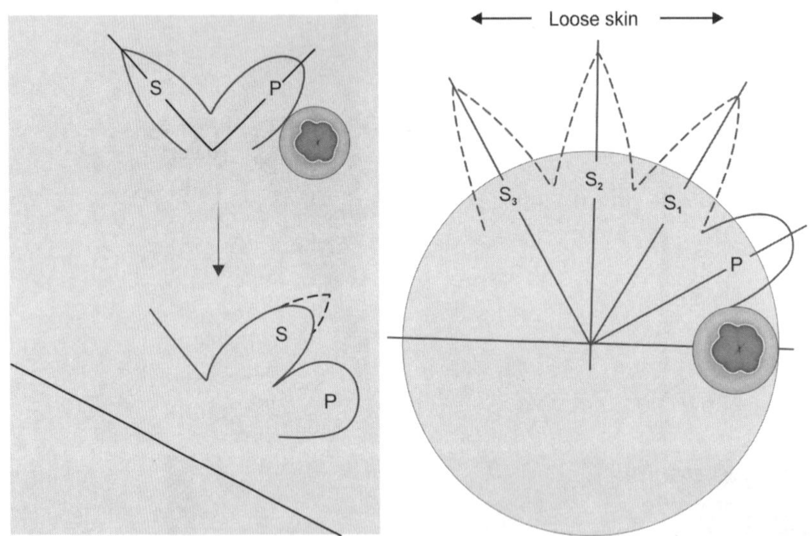

Bilobed flap. After the lesion is excised, the primary flap (P) is transposed into the initial defect, and the secondary flap (S) is moved to the site vacated by the primary flap. The bed of the secondary flap is then closed primarily. The primary flap is slightly narrower than the initial defect, whereas the secondary flap is half the width of the primary flap. To be effective, this must be planned in an area where loose skin surrounds the secondary flap site. Three choices for the secondary flap are shown (S_1, S_2, and S_3).

- *Rhomboid or Limberg flap:* The rhomboid defect must have 60 and 120° angles so that the length of the short diagonal is the same as the length of the sides. The short diagonal is extended by its own length to point E. The line EF is parallel to CD, and they are equal in length. There are four possible Limberg flaps for any rhomboid defect; the flap should be planned in an area where loose skin is available to close the donor defect primarily.

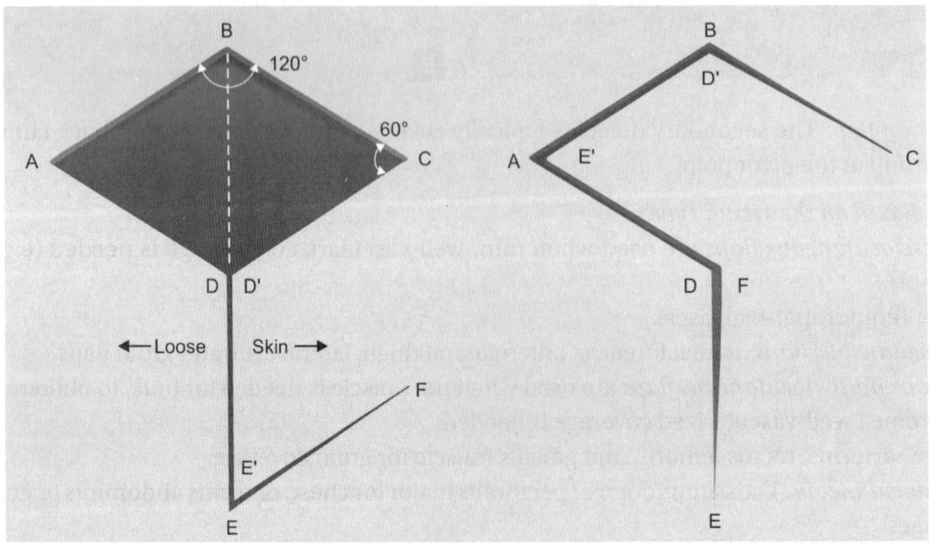

Principles of Skin Flap

- *Replace like-with-like:* This is a particularly important principle. When filling in a defect, replace like-with-like. Ralph Millard once said, "When a part of one's person is lost, it should be replaced in kind, bone for bone, muscle for muscle, hairless skin for hairless skin, an eye for an eye, a tooth for a tooth."
- *Think of reconstruction in terms of units:* According to Millard, human beings may be divided into seven main parts—the head, neck, body, and extremities. Each of these body parts can be further subdivided into units. The head, e.g., is composed of several regional units—scalp, face, and ears. Consider that each of these units has its own unique features, and each feature has, in turn, multiple subunits with their own special shapes. All of these different units and subunits must be considered and reproduced during reconstruction.
- *Always have a pattern and a backup plan:* As with all surgery, comparing the pros and cons of each surgical option is of the utmost importance. The reconstructive ladder is a mental exercise that provides the surgeon with options ranging from the simplest to the most complex. Usually, things should be kept as simple as possible. This benefits both the surgeon and the patient; the simplest plan is often the safest.
- *Steal from Peter to pay Paul:* Apply the principle "steal from Peter to pay Paul, but only when Peter can afford it." Using what the body has to reconstruct a deficit is essentially "robbing the bank." The goal to achieve is ultimate efficiency, or, according to Millard, "getting something for almost nothing."
- *Never forget the donor area:* Remember that donor areas are not limitless. One cannot continuously use tissue without paying back in some way. Carelessness or overuse of a donor area eventually causes damage that may be far greater than the original defect.

7. TRAM flap. ***WBUHS 2015***

Autologous Reconstruction

- *Pedicled flap:* Today, the gold standard in breast reconstruction with autogenous tissue is the transverse rectus abdominis myocutaneous (TRAM) flap because of the lower abdominal tissue's similarities in consistency with breast tissue.
- The first description of the TRAM flap used in breast reconstruction, by Robbins in 1979, was with a vertical skin island. The TRAM flap as we know it, with a horizontal lower abdominal skin paddle, was first described by Hartrampf in 1982. This orients the donor scar into a more acceptable abdominoplasty location.
- Although this location of the skin paddle provides for a better arc of rotation—the ensuing blood supply to this large volume of tissue is more distal and therefore tenuous.
- This donor area of skin and adipose tissue has a dual blood supply for the superior and inferior epigastric systems. Pedicled flaps are thus supplied by the proximal superior epigastric vessels and the inferior system must be divided for transfer.
- The small vessels connecting the superior and inferior systems, known as choke vessels, are then dilated to increase perfusion once the deep system is ligated.
- Studies by Moon and Taylor have further elucidated the perfusion zones of the lower abdomen skin territory. They found rich perforating blood vessels that arise out of the rectus to supply the overlying skin and fat. Perfusion is best overlying the rectus muscle (zone I) on the side (pedicle) used, followed by the region overlying the contralateral rectus muscle (zone II). Next is the ipsilateral outer region of tissue (zone III), and the region perfused the least is the farthest from the rectus pedicle (zone IV).
- This type of reconstruction is advantageous in that it replaces like-with-like tissue and provides an acceptable donor scar and improvement of abdominal contour.

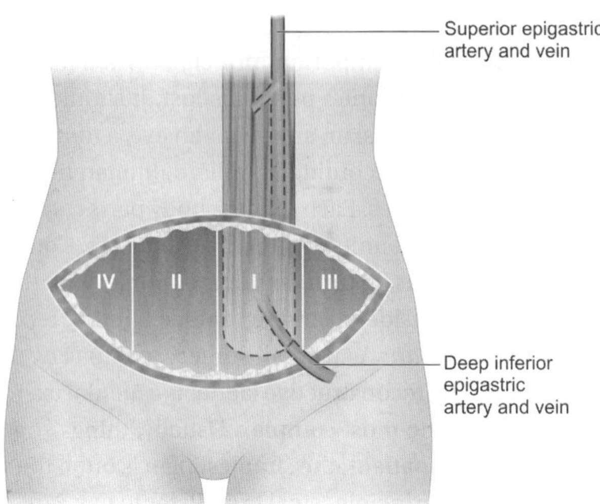

Vascular territories of the abdominal wall are provided by a unilateral TRAM flap (as determined by Moon and Taylor). Blood flow is best in zone I, followed by zones II, III, and IV, respectively.

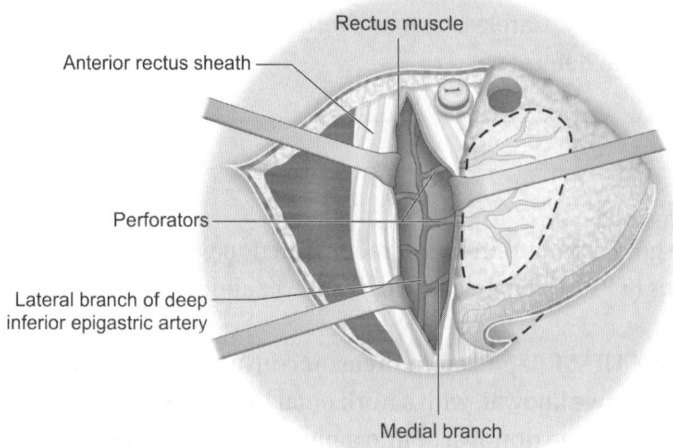

Deep inferior epigastric artery and vein.

The limitations include the following:

- This tissue has high metabolic demands that are sometimes not met so that portions of the flap go on to form fat necrosis or die.
- There is a longer recovery period after this surgery, with increased abdominal discomfort and risk for abdominal weakness and/or hernia formation.
- Its use can also be limited by previous abdominal operations and scars.
- Who are obese, smokers, or have medical comorbidities (especially diabetes) are at greater risk for these complications.

Transverse Rectus Abdominis Muscle Flap Reconstruction

Indications

Breasts of all sizes	Abdominal liposuction	Abdominal liposuction
Breast ptosis	Previous abdominal surgery	Previous abdominal surgery
Relative contraindications	Pulmonary disease	Pulmonary disease
Smoking	Obesity	Obesity

Contraindications

- Previous abdominoplasty
- Patient unable to tolerate a 4–6 weeks recovery period
- Patient unable to tolerate a longer procedure

8. Outline the principles of microsurgery. Discuss briefly the pectoralis major flap.

Principles of Microsurgery.

- Microsurgery is a surgical discipline that combines magnification with advanced diploscopes, specialized precision tools, and various operating techniques. These techniques are primarily used to anastomose small blood vessels (arteries and veins) and to coapt the nerves.
- Microsurgical reconstruction is used for complex reconstructive surgery problems when other options (e.g., primary closure, healing by secondary intention, skin grafting, and local or regional flap transfer) are not adequate.
- Microsurgery may not be the best solution for all reconstructive dilemmas and usually is not the first choice in the reconstructive ladder; however, it can offer the reconstructive surgeon an important tool for achieving complex reconstruction by proceeding with free tissue transfer from distant sites. Free tissue transfer includes flaps such as the following:
  - Isolated transfers
  - Composite tissue transfers
  - Functioning free muscle transfers
  - Vascularized bone grafts
  - Toe transplantation
    - In addition, specific tissue transfers such as neural grafts or vein grafts are also considered free tissue transfer.
    - In specific cases, such as large defects of the face after tumor resection and free tissue transfer may be the best option for the closure of the defect.
    - Reconstructive microsurgery has entered a stage where, because of continued developments in technology and a better understanding of the anatomy, anastomosis of very small vessels (0.3 mm) is possible.
    - These highly challenging procedures are referred to in the literature as supermicrosurgery.
    - They allow anastomosis of perforator flaps, such as the medial plantar flap to perforator recipient vessels.
    - Additional applications include complex digit reimplantation and lymphatic anastomosis.

Although microsurgery continues to develop, the basic principles of microsurgery remain the same:

- Select patients carefully
- Develop a careful preoperative plan and a backup plan
- Use a well-defined workhorse flap
- Obtain full patient consent
- Pay attention to intraoperative details
- Employ meticulous microsurgical technique
- Remain vigilant during postoperative care

Indications

Indications for tissue transfer utilizing microsurgical techniques include the following:

- Need to cover exposed vital structures, such as joint surfaces, tendons, vessels, and bone denuded of periosteum
- Need to restore shape, as in the breast after mastectomy
- Need to restore function, as in the muscles of the face

Technical Considerations

Vessel injury and regeneration:

Vessel injury and regeneration occur through the following steps:
- Formation of a platelet plug
- Pseudointima formation
- Endothelial regeneration

Classification of Flaps
Mathes and Nahai classified flaps as either random or axial on the basis of blood supply. A random flap is perfused by random small blood vessels without a proper name (e.g., local bilobed flap). An axial flap is based on a known, named blood vessel or set of blood vessels. Mathes and Nahai classified these flaps as follows:
- One vascular pedicle [e.g., tensor fasciae latae (TFL)]
- Dominant pedicle(s) and minor pedicle(s) (e.g., gracilis)
- Two dominant pedicles (e.g., gluteus maximus)
- Segmental vascular pedicles (e.g., sartorius)
- One dominant pedicle and secondary segmental pedicles (e.g., latissimus dorsi)

Pectoralis Major Flap
Anatomy of the pectoralis major:
- *Origin:*
  - Clavicle
  - Sternum (2–7 costal cartilages)
  - Abdominal rectus sheath
- *Insertion:* Greater tubercle of humerus
- *Arterial supply:* Pectoral branches of the thoracoacromial artery from the axillary and from the subclavian artery
- *Innervation:* Medial and lateral pectoral nerves
- *Mohrenheim's fossa:*
  - Fossa between the pectoralis major, deltoid, and clavicle
  - *Importance:* Cephalic vein passes here
- *Indications:*
  - *Pectoralis major myofascial flap:* A valuable tool in contemporary head and neck reconstruction
  - Pectoralis major musculocutaneous flap in oropharyngeal reconstruction
  - Pectoralis myofascial flap during salvage laryngectomy prevents pharyngocutaneous fistula
- *Strengths:*
  - Robust and highly reliable
  - Ease of harvest
  - Excellent color-texture match to neck and facial skin
- *Limitations:*
  - Bulky
  - Restricted reach
- *Preparation:*
  - Mark the thoracoacromial artery:
    - Draw a line from the acromial end of the clavicle to the xiphisternum
    - Draw a second line vertically from the midpoint of the clavicle to intersect the first line
  - Design the skin incision and skin paddle:
    - Consider any potential future or concurrent need for a deltopectoral flap
      - For men—plan a vertically oriented skin paddle, adjacent to but sparing the nipple
      - For women—plan a horizontally oriented inframammary skin paddle
    - Consider the secondary defect closure
    - Generally, chest skin defects of approximately 9 cm or less may be closed primarily
    - Use a sponge or towel to plan the skin paddle to make sure that it will reach the defect
      - Place the sponge on the clavicle and arc around

- Dr Fong designs the incision as a curvilinear line from lateral to just medial to the nipple in a man

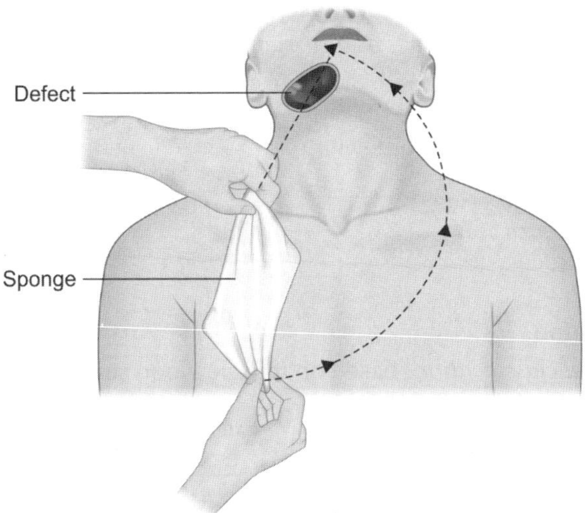

Procedure

- Incise through the skin to the fascia of the pectoralis major muscle.
- Expose the pectoralis major muscle by elevating skin flaps in the suprafascial plane
- *Transect the pectoralis major muscle:*
  - Transect the pectoralis major muscle laterally and bluntly elevate from the pectoralis minor muscle.
  - Continue to transect the pectoralis major muscle inferiorly to accommodate the skin paddle.
  - Transect the pectoralis major muscle medially to separate from the sternal attachments.
  - Continue to transect the pectoralis major muscle up to the clavicle.
- Identify and cauterize the intercostal vessels well since they will retract back into the chest.
- Elevate the pectoralis major muscle from the pec minor in the avascular plane
- Identify the thoracoacromial artery and cephalic vein on the deep surface of the pectoralis major muscle.
- Transect the pectoralis major muscle lateral attachment to the humerus—protect the pedicle with your fingers.
- *Optional:* Identify and denervate the flap by clipping and dividing the medial and lateral pectoral nerves.
  - Bluntly dissect the subplatysmal plane tunnel superficial to the clavicle superiorly into the neck.
  - Generally, about four fingerbreadths of space are needed to prevent ischemia of the pedicle.
  - Pass the flap into the neck:
    - Avoid shearing the skin paddle
    - Check the pedicle for twisting
- Close the secondary defect:
  - If needed, undermine adjacent skin to facilitate primary closure
  - If needed, harvest an STSG for closure
  - Two suction drains in the chest, exiting inferolaterally, secured with 2-0 Silk
  - 3-0 Polysorb interrupted buried deep dermal
  - 5-0 Fast or 5-0 Prolene simple running versus staples to approximate the epidermis

9. Myocutaneous flaps. ***NTRUHS, Vijayawada 2024***

Definition

A *myocutaneous flap* is a *composite flap* that includes:

- *Skin,*
- *Subcutaneous tissue,* and
- *Underlying muscle*

} All supplied by the *same vascular pedicle*

It is used for *reconstruction of soft-tissue defects,* especially where both *bulk and skin cover* are needed.

Principle

- The *muscle's vascular pedicle* supplies both the muscle and the overlying skin through *perforating vessels.*
- When the flap is transferred, the *muscle acts as a carrier* of the skin island, ensuring reliable blood supply.

Advantages	*Disadvantages*
• Excellent *vascularity* → better resistance to infection • Provides *bulk* to fill dead space • Can carry *skin of good quality* for coverage • Can be used in *irradiated or scarred beds* • Allows *single-stage reconstruction*	• *Donor site morbidity* (loss of muscle function) • *Bulky flap*—may need secondary contouring • Longer operative time

Vascular Basis and Classification

According to *Mathes and Nahai classification* (based on muscle blood supply):

Type	*Vascular pattern*	*Example*
I	Single dominant vascular pedicle	Gastrocnemius, tensor fascia lata
II	One dominant + minor pedicles	Gracilis
III	Two dominant pedicles	Gluteus maximus, rectus abdominis
IV	Segmental pedicles	Sartorius
V	One dominant + segmental	Latissimus dorsi

Common Myocutaneous Flaps and Uses

Flap	*Arterial supply*	*Common uses*
Pectoralis major	Thoracoacromial artery	Head and neck reconstruction, chest wall defects
Latissimus dorsi	Thoracodorsal artery	Chest wall, breast, back, shoulder reconstruction
Rectus abdominis (TRAM)	Deep inferior epigastric artery	Breast reconstruction
Gracilis	Medial circumflex femoral artery	Perineal, vaginal, lower limb defects
Gastrocnemius	Sural branches of popliteal artery	Knee, upper tibial defects
Soleus	Posterior tibial and peroneal arteries	Middle third leg defects
Tensor fascia lata (TFL)	Lateral circumflex femoral artery	Trochanteric and groin defects
Gluteus maximus	Inferior gluteal artery	Sacral pressure sore coverage

Types of Myocutaneous Flaps (by Transfer Method)

Type	*Description*	*Example*
Pedicled flap	Flap remains attached to its native blood supply and is rotated into nearby defect	Pectoralis major, gastrocnemius
Free flap	Flap completely detached and revascularized by *microvascular anastomosis* at recipient site	Free latissimus dorsi, free rectus abdominis

Indications

- Reconstruction of *complex soft tissue defects* (trauma, oncologic resections).
- *Coverage of exposed bone, tendon, or prosthesis.*
- *Filling dead space* (e.g., after osteomyelitis excision).
- *Pressure sore coverage* (sacral, ischial, trochanteric).
- *Breast reconstruction* (TRAM flap).

Complications
- *Partial or total flap necrosis* (vascular compromise).
- *Hematoma/seroma* formation.
- *Infection.*
- *Donor site morbidity* (muscle weakness, contour defect).

Advantages over Pure Cutaneous Flaps
- More *robust blood supply.*
- Better survival in *irradiated or infected fields.*
- Can obliterate *deep cavities* due to muscle bulk.

SKIN GRAFTING

10. Skin grafting and flaps.

Split-thickness Skin Grafts
- Thicker knife-gap settings give rise to fewer but brisker bleeding points on the donor site
- Thicker grafts heal with less contracture and are more durable.
- Thinner donor sites heal better
- Grafts are hairless and do not sweat (these structures are not transferred)

Full-thickness Skin Grafts
- Full-thickness grafts are harvested to incorporate the whole dermis, with the underlying fat trimmed away—unless elements of fat (or even cartilage as well) are deliberately left attached to form a composite graft.
- Full-thickness and composite grafts require the most careful handling and postoperative nursing to help ensure that they "take" in their transplanted site.

Grafts are tissues that are transferred without their blood supply, which therefore have to revascularize once they are in a new site.

They include the following:
- *STSGs (of varying thickness).* These are sometimes called Thiersch grafts. They are used to cover all sizes of wounds, are of limited durability, and will contract. They may be used to provide valuable temporary wound closure before better cosmetic secondary correction after rehabilitation.
- *Full-thickness skin grafts (Wolfe grafts).* Used for smaller areas of skin replacement where good elastic skin that will not contract is required (such as fingers, eyelids, and facial parts).
- *Composite skin grafts (usually skin and fat or skin and cartilage).* Often taken from the ear margin and useful for rebuilding missing elements of the nose, eyelids, and fingertips.
- *Nerve grafts:* Usually, taken from the sural nerve, but smaller cutaneous nerves may be used.
- *Tendon grafts:* Usually, taken from the palmaris longus or plantaris tendon (runs just anteromedial to the Achilles tendon) and used for injury loss or nerve damage correction.

Flaps

Flaps are tissues that are transferred with a blood supply. They therefore have the advantage of bringing vascularity to the new area. Flaps can be raised to consist of any specific tissue; for skin flaps, the following will illustrate the types that exist.
- *Random flaps:* Three sides of a rectangle, bearing no specific relationship to where the blood supply enters; the length-to-breadth ratio is no >1.5:1. This pattern can be lengthened by "delaying" the flap, a process in which the cuts are partially made and the flap is partly lifted at a first operation; it is then replaced, thus "training" the blood supply from a single border of the rectangle. At a second procedure, it is raised further and finally transferred.

- *Axial flaps:* Much longer flaps, based on known blood vessels supplying the skin. This technique was rediscovered in the 1960s and 1970s and enables many long thin flaps to be safely moved across large distances.
- *Pedicled/islanded flaps:* The axial blood supply of these flaps means that they can be swung round on a stalk or even fully "islanded" so that the business end of the skin being transferred can have the pedicle buried.
- *Free flaps:* The blood supply has been isolated, disconnected, and then reconnected using microsurgery at the new site.
- *Composite flaps:* Various tissues are transferred together, often skin with bone or muscle (osseocutaneous or myocutaneous flaps, respectively).
- *Perforator flaps:* This description refers to a whole new subgroup of axial flaps in which tissues are isolated on small perforating vessels that run from more major blood vessels to supply the surface.

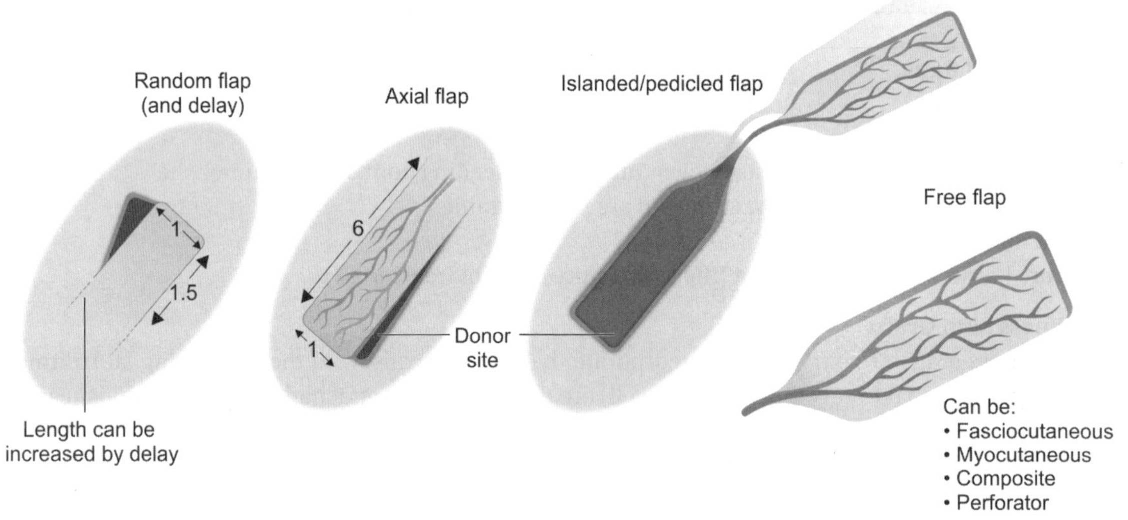

11. What is a skin graft take? What are the stages of skin graft take? What are the advantages of meshing a skin graft? ***WBUHS 2022***

Introduction

- Skin graft take refers to the successful attachment and survival of a skin graft after it has been transplanted to a recipient site.
- Skin grafting is a surgical procedure in which a piece of healthy skin, either from the patient's own body (autograft) or from a donor (allograft), is removed and transplanted to a site where there is damaged or missing skin, such as a burn, wound, and surgical incision.
- The success of a skin graft is measured by the extent to which the transplanted skin is able to integrate with the surrounding tissue and establish a blood supply, which is necessary for the survival of the graft.
- The percentage of skin graft take is determined by the amount of graft tissue that remains viable and adheres to the recipient site. A high percentage of skin graft take is important for the proper healing of the wound and to reduce the risk of infection or other complications.

The stages of skin graft take are:

- Skin graft adherence
- Imbibition
- Revascularization
- Remodeling

Skin Graft Healing Phases

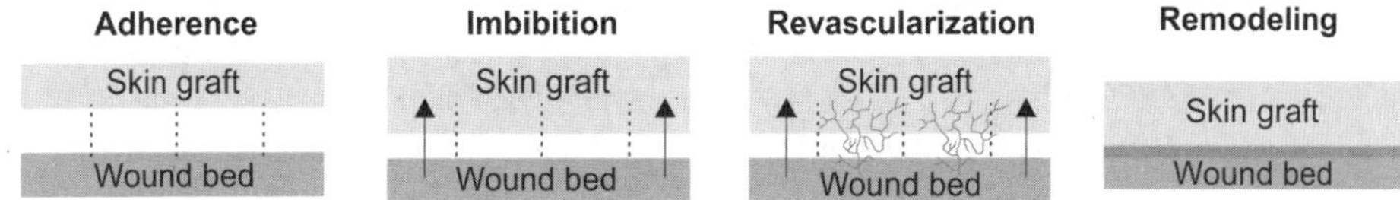

Skin Graft Adherence

- This occurs instantly if a suitable bed has been selected for the skin graft.
- Fibrin bonds form and the proliferation of fibroblasts replace the fibrin with collagen.

Serum Imbibition

- The graft absorbs fluids within 72 hours resulting in increased graft size.
- The fluid contains nutrition to keep the graft viable.

Revascularization

- A small vascular network starts to form in the fibrin layer connected to the graft and the wound bed after ~72 hours.
- This occurs through inosculation and neovascularization which allow the outgrowth of capillary buds.
- This brings "pinkness" to the graft.

Remodeling

Graft architecture returns to "normal skin"

Advantages of Meshing a Skin Graft

- In a meshed skin graft, the skin from the donor site is stretched to allow it to cover an area larger than itself. Healing occurs as the spaces between the mesh fill in with new skin growth. (The disadvantages of meshing are that it is less than a sheet graft and that the larger the mesh, the greater the permanent scarring.)
- It increases the flexibility of the graft so that it can conform to uneven recipient beds.
- Meshing allows blood and body fluids to drain from under the skin grafts, preventing graft loss, and it allows the donor skin to cover a greater burned area because it is expanded.
- It can be used in both split-thickness and full-thickness skin grafting.

TISSUE ENGINEERING AND REGENERATIVE SURGERY

12. Discuss principles and applications of tissue engineering and regenerative therapy in modern surgical practice. ***Rajasthan University of Health Sciences 2025***

Introduction

Tissue engineering and *regenerative therapy* are rapidly evolving fields that combine principles of *biology, engineering, and material science* to restore, maintain, or improve tissue and organ function.

They aim to *regenerate damaged tissues* rather than simply replace them—marking a paradigm shift from traditional reconstructive surgery to *biological restoration.*

Definitions

- *Tissue engineering:* The use of *cells, biomaterials (scaffolds), and bioactive molecules* to create functional tissues that can repair or replace damaged biological structures.
- *Regenerative therapy:* Broader term encompassing *cell-based therapies, gene therapy, stem cell therapy, and tissue engineering* aimed at restoring normal tissue structure and function.

Basic Principles (Triad of Tissue Engineering)

Successful tissue engineering depends on the interaction of three essential components:

Component	*Function*	*Examples*
Cells	Provide regenerative capacity	Stem cells (embryonic, mesenchymal, induced pluripotent), autologous chondrocytes
Scaffolds	Provide 3D structure for cell attachment and tissue growth	Collagen, polyglycolic acid, hydrogel, decellularized matrices
Signaling molecules (growth factors)	Stimulate cell proliferation, differentiation, angiogenesis	VEGF, BMPs, TGF-β, PDGF

Process of Tissue Engineering

- Cell source selection and culture (e.g., stem cells or autologous tissue-derived cells)
- Scaffold fabrication and seeding
- In vitro tissue growth under bioreactor conditions
- Implantation into patient
- Integration and remodeling with host tissue

Types of Cells Used

Cell type	*Characteristics*	*Applications*
Embryonic stem cells	Pluripotent, ethical issues	Research stage
Adult stem cells	Multipotent, less ethical concern	Bone marrow, fat, muscle
Mesenchymal stem cells (MSCs)	From bone marrow, adipose tissue	Bone, cartilage, wound healing
Induced pluripotent stem cells (iPSCs)	Reprogrammed adult cells	Organ engineering, gene correction

Scaffold Materials

- *Natural:* Collagen, fibrin, alginate, chitosan
- *Synthetic:* Polylactic acid (PLA), polyglycolic acid (PGA), polycaprolactone (PCL)
- *Properties desired:*
  - Biocompatibility
  - Biodegradability
  - Mechanical strength
  - Porosity for cell infiltration

Applications in Modern Surgical Practice

- *General surgery*
  - *Skin substitutes and wound healing*
    - Bioengineered skin (e.g., Integra, Apligraf) for burns and chronic ulcers
    - Growth factor gels (e.g., PDGF) enhance healing
  - *Bowel regeneration*: Research into bioengineered small intestine segments
- *Plastic and reconstructive surgery*
  - *Cartilage and bone tissue engineering* for facial reconstruction
  - *Fat-derived stem cells* for soft tissue augmentation
  - *Bioengineered skin grafts* for burns and scars
- *Orthopedic surgery*
  - *Bone graft substitutes* using MSCs and hydroxyapatite scaffolds
  - *Cartilage regeneration*—Autologous Chondrocyte Implantation (ACI) and matrix-assisted ACI (MACI)
  - *Tendon and ligament repair* using bioresorbable scaffolds

- *Cardiothoracic surgery*
  - *Tissue-engineered heart valves* and vascular grafts
  - *Myocardial regeneration* using stem cell therapy after infarction
  - *Bioengineered trachea* for airway reconstruction
- *Urology*
  - *Bladder reconstruction* using autologous urothelial cells on scaffolds (e.g., Atala's work)
  - *Urethral reconstruction* with tissue-engineered grafts
- *Neurosurgery*
  - *Nerve conduits* (biodegradable tubes) guiding axonal regeneration in peripheral nerve injuries
  - *Stem cell therapy* for spinal cord injury and Parkinson's disease (research stage)
- *Hepatobiliary and pancreatic surgery*
  - *Bioartificial liver devices* with hepatocyte scaffolds for temporary liver support
  - *Islet cell transplantation* or stem cell-derived beta cells for diabetes management

Recent and Emerging Advances

- *3D Bioprinting:* Layer-by-layer fabrication of tissues using cell-laden bioinks.
- *Organoids:* Miniature organ-like structures grown from stem cells for transplantation or drug testing.
- *Decellularized organ scaffolds:* Natural extracellular matrices repopulated with patient's own cells.
- *Gene-edited stem cells (CRISPR):* Correction of genetic defects before implantation.
- *Nanotechnology in scaffolds:* For controlled release of growth factors and enhanced integration.

Challenges and Limitations

- Limited vascularization in large constructs
- Risk of immune rejection or tumorigenesis (especially with pluripotent stem cells)
- Ethical issues (especially with embryonic stem cells)
- High cost and technical complexity
- Regulatory hurdles for clinical translation

Future Directions

- *Personalized regenerative medicine* using patient-specific stem cells and 3D bioprinting
- *Whole organ engineering* (e.g., kidney, liver)
- *Integration with AI and robotics* for precise tissue design and implantation
- *Hybrid constructs* combining synthetic and biological materials

TISSUE EXPANSION

13. Tissue expansion. ***WBUHS 2022***

Tissue expansion is a reconstructive technique that uses an inflatable silicone balloon to serially expand surrounding skin. This expansion adjacent to the wound provides donor tissue of similar color, texture, thickness, and sensation, with minimal scar formation and donor-site morbidity. The technique takes advantage of the skin's ability to accommodate a slowly enlarging mass beneath it by increasing its surface area. The idea is to create and develop donor tissue, harvest it, and leave the original donor site preserved.

Advantages	*Disadvantages*
The advantages include lower donor-site morbidity and the provision of donor tissue of similar quality to the recipient tissue. Tissue expansion is a simple and versatile technique that provides robust tissue	The disadvantages are that it is a staged technique, there is a visible deformity during the period of expansion, it requires frequent visits for expansion, and there is a relatively high rate of complications, including infection and extrusion

Technique

- Preoperative planning involves assessing the defect size, locating matching tissue to be expanded, and deciding where the final scars will be.
- Expander placement is usually performed through an incision at the junction of the lesion and the area of the proposed expansion.
- The length of the incision is controversial. Some authors propose one-third the length of the expander (it should be big enough to ensure full pocket creation).
- The filling port can be incorporated into the expander or placed in a separate pocket.
- In addition, the port may be externalized to minimize anxiety and pain during filling, especially in the pediatric population.
- Partially filling the expander on initial placement may reduce the duration of the expansion phase and reduce mechanical implant failure due to folding.
- The expansion phase begins 2–3 weeks after expander placement.
- The expander is inflated weekly with saline, using a sterile technique.
- The amount infused with each fill depends on patient comfort, skin tension, and blanching of overlying skin. A rough guide is 10% of expander volume per injection.
- The duration of the expansion phase can vary from 6 weeks to 3 months.
- Waiting 2–3 weeks after the desired volume is achieved allows the expanded skin to soften, decreasing the contraction at the time of flap transposition.
- Removal of the expander is straightforward; however, infection, exposure, or rupture may necessitate early explant.
- The expanded tissue is usually in the form of a random flap (rotation, advancement, or transposition). If more than one flap is necessary using expanded tissue, one must ensure that all flaps have adequate blood supply.

The Origin of the New Tissue

- The origin of the new tissue is not completely understood.
- One potential source is new tissue created in response to the expansion process.
- Alternatively, tissue may derive from the recruitment of adjacent tissues by stretching or creep and by stress relaxation.
- These possibilities are not mutually exclusive.
- Studies have shown that expansion gives rise to an increase in the thickness of the epidermis, a decrease in the thickness of the dermis, and atrophy of the underlying muscle and fat

Tissue Expanders are Indicated

- Tissue expanders are indicated for patients who cannot, or choose not to, tolerate the longer operative procedures or rehabilitation associated with more distant flaps.
- In areas where little suitable tissue is available (e.g., scalp), tissue expansion can be the aesthetically superior option.
- The patient must be motivated and understand the process.
- Common indications include burn alopecia, congenital nevi, male pattern baldness, and postmastectomy breast reconstruction.

Relative Contraindications

- Relative contraindications include malignancy or an open wound, active infection, and unwillingness to comply with multiple procedures.
- Similarly, tissue expanders cannot be placed under burned tissue, scar, skin graft, or a prior incision.
- In addition, tissue expanders are less effective in areas that will be irradiated because the skin in those areas thickens, scars, and contracts, minimizing the degree of expansion possible.

Complications

- Complications include pain, seroma, hematoma (rates widely variable), infection (1–5%), exposure or extrusion (5–10%), and skin necrosis.
- Less common complications include striae, resorption of the underlying bone, and neurapraxia.

14. Tissue expanders. *KGMU, Lucknow 2025*

Definition

A tissue expander is a temporary, inflatable prosthesis placed beneath the skin and/or muscle to gradually stretch existing tissue.

This creates additional skin of similar color, texture, and thickness, which can later be used to reconstruct defects (e.g., after tumor excision, burns, or trauma).

Principle

- Based on the concept of mechanical creep and biologic creep:
  - *Mechanical creep:* Immediate stretching of collagen and elastic fibers due to tension.
  - *Biologic creep:* Long-term tissue growth due to cellular proliferation and remodeling in response to sustained tension.

Repeated, controlled inflation of the expander causes the overlying skin and soft tissues to grow—providing new, vascularized tissue for reconstruction.

Components of a Tissue Expander

- Expandable silicone shell—flexible, biocompatible balloon.
- Injection port/reservoir—allows saline to be injected percutaneously; can be:
  - *Integral* (attached to the expander)
  - *Remote* (connected by a tube and placed nearby)
- *Filling solution:* Sterile normal saline (occasionally air in some designs).

Mechanism of Action

- Expander is surgically placed in a subcutaneous or submuscular pocket adjacent to the defect.
- Initial healing phase (~1–2 weeks).
- *Serial inflation phase:* Periodic injection of saline (typically weekly) through the port, gradually stretching overlying tissue.
- *Maturation phase:* Expanded tissue maintained for a short period to stabilize.
- *Second operation:* Expander is removed and expanded tissue is used to cover the defect.

Biological Changes in Expanded Tissue

Tissue	*Changes*
Epidermis	Hyperplasia but maintains normal keratinization
Dermis	Thinning of collagen bundles
Subcutaneous tissue	*Thinning and reorganization*
Vascularity	*Increased capillary density—tissue remains well perfused*
Underlying muscle	*Thinning and flattening over time*

Indications

Reconstructive Surgery

- Post-tumor excision (e.g., breast, scalp, face)
- Post-burn or trauma defects

- Congenital defects (e.g., giant congenital nevus, microtia)
- Scar revision (replacement with normal skin)

Common Sites
- Breast reconstruction (after mastectomy)
- Scalp (to replace hair-bearing skin)
- Neck and face (for color/texture match)

Advantages
- Provides tissue with identical color, texture, thickness, and sensation.
- Maintains hair-bearing qualities (useful for scalp).
- Creates well-vascularized flaps, reducing risk of necrosis.
- Reduces need for skin grafts or distant flaps.

Disadvantages/Complications

Category	*Examples*
Infection	May require removal of expander
Exposure/extrusion	Due to skin necrosis over expander
Hematoma/seroma	At implantation site
Pain or discomfort	During inflation
Expander failure/leakage	Mechanical problem
Overlying tissue problems	Ischemia, ulceration, thinning
Unfavorable scarring/distortion	Especially in facial areas

Contraindications
- Active infection or poor local tissue condition
- Irradiated or poorly vascularized skin (relative)
- Patient non-compliance (due to need for serial expansions)

Recent Developments
- *Self-inflating expanders:* Osmotic expanders using hydrogel that gradually absorb fluid and expand automatically.
- 3D-printed custom expanders for complex defects.
- Endoscopic-assisted placement in certain anatomical areas.

15. Discuss the types of skin substitutes and their role in management of surgical wound. ***AIIMS, Patna 2025***

Skin Substitutes

Definition: Skin substitutes are *biomaterials designed to temporarily or permanently replace the form and function of skin*, providing a *cover for wounds* when autologous skin grafting is not immediately possible or sufficient.

They aim to:
- Promote wound healing
- Prevent infection and fluid loss
- Reduce pain
- Decrease donor site morbidity

Classification of Skin Substitutes

Skin substitutes can be classified in several ways. The most common are *based on durability, composition, and structure.*

- *Based on durability*

Type	Examples	Features/indications
Temporary (biological or Synthetic)	• Human or animal-derived (xenograft, allograft) • Synthetic dressings (biobrane, hydrocolloids, films)	• Provide short-term coverage • Promote healing and prepare wound bed for definitive closure • Used in burns, trauma, donor sites
Permanent (composite/ tissue-engineered)	• Cultured epithelial autograft (CEA) • Dermal matrices (Integra®, AlloDerm®) • Composite substitutes (epidermal + dermal layers)	• Integrate with host tissue for long-term closure • Used when autograft area limited (major burns, chronic ulcers)

- *Based on material composition*

Category	Source/example	Description/role
Biological (Natural)	• *Autograft*: Patient's own skin (split/full-thickness graft) • *Allograft*: Cadaveric human skin • *Xenograft*: Animal skin (porcine, bovine)	• Excellent biocompatibility • Provide ECM proteins and growth factors • Temporary cover (except autograft)
Synthetic (Artificial)	• Polyurethane films, silicone membranes, nylon mesh, hydrocolloids, hydrogels	• Readily available, sterile, inexpensive • Barrier function and moisture control • No immunologic reaction
Biosynthetic/ Composite	• Biobrane (silicone + nylon mesh + collagen) • Integra (bovine collagen + chondroitin-6-sulfate + silicone) • Dermagraft (human fibroblast–derived)	• Combine benefits of biological and synthetic materials • Promote dermal regeneration and epithelialization

- *Based on structural compositio*

Type	Components	Examples	Function
Single-layer	Epidermal or dermal analog	• Epidermal: Cultured epithelial autograft (CEA) • Dermal: AlloDerm, Integra (dermal component)	Provides partial replacement; may require later grafting
Bi-layered/ Composite	Both epidermal & dermal components	• Apligraf (collagen + keratinocytes/fibroblasts) • OrCel	Closer to native skin structure; permanent or long-term cover

Commonly Used Skin Substitutes (Examples)

Product/type	Composition	Indication/use
Biobrane®	Silicone + nylon mesh + porcine collagen	Partial thickness burns, donor sites
Integra®	Bovine collagen + glycosaminoglycan + silicone	Deep burns, after excision; provides dermal matrix
Apligraf®	Human fibroblasts + keratinocytes in collagen	Chronic venous and diabetic ulcers
AlloDerm®	Acellular human dermal matrix	Reconstruction, burns, chronic wounds
Dermagraft®	Human fibroblast-seeded biodegradable scaffold	Diabetic foot ulcers
CEA (cultured epithelial autograft)	Patient's own keratinocytes cultured in vitro	Extensive full-thickness burns when donor sites limited
Porcine xenograft	Pig skin	Temporary biological dressing
Amniotic membrane	Human placental membrane	Burns, chronic ulcers, ocular surface defects

Role of Skin Substitutes in Surgical Wound Management

- *Temporary wound coverage*
  - Prevents infection and fluid/electrolyte loss in large burns or open wounds.
  - Protects underlying structures while preparing wound bed for definitive closure.
- *Permanent skin replacement:* Used when donor skin is unavailable (extensive burns, chronic non-healing wounds).
- *Promotion of healing*
  - Provide extracellular matrix (ECM) for cell migration.
  - Deliver growth factors and cytokines that stimulate angiogenesis and epithelialization.
- *Reduction of pain and infection*: Acts as a biological dressing; reduces exposure of nerve endings and bacterial contamination.
- *Reduction in donor site morbidity*: Minimizes need for repeated graft harvesting.
- *Improved aesthetic and functional outcomes*: Provide better pliability, pigmentation, and less contracture than conventional grafts in some cases.

Advantages and Disadvantages

Advantages	**Disadvantages**
• Readily available when donor sites limited • Reduce pain and infection • Promote faster healing • Can be tailored to wound type	• High cost • Limited availability (biological types) • Risk of immune reaction (xenografts/allografts) • Infection risk if integration fails • May require secondary procedures

Indications in Surgical Practice

- Extensive burns (>40–50% TBSA)
- Chronic non-healing ulcers (diabetic, venous, pressure)
- Large traumatic or surgical wounds with poor vascularity
- Exposed tendons, bone, or hardware
- Temporary cover after excision of malignancy or infection

SKIN SUBSTITUTES

16. Uses of bioengineered skin substitutes. ***WBUHS 2021***

Introduction

- Skin substitutes are heterogeneous group of wound coverage materials that aid in wound closure and replace the functions of the skin, either temporarily or permanently, depending on the product characteristics.
- These substances are alternatives to the standard wound coverage in circumstances when standard therapies are not desirable.

The need for supplements to autologous skin grafts has prompted the development and use of a wide variety of skin substitutes as biological and synthetic wound dressings.

Functions

- Permanent wound coverage
- Temporary coverage to promote healthy wound bed

Bioengineered Skin/Cultured Epidermal Autografts (CEA)

- Autografts are derived from the patient's own skin cells grown or cultured from very small amounts of skin or hair follicles.

- Production time is prolonged. One such product is grown on a layer of irradiated mouse cells, bestowing some elements of a xenograft.
- Wide-spread usage has not been available due to limited availability or access to the technology.

Bioengineered Skin Substitutes or Cellular and Tissue-based Products (CTPs)

- Products developed in an attempt to circumvent problems inherent with autografts, allografts, and xenografts.
- These constitute biological covers for refractory wounds with full-thickness skin loss secondary to third-degree burns or other disease processes, such as diabetic neuropathic ulcers and the skin loss of chronic venous stasis or venous hypertension.
- The production of these biological skin substitutes or CTPs varies by company and product, but generally involves the creation of immunologically inert biological products containing protein, hormones, or enzymes seeded into a matrix which may provide protein or growth factors proposed to stimulate or facilitate healing or promote epithelization.
- A variety of biosynthetic and tissue-engineered skin substitution products marketed as human skin equivalents (HSE) or cellular or tissue-based products (CTP) are manufactured under an array of trade names and marketed for a variety of indications.
- All are procured, produced, manufactured, processed, and promoted in sufficiently different manners to preclude direct product comparison for equivalency or superiority in randomized controlled trials.

Application of Bioengineered Skin Substitutes

- Alloderm is tissue from cadavers that are used to create an acellular dermal matrix that has been freeze-dried. The collagen framework acts as a strengthening scaffold for normal tissue remodeling. It can often be used for burns or full-thickness wounds.
- Apligraf is a bilayered skin substitute produced by combining bovine collagen and living cells derived from tissue-cultured human infant foreskins. It can be used in diabetic foot ulcers.
- Dermagraft is a human fibroblast-derived dermal substitute manufactured by seeding dermal fibroblasts onto a three-dimensional (3D) bioabsorbable scaffold. It has been marketed for use in the treatment of diabetic foot ulcers, venous ulcers, and pressure sores. A clinical trial showed improved healing rates in diabetic foot ulcers.
- Integra is a dual-layered membrane system with a porous matrix that cross-links bovine tendon collagen and glycosaminoglycans. It can be used for deep partial-thickness and full-thickness burns owing to the good barrier function of the system, but operative removal of the silicone layer is required.
- Oasis is a xenogeneic acellular collagen matrix derived from porcine small intestinal submucosa in such a way that an extracellular matrix and natural growth factors remain intact. This provides a scaffold for inducing wound healing.
- EZ Derm is a porcine-derived xenograft of collagen that has been chemically cross-linked with aldehyde to provide strength and durability. It can be used for venous stasis ulcers, diabetic ulcers, pressure ulcers, and partial-thickness burns; however, it does have the capacity to cause a potential immune response or disease transmission.
- Cultured epithelial autograft is an epidermal replacement that is grown in tissue culture from a skin biopsy taken from the recipient and is cocultured with mouse cells. Preparation of the graft requires about 2 weeks of culture time.
- EpiFix is a relatively new matrix scaffold used in wound healing. It is composed of a dehydrated human amnion/chorion membrane. EpiFix is a bioactive tissue matrix allograft, and the dehydrated human amnion/chorion membrane (dHACM) preserves and contains multiple extracellular matrix proteins, cytokines, growth factors, and other specialty proteins.

Use of Flap Closures

- Delayed primary closure of a chronic wound, as shown below, requires well-vascularized clean tissues and tension-free apposition.

- This usually requires undermining and mobilization of adjacent tissue planes by creating skin flaps or myocutaneous flaps.

CLEFT LIP AND CLEFT PALATE

17. Schematic diagram of development of face. ***WBUHS 2021 Supplementary***

18. Principles of cleft lip repair.

19. Discuss in brief about cleft palate.

20. Discuss the management of cleft palate. ***WBUHS 2021 Supplementary***

21. Classify cleft lip and palate. Enumerate the several, multiple procedures that are undertaken sequentially at specific times depending on the advancing age of the patient in managing complex cleft of lip and palate. ***WBUHS 2022***

22. Describe the principles of management of cleft lip and palate and the secondary management following surgery. ***RGUHS, Karnataka 2025***

- During week 3 of embryonic development, an oropharyngeal membrane initially appears at the site of the future face. It is comprised of ectoderm and endoderm—externally and internally, respectively.
- During the fourth week, the oropharyngeal membrane begins to break down in order to become the future oral cavity and sits at the beginning of the digestive tract.
- *The structures of the external face are derived from two sources:*
  1. Frontonasal prominence—formed by the proliferation of mesenchymal neural crest cells ventral to the forebrain.
  2. Mandibular and maxillary prominences—parts of the first pharyngeal arch
- A space lies between the maxillary prominences, covered by the oropharyngeal membrane; this is known as the stomatodeum, the precursor to the mouth and pituitary gland.
- Nasal development is instigated by the appearance of raised bumps called nasal placodes on both sides of the frontonasal prominence. These then invaginate to form nasal pits, with medial and lateral nasal prominences on either side.
- As the maxillary prominences expand medially, the nasal prominences are "pushed" closer to the midline. The maxillary prominences then fuse with the nasal prominences—and soon after fuse in the midline to form a continuous central structure.

Prominence	*Derivatives*
Frontonasal	Forehead, bridge of the nose, and medial and lateral nasal prominences
Medial nasal	Philtrum, primary palate, upper four incisors, and associated jaw
Lateral nasal	Sides of nose

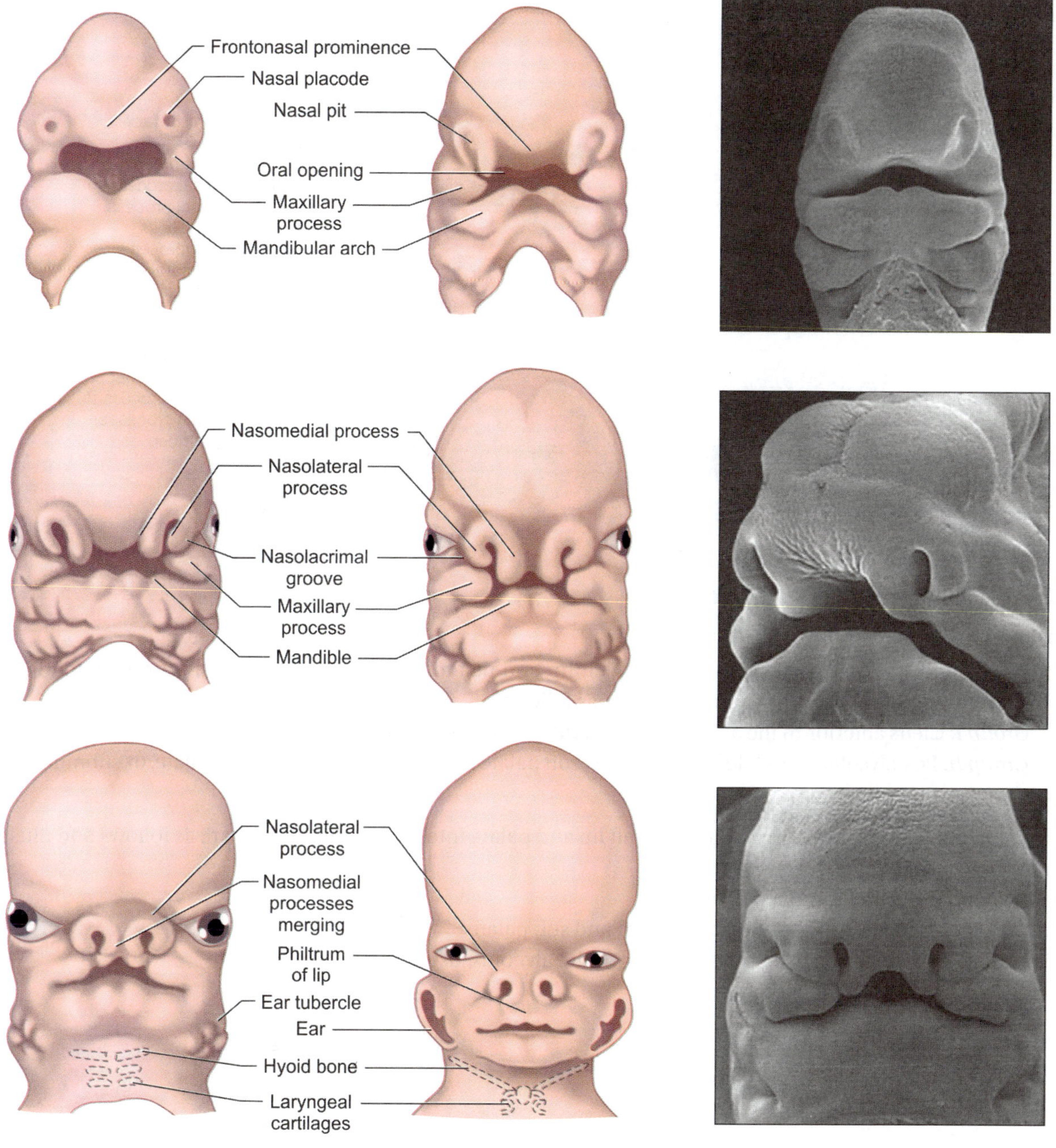

Development of face and nose.

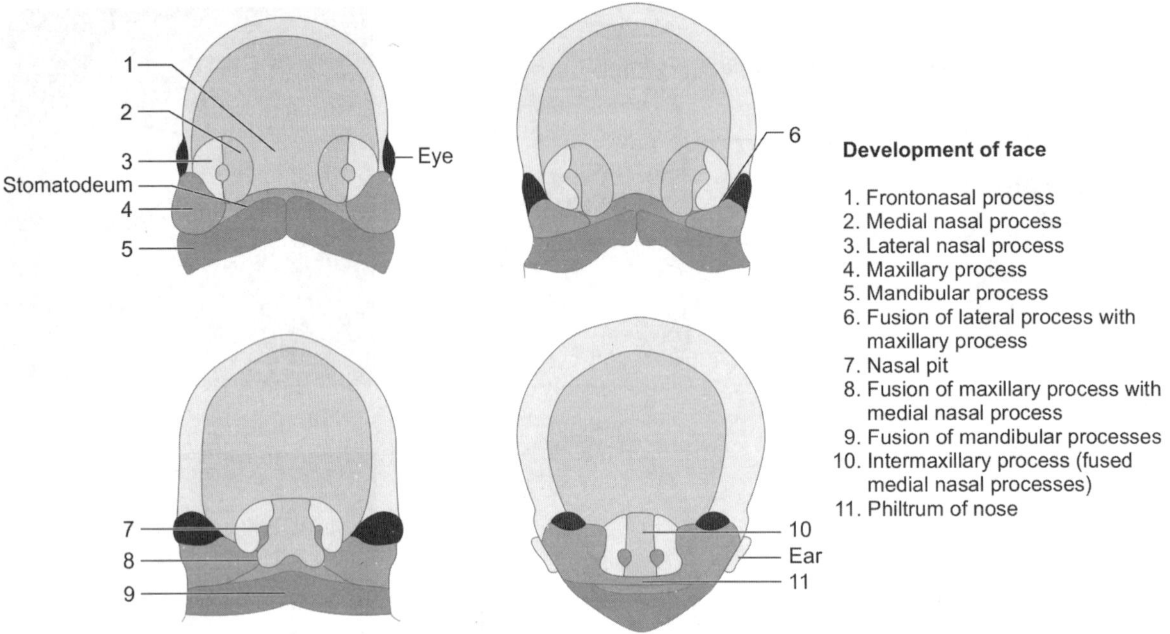

Classification of Cleft Lip and Palate

Davis and Ritchie Classification

The Davis and Ritchie classification divides cleft lip and palate into two groups, which are subdivided into the extent of the cleft (e.g., one-third and one-half), as follows:

- *Group I:* Clefts anterior to the alveolus (unilateral, median, or bilateral cleft lip)
- *Group II:* Postalveolar clefts (cleft palate alone, soft palate alone, soft palate and hard palate, or submucous cleft)

Veau Classification

The Veau classification system divides the cleft lip and palate into four groups, which are as follows and illustrated in the image below:

1. *Group I:* Defects of the soft palate only
2. *Group II:* Defects involving the hard palate and soft palate
3. *Group III:* Defects involving the soft palate to the alveolus, usually involving the lip
4. *Group IV:* Complete bilateral clefts

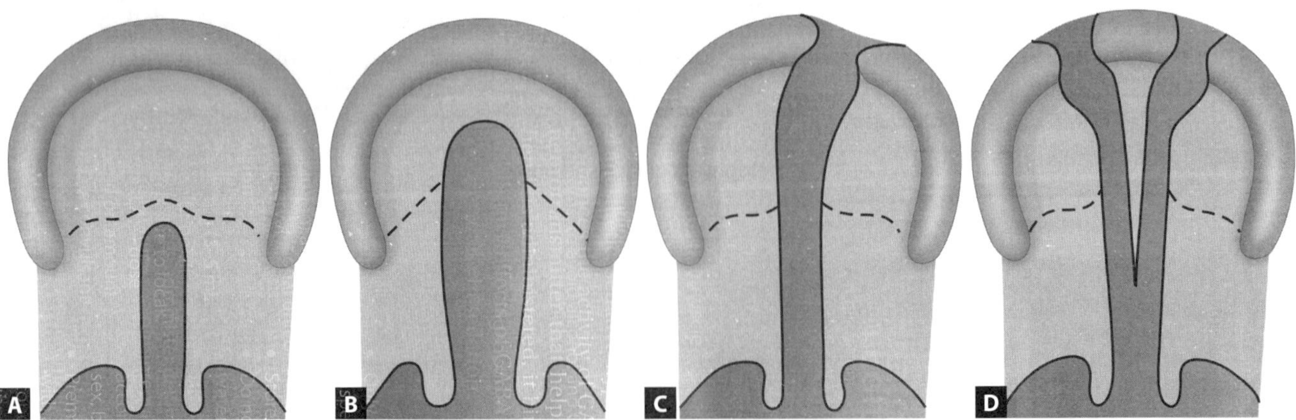

Veau classification of cleft lip and palate. (A) *Group I:* Defects of the soft palate only; (B) *Group II:* Defects involving the hard palate and soft palate; (C) *Group III:* Defects involving the soft palate to the alveolus, usually involving the lip; and (D) *Group IV:* Complete bilateral clefts.

Kernahan and Stark Symbolic Classification

The Kernahan and Stark classification highlight the anatomic and embryonic importance of the incisive foramen that is formed during weeks 4–7 gestational age (GA). The secondary palate forms the roof of the mouth from the incisive foramen to the uvula during weeks 7–12.

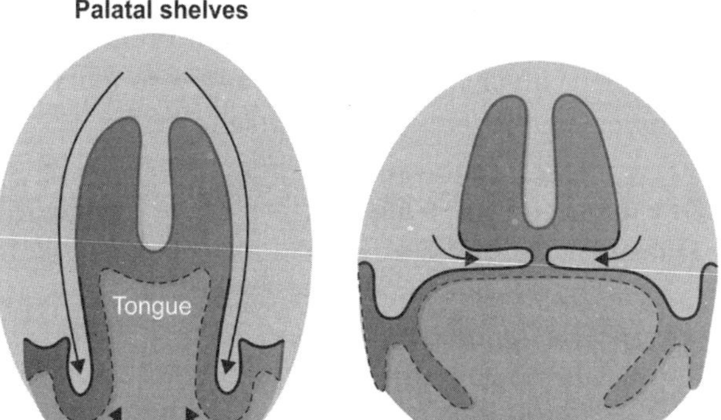

Formation of the secondary palate.

This system provides a graphic classification scheme using a Y-configuration, which can be divided into nine areas, as follows (see also the figure underneath):

- *Areas 1 and 4:* Lip
- *Areas 2 and 5:* Alveolus
- *Areas 3 and 6:* Palate between the alveolus and the incisive foramen
- *Areas 7 and 8:* Hard palate
- *Area 9:* Soft palate

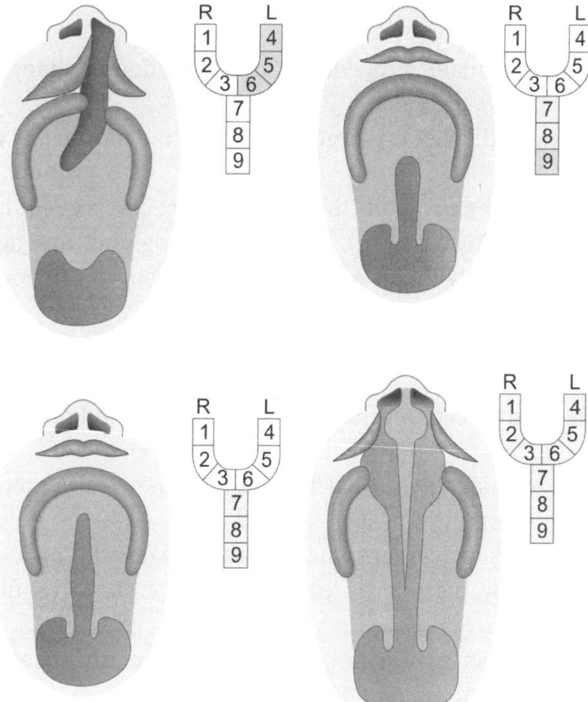

Kernahan and Stark symbolic classification of cleft lip and palate. (R: right; L: left)

International Confederation of Plastic and Reconstructive Surgery Classification

The International Confederation of Plastic and Reconstructive Surgery classification system uses an embryonic framework to divide clefts into three groups, with further subdivisions to denote unilateral or bilateral cases, as follows:

1. *Group I:* Defects of the lip or alveolus
2. *Group II:* Clefts of the secondary palate (hard palate, soft palate, or both)
3. *Group III:* Any combination of clefts involving the primary and secondary palates

   Timing of primary cleft lip and palate procedures (after Delaire)

- *Cleft lip alone:*
  - *Unilateral (one side):* One operation at 5–6 months
  - *Bilateral (both sides):* One operation at 4–5 months
- *Cleft palate alone:*
  - *Soft palate only:* One operation at 6 months
  - *Soft and hard palate:*
    - *Two operations:*
      1. Soft palate at 6 months
      2. Hard palate at 15–18 months
- *Cleft lip and palate:*
  - *Unilateral:*
    - *Two operations:* Cleft lip and soft palate at 5–6 months
    - Hard palate and gum pad with or without lip revision at 15–18 months
  - *Bilateral:*

    Two operations:

    i. Cleft lip and soft palate at 4–5 months

    ii. Hard palate and gum pad with or without lip revision at 15–18 months

Surgical Management

- Closure of the cleft lip is the first major procedure that tremendously changes children's future development and ability to thrive.
- Variations occur in the timing of the first lip surgery; however, the most usual time occurs at approximately age 3 months.
- Pediatricians used to strictly follow a rule of "three 10s" as a necessary requirement for identifying the child's status as suitable for surgery [i.e., 10 lb (4.5 kg), 10 g/dL of hemoglobin, and age 10 weeks)].
- Although pediatricians are presently much more flexible, and some surgeons may well justify a neonatal lip closure, considering the rule of three 10s is still very useful.
- Anatomic differences predispose children with cleft lip and palate (CLP) and those with isolated cleft palate (CP) to ear infections.
- Therefore, ventilation tubes are placed to ventilate the middle ear and prevent hearing loss secondary to otitis media with effusion.
- In multidisciplinary teams with significant participation of an otolaryngologist, the tubes are placed at the initial surgery and the second surgery routinely.
- The hearing is tested after the first placement when ears are clear with tubes.
- If no cleft surgery is planned early, placing the tubes early (e.g., by age 6 months) and monitoring hearing with repeated testing is recommended.
- Complications include eardrum perforation and otorrhea, particularly in patients with open secondary palates in which closure is planned for later.
- For preventive reasons, ear tubes are usually placed when the child is still under general anesthesia for cleft repair.

The most common surgical procedures for a child with a cleft lip palate anomaly are as follows:

- Repair of the CL
- Repair of the CP
- Revision of the CL
- Closure and bone grafting of the alveolar cleft
- Closure of palatal fistulae
- Palatal lengthening
- Pharyngeal flap
- Pharyngoplasty
- Columellar lengthening
- CL rhinoplasty and septoplasty
- Lip scar revision
- Le Fort I maxillary osteotomy

Maxillary distraction osteogenesis is increasingly being used as an alternative to conventional orthognathic surgery for the correction of maxillary hypoplasia in CLP patients.

Orthodontic treatment is highly specialized and varies from case to case. The two stages of orthodontic treatment of a child with CLP are as follows:

1. *Surgery-related orthodontics:* Early management (from birth until the time of surgical closure of the palate), orthodontics related to alveolar bone graft, and permanent dentition management
2. Cleft-related orthodontics (not related to surgical treatments)

Points to be Remembered in Cleft Lip Repair

- A cleft lip is characterized by a partial or complete lack of circumferential continuity of the lip.
- Most cleft lips occur at a typical location in the upper lip where one of the philtral columns normally lies, and they extend into the nose.
- The deformity involves the mucosa, orbicularis oris muscle, and skin.
- There are many techniques for the repair of a cleft lip, but most are a variation of the rotation-advancement repair.
- Millard introduced this technique of downward rotation of the medial portion of the lip and advancement of the lateral portion into the defect created by the rotation. The repair is based on the principle that existing elements need to be returned to their normal position to restore the normal anatomy while remaining cognizant of future growth and the effects of surgery on growth.

Principles of Cleft Lip Repair

- "Rule of 10" should be fulfilled
- It should be operated before 6 months
- Infection should not be present
- Millard advancement flap is commonly used for unilateral cleft lip repair
- Bilateral cleft lip repair can be done either in single or two stages (with a 6-month gap between each stage).
- One-stage bilateral cleft lip repair is done using the Veau III method/Millard's single stage/Black method
- Proper markings are made prior to surgery and the incision should be over full-thickness lip
- Often 1:2,00,000 adrenaline injection is used to achieve hemostasis
- Three-layer lip repair should be done (mucosa, muscle, and skin):
    1. Cupid's bow should be horizontal
    2. Continuity of the white line should be maintained
    3. Vermilion notching should not be there

Timing of the Cleft Surgery

- Unilateral/bilateral cleft lip alone, in a one-stage operation done in 4–6 months

- Cleft palate alone involving only the soft palate, is one stage surgery done in 6 months
- Cleft palate alone but involving both soft and hard palates—soft palate in 6 months; hard palate in 18 months.
- In combined cleft lip and palate, unilateral or bilateral, done in two stages—(1) cleft lip and (2) soft palate in 6 months; hard palate and gum pad with or without lip revision in 18 months.
- Revisional surgery should be delayed for 2 years after primary lip closure.

Treatment for Cleft Lip

Millard criteria are used to undertake surgery for cleft lip.

Millard criteria (Rule of "10"):

- 10 pounds in weight
- 10 weeks old
- 10 g% hemoglobin
  - Millard cleft lip repair by rotating the local nasolabial flaps
  - Management of associated primary or secondary cleft palate deformity
  - Proper postoperative management like control of infection, training for sucking, swallowing, and speech
  - Tenninson's "Z" plasty (Tennison-Randall triangular flap)

Unilateral Cleft Lip Repair

- Design a closure interface (scar) that closely mirrors the contralateral philtral ridge in shape and length limiting the total scar burden inherent in the design.
- Create a symmetric and natural Cupid's bow.
- Match the volume of vermilion on each side of the cleft.
- Restore muscular continuity such that normal lip movement results.
- Create a labial sulcus of normal depth.
- Create a normal nasal floor, nasal sill, and alar base.
- Centralize the columella and elevate the columella base.

Bilateral Cleft Lip Repair

- Maintain (or establish) symmetry
- Prepare the projecting premaxilla
- Anticipate future changes that will occur with growth (particularly in the design of the size and shape of the philtral flap)
- Construct a full central lip using lateral labial elements and discard prolabial vermilion
- Deepen the gingivolabial sulcus using premaxillary mucosa
- Establish muscular continuity primarily
- Address the nasal deformity synchronously

Cleft Palate

Introduction

- Cleft palate is a condition in which the two plates of the skull that form the hard palate (roof of the mouth) are not completely joined.
- The soft palate is in these cases cleft as well. In most cases, cleft lip is also present.
- Cleft palate occurs in about one in 700 live births worldwide.

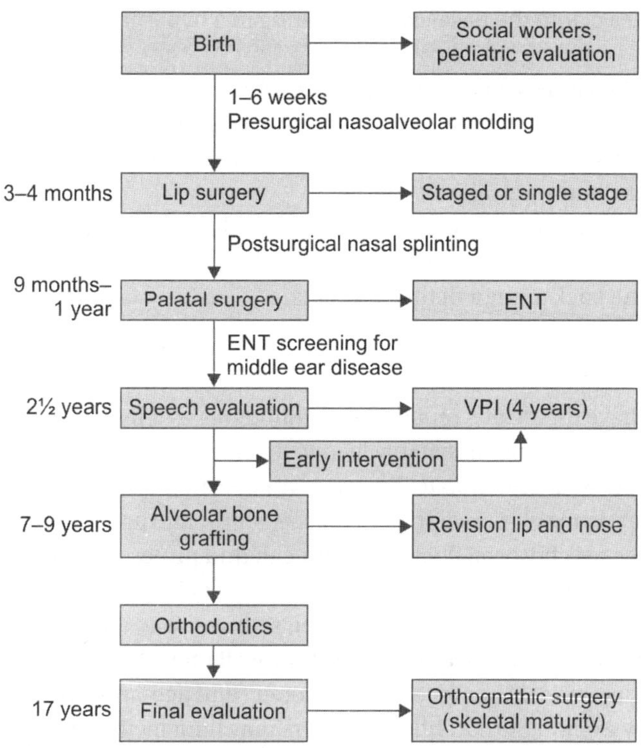

(ENT: ear, nose, and throat; VPI: velopharyngeal insufficiency)

- Palate cleft can occur as complete (soft and hard palate, possibly including a gap in the jaw) or incomplete (a "hole" in the roof of the mouth, usually as a cleft soft palate).
- When cleft palate occurs, the uvula is usually split. It occurs due to the failure of fusion of the lateral palatine processes, the nasal septum, and/or the median palatine processes (formation of the secondary palate).
- The hole in the roof of the mouth caused by a cleft connects the mouth directly to the nasal cavity.

Syndromes

- The Van der Woude syndrome is caused by a specific variation in the gene *IRF6* that increases the occurrence of these deformities threefold.
- Another syndrome, Siderius X-linked mental retardation, is caused by mutations in the *PHF8* gene (OMIM:300263); in addition to cleft lip and/or palate, symptoms include facial dysmorphism and mild mental retardation.

In some cases, cleft palate is caused by syndromes which also cause other problems.

- Stickler's syndrome can cause cleft lip and palate, joint pain, and myopia.
- Loeys–Dietz syndrome can cause cleft palate or bifid uvula, hypertelorism, and aortic aneurysm.
- Hardikar syndrome can cause cleft lip and palate, hydronephrosis, intestinal obstruction, and other symptoms.
- Cleft lip/palate may be present in many different chromosome disorders including
- Patau syndrome (trisomy 13)
- Malpuech facial clefting syndrome
- Hearing loss with craniofacial syndromes
- Popliteal pterygium syndrome
- Treacher Collins syndrome

Pathology

- A result of an open connection between the oral cavity and nasal cavity is called velopharyngeal inadequacy (VPI).

- Because of the gap, air leaks into the nasal cavity resulting in a hypernasal voice resonance and nasal emissions while talking.
- Secondary effects of VPI include speech articulation errors (e.g., distortions, substitutions, and omissions) and compensatory misarticulations and mispronunciations (e.g., glottal stops and posterior nasal fricatives).
- Possible treatment options include speech therapy, prosthetics, augmentation of the posterior pharyngeal wall, lengthening of the palate, and surgical procedures.
- Submucous cleft palate (SMCP) can also occur, which is a cleft of the soft palate with a classic clinical triad of a bifid, or split, uvula which is found dangling in the back of the throat, a furrow along the midline of the soft palate, and a notch in the back margin of the hard palate.

Problems

- *Psychosocial:*
  - Most children who have their clefts repaired early enough are able to have a happy youth and social life.
  - Having a cleft palate/lip does not inevitably lead to a psychosocial problem.
  - However, adolescents with cleft palate/lip are at an elevated risk for developing psychosocial problems especially those relating to self-concept, peer relationships, and appearance.
  - Adolescents may face psychosocial challenges but can find professional help if problems arise.
  - A cleft palate/lip may impact an individual's self-esteem, social skills, and behavior.
  - Children with clefts tend to report feelings of anger, sadness, fear, and alienation from their peers, but these children were similar to their peers in regard to "how well they liked themselves."
  - A child who is entering school should learn the proper (and age-appropriate) terms related to the cleft. The ability to confidently explain the condition to others may limit feelings of awkwardness and embarrassment and reduce negative social experiences.
  - As children reach adolescence, the period of time between the ages 13 and 19 years, the dynamics of the parent-child relationship change as peer groups are now the focus of attention.
  - An adolescent with cleft lip and or cleft palate will deal with the typical challenges faced by most of their peers including issues related to self-esteem, dating, and social acceptance.
  - Adolescent boys typically deal with issues relating to withdrawal, attention, thought, and internalizing problems and may possibly develop anxiousness depression and aggressive behaviors.
  - Adolescent girls are more likely to develop problems relating to self-concept and appearance. Individuals with cleft lip and or cleft palate often deal with threats to their quality of life for multiple reasons including—unsuccessful social relationships, deviance in social appearance, and multiple surgeries.
  - *Complications:* A baby being fed using a customized bottle. The upright sitting position allows gravity to help the baby swallow the milk more easily.
- *Cleft may cause problems with feeding, ear disease, speech, and socialization.*
  - Due to lack of suction, an infant with a cleft may have trouble feeding. An infant with a cleft palate will have greater success feeding in a more upright position. Gravity will help prevent milk from coming through the baby's nose if he/she has cleft palate.
  - *Speech and hearing:*
    - Children with cleft palate typically have a variety of speech problems. Some speech problems result directly from anatomical differences, such as velopharyngeal inadequacy.
    - Velopharyngeal inadequacy refers to the inability of the soft palate to close the opening from the throat to the nasal cavity, which is necessary for many speech sounds, such as /p/, /b/, /t/, /d/, /s/, and /z/.
    - This type of error typically resolves after palate repair.
  - Speech-language pathology can be very beneficial to help resolve speech problems associated with cleft palate.

Diagnosis

- Traditionally, the diagnosis is made at the time of birth by physical examination.
- Recent advances in prenatal diagnosis have allowed obstetricians to diagnose facial clefts in utero

Treatment

Often a cleft palate is temporarily covered by a palatal obturator (a prosthetic device made to fit the roof of the mouth covering the gap).

- Cleft palate can also be corrected by surgery, usually performed between 6 and 12 months.
- Approximately 20–25% only require one palatal surgery to achieve a competent velopharyngeal valve capable of producing normal, nonhypernasal speech.
- Combinations of surgical methods and repeated surgeries are often necessary as the child grows. One of the new innovations of cleft lip and cleft palate repair is the Latham appliance.
- The Latham is surgically inserted by use of pins during the child's fourth or fifth month.
- If the cleft extends into the maxillary alveolar ridge, the gap is usually corrected by filling the gap with bone tissue.
- The bone tissue can be acquired from the patient's own chin, rib, or hip.

Cleft Palate Surgery

- Cleft palate closure can be achieved by one- or two-stage palatoplasty.
- The surgical principle is mobilization and reconstruction of the aberrant soft palate musculature together with the closure of the residual hard palate cleft by minimal dissection and subsequent scar formation.
- Excess scar formation in the palate adversely affects the growth and development of the maxilla.
- The philosophy of two-stage closure encourages a physiological narrowing of the hard palate cleft to minimize surgical dissection at the time of the second procedure.

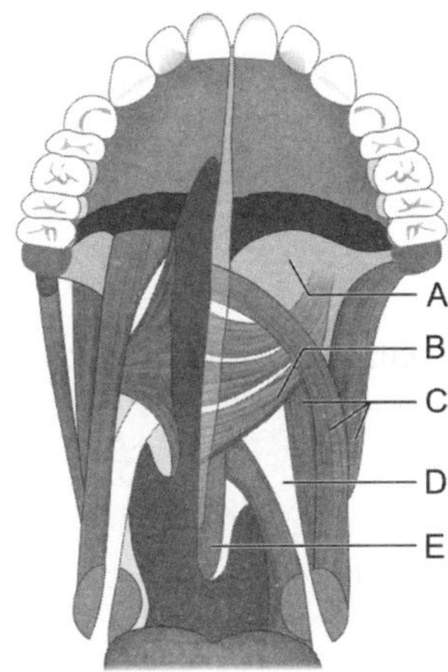

(a) Cleft of soft palate and incomplete cleft of hard palate. (b) Muscles of the soft palate: Left, cleft palate; right, normal anatomy. A: tensor palatini; B: levator palatini; C: palatopharyngeus; D: palatoglossus; E: musculus uvulae.

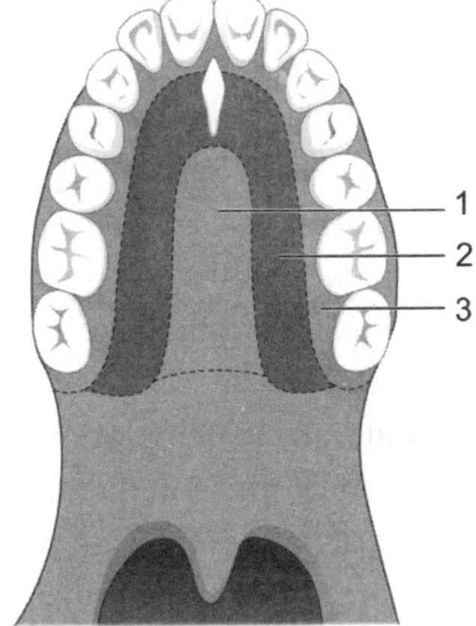

The three mucosal zones of the hard palate. (1) Palatal fibromucosa; (2) Maxillary fibromucosa; (3) Gingival fibromucosa.

Other Surgeries

- *Orthognathic surgery:*
  - Surgical cutting of bone to realign the upper jaw (osteotomy).
  - Single-piece osteotomy is carried out where there is sufficient alveolar continuity achieved from a successful bone graft.
  - Multipiece osteotomy is performed when there is a notable residual alveolar defect with a dental gap and oronasal fistula (communication between the oral and nasal cavities).
  - The goal of both single and multipiece osteotomy is to displace the maxilla forward to obtain adequate occlusion as well as to provide better support for the upper lip and the nose and to close any fistulae.
- *Distraction osteogenesis:*
  - Bone lengthening by gradual distraction

- This involves cutting bone and moving ends apart incrementally to allow new bone to form in the gap.
- This consists of several phases. After the attachment of the distracting device and the bone cuts, there is a latency phase of 3–7 days when a callus forms.
- In the activation phase distraction of the callus induces bony ingrowth which can last up to 15 days depending on the required distraction.
- Once the required bone length is reached, the distraction device is left to remain in situ as it acts as a rigid skeletal fixation device until the new bone has matured (known as the consolidation period).

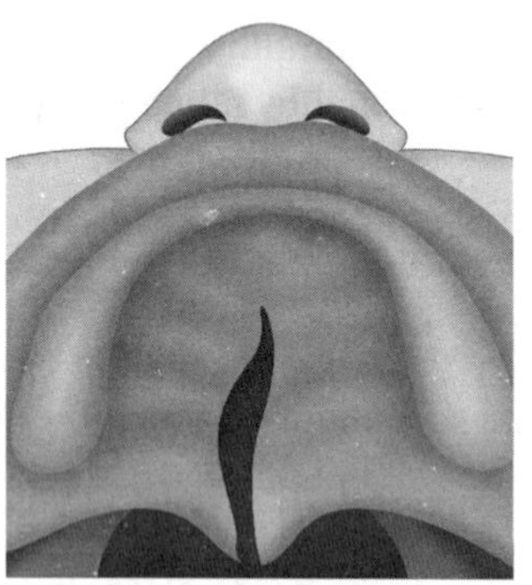
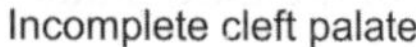
Incomplete cleft palate

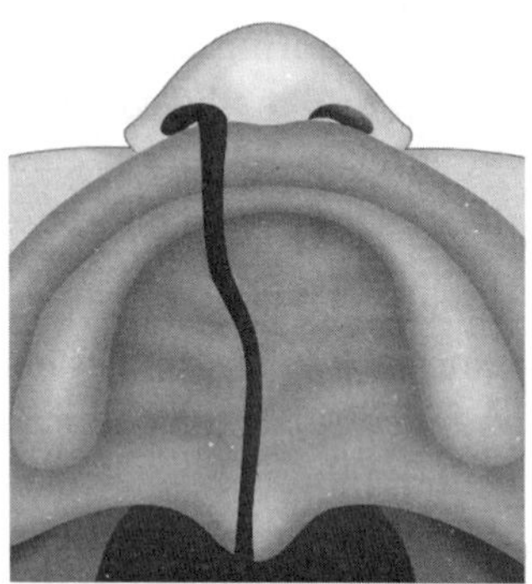
Unilateral complete lip and palate

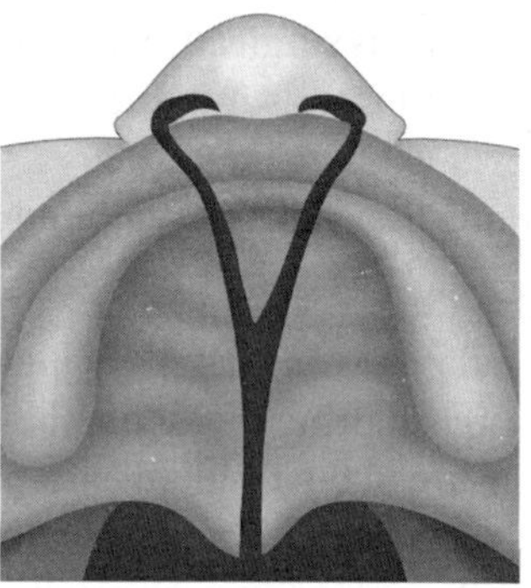
Bilateral complete lip and palate

Timing of Primary Cleft Lip and Palate Procedures (after Delaire)

- *Cleft lip alone:*
  - Unilateral (one side)—one operation at 5–6 months
  - Bilateral (both sides)—one operation at 4–5 months
- *Cleft palate alone:*
  - Soft palate only—one operation at 6 months
  - Soft and hard palate—two operations soft palate at 6 months, hard palate at 15–18 months
- *Cleft lip and palate:*
  - Unilateral—two operations:
    1. Cleft lip and soft palate at 5–6 months
    2. Hard palate and gum pad with or without lip revision at 15–18 months
  - Bilateral—two operations:
    1. Cleft lip and soft palate at 4–5 months
    2. Hard palate and gum pad with or without lip revision at 15–18 months

23. Describe the developmental malformation of face. ***WBUHS 2024***

Developmental Malformations of the Face

Facial development occurs between the 4th and 10th weeks of embryonic life through the fusion of five facial prominences: one frontonasal, two maxillary, and two mandibular. Disruption in this process leads to facial malformations. Common developmental malformations include:

1. *Cleft lip and cleft palate:*
   - *Cleft lip:* Failure of fusion between the maxillary and medial nasal processes.
   - *Cleft palate:* Incomplete fusion of the palatal shelves.
   - Can be unilateral or bilateral; isolated or associated.
2. *Hypertelorism:*
   - Abnormally wide spacing between the eyes.
   - Due to defective development of the frontonasal prominence.

3. *Holoprosencephaly:*
   - Failure of midline facial and brain structures to develop properly.
   - Can result in cyclopia, a single central incisor, or midline clefts.
4. *Mandibulofacial dysostosis (Treacher Collins syndrome):*
   - Abnormal development of the first and second branchial arches.
   - Features include underdeveloped zygoma, mandibular hypoplasia, and malformed ears.
5. *Hemifacial microsomia:*
   - Unilateral underdevelopment of the facial structures (usually the mandible and ear).
   - Caused by vascular disruption during development.
6. *Micrognathia/macrognathia:*
   - Abnormally small or large jaw, respectively.
   - Seen in syndromes like Pierre Robin sequence (micrognathia, cleft palate, glossoptosis).
7. *Craniofacial clefts:*
   - Rare anomalies resulting from failure of fusion along different facial lines.
   - May affect the lips, nose, orbits, and skull.
8. *Frontonasal dysplasia:*
   - Median facial cleft, wide-set eyes, and broad nasal root.
   - Due to abnormal development of the frontonasal prominence.

HAND INJURIES

24. Surgical options for fingertip reconstruction. *WBUHS 2022*

Treatment Options

- *Healing by secondary intention—open technique*
  - The open technique involves allowing the wound to heal by secondary intention with wound contraction, which pulls innervated pulp into the wound.
  - This technique applies to distal and volar-directed fingertip injuries without protruding bone.
  - Some small fingertip wounds with a minimal amount of protruding bone can be treated with the open technique if this bone is debrided with a rongeur.
  - The open technique is discouraged for wounds larger than 1 cm because the healing time exceeds 3–4 weeks and significantly delays return to work.
  - This approach is suitable for fingertip injuries in children because of their increased capacity to regenerate soft tissues.
  - The complications potentially encountered with the open technique include loss of volume and pulp.
- *Primary closure and revision amputation:*
  - Many fingertip injuries can be closed primarily or by recruiting adjacent soft tissues.
  - Viability of the remaining soft tissues must be ascertained before the application of a tourniquet.
  - Occasionally, the fillet flap principle can be applied in reconstructing these wounds.
  - Occasionally, bone shortening or revision amputation is required to allow tension-free primary closure of the soft tissues and adequate padding.
  - Furthermore, in an effort to minimize recovery time and hasten return to work, some fingertip injuries are treated with revision amputation.
- *Skin grafts:*
  - Skin graft application is considered for distally located and volar-directed fingertip wounds without exposed bone or tendon.
  - Controversy exists as to whether split- or full-thickness grafts are better.

    - Advocates for split grafts maintain the take is earlier and more reliable and wounds contract more, resulting in a smaller defect, while others favor full-thickness grafts for earlier reinnervation and more reliable, durable coverage.
    - In other words, split grafts may be preferable for wounds in which greater contraction is desirable.
    - Full-thickness grafts can be obtained from the amputated tip by merely defatting the underside.
    - However, when the amputated part is crushed and macerated, this should not be used as a graft.
    - Moreover, when the amputated tip is not available, a skin graft can be obtained from multiple areas.
    - Glabrous skin provides a better aesthetic appearance and match of texture and color. Glabrous skin can be harvested from the hypothenar eminence or feet.
    - Nonglabrous skin can be obtained from the wrist crease, forearm, medial upper arm, or groin.
    - Split-thickness skin can be harvested from the hypothenar eminence using a Weck blade after infiltrating with 1% lidocaine containing 1:100,000 epinephrine.
    - Full-thickness grafts are harvested in the configuration of an ellipse to allow for donor closure.
    - The graft is secured circumferentially with 3-0 nylon sutures, which are left long to tie over an Adaptic gauze and a bolus of cotton, creating a bolster/stent.
    - The finger is placed in a splint. This bolster dressing is removed at 5–7 days, and an active range of motion is begun immediately.
- *Composite tip grafts:*
    - Reapplication of composite tip grafts, amputated parts containing bone fat, or nail bed, can be considered for children younger than age 6 years.
    - As composite tip grafts must initially survive by plasmatic imbibition until neovascularization, revascularization is not reliable for adults and tip grafts should not be reapplied for adults.
    - The distal phalanx fracture is reduced and secured with internal fixation using a K-wire. The surrounding skin is approximated with an absorbable chromic suture to avoid the hassle of suture removal in a child.
    - Moreover, the child's upper extremity is placed in a soft splint using multiple Kerlix rolls from the hand to the upper arm. The splint is removed for a duration of 2 weeks.
- *Local flap options for the fingers:*
    - When a bone or tendon is exposed at the base of a fingertip wound, a local flap is required.
    - The various local flaps used to reconstruct fingertips include volar V-Y, bilateral V-Y flaps, cross-finger flap, and island flaps.
    - Flap choice depends on the orientation and configuration of the wound, injured finger, and sex of the patient.
    - Surgeons can optimize the reliability of these local flaps by avoiding tension on the suture line and preserving the traversing subdermal blood vessels into the flap.
- *Volar V-Y flap:*
    - The volar V-Y flap is a triangular-shaped volar advancement flap outlined with its tip at the distal interphalangeal crease.
    - The local flap is most applicable for transverse and dorsal avulsions when a relative abundance of pulp skin is present.
- *Bilateral V-Y flaps:*
    - These local V-Y advancement flaps are harvested from the ulnar and radial aspect of the injured fingertip and advanced distally to cover the defect.
    - This technique is best applied to volar and transverse avulsions with exposed bone when excess lateral skin is present.
    - These flaps are designed along the midlateral line and should not extend proximal to the distal interphalangeal joint.
- *Cross-finger flap:*
    - The cross-finger flap is commonly used for volar-directed tip injuries with exposed bone or tendon when insufficient pulp for the volar V-Y flap is present.

- Use of this flap is reserved for fingertip wounds associated with deficiency of local tissues, which would allow for a single-stage flap because the cross-finger flap involves two operations.
- Moreover, the fingers become stiff during the delay between these two stages. At the first stage, a template of the defect is fashioned from the Esmarch bandage and superimposed to the adjacent finger dorsum from which the flap will be harvested.
- Generally, the flap is harvested from the finger radial to the injury, except when reconstructing the index.
- The advantages of the cross-finger flap include a reliable and large flap that can even be innervated.

- *Thenar flap:*
  - The classic description of the thenar flap by Gatewood in 1926 was proximally based in 1976.
  - Smith and Albin described the H-shaped modification of the thenar flap.
  - With the H modification, both proximal and distal flaps are raised in the configuration of an H.
  - These flaps are both sutured to the injured finger, but, at flap division, one flap is inset to the finger while the other is advanced to repair the donor site.
  - The thenar flap was classically elevated from the thenar eminence, which placed a potentially tender scar where we rest the hand.
  - A better location for this donor scar is the metacarpophalangeal (MCP) joint flexion crease of the thumb.
  - A 2 × 4 cm thenar flap can be harvested from the MCP crease and still allow primary closure of the donor site with thumb flexion.
  - Care must be exercised in harvesting this thenar flap at the MCP crease to avoid injury to the neurovascular bundles and flexor pollicis longus tendon.
  - This flap can easily reach the index and long fingers and is preferred for women because it is hairless and does not scar the hand dorsum.
  - The thenar flap can be used for volar, transverse, and dorsal injuries.
  - The disadvantages of the thenar flap are that two operations are required with a 2–3 weeks delay and consequent risk for joint stiffness and contracture. Accordingly, the thenar flap is discouraged for older patients and the small and ring fingers.
- *Reverse homodigital arterial flap:*
  - The reverse digital flap is an arterialized homodigital flap described by Lai in 1989, which replaces injured tissue with like tissue from the same digit in a single stage.
  - The flap is harvested from the lateral aspect of the proximal phalanx of the same finger, preferably the nonopposition side.
  - The reverse digital flap is an axial flap based on collateral flow through the contralateral digital artery, thus it is only applicable to defects distal to the crossover communication from the contralateral digital artery.
- *Homodigital arterial flap:*
  - This flap is similar to the reverse digital artery flap, as it is an island flap harvested from the same injured finger in one stage.
  - This flap is harvested based on the dorsal branches of the proper digital artery and venous supply within a 5-mm wide bridge of fat of the dorsal branch of the proper digital artery at the distal finger crease.
  - This flap can be harvested with dorsal digital nerve branches to be a sensate flap.
  - The arc of motion of this flap makes it difficult to reach the fingertip.
- *Homodigital dorsal middle phalangeal neurovascular island flap:*
  - In fingers with large pulp defects, a homodigital dorsal middle phalangeal neurovascular island flap procedure showed good long-term outcomes.
  - The procedure is based on a single neurovascular pedicle and preserves the length of the finger.
- *Visor flap:*
  - The visor flap is a bipedicled dorsal finger skin flap that can be used to cover fingertip wounds after digital amputations proximal to the nail bed.

- Blood supply through this flap is provided through dorsal branches of the volar digital arteries and this is more reliable distal to the proximal phalanx.
- In elevating the visor flap it is critical to preserve the extensor peritenon to allow this donor site to be skin grafted.

Local Flaps for Thumb

- *Rectangular volar advancement flap:*
  - This is a rectangular volar flap based on both neurovascular bundles.
  - The flap is undermined in the distal to proximal direction to the MCP crease superficial to the flexor pollicis sheath and advanced in the distal direction.
  - This flap can usually be advanced 1.5 cm distally.
  - Other manipulations that can improve distal flap advancement include flexion of the interphalangeal joint.
  - The volar advancement flap is discouraged for the fingers because the inclusion of both neurovascular bundles jeopardizes blood supply to the dorsum of the fingers and causes severe flexion contractures of the fingers.
- *Littler flap:*
  - The neurovascular island flap was first described by Littler in 1960. He termed it the interdigital flap. It is most applicable for large defects of the volar thumb.
  - The neurovascular island flap is harvested from the ulnar aspect of the middle finger or the radial aspect of the ring finger, basically on the common neurovascular bundle to the third web space within the median nerve supply.
  - Before division of the distal branch of the proper digital artery, temporarily clamp to assess the blood supply to the donor's finger through what will be the remaining digital artery.
  - The advantage to the use of the Littler flap in thumb reconstruction is that it provides a large skin paddle with glabrous skin that is sensate, ultimately preserving thumb length.
  - The disadvantage is the donor site, which usually requires a skin graft and is prone to flexion contracture deformity.
- *First dorsal metacarpal artery flap:*
  - The first dorsal metacarpal artery flap is a neurovascular island flap raised from the dorsum of the index proximal phalanx based on the first dorsal metacarpal artery and branch of the superficial radial nerve.
  - The first dorsal metacarpal artery flap reaches defects on the volar thumb tip, thumb dorsum, first web space, the MCP joint of the small finger, and even the wrist and carpal joints.
  - A second dorsal metacarpal artery flap can be used for defects on the dorsum of the other fingers or the ulnar aspect of the hand.
  - The pedicle is fashioned by elevating a narrow skin flap over the first interosseous space and subcutaneous tissue to include subdermal veins to drain the flap.
  - The branch of the radial nerve to the index finger is frequently not visible as it courses at a slightly deeper plane than the subdermal vein plexus.
  - The radial border of the second metacarpal bone must be exposed while performing the elevation of the pedicle, dissecting close to the periosteum of the metacarpal shaft.
  - The plane of dissection for raising the first dorsal metacarpal artery pedicle is subfascial over the first dorsal interosseous muscle to include the fascia through which the first metacarpal artery can be visualized.
  - Distally, the skin flap should be elevated in the plane superficial to the paratenon over the dorsum of the proximal phalanx to provide a bed appropriate for skin grafting of the donor site.
  - Proximally, the pedicle is dissected from the paratenon of the tendon of the first dorsal interosseous muscle and then from the muscle itself in the distal to proximal direction. It is usually not necessary to skeletonize the first dorsal metacarpal artery back to its origin from the radial artery for the distal edge of the skin flap to reach the thumb volar tip.

  - The first dorsal metacarpal artery flap has several advantages over the Littler flap for sensate resurfacing of the thumb when the Moberg flap is not an option because the thumb tip defect is larger than 1.5 cm.
  - The dissection of the first dorsal metacarpal artery flap is easier than the Littler flap and contains a more reliable venous drainage plexus than the mere venae comitantes with the digital artery to the Littler flap.
  - A larger and more reliable skin paddle can be elevated with the first dorsal metacarpal artery flap than with the Littler flap. The donor site of the first dorsal metacarpal artery flap is more desirable compared to the Littler flap.
- *Cross-finger to thumb flap:*
  - On occasion, the Littler flap and first dorsal metacarpal artery flap are not available for sensate resurfacing of the thumb; a cross-finger flap from the dorsum of the index finger is required.
  - The disadvantage to the use of this flap is that it requires two stages and a neurorrhaphy of the radial nerve branch to the ulnar aspect digital nerve of the thumb.
  - Therefore, the Littler and first dorsal metacarpal artery flaps are preferred for larger thumb defects that cannot be reconstructed with the Moberg flap.
  - The flap is harvested superficially to the paratenon of the dorsum of the finger to allow for skin grafting of the donor.

Nail Bed Repairs
- Subungual hematomas result from the disruption of nail bed vessels.
- In the short term, even small hematomas can cause severe pain, requiring treatment with trephination.
- In performing nail trephination, a hole can be fashioned in the nail plate with cautery, a heated paper clip, or a drill to relieve this associated pain.
- In the long term, these small hematomas can become incorporated into the nail bed. Larger hematomas are associated with significant lacerations in the nail bed, which may result in significant scarring.
- Longitudinal scars in the nail bed can result in split-nail deformity.
- Transverse nail bed scars can result in nail nonadherence.
- Both split-nail deformities and nail nonadherence are risk factors for frequent paronychia infections, which may eventually require nail bed ablation.
- Occasionally, defects of the nail bed cannot be primarily approximated, and residual nail bed fragments can be found on the underside of the avulsed nail plate or harvested as a split-thickness graft from an uninjured area on this nail bed or from the second toe.

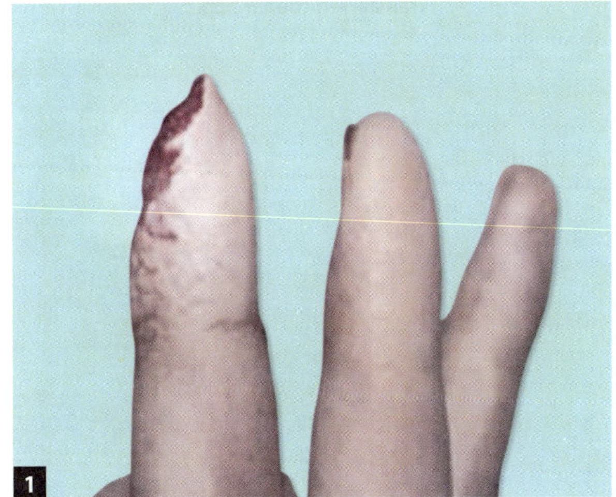

1 The most suitable cases for volar V-Y advancement techniques is dorsal oblique amputations.

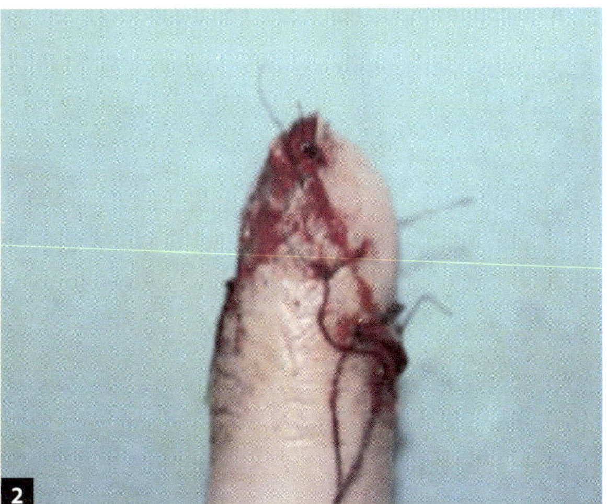

2 Length of middle leg of the Y can not be long as much as expected, yet it will give enough movements the flap that can cover the defect.

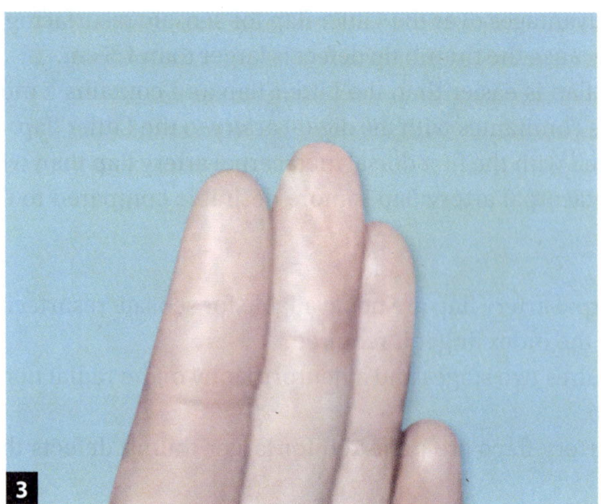
Late result, lateral aspect.

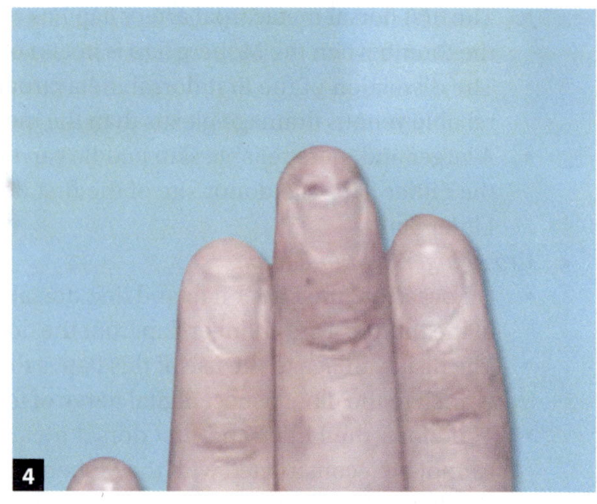
Concomitant nail bed injury can be repaired by skin grafting.

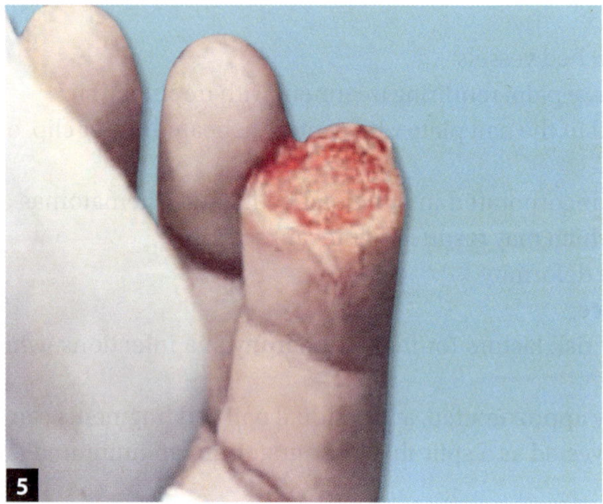
A guillotine amputation located on the index finger.

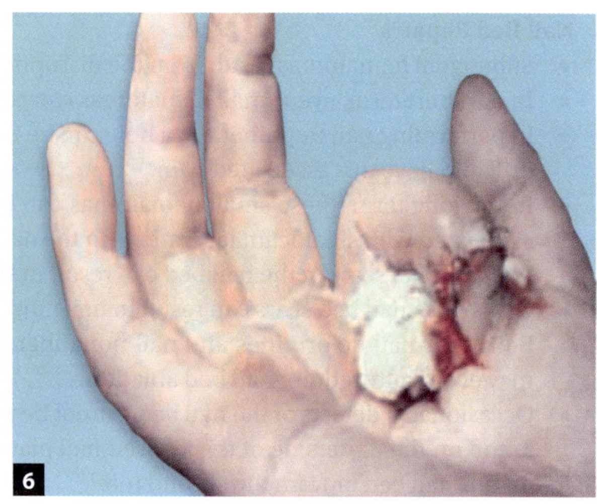
Transferred thenar flap.

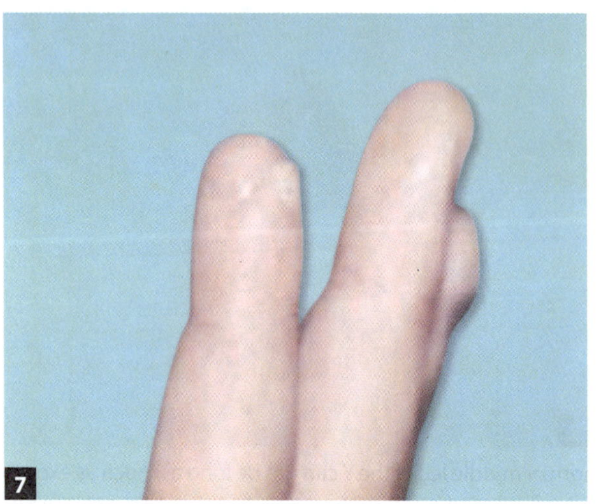
Late result with thenar flap, lateral view.

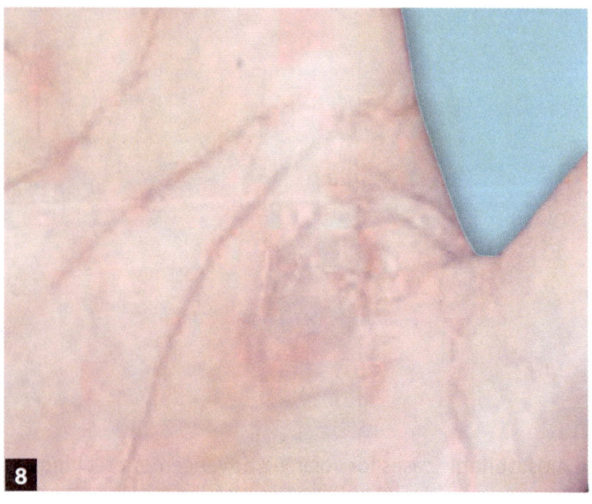
Postoperative appearance of donor area associated with thenar flap at 4th month.

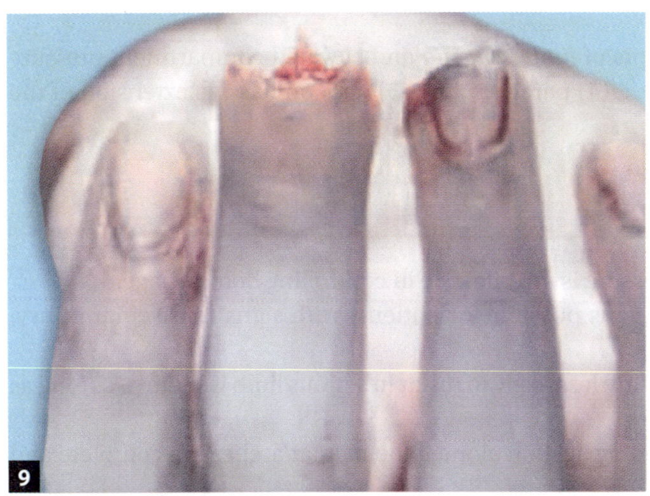

A composite grafting that ended with failure on the third finger tip. On the same hand, a V-Y advancement flap was done to close fingertip defects located on the 4th finger.

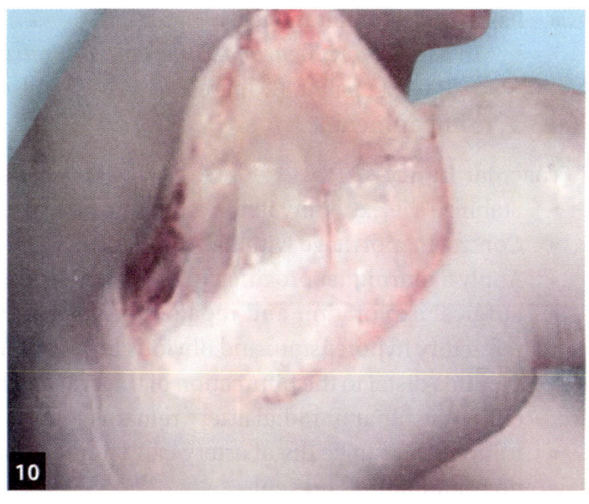

For third finger, a cross finger flap was prepared.

25. How will you proceed in a case of a glass cut injury wrist with bleeding attended to the emergency room?
WBUHS 2021 Supplementary

Glass Cut Injury Wrist with Bleeding

Points of Consideration

- Sharp clean cut and deep
- Depth may reach up to the bones
- Small area
- Even small lacerations may cause functional issues
- *Injuries:*
    - Vascular injuries
    - Muscle/tendon injuries
    - Nerve injuries

Look

- Tourniquet application
- Remove glass bits/foreign bodies
- Proper wash with normal saline
- Localize the source of bleed by frequent release of tourniquets
- Active or pulsatile hemorrhage/pulsatile/expanding hematoma
- Look for deformities
- *Documentation:*
    - Pulsatile or expanding hematoma
    - Pain on passive extension is the earliest and most sensitive physical finding

Feel

- Temperature and tenderness
- Pulsations
- Capillary refill time

Move

- Active—initiated and maintained by the patient

- Passive—examiner moves the limb
    - *To assess bony, neuronal, and tendon injuries:* Signs of *limb ischemia* and elevated compartment pressure 5 *"P's*—(1) pallor, (2) paresthesias, (3) pulse deficit, (4) paralysis, and (5) pain on passive extension of the compartment.

Vascular Injury

- Stabilize the extremity in the anatomic position.
- Control hemorrhage with direct pressure.
- Apply a tourniquet proximal to the injury if direct pressure is not effective in controlling hemorrhage.
- Surgical exploration and repair is performed as soon as possible for patients with signs of vascular injury, refractory hypotension, and obvious limb ischemia.
- Wounds distal to the bifurcation of the brachial artery are less likely to result in serious limb ischemia, as long as either the ulnar or radial artery remains intact.
- Injuries to a single distal artery can often be managed by ligation alone if the palmar arches are complete and no prior injury is present.
- A vascular surgeon must be consulted whenever a major vascular injury is a concern and facilities available
- Do not apply clamps or hemostats to vascular structures, since this may make definitive repair more difficult and damage surrounding tissues.

Tendon Injury

- *Extensor tendon injury:*
    - Divided into zones according to the anatomical location of the injury
    - In the hand and wrist there are seven extensor tendon zones
- *Flexor tendon injuries:* Five zones in the hand and the wrist
- Lacerated tendon when repaired takes 6–8 weeks of healing and hand therapy to recover

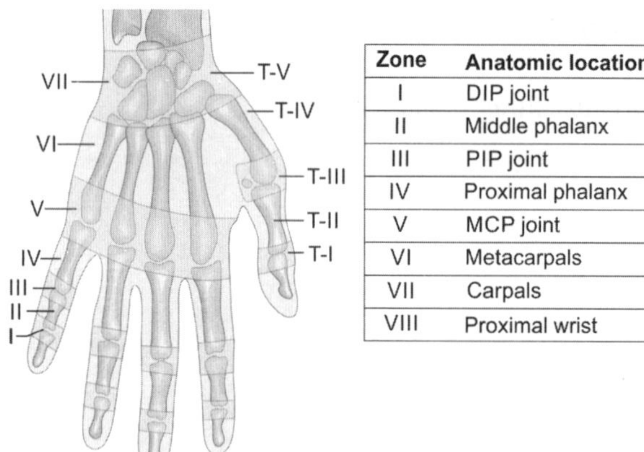

Zone	Anatomic location
I	DIP joint
II	Middle phalanx
III	PIP joint
IV	Proximal phalanx
V	MCP joint
VI	Metacarpals
VII	Carpals
VIII	Proximal wrist

Zones of extensor tendon injury

Zone	*Presentation*	*Management*
I	Mallet deformity	• *Closed:* Splinting 6–8 weeks • *Open:* Suture repair for fixation. Soft tissue reconstruction
III	Boutonniere's deformity	• *Closed:* Splinting MCP and PIPJ in hyperextension for 6 weeks • *Open:* Suture repair (figure-of-eight suture)
V	Fixed flexion of MCP	• *Closed:* Splinting—45° extension at wrist and 20° flexion at MCP • *Open:* Suture repair
VII	Fixed flexion of MCP	Suture repair followed by postoperative splinting

(MCP: metacarpophalangeal; PIPJ: proximal interphalangeal joint)

Flexor tendon injuries—five zones in the hand and the wrist

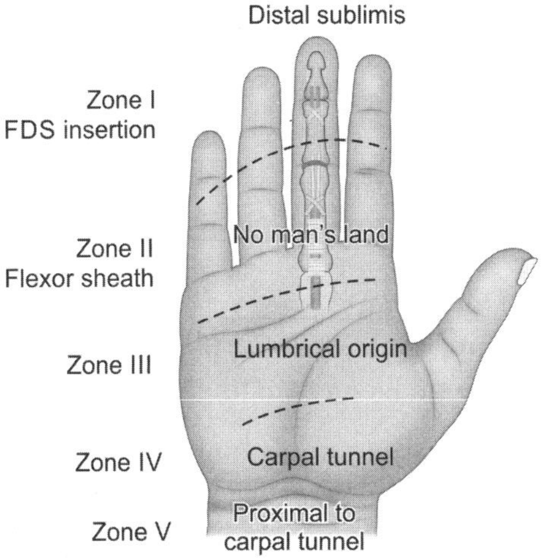

Distal sublimis
Zone I FDS insertion
Zone II Flexor sheath
No man's land
Zone III
Lumbrical origin
Zone IV
Carpal tunnel
Zone V
Proximal to carpal tunnel

Zone I: One tendon only (FDP) from middle of middle phalanx distally
Zone II: Two tendons (FDS and FDP) from MCP joints to middle of middle phalanx
Zone III: Central palm
Zone IV: Tendons in the carpal tunnel
Zone V: Tendons proximal to the carpal tunnel

(FDP: flexor digitorum profundus; FDS: flexor digitorum superficialis; MCP: metacarpophalangeal)

Classification

Zone	*Definition*	*Introduction*	*Treatment*
I	Distal to FDS insertion	Jersey finger	
II	FDS insertion to distal palmar crease	Zone is unique in that FDP and FDS in the same tendon sheath (both injured within the flexor retinaculum)	Direct repair of both tendons followed by early ROM (Duran and Kleinert). Be sure to preserve the A2 and A4 pulley. This zone historically had very poor results but results have improved due to advances in postoperative motion protocols
III	Palm	Often associated with neurovascular injury which carries a worse prognosis	Direct tendon repair. Good results from direct repair can be expected due to the absence of retinacular structures (if no neurovascular injury)
IV	Carpal tunnel	Often complicated by postoperative adhesions due to close quarters and synovial sheath of the carpal tunnel	Direct tendon repair. Transverse carpal ligament should be repaired in a lengthened fashion
V	Wrist to forearm	Often associated with neurovascular injury which carries a worse prognosis	Direct tendon repair
Thumb	TI, TII, and TIII	Outcomes are different than fingers. Early motion protocols do not improve long-term results and there is a higher re-rupture rate than flexor tendon repair in fingers	Direct end-to-end repair of FPL is advocated. Try to avoid zone III to avoid injury to the recurrent motor branch of the median nerve. Oblique pulley is more important than the AI pulley; however, both may be incised if necessary. Attempt to leave one pulley intact to prevent bowstringing

(FDP: flexor digitorum profundus; FDS: flexor digitorum superficialis; FPL: flexor pollicis longus; ROM: range of motion)

Nerve Injury

- Most common—median nerve
- *Low median nerve injuries:*
  - Injury in the distal third of the forearm with sparing of the forearm muscles of the hand paralyzed
  - Anesthesia over the median nerve distribution in the hand
  - Thenar eminence is wasted and thumb abduction and opposition are weak sensation lost over the radial three and a half digits and trophic changes.

Management

- *Direct injury:* Nerve repair
- *Long-standing cases:* Tendon transfers
  - *Low median nerve:* Rerouting of ring/middle finger superficial flexor around flexor carpi ulnaris (FCU) to abductor pollicis brevis (APB) to aid thumb opposition.
  - *High median nerve:* Suturing of profundus tendons to ring and small finger tendons for restoration of IP joint movements—ECU rerouting and attachment to dorsal radius/transfer of biceps insertion from medial to lateral radius for weak forearm pronation.

26. A 25-year-old male suffered a crush injury to his right hand while working in a factory. What is meant by mangled extremity? Describe the current algorithm for the management of finger trauma. ***WBUHS 2021***

- The mangled extremity is defined as massive anatomic disruption of the bone, muscle, tendon, nerve, vasculature, and/or soft tissue that threatens limb viability and functionality. The clinical team is left with the decision of whether to amputate or salvage and reconstruct.
- Mangled extremity severity score (MESS) is a scoring system that can be applied to mangled extremities and help one determine which mangled limbs will eventually come to amputation. The MESS is a graduated grading system based on skeletal and soft tissue injury, shock, ischemia, and age.
- Fingertip injuries can be classified by the mechanism of injury or the level of injury based on the frequently used Allen classification system. The most common mechanisms seen include the following:

Allen Classifications

- *Type 1:* Involves only the pulp
- *Type 2:* Involves the pulp and nail bed
- *Type 3:* Includes partial loss of the distal phalanx
- *Type 4:* Injury proximal to the germinal matrix

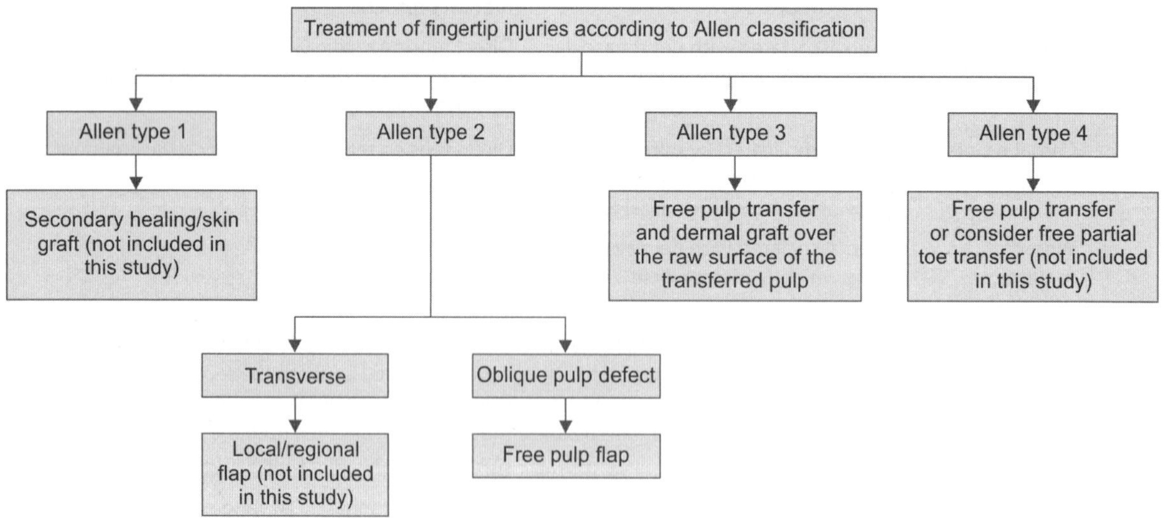

27. Classify flexor tendon injury of the hand and briefly mention its management. ***WBUHS 2017***

Flexor Tendon Injury of Hand

Anatomy

- Muscles:
  - Flexor digitorum profundus (FDP):
    - Functions as a flexor of the distal interphalangeal joint (DIP) joint

- Assists with proximal interphalangeal joint (PIPJ) and MCP flexion
- Shares a common muscle belly in the forearm
- Flexor digitorum superficialis (FDS):
  - Functions as a flexor of the PIPJ
  - Assists with MCP flexion
  - Individual muscle bellies exist in the forearm
  - FDS to the small finger is absent in 25% of people
- Flexor pollicis longus (FPL):
  - Located within the carpal tunnel as the most radial structure
- Flexor carpi radialis (FCR):
  - Primary wrist flexor
  - Inserts on the base of the second metacarpal
  - Closest flexor tendon to the median nerve
- FCU:
  - Primary wrist flexor
  - Inserts on the pisiform, hook of hamate, and the base of the fifth metacarpal

- Blood supply:
  - Two sources exist:

Zone	*Definition*	*Introduction*	*Treatment*
I	Distal to FDS insertion	Jersey finger	
II	FDS insertion to distal palmar crease	Zone is unique in that FDP and FDS in the same tendon sheath (both injured within the flexor retinaculum)	Direct repair of both tendons followed by early ROM (Duran and Kleinert). Be sure to preserve the A2 and A4 pulley. This zone historically had very poor results but results have improved due to advances in postoperative motion protocols
III	Palm	Often associated with neurovascular injury which carries a worse prognosis	Direct tendon repair. Good results from direct repair can be expected due to the absence of retinacular structures (if no neurovascular injury)
IV	Carpal tunnel	Often complicated by postoperative adhesions due to close quarters and synovial sheath of the carpal tunnel	Direct tendon repair. Transverse carpal ligament should be repaired in a lengthened fashion
V	Wrist to forearm	Often associated with neurovascular injury which carries a worse prognosis	Direct tendon repair
Thumb	TI, TII, and TIII	Outcomes are different than fingers. Early motion protocols do not improve long-term results and there is a higher re-rupture rate than flexor tendon repair in fingers	Direct end-to-end repair of FPL is advocated. Try to avoid zone III to avoid injury to the recurrent motor branch of the median nerve. Oblique pulley is more important than the Al pulley; however, both may be incised if necessary. Attempt to leave one pulley intact to prevent bowstringing

(FDP: flexor digitorum profundus; FDS: flexor digitorum superficialis; FPL: flexor pollicis longus; ROM: range of motion)

- Diffusion through synovial sheaths:
  - It occurs when flexor tendons are located within a sheath.
  - It is the more important source distal to the MCP joint.
- Direct vascular supply:
  - It nourishes flexor tendons located outside of synovial sheaths.

- *Camper's chiasm:* It is located at the level of the proximal phalanx where FDP splits FDS.

- *Pulley system:*
  - Digits 1–4 contain:
    - Five annular pulleys (A1 to A5)
    - Three cruciate pulleys (C1 to C3)
    - A2 and A4 are the most important pulleys to prevent flexor tendon bowstringing
  - Thumb contains:
    - Two annular pulley
    - Interposed oblique pulley (most important)

Classification

Flexor Tendons

Verdan described five zones of flexor tendon injury:

- *Zone 1:* Distal to FDS insertion
- *Zone 2:* Between proximal flexor sheath and FDS insertion
- *Zone 3:* Between distal flexor retinaculum and proximal flexor sheath
- *Zone 4:* Under the flexor retinaculum
- *Zone 5:* Proximal to the flexor retinaculum

Zone 2 Repair is Complicated by Having Two Tendons in a Tight Sheath

- *Thumb zones:*
  - *Zone T1:* Distal to interphalangeal joint (IPJ)
  - *Zone T2:* From A1 pulley to IPJ
  - *Zone T3:* In the thenar eminence
  - Zones T4 and T5 are the same as for the fingers.
- *FDP can be avulsed from its bony attachment:*
  - It is caused by a hyperextension force on an actively flexed distal interphalangeal joint (DIPJ).
  - It is known "rugger jersey finger"—a tackler grabs the opponent's Rugby shirt.
  - The ring finger is most commonly injured because it is the "longest" flexed finger.
- *Leddy and Packer classify FDP avulsions:*
  - *Type I:* Tendon retracts into the palm; rupture of both vincula
  - *Type II:* Tendon retracts to the PIPJ; long vinculum intact
  - *Type III:* A large bony fragment avulsed with the tendon prevents retraction beyond the A4 pulley.

Injury Pattern

- Injury patterns are differentiated into open or closed, sharp or blunt, traumatic, or degenerative lesions, as well as injury to the dorsal or palmar part.
- Further subdivisions are osseous tendon lesions, complex lesions with concomitant trauma or injury of the tendon sheath and pulley system.
- Closed tendon injuries are quite common.

Flexor Tendon Healing

Two forms:

1. *Intrinsic healing:* It occurs without direct blood flow to the tendon.
2. *Extrinsic healing:* It occurs by the proliferation of fibroblast from the peripheral epitenon, adhesion occurs because of extrinsic healing of the tendon and limits tendon gliding within the fibrous synovial sheath

Phase of Intrinsic Healing

- *Inflammatory (0–5 days):* Strain of the repair is reliant on the strength of the suture itself
- Fibroblastic (5–28 days) or so-called collagen-producing phase
- Remodeling (>28 days)

Signs and Symptoms

- Unable to bend one and more finger joints
- Pain when bending finger/s
- Open injury to hand
- Mild swelling over the joint close to the fingertip
- Tenderness along the effect finger/s on the palm side of the hand
- Complain of numbness proceeded by excessive bleeding—consider neurovascular insults

Examination

- *Inspection:*
  - There is a normal arcade to hand with the index finger showing the least and the little finger showing the maximum flexion
  - If the affected finger shows more extension than other digits, the chance of tendon injury is high
  - If the distal IP joint can be actively flexed while the proximal IP joint is stabilized, the profundus tendon has not been served.
  - If the proximal IP joint can be actively flexed while adjacent fingers are held completely extended.
  - Sublimis tendon has not been severed
  - *FPL:* Stabilized the MCP joint, ask the patients to flex the IP joint
- *Diagnosis of flexor tendon injuries:* History
- *Clinical examination:*
  - Use of bedside ultrasound (USG) in emergency room (more sensitive and specific than physical examination)
  - Wound exploration technique or magnetic resonance imaging (MRI)
  - Three-view X-ray to rule out foreign body or bony injury or dislocation
- *Flexor tendon repair type:*
  - *Primary repair:* First 24 hours of the injury
  - *Delayed primary:* 1–10 days
  - *Secondary repair:* 2–4 weeks
  - *Late secondary repair:* After 4 weeks
- *Primary repair:*
  - Emergency repair is needed if altered digital perfusion present
  - Clean wound caused by a sharp object
- *Secondary repair:* Indicated if associated with:
  - Extensive crushing with bony communication
  - Severe neurovascular injury
  - Severe joint injury and skin loss requiring a coverage procedure
  - Primary repair gives a better functional outcome than secondary repair.
    - No repair if <25% laceration
    - Only epitenon repair in 25–50% laceration
    - Core suture plus epitenon repair when >50% laceration
    - Dorsal blocking splint for 6–8 weeks as a conservative measure

Suture Technique

Flexor tendon repair

Skin Incision

- An extensive exposure is planned
- Popular approaches include the Brunner and midlateral

The Extensor Tendon Sheath

- A synovial-lined fibro-osseous tunnel in the fingers and thumb.

- Runs between the metacarpal neck and DIPJ
- Synovial portion contributes to tendon glide and nutrition
- Retinacular portion contributes mechanical efficiency
- Retinacular part consists of five annular (A) and three cruciform (C) pulleys:
  - A1, A3, and A5 originate from the volar plates of MCPJ, PIPJ, and DIPJ, respectively.
  - A2 and A4 originate from the proximal and middle phalanx, respectively.
  - Cruciform pulleys are collapsible; they "concertina" to allow flexion.
- Pulleys are ordered from proximal to distal as follows: A1–A2–C1–A3–C2–A4–C3–A5
- The thumb has two annular pulleys overlying the MCPJ (A1) and IPJ (A2).
- *An oblique pulley runs between the two:* From ulnar on the proximal phalanx to radial on the distal phalanx.
- The sheath usually needs to be opened for access to the tendon ends.
  - As much sheath as possible should be preserved to maintain function.
  - Function is usually adequate if either A2 or A4 is preserved.
- Closure of the sheath is controversial, particularly if it limits glide.

An Alternative to Venting Zone II Pulleys is Excising a Slip of FDS

The Tendon Repair

- Results are better when repair is done within the first few days of injury.
- The following principles apply to most techniques:
  - Handle tendon ends as little as possible.
  - Repair should be strong enough to allow early mobilization.
  - Strength of repair is dependent on:
    - Gauge of suture—3/0 is stronger than 4/0
    - Number of strands crossing the repair—four are stronger than two
    - Configuration of the peripheral suture
    - Tendon-suture interaction—grasping sutures pull through easily; locking sutures "lock" a bundle of tendon fibers, minimizing suture pullout.
  - Excessive suture bulk can increase resistance to tendon glide
  - No gapping of the tendon ends on mobilization
    - A 2 mm gap increases gliding resistance significantly
    - A 3 mm gap is unlikely to pass under the A2 pulley without rupture
  - Avoid shortening FDP >1 cm—quadriga may ensue:
    - The quadriga phenomenon was described by Verdan
    - Occurs when FDP excursion in an unaffected finger is reduced as a result of decreased FDP excursion in another finger due to stiffness, injury, or adhesion.
- Decreases global grip strength because all FDPs share a common muscle belly
- Most repairs use core and peripheral sutures
- No evidence that using 'cutting' needles gives a higher rupture rate
- *Examples of core sutures include:*
  - Two-strand repair:
    1. Kessler, with two knots on the outside of the tendon
    2. Modified Kessler, with a single knot within the repair site
  - Four-strand repair:
    1. Cruciate
    2. Adelaide (modified Savage)
    3. Six-strand repair
    4. Savage

Peripheral sutures do the following:

- Align tendon ends prior to core suture (back wall first)
- Tidy up tendon ends following core suture
- Contribute significant strength to the repair
- *Examples of peripheral sutures include:*
  - Strickland simple continuous suture
  - Halsted continuous horizontal mattress

Partial Injury

- Lacerations up to and beyond 75% of the cross-sectional tendon area maintains adequate strength at physiological loads.
- Partial lacerations may cause triggering—the triggering part should be trimmed.
- Placing epitendinous sutures into partial lacerations doubles the gliding resistance.
- This is unnecessary; may require sheath incisions for access.

Rehabilitation Following Repair of Flexor Tendons

- Tendons were historically immobilized in the belief that adhesions were necessary for healing
- Discovery of intrinsic healing allowed early mobilization to improve glide
- Most regimes require a dorsal blocking splint to protect the repair
- The splint is maintained for up to 6 weeks
- Heavy use is avoided for 12 weeks in total
- Common regimes are variations on the following:

Immobilization

Mainly for children or adults unsuitable for early mobilization.

Early Passive Mobilization

No active movement is permitted

Early Active Extension with Passive Flexion

- Advocated by Kleinert et al.
- Finger flexion is maintained by rubber-band traction
- Active extension is done against the recoil of the bands
- Passive flexion occurs by elastic recoil of the bands
- Critics state that PIPJ extension lag is a problem due to prolonged PIPJ flexion
- It is also regarded as a poor mobilizer of the DIPJ.

Early Active Mobilization

- Strength of repair is increased by early active flexion.
- The "Belfast" regime is widely used in the United Kingdom in modified forms.
- Active mobilization is started 48 hours after the operation.
- *Exercises are repeated 2-hourly throughout the day:*

Two passive movements, then two active movements of the finger(s)

- The aim is full passive flexion in the splint within the first week.
- Range of active motion is gradually increased.

Outcomes

- Rupture and adhesion affect 5% of flexor tendon repairs
- No consensus on ideal outcome measures:
  - Most measure range of motion
  - The commonly used systems have never been validated.

CHAPTER 55

Pediatric Surgery

LEARNING OBJECTIVES

- Branchial Fistula and Cystic Hygroma
- Development of Diaphragm and Congenital Diaphragmatic Hernia
- Patent Ductus Arteriosus
- Vascular Malformations in Childhood
- Tracheoesophageal Fistula
- Infantile Hypertrophic Pyloric Stenosis and Biliary Atresia
- Intestinal Atresias
- Abdominal Wall Defect, Gastroschisis, Omphalocele
- Umbilicus, Meckel's Diverticulum
- Midgut Volvulus
- Intussusceptions
- Hirschsprung's Disease and Congenital Megacolon
- Anorectal Malformations
- Prenatal Surgery

BRANCHIAL FISTULA AND CYSTIC HYGROMA

1. Outline the surgical anatomy and management of branchial fistula. ***WBUHS 2021 Supplementary***

Branchial Anomalies

- *Embryology:*
  - Branchial anomalies result from improper development of the branchial apparatus.
  - Branchial apparatus develops 2nd–6th week.
  - Neck is shaped like a hollow tube with circumferential ridges = Arches (mesoderm)
  - Ridges between arches = Clefts and pouches
  - Clefts = Outside (ectoderm); pouches = inside (endoderm)

Arches

- *Each arch:* Contains cartilage, cranial nerve, artery, muscle component, all neural crest origin
- Six arches, only five form structures in humans 1, 2, 3, 4, and 6, 5th fails to develop.

Branchial Clefts and Pouches

- Four clefts and four pouches
- 5th and 6th contribute to the 4th
- Clefts provide "covering" to structures of the corresponding arch and pouch

Branchial Cleft Anomalies

- *1st cleft:* Cysts, EAC atresia or stenosis, pits of lower lips, preauricular sinuses or tags
- *2nd cleft:* Cysts, cervical sinuses
- *3rd cleft:* Cysts (rare)—thymic cysts
- *4th cleft:* Cysts (extremely rare)—cysts on the vagus nerve—cough

Branchial Cleft Cysts

- Results from failed obliteration of branchial clefts
- 2–3% are bilateral
- 2nd cleft cyst is the most common type
- ~95% of cases

2nd Branchial Cleft Cyst

- Most common branchial cyst
- Presents as a mass just anterior and medial to the upper one-third of sternocleidomastoid (SCM) in the neck
- Tract—anterior neck—along carotid sheath—between external and internal carotid arteries—superficial to CNIX and -XII—opens into tonsillar fossa

Imaging

- *Ultrasound:* Round mass with uniform low echogenicity and lack of internal septations
    - *Advantages:* No radiation, no sedation for children, low cost
- *CT:* Homogeneous lesion with low attenuation centrally and a smooth enhancing rim. More radiation, higher cost, may require sedation (children)
- *MRI:* Hypointense on T1 and hyperintense on T2
- *Fluoroscopic fistulography or CT fistulography:* Inject radiopaque dye into the fistula or sinus to delineate course
- Barium swallow esophagography; help locate fistula tract in types 3 and 4 anomalies

Fine Needle Aspiration (FNA)

Usually only done if suspect cancer.

Treatment

- *Infected cyst:*
    - Antibiotics—should cover respiratory flora and *Staphylococcus aureus* (broad spectrum)—cover 2–4 weeks
    - Abscess—I and D
    - Once infection cleared, operate
    - *Surgical:* Complete excision of the tract and cyst

Branchial cleft fistulas (BCFs) originate from the 1st to 3rd branchial apparatus during embryogenesis of the head and neck.

- Anomalies of the 2nd branchial cleft are by far the most commonly found.
- They can be a cyst, a sinus tract, or fistulas.
- Fistulas (or sinus tract if they end blindly) display themselves as small cutaneous opening along the anterior lower third border of the sternocleidomastoid muscle, communicates proximally with the tonsillar fossae, and can drain saliva or a mucoid secretion.
- Management consists of excision since inefficient drainage may lead to infection.
    - 1st BCF are uncommon, located at the angle of the mandible, and communicating with the external auditory canal. They have a close association with the facial nerve.
    - 3rd BCF are very rare, run into the piriform sinus and may be a cause of acute thyroiditis or recurrent neck infections.

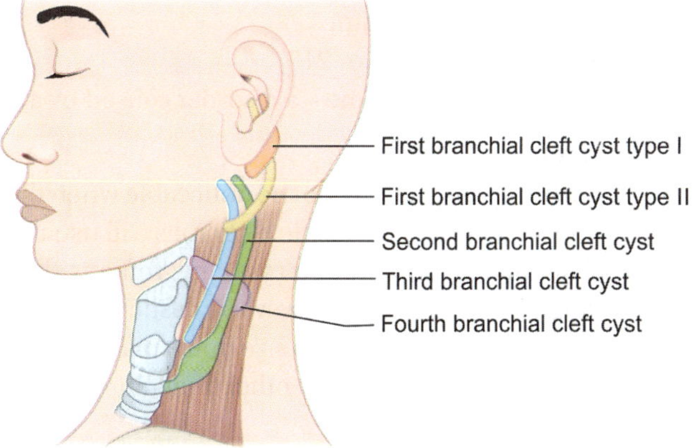

Management

Diagnosis

- *Fistulography:* Fistulography (opacifying the fistula with contrast media) delineates a smooth tract extending from the external cutaneous opening at the lateral neck superomedially passing between the ECA and ICA to the tonsillar fossa.
- *Ultrasound:* Ultrasound can demonstrate the fistulous tract as an anechoic linear structure filled with faint echogenic debris, comprising cellular material, cholesterol crystals, and keratin.
- *CT:* Usually combined with fistulography offers excellent anatomical delineation
- *MRI:* Less diagnostic value but T1-weighted images provide better soft tissue contrast of the upper half of the fistula at the level of carotid bifurcation.

Treatment

- Due to the risk of recurrent infection and even squamous cell carcinoma, obliteration of the tract is preferred.
- Options include—use of sclerosing agents, excision of the fistulous tract (Hockey stick type or Step Ladder incision), and pull through brachial fistulectomy.

---

2. Discuss cystic hygroma. ***WBUHS 2013***

Introduction

- Cystic hygromas are abnormal growths that usually appear on a baby's neck or head. They consist of one or more cysts and tend to grow larger over time. This disorder most often develops while the baby is still in the womb. However, a cystic hygroma can also appear after birth.
- Cystic hygromas are fluid-filled sacs caused by blockages in the lymphatic system. They usually form between the 9th and 16th week of pregnancy. Approximately half of all fetuses with a cystic hygroma have chromosomal abnormalities. The baby is unlikely to have a chromosomal abnormality if the cystic hygroma goes away by week 20.
- Cystic hygromas can also increase the risk of miscarriage and may even be life threatening.

Causes

- Cystic hygromas can develop due to genetic disorders or environmental factors. One or more growths may be present at the time of diagnosis.
- Common environmental causes of cystic hygromas are:
  - Viral infections passed from the mother to the baby during pregnancy
  - Exposure to drugs or alcohol during pregnancy
- Cystic hygromas are seen more often in infants with genetic diseases. They are particularly common in infants with chromosomal abnormalities. Some genetic conditions associated with hygromas include:
  - Turner's syndrome
  - Trisomy 13, 18, or 21
  - Noonan syndrome—a disorder caused by a mutation (change) in one of seven particular genes

Symptoms

- Cystic hygromas may not be noticeable when the baby is born. They can become visible as they grow larger and the child gets older. Cystic hygromas will usually appear by the time the child is 2-year-old.
- The main symptom of a cystic hygroma is the presence of a soft, spongy lump. This lump most commonly appears on the neck. However, a cystic hygroma can also form in the armpits and groin area.
- Cystic hygromas range in size from smaller than a quarter to as large as a baseball. Larger growths may interfere with movement or cause other difficulties.

Diagnosis

- Amniocentesis if cystic hygroma is found during an ultrasound. An amniocentesis can check for genetic abnormalities in your fetus.
- Other tests will be used to make a diagnosis if cystic hygromas are not found until after the child is born.

These include:
- Chest X-ray
- Ultrasound
- CT scan

Treatments
- Cystic hygromas are not treated while the baby is in the womb.
- A cystic hygroma is usually treatable if it is found after birth. The first step of treatment is surgery. The entire growth must be removed to prevent it from coming back.
- In some cases, other techniques may be used to shrink large cystic hygromas:
    - Sclerotherapy—bleomycin is injected into the cyst
    - Chemotherapy
    - Radiation therapy
    - Steroid medication

Long-term Outlook for Babies with Cystic Hygromas
The main potential complications of cystic hygromas are:
- Recurring growths
- Bleeding
- Infection in the affected area
- Damage to muscles, nerves, or tissues from surgery to remove the hygroma

However, the outlook for babies with cystic hygromas is generally good if the growths appear after birth. This is especially true if the growths can be completely removed. If they cannot be removed, cystic hygromas may return or spread to other areas.

CONGENITAL DIAPHRAGMATIC HERNIA

3. Congenital diaphragmatic hernia. ***WBUHS 2010***

4. Explain congenital diaphragmatic hernia and its treatment. ***RGUHS Karnataka 2025***

5. Development of diaphragm and management of diaphragmatic hernia. ***WBUHS 2017, RIMS-IMPHAL 2022***

6. Describe clinical features, diagnosis, and management of congenital diaphragmatic hernia. ***WBUHS 2019***

The diaphragm is a curved musculofibrous sheet that separates the thoracic from the abdominal cavity.
- Pierced by structures that pass between these two regions of the body
- Primary muscle of respiration
- Dome shaped and consists of a peripheral muscular part and central tendinous part
- Muscular part arises from the margins of the thoracic opening and gets inserted into the central tendon.
- Attachments to the thoracic wall are low posteriorly and laterally, but high anteriorly.
- Origin is vertebral, costal, and spinal attachments from which muscular fibers curve upward and inward from periphery to be inserted into the fibrous sheet called central tendon.

Develops from four sources:
1. Septum transversum
2. Pleuroperitoneal membrane
3. Medial dorsal portion of primary esophageal mesentery
4. Marginal ingrowths of the body wall

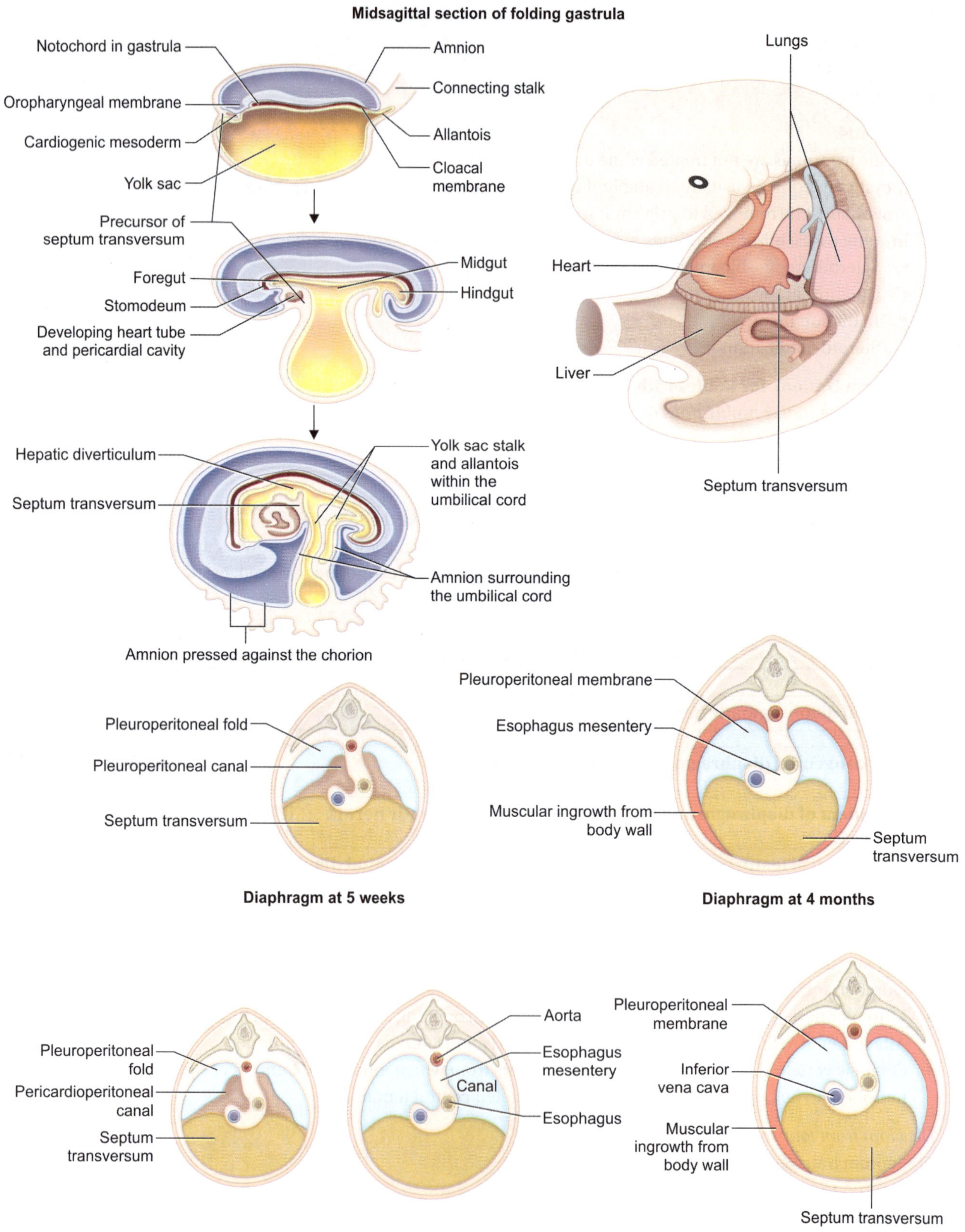

Midsagittal section of folding gastrula
Notochord in gastrula
Oropharyngeal membrane
Cardiogenic mesoderm
Yolk sac
Amnion
Connecting stalk
Allantois
Cloacal membrane
Precursor of septum transversum
Foregut
Stomodeum
Developing heart tube and pericardial cavity
Midgut
Hindgut
Hepatic diverticulum
Septum transversum
Yolk sac stalk and allantois within the umbilical cord
Amnion surrounding the umbilical cord
Amnion pressed against the chorion
Lungs
Heart
Liver
Septum transversum
Pleuroperitoneal fold
Pleuroperitoneal canal
Septum transversum
Diaphragm at 5 weeks
Pleuroperitoneal membrane
Esophagus mesentery
Muscular ingrowth from body wall
Septum transversum
Diaphragm at 4 months
Pleuroperitoneal fold
Pericardioperitoneal canal
Septum transversum
Aorta
Esophagus mesentery
Canal
Esophagus
Pleuroperitoneal membrane
Inferior vena cava
Muscular ingrowth from body wall
Septum transversum

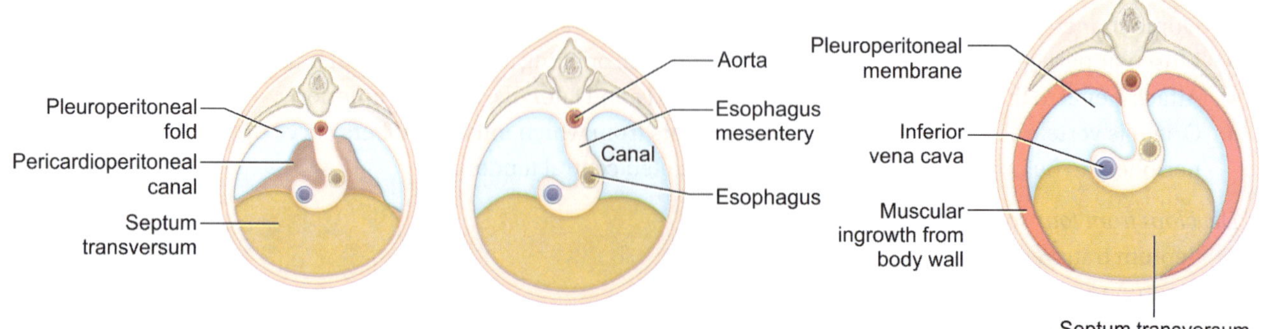

Septum Transversum

- Third week of development
- Mass of mesoderm situated cranially to the pericardial cavity
- Contributes to the ventral portion like the sternal and costal parts

Pleuroperitoneal Membrane

- It is a paired dorsolateral portion
- Fuses with dorsal mesentery of esophagus and dorsal portion of the septum transversum to complete the partition between thorax and abdomen
- Forms the primitive diaphragm at 7th week of development

Medial Portion of the Diaphragm

- From the medial dorsal portion of primary esophageal mesentery
- Fuses with septum transversum and pleuroperitoneal membrane
- Curves of diaphragm—develop from growth of muscle fibers into the dorsal mesentery of the esophagus.
  - At 9–12th week, the source is contributed by—the marginal outgrowth of the body wall.
  - These contributions from thoracic myotome contain nerve fibers of lower six or seven intercostal nerves—distribute the sensory fibers to periphery of diaphragm.
  - At the 5th week, nerve fibers from the 3rd, 4th, and 5th cervical segments of spinal cord grow into septum transversum, via the pleuropericardial membrane to form the phrenic nerve.
  - At the 8th week, diaphragm attached to dorsal body of 1st lumbar vertebrae, giving rise to the domed contour character of the diaphragm.

Origin of the Diaphragm

- Sternal part—arising from the posterior surface of the xiphoid process
- Costal part arising from the deep surfaces of the lower six ribs and their costal cartilages and forms the right and left domes.
- Vertebral/lumbar part arising from upper three lumbar vertebrae; forms the right and left crura and the arcuate ligaments.
- *Crura:* The right crus is from the bodies of first three lumbar vertebrae. The left crus originates from the bodies of first two lumbar vertebrae.

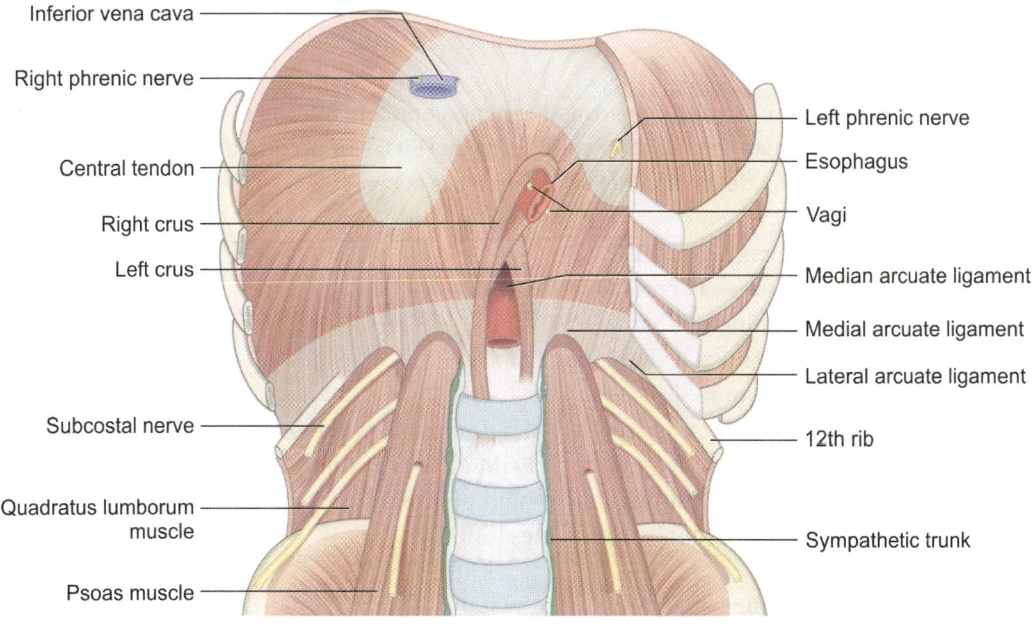

Etiology

- Incomplete diaphragm development at 8 weeks' gestation results in herniation of abdominal organs into the chest, preventing normal lung development.
- Left leaflet occurs in 90% of cases, and right leaflet in 10%.
- Bochdalek (posterolateral defect; 85% of cases); Morgagni (anterior, parasternal; fewer pulmonary and systemic complications)
- A 1:1 male-to-female ratio

Diagnosis

- Antenatal ultrasound and maternal–fetal magnetic resonance imaging (MRI); polyhydramnios is detected in up to 80% of cases.
- *Physical examination:*
  - Cardiorespiratory distress
  - Asymmetric "funnel" chest
  - Reduced breath sounds on the affected side
  - Scaphoid abdomen
- *Chest X-ray:*
  - Herniated abdominal viscera within the chest
  - Mediastinal shift
- *Mortality:*
  - Approximately 35%
  - May be higher in patients with severe pulmonary hypoplasia and hypertension or in the presence of associated congenital anomalies
- *Management:*
  - *Immediate postnatal care:*
    - Supplemental oxygen
    - Endotracheal intubation is indicated if significant respiratory distress is present. Avoid bag-mask ventilation, which exacerbates gastrointestinal (GI) distention and further impedes lung ventilation.
    - Intravenous access is necessary for the administration of fluids to maintain organ perfusion
    - GI decompression by orogastric or nasogastric intubation reduces distention of the stomach and within the thoracic cavity.
  - *Intensive care:*
    - Conventional ventilation utilizing permissive hypercapnia to minimize barotrauma
      - Once stabilized, wean fraction of inspired oxygen (FiO_2) for preductal oxygen saturation >90%.
      - Arterial carbon dioxide tension of 60–70 mm Hg is acceptable.
      - Maintain pH >7.20.
      - Peak airway pressures <25 cmH_2O.
      - Mean airway pressures <12 cmH_2O.
    - High-frequency oscillating ventilator (HFOV):
      - May be used if conventional ventilation failed
      - Possibly limit barotrauma
    - Inhaled nitric oxide may decrease severity of pulmonary hypertension.
    - Extracorporeal membrane oxygenation (ECMO) is considered for patients with severe preductal hypoxemia or right-to-left shunting due to high pulmonary hypertension. Patients with overwhelming pulmonary hypoplasia may not be candidates for ECMO.
  - *Operative intervention:*
    - Usually deferred until the patient's pulmonary status is stable

- A subcostal incision on the affected side allows the herniated abdominal contents to be replaced in the peritoneal cavity.
- Repaired primarily or with a synthetic patch, depending on the size of the defect

- *Complications:* Long-term respiratory insufficiency, gastrointestinal (GI) reflux, neurologic sequelae from prolonged hypoxia, recurrence of hernia.

PATENT DUCTUS ARTERIOSUS

7. Describe indications of cardiopulmonary bypass and treatment options in patent ductus arteriosus.
WBUHS 2019

Introduction

- Cardiopulmonary bypass with balloon occlusion provides a safe operation for adult patients with complicated patent ductus arteriosus.
- The majority of patent ductus arteriosus (PDA) patients undergo a surgical correction in childhood.
- However, some situations retard the operation until adulthood.

Complications of untreated PDA include bacterial endocarditis, late congestive heart failure (CHF), and the development of pulmonary vascular obstructive disease.

Surgical procedures in which cardiopulmonary bypass is used:

- Coronary artery bypass surgery
- Cardiac valve repair and/or replacement (aortic valve, mitral valve, tricuspid valve, and pulmonic valve)
- Repair of large septal defects (atrial septal defect, ventricular septal defect, and atrioventricular septal defect)
- Repair and/or palliation of congenital heart defects (tetralogy of Fallot, transposition of the great vessels)
- Transplantation (heart transplantation, lung transplantation, heart–lung transplantation, liver transplantation)
- Repair of some large aneurysms (aortic aneurysms, cerebral aneurysms), pulmonary thromboendarterectomy
- Pulmonary thrombectomy
- Isolated limb perfusion

Patent ductus arteriosus can complicate other circulatory or ventilatory abnormalities, such as the following:

- Aortic rupture
- Eisenmenger physiology
- Left heart failure
- Myocardial ischemia
- Necrotizing enterocolitis
- Pulmonary hypertension
- Right heart hypertrophy and failure

Treatment Options for PDA

- *Watchful waiting:* In a premature baby, a PDA often closes on its own.
- *Medications:* In a premature baby, nonsteroidal anti-inflammatory drugs (NSAIDs)—such as ibuprofen (Advil, Infant's Motrin, others) or indomethacin (Indocin)—might be used to help close a PDA.
- *Surgical closure:*
  - Surgical ligation or surgical ligation and division remain the standard treatment of large PDA that requires treatment in infancy. This is a particularly successful, low-risk procedure in the hands of an experienced pediatric cardiovascular surgeon. This is true even in the smallest premature babies.
  - *Ligation:* With or without division of the PDA without cardiopulmonary bypass can be performed through a left posterolateral thoracotomy. Video-assisted thoracoscopic surgery (VATS) ligation of PDA is less invasive than the posterolateral thoracotomy and also safe and effective.

- *Catheter procedures:*
  - *Cardiac catheterization:*
    - The use of the percutaneous route to close the PDA is becoming more common.
    - Most patients with an isolated PDA can have successful treatment by catheterization after the first few months of life.
    - After the first birthday, the most common treatment for a PDA is occlusion at cardiac catheterization.

VASCULAR MALFORMATIONS IN CHILDHOOD

8. Describe pathology of vascular malformations in childhood. ***WBUHS 2010***

Vascular Malformations

Key Facts

Classified broadly into two principal groups

Primary Hemangiomas (with Endothelial Hyperplasia)

- All congenital or idiopathic
- Mostly sporadic but may rarely be part of a familial syndrome, e.g., von Hippel-Lindau
- Pulmonary hemangiomas commonly seen in hereditary hemorrhagic telangiectasia are linked to a deficiency in endoglin (endothelial growth factor).

True Arteriovenous Malformations (AVM)

AVMs have three main causes:

1. *Congenital:* Origin/cause unknown. Mostly sporadic but may rarely be part of a congenital syndrome (e.g., Klippel-Trenaunay)
2. *Traumatic:* May follow relatively minor trauma
3. *Iatrogenic:* Following a variety of surgical/interventional procedures

Pathological Features

Vascular malformations are histologically categorized as capillary, venous, lymphatic, or mixed in type, depending on the predominant vessel type affected, and subdivided into low- or high-flow varieties.

Clinical Features

- Congenital AVMs are usually evident at birth and the superficial lesion may only represent a part of the overall abnormality.
- Symptoms are dependent on the size, site, and type of vessel affected, and whether the AVMs are high or low flow.

Low Flow

- May result in considerable cosmetic deformity if large (e.g., Klippel-Trenaunay)
- Pain may be a feature due to spontaneous thrombosis of some/all of the venous elements
- Classically the symptoms are worse after exercise when blood flow is maximized

High Flow

- These are largely asymptomatic but there may be a detectable venous hum or bruit.
- They may result in local hyperhidrosis, heat, ulceration or present with profuse bleeding.
- May lead to high-output cardiac failure if large and untreated

Go Through

Diagnosis and investigation:

- *Doppler duplex:* Diagnoses lesion, can estimate flow rate, and is useful for follow-up monitoring.
- MRI has replaced CT as the best imaging modality and gives both the extent and related anatomy for complex lesions
- Angiography is reserved for high-flow lesions when suitability for embolization

Treatment

Largely Conservative

- Congenital AVMs frequently reduce in size with growth of the child and treatment is rarely easy
- Adult AVMs only require treatment for complications or occasionally cosmesis

Interventional Radiology

- Percutaneous embolization using wire coils or foam sclerosant under radiological guidance
- *Risks include:*
    - Risks of percutaneous puncture (infection, false aneurysm formation, and embolization)
    - Inadvertent embolization of adjacent vessels
    - Tissue necrosis after successful lesion embolization
    - Postembolization syndrome may occur with pain at the site of embolization accompanied by malaise, fever, leukocytosis, and hyperkalemia. This usually settles with symptomatic treatment in 24–48 hours due to tissue necrosis and cytokine release.

Surgery

- Small lesions may be excised completely
- Obliteration of small superficial venous malformations can be undertaken by direct puncture and injecting a sclerosant such as STD (sodium tetradecyl sulfate).
- Open surgery is mostly confined to high-flow lesions after preoperative embolization.

TRACHEOESOPHAGEAL FISTULA

9. What are the types of tracheoesophageal fistula in newborn? Discuss the management of tracheoesophageal fistula. ***WBUHS 2022, 2025***

10. Management of tracheoesophageal fistula. ***Rajiv Gandhi University of Health Sciences 2019, Karnataka 2019***

11. Describe the clinical features, diagnosis, and management of tracheoesophageal fistula. ***DY Patil Education Society, Deemed to be University 2020, 2024***

Types of Tracheoesophageal Fistula

- Type A = Pure esophageal atresia
- Type B = Esophageal atresia with proximal tracheoesophageal fistula
- Type C = Esophageal atresia with distal tracheoesophageal fistula
- Type D = Esophageal atresia with proximal and distal tracheoesophageal fistula
- Type E = H-type tracheoesophageal fistula without esophageal atresia

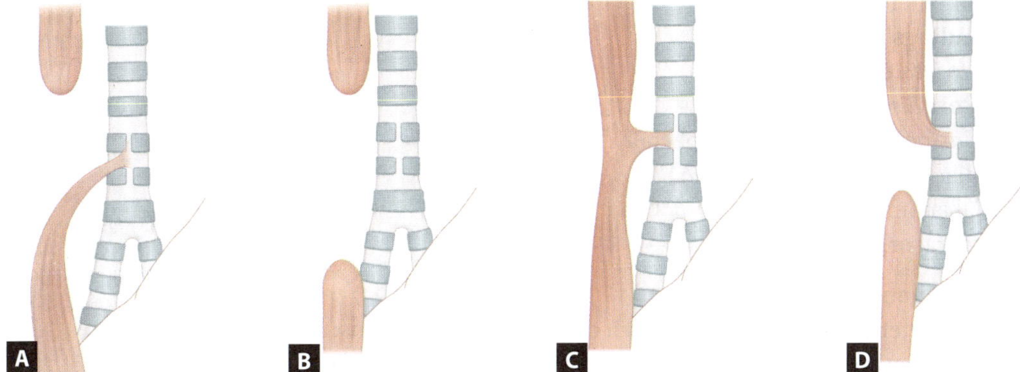

Esophageal atresia. (A) Esophageal atresia with distal tracheoesophageal fistula; (B) Proximal and distal blind pouches without fistula; (C) H fistula; (D) Esophageal atresia with proximal tracheoesophageal fistula

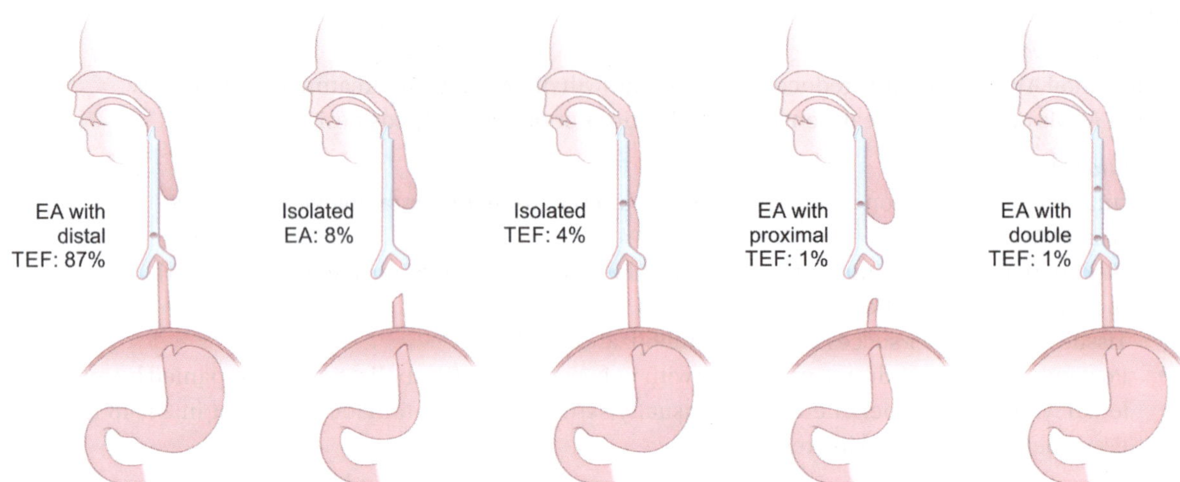

The diagnosis of esophageal atresia and tracheoesophageal fistula is usually made soon after birth, when the affected infant exhibits some form of respiratory distress.

Clinical Features

A. Immediately after birth

- *Excessive salivation and drooling*
  - Baby constantly produces frothy saliva or mucus at mouth and nose.
- *Coughing, choking, and cyanosis during first feed*
  - Due to aspiration of milk into trachea through the fistula.
- *Regurgitation of feeds through nose and mouth*
  - Because esophagus ends in a blind pouch.
- *Inability to pass nasogastric tube into stomach*
  - Tube meets resistance at 10–12 cm from gums.

B. Respiratory Symptoms

- *Choking and coughing on attempted feeding*
- *Cyanotic spells* that improve when feeding is stopped
- *Recurrent aspiration pneumonia*
  - Milk or secretions enter trachea through fistula.
- *Abdominal distension (in EA with distal TEF)*
  - Air passes from trachea to stomach through distal fistula.
- *Scaphoid abdomen (in pure EA without TEF)*
  - No air enters the stomach.

C. General Findings

- *Failure to feed or gain weight*
- *Respiratory distress*
- *Signs of associated anomalies,* especially:
  - Cardiac defects (e.g., VSD, PDA)
  - Renal anomalies
  - Vertebral or limb defects

Physical Examination

- Aspiration of material from the upper pouch causes some symptoms:
  - The infant may appear to be salivating excessively and may drool continuously.
  - The aspiration may also cause coughing spasms, intermittent choking, or cyanosis that develops when the infant is feeding.

- Continuous aspiration of gastric secretions occurs if a fistula is present. This aspiration is more severe and more harmful than that from the upper pouch.
- Tachypnea and signs of pneumonia may develop.
- A scaphoid abdomen due to the unused gastrointestinal tract accompanies pure atresia.
- Attempts to pass a tube through the nose into the stomach will fail, because the tube will stop in the blind pouch of the esophagus, thus confirming the suspicion of esophageal atresia.

Radiographs of Both the Chest and the Abdomen are Important in Order to Make a Diagnosis and to Prepare for Treatment

- The chest film will show the blind upper pouch and also the failure of passage by the gastric tube.
- A gas-free abdomen is characteristic of pure atresia.
- Hyperventilation, atelectasis, or pneumonia must be evaluated so that the proper surgical approach (i.e., immediate vs. delayed repair) can be chosen. Identification of the aortic arch is also necessary for proper surgical management. The use of echocardiography may also assist in determining not only the aortic anatomy but also any associated congenital heart anomalies.
- The length of the esophageal defect can be measured on a lateral film.

Preoperative Management

Several steps should be taken once the diagnosis is made:

- Decompression of the proximal pouch by means of a sump tube with constant suction (Replogle tube) is required.
- An upright position is maintained, using achalasia chair.
- Gastrostomy is performed if delayed repair is chosen.
- This procedure prevents further gastric aspiration.
- It also provides a route for preoperative feedings if surgery is delayed for an extended period.
- Stretching the proximal pouch daily in a pure atresia shortens the distance between the esophageal ends in preparation for eventual repair.

Operative Management

Primary repair at the time of presentation can be undertaken if the defect measures <2 cm and no signs of pneumonitis are present. Delayed repair may be needed if the defect is >2 cm or extends the length of 2½ vertebral bodies. At the time of surgery, the approach is the same for either immediate or delayed repair.

- Broad-spectrum antibiotic therapy is begun.
- If not previously undertaken, a gastrostomy may be performed, although this measure is controversial.
- An extrapleural dissection through the hemithorax opposite the aortic arch is currently favored to prevent empyema from occurring as the result of an anastomotic leak.
- The tracheoesophageal fistula is repaired.
- A primary esophagostomy is performed.
    - The distal esophagus must be carefully dissected because the blood supply is tenuous.
    - An adequate length of esophagus is necessary to create a tension-free anastomosis and is obtained by dissecting the proximal pouch. The use of myotomies may aid in gaining length for closure.
- A drain is placed in the extrapleural space.

Postoperative management is directed at potential pulmonary and esophageal problems.

- The infant is extubated as soon as possible to protect the tracheal repair.
    - Vigorous pulmonary toilet is necessary to clear up any previous pneumonia and to prevent the need for reintubation.
    - Reintubation may disrupt the esophageal repair, the tracheal repair, or both.
    - A degree of tracheal malacia compromises pulmonary function.
    - Chest percussion is mandatory to prevent early postoperative problems.
- The infant is kept upright, because esophageal function will not yet be adequate for swallowing oral secretions.

- Esophagotracheal suction is done carefully and with a specifically defined length of tubing. Disruptions of the esophagus can occur during placement of a suction catheter through the anastomotic line.
- The esophagus is evaluated after 7 days by means of a swallow study.
    - If no leak is present, oral feedings are started; if feedings are tolerated, the extrapleural drain is removed.
    - Before evaluation after 7 days, the gastrostomy (if present) may be used for continuous feedings.

Surgical follow-up is very important. Certain well-recognized problems sometimes develop and they can have a drastic effect on the outcome in these patients.

- Esophageal dysmotility and its concomitant problems are *major* concerns.
    - The patient may develop a dilated proximal pouch with resultant aspiration or tracheal compression.
    - The patient may also have severe gastroesophageal reflux and aspiration.
    - *Anastomotic stricture,* once thought to be solely related to ischemia at the suture line, is now considered to be a consequence of esophagitis from gastroesophageal reflux.
    - If gastroesophageal reflux is implicated in postoperative problems, an antireflux procedure (usually a Nissen fundoplication) is recommended.
    - Recurrent fistulas were formerly considered to be a relatively common potential problem, but in recent studies, they have occurred in. fewer than 10% of patients.
    - The prognosis is related to the size of the patient, the condition of the lungs, and the presence or absence of associated anomalies. Patients have been grouped into three categories:
        1. *Group A—100% survival:* Patients weigh >2,500 g, having no associated anomalies, and having no signs of pneumonitis.
        2. *Group B—80% survival:* Patients having one of the following conditions:
            - Patients weigh 1,800–2,500 g.
            - Patients weigh >2,500 g but have mild pneumonitis.
            - One or more associated anomalies is present but is not life threatening.
        3. *Group C—43% survival:* Patients having one of the following conditions:
            - Patients weigh <1,800 g
            - Patients having severe pneumonitis
            - Patients have a life-threatening anomaly

12. Describe surgical approach to tracheoesophageal fistula (TOF). ***WBUHS 2014***

Principle Objective

Closure of the fistula, maintain airway, and repair esophagus/trachea

Approach: Dependent on fistula size

- Small fistulas—direct suture closure of the membranous trachea and esophagus, interposition of strap muscle.
- Large fistulas—require tracheal resection and concomitant repair of the esophagus
    - Lateral or anterior cervical approach with a low cellar incision
    - Upper sternal spilt if distal exposure to the trachea is necessary
    - Distal tracheal, approach through the right posterolateral thoracotomy

Tracheal Management

- *Most common:* Tracheal resection or membranous tracheal closure
- Standard techniques for resection apply
- Long TEFs—alloderm—to recreate membranous trachea

Esophageal Management

- Small fistulas may be repaired by 1 or 2 layer closure.
- Large fistulas might require end-to-end esophageal anastomosis or fill thickness skin graft.

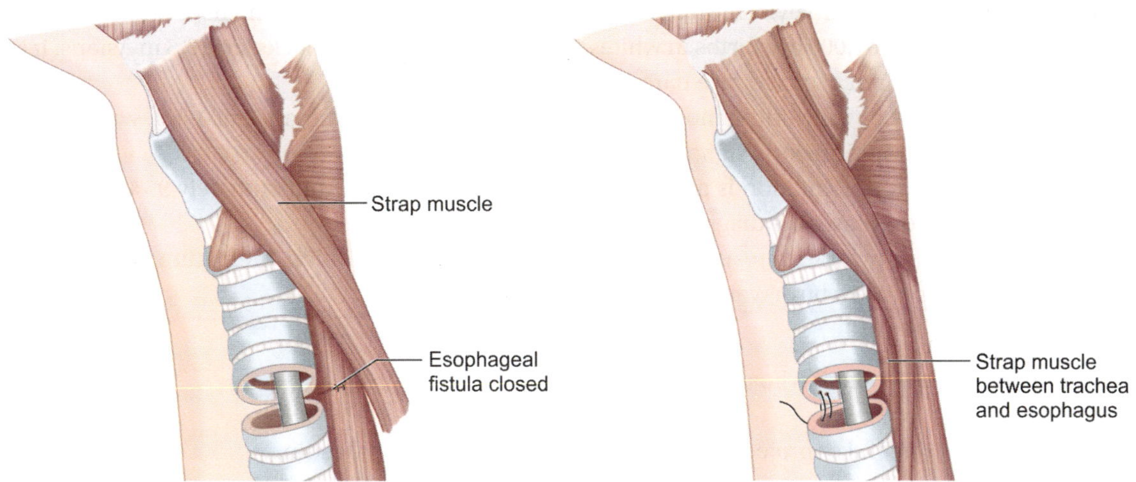

Definitive surgical repair of small tracheoesophageal fistula can be addressed through a lateral cervical approach with mobilization of the trachea and direct suture closure of the membranous trachea and esophagus with interposition of a strap muscle.

INFANTILE HYPERTROPHIC PYLORIC STENOSIS AND BILIARY ATRESIA

13. Infantile Hypertrophic pyloric stenosis. ***AIIMS, Bhopal 2023***

14. Clinical presentation diagnosis and management of congenital hypertrophic pyloric stenosis.
The Tamil Nadu Dr MGR Medical University 2025; WBUHS 2019, RIMS, Imphal 2022

15. Congenital hypertrophic pyloric stenosis.
Maharashtra University of Health Sciences 2025, Rajasthan University of Health Sciences 2025.

16. Clinical presentation diagnosis and management of infantile hypertrophic pyloric stenosis. ***DNB 2021 June***

Introduction

Infantile hypertrophic pyloric stenosis (IHPS) causes a functional gastric outlet obstruction as a result of hypertrophy and hyperplasia of the muscular layers of the pylorus. In infants, hypertrophic pyloric stenosis is the most common cause of gastric outlet obstruction and the most common surgical cause of vomiting.

Pathophysiology

- Marked hypertrophy and hyperplasia of the two (circular and longitudinal) muscular layers of the pylorus occurs, leading to narrowing of the gastric antrum.
- The pyloric canal becomes lengthened, and the whole pylorus becomes thickened.
- The mucosa is usually edematous and thickened. In advanced cases, the stomach becomes markedly dilated in response to near-complete obstruction.
- The causes of infantile hypertrophic pyloric stenosis are multifactorial.
- Both environmental factors and hereditary factors are believed to be contributory. Possible etiologic factors include deficiency of nitric oxide synthase containing neurons, abnormal myenteric plexus innervation, infantile hypergastrinemia, exposure to macrolide antibiotics, lack of exposure to vasoactive intestinal peptide in breast milk, and hypersensitivity to motilin.

Epidemiology

- The incidence of infantile hypertrophic pyloric stenosis is 2–4 per 1,000 live births.
- *Mortality/morbidity:* Death from infantile hypertrophic pyloric stenosis is rare and unexpected.

- *Race:* Infantile hypertrophic pyloric stenosis is more common in whites than Hispanics, Blacks, or Asians. The incidence is 2.4 per 1,000 live births in whites, 1.8 in Hispanics, 0.7 in blacks, and 0.6 in Asians. It is also less common among children of mixed race parents.
- *Sex:* Infantile hypertrophic pyloric stenosis has a male-to-female predominance of 4–5:1, with 30% of patients with infantile hypertrophic pyloric stenosis being first-born males.
- *Age:* The usual age of presentation is approximately 2–6 weeks of life. Approximately 95% of infantile hypertrophic pyloric stenosis cases are diagnosed in those aged 3–12 weeks.
- Infantile hypertrophic pyloric stenosis is rare in premature infants. In addition, premature infants have a delayed diagnosis secondary to low birth weight and atypical presentation.

Clinical Presentation

- Occurs generally in neonates who are 2–5 weeks of age
- Vomiting
- Characteristically forceful or projectile and occurs 30–60 minutes after feeding.
- Formula intolerance initially suspected but does not resolve with change of feeds
- The "olive" mass:
  - Mass palpated to the right and above the umbilicus
  - Approximately 2 cm in diameter, firm, and mobile

Laboratory Studies

- Electrolytes, pH, blood urea nitrogen (BUN), and creatinine levels should be obtained at the same time as intravenous access in patients with pyloric stenosis.
- Hypochloremic, hypokalemic metabolic alkalosis is the classic electrolyte and acid–base imbalance of pyloric stenosis. This constellation of electrolyte abnormalities is now present in <50% of cases given the prompt and timely diagnosis of most infants with pyloric stenosis. However, delayed presentations, or missed cases may lead to persistent emesis. This prolonged vomiting causes progressive loss of fluids rich in hydrochloric acid, which causes the kidneys to retain hydrogen ions in favor of potassium.
- The dehydration may result in hypernatremia or hyponatremia and may result in prerenal renal failure.
- Elevated unconjugated bilirubin levels may be present.

Imaging Studies

Diagnosis

Abdominal ultrasonography:

- Pyloric diameter >14 mm
- Macular thickness >4 mm
- Pyloric length >16 mm is diagnostic of pyloric stenosis.

Upper GI contrast study:

- Enlarged stomach
- Poor gastric emptying
- Elongated, narrow pyloric channel or "string sign"

Management

- *Preoperative fluid resuscitation:*
  - 20-mL/kg bolus
  - 5% dextrose in normal saline to achieve urine output of 2 mL/kg/h
  - Addition of potassium and changing to 5% dextrose in 0.45% normal saline occurs when urine output is adequate
- Correction of the hypochloremic hypokalemic metabolic alkalosis
- Operative intervention

- Indicated only after adequate resuscitation and correction of metabolic alkalosis
- Pyloromyotomy
- *Ramsted's pyloromyotomy is the treatment of choice:*
  - Division of the hypertrophied pyloric muscle, leaving the mucosa intact
  - Open or laparoscopic technique
- *Postoperative feeding:*
  - Begin electrolyte solution by mouth 6 hours after pyloromyotomy.
  - Over the next 12 hours, formula or pumped breast milk can be started and should reach goal within 24 hours.
  - Parents should be advised that vomiting may occur postoperatively as a result of swelling at the pyloromyotomy, but this problem is self-limited.
  - If the pyloric mucosa is perforated and repaired during surgery, nasogastric drainage recommended for 24 hours.

17. Describe biliary atresia. ***WBUHS 2009***

Introduction

- Most common cause of infantile jaundice that requires surgical correction.
- Etiology is unknown.
- Disease characteristics:
  - Progressive obliteration and sclerosis of the biliary tree
  - With age, obliteration of the extrahepatic bile ducts, proliferation of the intrahepatic bile ducts, and liver fibrosis progress at an unpredictable rate.

There are variants of BA ranging from fibrosis of the distal bile ducts with:

- Proximal patency (5%, considered correctable form)
- Fibrosis of the proximal bile ducts with distal patency (15%), or fibrosis of both proximal and distal bile ducts (80%).

Diagnosis

- Clinical and laboratory information is often nonspecific.
- Jaundice
- Alcoholic stools
- Dark urine
- Hepatomegaly

A serum direct bilirubin level of >2.0 mg/dL or >15% of the total bilirubin level defines cholestasis.

In addition to a careful history and physical examination, the following investigations are done:

- Blood and urine are obtained for bacterial and viral cultures.
- Reducing substances in the urine to rule out galactosemia
- Serum immunoglobulin M (IgM) titers for syphilis
- Cytomegalovirus, herpes, and hepatitis B
- Serum a_1-antitrypsin level and phenotype
- Serum thyroxine level
- Sweat chloride test done to exclude cystic fibrosis
- Percutaneous liver biopsy: Biopsy results range from classic biliary tree fibrosis to those unable to be differentiated from α1-antitrypsin deficiency or neonatal hepatitis.
- Technetium-99m iminodiacetic acid hepatobiliary imaging aids in differentiation between liver parenchymal disease and biliary obstructive disease. In biliary atresia, the liver readily takes up this tracer molecule, but no excretion into the extrahepatic biliary system or duodenum is seen.
- Ultrasonography: Shrunken extrahepatic ducts and a noncontractile or absent gallbladder

Management

- *Diagnosis:*
  - *Open liver biopsy and cholangiogram:*
  - The common bile duct is visualized by cholangiography in only 25% of patients with biliary atresia.
  - Cholangiography in the remaining 75% of patients demonstrates an atresia biliary tree.
- *Operative intervention:*
  - *Kasai procedure:*
  - "Hepatoportoenterostomy"
  - Excision of obliterated extrahepatic ducts with hepaticojejunostomy
  - When the distal common bile duct is patent, a choledochojejunostomy is constructed.
  - The overall results have shown that in children treated with a Kasai procedure, one-third show long-term improvement, one-third obtain temporary benefit, and one-third experience treatment failure.
  - *Postoperative management:*
    - Postoperatively, the use of oral choleretic bile salts such as ursodeoxycholic acid may facilitate bile flow.
    - In addition, methylprednisolone is employed as an anti-inflammatory agent.
    - Trimethoprim sulfamethoxazole is administered for long-term antimicrobial prophylaxis.
    - Cholangitis is a serious but common problem after hepatoportoenterostomy. Episodes of cholangitis are managed by hospitalization, rehydration, broad-spectrum IV antibiotics, steroids, and occasionally surgical exploration of the portoenterostomy.
  - *Liver transplant (living donor liver transplant is preferable):* Definitive management

INTESTINAL ATRESIAS

18. Intestinal Atresias. ***Ayush University Chhattisgarh 2025***

Intestinal atresias are *congenital obstructions of the intestinal lumen* caused by an absence or closure (atresia) of a portion of the intestine. They prevent the normal passage of intestinal contents and are a major cause of neonatal intestinal obstruction.

Classification by Location

Type	*Site*	*Common features*
Duodenal atresia	Duodenum (usually distal to ampulla of Vater)	"Double bubble" sign on X-ray, bilious vomiting, associated with Down syndrome
Jejunal atresia	Jejunum	Multiple air-fluid levels, "triple bubble," may have *apple-peel* (Christmas tree) appearance
Ileal atresia	Ileum	Distended abdomen, meconium ileus differential
Colonic atresia	Colon	Distention, failure to pass meconium, less common

Types (Pathologic Classification)

Based on Gross' classification:

Type	*Description*
Type I	Mucosal web or membrane; bowel continuity intact, but lumen obstructed
Type II	Two blind ends connected by a fibrous cord; mesentery intact
Type IIIa	Two blind ends separated by a mesenteric defect
Type IIIb ("Apple-peel" or "Christmas tree")	Jejunal atresia with distal small bowel coiled around a single artery
Type IV	Multiple atresias → "string of sausages" appearance

Pathogenesis

- *Vascular accident theory* (most accepted for jejunoileal atresia): intrauterine ischemia → necrosis → resorption → atresia.
- *Failure of recanalization* (duodenal atresia): occurs during embryonic development (around 8–10 weeks gestation).

Clinical Features

- *Bilious vomiting* (if obstruction distal to ampulla of Vater)
- *Abdominal distention*
- *Failure to pass meconium*
- *Antenatal findings:* Polyhydramnios, dilated bowel loops on fetal ultrasound

Diagnosis

- *Antenatal ultrasound:* polyhydramnios, dilated proximal bowel.
- *Plain abdominal X-ray:*
    - *Duodenal atresia:* "double bubble" (stomach + duodenum)
    - *Jejunoileal atresia:* multiple air-fluid levels; no gas distally
- **Contrast enema:** to delineate distal bowel and confirm diagnosis.

Management

I. Initial Stabilization

- Nasogastric tube decompression
- IV fluids and electrolyte correction
- Broad-spectrum antibiotics

II. Definitive Surgical Repair

- *Duodenal atresia:* Duodenoduodenostomy (side-to-side anastomosis)
- *Jejunoileal atresia:* Resection of atretic segment + end-to-end anastomosis
- *Colonic atresia:* Resection and primary anastomosis or temporary colostomy (depending on condition)

III. Postoperative Care

- Parenteral nutrition until bowel function returns
- Gradual introduction of enteral feeds

Associated Anomalies

- *Duodenal atresia:* ~30–40% associated with *Down syndrome (Trisomy 21)*, annular pancreas, cardiac defects.
- *Jejunoileal atresia:* Less commonly associated with chromosomal anomalies but may occur with *cystic fibrosis* or gastroschisis.

Prognosis

- Excellent with early diagnosis and surgical correction.
- Mortality mainly related to *prematurity, associated anomalies or short bowel syndrome* (if large resection required).

ABDOMINAL WALL DEFECT

19. Discuss the pediatric abdominal wall defects with its embryology with the specific emphasis on omphalocele and gastroschisis. ***WBUHS 2022***

Gastrointestinal Development in Utero

- *3rd week:* Rapid growth of ectoderm and mesoderm leads to ventral folding of the embryo around endoderm. This process involves four body walls: cranial, caudal, and two lateral, which normally approximate to form the umbilical ring.

- *6th week:* Physiologic herniation of the midgut through the umbilical ring, intestinal rotation counterclockwise 270°
- *10th week:* Spontaneous reduction of herniation

The two types of abdominal wall defects are gastroschisis and omphalocele.
Although the abdominal contents are located outside of the peritoneal cavity in each type, the similarities (both developmental and therapeutic) end at that point.

Gastroschisis is an opening in the abdominal wall, immediately adjacent to the right of the umbilicus, which is located in the normal position.

- During fetal development, the abdominal wall is completely formed, but the peritoneal cavity does not enlarge enough to hold the abdominal contents.
- The protruding viscera, which consist of the mid portion of the small intestine, the spleen, the stomach, the colon, and occasionally the liver, has no protective covering. The intestine is edematous, semi-rigid, leathery, and matted together as a result of chemical peritonitis.
- Associated anomalies and syndromes are rare, and intestinal atresia is the most frequent (10% of cases) anomaly.

Omphalocele is an opening in the abdominal wall at the umbilicus.

- It is caused by incomplete closure of the somatic folds of the anterior abdominal wall in the fetus.
- Unless ruptured, a sac covers the extruded visceral contents, and no signs of chemical peritonitis appear. The liver and small bowel are the organs that most commonly protrude through the defect.
- The omphalocele may be a part of the pentalogy of Cantrell, which also includes:
  - Diaphragmatic hernia
  - Cleft sternum
  - Absent pericardium
  - Intracardiac defects
- If the caudal folds are involved, exstrophy of the bladder or cloacal exstrophy is present.
- *Associated anomalies:* Approximately 50% of these infants have one or more associated anomalies, including trisomies 13 and 18; Beckwith's syndrome; and cardiac, neurologic, and genitourinary malformations.

Prenatal diagnosis may be made by the use of ultrasonography. This visualization of deep structures aids in the diagnosis of associated anomalies and in prenatal counseling as well as in early postdelivery management.

Preoperative management is similar in both disorders.

- Gastrointestinal decompression, intravenous fluids, and antibiotics are instituted.
- Protection of the abdominal contents is imperative, especially because the escape of moisture and heat is considerable in these patients.
  - The unruptured omphalocele is left intact and protected with a sterile dressing to prevent it from drying out.
  - Gastroschisis or a ruptured omphalocele is protected under a plastic covering (intestinal bag).
- When the patient with gastroschisis has a small defect and a swollen intestine, kinking of the vascular supply may occur at the edge of the defect. This vascular compromise may be prevented by placing the infant on his or her side. Occasionally, emergent enlargement of the defect may be necessary to protect the blood supply to the intestine.
- The outcome of gastroschisis is related to the condition of the intestines at the time of surgery.

Operative management differs slightly for the two disorders. However, the goal in both conditions is to cover the abdominal viscera either with prosthetic material or with the abdominal wall itself.

Gastroschisis: Closure is emergent, as there is no covering over the gastrointestinal tract to prevent heat and fluid losses. Primary closure involves decompressing the gastrointestinal tract and stretching the abdominal wall over the defect.

If the closure is too tight, the blood supply to the intestine, abdominal wall, or lower extremities is compromised. To avoid this complication, it is better to cover the exposed organs temporarily with prosthetic materials.

- Preconstructed silicon ventral wall defect silo bags are now available for staged closure. They eliminate suture lines that leak, and they also have a spring anchoring device for ease of application.
- Reduction can now usually be completed by days 5–7, thus minimizing the risk of infection. A nasogastric tube is placed for decompression with either method of treatment.

Omphalocele: A ruptured omphalocele, like a gastroschisis, must be covered emergently. If the sac is intact, workup for associated defects such as a cardiac anomaly can be performed.

The choice of procedures includes primary closure, staged repair, or, for an unruptured omphalocele, nonoperative management. The important factor is the size of the defect.

The greater the size of the defect, the less the peritoneal cavity has enlarged with adequate musculature of the abdominal wall; with a large defect, primary closure may involve too much tension.

- An alternative method of treatment is to cover the defect with skin flaps, leaving the resultant ventral hernia to be repaired later on.
- Silastic sheeting or preconstructed silo bags can be used to stage the repair; by keeping tension on the prosthetic sac, the Silastic sheet stretches the abdominal wall enough to accommodate the herniated viscera.
- As with a staged repair of gastroschisis, closure is usually accomplished within 10 days.
- A prosthetic material such as Alloderm can be used to close the defect.

Nonoperative management is an alternative in patients with associated anomalies.

- The sac is coated with silver sulfadiazine (Silvadene).
- An eschar forms with subsequent coverage by granulation tissue.
- The resultant ventral hernia can be repaired later on.
- The risks associated with this method are rupture of the sac, requiring subsequent repair in an infected area, sepsis, undiagnosed intestinal atresia, and prolonged hospitalization.
- As with gastroschisis, a nasogastric tube is placed for decompression.

Postoperative Management

- With primary closure, respiration may be inhibited if the reduced abdominal contents compress the diaphragm. Patients may require muscular paralysis and mechanical ventilation until the abdomen stretches enough to accommodate the viscera.
- Venous return may be compromised owing to compression of the inferior vena cava.
  - For vascular access, upper extremity veins should be used.
  - The legs may show signs of venous obstruction and resultant edema.
- With staged repair, the patient needs to be observed after each daily reduction for both respiratory compromise and decreased venous return due to increased abdominal pressure.
- Patients require hyperalimentation with both primary and staged repairs, because intestinal motility and absorption are slow to return.
- After an unruptured omphalocele has been repaired, intestinal function is not as delayed as gastroschisis; however, hyperalimentation may still be needed.

Prognosis

- Gastroschisis, although more difficult to manage initially, has very few long-term problems. Intestinal strictures may occur at the site of evisceration and will require resection later on.
- The mortality rate, approximately 30% in the past, has improved greatly with the use of hyperalimentation and is now approximately 5%. Mortality is related to sepsis and the viability of the gastrointestinal tract at the time of surgery.
- With resection for intestinal gangrene, short-bowel syndrome may develop.
- *Omphalocele:* The outcome for an omphalocele is related to the size and location of the defect.

UMBILICUS

20. Describe causes of discharging lesions of umbilicus.

21. Discuss vitelline duct abnormalities.

Urachal abnormalities	*Vitello intestinal duct abnormalities*	*Inflammatory and related disorders*
• Urachal sinus • Urachal diverticulum • Urachal cyst • Vesicoumbilical fistula • Alternating sinus	• Umbilical adenoma/polyp • Vitelline sinus • Umbilical fistula	• Umbilical granuloma • Omphalitis

Vitelline duct is connection between midgut and yolk sac.

- Usually involutes in 7th–9th weeks

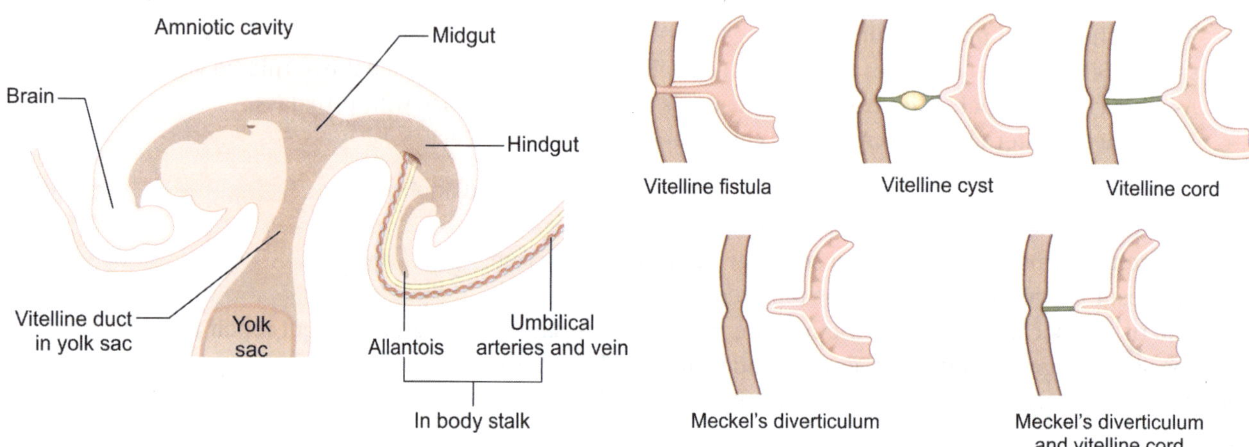

Treatment

- Symptomatic children with vitellointestinal or omphalomesenteric duct remnants should be resuscitated before intervention.
- Those with significant hemorrhage should be transfused. Patients with obstructive symptoms should be resuscitated as rapidly as possible to obviate the need for ischemic bowel resection.
- The incision chosen varies with the symptoms and the age of the patient. Children with feculent umbilical drainage or prolapse of the omphalomesenteric duct remnant can be explored by a small infraumbilical incision.
- When connected to the ileum, a patent vitellointestinal duct may have a wide lumen or be a high-output fistula. This may lead to fluid and electrolyte deficits, especially in neonates, and treatment should be expeditious. The treatment of a patent vitellointestinal is wedge or segmental resection.
- Children with Meckel's diverticulitis or a bleeding Meckel's diverticulum are operated on by using a transverse appendectomy incision with medial extension if necessary.
- Patients with suspected intestinal obstruction should be explored through a generous laparotomy incision.

22. Describe Meckel's diverticulum. *WBUHS 2009, The Tamil Nadu Dr MGR Medical University 2025*

Incidence and Etiology

- Meckel's diverticulum is the most commonly encountered congenital anomaly of the small intestine, occurring in about 2% of the population.
- Meckel's diverticulum is located on the antimesenteric border of the ileum 45–60 cm proximal to the ileocecal valve.
- It results from incomplete closure of the omphalomesenteric or vitelline duct.

- An equal incidence is found among men and women.
- Meckel's diverticulum may exist in different forms, ranging from a small bump that may be easily missed to a long projection that communicates with the umbilicus by a persistent fibrous cord or, much less commonly, a patent fistula. The usual manifestation is a relatively wide-mouth diverticulum measuring about 5 cm in length, with a diameter of up to 2 cm. Cells lining the vitelline duct are pluripotent; therefore, it is not uncommon to find heterotopic tissue within the Meckel's diverticulum, the most common of which is gastric mucosa (present in 50% of all Meckel's diverticula). Pancreatic mucosa is encountered in about 5% of diverticula; less commonly, these diverticula may harbor colonic mucosa.

Clinical Manifestations

- Most Meckel's diverticula are entirely benign and are incidentally discovered during autopsy, laparotomy, or barium studies.
- The most common clinical presentation of Meckel's diverticulum is gastrointestinal bleeding, which occurs in 25–50% of patients who present with complications. Hemorrhage is the most common symptomatic presentation in children aged 2 years or younger. The usual source of the bleeding is a chronic acid-induced ulcer in the ileum adjacent to a Meckel's diverticulum that contains gastric mucosa.
- Diverticulum associated with a fibrotic band attached to the abdominal wall, intussusception, or, rarely, incarceration of the diverticulum in an inguinal hernia (Littre's hernia).
- Volvulus is usually an acute event and, if allowed to progress, may result in strangulation of the involved bowel.
- In intussusception, a broad-based diverticulum invaginates and then is carried forward by peristalsis. This may be ileoileal or ileocolic and present as acute obstruction associated with an urge to defecate, early vomiting, and, occasionally, the passage of the classic currant-jelly stool. A palpable mass may be present. Although reduction of an intussusception secondary to Meckel's diverticulum can sometimes be performed by barium enema, the patient should still undergo resection of the diverticulum to negate subsequent recurrence of the condition.
- Diverticulitis accounts for 10–20% of symptomatic presentations. This complication is more common in adult patients. Meckel's diverticulitis, which is clinically indistinguishable from appendicitis, should be considered in the differential diagnosis of a patient with right lower quadrant pain. Progression of the diverticulitis may lead to perforation and peritonitis.
- Finally, much rarer complications of Meckel's diverticula include neoplasms, with the most common benign tumors reported as leiomyomas, angiomas, and lipomas. Malignant neoplasms include adenocarcinomas, which commonly originate from the gastric mucosa, sarcoma, and carcinoid tumor.

Diagnostic Studies

- The diagnosis of Meckel's diverticulum may be difficult.
- Plain abdominal radiographs, CT, and ultrasonography are rarely helpful.
- In children, the single most accurate diagnostic test for Meckel's diverticula is scintigraphy with sodium ^{99m}Tc-pertechnetate. The ^{99m}Tc-pertechnetate is preferentially taken up by the mucus-secreting cells of gastric mucosa and ectopic gastric tissue in the diverticulum.
- In adults, ^{99m}Tc-pertechnetate scanning is less accurate because of the reduced prevalence of ectopic gastric mucosa within the diverticulum. The sensitivity and specificity can be improved by the use of pharmacologic agents such as pentagastrin and glucagon or histamine-2 (H_2)-receptor antagonists (e.g., cimetidine).
- In adult patients, when nuclear medicine findings are normal, barium studies should be performed.
- In patients with acute hemorrhage, angiography is sometimes useful.

Treatment

- The treatment of a symptomatic Meckel's diverticulum should be prompt surgical intervention with resection of the diverticulum or resection of the segment of ileum bearing the diverticulum.
- Segmental intestinal resection is required for treatment of patients with bleeding because the bleeding site usually is in the ileum adjacent to the diverticulum.

- It is generally recommended that asymptomatic diverticula found in children during laparotomy have to be resected. The treatment of Meckel's diverticula encountered in the adult patient, however, remains controversial.
- The recommendation is that an incidentally found Meckel's diverticulum should be removed at any age up to 80 years as long as no additional conditions (e.g., peritonitis) made removal hazardous.

MALROTATION OF GUT AND MIDGUT VOLVULUS

23. Discuss malrotation of gut.

Malrotation and Volvulus

Key Facts and Clinical Features (Neonates)

Malrotation:

- This can present at birth or soon after and symptoms are due to rotation of the small bowel leading to duodenal obstruction. Intestine fails to undergo its normal rotation and fixation during embryologic development.
- Ladd's bands are occasionally the cause of the obstruction.
- Proximal duodenal distension leads to bile-stained vomiting.
- The cecum may be in an abnormally high or midline position.
- Incidence 1/500 to 1/6,000 live births
- Associated anomalies are present in 30–59% of patients.

Volvulus:

- Twisting, in clockwise direction, of malrotated, non-fixed midgut loop on its narrow-based mesentery through 360° or more.
- Results in obstruction of superior mesenteric blood vessels
- *Signs:* Sudden onset of abdominal pain; bile-vomiting; progression to shock; passage of blood per rectum.
- *May be less dramatic:* Most dangerous in newborn period because of delay in diagnosis and rapid development of gut ischemia
- Older children may present insidiously or as rapid onset of shock with less prominent other symptoms

Diagnosis and Investigations

History and Physical Examination

- Bilious emesis
- Hematemesis
- Abdominal distention
- Abdominal tenderness
- Hematochezia

If in doubt operate, viability of twisted bowel is very time-dependent delays in diagnosis can be very serious.

- *Plain abdominal X-ray:* Double bubble sign with some distal gas
- *Barium meal:* Obstruction of second part duodenum, nonrotation of duodenum/jejunum, and corkscrew appearance of proximal small bowel loops; absent C loop of duodenum.
- *Ultrasound scan:* Reversed relation of superior mesenteric artery and vein
- *Doppler ultrasound:* Absent or abnormal small bowel blood

Treatment

- Resuscitation including decompression with nasogastric tube
- Prompt surgery to avoid irreversible bowel damage
- Laparotomy may reveal:
    - Obstructed but viable bowel
    - Patchy ischemic changes
    - Established necrosis

- Resection of ischemic gut may risk short gut syndrome. Second look laparotomy (24–48 hours) allows reassessment prior to resection.

24. Describe intussusceptions in a child. *RIMS, Imphal Manipur 2012*

Introduction

- Intussusception is a serious disorder in which part of the intestine—either the small intestine or colon—slides into another part of the intestine. This "telescoping" often blocks the intestine, preventing food or fluid from passing through. Intussusception also cuts off the blood supply to the part of the intestine that is affected.
- Intussusception is the most common cause of intestinal obstruction in children. Intussusception is rare in adults. Most cases of adult intussusception are the result of an underlying medical condition. In contrast, most cases of intussusception in children have no demonstrable cause.

Intussusception

- Occurs most often in babies between 5 and 10 months of age (80% of cases occur before a child is 24 months old)
- Affects between 1 and 4 infants out of 1,000
- Is more common in boys than in girls
- With prompt attention, intussusception can often be successfully treated without lasting problems.

Causes

For most cases of intussusception in children, the cause is unknown. Possible triggers may be:

- Viral infection
- A noncancerous growth or a cancerous tumor in the intestine
- Meckel's diverticulum
- Polyp
- Duplication
- Appendix
- Hyperplasia of Peyer's patches
- Idiopathic

Risk Factors

- *Age:* Children are much more likely to develop intussusception than adults are. It is the most common cause of bowel obstruction in children between the ages of 3 months and 6 years, with the majority of cases occurring in children <1 year.
- *Sex:* Intussusception affects boys more often than girls.
- *Abnormal intestinal formation at birth:* Malrotation, a condition present at birth (congenital) in which the intestine does not develop correctly, also is a risk factor for intussusception.
- *A prior history of intussusception*

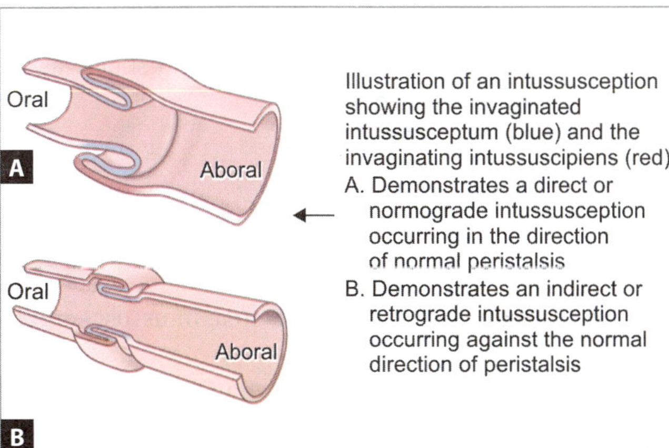

Illustration of an intussusception showing the invaginated intussusceptum (blue) and the invaginating intussuscipiens (red)
A. Demonstrates a direct or normograde intussusception occurring in the direction of normal peristalsis
B. Demonstrates an indirect or retrograde intussusception occurring against the normal direction of peristalsis

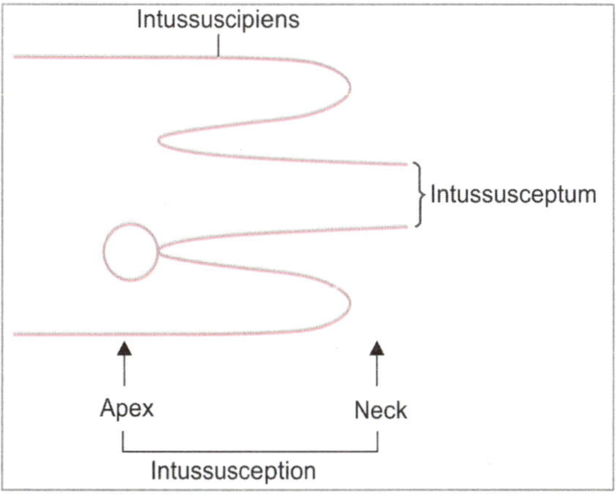

Classification

- *Ileoileal:* 5%
- *Ileocolic:* 77%
- *Ileo-ileo-colic:* 12%
- *Colocolic:* 2%
- *Multiple:* 1%
- *Retrograde:* 0.2%
- *Others:* 2.8%

Symptoms

Children: Signs and symptoms of intussusception in children include—

- Severe abdominal pain that comes and goes (intermittent pain)
- Stool mixed with blood and mucus (sometimes referred to as "currant jelly" stool because of its appearance
- A lump in the abdomen
- Swollen (distended) abdomen
- Vomiting, possibly vomiting bile (yellow-brown or greenish fluid)
- Diarrhea
- Fever
- Dehydration
- Lethargy
- The first sign of intussusception in an otherwise healthy infant may be sudden, loud crying caused by abdominal pain. Infants who have abdominal pain may pull their knees to their chests when they cry. The pain of intussusception comes and goes, usually every 15–20 minutes at first. These painful episodes last longer and happen more often as time passes.

Complications

- Intussusception can cut off the blood supply to the affected portion of the intestine. If left untreated, lack of blood causes tissue of the intestinal wall to die.
- Tissue death can lead to a tear (perforation) in the intestinal wall, which can cause peritonitis, an infection of the lining of the abdominal cavity.
- Peritonitis is a life-threatening condition that requires immediate medical attention.

Tests and Diagnosis

- Physical examination
- Blood or urine tests
- Ultrasound or other abdominal imaging
- Air or barium enema

Treatments

Emergency medical care is required to treat intussusception to avoid severe dehydration and shock, as well as prevent infection that can occur when a portion of intestine dies due to lack of blood.

Initial Care

- Intravenous (IV) fluids
- Nasogastric tube

Correcting the Intussusception

- *A barium or air enema:* This can correct the telescoping intestine and successfully treat intussusception. If an enema works, further treatment is usually not necessary.
- *Surgery:* In some cases, intussusception may be temporary and improve on its own without treatment. If no underlying medical condition is found that caused the intussusception, no further treatment is necessary.

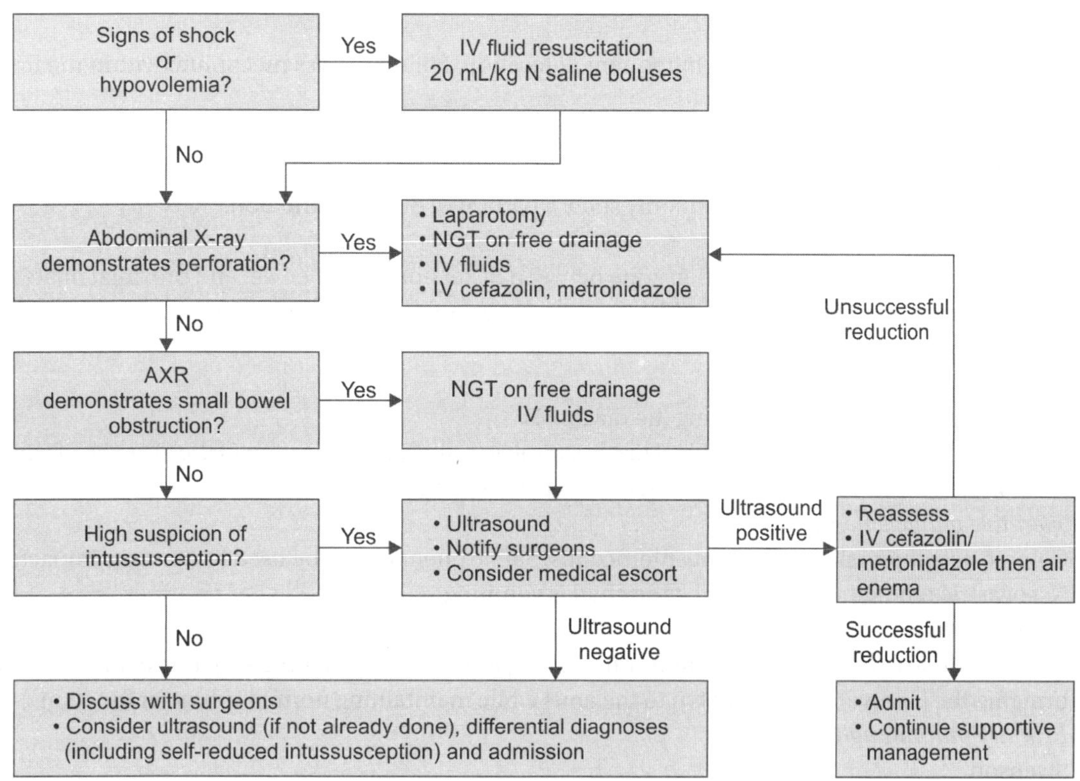

(IV: intravenous; NGT: nasogastric tube)

HIRSCHSPRUNG'S DISEASE AND CONGENITAL MEGACOLON

25. Describe Hirschsprung's disease. ***AIIMS, Raipur 2025***

Introduction

- Incidence 1 in 5,000 live births
- Commoner in males

Pathological Features

- Due to incomplete migration of neural crest cells into the hindgut resulting in distal aganglionosis and failure of coordinated peristaltic waves, abnormal anorectal relaxation, and loss of rectoanal inhibitory reflexes.
- *May involve:*
  - *Just the anorectal junction (ultrashort segment):* Often presents in adult life
  - *The rectum and rectosigmoid (short segment; 70%):* Presents in infancy or early childhood
  - *Extensive colonic involvement (long segment):* Rare
- *The proximal (normal) bowel becomes progressively distended due to buildup of fecal matter.*

Clinical Features

- There is failure to pass meconium within 24–48 hours, abdominal distension, and bile vomiting.

- It may be associated with Down's syndrome.
- It may present late with poor weight gain, offensive diarrhea, or enterocolitis.

Management

- *Diagnosis:*
  - *History:*
  - *Neonates:* Abdominal distention, infrequent defecation, failure to pass meconium within the first 48 hours of life, or enterocolitis with sepsis
  - Older infants and children present with chronic constipation or failure to thrive
  - *Radiology:*
  - Plain abdominal radiographs commonly show a pattern of distal obstruction.
  - *Barium enema:*
    - Usually demonstrates a transition zone between distal nondilated bowel and proximal dilated bowel.
    - Most common in the rectosigmoid, but may be seen anywhere in the colon.
    - Total colonic aganglionosis: No transition zone
  - *Pathology:*
  - Rectal biopsy is essential for making the diagnosis.
  - Full-thickness specimens are the ideal tissue samples to allow identification of the absence of ganglion cells.
  - In neonates, rectal suction biopsy often is sufficient for diagnosis.
- *Preoperative management:*
  - Colonic decompression to prevent enterocolitis. Saline enemas may be used to evacuate impacted stool.
  - Nasogastric tube should be placed if the child is vomiting.
- *Operative treatment:*
  - Goals of surgical management are removal of aganglionic bowel and reconstruction of the intestinal tract by bringing the innervated bowel down to the anus while maintaining normal sphincter function.
  - *Primary pull-through:*
  - Swenson
  - Duhamel
  - Soave
  - Laparoscopic endorectal pull-through (Georgeson)
  - Transanal endorectal pull-through (Langer)

Each of these operations has been modified to improve functional results and may be performed in the newborn period, although surgery may be delayed to allow for increased weight gain or resolution of enterocolitis.

- *Diverting colostomy:*
  - Performed proximal to aganglionic segment in patients who are unstable or who have massively dilated bowel.
  - Daily rectal irrigations may obviate the need for a colostomy.
- Currently, several different surgical approaches are used, which include the Swenson, Soave, Duhamel, and Boley procedures. The Swenson procedure leaves a small portion of the diseased bowel. The Soave procedure leaves the outer wall of the colon unaltered.
- The Boley procedure is a small modification of the Soave procedure, so the term "Soave-Boley" procedure is sometimes used. The Duhamel procedure uses a surgical stapler to connect the good and bad bowel.
  - For the 15% of children who do not obtain full bowel control, other treatments are available. Constipation may be remedied by laxatives or a high-fiber diet. In those patients, serious dehydration can play a major factor in their lifestyles. A lack of bowel control may be addressed by a stoma, similar to a colostomy.
  - If the affected portion of the lower intestine is restricted to the lower portion of the rectum, other surgical procedures may be performed, such as a posterior rectal myectomy.

Prognosis

- The prognosis is good in 70% of cases.
- Chronic postoperative constipation is present in 7–8% of the operated cases.
- Postoperative enterocolitis, a severe manifestation, is present in the 10–20% of operated patients.

26. Discuss congenital megacolon.

27. Describe the symptomatology and management of congenital megacolon. ***WBUHS 2023***

Introduction

- It is a developmental disorder characterized by the absence of ganglia in the distal colon, resulting in a functional obstruction.
- It is a rare condition similar to Hirschsprung's disease where abnormalities in the bowel muscles prevent it from contracting normally and pushing the fecal matter through.
- Congenital megacolon differs from Hirschsprung's disease in that the whole colon tends to be dilated.
- An infant with congenital megacolon is born with a rectum and colon that do not work properly because the nerves that stimulate the bowel are absent.
- Congenital megacolon causes dilation of the colon and rectum, as well as a build-up of stool in the colon and rectum.
- Congenital megacolon is usually inherited and may be associated with Down's syndrome.

Clinical Features

Signs and symptoms of congenital megacolon are as follows:

Constipation from birth	Blood-streaked stool	Intestinal colic	Short anal canal	Enlargement of colon
Large stool	Difficult bowel movements	Distended abdomen	Dilated rectum	Gas
Hard stool	Painful bowel movements	Palpable fecal masses	Dilated pelvic colon	Stomach noises

Conditions Mimicking Congenital Megacolon

- Hirschsprung's disease
- Intestinal immotility
- Intestinal obstruction
- Meconium
- Constipation

Complications of congenital megacolon include:

- Bacterial enterocolitis
- Intestinal perforation
- Gastrointestinal bleeding

Tests that may be used to evaluate congenital megacolon include:

- *Barium enema X-ray:* Can show findings of this condition
- *Intestinal biopsy:* Needed to confirm the diagnosis of congenital megacolon

Treatment for congenital megacolon may include:

- Intravenous fluids for dehydration
- Enemas for congenital megacolon
- Surgery for congenital megacolon:

- Resection anastomosis with or without colostomy
- Colostomy
- Swenson, Soave, Duhamel, and Boley procedures

ANORECTAL MALFORMATIONS

28. Classify anorectal malformations. Discuss investigations and management of various anorectal malformations. ***WBUHS 2016***

29. Describe imperforate anus.

Anorectal Embryology

- By 6 weeks of gestation, the urorectal septum moves caudally to divide the cloaca into the anterior urogenital sinus and posterior anorectal canal. Failure of this septum to form results in a fistula between the bowel and urinary tract (in boys) or the vagina (in girls).
- Complete or partial failure of the anal membrane to resorb results in an anal membrane or stenosis.
- The perineum also contributes to development of the external anal opening and genitalia by formation of cloacal folds, which extend from the anterior genital tubercle to the anus. The perineal body is formed by fusion of the cloacal folds between the anal and urogenital membranes.
- Breakdown of the cloacal membrane anywhere along its course results in the external anal opening being anterior to the external sphincter (i.e., anteriorly displaced anus).

Etiology

- Incidence ranges from 1 in 4,000 to 5,000 live births
- Slightly more common in boys
- The most common defect is an imperforate anus with a fistula between the distal colon and the urethra in boys or the vestibule of the vagina in girls.

Classification of congenital anomalies of the anorectum.

	Female	*Male*
High	• Anorectal agenesis with or without rectovaginal fistula • Rectal atresia	• Anorectal agenesis with or without rectoprostatic urethral fistula • Rectal atresia
Intermediate	• Anorectal agenesis with or without rectovaginal fistula • Anal agenesis	• Anorectal agenesis with or without rectobulbar urethral fistula • Anal agenesis
Low	• Anovestibular or anocutaneous fistula (anteriorly displaced anus) • Anal stenosis	• Anocutaneous fistula (anteriorly displaced anus) • Anal stenosis
Cloaca		

Classification as per therapeutic and prognostic point of view.

Male	*Female*

• Cutaneous (perineal fistula)
• Rectourethral fistula:
  – Bulbar
  – Prostatic
• Recto-bladder neck fistula
• Imperforate anus without fistula
• Rectal atresia
	• Cutaneous (perineal fistula)
	• Vestibular fistula
	• Imperforate anus without fistula
	• Rectal atresia
	• Cloaca
	• Complex malformations

- Rectal atresia refers to an unusual lesion in which the lumen of the rectum is either completely or partially interrupted, with the upper rectum being dilated and the lower rectum consisting of a small anal canal.
- A persistent cloaca is defined as a defect in which the rectum, vagina, and urethra all meet and fuse to form a single, common channel.
- In girls, the type of defect may be determined by the number of orifices at the perineum. A single orifice would be consistent with a cloaca.
- If two orifices are seen (i.e., urethra and vagina), the defect represents either a high imperforate anus or, less commonly, a persistent urogenital sinus comprising one orifice and a normal anus as the other orifice.

Associated Anomalies

- *Sacrum and spine:* Sacral deformities appear to be the most frequently associated defect.
- *Genitourinary defects:* The frequency of associated genitourinary defects varies from 20 to 54%.
- Anal atresia may occur as a part of the VACTERL group of anomalies:
  V—*V*ertebral body segmentation defect
  A—*A*nal atresia
  C—*C*ardiovascular (PDA and VSD)
  TE—*T*racheoesophageal fistula
  R—Unilateral *R*enal agenesis
  L—*L*imb anomaly (radial ray hypoplasia)
- *Cardiovascular system (CVS):* Tetralogy of Fallot or VSD
- *GI:* Tracheoesophageal abnormality, duodenal atresia, Hirschsprung's disease

Preoperative Evaluation

- Clinical evaluation includes plain radiographs of the spine as well as an ultrasound of the spinal cord.
- Genitourinary abnormalities other than the rectourinary fistula occur in 26–59% of patients.
- Vesicoureteral reflux and hydronephrosis are the most common, but other findings such as horseshoe, dysplastic, or absent kidney, as well as hypospadias or cryptorchidism, also must be considered.
- In general, the higher the anorectal malformation (ARM), the greater the frequency of associated urologic abnormalities
- Radiographic evaluation of the urinary tract includes renal ultrasonography and voiding cystourethrography; a rectourinary fistula (if present) likely will be demonstrated by the latter procedure.
- In addition to the other tests described previously, a plain chest radiograph and careful clinical evaluation of the heart are conducted. If a cardiac defect is suspected, echocardiography is performed before any surgical procedure.
- Before feeding, a nasogastric tube is placed and its presence within the stomach confirmed to exclude esophageal atresia.

Investigations for associated anomalies.

Investigations	*Purpose*
Plain X-ray abdomen in erect posture	To rule out pouch colon
X-ray lumbosacral spine	To rule out spinal (sacral) anomalies
2-D Echo	Cardiac anomaly
USG abdomen and pelvis	Urogenital anomaly
Micturating cystourethrogram (optional at birth, can be done later if needed)	Vesicoureteric reflex

(USG: ultrasonography)

Investigations for boys with anorectal anomalies.

Clinical features	***Investigation***	***Timing***	***Purpose***	***Details***
Absent anus + Bulge in perineum/anal site especially on crying				
Anus present – Perineal fistula/ anal stenosis				
Absent anus + No bulge in anal site on crying ± meconium stained urine ± meconium at the urethral meatus	• Invertogram (not preferred now) • Cross table prone lateral (CTPL) X-ray	• 18–24 hours after birth	• Delineate the level of gas filled rectum which gives information of level of atresia • Decisive for type of surgery	• *Invertogram:* Baby held upside down for 3–5 minutes and then lateral X-ray is taken centered at the greater trochanter • *CTPL:* Prone position with hips and knees flexed at 45° lateral X-ray centered at greater trochanter interpretation

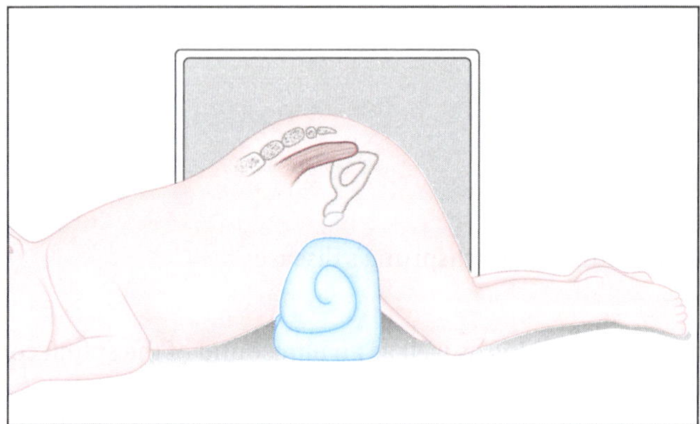

Positioning of the baby for cross table prone lateral X-ray.

Interpretation of invertogram or crossed table posterolateral (CTPL) X-ray.

Investigations for girls with anorectal anomalies.

Clinical features	***Investigation***	***Timing***	***Purpose***
Absent anus + 3 openings in vestibule	–	–	–
Absent anus + 2 openings in vestibule (high anomaly rectovaginal fistula most common)			
Absent anus + single opening in vestibule (cloaca)	Cloacagram + cystovaginoscopy	At birth	To plan for type of surgical intervention, either: a. Primary repair b. Colostomy
Anteposed anus	–	–	–

Low Lesions

The newborn infant with a low lesion can have a primary, single-stage repair procedure without need for a colostomy.

- Three basic approaches may be used. For anal stenosis in which the anal opening is in a normal location, serial dilation alone is usually curative.

- Dilations are performed daily by the caretaker, and the size of the dilator is increased progressively (beginning with 8–9 French and increased slowly to 14–16 French).
- If the anal opening is anterior to the external sphincter (i.e., anteriorly displaced anus) with a small distance between the opening and the center of the external sphincter, and the perineal body is intact, a cutback anoplasty is performed.
- This consists of an incision extending from the ectopic anal orifice to the central part of the anal sphincter, thus enlarging the anal opening.
- Alternatively, if there is a large distance between the anal opening and the central portion of the external anal sphincter, a transposition anoplasty is performed in which the aberrant anal opening is transposed to the normal position within the center of the sphincter muscles, and the perineal body is reconstructed.

High or Intermediate Lesions

Infants with intermediate or high lesions traditionally require a colostomy as the first part of a three-stage reconstruction.

- The colon is completely divided in the sigmoid region, with the proximal bowel as the colostomy and the distal bowel as a mucous fistula.
- Complete division of the bowel minimizes fecal contamination into the area of a rectourinary fistula, and it may lessen the risk for urosepsis.
- Furthermore, the distal bowel can be evaluated radiographically to determine the location of the rectourinary fistula.
- The second-stage procedure usually is performed 3–6 months later and consists of surgically dividing the rectourinary or rectovaginal fistula with pull-through of the terminal rectal pouch into the normal anal position.
- A posterior sagittal approach is the procedure most frequently performed. This consists of determination of the location of the central position of the anal sphincter by electrical stimulation of the perineum.
- An incision is then made in the midline extending from the coccyx to the anterior perineum and through the sphincter and levator musculature until the rectum is identified. The fistula from the rectum to the vagina or urinary tract is divided.
- The rectum is then mobilized and the perineal musculature reconstructed. The third and final stage is closure of the colostomy, which is performed a few months later. Anal dilations are begun 2 weeks after the pull-through procedure and continue for several months after the colostomy closure.

More recently, a single-stage procedure using a transabdominal laparoscopic approach has been described for treatment of intermediate and high imperforate anus anomalies. This technique offers the theoretic advantages of placement of the neorectum within the central position of the sphincter and levator muscle complex under direct vision and avoids the need to cut across these structures. The long-term outcome of this new approach when compared with the standard posterior sagittal method is presently unknown.

- Most of the morbidity in patients with anorectal malformations is related to the presence of associated anomalies.
- Fecal continence is the major goal regarding correction of the defect.
- Prognostic factors for continence include the level of the pouch and whether the sacrum is normal.
- Constipation is the most common sequela.
- A bowel management program consisting of daily enemas is an important postoperative plan to reduce the frequency of soilage and improve the quality of life for these patients.

Algorithm for Management of ARM in Newborn Male

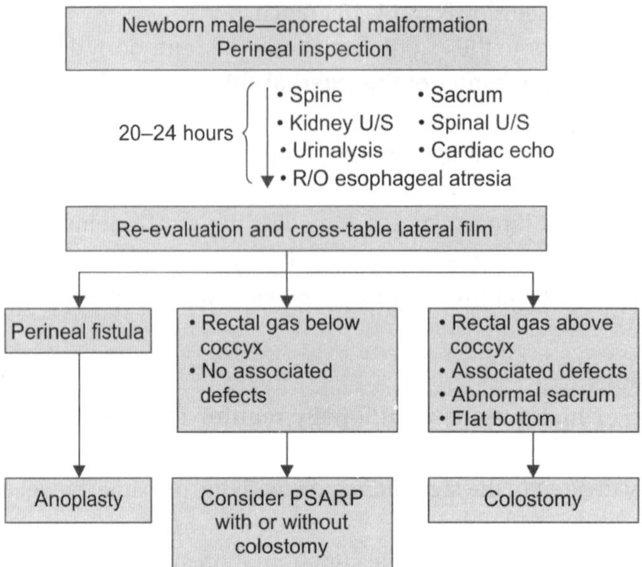

(PSARP: posterior sagittal anorectoplasty)

Posterior sagittal anorectoplasty (PSARP) involves:

- Stimulation of muscles to demonstrate the midline and sphincter
- Posterior sagittal incision—length depends on severity of abnormality and required extent of dissection
- Rectum identified. Abdominal approach may be required in addition in 10% of males and 40% of cloacae
- Rectum dissected
- Separation from genitourinary tract—often the most difficult part
- Repositioning the neoanus within the sphincteric mechanism

Algorithm for Management of ARM in Newborn Female

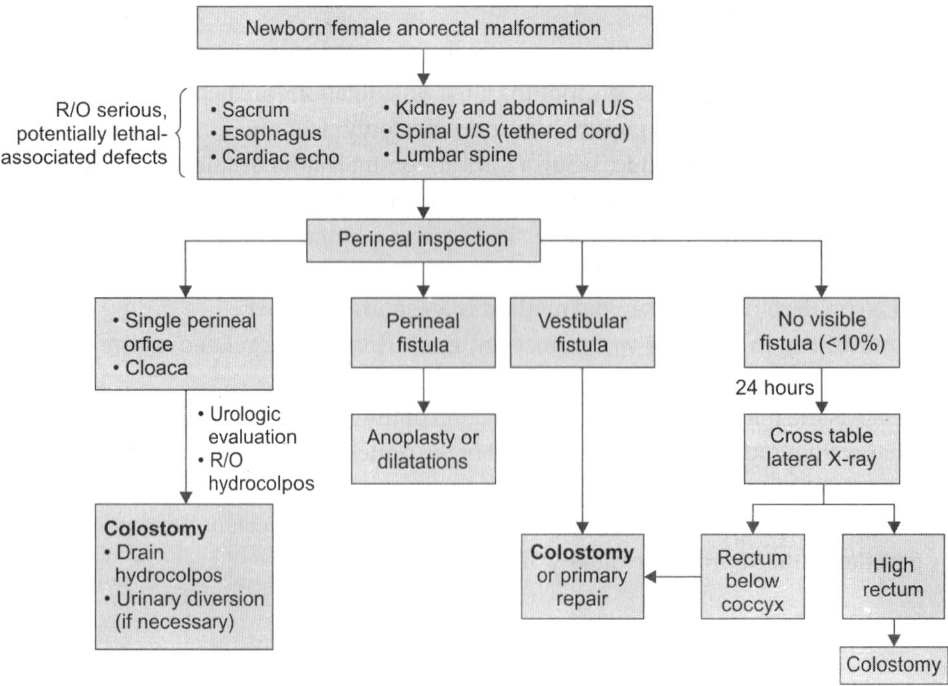

PRENATAL SURGERY

30. Discuss the principles of pre-natal surgery. ***Srimanta Sankaradeva University, Assam 2025***

Principles of Prenatal (Fetal) Surgery

Prenatal or fetal surgery refers to the surgical correction of congenital abnormalities before birth—while the fetus is still in the uterus. It is a specialized field combining obstetrics, pediatric surgery, and neonatology, aimed at preventing the progression of fetal disease and improving postnatal outcomes. The principles guiding prenatal surgery ensure *maternal safety, fetal benefit,* and *ethical justification.*

I. Careful Case Selection

Not every fetal anomaly is suitable for prenatal intervention. Candidates must be chosen based on:

- *Diagnosis:* The condition must be accurately diagnosed using high-resolution ultrasound, MRI, or genetic testing.
- *Natural history:* The abnormality should be one that will *worsen* or become *lethal* if left untreated until birth (e.g., severe spina bifida, twin-to-twin transfusion syndrome, congenital diaphragmatic hernia).
- *Potential for Benefit:* The surgery should *significantly improve survival or quality of life* compared with postnatal treatment.
- *Absence of lethal or syndromic anomalies:* There should be no major associated anomalies incompatible with life.

II. Maternal Safety and Informed Consent

- The **mother's health and autonomy** are paramount.
- She must receive full counseling regarding:
  - Risks to her own health (bleeding, infection, preterm labor, uterine rupture, complications in future pregnancies).
  - Risks and potential benefits to the fetus.
  - Ethical implications and experimental nature (if applicable).
- Informed consent should be thorough, voluntary, and documented.

III. Multidisciplinary Approach

Prenatal surgery requires coordination among:

- Maternal-fetal medicine specialists
- Pediatric surgeons
- Anesthetists (maternal and fetal)
- Neonatologists
- Geneticists, radiologists, and ethicists

A multidisciplinary team ensures appropriate selection, planning, and postoperative management.

IV. Accurate Imaging and Planning

- Detailed *ultrasound and fetal MRI* guide diagnosis, timing, and surgical approach.
- Planning includes assessing:
  - Placental location
  - Fetal position
  - Uterine wall thickness
  - Vascular anatomy
- Computer-assisted or image-guided systems may aid in minimally invasive access.

V. Minimally Invasive Techniques

- Preference for *fetoscopic (endoscopic)* or *percutaneous* techniques over open fetal surgery to reduce maternal and fetal risk.
  - *Examples:* Fetoscopic laser ablation for twin-to-twin transfusion syndrome.
- *Open fetal surgery* (via hysterotomy) is reserved for specific, well-defined indications (e.g., myelomeningocele repair).

VI. Maintenance of Uteroplacental Integrity

- The *uterus and placenta* must remain functional throughout the procedure.
- Avoid placental injury and minimize uterine bleeding.
- Use of tocolytics to prevent preterm contractions.
- Maintain maternal oxygenation, uterine relaxation, and temperature.

VII. Fetal Anesthesia and Monitoring

- Fetus receives anesthesia either through maternal administration or direct fetal injection.
- Continuous monitoring of fetal heart rate, oxygenation, and movement is essential.
- Fetal well-being determines continuation or termination of the procedure.

VIII. Prevention of Preterm Labor and Membrane Rupture

- Surgical entry and closure techniques should minimize trauma to membranes and uterus.
- *Amniotic fluid* may need to be replenished (amnioinfusion).
- *Tocolytic agents* are used before and after the procedure.

IX. Postoperative Care

- *Maternal monitoring:* Uterine activity, infection, bleeding.
- *Fetal monitoring:* Growth, well-being, and continuation of normal development.
- Delivery is often planned via cesarean section, especially after open fetal surgery, to prevent uterine rupture.

X. Ethical and Legal Considerations

- Interventions must be ethically justified — *maternal risk must be proportionate to fetal benefit.*
- Institutional ethics committee approval is often required.
- Procedures should be conducted in *accredited centers* with facilities for emergency maternal and neonatal care.

---

31. Describe the history of development of fetal surgery. What are the multidisciplinary approaches in fetal surgery? ***Tripura University 2025.***

History of Development of Fetal Surgery

Fetal surgery evolved gradually through *animal research, technological innovation*, and *careful clinical application.* It represents one of the most remarkable advances in perinatal medicine.

I. Early Experimental Era (1940s–1970s)

- *1940s–1950s:* Basic understanding of fetal physiology and circulation (by *Liley, Creasy,* and others) established the scientific foundation.
  - *Liley (1963)* performed the first *intrauterine transfusion* for rhesus isoimmunization — often regarded as the *first successful fetal therapy.*
- These interventions were *percutaneous* and not open surgeries.

II. Pioneering Animal Studies (1970s)

- Researchers began experimenting on animal models (mainly sheep and monkeys) to explore the feasibility of *in utero surgery.*

- Key contributors:
  - *Dr. Michael R. Harrison* (University of California, San Francisco)—widely recognized as the *father of fetal surgery.*
- *He and his team studied techniques to:*
  - Maintain uteroplacental circulation
  - Prevent preterm labor
  - Ensure fetal survival after open surgery
- Development of *hysterotomy closure techniques* and *tocolytic regimens* were crucial achievements.

III. First Human Fetal Surgery (1981)

- *1981 - UCSF (Dr Harrison's team):*
  - First successful *open fetal surgery for severe obstructive uropathy* (urinary tract obstruction leading to renal failure).
  - Procedure done via *maternal laparotomy and hysterotomy,* repair performed directly on the fetus.
- This marked the beginning of *clinical fetal surgery.*

IV. Evolution of Techniques (1980s–1990s)

- *Early open procedures were associated with:*
  - High maternal morbidity
  - Preterm labor
  - Limited survival benefits
- Advances in *imaging (ultrasound, MRI)* and *fetal monitoring* improved safety and accuracy.
- Introduction of *minimally invasive (fetoscopic)* and *image-guided techniques* reduced maternal risks.
- *1990s:*
  - *Fetoscopic laser ablation* for *twin-to-twin transfusion syndrome (TTTS)* developed by *Quintero et al.*
  - *Shunt placement* for fetal hydrothorax and urinary obstruction refined.

V. Modern Era (2000s–Present)

- *2003 - MOMS (Management of Myelomeningocele Study):*
  - Landmark multicenter randomized trial comparing prenatal vs postnatal repair of *spina bifida (myelomeningocele).*
  - Showed significant reduction in need for shunt placement and improved motor outcomes — with acceptable maternal risks.
  - Established *open fetal surgery for myelomeningocele* as standard of care in selected cases.
- *Current developments:*
  - *Fetoscopic spina bifida repair* (less invasive approach).
  - *Gene therapy, stem cell therapy,* and *tissue engineering* are being explored.
  - Increasing collaboration between *maternal-fetal medicine specialists, pediatric surgeons,* and *neurosurgeons.*

Multidisciplinary Approaches in Fetal Surgery

Fetal surgery is inherently *multidisciplinary,* requiring collaboration among several specialties to ensure optimal maternal and fetal outcomes.

I. Obstetrician/Maternal-Fetal Medicine Specialist

- Leads *prenatal diagnosis, case selection,* and *pregnancy management.*
- Monitors maternal and fetal condition before, during, and after surgery.
- Ensures maternal safety, counseling, and informed consent.

II. Pediatric Surgeon/Fetal Surgeon

- Performs the surgical procedure (open or fetoscopic).
- Determines the best operative technique to correct the anomaly.
- Coordinates intraoperative fetal handling and repair.

III. Anesthesiologists

- *Maternal anesthetist:* Provides uterine relaxation, analgesia, and maintains maternal-fetal hemodynamic stability.
- *Fetal anesthetist:* Delivers fetal anesthesia (transplacentally or directly) and monitors fetal vital parameters.

IV. Neonatologist

- Manages the *postnatal care* of the newborn.
- Prepares for possible preterm delivery and neonatal complications.
- Coordinates NICU management.

V. Radiologist/Fetal Imaging Specialist

- Provides detailed *prenatal imaging* (ultrasound, MRI) for diagnosis and surgical planning.
- Assists in image-guided procedures (e.g., needle or fetoscopic interventions).

VI. Geneticist and Genetic Counselor

- Evaluates for chromosomal or syndromic associations.
- Provides risk assessment and genetic counseling for the family.

VII. Nursing and Perioperative Team

- Specialized nurses assist in pre-, intra-, and postoperative care.
- Support patient education, infection control, and monitoring.

VIII. Psychologist/Ethicist/Social Worker

- Provide emotional support and counseling to the parents.
- Ethics consultants review indications, ensuring that maternal autonomy and fetal benefit are balanced.

IX. Biomedical Engineers and Technicians

Develop and maintain fetoscopic instruments, imaging systems, and fetal monitoring technologies.

CHAPTER 56

Investigations in Urology

LEARNING OBJECTIVES

- Uroflowmetry
- MCU

1. Uroflowmetry. *WBUHS 2012*

Uroflowmetry is a simple, diagnostic screening procedure used to calculate the flow rate of urine over time. The test is noninvasive (the skin is not pierced) and may be used to assess bladder and sphincter function.

Uroflowmetry is performed by having a person urinate into a special funnel that is connected to a measuring instrument. The measuring instrument calculates the amount of urine, rate of flow in seconds, and length of the time until completion of the void. This information is converted into a graph and interpreted by a physician. The information helps evaluate the function of the lower urinary tract or helps determine if there is an obstruction of normal urine outflow.

During normal urination, the initial urine stream starts slowly but almost immediately speeds up until the bladder is nearly empty. The urine flow then slows again until the bladder is empty. In persons with a urinary tract obstruction, this pattern of flow is altered, and increases and decreases more gradually. The uroflowmeter graphs this information, taking into account the person's gender and age.

Indications

Uroflowmetry is a quick, simple diagnostic screening test that provides valuable feedback about the health of the lower urinary tract. It is commonly performed to determine if there is an obstruction to normal urine outflow. Benign prostatic hypertrophy (BPH)—a benign enlargement of the prostate gland that usually occurs in men over the age of 50 years. Enlargement of the prostate interferes with the normal passage of urine from the bladder. If left untreated, the enlarged prostate can obstruct the bladder completely.

- Cancer of the prostate, or bladder tumor
- Urinary incontinence—involuntary release of urine from the bladder
- Urinary blockage—obstruction of the urinary tract can occur for many reasons along any part of the urinary tract from the kidneys to the urethra. Urinary obstruction can lead to a backflow of urine causing infection, scarring, or kidney failure if untreated.
- Neurogenic bladder dysfunction—improper function of the bladder due to an alteration in the nervous system such as a spinal cord lesion or injury
- Frequent urinary tract infections (UTIs)

Uroflowmetry may be performed in conjunction with other diagnostic procedures, such as cystometry and cystography.

Normal results: Normal values vary depending on age and sex. In men, urine flow declines with age. Women have less change with age:

- *Ages 4–7 years:* The average flow rate for both males and females is 10 mL/s.
- *Ages 8–13 years:*
  - The average flow rate for males is 12 mL/s.
  - The average flow rate for females is 15 mL/s.
- *Ages 14–45 years:*
  - The average flow rate for males is 21 mL/s.
  - The average flow rate for females is 18 mL/s.
- *Ages 46–65 years:*
  - The average flow rate for males is 12 mL/s.
  - The average flow rate for females is 18 mL/s.
- *Ages 66–80 years:*
  - The average flow rate for males is 9 mL/s.
  - The average flow rate for females is 18 mL/s.
- Results are compared with your symptoms and physical exam. A result that may need treatment in one patient may not need treatment in another patient.
- Several circular muscles normally regulate urine flow. If any of these muscles become weak or stop working, you may have an increase in urine flow or urinary incontinence.
- If there is a bladder outlet obstruction or if the bladder muscle is weak, you may have a decrease in urine flow. The amount of urine that remains in your bladder after urinating can be measured with ultrasound.
- *Risks of the procedure:* Because uroflowmetry is a noninvasive procedure, it is safe for most persons. The test is usually done in privacy to ensure that the person voids in a natural setting. There may be risks depending on your specific medical condition. Be sure to discuss any concerns with your doctor before the procedure. Certain factors or conditions may interfere with the accuracy of uroflowmetry. These factors include, but are not limited to, the following:
  - Straining with urination
  - Body movement during urination
  - Certain medications that affect bladder and sphincter muscle tone.

2. Micturating cystourethrography (MCU).

Introduction

- Voiding cystourethrography (VCUG), also known as an MCU
- It is a fluoroscopic study of the lower urinary tract in which contrast is introduced into the bladder via a catheter.
- It is done to assess the bladder, urethra, postoperative anatomy, and micturition in order to determine the presence or absence of bladder and urethral abnormalities.
- Good investigation for vesicoureteric reflux (VUR)
- It is more commonly performed in the pediatric population than in adults.

Indications

- Urinary tract infection
- Dysuria
- Dysfunctional voiding
- Hydronephrosis and/or hydroureter
- Bladder outlet obstruction
- Hematuria
- Trauma
- Urinary incontinence
- Neurogenic dysfunction of the bladder, e.g., spinal dysraphism

- Congenital anomalies of the genitourinary tract
- Postoperative evaluation of the urinary tract

Technique

- The bladder of the patient should be emptied before the operation.
- A urinary catheter is inserted into the bladder.
    - An infant feeding tube can be inserted under aseptic precautions for infants or young children
    - A Foley catheter can be used for older children.
- Contrast medium is slowly infused through the catheter into the bladder. The contrast is monitored initially to confirm the position of the catheter.
- Intermittent screening images can be taken while distending the bladder with contrast to check for a ureterocele or VUR.
- When the bladder is filled to its capacity (which will vary as per the age of the patient), the catheter is removed and the patient is asked to void:
    - Younger children can void on an absorbent pad
    - Older children can urinate into a urine receiver
    - Suprapubic pressure may be applied to increase the rate of voiding.
    - The catheter should only be removed when it is assured that the patient is able to urinate, the patient is unable to tolerate further infusion, or there is no more contrast medium for infusion.
    - Spot images are taken to look for vesicoureteric junction (VUJ) obstruction.
    - The lower ureter is best seen in the anterior oblique position
    - Oblique or lateral positions are also useful to visualize the whole of the urethra.
    - An abdominal view is taken to look for any reflux into the kidneys or record the postmicturition volume of the bladder.
    - Lateral view is useful to determine and delineate fistula formation into the rectum or vagina.

The following projections should be acquired keeping within the ALARA (as low as reasonably achievable) principle:

- Antegrade pyelogram (AP) with a full bladder for demonstration of the presence or absence of VUR
- Left and right oblique images for demonstrating bilateral VUJs
- Postvoid films are taken to check for a ureterocele

Voiding cystourethrogram/MCU versus retrograde urethrogram (RUG)/ascending urethrography (ASU):

- While, the urethra is well visualized in both procedures, RUG/ASU is better for visualizing anterior urethral abnormalities and VCUG is better for posterior urethral abnormalities.
- Additionally, VCUG is performed for the detection of bladder abnormalities and VUR.
- VCUG is the initial investigation of choice after metoidioplasty or phalloplasty in transgender males.

Kidney and Ureter

LEARNING OBJECTIVES

- Urinary Stones: Pathogenesis, Clinical Features, Management
- ESWL, PCNL
- Hematuria
- Vesicoureteric Reflux
- Hydronephrosis
- Polycystic Kidney Disease
- Renal Cyst
- Renal Cell Carcinoma
- Nephron-sparing Surgery
- Obstructive Uropathy

URINARY STONES

1. Discuss the pathogenesis of urinary stones. What are the features of stones in the renal pelvis? How do you manage such a patient? ***WBUHS 2009, 2012***

2. Discuss aetiology, types, clinical features and management of renal calculi. ***NTRUHS Vijayawada 2025***

3. Discuss etiology and management of urolithiasis. ***DY Patil Educational Society, Deemed to be University 2024.***

Introduction

- The formation of kidney stones is the result of a combination of factors.
- Stones are formed when urine does not have the right balance of fluids and a combination of minerals and acids. If the urine contains more crystal-forming substances than the liquid can dissolve, crystals can form.
- Urine usually contains compounds that prevent these crystals from clumping together.
- When these substances are classified below their normal ratio, stones can form from the accumulation of crystals.

Etiology

Phosphate Calculi

- *Diet:*
  - Vitamin A deficiency causes epithelial damage.
  - Cells will form nidus to form stones.
  - Whether this mechanism is important beyond the formation of the gallbladder is not known.
- *Altered urinary solutes and colloids:*
  - Urine solution with modified colloids
  - Dehydration increases urine solutes leading to precipitation.
  - Dehydration can reduce the amount of colloids in urine that absorb solutes or calcium deposits, leading to crystals and stone formation.

- *Decreased urinary citrate:*
  - Urine citrate levels are low (300–900 mg/24 hours) due to the presence of citric acid in urine to keep the solution slightly insoluble.
  - The amount of citrate released is hormonal and decreases during menstruation.
- *Kidney infection:*
  - Infection can cause urinary calculus and stone formation in clinical and experimental studies.
  - *Staphylococcus aureus*, *Streptococcus pneumoniae*, and *Proteus species* are the most common bacteria in urine.
  - Lack of urinary drainage can lead to the formation of stones when urine cannot pass freely.
- *Prolonged immobilization:* Prolonged immobilization can lead to increased urinary calcium, which promotes skeletal decalcification and the formation of calcium.
- *Hyperparathyroidism:*
  - About 5% of people with radiopaque calculi will have hypercalcemia, which is excessive excretion of calcium in the urine.
  - This is called "peeing your skeletons in your urine" and should be ruled out as a cause of kidney stones.
  - It can cause hyperparathyroidism, hypercalcemia, and hypercalciuria.
  - If kidney stones are recurrent or large, an endoscopy may be necessary to eliminate the cause.
  - In this case, the patient should have the parathyroid adenoma removed before proceeding with treatment for renal calculus.

Clinical Features

- *Pain:*
  - In three quarters of people with urinary stones, pain is the main symptom.
  - Pain in the kidney (at the corner of the kidney), in the anterior hypochondrium, or both
  - May be worse with movement, especially climbing stairs
- *Hematuria:*
  - Hematuria is sometimes the main symptom of urolithiasis
  - Sometimes, it can be a single symptom.
- *Pyuria:*
  - Infection is most likely to occur if there are stones present.
  - Pyuria is more likely to occur if the kidney is obstructed.
  - The mechanical action of the stones that irritate the urinary bladder may also cause pyuria if there are no stones present.

Investigation of Suspected Urinary Stone Disease

X-ray: The "KUB" film shows the kidney, ureter, and gallbladder. If the kidney stones are bilobular, there is no doubt about the diagnosis. Inhalation, which holds its position in relation to the urinary tract, seems to be a stone. Lateral radiographs can sometimes show calcified mesenteric nodules and symptoms in the anterior gastro- intestinal tract of the vertebral body and thus outside the urinary tract.

Features on Abdominal Radiographs that may be Confused with Kidney Stones

- It is a calcified mesenteric lymph node
- Cobblestone or concrete in aggregate
- Tablets or foreign bodies in the digestive tract (cyclopenthiazide)
- Phleboliths—calcifications in the walls of arteries, especially in the pelvis
- Ossified tip of the 12th rib
- Calcified tuberculous lesion in the kidney
- Calcified adrenal gland
- *Contrast-enhanced computed tomography:* Spiral CT has become the mainstay of research for acute urinary colic.

- *Excretion urography:* Urography will determine the presence and anatomical location of calculus. It also provides important information about other kidney functions.
- *Ultrasound:* Ultrasound is most important in locating stones for treatment with extracorporeal shock wave lithotripsy (ESWL).

Treatment

Conservative Management

- Calculus <0.5 cm resolves spontaneously if not affected.
- Any surgical intervention has a risk of complications and unnecessary interventions should be avoided.
- A small kidney calculus can block the calculus or act as a secondary site of infection, causing symptoms.

However, most of them can be watched safely until they pass.

Management of Small Stones

- Most small urinary calculi will pass spontaneously and can be treated conservatively.
- The presence of infection in an upper urinary tract obstructed by stone is dangerous and is an indication for urgent surgical intervention.

Preoperative Treatment

In case of urinary tract infection, appropriate antibiotic therapy should be started and continued during and after surgery if necessary.

Treatment for Stone

- Most stones are treated with minimal access and minimally invasive techniques.
- Open operations are performed when there is no relevant experience or when newer methods cannot refine the calculations.

Modern Methods of Stone Removal

- *Kidney stone removal:* Most urinary calculi can be treated with minimally invasive procedures.
- *Percutaneous nephrolithotomy:*
  - This includes placing a hollow needle through the soft tissue of the pelvis and renal parenchyma into the renal collecting system.
  - A wire inserted into a needle is used to guide a set of dilators that widen the path to the kidney until the nephroscope is used to take pictures of stones.
  - Small stones can be visualized and removed whole.
  - Large stones must be fragmented with ultrasound, laser, or electrohydraulic probe.
  - The goal is to remove as many parts as possible, and this may take some time if the calculation is large.
  - A nephrostomy drain remains in the system after the procedure. This breaks up the kidney and allows stone particles to re-enter if they persist.
  - Tuberculosis nephrolithotomy is sometimes combined with ESWL in the treatment of complex (diaphragmatic) calculus. The surgeon simply removes the central part of the stone and the more peripheral part is treated with ESWL.
- *Extracorporeal shock wave lithotripsy:*
  - When ESWL is successful, stone fragments must pass through the urethra.
  - Ureteric colic is common after ESWL, and the patient needs analgesia, usually in the form of nonsteroidal anti-inflammatory drugs.
  - Large pieces of stones can block the flow of urine.
  - To prevent this, the stent should be placed in the ureter as the kidney stone fragments pass.
  - Occasionally, the affected part must be removed ureteroscopically.
  - There is currently considerable interest in the long-term outcomes of patients treated with ESWL. Of course, some stones recur, especially if small fragments remain after treatment.

Open Kidney Surgery

Indications:

- Complex stone burden (projection of stone into multiple calyces, such that multiple PCNL tracks would be required to gain access to all the stone)
- Failure of endoscopic treatment (technical difficulty gaining access to the collecting system of the kidney)
- Anatomic abnormality that precludes endoscopic surgery (e.g., retrorenal colon)
- Body habitus that precludes endoscopic surgery (e.g., gross obesity, kyphoscoliosis open stone surgery can be difficult)
- Patient request for a single procedure where multiple PCNLs might be required for stone clearance
- Nonfunctioning kidney

Pyelolithotomy

- Pyelolithotomy is indicated for stones in the renal pelvis.
- Peripheral stone fragments can be detected by direct palpation or by intraoperative radiography or nephroscopy.
- If there is no infection, the pelvic incision is closed with stitches.
- If gross sepsis is present, nephrostomy is needed to decompress the system.

Extended Pyelolithotomy

- *Extended pyelolithotomy:*
  - The plane between the renal sinus and the wall of the collecting system is developed on the posterior surface of the kidney.
  - This avoids major vessels and allows incisions to be made into the calyces so that even large staghorn stones can be removed intact.

Nephrolithotomy

- If there is a complex calculus branching into the most peripheral calyces, it may be necessary to make incisions into the renal parenchyma to clear the kidney.
- Nephrolithotomy may also be necessary when the adhesions resulting from previous surgery make access to the renal pelvis difficult.
- *Treatment of bilateral renal stones:*
  - Usually the kidney with better function is treated first unless the other kidney is more painful or there is pyonephrosis, which needs urgent decompression.
  - Silent bilateral staghorn calculi in the elderly and infirm may be treated conservatively.
  - The patient should be encouraged to maintain a high fluid intake.
- *To prevent recurrence:*
  - Ideally, all former stones should be investigated to rule out metabolic factors, but the diagnostic yield in patients with single small stones is low. The urine of stone patients should be checked for infection. The following studies are suitable for bilateral and repetitive masons:
    - Serum calcium, measured fasting on three occasions to exclude hyperparathyroidism
    - Serum uric acid
    - Urinary urate, calcium and phosphate in a 24-hour collection; the urine should also be screened for cystine
    - *Analysis of any stone that passes:*
      - Dietary advice is usually not helpful in preventing stone recurrence in people who eat a balanced diet.
      - Patients with hyperuricemia should avoid red meats, offal, and fish, which are rich in purines, and should be treated with allopurinol. Eggs, meat, and fish are high in sulfur-containing proteins and should be restricted in cystinuria.
  - Stone sufferers should drink plenty to keep their urine dilute. Fluid intake should be increased appropriately to take account of increased losses.
  - Drug treatment is largely ineffective except in those few patients who are shown to have idiopathic hypercalciuria. Bendroflumethiazide (5 mg) and a calcium-restricted diet reduce urinary calcium.

4. What are the indications of metabolic evaluation in patients with urinary lithiasis? What are the components of such evaluation? Discuss the different management options for a 1.5-cm lower pole renal calculus. ***WBUHS 2023***

High-risk Stone Formers

General factors	*Diseases associated with stone formation*
• Early onset of urolithiasis (especially in children) • Familial stone formation • Brushite-containing stones (calcium hydrogen phosphate; $CaHPO_4.2H_2O$) • Uric acid and urate-containing stones • Infected stones • Solitary kidney (the solitary kidney itself does not particularly increase risk of stone formation, but prevention of stone recurrence is of more importance)	• Hyperparathyroidism • Nephrocalcinosis • Gastrointestinal diseases (e.g., jejunoileal bypass, intestinal resection, Crohn's disease, malabsorptive conditions, enteric hyperoxaluria after urinary diversion) and bariatric surgery • Sarcoidosis

Indications for Metabolic Evaluations

- Recurrent stone formers
- Strong family history of stones
- Intestinal disease (particularly chronic diarrhea)
- Pathologic skeletal fractures
- Osteoporosis
- History of urinary tract infection (UTI) with calculi
- Personal history of gout
- Infirm health (unable to tolerate repeat stone episode)
- Solitary kidney
- Anatomic abnormalities
- Renal insufficiency
- Stones composed of cystine, uric acid, and struvite
- Children
- Bad eating habits that contribute to the development of kidney stones include:
  - Low fluid intake or high fluid loss (for example, from sweat or gastrointestinal losses), which leads to a decrease in urine output and thus a higher concentration of lithogenic factors
  - High levels of animal protein can cause increased calcium and uric acid excretion and reduced urinary citrate excretion
  - A high-sodium diet that increases urinary calcium excretion
  - Increase the consumption of foods that contain oxalate, especially spinach. The amount of dietary oxalate contribution to urinary oxalate is controversial and may vary from person to person due to differences in gastrointestinal absorption.
  - Low calcium intake affects dietary oxalate absorption and higher urinary oxalate excretion due to decreased calcium oxalate complex formation in the intestinal lumen. The effect of low calcium intake on raising low urinary oxalate is reduction in calcium absorption and excretion.
  - Too much vitamin C and D, which can increase urinary oxalate or calcium, respectively
  - Excessive sugar intake (sucrose and fructose), which can increase calcium and/or oxalate excretion

Metabolic Abnormalities

- Hypercalciuria (>5 mmol/day)
- Hyperoxaluria (oxalate >0.5 mmol/day)
- Hyperuricosuria (>4 mmol/day in women and 5 mmol/day in men)

- Hypomagnesuria (<3 mmol/day)
- Hyperphosphaturia (phosphate level >1.3 g/dL)
- High PTH (>65 pg/mL)
- Hypercalcemia (ionized calcium >1.32 mmol/L)

Objectives of Metabolic Assessment

- Prevent the formation of recurrent stones in high-risk stone massage.
- Prevent emergencies related to network outages.

Complete Metabolic Assessment

- A complete metabolic evaluation for nephrolithiasis consists of blood and urine tests, including at least 2 hours of urine collection.
- *Urinalysis:*
  - Urinalysis should be performed on voided urine samples.
  - Urinalysis should include the determination of pH, because a pH >7.5 increases the risk of stone formation due to urea-producing bacteria, while a pH <5.5 favors uric acid lithiasis.
  - Urine sediment should also be checked for crystalluria, because specific types of crystals can provide information about stone composition.
  - *Uric acid crystals:* Uric acid crystals are present in acidic urine (usually pH <5.5), which supports the conversion of slightly soluble uric acid to insoluble uric acid.
  - *Calcium phosphate or calcium oxalate crystals:* Formation of calcium oxalate crystals does not depend on urine pH, while calcium phosphate crystals are only formed in stomach urine (usually pH ≥6.5).
  - *Cystine crystals:* The typical hexagonal shape cystine crystals are diagnostic of cystinuria.
  - *Magnesium ammonium phosphate crystals:* Magnesium ammonium phosphate (struvite) and calcium carbonate apatite are constituents of struvite stones.
    - Normal urine is not coated with magnesium ammonium phosphate and struvite stone formation occurs only when ammonia production increases and urine pH increases.
    - Both of these requirements are met only when upper urinary tract infections are caused by urea-producing bacteria such as *Proteus* or *Klebsiella*.
- *Blood test:*
  - Routine chemistry profiles should be obtained, including measurements of serum electrolytes, serum creatinine, and serum calcium.
  - The results may aid in the diagnosis of certain disorders such as distal renal tubular acidosis associated with primary hyperparathyroidism, hyperuricemia, and nephrolithiasis.
  - Blood calcium concentration should be measured to detect hypercalcemia; if above normal, serum calcium should be repeated.
  - Measurement of circulating parathyroid hormone is required in patients with serum calcium values in the upper normal range or high urinary calcium, because primary hyperparathyroidism is often associated with only intermittent and mild increases in serum calcium concentration.
  - Although usually in the middle of the reference range, the presence of low serum bicarbonate concentration raises the possibility of distal renal tubular acidosis or chronic diarrhea.
- *24-hour urine collections:* An important component of the evaluation of patients at moderate to high risk for recurrent stone disease is the assessment of urine composition
- *Number of collections:* At least two 24-hour urine collections should be obtained in the outpatient setting, with the patient following their usual diet, fluid intake, and physical activity. The differences among the collections are often substantial, so an important contributor may be missed in many patients if only one sample is collected.
- *Timing of collections:* The urine collections should be obtained while the patient is on their usual diet. Values should not be measured immediately after the acute stone episode

- *Tests to include:*
  - The urine volume and excretion of calcium, uric acid, citrate, oxalate, creatinine (to assess the completeness of the collection), pH, sodium, potassium, and magnesium should all be measured. Ideally, the supersaturation of lithogenic substances should be calculated.
  - Measurement of sodium excretion is also important. Higher sodium intake can contribute to increased calcium excretion and will affect the response to a thiazide diuretic when prescribed to reduce urine calcium.
    - *A variety of definitions for "normal" are used by different laboratories for each of the urinary parameters. Below are some more common definitions.*
      - *Calcium:* Less than 200 mg (5.0 mmol) per day in females or <250 mg (6.25 mmol) per day in males
      - *Uric acid:* Less than 750 mg (4.5 mmol) per day in females or <800 mg (4.8 mmol) per day in male
      - *Oxalate:* Less than 40 mg (0.44 mmol) per day in both females and males
      - *Citrate:* Greater than or equal to 450 mg per day in both females and males

Different Management Methods for Lower Pole Renal Calculus 1.5 cm

Diagnostic Tests

- *Abdominal X-ray:* Radiodense calcium-containing calculi. Stones that contain sulfur (cystine) are slightly radiating in plain radiographs.
- Totally reflective stones (such as uric acid, triamterene, indinavir) are suspected based on the patient's history and/or urine pH (pH <6; drug history—triamterene and indinavir), and the diagnosis can be confirmed by ultrasound, computerized tomography urography (CTU), or magnetic resonance urography (MRU).
- *Renal ultrasound:* ~95% sensitivity for detecting renal calculi. A combination of open abdominal radiography and renal ultrasonography is a useful screening test for renal calculi.
- *IVU:* Increasingly replaced by CTU. Useful in patients with suspected indinavir stones (not visible on CT)
- *CTU:* Highly accurate method for detecting all but indinavir stones. This allows for accurate determination of stone size and location with good pelvic anatomy.
- *MRU:* It cannot visualize stones but can indicate hydronephrosis.

Treatment

- *Acute presentation (renal colic):*
  - Take analgesia, for example diclofenac; IV fluid.
  - Small stones (<0.5 cm) can be managed spontaneously because most of them will pass spontaneously.
  - If pain or obstruction persists, emergency treatment with percutaneous nephrostomy
  - Common symptoms of infection are pain, infection, and obstruction
- *Elective presentations:*
  - *Extracorporeal shock-wave lithotripsy (ESWL):*
    - Focused, externally generated electrohydraulic or ultrasonic shock waves
    - Targeted on to the calculus using ultrasound, X-ray, or a combination
    - Causes stone disintegration and the fragments are then voided—effective for stones up to 1 cm.
  - *Percutaneous nephrolithotomy (PCNL):*
    - For stones in the renal pelvis or calyces
    - Percutaneous track into the renal pelvis using fluoroscopic guidance
    - Nephroscope is inserted and the calculus visualized
    - Removed either in total or, if large, following fragmentation
  - URS (ureteroscopic retrieval can also be tried)
  - *Open nephrolithotomy:*
    - For large staghorn calculi or complex stones
- *Prevention of recurrence:*
  - Increase oral fluid intake and reduce calcium intake
  - Correct metabolic abnormalities

- Treat infection promptly
- Urinary alkalization, e.g., sodium (mainly for cystine and urate stones)
- Thiazide diuretics (for idiopathic hypercalciuria)

Remember

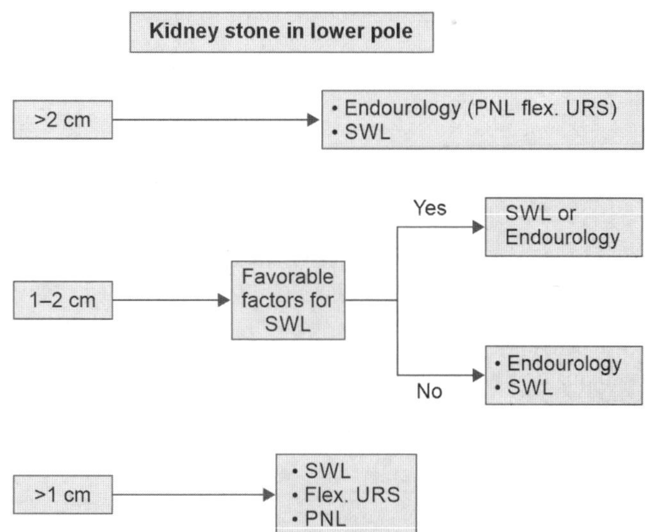

(PNL: percutaneous nephrolithotomy; URS: ureterorenoscopy; SWL: shock-wave lithotripsy)

5. Discuss in brief the following interventional procedures for the treatment of urolithiasis, with their indications and complications: (a) dietary modifications for calciumbased stones, (b) ESWL, (c) endoscopic (ureteroscope), (d) PCNL. ***WBUHS 2022***

Interventional procedure	*Indications*	*Complications*
Dietary modifications for calcium-based stones	• *Reduce simple sugars Intake while preferring complex carbohydrates:* An acute load of glucose causes an Increase of calcium urinary excretion in normal subjects which Is greater in calcium stone formers. Furthermore, diets with different content of carbohydrates at equal supply of other nutrients causes an Increase In calcium excretion directly proportional to carbohydrates intake • Reduce saturated fats while preferring vegetable, mono- and polyunsaturated fats. Stone formers have a high prevalence of hypercholesterolemia and the amount of fat Introduced Is directly proportional to oxalate excretion • Reduce the amount of salt and preserved foods. High salt Intake Is associated with an Increase of urine calcium excretion. It has been estimated that an Increase of 100 mmol of sodium chloride (6 grams of salt) Increases urinary calcium of 1 mmol In normal subjects and a twofold Increase In hypercalciuric stone formers • Increase the consumption of fruit, vegetables, and food rich In fiber • Reduce animal protein Intake while preferring plant-derived proteins. Restrict foods like rhubarb, beets, okra, spinach, Swiss chard, sweet potatoes, nuts, tea, chocolate, black pepper, and soy products. Choose a diet low In salt and animal protein	

Contd...

Contd...

Interventional procedure	*Indications*	*Complications*
ESWL	• ESWL, the least Invasive of the surgical methods of stone removal, utilizes high-energy sound waves focused on the stone to shatter It Into passable fragments • It Is especially suitable for stones that are smaller than 2 cm and lodged In the upper or middle calyx	• It Is contraindicated In pregnancy, patients with untreatable bleeding disorders, tightly Impacted stones, or In cases of ureteral obstruction distal to the stone • In addition, the effectiveness Is limited for very hard stones (which tend to be dense on CT scan), cystine stones, and In very obese patients
Endoscopic (ureteroscope)	• Ureteroscopy Is especially suitable for removal of stones that are 1–2 cm, lodged In the lower calyx or below, cystine stones, and high attenuation ("hard") stones • It is also useful in patients who have multiple small calculi or pre-existing nephrostomy tubes, and following an UTI. The typical patient has acute symptoms caused by a distal ureteral stone, usually measuring 5–8 mm	• One of the drawbacks to use rigid or semirigid ureteroscopes for the management of kidney stones Is the limited visualization of the entire renal system. This Is avoided with the use of a flexible ureteroscope, which allows for visualization of the entire collecting system • The fragility of the fiber optic Instrument Is also a concern, with some studies reporting that repairs (often very expensive) were required every 6–15 procedures • With regard to the actual stone removal, this procedure requires small stone fragments to allow for retrieval by stone basket • There Is also the risk of ureteral Injury, which can be reduced with the use of preoperative double-J stenting
PCNL	• PCNL allows fragmentation and removal of large calculi from the kidney and ureter • Percutaneous nephrostolithotomy Is especially useful for stones >2 cm In diameter • Normal saline should be used for Irrigation, as opposed to sterile water, to prevent electrolyte disturbances and hemolysis • Stone-free rates for PCNL monotherapy have been shown to be about 56% • In some cases, a combination of ESWL and a percutaneous technique is necessary to completely remove all stone material from a kidney. This technique, called sandwich therapy, Is reserved for staghorn or other complicated stone cases • Minimally Invasive PCNL Is associated with fewer complications compared with standard PCNL but Its efficacy may be limited to stones <2 cm; management of larger stones Is especially difficult • Ultra-mini percutaneous nephrolithotomy, which Involves use of a small access sheath, has been shown to be safe and effective for the management of renal stones In children	• Percutaneous procedures have higher morbidity than ESWL and ureteroscopy and so are generally reserved for large and/or complex renal stones and cases In which the other two modalities have failed • Multiple sessions of PCNL may be necessary to achieve high stone-free rates. This can result In Increased tract-related complications • Efficacy of minimally Invasive PCNL limited to stones <2 cm; management of larger stones Is especially difficult

(ESWL: extracorporeal shock wave lithotripsy; PCNL: percutaneous nephrolithotomy)

6. What are the current trends in the management of urolithiasis? *WBUHS 2011, 2025*

Risk factors for the development of urinary calculi.

Risk factor	*Mechanisms*
Bowel disease	Promotes low urine volume; acidic urine depletes available citrate; hyperoxaluria
Excess dietary meat (including poultry)	Creates acidic urinary milieu, depletes available citrate; promotes hyperuricosuria
Excess dietary oxalate	Promotes hyperoxaluria
Excess dietary sodium	Promotes hypercalciuria
Family history	Genetic predisposition
Insulin resistance	Ammonia mishandling; alters pH of urine
Gout	Promotes hyperuricosuria
Low urine volume	Allows stone constituents to supersaturate
Obesity	May promote hypercalciuria; other results similar to excess dietary meat
Primary hyperparathyroidism	Creates persistent hypercalciuria
Prolonged immobilization	Bone turnover creates hypercalciuria
Renal tubular acidosis (type 1)	Alkaline urine promotes calcium phosphate supersaturation; loss of citrate

Clinical clues to the diagnosis of urinary calculi.

Evaluation	*Possible findings*
Laboratory evaluations	
Complete blood count	Leukocytosis with struvite calculi
Serum chemistry	Elevation in creatinine levels with obstructing calculi; hypokalemia and hyperchloremia with renal tubular acidosis; elevated serum calcium levels with parathyroid disease
Serum parathyroid hormone levels	Elevated in hyperparathyroidism
Urinalysis	Microscopic or gross hematuria; acidic urine; alkaline urine (with struvite calculi); pyuria; crystals from involved calculi
24-hour urinalysis	Elevated urinary calcium, oxalate, and sodium levels; decreased urinary volume and citrate levels
Radiographic evaluations	
Abdominal, kidney, and upper bladder radiography	Urinary calculi >2 mm may be visible
CT (stone protocol)	Nearly all calculi are visible on CT. Evaluates renal parenchyma, hydronephrotic changes, and surrounding organs for other etiologies of abdominal pain
Intravenous pyelography	Calculi visible on scout film. Delay in contrast excretion if obstruction is present. Calculi may appear as filling defect
MRI	Conventional MRI is not useful for imaging calculi
Ultrasonography	Calculi appear as hyperechoic lesions that cast acoustic shadows. Not reliable for ureteral calculi. May demonstrate dilation of collecting system

Treatment

- If the stone is asymptomatic, watchful waiting is the right choice.
- For symptomatic stones, pain control is usually the first step, using medications such as anti-inflammatory steroids or opioids.
- More severe cases may require surgical intervention.
  - For example, some stones can be broken into small pieces using extracorporeal shock wave lithotripsy.
  - In some cases, a more complex type of surgery is required. Examples include cystoscopic procedures such as laser lithotripsy or percutaneous techniques such as percutaneous nephrolithotomy.

- Sometimes, a ureteral tube (ureteral stent) may be inserted to remove the obstruction and relieve symptoms, as well as to prevent urinary leakage after ureteroscopy stone removal.

Conservative Management

- Most urethral calculi are benign and do not require intervention. Spontaneous passage depends on the size of the stone, shape, location, and urine output (which depends on how long the stone does not pass). Ureteral calculus 4–5 mm has a 40–50% chance of spontaneous resolution. On the other hand, calculi >6 mm have the potential to pass spontaneously.
- Most stones pass within 6 weeks from the onset of symptoms. Urethral calculi detected in the distal urethra at presentation have a 50% chance of spontaneous resolution, as opposed to a 25% and 10% chance in the middle and proximal urethra, respectively.

Medical Agents

Tamsulosin and nifedipine are safe and effective in distal urolithiasis patients with renal colic. However, tamsulosin is better than nifedipine in relieving renal colic and facilitating and accelerating urination.

Chemolytic Stone Dissolution

- Oral or percutaneous irrigation chemolysis of stones or their fragments can be useful first-line therapy. It may also be an adjunct to ESWL, percutaneous nephrolithotomy (PNL), ureterorenoscopy (URS) or open surgery to support elimination of small residual fragments, considering that its use as first-line therapy may take several weeks to be effective.
- Combined treatment with ESWL and chemolysis is a minimally invasive option for patients with partial or complete infection staghorn stones who are not eligible for PNL.
- Stone fragmentation leads to increased stone surface area and improved efficacy of chemolitholysis.
- Chemolysis is possible only for the stone compositions listed below; therefore, knowledge of stone composition is mandatory before treatment.

Oral Chemolysis

Oral chemolitholysis is efficient only for uric acid calculi, and is based on alkalinization of urine by application of alkaline citrate or sodium bicarbonate.

ESWL

Indications

- Kidney stones of <2.5 cm in size
- Proximal ureter stones
- Distal ureter stones

URS

- Ureteroscopy can be employed to treat ureteral stenosis/stricture and ureteropelvic junction obstruction.
- It is useful for retrieval of distal ureteric and ureterovesical junction stones.
- Ho:YAG laser lithotripsy is the preferred method for (flexible) URS.

PCNL

Indications

- Stones >1.5 cm in the kidneys or the ureter
- Stones >1 cm in the lower pole of the kidney
- Staghorn-shaped stones
- Patient choice

Open and Laparoscopic Surgery for Removal of Renal Stones

- *Open surgery:* Advances in ESWL and endourological surgery (URS and PNL) have significantly decreased the indications for open stone surgery.

- The incidence of open stone surgery is ~1.5% of all stone removal interventions in developed countries, and in developing countries, it has dropped from 26 to 3.5% in recent years.

Open Surgery for Renal Calculi

- Operations for kidney stone are usually performed via a loin or lumbar approach. All of the procedures are difficult unless the kidney is fully mobilized and its vascular pedicle controlled. A sling should be placed around the upper ureter to stop stones migrating downwards.
- Surgical techniques such as extended pyelolithotomy, pyelonephrolithotomy, anatrophic nephrolithotomy, multiple radial nephrotomy, partial nephrectomy, and renal surgery under hypothermia

Indications

- Complex stone burden (projection of stone into multiple calyces, such that multiple PCNL tracks would be required to gain access to all the stone)
- Failure of endoscopic treatment (technical difficulty gaining access to the collecting system of the kidney)
- Anatomic abnormality that precludes endoscopic surgery (e.g., retrorenal colon)
- Body habitus that precludes endoscopic surgery (e.g., gross obesity, kyphoscoliosis open stone surgery can be difficult)
- Patient request for a single procedure where multiple PCNLs might be required for stone clearance
- Nonfunctioning kidney

---

7. Discuss on prevention of recurrence of urolithiasis. ***WBUHS 2024***

Prevention of Recurrence of Urolithiasis

Urolithiasis refers to the formation of stones (calculi) in the urinary tract, which can occur in the kidneys, ureters, bladder, or urethra. The recurrence of urolithiasis is a common problem, as once a person has developed kidney stones, the likelihood of developing them again is high. Preventing recurrence is crucial to improving the patient's quality of life, reducing complications, and avoiding the need for repeated treatments or surgeries.

Factors Contributing to Urolithiasis Recurrence

The recurrence of urolithiasis is influenced by several factors, including:

- *Metabolic abnormalities:* Imbalances in calcium, uric acid, oxalate, or phosphate levels in the urine.
- *Dehydration:* Low fluid intake can lead to concentrated urine, which promotes stone formation.
- *Dietary factors:* High intake of certain foods, like sodium, animal proteins, or oxalate-rich foods, can contribute to stone formation.
- *Family history:* Genetic predisposition can make individuals more susceptible to developing kidney stones.
- *Medical conditions:* Diseases such as hyperparathyroidism, gout, diabetes, and obesity can increase the risk of stone formation.
- *Medications:* Some medications, such as diuretics or calcium-based supplements, may increase the likelihood of stones forming.

Preventive Measures for Recurrence of Urolithiasis

Increase fluid intake

- *Hydration:* The most important preventive measure is to increase fluid intake, especially water, to produce at least 2 to 2.5 liters of urine daily. This helps dilute the urine and prevents supersaturation of stone-forming substances.
- *Water:* Drinking water is preferred over sugary or caffeinated drinks. People with a history of stones are often advised to drink water throughout the day, aiming for clear or light yellow urine.
- *Lemonade or citrusy drinks:* Citrus fruits, especially lemons, contain citrate, which can help prevent stone formation by binding calcium in the urine.

Dietary modifications

- *Calcium intake:* Contrary to what some might think, a low-calcium diet is not always recommended. Adequate dietary calcium intake from food sources like dairy products helps bind oxalate in the intestines and reduces its absorption into the bloodstream, thereby reducing kidney stone formation. Calcium supplements should only be taken under a doctor's guidance.

- *Limit oxalate-rich foods:* Oxalate can combine with calcium to form calcium oxalate stones, the most common type of kidney stones. Foods like spinach, beets, nuts, chocolate, and tea are high in oxalate. Limiting these foods can reduce the risk.
- *Reduce sodium intake:* High salt intake increases calcium excretion in the urine, which can promote stone formation. A low-sodium diet helps reduce the risk of stones.
- *Moderate animal protein:* Excessive intake of animal protein (red meat, poultry, eggs) can increase uric acid and calcium levels in the urine, promoting stone formation. Reducing animal protein intake can help decrease this risk.
- *Limit Sugary Beverages:* Soda and other sugar-sweetened drinks can increase the risk of kidney stones due to their high fructose content, which can raise uric acid levels in the urine.

Medications and supplements

- *Thiazide diuretics:* These medications help lower calcium levels in the urine and are often prescribed to prevent calcium-containing stones.
- *Citrate supplements:* Potassium citrate or magnesium citrate may be prescribed to increase urinary citrate levels, which helps prevent stone formation, especially calcium oxalate stones.
- *Allopurinol:* For patients with uric acid stones or high levels of uric acid, allopurinol can be used to reduce the production of uric acid.
- *Phosphate binders:* In cases of calcium phosphate stones, phosphate binders may be used to decrease phosphate levels in the urine.

Management of underlying health conditions

- *Hyperparathyroidism:* If a parathyroid gland disorder is causing calcium imbalance, surgery or medication may be necessary to regulate calcium levels.
- *Gout:* Managing gout with medications like allopurinol or febuxostat can lower uric acid levels and prevent uric acid stone formation.
- *Obesity:* Obesity is linked to a higher risk of stone formation. Maintaining a healthy weight through diet and exercise can reduce the risk.
- *Diabetes management:* Proper control of blood sugar and avoiding metabolic changes that lead to kidney stone formation is essential for diabetic patients.

Regular monitoring and follow-up

- *Urine testing:* Regular urine tests (such as 24-hour urine collection) can help assess urine composition, identify risk factors, and guide treatment plans.
- *Blood tests:* Monitoring calcium, uric acid, phosphate, and parathyroid hormone levels can help detect metabolic abnormalities that predispose to stone formation.
- *Imaging:* Periodic imaging tests, like ultrasounds or CT scans, may be recommended to monitor for the development of new stones.

Lifestyle modifications

- *Physical activity:* Regular exercise can help maintain a healthy weight and reduce the risk of stone formation.
- *Avoid dehydration:* During hot weather or exercise, it is essential to drink plenty of fluids to avoid dehydration, which increases the risk of stone formation.
- *Avoid excessive use of calcium supplements:* Unless prescribed by a healthcare provider, avoid taking large amounts of calcium supplements, as they may increase the risk of developing stones.

8. Describe extracorporeal shock wave lithotripsy.

Tips and Techniques

- Urinary calculus has a crystalline structure.
- It breaks into fragments bombarded by a shock wave of sufficient energy.

- The principle is that in the simplest Dornier device, a shock wave is generated from an electric current placed at a point on an ellipsoid mirror.
- Stone fragments must pass through the urethra when ESWL is successful. Ureteric colic is common after ESWL and patients require analgesia, usually in the form of steroidal anti-inflammatory drugs such as diclofenac.
- Large stones can block the flow of urine. To prevent this, the ureteric stent should be inserted when the kidney stones flow.
- Occasionally, the affected part must be removed ureteroscopically.

Indications

- Kidney stones of <2.5 cm in size
- Proximal ureter stones
- Distal ureter stones

Complications and Limitations

- The main challenge of ESWL is infection.
- Most calculi contain bacteria that come out of broken stones.
- It is wise to administer prophylactic antibiotics before ESWL, and the obstructing system should be compressed by placing a ureteral stent or percutaneous nephrostomy before treatment.
- Results are not satisfactory with harder stones, especially cystine stones. When treating gallstones, patients should be warned that it may take several months to clear the pieces.
- There is now considerable interest in the long-term outcomes of patients treated with ESWL. Of course, some stones recur, especially if small fragments remain after treatment.

---

9. Describe PCNL. ***WBUHS 2006***

Percutaneous Nephrolithotomy (PCNL)

Indications for PCNL

PCNL is usually recommended:

- Stone diameter >3 cm
- Attempts at invasive and/or flexible ureteroscopy and laser therapy were unsuccessful
- First line for staghorn calculus when using ESWL and/or repeat PCNL for residual stone fragments
- ESWL (with JJ stent in place), flexible ureteroscopy and laser therapy, and PCNL are available for stones 2–3 cm in diameter. PCNL offers the best chance for complete stone clearance in a single procedure, but this is achieved at a high-morbidity risk.

Technique

- PCNL is the removal of kidney stones through an advanced path between the surface of the skin and the kidney collecting system.
- The first step requires inflation of the kidney collecting system (pelvis and calyx) with fluid or air through a cystoscopically inserted urinary catheter.
- This facilitates subsequent percutaneous puncture of the remaining kidney with a nephrostomy needle.
- Once the nephrostomy needle is in the calyx, a guidewire is inserted into the renal pelvis to act as an extension guide. Sheath entrance through the channel and calyx, and through this nephroscope can grow into the kidney.
- An ultrasound lithotripsy scan is used to break up stones and remove debris.
- The lateral approach is often used; below the 12th rib (away from the ribs to avoid the pleura and avoid the intercostals, tendons, and nerves).
- The best approach is through the posterior calyx instead of the renal pelvis, because this avoids damage to the posterior branch of the renal artery, which is closely related to the renal pelvis. General anesthesia can be used with general, regional, or local anesthesia (with sedation).

Results

- For small stones, the stone-free rate after PCNL is in the order of 90–95%.
- Stone-free PCNL rates for gallstones are in the order of 80–85% when combined with postoperative ESWL for residual stone fragments.

Complications

- Hemorrhage from the perforated renal parenchyma—this is very useful and can be difficult to control
- Perforation of the collection system by saline irrigation wells
- Perforation of bowel or pleural space during percutaneous catheter placement

10. PUJ obstruction. *AIIMS, Patna 2025*

Definition: *A functional or anatomical blockage* at the pelviureteric junction (PUJ), causing *impaired drainage of urine* from the renal pelvis into the ureter.

- **Causes**
  - **Congenital (most common)**
    - Intrinsic narrowing of the PUJ due to abnormal muscle development or fibrosis.
    - Presence of aberrant crossing blood vessel compressing the PUJ externally.
    - High insertion of the ureter.
  - **Acquired**
    - Secondary to scarring from stones, infection, trauma, or prior surgery.
    - Post-inflammatory or ischemic changes.
    - Ureteral or pelvic tumors (rare).

Epidemiology

- Can present in *infants and children* (often detected on prenatal ultrasound as hydronephrosis)
- May also present in *adults*, often discovered incidentally or due to symptoms.

Clinical Features

- Flank or loin pain (especially after drinking fluids).
- Recurrent urinary tract infections.
- Hematuria (blood in urine).
- Palpable renal mass in infants.
- Deteriorating renal function or hydronephrosis on imaging.

Investigations

- *Ultrasound (USG):* It shows hydronephrosis (dilated pelvis and calyces).
- *Diuretic renogram (MAG3 or DTPA scan):* It assesses drainage and split renal function.
- *CT urography or MR urography:* It defines anatomy and presence of crossing vessels.
- *Intravenous urography (IVU):* (less common now) shows delayed drainage.

Management

Depends on *severity and renal function*:

Conservative (Observation)

- For mild cases with good renal function and no symptoms.
- Regular ultrasound and renal scans to monitor.

Surgical

- *Pyeloplasty (Anderson-Hynes dismembered pyeloplasty):* Gold standard; can be open, laparoscopic, or robotic.
- *Endopyelotomy:* Incision of the PUJ endoscopically (for selected cases).
- *Nephrectomy:* For non-functioning kidneys.

Prognosis
- Excellent after surgical correction.
- Early detection and treatment preserve renal function.

HEMATURIA

11. Enumerate causes of painless hematuria in a 60-year-old aged man. Discuss its investigation and treatment protocol. ***WBUHS 2012***

12. Describe the causes, investigations and principles of management of hematuria. ***Maharashtra University of Health Sciences 2025***

Introduction
- Hematuria is usually divided into macroscopic (where urine is stained) and microscopic (where blood is only present on smear or microscopic examination).
- There are clinical differences between painful and painless hematuria and between glomerular and postglomerular hematuria.

Causes of Benign Hematuria
- *Renal tumors:*
  - The most common primary renal tumor is renal cell carcinoma, an adenocarcinoma of collecting tubule origin. Diagnosis is made by CT scanning and treatment is by surgical excision.
  - Transitional cell carcinoma of the renal collecting system is usually present with hematuria. Diagnosis can be difficult, requiring retrograde imaging and ureteroscopy. Treatment is done by local excision or nephroureterectomy for high grade or large lesions. Immunotherapy has been used for metastases with limited success.
  - Kidney tumors can cause bleeding and diagnostic complications. Incidental and usually asymptomatic renal cysts are excluded.
- *Kidney stones:*
  - Stone disease is very common, cysts form in the renal papilla, then a nidus forms for stone formation in the collecting system. Kidney stones are usually asymptomatic, but mucosal infection or direct irritation may cause hematuria.
  - Diagnosis is usually made by imaging with vascular urography. Kidney stones can usually be treated with extracorporeal shock wave lithotripsy, but large or complex stones may require continuous or open surgical removal.
- *Glomerulonephritis:* Glomerulonephritis presents with microscopic hematuria, which, although associated with pain, is often asymptomatic or may present with symptoms of kidney failure.
- *Pyelonephritis (ascending urinary tract infection):* Acute bacterial pyelonephritis caused by direct spread from the bladder (vesicoureteric reflex) or by periureteric lymphadenopathy. Painless hematuria can occur, but a complex of symptoms usually includes abdominal pain, fever, and septicemia.
- *Papillary necrosis:* This condition occurs in diabetes and in patients with lack of oxygen, especially sickle cell disease. Reflective filling defects in IVU are identified and usually estimated.
- *Ureteric stones:* These are almost always painful, but may have hematuria as the only symptom. The presence or absence of defects and the size of the stone requires management.
- *Cystitis:* Cystitis is usually painful and, in men, often associated with gallstones. Schistosomiasis, interstitial cystitis, and drug-related cystitis are rare causes of gallbladder bleeding. Diagnosis is by cystoscopy and urine microscopy and culture. A fluid biopsy may be necessary.
- *Bladder tumors:*
  - Most of the interest in painless hematuria stems from the desire to diagnose bladder tumors at an early stage. Nearly all are transitional cell cancers, with smoking and aromatic hydrocarbon exposure being risk

factors. Rarer bladder tumors include adenocarcinoma (usually arising from the urachus) and squamous cancer (associated with chronic inflammation and schistosomiasis).

- *Diagnosis is as outlined above with management depending on the stage and grade:* 70% are superficial at presentation and are managed by transurethral surgery with or without the use of intravesical therapy. For invasive tumors, the choice lies between radical cystectomy or radiotherapy. Metastatic disease may respond to platinum-based chemotherapy.

- *Prostate tumors:*
  - *Benign prostatic hyperplasia is ubiquitous but can bleed on its own:* It may also cause bacterial cystitis. Diagnosis is by urinary flow assessment and bladder residual volume measurement. Assuming that other causes of hematuria have been ruled out, treatment is tailored to the individual.
  - Prostate specific antigen levels should be checked (after any UTI has been treated) to rule out prostate cancer, which may cause hematuria directly or by urinary tract infection. Diagnosis is by prostatic biopsy, usually with ultrasound control. Treatment depends on the stage and outlook, but local disease may be suitable for radical prostatectomy or radiotherapy while advanced disease responds to hormonal manipulation.
- *Rare causes of hematuria:*
  - Arteriovenous disorders, tuberculosis, and arteritis can cause hematuria.
  - Patients on controlled anticoagulants in the standard therapeutic range who develop hematuria should be fully investigated as above, as hematuria is not a common consequence of anticoagulation.

Investigations of Hematuria

- General physical examination (not forgetting blood pressure, the prostate in a male and the gynecological organs in a female)
- *Urinary examination:*
  - This must include microscopy for red and white blood cells and bacteria.
  - The presence of any crystals, ova or parasites should be noted and culture of a mid-stream specimen carried out.
  - If schistosomiasis or tuberculosis is suspected, a first void urine sample is usually requested.
  - The level of protein in the urine must be assessed, but in heavy hematuria, it may be difficult to be sure if light proteinuria is due to the hemoglobin present.
  - If no red blood cells are found in the urine but hemoglobin is present, the patient should be investigated for causes of hemoglobinuria.
- Complete blood count with an erythrocyte sedimentation rate
- Serum urea, creatinine, and electrolytes should be measured, along with albumin, calcium, and liver function tests if the patient is unwell or in renal failure.
- Coagulation studies are not routine.
- Assuming microscopic amounts of blood are found, the presence or absence of proteinuria may guide initial investigation. In this event, C-reactive protein and 24-hour urine protein excretion will be informative, as may serum electrophoresis and autoantibodies. Ultrasound will show renal cortical thickness and density.
- In the majority of cases, a renal biopsy with immunoglobulin histochemistry will be necessary to make a definitive diagnosis.
- In cases of microscopic hematuria without proteinuria, and all macroscopic cases, a "surgical" investigation plan can be followed. This is based around the exclusion of malignant or stone disease, and centers on cystoscopy to directly inspect the bladder.
- *Imaging:*
  - Intravenous urography
  - Combination of plain abdominopelvic radiography and ultrasound of the urinary tract
  - If no abnormality is found then a flexible cystoscopy under local anesthetic may be performed
  - If either the imaging or this endoscopic examination suggests a bladder lesion, the patient will require a transurethral biopsy and examination under anesthetic for both treatment and diagnosis.

- In any of the above scenarios, it is important to remember that if a particular investigation pathway leads to a negative result, consideration should be given to carry out the test of the other pathways, thus flexible cystoscopy for a patient with persistent microscopic hematuria in whom no renal cause is found, and ultrasound in a patient with a normal bladder and intravenous urogram.

VESICOURETERAL REFLUX

13. Vesicoureteral reflux. ***KNRUHS, Telangana 2022***

Introduction

Vesicoureteral reflex (VUR) is the abnormal movement of urine from the ureter to the ureter or kidney. Urine is usually excreted from the kidneys and passed into the bladder. In the vesicoureteral reflex, the direction of urine flow is reversed (retrograde).

Markings

Prenatal hydronephrosis of the vesicoureteral reflex can occur with abnormal dilatation of the ureter or with urinary tract infection or acute pyelonephritis.

- Symptoms such as painful urination or colic/renal flank pain are not symptoms related to the vesicoureteral reflex.
- Neonates can present with lethargy, infants and small children usually present with pyrexia, dysuria, urinary frequency, noxious urine, and gastrointestinal tract (GIT) symptoms, but only urinary tract infection is the initial presentation of VUR.

Reason

- In healthy individuals, the ureter penetrates the urethra significantly and runs submucosa for some time.
- It helps to protect and support the muscles of the urinary tract in addition to protect them.
- Together, these features create a valve-like effect that regulates the flow of urine during retention and voiding.
- In people with VUR, there is a disruption of this mechanism with retrograde flow of urine.

Features

- *Primary VUR:* Submucosal length compared to the diameter of the ureter, leading to valve mechanism insufficiency. It is caused by a congenital defect/absence of the internal urethral longus muscle, resulting in anomalous urethral stricture [ureterovesical junction (UVJ)].
- *Secondary VUR:* In this category, the valve mechanism is intact and healed early, but becomes excessive due to increased vesicular pressure associated with obstruction that disrupts the urinary system. Impairments can be anatomical or functional. Secondary VUR can be further divided into anatomical and functional groups:
  - *Anatomical:* Lateral excretory valve; ureteral or meatal stenosis

  This cause is treated with surgery whenever possible.
  - *Functional:* Bladder gland instability, neurogenic bladder and neuropathic bladder
  - Urinary tract infections can cause reflexes due to high pressure associated with swelling.

Treatment

- Resolution of functional VUR usually occurs if the underlying cause is treated and resolved.
- Medical and/or surgical treatment may be indicated.
  - *Age:* Children are more susceptible to VUR due to the shortness of the submucosal ureter. As children grow, this sensitivity decreases as the length of the urethra increases. 70% of children under 1 year of age with a urinary tract infection have VUR. This number drops to 15% by age 12.
  - *Gender:* Although vesicoureteric reflux (VUR) is more common in males antenatally, 85% are females in later life, with definite female predominance.

International Classification of Vesicoureteral Reflex

- Class I—reflex to void urine
- Class II—renal pelvis without reflex or dilatation

- Class III—mild/moderate dilatation with minimal prolapse of the ureter, renal pelvis, and pelvis
- Class IV—cutting with dilatation of the renal pelvis and middle ureter
- Class V—general dilatation of the ureter, pelvis and pelvis; urination; loss of papillary effects
- The younger the patient and the lower the presentation, the higher the chance of spontaneous resolution
- *Diagnosis:* VCUG shows grade III vesicoureteral reflex.
- *The following procedures can be used to diagnose VUR:*
  - Renal cystogram (RNC)
  - Fluoroscopic ultrasound cystourethrogram (VCUG)
  - Ultrasound cystography
  - Abdominal ultrasound

Abdominal ultrasound may suggest VUR if urine output is present; however, sonograms may be normal in most cases of mild to moderate VUR, so they may not be of sufficient value as a single diagnostic test in the evaluation of children with suspected VUR, such as those presenting with prenatal hydronephrosis or urinary tract infection (UTI).

- *VCUG (voiding cystourethrogram)* is the method of choice for evaluation and initial work-up, RNC is preferred for further evaluation due to less radiation exposure. A high index of suspicion should be added if anatomic causes are excluded in pediatric urinary tract infections. In this case, VCUG and abdominal ultrasound should be done. Early diagnosis in children is important because studies have shown that children with UTI and associated acute pyelonephritis are more likely to develop permanent renal cortical scarring than children without VUR. Thus, VUR not only increases the frequency of UTIs, but also increases the risk of damage to the upper urinary tract.

Treatment

- *Medical treatment:*
  - Medical treatment is the preferred method, but surgical intervention may be necessary.
  - Medical management is recommended for children with grades I-III VUR, as most cases will resolve spontaneously.
  - A trial of medical therapy is indicated in patients with VUR stage IV, especially in young patients or patients with unilateral disease.
  - Of patients with VUR grade V, only infants are tested for a medical approach before surgery is indicated, in elderly patients surgery is the only option.
  - Medical treatment requires low-dose antibiotic prophylaxis until VUR resolves. Antibiotics are given in half the usual therapeutic dose at night. The specific antibiotics used vary depending on the age of the patient and include:
    - Amoxicillin or ampicillin—babies <6 weeks
    - Trimethoprim-sulfamethoxazole (co-trimoxazole): 6 weeks to 2 months
  - After 2 months, the following antibiotics are suitable:
    - Nitrofurantoin dose (5–7 mg/kg/24 hours)
    - Nalidixic acid
    - Bactrim
    - Trimethoprim
    - Cephalosporins
  - Urine cultures are performed three times a month to rule out advanced infections.
  - Annual radiological studies are also indicated. Good, periodic, and double sound perineal hygiene is an important aspect of medical care. Dehydration is treated with anticholinergics.
  - *Endoscopic injection:* Deflux is a gel used in endoscopic injection to treat VUR
- *Surgical management:*
  - A surgical approach is necessary in cases where a breakthrough infection results despite prophylaxis, or there is noncompliance with the prophylaxis.
  - Similarly if the VUR is severe (Grade IV and V), there are pyelonephritic changes or congenital abnormalities.
  - Other reasons necessitating surgical intervention are failure of renal growth, formation of new scars, renal deterioration, and VUR in girls approaching puberty.

- There are three types of surgical procedure available for the treatment of VUR:
  1. Endoscopic (STING/HIT procedures)
  2. Laparoscopic
  3. Open procedures (Cohen procedure, Leadbetter-Politano procedure)
- *Follow-up:*
  - 2010 guidelines from the American Urological Association recommend ongoing monitoring of children with VUR until the abnormality resolves or is no longer clinically significant.
  - The recommendations are for annual evaluation of blood pressure, height, weight, urinalysis, and renal ultrasonography.

HYDRONEPHROSIS

14. Describe investigation and treatment of 5-year-old boy with bilateral hydronephrosis. ***WBUHS 2021***

Disorders Associated with Bilateral Hydronephrosis
- Uterine bilateral obstructive uropathy—sudden blockage of the kidneys
- Biliary obstruction—a blockage in the gallbladder that prevents drainage
- Posterior urethral valve—urinary system that causes decreased urine flow (in men)
- Abdominal dissection syndrome—gallbladder causes abdominal distension
- Ureteropelvic junction obstruction—blockage in the kidney where the ureter enters the kidney
- Vesicoureteric reflex—backs up urine from kidney to kidney

The Following Tests may Indicate Bilateral Hydronephrosis
- CT scan of the abdomen or kidneys
- Intravenous pyelogram (IVP), less often used
- Check for kidney stones
- Abdominal or kidney ultrasound
- If ultrasonography shows persistent hydronephrosis, voiding cystourethrography (VCUG) should be performed. In male infants, a thorough evaluation of the posterior urethra should be performed to detect possible PUVs.

Treatment
Inserting a tube into the bladder (a Foley catheter) can open the blockage. Other treatments include:
- Breastfeeding
- Insert a tube through the skin into the kidney to relieve pressure
- Placing a ureteral tube (stent) to allow urine to flow from the kidney to the bladder

The cause of the blockage must be found and treated after the urethra is established.

POLYCYSTIC KIDNEY DISEASE

15. Write about developmental anatomy of kidney. Write about adult polycystic kidney disease. ***KIIT University Odisha 2025***

Stages of Kidney Development
Kidney development occurs in *three successive stages*, each more advanced than the previous one:

Stage	*Structure*	*Time of appearance*	*Fate*
Pronephros	Primitive, non-functional	4th week	Regresses completely
Mesonephros	Interim kidney	Late 4th–5th week	Mostly degenerates; part forms male genital ducts
Metanephros	Permanent kidney	Begins in 5th week, functional by 10–12th week	Becomes the definitive kidney

Development of the Metanephros (Permanent Kidney)

The **metanephros** develops from two embryological sources:

Structure	*Origin*	*Develops into*
Metanephric diverticulum (ureteric bud)	Outgrowth from the mesonephric duct	Collecting system (ureter, renal pelvis, calyces, collecting ducts)
Metanephric blastema (metanephric mesenchyme)	Intermediate mesoderm in sacral region	Excretory system (nephrons: Bowman's capsule, PCT, loop of Henle, DCT)

Inductive Interaction

- The *ureteric bud* and *metanephric blastema* interact reciprocally.
- The bud *induces* the metanephric tissue to form nephrons.
- The blastema *induces* branching of the ureteric bud to form the collecting system. This mutual induction is essential for normal kidney development.

Development of the Nephron

- Each nephron is derived from the *metanephric mesenchyme.*
- The *blind end* of a metanephric tubule enlarges to form *Bowman's capsule,* which invaginates the *glomerular capillaries.*
- The tubule elongates and differentiates into *proximal convoluted tubule, loop of Henle,* and *distal convoluted tubule.*
- The *distal tubule* joins a *collecting duct* from the ureteric bud.

Ascent of the Kidney

- The metanephric kidneys initially lie in the *pelvic region.*
- As the embryo grows, they *ascend* to the *lumbar region* due to differential growth of the caudal part of the embryo.
- During ascent, the kidneys receive blood from successively higher levels of the aorta; lower vessels degenerate.

Rotation of the Kidney

- During ascent, the kidneys *rotate medially* by about 90°, so that the renal hilum faces *anteromedially.*
- Failure of rotation or abnormal rotation can lead to *malrotated kidneys.*

Formation of the Ureter

- The *ureter* develops from the *stalk of the ureteric bud.*
- It connects the developing kidney to the *urinary bladder.*

Blood Supply

- Initially, the kidneys are supplied by pelvic branches of the common iliac arteries.
- As they ascend, they receive new branches from the aorta, while lower ones usually regress.
- Occasionally, accessory renal arteries persist.

Clinical Correlations

- *Renal agenesis:* Absence of ureteric bud or its failure to interact with metanephric blastema.
- *Duplicated ureter:* Early branching of the ureteric bud.
- *Polycystic kidney disease:* Abnormal interaction between ureteric bud and metanephric blastema.
- *Ectopic kidney:* Failure of ascent (pelvic kidney).
- *Horseshoe kidney:* Fusion of lower poles preventing normal ascent.

Adult Polycystic Kidney Disease (APKD)

(Autosomal Dominant Polycystic Kidney Disease – ADPKD)

Definition

Adult polycystic kidney disease is a *hereditary disorder* characterized by the *progressive development of multiple cysts* in both kidneys, leading to *enlargement* of the kidneys and *gradual loss of renal function.*

Genetics

- *Inheritance:* Autosomal dominant (hence "adult" form).
- *Incidence:* ~1 in 400–1000 live births.
- *Genes involved:*
  - *PKD1* gene on chromosome *16p13.3* (~85% cases) → codes for *polycystin-1.*
  - *PKD2* gene on chromosome *4q21* (~15% cases) → codes for *polycystin-2.*
- Mutations lead to *abnormal tubular epithelial cell growth and cyst formation.*

Pathogenesis

- Cysts arise from *any part of the nephron,* mainly the *distal tubule and collecting ducts.*
- Progressive cyst enlargement compresses adjacent normal renal tissue → *ischemia and fibrosis* → *renal failure.*
- Cysts may also occur in *other organs* (liver, pancreas, spleen, etc.).

Gross Pathology

- *Both kidneys enlarged,* may weigh up to 3–4 kg each.
- External surface - irregular, *covered with numerous cysts* of varying sizes (up to several cm).
- *Cysts contain* clear, turbid, or hemorrhagic fluid.
- *Normal parenchyma* is markedly reduced and compressed between cysts.

Microscopic Features

- Cysts lined by *flattened or cuboidal epithelium.*
- *Interstitial fibrosis* and *chronic inflammation* in remaining parenchyma.
- *Arteriolar sclerosis* and *glomerular changes* due to ischemia.

Clinical Features

Usually presents in *adults (30–50 years).* Common features include:

- *Flank or abdominal pain:* Due to cyst distension or infection.
- *Palpable enlarged kidneys:* Often bilateral.
- *Hematuria:* Microscopic or gross, due to rupture of cysts.
- *Hypertension*: Common and early sign.
- *Recurrent urinary tract infections.*
- *Progressive renal failure* → chronic kidney disease (CKD).

Extrarenal Manifestations

- *Liver cysts* (most common extrarenal feature).
- *Pancreatic and splenic cysts.*
- *Intracranial (berry) aneurysms* → risk of *subarachnoid hemorrhage.*
- *Mitral valve prolapse* and other valvular defects.
- *Colonic diverticulosis.*

Investigations

- *Ultrasound:* Multiple bilateral cysts, enlarged kidneys.
- *CT/MRI:* Defines size, number, and distribution of cysts.
- *Genetic testing:* Identifies PKD1/PKD2 mutations.
- *Renal function tests:* Elevated urea and creatinine in advanced stages.

Complications

- *Hypertension* (renin-mediated).
- *Chronic renal failure.*
- *Infected cysts.*
- *Hemorrhage into cysts.*
- *Nephrolithiasis.*
- *Subarachnoid hemorrhage* from ruptured berry aneurysm.

Treatment

- *No definitive cure* — management is supportive and aimed at slowing progression.
- *Control blood pressure* — ACE inhibitors/ARBs.
- *Treat infections* promptly.
- *Pain management* — avoid trauma.
- *Tolvaptan* (vasopressin V2 receptor antagonist) — slows cyst growth and decline in renal function.
- *Dialysis or renal transplantation* — in end-stage renal disease (ESRD).

Prognosis

- Progressive disease → *renal failure typically by 50–70 years.*
- *PKD1* mutation → earlier and more severe course than PKD2.

RENAL CYST

16. Classify renal cyst based on CT. ***DY Patil Educational Society, Deemed to be University 2024***

Classify renal cyst based on CT

CT-Based Classification of Renal Cysts (Bosniak Classification)

The Bosniak classification (developed by Morton Bosniak) is the standard system used to categorize renal cystic lesions on contrast-enhanced CT based on their imaging features. It helps in assessing the risk of malignancy and guiding management.

Bosniak Classification (CT Criteria)

Class	*CT Features*	*Risk of malignancy*	*Management*
I – Simple cyst	• Thin, smooth wall • Water density (0–20 HU) • No septa, calcification, or enhancement	~0% (benign)	No treatment or follow-up needed
II – Minimally complex cyst	• Few thin (<1 mm) septa • Fine or thin calcification • Hyperdense (<3 cm), well-marginated cysts without enhancement	~0% (benign)	No follow-up needed
IIF – "Follow-up" cyst	• Multiple thin septa • Minimal wall/septal thickening • May have thick or nodular calcification • No measurable enhancement • >3 cm hyperdense cysts	<5% (low malignant potential)	Periodic imaging follow-up
III – Indeterminate cystic mass	• Thickened or irregular walls/septa • Measurable enhancement after contrast	~50% malignant	Surgical exploration or excision
IV – Clearly malignant cystic mass	All features of Bosniak III plus enhancing soft-tissue components independent of wall or septa (solid nodules)	>90% malignant	Surgical removal (nephrectomy/partial nephrectomy)

RENAL CELL CARCINOMA

17. Classify tumors of the kidney. Discuss about Clinical features. ***WBUHS 2007***

18. TNM staging and management of renal cell carcinoma.
WBUHS 2021 Supplementary; Srimanta Sankaradeva University, Assam 2025

19. Discuss the management of a case of renal cell carcinoma with particular reference to different surgical approaches and their steps appropriate for such a patient. ***WBUHS 2007***

20. Describe clinical features and management of renal cell carcinoma. ***RIMS, Imphal 2022***

21. Describe clinical features, diagnostic and staging investigations and management of renal cell carcinoma. ***Gujarat University 2025***

WHO Classification of Kidney Tumors

Familial Renal Cancer

- *Renal cell tumors:*
  - *Malignant:*
    - Clear cell renal cell carcinoma
    - Multilocular clear cell renal cell carcinoma
    - Papillary renal cell carcinoma
    - Chromophobe renal cell carcinoma
    - Carcinoma of the collecting ducts of Bellini
    - Renal medullary carcinoma
    - Xp11 translocation carcinomas
    - Carcinoma associated with neuroblastoma
    - Mucinous tubular and spindle cell carcinoma
    - Renal cell carcinoma unclassified
  - *Benign:*
    - Papillary adenoma
    - Oncocytoma
- *Metanephric tumors:*
  - Metanephric adenoma
  - Metanephric adenofibroma
  - Metanephric stromal tumors
- *Mixed mesenchymal and epithelial tumors:*
  - Cystic nephroma
  - Mixed epithelial and stromal tumor
  - Synovial sarcoma
- *Nephroblastic tumors:*
  - Nephrogenic rests
  - Nephroblastoma
  - Cystic partially differentiated nephroblastoma
- *Neuroendocrine tumors:*
  - Carcinoid
  - Neuroendocrine carcinoma
  - Primitive neuroectodermal tumor
  - Neuroblastoma
  - Pheochromocytoma
- *Other tumors:*
  - Mesenchymal tumors
  - Hematopoietic and lymphoid tumors
  - Germ cell tumors
  - Metastatic tumors

Pediatric Patients

Wilm's tumor.

Clinical Features

Signs and Symptoms

- The classical presentation is described as triad of gross hematuria, flank pain, and a palpable mass that occurs in only 7–10% of patients.
- Frequently manifests as advanced disease.
- Patients may also present with hematuria, dyspnea, cough, and bone pain which are typically symptoms secondary to metastases.
- With the routine use of CT scanning for evaluation of nonspecific findings, asymptomatic renal tumors are increasingly detected incidentally (>50%).
- *Paraneoplastic syndromes:* Renal cell carcinoma (RCC) is associated with a wide spectrum of paraneoplastic syndrome.

Paraneoplastic syndromes.

Syndrome associated with RCC	*Cause*
Anemia	Hematuria, chronic disease
Polycythemia	Ectopic secretion of erythropoietin
Hypertension (25%)	Ectopic secretion of renin, renal artery compression, or AV fistula
Hypoglycemia	Ectopic secretion of insulin
Cushing's syndrome	Ectopic secretion of ACTH
Hypercalcemia	Ectopic secretion of parathyroid hormone-like substance
Gynecomastia, amenorrhea, reduced libido, baldness	Ectopic secretion of gonadotropins
Stauffer's syndrome: hepatic dysfunction, fever, anorexia	Unknown; resolves in 60–70% of patients postnephrectomy

Investigations

- The diagnosis of renal cell carcinoma is often made by CT (and, less frequently, by intravenous urography) performed as an initial step in the workup of hematuria, an enigmatic metastatic lesion, or suspicious laboratory findings.
- The diagnosis of renal cell carcinoma is often made by CT (and less frequently by vascular urography) as the initial step of hematuria, a primary metastatic lesion, or suspicious laboratory findings.

Laboratory Results

- Microscopic urinalysis reveals hematuria in most patients.
- Erythrocyte sedimentation rate may be increased but is unknown.
- Elevations in hematocrit and serum calcium, alkaline phosphatase, and aminotransferase levels occur in <10% of patients.
- These findings almost always resolve with curative nephrectomy and are therefore usually not indicative of metastasis.
- Bleeding related to blood loss occurs in 20–40% of patients, especially those with advanced disease.

Imaging

- The diagnosis of renal cell carcinoma is often made by CT (and rarely by vascular urography) as an initial step for hematuria, primary metastatic lesions, or suspicious laboratory findings.
- Ultrasound and CT scans often detect renal masses, which now account for 50% of early kidney cancer diagnoses in patients with unknown kidney disease.
- Abdominal X-ray can show calcified kidney mass, but only 20% of kidney mass has visible calcification (20% of masses with malignant peripheral calcification; more than 80% with malignant central calcification)
- The main method to work on hematuria is now CT urography; vascular urography alone detects only 75% of renal mass lesions.
- Differentiation of the most common renal mass (i.e., a simple benign cyst) can be done by finding a radiating center with a thin wall and a sharp interface between the mass and the renal cortex (typical "beak sign" cortical cyst).

- *Ultrasonography:* Additional determination of all renal masses seen in venous urography is required. Occasionally, some masses detected on CT require further characterization by ultrasound. Abdominal ultrasound can detect venous thrombus and cyst extent.
- *CT scan:*
  - CT scanning is the diagnostic modality of choice when a solid renal mass is identified on ultrasound.
  - CT scans are >95% accurate in detecting renal cell carcinoma. >80% of lesions are enhanced with iodinated contrast medium, which shows higher blood vessels.
  - CT scanning is also useful in local staging and can show perinephric fatty tumor infiltration; local hilar lymph node enlargement indicates metastases; or tumor thrombus in the renal vein or inferior vena cava.
  - CT angiography can determine the renal vasculature useful in the surgical planning of partial nephrectomies.
- *MRI:*
  - MRI is less accurate and more expensive than CT.
  - However, it is the most accurate way to identify renal vein or venous thrombi.
  - Magnetic resonance angiography (MRA) has been particularly useful for mapping the blood supply and the relationship with adjacent structures in candidates for partial nephrectomy.
- *Isotope scan:*
  - Sometimes a renal mass is suspected on vascular urography but not seen on equivalent or ultrasound.
  - Renal cortical isotope scan agent such as technetium-99m dimercaptosuccinic acid (DMSA) is useful in this case. Isotope scans of kidneys or cysts show areas of degeneration, while areas of proliferation show renal "pseudotumors" or hypertrophied columns of Bertie.
- *Other diagnostic or staging methods:*
  - Isotope bone scan is useful in patients with bone pain, increased gastric phosphatase, or known metastases.
  - Chest X-ray is negative enough, but if equivalent, chest CT scan can be used to detect metastases.
  - Currently, there are no specific tumor markers for renal cell carcinoma
  - Occasionally, mass aspiration cytology may be useful in interesting situations.
  - Diagnosis is often made by noninvasive methods and needle aspiration is required only in undiagnosed cases (<10%).
  - *Treatment:* Staging is the key to design the treatment plan.

TNM staging classification and prognosis of renal cell cancer.

Robson stage	*T*	*N*	*M*	*5-year survival (%)*
I. Tumor confined by renal capsule	T1 (<7.0 cm tumor) T2 (>7.0 cm tumor)	N0 (nodes negative)	M0 (no distant metastases)	80–100
II. Tumor extension to perirenal fat or Ipsilateral adrenal but confined by Gerota's fascia	T3a	N0	M0	50–60
IIIa. Renal vein or Inferior vena cava involvement	T3b (renal vein involvement)	N0	M0	50–60 (renal vein)
	T3c (renal vein and caval involvement below the diaphragm)			25–35 (vena cava)
	T4b (caval Involvement above the diaphragm)			
IIIb. Lymphatic involvement	T1–3	N1 (single regional node involved)	M0	15–35
		N2 (multiple regional, contralateral, or bilateral nodes involved)		
IIIc. Combination of IIIa and IIIb	T3–4	N1–2	M0	15–35
IVa. Spread to contiguous organs except Ipsilateral adrenal	T4	N1–2	M0	0–5
IVb. Distant metastases	T1–4	N0–2	M1	0–5

Surgical Treatment

- Patients with tumor thrombus (stage T1, T2, and T3a) confined to the kidney (Gerota's fascia) or confined to the intact renal artery or vein are best treated by radical nephrectomy.
- This includes blocking the kidneys and Gerota's fascia (including the ipsilateral adrenal), renal hilar lymph nodes, and approximately half of the urinary tract.
- Para-aortic node dissection has not been proven useful and is not routinely performed.
- If the tumor is very large and the contralateral kidney is normal, radical nephrectomy is recommended.
- If the renal vein or inferior vena cava is dilated, initial monitoring is performed above and below the tumor. If there is an enlargement of the chest, the cardiac team may be required to put the patient on cardiac bypass, and if necessary, the tumor is removed from the right side of the heart.
- Patients with small kidney tumors, diabetes or kidney failure, and tumors <4 cm (even with a normal contralateral kidney) should be considered partial nephrectomy, because in such cases the prognosis (if negative surgical margins are obtained) is same as radical nephrectomy:
  - *Radical laparoscopic or partial nephrectomy:* Introduced as equal to the open approach with the advantage of less blood loss, shorter hospital stay, and earlier return to normal activity.
  - *Laparoscopic or percutaneous renal ablation* has also shown great promise. Alternatively, radiofrequency ablation has been used for small kidney tumors, but this procedure requires further study and longer follow-up in treated patients.
  - *Nephrectomy* is not associated with improved survival in patients with multiple distant metastases (stage IV) and is not recommended unless patients are symptomatic or promising treatment protocols have been explored.
  - Patients with solitary lung metastases benefited from combined surgical resection of primary lesions and metastatic lesions (30% survival in 5 years).

Embolization

Operative arterial embolization in patients with or without metastases does not improve survival, but may be beneficial as a single treatment option in patients with symptomatic but unresectable primary lesions.

Radiation Therapy

Radiation therapy has no benefit other than treating symptomatic bone metastases.

Chemotherapy

- Medroxyprogesterone for metastatic renal cell carcinoma has a short-term response rate of 5–10%.
- Vinblastine, the minimum duration is about 20%. There are no other cytotoxic chemotherapy agents.

Immunotherapy

- 15–20% respond to immunotherapy with alpha interferon. Interferon alone (interferon beta, interferon gamma) or in combination with chemotherapy agents is less effective than interferon alpha.
- Induction immunotherapy—uses lymphocytes (lymphokine-activated killer cells) to expose the patient's own peripheral blood lymphocytes to interleukin-2 (IL-2) in vitro, then infuses the patient with a systemic high-dose intravenous IL-2 agent. Deep capillary leak syndrome and acute toxicity

Molecularly Targeted Therapy

- Recent advances in the Von Hippel–Lindau tumor suppressor gene have led to the identification of growth factors, including vascular endothelial growth factor (VEGF) and platelet-derived growth factor, in the treatment of advanced kidney cancer.
- Early studies using bevacizumab, an antibody to vascular endothelial growth factor, have shown promising results.
- Sorafenib, a tyrosine kinase inhibitor that blocks the pathway leading to the production of several growth factors, was studied in patients with metastatic renal cell carcinoma and showed a median progression-free survival of placebo (24 weeks vs. 6 weeks).
- Sunitinib, another tyrosine kinase inhibitor, has shown longer progression-free survival and higher response rates than interferon alpha in patients with metastatic kidney disease. These oral agents are currently used as first-line therapy in this patient group.

- Temsirolimus, a specific inhibitor of the mammalian kinase of rapamycin (mTOR inhibitor), is another targeted agent showing promising results. It is currently used as first-line therapy in patients with poor prognosis. Many other agents are currently under investigation.

Prognosis

- Patients with localized renal cancer (stages T1, T2, and T3a) treated surgically have 5-year survival rates of approximately 70–80%, whereas rates for those with local nodal extension or distant metastases are 15–25% and <10%, respectively.
- Most patients who present with multiple distant metastases succumb to disease within 15 months. The advent of new agents for renal cancer may improve the outcome in these patients.

Different surgical approaches: Most common operation for renal cell carcinoma is nephrectomy.

- The transperitoneal abdominal approach is usually considered superior in renal malignancy for the better access it gives to the great vessels.
- For very large upper renal tumors, or for retroperitoneal sarcomas, a thoracoabdominal approach, with or without liver mobilization provides very extensive access.
- Alternatively retroperitoneal loin approach may also be preferable.
- Nephrectomy may involve removing either an entire organ and surrounding tissue or a small part of the kidney.

Partial nephrectomy: In partial nephrectomy, which is also referred to as kidney-sparing surgery, only the diseased or infected portion of the kidney is removed. The healthy kidney tissue is left in place as much as possible.

Radical nephrectomy: Radical nephrectomy involves the removal of the entire kidney, the adrenal gland, the ureter and the fatty tissue that surrounds the kidney.

Simple nephrectomy: Simple nephrectomy is done for a living donor transplant purposes that requires the removal of the kidney and a section of the attached ureter.

Open nephrectomy: This is the traditional surgery and the donor or patient may be under general anesthesia. A 10–20-inch incision is done in the side or abdomen and a lower rib may be removed.

Laparoscopic nephrectomy: This is a minimally invasive surgery. This type of nephrectomy may last longer than the open nephrectomy, but studies have shown that it promotes faster recovery time and less postoperative pain.

Nephrectomy

Steps

- Abdomen is opened through midline incision.
- The gonadal vein runs superiorly between the transversalis fascia and psoas major. The ureter runs parallel with the gonadal vein, but straight to the hilum of the kidney. It can be seen running superiorly inside the renal fascia, on the surface of paranephric fat.

  Step 1: Identify the gonadal vein and the ureter. Visually identify the gonadal vein running inferiorly on psoas major. Visually identify the ureter inferiorly of the inferior pole and verify that it is the ureter by prodding it with the ultrasonic dissector and observing wormlike movement.

  Step 2: Free the ureter.

  Step 3: Ligate and cut the ureter. Dissect the hilum. The kidney is connected to the vena cava and the abdominal aorta by the renal vein and renal artery. These vessels run medially inside the medial perinephric fat and attach to the kidney at the hilum.

  Clear vessel, push the kidney anterior keep fatty tissue in the hilum under tension. Dissect surface layer of tense fatty tissue in hilum region using the ultrasonic dissector until vessel structure becomes apparent in tissue.

  - Ligate and cut vessel.
  - Freeing the superior pole and peritoneum: The renal hilum is now dissected; the kidney is still connected by binding tissue to the diaphragm, the abdominal wall, and the peritoneum

- Freeing the superior pole
- Freeing part of the peritoneum
- Take out the kidney

NEPHRON-SPARING SURGERY

22. Role of nephron sparing surgery in the management of renal cell carcinoma. ***WBUHS 2021 Supplementary***

23. Discuss the role of conservative surgery for RCC.

24. Nephron sparing surgery. ***WBUHS 2025 Supplementary***

25. What is nephron sparing surgery? ***WBUHS 2025***

Introduction

Nephron-sparing surgery (NSS), consists of complete excision of the tumor, while preserving as much of the normal functional parenchyma of the affected kidney as possible

- Nephron-sparing surgery (NSS) provides effective curative treatment for patients with renal cell carcinoma. It represents an alternative to renal replacement therapy in patients with critical indications. For selected patients with systemic disease threatening global kidney function, NSS preserves unaffected nephrons with excellent cancer survival.
- Nephron-sparing surgery is indicated
- When radical nephrectomy renders the patient functionally anephric, dialysis is required.
- These settings include:
  - Renal cell carcinoma
  - RCC with insufficient kidney function
  - Bilateral synchronous RCC
- Nephron-sparing surgery is better in this situation for patients with tumors >4 cm located in the upper or lower pole or in the periphery.
- Nephron-sparing surgery is also used for small tumors with normal contralateral kidneys.
- Patients with hereditary forms of RCC such as von Hippel–Lindau syndrome should also be considered for nephron-sparing therapy.
- After nephron-sparing surgery, local recurrence in the operated kidney occurs in <5% of patients.
- Cancer survival after partial nephrectomy is 90–100% in patients with a single tumor 4 cm or less.

Operational Considerations

Preoperative Assessment

- Initial evaluation of RCC patients should include assessment of local tumor location and grade, as well as the presence of local or distant metastases.
- Renal arteriography represents the internal vasculature. For patients with large or central tumors, renal venography should also be performed to rule out internal venous thrombosis.
- Preoperative hydration and administration of mannitol is also necessary to ensure renal recovery during surgery.

Intraoperative Ultrasonography (USG)

- Recently, intraoperative sonography has served as a useful adjunct in nephron-sparing surgery by guiding the surgical approach and excision of the tumor.
- Intraoperative ultrasound can provide important insight into the extent of the tumor as well as the relationship of the tumor to the renal vessels and other important adjacent structures.
- This internal imaging technique is more useful in cases where deep internal lesions cannot be detected and cannot be visualized during surgery.

Surgical Technique

- Once the size of the tumor has been determined, several surgical techniques can be used depending on the characteristics of the tumor.
- Tumor confined to the upper or lower pole of the kidney is usually removed by polar segmental nephrectomy.
- Transverse resection is used for large tumors that extend into the upper or lower pole of the kidney. For tumors that are not located in the upper or lower pole of the kidney, surgical resection is used.
- Regardless of the surgical technique, general principles such as a 1 cm tumor-free margin, early vascular control, proper hemostasis, occlusion of the collecting system, and avoidance of renal ischemia.
- Once the tumor is inflated, monitoring the blood flow is imperative.
  - Given the increasing complexity of nephron-sparing surgery, intraoperative and postoperative bleeding is a common complication.
  - Therefore, blood flow control is an integral part of the surgical procedure.
  - The main way to control severe bleeding involves temporary clamping of the renal artery while controlling the blood supply.
  - If such measures are anticipated for a long time, cooling the kidney with ice wash and mannitol infusion can provide safe ischemia and prevent permanent ischemic injury to the kidney.
  - Other methods of effective hemostasis include ultrasound aspiration, laser photocoagulation, microwave coagulation, and fibrin glue.
- Except in the case of nephron-sparing surgery, some advocate an extracorporeal approach, especially for RCC tumors that require a very complex excision. Such procedures involve total nephrectomy, tumor resection, and kidney transplantation, followed by autologous kidney transplantation. This procedure is useful in cases where large RCC lesions are associated with extravasation or renal artery disease, as it provides a better opportunity for surgery.

Disadvantages

- *Tumor recurrence in the preserved kidney:*
  - The main disadvantage of NSS in the treatment of RCC is the risk of recurrence in the ipsilateral kidney (ipsilateral recurrence)
  - Ipsilateral recurrence is often associated with multifocality of the tumor instead of complete resection of the tumor leaving a positive surgical margin.
  - Although the disease-specific and overall survival rates of patients undergoing NSS are comparable to those of patients undergoing RN, the presumed higher risk of postoperative local recurrence after NSS mandates a more intensive surveillance than that proposed in the European Association of Urology guidelines. Regular ultrasound and/or annual CT scan of both the ipsilateral and contralateral kidney are considered appropriate.
- *Complications and morbidity associated with nephron-sparing surgery:*
  - Another argument that was initially used against expanding the indications for NSS was the greater risk of complications with NSS compared with RN.
  - Partial nephrectomy is a more complicated operation than RN. Hemorrhage is the most common complication, with an incidence between 0 and 5% in NSS. Less-frequent complications include urinary leakage or fistula formation, renal artery thrombosis, and acute renal failure.
    - Complications in patients undergoing open NSS are related to the level of experience the surgeon has with the procedure. Complications in these patients are rare, therefore, in experienced hands, and when they do occur, they can mostly be managed conservatively.
    - Laparoscopic partial nephrectomy is an emerging minimally invasive approach for the treatment of RCC.
    - The laparoscopic approach had a longer renal warm-ischemia time compared with the open approach and was associated with more frequent and more severe intraoperative complications and more postoperative urological complications than open NSS.
- *Elevation of the hematocrit and levels of serum calcium, alkaline phosphatase, and amino acids.*

CHAPTER 58

Prostate and Urethra

LEARNING OBJECTIVES

- ➢ Hypospadias
- ➢ Benign Hypertrophy of Prostate
- ➢ Carcinoma Prostate

1. Write in short, the development of urethra. Describe the clinical features and management of hypospadias. ***WBUHS 2023***

2. Define hypospadias. What are the different types of hypospadias? Outline the management of hypospadias. ***WBUHS 2021 Supplementary; RGUHS, Karnataka 2024***

3. Outline the classification and surgical management of hypospadias in adults. ***WBUHS 2025***

4. Write in brief about repair of hypospadias.

Development of Urethra

Development of male urethra

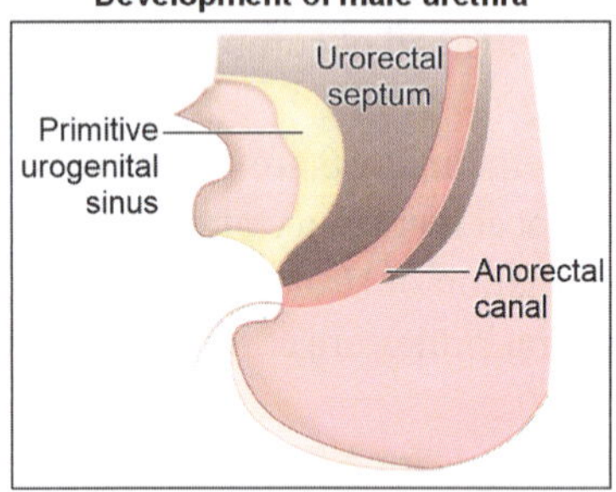

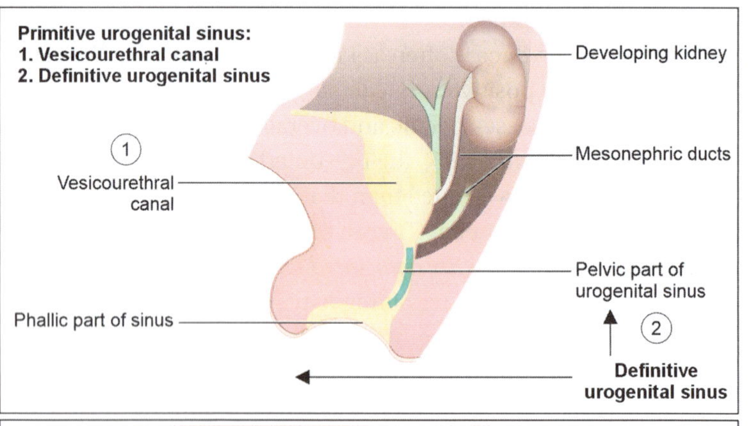

- **The upper part of the prostatic urethra** (till the opening of the ejaculatory duct) derives from **endoderm** of the distal end of the vesicourethral part of the cloaca + absorbed part of the **mesonephric** duct
- **The lower part of the prostatic urethra + membranous urethra** derives from the endoderm of the *upper pelvic part of the definitive urogenital sinus*
- **Spongy (penile) urethra** derives from the *phallic (distal) part of the definitive urogenital sinus* **(endoderm)** + migrating **ectoderm** of the glans phallus (penis)

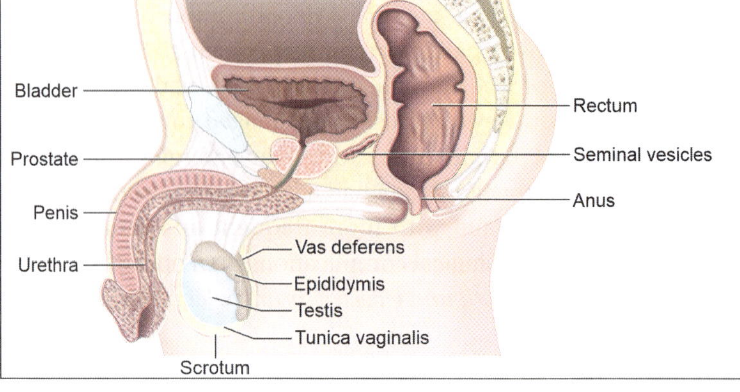

- During the 4th–7th weeks of development, the cloaca divides into the urogenital sinus anteriorly and the anal canal posteriorly. The urorectal septum is a layer of mesoderm between the primitive anal canal and the urogenital sinus. The tip of the septum will form the perineal body.
- Three portions of the urogenital sinus can be distinguished:
  1. The upper and larger part is the urinary bladder—initially, the bladder is continuous with the allantois, but when the lumen of the allantois is obliterated, a thick fibrous cord, the urachus, remains and connects the apex of the bladder with the umbilicus (in the adult—median umbilical ligament).
  2. The pelvic part of the urogenital sinus is a narrow canal, which, in the male gives rise to the prostatic and membranous parts of the urethra.
  3. The phallic part of the urogenital sinus—it is flattened from side to side, and as the genital tubercle grows, this part of the sinus will be pulled ventrally (differs greatly between the two sexes).
- During differentiation of the cloaca, the caudal portions of the mesonephric ducts are absorbed into the wall of the urinary bladder. Consequently, the ureters, initially outgrowths from the mesonephric ducts, enter the bladder separately.
- As a result of ascent of the kidneys, the orifices of the ureters move farther cranially; those of the mesonephric ducts move close together to enter the prostatic urethra and, in the male, become the ejaculatory ducts.
- Since both the mesonephric ducts and the ureters originate in the mesoderm, the mucosa of the bladder formed by incorporation of the ducts (the trigone of the bladder) is also mesodermal.
- With time, the mesodermal lining of the trigone is replaced by endodermal epithelium, so that finally, the inside of the bladder is completely lined with endodermal epithelium.
- The epithelium of the urethra in both sexes originates in the endoderm; the surrounding connective and smooth muscle tissue is derived from visceral mesoderm.
- At the end of the third month, epithelium of the prostatic urethra begins to proliferate and forms a number of outgrowths that penetrate the surrounding mesenchyme.
- In the male, these buds form the prostate gland. In the female, the cranial part of the urethra gives rise to the urethral and paraurethral glands.

Hypospadias

Definition

Hypospadias is a congenital deformity where the opening of the urethra (the meatus) occurs on the underside (ventral) part of the penis, anywhere from the glans to the perineum.

- It is often associated with hooded foreskin and chordae (ventral curvature of the penile shaft).

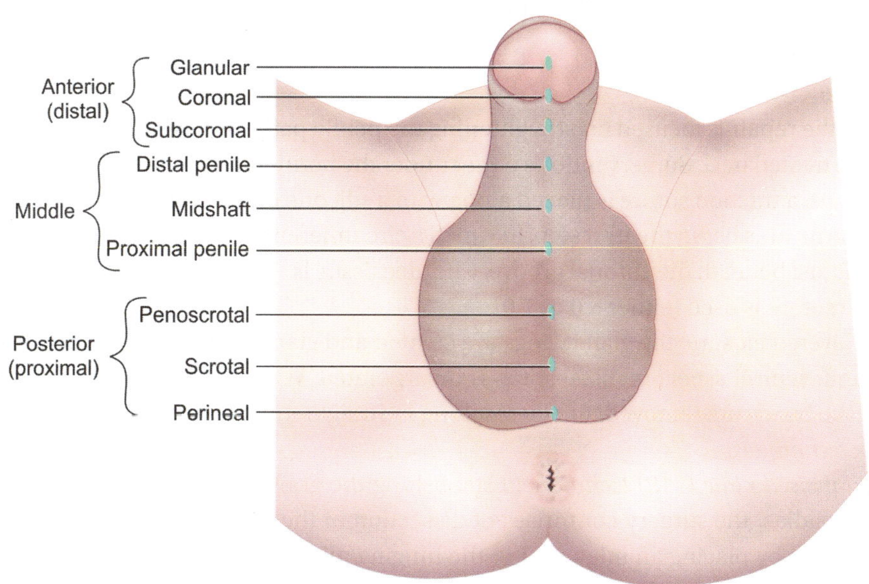

Classification

Hypospadias can be classified according to the anatomical location of the urethral meatus:

- *Anterior (or distal):* Glandular, coronal, and subcoronal (~50%)
- *Middle:* Distal penile, midshaft, and proximal penile (~30%)
- *Posterior (or proximal):* Penoscrotal, scrotal, and perineal (~20%)

Clinical features

- Abnormal ventral meatus
- Hooded prepuce
- Chordae (15% anterior cases, >50% posterior cases)
- Meatal dystopia
- Paraurethral sinuses
- Flattened glans with a cleft
- Scrotum may be bifid
- Penile torsion
- *Associated with:*
    - Inguinal hernia
    - Hydrocele
    - Urethral valves/vesicoureteral reflux (VUR)
- Very rarely may be the part of disorder of sex development (DSD) spectrum

Treatment

- Surgery is indicated where deformity is severe, interferes with voiding, or is predicted to interfere with sexual function.
- Surgery is now performed between 6 and 12 months of age.
- Local application of testosterone for 1 month preoperatively can help increase tissue size.
- Surgery aims to correct penile curvature (orthoplasty), reconstruct a new urethra, and bring the new meatus to the tip of the glans using urethroplasty, glanuloplasty, and meatoplasty techniques. Severe cases may require staged procedures.
- Common operations for anterior hypospadias include meatal advancement and glanuloplasty (MAGPI), meatal-based flaps (Mathieu procedure), and tubularization of the urethral plate. Posterior defects require free grafts (buccal mucosa), onlay grafts, and preputial transfer flaps.

Types of Single-stage Repair

- *MAGPI technique:*
    - In this stage, the repair is focused on straightening the penile path, while defects examined in the degree of curvature are treated next. Surgery is done either under the perineum or in the scrotum skin. In the first step, inside the glans, a traction suture is placed along with a silicone catheter tube inside the bladder of meatus.
    - Degloving the meatus lies in the next step, in which a circumferential incision is carried out around the penis skin, which is just beneath the coronal groove. Chordee tissue is then resected in the junction of penoscrotal. A resorbable suture is used (either 6.0 or 7.0).
    - With a two-layered closure, the glans wings are created and glanuloplasty is then performed. For a normal conical strand, ventral aspect of distal stitch is incorporated. When the skin gets peeled off from the shaft, tethered tissue bands are removed, finally resulting in straightening of the penis.
- *Tubularization techniques:*
    - *Tubularized incised plate (TIP) technique:* Establishing the graft is done via tubularization technique. For severe hypospadias, the surgery comprises of dissection of the lining of the penis erectile path. The graft can be processed by placing an inlay next to the hinging midline. Glansplasty is usually performed for the creation of meatus and deep placement of the neomeatus. Dissection is performed at the bottom of the penis

and in some complex redo cases; tunica vaginalis flap acts as a possible graft to interpret this additional layer. A transurethral indwelling catheter is left after this stage and later removed after a week.

- *GAP repair technique:* This technique is based on the Thiersch–Duplay techniques, with the same procedure as in TIP. In this technique, wide urethral plate has been closed alongside the dorsal aspect without relaxing incision.
- *Flap technique—Mathieu procedure:* This process starts with the measurement of defective location from glans tip to meatus. On the shaft skin of the penis, equal markings are done to make cautious dissection of flaps on subcutaneous tissue.

  The flap is then flipped approximately (around 7–8 mm) to the lateral lines of urethral plate. The width of the flaps is tapered to 5–6 mm at the lateral point of glans. The fibrous joint (suture) is then covered using a flap tissue, and finally lateral stitching is done. The meatus gets developed up to the glans.

  The wings of the glans are approximated and the suture gets covered by dartos flap, a connection tissue found in the penis. Finally, the adjacent blood vessels are dressed appropriately.

Treating Proximal Hypospadias

Single-stage repairs

- Under single-stage repair, the following techniques are performed:
  - *Transverse island flap (TIP):* The process starts with penis degloving and chordee correction. The inner foreskin is inflated like a pedicle graft and then encovering urethral plate using ventral transpose, like onlay flap. Stitching can be done by ignoring regular anastomosis in order to avoid a baggy-like structure; however, it is dressed to prevent urethral diverticulum.
  - *One-stage repair with Koyanagi–Nonomura:* In this technique, from the shaft skin, a wide graft is harvested so as to make proper stitching in preputial hood. Harvested graft is then tubularized for single-stage correction. This technique is an essence of two stages accomplished in a single stage.
  - *TIP urethroplasty:* This is a successful treatment in distal hypospadias that can be used in treatment even in the absence of chordee. The process can be carried out in some complicated operations, as mentioned in distal TIP. Not all the attempts in TIP are as good as acknowledged but show compromising results after redo.

---

5. Principles of surgery for midpenile hypospadias. ***WBUHS 2010***

Hypospadias can be classified according to the anatomical location of the urethral meatus:

- *Anterior (or distal):* Glandular, coronal, and subcoronal (~50%)
- *Middle:* Distal penile, midshaft, and proximal penile (~30%)
- *Posterior (or proximal):* Penoscrotal, scrotal, and perineal (~20%)

Diagnosis

- A full clinical examination will make the diagnosis.
- However, it is also important to seek out associated abnormalities which will need treatment (undescended testes, inguinal hernias, and hydroceles).
- Patients with absent testes and severe hypospadias should undergo chromosomal and endocrine investigation to exclude intersex conditions.

Treatment

- Surgery is indicated where deformity is severe, interferes with voiding, or is predicted to interfere with sexual function.
- Surgery is now performed between 6 and 12 months of age. Local application of testosterone for 1 month preoperatively can help increase tissue size.
- Surgery aims to correct penile curvature (orthoplasty), reconstruct a new urethra, and bring the new meatus to the tip of the glans using urethroplasty, glanuloplasty, and meatoplasty techniques.
- Severe cases may require staged procedures.

- Common operations for anterior hypospadias include MAGPI, meatal-based flaps (Mathieu procedure), and tubularization of the urethral plate. Posterior defects require free grafts (buccal mucosa), onlay grafts, and preputial transfer flaps.
- The onlay island flap is a variation of the transverse preputial island flap for hypospadias repair. It is useful in patients without fibrous chordee whose meatus is midpenile or subcoronal.
- The cosmetic results with the onlay island flap were quite satisfactory and the complication rate was 6%, which was identical to that observed with the Mathieu repair.
- The onlay island flap is applicable particularly in patients with midshaft hypospadias without chordee, if the meatus is too proximal for a Mathieu repair, and in patients with distal penile hypospadias with deficient ventral skin.
- Tabularized incised plate urethroplasty was found to be a successful method for treating distal hypospadias and encouraging results were obtained in midpenile hypospadias cases.
- *The Mathieu–Righini technique for mid-distal hypospadias repair:*
  - This technique employs a meatal flap in which the prepuce is preserved and reconstructed.
  - This technique provides very good cosmetic and functional results—the penis is normal in appearance as well as function. In the author's opinion, the Mathieu–Righini technique is the procedure of choice for mid-distal hypospadias without chordae repair.

6. Pharmacotherapy of benign prostatic hyperplasia.

Introduction

Benign prostatic hyperplasia is most commonly treated medically with α-blockers, such as doxazosin, terazosin, tamsulosin, and alfuzosin. Another class of medications, 5-α-reductase inhibitors, such as finasteride or dutasteride, are also used to treat BPH.

Drugs used are:

- *Alpha-blockers* are categorized by their selectivity for the androgen receptor (AR) and by their elimination half-life.
  - *Nonselective:* Phenoxybenzamine for effective symptom control but high side-effect profile
  - *Short-acting:* Prazosin, alfuzosin, and indoramin
  - *Long-acting:* Terazosin, doxazosin, and alfuzosin SR
  - *Subtype selective:* Tamsulosin relatively selective for (1a-AR subtype compared to the 1 ± 1b subtype)

  No study has directly compared one alpha-blocker with another in terms of efficacy or side effects.

Indications for Treatment

Bothersome lower urinary tract symptoms (LUTS) where watchful waiting (WW) has failed or the patient wishes to have treatment.

- *5-alpha-reductase inhibitors* inhibit the conversion of testosterone to dihydrotestosterone (DHT), the more potent androgen in the prostate. This causes shrinkage of the prostatic epithelium and therefore a reduction in prostate volume, thereby reducing the component of benign prostatic enlargement. This takes some months to occur, so urinary symptoms will not improve initially.
  - Finasteride is a competitive inhibitor of the enzyme 5-alpha-reductase (type II isoenzyme) which converts testosterone to DHT. Finasteride therefore lowers serum and intraprostatic DHT levels.
  - Dutasteride can also be used.
  - Epristeride is a dual inhibitor of 5-alpha-reductase—whether it has any clinically significant advantages over finasteride remains to be established.
- *Combination therapy:* A combination of an alpha-blocker and a 5-alpha-reductase inhibitor. Most studies, suggest that combination therapy is no more useful than an alpha-blocker alone.

- *Alternative drug therapy:*
  - *Anticholinergics:* For a man with frequency, urgency, and urge incontinence symptoms suggestive of an overactive bladder consider prescribing an anticholinergic (e.g., oxybutynin, tolterodine, trospium chloride, or flavoxate). There is the concern that these drugs could precipitate urinary retention in men with bladder outlet obstruction (BOO) (because they block parasympathetic/cholinergic-mediated contraction of the detrusor), but the risk of this occurring is probably very low, even in men with urodynamically proven BOO.
  - *Phytotherapy:* It is an alternative drug treatment for BPH symptoms. These agents are derived from plants and include the African plum (*Pygeum africanum*), purple coneflower (*Echinacea purpurea*), South African star grass (*Hypoxis rooperi*), and saw palmetto berry (*Serenoa Repens*, Permixon).

---

7. What is the etiology of benign prostatic hyperplasia (BPH)? Describe the nonsurgical and minimally invasive surgical management of BPH. ***WBUHS 2023***

---

8. Mention the merits and demerits of conservative and surgical treatment options for BPH. ***WBUHS 2018***

---

9. Outline the surgical management of benign hyperplasia prostate. ***WBUHS 2025 Supplementary***

---

10. Discuss clinical features and management of benign hypertrophy of prostate.
Rajiv Gandhi University of Health Sciences, Karnataka 2019; Ayush University, Chhattisgarh 2025

---

11. What are lower urinary tract symptoms (LUTS)? Describe principles of management of BPH.
Rajiv Gandhi University of Health Sciences, Karnataka 2024

---

12. Management of BPH with overactive bladder. ***Gujarat Health University 2025***

Etiology of BPH

- Idiopathic
- Aging along with endocrine factors
- Accumulation of DHT
- Cancer of prostate
- *Others:*
  - Obesity
  - Inflammation
  - Alcohol consumption

Merits and demerits of conservative and surgical treatment options for BPH.

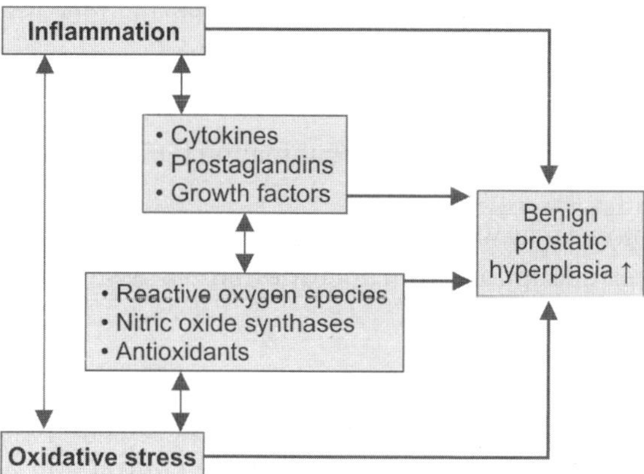

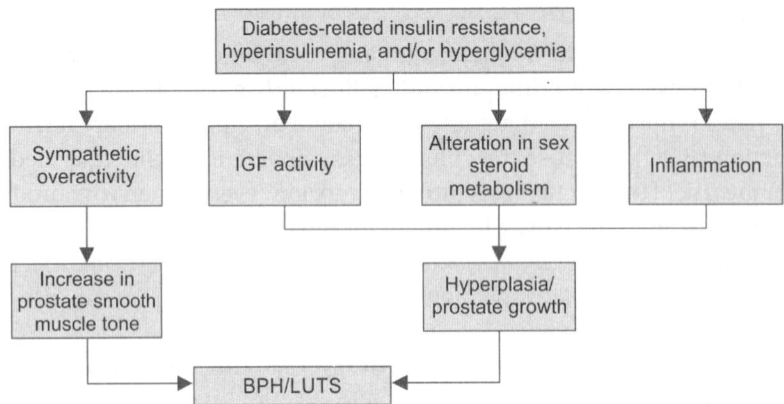

(BPH: benign prostatic hyperplasia; IGF: insulin-like growth factor; LUTS: lower urinary tract symptoms)

Clinical Features of BPH

Lower Urinary Tract Symptoms (LUTS)

BPH symptoms are typically categorized into *obstructive* (voiding) and *irritative* (storage) symptoms:

- *Obstructive symptoms (due to prostate enlargement obstructing urine flow)*
    - *Weak urine stream:* Reduced force or caliber of the urinary stream.
    - *Hesitancy:* Difficulty initiating urination, with a delay before the flow starts.
    - *Intermittency:* Urine flow that stops and starts during voiding.
    - *Straining*: Need to push or strain to urinate.
    - *Incomplete bladder emptying:* Feeling that the bladder is not fully emptied after urination.
    - *Dribbling:* Postvoid dribbling or leakage after urination.
- *Irritative symptoms (due to bladder overactivity or irritation)*
    - *Urgency:* Sudden, compelling need to urinate.
    - *Frequency:* Needing to urinate more often, typically more than 8 times per day.
    - *Nocturia*: Waking up at night to urinate, often multiple times.
    - *Urge incontinence:* Involuntary leakage of urine due to urgent need to void.

Other Clinical Features

- *Bladder changes:* Over time, the bladder may become overactive or less compliant, worsening symptoms.
- *Acute urinary retention (AUR):* Sudden inability to urinate, requiring catheterization (a severe complication).
- *Chronic urinary retention:* Gradual buildup of residual urine, potentially leading to overflow incontinence.
- *Hematuria:* Blood in the urine, though less common, may occur due to bladder irritation or vascular prostate tissue.
- *Recurrent urinary tract infections (UTIs):* Caused by incomplete bladder emptying.
- *Bladder stones:* Formation due to stagnant urine in the bladder.

Associated Features

- *Prostate enlargement:* Detected via digital rectal examination (DRE), though size does not always correlate with symptom severity.
- *Symptom variability:* Symptoms may wax and wane, and severity varies widely among individuals.
- *Impact on quality of life:* Sleep disruption (from nocturia), embarrassment, or activity limitations due to frequent urination.

Medical Management of BPH

Alpha-blockers: The rationale for alpha-blocker therapy in BPH. Benign prostatic hyperplasia is caused partly by alpha-1-adrenoceptor-mediated prostatic smooth muscle contraction and this is the rationale for alpha 1-adrenoceptor-blocker treatment for symptomatic benign prostatic obstruction (BPO).

Alpha-blocker classification:
Alpha-blockers are categorized by their selectivity for the AR and by their elimination half-life.

- *Nonselective:* Phenoxybenzamine—effective in symptom control but high side-effect profile
- *Alpha-1, short-acting:* Prazosin 2 mg twice a day
- *Alpha-1, long-acting:* Terazosin 5 or 10 mg daily, doxazosin 4 or 8 mg daily
- *Alpha-1a selective:* Tamsulosin 0.4 or 0.8 mg daily, alfuzosin 10 mg daily, silodosin 4 or 8 mg daily.

Indications for treatment: Bothersome LUTS where WW has failed or the patient wishes to have treatment.

Efficacy: Percentage of patients who respond to alpha-blockers:

- >25% improvement in symptoms relative to placebo
- The mean probability for improvement in symptom score after transurethral resection of the prostate (TURP) is in the order of 80% (i.e., 8 out of 10 men will notice an improvement in their symptoms after TURP).

Improvements in symptom score in men who respond to alpha-blockers: The average improvement in symptom score after TURP is about 85%.

Side effects:

- A substantial proportion of men stop taking their medication either because of side effects or because of a perceived lack of effectiveness.
- *Side effects:* Asthenia (weakness, in 5%), dizziness (6%), headache (2%) and postural hypotension (1%), and retrograde ejaculation (8%)

Medical Management of BPH

5-alpha-reductase inhibitors

- 5-alpha-reductase inhibitors inhibit the conversion of testosterone to DHT, the more potent androgen in the prostate. This causes shrinkage of the prostatic epithelium and therefore a reduction in prostate volume, thereby reducing the static component of benign prostatic enlargement. This takes some months to occur, so urinary symptoms will not improve initially. Finasteride is a competitive inhibitor of the enzyme 5-alpha-reductase (type II isoenzyme) which converts testosterone to DHT.
- Finasteride therefore lowers serum and intraprostatic DHT levels. Epristeride is a dual inhibitor of 5-alpha-reductase. Whether it has any clinically significant advantages over finasteride remains to be established.

Efficacy

- A small reduction in the risk of urinary retention
- Substantial reduction in the risk of urinary retention
- Shrinking large vascular prostates probably helps to reduce the frequency of hematuria in men with BPH.

Side effects: Sexual problems (e.g., loss of libido 5%; impotence 5%; and reduced volume of ejaculate in a few percent).

Combination Therapy

A combination of an alpha-blocker and a 5-alpha-reductase inhibitor.

- Combination prevented progression of BPH (progression being defined as a worsening of symptom score by 4 or more, or the development of complications such as urinary tract infection (UTI) or acute urinary retention).

Medical Management of BPH

Alternative Drug Therapy

- *Anticholinergics:* For a man with frequency, urgency, and urge incontinence symptoms suggestive of an overactive bladder consider prescribing an anticholinergic (e.g., oxybutynin, tolterodine, trospium chloride, or flavoxate).
- *Phytotherapy:* An alternative drug treatment for BPH symptoms, and one which is widely used in Europe and increasingly in North America, is phytotherapy. 50% of all medications consumed for BPH symptoms are phytotherapeutic ones.

Surgical Treatment of BPH

- *Minimally invasive management of BPH: Surgical alternatives to TURP:*
  - *Transurethral radiofrequency needle ablation (TUNA) of the prostate:*
    - Low-level radiofrequency is transmitted to the prostate via a transurethral needle delivery system; the needles transmit the energy being deployed in the prostatic urethra once the instrument has been advanced into the prostatic urethra. It is done under local anesthetic, with or without intravenous sedation. The resultant heat causes localized necrosis of the prostate.
    - Improvements in symptom score and flow rate are modest. Side effects include bleeding (one third of patients), UTI (10%), and urethral stricture (2%).
    - No adverse effects on sexual function have been reported.
  - *Transurethral microwave thermotherapy (TUMT):*
    - Microwave energy can be delivered to the prostate via an intraurethral catheter (with a cooling system to prevent damage to the adjacent urethra), producing prostatic heating and coagulative necrosis. Subsequent shrinkage of the prostate and thermal damage to adrenergic neurons (i.e., heat-induced adrenergic nerve block) relieves obstruction and symptoms.
    - Compared with TURP, TUMT results in symptom improvement in 55% of men and TURP in 75%. Sexual side effects after TUMT (e.g., impotence and retrograde ejaculation) are less frequent than after TURP, but catheterization period is longer and UTI and irritating urinary symptoms are more common.
    - *High-intensity focused ultrasound (HIFU):* A focused ultrasound beam can be used to induce a rise in temperature in the prostate or indeed in any other tissue to which it is applied. For HIFU treatment of the prostate, a transrectal probe is used. A general anesthetic or heavy intravenous sedation is required during the treatment. It is regarded as an investigational therapy.
- *Invasive surgical alternatives to TURP:*
  - *Transurethral electrovaporization of the prostate (TUVP):* Vaporizes and desiccates the prostate. TUVP seems to be as effective as TURP for symptom control and relief of BOO, with durable (5 years) results. Operating time and inpatient hospital stay are equivalent. Requirement for blood transfusion may be slightly less after TUVP. TUVP does not provide tissue for histological examination so prostate cancers cannot be detected.
    - *Laser prostatectomy:*
      - *Transurethral ultrasound-guided laser-induced prostatectomy (TULIP):* Performed using a probe consisting of a Nd:YAG (neodymium-doped yttrium–aluminum–garnet) laser adjacent to an ultrasound transducer.
      - *Visual laser ablation of the prostate (VLAP):* This side-firing system uses a mirror to reflect or a prism to refract the laser energy at various angles (usually 90°) from a laser fiber located in the prostatic urethra onto the surface of the prostate. The principle tissue effect was one of coagulation with subsequent necrosis.
      - *Contact laser prostatectomy:* Produces a greater degree of vaporization than VLAP, allowing the immediate removal of tissue
      - *Interstitial laser prostatectomy (ILP):* Performed by transurethral placement of a laser fiber directly into the prostate which produces a zone of coagulative necrosis some distance from the prostatic urethra.
      - TULIP, VLAP, contact laser prostatectomy, and ILP have been succeeded by holmium laser prostatectomy.
      - *Holmium laser prostatectomy:* The wavelength of the holmium:YAG laser is such that it is strongly absorbed by water within prostatic tissue. It produces vaporization at the tip of the laser fiber. Its depth of penetration is <0.5 mm and thus, it can be used to produce precise incisions in tissue.

      It can be used with normal saline, thus avoiding the possibility of TURP syndrome.

Three techniques holmium laser prostatectomy developed in progression:

1. Vaporization (holmium-only laser ablation of the prostate, HoLAP); time-consuming, suitable only for small prostates
2. Resection (holmium laser resection of the prostate, HoLRP); similar symptomatic outcome to TURP
3. Enucleation (holmium laser enucleation of the prostate, HoLEP); lobes of the prostate are dissected off the capsule of the prostate and then pushed back into the bladder.

- *TURP and open prostatectomy*
  - *TURP:* Removal of the obstructing tissue of BPH or obstructing prostate cancer from within the prostatic urethra, leaving the compressed outer zone intact.

  Indications for TURP:
  - Bothersome LUTS which fail to respond to changes in lifestyle or medical therapy
  - Recurrent acute urinary retention
  - Renal impairment due to BOO (high-pressure chronic urinary retention)
  - Recurrent hematuria due to benign prostatic enlargement
  - Bladder stones due to prostatic obstruction

Open Prostatectomy

Indications

- Large prostate (>100 g)
- TURP not technically possible (e.g., limited hip abduction)
- Failed TURP (e.g., because of bleeding)
- Urethra too long for the resectoscope to gain access to the prostate
- Presence of bladder stones which are too large for endoscopic cystolitholapaxy, combined with marked enlargement of the prostate.

Contraindications

- Small fibrous prostate
- Prior prostatectomy in which most of the gland has been resected or removed; this obliterates the tissue planes.
- Carcinoma of the prostate

Complications: Hemorrhage; urinary infection; rectal perforation (close and cover with a colostomy)

Management of *benign prostatic hyperplasia (BPH)* with *overactive bladder (OAB)* symptoms requires a *careful, combined approach*—since both conditions affect lower urinary tract function but respond to different treatments.

Overview

- *BPH* → obstruction at the bladder outlet due to enlarged prostate.
- *OAB* → urgency, frequency, nocturia, ± urge incontinence due to detrusor overactivity.

Many men have *both*, especially older patients—this is often called *LUTS (Lower Urinary Tract Symptoms)* with a mix of *voiding* and *storage* symptoms.

Assessment

History and Symptom Scoring

- International prostate symptom score (IPSS) or AUA symptom index
- Evaluate storage vs voiding symptoms

Physical Examination

- Digital rectal examination (DRE)
- Neurological assessment (if needed)

Investigations

- Urinalysis (rule out infection)
- Serum PSA (prostate cancer screening if indicated)

- Post-void residual (PVR) volume (important before adding OAB drugs)
- *Optional:* Uroflowmetry, bladder diary, ultrasound

Management Approach

Step 1: Lifestyle and Behavioral Measures

- Limit caffeine, alcohol, and evening fluids
- Timed voiding and bladder training
- Weight reduction and physical activity
- Manage constipation (it worsens urinary symptoms)

Step 2: Pharmacologic Therapy

- *Treat the BPH (obstruction)*
  - *α-adrenergic blockers*
    - e.g., *Tamsulosin, Alfuzosin, Silodosin, Doxazosin, Terazosin*
    - *Mechanism:* Relax smooth muscle in the prostate and bladder neck → improve flow.
    - *Onset:* Days to weeks.
    - *Side effects:* Dizziness, hypotension, retrograde ejaculation.
  - *5-α reductase inhibitors (5-ARI)*
    - E.g., *Finasteride, Dutasteride*
    - *Mechanism:* Shrink prostate by reducing DHT.
    - *Onset:* Months.
    - Useful if prostate >40 mL or PSA >1.5 ng/mL.
    - *Side effects:* Decreased libido, erectile dysfunction.
  - *Combination therapy:* α-blocker + 5-ARI → greater symptom relief and reduced progression risk (MTOPS trial).
- *Treat the overactive bladder (storage symptoms)*
  If urgency/frequency persist *after α-blocker optimization* and *PVR <150 mL:*
  - *Antimuscarinics*
    - e.g., *Solifenacin, Tolterodine, Oxybutynin, Fesoterodine, Trospium*
    - Decrease detrusor overactivity.
    - Monitor for urinary retention (especially if baseline PVR high).
  - *α3-adrenergic agonist*
    - e.g., *Mirabegron or Vibegron*
    - Relax detrusor muscle during filling phase.
    - Can be safely combined with α-blockers.
    - Fewer anticholinergic side effects.
  - *Combination therapy*
    - α-blocker + antimuscarinic (e.g., *Tamsulosin + Solifenacin*)
    - α-blocker + β3 agonist (e.g., *Tamsulosin + Mirabegron*)

    Combination therapy improves storage symptoms without significantly increasing risk of urinary retention in men with low PVR.

Step 3: Refractory or Severe Cases

If symptoms persist despite optimal medication:

- *Minimally invasive BPH procedures:*
  - UroLift (prostatic urethral lift)
  - Rezūm (water vapor therapy)
  - TUMT, TUNA (less common now)

- *Surgical interventions:*
    - TURP (Transurethral Resection of Prostate)
    - HoLEP (Holmium Laser Enucleation)
    - Open or robotic simple prostatectomy (for very large glands)

Step 4: Follow-up

- Reassess IPSS, QOL, and PVR after 4–12 weeks.
- Monitor for retention or side effects (especially from antimuscarinics).

---

13. Describe the recent trends in diagnosis and management of carcinoma of prostate.
WBUHS 2016, 2017; RIMS, Imphal 2022

---

14. Recent advances in management of carcinoma prostate. ***RIMS, Imphal 2022***

---

15. Discuss the current trend in management of prostatic carcinoma with special reference to robotic surgery.
WBUHS 2011

Screening

- The incidence of prostate cancer increases with age and postmortem data demonstrates histological prostate cancer in approximately 30% of all men in their 40s and in up to 90% of men in their 80–90s.
- The multicenter European Randomized Study of screening for prostate cancer in 1994 is the only study to show a significant benefit from screening with 0.4% of the patients assigned to prostate-specific antigen (PSA) screening dying from prostate cancer, compared to 0.5% in the control group.
- The United States Preventative Services Task Force recommended against PSA testing in men aged ≥75 years.
- The Urological Association recommends screening in the 55–69 years age groups only after an informed shared decision, discussing potential benefits and risks have taken place.

Diagnosis

Transrectal Ultrasound-guided Biopsies

- The most common diagnostic modality for prostate cancer is currently transrectal ultrasonography (TRUS) with guided biopsies. There have been many criticisms of this technique. Analysis of radical prostatectomy specimens has found that 20–25% of patients may harbor anterior tumors which can be missed by the transrectal approach.
- In addition, over 30% of patients will be found to have a tumor after rebiopsy with a negative initial biopsy and persistent concern for prostate cancer.
- Another concern with TRUS biopsies has been associated sepsis rate up to 6% due to the passage of the needle through rectal flora.

Indications for TRUS Alone

- Accurate measurement of prostate volume
- Male infertility with azoospermia, to look for seminal vesicle and ejaculatory duct obstruction due to calculus or Müllerian cyst
- Suspected prostatic abscess (can be drained by needle aspiration)
- Investigation of chronic pelvic pain, looking for prostatic cyst or calculi

Indications for TRUS with Biopsies

- An abnormal digital rectal examination (DRE) and/or an elevated PSA (exceptions include very elderly men with massively elevated PSA and abnormal DRE, or those in whom a TURP is indicated for BOO with severe LUTS/retention where histology will be obtained). Previous biopsies showing isolated prostatic intraepithelial neoplasia (PIN) or atypical small acinar proliferation (ASAP).
- Previous biopsies normal, but PSA rising or DRE abnormal

- To confirm viable prostate cancer following treatment if further treatment is being considered
  - *Transperineal biopsies:*
    - It has improved accuracy with sepsis rate <1%.
    - Acute urinary retention is more common.

Radiographic Features

Ultrasound

- TRUS is often initially performed to detect abnormalities and to guide biopsy, usually following an abnormal PSA level or DRE.
- Ultrasound is used to direct biopsy of suspicious, hypoechoic regions, usually in the peripheral zone. Because of the high incidence of multifocality, systematic sextant biopsies are recommended.
- On ultrasound, prostate cancer is usually seen as a hypoechoic lesion (60–70%) in the peripheral zone of the gland but can be hyperechoic or isoechoic (30–40% of lesions).
- Transrectal ultrasound is also the modality of choice for directing brachytherapy (BT) seeds into the prostate gland.

Magnetic Resonance Imaging (MRI)

The primary indication for MRI of the prostate is in the evaluation of prostate cancer after an ultrasound-guided prostate biopsy has confirmed cancer in order to determine if there is extracapsular extension. Increasingly, MRI is also being used to detect and localize cancer when the PSA is persistently elevated, but routine TRUS biopsy is negative. Both the American College of Radiology (ACR) and the European Society of Uroradiology (ESUR) advocate the use of multiparametric.

MRI-guided prostate biopsy is also being used, particularly in those cases where TRUS biopsy is negative, but clinical and PSA suspicion remains high. Following radical prostatectomy, patients with elevated PSA should also be examined using MRI.

MR Spectroscopy

MR spectroscopy in prostate cancer: Increased choline:citrate or choline + creatine:citrate ratios is seen in prostate cancer (see further for more details).

Routine use of body 3T magnets now means that endorectal coils have become unnecessary for prostate imaging due to the improved signal-to-noise and spatial resolution associated with higher field strength. MRI parameters routinely assessed include the presence of a mass with a low T2 signal, restricted diffusion with reduced apparent diffusion coefficient (ADC), and increased tissue capillary permeability using dynamic gadolinium contrast-enhanced imaging and calculation of the so-called Ktrans (a calculated time constant for permeability). These so-called multiparametric techniques are increasingly being used in the assessment of prostate malignancy with MRI.

Extracapsular extension carries a poor prognosis. Assess for:

- Asymmetry/extension into the neurovascular bundles
- Obliteration of the rectoprostatic angle
- Involvement of the urethra
- Extension into the seminal vesicles (normal seminal vesicles have high signal on T2) Lymphadenopathy is best appreciated on T1-weighted images.

Multiparametric MRI

- Negative predictive value is between 80 and 90%.
- Targeted biopsies can be performed.

Computed Tomography (CT)

- Not accurate at detecting in situ prostate cancer. Scans of the abdomen and pelvis are commonly obtained before the onset of radiation therapy to identify bony landmarks for planning.
- In advanced disease, CT scan is the test of choice to detect enlarged pelvic and retroperitoneal lymph nodes, hydronephrosis, and osteoblastic metastases.

Nuclear medicine: Tc-99m methylene diphosphonate (MDP) bone scans are usually used to detect metastases.

PSA is currently used as a tumor marker for prostate adenocarcinoma. Its normal physiologic role is as a liquifying agent for seminal fluid and the normal amount in human serum is usually very low. Elevated serum levels of PSA have been associated with prostate carcinoma.

PSA can exist in two forms:

1. *Bound/complexed (to serum protein):* Elevated levels are associated with prostate cancer.
2. *Free PSA (fPSA):* Elevated levels are associated with benign prostatic hyperplasia (BPH).

PSA levels: Although an increased PSA level is associated with prostate cancer, a low level cannot exclude prostate cancer. Although exact cut-off values are continually in flux, subject to the most recent data:

- *2–4 ng/mL:* 15–25% change in a man >50 years old of having prostate cancer
- *4–10 ng/mL:* Imaging screening/biopsy indicated

The absolute level may also be misleading if there is a trend in the data upward (or downward) over time. Men with enlarged glands from BPH may also have elevated PSA levels. False-positive levels have been associated with:

- Benign prostatic hyperplasia
- Prostate infection/prostatitis
- UTI
- Manipulation (e.g., DRE or TRUS)
- Recent ejaculation

An upward trend in a patient's PSA value may also be concerning after a prostatectomy, and it may indicate recurrent or metastatic disease.

Prostate cancer staging can be thought of in terms of physical location or grading histologically. The tumor, node, and metastasis (TNM) classification is used to determine spread and the Gleason score is used to determine the histological type. Another staging system is the Jewett-Whitmore staging system.

Additionally, there is some overlap with prebiopsy imaging assessment using prostate imaging reporting and data system (PIRADS).

TNM Staging

Primary Tumor Staging (T)

- *T1:* Not palpable via DRE or seen using TRUS
  - *T1a:* Cancer found incidentally during TURP, <5% of the gland.
  - *T1b:* Cancer found incidentally, but over 5% of the gland is involved.
  - *T1c:* Found by needle biopsy for a raised PSA
- *T2:* Palpable on DRE but confined to the prostate
  - *T2a:* Less than half of one lobe
  - *T2b:* More than half of one lobe
  - *T2c:* Cancer in both lobes of the prostate
- *T3:* Spread outside the prostate
  - *T3a:* Extracapsular extension (one or both sides)
  - *T3b:* Tumor invades the seminal vesicles.
- *T4:* Spread into the adjacent tissues (other than seminal vesicles)
  - For example, bladder sphincter, rectum, levator ani, or pelvic side wall

Nodal Status (N)

On CT, a 1-cm short-axis diameter cut-off is used if it is purely on size grounds.

- *N0:* No spread to lymph nodes
- *N1:* One or more nearby lymph nodes involved

Metastases (M)

- *M0:* No spread beyond regional lymph nodes
- *M1:* Spread beyond local nodes
  - *M1a:* Distant lymph nodes outside the pelvis
  - *M1b:* Bony metastasis
  - *M1c:* Other organ involvement independent of bone involvement
  - For example, lungs, liver, and brain

Histopathologic Grading

Gleason scores can be then grouped into a variety of grades as follows:

- *Gx:* Grade cannot be assessed.
- *G1:* Well-differentiated (slight anaplasia) (Gleason score of 2–4)
- *G2:* Moderately differentiated (moderate anaplasia) (Gleason score of 5–6)
- *G3–4:* Poorly differentiated or undifferentiated (marked anaplasia) (Gleason score of 7–10)

Stage I	Stage II	Stage III	Stage IV
T1a, N0, M0, G1	• T1a, N0, M0, G2-4 • T1 b, N0, M0, any G • T1c, N0, M0, any G • T1, N0, M0, any G • T2, N0, M0, any G	T3, N0, M0, any G	• T4, N0, M0, any G • Any T, N1, M0, any G • Any T, any N, M1, any G

Selection of Patients for WW

Watchful waiting is the best option for patients with localized prostate cancer and:

- Gleason score 2–4 disease (in which the results of the more aggressive treatments described below are no better); any age
- Gleason score 5 and 6 disease; >75 years old
- Significant comorbidity; life expectancy considered to be <10 years
- Stage T1a disease with normal PSA (only 17% T1a will progress, compared to 68% with T1b)

However, WW should be considered and discussed with all who have Gleason score <7, when small-volume disease is predicted by DRE and the biopsy report.

- *Active surveillance:*
  - Active surveillance protocols were implemented in an attempt to defer radical treatment patients and thus avoid their potential significant side effects.
  - Most protocols involve repeat biopsy and PSA-doubling time.

Management of Localized Prostate Cancer

Radical Prostatectomy

- *Inclusion criteria:*
  - Patient's age <75 years
  - Clinical T1 or T2 disease
  - A life expectancy >10 years
  - PSA <50 years

Radical (total) prostatectomy (RP) is excision of the entire prostate, including the prostatic urethra, with seminal vesicles. It may be performed by open retropubic, perineal, or laparoscopic approaches. The perineal approach does not allow a simultaneous pelvic lymph node dissection. Following excision of the prostate, reconstruction of the bladder neck and vesicourethral anastomosis completes the procedure.

- Comparing the surgical methods for robotic, laparoscopic, or open-radical prostatectomy, a significant difference in oncological outcomes has not been shown.

Radiotherapy

- The current standard of care is intensity-modulated radiotherapy (IMRT).
  BT: Generally accepted patient selection criteria for low-dose BT include:
  - Stage c T1b–T2a, N0, M0
  - Gleason score <6
  - PSA <10 ng/dL
  - <50% biopsy cores involved with cancer
  - Prostate volume of <50 cc
  - International Prostatic Symptom Score <12

Management of localized prostate cancer: Radical external beam radiotherapy (EBRT):
EBRT is administered with curative intent, often accompanied by 3 months of neoadjuvant hormone therapy in high-risk cases.

Management of localized prostate cancer: BT
This is ultrasound-guided transperineal implantation of radioactive seeds, usually I^{125}, into the prostate. The treatment is expensive due to the cost of the consumables.

Management of localized and radiorecurrent prostate cancer: Cryotherapy and HIFU:

- *Management of locally advanced nonmetastatic prostate cancer:* ERBT, hormone therapy.
- *Management of advanced prostate cancer:* Hormone therapy

Mechanisms of androgen deprivation:

- *Surgical castration:* Bilateral orchidectomy
- *Medical castration:* Luteinizing hormone-releasing hormone (LH-RH) agonists, estrogens; also termed androgen ablation or androgen deprivation
- *Antiandrogens (steroidal or nonsteroidal):* AR blockade at target cell
- *Maximal androgen blockade (MAB):* Medical or surgical castration plus antiandrogen
- 5-alpha reductase inhibition (5-ARI) with finasteride or dutasteride

Management of localized and radiorecurrent prostate cancer: Cryotherapy and HIFU:
Two minimally invasive treatments for localized prostate cancer are in development. Proponents claim they are viable alternatives to radical surgery or radiotherapy and that they are the only current options for salvage treatment of organ-confined recurrent disease following radical radiotherapy.

Metastatic prostatic cancer:

- Treatment of advanced and metastatic prostate cancer has largely been with hormonal manipulation/androgen-deprivation therapy by either blockade of the AR, by disrupting the hypothalamic–pituitary–gonadal axis (LH-RH antagonists/agonists) or by preventing secretions with bilateral orchidectomy.
- Surgical or chemical castration is the ultimate goal, where currently the aim for a testosterone level of <20 ng/mL (0.7 nmol/L).
- After 18–24 months, patients eventually develop a castrate resistance state where PSA continues to rise despite castrate testosterone levels. The current definition is three consecutive rises, 1 week apart, with two PSAs rising >50% over the nadir.
- Classically, initial treatment has been the use of maximum androgen blockade with the addition of antiandrogens such as bicalutamide to the LH-RH agonist.
- Chemotherapy with docetaxel + prednisolone can also be used.
- Recently, although newer treatments such as abiraterone, enzalutamide, and cabazitaxel have become available, which have been assessed in the pre- and postdocetaxel setting.
- Abiraterone is a CYP17 inhibitor which prevents intracellular testosterone synthesis and is usually administered alongside prednisolone.

- Enzalutamide is a new antiandrogen which blocks the AR and also prevents its translocation and transcription.
- Cabazitaxel is a taxane derivative.

Palliative management of prostate cancer: The involvement of the acute pain team, palliative care physicians, and nurses is often necessary in the terminal phase of the illness to optimize quality of life.

- *Pain:* It is undoubtedly the most debilitating symptom of advanced prostate cancer. The pathogenesis of this pain is poorly understood, but there is known to be increased osteoclastic and osteoblastic activity.
- Spinal cord compression
- *LUTS/urinary retention:*
  - A TURP may be required for BOO or retention.
  - A long-term urethral or suprapubic catheter may be required for difficult voiding symptoms or recurrent retention.

BOO

- This is a uro-oncological emergency.
- Locally advanced prostate cancer and bladder cancer may cause bilateral ureteric obstruction.
- The patient presents either with symptoms and signs of renal failure or is anuric without a palpable bladder.
- Renal ultrasound will demonstrate bilateral hydronephrosis and an empty bladder.
- After treating any life-threatening hyperkalemia, the treatment options include bilateral percutaneous nephrostomies or ureteric stents.
- A clotting screen is required prior to nephrostomy insertion. Insertion of retrograde ureteric stents in this scenario is usually unsuccessful because tumor on the trigone obscures the location of the ureteric orifices.
- Antegrade ureteric stenting following placement of nephrostomies is usually successful.

Hormone therapy should be commenced if not previously used; even in patients with androgen-independent disease, there are reports of high-dose intravenous estrogens (Honvan) unobstructing ureters.

Unilateral ureteric obstruction: It is occasionally observed at presentation or on progression. If asymptomatic, this may be managed conservatively, provided there is a normal contralateral kidney.

Anemia, thrombocytopenia, and coagulopathy.

For some patients, their hemoglobin levels drop rapidly and they become symptomatic on a regular basis. This tends to be normochromic and normocytic and often occurs without other symptoms and with normal renal function. Such patients require regular transfusions. Platelet transfusions are rarely required for bleeding. Terminal patients may develop a clinical picture similar to disseminated intravascular coagulation (DIC), leading to problematic hematuria.

16. Prostate cancer: Prevention; complementary and alternative therapies. ***WBUHS 2011***

Introduction

The diagnosis of prostate cancer is on the increase, probably as a result of increasing use of serum *PSA* testing for both symptomatic and asymptomatic men and the use of more extensive prostatic biopsy protocols.

PSA and Prostate Cancer

- PSA has revolutionized the diagnosis and management of prostate cancer, although its use in screening and early detection remains controversial.
- In addition to its use as a serum marker for the diagnosis of prostate cancer, PSA elevations may help in staging, counseling, and monitoring prostate cancer patients.
- PSA generally increases with advancing stage and tumor volume, although a small proportion of poorly differentiated tumors fail to express PSA.
- *PSA* is used, along with clinical *(DRE)*, T stage, and Gleason score, to predict pathological tumor staging and outcome after radical treatments using statistically derived nomograms and artificial neural networks.

- >50% of patients have extraprostatic disease if PSA >10 ng/mL.
- <5% of patients have lymph node metastases and only 1% have bone metastases if PSA <20 ng/mL.
- 66% of patients have lymphatic involvement and 90% have seminal vesicle involvement if PSA >50 ng/mL.

- PSA should be virtually undetectable following radical prostatectomy for gland-confined disease.
- PSA rise after radical prostatectomy precedes the development of clinical metastatic disease by a mean time of 8 years.
- PSA falls within the normal range in 80% of patients with metastatic disease on hormone therapy within 4 months; the PSA rises in a mean time of 18 months after starting hormone therapy, signaling progressing disease.

In the presence of infection or instrumentation, PSA should not be requested until at least 28 days after the event to avoid a false-positive result, causing unnecessary concern to doctor and patient. Ideally, PSA should not be requested within 2 days of ejaculation or DRE, but in practice, it makes negligible difference to the result.

PSA Derivatives: Free-to-total Ratio (F:T), Density, and Velocity

- Measurement of the F:T PSA ratio increases the specificity of total PSA because the ratio is lower in men with prostate cancer than in men with benign hyperplasia. This may be helpful in deciding whether to rebiopsy a patient with previous benign biopsies.
- Consideration may be given to the prostate volume, since large benign prostates are the most common cause of mildly elevated PSA. Serum PSA/prostate volume = PSA density, and serum PSA/prostate transition-zone volume = PSA-TZ density. Various cut-off densities have been proposed to raise the specificity of total PSA, possibly to reduce the need for prostatic biopsy, but the issue remains controversial.
- Short-term variations in serum PSA occur in the presence or absence of cancer, the cause of which may be technical or physiological. Longer term, the PSA tends to rise slowly due to BPH and faster due to prostate cancer PSA velocity.
- A PSA velocity >0.75 ng/mL per year over at least 18 months in total PSA range 10 ng/mL is suggestive of the presence of prostate cancer, given that only 5% of men without cancer exhibit such a velocity. A PSA velocity >20% per year should also prompt the recommendation of a biopsy, although a slower velocity does not exclude the presence of cancer. The use of PSA velocity is an option for the patient who wishes to avoid an initial or repeat prostatic biopsy.

Robotic radical prostatectomy is the most preferred way of treating localized prostate cancer. Robotic prostatectomy is performed with the help of a surgical robot (da Vinci) through 4–5 small, 1-cm keyhole incisions across the abdomen. Through these small incisions, the robotic arms enter the abdomen. The operating surgeon sitting at the operating console controls the robotic instruments to precisely dissect the prostate gland, seminal vesicles, and vas deferens from the urethra and bladder.

Once the prostate gland is dissected free from the bladder, rectum, and urethra, it is placed in a small plastic bag and eventually removed intact by extending one of the keyhole incisions.

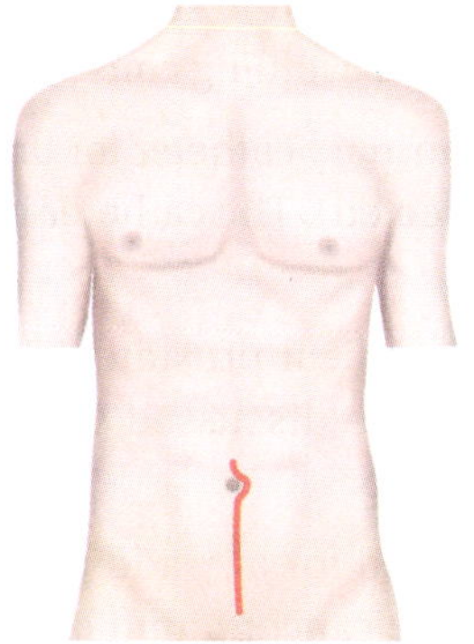

Scar in open surgery

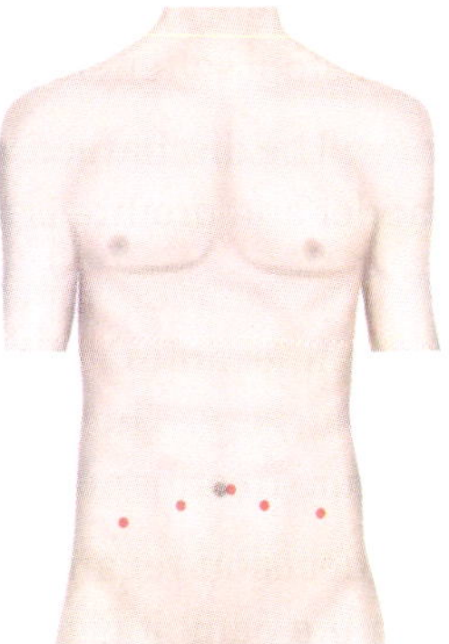

Robotic surgery scar

The complete prostate along with the lymph nodes are then sent to the histopathologist for detailed examination. The bladder is sewn back to the urethra to restore continuity of the urinary tract using robotic instruments and absorbable suturing material. A Foley catheter is placed through the penis to drain the bladder and allow healing of the bladder-urethra connection. In addition, a small drain is placed around the surgical site, exiting one of the keyhole incisions.

Robotic surgery is performed adhering to the same anatomic principles of open surgery but without the surgeon's hands entering into the patient's body cavity. Especially designed EndoWrist instruments allow seven degrees of motion that mimic the dexterity of the human hand and wrist. The result is a better anastomosis when the bladder and the urethra are sewn together after removal of the prostate. Thus, the quality of open surgery is achieved without giving a big surgical incision and its associated complications. In fact, during robotic surgery, a high-resolution three-dimensional (3-D) vision along with 10–12 folds magnification provides true-to-life view of the surgical field and gives the surgeon an excellent visualization and details of the prostate gland and the surrounding neurovascular structures, allowing for precise dissection of the prostate and suturing of blood vessels.

The average *length of surgery* is 2.5–3 hours, but it varies from patient to patient (2.5–4.5 hours) depending on the size of the prostate gland, shape of the pelvis, weight of the patient, and presence of scarring or inflammation within the pelvis due to infection or prior abdominal/pelvic surgery.

Blood loss during robotic prostatectomy is routinely <300 cc. Transfusions are rarely required. Donation of blood prior to surgery for autologous blood transfusion can be arranged if the patient desires, but it is not recommended.

Pain: Another advantage of robotic surgery is much less pain compared to open surgery. Immediate postsurgery pain medication can be controlled and delivered by the patient via an intravenous patient-controlled analgesia (PCA) pump or by injections by the nursing staff. Minor transient shoulder pain may be experience related to carbon dioxide gas used to inflate the abdomen during surgery.

Bladder spasms are experienced after prostatectomy as a cramping sensation in the lower abdomen. These spasms are transient and decrease over time. If severe, medication can be prescribed.

Gas cramps: One may experience sluggish bowels and gas cramps for initial 2–3 days after surgery. Pain medications and effect of anesthetic drugs also prolong the recovery of bowel functions. Getting out of bed, walking, more fluids, and stool softeners help in the recovery.

Hospital stay: Typically, a patient stays for 1–2 nights in the hospital.

Back to normal activities: One of several advantages of robotic surgery is earlier return to normal activity. Driving should be avoided for 2 weeks after surgery. Most patients return to full activity at an average of 3–4 weeks after surgery. Lifting heavy weights and strenuous exercises (jogging, biking, contact sports, etc.) should be deferred for 6 weeks or until instruction by doctor.

Diet and bowel functions: Oral liquids are allowed once you recover from the effect of anesthetic drugs. It is advised to take liquids and avoid high fiber diet in the beginning (till you have a normal bowel movement). It may take 2–3 days for the intestines to recover from the surgery and anesthesia. Pain medication, decreased physical activity, and dehydration may cause constipation. Therefore, pain medication should be discontinued as soon as possible. Lots of fluids and mild laxatives or stool softeners may help in avoiding constipation.

Follow-up appointment: Patient will be discharged with a urinary catheter for draining the bladder and supporting the anastomosis (where the bladder and urethra is reconnected). The catheter is typically removed after 7–10 days following surgery.

Pathology results: The result of the examination of the radical prostatectomy specimen is usually available approximately 7 days following surgery. The results will be discussed with you in the office along with the implications of the findings on future treatment and follow-up.

Need for further treatment: The decision regarding the need for any additional treatment such as radiation or hormonal therapy is based upon the pathologic stage of the cancer found on radical prostatectomy specimen as well as the trend of PSA values following surgery.

Long-term follow-up: First PSA test is drawn 6 weeks after surgery. Subsequently, PSA is evaluated every 3 months.

Urinary incontinence: Most men will experience some degree of stress urinary incontinence. This generally improves with time. Most men experience improvement within 3–6 months. Approximately, 70% of the patients are dry at 6 months and >90% at 12 months. Pelvic floor muscle exercise (Kegel exercise) may help in faster recovery of bladder control. Avoid excessive caffeine, alcohol, or fluid intake during the recovery period as this will exacerbate urinary leakage.

Erectile function: The return of erectile function following surgery depends upon age of patient, preoperative potency, and nerve-sparing surgery. Whether one or both side's erectile nerve bundles can be spared depends upon the tumor volume, Gleason score, and proximity of the tumor-to-prostate capsule. Discuss the issues related to return of erectile function with your doctor.

Robotic prostatectomy is a radical prostatectomy that is also known as robotic-assisted laparoscopic prostatectomy (RALP). It is a minimally invasive prostate removal and cancer treatment surgery.

SMART (Samadi Modified Advanced Robotic Technique)

- Dr Samadi developed his signature *SMART (Samadi Modified Advanced Robotic Technique)* surgery which incorporates oncologic principles, combines it with open radical prostatectomy skills, and builds upon it with a robotic approach.
- SMART is a revolutionary and advanced prostate cancer surgery and prostate cancer treatment method, which drastically reduces blood loss, pain, hospital stay, recovery time, and the side effects of other types of prostate cancer treatments.
- SMART is also known as bloodless prostate surgery.
- SMART does not require opening the endopelvic fascia or cutting the dorsal vein complex. This results in no sutures and less damage to the neurovascular bundle.

17. Medical management of carcinoma prostate. ***DNB 2021 June***

The *medical management of prostate cancer (carcinoma of the prostate)* depends on the *stage of the disease, Gleason score, PSA levels, patient age, comorbidities*, and *patient preference*. Here's an organized overview:

Risk Stratification

Prostate cancer is stratified into:

- Low-risk
- Intermediate-risk
- High-risk
- Locally advanced
- Metastatic

Management varies accordingly.

Medical Management Options

1. *Active surveillance*
    - For *low-risk*, localized prostate cancer (e.g., low PSA, low Gleason score, small tumor)
    - Involves regular:
        - PSA testing
        - Digital rectal examination (DRE)
        - Repeat biopsies or MRI
2. *Androgen deprivation therapy (ADT):* Suppresses testosterone, which fuels prostate cancer growth.
    a. *LHRH agonists:*
        - Leuprolide, Goserelin
        - Initially cause testosterone flare
    b. *LHRH antagonists:*
        - Degarelix, Relugolix
        - Avoid testosterone flare

c. *Antiandrogens:*
   - Bicalutamide, Flutamide, Enzalutamide
   - Often combined with LHRH analogs

d. *Orchiectomy (Surgical Castration):* Rarely used now due to irreversible nature

Used in:
- Advanced/metastatic disease
- As neoadjuvant/adjuvant with radiation

3. *Chemotherapy*
   Mainly used for:
   - Castration-resistant prostate cancer (CRPC)
   - High-volume metastatic hormone-sensitive disease

   Common agents:
   - Docetaxel (first-line for mCRPC)
   - Cabazitaxel (post-docetaxel failure)

4. *Novel hormonal agents:* Used in mCRPC or advanced non-metastatic CRPC.
   - *Abiraterone* (CYP17 inhibitor, blocks androgen synthesis): Requires co-administration with prednisone
   - *Enzalutamide, Apalutamide, Darolutamide:* Androgen receptor inhibitors

5. *Radiopharmaceuticals:*
   Used for bone-predominant metastatic CRPC.
   - *Radium-223 dichloride*: Alpha-emitter targeting bone metastases

6. *Immunotherapy/Targeted Therapy:* Still evolving and used in select patients:
   a. *Sipuleucel-T (autologous cellular immunotherapy):*
      - For asymptomatic/minimally symptomatic mCRPC

   b. *PARP Inhibitors (e.g., Olaparib, Rucaparib):*
      - For patients with *BRCA1/2* or other homologous recombination repair (HRR) gene mutations

Combination Strategies
- *ADT + Novel Hormonal Therapy* (e.g., Enzalutamide or Abiraterone)
- *ADT + Chemotherapy* (e.g., Docetaxel) for high-risk metastatic disease

Monitoring:
- Regular *PSA* levels
- Imaging (bone scan, CT/MRI, PSMA PET where available)
- Watch for progression to castration-resistant prostate cancer (CRPC)

---

18. PSA (Prostate specific antigen). ***Gujarat Health University 2024***

Prostate-specific Antigen (PSA)

PSA is a *glycoprotein enzyme* (a serine protease) produced almost exclusively by the *epithelial cells of the prostate gland.* It is secreted into seminal fluid to help liquefy semen but small amounts enter the bloodstream—where it is measurable by a blood test.

Clinical Importance of PSA

PSA is widely used as a *biomarker* for:
- *Screening* for prostate cancer (with limitations)
- *Diagnosis* and *staging* of prostate cancer
- *Monitoring* response to treatment
- *Detecting* recurrence or progression after therapy

Normal PSA Levels

Age group	*Approximate normal upper limit*
40–49 years	<2.5 ng/mL
50–59 years	<3.5 ng/mL
60–69 years	<4.5 ng/mL
≥70 years	6.5 ng/mL

There is *no absolute cutoff*, but PSA >4 ng/mL often prompts further evaluation. Age-specific ranges and PSA kinetics (velocity, doubling time) are more informative.

Forms of PSA in Blood

- *Free PSA* (unbound)
- *Complexed PSA* (bound to proteins like α1-antichymotrypsin)

The *ratio of free to total PSA* helps distinguish *benign* from *malignant* causes:

- *Lower free/total PSA ratio (<15–20%)* → higher risk of prostate cancer
- *Higher ratio (>25%)* → more likely benign (e.g., BPH)

Causes of Elevated PSA

- *Malignant causes: Prostate cancer*
- *Benign/nonmalignant causes*
  - BPH (Benign Prostatic Hyperplasia)
  - Prostatitis (infection or inflammation)
  - Urinary retention
  - Recent ejaculation
  - Prostate manipulation (DRE, biopsy, catheterization)
  - Vigorous exercise or cycling

PSA Kinetics

These are important for prognosis and monitoring:

Parameter	*Meaning*	*Interpretation*
PSA velocity	Rate of PSA rise over time	>0.75 ng/mL/year → higher cancer risk
PSA doubling time	Time for PSA to double	Shorter doubling time → more aggressive disease
PSA density	PSA ÷ prostate volume	>0.15 ng/mL/cm^3 → suspicious for cancer

Clinical Uses

Screening

- Typically combined with *Digital Rectal Exam (DRE).*
- Controversial due to *false positives* (overdiagnosis) and *false negatives.*
- *Current approach: Shared decision-making* for men aged 50–70, or earlier if high-risk (e.g., African ancestry, family history).

Diagnosis

Elevated PSA → further evaluation with *multiparametric MRI* and *targeted prostate biopsy.*

Staging/Prognosis

- Very high PSA (>20 ng/mL) often indicates *locally advanced* or *metastatic* disease.
- PSA combined with *Gleason score* and *tumor stage* helps risk-stratify patients.

Monitoring After Treatment

- After *radical prostatectomy:*
  - PSA should fall to *undetectable (<0.1 ng/mL)* within weeks.
  - Rising PSA indicates *biochemical recurrence.*
- After *radiotherapy:* PSA declines more gradually; a *rise of ≥2 ng/mL* above the nadir defines recurrence

19. Medical and Surgical castration in carcinoma prostate. ***Gujarat Health University 2024***

Prostate cancer is an *androgen-dependent malignancy.*

The *testosterone* produced mainly by the *testes (≈90–95%)* and to a lesser extent by the *adrenal glands (≈5–10%)* stimulates the growth of prostate cancer cells.

Therefore, *androgen deprivation therapy (ADT)*—also known as *castration*—is a cornerstone in the management of advanced or metastatic prostate cancer.

Goal of Castration

To reduce serum testosterone to *castrate levels*:

- *<50 ng/dL (1.7 nmol/L)*—traditional definition
- *<20 ng/dL*—now considered optimal ("modern" castrate level)

Types of Castration

Surgical Castration (Orchiectomy)

Permanent and immediate reduction in testosterone.

- *Bilateral simple orchiectomy*
  - Removal of both testes through scrotal incisions.
  - Commonly performed under local or general anesthesia.

  Advantages:
  - Rapid testosterone reduction within hours (lowest nadir within 12 hours)
  - One-time procedure, low cost
  - No compliance issues

  Disadvantages:
  - Irreversible
  - Psychological impact ("loss of masculinity")
  - Cosmetic concern (can insert testicular prostheses if desired)
- *Subcapsular orchiectomy*
  - Removal of testicular parenchyma while leaving tunica albuginea and epididymis.
  - Same hormonal result, better cosmetic outcome.

Medical Castration (Pharmacologic Androgen Deprivation)

Reversible suppression of testosterone production using drugs that act on the hypothalamic-pituitary-gonadal axis.

- *LHRH (GnRH) agonists*
  - Leuprolide, Goserelin, Triptorelin, Buserelin
  - Mechanism:
    - Initial stimulation of LH/FSH → transient *testosterone surge (flare)* for ~1 week
    - Continuous stimulation → **downregulation of pituitary receptors

Urinary Bladder

LEARNING OBJECTIVES

- Exstrophy of Bladder
- Neurogenic Bladder
- Transrectal Ultrasound (TRUS)
- Carcinoma Urinary Bladder
- Vesicovaginal Fistula

1. Exstrophy of bladder. *WBUHS 2013*

Bladder exstrophy (also known as *ectopia vesicae*) refers to a herniation of the urinary bladder through an anterior abdominal wall defect. The severity of these defects is widely variable.

Epidemiology

- The estimated incidence of bladder exstrophy is 1:10,000–50,000 live births.
- There is a recognized male predilection with a male-to-female ratio of ~3:1.
- Most cases are sporadic.

Pathology

- Bladder exstrophy is thought to be caused by a developmental defect of the cloacal membrane, which results in a subsequent eversion of the bladder mucosa.
- This then protrudes out as a mass-like lesion.

Associations

General	*In females*
• Extension of the bladder defect into the urethra • Cryptorchidism • Bilateral inguinal herniation • OEIS (omphalocele-exstrophy-imperforate anus-spinal defects) complex • Epispadias	• Vaginal duplication • Clitoral cleft

Serological Markers

Raised maternal alpha-fetoprotein levels.

Radiographic Features

- Imaging findings include a soft-tissue mass, extending from a large infraumbilical anterior wall defect which may be close to the umbilical arterial exits.
- The absence of a normal urinary bladder and a low-lying umbilical cord insertion may also indicate the diagnosis.
- Failure of the pubic bones to meet in the midline (widened pubic symphysis).
- Amniotic fluid volumes are often normal.

Treatment and Prognosis

Treatment is with surgical intervention (primary closure/excision with urinary diversion) and prognosis is generally good.

Complications

- Urinary incontinence
- Infertility
- Acute pyelonephritis
- Increased incidence of malignancy in the extruded bladder

---

2. What are the conditions collectively described as neurogenic bladder? How are patients of neurogenic bladder evaluated and treated? ***WBUHS 2008, 2021***

Introduction

- There are two main types of bladder-control problems associated with neurogenic bladder.
- Depending on the nerves involved and the nature of the injury, the bladder can be overactive (spastic or hyper-reflexive) or inactive (flaccid or hypotonic).

Reasons

- Neurogenic bladder is often associated with spinal cord disease (syringomyelia/hydromyelia), trauma, and neural tube defects such as spina bifida.
- Brain tumors and other brain disorders can also be caused by peripheral nerve disease.
- This is a common complication of major pelvic surgery such as removal of sacrococcygeal teratoma and other tumors.
- Other disorders such as syphilis, diabetes, stroke, or ruptured intervertebral disk.
- Degenerative neurological diseases such as multiple sclerosis and amyotrophic lateral sclerosis
- Long-term effects of alcohol

Types of Neurogenic Bladder

Types of neurogenic bladder can be classified according to the anatomical location of the lesion as follows:

- Supraspinal lesions
- Spinal cord injury
- Peripheral nerve damage

There are several types of neurogenic bladder depending on the cause. Many of these can have similar symptoms.

- *Uninhibited:*
  - Urinary incontinence is usually related to brain damage from stroke or brain tumors.
  - This can lead to fullness of the gallbladder, low gallbladder, and urinary incontinence.
  - Unlike other types of neurogenic bladder, it does not cause bladder pressure that can cause kidney damage.
- *Spastic:*
  - In spastic neurogenic bladder (also called upper motor neuron or hyper-reflexive bladder), the bladder (detrusor) and urethral sphincter muscles do not work together and usually contract tightly at the same time.
  - This phenomenon is also known as detrusor external sphincter dyssynergia (DESD).
  - This leads to urinary retention with high pressure in the bladder which can damage the kidneys.
  - Bladder volume is smaller than normal due to increased muscle tone in the fluid.
  - Spastic neurogenic neuropathy is usually the result of a spinal cord injury above the level of the 10th thoracic vertebra (T10).
- *Flaccid:*
  - In hypotonic bladder (also called lower motor neuron or hypotonic bladder), the bladder muscles lose their ability to contract normally.

- This can cause emptying of the bladder even when the bladder is full and can lead to an enlarged bladder.
- The internal urethral sphincter may be palpable normally, but urinary incontinence is normal.
- Neurogenic bladder is caused by damage to the peripheral nerves that run from the spinal cord to the bladder.

- *Mixed:*
  - Mixed forms of neurogenic bladder can cause a combination of the abovementioned manifestations.
  - In mixed type A, the bladder muscle is smooth, but the sphincter is hyperactive.
  - This results in an enlarged bladder, low pressure, and inability to empty but does not carry the risk of kidney damage like a spastic bladder.
  - *Mixed type is characterized by spastic bladder with external sphincter and distension.*

Symptoms

- Urinary incontinence is characterized by the involuntary release of large amounts of urine or the continuous flow of small amounts of urine. There may be dampness in the bed.
- Frequent urination
- Constant urge to urinate despite the last voiding; constant feeling that the urine is not empty.
- Pain or burning during urination.

Laboratory Studies

- These include the following:
  - Urinalysis and urine culture—urinary tract infection (UTI) can cause irritative voiding symptoms and urge incontinence.
  - Urine cytology—irritative voiding symptoms out of proportion to the overall clinical picture and/or hematuria warrant urine cytology and cystoscopy, as these may indicate carcinoma in situ of the urinary bladder.
  - Kidney function studies—blood urea nitrogen (BUN) and creatinine (Cr) are checked if compromise of kidney function is suspected.
- *Other tests:*
  - A voiding diary is a daily record of the patient's bladder activity. It is an objective documentation of the patient's voiding pattern, incontinent episodes, and inciting events associated with urinary incontinence.
  - The pad test is an objective test that documents and can quantify urine loss. It may be helpful to assess the severity of incontinence.

Diagnostic Procedures

Procedures	*Comments*
Postvoid residual (PVR) bladder volume	• PVR measurement is a part of the basic evaluation for urinary incontinence • If the PVR is high, the bladder may be poorly contractile or the bladder outlet may be obstructed • Both of these conditions can cause urinary retention with overflow incontinence
Uroflow rate	• Uroflow rate is a useful screening test used mainly to evaluate bladder outlet obstruction but will also identify detrusor weakness • Uroflow rate is volume of urine voided per unit of time • Low uroflow rate may reflect urethral obstruction, a weak detrusor, or a combination of both • This test alone cannot distinguish an obstruction from a contractile detrusor
Filling cystometrogram (CMG)	• A filling CMG assesses the bladder capacity, compliance, and the presence of phasic contractions (detrusor instability). Most commonly, liquid-filling medium is used • An average adult bladder holds approximately 50–500 mL of urine. During the test, provocative maneuvers help to unveil bladder instability

Contd...

Contd...

Procedures	Comments
Voiding CMG (pressure–flow study)	• Pressure–flow study simultaneously records the voiding detrusor pressure and the rate of urinary flow • This is the only test able to assess bladder contractility and the extent of a bladder outlet obstruction • Pressure–flow studies can be combined with voiding cystogram and videourodynamic study for complicated cases of incontinence
Cystogram	• A static cystogram (anteroposterior and lateral) helps to confirm the presence of stress incontinence, the degree of urethral motion, and the presence of a cystocele. Intrinsic sphincter deficiency will be evident by an open bladder neck • The presence of a vesicovaginal fistula or bladder diverticulum also may be noted • A voiding cystogram can assess bladder neck and urethral function (internal and external sphincter) during filling and voiding phases • A voiding cystogram can identify a urethral diverticulum, urethral obstruction, and vesicoureteral reflux
Electromyography (EMG)	• EMG helps to ascertain whether voiding is coordinated or uncoordinated • Failure of urethral relaxation during bladder contraction results in uncoordinated voiding (detrusor sphincter dyssynergia) • EMG allows accurate diagnosis of the detrusor sphincter dyssynergia that is common in spinal cord injuries
Cystoscopy	• The role of cystoscopy in the evaluation of neurogenic bladder is to allow discovery of bladder lesions (e.g., bladder cancer and bladder stone) that would remain undiagnosed by urodynamics alone • Cystoscopy is indicated for patients complaining of persistent irritative voiding symptoms or hematuria
Videourodynamics	• It is the criterion standard for evaluation of a patient with incontinence. Videourodynamics combines the radiographic findings of voiding cystourethrogram (VCUG) and multichannel urodynamics • Videourodynamics enables documentation of lower urinary tract anatomy, such as vesicoureteral reflux and bladder diverticulum, as well as the functional pressure–flow relationship between the bladder and the urethra

Management

Medical Care

Treatment of urinary incontinence varies by type, as follows:

- Stress incontinence may be treated with surgical and some nonsurgical approaches.
- Urge incontinence may be treated with behavioral modification, pharmacotherapy, or third-line procedures.
- Mixed incontinence may require medications as well as surgery.
- Overflow incontinence is generally treated by emptying the bladder with a catheter.
- Other forms of incontinence may be resolved by treating the underlying cause (e.g., UTI and constipation).

Absorbent pads and internal and external collecting devices have an important role in the management of chronic incontinence. The criteria for use of these products are fairly straightforward, and they are beneficial in certain situations:

- Failure of all other treatments and persistent incontinence
- Illness or disability that prevents participation in care
- Inability to benefit from medications
- Incontinence disorders that cannot be corrected by surgery
- Awaiting surgery

Surgical Care

- Periurethral bulking therapy
- Sling procedures
- Artificial urinary sphincter

Surgical care for urge incontinence involves procedures that improve bladder compliance or bladder capacity, which include the following:

- Sacral neuromodulation
- Botulinum toxin injections

3. Transrectal ultrasound (TRUS). ***WBUHS 2006***

TRUS

It is an ultrasound technique used to visualize the human prostate and surrounding tissue. An ultrasound transducer (probe) sends sound waves through the rectal wall directly into the prostate gland. TRUS may also be called a prostate sonogram or endorectal ultrasound.

Indications

- Measure the size of the prostate [prostatic enlargement is suspected based on digital rectal examination (DRE) and surgery in the form of open prostatectomy is considered.]
- Aid in prostate biopsy (allows biopsy of hypoechoic or hyperechoic lesions)
- Azoospermia test (can determine the obstruction of the ejaculation channel)
- Helps to guide prostate cancer treatment.
- TRUS is used to place implants during brachytherapy.
- It can help doctors perform cryosurgery.
- TRUS can be used to deliver high-intensity focused ultrasound (HIFU).

TRUS is usually performed as an outpatient procedure in a doctor's office, clinic, or hospital. The test usually lasts 15–30 minutes.

Some special preparation is required before TRUS:

Aspirin: Avoid taking aspirin and other medicines that can thin the blood for 7–10 days before the test.

Vomiting is induced 1–2 hours before the procedure to help cleanse the bowels. Many people may be told to urinate to empty the bladder before the procedure.

CARCINOMA URINARY BLADDER

4. Mention TNM (tumor, node, and metastasis) classification of urinary bladder tumor. Discuss management of muscle-invasive urinary bladder tumor. ***WBUHS 2010***

5. Discuss the investigations and management of carcinoma urinary bladder. ***WBUHS 2016***

6. Describe clinical features of urinary bladder cancer. Evaluation and management of muscle invasive bladder cancer. ***RGUHS, Karnataka 2025***

Clinical Features of Urinary Bladder Cancer

- *Hematuria (most common symptom)*
  - *Painless gross (visible) hematuria* is the hallmark feature.
  - May be *intermittent* initially.
  - *Microscopic hematuria* may be detected incidentally.
  - Blood typically appears *throughout micturition* (total hematuria).

- *Irritative (voiding) symptoms*
  Occur when the tumor involves the bladder mucosa or irritates it.
  - *Frequency* (increased urge to urinate)
  - *Urgency*
  - *Dysuria* (burning sensation during urination)
  - These symptoms can mimic *urinary tract infection (UTI)* but *urine cultures are sterile.*
- *Pain*
  - *Suprapubic pain* if the tumor invades the bladder wall.
  - *Flank pain* if there is ureteric obstruction from tumor spread to the ureteric orifice, leading to *hydronephrosis.*
  - *Pelvic pain* in advanced or locally invasive disease.
- *Constitutional symptoms (late stages)*
  - *Weight loss*
  - *Anorexia*
  - *Fatigue*
  - *Bone pain* (if metastasis to bone)
  - *Cough or dyspnea* (if pulmonary metastases)
- *Findings on physical examination*
  Usually normal in early disease; in advanced cases:
  - *Palpable suprapubic mass* (locally advanced tumor)
  - *Pelvic mass* on bimanual examination under anesthesia
  - *Lower limb edema* (if pelvic lymph node involvement compresses veins)

TNM Staging of Bladder Carcinoma

Tx Primary tumor cannot be assessed.

T0 No evidence of primary tumor

Ta Noninvasive papillary carcinoma.

Tis Carcinoma in situ

T1 Tumor invades subepithelial connective tissue.

T2 Tumor invades muscularis propria (detrusor): T2a inner half; T2b outer half.

T3 Tumor invades beyond muscularis propria into perivesical fat: T3a = microscopic; T3b = macroscopic

T4a Tumor invades any of: prostate, uterus, vagina, or bowel.

T4b Tumor invades pelvic or abdominal wall.

Nx Regional (iliac and para-aortic) lymph nodes cannot be assessed.

N0 No regional lymph node metastasis

N1 Metastasis in a single lymph node <2 cm in greatest dimension

N2 Metastasis in a single lymph node 2–5 cm or multiple nodes <5 cm

N3 Metastasis in a single lymph node or multiple nodes >5 cm in greatest dimension

Mx Distant metastasis cannot be assessed.

M0 No distant metastasis

M1 Distant metastasis present

Diagnosis

- After a UTI has been excluded or treated, all patients with microscopic or macroscopic hematuria require investigation of their upper tracts, bladder, and urethra.

- Renal *ultrasound* and *flexible cystoscopy*, performed under local anesthetic, are first-line investigations.
- If these fail to find a cause, an *intravenous urogram (IVU)* or *computed tomography urography (CTU)* and *urine cytology* are justified second-line investigations.
  - Patients with predominantly filling-type lower urinary tract symptoms (LUTS), suprapubic pain, or recurrent UTI/pneumaturia should also be treated with *urine cytology* and *cystoscopy*.
  - *CTU* before and after intravenous (IV) contrast is becoming *the first-line radiological investigation of hematuria*.
    - It is faster and more sensitive than ultrasound or IVU in the detection of renal (parenchymal and urothelial) and ureteric tumors.
    - CTU also detects some bladder tumors but may overcall bladder wall hypertrophy as tumor and will miss flat carcinoma in situ (CIS) and urethral pathology.
    - Thus, it cannot replace cystoscopy.

If all investigations are normal, consideration should be given to nephrological disorders that may cause hematuria, such as glomerulonephritis. *Cross-referral to a renal physician is advised in patients with persisting microscopic hematuria, especially those with associated proteinuria or hypertension.*

- *Transurethral resection of bladder tumor (TURBT)* usually provides definitive histological diagnosis.
  - This is usually undertaken under general or spinal anesthesia.
  - Bimanual examination is mandatory before and after bladder tumor resection to assess size, position, and mobility.
  - The pathologist should report on the tumor type, grade, and stage; in particular, the presence or absence of muscularis propria should be noted, since its absence will preclude reliable T staging.
  - Red patches are biopsied separately; the prostatic urethra is biopsied if radical reconstructive surgery is under consideration.
  - Care is taken in resecting tumors at the dome, since intraperitoneal bladder perforation may occur, especially in women with thin-walled bladders.

Staging investigations are usually reserved for patients with biopsy-proven muscle-invasive bladder cancer unless clinically indicated, since superficial transitional cell carcinomas (TCC) and CIS disease are rarely associated with metastases.

- Pelvic CT or MRI may demonstrate extravesical tumor extension or iliac lymphadenopathy, reported if *>8 mm* in maximal diameter.
- Chest X-ray
- Isotope bone scan (positive in 5–15% of patients with muscle-invasive TCC) is obtained in cases being considered for radical treatment.
- Staging lymphadenectomy (open or laparoscopic) may be indicated in the presence of CT-detected pelvic lymphadenopathy if radical treatment is under consideration.

Muscle-invasive Bladder Cancer

Surgical management of localized (pT2/3a) disease: This is a dangerous disease; untreated 5-year survival is 3%. In the absence of prospective randomized trials comparing the surgical and nonsurgical treatments, the options for a patient with newly diagnosed confined muscle-invasive bladder cancer are:

Bladder Preserving

- *Radical TURBT plus systemic chemotherapy:* Little data, not mainstream.
- *Palliative TURBT + palliative radiotherapy (RT):* For elderly/unfit patients
- Partial cystectomy ± neoadjuvant systemic chemotherapy
- *TURBT plus definitive RT:* Poor options for squamous cell carcinoma (SCC) and adenocarcinoma as they are seldom radiosensitive.

Treatment Algorithm for Muscle-invasive Bladder Cancer showing Bladder-sparing Approach

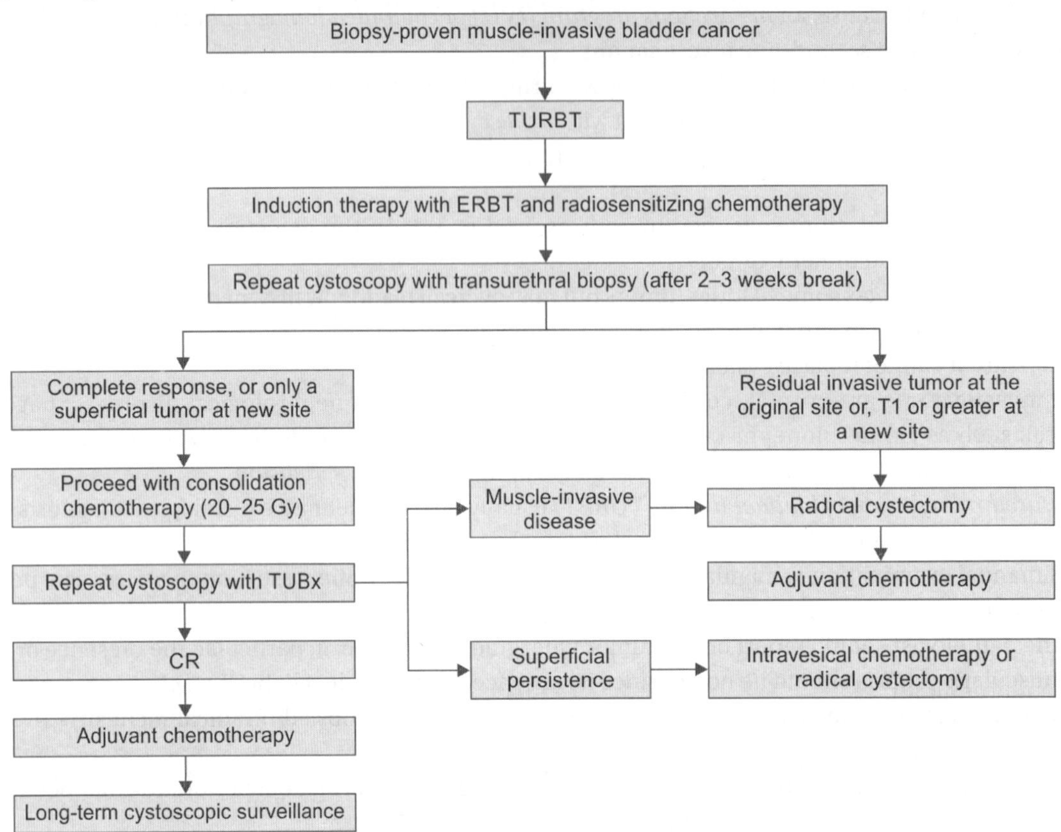

(CR: complete remission; ERBT: en bloc resection of bladder tumor; TUBx: transurethral biopsy; TURBT: transurethral resection of bladder tumor)

Radical cystectomy with:
- Ileal conduit urinary diversion
- Ureterosigmoidostomy urinary diversion
- Continent urinary diversion
- Neoadjuvant chemotherapy: Some evidence of benefit
- Neoadjuvant RT: Some evidence of benefit

Postoperative Care
- *Many patients* will spend the first 24 hours in the high-dependency unit or intensive therapy unit (ITU).
- Daily clinical evaluation, including inspection of the wound (and stoma if present), plus monitoring of blood count and Cr/electrolytes, is mandatory.
- Broad-spectrum antimicrobial prophylaxis and thromboembolic prophylaxis with thromboembolic-deterrent (TED) stockings, pneumatic calf compression, and subcutaneous heparin are standard.
- Mobilization after 24 hours is ideal.
- Chest physiotherapy and adequate analgesia are especially important in smokers and patients with chest comorbidity.
- Oral intake is restricted until bowel sounds are present; some patients may require parenteral nutrition in the presence of gastrointestinal complications.
- Drains are usually sited in the pelvis and near the uretero-diversion anastomosis, plus ureteric catheters passing from the renal pelvis through the diversion and exiting percutaneously, plus a catheter draining the diversion (except in the case of ileal conduit) exiting urethrally or suprapubically.

- Most patients stay in hospital for 10–14 days.

Salvage radical cystectomy is technically a more difficult and slightly more morbid procedure. Relatively few patients who have failed primary RT are suitable for this second chance of a cure; fit patients with clinically localized disease.

7. Vesicovaginal fistula (VVF). *WBUHS 2006*

Introduction

VVF is a subtype of female urogenital fistula (UGF). VVF is an abnormal fistulous tract extending between the bladder and the vagina that allows the continuous involuntary discharge of urine into the vaginal vault.

Etiology

Developing Countries

- Numerous factors contribute to the development of VVF in developing countries.
- Marriage and conception at a young age, often before full pelvic growth has been achieved.
- Chronic malnutrition increases the risk of cephalopelvic disproportion and malpresentation.
- Few women are attended by qualified healthcare professionals or have access to medical facilities during childbirth; their obstructed labor may be protracted for days or weeks.
- Other cultural factors that increase the likelihood of obstetrical UGFs include outlet obstruction due to female circumcision and the practice of harmful traditional medical practices.

Developed Countries

- VVFs in developing countries are attributed predominantly to inadvertent bladder injury during pelvic surgery (90%). Such injuries include unrecognized intraoperative laceration of the bladder, bladder wall injury from electrocautery or mechanical crushing, and the dissection of the bladder into an incorrect plane, causing avascular necrosis.
- Suture placement through the bladder wall in itself may not play a significant role in VVF development.
- Gynecologic procedures are the most common iatrogenic factor.
- Also occurred after RT.
- Obstetric UGFs in modern centers include vaginal lacerations from forceps rotations, cesarean delivery, hysterectomy, and ruptured uterus.
- Other types of pelvic surgery (e.g., urologic, gastrointestinal surgery) also contribute to the incidence of VVFs; such surgeries include suburethral sling procedures, surgical repair of urethral diverticulum, electrocautery of bladder papilloma, and surgery for pelvic carcinomas.
- Other less common causes of VVFs include pelvic infections (e.g., tuberculosis, syphilis, and lymphogranuloma venereum), vaginal trauma, and vaginal erosion with foreign objects (e.g., neglected pessary). Lastly, a congenital urogenital abnormality may exist that includes a VVF.
- Risk factors that predispose to VVFs include prior pelvic or vaginal surgery, previous pelvic inflammatory disease (PID), ischemia, diabetes, arteriosclerosis, carcinoma, endometriosis, anatomic distortion by uterine myomas, and infection, particularly postoperative cuff abscess.

Presentation

- The uncontrolled leakage of urine into the vagina is the hallmark symptom of patients with UGFs.
- Patients may complain of urinary incontinence or an increase in vaginal discharge following pelvic surgery or pelvic RT with or without antecedent surgery.
- The drainage may be continuous; however, in the presence of a very small UGF, it may be intermittent. Increased postoperative abdominal, pelvic, or flank pain; prolonged ileus; and fever should alert the physician to possible urinoma or urine ascites and mandates expeditious evaluation.
- Recurrent cystitis or pyelonephritis, abnormal urinary stream, and hematuria also should initiate a workup for UGF.

- Patients with radiation-induced VVFs initially present with symptoms of radiation cystitis, hematuria, and bladder contracture.

Management

Symptomatic VVF merits appropriate treatment. Further details regarding the indications for a specific procedure are described in surgical objectives or principles.

In general, no absolute contraindications exist for the attempted correction of a VVF in patients who can medically tolerate a surgical procedure.

Laboratory Investigations

- Upon examination of the vaginal vault, any fluid collection noted can be tested for urea, Cr, or potassium concentration to determine the likelihood of a diagnosis of VVF as opposed to a possible diagnosis of vaginitis.
- Indigo carmine dye can be given intravenously and if the dye appears in the vagina, a fistula is confirmed.
- Once the diagnosis of urine discharge is made, the source should be identified.

Imaging Studies

- *Radiologic studies should be used before surgical treatment of VVF:*
    - IVU is necessary to rule out urethral prolapse or fistula because 10% of VVFs are related to ureteral fistula.
    - If there is a high suspicion of urinary leakage or fistula and IVU results are negative, retrograde uretero-pyelography should be performed during cystoscopy and anesthesia examination.
    - A Trattner catheter can be used to evaluate urinary fistulas.
    - Fibrin occlusion therapy is used to treat various fistulas including enterocutaneous, anorectal, bronchopleural, uretero-cutaneous, and more recently, VVF. Fistulograms are a valuable adjunct to fibrin occlusion therapy.
- *Diagnostic procedure:*
    - Operative evaluation for fluid injury or urinary tract can be done with IV indigo carmine and close observation of the excretion of the dye into the pelvis.
        - Cystourethroscopy has been advocated by some authors as a standard-of-care for some pelvic surgery to ensure bilateral voiding and no placement of sutures in the urethra or in the urethral orifice.
        - Alternatively, filling the bladder with methylene blue or sterile milk before completing abdominal or pelvic surgery can help detect a gallbladder leak.
        - Retrograde filling of the mammary gland can be used intraoperatively to better define the fundus of the gallbladder in more difficult cases.
    - Evaluation must include a complete physical examination and a complete review of the system. Noninvasive cystoscopy can be used to identify VVF in the bladder or urinary tract, determine the number, location, and distance of ureters, and to identify and rule out abnormalities such as calculi or sutures in the bladder.
    - Water cystoscopy may be inadequate in the presence of large or multiple fistulas.
    - Cystoscopy using carbon dioxide can be used with the patient in the genupectoral position.
    - Combined vaginoscopy–cystoscopy.
    - Color Doppler ultrasonography can be considered in cases where cystoscopic assessment is not optimal, such as patients with changes in the bladder wall such as cysts or diverticula.

Treatment

- *Medical therapy:*
    - *Conservative management:* If VVF is diagnosed within the first few days of surgery, a transurethral or suprapubic catheter should be placed and maintained for up to 30 days. Small fistulas (<1 cm) may resolve or decrease during this period if caution is used to ensure proper continuous drainage of the catheter.
- *Surgical therapy:*
    - *Surgical objectives or principles:*
        - Adequate exposure of the operative field should be obtained to avoid inadvertent organ injury and to ensure prompt identification of any injury incurred.

    - Minimize bleeding and hematoma formation. The closure of dead space at the anterior vaginal wall upon completion of an anterior colporrhaphy will prevent hematoma formation.
    - This technique employs intermittently incorporating pubocervicovaginal fascia with the vaginal mucosal layer as the vaginal wall is sutured.
    - Widely mobilize the bladder from the vagina during hysterectomy to diminish the risk of suture placement into the bladder wall. A minimum of 1–2 cm margin of dissection of the bladder from the vaginal cuff should be developed prior to cuff closure.
    - Dissect the pubocervicovaginal endopelvic fascia between the vagina and the bladder in the appropriate plane.
    - Dissection may be easier with a sharp technique compared to a blunt technique; the key is to prevent trauma and separation of bladder wall fibers as the bladder is mobilized off the anterior vaginal wall.
    - The principle of traction and countertraction of the bladder and uterus works well to effect a bloodless dissection at the areolar pubocervicovaginal fascial plane.
    - If scarring is present at the pubocervicovaginal fascia and dissection is difficult, consider performing an intentional anterior extraperitoneal cystotomy.
    - This technique enables the surgeon to assess the anatomic boundaries of the bladder wall with digital palpation.
    - If scarring is present at the pubocervicovaginal fascia and dissection is difficult, consider employing an intrafascial technique of hysterectomy to best dissect the endopelvic fascial plane.
    - Intraoperative retrograde filling and emptying of the bladder or mild traction on a temporarily placed small Foley catheter inserted into the fistula itself are helpful to optimally identify anatomical planes and reveal intraoperative bladder lacerations.
    - Consider supracervical abdominal hysterectomy instead of TAH. The incidence of UGF formation is lower for supracervical versus total hysterectomy.
- If an intraoperative bladder injury does occur, it is better to widely mobilize the bladder from the underlying structures (fascia and vagina, cervix, or uterus). In doing so, the surgeon can effect a VVF closure under no tension.
- For repairing a cystotomy at the trigonal area, a transverse closure is preferable over a vertical one. Vertical closure would be more likely to produce ureteral obstruction because the ureteral orifices would be drawn inward toward each other. Ureteral catheters should be considered in repair of a cystotomy involving or encroaching on ureteric orifices.
- Consider performing cystourethroscopy when performing pelvic surgery. Cystourethroscopy to assure bilateral ureteral patency and the absence of suture placement in the bladder or the urethra has been advocated by some authors as a standard for all pelvic surgery.

CHAPTER 60

Penis

LEARNING OBJECTIVES

- Paraphimosis and Circumcision
- Carcinoma Penis
- Partial Amputation of Penis
- Ilioinguinal Block Dissection
- Nonerectile Dysfunction

1. Paraphimosis.

Introduction

It is a common medical condition in which the prepuce is trapped behind and cannot be reduced. If this condition persists for several hours or if there are signs of lack of circulation, medical attention should be considered as paraphimosis can lead to gangrene.

Reason

Paraphimosis is usually found by well-intentioned medical professionals or parents who mishandle the skin: The skin can be pulled back during penile examination, penile cleansing, urinary catheterization, or cystoscopy; if the skin is pulled for a long time, some skin tissues may swell (swell with fluid), making it difficult for the skin to shrink later.

Treatment

- Phimosis (pathological and normal physiological forms of childhood) is a risk factor for paraphimosis.
- Physiological phimosis resolves naturally as the child grows, but pathological phimosis may be recommended to be treated with prolonged or elective long-term surgical procedures (for example, preputioplasty for circumcision to partially or completely remove the foreskin).
- Paraphimosis can often be effectively treated by manual manipulation of the inflamed skin tissue. This involves compressing the gland and repositioning the skin, possibly with the help of massage, cold compresses, and if necessary, local anesthesia.
- Failing this, the hard tissue can be surgically removed with skin or circumcision.
- An alternative method, the Dundee method, involves making several punctures in the inflamed skin with a fine needle, followed by manual pressure to drain the edema fluid.
- Some recommend postponing elective circumcision until the paraphimosis resolves.

2. Circumcision. *WBUHS 2008*

Male circumcision is the removal of part or all of the private parts.

Indications

- The prevalence of circumcision varies mainly based on religion and sometimes by culture.
- Most circumcisions are performed at puberty for cultural or religious reasons; in some countries, it is often done during childhood.

- Circumcision is also used therapeutically as a form of treatment in:
  - Balanitis xerotica obliterans (BXO)
  - Paraphimosis
  - Balanitis
  - Posthitis
  - Balanoposthitis
  - Urinary tract infection

Advantages

- Many older men with prostate or prostate problems have problems with their skin due to surgery, cleaning, and the use of instruments by the surgeon. Some of these patients need to be circumcised.
- Some older men develop prostate cancer—one in 1,000—very rare, but if you or your son is in this small statistic. Infant circumcision is almost 100% protective, and young adult circumcision is very protective.
- Cervical warts in women are caused by the human papillomavirus (HPV). It grows under and on the skin where it can be sexually transmitted.
- Protection against human immunodeficiency virus (HIV) and acquired immunodeficiency syndrome (AIDS).
- As with HIV, there is some protection against other sexually transmitted infections.
- Many men and their partners like the appearance of their private parts after circumcision, they feel odorless and cleaner and enjoy better sex. Understanding good body image is an important factor in building self-confidence.
- *Balanitis*—an unpleasant, often recurring, swelling of the glans. This is normal and can be prevented by circumcision.
- Urinary tract infections sometimes occur in babies and can be very serious. Childhood circumcision makes it 10 times less likely.

Direct Challenge

- *Infection:*
  - Infections are usually minor and localized, but can sometimes lead to urinary tract infections, life-threatening systemic infections, meningitis, or death.
  - Staphylococcal infections are a growing problem for hospital operations, and methicillin-sensitive *Staphylococcus aureus* (MSSA) (methicillin-susceptible) strains have affected neonatal intensive care units.
  - Herpes
- *Bleeding:* Bleeding after circumcision is usually minor and easy to control, but rarely leads to blood loss (hypovolemic shock) or death (exsanguination). Digestive disorders affect 2–4% of the population and are diagnosed with the condition. Heavy bleeding after circumcision can be a sign of hemophilia.
- *Surgical complications:* Complications can occur with any surgery. Surgical complications of circumcision include all injuries associated with penile denudation, amputation of part or all of the genital tissue, urethral fistula, various types of circumcision clamps used, and penile necrosis.
- *Anesthetic risks:* Anesthetic risks include methemoglobinemia.

Delayed Complications

- Meatal stenosis may be a common longer-term complication from circumcision.
- The opening to the urethra (meatus) may also be affected, leading to inflammation and meatal ulceration.
- Urinary retention
- Venous stasis is the slowing down of venous blood flow.
- Concealed penis
- Adhesions
- Skin bridges, when the cut skin attaches to the glans penis. Skin bridges do not commonly require surgical correction; rather, a brief, simple office procedure may be performed.
- Painful erections

3. Pyronie disease. ***Gujarat Health University 2025***

Peyronie's disease (sometimes spelled *Pyronie's*) is a medical condition that affects the *penis,* causing *curvature, pain, and sometimes erectile dysfunction* due to the formation of *fibrous scar tissue (plaque)* inside the penis.

- Normally, the penis contains elastic tissue that expands evenly during an erection.
- In Peyronie's disease, *fibrous plaques* (scar tissue) develop under the skin of the penis, usually on one side.
- When the penis becomes erect, the plaque area does not stretch as much, causing *curvature or bending* toward that side.

Symptoms

- *Curved or bent erections* (up, down, or to the side)
- *Pain* during erections (especially early in the disease)
- *Palpable lumps or plaques* under the skin
- *Shortening* of the penis
- *Erectile dysfunction* (in some cases)

Phases

I. *Acute (active) phase*—lasts 6–18 months
  - Plaque forms
  - Pain and progressive curvature may occur

II. *Chronic (stable) phase*—curvature stabilizes
  - Pain often lessens
  - Deformity may persist

Causes and Risk Factors

- Repeated *microtrauma* to the penis (during sex or sports)
- Genetic predisposition
- Connective tissue disorders (like *Dupuytren's contracture*)
- Aging
- Certain medical conditions (e.g., *diabetes, hypertension*)

Treatment Options

Treatment depends on the *severity* and whether it's in the acute or chronic phase.

Nonsurgical (first-line):

- *Observation:* Mild cases may improve on their own.
- *Oral medications:* Limited benefit (vitamin E, pentoxifylline).
- *Injectable medications:*
  - *Collagenase Clostridium histolyticum* (brand: *Xiaflex*)—FDA-approved and can help dissolve the plaque.
  - *Verapamil or interferon-alpha* injections—reduce plaque formation.
- *Penile traction therapy:* Mechanical devices can gently stretch the penis over time to reduce curvature.

Surgical (for severe or stable cases):

- *Plication:* Shortens the longer side to straighten the penis.
- *Plaque incision/excision with grafting:* Removes or cuts the scar and replaces it with a graft.
- *Penile prosthesis:* For men with significant erectile dysfunction

4. Premalignant conditions and risk factors of penile carcinoma.

5. What are the premalignant lesions of penis? ***RGUHS, Karnataka 2025; AIIMS, Bhubaneswar 2024***

Precancerous conditions of the penis can develop into penile cancer.

The most common premalignant conditions of carcinoma penis are:

- *Penile intraepithelial neoplasia (PeIN):* PeIN is the most common condition of the genitals. PeIN is a general term used to describe cases of genital warts that may progress to invasive squamous cell carcinoma (SCC) in the absence of curative treatment.
- *BXO:* It is an inflammatory skin condition that affects the skin and glans penis (penis or glans). It is also called penile lichen sclerosus.
- *Buschke–Löwenstein tumor:* This tumor usually occurs in the glans (glans or head of the penis). A Buschke-Lowenstein tumor has been suggested to be a low-grade cancer associated with genital carcinoma. A tumor that grows slowly that can grow up to 15 cm.
- *Bowenoid papulosis:* It has a very low chance of becoming cancerous. It affects young men more often than older men.
- The following risk factor may increase a person's chance of developing bowenoid papulosis—HPV infection.
- *Leukoplakia:* Leukoplakia has the potential to become SCC.

Risk factors for SCC of the penis include:

- *Age:* The incidence of penile cancer increases in the sixth decade and peaks in the eighth decade. It is rare in people <40 years old but has been reported in children.
- *Premalignant lesions:* About 42% of the penile SCC patients are reported to have preexisting penile lesions.
- *Penile (skin):* Penile cancer is rare in men who are circumcised at a young age. Almost nothing in Israel. It is thought to contribute to chronic irritation with smegma and inflammation (balanitis).
- HPV wart infection, especially with types 16, 18, and 21.
- Cigarettes and tobacco products

6. Discuss clinical features, staging, and treatment outline of carcinoma penis.
WBUHS 2020 , Gujarat Health University 2025

7. TNM staging for carcinoma penis. ***DNB 2021 June***

Presentation

- A hard, painless lump on the glans penis is the most common presentation.
- A bloody discharge may be confused with hematuria.
- Rarely, a groin mass or urinary retention are presenting symptoms.
- Examination reveals a solid nontender mass or ulcer beneath or involving the foreskin.
- There is usually evidence of local infection.
- In more advanced diseases, the prepuce, glans, shaft, scrotum, and even perineum are replaced by tumors.
- The inguinal lymph nodes (LNs) are examined. They may be enlarged, fixed, or even ulcerate overlying skin.

Staging of Penile SCC

Tumor (T)

- *TX:* The primary tumor cannot be evaluated.
- *T0:* There is no tumor.
- *Tis:* An early, noninvasive precancerous growth. This is also called *carcinoma in situ.*
- *Ta:* A noninvasive squamous cell carcinoma located in only one area.
- *T1:* The tumor has grown into one of more outer layers of the penis. Depending on where on the penis the cancer is growing, these may include the lamina propria, the layer of skin called the dermis, dartos fascia, or connective tissue underneath the skin. This stage may also be divided into two substages based on the grade of the tumor and whether it has grown into blood vessels, lymph vessels, or nerves:
  - *T1a:* The tumor has not grown into blood vessels, lymph vessels, or nerves and is not high-grade or G3 (see earlier).
  - *T1b:* The tumor has grown into blood vessels, lymph vessels, and/or nerves and is high-grade (G3).

- *T2:* The tumor has grown into the corpus spongiosum, an internal chamber of the penis. It may or may not have grown into the urethra.
- *T3:* The tumor has grown into the corpora cavernosum, an internal chamber of the penis. It may or may not have grown into the urethra.
- *T4:* The tumor has grown into other nearby structures, such as the pubic bone, scrotum, and prostate.

Node (N)

- *NX:* The regional lymph nodes cannot be evaluated.
- *N0:* Cancer has not spread to the regional lymph nodes.
- *N1:* Cancer has spread to two or fewer inguinal lymph nodes on the same side of the body. The inguinal lymph nodes are located in the groin.
- *N2:* Cancer has spread to three or more inguinal lymph nodes on one or both sides of the body.
- *N3:* The cancer has grown from the inguinal lymph nodes into the surrounding tissue in the groin, and/or the cancer has spread to lymph nodes in the pelvis.

Metastasis (M)

- *M0:* There is no distant metastasis.
- *M1:* There is metastasis to parts of the body other than the penis and the regional lymph nodes.

Cancer Stage Grouping

- *Stage I:* A low-grade cancer that has grown just below the surface layer of skin but not to nerves, lymph vessels, or blood vessels. It has not spread to lymph nodes or distant parts of the body (T1a, N0, and M0)
- *Stage IIA:* The cancer is high grade or has grown into blood vessels, lymph vessels, or nerves; or, it has grown into the corpus spongiosum and may or may not have grown into the urethra. It has not spread to lymph nodes or distant parts of the body (T1b or T2; N0 and M0).
- *Stage IIB:* The cancer has grown into the corpora cavernosum and may or may not have grown into the urethra. It has not spread to lymph nodes or distant parts of the body (T3, N0, and M0)
- *Stage IIIA:* The tumor has not grown beyond the penis and urethra. It has spread to one to two groin lymph nodes but not to the distant parts of the body (T1, T2, or T3; N1 and M0).
- *Stage IIIB:* The tumor has not grown beyond the penis and urethra but has spread to three or more groin lymph nodes. It has not spread outside the groin lymph nodes, to the pelvic lymph nodes, or to distant parts of the body (T1, T2, or T3; N2 and M0).
- *Stage IV:* Any of the following—
  - The cancer has grown into nearby tissues, such as the pubic bone, scrotum, or prostate (T4, any N, and any M).
  - The cancer has grown from the groin lymph nodes into the surrounding tissue (any T, N3, and any M).
  - The cancer has spread to one or more of the pelvic lymph nodes (any T, N3, and any M).
  - The cancer has spread to distant parts of the body (any T, any N, and M).

Investigations

A biopsy is indicated	Chest radiology	Pelvic computed tomography (CT) scan	Serum calcium	Liver function tests

Treatment

The Primary Tumor

- The first-line treatment of penile cancer, regardless of the inguinal node status, is surgery.
- Circumcision is appropriate for preputial lesions, but local recurrence is observed in.
- Penis-preserving wide excision of glandular lesions with skin graft glandular reconstruction may be suitable for smaller tumors, giving good cosmetic and functional results.

- Alternatives to surgery include laser or cryoablation, radiotherapy or brachytherapy, photodynamic therapy, or topical 5-fluorouracil.
- For more advanced tumors, partial or total penile amputation is required, depending on the extent of the tumor. Partial amputation is preferable, provided a 2-cm margin of palpably normal shaft can be obtained.
- Local recurrence occurs in 10% if the excision margin is positive.
  - Total amputation involves the excision of the scrotum and its contents, with the formation of a perineal urethrostomy. The most common complication is urethral meatal stenosis.
  - Radiotherapy remains an alternative, but disadvantages include radioresistance, leading to reported recurrence rates of 30–60%; tissue necrosis and damage leading to urethral stricture, fistula, and pain.
  - *Lymphadenopathy:*
    - For about 6 weeks broad-spectrum antimicrobials are given after the primary tumor has been removed. Nodes become clinically insignificant in 50% of the patients, who may then be followed up.
    - For those with persistent inguinal lymphadenopathy, in the absence of demonstrable pelvic or metastatic disease, bilateral inguinal lymphadenectomy should be considered.
      Radiotherapy and chemotherapy are alternative or adjuvant treatments for metastatic nodal disease in unfit, elderly, or inoperable patients.
- Prophylactic lymphadenectomy is currently practiced for tumors exhibiting vascular invasion, high grade, or stages T2–4.
- Distant metastatic disease is treated using single-agent systemic chemotherapy—cisplatin, bleomycin, or methotrexate.
- Experience with combination chemotherapy is increasing.

8. Partial amputation of the penis—steps. ***RGUHS, Karnataka 2025; WBUHS 2011***

This procedure is indicated when the enlargement is limited to the glans and does not spread to the penis.

- Spinal anesthesia
- Patient is at a high level.
- Atrial septal defect (ASD)
- A thin catheter is used as a tourniquet in the bottom of the woman.
- A long ventral flap with a width equal to half the circumference of the penis and a length equal to the diameter of the penis is made.
- A short flap 1.25 cm long is made on the dorsal side. Flaps are divided into bases. The corpus spongiosum is isolated from the corpora cavernosa by placing a fine scalpel on both sides of the corpus spongiosum and dissecting 1.25 cm at the recommended level of the corpora cavernosa.
- The corpora cavernosa is now divided at the level of the flap. The competition has now been eliminated, and the bleeding points have been secured.
- A small opening is made in the ventral flap and the corpus spongiosum is exposed.
- Two loops are now sewn at the base of the penis.
- Sutures should be well separated for adequate drainage that may form beneath the hematoma.
- The end of the urinary catheter is divided by 1 cm, and each half is sewn to the skin. This is done to prevent further hardening. The catheter is self-retaining and inserted.

WRITE SHORT NOTES ON

9. Anatomical limits of ilioinguinal block dissection. ***WBUHS 2020***

10. Describe the steps of ilioinguinal block dissection. ***RGUHS, Karnataka 2025***

11. Enumerate the complications of ilioinguinal block dissection. ***WBUHS 2020***

Inguinal Anatomy

Inguinal lymph nodes are divided into superficial and deep groups separated by fascia lata of the thigh.

Superficial Group Composed of 4–25 Lymph Nodes

Five Anatomic Groups

1. Central nodes around the saphenofemoral junction (SFJ)
2. Superolateral nodes around the superficial circumflex vein
3. Inferolateral nodes around lateral femoral cutaneous vein
4. Superomedial nodes around the superficial external pudendal vein
5. Inferomedial nodes around the great saphenous vein

Deep Group

- Lies medial to femoral vein in the femoral canal.
- Node of Cloquet is the most cephalad of the group.
- External iliac lymph nodes receive drainage from the deep inguinal, obturator, and hypogastric groups, and it drains to common iliac and paraaortic nodes.
    - The inguinofemoral dissection is designed to cover an area outlined superiorly by a line drawn from the superior margin of the external ring to the anterior superior iliac spine, laterally by a line drawn from the anterior superior iliac spine extending 20 cm inferiorly, and medially by a line drawn from the pubic tubercle 15 cm down the medial thigh.

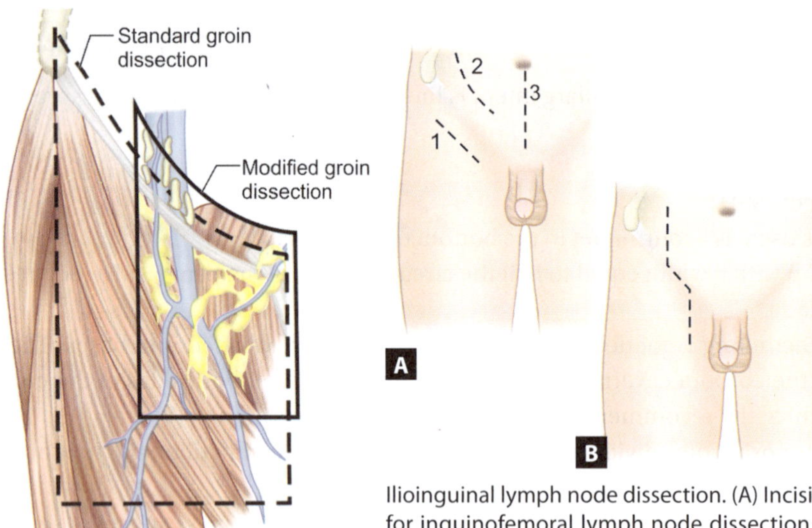

Limits of standard and modified groin dissection.

Ilioinguinal lymph node dissection. (A) Incisions for inguinofemoral lymph node dissection (1), unilateral pelvic lymph node dissection (2), and bilateral pelvic lymph node dissection (3); (B) Single-incision approach for ilioinguinal lymph node dissection.

- An oblique incision approximately 3 cm below and parallel to the inguinal ligament and extending from the lateral to the medial limit of the dissection.
- Superior and inferior skin flaps are developed in the plane just below the Scarpa's fascia.
- The superior flap is elevated cephalad to a point 4 cm above the inguinal ligament, and the inferior flap to the limit of the dissection.
- The fat and areolar tissues are dissected from the external oblique aponeurosis and the spermatic cord to the inferior border of the inguinal ligament, forming the superior boundary of the lymph node packet.

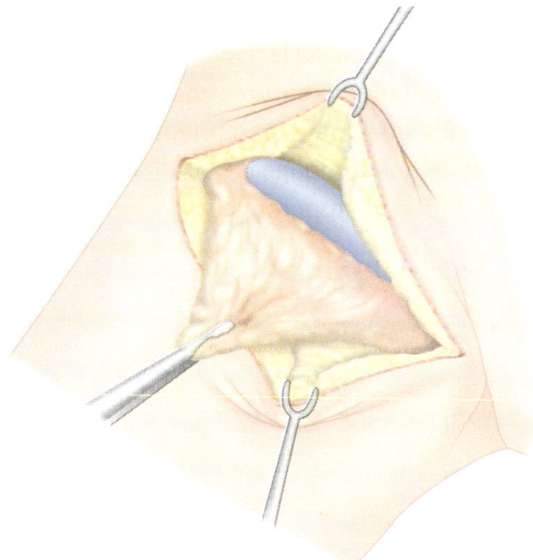

Initial dissection for radical inguinofemoral lymph node dissection with exposure of superior border defined by the external oblique fascia.

- The inferior angle of the inguinofemoral exposure is at the apex of the femoral triangle, where the long saphenous vein is identified and divided.
- The saphenous vein is divided at the saphenofemoral junction, and the dissection is continued superiorly to include the deep inguinal nodes medial and lateral to the femoral vein until continuity with the pelvic dissection is attained at the femoral canal.

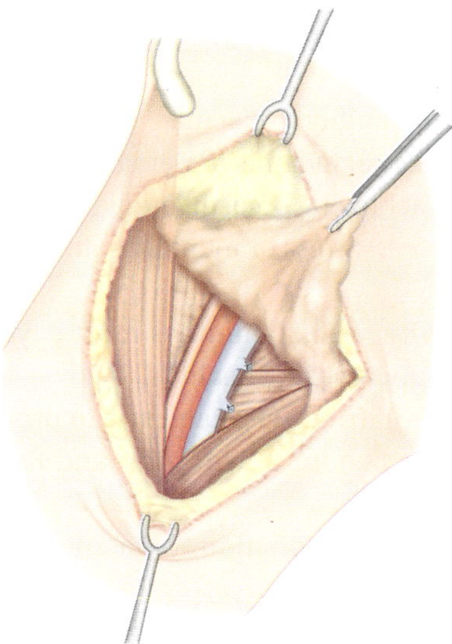

Inferior dissection during radical inguinofemoral lymph node dissection with removal of lymph node packet from the inferior border of the femoral triangle. After further lateral and medial dissection, the packet remains in continuity with the pelvic dissection in the area of the femoral canal.

- After the femoral triangle is dissected, the sartorius muscle is mobilized from its origin at the anterior superior iliac spine and either transposed or rolled 180° medially to cover the femoral vessels.
- The muscle is sutured to the inguinal ligament superiorly, and its margins are sutured to the muscles of the thigh immediately adjacent to the femoral vessels.
- The femoral canal is closed, if necessary, by suturing the shelving edge of the inguinal ligament to the Cooper's ligament.

- Closed-suction drains are placed under the subcutaneous tissue and brought out inferiorly.
- During closure, the skin flaps are sutured to the surface of the exposed musculature to decrease dead space.
- The skin is closed with absorbable subcutaneous sutures and staples.
- The patient is maintained at bed rest for 2 or 3 days, and pneumatic compression stockings are used.
- The drains are removed after 5–7 days when drainage is <30–40 mL/day.
- Compression stockings are recommended postoperatively.

Complications of Ilioinguinal Block Dissection
- Lymphedema—may be debilitating.
- Deep venous thrombosis (DVT)
- Wound infection
- Skin flap necrosis—occurs in 5–21% of patients.
- Lymphocele
- Lymphorrhea
- Seroma
- Temporary lower extremity edema

12. Nonerectile dysfunction management. ***Gujarat Health University 2024***

Managing nonerectile dysfunction (non-ED) sexual health concerns involves addressing various issues that affect sexual function, libido, or overall sexual well-being, excluding erectile dysfunction. Below is a concise overview of strategies and considerations based on general medical and lifestyle approaches:

- *Common non-ED sexual health issues:*
  - *Low libido:* Reduced sexual desire due to hormonal imbalances, stress, or relationship issues.
  - *Premature ejaculation (PE):* Ejaculation occurring too quickly, often linked to psychological or neurological factors.
  - *Delayed ejaculation:* Difficulty or inability to ejaculate despite adequate stimulation.
  - *Painful intercourse:* Conditions like vaginismus or penile discomfort due to infections or anatomical issues.
  - *Orgasmic dysfunction:* Difficulty achieving orgasm, often tied to psychological or medical factors.
  - *Sexual anxiety or performance issues:* Stress or mental health concerns impacting sexual performance.
- *Lifestyle and behavioral approaches:*
  - *Exercise regularly:* Physical activity (e.g., 30 minutes most days) improves blood flow, boosts mood, and enhances stamina, which can support sexual health.
  - *Healthy diet:* A balanced diet rich in fruits, vegetables, lean proteins, and whole grains supports hormonal balance and energy levels. Foods like nuts, avocados, and fish (rich in omega-3s) may promote sexual wellness.
  - *Stress management:* Techniques like meditation, yoga, or mindfulness can reduce anxiety and improve sexual confidence.
  - *Sleep hygiene:* Aim for 7–9 hours of quality sleep nightly to regulate hormones like testosterone and reduce fatigue.
  - *Limit alcohol and avoid smoking:* Excessive alcohol and smoking can impair libido and sexual response.
- *Psychological and relational strategies:*
  - *Therapy or counseling:* Cognitive-behavioral therapy (CBT) or sex therapy can address performance anxiety, low libido, or relationship conflicts.
  - *Communication with partner:* Open discussions about desires, boundaries, and concerns can improve intimacy and reduce performance pressure.
  - *Sensate focus exercises:* Gradual, non-sexual touch exercises with a partner can reduce anxiety and rebuild intimacy.

- *Medical and professional interventions:*
  - *Hormonal evaluation:* Low testosterone or thyroid issues can affect libido. Consult a healthcare provider for blood tests and possible treatments like hormone therapy.
  - *Medications for specific issues:*
    - For premature ejaculation, selective serotonin reuptake inhibitors (SSRIs) or topical anesthetics may be prescribed.
    - For painful intercourse, infections (e.g., yeast or STIs) or conditions like Peyronie's disease should be evaluated.
  - *Pelvic floor therapy:* Strengthening pelvic muscles through exercises (e.g., Kegels) can help with ejaculation control or pelvic pain.
  - *Address underlying conditions:* Diabetes, depression, or neurological disorders can impact sexual function. Managing these is key.
- *Natural and supplemental options:*
  - *Supplements:* Some evidence suggests supplements like L-arginine, zinc, or maca root may support libido, but consult a doctor before use.
  - *Avoid unproven treatments*
- *When to seek help:*
  - Persistent issues (e.g., lasting over 3 months) warrant a visit to a urologist, endocrinologist, or sex therapist.
  - Sudden changes in sexual function may indicate underlying health issues (e.g., cardiovascular or neurological conditions).

CHAPTER 61

Scrotum and Testis

LEARNING OBJECTIVES

- Development and Descent of Testis
- Undescended and Ectopic Testis
- Acute Scrotum
- Testicular Torsion and Varicocele
- Testicular Tumors

TESTIS

1. Describe the development and descent of testis. ***WBUHS 2013, 2019***

2. Discuss the medical and surgical management of undescended testis. ***WBUHS 2016***

3. Imperfectly descended testis. ***WBUHS 2012***

4. Surgery for maldescended testis. ***WBUHS 2010***

5. Explain testicular development, evaluation, and management of undescended testis. ***DNB 2024 October***

Testicular Differentiation

- The male gonad develops into the testis toward week 7 of the development. Until then, it is undifferentiated. The differentiation is determined by the XY genetic constitution and proceeds as follows:
    - The primary sex cords, proliferating from the coelomic epithelium, condense and extend into the medulla of the gonad.
        - In the medulla, the cords branch, their deep ends anastomose, and they form the rete testis.
        - The prominent sex cords become the seminiferous or testicular cords which soon lose their connections with the germinal epithelium because of the development of a thick fibrous capsule, the tunica albuginea.
            - The tunica albuginea is a layer of connective tissue that is interposed early, between the coelomic epithelium (parietal peritoneum) and the rest of the gland. It produces partitions that compartmentalize the gland, closing off the seminiferous ducts, about day 50, into testes cords.
            - Development of the tunica albuginea is a characteristic and diagnostic feature of testicular development.
    - The seminiferous or testicular cords develop into the seminiferous tubules, whose deep portions narrow to form the tubuli recti, which converge on the rete testis.

- The seminiferous tubules become separated by mesenchyme which gives rise to the interstitial cells of Leydig:
  - It is here that the androgenic hormones are secreted which help in the differentiation of the genital tract and the external genital organs.
  - The interstitial cells of Leydig reach their maximum development between 3.5 and 4 months.
- The walls of the seminiferous tubules, as a result of their cellular duality of origin, are composed of two types of cells—(1) supporting or (2) sustentacular cells of Sertoli, derived from the germinal epithelium, and the spermatogonia, derived from the primordial germ cells (unlimited in number, in contrast to the oogonia):
  - The cells of Sertoli make up most of the seminiferous epithelium in the fetal testis.
  - Gradually, the enlarging testis separates from the regressing mesonephros and is suspended by its own mesentery, the mesorchium.

- In later development, the germinal epithelium flattens to form the mesothelium on the surface of the testis and the rete testis becomes continuous with the 15–20 adjacent persistent mesonephric tubules:
  - The persistent mesonephric tubules, after regression of the mesonephric (Wolffian) body, participate in the formation of the excretory tracts of the testis, forming the vasa efferentia or efferent ductules
  - The efferent ductules open into the adjacent mesonephric duct which becomes the ductus epididymidis (epididymis).
  - Thus, the vasa efferentia and the epididymis are of mesonephric origin.

Testicular Descent

Various theories have been propounded to explain the phenomenon of testicular descent:

- Traction by gubernaculums and/or cremaster muscle
- Force of abdominal pressure
- *Hormonal theory:*
  - Role of androgens by action on gubernaculum
  - Estrogens may hinder testicular descent.
  - Müllerian inhibiting substance (MIS)—facilitates testicular descent by causing regression of Müllerian structures
- Calcitonin gene-related peptide
- Role of nerves, e.g., genitofemoral nerve

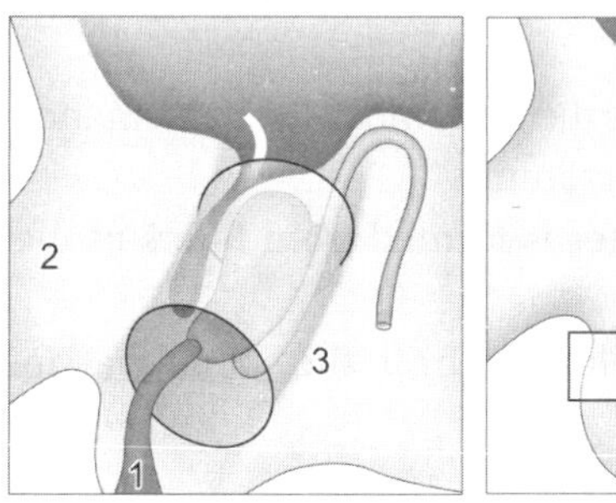

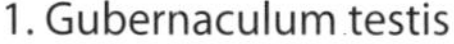

1. Gubernaculum testis
2. Penis
3. Inguinal canal
4. Testis
5. Peritoneal cavity
6. Deferent duct

Descent of testis.

Between the third and seventh month of pregnancy, the testes remain near the inguinal canal in order to pass through it. The vaginal process lengthens while the gubernaculum shortens, thereby drawing the testis, the deferent duct, and its vessels on both sides downward.

In the ninth month of pregnancy (but also sometimes only after birth) the testes reach the scrotum. The vaginal process forms now a serous bilaminar structure on the front side of the testis.

Section through the scrotum at the time of birth

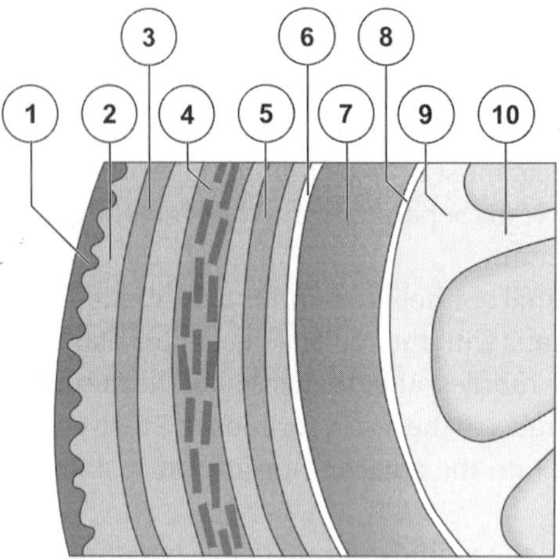

Section of the scrotum.

1. Epidermis
2. Dermis (tunica dartos)
3. External spermatic fascia
4. Musculus cremaster
5. Internal spermatic fascia
6. Parietal lamina of the tunica vaginalis
7. Virtual cavity between the two layers of the tunica vaginalis
8. Visceral lamina of the tunica vaginalis
9. Tunica albuginea
10. Interlobular septum of the testis

In that the vaginal process lengthens downwardly, it takes the muscle fibers of the oblique internal muscle and the transverse muscle with it.

The muscle fascia of the transverse muscle is the innermost layer and in the scrotal region, it forms the internal spermatic fascia of the spermatic cord and the scrotum.

The muscle layer of the musculus cremaster is formed from fibers of the oblique internal and transverse muscles.

Externally, the external spermatic fascia is formed from the superficial aponeurosis of the oblique external abdominal muscle.

Detail of the various layers that have formed in the scrotum by the end of the pregnancy:

- Between the 7th and 12th week the gubernaculum shortens and pulls the testes, deferent duct, and its vessels downward.
- Between the third and seventh month the testes stay in the area of the inguinal canal so they can enter into it. They reach the scrotum at roughly the time of birth under the influence of the androgen hormone.
- While in the first year of life, the upper part of the vaginal process becomes obliterated, there remains only the peritoneovaginal ligament. The lower portion persists as the tunica vaginalis testis, which consists of a parietal and a visceral layer.

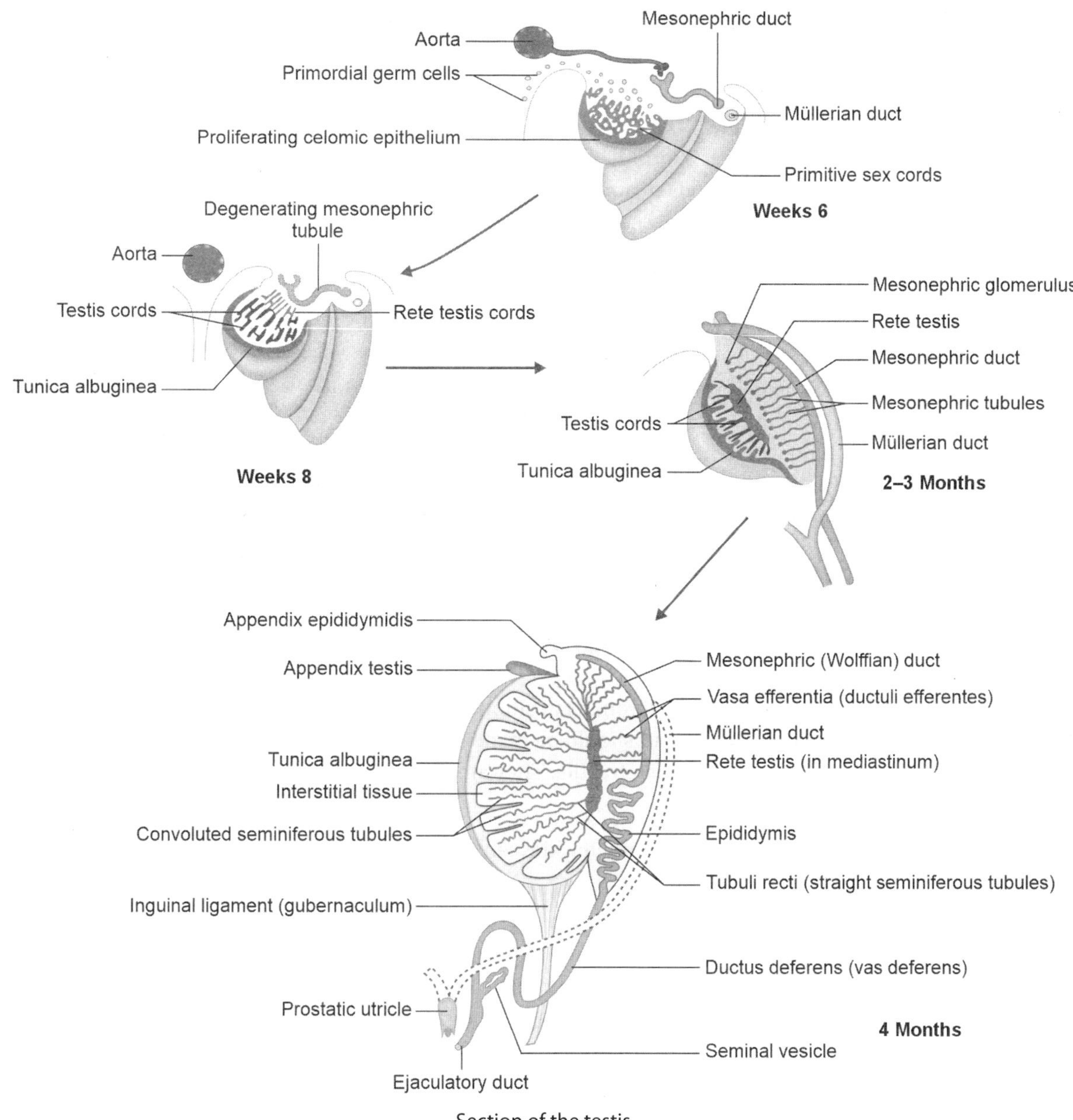

Section of the testis.

Imperfectly Descended Testis

Imperfectly/incompletely descended testis.

Incidence

- About 4% of the boys are born with one or both testes incompletely descended.
- About half of these reach the scrotum during the first month of life, but full descent after that is uncommon.
- The condition is sometimes missed at birth and discovered later in life. In a few cases, the presence of a hernia, testicular pain, or acute torsion directs attention to the abnormality.
- In 10% of the unilateral cases there is a family history.

Pathology

- Incompletely descended testes are often macroscopically normal in early childhood but by puberty, the testis is poorly developed compared with its intrascrotal counterpart.

- The epithelial elements are immature histologically and by late puberty irreversible destructive changes halt spermatogenesis and limit the production of androgens.
- An incompletely descended testis brought down in early childhood often functions satisfactorily.

Undescended Testis

- Testes absent from the scrotum after 3 months of age are unlikely to descend fully.
- An incompletely descended testis tends to atrophy as puberty approaches
- Early repositioning of an incompletely descended testis can preserve function.

Clinical Features

- The condition is more common on the right and is bilateral in 20% of the cases.
- Secondary sexual characteristics are typically normal.
- *The testis may be:*
    - Intra-abdominal, lying extraperitoneal above the internal inguinal ring
    - Inguinal, in which case it may or may not be palpable.
    - In the superficial inguinal pouch, in which case it must be distinguished from retractile testis.
    - During childhood the testes are mobile and the cremasteric reflex is active.
    - In some boys, any stimulation of the skin of the scrotum or thigh causes the testis to disappear into the inguinal canal.
    - Simply exposing the parts can also do this so that the testis is never seen in an intrascrotal position.
    - The scrotum is normal as opposed to underdeveloped, which is usually seen with true incomplete descent.
    - When the cremaster relaxes, the telltale bulge of the testis reappears only to vanish when the scrotal skin is touched again.
    - A retractile testis can be gently milked from its position in the inguinal region to the bottom of the scrotum.
    - A diagnosis of true incomplete descent should be made only if this is not possible.
    - In infancy, most inapparent testes are retractile. They are normal and require no treatment.

Retractile Testis

Retractile testes are more common than incompletely descended testes and require no treatment.

Ectopic Testis

The sites of ectopic testis are:

- At the superficial inguinal ring
- In the perineum
- At the root of the penis
- In the femoral triangle

  An ectopic testis is usually fully developed. The main hazard is liability to injury.

Hazards of incomplete descent are:

- Sterility in bilateral cases (especially intra-abdominal testes)
- Pain as a result of trauma
- An associated indirect inguinal hernia is often present and may cause symptoms
- Torsion
- Epididymo-orchitis in an incompletely descended right testis can mimic appendicitis; atrophy of an inguinal testis before puberty may possibly be caused by recurrent minor trauma
- Increased liability to malignant disease; cancer is more common in incompletely descended testes—orchidopexy may or may not diminish the risk but it does improve the prospect of early diagnosis.

Treatment of UDT

- The aim of the treatment is to fix the testis in the scrotum.
- This is done to prevent the potential complications of UDT which are, testicular torsion, risk of trauma, and testicular tumors.

- It is hoped that the endocrine and germ cell functions of such a testis will show improvement, especially if orchidopexy is done early.

Treatment Options

- Hormonal treatment
- Surgical treatment

Hormonal Treatment

- The starting point of hormone therapy is that the lack of hormones in the hypothalamic-pituitary-testicular axis prevents testicular descent and is responsible for such testicular dysfunction.
- Direct androgen therapy has been associated with many side effects (early puberty and growth retardation) and is being replaced by human chorionic gonadotropin (hCG) and luteinizing hormone-releasing hormone (LH-RH) therapy. It is now understood that these hormonal treatments are of little use in promoting the descent of a truly undescended testicle; while the acquired variants of the undescended testicle (retracted testicle, ascending testicle) respond quite well to this treatment.
- The general success rate is 10–50%. The success of hormone therapy depends directly on age and inversely on the position of the testicle.
- Hormone therapy appears to be more effective in older children (<5 years), boys with bilateral pathology, and those with undescended testes.
- Hormone therapy is thought to improve fertility by improving gamete maturation and increasing the number of gametes.
- Therefore, hormone therapy may be recommended before surgery, but only for bilateral nonpalpable testicles.
- Hormone therapy should not be used in patients with inguinal hernia, ectopic testes, obstructive dystrophy, or previous surgery.
- Up to 20% of the patients may experience testicular retraction as a result of hormone therapy.

hCG therapy dosages	250 IU/dose—young infants 500 IU/dose—up to 6 years 1000 IU/dose—older children hCG is administered in two doses/week for 5 weeks 1,500 IU/m^2 as nine injections
Intranasal LHRH therapy	100 mg intranasally in each nostril six times a day for 3–4 weeks
Combined therapy	400 µg of LHRH as nasal spray three times daily for 4 weeks followed by hCG 1,500 IU/week for 3 weeks

(hCG: human chorionic gonadotropin; LHRH: luteinizing hormone-releasing hormone)

- The side effects of hormonal treatment include increased scrotal rugosities and pigmentation, and premature epiphyseal closure. Growth retardation, penile/pubic hair growth, and higher doses can make testis refractory to hormonal stimulation.

Surgical Treatment

- Conventional orchidopexy is usually performed on a unilateral UDT and requires a standard inguinal incision, with lateral extension if necessary.
- Most patients with UDT present with an indirect hernia sac that must be separated from the umbilical structures to mobilize them.
- Some patients require extensive retroperitoneal dissection, including division of the retroperitoneal zones (Browne's zones) to the kidney to bring the testicle into the scrotum.
- The testicle is then passed through the outer ring and attached to the scrotum. Some surgeons prefer to take a suture from the tunica vaginalis to the lowest scrotum, while others prefer to fit the scrotum with the extradartotic bag (Lattimer) technique.
- If no stone inguinal canal is found, the internal inguinal ring is immediately opened.
- A "squealing testicle" can often be made more visible by applying abdominal pressure over the incision.

- If the testicle is high in the abdominal position or close to the bladder, the groin approach may not provide a wide enough view of the abdomen to correctly locate the testicle, and abdominal insertion should be performed for greater certainty.
- This approach is mandatory if the stone is not found in the inguinal examination, but the patent process occurs vaginally.
- Testicular blood flow should be maintained if possible.
- Although the main blood supply to the testicle is from the testicular vein, which is a direct branch of the aorta, additional blood supply is provided by several anastomoses of the vascular artery (branch of the inferior vesical artery and the cremasteric artery and branch of inferior epigastric artery); most of which are 3–4 cm from the testicular poles.
- Therefore, despite the extensive mobilization of cord structures, the testicle survives.
- Approximately 4 cm above the superior pole of the testicle, the testicular artery divides into two main branches, and these anatomical considerations are important for staged orchidopexy with the division of the testicular vein.
- If the testicular vessels are too short, a two-stage orchidopexy is recommended without cutting the vessels and involves mobilizing the testicle into the abdominal cavity and securing it as low as possible (e.g., to the pubic tubercle or the inguinal ligament).
- In such patients, few surgeons prefer to wrap the testicle in an inert bag to avoid multiple attachments to the surrounding tissues and to prevent possible damage to the reproductive tract in the second stage.
- The second stage is done after 6–12 months. In some patients, retraction of the umbilical cord can achieve successful repositioning of the testicular scrotum (forming a new internal inguinal ring medial to the lower abdominal vessels).

Fowler–Stephens Orchidopexy

- This procedure is used in boys with intra-abdominal testes whose testicular artery and veins are too short for the testicle to reach the scrotum with a standard orchidopexy.
- These are usually patients whose testis is >3 cm beyond the ipsilateral internal inguinal ring.
- The Fowler–Stephens technique involves dissection and dissection of testicular vessels and can be performed as a one- or two-stage open or laparoscopic procedure.
- As previously stated, excess arterial flow through the deferent (vasal) artery allows the testis to survive.
- When this technique is performed as a one-stage procedure, the vas deferens is isolated, ligated (or cut), and cut at least 3–4 cm from the testicle, allowing the testicle to be pushed into the scrotum without tension.
- The main disadvantage of this one-stage procedure is that the vein can be so small that if it spasms, there is a high probability of testicular atrophy.
- One of the requirements of this procedure is that the vein must be long enough to allow the testicle to be repositioned into the scrotum. Another important point is this Fowler's decision
- Stephen's open orchidopexy procedure should be done early enough to disturb the epididymis as little as possible.
- This means minimal or no surgery of the spermatic cord structures and uniform preservation of the peritoneum.
- Therefore, most pediatric surgeons prefer to perform this procedure in stages. In the first stage, the sperm vessels are cut at a distance of 3–4 cm from the testicle.
- The second stage of the Fowler–Stephen's procedure is performed 3–6 months later.
- This interval is necessary to improve collateral circulation in late blood vessels.
- Both stages can be performed as a laparoscopic procedure.
- In the second step, the spermatic vessels are divided between the clamps, and the testicle is moved down into the scrotum.

Bianchi Technique

- This technique involves surgical treatment of palpable and ascending or descending testicles in infants.
- A transverse incision is made in the neck of the scrotum, and the Tunica vaginalis is exposed and delivered through the wound (under tension).

- The attachment sites of the spermatic cord are divided and the fibrous thread remaining from the removed vaginal process is identified and divided to release the blood vessels and vessels to reach a sufficient length to transfer the testicle to the scrotum.
- In small children, the hernia sac can be treated with the same incision, because their inguinal canal is very short.
- Cosmesis is great.

Laparoscopic Orchidopexy

- Laparoscopic assisted orchidopexy preserves the spermatic vessels and the technique essentially consists of dividing the gubernacular appendage and mobilizing the testicular vessels and subsequent peritoneal vessels to a certain distance so that the testicle can be moved to the scrotum.
- One simple test to evaluate the success of laparoscopic orchidopexy is that the mobilized testicular stalk can easily reach the contralateral internal inguinal ring.
- Sometimes a neo-inguinal ring forms medial to the lower abdominal vessels and umbilical artery, especially if there is a short cord (Prentiss maneuver).

Microvascular Orchidopexy

- Silber and Kellyand introduced a microsurgical testicular autotransplantation technique in which a microscopic anastomosis of the testicular artery and vein is performed to the inferior epigastric vessels when the testicular vessels and vessels are too short for successful orchidopexy.
- However, the popularity of this technique was limited due to the long duration of the operation and the need for microsurgical skills and special instruments. In experienced hands, microvascular orchiopexy is approximately 80% successful.

Orchiectomy

- If the surgeon detects a hypotrophic or atrophic intra-abdominal testis during an inguinal or laparoscopic examination, laparoscopic orchiectomy is the best therapeutic option, especially if there is a normal contralateral descending testis.
- This is to avoid the need to constantly monitor testicular remnants, which can become malignant over time.
- Laparoscopic orchidectomy involves extracting the spermatozoa from the posterior part of the peritoneum and then cauterizing/ligating them followed by their division.
- For cosmetic reasons, age-appropriate testicular implants can be placed in the empty scrotum at a later operation.

Surgical management of bilateral intra-abdominal testis:

- The principle of surgical management generally remains the same, except that preoperative karyotyping and hormonal work-up is necessary to confirm the presence or absence of testicular tissue and rule out intersex disorder.
- Bilateral orchidopexy is generally preferred in the same sitting though few may like to stage the procedure.
- When no testicular structures are evident on laparoscopy, the patient should be referred to a pediatric endocrinologist for hormone replacement therapy.

SPECIAL NOTE: METHODS OF ORCHIDOPEXY

These are as follows:

- *Extradartos pouch*—conventional orchidopexy: high ligation of the sac is done through an inguinal approach, testis is placed in an extradartos pouch in the scrotum.
- *Prentiss maneuver*—if the testis does not reach the scrotum easily then the inferior epigastric artery and vein can be ligated and the testis is brought directly through the transversalis fascial floor.
- *Transscrotal orchidopexy*—it is high ligation of processus vaginalis, dissection of spermatic cord, and placement of testis in an ipsilateral subdartos pouch.

- *Fowler-Stephen's technique*—a division of the main testicular vessels, thus relies on a delicate vessel and cremasteric collaterals for testicular survival and growth.
- *Staged Fowler-Stephen's technique*—is a second staged procedure. In stage 1 ligation of the spermatic vessels to gain length is done to allow the collateral blood supply to develop without mobilizing the testis. After 6 months at the second stage, the testis is brought into the scrotum by inguinal exploration. The testicular blood supply is supported by the artery to the vas.
- *Multistage orchiopexy*—the testis is mobilized and brought into the inguinal canal as far as possible. The testis and spermatic cord are wrapped with a silicone sheath to prevent adhesions. After 1 year of waiting, at the second stage, the testis is brought down to the scrotum.
- *Microvascular orchiopexy (testicular autotransplantation)*—the best procedure to avoid testicular atrophy. This involves high mobilization of the testicular vascular pedicle, transfer of the testis to the scrotum, and immediate revascularization of one arterial and one or two venous anastomoses to the inferior epigastric vessels.
- *Refluo technique*—consists of full venous drainage by microvascular anastomosis of the testicular vein to the inferior epigastric vein, but relies on the arterial input from the vassal collaterals.
- *Qmbredaanne's procedure*—testis is placed into the contralateral scrotal sac through the scrotal septum.

6. Write down the clinical evaluation and management principle of impalpable undescended testis.
WBUHS 2025

Clinical Evaluation

An impalpable undescended testis is a testis that cannot be felt on physical examination. It may be intra-abdominal, atrophic, or absent.

History

- *Perinatal history:* Prematurity, low birth weight
- Family history of UDT or genitourinary anomalies
- History of prior inguinal/scrotal surgery or trauma
- Any hormonal treatment given previously

Physical Examination

- Perform in a warm room with a relaxed child
- Palpate from iliac crest to scrotum, in both supine and frog-leg positions
- Look for:
  - Empty hemiscrotum
  - Compensatory hypertrophy of the contralateral testis (suggestive of absent testis on affected side)
  - Inguinal fullness or bulge

Distinguishing Palpable versus Impalpable

- If not confidently palpable → consider it impalpable
- Examination under anesthesia (EUA) can help confirm impalpable status

Imaging (Not routinely recommended)

- Ultrasound has low sensitivity for intra-abdominal testes
- MRI/CT not routinely used due to cost, radiation, and limited additional value
- Imaging may be used in select cases, especially when the diagnosis is uncertain or for surgical planning

Management Principles

Management aims to locate, assess viability, and reposition (or remove) the testis as appropriate.

Timing of Intervention

- Ideally performed between 6 and 18 months of age
- No later than 2 years, to reduce risks of infertility and malignancy

Surgical Exploration

- *Diagnostic laparoscopy—gold standard*
  - Confirms presence/absence and location of testis
  - Determines further management path
- *Findings and corresponding management*

Laparoscopic finding	*Interpretation*	*Management*
Intra-abdominal testis	Viable testis seen intra-abdominally	Proceed with orchidopexy (1 or 2-stage)
Testicular nubbin or remnant	Atrophic or nonfunctional testis	Orchidectomy (removal)
Blind-ending vas and vessels	Suggests vanishing/absent testis	No further surgery needed
Peeping testis (seen at internal ring)	Testis may be canalicular	May convert to open inguinal exploration for orchidopexy

Surgical Techniques

- *Single-stage orchidopexy*
  - For low intra-abdominal testis (<2 cm from internal ring)
  - Mobilize and bring testis into scrotum via standard or Prentiss maneuver
- *Two-stage Fowler-Stephens orchidopexy*
  - For high intra-abdominal testis
  - *Stage 1:* Clip/ligate testicular vessels (collateral blood flow develops)
  - *Stage 2 (6 months later):* Mobilize and bring testis into scrotum
- *Orchidectomy*
  - If testis is atrophic or nonviable
  - Consider testicular prosthesis later for cosmetic reasons (usually at puberty)

Postoperative Follow-up

- Clinical exam at 6 weeks and then periodically
- Assess:
  - Testis position
  - Testicular size and consistency
- Long-term surveillance for testicular function and malignancy risk

Key Considerations

- Early intervention reduces risks of subfertility and testicular cancer.
- Always consider bilateral impalpable testes as a possible sign of Disorders of Sex Development (DSD) → requires urgent endocrine and genetic evaluation.
- Hormonal therapy (e.g., hCG, GnRH) is not recommended as first-line treatment.

7. Ectopic testis. ***Gujarat Health University 2024***

Definition

An *ectopic testis* is a testicle that *has deviated from its normal path of descent* and is located *outside the normal scrotal or inguinal canal route*, unlike an undescended (cryptorchid) testis which is along the normal path.

Etiology/Pathophysiology

- During fetal development, the testis *descends from the abdomen into the scrotum* guided by the gubernaculum.
- In ectopic testis, the testis *leaves the normal path* due to:
  - Misguided gubernacular attachment
  - Abnormal mechanical obstruction
  - Hormonal or genetic factors

Common Sites of Ectopic Testis

Site	Frequency/features
Superficial inguinal pouch	Most common (~75%); just lateral to scrotum
Femoral	Rare; below inguinal ligament
Perineal	Posterolateral perineum
Penile/prepubic	Anteriorly, along shaft of penis or pubis
Contralateral scrotum (crossed)	Extremely rare; may mimic hernia

Unlike cryptorchid testis, an *ectopic testis cannot be manipulated into the scrotum* easily because its location is "off the normal path."

Clinical Features

- *Empty scrotum* on the affected side
- *Palpable mass* at ectopic site (usually firm, movable)
- *Normally descended contralateral testis*
- May present with:
  - Inguinal or perineal mass
  - Cosmetic concern
  - Complications if untreated: *Infertility, malignancy, torsion, trauma*

Diagnosis

- *Clinical examination:* Palpable ectopic testis; empty scrotum
- *Ultrasound/Doppler:* Confirms location and vascularity (especially if impalpable)
- *MRI/CT:* Rarely needed for deep or non-palpable testis
- *Differential:* Cryptorchid testis, inguinal hernia, lipoma, hydrocele

Complications

- *Infertility:* Due to abnormal temperature exposure
- *Malignancy risk:* Seminoma or non-seminomatous germ cell tumor (risk increased in ectopic and undescended testes)
- *Testicular torsion:* Due to abnormal fixation
- *Trauma:* Especially perineal or superficial ectopic testes

Management

- *Timing: Surgery recommended early:* Ideally *between 6 and 18 months* to preserve fertility and reduce malignancy risk.
- *Surgical approach:*
  - *Orchidopexy (testis fixation in scrotum):*
    1. Incision over ectopic site
    2. Mobilize spermatic cord and testis
    3. Divide or lengthen cord if necessary
    4. Create subdartos pouch in scrotum
    5. Fix testis without tension
  - *Laparoscopic approach:* Rarely required; mainly for impalpable ectopic testis
- *Special considerations:*
  - Always check *contralateral testis*
  - *Testis biopsy* generally not indicated unless suspicious lesion
  - *Postoperative follow-up:* Monitor for position, viability, and growth

Prognosis
- Good if *orchidopexy done early*
- Fertility may be partially reduced depending on duration of ectopia
- Malignancy risk remains slightly higher than normal testes, but early orchidopexy allows easier surveillance

ACUTE SCROTUM

8. Discuss the causes of the "acute scrotum." Outline its management. ***WBUHS 2023***

Definition
Acute scrotum pain is defined as "the constellation of new-onset pain, swelling, and/or tenderness of the intra-scrotal contents." Patients may describe the onset of symptoms as rapidly as occurring within minutes or up to 1–2 days, depending on the etiology.

Causes
It is difficult to describe the causes of acute scrotum pain in subgroups, as many conditions are chronic but have an acute presentation.

The causative etiologies of acute scrotum pain are broad. These include ischemic, traumatic, infectious, inflammatory, referred pain, acute or chronic, or idiopathic.

Ischemic/traumatic
- Torsion of testes
- Torsion of testicular appendages
- Testicular hematoma
- Thrombosed varicocele
- Inguinoscrotal hernia (obstructed/strangulated)

Infective/inflammatory
- Epididymitis
- Epididymo-orchitis

Neuropathic/Referred and Physical Pain
- Midureteral stone
- Inguinal hernias (obstructed/strangulated)
- Aortic/common iliac artery aneurysm
- Nerve entrapment
- Diabetic neuropathy (chronic presentation is more common)
- Sexual abuse

By far the most common causes are epididymitis/epididymo-orchitis, testicular appendage torsion, spermatic cord torsion (commonly referred to as testicular torsion), varicoceles, and obstructed or strangulated inguinal hernias. The incidence and frequency of these etiologies are highly variable by age group. Acute scrotal pain in children is much more likely to represent torsion of the spermatic cord or testicular appendages whereas patients older than 25 years of age are much more likely to have epididymitis.

History
A focused history and physical examination are essential in the evaluation of the acute scrotum.
- Characterize the pain
- *Location:* Testes, epididymis (posterolateral aspect of the testicle), and the upper pole of the testes
- *Onset:* Sudden or gradual
- Frequency of pain
- Radiation, intensity, and duration

- *Events associated:* Trauma; dysuria, urethral discharge, and urinary frequency; sexual history
- Constitutional symptoms
- *Medical history:* Genitourinary (GU) abnormalities, recurrent urinary tract infections (UTIs), diabetes, alcoholism, and steroid use
- Recent catheterization or instrumentation of the urinary tract

Physical Examination for the Acute Scrotum

- *Inspection:*
  - Symmetry and size of testicles
  - Skin erythema
  - Blue dot at the upper pole of the testicle
  - Urethral discharge
  - Unilateral vein engorgement
- *Palpation:* Determine the site of maximal tenderness and check for masses
  - Testes
  - Epididymis
  - Upper pole of testes
  - Inguinal canal
  - Scrotum
  - McBurney's point, costovertebral angle, or another abdominal or flank location
  - Look bilaterally for the presence of a cremasteric reflex
    - A "high-riding" asymmetrical testicle with an abnormal lay and loss of ipsilateral cremasteric reflex is historically described as the classic presentation of acute testicular torsion. If there is pain relief on lifting the affected testicle, this is suggestive of epididymitis, but if there is no pain relief then this suggests testicular torsion. This is called *Prehn's sign.* However, this dogmatic description of the classic presentation is not universally observed in all cases and may lead to misdiagnosis or delay in definitive treatment.

Evaluation

- It first begins with a detailed history and physical examination.
- If the diagnosis of spermatic cord torsion is strongly suspected, then an emergency surgical consultation is warranted without further delay.
- The "classic" cutoff for salvage of testicular torsion is surgical exploration and detorsion within 6 hours of the onset of symptoms.
- Provided it does not delay definitive surgical consultation, additional studies that may be useful include complete blood counts, urinalysis with microscopy, urine culture, and urethral swabs for gonorrhea and chlamydia.
- For systemically ill patients or those presenting with sepsis, blood cultures, inflammatory markers, and cross-sectional imaging of the pelvis through the mid-thighs may be considered.
- Doppler ultrasonography (USG) is the most appropriate imaging modality for the evaluation of the acute scrotum. The sensitivity of color Doppler ultrasound is reported to range from 96 to 100% with a specificity of 84–95%.
- Other imaging modalities are also available
- Radionuclide scrotal imaging (RNSI)—this modality is prone to false positives, particularly in cases of spermatocele, hydrocele, and inguinal hernias, and may lead to unnecessary surgical exploration when compared to modern USG.
- Magnetic resonance imaging (MRI) had 93% sensitivity and 100% specificity for diagnosing torsion; however, availability and length of time required to complete may limit its appropriateness.
- Computed tomography (CT) imaging is useful when there is a concern for necrotizing skin and soft tissue infections and Fournier gangrene.

Treatment

- The definitive treatment of testicular torsion is surgical exploration and detorsion, usually followed by orchiopexy to prevent recurrent torsion.
- Manual detorsion can and often should be attempted at the bedside; although, its success rate is widely variable and has been reported to range from 25 to 80%.
- Manual detorsion is contraindicated if pain and/or suspected torsion have been present for longer than 6 hours.
- The ultrasound may be useful in evaluating the direction and effectiveness of this maneuver.
- Treatment of epididymitis is conservative.

Pathology	*Symptoms and signs*	*Management*
Testicular torsion	• *Age:* Typically, perinatal or adolescent • Abdominal, flank, or scrotal pain • Nausea/vomiting • Testicular swelling • Testicular hardness • High-riding testicle	• Any suspicion at all requires a color Doppler ultrasound • If torsion is obvious, attempt the open-book technique to detort the testicle • Requires surgical management
Epididymitis epididymo-orchitis	• Can occur at any age • Dysuria, frequency, and urethral discharge [thick and yellow suggests *Neisseria gonorrhoeae (N. gonorrhea)*] • Aching pain radiating to the flank, abdomen, or groin • Tender along epididymis • An inflammatory hydrocele • Manual elevation of the testicle will decrease pain (Prehn's sign) • Also, tender on testicle is equal to epididymo-orchitis; should consider mumps	• Urinalysis plus urine culture • Ultrasound to rule out torsion. Ultrasound typically shows increased blood flow with epididymitis • In men under 35 years of age give 1 g of azithromycin and cover for *N. gonorrhea* based on local resistance patterns • In children and men over 35 years of age treated like a UTI • NSAIDs can help reduce symptoms • If no response to treatment in 3 days, then require further follow-up
Fournier's Gangrene	• *Immunosuppressed patient:* Diabetic, alcoholic, liver disease, etc. • Severe pain in the perineum and scrotum • Feeling unwell for 2–5 days prior to presentation • Fever, chills, and sweats • Tachycardia • Skin can be erythematous, edematous, blistered, or gangrenous • Crepitus may be present • Testicles will be spared due to separate blood supply	• IV broad-spectrum antibiotics • CT scan • Consult urology
Testicular rupture	• Typically, a very clear history of trauma. If not, then consider carcinoma. • Immediate swelling after trauma is equal to rupture • *On examination:* Tender, swollen, and mass that does not transilluminate	• Pain control • Ultrasound to delineate injury • Consult urology, will need orchiectomy
Testicular hematoma	Like rupture; however, swelling will be gradual and not instant	Pain control, elevation, and ice packs

(CT: computed tomography; IV: intravenous; NSAIDs: nonsteroidal anti-inflammatory drugs; UTI: urinary tract infection)

Algorithm for Management of Impalpable Undescended Testis

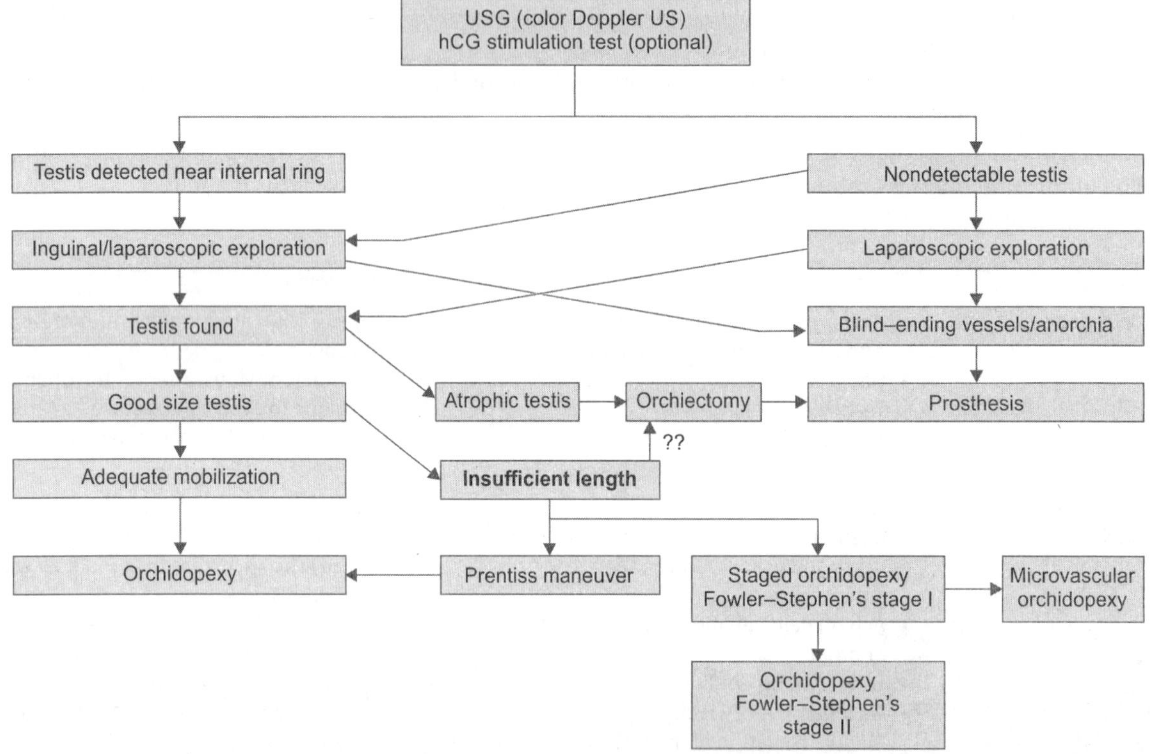

(hCG: human chorionic gonadotropin; USG: ultrasonography)

TESTICULAR TORSION

9. A 20-year-old medical student complains of sudden onset scrotal pain, the exact time of which he can recall, along with scrotal erythema, nausea, vomiting, and fever. How would you proceed to examine physically, do a quick workup, and plan urgent management to ensure the safe salvage of the testes? Give any recommended scoring system for the diagnosis of the condition. ***WBUHS 2022***

10. Discuss management of torsion of testis in an adolescent. ***Rajiv Gandhi University of Health Sciences 2019***

The constellation of symptoms encompassing the acute scrotum includes new-onset pain, tenderness, and swelling. The differential diagnosis of this presentation includes the following:

- Appendage torsion (appendix testis, epididymis, paradidymis, and vas aberrans)
- Spermatic cord torsion—intravaginal (acute or intermittent) versus extravaginal
- Epididymitis—infectious (viral, sexually transmitted infection, and urinary tract infection) versus sterile/traumatic
- Scrotal edema or erythema
- Orchitis—associated with epididymitis or abscess, vasculitis, or viral infection (mumps orchitis)
- Trauma
- Hernia
- Hydrocele or intrascrotal mass
- Varicocele
- Inguinal tendonitis or muscle strain
- Referred pain (ureteral calculi)

Differential Diagnoses

- Epididymitis
- Hydrocele
- Orchitis
- Prepubertal testicular and paratesticular tumors
- Testicular trauma
- Varicocele

Clinical Evaluation

- In the adolescent presenting with scrotal pain, the physical examination should begin with visual inspection for swelling or discoloration, followed by evaluation of the cremasteric reflex, and finally palpation for assessment of testicular orientation or tenderness.
- There is often swelling and erythema of the ipsilateral scrotum.
- The cremasteric reflex is assessed by scratching the superomedial surface of the thigh.
- A normal response is for the ipsilateral testis to rise cranially due to contraction of the cremasteric muscle fibers in the spermatic cord.
- The testis may have an aberrant lie within the scrotum, often cranially displaced toward the inguinal ring, and horizontally oriented.
- A significant generalized tenderness of the affected testis is expected.

The Testicular Workup for Ischemia and Suspected Torsion (TWIST)

- This score has been developed to assist non-expert physicians in identifying those patients most likely to have torsion.
- This is based on scoring clinical variables including edema, hard mass, absent cremasteric reflex, high-riding testis, nausea, and vomiting.
- In those patients demonstrating all of the clinical variables, torsion was noted in 100%.

Ultrasound

- Testicular torsion is a clinical diagnosis.
- If the history and physical examination strongly suggest testicular torsion, the patient should proceed directly to surgery without delaying imaging studies.
- If there is a little suspicion of testicular torsion, color Doppler and power Doppler USG can demonstrate arterial blood flow to the testicle while providing information about scrotal anatomy and other testicular abnormalities.

Doppler Ultrasound

- It can alone be less accurate than color Doppler in assessing testicular blood flow.
- In fact, in the early stages of testicular torsion, a grayscale ultrasound may be completely normal.
  Ultrasound findings suggestive of acute testicular torsion include:
  - Lack or reduction of blood circulation in the affected testicle
  - Decreased flow velocity in intratesticular arteries
  - Increase in resistance indices of intratesticular arteries
  - Hypervascularity with low resistance flow (after partial torsional torsion)
- The sensitivity of color Doppler examination with newer ultrasound devices in detecting acute testicular torsion in children is 90–100%.

MRI

- As a second-line imaging option, MRI has been utilized to diagnose incomplete or delayed torsion.
- It is also useful in differentiating between scrotal abscess and testicular torsion.
- However, the use of MRI is limited because it is not always immediately available in urgent settings.

Radionuclide Scans

If the diagnosis is equivocal, a radionuclide scan of the testicles can be helpful to assess blood flow and to differentiate torsion from other conditions.

Near-infrared Spectroscopy

- Near-infrared spectroscopy (NIRS) is an emerging tool to assess testicular torsion.
- It can measure oxygen saturation 3–4 cm deep in the skin, is rapid (lasting 20 seconds), and is noninvasive.

Treatment

- *Manual detorsion:*
  - During the initial examination, manual detorsion may be attempted.
  - This is done by elevating the testis toward the ipsilateral inguinal ring, stabilizing the cranial portion of the spermatic cord, and rotating the testis laterally.
  - If successful, there will be a lengthening of the spermatic cord and immediate relief of pain.
  - If the first attempt is unsuccessful, a second attempt could be made using the medial rotation of the testis.
  - Regardless of the outcome of manual detorsion, surgical exploration, and testicular fixation should be performed prior to the patient being discharged from the hospital.
  - Success of manual detorsion can be assessed with the use of Doppler sonography and resolution of symptoms.
- *Surgical detorsion:*
  - Surgical detorsion and subsequent orchidopexy or orchiectomy is the definitive management strategy and should proceed immediately in patients whose clinical findings suggest torsion.
  - The patient and/or caregiver should be counseled on the risk of immediate or delayed testicular loss.
  - Additionally, they should be advised that the impact of torsion on later fertility, even if testicular salvage occurs, cannot be assured.
- *Extravaginal torsion:*
  - In newborns presenting with torsion at birth, the timing of surgical exploration remains controversial, since testicular salvage rates are low and anesthetic risk is increased.
  - Additionally, asynchronous torsion remains uncommon.
  - Despite those concerns, most of the literature supports immediate exploration and fixation of the contralateral testis to prevent the potentially devastating outcome of asynchronous testis loss.
- *Intravaginal torsion:*
  - Immediate surgical exploration with detorsion and orchidopexy or orchidectomy is the recommended and accepted management strategy for males presenting with clinical signs of testis torsion.
  - Surgical exploration should not be delayed to obtain confirmatory radiologic studies in patients who present with suggestive clinical signs of torsion.
- *The surgical approach:*
  - It is through a midline longitudinal or bilateral transverse scrotal incision.
  - On entry into the affected hemi-scrotum, the surgeon should perform immediate detorsion of the affected testis, while noting color, degree of torsion, and anatomy of the tunica vaginalis.
  - After the testis is untwisted, it is wrapped in warm wet gauze.
  - Exploration of the contralateral hemiscrotum and orchidopexy of the unaffected testis is then performed to reduce the risk of asynchronous torsion.
  - The affected testis is reexamined for viability.
  - If blood flow remains questionable, intraoperative Doppler can be utilized, or an incision can be made into the tunica albuginea. If the testis appears viable, orchidopexy is performed.
  - If the decision is made to perform an orchiectomy, a prosthesis can be placed at this time, but insertion is often deferred for the nonacute setting.

Approach Considerations

- If testicular torsion is clinically indicated, perform immediate surgical exploration regardless of laboratory testing, as a negative scrotal exam is more acceptable than the loss of a salvageable testicle.
- Laboratory tests are probably not appropriate. However, if there is a strong suspicion of an alternative diagnosis, laboratory tests may be useful.
- Imaging studies are usually not necessary.
- However, imaging studies (e.g., ultrasound and core scan) may be useful if there is a low suspicion of testicular torsion.
  - The *TWIST* scoring system was developed for the purpose of determining the risk of testicular torsion on clinical grounds, thus decreasing the indication for ultrasound. TWIST has been validated when scored by nonurological nonphysician providers as well as urologists.

TWIST consists of the following urological history and physical examination parameters:

- Testis swelling (two points)
- Hard testis (two)
- Absent cremasteric reflex (one)
- Nausea/vomiting (one)
- High-riding testis (one)

TWIST scores and risk groups are as follows:

- *0–2 points:* Low risk
- *3–4 points:* Intermediate risk
- *5–7 points:* High risk

Analysis of result in TWIST score:

- 'TWIST has shown 100% negative predictive value when scored by a urologist, using a cutoff value of two to identify low-risk patients, and when scored by trained emergency medical technicians (EMTs) using a cutoff of 0 in children.
- Cutoff values of five (scored by a urologist) and six (EMTs) have been used to identify high-risk patients.
- Ultrasound evaluation is indicated for intermediate-risk patients; low-risk patients do not require ultrasound to rule out torsion, and patients at high risk can proceed directly to surgery, with >50% avoiding ultrasound.

VARICOCELE

11. Varicocele.

Definition

A varicocele is an abnormal enlargement of the pampiniform venous plexus in the scrotum. This plexus of veins drains the testicles.

Pathogenesis

- The testicular blood vessels originate in the abdomen and course down through the inguinal canal as part of the spermatic cord on their way to the testis.
- Upward flow of blood in the veins is ensured by small one-way valves that prevent backflow.
- Defective valves, or compression of the vein by a nearby structure, can cause dilatation of the testicular veins near the testis, leading to the formation of a varicocele.

Causative Factors

- 8–10 cm longer left testicular vein → increased hydrostatic pressure in an upright position
- Entry of left testicular vein into the renal vein at 90°
- "Nutcracker phenomenon" due to passage of the left testicular vein between the superior mesenteric artery (SMA) and aorta
- Congenital absence of valve in a left vein in 40%

- Intrinsic ectasia of the plexus due to cremaster atrophy
- Loaded left colon
- Left-sided renal cell carcinoma (RCC)

Clinical Features

- A varicocele often produces no signs or symptoms.
- Rarely, it may cause pain. The pain may:
    - Vary from sharp to dull discomfort
    - Increase with standing or physical exertion, especially over long periods
    - Worsen over the course of a day
    - Be relieved when lying on your back
- Visible or palpable (able to be felt) enlarged vein
- Feeling of heaviness in the testicle(s)
- Atrophy (shrinking) of the testicle(s)
- Alteration of testosterone levels
- Benign prostatic hyperplasia (BPH) and related urinary problems

Clinical Examinations

- Increases on standing.
- "Bag of worms" feel
- *Grades of varicocele:*
  Grade I: Palpable only during the Valsalva maneuver
  Grade II: Palpable without Valsalva in standing upright position
  Grade III: Visible through scrotal skin
- *Subclinical:* Detected during USG

Investigations

- Doppler stethoscope (5.3 MHz probe)—audible rush of blood on Valsalva
- Color Doppler—detects subclinical varicocele also
- Ultrasound of the abdomen
- Semen examination

Treatment

Expectant treatment—in adolescent males who are asymptomatic with normal size of testis.

Indications of Intervention

- Asymptomatic varicocele with >20% volume loss of the testis (>2 mL)
- Symptomatic varicocele
    - Impaired sperm quality
    - Pain
    - Cosmetic reasons
- Medically unfit

TESTICULAR TUMORS

12. Classify testicular tumors. Discuss the investigation necessary to plan the treatment for a suspected testicular tumor. What are the treatment options available?

The World Health Organization (WHO) histopathological classification of testicular tumors:

- Germ cell tumors (GCTs) (90%)
    - *Seminoma (48%):* Spermatocytic, classical, and anaplastic subtypes

- *Nonseminomatous germ cell tumor (NSGCT) (42%):*
  - *Teratoma:*
    - Differentiated/mature
    - Intermediate/immature
    - Undifferentiated/malignant
  - Yolk sac tumor
  - Choriocarcinoma
  - Mixed NSGCT
- Mixed GCT (10%)

- Other tumors (7%)
  - Epidermoid cyst (benign)
  - Adenomatoid tumor
  - Adenocarcinoma of the rete testis
  - Carcinoid
  - Lymphoma (5%)
  - Metastatic, from another site (1%)
- Sex cord-stromal tumors (3%) (10% malignant)
  - Leydig cell
  - Sertoli cell
  - Mixed or unclassified
- Mixed germ cell/sex cord tumors (rare)

Tumorigenic Model for Germ Cell Tumors of the Testis

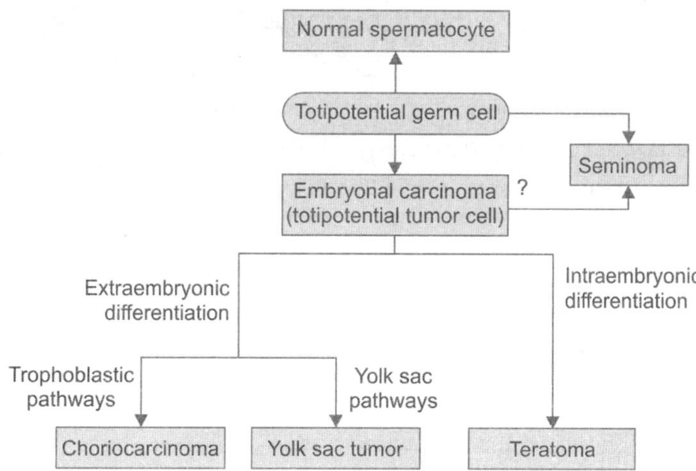

Investigations

- *Investigation and staging:*
  - *USG:* The diagnosis is confirmed by ultrasound scanning of the testis.
  - *Tumor markers:* In confirmed cases, staging is an essential step in planning treatment.
    - Blood is taken prior to orchidectomy to measure the levels of tumor markers
      - Which are raised in around 50% of the cases.
      - A rise in α-fetoprotein (AFP) is seen in around 50–70% of NSGCTs
      - A rise in hCG is seen in 40–60% of NSGCTs and around 30% of seminomas.
      - When raised, these markers are used to monitor the response to treatment.

- The mean serum half-lives of AFP and hCG are 5–7 days and 2–3 days, respectively
- *Reassessment of the markers following orchidectomy:*

It can indicate whether all the tumor tissue has been removed.

Incidence of Elevated Tumor Markers by Histologic Type in Testicular Cancer

Tumor	*hCG (%)*	*AFP (%)*
Seminoma	7	0
Teratoma	25	38
Teratocarcinoma	57	64
Embryonal cell carcinoma	60	70
Choriocarcinoma	100	0

(AFP: α-fetoprotein; hCG: human chorionic gonadotropin)

Imaging Studies

- *X-ray and CT scan:* While a chest X-ray will occasionally demonstrate the "classical cannonball" metastases computed tomography (CT) of the chest and abdomen has taken over as the most useful means of detecting metastatic disease and for monitoring the response to therapy.
- Routine chest X-rays can detect 85–90% of pulmonary metastasis.
- CECT abdomen can detect retroperitoneal nodes.
- PET - No apparent advantage over CT.
- MRI - No apparent advantage over CT.

Treatment

Principles of treatment	
Treatment should be aimed at one stage above the clinical stage	Radical inguinal orchidectomy is the standard first line of therapy
Seminomas—radiosensitive: Treat with radiotherapy	Lymphatic spread initially goes to retroperitoneal nodes
Nonseminomas are radioresistant and best treated by surgery	Early hematogenous spread is rare
Advanced disease or metastasis—responds well to Chemotherapy	Bulky Retroperitoneal tumors or metastatic tumors are initially "down-staged" with chemotherapy

T—primary tumor	
TX	Cannot be assessed
T0	No evidence of a primary tumor
Tis	Intratubular cancer (CIS)
T1	Limited to testis and epididymis, no vascular invasion
T2	Invades beyond tunica albuginea or has vascular invasion
T3	Invades spermatic cord
T4	Invades scrotum
N—regional lymph nodes	
NX	Cannot be assessed
N0	No regional lymph node metastasis
N1	Lymph node metastasis ≤ 2 cm, or multiple nodes, none > 2 cm, and less than six nodes positive
N2	Nodal mass > 2 cm and ≤5 cm or more than equal to six nodes positive
N3	Nodal mass > 5 cm

Contd...

Contd...

M—distant metastasis	
MX	Cannot be assessed
M0	No distant metastasis
M1	Distant metastasis presents in nonregional lymph nodes or lungs
M2	Nonpulmonary visceral metastases
S—serum tumor markers	
SX	Markers not available
S0	Marker levels within normal limits
S1	Lactic acid dehydrogenase (LDH) < 1.5 × normal and hCG < 5,000 mIU/mL and AFP < 1,000 ng/mL
S2	LDH 1.5–10 × normal or hCG 5,000–50,000 mIU/mL or AFP 1,000–10,000 ng/mL
S3	LDH > 10 × normal or hCG > 50,000 mIU/mL or AFP > 10,000 ng/mL

TNM Classification of Testicular Tumor: (Try to Remember)

Treatment

Treatment for seminomas		***Treatment for nonseminomas***
Stage I, IIA, and IIB (?): Radical inguinal orchidectomy followed by radiotherapy to ipsilateral retroperitoneum and ipsilateral iliac group of lymph nodes (2,500-3,000 rads)	*Bulky stage II and III seminomas:* Radical inguinal orchidectomy followed by chemotherapy	*Stage I and IIA:* Radical orchidectomy followed by retroperitoneal lymph node dissection *Stage IIB:* Retroperitoneal lymph node dissection (RPLND) with possible adjuvant chemotherapy *Stage IIC and III:* Initial chemotherapy followed by surgery for residual disease

Standard Chemotherapy for NSGCTs

Chemotherapy (BEP)	***Toxicity***
Bleomycin	Pulmonary fibrosis
Etoposide (VP-16)	Myelosuppression, alopecia, mild renal insufficiency, and secondary leukemia
Cisplatin	Renal insufficiency, nausea, vomiting, and neuropathy

(BEP: bleomycin, etoposide, and platinum; NSGCTs: nonseminomatous germ cell tumors)

13. Seminoma testes. ***RIMS, Imphal 2012***

14. Describe diagnosis and management of seminoma testis. ***Gujarat Health University 2024***

Introduction

- Seminoma (also known as pure seminoma or classical seminoma) is a germ cell tumor (cancer) of the testis.
- It is one of the most treatable and curable cancers, with survival >95% in the early stages.
- Treatment usually requires the removal of one testis, but this does not affect fertility or other sexual functioning.

Types of Seminoma

- Classic (typical)
- Anaplastic (atypical)
- Spermatocytic

Presentation

- The average age of diagnosis is 40 years.
- This is about 5–10 years older than men with other germ cell tumors of the testes.
- In most cases, they produce masses that are readily felt on testicular self-examination; however, in up to 11% of the cases, there may be no mass able to be felt, or there may be testicular atrophy.
- Testicular pain is reported in up to one-fifth of the cases. Low back pain may occur after metastasis to the retroperitoneum.

Points to Remember

- *Seminomas—radiosensitive:* Treat with radiotherapy
- Advanced disease or metastasis—responds well to chemotherapy
- Radical inguinal orchidectomy is the standard first line of therapy
- Lymphatic spread initially goes to retroperitoneal nodes
- Early hematogenous spread rare
- Bulky retroperitoneal tumors or metastatic tumors initially "down-staged" with chemotherapy

Diagnosis

- *Tumor markers:*
    - Blood tests may detect the presence of placental alkaline phosphatase (PLAP) in fifty percent of cases.
    - hCG may be elevated in some cases, but this correlates more to the presence of trophoblast cells within the tumor than to the stage of the tumor.
    - Serum alpha-fetoprotein is not elevated in classical seminoma.
    - Serum LDH concentrations are elevated in 30–80% of men with pure seminoma and in 60% of those with nonseminomatous tumors.
    - POU domain, class 2, associating factor 1 (POU2AF1), and prominin 1 (PROM1) have been proposed as possible markers.
- *HPE and microscopy:*
    - The cut surface of the tumor is fleshy and lobulated, and varies in color from cream to tan to pink. The tumor tends to bulge from the cut surface, and small areas of hemorrhage may be seen. These areas of hemorrhage usually correspond to trophoblastic cell clusters within the tumor.
    - Microscopic examination shows that seminomas are usually composed of either a sheet-like or lobular pattern of cells with a fibrous stromal network.
    - The fibrous septa almost always contain focal lymphocyte inclusions, and granulomas are sometimes seen.
    - The tumor cells themselves typically have abundant clear to pale pink cytoplasm containing abundant glycogen, which is demonstrable with a periodic acid–Schiff (PAS) stain.
    - The nuclei are prominent and usually contain one or two large nucleoli, and have prominent nuclear membranes.
    - Foci of syncytiotrophoblastic cells may be present in varied amounts.
    - The adjacent testicular tissue commonly shows intratubular germ cell neoplasia, and may also show variable spermatocytic maturation arrest.

Treatment

- A radical inguinal orchiectomy with high ligation of the spermatic cord near the internal inguinal ring is performed to permit histologic evaluation of the primary tumor and to provide local tumor control. Scrotal violation through a scrotal incision or an attempt to biopsy the testicle must be avoided because of concern for changing the lymphatic channels available to the testis tumor and the potential for a poorer outcome.
- *Seminomas metastasize via the lymphatics and hematogenous spread is uncommon:* After the determination of the histologic subtype of testis cancer, several parameters may identify patients at high risk for metastasis to the retroperitoneum despite the absence of lymphadenopathy on the staging CT scan. Treatment should be aimed at one stage above the clinical stage.

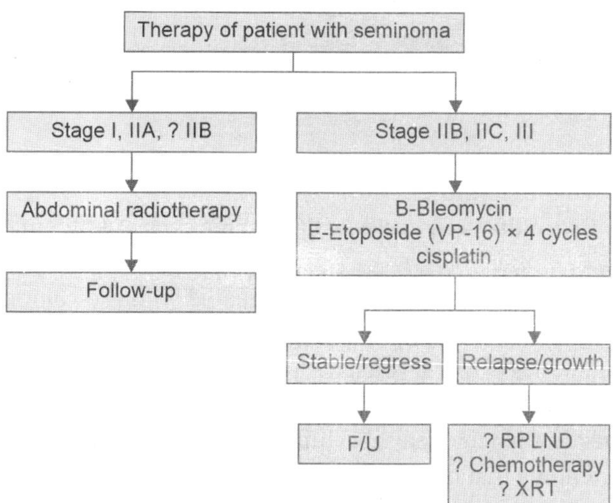

(RPLND: retroperitoneal lymph node dissection; VP-16: etoposide; XRT: external beam radiation therapy)

Prognosis for Seminoma (5-year Survival Rate)

- *Stage I:* 99%.
- *Stage II:* 70–92%
- *Stage III:* 80–85%

15. Chemotherapy in the testicular tumor.

Chemotherapy in Testicular Tumor—for

- *Seminomas:*
  - *Stage I seminomas:*
    - *Chemotherapy:* An option that works as well as radiation is one or two cycles of chemotherapy with the drug carboplatin after surgery. Many experts prefer chemo over radiation because it seems to be easier to tolerate.
  - *Stage IIA seminomas:*
    - *Chemotherapy:* Another option is chemo, with either four cycles of etoposide and cisplatin (EP) or three cycles of bleomycin, etoposide, and cisplatin (BEP).
  - *Stage IIB seminomas:*
    - *Chemotherapy:* This is the preferred treatment. Patient can be given either four cycles of EP or three cycles of BEP.
  - *Stage IIC seminomas:*
    - *Chemotherapy* with four cycles of EP or three or four cycles of BEP. Radiation therapy is generally not used for stage IIC seminoma.
- *Nonseminomas:*
  - *Stage IA nonseminomas:*
    - *Chemotherapy:* Instead of surgery, the patient may get one cycle of the BEP regimen. This helps to reduce the risk of relapse.
  - *Stage IB (T2, T3, or T4):*
    - *Chemotherapy:* Instead of surgery, one cycle of the BEP regimen can be given. If cancer was found in lymph nodes after surgery, 2–4 cycles of BEP or EP can be given.
  - *Stage IS nonseminoma:* If tumor marker levels (such as AFP and hCG) are still high even after the cancer has been removed, but the CT scan does not show a tumor, chemotherapy is recommended. Patient may get either three cycles of BEP or four cycles of EP.

- *Stage IIA nonseminomas:*
  - If tumor marker levels are normal:
    - *Chemotherapy:* If cancer was found in many lymph nodes, give either four cycles of EP or three cycles of BEP.
- *Stage IIB nonseminomas:*
  - *If tumor marker levels are elevated:*
    - *Chemotherapy:* Give either four cycles of EP or three cycles of BEP may be used
- *Stage III seminomas and nonseminomas:*
  Both stage III seminomas and nonseminomas are treated with radical inguinal orchiectomy followed by chemotherapy with either four cycles of EP or three or four cycles of BEP.
  - Patient may get four cycles of BEP if you have an intermediate or poor risk nonseminoma. (This depends on the spread to distant areas and tumor marker levels.) If there are medical reasons that make treatment with bleomycin unsafe, then one may get vinblastine, ifosfamide, and cisplatin (VIP) instead.
  - If the cancer is seminoma that has spread to bones, liver, or brain, it is intermediate risk—then give VIP (etoposide, mesna, ifosfamide, and cisplatin).
  - If the patient has high levels of the tumor marker hCG, the distant spread of cancer is seen on scans, and there is a high suspicion that he might have a testicular choriocarcinoma, chemotherapy may be started without a biopsy or surgery to remove the testicle.

16. Principles of RPNLD (Retroperitoneal lymph node dissection). ***Gujarat Health University 2024***

17. RPNLD. ***Tripura University 2023***

Retroperitoneal Lymph Node Dissection (RPLND)

Definition: RPLND is a *surgical procedure to remove lymph nodes from the retroperitoneum* (between the renal vessels and iliac vessels) for *diagnostic, staging, or therapeutic purposes,* most commonly in *testicular cancer.*

Principles of RPLND

- *Oncological principles*
  - *Complete removal of involved nodes:* All lymphatic tissue in the defined template (paracaval, para-aortic, interaortocaval) must be excised to *minimize recurrence.*
  - *Follow lymphatic drainage patterns:*
    - *Right testis:* Drains mainly to *paracaval and interaortocaval nodes*
    - *Left testis:* Drains mainly to *para-aortic and interaortocaval nodes*
  - *Avoid leaving residual disease:* Especially in postchemotherapy patients with fibrotic or necrotic nodes.
- *Anatomical principles:*
  - *Respect major retroperitoneal structures:* Aorta, inferior vena cava (IVC), renal vessels, ureters.
  - *Template-based dissection:*
    - Standard vs. modified (nerve-sparing) templates
    - Extended dissection for bulky or high-risk disease
  - *Nerve preservation:* Preserve *sympathetic fibers* running along aorta and IVC to maintain *ejaculatory function.*
- *Technical principles:*
  - *Systematic and methodical dissection:* Work from known anatomical landmarks; avoid blind clamping.
  - *Adequate exposure:* Mobilize bowel to visualize retroperitoneum fully.
  - *Hemostasis:* Carefully ligate vessels; control lymphatic channels to prevent chylous leak.
  - *Use of intraoperative adjuncts:* Nerve-sparing techniques, magnification, and sometimes intraoperative Doppler or ultrasound.

- *Perioperative principles:*
  - *Patient selection:* Ideal in NSGCT stage I with high-risk features, or residual masses post-chemotherapy.
  - *Multidisciplinary care:* Collaboration with oncology, anesthesiology, and critical care.
  - *Postoperative monitoring:* Tumor markers, renal function, electrolytes, and early detection of complications (bleeding, lymphocele, nerve injury).

Indications

- *Testicular cancer:*
  - *Nonseminomatous germ cell tumors (NSGCT):*
    - *Primary RPLND:* For clinical stage I with high-risk features (e.g., lymphovascular invasion)
    - *Postchemotherapy RPLND:* For residual masses after cisplatin-based chemotherapy
  - *Seminomatous germ cell tumors (SGCT):* Rarely used; mainly for residual masses after chemotherapy if PET-positive
- *Other indications:*
  - Retroperitoneal metastases from *renal cell carcinoma, adrenocortical carcinoma,* or *melanoma*
  - Lymphoma (rare; usually biopsy only)

Anatomy of Retroperitoneal Lymph Nodes

Region	Boundaries	Clinical relevance
Paracaval	Right side of IVC	Common site for right testis tumors
Interaortocaval	Between aorta and IVC	Midline drainage; frequent metastasis
Para-aortic	Left side of aorta	Common site for left testis tumors
Renal hilum/suprarenal	Superior boundary	Rarely involved; careful dissection required
Iliac/pelvic	Inferior boundary	Usually included in extended dissection

Surgical Technique

- *Patient position:* Supine with slight *Trendelenburg* tilt
- *Incision*
  - Midline laparotomy from *xiphoid to pubic symphysis* (or modified transperitoneal approach)
  - Laparoscopic and robotic approaches are increasingly used in select centers.
- *Steps*
  1. *Mobilize the intestines* to expose retroperitoneum.
  2. *Identify major vessels*: Aorta, IVC, renal vessels, ureters.
  3. *Dissect lymph nodes* systematically:
     - *Right-sided RPLND:* Paracaval, interaortocaval
     - *Left-sided RPLND:* Para-aortic, interaortocaval
  4. *Preserve sympathetic nerves* where possible to maintain *ejaculatory function* (nerve-sparing RPLND).
  5. *Hemostasis and drainage.*

Types of RPLND

Type	Description
Primary RPLND	Performed for staging and treatment of stage I NSGCT
Post-chemotherapy RPLND	Removes residual masses after chemotherapy; technically more difficult due to fibrosis
Modified (nerve-sparing) RPLND	Preserves sympathetic fibers → maintains antegrade ejaculation
Extended RPLND	Includes additional nodes (paracaval + para-aortic + interaortocaval) for higher-risk cases

Complications

Early/Intraoperative	*Late/Postoperative*
Bleeding (IVC or aorta injury)	Retrograde ejaculation (nerve injury)
Injury to ureter	Infertility (if bilateral orchiectomy)
Bowel injury	Lymphocele/chylous ascites
Infection/wound complications	Recurrence in residual nodes
Pulmonary embolism	Adhesion-related bowel obstruction

Postchemotherapy RPLND has *higher morbidity* due to fibrosis.

Postoperative Care

- Monitor *renal function, electrolytes, hemoglobin*
- Early ambulation to prevent DVT
- Diet advanced as tolerated
- Follow-up: *Tumor markers (AFP, β-hCG, LDH), imaging*

Outcomes

- *Curative in stage I NSGCT* with high-risk features
- *Postchemotherapy RPLND* can remove chemo-resistant residual disease
- *Nerve-sparing technique* preserves fertility in most patients.

Index

Page numbers followed by *f* refer to figure.

B

C

D

E

F

G

H

I

J

K

L

M

N

O

S

T

U

V

W

Y

Z